current Medical Diagnosis & Treatment 1985

From inability to let well alone; from too much zeal for the new and contempt for what is old; from putting knowledge before wisdom, science before art and cleverness before common sense; from treating patients as cases; and from making the cure of the disease more grievous than the endurance of the same, Good Lord, deliver us.

–Sir Robert Hutchison

current Medical Diagnosis & Treatment —1985

Edited By

MARCUS A. KRUPP, MD

Clinical Professor of Medicine Emeritus
Stanford University School of Medicine (Stanford)
Director of Research Institute
Palo Alto Medical Foundation (Palo Alto)

MILTON J. CHATTON, MD

Clinical Professor of Medicine Emeritus
Stanford University School of Medicine (Stanford)
Senior Attending Physician
Santa Clara Valley Medical Center (San Jose)
Research Associate
Palo Alto Medical Foundation (Palo Alto)

DAVID WERDEGAR, MD, MPH

Professor and Chairman
Family and Community Medicine
University of California School of Medicine (San Francisco)

With Associate Authors

Lange Medical Publications
Los Altos, California 94022

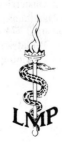

Current Medical Diagnosis & Treatment

Copyright © 1962, 1963, 1964, 1965, 1966, 1967, 1968, 1969, 1970, 1971, 1972,
1973, 1974, 1975, 1976, 1977, 1978, 1979, 1980, 1981, 1982, 1983, 1984

A Concise Medical Library for Practitioner and Student

Current Pediatric Diagnosis & Treatment, 8th ed. Edited by C.H. Kempe, H.K. Silver,   1984
and D. O'Brien. 1164 pp, *illus.*

Current Surgical Diagnosis & Treatment, 6th ed. Edited by L.W. Way. 1221 pp, *illus.*   1983

Current Obstetric & Gynecologic Diagnosis & Treatment, 5th ed. Edited by R.C. Benson.   1984
1082 pp, *illus.*

Current Emergency Diagnosis & Treatment. Edited by J. Mills, M.T. Ho, and D.D. Trunkey.   1983
738 pp, *illus.*

Harper's Review of Biochemistry, 19th ed. D.W. Martin, Jr., P.A. Mayes, and   1983
V.W. Rodwell. 638 pp, *illus.*

Review of Medical Physiology, 11th ed. W.F. Ganong. 643 pp, *illus.*   1983

Review of Medical Microbiology, 16th ed. E. Jawetz, J.L. Melnick, and E.A. Adelberg.   1984
557 pp, *illus.*

Basic & Clinical Endocrinology. Edited by F.S. Greenspan and P.H. Forsham. 646 pp, *illus.*   1983

Basic & Clinical Immunology, 5th ed. Edited by D.P. Stites, J.D. Stobo, H.H. Fudenberg,   1984
and J.V. Wells. 803 pp, *illus.*

Basic & Clinical Pharmacology, 2nd ed. Edited by B.G. Katzung. 888 pp, *illus.*   1984

Basic Histology, 4th ed. L.C. Junqueira and J. Carneiro. 510 pp, *illus.*   1983

Clinical Cardiology, 3rd ed. M. Sokolow and M.B. McIlroy. 763 pp, *illus.*   1981

General Urology, 11th ed. D.R. Smith. 661 pp, *illus.*   1984

General Ophthalmology, 10th ed. D. Vaughan and T. Asbury. 407 pp, *illus.*   1983

Correlative Neuroanatomy & Functional Neurology, 18th ed. J.G. Chusid. 476 pp, *illus.*   1982

Principles of Clinical Electrocardiography, 11th ed. M.J. Goldman. 438 pp, *illus.*   1982

Electrocardiography: Essentials of Interpretation. N. Goldschlager and M.J. Goldman.   1984
236 pp, *illus.*

Review of General Psychiatry. Edited by H.H. Goldman. 696 pp, *illus.*   1984

Handbook of Obstetrics & Gynecology, 8th ed. R.C. Benson. 804 pp, *illus.*   1983

Physician's Handbook, 20th ed. M.A. Krupp, L.M. Tierney, Jr., E. Jawetz, R.L. Roe, and   1982
C.A. Camargo. 774 pp, *illus.*

Handbook of Pediatrics, 14th ed. H.K. Silver, C.H. Kempe, and H.B. Bruyn. 883 pp, *illus.*   1983

Handbook of Poisoning: Prevention, Diagnosis, & Treatment, 11th ed. R.H. Dreisbach.   1983
632 pp.

Table of Contents

The Authors

Michael J. Aminoff, MD
Professor of Neurology, University of California School of Medicine (San Francisco).

Ralph C. Benson, MD
Professor and Chairman Emeritus of Department of Obstetrics & Gynecology, Oregon Health Sciences University (Portland).

R. Laurence Berkowitz, MD
Clinical Assistant Professor of Plastic & Reconstructive Surgery, Stanford University School of Medicine (Stanford). ·

Lloyd L. Brandborg, MD
Staff Physician, Veterans Administration Hospital (San Francisco); Clinical Professor of Medicine, University of California School of Medicine (San Francisco).

James J. Brophy, MD
Associate Clinical Professor of Psychiatry, University of California School of Medicine (San Diego).

Carlos A. Camargo, MD
Associate Professor of Clinical Medicine, Stanford University School of Medicine (Stanford); Director of Endocrine Clinic, Stanford University Hospital (Stanford).

John V. Carbone, MD
Professor of Medicine, University of California School of Medicine (San Francisco).

Milton J. Chatton, MD
Clinical Professor of Medicine Emeritus, Stanford University School of Medicine (Stanford); Senior Attending Physician, Santa Clara Valley Medical Center (San Jose); Research Associate, Palo Alto Medical Foundation (Palo Alto).

Wayne W. Deatsch, MD
Clinical Professor of Otorhinolaryngology, University of California School of Medicine (San Francisco).

Robert H. Dreisbach, MD, PhD
Clinical Professor of Environmental Health, School of Public Health and Community Medicine, University of Washington (Seattle).

Ephraim P. Engleman, MD, FACP
Clinical Professor of Medicine and Director of Rosalind Russell Medical Research Center for Arthritis, University of California School of Medicine (San Francisco).

John M. Erskine, MD
Associate Clinical Professor of Surgery, University of California School of Medicine (San Francisco); Associate in Surgery, Stanford University School of Medicine (Stanford).

Lawrence Z. Feigenbaum, MD
Clinical Professor of Medicine, University of California School of Medicine (San Francisco); Director of Professional Services and Medical Education and Director of Geriatric Center, Mount Zion Hospital and Medical Center (San Francisco).

Steven S. Fountain, MD
Clinical Associate Professor of Surgery, Orthopedics, Stanford University School of Medicine (Stanford).

Armando E. Giuliano, MD
Associate Professor of Surgery, University of California School of Medicine (Los Angeles).

Robert S. Goldsmith, MD, MPH, DTM&H
Professor of Tropical Medicine and Epidemiology, University of California School of Medicine (San Francisco).

Sadja Greenwood, MD, MPH
Assistant Clinical Professor of Obstetrics, Gynecology, and Reproductive Sciences, University of California School of Medicine (San Francisco).

Moses Grossman, MD
Professor of Pediatrics, University of California School of Medicine (San Francisco); Chief of Pediatrics, San Francisco General Hospital.

F. Carl Grumet, MD
Associate Professor of Pathology, Stanford University School of Medicine (Stanford).

Carlyn Halde, PhD
Associate Professor of Microbiology and Immunology, University of California School of Medicine (San Francisco).

Ernest Jawetz, MD, PhD
Professor of Microbiology and Medicine Emeritus, University of California School of Medicine (San Francisco).

Floyd H. Jergesen, MD
Clinical Professor of Orthopedic Surgery Emeritus, University of California School of Medicine (San Francisco).

John H. Karam, MD
Associate Professor of Medicine, Co-director of Diabetes Clinic, and Chief of Clinical Endocrinology, University of California School of Medicine (San Francisco).

C. Michael Knauer, MD
Chief of Division of Gastroenterology, Santa Clara Valley Medical Center (San Jose); Clinical Professor of Medicine, Stanford University School of Medicine (Stanford).

Felix O. Kolb, MD
Clinical Professor of Medicine, University of California School of Medicine (San Francisco).

Margaret S. Kosek, MD
Staff Physician, Palo Alto Medical Foundation (Palo Alto).

Marcus A. Krupp, MD
Clinical Professor of Medicine Emeritus, Stanford University School of Medicine (Stanford); Director of Research Institute, Palo Alto Medical Foundation (Palo Alto).

R. Morton Manson, MD
Clinical Associate Professor of Medicine, Stanford University School of Medicine (Stanford); Chief of Medicine, Lockheed Missiles and Space Company (Sunnyvale, California).

Alan J. Margolis, MD
Professor of Obstetrics, Gynecology, and Reproductive Sciences, University of California School of Medicine (San Francisco).

Rees B. Rees, Jr., MD
Clinical Professor of Dermatology Emeritus, University of California School of Medicine (San Francisco).

James L. Rushing, MD
Department of Anesthesia, Stanford University School of Medicine (Stanford), and *formerly* Assistant Professor of Medicine, Stanford University School of Medicine (Stanford); Chief of Respiratory Medicine, Santa Clara Valley Medical Center (San Jose).

Sydney E. Salmon, MD
Professor of Internal Medicine, Hematology and Oncology, University of Arizona College of Medicine (Tucson); Director of Arizona Cancer Center.

Martin A. Shearn, MD
Clinical Professor of Medicine, University of California School of Medicine (San Francisco); Chief of Department of Medicine, Kaiser-Permanente Medical Center (Oakland).

Sol Silverman, Jr., DDS
Professor of Oral Medicine and Chairman of the Department, University of California School of Dentistry (San Francisco).

Maurice Sokolow, MD
Professor of Medicine Emeritus and Senior Staff Member, Cardiovascular Research Center, University of California School of Medicine (San Francisco).

Samuel Strober, MD
Professor of Medicine and Chief of Division of Immunology, Stanford University School of Medicine (Stanford).

Phyllis M. Ullman, MA, RD
Senior Dietitian, Stanford Heart Disease Prevention Program, Stanford University Department of Medicine (Stanford).

Daniel Vaughan, MD
Clinical Professor of Ophthalmology, University of California School of Medicine (San Francisco); Member, Francis I. Proctor Foundation for Research in Ophthalmology.

Ralph O. Wallerstein, MD
Clinical Professor of Medicine, University of California School of Medicine (San Francisco).

David Werdegar, MD, MPH
Professor and Chairman of Family and Community Medicine, University of California School of Medicine (San Francisco).

Preface

Current Medical Diagnosis & Treatment 1985 is intended to serve health practitioners as a useful desk reference on widely accepted methods currently available for diagnosis and treatment. It is not intended to be used as a textbook of medicine. Selected current references to the clinical literature and general bibliographies—emphasizing material published within the last 5 years—are included as a guide to further study.

The book has been revised annually since its first appearance in 1962, and its continued wide acceptance has been most gratifying. Over 1.3 million volumes of the book have been purchased in the course of 23 revisions. The widespread dissemination of this book overseas, both in translation and in its English language editions, has been a particular source of satisfaction to all of us who have worked on it over the years. A Spanish edition is available from El Manual Moderno (Mexico City), an Italian edition from Piccin Nuova Libraria (Padua), a Serbo-Croatian edition from Savremena Administracija (Belgrade), a Portuguese edition from Atheneu Editora (São Paulo), a German edition from Springer-Verlag (Heidelberg), a Greek edition from Gregory Parisianos (Athens), and a Dutch edition from Kooyker (Leiden). French and Turkish translations are in preparation. An English edition for distribution in Asia is printed in Singapore by Maruzen, and a Middle East edition (in English) is available under the imprint of Librairie du Liban (Beirut). English editions are also produced in Taiwan, the Philippines, and Korea.

A new title-page editor and several new authors have joined us in this latest revision.

The editors wish to express their sincere thanks to their associate authors for participating so effectively in this venture, and to the many students and physicians who have contributed suggestions and criticisms for this and previous editions. We continue to solicit comments and recommendations for future editions. These should be addressed to us, care of Lange Medical Publications, Drawer L, Los Altos, CA 94022.

Marcus A. Krupp
Milton J. Chatton
David Werdegar

January, 1985

General Symptoms | 1

Milton J. Chatton, MD

PAIN

Pain in its myriad forms, including aching, soreness, and tenderness, is the most common symptom for which patients seek relief. Acute pain is an unpleasant experience primarily associated with tissue injury, and the protective response patients have to pain provides the clinician with critical diagnostic information. In taking a history from the patient with pain, there should be a careful suggestion-free elicitation of characteristics such as chronology, nature, location, radiation, and aggravating and alleviating factors that influence the pain. Because pain is a subjective phenomenon, it is not surprising that the description of pain by the patient may be difficult to interpret.

The reaction to pain, a function of the higher centers, is extremely variable and influenced by many factors depending upon the individual patient (the affective component) and the situation (the sensory component). When pain becomes chronic, the multifactorial influences (eg, anxiety; depression; social, cultural, and economic factors; and secondary gain) play an even larger role. It is therefore essential to determine, whenever possible, the primary cause (eg, infection), the pathogenesis (eg, inflammation, ulceration, anoxia), and the secondary or contributing factors.

Principles of Pain Relief

Measures directed at correcting the cause of pain deserve first consideration. The relief of pain is achieved by removal of the primary cause (eg, cure of infection), neutralization of the effect of the stimulus (eg, antacids for peptic ulcer), physical relief of discomfort (eg, rest), suppression of the disease process (eg, anti-inflammatory drugs), and, when these are not feasible, by dulling or obliterating the sense of pain (eg, analgesic drugs).

The hazards of administering analgesics without first attempting to establish a diagnosis cannot be overemphasized (eg, acute abdominal pain). Analgesics, particularly narcotics, may mask the symptoms of serious acute or chronic illness.

Pain may be treated nonspecifically with drugs (which may act at the receptor, spinal cord, or brain levels), physical measures (eg, heat, cold, immobilization), nerve block (eg, local anesthesia), surgery (eg, chordotomy), and by other measures of uncertain mechanism (eg, acupuncture). There is evidence that endogenous opioid peptides in the brain—the endorphins—may be released by stress and other stimuli to produce analgesia. (This form of analgesia can be antagonized by the relatively specific opiate antagonist naloxone.) It is postulated that the release of these morphinelike endogenous brain chemicals is responsible for the absence of pain in some instances of extensive trauma and for the remarkable relief of pain provided by such divergent therapeutic measures as acupuncture, placebos, hypnosis, and electrical stimulation.

Because psychologic factors may greatly influence the pain threshold, it is important to consider the "placebo" role of all therapeutic measures for the control of pain. Pharmacologically inactive drugs may be surprisingly effective in alleviating the pain of organic as well as functional disorders. The use of the placebo for differentiation of organic from functional pain is therefore unreliable. Reassurance and explanation are thus important factors in relieving pain with or without analgesic drugs.

Concern about the widespread use of addictive and abused drugs—and the inconvenience resulting from official restrictions placed upon their medicinal use—may sometimes lead to reluctance to prescribe narcotic analgesics when they are badly needed for pain relief. Familiarity with the pharmacology of the several available analgesics—their relative potency, duration of action, and addiction and abuse liability—is essential (Table 1–1). It must not be assumed that the average patient is addiction-prone. It is a good rule to give the lowest effective dose of the appropriate agent for the given clinical circumstance to provide adequate symptomatic relief for only as long as is necessary; this implies adequate clinical monitoring. It may be necessary to give the narcotic on a "once only" or "twice only" or interim basis. When severe pain is anticipated, around-the-clock administration may lower the required total daily dose. Remember that with development of drug tolerance the analgesic effect is lessened, so that increased dosage or alternative analgesics may be required. When pain is severe and intractable, however, as in terminal cancer, it is inhumane to permit unnecessary suffering. These general concepts or attitudes should be made clear to all individuals (eg, nurses, relatives) who may be responsible for the administration of narcotic drugs to patients under the physician's care.

Table 1–1. Useful narcotic analgesics.*

Generic Name	Proprietary Name	Approximate Equivalent Dose (mg)	Oral:Parenteral Potency Ratio	Duration of Analgesia (hours)	Maximum Efficacy	Addiction/Abuse Liability
Morphine		10	Low	4–5	High	High
Hydromorphone	Dilaudid	1.5	Low	4–5	High	High
Oxymorphone	Numorphan	1.5	Low	3–4	High	High
Methadone	Dolophine	10	High	4–6	High	High
Meperidine	Demerol	60–100	Medium	2–4	High	High
Alphaprodine	Nisentil	30–50	Parenteral use only	1–2	High	High
Fentanyl	Sublimaze	0.2	Parenteral use only	1–1½	High	High
Levorphanol	Levo-Dromoran	1.5–3	High	4–5	High	High
Codeine		30–60‡	High	3–4	Low	Medium
Oxycodone†	Percodan	4.5‡	Medium	3–4	Moderate	Medium
Dihydrocodeine†	Drocode	16‡	Medium	3–4	Moderate	Medium
Propoxyphene	Darvon	60–120‡	Oral use only	4–5	Very low	Low
Pentazocine	Talwin	30–50‡	Medium	3–4	Moderate	Low
Nalbuphine	Nubain	0.5–1	Parenteral use only	3–6	High	Low
Buprenorphine§	Temgesic	0.3	Parenteral use only	4–8	High	Low
Butorphanol	Stadol	2	Parenteral use only	3–4	High	Low

*Modified and reproduced, with permission, from Katzung BG (editor): *Basic & Clinical Pharmacology,* 2nd ed. Lange, 1984.
†Available only in tablets containing aspirin or acetaminophen.
‡Analgesic efficacy at this dose not equivalent to 10 mg of morphine. See text for explanation.
§Not yet available in the USA.

Chronic Pain (See also p 654.)

The relief of chronic pain can be one of the most perplexing and difficult problems encountered in medicine, since the cause of chronic pain is often obscure. Measures useful for the treatment of acute pain are often ineffective in managing the chronic pain syndromes. It is often necessary to resort to a combination of indirect and multidisciplinary therapeutic methods.

Numerous psychologic techniques such as operant conditioning, biofeedback, progressive relaxation, distraction, and placebo have had varying degrees of success in relieving pain. Hypnosis as a means of controlling chronic pain has a fluctuating history of acceptability and practice. Hypnosis may relieve sensory pain in some responsive patients through both tranquilizing and placebo effects.

Transcutaneous electrical nerve stimulation is a simple and effective means of relieving well-localized chronic pain in some patients.

Acupuncture as a means of providing pain relief has been used in the Orient for centuries, but the method has not had widespread acceptance in the USA. The mechanism of acupuncture analgesia remains uncertain.

Neurosurgical procedures (eg, chordotomy, deep brain electrical stimulation), although generally considered as a last resort for chronic pain relief, should not be unnecessarily delayed to the point of hopeless invalidism and addiction.

Nonaddictive Analgesics

The systemic nonnarcotic analgesics act peripherally to block pain; their mechanism of action is probably due to their ability to inhibit the synthesis of prostaglandins and other inflammation mediators.

A. Salicylates: The salicylate drugs are analgesic, anti-inflammatory, uricosuric, and antipyretic. They are useful in relieving myalgias, neuralgias, arthralgias, headaches, and dysmenorrhea. Untoward reactions are usually mild, consisting of dizziness and dyspepsia, but large doses may cause tinnitus, deafness, blurring of vision, nausea and vomiting, diarrhea, gastrointestinal hemorrhage, hepatitis, renal impairment, diaphoresis, headache, and delirium. In sensitive patients, salicylates may cause urticaria, asthma, and acute laryngeal edema.

1. Aspirin–Aspirin, the standard anti-inflammatory analgesic, is the drug of initial choice for treating mild to moderate pain of varied origin. Aspirin is available as plain, buffered, or enteric-coated 0.3-g tablets. The usual dose is 0.3–0.6 g with a full glass of water every 4 hours as needed. Gastrointestinal irritation may sometimes be reduced by administration of the drug with food or an antacid. Enteric-coated aspirin is slower-acting, but it prevents gastric irritation and is also useful for patients who might be skeptical of the analgesic value of "ordinary aspirin."

Aspirin can cause gastric irritation and increased microscopic blood loss from the gut in otherwise healthy individuals and is an occasional cause of massive gastrointestinal hemorrhage. It should not be used in patients with acute or chronic gastrointestinal problems—especially gastrointestinal bleeding. The incidence of aspirin-induced gastric ulceration and bleeding may be increased when there is concurrent use of alcohol or corticosteroids.

Hypersensitivity or intolerance to aspirin does occur, although uncommonly in view of the widespread use of the drug, and in rare instances the consequences may be very serious. Aspirin intolerance may be due to allergy but is more frequently unexplained in certain susceptible patients. Intolerance to aspirin often develops spontaneously in young or middle-aged adults who were formerly able to take aspirin without difficulty. Intolerance may be manifested by rhinorrhea, nasal polyposis, asthma, prolonged bleeding time, and anaphylactic shock. Further use of the drug is contraindicated in aspirin-intolerant patients. The incidence of true aspirin allergy (ie, with an immunochemical basis) is probably less than 0.1%, although it may be as high as 2–5% in known asthmatics.

Salicylates may cause a reversible decrease of glomerular filtration rate; it is therefore advisable to perform periodic tests of renal function in patients who are taking large amounts of aspirin or who have underlying renal disease. Aspirin may cause mild hepatitis in patients with underlying systemic disorders (eg, collagen diseases) and should not be used if there is active hepatic disease. Aspirin is not recommended for pregnant women, particularly during the last trimester of pregnancy.

Aspirin slightly prolongs the bleeding time by inhibiting platelet aggregation. This can increase the bleeding tendency in patients with a wide variety of bleeding problems (eg, anticoagulant therapy, hemophilia).

Aspirin may interact adversely with the anticoagulant drugs and with phenylbutazone, probenecid, and spironolactone; patients who are taking these drugs should be advised against the use of aspirin in all forms.

2. Other salicylate preparations–Aspirin is widely employed in combination with caffeine or with caffeine and phenacetin (APC) for synergistic effects. Although caffeine does enhance the analgesic effect of aspirin, it is doubtful that the addition of phenacetin provides any pharmacologic advantage. The large amounts of phenacetin ingested by habitual users of some of these combinations may cause nephropathy.

Sodium salicylate, enteric-coated, 0.3–0.6 g every 4 hours, may be used by patients with gastric intolerance to aspirin. It is less effective than aspirin.

B. Acetaminophen: Acetaminophen in a dosage of 325–650 mg orally 3–4 times daily has an analgesic and antipyretic potency comparable to aspirin. It has no anti-inflammatory actions and is therefore ineffective in rheumatoid arthritis and other inflammatory disorders. Acetaminophen may be especially useful as a mild analgesic and antipyretic agent in patients intolerant of aspirin and in those with bleeding disorders, peptic ulceration, and gout. It does not produce coagulation defects or cause gastric irritation and does not affect blood uric acid levels. Hypersensitivity reactions and hematologic abnormalities are quite rare. Large doses of acetaminophen taken over a prolonged period may cause hepatotoxicity. Simultaneous use of the drug with alcohol is inadvisable. Very large doses of acetaminophen taken accidentally or with suicidal intent can cause fulminant hepatic failure.

C. Newer Nonsteroidal Anti-inflammatory Drugs (NSAIDs): Several newer antipyretic, anti-inflammatory analgesic drugs are available largely for the treatment of arthritic disorders in patients who are intolerant of aspirin. Patients who fail to respond to one class of NSAIDs may at times respond to an agent of another class. A wide range of clinical renal syndromes may be caused by the newer NSAIDs, including acute renal failure, papillary necrosis, nephrotic syndrome, and interstitial nephritis. Renal complications are most apt to occur in patients with preexisting chronic renal disease, heart failure, volume depletion, and liver disease. Patients who are to be given these NSAIDs, particularly the elderly, should have an initial and periodic assessment of renal function. Gastric irritation seems to be less than with aspirin, but the drugs should still be used cautiously in patients with a history of peptic ulcer; severe gastrointestinal bleeding reportedly due to the drugs completely precludes their use in patients known to have active peptic ulcers. The drugs, like aspirin, can interfere with blood coagulation and may cause bleeding in patients with a hemorrhagic diathesis.

These agents should not be used concomitantly with aspirin or in patients with a history of nasal polyps, rhinitis, urticaria, or bronchospasm associated with aspirin use. They should not be taken during pregnancy and lactation.

Other side effects may include skin rashes, headaches, dizziness, drowsiness, visual disturbances, tinnitus, palpitation, dyspnea, and sodium retention.

The recommended oral dosages are as follows:
Diflunisal (Dolobid), 500 mg twice daily.
Fenoprofen (Nalfon), 300–600 mg 4 times daily.
Ibuprofen (Motrin, Rufen), 300–400 mg 3–4 times daily.
Meclofenamate sodium (Meclomen), 100 mg 3 times daily.
Naproxen (Naprosyn), 250 mg twice daily.
Piroxicam (Feldene), 20 mg once daily.
Sulindac (Clinoril), 200 mg twice daily.
Tolmetin (Tolectin), 400 mg 3 times daily.

D. Indomethacin: This anti-inflammatory analgesic is usually reserved for treatment of pain due to ankylosing spondylitis, acute gouty arthritis, and osteoarthritis of the hip. The usual dose is 25 mg 2–4 times daily; if tolerated, the dose is increased up to no more than 200 mg daily. Untoward effects include headache, dizziness, light-headedness, tinnitus, depression, psychosis, drug rash, stomatitis, anorexia, nausea and vomiting, peptic ulceration, gastrointestinal bleeding, diarrhea, fluid retention, and renal insufficiency. Because visual disturbances may occur (corneal deposits, retinopathy), periodic ophthalmologic evaluation is recommended. Psychiatric disorders, epilepsy, and parkinsonism may be aggravated by the drug. Patients receiving indomethacin should be observed carefully for any evidence of toxicity.

E. Phenylbutazone (Butazolidin): Phenylbutazone is a potent anti-inflammatory analgesic and is usually reserved for treatment of pain due to gouty arthritis, active ankylosing spondylitis, and superficial thrombophlebitis. Serious adverse reactions to long-term use of the drug—notably aplastic anemia, agranulocytosis, hemolytic anemia, hepatic and renal necrosis, and exfoliative dermatitis—limit application of the drug largely to short-term treatment of acute disorders. The recommended dosage is usually 300–400 mg/d (or less) in divided doses. If the drug fails to produce a favorable response within one week, therapy should be discontinued. When it is necessary to use phenylbutazone for prolonged periods, blood checks should be carried out monthly and patients should be observed frequently for evidence of toxicity.

F. Carbamazepine (Tegretol): This tricyclic compound is effective in relieving pain in about 75% of patients with trigeminal neuralgia and in some cases may induce prolonged remissions (see p 584). Carbamazepine has been used unpredictably and less effectively in other severe neuralgias and in pain due to tabes dorsalis.

Moderately or Potentially Addictive Analgesics

A. Codeine: Codeine is pharmacologically similar to morphine but is less potent. Codeine diminishes the cough reflex and decreases bowel motility (constipating). It is preferred to morphine for relief of moderate degrees of pain because it is much less habit-forming and causes fewer untoward reactions (urticaria, nausea and vomiting, pruritus, dermatitis).

The dosage of codeine phosphate is 8–65 mg orally or subcutaneously every 3–4 hours as needed. If 65 mg is ineffective, stronger narcotics should be used rather than larger doses of codeine, which only cause more severe side effects without enhanced analgesic effect.

Codeine in doses ranging from 8 to 65 mg is often used in combination with aspirin or acetaminophen to produce an additive analgesic effect. The dosage is 1 tablet orally 3–4 times daily as necessary.

B. Propoxyphene: Propoxyphene (Darvon), given in doses of 30–65 mg orally every 6 hours as needed, has about the same analgesic potency as aspirin. The drug is related chemically to the narcotics and, although considerably less potent in all respects, may be addictive. It is a Schedule IV controlled mild narcotic.

C. Agonist-Antagonist Opioids: The agonist-antagonist opioids have both morphinelike and narcotic antagonist properties. Although these drugs approach the analgesic effectiveness of morphine, special anticipated benefits have not yet been completely realized.

Tolerance develops more slowly to agonist-antagonist analgesics than to morphine. Although dependence liability is less than with conventional narcotics, caution should be exercised with addiction-prone individuals; the drugs can induce withdrawal symptoms in narcotics addicts. Sedation is a common side effect; dizziness, nausea, and vomiting can occur.

Pentazocine may cause psychotomimetic reactions and produce skin ulceration and fibrous myopathy at injection sites after long-term use.

The dosages are as follows: butorphanol (Stadol), 1–2 mg intramuscularly or intravenously every 4 hours as needed; nalbuphine (Nubain), 10 mg intramuscularly or intravenously every 3–6 hours as needed; pentazocine (Talwin), 30 mg intramuscularly, intravenously, or subcutaneously every 3–4 hours as needed.

Strongly Addictive Analgesics

The strongly addictive narcotic analgesics alter the perception of pain by their effects on the central nervous system. They are indicated for the relief of pain that is too intense to be controlled with nonnarcotic drugs or when pain is of a type not relieved by the salicylates (eg, visceral pain).

The narcotics are also mildly sedative in small doses; larger doses produce sleep, stupor, and respiratory depression. Adjunctive drugs such as aspirin, acetaminophen, and antidepressants may enhance the effect of narcotic drugs and reduce the doses needed for pain control. Narcotics should be used with great caution and with reduced dosage in patients who are receiving any type of central nervous system depressant, including alcohol. They are addictive and should be used with careful attention to federal and state laws. Except for codeine, the narcotics should not be used for chronic illnesses unless necessary for the control of intractable pain in terminal illness.

Addiction and withdrawal and the specific treatment of intoxication with these drugs are discussed in Chapter 18.

A. Morphine: This drug is the most valuable of the potent narcotics for general clinical use. It causes central nervous system depression that results in powerful analgesia associated with sedation, euphoria, and hypnosis; selective respiratory center depression; and dulling or abolition of the cough reflex. It increases intracranial pressure. Morphine is useful for the relief of almost every type of severe pain. It is the drug of choice for the pain of myocardial infarction and is also valuable in the treatment of severe cardiac dyspnea (eg, pulmonary edema or cardiac asthma of left ventricular failure).

Morphine is a valuable drug for the treatment of severe chronic pain in terminal illness. Appropriate, frequent dosages can usually provide sustained comfort without producing fluctuation between distress and unconsciousness. Heroin (diacetylmorphine), a potent and fast-acting narcotic with euphoriant properties, is prohibited by legislation in the USA. Attempts are being made to legalize heroin for treating intractable pain of terminal cancer.

Morphine is contraindicated in morphine sensitivity, bronchial asthma, undiagnosed surgical abdominal disease, hepatic insufficiency, hypothyroidism, morphinism, head injury, Addison's disease, and whenever the possibility of vomiting may be dangerous. The hypnotic effect associated with the analgesia produced by morphine may be undesirable. Side effects include respiratory depression, shock, nausea and vomiting, severe constipation, urticaria, and pruritus.

1. Morphine sulfate–The dosage of morphine sulfate is 8–15 mg orally or subcutaneously. In cases of severe agonizing pain—especially pain associated with impending neurogenic shock—morphine may be given slowly intravenously in 5 mL of physiologic saline. It is probable that only increased duration of effect is gained by increasing the dose above 10 mg.

2. Morphine adjuncts–Belladonna alkaloids such as atropine and scopolamine, 0.3–0.6 mg subcutaneously along with morphine, may reduce some of the untoward effects of morphine. The phenothiazine tranquilizers may enhance the sedative effect of morphine, making it possible to give the latter in smaller doses. **Brompton mixture,** an elixir containing morphine and cocaine, is used for the relief of chronic pain in inoperable cancer. It should be given on an individualized regular schedule with a phenothiazine in appropriate dosage to prevent pain while preserving a normal sensorium.

B. Morphine Congeners: The drugs in this category are equivalent to morphine but have no appreciable advantages. The following subcutaneous doses are equivalent to 10 mg of morphine: hydromorphone (Dilaudid), 1.5 mg; levorphanol (Levo-Dromoran), 1.5–3 mg; oxymorphone (Numorphan), 1.5 mg.

C. Methadone: Methadone has powerful addictive properties. The only situation in which methadone is preferred is in the authorized treatment of narcotic addiction; withdrawal symptoms are ameliorated if methadone is first substituted for heroin or other opiates (see Chapter 18). Methadone, 2.5–10 mg subcutaneously or intramuscularly, is also used as a morphinelike analgesic. Given orally, the drug is only one-half as effective as morphine, its onset is slower, and its effect is more prolonged.

D. Meperidine (Demerol): Meperidine, 75–150 mg orally or intramuscularly (not subcutaneously) every 3–4 hours, provides analgesia and causes less intense side effects than morphine. It is less addictive than morphine, but addiction to meperidine is very common nonetheless.

E. Alphaprodine (Nisentil): Alphaprodine, a meperidine congener, given 30–40 mg subcutaneously or 30 mg intravenously, has a more rapid onset and shorter duration of effect than meperidine or morphine.

Cassell EJ: The relief of suffering. *Arch Intern Med* 1983; **143:**522.

Chan WY: Prostaglandins and nonsteroidal anti-inflammatory drugs in dysmenorrhea. *Annu Rev Pharmacol Toxicol* 1983; **23:**131.

Clive DM, Stoff JS: Renal syndromes associated with nonsteroidal antiinflammatory drugs. *N Engl J Med* 1984;**310:**563.

Cooper SA: New peripherally-acting oral analgesic agents. *Annu Rev Pharmacol Toxicol* 1983;**23:**617.

Goodman CE: Pathophysiology of pain. *Arch Intern Med* 1983; **143:**527.

Graves DA et al: Patient-controlled analgesia. *Ann Intern Med* 1983;**99:**360.

Health and Public Policy Committee, American College of Physicians: Drug therapy for severe, chronic pain in terminal illness. *Ann Intern Med* 1983;**99:**870.

Inturrisi CE: Narcotic drugs. *Med Clin North Am* 1982;**66:**1061.

Lasagna L, McMahon FG (editors): New perspectives on aspirin therapy. *Am J Med* (June 14) 1983;**74(Suppl):**1.

Laska EM et al: Caffeine as an analgesic adjuvant. *JAMA* 1984;**251:**1711.

Levine J: Pain and analgesia: The outlook for more rational treatment. *Ann Intern Med* 1984;**100:**269.

McGivney WT, Crooks GM: The care of patients with severe, chronic pain in terminal illness. *JAMA* 1984;**251:**1182.

Mendelson G et al: Acupuncture treatment of chronic back pain: A double-blind placebo-controlled trial. *Am J Med* 1983; **74:**49.

Miles J: Neurological advances in the relief of pain. *Br J Hosp Med* 1983;**30:**348.

Skrabanek P: Acupuncture and the age of unreason. *Lancet* 1984;**1:**1169.

Solomon RA, Viernstein MC, Long DM: Reduction of postoperative pain and narcotic use by transcutaneous electrical nerve stimulation. *Surgery* 1980;**87:**142.

Sriwatanakul K et al: Analysis of narcotic analgesic usage in the treatment of postoperative pain. *JAMA* 1983;**250:**926.

Stillman MT, Napier J, Blackshear JL: Adverse effects of antiinflammatory drugs on the kidney. *Med Clin North Am* 1984;**68:**371.

Way WL, Way EL: Narcotic analgesics and antagonists. Chapter 29 in: *Basic & Clinical Pharmacology*, 2nd ed. Katzung BG (editor). Lange, 1984.

Winchester JF (editor): Georgetown University Symposium on Analgesics: Aspirin and acetaminophen. *Arch Intern Med* 1981;**141:**271. [Special issue.]

FEVER & HYPERTHERMIA

Fever was well known to the ancients as an important manifestation of illness, but it remained for modern medical science to provide a better understanding of the significance of body temperature variations in health and disease. As the large number of specific causes of fever were being identified over the past century, interest also turned toward the pathogenesis of fever. It is now believed that fever, or pyrexia, represents regulation of body temperature at an elevated thermoregulatory "set point" (ie, to a new point above 37 °C). The thermoregulatory center is in the hypothalamus. When bacterial toxins or other stimuli act on the body's bone marrow–derived phagocytic cells (eg, leukocytes), they produce endogenous pyrogens that circulate to the thermoregulatory center and cause an elevation of the set point. This rarely exceeds 41.1 °C (106 °F). The elevation may result from either increased heat production (eg, shivering) or decreased heat loss (eg, peripheral vasoconstriction).

Hyperthermia, usually an exogenous process, differs from fever in that it occurs when the body temperature is higher than the thermoregulatory set point; temperatures may rise to lethal levels. Hyperthermia occurs when body metabolic heat production or environmental heat load exceeds normal heat loss capacity or when there is impaired heat loss.

The body temperature is normally subject to individual variation as well as to fluctuation due to physiologic factors, eg, exercise, digestion, sudden increase in environmental temperature, and excitement. The normal diurnal variation may be as much as 1 °C, being lowest in the early morning and highest in the late afternoon. There is a slight sustained temperature rise following ovulation during the menstrual cycle and in the first trimester of pregnancy.

The average normal oral body temperature is 37 °C (range 36–37.4 °C), or 98.6 °F (range 96.8–99.3 °F). The normal rectal or vaginal temperature is 0.5 °C (1 °F) higher than the oral temperature, and the normal axillary temperature is correspondingly lower. Rectal temperature measurement is more reliable than oral temperature—particularly in the case of patients who are mouth-breathers or who are tachypneic.

While fever as a symptom should generally be regarded with appropriate concern, in some circumstances it may play a beneficial role. Experimental evidence and clinical observation suggest that host defense response may be enhanced in the presence of fever, and, conversely, inability of a patient to produce fever may carry a grave prognosis. In the preantibiotic era, fever was employed with limited success as nonspecific therapy for chronic infections (eg, central nervous system syphilis). Hyperthermia has also been used with limited success in treatment of certain neoplastic diseases. Markedly elevated or prolonged fevers may result in profound metabolic disturbances. High fever during the first trimester of pregnancy may cause birth defects that are apparently unrelated to the cause or treatment of the fever. Fever per se may increase insulin requirements and also alter the metabolism and disposition of drugs used for the treatment of the diverse diseases associated with fever. Prolonged elevation of rectal temperature over 41 °C (105.8 °F) may result in permanent brain damage; when the rectal temperature is over 43 °C (109.4 °F), heat stroke occurs and death is common.

The body temperature may provide important information about the presence of illness and about changes in the clinical status of the patient. The fever pattern (graphic record), however, is of rather limited use for specific diagnosis. Furthermore, the degree of temperature elevation does not necessarily correspond to the severity of the illness. In general, the febrile response tends to be greater in children than in adults; in elderly persons, the febrile response is less marked than in younger adults. A sudden fall in temperature in the febrile patient is not necessarily a favorable sign; unless there is a corresponding clinical improvement, it may portend a serious complication such as shock.

Diagnostic Considerations

The outline below illustrates the wide variety of clinical disorders that may cause fever. Most febrile illnesses are due to common infections, are short-lived, and are relatively easy to diagnose. In certain

instances, however, the origin of the fever may remain obscure ("fever of undetermined origin," FUO) after careful diagnostic examination. Meticulous history taking (including history of exposure to infection, travel, drugs), careful physical examination, extensive laboratory and x-ray studies, and even exploratory surgical procedures may be required (see Chapter 22).

In about 40% of cases, the cause of FUO is infectious disease. About 20% of cases of FUO are due to neoplastic disease, about 25% to connective tissue disease, and the remainder to miscellaneous causes. In 5–10% of cases, the diagnosis is never established.

Use of the so-called therapeutic test for the diagnosis of a febrile disorder is justified only when a specific disease is strongly suspected and when a diagnosis cannot be established by other means (eg, chloroquine for malaria). Hasty, empiric use of polypharmaceutic measures (eg, multiple antimicrobials, corticosteroids, antipyretics, analgesics) may seriously interfere with rational diagnosis and therapy and may actually be hazardous. The possibility of factitious or self-induced fever should be considered in patients with underlying psychiatric disorders.

Clinical Classification of Causes of Fever (With Examples)

(1) Infections: Viral, rickettsial, bacterial, fungal, and parasitic infections are the commonest causes of fever. (a) Generalized infections without localizing signs (eg, septicemia). (b) Generalized infections with localizing signs (eg, scarlet fever). (c) Localized infections (eg, pyelonephritis).

(2) Collagen diseases: Systemic lupus erythematosus, polyarteritis nodosa, dermatomyositis, rheumatoid arthritis, rheumatic fever.

(3) Central nervous system disease: Cerebral hemorrhage, head injuries, brain and spinal cord tumors, degenerative central nervous system disease (eg, multiple sclerosis), spinal cord injuries.

(4) Malignant neoplastic disease: Primary neoplasms (eg, of thyroid, lung, liver, pancreas, and genitourinary tract). Secondary neoplasms, carcinoid.

(5) Hematologic disease: Lymphomas, leukemias, pernicious anemia, hemolytic anemias, hemorrhagic disease (eg, hemophilia).

(6) Cardiovascular disease: Myocardial infarction, thromboembolic diseases, infective endocarditis, pulmonary embolism, paroxysmal tachycardias.

(7) Gastrointestinal disease: Inflammatory bowel disease, cirrhosis (necrotic phase), liver abscess.

(8) Endocrine disease: Hyperthyroidism, pheochromocytoma.

(9) Diseases due to physical agents: Heat stroke, radiation sickness, trauma (eg, surgery).

(10) Diseases due to chemical agents: Drug reactions, anesthesia (malignant hyperpyrexia), anaphylactic reactions, serum sickness, chemical poisoning, pyrogen reactions (following intravenous fluids).

(11) Disorders of fluid balance: Dehydration, acidosis.

(12) Other miscellaneous diseases: Sarcoidosis, amyloidosis.

(13) Psychogenic fever.

(14) Factitious, or "false," fever.

(15) Unknown causes.

Treatment

A. Removal of the Specific Cause of the Fever: The principal problem is to determine and eradicate the cause of the fever. Symptomatic measures directed solely toward depression of elevated body temperature are not indicated except for high, prolonged fevers.

Prevention of the serious "malignant hyperpyrexia" that may follow certain types of anesthesia (succinylcholine and potent inhalation anesthetics) can best be accomplished by recognizing the patient who is predisposed by virtue of heredity (past personal or family history of difficult anesthesia) and by choosing the proper anesthetic agent, with temperature monitoring during the entire course of anesthesia. As soon as the syndrome is detected, emergency treatment is required. Prompt and vigorous body cooling (see below), hyperventilation with 100% oxygen, intravenous dantrolene, and measures to correct metabolic acidosis and renal failure are instituted.

B. Reduction of Fever by Nonspecific Means: Use measures given below when the body temperature is greater than 40 °C (104 °F), particularly if prolonged, symptomatic treatment may be required (Table 1–2). Since moderately high fevers are usually well tolerated by the body, with little direct tissue damage, aggressive symptomatic treatment should be avoided. *Extreme pyrexia (hyperpyrexia) — temperatures in excess of 41 °C (105.8 °F) — is a medical emergency.* (See Heat Stroke, p 984.)

1. Measures for removal of heat–Alcohol sponges, cold sponges, ice bags, and ice-water enemas will reduce fever and provide physical comfort for patients who complain of feeling *hot.* Use of these measures should be appropriate to the degree of fever and discomfort and is to be avoided when the febrile patient feels and looks *cold.*

2. Antipyretic drugs–Aspirin or acetaminophen, 0.3–0.6 g every 4 hours as needed, is quite effective in reducing fever due to diseases that act upon the hypothalamic thermoregulatory center. The drugs may occasionally obscure the clinical picture and cause undesirable side effects such as excessive sweating, nausea and vomiting, skin eruptions, and hematologic changes (see p 2).

3. Fluid replacement–Oral or parenteral fluids must be administered in amounts sufficient to compensate for the extra fluid and electrolyte losses from perspiration and all other causes.

Atkins E: Fever: New perspectives on an old problem. (Editorial.) *N Engl J Med* 1983;**308**:958.

Dinarello CA, Wolff SM: Molecular basis of fever in humans. *Am J Med* 1982;**72**:799.

Donaldson JF: Therapy of acute fever: A comparative approach. *Hosp Pract* (Sept) 1981;**16**:125.

Hurley DL: Fever in adults: What to do when the cause is not obvious. *Postgrad Med* (Nov) 1983;**74**:232.

Kauffman CA et al: Diagnosing fever of unknown origin in older patients. *Geriatrics* (Feb) 1984;**39**:46.

Murray HW (editor): *FUO: Fever of Undetermined Origin.* Futura, 1983.

Nelson TE, Flewellen EH: The malignant hyperthermia syndrome. *N Engl J Med* 1983;**309**:416.

Rodbard D: The role of regional body temperature in the pathogenesis of disease. *N Engl J Med* 1981;**305**:808.

Tandberg D, Sklar D: Effect of tachypnea on the estimation of body temperature by an oral thermometer. *N Engl J Med* 1983;**308**:945.

WEIGHT LOSS

Marked unexplained weight loss is often an indication of serious physical or psychologic illness. If the weight loss is immediately discernible from the patient's physical appearance, the clinician should pro-

Table 1–2. Pathophysiology, clinical findings, and treatment of fever and hyperthermia.[*]

Pathophysiologic Basis for Fever	Clinical Findings	Treatment
Endogenous pyrogens act on hypothalamus to induce fever (eg, infection, collagen disease, allergy).	Patient complains of feeling cold. Shivering. "Gooseflesh."	Antipyretic drugs: aspirin or acetaminophen, 300–600 mg 4 times daily. Supply clothing and covers just sufficient for maximal comfort.
Agent or illness acts on hypothalamus to induce fever (eg, central nervous system lesions, toxins, radiation).	Cold extremities. Minimal sweating.	*Avoid* measures for physical removal of heat (eg, sponging, ice bags).
Heat production exceeds normal heat loss mechanisms (eg, malignant hyperthermia, thyroid storm).	Patient complains of feeling hot. Hot extremities. Active sweating (except in cases where there is defective heat loss mechanism).	Remove excessive clothing or covers. Eliminate excess environmental heat source. Employ measures for physical removal of heat (eg, sponging, ice bags, ice-water enemas).
Environmental heat load exceeds normal heat loss mechanisms (eg, exposure to industrial heat, overuse of sauna).		
Defective heat loss mechanisms cannot cope with normal heat load (eg, heat stroke, burns, sweat gland disorders).		*Avoid* antipyretic drugs.

*Modified and reproduced, with permission, from Stern RC: Pathophysiologic basis for symptomatic treatment of fever. *Pediatrics* 1977;**59**:92.

ceed promptly with appropriate (but not necessarily exhaustive) diagnostic studies based upon the findings of a careful history, physical examination, and routine laboratory studies.

Weight loss may be due to a wide variety of acute and chronic disease processes (eg, malignancy, infection, toxins) of any organ system of the body, as well as to psychiatric disorders. If the initial evaluation is done with discernment, many of the physical causes of weight loss can be relatively quickly uncovered. It is important early to correlate weight change with a history of significant change in appetite, physical activity, and psychosocial factors.

When the patient complains of weight loss but appears to be adequately nourished, inquiry should be made about exact weight changes (with approximate dates) and about changes in clothing size. Family members may provide confirmation of weight loss.

Once it has been established that the patient has marked weight loss, further methodical laboratory and radiologic investigation may be indicated. For unexplained reasons, marked weight loss can sometimes occur in the absence of serious physical illness. Psychiatric consultation should be considered when there is evidence of depression, anorexia nervosa, or other psychologic problems.

Botoman VA, Black HR: Weight loss: Guide to evaluating patients. Consultant (Jan) 1984;**28**:258.
Marton KI, Sox HC, Krupp JR: Involuntary weight loss: Diagnostic and prognostic significance. *Ann Intern Med* 1981;**95**:568.

FATIGUE

Fatigue and the closely related complaints of weakness, tiredness, and lethargy are most often readily explained by apparent common factors such as overexertion, poor physical conditioning, inadequate rest, marked obesity, inadequate nutrition, and emotional problems. The possibility that excessive fatigue may be due to physical illness, particularly in its incipient phase, sometimes makes it necessary to search for a wide variety of organic causes (see below).

A carefully elicited history of the patient's daily living habits and working environment may obviate the need for extensive and unproductive medical studies. The presence of fatigue on arising in the morning (that clears as the day progresses) and a history of emotional stress or of recurrent episodes of anxiety or depression lend support to a functional diagnosis.

Some of the organic causes of fatigue that might be considered are the following:

(1) Endocrine disorders: Addison's disease, hypothyroidism, hyperthyroidism, diabetes mellitus.

(2) Neurologic disorders: Myasthenia gravis.

(3) Infectious disease: Hepatitis, tuberculosis, brucellosis, infective endocarditis, intestinal parasites.

(4) Respiratory disorders: Emphysema, asthma.

(5) Hematologic disorders: Anemia, infectious mononucleosis.

(6) Collagen disorders: Rheumatoid arthritis, systemic lupus erythematosus.

(7) Cancer: Any type.

(8) Drugs and toxins: Alcohol, sedatives and tranquilizers, environmental toxins.

Massey EW, Scherokman B: The many causes of acute weakness. *Emergency Med* (Feb 15) 1984;**16**:181.
Morrison JD: Fatigue as a presenting complaint in family practice. *J Fam Pract* 1980;**10**:795.

SHOCK SYNDROME
(Circulatory Shock)

"Shock" is a complex group of acute cardiovascular syndromes that defy precise definition because of their varied origins. It is practical, however, to consider shock as a disturbance of circulation resulting in reduction of perfusion of tissues of vital organs with hypoxia and a wide range of systemic effects. The term is descriptive of a "classic" but highly variable pattern of signs and symptoms that usually includes arterial hypotension, altered sensorium, ashen pallor, clammy skin, rapid and weak pulse, air hunger, thirst, oliguria, and a tendency to steadily progress toward a refractory and so-called irreversible phase. Recognition of early shock may be obscured by factors such as anxiety, complicating medical problems, and surrounding circumstances. The "classic" signs of shock may appear suddenly and often represent fully developed shock.

In so-called warm shock, such as may be seen in the early phase of septic shock, the skin is pink and warm and the urine volume is adequate despite the arterial hypotension and peripheral pooling.

The 3 major pathophysiologic mechanisms involved in the production of shock are (1) hypovolemia (decreased effective blood volume), (2) cardiac insufficiency (pump failure), and (3) altered vascular resistance (vasoconstriction or vasodilatation).

Alteration of one or more of these factors may result in diminished microcirculatory flow. It is the adaptation or failure of adaptation of the microcirculation that is responsible for arteriovenous shunting, decreased urine output, fluid loss from the capillaries, sludging of red blood cells, disseminated intravascular coagulation, stagnant tissue hypoxia, acidosis, hyperlacticacidemia, and cellular injury, all of which occur in the shock syndrome.

Debility, malnutrition, senility, temperature extremes, alcoholism, hypotensive drugs, anesthetics, autonomic disorders, diabetes, and adrenocortical disorders are factors that can predispose to shock. Acute alcoholism may cause a misleading and unexplainable severe hypotension of several hours' duration without other evidence of clinical shock (ie, organ ischemia) in trauma patients. A rapid and thorough search for a cause is essential.

Factors that unfavorably influence the prognosis in shock states include coma, acidosis (pH < 7.30), $Pa_{CO_2} > 45$ mm Hg, serum lactate > 2 mmol/L, severe sepsis, anuria, heart disease, hepatic disease, and advanced age (> 70 years).

Classification

No classification of shock is completely satisfactory, but one that is based upon the predominant hemodynamic changes in the various types of shock is clinically the most useful (Table 1–3). It should be apparent that in a given patient with shock, several hemodynamic mechanisms are at work simultaneously, so that continuous monitoring of multiple parameters of cardiovascular function is required. For example, hypovolemia and altered peripheral resistance may be significant factors in cardiogenic shock, and pump failure may be an important feature of hypovolemic shock. Therapeutically, this implies a real hazard in focusing on only a single deranged mechanism in treating a so-called specific type of shock.

A. Hypovolemic Shock (Oligemic, Hemorrhagic, Traumatic, Burn, or Surgical Shock): In this form of shock there is a true diminution of blood volume owing to loss of whole blood or plasma from the circulation. Compensatory vasoconstriction temporarily reduces the size of the vascular bed and may temporarily maintain the blood pressure, but if fluid is not replaced immediately, hypotension occurs, peripheral resistance increases, capillary and venous beds collapse, and the tissues become progressively more hypoxic. Since the vascular space is the smallest of the body fluid compartments, even a moderate sudden loss of circulating fluids can result in severe and sometimes irreversible damage to vital centers. Rapid loss of 50% of blood volume is usually fatal.

Hypovolemic shock may result from (1) loss of

Table 1–3. Classification of shock.

I. **Hypovolemic shock (decreased effective blood volume)**
  A. Exogenous (external) loss of fluid
    I. Whole blood (eg, hemorrhage)
    2. Plasma (eg, burns)
    3. Fluid and electrolytes (eg, vomiting, diarrhea)
  B. Endogenous (internal) loss of fluid
    I. Exudative (eg, peritonitis)
    2. Traumatic (eg, hematoma)
II. **Cardiogenic shock (pump failure)**
  A. Intrinsic myocardial disorders (eg, decreased myocardial contractility)
    I. Focal damage (eg, myocardial infarction)
    2. Generalized disorder (eg, dysrhythmia, myocarditis)
  B. Extrinsic disorders
    I. Cardiac tamponade (eg, pericardial disease)
    2. Obstruction of major blood channels (eg, pulmonary embolism)
III. **Vascular (vasomotor, distributive, low-resistance) shock (altered vascular resistance and capacity)**
  A. Increased venous capacitance (pooling) (eg, bacterial endotoxin)
  B. Decreased arteriolar resistance (eg, fright, pain, vasodilative drugs)

whole blood by hemorrhage due to external or internal injuries, (2) loss of whole blood through nontraumatic internal hemorrhage (eg, bleeding peptic ulcer, ruptured varices), (3) loss of blood and plasma in extensive fractures and crushing injuries, (4) loss of plasma and hemolysis of red cells in extensive burns, (5) loss of plasma into serous body cavities (eg, peritonitis), (6) loss of plasma due to nephrotic syndrome, or (7) loss of fluid and electrolytes (eg, vomiting, diarrhea, endocrine disturbances).

B. Cardiogenic Shock: Shock due to inability of the left ventricle to perform effectively as a pump in maintaining an adequate cardiac output occurs most frequently following myocardial infarction, but it also occurs in serious cardiac arrhythmias, pulmonary embolism, cardiac tamponade, terminal congestive failure, or as a complication of other forms of severe shock. Shock associated with myocardial infarction or other serious cardiac disease carries a very high mortality rate (75–80%) despite therapy.

Clinical findings are of limited value in predicting the course or determining the prognosis of myocardial shock. Major myocardial infarction as determined by electrocardiography, enzyme studies, and sophisticated indices of cardiovascular function may provide reasonably reliable evidence of impending shock.

C. Vascular Shock (Vasomotor, Distributive, Low-Resistance Shock): In this type of shock, the available circulating volume of blood may be unaltered, but the blood volume is inadequate because the capacity of the vascular system is expanded. The increased vascular capacity may result from widespread dilatation of arteries and arterioles, from arteriovenous shunting, or from venous pooling. Often the skin is warm and the venous pressure normal.

1. Septic shock–The most common form of vascular, or low-resistance, shock is that due to gram-negative bacillemia, or so-called septic shock. The toxemia of overwhelming infection is characterized by an initial short period of vasoconstriction followed by vasodilatation, with venous pooling of blood in the microcirculation. There is often a direct toxic action on the heart and adrenals. The mortality rate is high (40–80%). Septic shock is most commonly caused by infection due to gram-negative organisms (*Escherichia coli, Klebsiella, Proteus, Pseudomonas*). Gram-negative anaerobes (eg, *Bacteroides*) are increasingly recognized as a cause of septic shock. Septic shock occurs more often in the very young and the very old; in diabetes, hematologic cancers, and diseases of the genitourinary, hepatobiliary, and intestinal tracts; in meningitis or pneumonia; and with corticosteroid, immunosuppressive, or radiation therapy. Immediate precipitating factors may be urinary, biliary, or gynecologic manipulations. Septic shock may be obscured by ineffective antibiotic therapy.

Septic shock should always be suspected when a febrile patient has chills associated with hypotension. Early, the skin may be warm and the pulse full. Hyperventilation may occur and result in respiratory alkalosis. The sensorium and urinary output are often initially normal. The classic signs of shock become manifest later. The symptoms and signs of the inciting infection are not invariably present. (See Chapter 24.)

2. Neurogenic shock–Neurogenic or psychogenic factors, eg, spinal cord injury, pain, trauma, fright, gastric dilatation, or vasodilator drugs, may also cause vascular shock. Sudden autonomic overactivity results in vasodilatation or inhibition of constriction of the arterioles and rapid peripheral and splanchnic pooling of blood. Following a period of anxiety and signs of epinephrine release (tachycardia, tremors, and pallor), there is a sudden reflex vagal stimulation with decreased cardiac output, hypotension, and decreased cerebral blood flow. Simple fainting in response to strong emotion is the most common example. In the absence of spinal cord injury or other complicating factors, the patient usually revives promptly in the recumbent position or following the administration of simple forms of treatment (eg, spirits of ammonia, physical stimuli), but observation is necessary to prevent recurrence and possible progression.

Vascular shock may also be due to anaphylaxis, histamine response, ganglionic blockade, and hypnotic drug intoxication.

Treatment

It is of vital importance to determine the specific cause or causes, contributing factors (eg, age, prior physical status, complications), severity, and duration of shock. Prompt, rational, and decisive action is essential. Prevention or early recognition of shock and of contributing medical factors is simpler and considerably more effective than the treatment of established shock. Observe and record vital signs (pulse, temperature, respiration, and blood pressure), color and texture of skin, and level of consciousness. Careful monitoring of the patient through close observation and examination by the clinician is of first importance, but additional physiologic and laboratory studies are often required.

A. General Measures:

1. Position–Place the patient with the head and torso in the horizontal or slightly elevated position with moderate (30-degree) elevation of the legs. Avoid the so-called shock position. Simple elevation of the legs is considered to be more desirable, since it is less apt to interfere with cerebral blood flow, although this too should be avoided if dyspnea is present.

2. Oxygen–Clear the airway of obstructions and secretions and, if necessary, insert an oropharyngeal or endotracheal airway. Start oxygen by mask or nasal catheter as soon as possible. Frequent monitoring of blood gases is of the greatest importance. If arterial P_{O_2} (Pa_{O_2}) is below 60 mm Hg or if dyspnea or cyanosis is present, increased oxygen is usually required. Positive pressure ventilation may be required to maintain adequate oxygen exchange. If Pa_{O_2} fails to show a prompt rise, suspect pulmonary shunting or so-called shock lung (see p 167). When positive end-expiratory pressure (PEEP) is employed, constant monitoring of cardiopulmonary physiology is required. If there is evidence of depression of cardiac output and depleted blood volume as the PEEP is increased, fluids and inotropic agents are given.

3. Temperature–Keep the patient comfortably warm. Avoid chilling (to prevent heat loss) and excessive externally applied heat, which will further dilate the peripheral vessels.

4. Analgesics–Control severe pain promptly with first aid measures and analgesic drugs. Give morphine sulfate, 8–15 mg subcutaneously, for pain. Since subcutaneous absorption is poor in patients in shock, morphine sulfate, 4–8 mg slowly intravenously, may be used for severe pain. *Caution:* Do not give morphine to unconscious patients, to patients who have head injuries, or to those with respiratory depression.

5. Laboratory studies–Determine blood hemoglobin, hematocrit, and red cell count immediately for baseline and follow-up values. Obtain blood for typing and cross-matching. Laboratory studies for rapid serial determination of serum electrolytes, pH, Pa_{O_2}, and Pa_{CO_2} may be invaluable. Present methods of blood volume determination are of limited value in monitoring the treatment of shock. Blood lactate levels are a measure of the severity of perfusion failure; a disproportionate rise in lactate indicates a poor prognosis.

6. Urine flow–In the patient without preexisting renal disease, urine output is a reliable indication of vital organ perfusion and is perhaps the best single criterion of shock. Insert an indwelling catheter to monitor urine flow (which should be kept above 0.5 mL/kg/h). Urine flow of less than 25 mL/h indicates inadequate renal circulation, which, if not corrected, can result in renal tubular necrosis.

7. Central venous pressure (CVP) or pulmonary artery wedge pressure (PAWP)–Monitoring of central venous pressure or pulmonary artery wedge pressure may be helpful in evaluating and treating the patient in shock. Central venous pressure determination is relatively simple and may be useful when serial measurements are made and are correlated with simultaneous clinical and laboratory observations. Central venous pressure is not as reliable as determinations of the pulmonary artery wedge pressure by the Swan-Ganz catheter technique, which provides a better index of left ventricular function.

In central venous pressure determination, a catheter is inserted percutaneously (or by cutdown) through the antecubital vein or through a major vein (eg, superior or inferior vena cava) and is connected to a saline manometer. Normal values range from 5 to 8 cm of water. A low central venous pressure in the presence of intense peripheral vasospasm (pale, clammy skin) suggests a low blood volume and need for fluid replacement, whereas a high central venous pressure (about 15 cm of water) suggests fluid overload or insufficient cardiac output. The central venous pressure, however, may be normal in left ventricular failure and neurogenic shock. Spuriously high central venous pressure readings may occur when the left ventricular end-diastolic pressure (LVEDP) is low in chronic obstructive pulmonary disease; low readings may be found when the LVEDP is high in aortic stenosis and acute left ventricular failure. Pressure changes in response to cautious administration of small amounts of intravenous fluids may increase the value of central venous pressure as an indicator of blood volume and cardiac efficiency.

Pulmonary artery wedge pressure determinations are considerably more reliable than central venous pressure for assessing adequacy of restoration of fluid volume and should therefore be used whenever possible. A mean pressure of 12 mm Hg is considered to be the upper limit of normal. An elevated pulmonary artery wedge pressure (> 14 mm Hg) may serve as a warning of impending pulmonary edema and of the hazard of fluid overload. In critically ill patients, the pulmonary artery wedge pressure may correlate poorly with left ventricular preload, probably because of abnormal left ventricular compliance.

8. Volume replacement–*Replace and maintain adequate blood volume.* Initial or emergency needs may be determined by the history, general appearance, vital signs and other physical findings, hemoglobin, and hematocrit, although these are not reliable guides for volume replacement. Under ordinary clinical conditions, determination of effective blood volume may be difficult and is subject to considerable variation. There is no simple technique or rule by which to accurately judge the fluid requirements. An estimate of total fluid losses is an essential first step. Continuous central venous pressure or pulmonary artery wedge pressure monitoring may be useful as a guide to safe fluid replacement. Response to therapy—particularly the effect of carefully administered, gradually increasing amounts of intravenous fluids on the central venous pressure or pulmonary artery wedge pressure—is a valuable index.

Selection of the proper fluid for restoration and maintenance of hemodynamic stability and other needs of patients in various stages and types of shock is often difficult and controversial. Consideration must be given to the type of fluid that has been lost (whole blood, plasma, water, electrolytes), associated medical problems, availability of the various replacement solutions, clinical and laboratory monitoring facilities, and, to a lesser extent, expense.

The most effective replacement fluid in case of gross hemorrhage is usually packed red cells in saline or whole blood, but other readily available crystalloid or colloid fluids should be given immediately pending the results of preliminary laboratory work and the procurement of whole blood. Rapid volume replacement in the case of blood loss will often prevent shock, and the amount of fluid required is more nearly equivalent to actual fluid loss. Delayed or inadequate volume replacement permits shock to develop and become progressively worse, so that the fluid volumes required for replacement are disproportionately large and more difficult to determine. If the central venous pressure or pulmonary artery wedge pressure is low and the hematocrit greater than 35%—and if there is no clinical evidence to suggest occult blood loss—replace blood volume with crystalloid solutions or colloids.

a. Crystalloid solutions–Crystalloid solutions available include sodium chloride injection (physiologic saline, 0.9%) or lactated Ringer's injection. Immediately give 500–2000 mL of the selected solutions rapidly intravenously under central venous pressure or pulmonary artery wedge pressure monitoring while making preparations for use of colloids or whole blood. The crystalloids can be used without the delay caused by the need for cross-matching and are readily available for emergencies and mass casualties. They may obviate the need for blood or colloids. They are remarkably effective when given in adequate doses, but the restoration of plasma volume is usually not sustained as it is in the case of the colloids, and there may be an undesirable overexpansion of the interstitial water. When large volumes of crystalloids are given, patients should be carefully monitored and examined frequently for evidence of water overload and pulmonary complications. If shock persists after prompt infusion of 2 L of crystalloids, it is necessary to give blood or other colloids.

b. Blood–(See above.) Packed red blood cells or whole blood is used for patients who require an increase in the oxygen-carrying capacity of the blood, as in hemorrhagic shock. Use of packed or frozen red cells is preferred over that of whole blood, because the red cells contain the same valuable components as whole blood but are not associated with many of the hazards of whole blood transfusions (eg, hemolytic reactions, allergic reactions, circulatory overload, citrate-induced alkalosis). The packed red cells can usually be obtained more promptly than whole blood, and they can be administered with sufficient volumes of crystalloids to correct volume deficits. If whole blood is used, it should be group- and type-specific and, whenever possible, the blood should be cross-matched. The amount of blood to be given will depend upon the clinical course, hematocrit, and hemodynamic findings.

c. Plasma fractions–Group-specific frozen plasma is a satisfactory colloidal volume expander that is usually readily available and may be used to correct specific coagulation defects. Whenever possible, unit-bagged plasma should be used rather than pooled plasma. Albumin 5% in saline, albumin 25% concentrate, or plasma protein fraction (containing 80–85% albumin) may be rapidly set up for emergencies, and blood typing is not required. These substances have been heat-treated to minimize the risk of infectious hepatitis. Purified albumin preparations are expensive and in limited supply. The use of plasma fractions is not advisable in profound, prolonged hypovolemic shock; because of impaired capillary permeability, there is an escape of protein into the interstitial tissues of vital organs that often results in serious adverse effects on pulmonary and cerebral function.

d. Dextrans–Dextrans are high-molecular-weight polysaccharide colloids that are fairly effective plasma expanders or "substitutes" for the treatment of shock. They have the advantage of being sterile and readily available for emergency use when blood or plasma fractions are not at hand. Dextrans may also be required because of a patient's rare blood type or religious belief. Low-molecular-weight dextran (dextran 40) has a comparatively short action as a colloid—about 8–10 hours. Furthermore, dextrans can impair blood coagulation, decrease the already impaired immune mechanism, and interfere with blood typing and may cause infrequent (but serious) anaphylactoid reactions. Dextrans are used infrequently now.

9. Vasoactive drugs–Because of their remarkable ability to raise the blood pressure, several of the adrenergic drugs have been used extensively, on a largely empiric basis, for the treatment of all types of shock. It is now known that simple blood pressure elevation produced by the vasopressor drugs has little beneficial effect on the underlying disturbances, and there is good evidence that in many instances that effect may be detrimental. Their routine use in all cases of shock is to be deplored.

Although the pharmacologic effects of the various adrenergic drugs cannot always be clearly explained and although their action in different disease states is not always predictable, certain of the known pharmacologic effects of available agents can be selectively utilized in the adjunctive therapy of shock (Table 1–4). Selection of the proper agent obviously depends upon the carefully determined particular pathophysiologic derangement in any given patient. *The adrenergic drugs should not be considered a primary form of therapy in shock.* Immediate restoration of blood volume, correction of hypoxia and fluid and electrolyte disturbances, and a search for treatable causes deserve first consideration. Continuous monitoring of vital signs, sensorium, central venous pressure or pulmonary artery wedge pressure, and urinary output is essential to determine if, when, how much, and for how long the adrenergic drugs are to be used.

The purely alpha-adrenergic stimulating drugs have little or no value in the treatment of shock. The mixed alpha- and beta-adrenergic agents are used most frequently, depending upon the need for adequate tissue perfusion pressure. Currently, dopamine is enjoying widespread use because of a uniquely favorable effect on renal and splanchnic blood flow, but its ultimate relative value in the treatment of shock remains to be determined. Epinephrine, of course, has a favored place among the adrenergic drugs because of its great value in the treatment of anaphylaxis, but its use is not recommended in other forms of shock. The beta-adrenergic stimulating agent isoproterenol has some value as a potent vasodilator and inotropic agent, but it is particularly apt to cause serious dysrhythmias. The alpha- and beta-adrenergic blocking agents have been largely limited to investigational use for the treatment of shock.

The principal vasoactive drugs currently used for shock are the following:

a. Metaraminol bitartrate is both an alpha- and a beta-mimetic agent with cardiotonic as well as vasopressor effects. Give 2–10 mg intramuscularly, or 0.5–5 mg cautiously intravenously, or 15–100 mg by slow intravenous infusion in 250–500 mL of 5% dextrose solution.

b. Isoproterenol, a beta-adrenergic stimulator, increases cardiac output by its action on the myocardial contraction mechanism and produces peripheral vasodilatation. Give 1–2 mg in 500 mL of 5% dextrose in water intravenously. Because of its inotropic effect, an increased incidence of cardiac arrhythmias precludes its use if the cardiac rate is greater than 120/min.

c. Dopamine hydrochloride (Intropin) is an endogenous catecholamine that has an added advantage over other adrenergic drugs because it has a beneficial effect on renal blood flow and also increases cardiac output and blood pressure. Dopamine hydrochloride, 200 mg in 500 mL of sodium chloride injection USP (400 μg/mL), is given initially at a rate of 2.5 μg/kg/min. This dosage stimulates both the dopaminergic receptors, which increase the renal blood flow and urinary output, and the beta-adrenergic cardiac receptors, which increase the cardiac output. If the shock is profound, gradually increasing doses of dopamine in excess of 20 μg/kg/min may be required. At these

Table 1–4. Adrenergic stimulating drugs used in hypotensive states.
(Effects graded on a scale of 0–5.)

Drug	Vasomotor Effect		Cardiac Stimulant (Inotropic Effect)	Cardiac Output	Renal and Splanchnic Blood Flow
	Vasoconstriction	Vasodilatation			
Mixed alpha- and beta-adrenergic					
Metaraminol (Aramine)	3	2	1	Reduced	Reduced
Epinephrine (Adrenalin)	4	3	4	Increased	Reduced
Dopamine (Intropin)*	2	2	2	Usually increased	Increased
Dobutamine (Dobutrex)	0–1	2–4	4	Usually increased	May be increased (due to increased cardiac output)
Norepinephrine (Levophed)	4	0	2	Reduced	Reduced
Beta-adrenergic					
Isoproterenol (many trade names)	0	5	4	Increased	Usually reduced

*Claimed to have special (dopaminergic) receptor.

higher levels, alpha-receptors may be stimulated, causing systemic vasoconstriction and a reversal of the vasodilatation of the renal vessels achieved at lower levels. After an effective dosage level has been reached, the infusion rate should be adjusted periodically to the lowest point necessary to maintain adequate organ perfusion. Dopamine alone may fail to maintain adequate perfusion pressure or to relieve intense vasoconstriction, and it may sometimes be necessary to use it in combination with another appropriate adrenergic drug. Patients with established shock in whom perfusion failure is associated with a substantial elevation in arterial blood lactate fail to respond to dopamine.

Adverse reactions include ventricular arrhythmias, anginal pain, nausea and vomiting, headache, hypotension, azotemia, and rare cases of peripheral gangrene. Special care should be exercised when dopamine is used in the treatment of shock following myocardial infarction, because the drug's inotropic effect may cause poorer myocardial metabolism. Dopamine should not be used in patients with pheochromocytoma or uncorrected tachyarrhythmias or in those who are receiving monoamine oxidase inhibitors.

d. Dobutamine, a synthetic catecholamine pharmacologically similar to dopamine but with greater inotropic effect, has been reported to be especially useful when filling pressures are high because of fluid overload or heart failure, as in septic shock.

e. The vasodilator phenoxybenzamine has been recommended as a safe, effective agent for increasing tissue perfusion in patients with severe shock who have failed to respond to adequate volume replacement and other conventional treatment. Correction of hypovolemia is mandatory prior to vasodilator therapy.

10. Corticosteroids–The beneficial effects of large doses of corticosteroids in shock are not completely understood, and their efficacy in the many types of shock syndromes is controversial. They may be related to improved cardiac efficiency or to increased blood flow to vital tissues. In the case of septic shock, they may decrease sensitivity to endotoxin, but it is questionable whether adrenocorticosteroids should be used for that condition, since they suppress the immune response and increase the likelihood that bacteremia will develop from a site infected with gram-negative rods (eg, urinary tract infections).

Those who express enthusiasm for corticosteroid therapy in the management of shock have suggested that corticosteroids should be administered as soon as shock is suspected—making it difficult to appraise the real value of the treatment. Dosage recommendations vary widely. Massive doses have been employed by some (eg, methylprednisolone, 30 mg/kg intravenously). Treatment should be discontinued immediately if there is any evidence of gastrointestinal bleeding.

11. Diuretics–The cautious early administration of mannitol as a 10–25% solution in 500–1000 mL of normal saline or Ringer's injection has been recommended (in association with other treatment measures) in selected patients in whom oliguria is present or impending. Furosemide, 20 mg intravenously, has also been recommended for this purpose. Urine flow and central venous pressure must be carefully monitored. The effectiveness of these agents in shock is still unknown.

Prior to the use of diuretics, it may be helpful to determine the urinary sodium; values greater than 30 meq/L suggest acute tubular necrosis and the possible advantage of diuretic therapy.

12. External pneumatic pressure–Careful application of external pneumatic pressure to the patient's legs and buttocks using specially designed inflatable garments such as military antishock trousers (MAST suits) or anti-G suits may be effective for temporary stabilization of patients with hypovolemic shock. Counterpressure has also been reported to be of value in controlling intractable abdominal bleeding to sustain vital signs until corrective surgery can be performed.

13. Heparin–(See Disseminated Intravascular Coagulation, p 345.)

B. Specific Measures:

1. Hemorrhage and anemia–Although crystalloids, plasma, or other volume expanders may be given as an emergency measure in shock complicating hemorrhage, severe anemia must be corrected by replacement with type-specific whole blood or packed red cells to prevent hypoxia. The quantity of blood to be given depends on clinical response, hematocrit, and hemodynamic studies.

2. Fluid and electrolyte balance–Abnormalities of fluid, electrolyte, and acid-base balance should be corrected. If acidosis fails to respond to adequate fluid replacement as evidenced by an arterial blood pH of less than 7.35, cautiously give sodium bicarbonate, 40–100 meq intravenously, and gauge further therapy by serial arterial pH determinations. Avoid alkalosis.

3. Cardiac disorders–Digitalis glycosides are indicated only for those patients with preexisting or presenting evidence of cardiac failure, digitalis-responsive arrhythmias, and, very controversially, in some patients with myocardial infarction. Atropine may be of value in treating selected postmyocardial infarction bradycardias associated with hemodynamic abnormalities predisposing to cardiogenic shock. Parenteral fluid for volume expansion may be necessary if there is evidence of hypovolemia as suggested by a low central venous pressure but should be given cautiously (especially sodium-containing solutions). Phlebotomy is sometimes useful in case of cardiac failure. The use of vasopressor drugs in myocardial infarction is controversial; if there is evidence of clinical shock (not merely mild hypotension), many physicians feel that the mortality rate can be reduced by maintaining the systolic blood pressure at levels of approximately 85 mm Hg (no more than 100 mm Hg). Continuous cardiac monitoring is required (especially when using beta-mimetic adrenergic drugs). The hemodynamic effectiveness of vasodilator drugs in reducing preload and outflow resistance in patients with left ventricular failure and cardiogenic shock is the subject of ongoing investigation. (See p 225.) The use of parenteral corticosteroids needs further evaluation.

Following myocardial infarction, mechanical circulatory assistance that reduces myocardial work and increases coronary perfusion—utilizing intra-aortic balloon counterpulsation on an emergency basis—may be temporarily helpful, though the effects on overall survival are not known. Emergency coronary bypass operations; infarctectomies; and repair of ventricular aneurysms, chordae tendineae, and septal defects following myocardial infarctions offer hope for some patients. It is difficult to assess the true value of these procedures at this time. (See Chapter 8.)

4. Infection–Immediate measures should be taken to combat infection, if present. Early recognition of incipient shock is critical, since death often occurs in less than 48 hours. The mortality rate in gram-negative shock remains at about 50% despite advances in treatment. Bacteriologic studies should be started immediately—before therapy if possible. If there are any indications of shock, institute preliminary broad-spectrum antibiotic therapy until bacteriologic studies reveal the identity of the organism. "Prophylactic" antibiotics, when there is no evidence of infection, are not indicated except when the hazard of infection is great (eg, extensive burns).

5. Andrenocortical failure–See p 729.

6. Anaphylactic reactions–See p 15.

C. Evaluation of Therapy: Constant observation of the patient is imperative. The vital signs, central venous pressure, urinary output, and laboratory studies must be monitored at appropriate intervals until the patient's condition has stabilized.

Barach EM et al: Epinephrine for treatment of anaphylactic shock. *JAMA* 1984;**251:**2118.

Calvin JE, Driedger AA, Sibbald WJ: Does the pulmonary capillary wedge pressure predict left ventricular preload in critically ill patients? *Crit Care Med* 1981;**9:**437.

Cullen DJ et al: Objective, quantitative measurement of severity of illness in critically ill patients. *Crit Care Med* 1984;**12:**155.

Ellenbogen C: Treatment priorities for septic shock. *Am Fam Physician* 1982;**25:**163.

Gaffney FA et al: Hemodynamic effects of medical antishock trousers (MAST garment). *J Trauma* 1981;**21:**931.

Holcroft JW: Shock. Chapter 15 in: *Current Surgical Diagnosis & Treatment*, 6th ed. Way LW (editor). Lange, 1983.

Ledingham IM, Cowan BN, Burns HJG: Prognosis in severe shock. *Br Med J* 1982;**284:**443.

Leier CV, Unverferth DV: Drugs five years later: Dobutamine. *Ann Intern Med* 1983;**99:**490.

Parker MM, Parrillo JE: Septic shock. *JAMA* 1983;**250:**3324.

Parker MM et al: Profound but reversible myocardial depression in patients with septic shock. *Ann Intern Med* 1984;**100:**483.

Pierson DJ, Hudson LD: Monitoring hemodynamics in the critically ill. *Med Clin North Am* 1983;**67:**1343.

Pinsky MR: Cause-specific management of shock. *Postgrad Med* (April) 1983;**73:**127.

Poole GV et al: Comparison of colloids and crystalloids in resuscitation from hemorrhagic shock. *Surg Gynecol Obstet* 1982;**154:**577.

Shoemaker WC: Pathophysiology and therapy of shock syndromes. In: *Textbook of Critical Care*. Shoemaker WC et al (editors). Saunders, 1984.

Shoemaker WC et al: Clinical trial of algorithm for outcome prediction in acute circulatory failure. *Crit Care Med* 1982; **10:**390.

Smith JA et al: The fluid of choice for resuscitation of severe shock. *Br J Surg* 1982;**69:**702.

Swan HJC, Ganz W: Measurement of right atrial and pulmonary arterial pressures and cardiac output: Clinical application of hemodynamic monitoring. *Adv Intern Med* 1982;**27:**453.

Swedberg J, Driggers D, Johnson R: Hemorrhagic shock. *Am Fam Physician* (July) 1983;**28:**173.

Wolff SM: The treatment of gram-negative bacteremia and shock. (Editorial.) *N Engl J Med* 1982;**307:**267.

SYSTEMIC ALLERGIC REACTIONS

Allergic, or hypersensitivity, disorders may be manifested by generalized systemic reactions as well as by localized reactions in any organ system of the body. The reactions may be acute, subacute, or chronic, immediate or delayed, and may be caused by an endless variety of offending agents (antigens)—pollens, molds, dusts, feathers, fur, venoms, food, drugs, etc. Many hypersensitive patients have a positive family history of allergy. It is felt that abnormal autonomic nervous system responsiveness may contribute to the pathogenesis of allergy.

A true allergic reaction is one that is immunologically mediated (ie, by an antibody following reexposure to an antigen). This is to be distinguished from a simple chemical reaction in an individual with an altered, damaged, or otherwise abnormal chemoreceptor system. An allergic response is particularly to be differentiated from unfavorable responses such as are produced by psychologic dislikes, overindulgence, and—in the case of drugs—overdosage, side reactions, and known adverse pharmacologic effects.

Several of the immunologic factors underlying hypersensitivity reactions have been identified. IgE is a humoral immunoglobulin which contains the reaginic antibody that plays a primary role in mediating many allergic reactions of the "immediate" hypersensitivity type (eg, asthma, acute urticaria, hay fever, anaphylaxis). When IgE antibody fixed to mast cells combines with antigen, the resulting complex disrupts the mast cell or basophil membranes, releasing histamine, slow-reacting substance of anaphylaxis (SRS-A; leukotrienes C and D_5), eosinophilic chemotactic factor of anaphylaxis (ECF-A), kinins, and prostaglandins. These chemical mediators act on the shock organs (eg, skin, bronchioles) and are responsible for the clinical manifestations of the immediate type of allergy.

Atopic, "natural or spontaneous," allergies occur in about 10% of the population, often with a family history of similar disorders. Determination of the allergens in the atopic patient is difficult, since complete reliance cannot be placed upon clinical history, skin tests, or elimination diets. Positive skin tests to multiple antigens are found frequently in atopic individuals. Skin testing often can help differentiate atopic from nonatopic individuals, but the relevance of scientific tests rests upon correlation with a careful history and physical examination. It has some degree of reliability in testing for certain drugs but is of no value in testing for food allergies. Eosinophilia and increased serum IgE levels are characteristic but not pathognomonic of atopic disorders. The serum IgE levels do not necessarily parallel the clinical degree of allergic response. The radioallergosorbent test (RAST) is an in vitro method of measuring allergen-specific IgE in patients in whom intradermal testing is inappropriate, hazardous, or equivocal. The test, purported to be of special value in testing for atopy, is not generally suitable for clinical practice. The atopic disorders include hay fever (allergic rhinitis), atopic dermatitis, allergic eczema, allergic asthma, and anaphylactic reactions.

Other protective body mechanisms at work include cellular immunity, the inflammatory response, other immunoglobulins (IgG, IgA, IgM), and the complement system. A useful classification of allergic reactions that embodies the immunopathologic mechanisms in the various allergic disorders is shown in Table 1–5.

"Delayed" hypersensitivity reactions—based upon a longer interval for the reaction to occur following a challenging antigen dose—are due largely to cell-mediated immunity and include most immunologic responses not dependent upon circulating immune globulins. Sensitized T lymphocytes react directly with antigen, producing inflammation through the action of soluble lymphokines. The tuberculin response and the various types of contact dermatitis are examples of the delayed reactions, which usually take hours or days to occur. Anergy, primarily a deficiency in the lymphocyte-mediated response, may be of importance in skin testing, viral infections, malignant disease, malnutrition, organ transplantation, and immunosuppressive therapy.

Adkinson NF Jr et al: Keeping current on allergic reactions. *Patient Care* (Nov) 1983;**17**:20.

Buisseret PD: Allergy. *Sci Am* (Aug) 1982;**247**:86.
Kaliner M et al: Autonomic nervous system abnormalities and allergy. *Ann Intern Med* 1982;**96**:349.
Marquardt DL, Wasserman SJ: Allergy: Choosing the right diagnostic procedure. *Consultant* (Jan) 1984;**28**:151.
Salvaggio JE (editor): Primer on allergic and immunologic diseases. *JAMA* 1982;**248**:2579. [Entire issue.]
Schaeffer M Jr, Sisk LC: Allergic extracts: A review of their safety and efficacy. *Ann Allergy* 1983;**52**:2.
Stites DP et ll (editors): *Basic & Clinical Immunology*, 5th ed. Lange, 1984.
VanArsdel PP Jr: Diagnosing drug allergy. *JAMA* 1982;**247**:2576.

1. ANAPHYLACTIC & ANAPHYLACTOID REACTIONS

Anaphylactic reactions are the immediate shock-like and frequently fatal reactions that occur within minutes after administration of foreign sera or drugs (especially penicillin and aspirin). Anaphylactic reactions may occur following the injection of sera, penicillin and other antibiotics, and practically all repeatedly administered parenteral diagnostic and therapeutic agents. *Note:* Drugs having a relatively high sensitizing risk (see below) should not be administered indiscriminately by oral, topical, or parenteral routes. Emergency drugs should be available whenever injections are given.

Anaphylactoid reactions, which mimic true anaphylaxis, are idiosyncratic reactions that occur generally when the patient is first exposed to a particular drug or agent. Although not immunologically mediated, their emergency management is the same.

Symptoms of anaphylaxis include apprehension, paresthesias, generalized urticaria or edema, choking, cyanosis, wheezing, cough, incontinence, shock, fever, dilatation of pupils, loss of consciousness, and convulsions. Death may occur within 5–10 minutes.

Emergency Treatment

(1) Epinephrine solution, 0.4–1 mL of 1:1000 solution (0.4–1 mg) intramuscularly, repeated in 5–10 minutes and later as needed. *Note:* This is the first measure to be employed. If the patient does not re-

Table 1–5. Classification of allergic diseases (after Coombs and Gell).

Type	Mechanism	Principal Antibody	Examples
I	Anaphylactic (immediate, homocytotropic, antigen-induced, antibody-mediated)	IgE	Anaphylaxis (drugs, insect venom, antisera), atopic bronchial asthma, allergic rhinitis, urticaria, angioedema
II	Cytotoxic (antimembrane)	IgG, IgM (activate complement, causing cell lysis)	Transfusion reactions, Goodpasture's syndrome, autoimmune hemolysis, hemolytic anemia, certain drug reactions
III	Immune complex (serum sickness–like)	IgG, IgM (form complexes with complement, injuring vessels and basement membranes)	Serum sickness, lupus nephritis, occupational allergic alveolitis, allergic contact dermatitis
IV	Cell-mediated (delayed) or tuberculin type response	. . .	Allergic contact dermatitis, infectious granulomas (tuberculosis, mycoses), tissue graft rejection

spond immediately, give 0.1–0.2 mL of 1:1000 solution diluted in 10 mL saline *slowly* intravenously.

(2) Place in recumbent position.

(3) Maintain adequate airway with oral airway or endotracheal tube. If respirations have ceased, provide artificial respiration by mouth-to-mouth or endotracheal techniques. Emergency tracheostomy may be necessary for laryngeal edema.

(4) Diphenhydramine hydrochloride, aqueous, 5–20 mg intravenously, if epinephrine response is not rapid and sustained.

(5) Oxygen at 4–6 L/min.

(6) Aminophylline injection, 250–500 mg in 10–20 mL of saline *slowly* intravenously, for severe bronchospasm (without shock). Repeat in 3–4 hours as needed.

(7) Intravenous fluids may be used to correct hypovolemia. If arterial hypotension is severe, vasopressor agents (eg, dopamine, 200 mg in 500 mL of dextrose in water) may be given slowly by intravenous infusion.

(8) Hydrocortisone sodium succinate, 100–250 mg in water or saline intravenously over a period of 30 seconds, after epinephrine or diphenhydramine, to prevent prolonged reactions.

Prevention

A. Precautions: Be aware of the danger. Do not use potentially dangerous drugs unless there is no reasonable alternative. Use special precautions in giving drugs to patients with a history of hay fever, asthma, or other allergic disorders. Whenever possible, determine by inquiry whether the patient has been previously given the drug that is about to be administered. If there is a report of any allergic reaction on prior administration, the hazard of giving the drug, *either orally or by injection,* must be carefully considered. Scratch, intradermal, or conjunctival tests with dilute solutions of the test substance are unreliable and not without hazard.

One of the most common forms of drug anaphylaxis reported is that due to penicillin. Avoidance of use of penicillin is the only sure method of avoiding allergic reactions. Semisynthetic penicillins and related compounds are, in varying degrees, cross-allergenic with natural penicillins. Oral administration of penicillin seems to be safer than parenteral. Specific penicillin antigen tests can be done with "major" and "minor" determinants but are not routinely available. A negative history or a negative skin test does not always assure safety, but a history of penicillin reaction or a positive skin test—despite the fact that allergy to penicillin is known to wax and wane in some individuals—should warn the physician not to use penicillin if another effective drug can be safely substituted. In extremely rare instances where penicillin alone or in combination is the only effective regimen, progressive desensitization may be cautiously attempted. Since this involves irreducible risks, after written informed consent has been obtained, desensitization must be done under close supervision in a hospi-

tal with adequate resuscitation measures at hand. (See Patterson and Anderson reference, below.)

Other drugs besides penicillin that are likely to induce anaphylaxis are immune antisera (eg, tetanus, snake antivenin), protein drugs (eg, chymotrypsin), dehydrocholate sodium, demeclocycline, nitrofurantoin, sulfobromophthalein (BSP), streptomycin, water-soluble iodine radiographic contrast media for parenteral use, and, rarely, vaccines.

Hymenoptera (honey bees, hornets, yellow jackets, and wasps) are the most common causes of allergic emergencies due to stinging in the USA, although there has been an increasing menace from stings of fire ants *(Solenopsis).* Patients who are known to be sensitive to insect bites should avoid areas where such insects are apt to be present. Protective garments (eg, gloves, netting, full-length clothing) may be necessary. Sensitized patients should always carry an insect-sting first aid kit containing a preloaded syringe of epinephrine, 1:1000 (the solution should not be more than 1 year old); ephedrine sulfate tablets (25 mg); antihistamine tablets; and a tourniquet and should be familiar with the use of these items.

Individuals with known sensitivity to drugs and stings should wear a medical identification bracelet or tag (Medic-Alert) or carry an identification card.

B. Prior Administration of Antihistamines and Corticosteroids: Antihistamines, corticotropin, and corticosteroids have been given before cautious administration of important drugs to which the individual is sensitive in an attempt to anticipate hypersensitivity reactions, but the results are unpredictable and the procedure is hazardous.

C. Desensitization: (See p 834.) Hypersensitivity to insect allergens may be extreme, and desensitization of suspected insect-sensitive patients, although effective, may be hazardous and is best performed by an experienced allergist. It is felt that patients with a history of bee sting anaphylaxis should be desensitized, preferably with venom immunotherapy.

Beeley L: Allergy to penicillin. *Br Med J* 1984;**288:**511.

deShazo RD, Salvaggio JE: Anaphylactic emergencies: Update on changing picture. *Mod Med* (April) 1982;**50:**112.

Haupt MT, Carlson RW: Anaphylaxis and anaphylactoid reactions. Pages 72–81 in: *Textbook of Critical Care.* Shoemaker WC et al (editors). Saunders, 1984.

Insect venoms. *Med Lett Drugs Ther* 1983;**25:**53.

Patterson R, Anderson J: Allergic reactions to drugs and biologic agents. *JAMA* 1982;**248:**2637.

Patterson R, Valentine M: Anaphylaxis and related allergic emergencies including reactions to insect stings. *JAMA* 1982;**248:**2632.

2. SERUM SICKNESS-LIKE REACTIONS

"Serum sickness" is a systemic allergic reaction that can occur within 1–2 weeks after administration of any foreign serum or drug and even more frequently as a result of administration of many widely prescribed drugs. The vasculitic type of response in the serum sickness syndrome is due primarily to circulating immune complexes induced by the offending agent. It is characterized by malaise, fever, urticaria, patchy or generalized rash, lymphadenopathy, musculoskeletal aches and pains, nausea and vomiting, and abdominal pain. Serious neuropathy, vasculitis, and glomerulonephritis occur very rarely. In previously sensitized individuals, the reaction may be severe or even fatal; the onset may occur immediately or after a latent period of hours to days.

Prevention & Treatment

Recognition of individual hypersensitivity is based upon a history of allergic diathesis or previous drug or serum reactions. It warrants special preliminary testing for sensitivity and careful precautions in administering immunizing sera.

Antihistamines or salicylates may be given as needed for mild reactions. Epinephrine, ephedrine, or the corticosteroids may also be required for moderate or prolonged reactions. Severe reactions should be treated as for anaphylaxis.

•   •   •

DRUGS USED IN ALLERGIC DISORDERS

Drugs are useful for the symptomatic treatment of allergic disorders but should not be used as a substitute for accurate diagnosis, except for allergic emergencies.

The ideal management of the allergic patient is to identify and prevent exposure to the offending agent, and this should be attempted whenever possible. In practice, however, it is often difficult to determine the exact allergen, and there may be multiple allergens. Furthermore, it is frequently impossible to incriminate the many possible sources of the allergens or to anticipate exposure, even when the allergens have been properly identified.

Desensitization (immunotherapy) of some allergic patients may sometimes be accomplished by cautious administration of progressively larger doses of the allergenic substances, especially when the allergic reaction is due to demonstrable extrinsic causes (eg, pollens, environmentals).

Many manifestations of allergic reactions are due to the liberation of histamine and other chemical mediators of the hypersensitivity reactions from storage sites in the body—tissue mast cells and circulating blood basophils. The treatment of allergies may thus consist of drugs that (1) block some of the effects of histamine (antihistamines; see below); (2) inhibit release of histamine by increasing intracellular levels of cyclic nucleotides (beta-adrenergic drugs [see p 129] and prostaglandin E_2); (3) inhibit release of histamine by blocking the enzyme that inactivates intracellular cAMP (theophylline; see p 128); (4) prophylactically inhibit release of histamine by an unknown mechanism (cromolyn; see p 130); or (5) suppress the allergic inflammatory reaction (corticosteroids; see p 129 and Table 19–17).

The Antihistamines

These drugs, besides blocking the effects of histamine, also have sedative and atropinelike effects. There are 5 chemical classes of antihistamines: ethanolamines (eg, diphenhydramine), ethylenediamines (eg, tripelennamine), alkylamines (eg, brompheniramine), piperazines (eg, hydroxyzine), and phenothiazines (eg, promethazine). The several dozen available antihistamine drugs differ from each other principally in potency, duration of action, degree of sedation, and incidence of side effects. It is doubtful that any given drug will be suitable for all patients. Selectivity is important, and it may be necessary to try different types of antihistamines to determine optimal effectiveness for a given patient.

The antihistamines are most useful in the symptomatic treatment of seasonal allergic rhinitis, urticaria, angioneurotic edema, insect stings, and serum sickness. They are less predictably useful in vasomotor or perennial rhinitis and are least apt to be effective in atopic dermatitis and bronchial asthma. By themselves, even when used intravenously, they fail to protect against the physiologic disturbances of severe allergic reactions (eg, anaphylaxis). Topical application of antihistamines to the skin should be avoided in the treatment of dermatoses.

Some commonly used antihistaminic drugs and their usual oral dosages are as follows:

A. Sedation Infrequent:
   *Chlorpheniramine (Chlor-Trimeton), 4 mg 3–4 times daily.
   *Brompheniramine (Dimetane), 4 mg 3–4 times daily.

B. Sedation Often Prominent:
   *Diphenhydramine (Benadryl), 25–50 mg 3–4 times daily.
   *Hydroxyzine (Atarax, Vistaril), 25–100 mg 3–4 times daily.
   *Tripelennamine (Pyribenzamine), 25 mg 3–4 times daily.
   *Promethazine (Phenergan), 12.5–25 mg twice daily.

Allergy and Immunology Committee, American College of Physicians: Allergy and immunology: An annotated bibliography of recent literature. *Ann Intern Med* 1982;**97**:791.

Antiallergic, antiviral and immunologic agents. Chapter 9 in: *AMA Drug Evaluations*, 5th ed. American Medical Association, 1983.

Foreman JC: The pharmacological control of immediate hypersensitivity. *Annu Rev Pharmacol Toxicol* 1981;**21**:63.

Hiller FC, Wilson FJ Jr: Evaluation and management of asthma. *Med Clin North Am* 1983;**67**:669.

Lichtenstein LM, Fauci AM: *Current Therapy of Allergy and Immunology*. Mosby, 1983.

Matthews KP: Respiratory atopic disease. *JAMA* 1982;**248**: 2587.

*Parenteral preparation available.

2 | Geriatric Medicine & the Elderly Patient

Lawrence Z. Feigenbaum, MD

The biologic changes associated with aging are influenced by hereditary and environmental factors. A distinction should be made between physiologic aging—the normal wear and tear that occurs with the passage of time—and pathologic phenomena occurring in old people that are the result of disease or adverse features of the individual's life-style. The roles of disuse and physical deconditioning are other factors that should logically be considered apart from the physiologic aging process.

Aging ordinarily occurs gradually throughout life, but quite unevenly from individual to individual; some persons age more rapidly than others. Specific chronologic age criteria for designating older individuals as a group are unavoidably arbitrary and may be harmful. The terms "elderly" and "senior citizen" are better defined in terms of functional status rather than by chronologic age, though for purposes of administrative convenience, age 65, age 75, etc, are often used. Some writers now subclassify the elderly into the "young-old" (ages 65–74) and the most rapidly growing group, the "old-old" (over 85).

Some of the consequences of aging that determine the nature and degree of functional impairment are listed below:

(1) Decreased function of one or more organ systems. The following are examples of changes that occur as a result of "normal" aging.

Skin: Decrease in subcutaneous fat, increase in wrinkling, atrophy of sweat glands.

Eyes: Decrease in pupil size, presbyopia with marked decrease in accommodation, lens opacification and discoloration.

Ears: Decrease in hearing of high frequencies and sensitivity to loud noise.

Cardiovascular system: Decrease in cardiac output, decrease in response of heart rate to stress, decrease in elasticity and compliance of peripheral vessels.

Respiratory system: Decrease in elasticity and ciliary activity, less sensitive cough reflex.

Gastrointestinal system: Decrease in hydrochloric acid and saliva flow, decrease in absorption of calcium, decrease in colon motility.

Genitourinary system: Drying and atrophy of vaginal mucous membranes, slower sexual response, enlargement of prostate with bladder outflow obstruction, decrease in renal blood flow, decrease in maximum urine osmolality.

Nervous system: Slower psychomotor performance, slower righting reflexes, fewer hours of REM sleep.

Musculoskeletal system: Decrease in bone mass, decrease in lean body mass.

Endocrine system: Glucose intolerance due to decreased peripheral utilization, increase in ADH response, decrease in estrogen secretion.

Immune system: Absent thymic hormone secretion, diminished T cell function.

(2) Decreased stress tolerance, eg, temperature extremes, trauma.

(3) Increased psychologic stress due to personal losses, eg, loss of physical vigor, deaths of friends and family members, retirement, reduced income, loss of sense of identity and self-worth.

(4) Impaired immunity, eg, greater susceptibility to infection, neoplastic disease.

(5) Increased susceptibility to disease, often to multiple diseases.

(6) Increased frequency of atypical presentation of disease.

(7) Altered pharmacokinetics, eg, adverse drug reactions.

(8) Decreased physical conditioning, eg, loss of muscle tone.

This list of age-related psychophysiologic changes is intended only to emphasize the variety of problems that may require special consideration in the medical management of elderly patients. Stereotypic concepts of hopelessness or progressive physical and mental deterioration must be avoided, since most older patients do enjoy good health and respond well to proper medical care.

An awareness of special problems of the elderly; a willingness to listen; a realistic, understanding attitude in dealing with older patients; and a knowledge of community support services can help the elderly function independently and actively as long as possible.

HISTORY TAKING WITH ELDERLY PATIENTS

It must not be assumed that an older patient is unable to provide a reliable medical history. At the initial interview, the examiner should note any impairment of hearing or speech, mood disturbance, or apparent difficulty with thought processes, any of which may interfere with the history-taking process. The elderly patient, just as any other patient, should be interviewed in an unhurried, reassuring manner in quiet, pleasant surroundings. If the patient is unable to comprehend or communicate, data should be sought from family and friends. The history should include pertinent information about daily living activities and socioeconomic circumstances.

Drug History

It is essential to review *all* drugs the patient has been taking. Have the patient or family bring in both prescription and over-the-counter drugs. Review them one by one by name, inquiring about the reason for taking the drug, its dosage and frequency of administration, and any adverse side effects the patient may attribute to the drug. Repeat this important exercise as often as necessary to make certain the patient's drug intake is both rational and minimal.

Dietary History

Many elderly patients have limited nutritional intake. It is important to inquire about the diet, asking specifically about adequacy of income, problems with shopping or preparing meals, eating habits, impaired senses of taste and smell, and difficulties with dentures.

Psychiatric History

Depression and anxiety resulting from severe psychologic stress or organic disease are common in the elderly. (The highest incidence of suicide in the USA is in white men over age 75.) Depression is a treatable condition that may be overlooked unless one is alert to its possibility. Loss of appetite, change in sleep patterns, and constipation are common in the well elderly but may also be signs of depression. Ask openly about suicidal thoughts and crying spells and any past history of mental illness. Psychiatric illness in old people can often be successfully treated, and psychiatric consultation should be recommended without hesitation if the history arouses concern about the patient's emotional status.

Do not avoid questions about sexual feelings or problems, since elderly patients may welcome an opportunity to discuss such matters. Many elderly people worry that it is abnormal for them to still have sexual feelings. Impotence or unreliable erections may be a significant problem for elderly men, and dryness of the vagina with a history of dyspareunia for elderly women.

Be aware of the possibility of drug abuse and alcoholism; they are more common than is generally recognized in the elderly.

PHYSICAL EXAMINATION OF ELDERLY PATIENTS

A complete physical examination, including pelvic examination in women and rectal examination in both sexes, is essential. Note abnormalities of gait and steadiness on standing. Examine the patient completely undressed (with gown) so that the skin can be carefully inspected. Test and record hearing and vision. Remove excess cerumen from the external auditory canals, look for cataracts, test ability to read, and check visual fields. Note redness or tenderness over the temporal artery. Look to see if dentures fit well, and inspect the oral cavity carefully with dentures removed, remembering that malignant lesions of the mouth are more often red than white. In auscultating the chest, bear in mind that the presence of an S_4 in an elderly patient does not imply clinically significant cardiac disease. Check muscle strength and range of motion of joints, and observe for neurologic deficit. Careful examination of the feet, including how well the shoes are fitted, is important in the patient with gait disturbance. In the chair-bound or bed-bound patient, great care must be taken to examine the skin for reddening or evidence of early ulceration over pressure points.

Mental Status Examination

Some form of cognitive testing is desirable with all elderly patients. Remember that patients with mild degrees of dementia may mask intellectual impairment by a cheerful and cooperative manner. If the patient appears mentally competent, the physician should explain that a mental status evaluation is part of every complete examination, so that the patient will not feel singled out and insulted. An examination that tests only orientation as to person, place, and time is often not sufficient to detect intellectual impairment. Many practical mental status tests are available (eg, Jacobs Cognitive Capacity Screening Test, the Short Portable Mental Status Questionnaire [SPMSQ], Mini-Mental Status Examination of Folstein).

Emphasis on Functional Capacity & Rehabilitation

Simply taking a history, performing a physical examination, and listing medical diagnoses are not sufficient for a frail elderly patient at high risk for institutional care. A clear description of the patient's degree of fitness or functional incapacity based on both medical and psychosocial problems is essential. Before nursing home placement is recommended, a thorough multidisciplinary geriatric functional assessment should be done in most instances. In addition to the physician, the assessment team usually includes the following:

(1) A social worker who assesses the ability of the family, friends, and community agencies to provide those supports which will allow the patient to remain in his or her home.

(2) An occupational therapist who assesses the patient's ability to perform the activities of daily living. The Katz Index of Activities of Daily Living is the most commonly used instrument (Katz S et al: *JAMA* 1963;**185**:94). It classifies patients according to their functional independence or dependence in the follow-

ing areas: bathing, dressing, feeding, transferring, using the toilet, and continence. For those patients who are less incapacitated, testing of more complex functions requiring both physical and cognitive ability should be done. These instrumental activities of daily living include reading, writing, cooking, shopping, using the telephone, and managing money and medications. Assessment of these functions and careful consideration of what steps can be taken to help the patient become more independent are often the most important contributions the health team can make in improving the patient's quality of life and preventing or delaying institutionalization. The occupational therapist is also helpful in detecting perceptual disorders and apraxias.

(3) A speech pathologist who may detect speech, hearing, and communication problems that might otherwise be overlooked.

(4) A psychiatrist or psychologist who may help differentiate depression from dementia, as well as organic from psychogenic symptoms.

Other consultants may be required, eg, physiatrist, neurologist, urologist, gynecologist, dentist, and nutritionist.

A home visit is of great value in assessing the patient's ability to function in his or her own environment.

About 25% of patients on waiting lists for nursing home care can remain in their homes if a multidisciplinary functional assessment is carried out.

LABORATORY EXAMINATIONS

Standard normal laboratory values are essentially the same for the elderly as for younger adults. (There is, for example, no "anemia of old age.") An elevated sedimentation rate should arouse a suspicion of polymyalgia rheumatica, cranial arteritis, infection, or cancer. The fasting blood glucose is not significantly altered by age, but the postprandial blood glucose may be higher than normal. Serum creatinine is not a good index of renal sufficiency in the elderly, since creatinine levels may be low because of the decrease in lean body mass. An age-corrected creatinine clearance can be used as a guide for dosage of ototoxic and nephrotoxic antibiotics. Since "apathetic" hyperthyroidism is commoner in the aged, thyroid function tests may be indicated. In the confused elderly patient, urinalysis; serum electrolytes; renal, thyroid, and hepatic function tests; blood gases; and serum vitamin B_{12} and red blood cell folate levels may be of diagnostic value.

THE FRAIL ELDERLY & THE FIVE *I's*

Frail elderly patients are subject to certain problems that are referred to as the "five *I's*" of geriatrics: (1) intellectual impairment, (2) immobility, (3) insta-

bility, (4) incontinence, and (5) iatrogenic drug reactions.

INTELLECTUAL IMPAIRMENT
(Senile Dementia)

Senile dementia is probably the most feared condition among the aging population. It is important to reassure elderly patients who may have some degree of benign forgetfulness that senile dementia is not inevitable. Clinically significant intellectual impairment affects an estimated 5% of people over age 65 and only 20% of people over age 80. About 60% of cases of senile dementia are of the Alzheimer type, and 15–20% are what is called multi-infarction dementia. Another 15–20% show evidence of both forms of the disorder.

Clinical Features

Early manifestations of senile dementia include decrease in attention span, impaired powers of concentration, some personality change, and forgetfulness. These changes will often be noted by the family during periods of physical or emotional stress. Many patients with dementia maintain their social graces even in the face of significant cognitive impairment; thus, a clinical impression without mental status testing may miss the diagnosis. As the disease progresses, there is loss of computational ability, further memory loss, and, ultimately, complete disorientation and social withdrawal. Senile dementia of the Alzheimer type has an insidious onset and is steadily progressive. Multi-infarction dementia is more likely to progress in a series of recognizably distinct steps.

Diagnosis

Diagnosis is based on the history and the physical, laboratory, and mental status examinations. CT scan is useful only to rule out structural brain disorders, such as hematomas, tumors, hemorrhage, hydrocephalus, and infarction. The scan may show minimal or no cerebral atrophy or ventricular enlargement in patients with severe dementia; conversely, these abnormalities may be incidental findings of no clinical significance in the normal elderly.

Differential Diagnosis

One of the most important tasks of the physician dealing with older people is to rule out treatable causes of confusional states that may mimic dementia. The following common causes of confusional states may be missed if not specifically looked for.

A. Drugs: A wide variety of agents may cause confusion in the elderly. The most common are sedatives, hypnotics, neuroleptics, antidepressants, anticholinergics, antihypertensives, and antiarthritic drugs. If, as sometimes happens, the patient is receiving the same drug under different brand names, there is an increased likelihood of drug-induced confusion. Chronic alcoholism is not rare in the elderly.

B. Depression: Depression in the elderly can mimic dementia or may be superimposed on mild dementia. Differentiation may be difficult and may warrant a therapeutic trial of antidepressant drugs.

C. Other Psychiatric Problems: Confusion may result from the anxiety and disorienting effect of being in a hospital or other unfamiliar surroundings. Severe anxiety over normal forgetfulness or psychotic behavior may be misdiagnosed as dementia.

D. Sensory Loss: Hearing loss not only leads to social isolation but results in inappropriate answers that may be misinterpreted as evidence of dementia. Abnormalities of perception in patients with lesions of the nondominant parietal lobe may be mistaken for dementia.

E. Metabolic Disturbances: Hyponatremia is a common cause of confusional state in hospitalized elderly people because of the age-related increase in ADH responsiveness to stress (eg, hypovolemia, morphine, trauma) and the syndrome of inappropriate antidiuretic hormone (SIADH) secretion, many of whose causes are common in the elderly (eg, tuberculosis, carcinoma of the lung and prostate, head injury, brain tumor). Other metabolic derangements such as liver failure, renal failure, and cardiopulmonary failure can also cause metabolic confusional states. Confusion due to hypercalcemia is particularly apt to occur in bone disorders that are more often seen in elderly patients (eg, Paget's disease, multiple myeloma, metastatic carcinoma).

F. Endocrine Abnormalities: Hypothyroidism and hyperparathyroidism may cause confusion and be interpreted as senile dementia.

G. Nutritional Deficiencies: Cognitive impairment can be produced by folate, niacin, riboflavin, and thiamine deficiencies. Many factors including poor appetite, loss of taste and smell, poorly fitting dentures, and difficulty in shopping for and preparing meals increase the likelihood of nutritional problems.

H. Trauma: Subdural hematoma must always be considered as a possible cause of confusion. Falls with head injury may be forgotten or not reported by the patient and unknown to the family.

I. Brain Tumor: Metastatic lesions and gliomas are the most common brain tumors in old people.

J. Infections: Acute infection in the elderly may cause confusion. Suspect acute infection (eg, pneumonia, pyelonephritis) when an older patient without fever or neurologic deficit suddenly becomes confused. Chronic infections of lung, bone, kidneys, skin (associated with pressure sores), and the central nervous system may also present as dementia.

K. Cardiovascular or Cerebrovascular Accidents: Acute myocardial infarction, acute congestive heart failure, or pulmonary embolism may present as an acute confusional state. Strokes that result in fluent or receptive aphasias are often mistaken for dementia.

Treatment

A. General Measures: The important first step in management of a "demented" elderly patient is the search for treatable factors contributing to the confusional state (see above).

1. Discontinue nonessential medications, particularly sedatives and hypnotics.

2. Provide for the patient's comfort and safety. Whenever possible, allow patients to remain in their own living quarters to minimize confusion and disorientation. Remember that the patient who becomes confused for the first time during a hospital stay is likely to recover at home. The adverse consequences of isolation must be balanced against the normal desire for an appropriate degree of privacy.

3. Provide adequate nutrition and hydration, and treat associated medical problems.

4. Remember that no drug treatment has been shown to alter the course of dementia.

5. Help the patient's family cope with this devastating condition.

B. Management of Depression: The elderly patient with early dementia deserves evaluation for possible depression. Since early dementia and depression may be indistinguishable, a cautious therapeutic trial of antidepressant medication may be required.

There is no ideal antidepressant drug. All of the tricyclic antidepressants seem about equally effective, but there are significant differences in side effects (see Chapter 18) that must be considered. Initial dosage should be low, and drug increases should be made slowly. Careful follow-up supervision is required in order to anticipate and minimize anticholinergic side effects, orthostatic hypotension, sedating effects, confusion, bizarre mental symptoms, cardiovascular complications, and drug overdose with suicidal intent. Provide the patient and family with all of the necessary information and warnings, so that adverse drug reactions are not assumed to be due to the aging process.

Experience in the elderly with the tetracyclic agents and other new antidepressants has been limited. The monoamine oxidase inhibitors, used cautiously, are sometimes of benefit when other antidepressants are ineffective. Monoamine oxidase inhibitors should not be used in combination with the cyclic compounds. Electroconvulsive therapy has been successfully used and is usually tolerated well by elderly patients who remain severely depressed despite drug treatment.

IMMOBILITY
(Chair- or Bed-bound)

The main causes of immobility in the elderly are weakness, stiffness, pain, imbalance, and psychologic problems. Weakness may result from disuse of muscles, malnutrition, electrolyte disturbances, anemia, neurologic disorders, or myopathies. The commonest cause of stiffness in the elderly is osteoarthritis, but rheumatoid arthritis, gout, and pseudogout also occur in this age group. Polymyalgia rheumatica should not be overlooked in the elderly patient with pain and stiffness, particularly of the pelvic and shoulder girdle, and with associated systemic symptoms (see Chapter 14).

Pain, whether from bone (eg, osteoporosis, osteomalacia, Paget's disease, metastatic bone cancer, trauma), joints (eg, osteoarthritis, rheumatoid arthritis, gout), or muscle (eg, polymyalgia rheumatica, intermittent claudication), may immobilize the patient. Foot problems are common and include plantar warts, ulceration, bunions, corns, and ingrown toenails. Poorly fitting shoes are a frequent cause of these disorders.

Imbalance and fear of falling are major causes of immobilization. Imbalance may result from general debility, neurologic causes (eg, stroke, loss of postural reflexes, peripheral neuropathy due to diabetes, alcohol, or malnutrition, vestibulo-cerebellar abnormalities), anxiety, or drugs or may occur following prolonged bed rest (see Instability, below).

Psychologic conditions such as severe anxiety, depression, or catatonia may produce or contribute to immobilization.

Iatrogenic factors, particularly excessive bed rest and drugs (eg, haloperidol), may immobilize the patient.

Treatment

A. General Measures: Treatment should be directed toward correction of malnutrition, anemia, and electrolyte disturbances that may be responsible for the patient's immobilized status. Installing handrails, lowering the bed, and providing chairs of proper height with arms and rubber skid guards may allow the patient to be safely mobile in the home. A properly fitted cane or walker may be necessary for getting the patient out for walks. (These aids should not be encouraged if the patient can manage without them.) Podiatric care, including proper footwear, is often essential.

In treating arthritis in the elderly, it must be remembered that nonsteroidal anti-inflammatory drugs, especially indomethacin, may cause central nervous system side effects with resultant confusion.

The hazards of bed rest must be recognized and avoided. Prevention is the best means of dealing with the serious and sometimes life-threatening complications of immobilization. Appropriate active exercises, no matter how limited the patient's capacity, should be encouraged on a regular basis when the patient is chair- or bed-bound.

B. Management of Specific Complications:

1. Bedsores (decubitus ulcers)–Prevention requires frequent and careful observation of the skin, particularly over pressure points. Keep the skin clean and dry. A special mattress (eg, foam-rubber egg-crate mattress) or water bed may be required for the very debilitated patient. If the patient is chair-bound, the skin over the coccyx and ischial tuberosities must be inspected daily. Correction of malnutrition and anemia is essential (see Chapter 4).

2. Muscle weakness and wasting and osteoporosis–Graded exercises and early ambulation are important.

3. Contractures–These may be avoided by early institution of range-of-motion exercises.

4. Venous thrombosis–(See Chapter 9.) Frequent ankle flexion while in bed, elastic stockings, correction of dehydration, and early ambulation are important.

5. Incontinence–Spurious urinary incontinence is a common problem in immobilized elderly patients who cannot get to the bathroom if the bedpan or urinal is not made easily available. Incontinence must be avoided because of its devastating psychologic effect as well as the potential for skin maceration, bedsores, and secondary skin infections. The patient should be toileted frequently, preferably in the bathroom or on a bedside commode rather than a bedpan. Avoid restraints and side rails whenever possible. (See Urinary Incontinence, below.)

INSTABILITY
(Physical Instability, Falls, Unstable Gait)

Falls are a major problem for elderly people and are often the major cause of loss of independence. It is often difficult to tell from the history what caused a fall. The patient who is uncertain about what happened will often say, "I must have tripped."

Causes of Falls

General physiologic impairments associated with aging that may increase the risk of falling include reduced vision, general debility and excessive bed rest, impaired "righting" reflexes, and increased body sway when the patient assumes the upright posture. Some specific factors that cause old people to fall are the following:

A. Environmental: The home environment can pose hazards, especially for a patient with poor vision, weakness, confusion, or problems of mobility. These consist of slippery floors or loose or worn carpeting, loose appliance and telephone cords, poor lighting, steep stairs, and absence of handrails in halls and bathrooms and on stairways. All of these are an even greater hazard if the patient wears loose-fitting slippers or walks in stocking feet.

B. "Drop Attacks": These occur without warning and without loss of consciousness, possibly as a result of sudden loss of antigravity reflexes. The patient usually falls backward. Pressure on the soles of the feet is one stimulus that often helps the patient to get up again.

C. Loss of Consciousness, Syncope, Vertigo: (See Chapters 6 and 17.) Such episodes may be due to cerebrovascular or cardiovascular disease (eg, arrhythmias, aortic stenosis, postural hypotension). Leading questions should be avoided, since many patients will say they were "dizzy," if asked.

D. Spasticity and Rigidity: These may be due to pyramidal or extrapyramidal disease. Patients with Parkinson's disease may fall because of their spasticity

Abramson JS et al: Antistaphylococcal IgE in patients with atopic dermatitis. *J Am Acad Dermatol* 1982;**7**:105.

Dahl MV: *Staphylococcus aureus* and atopic dermatitis. *Arch Dermatol* 1983;**119**:840.

Hanifin JM: Atopic dermatitis. *J Am Acad Dermatol* 1982;**6**:1.

LICHEN SIMPLEX CHRONICUS
(Localized Neurodermatitis)

Essentials of Diagnosis

- Chronic itching associated with pigmented lichenified skin lesions.
- Exaggerated skin lines overlying a thickened, well-circumscribed scaly plaque.
- Predilection for nape of neck, wrists, external surfaces of forearms, inner thighs, genitalia, postpopliteal and antecubital areas.

General Considerations

Lichen simplex chronicus is a persistent, usually well-localized plaque several centimeters in diameter, commonly located on the side of the neck, the flexor aspect of the wrist, or the ankle. A "scratch-itch" cycle is a prominent feature. The lesions may arise out of normal skin, or the disease may occur as a complication of contact dermatitis or any irritative dermatitis. It is particularly common in persons of Oriental extraction living in the USA but is said to be rare in their countries of origin. It is more common in women over 40 years of age. Only one person in 5 is born with skin that has the ability to lichenify following chronic manipulation or scratching. Atopic subjects become lichenified more readily than others.

Clinical Findings

Intermittent itching incites the patient to manipulate the lesions. Dry, leathery, hypertrophic, lichenified plaques appear on the neck, wrist, perineum, thigh, or almost anywhere. The patches are well-localized and rectangular, with sharp borders, and are thickened and pigmented. The lines of the skin are exaggerated and divide the lesion into rectangular plaques.

Differential Diagnosis

Differentiate from other plaquelike lesions such as psoriasis, lichen planus, seborrheic dermatitis, and nummular dermatitis.

Treatment

The area should be protected and the patient encouraged to avoid stressful and emotionally charged situations if possible. Topical corticosteroids give relief. The injection of dilute triamcinolone acetonide suspension into the lesion may occasionally be curative. Application of triamcinolone acetonide 0.1%, fluocinolone 0.025%, betamethasone valerate 0.1%, or fluocinonide 0.05% cream nightly with occlusive plastic wrap (eg, Saran Wrap) covering may be helpful. One may paint equal parts of crude coal tar, acetone, and flexible collodion on affected areas daily. Stimulants (caffeine, etc) should be avoided.

Prognosis

The disease tends to be chronic and will disappear in one area only to appear in another. Itching may be so intense as to interfere with sleep.

DERMATITIS MEDICAMENTOSA
(Drug Eruption)

Essentials of Diagnosis

- Usually abrupt onset of widespread, symmetric erythematous eruption.
- May mimic any inflammatory skin condition.
- Constitutional symptoms (malaise, arthralgia, headache, and fever) may be present.

General Considerations

As is well recognized, only a minority of cutaneous drug reactions result from allergy. Such factors as overdose, toxic side effects, neoplastic disease, superinfection, drug interaction, impaired degradation or excretion, conditions mimicking allergic reactions (eg, Jarisch-Herxheimer reaction), ampicillin reactions with infectious mononucleosis, Stevens-Johnson syndrome, intolerance with low doses, and idiosyncrasy may be operative. True allergic drug reactions involve prior exposure, an "incubation" period, reactions to doses far below the therapeutic range, manifestations different from the usual pharmacologic effects of the drug, involvement of only a small portion of the population at risk, restriction to a limited number of syndromes (anaphylactic and anaphylactoid, urticarial, vasculitic, etc), occasional identification of antibodies or T lymphocytes that react specifically with the drug or a metabolite, and reproducibility.

Clinical Findings

A. Symptoms and Signs: The onset is usually abrupt, with bright erythema and often severe itching, but may be delayed (penicillin, serum). Fever and other constitutional symptoms may be present. The skin reaction usually occurs in symmetric distribution. In a given situation the physician may suspect one specific drug (or one of several) and must therefore inquire specifically whether it has been used or not.

Drug eruptions may be briefly classified, with examples, as follows:

1. Toxic erythema–(Commonest skin reaction to drugs; causes many patterns of erythema.) Often more pronounced on the trunk than on the extremities. In previously exposed patients, the rash may start in 2–3 days. In the first course of treatment, the eruption often appears about the ninth day. Fever may be present. Common offenders include the following: antibiotics (especially ampicillin), sulfonamides and related compounds (including thiazide diuretics, furosemide, and sulfonylurea hypoglycemics), barbiturates, phenylbutazone, aminosalicylic acid.

2. Erythema multiforme–The targetlike lesions appear mainly on the extensor aspect of the limbs. Bullae may occur. The commonest offenders are the sulfonamides, barbiturates, phenylbutazone, sulindac, and fenoprofen.

3. Erythema nodosum–Oral contraceptives.

4. Allergic vasculitis–Inflammatory changes most severe around veins and venules. Lesions range from urticaria to necrotic ulcers. Common offenders: sulfonamides, phenylbutazone, indomethacin, phenytoin, and ibuprofen.

5. Purpura–(Results from thrombocytopenia, by damage to blood vessel or by affecting blood coagulation.) Itchy, brownish, petechial rash on dependent areas. Common offenders: thiazides, sulfonamides, phenylbutazone, sulfonylureas, barbiturates, quinine, sulindac, zomepirac.

6. Eczema–Rare epidermal reaction similar to contact dermatitis in patients previously sensitized by external exposure who are given the same or a related substance systemically: penicillin, neomycin, phenothiazines, local anesthetics.

7. Exfoliative dermatitis and erythroderma–(Entire skin surface is red and scaly.) Phenylbutazone, aminosalicylic acid, isoniazid, gold, carbamazepine.

8. Photosensitivity–(An exaggerated response to ultraviolet light.) Affects the exposed skin of the face, neck, and backs of the hands, and also, in women, the lower legs. On occasion, the ultraviolet emission from fluorescent lighting may be sufficient. Common offenders are sulfonamides and sulfonamide-related compounds (thiazide diuretics, furosemide, sulfonylurea hypoglycemics), tetracyclines (especially demeclocycline), phenothiazines, and nalidixic acid.

9. Drug-related lupus erythematosus–May present with a photosensitive rash accompanied by fever, polyarthritis, myalgia, and serositis (pleural and pericardial). Less severe than systemic lupus erythematosus, and recovery often follows drug withdrawal. Common offenders are hydralazine, isoniazid, procainamide, and phenytoin, as well as many other drugs.

10. Lichenoid eruptions–Flat-topped papules, often with scaling and dermatitic change. The mouth is seldom affected. Some of the drugs known to cause this reaction are chloroquine, quinacrine (mepacrine), gold, arsenic, phenothiazines, and aminosalicylic acid.

11. Fixed eruptions–Demarcated, round, erythematous plaques that recur at the same site when the drug is repeated. Pigmentation remains after healing. Fixed drug eruptions have been described with at least 69 drugs, including antimicrobials, analgesics, cardiovascular drugs, heavy metals, antiparasitics, antihistamines, and a large miscellaneous group. Immunologic studies strongly indicate that the immune system plays a major role in pathogenesis.

12. Toxic epidermal necrolysis–(Rare.) Large sheets of erythema develop, followed by separation, which looks like scalded skin. In adults, the eruption has occurred after administration of the following drugs: barbiturates, phenytoin, sulfonamides, phenylbutazone, oxyphenbutazone, penicillin, sulindac, and methotrexate.

13. Urticaria–(Rare in chronic form.) The penicillins and salicylates may be responsible.

14. Pruritus–Itchy skin without rash may be due to a wide variety of drug reactions. Pruritus ani may be due to overgrowth of *Candida* after systemic antibiotic treatment. The following drugs may produce this symptom due to biliary stasis: contraceptive pills, phenothiazines, and rifampin.

15. Hair loss–Predictable side effect of cytotoxic agents and oral contraceptives. Diffuse hair loss also occurs unpredictably with anticoagulants (heparin, coumarins, phenindione) and antithyroid drugs (carbimazole and thiouracil).

16. Pigmentation–Drugs can cause many types of pigmentary disturbances.

a. Flat hyperpigmented areas on the forehead and cheeks (chloasma) is the most common pigmentary disorder associated with drug ingestion. Improvement is slow despite stopping the drug. Oral contraceptives are the usual cause.

b. A blue-gray discoloration on light-exposed areas may occur with chlorpromazine and related phenothiazines.

c. A generalized brown or blue-gray pigmentation may occur with heavy metals (silver, gold, bismuth, and arsenic).

d. A generalized yellow color is usually due to quinacrine (Atabrine).

e. Blue-black patches on the shins, pigmentation of the nails and palate, and depigmentation of the hair may be due to chloroquine or minocycline.

B. Laboratory Findings: The complete blood count may show leukopenia, eosinophilia, agranulocytosis, or evidence of aplastic anemia. Patch tests performed with the suspect drug, although not routinely useful, may detect an offending drug when contact sensitivity is also present.

Differential Diagnosis

Distinguish from other eruptions, usually by history and subsidence after drug withdrawal, although fading may be slow.

Complications

Blood dyscrasias, anaphylaxis, laryngeal edema, photosensitivity, and hepatic, renal, ocular, central nervous system, and other complications may occur with dermatitis medicamentosa.

Prevention

People who have had dermatitis medicamentosa should avoid analogs of known chemical "allergens" as well as known offenders. The physician should pay careful attention to a history of drug reaction.

Treatment

A. General Measures: Treat systemic manifestations as they arise (eg, anemia, icterus, purpura). Antihistamines may be of value in urticarial and angioneurotic reactions (see p 64), but epinephrine, 1:1000, 0.5–1 mL intravenously or intramuscularly, should be used as an emergency measure. Corticosteroids may be used as for acute contact dermatitis in severe cases. Dialysis may speed drug elimination.

B. Specific Measures: Stop all drugs, if possible, and hasten elimination from the body by increasing fluid intake. Dimercaprol (BAL) or other chelating agents such as calcium disodium edetate may be tried in cases due to heavy metals (eg, arsenic, mercury, gold). Sodium chloride, 5–10 g daily orally, may hasten elimination of bromides and iodides in cases due to those drugs. (See Chapter 31.)

C. Local Measures: Treat the varieties and stages of dermatitis according to the major dermatitis simulated. Watch for sensitivity.

Prognosis

Drug rash usually disappears upon withdrawal of the drug and proper treatment. If systemic involvement is severe, the outcome may be fatal.

Bruinsma W: *A Guide to Drug Eruptions.* Excerpta Medica, 1982.

Korkij W, Soltani K: Fixed drug eruption: A brief review. *Arch Dermatol* 1984;**120**:520.

Millikan LE: Cutaneous adverse drug reactions. *Curr Concepts Skin Disorders* (Spring) 1984;**5**:5.

EXFOLIATIVE DERMATITIS
(Generalized Erythroderma)

Essentials of Diagnosis

- Scaling and erythema over large area of body.
- Itching, malaise, fever, weight loss.
- Primary disease or exposure to toxic agent (contact, oral, parenteral) may be evident.

General Considerations

As a causative factor, a preexisting dermatosis may be found in half of cases, including psoriasis, atopic dermatitis, seborrheic dermatitis, photosensitivity, nummular eczema, and ichthyosis. Reactions to external and internal drugs account for perhaps one-fourth of cases, and cancer for 4–8%. Causation of the remainder is undeterminable.

Clinical Findings

A. Symptoms and Signs: Symptoms include itching, weakness, malaise, fever, and weight loss. Exfoliation may be generalized or universal and sometimes includes loss of hair and nails. Generalized lymphadenopathy may be due to lymphoma or leukemia or may be part of the clinical picture of the skin disease (dermatopathic lymphadenitis). There may be mucosal sloughs.

B. Laboratory Findings: Blood and bone marrow studies and lymph node biopsies may show evidence of lymphoma or leukemia. There may be pathologic serum electrophoresis, elevated erythrocyte sedimentation rate, eosinophilia, elevated serum IgE, elevated white blood count, anemia, and peripheral blood lymphocytosis.

Differential Diagnosis

It is often impossible to delineate exfoliative dermatitis early in the course of the disease, so careful follow-up is necessary. Differentiate from other scaling eruptions such as psoriasis, lichen planus, severe seborrheic dermatitis, and dermatitis medicamentosa, which may themselves develop into exfoliative dermatitis.

Complications

Septicemia, debility (protein loss), pneumonia, high-output cardiac failure, masking of fever, hypermetabolism, thermoregulatory disorders, and anemia.

Prevention

Patients receiving sensitizing drugs should be watched carefully for the development of skin reactions of all types. The drug should be withheld until the nature of the skin reaction is determined. Proved sensitization should be considered an absolute contraindication to further administration of the drug. Dermatitis or dermatoses should not be overtreated.

Treatment

A. General Measures: Hospitalize the patient at bed rest with talc on bed sheets. Keep room at warm, constant temperature and avoid drafts. Transfusions of whole blood or plasma may be required. Avoid all unnecessary medication.

Systemic corticosteroids may provide spectacular improvement in severe or fulminant exfoliative dermatitis, but long-term therapy should be avoided if possible (see Chapter 19). Suitable antibiotic drugs should be given when there is evidence of bacterial infection; pyoderma is a common complication of exfoliative dermatitis.

B. Specific Measures: Stop all drugs, if possible, and hasten elimination of the offending drug by all means, eg, by increasing fluid intake. Dimercaprol (BAL) may lessen the severity or duration of reactions due to arsenic or gold (see Chapter 31).

C. Local Measures: Observe careful skin hygiene and avoid irritating local applications. Treat skin as for acute extensive dermatitis first with wet dressings, soothing baths (see p 48), powders, and calamine or starch shake lotions; and later with soothing oily lotions and ointments. Topical anti-infective drugs may be used when necessary.

Prognosis

Most patients recover completely or improve greatly over time. Deaths have been reported but are rare unless there is an underlying malignancy. A minority will suffer from undiminished erythroderma for indefinite periods of time.

Hasan T, Jansen CT: Erythroderma: A follow-up of fifty cases. *J Am Acad Dermatol* 1983;**8**:836.

PHOTODERMATITIS
(Dermatitis Actinica, Erythema Solare or Sunburn, Polymorphous Light Sensitivity, Contact Photodermatitis)

Essentials of Diagnosis

- Painful erythema, edema, and vesiculation on sun-exposed surfaces.
- Fever, gastrointestinal symptoms, malaise, or prostration may occur.
- Proteinuria, casts, and hematuria may occur.

General Considerations

Photodermatitis is an acute or chronic inflammatory skin reaction due to overexposure or hypersensitivity to sunlight or other sources of actinic rays, photosensitization of the skin by certain drugs, or idiosyncrasy to actinic light as seen in some constitutional disorders including the porphyrias and many hereditary disorders (phenylketonuria, xeroderma pigmentosum, and others). Contact photosensitivity may occur with perfumes, antiseptics, and other chemicals.

Clinical Findings

A. Symptoms and Signs: The acute inflammatory skin reaction is accompanied by pain, fever, gastrointestinal symptoms, malaise, and even prostration. Signs include erythema, edema, and possibly vesiculation and oozing on exposed surfaces. Exfoliation and pigmentary changes often result.

B. Laboratory Findings: Proteinuria, casts, hematuria, and hemoconcentration may be present. Look for porphyrins in urine and stool, protoporphyrins in blood, and findings in other inborn errors of metabolism. Elaborate testing for photosensitivity may be performed by experts.

Differential Diagnosis

Differentiate from contact dermatitis that may develop from one of the many substances in suntan lotions and oils. Sensitivity to actinic rays may also be part of a more serious condition such as porphyria, erythropoietic protoporphyria, lupus erythematosus, or pellagra. Phenothiazines, sulfones, chlorothiazides, griseofulvin, oral antidiabetic agents, and antibiotics may photosensitize the skin. Polymorphous light eruption appears to be an idiopathic photodermatosis that affects both sexes equally, frequently starts in childhood, and lasts into late adult life. The action spectrum often lies in both long (320–400 nm) and short (below 320 nm) ultraviolet wavelengths. Contact photodermatitis may be caused by halogenated salicylanilides (weak antiseptics in soaps, creams, etc).

Complications

Delayed cumulative effects in fair-skinned people include keratoses and epitheliomas. Some individuals become chronic light-reactors even when they apparently are no longer exposed to photosensitizing or phototoxic drugs.

Prevention

Persons with very fair, sensitive skins should avoid prolonged exposure to strong sun or ultraviolet radiation. Preliminary conditioning by graded exposure and protective clothing is advisable.

Protective sunscreening agents (eg, those containing PABA and oxy- or dioxybenzone) may be applied before exposure, although PABA itself may cause photosensitivity dermatitis.

The use of psoralens orally is controversial.

In those photodermatoses in which the action spectrum involves wavelengths beyond the short ultraviolet range (320 nm), sunshades that contain titanium dioxide (Maxafil, Reflecta) must be used. RVPaque, which contains zinc oxide, may also be used.

Treatment

A. General Measures: Treat constitutional symptoms by appropriate supportive measures. Control pain, fever, and gastrointestinal and other symptoms as they arise. Aspirin may have some specific value. Corticosteroids, both systemically and topically, may be required for severe reactions. Beta carotene (Solatene), 60 mg daily by mouth, is effective treatment for erythropoietic protoporphyria. Doses of 90–300 mg of beta carotene by mouth may be tried in adults with photosensitive eczema, polymorphic light eruptions, or solar urticaria, although double-blind studies have not been done because of unavoidable skin staining. Chloroquine, 125 mg orally twice weekly for 3–9 months, is effective in treating porphyria cutanea tarda. Patients must be followed clinically and ophthalmologically and with laboratory uroporphyrin determinations. This is not suitable if the patient has hepatitis or cirrhosis. Phlebotomy, letting 500 mL of blood every 2 weeks, is an alternative mode of therapy but is often complicated by anemia, other hematologic disorders, hypoproteinemia, or vasomotor dysfunction. Liver toxins, including alcohol, should be interdicted. Neocytopheresis (twice weekly autotransfusion with the supernatant of the patient's centrifuged blood, containing neocytes) apparently is effective for all types of porphyria (personal communication from Charles Lewis, MD, San Antonio, Texas).

Triamcinolone acetonide suspension, 30–40 mg, may be given deep in the gluteal muscle once yearly for flare-ups of polymorphous light eruption.

Trioxsalen (Trisoralen), 25–30 mg, orally, followed by sunlight exposure 2 hours later, may control polymorphous light eruption. Treatment may be given for 4 days each month if needed. Initial flare-ups may occur.

B. Local Measures: Treat as for any acute dermatitis (see p 47). First use cooling and soothing wet dressings with saline, bicarbonate, or aluminum subacetate solutions, and follow with calamine or starch lotions. Greases must be avoided because of the occlusive effect.

For maximum protection, sunscreens with a sun protective factor (SPF) of 15 should be used. These aid in delaying sun damage and aging of fair skin and in the management of photodermatoses. Unfortunately, contact or photoallergy may be caused by sunscreens themselves, in which case sunshades containing titanium dioxide, zinc oxide, or talc may be used instead.

Prognosis

Dermatitis actinica is usually benign and self-limiting unless the burn is severe or when it occurs as an associated finding in a more serious disorder.

Frain-Bell W (guest editor): Photodermatoses. *Semin Dermatol* 1982;**1**:153. [Entire issue.]

Malkinson FD, Levitt L: Hydroxychloroquine treatment of porphyria cutanea tarda. *Arch Dermatol* 1980;**116**:1147.

Rapaport M: Sunlight and sunscreens. *Dermatology and Allergy* 1982;**5**:34.

LICHEN PLANUS

Essentials of Diagnosis

- Pruritic, violaceous, flat-topped papules with fine white streaks and symmetric distribution.
- Commonly seen along linear scratch mark (Koebner phenomenon).
- Anterior wrists, sacral region, penis, legs, mucous membranes.
- Usually occurs in an otherwise healthy but emotionally tense person.
- Histopathology is diagnostic.

General Considerations

Lichen planus may be an "allergic" reaction pattern, particularly following exposure to dyes, color film developers, and gold. The 3 cardinal findings are typical skin lesions, histopathologic features of band infiltration of T cells in the dermis, and fluorescence with IgG and C3 at the basement membrane. Links have been seen with bullous pemphigoid, alopecia areata, vitiligo, chronic ulcerative colitis, hypogammaglobulinemia, and graft-versus-host reactions. Drugs associated with lichen planus include gold, demeclocycline, streptomycin, tetracycline, arsenic, iodides, chloroquine, quinacrine, quinidine, and paraphenylenediamine. Antimony, phenothiazine, aminosalicylic acid, chlorothiazide, hydrochlorothiazide, and amiphenazole have also been incriminated. Colloid bodies appear in the upper dermis and may contain IgM as well as small amounts of IgG. Fibrin may be found in the upper dermis. These findings are not highly specific.

Clinical Findings

Itching is mild to severe. The lesions are violaceous, flat-topped, angulated papules, discrete or in clusters, on the flexor surfaces of the wrists and on the penis, lips, tongue, and buccal and vaginal mucous membranes. Mucosal lichen planus has been reported in the genital and anorectal areas, the gastrointestinal tract, the bladder, the larynx, and the conjunctiva. The papules may become bullous or ulcerated. The disease may be generalized. Mucous membrane lesions have a lacy white network overlying them that is often confused with leukoplakia. Papules are 1–4 mm in diameter, with white streaks on the surface (Wickham's striae).

Differential Diagnosis

Distinguish from similar lesions produced by quinacrine or bismuth sensitivity and other papular lesions such as psoriasis, papular eczema, and syphiloderm. Lichen planus on the mucous membranes must be differentiated from leukoplakia. Certain photodeveloping or duplicating solutions may produce eruptions that mimic lichen planus.

Treatment

A. General Measures: Patients with lichen planus are sometimes tense and nervous, and episodes of dermatitis may be temporally related to emotional crises. Measures should be directed at relieving anxiety, and judicious use of sedatives or hydroxyzine may be helpful. Corticosteroids (see Chapter 19) may be required in severe cases. Isotretinoin (Accutane) apparently is effective for oral lichen planus as well as generalized pruritic lichen planus. Begin with a dosage of 0.25 mg/kg/d (approximately 10 mg twice daily) for 2 months. Side effects are minimal with this dosage; at the very worst, chapped lips. The drug must not be used if there is any possibility of pregnancy. (See Acne Vulgaris, below, for side effects and precautions.)

B. Local Measures: Use shake lotions containing tar. X-ray or grenz ray therapy (by a specialist) may rarely be used when involvement is particularly severe. Intralesional injection of triamcinolone acetonide is useful for localized forms. Corticosteroid cream or ointment may be used nightly under thin pliable plastic film.

Application of tretinoin cream (retinoic acid; vitamin A acid), 0.05%, to mucosal lichen planus, followed by a corticosteroid ointment, may be helpful. For disabling hypertrophic lichen planus of the soles, tretinoin cream applied and covered with thin, pliable polyethylene film nightly is said to be effective.

Prognosis

Lichen planus is a benign disease, but it may persist for months or years and may be recurrent. Oral lesions tend to be especially persistent, and neoplastic degeneration has been described.

Handler HL: Isotretinoin for oral lichen planus. (Letter.) *J Am Acad Dermatol* 1984;**10**:674.

PSORIASIS

Essentials of Diagnosis

- Silvery scales on bright red plaques, usually on the knees, elbows, and scalp.
- Stippled nails.
- Itching is mild unless psoriasis is eruptive or occurs in body folds.
- Psoriatic arthritis may be present.
- Histopathologic features are specific.

General Considerations

Psoriasis is a common benign, acute or chronic inflammatory skin disease that apparently is based upon genetic predisposition. A genetic error in the mitotic control system has been postulated. For the relationship of psoriasis to histocompatibility (HLA) antigens, see Chapter 34. The decreased responsiveness of the cAMP system in psoriatic epidermis to prostaglandin E_1 suggests that altered response of the epidermis to prostaglandins may be one of the factors in the pathophysiology of psoriasis. Injury or irritation of psoriatic skin tends to provoke lesions of psoriasis in the site. Psoriasis occasionally is eruptive, particularly in periods of stress or after streptococcal pharyngitis. Grave, life-threatening forms may occur. There is some evidence that immunologic factors may play a part in the pathogenesis of psoriasis, but this is inadequately confirmed.

Clinical Findings

There are usually no symptoms. Eruptive psoriasis may itch, and psoriasis in body folds itches severely ("inverse psoriasis"). The lesions are dull red, sharply outlined plaques covered with silvery scales. The elbows, knees, and scalp are the most common sites. Nail involvement may resemble onychomycosis. Fine stippling in the nails is highly suggestive of psoriasis. There may be associated arthritis that resembles the rheumatoid variety but with a negative latex fixation test (see p 514).

Differential Diagnosis

Differentiate in the scalp from seborrheic dermatitis; in body folds from intertrigo and candidiasis; and in the nails from onychomycosis.

Treatment

A. General Measures: Desert climates seem to exert a favorable effect. Severe psoriasis calls for treatment in the hospital or a day-care center with the Goeckerman regimen.

Corticotropin or corticosteroids may be necessary to give relief in fulminating cases. Parenteral corticosteroids should not be used except in the most severe cases, because of the possibility of changing plaques to pustular lesions. Methotrexate is available for severe psoriasis. FDA guidelines must be followed.

Reassurance is important, since these patients are apt to be discouraged by the difficulties of treatment. An attempt should be made to relieve anxieties.

B. Local Measures:

1. Acute psoriasis – Avoid irritating or stimulating drugs. Begin with a calamine or starch lotion or bland ointment containing 10% solution of coal tar. As the lesions become less acute, gradually incorporate mild keratolytic agents into lotions and hydrophilic ointments. Betamethasone dipropionate, 0.05% in a glycol formulation (Diprolene ointment), rubbed into the skin once daily so that 45 g lasts 1 week, is sometimes highly effective in treating resistant psoriasis and other dermatoses; adrenal function remains relatively unaffected. It is best to restrict the ointment to 3 weeks' use until more is known about topical and systemic side effects.

2. Subacute psoriasis – Give warm baths daily, scrubbing the lesions thoroughly with a brush, soap, and water. Apply increasing concentrations of keratoplastic or stimulating agents incorporated in lotions and hydrophilic ointments. Solar or ultraviolet irradiations may be applied in gradually increasing doses.

3. Chronic psoriasis – The Goeckerman regimen in psoriasis day-care centers is highly effective and cost-effective and has high patient compliance. With treatment for 6 days a week for 6 or 7 hours daily, a remission rate of 90% clearing of the skin occurs in an average of 18 days. Long remissions occur. Intensive exposure to 2–5% crude coal tar in petrolatum to which 2.5% polysorbate 80 is added, coupled with exposure to ultraviolet light in the B range (UVB in 290- to 310-nm wavelength range), with the addition of 2% or 5% salicylic acid to the tar ointment for thick plaques, are the essentials of the treatment; mild corticosteroid creams are added, plus a 10% solution of coal tar USP in a skin oil for the scalp.

Estargel and Psorigel tar gels are elegant substitutes for crude coal tar. Anthralin ointment 0.1% may be helpful. It tends to be irritating, however, and it discolors white or gray hair. It should not be used near the eyes.

Experimental work suggests that exposure to sunlamps or blacklight lamps, without systemic or topical therapy, may benefit chronic psoriasis.

PUVA* tends to be a long-term form of treatment, as maintenance therapy is usually required. The ultraviolet dose is cumulative, and the relapse rate is about 63% in 1–6 months. The total safe dose is unknown, and the incidence of skin cancer is 9 times the normal incidence, with a reversal of the usual basal cell to squamous cell carcinoma ratio. Epidermal dystrophy by light microscopy is seen in 50% of patients treated with PUVA, and there is rapid aging of the skin. Cataracts are a potential threat, and there may be immunologic changes. Treatment now has FDA approval.

Simple application twice daily of commercial tar topical corticosteroids.

For recalcitrant scalp lesions, one may rub in,

---

*PUVA = psoralen plus ultraviolet-A, ie, ultraviolet light in 320- to 400-nm wavelength range. Same as black light.

nightly, a cream or ointment containing 0.5% anthralin, followed at once by Neutrogena T/Derm oil. This treatment stains pillowcases and may irritate the eyes.

Etretinate (aromatic retinoid), 0.3–1 mg/kg/d, appears to be the first choice in the treatment of severe pustular psoriasis. It is also useful for psoriatic erythroderma, psoriasis vulgaris, and psoriatic arthritis. Liver enzymes must be checked periodically. The drug is not yet approved for use in the USA. It has a prolonged half-life. An ominous finding is that of diffuse idiopathic skeletal hypertrophy (DISH syndrome) from long-term, high-dose therapy, eg, 4 mg/kg/d by mouth for many months.

Isotretinoin works on occasion. Side effects are dose-related and include mucocutaneous lesions and abnormalities of blood lipids and liver function tests.

Prognosis

The course tends to be chronic and unpredictable, and the disease may be refractory to treatment.

Gip L, Hamfelt A: Studies on the efficacy and adrenal effects of Diprolene ointment 0.05% and Dermolate ointment 0.05% in patients with psoriasis or other resistant dermatoses. *Cutis* 1984;**33**:215.

Menter A, Cram DL: The Goeckerman regimen in two psoriasis day care centers. *J Am Acad Dermatol* 1983;**9**:59.

Roelandts R: Mutagenicity and carcinogenicity of methoxsalen plus UV-A. *Arch Dermatol* 1984;**120**:662.

Roenigk HH Jr et al: Methotrexate guidelines: Revised. *J Am Acad Dermatol* 1982;**6**:145.

Wolska H, Jablonska S, Bounameaux Y: Etretinate in severe psoriasis. *J Am Acad Dermatol* 1983;**9**:883.

PITYRIASIS ROSEA

Essentials of Diagnosis

- Oval, fawn-colored, scaly eruption following cleavage lines of trunk.
- Herald patch commonly precedes eruption by 1–2 weeks.
- Occasional pruritus.

General Considerations

This is a common, mild, acute inflammatory disease which is 50% more common in females. Young adults are principally affected, mostly in the spring or fall. Concurrent household cases have been reported, and recurrences may take place over a period of years. The cause is unknown, but it is speculated that a picornavirus may be causative.

Clinical Findings

Occasionally, there is severe itching. The lesions consist of oval, fawn-colored macules 4–5 mm in diameter following cleavage lines on the trunk. Exfoliation of the lesions causes a crinkly scale that begins in the center. The proximal portions of the extremities are involved. An initial lesion ("herald patch") usually precedes the later efflorescence by 1–2 weeks. Attacks usually last 4–8 weeks.

Differential Diagnosis

Differentiate from secondary syphilis, especially when lesions are numerous, or smaller than usual. Tinea corporis, seborrheic dermatitis, tinea versicolor, and drug eruptions may simulate pityriasis rosea.

Treatment

Acute irritated lesions (uncommon) should be treated as for acute dermatitis with wet dressings or shake lotions. Apply coal tar solution, 5% in starch lotion, twice daily. Ultraviolet light is helpful.

Prognosis

Pityriasis rosea is usually an acute self-limiting illness that disappears in about 6 weeks.

Arndt KA et al: Treatment of pityriasis rosea with UV radiation. *Arch Dermatol* 1983;**119**:381.

Chuang T-Y et al: Pityriasis rosea in Rochester, Minnesota, 1969 to 1978: A 10-year epidemiologic study. *J Am Acad Dermatol* 1982;**7**:80.

SEBORRHEIC DERMATITIS & DANDRUFF

Essentials of Diagnosis

- Dry scales or dry yellowish dandruff with or without underlying erythema.
- Scalp, central face, presternal, interscapular areas, umbilicus, and body folds.

General Considerations

Seborrheic dermatitis is an acute or chronic papulosquamous dermatitis. It is based upon a genetic predisposition mediated by an interplay of such factors as hormones, nutrition, infection, and emotional stress. The role of *Pityrosporon* organisms is unclear in a causative, contributory, common, or even occasional sense. Dandruff per se is merely an intensification of the physiologic process of desquamation.

Clinical Findings

Pruritus may be present but is an inconstant finding. The scalp, face, chest, back, umbilicus, and body folds may be oily or dry, with dry scales or oily yellowish scurf. Erythema, fissuring, and secondary infection may be present.

Differential Diagnosis

Distinguish from other skin diseases of the same areas such as intertrigo and fungal infections; and from psoriasis (location).

Treatment

A. General Measures: Hygienic habits of living, with an adequate diet, regular working hours, recreation, sleep, and simple cleanliness are recommended. Treat aggravating systemic factors such as infections and emotional stress.

Pityrosporin ovale folliculitis of the scalp, previously resistant to treatment, responds to a brief course of ketoconazole by mouth (200 mg/d for 1 week).

B. Local Measures:

1. Acute, subacute, or chronic eczematous lesions–Treat as for dermatitis or eczema (see p 53). An emulsion base containing 0.5% hydrocortisone and 10% sodium sulfacetamide is useful. Corticosteroid creams, lotions, or solution may be used in all stages. Potent fluorinated corticosteroids used regularly on the face may produce steroid rosacea.

2. Seborrhea of the scalp–Use one of the following: (1) Selsun (selenium sulfide) suspension or Exsel once a week after shampoo. Fostex cream (containing soapless cleansers, wetting agents, sulfur, and salicylic acid) or Sebulex may be used as a weekly shampoo for oily seborrhea. The patient should be instructed to shampoo vigorously once and then shampoo again, leaving on for 5–10 minutes to loosen the scales. (2) Neutrogena T/Gel shampoo, containing tar, may succeed where others fail. (3) Shampoos containing zinc pyrithione may be helpful. (4) Betamethasone valerate (Valisone), 0.1% lotion, is excellent.

An alcoholic solution of aluminum chloride (see p 72) plus an antibiotic topical lotion (see below), rubbed in once or twice daily, may work where other measures fail.

3. Seborrhea of nonhairy areas–Mild stimulating coal tar lotion, mild sulfur–salicylic acid ointment, or 3–5% sulfur in hydrophilic ointment may be used. (The addition of 1% salicylic acid to these preparations aids in removing scales.)

4. Seborrhea of intertriginous areas–Avoid greasy ointments. Apply astringent aluminum subacetate wet dressings followed by 3% iodochlorhydroxyquin and 1% hydrocortisone in an emulsion base.

Prognosis

The tendency is to lifelong recurrences. Individual outbreaks may last weeks, months, or years.

Luppino M, Burkhart CG: Seborrheic dermatitis. *Dermatol Allergy* 1982;**5**:28.

ACNE VULGARIS

Essentials of Diagnosis

- Pimples (papules or pustules) over the face, back, and shoulders occurring at puberty.
- Open and closed comedones.
- Cyst formation, slow resolution, scarring.
- The most common of all skin conditions.

General Considerations

Acne vulgaris is a common inflammatory disease of unknown cause that is apparently activated by androgens in those who are genetically predisposed. It may occur from puberty through the period of sex hormone activity. Eunuchs are spared. Similar involvement may occur in identical twins.

The disease is more common and more severe in males. Contrary to popular belief, it does not always clear spontaneously when maturity is reached. If untreated, it may persist into the fourth and even sixth decade of life. The skin lesions follow sebaceous overactivity, plugging of the infundibulum of the follicles, retention of sebum, overgrowth of the acne bacillus *(Corynebacterium acnes)* in incarcerated sebum, irritation by accumulated fatty acids, and foreign body reaction to extrafollicular sebum. The role of antibiotics in controlling acne is not clearly understood, but they may work because of their antianabolic effect on the sebaceous gland. (Topical occlusive corticosteroids may produce acne.)

When a resistant case of acne is encountered in a woman, hyperandrogenism may be suspected. Look for hirsutism, irregular menses, or other signs of virilism. Dexamethasone, 0.5 mg nightly, may help.

Clinical Findings

There may be mild soreness, pain, or itching; inflammatory papules, pustules, ectatic pores, acne cysts, and scarring. The lesions occur mainly over the face, neck, upper chest, back, and shoulders. Comedones are common.

Self-consciousness and embarrassment may be the most disturbing symptoms.

Differential Diagnosis

Distinguish from acneiform lesions caused by bromides, iodides, and contact with chlorinated naphthalenes and diphenyls.

Complications

Cyst formation, severe scarring, and psychic trauma.

Treatment

A. General Measures:

1. Education of the patient–It should be explained that treatment is essential not only to produce an acceptable cosmetic result while the condition is active but also to prevent permanent scarring.

2. Diet–Specific dietary factors are less important than formerly thought in causing acne.

3. Eliminate all possible medication, especially bromides or iodides.

4. Avoid exposure to oils and greases.

5. Treat anemia, malnutrition, infection, gastrointestinal disorders, or other factors which may aggravate acne.

6. Aggravating or complicating emotional disturbances must be taken into consideration and treated appropriately.

7. Antibiotics–Minocycline, 200 mg daily by mouth, is more effective than 1000 mg of tetracycline. Tetracycline or minocycline may discolor growing teeth. Minocycline causes blackening of the thyroid gland.

Blood counts, blood chemistries, and urinalyses give essentially normal findings in persons on long-term low-dose tetracycline or erythromycin therapy for acne. Gram-negative folliculitis supervening in acne during broad-spectrum antibiotic therapy will respond to stopping the antibiotic. Chloramphenicol should not be used. Minocycline, 50 mg twice daily by mouth, is used as adjunctive therapy in severe acne. A number of commercial topical antibiotic lotions are available. The most effective are erythromycin or clindamycin, in hydroalcoholic or other special vehicles. There is a remote possibility of pseudomembranous colitis developing from the absorption of clindamycin (see p 392). Clindamycin phosphate should be used topically instead of the hydrochloride.

8. Oral contraceptives help some young women with acne. High-estrogen oral contraceptives have the most complications. Hyperpigmentation (melasma) is an occasional complication.

9. Isotretinoin (Accutane; 13-*cis*-retinoic acid), a vitamin A analog, is approved for treatment of severe cystic acne in the USA. A dosage of 0.5 mg/kg/d for 4 months is usually adequate for severe cystic acne. The drug is *absolutely contraindicated during pregnancy,* because of teratogenicity, and therapeutic abortion must be considered if the patient takes the drug during pregnancy. Side effects occur in most patients, usually related to dry skin and mucous membranes (dry lips, nosebleed, and dry eyes). If headache occurs, pseudotumor cerebri must be ruled out. At double the dose described above, about 25% of patients will develop hypertriglyceridemia, 15% hypercholesterolemia, and 5% lowering of high-density lipoproteins. Miscellaneous adverse reactions, usually not seen with doses of 0.5 mg/kg/d, include musculoskeletal or bowel symptoms, rash, thinning of hair, exuberant granulation tissue in lesions, and bony hyperostosis (seen only with very high doses). No serious liver or hematologic disturbances have been reported.

Serious adverse effects with isotretinoin include fetal abnormalities in women taking the drug during pregnancy, pseudotumor cerebri, hyperuricemia, regional ileitis, and reversible corneal opacities.

B. Local Measures: Desquam-X wash or Benzac W wash may be used. Avoid greasy cleansing creams and other cosmetics. Shampoo the scalp 1–2 times a week. Extract blackheads with a comedo extractor. Incise and drain fluctuant cystic lesions with a small sharp scalpel.

1. Keratoplastic and keratolytic agents–A sulfur-zinc acne lotion may be applied locally to the skin at bedtime and washed off in the morning. Tretinoin (Retin-A) liquid, cream, or gel has been recommended for comedo acne, but it is irritating.

2. Commercial preparations for acne include Fostex cream and cake; Acne-Dome cleanser, cream, and lotion; Benzac W wash and Benzac W gel; Desquam-X gel and wash; Benzagel; and Xerac BP. All of these gels contain benzoyl peroxide.

3. Dermabrasion–Cosmetic improvement may be achieved by abrasion of inactive acne lesions, particularly flat, superficial scars. The skin is first frozen and anesthetized with ethyl chloride or Freon and then carefully abraded with fine sandpaper, special motor-driven abrasive brushes, or diamond fraises. The technique is not without untoward effects, since hyperpigmentation, grooving, and scarring have been known to occur. Dark-skinned individuals do poorly.

4. Irradiation–Simple exposure to sunlight in graded doses is often beneficial. Ultraviolet irradiation may be used as an adjunct to other treatment measures. Use suberythema doses in graded intervals up to the point of mild erythema and scaling.

5. Liquid nitrogen spray is useful for blanching cysts and papules.

6. Intralesional triamcinolone acetonide suspension, 3 mg/mL, is helpful for acne cysts.

Prognosis

Untreated acne vulgaris often remits spontaneously, but the condition may persist throughout adulthood and may lead to severe scarring. The disease is chronic and tends to recur in spite of treatment. Remissions following systemic treatment with isotretinoin tend to be lasting.

Adverse effects with isotretinoin. *FDA Drug Bull* 1983;**13**:21.

Bruno MP, Beacham BE, Burnett JW: Adverse effects of isotretinoin therapy. *Cutis* 1984;**33**:484.

Pittsley RA, Yoder FW: Retinoid hyperostosis: Skeletal toxicity associated with long-term administration of 13-*cis*-retinoic acid for refractory ichthyosis. *N Engl J Med* 1983;**308**:1012.

Pochi PE: Hormones, retinoids and acne. (Editorial.) *N Engl J Med* 1983;**308**:1024.

Strauss JS et al: Isotretinoin therapy for acne: Results of a multicenter dose-response study. *J Am Acad Dermatol* 1984;**10**:490.

ROSACEA

Essentials of Diagnosis

- A chronic face disorder of middle-aged and older people.
- There is a large vascular component (erythema and telangiectasis).
- An acneiform component (papules, pustules, and seborrhea) is present.
- There is a glandular component accompanied by hyperplasia of the soft tissue of the nose (rhinophyma).

General Considerations

Aside from obvious genetic overtones, no single factor adequately explains the pathogenesis of this disorder. Emotional disturbances, a seborrheic diathesis, and a dysfunction of the gastrointestinal tract may be significant associated factors. A statistically significant incidence of migraine headaches accompanying rosacea has been reported.

A variant of rosacea is so-called demodex acne (demodicidosis), in which large numbers of the mite *Demodex folliculorum* are found in pores. These may be demonstrated under the microscope when squeezings from pores are examined in glycerin on a microscope slide.

Strong topical steroids can change trivial dermatoses of the face into a recognizable entity called perioral dermatitis. This occurs predominantly in young women and may be confused with acne rosacea. It yields to 1% hydrocortisone cream topically, plus tetracycline by mouth.

Clinical Findings

These are described above. The entire face may have a rosy hue. One sees few or no comedones. Inflammatory papules are prominent, and there may be pustules. Associated seborrhea may be found. The patient often complains of burning or stinging with episodes of flushing.

Differential Diagnosis

Distinguish from acne, bromoderma, iododerma, and demodicidosis, as described above. The rosy hue of rosacea generally will pinpoint the diagnosis.

Treatment

A. General Measures: Tetracycline, 250 mg orally daily on an empty stomach, when used in conjunction with the topical treatment described below, may be very effective.

Isotretinoin (13-*cis*-retinoic acid; Accutane) by mouth may succeed where other measures fail. A large-scale cooperative study in West Germany has shown excellent response of rosacea to isotretinoin by mouth in a dosage of 0.5–1 mg/kg/d orally for 12–28 weeks, with minimal side effects. Pregnancy must be avoided during treatment.

B. Local Measures: Hydrocortisone cream 0.5–1% or desonide cream 0.05% used morning and night, along with tetracycline orally, is a very effective regimen. Topical antibiotics in special vehicles may be helpful (see Acne). Benzoyl peroxide, 5–10% in an acetone gel, apparently will clear erythema, papules, pustules, and nodules but not telangiectasia of rosacea. Five to 8 weeks of treatment are needed for significant response. About one person in 6 or 7 experiences irritation, burning, edema, and erythema from the applications.

Prognosis

In the past, rosacea tended to be a stubborn and persistent process. With the regimens described above, it can usually be controlled adequately. Complicating rhinophyma may require surgical correction.

Montes L et al: Topical treatment of acne rosacea with benzoyl peroxide acetone gel. *Cutis* 1983;**32**:185.

Plewig G, Nikolowski J, Wolff HH: Action of isotretinoin in acne rosacea and gram-negative folliculitis. *J Am Acad Dermatol* 1982;**6**:766.

URTICARIA & ANGIOEDEMA

Essentials of Diagnosis

- Eruptions of evanescent wheals or hives.
- Itching is usually intense but may on rare occasions be absent.
- Special forms of urticaria have special features (hereditary angioedema, dermographism, cholinergic urticaria, solar urticaria, or cold urticaria).
- Most incidents are acute and self-limited over a period of 1--2 weeks.
- Chronic urticaria may defy the best efforts of the clinician to find and eliminate the cause.

General Considerations

Urticaria can result from many different stimuli. The pathogenetic mechanism may be either immunologic or nonimmunologic. The most common immunologic mechanism is the type I hypersensitivity state mediated by IgE. Another immunologic mechanism involves the activation of the complement cascade, which produces anaphylatoxins. These in turn can release histamine. Whether the pathogenesis is allergic or nonallergic, modulating factors affect mast cells and basophils to release mediators capable of producing urticarial lesions. These mediators include histamine, serotonin, kinins, slow-reacting substance of anaphylaxis, prostaglandins, acetylcholine, degradation products of fibrin, and anaphylatoxins that increase vascular permeability, producing wheals. Intracellular levels of cAMP have a modulating role in the secretory release of histamine from mast cells and basophils.

Clinical Findings

A. Symptoms and Signs: Itching is the classic presenting symptom but (paradoxically) may be absent in rare cases. Lesions are acute, with pseudopods and intense swelling. The morphology of the lesions may vary over a period of minutes to hours. There may be involvement of the lips, tongue, eyelids, larynx, palms, soles, and genitalia. Papular urticaria resulting from insect bites may persist for long periods and may occasionally be mistaken for lymphoma or leukemia cutis on the basis of histologic findings. A central punctum can usually be seen as with flea or gnat bites. Streaked urticarial lesions may be seen in acute allergic plant dermatitis, eg, poison ivy, oak, or sumac.

In familial angioedema, there is generally a positive family history, and the urticarial lesions may be massive. Death may occur from laryngeal obstruction.

Contact urticaria may be caused by a host of substances varying from chemicals to foods to medications on a nonimmunologic basis, or it may be due to allergy.

Seventeen patients (12.1% of 140 cases of chronic urticaria) showed thyroid autoimmunity with thyroid microsomal antibodies in serum titers at or above 1:1600. All 17 patients had angioedema, and 8 had goiter or thyroid dysfunction.

B. Laboratory Findings: Laboratory studies are not likely to be helpful in the evaluation of chronic urticaria unless there are suggestive findings in the history and physical examination. Sinus x-rays may be an exception.

Differential Diagnosis

Distinguish from contact dermatitis and from dermographism, which are different diseases.

Treatment

A. Systemic Treatment: Look for and eliminate the cause if possible. The chief nonallergic causes are drugs, eg, atropine, pilocarpine, morphine, codeine; arthropod bites, eg, insect bites and bee stings (although the latter may cause anaphylaxis as well as angioedema); physical factors such as heat, cold, sunlight, injury, and pressure; and, presumably, neurogenic factors such as tension states and cholinergic urticaria induced by physical exercise, excitement, hot showers, etc.

Allergic causes may include penicillin reactions, inhalants such as feathers and animal danders, ingestion of shellfish or strawberries, injections of sera and vaccines as well as penicillin, external contactants including various chemicals and cosmetics, and infections such as viral hepatitis.

A few patients with chronic urticaria may respond to a salicylate- and tartrazine-free diet. Although salicylates are ubiquitous in nature, drugs and food are the most obvious sources.

Systemic treatment includes antihistamines orally. Hydroxyzine, 10 mg twice daily to 25 mg 3 times daily, may be very useful. Cyproheptadine, 4 mg 4 times daily, may work where hydroxyzine fails and is especially useful for cold urticaria. Enthusiasm for antihistamines has lessened. Clinicians no longer claim 95% symptomatic relief; 35% may be closer to the mark. It may be necessary to give a burst of oral prednisone in a dose of 40 mg daily for 10 days. Epinephrine 1:1000, a few minims given subcutaneously sequentially, may be very useful.

For hereditary angioedema, methyltestosterone buccal tablets, 10 mg once or twice daily, may reduce the episodes. Danazol is effective for hereditary angioedema but is expensive. Stanozolol is a cheaper anabolic agent and is effective. Lyophilized, partially purified C1-inhibitor concentrate, in 5% dextrose, given intravenously in 10–45 minutes, may be lifesaving during an acute attack.

There is a continued search for effective treatment for chronic idiopathic urticaria. The combined use of H_1 and H_2 receptor blockers, such as chlorpheniramine and cimetidine, has given inconsistent results.

We need agents to counteract the kinins, the slow-reacting substance of anaphylaxis leukotrienes, the prostaglandins, the components of complement, and the potent factor that activates platelets.

When urticarial lesions persist indefinitely, biopsy is necessary to rule out vasculitis, and it may be desirable to determine the erythrocyte sedimentation rate, quantitative immunoglobulins, cryoglobulins, cryofibrinogens, antinuclear antibodies, total hemolytic complement, and circulating immune complexes.

Hepatitis B is one factor that may cause persisting lesions.

B. Local Treatment: Starch baths twice daily or Aveeno baths may be very useful. One cupful of finely refined cornstarch or a packet of Aveeno may be used in a comfortably warm bath. Alternatively, one may use calamine liniment with 0.25% menthol and 0.5% phenol topically or in addition to the bathing.

Solar urticaria is treated by graded exposure to sunlight or with cyproheptadine, 4 mg 4 times daily.

Prognosis

Acute urticaria usually lasts only a few days. The chronic form may persist for years.

Jacobson KW, Branch LB, Nelson HS: Laboratory tests in chronic urticaria. *JAMA* 1980;**243**:1644.

Leznoff A et al: Association of chronic urticaria and angioedema with thyroid autoimmunity. *Arch Dermatol* 1983;**119**:636.

Monroe EW et al: Vasculitis in chronic urticaria: An immunopathologic study. *J Invest Dermatol* 1981;**76**:103.

Shelley WB: Commentary: Antihistamines and the treatment of urticaria. *Arch Dermatol* 1983;**119**:442.

Winton GB, Lewis CW: Contact urticaria. *Int J Dermatol* 1982;**21**:573.

INTERTRIGO

Intertrigo is caused by the macerating effect of heat, moisture, and friction. It is especially likely to occur in obese persons and in humid climates. Poor hygiene is an important etiologic factor. There is often a history of seborrheic dermatitis. The symptoms are itching, stinging, and burning. The body folds develop fissures, erythema, and sodden epidermis, with superficial denudation. Urine and blood examination may reveal diabetes mellitus, and the skin examination may reveal candidiasis. A direct smear may show abundant cocci. "Inverse psoriasis," tinea cruris, erythrasma, and candidiasis must be ruled out.

Treat as for tinea cruris (see p 76), but do not use fungicidal agents. Recurrences are common.

MILIARIA
(Heat Rash)

Essentials of Diagnosis

- Burning, itching, superficial aggregated small vesicles or papules on covered areas of the skin.
- Hot, moist climate.
- May have fever and even heat prostration.

General Considerations

Miliaria is an acute dermatitis that occurs most commonly on the upper extremities, trunk, and intertriginous areas. A hot, moist environment is the most frequent cause, but individual susceptibility is important, and obese persons are most often affected. Plugging of the ostia of sweat ducts occurs, with consequent ballooning and ultimate rupture of the sweat duct, producing an irritating, stinging reaction. Increase in numbers of resident aerobes, notably cocci, apparently plays a role.

Clinical Findings

The usual symptoms are burning and itching. In severe cases, fever, heat prostration, and even death may result. The lesions consist of small, superficial, reddened, thin-walled, discrete but closely aggregated vesicles, papules, or vesicopapules. The reaction occurs most commonly on covered areas of the skin.

Differential Diagnosis

Distinguish from similar skin manifestations occurring in drug rash.

Prevention

Provide favorable working conditions when possible, ie, controlled temperature, ventilation, and humidity. Avoid overbathing and the use of strong, irritating soaps. Graded exposure to sunlight or ultraviolet light may benefit persons who will later be subjected to a hot, moist atmosphere. Susceptible persons should avoid exposure to adverse atmospheric conditions.

Treatment

An antipruritic cooling lotion such as the following should be applied 2–4 times daily:

℞	Menthol	0.5
	Phenol	0.5
	0.1% triamcinolone acetonide	30.0
	Lubriderm lotion, qs ad	120.0
	(unscented preferred)	

Alternative measures that have been employed with varying success are drying shake lotions and antipruritic powders or other dusting powders. Treat secondary infections (superficial pyoderma) with erythromycin or cloxacillin, 1 g daily by mouth. Tannic acid, 10% in 70% alcohol, applied locally twice daily, serves to toughen the skin. Anticholinergic drugs given by mouth may be very helpful in severe cases, eg, glycopyrrolate, 1 mg twice daily.

Prognosis

Miliaria is usually a mild disorder, but death may result in the severe forms (tropical anhidrosis and asthenia) as a result of interference with the heat-regulating mechanism. The process may also be irreversible to some extent, requiring permanent removal of the individual from the humid or hot climate.

ANOGENITAL PRURITUS

Essentials of Diagnosis

- Itching, chiefly nocturnal, of the anogenital area.
- There may be no skin reactions; or inflammation of any degree may occur up to lichenification.

General Considerations

Most cases have no obvious cause, but multiple specific causes have been identified. Anogenital pruritus may have the same causes as intertrigo, lichen simplex chronicus, or seborrheic or contact dermatitis (from soaps, colognes, douches, contraceptives) or may be due to irritating secretions, as in diarrhea, leukorrhea, or trichomoniasis, or local disease (candidiasis, dermatophytosis, erythrasma). Diabetes mellitus must be ruled out. Psoriasis or seborrheic dermatitis may be present. Uncleanliness may be at fault. It has been postulated that fecal bacterial endopeptidases play a causative role in pruritus ani.

Up to 10% of gynecologic patients may present with pruritus vulvae. In women, pruritus ani by itself is rare, and pruritus vulvae does not usually involve the anal area, although anal itching will usually spread to the vulva. In men, pruritus of the scrotum is less common than pruritus ani. When all possible known causes have been ruled out, the condition is diagnosed as idiopathic or essential pruritus—by no means rare.

Clinical Findings

A. Symptoms and Signs: The only symptom is itching, which is chiefly nocturnal. Physical findings are usually not present, but there may be erythema, fissuring, maceration, lichenification, excoriations, or changes suggestive of candidiasis or tinea.

B. Laboratory Findings: Urinalysis and blood glucose determination may lead to a diagnosis of diabetes mellitus. Microscopic examination or culture of tissue scrapings may reveal yeasts, fungi, or parasites. Stool examination may show intestinal parasites.

Differential Diagnosis

The etiologic differential diagnosis consists of *Candida* infection, parasitosis, local irritation from contact with drugs and irritants, and other primary skin disorders of the genital area such as psoriasis, seborrhea, or intertrigo.

Prevention

Treat all possible systemic or local causes. Instruct the patient in proper anogenital hygiene.

Treatment (See also Pruritus, p 48.)

A. General Measures: Avoid "hot" (spicy) foods, and drugs that can irritate the anal mucosa. Treat constipation if present (see p 353). Instruct the patient to use very soft or moistened tissue or cotton after a bowel movement and to clean the perianal area thoroughly. Women should use similar precautions after urinating. Anal douching is the best cleansing method for all types of pruritus ani. Instruct the patient regarding the harmful and pruritus-inducing effects of scratching.

B. Local Measures: Hydrocortisone or iodochlorhydroxyquin-hydrocortisone creams are quite useful. Potent fluorinated topical corticosteroids may lead to atrophy and striae. Sitz baths twice daily using silver nitrate, 1:10,000–1:200; potassium permanganate, 1:10,000; or aluminum subacetate solution, 1:20, are of value if the area is acutely inflamed and oozing. Underclothing should be changed daily. Paint affected areas with Castellani's solution. Balneol Perianal Cleansing Lotion or Tucks premoistened pads, ointment, or cream (all Tucks preparations contain witch hazel) may be very useful for pruritus ani.

Prognosis

Although usually benign, anogenital pruritus may be persistent and recurrent.

CALLOSITIES & CORNS (OF FEET OR TOES)

Callosities and corns are caused by pressure and friction due to faulty weight-bearing, orthopedic deformities, or improperly fitting shoes. Some persons are hereditarily predisposed to excessive and abnormal callus formation. It is crucial to provide optimal foot care for diabetics (see p 773) and those with insensitive extremities.

Tenderness on pressure and "after-pain" are the only symptoms. The hyperkeratotic well-localized overgrowths always occur at pressure points. On paring, a glassy core is found (which differentiates these disorders from plantar warts, which have multiple capillary bleeding points when cut). A soft corn often occurs laterally on the proximal portion of the fourth toe as a result of pressure against the bony structure of the interphalangeal joint of the fifth toe.

Treatment consists of correcting mechanical abnormalities that cause friction and pressure. Shoes must be properly fitted and orthopedic deformities corrected. Callosities may be removed by careful paring of the callus after a warm water soak or with keratolytic agents, eg, Keralyt gel (Westwood), which contains 6% salicylic acid. Apply locally to callus every night and cover with a polyethylene plastic film (Saran Wrap); remove in the morning. Repeat until the corn or callus is removed.

Extensive and severe palmar and plantar hyperkeratosis can be treated successfully by applying equal parts of propylene glycol and water nightly and covering with thin polyethylene plastic film (Baggies).

A metatarsal leather bar, 1.25 cm (½ inch) wide and 0.65 cm (¼ inch) high, may be placed on the outside of the shoe just behind the weight-bearing surface of the sole. "Ripple-sole" shoes may be effective.

Women who tend to form calluses and corns should not wear confining footgear.

Gibbs RC, Boxer MC: Abnormal biomechanics of feet and their cause of hyperkeratoses. *J Am Acad Dermatol* 1982;**6**:1061.

CHRONIC DISCOID LUPUS ERYTHEMATOSUS

Essentials of Diagnosis

- Red, asymptomatic, localized plaques, usually on the face, often in butterfly distribution.
- Scaling, follicular plugging, atrophy, and telangiectasia of involved areas.
- Histology distinctive.

General Considerations

Lupus erythematosus is a superficial, localized discoid inflammation of the skin occurring most frequently in areas exposed to solar or ultraviolet irradiation. The cause is not known. The disseminated type is discussed in Chapter 14.

Clinical Findings

A. Symptoms and Signs: There are usually no symptoms. The lesions consist of dusky red, well-localized, single or multiple plaques, 5–20 mm in diameter, usually on the face and often in a "butterfly pattern" over the nose and cheeks. There is atrophy, telangiectasia, and follicular plugging. The lesion is usually covered by dry, horny, adherent scales.

Where indicated, a complete medical study should be made to rule out systemic lupus erythematosus.

B. Laboratory Findings: There are usually no significant routine laboratory findings in the chronic discoid type. If there is leukopenia or proteinuria, with or without casts, one must suspect the disseminated or systemic form of the disease. Histologic changes are distinctive. The antinuclear antibody test is perhaps best for ruling out systemic lupus erythematosus. A direct immunofluorescence microscopy test reveals basement membrane antibody. "Uninvolved" skin adjacent to a lesion tends to be negative to direct immunofluorescence testing in discoid lupus erythematosus but positive in the systemic form of the disease.

One may also obtain a complete blood count, sedimentation rate, urinalysis, and anti-DNA, CH50, and C3 tests.

Differential Diagnosis

The scales are dry and "tacklike" and can thus be distinguished from those of seborrheic dermatitis. Differentiate also from the morphea type of basal cell epithelioma and, by absence of nodules and ulceration, from lupus vulgaris.

Complications

Dissemination may occur. There may be scarring.

Treatment

A. General Measures: Treat chronic infections. Provide protection from sunlight and all other powerful radiation. *Caution:* Do not use any form of radiation therapy.

Maintain optimal general health by providing a well-balanced diet with supplementary vitamins and iron as indicated. d-Alpha tocopheryl acetate (vitamin E) may be tried in doses of 400–2000 IU daily by mouth. Vitamin E is inactivated by iron and may potentiate the effect of insulin and digitalis. Ensure adequate rest. Prescribe bed rest for fever.

B. Medical Treatment: (For discoid type only.) *Caution:* The following drugs may cause serious eye changes. If the medication is continued, ophthalmologic examination should be done every 3 months. Chloroquine, 250 mg/d, or hydroxychloroquine, no more than 400 mg/d, is unlikely to cause retinopathy or other eye damage. Wherever possible, chronic discoid lupus erythematosus should be considered a cosmetic defect only and treated topically or with camouflaging agents.

1. Chloroquine phosphate, 0.25 g daily for 1 week, then 0.25 g twice weekly. Watch for signs of toxicity.

2. Hydroxychloroquine sulfate, 0.2 g orally daily and then twice weekly, may occasionally be effective when chloroquine is not tolerated.

3. Quinacrine (Atabrine), 100 mg daily, may be the safest of the antimalarials, since eye damage has not been reported. It colors the skin yellow.

C. Local Infiltration: Triamcinolone acetonide suspension, 2.5 mg/mL, may be injected into the lesions once a week or once a month. This should be tried before internal treatment (see above).

D. Corticosteroids: Corticosteroid creams applied each night and covered with airtight, thin, pliable plastic film may be useful.

Prognosis

The disease is persistent but not life-endangering, unless it turns into the disseminated variety.

Olansky AJ: Antimalarials and ophthalmologic safety. *J Am Acad Dermatol* 1982;**6**:19.

Tuffanelli DL: Lupus erythematosus. *J Am Acad Dermatol* 1981; **4**:127.

Zuehlke RL, Lillis PJ, Tice A: Antimalarial therapy for lupus erythematosus: An apparent advantage of quinacrine. *Int J Dermatol* 1981;**20**:57.

VIRAL INFECTIONS OF THE SKIN

HERPES SIMPLEX
(Cold or Fever Sore)
(See also p 829 and Chapters 23 and 29.)

Essentials of Diagnosis

- Recurrent small grouped vesicles on an erythematous base, especially around oral and genital areas.

- May follow minor infections, trauma, stress, or sun exposure.
- Regional lymph nodes may be swollen and tender.
- Tzanck smear is positive for large multinucleated epithelial giant cells surrounded by acantholytic balloon cells.

General Considerations

Although approximately 90% of the population acquire herpes simplex infection before the age of 4 or 5 years based on antibody studies, it is generally type 1 infection, following which the virus may remain in some form in the regional ganglia for life. No present means of treatment can eliminate the hidden foci of infection. The disease may manifest itself as severe gingivostomatitis in small children, or the initial infection may be subclinical. Thereafter, the subject may have recurrent attacks, provoked by fever, a cold, fatigue, menstruation, and other triggering factors such as sun and wind. *Herpes simplex virus type 1 is a major cause of fatal sporadic encephalitis.*

A 9-fold increase in the number of ambulatory patients with genital herpes simplex infections, usually caused by type 2, took place from 1966 to 1979. In addition to fever blisters, the virus may cause encephalitis, with a high morbidity and fatality rate, ophthalmitis, and a virulent infection in neonates.

Herpes simplex virus antibodies are found in 85% of young adults in lower economic classes.

A 15-year population study in Rochester, Minnesota, indicated an annual average incidence rate of herpes progenitalis of 50:100,000 population, with a peak of 128:100,000 in 1979. Females predominated by 1.5:1. Although there were 15 pregnancies in affected women, no neonatal herpes was noted, nor was there any invasive or in situ genital carcinoma.

Clinical Findings

The principal symptoms are burning and stinging. Neuralgia may precede and accompany attacks. The lesions consist of small, grouped vesicles which can occur anywhere but which most often occur on the lips, mouth, and genitals. Regional lymph nodes may be swollen and tender.

Differential Diagnosis

Lesions clinically diagnosed as chancroid, syphilis, pyoderma, or trauma have been found to be herpes simplex virus infections on culture. Viral culture is most helpful in confirming the clinical diagnosis and for showing viral shedding in asymptomatic patients. Although not completely sensitive, it is the most sensitive technique available. Other methods rely on detection of viral particles by electron microscopy, detection of viral antigen by immunologic methods (immunoperoxidase or immunofluorescence), or demonstration of multinucleated cells or intranuclear inclusion cells. The latter (Tzanck test) is the least sensitive.

Complications

Complications include pyoderma, eczema herpeticum, encephalitis, and keratitis.

Treatment

For persistent or severe, recurrent herpes:

A. General Measures: Eliminate precipitating agents when possible.

Acyclovir is effective systemically (intravenously, subcutaneously, intramuscularly, or orally) and is practically nontoxic, but experience has been relatively limited. It may prove more useful than intravenous vidarabine for herpes simplex encephalitis. However, although acyclovir will prevent local cutaneous recurrences if given continuously by mouth, attacks will recur when it is stopped; if the drug is used intermittently, resistance will develop rapidly.

B. Local Measures: Apply a moistened styptic pencil several times daily to abort lesions. Zinc sulfate solution, 0.025–0.05%, may be used as a warm compress, 10 minutes twice daily. Or one may apply epinephrine, 1:100 solution, frequently. Topical corticosteroids are contraindicated. Applied topically, toluidine blue has an anesthetic effect and appears to hasten drying of vesicles.

If there is associated cellulitis and lymphadenitis, apply cool compresses. Treat stomatitis with water and milk of magnesia mouthwashes.

There is no really safe and effective systemic approach to cure recurrent herpes simplex infections of the skin. It is strongly urged that topical use of 5% acyclovir ointment (Zovirax) be limited to the restricted indications for which it has been approved, namely, initial herpes genitalis and mucocutaneous herpes simplex infections in immunocompromised patients, because of promotion of resistant strains of the virus and the mild mutagenicity of the drug.

Future studies will include use of interferons and trials with lymphokines.

Prognosis

Aside from the dread complications described above, recurrent attacks last 1–2 weeks. A retrospective study indicated that 50% of those with genital herpes were found to be essentially free of frequently recurring episodes 7 years after onset.

Bierman SM: A retrospective study of 375 patients with genital herpes simplex infections seen between 1973 and 1980. *Cutis* 1983;**31:**548.

Chuang T-Y et al: Incidence and trend of herpes progenitalis: A 15-year population study. *Mayo Clin Proc* 1983;**58:**436.

Corey L et al: Intravenous acyclovir for the treatment of primary genital herpes. *Ann Intern Med* 1983;**98:**914.

Felman YM, Nikitas JA: Genital ulcers caused by sexually transmitted diseases. *Cutis* 1983;**32:**228.

Reichman RC et al: Treatment of recurrent genital herpes simplex infections with oral acyclovir: A controlled trial. *JAMA* 1984;**251:**2103.

HERPES ZOSTER
(Shingles)

Essentials of Diagnosis

- Pain along course of a nerve followed by painful grouped vesicular lesions.
- Involvement is unilateral. Lesions are usually on face and trunk.
- Swelling of regional lymph nodes (inconstant).

General Considerations

Herpes zoster is an acute vesicular eruption due to a virus that is morphologically identical with the virus of varicella. It usually occurs in adults. With rare exceptions, one attack of zoster confers lifelong immunity. Persons in anergic states (Hodgkin's disease, lymphomas, or those taking immunosuppressive drugs) are at greater risk, and generalized, life-threatening dissemination (varicella) may occur.

Clinical Findings

Pain usually precedes the eruption by 48 hours or more and may persist and actually increase in intensity after the lesions have disappeared. The lesions consist of grouped, tense, deep-seated vesicles distributed unilaterally along the neural pathways of the trunk. The commonest distributions are on the trunk or face. Regional lymph glands may be tender and swollen.

Differential Diagnosis

Since poison oak and poison ivy dermatitis may be produced unilaterally and in a streak by a single brush with the plant, it must be differentiated at times from herpes zoster. Differentiate also from similar lesions of herpes simplex, which is usually less painful.

Complications

Persistent neuralgia, anesthesia of the affected area following healing, facial or other nerve paralysis, and encephalitis may occur.

Treatment

A. General Measures: Sedatives may be required to control tension and nervousness associated with neuralgia. Aspirin with or without codeine phosphate, 30 mg, usually controls pain. A single intragluteal injection of 40 mg of triamcinolone acetonide suspension may give prompt relief. Prednisone, 60 mg orally for 10 days, may be the treatment of choice. Steroid therapy may decrease the incidence of postherpetic neuralgia. Ophthalmologic consultation should be considered for supraorbital involvement to avoid serious ocular complications. Hospitalization may be necessary in serious cases. Zoster has developed despite normal varicella-zoster antibody levels, indicating that cell-mediated immunity is more important in preventing zoster than are circulating antibodies. Zoster immune globulin (ZIG) can prevent chickenpox but has no effect on existing zoster lesions. (See Chapters 22, 23, and 29.)

Vidarabine, in a double-blind study, shortened the course of zoster and appeared to lessen the duration of postzoster neuralgia in immunosuppressed patients. This drug is now also available as ophthalmic ointment. Intravenous acyclovir, as compared to placebo, will shorten the course of herpes zoster but will not affect the occurrence of postzoster neuralgia. (See also p 829 and Chapter 29.)

B. Local Measures: Calamine or starch shake lotions are often of value. Apply lotion liberally and cover with a layer of cotton. Do not use greases.

C. Postzoster Neuralgia: Infiltration of skin with triamcinolone acetonide and lidocaine has been disappointing. High doses of systemic corticosteroids early in the disease may reduce the incidence of post-herpetic neuralgia. Vitamin E (d-alpha tocopheryl acetate), 800 units daily, should be tried. Intercostal nerve block and sympathetic ganglion block, repeated daily until the symptoms subside, have been recommended. Amitriptyline, 25 mg orally 3 times daily, and perphenazine, 4 mg orally 3 times daily, or fluphenazine, 1 mg 4 times daily, has also been suggested. Somnolence may occur with either type of drug. Pimozide (not available in the USA) may help most cases.

Prognosis

The eruption persists 2–3 weeks and does not recur. Motor involvement may lead to temporary palsy. No age group is exempt from the possibility of postzoster neuralgia persisting for a year or more, but the likelihood is greater in the 60- to 69-year age group (20%) and in those over 70 (30%). Ocular involvement may lead to blindness.

Bean B, Braun C, Balfour HH: Acyclovir therapy for acute herpes zoster. *Lancet* 1982;**2**:118.

Keczkes K, Basheer AM: Do corticosteroids prevent post-herpetic neuralgia? *Br J Dermatol* 1980;**102**:551.

Lowy DR: HPV: A large and sometimes lethal family. *Dermatol Forum* 1983;**1**:1.

Ogata A et al: Local anesthesia for herpes zoster. *J Dermatol* 1980;**7**:161.

Whitley RJ et al: Early vidarabine therapy to control the complications of herpes zoster in immunosuppressed patients. *N Engl J Med* 1982;**307**:971.

WARTS

Essentials of Diagnosis

- Warty elevation anywhere on skin or mucous membranes, usually no larger than 0.5 cm in diameter.
- Prolonged incubation period (average 2–18 months).
- Spontaneous "cures" are frequent (50%), but warts are often unresponsive to any form of treatment.
- "Recurrences" (new lesions) are frequent.

General Considerations

Nearly a million visits to physicians for warts took place in 1981, nearly triple the incidence for genital herpes. Almost 30 different subtypes of human papilloma viruses have been identified by serologic typing of viral proteins, molecular hybridization of viral DNA, and monoclonal antibody assays, using immunoperoxidase staining. About 25% of abnormal Papanicolaou smears are associated with the presence of human papilloma viruses, and 80% of cases of carcinoma of the cervix have similar associations, indicating that wart viruses may be more important than herpes simplex virus. Five oncogenic types of human papilloma viruses have been identified. Types 16 and 18 have been implicated in cervical carcinoma, and types 5, 8, and 14b in squamous cell carcinoma other than cervical. A number of children with laryngeal papillomas (types 11 and 6) treated with x-rays have developed squamous cell carcinoma of the larynx.

Clinical Findings

There are usually no symptoms. Tenderness on pressure occurs with plantar warts; itching occurs with anogenital warts. Occasionally a wart will produce mechanical obstruction (eg, nostril, ear canal).

Warts vary widely in shape, size, and appearance. Flat warts are most evident under oblique illumination. Subungual warts may be dry, fissured, and hyperkeratotic and may resemble hangnails or other nonspecific changes. Plantar warts resemble plantar corns or calluses.

Prevention

Avoid contact with warts. A person with flat warts should be admonished not to scratch the areas. Using an electric shaver will in occasional cases prevent the spread of warts in razor scratches. Anogenital warts may be transmitted venereally.

Treatment

A. Removal: Remove the warts whenever possible by one of the following means:

1. Surgical excision–Inject a small amount of local anesthetic into the base and then remove the wart with a dermal curet or scissors or by shaving off at the base of the wart with a scalpel. Trichloroacetic acid or Monsel's solution on a tightly wound cotton-tipped applicator may be painted on the wound, or electrocautery may be applied.

2. Liquid nitrogen applied for a few seconds may be used every 2 weeks for a period of 3 months if necessary.

3. Keratolytic agents–Either of the following may be used:

℞	Salicylic acid	2.5
	Lactic acid	2.5
	Flexible collodion, qs ad	15.0
	(Duofilm, Veruka, Viranol)	

Sig: Paint on warts each night with glass rod.

℞   Salicylic acid   3.6
     Alcohol, 40% qs ad   120.0

Sig: Paint on *flat* warts with cotton swab daily.

4. Anogenital warts are best treated by painting them weekly with 25% podophyllum resin in compound tincture of benzoin *(caution)*.

5. Plantar warts may be treated by applying a mixture of 1 g of trichloroacetic acid and 6 g of salicylic acid in sufficient glycerine to make a paste. The wart is pared and then rimmed with compound tincture of benzoin. The paste is applied by the physician and covered with an occlusive dressing. The wart may be pared 3–5 days later and the treatment repeated if necessary.

Bleomycin diluted to 0.1% with physiologic saline may be injected under warts, not exceeding 0.1 mL per puncture; with multiple punctures, it has been shown to have a high cure rate for plantar and common warts.

B. Immunotherapy: Dinitrochlorobenzene (DNCB) is useful for resistant warts. Initially, 400 μg of freshly prepared dinitrochlorobenzene is applied as a sensitizing dose to 2 or 3 sites on the forearm. Then the warts are painted with an Eppendorf pipette with precisely 20 μL of dinitrochlorobenzene at 2-week intervals until they recede.

Persistent, conservative application of topical irritants may cure warts by nonspecific boosting of wart antibodies. Specific wart antibodies (especially IgG) have been found in the serum of individuals with regressing warts.

C. Laser Therapy: The carbon dioxide laser is particularly effective for treating recurrent warts, plantar warts, and condylomata acuminata. The wart tissue is vaporized under magnified vision in a bloodless procedure without damage to surrounding areas.

D. Retinoids: Extensive warts have been reported to disappear when etretinate was given by mouth for a month. This drug is not available for use in the USA.

Prognosis

There is a striking tendency to the development of new lesions. Warts may disappear spontaneously or may be unresponsive to treatment.

Bailin PL: Lasers in dermatology: 1983. (Editorial.) *Cleve Clin Q* 1983;**50**:53.

Bunney MH: *Viral Warts: Their Biology and Treatment.* Oxford Univ Press, 1982.

Donagin WG, Millikan LE: Dinitrochlorobenzene immunotherapy for verrucae resistant to standard treatment modalities. *J Am Acad Dermatol* 1982;**6**:40.

Mackie RM: Extensive warts treated with etretinate. *Br J Dermatol* 1982;**107(Suppl 22)**:97.

BACTERIAL INFECTIONS OF THE SKIN

IMPETIGO

Impetigo is a contagious and autoinoculable infection of the skin caused by staphylococci or streptococci or both. The infected material may be transmitted to the skin by dirty fingernails. In children, the source of infection is often another infected child.

Itching is the only symptom. The lesions consist of macules, vesicles, pustules, and honey-colored gummy crusts (streptococcal) that when removed leave denuded red areas. The face and other exposed parts are most often involved.

Ecthyma is a deeper form of impetigo, with ulceration and scarring. It occurs frequently on the legs and other covered areas, often as a complication of debility and infestations.

Impetigo neonatorum is a highly contagious, potentially serious form of staphylococcal impetigo occurring in infants. It requires prompt systemic treatment and protection of other infants (isolation, exclusion from the nursery of personnel with pyoderma, etc). The lesions are bullous and massive and accompanied by systemic toxicity. Death may occur.

Impetigo must be distinguished from other vesicular and pustular lesions such as herpes simplex, varicella, and contact dermatitis (dermatitis venenata). A Gram stain and a Tzanck smear may be useful in differentiating the organisms.

Treatment is as for folliculitis. Some question has been raised about the efficacy of topical antibiotics. If there is fever or toxicity, or any concern over the possibility of a nephritogenic strain of *Streptococcus* being causative, systemic antibiotics may be given. Either erythromycin or dicloxacillin, 1 g daily, is usually effective, or one may use cephalexin, 50 mg/kg/24 h.

Dillon HC Jr: Treatment of staphylococcal infections: A comparison of cephalexin and dicloxacillin. *J Am Acad Dermatol* 1983;**8**:177.

Levine N: Bacterial skin infections: Telling them apart and treating them. *Mod Med* (Apr) 1981;**49**:26.

FOLLICULITIS
(Including Sycosis Vulgaris or Barber's Itch; Pseudofolliculitis)

Essentials of Diagnosis

- Itching and burning in hairy areas.
- Pustules in the hair follicles.
- In sycosis, inflammation of surrounding skin area.

General Considerations

Folliculitis is caused by staphylococcal infection

of a hair follicle. When the lesion is deep-seated, chronic, and recalcitrant, it is called sycosis. Sycosis is usually propagated by the autoinoculation and trauma of shaving. The upper lip is particularly susceptible to involvement in men who suffer with chronic nasal discharge from sinusitis or hay fever.

Bockhart's impetigo is a staphylococcal infection that produces painful, tense, globular pustules at the follicular orifices. It is a form of folliculitis.

Clinical Findings
The symptoms are slight burning and itching, and pain on manipulation of the hair. The lesions consist of pustules of the hair follicles. In sycosis, the surrounding skin becomes involved also and so resembles eczema, with redness and crusting.

Differential Diagnosis
Differentiate from acne vulgaris and infections of the skin such as impetigo or fungal infections.

Complications
Abscess formation.

Prevention
Correct any precipitating or aggravating factors: systemic (eg, diabetes mellitus) or local causes (eg, irritations of a mechanical or chemical nature, discharges).

Treatment
A. Specific Measures: Systemic anti-infectives may be tried if the skin infection is resistant to local treatment; if it is extensive or severe and accompanied by a febrile reaction; if it is complicated; or if it involves the so-called "danger areas" (upper lip, nose, and eyes).

Local anti-infective agents should be tried in sequence until a favorable response is obtained (allowing 3–4 days for evaluation in each case). These include polymyxin B in combination with bacitracin or oxytetracycline, and erythromycin. They should be applied initially at night and protected by dressings; soaks should be applied during the day. After the area has cleared, any of the following preparations may be applied 2–4 times daily: (1) Iodochlorhydroxyquin, 3% in cream or ointment form, locally twice daily. (2) Antibiotics, alone or in combination, as ointments locally 2–4 times daily.

Penicillin and sulfonamides should not be used topically.

B. Local Measures: Cleanse the area gently with a weak soap solution and apply saline or aluminum subacetate soaks or compresses to the involved area for 15 minutes twice daily. When skin is softened, gently open the larger pustules and trim away necrotic tissue.

Anhydrous ethyl alcohol containing 6.25% aluminum chloride (Xerac AC), applied to lesions and environs and followed by an antibiotic ointment (see above), may be very helpful. It is especially useful for chronic folliculitis of the buttocks.

Prognosis
Folliculitis is often stubborn and persistent, lasting for months and even years.

Shelley WB, Hurley HJ: Anhydrous formulation of aluminum chloride for chronic folliculitis. *JAMA* 1980;**244**:1956.

FURUNCULOSIS (BOILS) & CARBUNCLES

Essentials of Diagnosis
- Extremely painful inflammatory swelling of a hair follicle that forms an abscess.
- Primary predisposing debilitating disease sometimes present.
- Coagulase-positive *Staphylococcus aureus* is the causative organism.

General Considerations
A furuncle (boil) is a deep-seated infection (abscess) involving the entire hair follicle and adjacent subcutaneous tissue. The most common sites of occurrence are the hairy parts exposed to irritation and friction, pressure, or moisture or to the plugging action of petroleum products. Because the lesions are autoinoculable, they are often multiple. Thorough investigation usually fails to uncover a predisposing cause, although an occasional patient may have uncontrolled diabetes mellitus, nephritis, or other debilitating disease. Groups may be subject to epidemics.

A carbuncle is several furuncles developing in adjoining hair follicles and coalescing to form a conglomerate, deeply situated mass with multiple drainage points.

Clinical Findings
A. Symptoms and Signs: The extreme tenderness and pain are due to pressure on nerve endings, particularly in areas where there is little room for swelling of underlying structures. The pain, fever, and malaise are more severe with carbuncles than with furuncles. The follicular abscess is either rounded or conical. It gradually enlarges, becomes fluctuant, and then softens and opens spontaneously after a few days to 1–2 weeks to discharge a core of necrotic tissue and pus. The inflammation occasionally subsides before necrosis occurs.

Infection of the soft tissue around the nails (paronychia) is usually due to staphylococci when it is acute. This is a variant of furuncle. Other organisms may be involved.

B. Laboratory Findings: There may be slight leukocytosis.

Differential Diagnosis
Differentiate from deep mycotic infections such as sporotrichosis and blastomycosis; from other bacterial infections such as anthrax and tularemia; and from acne cysts and infected epidermal or pilar cysts.

Complications

Serious and sometimes fatal cerebral thrombophlebitis may occur as a complication of a manipulated furuncle on the central portion of the upper lip or near the nasolabial folds. Perinephric abscess, osteomyelitis, and other hematogenous staphylococcal infections may also occur.

Treatment

A. Specific Measures: Systemic anti-infective agents are indicated (chosen on the basis of cultures and sensitivity tests if possible). Sodium cloxacillin or erythromycin, 1 g daily by mouth for 10 days, is usually effective. Cephalexin is an effective alternative drug. Minocycline may be effective against strains of staphylococci resistant to other antibiotics.

Strains of pathogenic staphylococci may carry a plasmid, or episome, causing resistance to antibiotics such as erythromycin.

B. Local Measures: Immobilize the part and avoid overmanipulation of inflamed areas. Use moist heat to help larger lesions "localize." Use surgical incision and debridement *after* the lesions are "mature." Do not incise deeply. Apply anti-infective ointment and bandage the area loosely during drainage. It is not necessary to incise and drain an acute staphylococcal paronychia. Inserting a flat metal spatula or sharpened hardwood stick into the nail fold where it adjoins the nail will release pus from a mature lesion.

Prognosis

Recurrent crops may harass the patient for months or years. Carbunculosis is more severe and more hazardous than furunculosis.

An alcoholic aluminum chloride solution (see above) may be very useful in controlling repeated attacks of furuncles.

ERYSIPELAS

Essentials of Diagnosis

- Edematous, spreading, circumscribed, hot, erythematous area, with or without vesicle or bulla formation.
- Pain, malaise, chills and fever.
- Leukocytosis, increased sedimentation rate.

General Considerations

Erysipelas is an acute inflammation of the skin and subcutaneous tissue caused by infection with beta-hemolytic streptococci. It occurs classically on the cheek.

Clinical Findings

A. Symptoms and Signs: The symptoms are pain, malaise, chills, and moderate fever. A bright red spot appears first, very often near a fissure at the angle of the nose. This spreads to form a tense, sharply demarcated, glistening, smooth, hot area. The margin characteristically makes noticeable advances from day to day. The patch is somewhat edematous and can be pitted slightly with the finger. Vesicles or bullae occasionally develop on the surface. The patch does not usually become pustular or gangrenous and heals without scar formation. The disease may complicate any break in the skin that provides a portal of entry for the organism.

B. Laboratory Findings: Leukocytosis and increased sedimentation rate almost invariably occur.

Differential Diagnosis

Distinguish from cellulitis, with its less definite margin and involvement of deeper tissues; and from erysipeloid, a benign bacillary infection producing redness of the skin of the fingers or the backs of the hands in fishermen and meat handlers.

Complications

Unless erysipelas is promptly treated, death may result from extension of the process and systemic toxicity, particularly in the very young and in the aged.

Treatment

Place the patient at bed rest with the head of the bed elevated, apply hot packs, and give aspirin for pain and fever. Penicillin is specific for beta-hemolytic streptococcal infections. Erythromycin is a good alternative.

Prognosis

Erysipelas formerly was very dangerous to life, particularly in the very young and in the aged. It can now usually be quickly controlled with systemic penicillin or erythromycin therapy. Prompt and adequate treatment usually will limit it to one attack.

CELLULITIS
(See also p 300.)

Cellulitis, a diffuse spreading infection of the skin, must be differentiated from erysipelas (a superficial form of cellulitis) because the 2 conditions are quite similar. Cellulitis involves deeper tissues and may be due to one of several organisms, usually cocci. The lesion is hot and red but has a more diffuse border than does erysipelas. Cellulitis usually occurs after a break in the skin. Recurrent attacks may sometimes affect lymphatic vessels, producing a permanent swelling called "solid edema."

The response to systemic anti-infective measures (penicillin or broad-spectrum antibiotics) is usually prompt and satisfactory.

ERYSIPELOID

Erysipelothrix rhusiopathiae infection must be differentiated from erysipelas and cellulitis. It is usually a benign infection commonly seen in fishermen and meat handlers and characterized by redness of the skin, most often of a finger or the back of the hand, which gradually extends over a period of several days. Systemic involvement occurs rarely and is manifested by reversal of the albumin/globulin ratio and other serious changes. Endocarditis may occur.

Penicillin is usually promptly curative. Broad-spectrum antibiotics may be used instead.

DECUBITUS ULCERS
(Bedsores, Pressure Sores)

Bedsores (pressure sores) are a special type of ulcer caused by impaired blood supply and tissue nutrition due to prolonged pressure over bony or cartilaginous prominences. The skin overlying the sacrum and hips is most commonly involved, but bedsores may also be seen over the occiput, ears, elbows, heels, and ankles. They occur most readily in aged, paralyzed, debilitated, and unconscious patients. Low-grade infection may occur.

Good nursing care and nutrition and maintenance of skin hygiene are important preventive measures. The skin and the bed linens should be kept clean and dry. Bedfast, paralyzed, moribund, or listless patients who are candidates for the development of decubiti must be turned *frequently* (at least every hour) and must be examined at pressure points for the appearance of small areas of redness and tenderness. Water-filled mattresses, rubber pillows, alternating pressure mattresses, and thick papillated foam pads are useful in prevention and in the treatment of early lesions.

Early lesions should also be treated with topical antibiotic powders and adhesive absorbent bandage (Gelfoam). Established lesions require surgical consultation and care. A spongy Feathersoft pad placed under the patient may work best in some cases. It may be laundered often. A continuous dressing of 1% iodochlorhydroxyquin (Vioform) in Lassar's paste may be effective.

Andersen KE, Kvoming SA: Medical aspects of the decubitus ulcer. *Int J Dermatol* 1982;**21**:265.

Cooney TG, Reuler JB: Pressure sores. *West J Med* 1984; **140**:622.

FUNGAL INFECTIONS OF THE SKIN

Mycotic infections are traditionally divided into 2 principal groups: superficial and deep. In this chapter we will discuss only the superficial infections: tinea capitis, tinea corporis, and tinea cruris; dermatophytosis of the feet and dermatophytid of the hands; tinea unguium (onychomycosis, or fungal infection of the nails); and tinea versicolor. Candidiasis belongs in an intermediate group but will be considered here as well as with the deep mycoses.

The diagnosis of fungal infections of the skin is usually based on the location and characteristics of the lesions and on the following laboratory examinations: (1) Direct demonstration of fungi in 15% potassium hydroxide preparations of scrapings from suspected lesions. (2) Cultures of organisms. Dermatophytes responsive to griseofulvin are easily detectable, with color change from yellow to red on dermatophyte test medium (DTM); or one may use a microculture slide that produces color change and allows for direct microscopic identification (Oricult-DTM). (3) Skin tests, eg, trichophytin (not reliable) for superficial mycoses. (This test has exclusion value in suspected dermatophytid.) (4) Examination with Wood's light (an ultraviolet light with a special filter), which causes hairs to fluoresce a brilliant green when they are infected by *Microsporum* organisms. The lamp is also invaluable in following the progress of treatment. Ringworm of the scalp may be totally unsuspected yet discovered easily with Wood's light in mass surveys of schoolchildren. *Trichophyton*-infected hairs do not fluoresce. (5) Histologic sections stained with periodic acid–Schiff (Hotchkiss-McManus) technique. Fungal elements stain red and are easily found.

Serologic tests are of no value in the diagnosis of superficial fungal infections.

Delayed sensitivity to intradermal trichophytin appears to be a correlate of immunity, whereas immediate trichophytin reactivity is associated with chronic tinea infections.

Principles of Treatment

Treat acute active fungal infections initially as for any acute dermatitis (see p 47). *Note:* It may be necessary to treat the dermatitis before applying topical fungicidal medication.

Many topical fungicidal agents are strong skin irritants. *It is easy to overtreat.*

In 1981, ketoconazole was approved in the USA for treatment of candidiasis, chronic mucocutaneous candidiasis, oral thrush, candiduria, coccidioidomycosis, histoplasmosis, chromomycosis, and paracoccidioidomycosis. Dermatophytosis was not included, but the FDA allows for usage of an approved drug for unlisted indications if the physician judges it necessary. Prior to approval, more than 2000 patients had received ketoconazole for varying periods. Chief concerns are abnormal levels of liver enzymes, gynecomastia, nausea, and urticaria. Additional clinical experience will be required to determine the drug's efficacy, adverse effects, and long-term safety.

One person in 10–15 thousand may have liver damage. It is critical to warn patients to stop the drug at the first onset of nausea, indigestion, dark urine, clay-colored stools, or jaundice. Of those who developed jaundice, 82% did so within 11–168 days of treatment (average, 49 days). Liver function tests rapidly return to normal when the drug is stopped. Tests may be done every 2–4 weeks, though clinical signs and symptoms are more reliable. Gynecomastia can be avoided by giving the total dose once daily. It is best to avoid giving more than 200 mg/d (one tablet) if possible.

General Measures & Prevention

Keep the skin dry, since moist skin favors the growth of fungi. A cool climate is preferred. Reduce exercise and activities to prevent excessive perspiration. Dry the skin carefully after bathing or after perspiring heavily. Loose-fitting underwear is advisable. Socks and other clothing should be changed often. Sandals or open-toed shoes should be worn. Skin secretions should be controlled with talc or other drying powders or with drying soaks. Sedatives (eg, phenobarbital) may be effective in reducing skin secretions in tense, nervous people. Graded daily sunbaths or quartz lamp exposure may be helpful.

Duarte PA et al: Fatal hepatitis associated with ketoconazole therapy. *Arch Intern Med* 1984;**144**:1069.

Hanifin JM: Adverse reactions. Page 157 in: *Ketoconazole in the Management of Fungal Disease.* Levine HB (editor). ADIS Press, 1983.

Lewis JH et al: Hepatic injury associated with ketoconazole therapy. *Gastroenterology* 1984;**88**:503.

TINEA CAPITIS
(Ringworm of Scalp)

Essentials of Diagnosis

- Round, gray, scaly "bald" patches on the scalp.
- Usually in prepubertal children.
- Often fluorescent under Wood's lamp.
- Microscopic examination or culture identifies the fungus.

General Considerations

This persistent, contagious, and sometimes epidemic infection occurs almost exclusively in children and disappears spontaneously at puberty. Two genera *(Microsporum* and *Trichophyton)* cause ringworm infections of the scalp. *Microsporum* accounts for many of the infections, and hairs infected with this genus fluoresce brilliantly under Wood's light. *Trichophyton* species account for some of the very resistant infections, which may persist into adulthood.

Clinical Findings

A. Symptoms and Signs: There are usually no symptoms, although there may be slight itching. The lesions are round, gray, scaly, apparently bald patches on the scalp. (The hairs are broken off, and the patches are not actually bald.) Scalp ringworm may be undetectable with the naked eye, becoming visible only under Wood's light, in which case the hairs exhibit a brilliant green fluorescence extending down into the hair follicle.

B. Laboratory Findings: Microscopic or culture demonstration of the organisms in the hairs may be necessary.

Differential Diagnosis

Differentiate from other diseases of scalp hair such as pediculosis capitis, pyoderma, alopecia areata, and trichotillomania (voluntary pulling out of one's own hair).

Prevention

Exchange of headgear must be avoided, and infected individuals or household pets must be vigorously treated and scrupulously reexamined for determination of cure. The scalp should be washed after haircuts.

Complications

Kerion (a nodular, exudative pustule), possibly followed by scarring, is the only complication. It responds dramatically to saturated solution of potassium iodide orally.

Treatment

Microcrystalline griseofulvin, 0.25–0.5 g by mouth daily or twice daily for 2 weeks, will cure most cases. Selenium sulfide has a sporicidal effect when used as an adjunct to oral griseofulvin; it is used as a shampoo (Selsun, Exsel) twice weekly.

Prognosis

Tinea capitis may be very persistent but usually clears spontaneously at puberty. Most ringworm infections of the scalp will clear spontaneously in 1–2 years even if not treated, but follow-up is advisable to prevent occurrence of kerion. Kerion responds promptly to saturated solution of potassium iodide by mouth.

Allen HB et al: Selenium sulfide: Adjunctive therapy for tinea capitis. *Pediatrics* 1982;**69**:81.

Shelley WB, Wood MG: New technic for instant visualization of fungi in hair. *J Am Acad Dermatol* 1980;**2**:69.

TINEA CORPORIS OR TINEA CIRCINATA
(Body Ringworm)

Essentials of Diagnosis

- Pruritic, ringed, scaling, centrally clearing lesions; small vesicles in a peripherally advancing border.
- On exposed skin surfaces.
- History of exposure to infected domestic animal.
- Laboratory examination by microscope or culture confirms diagnosis.

General Considerations

The lesions are often on exposed areas of the body such as the face and arms. A history of exposure to an infected cat may be obtained. All species of dermatophytes may cause this disease, but some are more common than others.

Clinical Findings

A. Symptoms and Signs: Itching is usually intense, which distinguishes the disease from other ringed lesions. Rings of vesicles with central clearing are grouped in clusters and distributed asymmetrically, usually on an exposed surface.

B. Laboratory Findings: Hyphae can be demonstrated by removing the cap of a vesicle and examining it microscopically in a drop of 15% potassium hydroxide. The diagnosis may be confirmed by culture.

Differential Diagnosis

Itching distinguishes tinea corporis from other skin lesions with annular configuration, such as the annular lesions of psoriasis, erythema multiforme, and pityriasis rosea.

Complications

Complications include extension of the disease to the scalp hair or nails (in which case it becomes much more difficult to cure), overtreatment dermatitis, pyoderma, and dermatophytid.

Prevention

Avoid contact with infected household pets and exchange of clothing without adequate laundering.

Treatment

A. Specific Measures: Griseofulvin (microcrystalline), 0.5 g orally daily for children and 1 g orally daily for adults. Dermatophytosis is an unlisted indication for ketoconazole (see p 74), but griseofulvin and topical antifungals are preferred therapy.

B. Local Measures: One percent salicylic acid and 3% precipitated sulfur in hydrophilic ointment may be rubbed into lesions twice daily. *Caution:* Do not overtreat.

Compound undecylenic acid ointment may be used in the less chronic and nonthickened lesions.

Tolnaftate (Tinactin) solution or cream applied topically is effective against dermatophyte infections other than of the nails. Haloprogin, 1% cream or solution, may be used. Miconazole, 2% cream, is effective. Clotrimazole, an imidazole similar to miconazole, is available, as a 1% liquid or cream. Sulconazole, 1% cream, is now available as is 1% ciclopirox cream.

Prognosis

Body ringworm usually responds promptly to griseofulvin by mouth or to conservative topical therapy.

Conti-Diaz IA, Civila E, Asconegui F: Treatment of superficial and deep-seated mycoses with oral ketoconazole. *Int J Dermatol* 1984;**23**:207.

Tanenbaum L et al: Sulconazole nitrate 1.0 percent cream: A comparison with miconazole in the treatment of tinea pedis and tinea cruris/corporis. *Cutis* 1982;**30**:105.

TINEA CRURIS
(Jock Itch)

Essentials of Diagnosis

- Marked itching in intertriginous areas.
- Peripherally spreading, sharply demarcated, centrally clearing erythematous macular lesions, with or without vesicle formation.
- May have associated tinea infection of feet.
- Laboratory examination with microscope or culture confirms diagnosis.

General Considerations

Tinea cruris lesions are confined to the groin and gluteal cleft and are as a rule more indolent than those of tinea corporis and tinea circinata. The disease often occurs in athletes as well as in persons who are obese or who perspire a great deal. Any of the dermatophytes may cause tinea cruris, and it may be transmitted to the groin from active dermatophytosis of the foot. Intractable pruritus ani may occasionally be caused by tineal infection.

Clinical Findings

A. Symptoms and Signs: Itching is usually more severe than that which occurs in seborrheic dermatitis or intertrigo. Inverse psoriasis, however, may itch even more than tinea cruris. The lesions consist of erythematous macules with sharp margins, cleared centers, and active, spreading peripheries in intertriginous areas. There may be vesicle formation at the borders, and satellite vesicular lesions are sometimes present.

B. Laboratory Findings: Hyphae can be demonstrated microscopically in 15% potassium hydroxide preparations. The organism may be cultured readily.

Differential Diagnosis

Differentiate from other lesions involving the intertriginous areas, such as candidiasis, seborrheic dermatitis, intertrigo, psoriasis of body folds ("inverse psoriasis"), and erythrasma.

Treatment

A. General Measures: (See also p 47.) Drying powder should be dusted into the involved area 2–3 times a day, especially when perspiration is excessive. Keep the area clean and dry but avoid overbathing. Prevent intertrigo or chafing by avoiding overtreatment, which predisposes to further infection and complications. Underwear should be loose-fitting. Rough-textured clothing should be avoided.

B. Specific Measures: Griseofulvin is indicated for severe cases. Give 1 g orally daily for 1–2 weeks.

C. Local Measures: Treat the stage of dermatosis (see p 47). Secondarily infected or inflamed lesions are best treated with soothing and drying solutions, with the patient at bed rest. Use wet compresses of potassium permanganate, 1:10,000 (or 1:20

aluminum acetate solution), or, in case of anogenital infection, sitz baths.

Fungicidal preparations. Any of the following may be used: (1) Weak solutions of iodine (not more than 1% tincture) twice daily. (2) Carbolfuchsin solution (Castellani's paint), one-third strength, once a day. (3) Compound undecylenic acid ointment twice daily. (4) Sulfur–salicylic acid ointment. (5) Tolnaftate (Tinactin) solution or cream. (6) Haloprogin (Halotex), 1% cream or solution. (7) Miconazole, 2% cream. (8) Clotrimazole, 1% liquid or cream. (9) Sulconazole, 1% cream.

Prognosis

Tinea cruris usually responds promptly to topical or systemic treatment.

TINEA MANUUM & TINEA PEDIS
(Dermatophytosis, Tinea of Palms & Soles, "Athlete's Foot")

Essentials of Diagnosis

- Itching, burning, and stinging of interdigital webs, palms, and soles.
- Deep vesicles in acute stage.
- Exfoliation, fissuring, and maceration in subacute or chronic stages.
- Skin scrapings examined microscopically or by culture may reveal fungus.

General Considerations

Tinea of the feet is an extremely common acute or chronic dermatosis. It is possible that the causative organisms are present on the feet of most adults at all times. Certain individuals appear to be more susceptible than others. Most infections are caused by *Trichophyton* and *Epidermophyton* species.

Clinical Findings

A. Symptoms and Signs: The presenting symptom is usually itching. However, there may be burning, stinging, and other sensations, or frank pain from secondary infection with complicating cellulitis, lymphangitis, and lymphadenitis. Tinea pedis often appears as a fissuring of the toe webs, perhaps with denudation and sodden maceration. Toe web "tinea" may not be tinea at all but rather an intertrigo that may be called "athlete's foot." It may respond better to 30% aqueous aluminum chloride or to carbolfuchsin paint or a keratolytic agent (Keralyt gel) than to antifungal agents. However, there may also be grouped vesicles distributed anywhere on the soles or the palms, a generalized exfoliation of the skin of the soles, or destructive nail involvement in the form of discoloration and hypertrophy of the nail substance with pithy changes. Acute reddened, weeping vesicular lesions are seen on the skin in the acute stages.

B. Laboratory Findings: Hyphae can often be demonstrated microscopically in skin scales treated with 15% potassium hydroxide. Culture with Sabouraud's medium is simple and often informative but does not always demonstrate pathogenic fungi.

Differential Diagnosis

Differentiate from other skin conditions involving the same areas such as interdigital intertrigo, candidiasis, psoriasis, contact dermatitis (from shoes, powders, nail polish), atopic eczema, and scabies.

Prevention

The essential factor in prevention is personal hygiene. Rubber or wooden sandals should be used in community showers and bathing places. Open-toed shoes and sandals are best for general wear. Careful drying between the toes after showering is recommended. Socks should be changed frequently. Apply dusting and drying powders as necessary, and place small wads of cotton between the toes at night.

Treatment

A. Specific Measures: Griseofulvin has been disappointing in the treatment of dermatophytosis of the feet and should be used only for severe cases or those that are recalcitrant to topical therapy.

Ketoconazole, 200 mg daily by mouth, is an effective agent for griseofulvin-resistant dermatophytosis, although relapse may occur after discontinuing therapy. The drug is well tolerated; hepatotoxicity has been reported from its use.

B. Local Measures: *Caution:* Do not overtreat.

1. Acute stage (lasts 1–10 days) – Give aluminum subacetate solution soaks for 20 minutes 2–3 times daily. If secondary infection is present, use soaks of 1:10,000 potassium permanganate. If secondary infection is severe or complicated, treat as described on p 47.

2. Subacute stage – Any of the following may be used: (1) Miconazole cream, 2%. (2) Clotrimazole cream or lotion, 1%. (3) Solution of coal tar, 5% in starch lotion. (4) Coal tar, 1–2% in Lassar's paste.

3. Chronic stage – Use any of the following: (1) Sulfur–salicylic acid ointment or cream. (2) Whitfield's ointment, one-fourth to one-half strength. (3) Compound undecylenic acid ointment twice daily. (4) Alcoholic Whitfield's solution. (5) Carbolfuchsin solution (Castellani's paint). (6) Tolnaftate (Tinactin) solution or cream. (7) Haloprogin, 1% cream or solution. (8) Miconazole, 2% cream. (9) Clotrimazole (Lotrimin or Mycelex), 1% cream or lotion.

C. Mechanical Measures: Carefully remove or debride dead or thickened tissues after soaks or baths.

Prognosis

Tinea of the hands and feet usually responds well to treatment, but recurrences are common in strongly predisposed persons.

Fuerst JF et al: Comparison between undecylenic acid and tolnaftate in the treatment of tinea pedis. *Cutis* 1980;**25**:544.

Robertson MH et al: Ketoconazole in griseofulvin-resistant dermatophytosis. *J Am Acad Dermatol* 1982;**6**:224.

DERMATOPHYTID
(Allergy or Sensitivity to Fungi)

Essentials of Diagnosis

- Pruritic, grouped vesicular lesions involving the sides and flexor aspects of the fingers and the palms.
- Fungal infection elsewhere on body, usually the feet.
- Trichophytin skin test positive. No fungus demonstrable in lesions.

General Considerations

Dermatophytid is a sensitivity reaction to an active focus of dermatophytosis elsewhere on the body, usually the feet. Fungi are present in the primary lesions but are not present in the lesions of dermatophytid. The hands are most often affected, but dermatophytid may occur on other areas also.

Clinical Findings

A. Symptoms and Signs: Itching is the only symptom. The lesions consist of grouped vesicles, often involving the thenar and hypothenar eminences. Lesions are round, up to 15 mm in diameter, and may be present on the side and flexor aspects of the fingers. Lesions occasionally involve the backs of the hands or may even be generalized.

B. Laboratory Findings: The trichophytin skin test is positive, but it may also be positive with other disorders. A negative trichophytin test rules out dermatophytid. Repeated negative microscopic examination of material taken from the lesions is necessary before the diagnosis of dermatophytid can be established. Culture from the primary site tends to reveal *Trichophyton mentagrophytes* organisms rather than *Trichophyton rubrum*. There appears to be selective anergy in patients with chronic *T rubrum* infections.

Differential Diagnosis

Differentiate from all diseases causing vesicular eruptions of the hands, especially contact dermatitis, dyshidrosis, and localized forms of atopic dermatitis.

Prevention

Treat fungal infections early and adequately, and prevent recurrences (see p 74).

Treatment

General measures are as outlined on p 47. The lesions should be treated according to type of dermatitis. The primary focus should be treated with griseofulvin or by local measures as described for dermatophytosis (see above). A single injection of triamcinolone acetonide suspension, 30 mg intraglutually, may suppress the eruption until the causative focus is controlled.

Prognosis

Dermatophytid may occur in an explosive series of episodes, and recurrences are not uncommon; however, it clears with adequate treatment of the primary infection elsewhere on the body.

TINEA UNGUIUM
& CANDIDAL ONYCHOMYCOSIS

Essentials of Diagnosis

- Lusterless, brittle, hypertrophic, friable nails.
- Fungus demonstrated in nail section or nail dust by microscope or culture.

General Considerations

Tinea unguium is a destructive *Trichophyton* or *Epidermophyton* infection of one or more (but rarely all) fingernails or toenails. The species most commonly found are *Trichophyton mentagrophytes, Trichophyton rubrum,* and *Epidermophyton floccosum. Candida albicans* causes candidal onychomycosis. "Saprophytic" fungi may cause onychomycosis.

Clinical Findings

A. Symptoms and Signs: There are usually no symptoms. The nails are lusterless, brittle, and hypertrophic, and the substance of the nail is friable and even pithy. Irregular segments of the diseased nail may be broken.

B. Laboratory Findings: Laboratory diagnosis is mandatory. Portions of the nail should be cleared with 15% potassium hydroxide and examined under the microscope for branching hyphae or collections of spores. Fungi may also be cultured, using Sabouraud's medium. Periodic acid–Schiff stain of a histologic section will also demonstrate the fungus readily.

Differential Diagnosis

Distinguish from nail changes caused by contact with strong alkalies and certain other chemicals and from those due to psoriasis, lichen planus, and candidiasis.

Treatment

A. General Measures: See p 47.

B. Specific Measures: Onychomycosis is an unlisted indication for ketoconazole. Griseofulvin ultramicrosize, 1000 mg/d, is about as effective as ketoconazole, 200 mg/d. Increasing ketoconazole to 400 mg/d will substantially increase the cure rate of onychomycosis, but the side effects of ketoconazole (liver abnormalities, effects on the adrenal cortex, and antiandrogenic activity) must be taken into account.

C. Local Measures: Sandpaper or file the nails daily (down to nail bed if necessary). Ciclopirox (Loprox) is a topical fungicidal cream that contains a pyridone-ethanolamine salt and seems to penetrate nails better than other topical agents. Early reports indicate this might be the most effective topical agent in the treatment of dermatophyte infections of the fingernails and toenails (onychomycosis).

Prognosis

Cure is difficult, even with microcrystalline griseofulvin by mouth in a dose of 1–2 g daily for months, or with miconazole or clotrimazole, topically.

Smith EB: Topical antifungal agents. *Dermatol Clin* (Jan) 1984;**2**:109.

Zaias N, Drachman D: A method for the determination of drug effectiveness in onychomycosis: Trials with ketoconazole and griseofulvin ultramicrosize. *J Am Acad Dermatol* 1983;**9**:912.

TINEA VERSICOLOR
(Pityriasis Versicolor)

Essentials of Diagnosis

- Pale macules that will not tan.
- Velvety, chamois-colored macules that scale with scraping.
- Trunk distribution the most frequent site.
- Fungus observed on microscopic examination of scales.

General Considerations

Tinea versicolor is a mild, superficial *Pityrosporon orbiculare (Malassezia furfur)* infection of the skin (usually of the trunk). The eruption is called to the patient's attention by the fact that the involved areas will not tan, and the resulting pseudoachromia may be mistaken for vitiligo. The disease is not particularly contagious and is apt to occur more frequently in those who wear heavy clothing and who perspire a great deal. Epidemics may occur in athletes.

Clinical Findings

A. Symptoms and Signs: There may be mild itching. The lesions are velvety, chamois-colored macules that vary from 4 to 5 mm in diameter to large confluent areas. Scales may be readily obtained by scraping the area. Lesions may appear on the trunk, upper arms, neck, and face.

B. Laboratory Findings: Large, blunt hyphae and thick-walled budding spores may be seen under the low power objective when skin scales have been cleared in 15% potassium hydroxide. *M furfur* is difficult to culture.

Differential Diagnosis

Distinguish from vitiligo on basis of appearance. Differentiate also from seborrheic dermatitis of the same areas.

Treatment & Prognosis

Encourage good skin hygiene. Topical treatments include Selsun suspension or Exsel lotion (both contain selenium sulfide), which may be applied daily and left on for 5 minutes; or one may use equal parts of propylene glycol and water topically, diluting with water if there is irritation. Other choices are 3% salicylic acid in rubbing alcohol and Tinver lotion (contains sodium thiosulfate). Relapses are common.

Sulfur-salicylic acid soap (marketed by Stiefel) or shampoo (Sebulex) used on a continuing basis may be effective.

Ketoconazole, 200 mg daily orally for 1 week, apparently results in cure of 90% of cases. (Use caution because of possible hepatotoxicity.)

Bamford JTM: Treatment of tinea versicolor with sulfur-salicylic shampoo. *J Am Acad Dermatol* 1983;**8**:211.

Faergemann J, Fredriksson T: Propylene glycol in the treatment of tinea versicolor. *Acta Derm Venereol (Stockh)* 1980; **60**:92.

Savin RC: Systemic ketoconazole in tinea versicolor: A double-blind evaluation and 1-year follow-up. *J Am Acad Dermatol* 1984;**10**:824.

CUTANEOUS CANDIDIASIS
(Moniliasis)

Essentials of Diagnosis

- Severe pruritus of vulva, anus, or body folds.
- Superficial denuded, beefy-red areas with or without satellite vesicopustules.
- Whitish curdlike concretions on the surface.
- Fungus on microscopic examination of scales or curd.

General Considerations

Cutaneous candidiasis is a superficial fungal infection that may involve almost any cutaneous or mucous surface of the body. It is particularly likely to occur in diabetics, during pregnancy, and in obese persons who perspire freely. Antibiotics and oral contraceptive agents may be contributory. When the patient presents with chronic mucocutaneous candidiasis, baseline and yearly follow-up tests will screen for development of endocrinopathy. Tests for diabetes are glycosylated hemoglobin (hemoglobin A_{1c}), fasting and 2-hour postprandial glucose, and insulin antibody tests; for thyroid function, TSH, T_4, resin T_3 uptake, thyroglobulin, and microsomal antibody tests; for parathyroid function, calcium, phosphorus, and alkaline phosphatase tests; for adrenal function, electrolyte, blood glucose, and adrenal antibody tests and ACTH and cortisol levels.

Clinical Findings

A. Symptoms and Signs: Itching may be intense. Burning sensations are sometimes reported, particularly around the vulva and anus. The lesions consist of superficially denuded, beefy-red areas in the depths of the body folds such as in the groin and the intergluteal cleft, beneath the breasts, at the angles of the mouth, and in the umbilicus. The peripheries of these denuded lesions are superficially undermined, and there may be satellite vesicopustules. Whitish, curdlike concretions may be present on the surface of the lesions (particularly in the oral and vaginal mucous membranes). Paronychia and interdigital erosions may occur.

B. Laboratory Findings: Clusters of budding cells and short hyphae can be seen under the high-power lens when skin scales or curdlike lesions have been cleared in 15% potassium hydroxide. The organism may be isolated on Sabouraud's medium. In the more severe forms of mucocutaneous candidiasis, there may be negative skin tests to all common antigens including *Candida,* as well as inability to be sensitized to dinitrochlorobenzene.

Differential Diagnosis

Differentiate from intertrigo, seborrheic dermatitis, tinea cruris, and erythrasma involving the same areas.

Complications

In the debilitated or immunosuppressed patient, candidiasis may spread from the skin or mucous membranes to the bladder, lungs, and other internal organs.

Treatment

A. General Measures: Treat associated diabetes, obesity, or hyperhidrosis. Keep the parts dry and exposed to air as much as possible. If possible, discontinue systemic antibiotics; if not, give nystatin by mouth concomitantly in a dose of 1.5 million units 3 times daily. Ketoconazole, 200 mg daily by mouth, will eradicate lesions with minimal side effects except for rare instances of liver damage. Liver function must be monitored, and clinical signs of hepatotoxicity should be uppermost in the mind of the patient and physician. Recurrences follow discontinuation of therapy. Immune enhancers such as thymosin, transfer factor, levamisole, and cimetidine may play a role in maintaining control, as may supplemental iron.

B. Local Measures:

1. Nails and skin–Apply 1% ciclopirox cream, nystatin cream, 100,000 units/g, or miconazole or clotrimazole cream or lotion, 3–4 times daily. Gentian violet, 1%, or carbolfuchsin paint (Castellani's paint) may be applied 1–2 times weekly as an alternative.

2. Vulva, anal mucous membranes–For vaginal candidiasis, one may use miconazole cream (Monistat 7), one applicatorful vaginally at bedtime for 7 days; or clotrimazole (Gyne-Lotrimin, Mycelex-G), one suppository vaginally per day for 7 days; or nystatin, one tablet (100,000 units) vaginally twice daily for 7 days. Gentian violet or carbolfuchsin (see above) can also be used. Clotrimazole troches have proved effective in controlling chronic oral candidiasis.

Prognosis

Cutaneous candidiasis may be intractable and prolonged, particularly in children, in whom the disturbance may take the form of a granuloma that resists all attempts at treatment.

Dolen J, Varma SK, South MA: Chronic mucocutaneous candidiasis: Endocrinopathies. *Cutis* 1981;**28**:592.

Jorizzo JL: Chronic mucocutaneous candidiasis: An update. *Arch Dermatol* 1982;**18**:963.

Tkach JR, Rinaldi MG: Severe hepatitis associated with ketoconazole therapy for chronic mucocutaneous candidiasis. *Cutis* 1982;**29**:482.

PARASITIC INFESTATIONS OF THE SKIN

SCABIES

Essentials of Diagnosis

- Nocturnal itching.
- Pruritic vesicles and pustules in "runs" or "galleries," especially on the sides of the fingers and the heels of the palms.
- Mites, ova, and black dots of feces visible microscopically.

General Considerations

Scabies is a common dermatitis caused by infestation with *Sarcoptes scabiei.* An entire family may be affected. The infestation usually spares the head and neck (although even these areas may be involved in infants). The mite is barely visible with the naked eye as a white dot. Scabies is usually acquired by sleeping with an infested individual or by other close contact. This infestation is on the increase worldwide.

Clinical Findings

A. Symptoms and Signs: Itching occurs almost exclusively at night. The lesions consist of more or less generalized excoriations with small pruritic vesicles, pustules, and "runs" or "galleries" on the sides of the fingers and the heels of the palms. The run or gallery appears as a short irregular mark (perhaps 2–3 mm long), as if made by a sharp pencil. Characteristic lesions may occur on the nipples in females and as pruritic papules on the scrotum in males. Pruritic papules may be seen over the buttocks. Pyoderma is often the presenting sign.

B. Laboratory Findings: The adult female mite may be demonstrated by probing the fresh end of a run or gallery with a pointed scalpel. The mite tends to cling to the tip of the blade. One may shave off the entire run or gallery (or, in the scrotum, a papule) and demonstrate the female mite, her ova, and small black dots of feces. The diagnosis should be confirmed by microscopic demonstration of the organism, ova, or feces in a mounted specimen in glycerin or mineral oil. The diagnosis can be confirmed in most cases with the burrow ink test. Apply ink to the burrow and then do a superficial shave biopsy by sawing off the burrow with a No. 15 blade, painlessly and bloodlessly. The mite, ova, and feces can be seen under the light microscope.

Differential Diagnosis

Distinguish from the various forms of pediculosis and from other causes of pruritus.

Treatment & Prognosis

Unless the lesions are complicated by severe secondary pyoderma (see p 47), treatment consists primarily of disinfestation. If secondary pyoderma is present, it should be treated with systemic and topical antibiotics.

Disinfestation with lindane (gamma benzene hexachloride), 1% in cream or lotion base, applied from the neck down overnight, is a popular treatment. A warning has been issued by the FDA regarding potential neurotoxicity, and any use in infants and pregnant women, as well as overuse in adults, is discouraged. Bedding and clothing should be laundered or cleaned. This preparation can be used before secondary infection is controlled. An alternative drug is crotamiton (Eurax) cream or lotion, which may be applied in the same way as gamma benzene hexachloride. The old-fashioned medication consisting of 5% sulfur in petrolatum may still be used, applying it nightly from the collarbones down, for 3 nights, but one must be prepared to treat irritative, defatted dermatitis (see p 47). Benzyl benzoate may be compounded as a lotion or emulsion in strengths from 20% to 35% and used as generalized (from collarbones down) applications overnight for 2 treatments 1 week apart. The NF XIV formula is 275 mL benzyl benzoate (containing 5 g of triethanolamine and 20 g of oleic acid) in water to make 1000 mL. It is cosmetically acceptable, clean, and not overly irritating. Persistent pruritic postscabietic papules may be painted with undiluted crude coal tar or Estargel.

Unless treatment is aimed at all infected persons in a family, reinfestations will probably occur.

Resistant forms requiring multiple forms of treatment are appearing.

Davies JH et al: Lindane poisonings. *Arch Dermatol* 1983; **119:**142.

Felman YM, Nikitas JA: Scabies. *Cutis* 1984;**33:**266.

Orkin M, Maibach HI: Current views of scabies and pediculosis. *Cutis* 1984;**33:**85.

Taplin D et al: Eradication of scabies with a single treatment schedule. *J Am Acad Dermatol* 1983;**9:**546.

PEDICULOSIS

Essentials of Diagnosis

- Pruritus with excoriation.
- Nits on hair shafts; lice on skin or clothes.
- Occasionally, sky-blue macules (maculae caeruleae) on the inner thighs or lower abdomen in pubic louse infestation.

General Considerations

Pediculosis is a parasitic infestation of the skin of the scalp, trunk, or pubic areas. It usually occurs among people who live in overcrowded dwellings with inadequate hygiene facilities, although pubic lice may be acquired by anyone sitting on an infested toilet seat. There are 3 different varieties: (1) pediculosis pubis, caused by *Pthirus pubis* (pubic louse, "crabs"); (2) pediculosis corporis, by *Pediculus humanus* var *corporis* (body louse); (3) pediculosis capitis, by *Pediculus humanus* var *capitis* (head louse).

Head and body lice are similar in appearance and are 3–4 mm long. Head louse infestations may be transmitted by shared use of hats or combs. The body louse can seldom be found on the body, because the insect comes onto the skin only to feed and must be looked for in the seams of the underclothing.

Trench fever, relapsing fever, and typhus may be transmitted by the body louse.

Clinical Findings

Itching may be very intense in body louse infestations, and scratching may result in deep excoriations over the affected area. The clinical appearance is of gross excoriation. Pyoderma may be present and may be the presenting sign in any of these infestations. Head lice can be found on the scalp or may be manifested as small nits resembling pussy-willow buds on the scalp hairs close to the skin. They are easiest to see above the ears and at the nape of the neck. Body lice may deposit visible nits on the vellus hair of the body. Pubic louse infestations are occasionally generalized, particularly in a hairy individual; the lice may even be found on the eyelashes and in the scalp.

Differential Diagnosis

Distinguish head louse infestation from seborrheic dermatitis, body louse infestation from scabies, and pubic louse infestation from anogenital pruritus and eczema.

Treatment

For all types of pediculosis, lindane lotion (Kwell, Scabene) is used extensively. A thin layer is applied to the infested and adjacent hairy areas. It is removed after 12 hours by thorough washing. Remaining nits may be removed with a fine-toothed comb or forceps. Sexual contacts should be treated. Synergized pyrethrins (RID, A-200 Pyrinate, Pyrinyl) are over-the-counter products that are applied undiluted until the infested areas are entirely wet. After 10 minutes, the areas are washed thoroughly with warm water and soap and then dried. Nits may be treated as indicated above. For involvement of eyelashes, petrolatum is applied thickly twice daily for 8 days, and remaining nits are then plucked off. Reports of lindane resistance in pediculosis capitis probably represent reinfestation or treatment failures due to noncompliance.

Prognosis

Pediculosis responds to topical treatment.

Orkin M, Maibach HI: Current views of scabies and pediculosis pubis. *Cutis* 1984;**33:**85.

Parish LC, Witkowski JA, Kucirka SA: Lindane resistance and pediculosis capitis. *Int J Trop Dermatol* 1983;**22:**572.

SKIN LESIONS DUE TO OTHER ARTHROPODS

Essentials of Diagnosis

- Localized rash with pruritus.
- Furunclelike lesions containing live arthropods.

- Tender erythematous patches that migrate ("larva migrans").
- Generalized urticaria or erythema multiforme.

General Considerations

Some arthropods (eg, most pest mosquitoes and biting flies) are readily detected as they bite. Many others are not, eg, because they are too small, because there is no immediate reaction, or because they bite during sleep. Reactions may be delayed for many hours; many severe reactions are allergic. Patients are most apt to consult a physician when the lesions are multiple and pruritus is intense. Severe attacks may be accompanied by insomnia, restlessness, fever, and faintness or even collapse. Rashes may sometimes cover the body.

Many persons will react severely only to their earliest contacts with an arthropod, thus presenting pruritic lesions when traveling, moving into new quarters, etc. Body lice, fleas, bedbugs, and local mosquitoes should be borne in mind. Spiders are often incorrectly believed to be the source of bites; they rarely attack humans, although the brown spider *(Loxosceles laeta, Loxosceles reclusa)* may cause severe necrotic reactions and death due to intravascular hemolysis, and the black widow spider *(Latrodectus mactans)* may cause severe systemic symptoms and death.

In addition to arthropod bites, the most common lesions are venomous stings (wasps, hornets, bees, ants, scorpions) or bites (centipedes), dermatitis due to urticating hairs of caterpillars, dermatitis due to vesicating furunclelike lesions due to fly maggots or sand fleas in the skin, and a linear creeping eruption due to a migrating larva.

Clinical Findings

The diagnosis may be difficult when the patient has not noticed the initial attack but suffers a delayed reaction. Individual bites are frequently in clusters and tend to occur either on exposed parts (eg, midges and gnats) or under clothing, especially around the waist or at flexures (eg, small mites or insects in bedding or clothing). The reaction is often delayed for 1–24 hours or more. Pruritus is almost always present and may be all but intolerable once the patient starts to scratch. Secondary infection, sometimes with serious consequences, may follow scratching. Allergic manifestations, including urticarial wheals, are common. Papules may become vesicular. The diagnosis is aided by searching for exposure to arthropods and by considering the patient's occupation and recent activities. The principal arthropods are as follows:

(1) Bedbugs: In crevices of beds or furniture; bites tend to occur in lines or clusters. It is thought that *Cimex lectularius* (bedbug) may play a significant role in the transmission of hepatitis B. The closely related kissing bug has been reported with increasing frequency as attacking humans.

(2) Fleas: Fleas are blood-sucking ectoparasites that feed on dogs, cats, humans, and other species.

Flea saliva produces papular urticaria in sensitized individuals. *Ctenocephalides felis* and *Ctenocephalides canis* are the most common species found on cats and dogs, and both species attack humans. The human flea, *Pulex irritans,* is not commonly recognized by veterinarians as a pet animal problem.

To break the life cycle of the flea, one must treat the home, pets, and outside environment, using quick-kill insecticides, residual insecticides, and a growth regulator. Obviously, this is a repetitive job for the exterminator. Home foggers and flea collars are not adequate. Birds and fish are especially sensitive and must be protected during disinfestation.

(3) Ticks: Usually picked up by brushing against low vegetation. Larval ticks may attack in large numbers and cause much distress; in Africa and India they have been confused with chiggers. Ascending paralysis may occasionally be traced to a tick bite, and removal of the embedded tick is essential.

(4) Chiggers or **redbugs** are larvae of trombiculid mites. A few species confined to particular countries and usually to restricted and locally recognized habitats (eg, berry patches, woodland edge, lawns, brush turkey mounds in Australia, poultry farms) attack humans, often around the waist, on the ankles, or in flexures, raising intensely itching erythematous papules after a delay of many hours. The red chiggers may sometimes be seen in the center of papules that have not yet been scratched. Chiggers are the commonest cause of distressing multiple lesions associated with arthropods.

(5) Bird mites: Larger than chiggers, infesting chicken houses, pigeon lofts, or nests of birds in eaves. Bites are multiple anywhere on the body, although poultry handlers are most often attacked on the hands and forearms. Room air conditioning units may suck in bird mites and infest the inhabitants of the room. Rodent mites from mice or rats may cause similar effects.

The diagnosis of bird mites or rodent mites may readily be overlooked and the patient treated for other dermatoses or for psychogenic dermatosis. Intractable "acarophobia" (delusions of parasitosis) may result from early neglect or misdiagnosis.

(6) Mites in stored products: These are white and almost invisible and infest products such as copra ("copra itch"), vanilla pods ("vanillism"), sugar, straw, cotton seeds, and cereals. Persons who handle these products may be attacked, especially on the hands and forearms and sometimes on the feet. Infested bedding may occasionally lead to generalized dermatitis.

(7) Caterpillars of moths with urticating hairs: The hairs are blown from cocoons or carried by emergent moths, causing severe and often seasonally recurrent outbreaks after mass emergence, eg, in some southern states of the USA.

(8) Tungiasis is due to the burrowing flea known as *Tunga penetrans* (also known as chigoe, jigger; not the same as chigger), found in Africa, the West Indies, and South America. The female burrows under the skin, sucks blood, swells to 0.5 cm, and then ejects her eggs onto the ground. Ulceration, lymphangitis, gangrene, and septicemia may result, possibly with fatality. Ethyl chloride spray will kill the insect when applied to the lesion, and disinfestation may be accomplished with insecticide applied to the terrain.

Differential Diagnosis

Arthropods should be considered in the differential diagnosis of skin lesions showing any of the above symptoms.

Prevention

Arthropod infestations are best prevented by avoidance of contaminated areas, personal cleanliness, and disinfection of clothing, bedclothes, and furniture as indicated. Lice, chiggers, red bugs, and mites can be killed by lindane (gamma benzene hexachloride; Gammexane, Kwell, Scabene) applied to the head and clothing. (It is not necessary to remove clothing.) Benzyl benzoate and dimethylphthalate are excellent acaricides; clothing should be impregnated by spray or by dipping in a soapy emulsion.

Treatment

Caution: Avoid local overtreatment.

Living arthropods should be removed carefully with tweezers after application of alcohol. Preserve in alcohol for identification. (*Caution:* In endemic Rocky Mountain spotted fever areas, do not remove ticks with the bare fingers for fear of becoming infected.) Children in particular should be prevented from scratching.

Apply corticosteroid lotions or creams. Crotamiton (Eurax) cream or lotion may be used; it is a miticide as well as an antipruritic. Calamine lotion or a cool wet dressing is always appropriate. Antibiotic creams, lotions, or powders may be applied if secondary infection is suspected.

Localized persistent lesions may be treated with intralesional corticosteroids. Avoid exercise and excessive warmth. Codeine may be given for pain. Creams containing local anesthetics are not very effective and may be sensitizing.

Stings produced by many arthropods may be alleviated by applying papain powder (Adolph's Meat Tenderizer) mixed with water, or Xerac A C.

Extracts (expensive) from venom sacs of bees, wasps, yellow jackets, and hornets are now available for immunotherapy of patients at risk for anaphylaxis. Approximately 5% of patients fail to respond.

Chipps BE et al: Diagnosis and treatment of anaphylactic reactions to Hymenoptera stings in children. *J Pediatr* 1980; **97**:177.

Crissey JT: Bedbugs: An old problem with a new dimension. *Int J Dermatol* 1981;**20**:411.

Medleau L, Miller WH Jr: Flea infestation and its control. *Int J Dermatol* 1983;**22**:378.

Pien FD, Grekin JL: Common ectoparasites. *West J Med* 1983;**139**:382.

TUMORS OF THE SKIN

Excessive exposure of fair skin to sun radiation is a cancer risk of major degree. Inculcation of new attitudes about sunbathing and development of measures to counteract the adverse effects of sun damage are important public health objectives. Sunlight on sandy complexions can induce actinic (solar) keratoses, nevi, basal and squamous cell carcinoma, and melanoma. The best protection is shelter, but protective clothing, avoidance of direct sun exposure during the 4 peak hours of the day, and the assiduous use of commercially available chemical sunscreens or sunshades are helpful. The most effective sunscreens are PreSun 15 lotion (contains 5% aminobenzoic acid, 5% Padimate O, and 3% oxybenzone), Super Shade 15 (contains octyl dimethyl PABA), SolBar Plus 15 (oxybenzone and ethyldihydroxypropyl PABA), and Total Eclipse (glyceryl PABA, octyl dimethyl PABA, and oxybenzone). The sunshades include those containing opaque materials such as titanium dioxide or zinc oxide.

Classification

The following classification is admittedly oversimplified; almost any tumor arising from embryonal tissues in the various stages of their development can be found in the skin.

A. Benign: Seborrheic warts, considered by some to be nevoid, consist of benign overgrowths of epithelium that have a pigmented velvety or warty surface. They are relatively common, both on exposed and covered parts, and are commonly mistaken for melanomas or other types of cutaneous neoplasms.

B. Nevi: Any of the following (except freckles) may be excised if there are suspicious features.

1. Nevus cell nevi are almost always benign, and almost everyone has at least a few of these lesions. They usually appear in childhood and tend to undergo spontaneous fibrosis in old age. Pigmented nevi that are present at birth show a greater tendency toward the development of melanoma than those developing in later years and should be excised wherever possible. This is especially true of bathing trunk nevi, which should be excised in decrements if possible.

2. Junctional nevi, which consist of clear nevus cells and usually some melanin, have nevus cells on both sides of the epidermal junction. They are possible forerunners of malignant melanoma, although most melanomas arise de novo. If a nevus grows rapidly, darkens, or bleeds, the possibility of melanomatous degeneration should be considered.

3. Compound nevi, composed of junctional elements as well as clear nevus cells in the dermis, also tend to develop into malignant melanoma. Dermal cellular nevi are quite benign.

4. Dysplastic nevi are usually larger than most other nevi and irregular in outline and pigmentation. Changes in the macular portion are of greatest concern, particularly the development of black or blue-black pigmentation where none was present previously.

Complete cure can be obtained with minor surgery, forestalling the development of invasive melanoma. These lesions may be familial or sporadic.

5. Blue nevi are benign, although in some instances they behave in an invasive manner requiring multiple excisions. These lesions in the pristine state are small, slightly elevated, and blue-black.

6. Epithelial nevi include several types of verrucous epithelial overgrowths, usually in linear distribution. Microscopically, cells found normally in the epidermis are present. Such lesions rarely degenerate into squamous or basal cell carcinomas. The nevus sebaceus of Jadassohn, which occurs commonly in the scalp, is composed of a number of embryonal elements and is considered to be particularly likely to give rise to carcinomas.

7. Freckles, which in the juvenile form are called ephelides and in the adult delayed form are called lentigines, consist of excess amounts of melanin in the melanocytes in the basal layer of the epidermis. Juvenile freckles tend to disappear with time, whereas lentigines come on in later life and are more persistent.

C. Premalignant: Actinic or solar keratoses are flesh-colored and feel like little patches of sandpaper when the finger is pulled over them. When they degenerate they become squamous cell carcinomas. They occur on exposed parts of the body in persons of fair complexion, and nonactinic keratoses may be provoked by exposure to arsenic systemically or occupational irritants such as tars. In keratoses the cells are atypical and similar to those seen in squamous cell epitheliomas, but these changes are well contained by an intact epidermal-dermal junction. These lesions may be excised or removed superficially with a scalpel followed by cautery or fulguration. An alternative treatment is the use of 1–5% fluorouracil in propylene glycol or in a cream base. This agent may be rubbed into lesions morning and night until they become briskly sore (usually 1–3 weeks); the treatment should then be continued for several days longer and then stopped. The eyes and the mouth should be avoided. Any lesions that persist may then be excised for histologic examination.

D. Malignant:

1. Squamous cell carcinoma usually occurs on exposed parts in fair-skinned individuals who sunburn easily and tan poorly. They may arise out of actinic or solar keratoses. They tend to develop very rapidly, attaining a diameter of 1 cm within 2 weeks. These lesions appear as small red, conical, hard nodules that quickly ulcerate. Metastases may occur early, although they are said to be less likely with squamous cell carcinoma arising out of actinic keratoses than in those that arise de novo. Keratoacanthomas are benign growths that resemble squamous cell carcinoma but which for all practical purposes should be treated as though they were skin cancers. The preferred treatment of squamous cell carcinoma is excision. X-ray radiation may be used instead, and Mohs' fresh tissue microscopically controlled excision, where available, is excellent treatment also.

2. Basal cell carcinoma occurs mostly on exposed parts. These lesions grow slowly, attaining a size of 1–2 cm in diameter only after a year's growth. There is a waxy appearance, with telangiectatic vessels easily visible. Metastases almost never occur. Neglected lesions may ulcerate and produce great destruction, ultimately invading vital structures. It is important to widely excise basal cell carcinomas where possible. Excision and suturing may be used, or one may carve out the entire growth (called a "shave biopsy" by some physicians), following which the base of the wound is treated with curettage and electrodesiccation. If the growth is in areas such as embryonal cleavage planes where pockets of extension may occur, fresh tissue microscopically controlled extirpation may be done (modified Mohs' technique). X-ray therapy and cryosurgery are alternative methods of treatment.

3. Bowen's disease (intraepidermal squamous cell epithelioma) is relatively uncommon and resembles a plaque of psoriasis. The course is relatively benign, but malignant progression may occur and it is best to excise the lesion widely if possible.

4. Paget's disease, considered by some to be a manifestation of apocrine sweat gland carcinoma, may occur around the nipple, resembling chronic eczema, or may involve apocrine areas such as the genitalia. There seems to be less likelihood of an underlying sweat gland carcinoma if the lesions are on the vulva than if they are on the nipple or perianal area.

5. Malignant melanoma–The estimated incidence of new melanomas in the USA in 1984 is 17,700, based on the National Cancer Institute's SEER program 1973–1979 rates. Melanoma deaths for the same period are estimated at 5500, a death rate of 31%. This percentage is misleading, however, since the increased incidence of new melanomas will ultimately lead to a much higher cumulative death rate. Melanomas cause most of the deaths from skin cancer. The mean age of those dying from melanomas is less than that of those dying from other skin cancers. There is a trend toward a younger age incidence each year. Primary malignant melanomas may be classified into 6 clinicohistologic types, including lentigo maligna melanoma, a preinvasive lesion; superficial spreading malignant melanoma (the most common type, occurring in two-thirds of individuals developing melanoma); nodular malignant melanoma; acral-lentiginous melanomas; malignant melanomas on mucous membranes; and miscellaneous forms such as those arising from blue nevi, congenital and giant nevocytic nevi, and the dermal component of acquired compound and intradermal nevi in the central nervous system and viscera.

True melanomas vary from macules to nodules, with a surprising play of colors from flesh tints to pitch black and a frequent admixture of white, blue, purple, and red. The border tends to be irregular, and growth may be rapid.

Treatment of melanoma consists of wide excision, with lymph node dissection varying with the depth and location of the lesions and the background of the surgeon. Deaths from melanoma are increasing at a rate of 2% per year for females and 3% for males. Depth of invasion is the single most important prognostic factor (according to Breslow; see Balch reference, below).

6. Kaposi's sarcoma—Until recently in the USA, this rare malignant skin lesion was seen mostly in elderly white men, had a chronic clinical course, and was rarely fatal. Kaposi's sarcoma occurs endemically in an often aggressive form in young black men of equatorial Africa, but it is rare in American blacks. Within the past few years, epidemic clusters of Kaposi's sarcoma, predominantly in homosexual men, have been found in various large cities of the USA. Disseminated Kaposi's sarcoma in the homosexual population recurs as one feature of the new unexplained acquired immunodeficiency syndrome (AIDS). The disease has also been described in intravenous drug abusers, patients who have received multiple blood transfusions, and very infrequently in others. Many patients have serious associated infections such as cytomegalovirus infection, *Pneumocystis carinii* pneumonia, toxoplasmosis, recurrent herpes simplex, venereal disease, other infections, and cancer.

The cause of AIDS is unknown, but the possibility of a new virus or viral mutation seems strong. (See pp 824 and 1084.) Current methods of treatment are ineffective. Fever, adenopathy, and gastrointestinal complaints associated with red, purple, or dark plaques or nodules on cutaneous or mucosal surfaces should alert the clinician to the possibility of the disease. Both T and B cell deficiencies have been found.

Amman AJ et al: B-cell immunodeficiency in acquired immune deficiency syndrome. *JAMA* 1984;**251**:1447.

Balch CM: Measuring melanomas: A tribute to Alexander Breslow. *J Am Acad Dermatol* 1981;**5**:96.

Brooks NA: Curettage and shave excision: A tissue-sparing technic for primary cutaneous carcinoma worthy of inclusion in graduate training programs. *J Am Acad Dermatol* 1984; **10**:279.

Conte JE Jr et al: The acquired immune deficiency syndrome: A multidisciplinary enigma. *West J Med* 1984;**140**:66.

Greene MH et al: For the record: The history of precursors to malignant melanoma. (Letter.) *Arch Dermatol* 1984;**120**:18.

Salasche SJ: Status of curettage and desiccation in the treatment of primary basal cell carcinoma. *J Am Acad Dermatol* 1984;**10**:285.

Silverberg E: Cancer statistics, 1984. *CA* (Jan/Feb) 1984;**34**:7.

MISCELLANEOUS SKIN, HAIR, & NAIL DISORDERS

PIGMENTARY DISORDERS

Melanin is formed in the melanocytes in the basal layer of the epidermis. Its precursor, the amino acid tyrosine, is slowly converted to dihydroxyphenylalanine (dopa) by tyrosinase, and there are many further chemical steps to the ultimate formation of melanin. This system may be affected by external influences such as exposure to sun, heat, trauma, ionizing radiation, heavy metals, and changes in oxygen potential. These influences may result in hyperpigmentation, hypopigmentation, or both. Local trauma may destroy melanocytes temporarily or permanently, causing hypopigmentation, sometimes with surrounding hyperpigmentation as in eczema and dermatitis. Hypermelanosis appears to be associated with increased plasma immunoreactive β-MSH (melanocyte-stimulating hormone from the pituitary) only in Addison's disease. Melatonin, a pineal hormone, regulates pigment dispersion and aggregation.

Other pigmentary disorders include those resulting from exposure to exogenous pigments such as carotenemia, argyria, deposition of other metals, and tattooing. Other endogenous pigmentary disorders are attributable to metabolic substances, including hemosiderin (iron), in purpuric processes and in hemochromatosis; mercaptans, homogentisic acid (ochronosis), bile pigments, and carotenes.

Classification

Pigmentary disorders may be classified as primary or secondary and as hyperpigmentary or hypopigmentary.

A. Primary Pigmentary Disorders: These are nevoid or congenital, and include pigmented nevi, Mongolian spots, and incontinentia pigmenti, vitiligo, albinism, and piebaldism. In vitiligo, pigment cells (melanocytes) are destroyed. The greater the pigment loss, the fewer the number of melanocytes. At the borders of lesions, the melanocytes are often large and have long dendritic processes, and they resemble pigment cells in tissue cultures that are blocked in the G phase of the cell cycle. Loss of pigment surrounding nevi, and in melanomas, may represent immune responses. Vitiligo, found in approximately 1% of the population, may be associated with hyperthyroidism and hypothyroidism, pernicious anemia, diabetes mellitus, addisonism, and carcinoma of the stomach. Albinism, partial or total, occurs as a genetically determined recessive trait. Piebaldism, a localized hypomelanosis, is an autosomal dominant trait.

B. Secondary Pigmentary Disorders: Hyper- or hypopigmentation may occur following overexposure to sunlight or heat or as a result of excoriation or direct physical injury. Hyperpigmentation occurs in arsenical melanosis or in association with Addison's disease (due to lack of the inhibitory influence of hydrocortisone on the production of MSH by the pituitary gland). Several disorders of clinical importance are as follows:

1. Melasma—This occurs as patterned hyperpigmentation of the face. The localized pigmentation of chloasma may be a direct effect of certain steroid hormones, estrogens, and progesterones in predisposed clones of melanocytes. It occurs not only during pregnancy but also in 30–50% of women taking oral contraceptives.

2. Berlock hyperpigmentation can be provoked by hypersensitivity to essential oils in perfumes, and these should be excluded wherever possible.

3. Leukoderma or secondary depigmentation may complicate atopic dermatitis, lichen planus, psoriasis, alopecia areata, lichen simplex chronicus, and such systemic conditions as myxedema, thyrotoxicosis, syphilis, and toxemias. It may follow local skin trauma of various sorts, or may complicate dermatitis due to exposure to gold or arsenic. Antioxidants in rubber goods, such as monobenzyl ether of hydroquinone, cause leukoderma from the wearing of gauntlet gloves, rubber pads in brassieres, etc. This is most likely to occur in blacks.

4. Ephelides (juvenile freckles) and **lentigines** (senile freckles)–The number of functioning melanocytes decreases by about 10% per decade. The loss is often blotchy, particularly in areas of solar degeneration. Compensatory hypertrophy of some melanocytes gives rise to lentigines.

5. Drugs–Pigmentation may be produced by chloroquine, chlorpromazine, and minocycline.

Differential Diagnosis

One must distinguish true lack of pigment from pseudoachromia, such as occurs in tinea versicolor, pityriasis simplex, and seborrheic dermatitis. It may be difficult to differentiate true vitiligo from leukoderma and even from partial albinism.

Complications

Solar keratoses and epitheliomas are more likely to develop in persons with vitiligo and albinism. Vitiligo tends to cause pruritus in anogenital folds. There may be severe emotional trauma in extensive vitiligo and other types of hypo- and hyperpigmentations, particularly when they occur in naturally dark-skinned persons.

Treatment & Prognosis

There is no increase of pigment in partial or total albinism; return of pigment is rare in vitiligo; in leukoderma, repigmentation may occur spontaneously. Therapy of vitiligo is long and tedious. The patient must be strongly motivated. If less than 20% of the skin is involved (most cases), topical methoxsalen, 0.1% in ethanol and propylene glycol or in Acid Mantle cream or Unibase, is used, with cautious exposure to long wavelength ultraviolet light (UVA), followed by thorough washing, application of an SPF 15 sunscreen, and wearing of UVA-protective goggles for 48 hours (Noir Co.). With 20% to 50% involvement, oral methoxsalen, 0.6 mg/kg 2 hours before UVA exposure, is best. Severe phototoxic response may occur with topical or oral psoralens plus UVA. For more than 50% skin involvement, the use of 5% monobenzone cream to totally depigment the skin has been reported.

Potent topical corticosteroids have been advocated for the treatment of vitiligo. Betamethasone dipropionate ointment may be rubbed thoroughly into the moistened skin once daily for 10 days, followed by 10 days' rest, then repetition, over a period of time. Caution must be exercised, especially on the face and on thin skin, to avoid pseudoatrophy and other changes.

Localized ephelides and lentigines may be destroyed by careful application of a saturated solution of liquid phenol on a tightly wound cotton applicator. Chloasma and other forms of hyperpigmentation may be treated by protecting the skin from the sun and with cosmetics such as Covermark (Lydia O'Leary Company) or Maxafil (Cooper Laboratories, Inc.). Cosmetics containing perfumes should not be used.

Bleaching preparations generally contain hydroquinone or its derivatives. This is not without hazard, and it is best to start with the weakest preparation offered by the manufacturer. The use of this kind of bleach may result in unexpected hypopigmentation, hyperpigmentation, and even ochronosis and pigmented milia, particularly with prolonged use.

Treatment of other pigmentary disorders should be directed toward avoidance of the causative agent if possible (as in carotenemia) or treatment of the underlying disorder. Melasma, ephelides, and postinflammatory hyperpigmentation may be treated with 3–4% hydroquinone solution or cream and a sunscreen with an SPF (sun protection factor) of 15. Tretinoin cream, 0.01%, may be added. The superficial melasma responds well, but if there is predominantly dermal deposition of pigment, the prognosis is poor. Senile lentigines are resistant.

Fisher AA: Hydroquinone uses and abnormal reactions. *Cutis* 1983;**31**:240.

Kenney JA Jr., Grimes P: How we treat vitiligo. *Cutis* 1983;**32**:347.

Kumari J: Vitiligo treated with clobetasol propionate. *Arch Dermatol* 1984;**120**:631.

BALDNESS
(Alopecia)

Baldness Due to Scarring

Cicatricial baldness may occur following chemical or physical trauma, lichen planopilaris, severe bacterial or fungal infections, severe herpes zoster, chronic discoid lupus erythematosus, scleroderma, and excessive ionizing radiation. The specific cause is often suggested by the history, the distribution of hair loss, and the appearance of the skin, as in lupus erythematosus and other infections. Biopsy may be necessary to differentiate lupus from the others.

Scarring alopecias are irreversible and permanent. There is no treatment, except for surgical hair transplants.

Baldness Not Due to Scarring

Noncicatricial baldness may be classified according to distribution as alopecia universalis (generalized but not total hair loss), alopecia totalis (complete hair loss), and alopecia areata (patchy baldness).

Nonscarring alopecia may occur in association

with various **systemic diseases** such as disseminated lupus erythematosus, cachexia, lymphomas, uncontrolled diabetes, severe thyroid or pituitary hypofunction, and dermatomyositis. The only treatment necessary is prompt and adequate control of the underlying disorder, in which case hair loss may be reversible.

Male pattern baldness, the most common form of alopecia, is of genetic predetermination. The earliest changes occur at the anterior portions of the calvarium on either side of the "widow's peak." Associated seborrhea is evident as excessive oiliness and erythema of the scalp, with scaling. Premature loss of hair in a young adult male may give rise to a severe neurotic reaction. The extent of hair loss is variable and unpredictable. Investigative studies are under way regarding topical use of minoxidil in 1–5% concentrations or less for alopecia areata and androgenetic alopecia. Results are encouraging, although at higher concentrations, hair growth may occur in undesired locations, suggesting a systemic side effect. Response takes several months. Clinical use is unwarranted at this time. Seborrhea may be treated as described on p 61.

Hair loss or thinning of the hair in women results from the same common baldness that affects men (androgenic alopecia). Treatment is aimed at antagonizing the follicular effects of androgens. Cyproterone acetate is the only widely available antiandrogen in Europe; it is not available in the USA. A "reversed sequential regimen" of cyproterone acetate, 100 mg daily from days 5 to 14 of the menstrual cycle, and an estrogen, ethinyl estradiol, 50 mg from days 5 to 25, are given orally. Side effects are the same as for anovulatory medications. Oral corticosteroids have been recommended to suppress adrenal androgen production; give prednisolone, 2.5–7.5 mg/d plus oral antiandrogens. There are no well-documented studies to prove efficacy of these approaches. Topical estrogens are of doubtful value.

Women who complain of thin hair but show little evidence of alopecia may have unrelated psychiatric difficulties that would explain this disproportionate anxiety.

Telogen effluvium may be the cause of temporary hair loss in some women. A transitory increase occurs in the number of hairs in the telogen (resting) phase of the hair growth cycle. This may occur spontaneously, may appear at the termination of pregnancy, may be precipitated by "crash dieting" or malnutrition, or may be provoked by hormonal contraceptives, especially the monophasic contraceptives. If an abnormally high proportion of telogen hairs is present before taking the contraceptive, lasting improvement in hair growth may be expected. In one study, the only cause of telogen effluvium was found to be iron deficiency, and the hair counts bore a clear relationship to serum iron levels.

Alopecia areata is of unknown cause. Histopathologically, there are numerous small anagen hairs and a lymphocytic infiltrate. The bare patches may be perfectly smooth, or a few hairs may remain. Severe forms may be treated by systemic corticosteroid therapy, although systemic therapy is rarely justified unless the disease is of serious emotional or economic significance.

Anthralin, 0.5% ointment applied daily, may provoke hair growth *(caution)*. Intralesional corticosteroids are frequently effective. Triamcinolone acetonide, in a concentration not to exceed 5 mg/mL, is injected in aliquots of 0.1 mL at approximately 1- to 2-cm intervals, not exceeding a total dose of 50 mg per month for adults. Alopecia areata is usually self-limiting, with complete regrowth of hair, but some mild cases are permanent and the extensive forms are usually permanent, as are the totalis and universalis types. Both topical dinitrochlorobenzene (see p 71) and an experimental topical allergen, squaric acid dibutylester, have been used to treat persistent alopecia areata. The principle is to sensitize the skin, then intermittently apply weaker concentrations to produce and maintain a slight dermatitis. Hair regrowth in 3-6 months in some patients has been reported to be remarkable. Long-term safety and efficacy have not been established.

Cataracts may complicate extensive alopecia areata.

In trichotillomania (the pulling out of one's own hair), the patches of hair loss are irregular, and growing hairs are always present, since they cannot be pulled out until they are long enough.

Drug-induced alopecia is becoming increasingly important. Such drugs include thallium, excessive and prolonged use of vitamin A, antimitotic agents, anticoagulants, clofibrate (rarely), antithyroid drugs, oral contraceptives, trimethadione, allopurinol, amphetamines, salicylates, gentamicin, and levodopa.

Case PC et al: Topical therapy of alopecia areata with squaric acid dibutylester. *J Am Acad Dermatol* 1984;**10**:447.

Dawber RPR: Common baldness in women. *Int J Dermatol* 1981; **20**:647.

Weiss VC et al: Alopecia areata treated with topical minoxidil. *Arch Dermatol* 1984;**120**:457.

HIRSUTISM

Hirsutism is not curable except in rare surgically treatable Cushing's syndrome, prolactinoma, or androgen-secreting tumors of ovary or adrenal glands. Androgen levels can be reduced by a low-dose corticosteroid, eg, prednisolone, 5 mg nightly and 2.5 mg in the morning, or dexamethasone (not as good for suppression). A combined estrogen and nonandrogenic progestogen may help. However, these chemical treatments do not often suppress terminal hair growth enough to justify the long-term side effects. Dark facial and abdominal hair may be bleached with 5% hydrogen peroxide solution or commercial preparations, and hair removal may be done with chemical depilatories *(caution)* or by electrolysis.

Screening tests for hirsutism include levels of

serum testosterone, androstenedione (peripheral conversion of which accounts for 40–60% of circulating testosterone levels), luteinizing and follicle-stimulating hormones, and prolactin. Second-line tests might include dexamethasone suppression, ovarian ultrasound scan, adrenal CT scan, pituitary fossa x-ray, and visual field tests.

Rentoul J: Management of the hirsute woman. *Int J Dermatol* 1983;**22**:265.

KELOIDS & HYPERTROPHIC SCARS

Keloids are tumors consisting of actively growing fibrous tissue that occur as a result of trauma or irritation in predisposed persons, especially those of dark-skinned races. The trauma may be relatively trivial, such as an acne lesion. Keloids behave as neoplasms, although they are not malignant. Spontaneous digitations may project from the central growth, and the tumors may become large and disfiguring. There may be itching and burning sensations with both types of tumor.

Hypertrophic scars, usually seen following surgery or accidental trauma, tend to be raised, red, and indurated. After a few months or longer, they lose their redness and become soft and flat. Removal should not be attempted until all induration has subsided.

Intralesional injection of a corticosteroid suspension is effective against hypertrophic scars. The treatment of keloids is less satisfactory; surgical excision, x-ray therapy, and freezing with solid CO_2 or liquid nitrogen are used, as well as injection of corticosteroid suspensions into the lesions. They tend to involute in older age groups.

Stegman SJ, Tromovitch TA: Cosmetic dermatologic surgery. *Arch Dermatol* 1982;**21**:50.

NAIL DISORDERS

Nail changes are generally not diagnostic of a specific systemic or cutaneous disease. All of the nail manifestations of systemic disorders may be seen also in the absence of any systemic illness.

Nail dystrophies cannot usually be related to changes in thyroid function, hypovitaminosis, nutritional disturbances, or generalized allergic reactions.

Classification
Nail disorders may be classified as (1) local, (2) congenital or genetic, and (3) those associated with systemic or generalized skin diseases.

A. Local Nail Disorders:
1. Onycholysis (distal separation of the nails, usually of the fingers) is caused by excess exposure to water, soaps, detergents, alkalies, and industrial keratolytic agents. Nail hardeners and demeclocycline may cause onycholysis. Hypothyroidism is said to play a part.

2. Distortion of the nail occurs as a result of chronic inflammation of the nail matrix underlying the eponychial fold.

3. Discoloration and pithy changes, accompanied by a musty odor, are seen in ringworm infection.

4. Grooving and other changes may be caused by warts, nevi, synovial (myxomatous) cysts, etc, impinging on the nail matrix.

5. Allergic reactions (to formaldehyde and resins in undercoats and polishes) involving the nail bed or matrix formerly caused hemorrhagic streaking of the nails, accumulation of keratin under the free margins of the nails, and great tenderness of the nail beds.

6. Beau's lines (transverse furrows) may be due to faulty manicuring.

B. Congenital and Genetic Nail Disorders:
1. A longitudinal single nail groove may occur as a result of a genetic or traumatic defect in the nail matrix underlying the eponychial fold.

2. Nail atrophy may be congenital.

3. Hippocratic nails (club fingers) may be congenital.

C. Nail Changes Associated With Systemic or Generalized Skin Diseases:
1. Beau's lines (transverse furrows) may follow any serious systemic illness.

2. Atrophy of the nails may be related to trauma or vascular or neurologic disease.

3. Hippocratic nails (club fingers) are occasionally related to prolonged hypoxemia brought about by cardiopulmonary disorders.

4. Spoon nails are often seen in anemic patients.

5. Stippling of the nails is seen in psoriasis.

6. Nail changes may be seen also with alopecia areata, lichen planus, and keratosis follicularis.

Differential Diagnosis
It is important to distinguish congenital and genetic disorders from those caused by trauma and environmental disorders. Nail changes due to dermatophyte fungi may be difficult to differentiate from onychia due to *Candida* infections. Direct microscopic examination of a specimen cleared with 15% potassium hydroxide, or culture on Sabouraud's medium, may be diagnostic. Onychomycosis may be closely similar to the changes seen in psoriasis and lichen planus, in which case careful observation of more characteristic lesions elsewhere on the body is essential to the diagnosis of the nail disorders. Suspect malignancy with any persistent solitary subungual or periungual lesion.

Complications
Secondary bacterial infection occasionally occurs in onychodystrophies and leads to considerable pain and disability and possibly more serious consequences if circulation or innervation is impaired. Toenail

changes may lead to ingrown nail, in turn often complicated by bacterial infection and occasionally by exuberant granulation tissue. Poor manicuring and poorly fitting shoes may contribute to this complication. Cellulitis may result.

Treatment & Prognosis

Treatment consists usually of careful debridement and manicuring and, above all, reduction of exposure to irritants (soaps, detergents, alkali, bleaches, solvents, etc). Antifungal measures may be used in the case of onychomycosis and candidal onychia; antibacterial measures may be used for bacterial complications. Congenital or genetic nail disorders are usually uncorrectable. Longitudinal grooving due to temporary lesions of the matrix, such as warts, synovial cysts, and other impingements, may be cured by removal of the offending lesion. Intradermal triamcinolone acetonide suspension, 2.5 mg/mL, may be injected in the area of the nail matrix at intervals of 2–4

weeks for the successful management of various types of nail dystrophies (psoriasis, lichen planus, onycholysis, longitudinal splitting, grooving from synovial cysts, and others).

If it is necessary to remove nails for any reason (eg, fungal nails or severe psoriasis), one may apply urea 40%, anhydrous lanolin 20%, white wax 5%, white petrolatum 25%, and silica gel type H. The nail folds are painted with compound tincture of benzoin and then covered with cloth adhesive tape. Apply the urea ointment generously to the nail surface, and cover with plastic film and then adhesive tape. Avoid water. Leave the ointment on for 5–10 days; then lift off the nail plate. Medication can then be applied that is appropriate for the condition being treated.

Norton LA: Nail disorders. *J Am Acad Dermatol* 1980;**2**:451.

South DA, Farber EM: Urea ointment in the nonsurgical avulsion of nail dystrophies. *Cutis* 1980;**25**:609.

•   •   •

References

Arndt KA: *Manual of Dermatologic Therapeutics With Essentials of Diagnosis,* 3rd ed. Little, Brown, 1983.

Callen JP (editor): Symposium on the treatment of skin diseases. *Med Clin North Am* 1982;**66**:767.

Dermatology Committee, American College of Physicians: Dermatology: An annotated bibliography of recent literature. *Ann Intern Med* 1983;**98**:117.

Domonkos AN, Arnold HL Jr, Odom RB: *Andrews' Diseases of the Skin.* Saunders, 1982.

Fitzpatrick TB et al: *Update: Dermatology in General Medicine.* McGraw-Hill, 1983.

Landow RK: *Handbook of Dermatologic Treatment.* Jones Medical Publications, 1983.

Lever WF, Schaumberg-Lever G: *Histopathology of the Skin,* 6th ed. Lippincott, 1983.

Pillsbury DM, Heaton CL: *A Manual of Dermatology,* 2nd ed. Saunders, 1980.

Pinkus H, Mehregan AH: *A Guide to Dermatohistopathology,* 3rd ed. Appleton-Century-Crofts, 1981.

Sauer GC: *Manual of Skin Disease,* 4th ed. Lippincott, 1980.

Sherertz EF, Flowers FP: Rational use of topical corticosteroids. *Am Fam Physician* (Jan) 1984;**29**:262.

5 | Eye

Daniel Vaughan, MD

NONSPECIFIC MANIFESTATIONS OF EYE DISEASES

Redness

Redness is the most frequently encountered symptom in ocular disorders. It is due to hyperemia of the conjunctival, episcleral, or ciliary vessels. Redness is caused by irritation, infection, inflammation, trauma, tumors, dryness, or increased intraocular pressure (Table 5–1).

Dryness

Scratchiness, itching, and burning due to dryness of the eyes is a common complaint of older individuals, but it may occur at any age. The condition may arise from many causes, including dry environment, local ocular disease, systemic disorders, and drugs that lead to a deficiency of any of the tear film components. (See p 95.)

Pain

Ocular pain may be caused by trauma (chemical, mechanical, or physical), infection, inflammation, or sudden increase in intraocular pressure. Common eye disorders that cause pain include corneal injuries, foreign bodies, infections, iritis, and acute glaucoma.

Conjunctival Discharge

Discharge is usually caused by bacterial or viral conjunctivitis. A purulent discharge usually indicates bacterial infection. If the discharge is watery and is accompanied by photophobia or burning, viral conjunctivitis or keratoconjunctivitis may be present.

Obstruction of the lacrimal drainage system may also cause tearing, and infections of the lacrimal sac may lead to purulent discharge. Allergic conjunctivitis usually causes tearing and ropy discharge associated with itching. Any disruption of the corneal surface causes tearing.

Visual Impairment & Blindness

An individual may be considered to be visually impaired if the best corrected distant visual acuity in the better eye is less than 20/70 (6/21) or if visual fields are significantly restricted. Legal blindness (partial) in the USA is defined for practical purposes as visual acuity for distant vision of 20/200 (6/60) or less in the better eye with best correction, or widest diameter of the visual field subtending an angle of less than 20 degrees. WHO estimates that at least 10 million of the world's population are totally blind, and millions more have loss of sight sufficient to interfere with normal living.

A wide variety of causative factors, including infection, malnutrition, degenerative changes, immunologic reactions, neoplasms, hereditary factors,

Table 5–1. Differential diagnosis of common causes of inflamed eye.

	Acute Conjunctivitis	Acute Iritis*	Acute Glaucoma†	Corneal Trauma or Infection
Incidence	Extremely common	Common	Uncommon	Common
Discharge	Moderate to copious	None	None	Watery or purulent
Vision	No effect on vision	Slightly blurred	Markedly blurred	Usually blurred
Pain	None	Moderate	Severe	Moderate to severe
Conjunctival injection	Diffuse; more toward fornices	Mainly circumcorneal	Diffuse	Diffuse
Cornea	Clear	Usually clear	Steamy	Clarity change related to cause
Pupil size	Normal	Small	Moderately dilated and fixed	Normal
Pupillary light response	Normal	Poor	None	Normal
Intraocular pressure	Normal	Normal	Elevated	Normal
Smear	Causative organisms	No organisms	No organisms	Organisms found only in corneal ulcers due to infection

*Acute anterior uveitis.
†Angle-closure glaucoma.

and trauma that may involve any portion of the visual apparatus, can result in visual impairment. The most frequent causes of preventable blindness in the world are trachoma, leprosy, onchocerciasis, and xerophthalmia. Glaucoma, diabetic retinopathy, and other retinal disorders (many of which are related to the aging process) are leading causes of blindness in the USA and Western world. There are approximately 500,000 legally blind persons in the USA; about half are over age 65.

Blurred Vision

The most important causes of blurred vision are refractive error, corneal opacities, cataract, vitreous clouding, retinal detachment, macular degeneration, central retinal vein thrombosis, central retinal artery occlusion, optic neuritis, and optic atrophy.

"Eyestrain"

This is a common ocular complaint that usually means eye discomfort associated with prolonged reading or close work. Significant refractive error, early presbyopia, inadequate illumination, or phoria (usually exophoria with poor convergence) should be ruled out.

Photophobia

Photophobia is commonly due to corneal inflammation, aphakia, iritis, and ocular albinism. A less common cause is fever associated with viral infections (eg, influenza, dengue, pneumonia), which characteristically produces aching of the eyes along with photophobia.

"Spots Before the Eyes"

"Spots" are vitreous opacities that usually have no clinical significance though in some cases they signify impending retinal detachment or posterior uveitis.

Headache

Headache is only occasionally due to ocular disorders. The causes of ocular headache are in general the same as those of "eyestrain" (above).

Diplopia

Double vision is due to muscle imbalance or to paralysis of one or more of the extraocular muscles as a result of inflammation (including thyroid myopathy), hemorrhage, increased intracranial pressure, trauma, tumefaction, or inflammation of the third, fourth, or sixth nerves. In diplopia, the sixth nerve is most commonly affected.

Proptosis (Exophthalmos)

The most frequent cause of proptosis in the adult is thyroid disease. Other causes of (usually unilateral) proptosis include orbital tumors and inflammatory disorders, hemorrhage, cysts, and cavernous sinus syndrome.

OCULAR EMERGENCIES*

SUDDEN LOSS OF VISION

Sudden loss of vision (over a period of seconds) is a serious symptom requiring emergency ophthalmologic consultation. It may occur in optic disk edema associated with accelerated hypertension or severe papilledema due to raised intracranial pressure. Loss of vision for several minutes followed by return of vision is usually associated with retinal emboli from the heart or carotid arteries, although septic emboli from intravenous drug abuse have also been reported.

Sudden sustained loss of vision is generally due to vascular occlusion either in the central retinal artery or in the short posterior ciliary arteries supplying the optic nerve head which may be involved in cranial arteritis. Sudden visual loss with associated headache in an elderly patient is likely to be due to cranial arteritis. Diagnostic blood sedimentation rate, temporal artery biopsy, and treatment with steroids in high doses (eg, prednisolone, 80 mg orally) are mandatory to preserve vision in the fellow eye (see p 511).

Other causes of sudden severe visual loss are rare, but retinal detachment and retinal hemorrhage from any cause, especially if the macula is involved, are important.

Optic neuritis, usually from demyelinating disease but also from inflammatory conditions such as sarcoidosis, may cause sudden severe visual loss. These may be associated with pain on eye movement due to traction on the inflamed optic nerve sheath.

Bilateral sudden visual loss is rare from ocular causes. Migraine or vertebrobasilar disease may cause hypoperfusion of visual pathways or visual cortex with associated bilateral symptoms. Patients with homonymous hemianopia sometimes notice only the blind temporal field and claim uniocular symptoms. Normal pupillary reactions in the presence of visual loss suggest that the lesion is posterior to the lateral geniculate body.

ACUTE (ANGLE-CLOSURE) GLAUCOMA

Acute glaucoma can occur only with the closure of a preexisting narrow anterior chamber angle. If the pupil dilates spontaneously or is dilated with a mydriatic or cycloplegic, the angle will close and an attack of acute glaucoma is precipitated; for this reason, it is a wise precaution to examine the anterior chamber angle before instilling these drugs. Dilation of the pupil should be avoided if the anterior chamber is shallow (readily determined by oblique illumination of the an-

*Ophthalmologic consultation should be considered for all patients with ocular emergencies.

terior segment of the eye). About 1% of people over age 35 have narrow anterior chamber angles, but many of these never develop acute glaucoma; thus, the condition is very uncommon.

A quiet eye with a narrow anterior chamber angle may convert spontaneously to angle-closure glaucoma. The process can be precipitated by anything that will dilate the pupil, eg, indiscriminate use of mydriatics or cycloplegics by the patient or the physician. The cycloplegic can be administered in the form of eye drops or systemically, eg, by an anesthetist ordering scopolamine or atropine in preparation for cholecystectomy, or by a physician prescribing an atropinelike drug for any disorder. Increased circulating epinephrine in times of stress can also dilate the pupil and cause acute glaucoma. Sitting in a darkened movie theater can have the same effect.

Patients with acute glaucoma seek treatment immediately because of extreme pain and blurring of vision. The eye is red, the cornea is steamy, and the pupil is moderately dilated and does not react to light. Tonometry reveals elevated intraocular pressure.

Acute glaucoma must be differentiated from conjunctivitis and acute iritis and from corneal abrasion—especially after a general anesthetic.

Laser or surgical peripheral iridectomy within 12–48 hours after onset of symptoms will usually result in a permanent cure. Untreated acute glaucoma results in complete and permanent blindness within 2–5 days after onset of symptoms. Before surgery, the intraocular pressure must be lowered by means of miotics instilled locally and osmotic agents and carbonic anhydrase inhibitors administered systemically. Laser iridectomy is an effective new therapeutic approach that may eventually replace surgical iridectomy.

Three different osmotic agents (urea, mannitol, and glycerol) are available for lowering intraocular pressure preoperatively in angle-closure glaucoma. Urea and mannitol are administered intravenously, and glycerol is given orally. The usual dosage of all 3 of these osmotic drugs is 1.5 g/kg.

Arruga J, Sanders M: Ophthalmologic findings in 70 patients with evidence of retinal embolism. *Ophthalmology* 1982;**89**:1336.
Behrendt T: Eye emergencies: Treatment. *Fam Pract Recertification* (July) 1982;**4**:23.
Keltner J: Giant cell arteritis. *Ophthalmology* 1982;**89**:1101.
Kolker AE, Hetherington J: *Becker-Shaffer's Diagnosis and Therapy of the Glaucomas,* 5th ed. Mosby, 1982.
Wise J: Long-term control of adult open-angle glaucoma by argon laser treatment. *Ophthalmology* 1981;**88**:197.

FOREIGN BODIES

If a patient complains of "something in my eye" and gives a consistent history, a foreign body is usually present even though it may not be readily visible. Almost all foreign bodies, however, can be seen under oblique illumination with the aid of a hand flashlight and loupe.

Note the time, place, and other circumstances of the accident. Test visual acuity before treatment is instituted as a basis for comparison in the event of complications.

Conjunctival Foreign Body

Foreign body of the upper tarsal conjunctiva is suggested by pain and blepharospasm of sudden onset in the presence of a clear cornea and by less pain on blinking when the eye is turned (right or left) so that the cornea is away from the foreign body location. After instilling a local anesthetic, evert the lid by grasping the lashes gently and exerting pressure on the mid portion of the outer surface of the upper lid with an applicator. If a foreign body is present, it can be easily removed by passing a sterile wet cotton applicator across the conjunctival surface.

Corneal Foreign Body

When a corneal foreign body is suspected but is not apparent on simple inspection, instill fluorescein into the conjunctival sac and examine the cornea with the aid of a magnifying device and strong illumination. The foreign body may then be removed with a sterile wet cotton applicator. An antibiotic should be instilled, eg, gentamicin ointment. It is not necessary to patch the eye, but the patient must be examined 24 hours later for secondary infection of the crater. If a corneal foreign body cannot be removed in this manner, it should be removed by an ophthalmologist. Steel foreign bodies usually leave a diffuse rust ring. This requires excision of the affected tissue and is best done under local anesthesia using a slit lamp. *Caution:* Anesthetic drops should not be given to the patient for self-administration. If there is no infection, a layer of corneal epithelial cells will line the crater within 24 hours. It should be emphasized that the intact corneal epithelium forms an effective barrier to infection. Once the corneal epithelium is disturbed, the cornea becomes extremely susceptible to infection.

Early infection is manifested by a white necrotic area around the crater and a small amount of gray exudate. These patients should be referred immediately to an ophthalmologist.

Untreated corneal infection may lead to severe corneal ulceration, panophthalmitis, and loss of the eye.

Intraocular Foreign Body

A patient with an intraocular foreign body should be referred immediately to an ophthalmologist. With delay, the ocular media become progressively more cloudy, and a foreign body visible shortly after the injury may not be visible several hours later. The foreign body can often be removed with a magnet through the point of entry or through an incision in the sclera near its site of lodgment.

Brinton GS et al: Posttraumatic endophthalmitis. *Arch Ophthalmol* 1984;**102**:68.

Holt JE, Holt GR, Blodgett JM: Ocular injuries sustained during blunt facial trauma. *Ophthalmology* 1983;**90**:14.

Winthrop S et al: Penetrating eye injuries: A histopathological review. *Br J Ophthalmol* 1980;**64**:809.

CORNEAL ABRASIONS

A patient with a corneal abrasion complains of severe pain and photophobia.

Record the history and visual acuity. Examine the cornea and conjunctiva with a light and loupe to rule out a foreign body. If an abrasion is suspected but cannot be seen, instill sterile fluorescein into the conjunctival sac; the area of corneal abrasion will stain a deeper green than the surrounding cornea.

Instill gentamicin ophthalmic ointment and apply a bandage with firm pressure to prevent movement of the lid. The patient should rest at home, keeping the fellow eye closed, and should be observed on the following day to be certain that the cornea has healed. Recurrent corneal erosion may follow corneal abrasions, and all such cases should be referred to an ophthalmologist.

Niiranen M et al: Eye injuries in children. *Br J Ophthalmol* 1981;**65**:436.

CONTUSIONS

Contusion injuries of the eye and surrounding structures may cause ecchymosis ("black eye"), subconjunctival hemorrhage, edema or rupture of the cornea, hemorrhage into the anterior chamber (hyphema), rupture of the root of the iris (iridodialysis), paralysis of the pupillary sphincter, paralysis of the muscles of accommodation, cataract, subluxation or luxation of the lens, vitreous hemorrhage, retinal hemorrhage and edema (most common in the macular area), detachment of the retina, rupture of the choroid, fracture of the orbital floor ("blowout fracture"), and optic nerve injury. Many of these injuries are immediately apparent; others may not become apparent for days or weeks. Patients with moderate to severe contusions should be seen by an ophthalmologist.

Any injury severe enough to cause hyphema involves the danger of secondary hemorrhage, which may cause intractable glaucoma with permanent visual loss. Any patient with traumatic hyphema should be put at bed rest for 6–7 days with both eyes bandaged to lessen the chance of secondary hemorrhage. Secondary hemorrhage rarely occurs after this time.

Holt JE, Holt GR, Blodgett JM: Ocular injuries sustained during blunt facial trauma. *Ophthalmology* 1983;**90**:14.

Maltzman BA et al: A survey of ocular trauma. *Surv Ophthalmol* 1976;**21**:285.

Vinger PF: Sports eye injuries: A preventable disease. *Ophthalmology* 1981;**88**:108.

ULTRAVIOLET KERATITIS
(Actinic Keratitis)

Ultraviolet burns of the cornea are usually caused by use of an ultraviolet sunlamp without proper eye protection, exposure to a welding arc, or exposure to the sun when skiing ("snow blindness"). There are no immediate symptoms, but about 6–12 hours later the patient complains of agonizing pain and severe photophobia. Slit lamp examination after instillation of sterile fluorescein shows diffuse punctate staining of both corneas.

Treatment consists of binocular patching, systemic analgesics, and sedatives as indicated. All patients recover within 24–48 hours without complications. Local anesthetics should not be prescribed.

See reference under Corneal Abrasions, above.

CORNEAL ULCER

Corneal ulcers constitute a medical emergency. The typical gray, necrotic corneal ulcer may be preceded by trauma, usually a corneal foreign body. The eye is red, with lacrimation and conjunctival discharge, and the patient complains of blurred vision, pain, and photophobia.

Prompt treatment is essential to help prevent complications. Visual impairment may occur as a result of corneal scarring or infection.

Corneal ulcers have many causes, including bacterial, viral, and fungal infections and allergic disorders. Only the most common types will be discussed here.

Pneumococcal ("Acute Serpiginous") Ulcer

Streptococcus pneumoniae is a common bacterial cause of corneal ulcer. The early ulcer is gray and fairly well circumscribed; hypopyon is often present.

Since the pneumococcus is sensitive both to sulfonamides and to antibiotics, local therapy is usually effective. If untreated, the cornea may perforate. Concurrent dacryocystitis, if present, should also be treated; later, dacryocystorhinostomy must be considered to prevent recurrence of the ulcer.

Pseudomonas Ulcer

A common and devastating cause of corneal ulcer is *Pseudomonas aeruginosa*. The ulceration characteristically starts in a traumatized area and spreads rapidly, often causing perforation of the cornea and loss of the eye within 48 hours. *P aeruginosa* usually produces a pathognomonic bluish-green pigment.

Early diagnosis and vigorous treatment with local application and subconjunctival injection of antibiotics (gentamicin, carbenicillin, colistin, tobramycin) are essential to save the eye.

Herpes Simplex (Dendritic) Keratitis

Corneal ulceration caused by herpes simplex

virus is more common than any bacterial ulcer. It is almost always unilateral and may affect any age group of either sex. It is often preceded by upper respiratory tract infection with fever and facial "cold sores."

The commonest finding is of one or more dendritic ulcers (superficial branching gray areas) on the corneal surface. These are composed of clear vesicles in the corneal epithelium; when the vesicles rupture, the area stains green with fluorescein. Although the dendritic figure is its most characteristic manifestation, herpes simplex keratitis may appear in a number of other configurations.

Treatment consists of removing the virus-containing corneal epithelium without disturbing Bowman's membrane or the corneal stroma. This is best done by an ophthalmologist. *Caution:* Do not give local corticosteroids, as they enhance the activity of the virus by suppressing the local immune mechanisms. This may lead to perforation of the cornea and loss of the eye. (See also Chapter 22 and p 69.)

Idoxuridine (IUDR; 5-iodo-2′-deoxyuridine) is commonly used against herpes simplex keratitis. It is instilled locally as 0.1% solution.

Newer antiviral agents such as vidarabine (Vira-A) and trifluridine (Viroptic) may be effective against superficial epithelial herpetic infections of the cornea, but many ophthalmologists still prefer to remove the affected corneal epithelium mechanically and apply a pressure bandage for a few days until the epithelium regenerates.

Coster DJ et al: A comparison of acyclovir and idoxuridine as a treatment for ulcerative herpetic keratitis. *Br J Ophthalmol* 1980;**64:**763.

Lemp MA: Cornea and sclera: Annual review. *Arch Ophthalmol* 1976;**94:**473.

McGill J, Chapman C: A comparison of topical acyclovir with steroids in the treatment of herpes zoster keratouveitis. *Br J Ophthalmol* 1983;**67:**746.

Ostler HB, Thygeson P, Okumoto M: Infectious diseases of the eye. 3. Infections of the cornea. *J Cont Educ Ophthalmol* (Sept) 1978;**40:**13.

Pavan-Langston D et al: Ganglionic herpes simplex and systemic acyclovir. *Arch Ophthalmol* 1981;**99:**1417.

Wilhelmus K et al: Bilateral herpetic keratitis. *Br J Ophthalmol* 1981;**65:**385.

Wilson LA et al: Corneal ulcers and soft contact lenses. *Am J Ophthalmol* 1981;**92:**546.

CHEMICAL CONJUNCTIVITIS & KERATITIS

Chemical burns are treated by irrigation of the eyes with saline solution or plain water as soon as possible after exposure. Do *not* neutralize an acid with an alkali or vice versa, as the heat generated by the reaction may cause further damage. Alkali injuries are more serious and require prolonged irrigation, since alkalies are not precipitated by the proteins of the eye as are acids. The pupil should be dilated with 0.2% scopolamine or 2% atropine. Complications include

mucus deficiency, scarring of the cornea or conjunctiva (or both), symblepharon, tear duct obstruction, and secondary infection. Alkali burns have a poorer prognosis than acid burns.

Pfister RW: Chemical injuries of the eye. *Ophthalmology* 1983; **90:**1246.

GONOCOCCAL CONJUNCTIVITIS

Gonococcal conjunctivitis, which may cause corneal ulceration, is manifested by a copious purulent discharge. The diagnosis may be confirmed by a stained smear and culture of the discharge. Prompt treatment with both local and systemic penicillin is required (see p 880).

SYMPATHETIC OPHTHALMIA
(Sympathetic Uveitis)

Sympathetic ophthalmia is a rare type of severe bilateral granulomatous uveitis. The cause is not known, but the disease may occur at any time from 1 week to many years after a penetrating injury through the ciliary body. The injured (exciting) eye becomes inflamed first and the fellow (sympathizing) eye second. Symptoms and signs include blurred vision, light sensitivity, and redness.

The best treatment of sympathetic ophthalmia is prevention by enucleating the injured eye. Any severely injured eye (eg, one with perforation of the sclera and ciliary body, with loss of vitreous) can incite sympathetic uveitis. Early enucleation may prevent this. The decision about whether or not enucleation should be performed—and, if so, when—is controversial and requires the most careful consideration. In established cases of sympathetic ophthalmia, systemic corticosteroid therapy may be helpful. Without treatment, the disease progresses gradually to bilateral blindness.

Kinyoun JL, Bensinger RE, Chuang EL: Thirty-year history of sympathetic ophthalmia. *Ophthalmology* 1983;**90:**59.

Sharp DC et al: Sympathetic ophthalmia. *Arch Ophthalmol* 1984;**102:**232.

LACERATIONS

Lids

If the lid margin is lacerated, the patient should be referred for specialized care, since permanent notching may result. Lacerations of the lower eyelid near the inner canthus often sever the lower canaliculus. These require treatment by an ophthalmologist to attempt to restore the function of the torn canaliculus. Lid lacerations not involving the margin may be sutured just as any other skin laceration.

Conjunctiva

In superficial lacerations of the conjunctiva, sutures are not necessary. In order to prevent infection, instill a broad-spectrum antibiotic or sulfonamide into the eye until the laceration is healed.

Cornea or Sclera

Keep examination and manipulation at an absolute minimum, since pressure may result in extrusion of the intraocular contents. Bandage the eye lightly and cover with a metal shield that rests on the orbital bones above and below. The patient should be instructed not to squeeze the eyes shut and to remain as quiet as possible and should be transferred to an ophthalmologist. Always x-ray the eye to exclude the presence of foreign bodies.

McKinley RT, Cohen DN: Ophthalmic injuries: Handbook of initial evaluation and management. *Trans Am Acad Ophthalmol Otolaryngol* 1975;**79**:op880.

Sharkey TG, Brown SI: Transplantation of lacerated corneas. *Am J Ophthalmol* 1981;**91**:721.

ORBITAL CELLULITIS

Orbital cellulitis is manifested by an abrupt onset of fever, proptosis, and swelling and redness of the lids. It is usually caused by a pyogenic organism. Immediate treatment with systemic antibiotics is indicated to prevent brain abscess. The response to antibiotics is usually excellent. Patients with orbital cellulitis may need to be admitted to the hospital.

Check WA: Many misjudge severity of orbital cellulitis. *JAMA* 1982;**247**:1236.

Friberg TR: Advances in the treatment of vitreous disease. *JAMA* 1982;**247**:1623.

Jones IS, Jakobiec FA: *Diseases of the Orbit.* Harper & Row, 1979.

Weiss A et al: Bacterial periorbital and orbital cellulitis in childhood. *Ophthalmology* 1983;**90**:195.

VITREOUS HEMORRHAGE

Hemorrhage into the vitreous body may obscure a retinal detachment. Treatment by an ophthalmologist is indicated. The commonest causes of vitreous hemorrhage are diabetes, severe hypertension, blood dyscrasias, and trauma.

Boyd BF (editor): Chaps 1–4, pp 46–214, in: *Highlights of Ophthalmology.* 2 vols. Highlights of Ophthalmology Press, 1981.

Winslow RL, Taylor BC: Spontaneous vitreous hemorrhage: Etiology and management. *South Med J* 1980;**73**:1450.

COMMON OCULAR DISORDERS

CONJUNCTIVITIS

Conjunctivitis is the most common eye disease. It may be acute or chronic. Most cases are exogenous and due to bacterial, viral, or chlamydial infection, although endogenous inflammation may occur (eg, phlyctenular conjunctivitis, a delayed hypersensitivity response to circulating tuberculoprotein). Other causes are allergy, chemical irritations, and fungal or parasitic infection. The mode of transmission of infectious conjunctivitis is usually direct contact via fingers, towels, handkerchiefs, etc, to the fellow eye or to other persons.

Conjunctivitis must be differentiated from iritis, glaucoma, corneal trauma, and keratitis.

Bacterial Conjunctivitis

The organisms found most commonly in bacterial conjunctivitis are *Streptococcus pneumoniae, Staphylococcus aureus,* Koch-Weeks bacillus, and Morax-Axenfeld bacillus. All may produce a copious purulent discharge. Examination of stained conjunctival scrapings for white blood cells and bacteria is helpful; if the disease is purulent or membranous, culture studies are recommended. There is no pain or blurring of vision. The disease is usually self-limited, lasting about 10–14 days if untreated. A sulfonamide (eg, sulfacetamide, 10% ophthalmic solution or ointment) instilled locally 3 times daily will usually clear the infection in 2–3 days. Topical antibiotics are usually to be avoided for minimal infections and limited to those unlikely to be used systemically (see p 102).

Viral Conjunctivitis

One of the commonest causes of viral conjunctivitis is adenovirus type 3, which is usually associated with pharyngitis, fever, malaise, and preauricular adenopathy. Locally, the palpebral conjunctiva is red, and there is a copious watery discharge and scanty exudate. Children are more often affected than adults, and contaminated swimming pools are sometimes the source of infection. Epidemic keratoconjunctivitis (EKC) is caused by adenovirus types 8 and 19. There is no specific treatment, although local sulfonamide therapy may prevent secondary bacterial infection. The disease usually lasts at least 2 weeks. (See p 852.)

Keratoconjunctivitis Sicca
(Dry Eye Syndrome)

This is a common disorder, particularly in elderly women. The patient complains of dryness, redness, or a scratchy feeling of the eyes. A wide range of conditions predispose to or are characterized by dry eyes. Hypofunction of the lacrimal glands may be due to aging, hereditary disorders, systemic disease (eg, rheumatoid arthritis and other connective tissue disorders), and systemic and topical drugs. Excessive evaporation of tears may be due to environmental exposure (eg, a hot, dry, or windy climate). Mucin deficiency may be due to malnutrition, infection, burns, or drugs.

Treatment depends upon the cause. In most early cases, the corneal and conjunctival epithelial changes are reversible.

Aqueous deficiency can be treated by replacement of the aqueous with various types of artificial tears. Mucin deficiency can be partially compensated for by the use of ophthalmic vehicles of high molecular weight—eg, water-soluble polymers—or by the use of the patient's own serum as local eye drops. Serum used for this purpose must be kept refrigerated at all times. It acts by lowering the surface tension of the tears, assisting in the spreading of the tears, and wetting the epithelium. If the mucus is tenacious, as in Sjögren's syndrome, mucolytic agents (eg, acetylcysteine, 20%) may provide some relief.

Chlamydial Keratoconjunctivitis

A. Trachoma: Trachoma is a major cause of blindness worldwide. In endemic areas, it is contracted in childhood. In children, trachoma is usually insidious, with minimal symptoms. In adults, the disease is acute and is manifested by redness, itching, tearing, and slight discharge. The clinical picture consists of bilateral follicular conjunctivitis, epithelial keratitis, and corneal vascularization (pannus). Cicatrization of the conjunctiva occurs in the later stages of trachoma and usually follows necrosis of the conjunctival follicles. Scarring of the tarsal conjunctiva may result in entropion and trichiasis. Scarring of the limbal follicles results in round peripheral depressions with a clear central epithelium known as Herbert's pits. Superficial vascularization and scarring of the cornea cause decrease in vision. In endemic areas, superimposed bacterial conjunctivitis may aggravate the process.

The specific diagnosis can be made in Giemsa-stained conjunctival scrapings by the presence of typical cytoplasmic inclusions in epithelial cells. In active trachoma, the smear may also include polymorphonuclear leukocytes, plasma cells, and debris-filled macrophages (Leber cells).

Trachoma is transmitted from eye to eye by contact with contaminated fingers, towels, eye cosmetics, or other objects.

Treatment should be started on the basis of clinical findings without waiting for laboratory confirmation. Medical treatment consists of oral tetracycline given in full doses for 3–5 weeks. Local treatment is not necessary. *Caution:* Do not give tetracyclines during pregnancy or to young children, and do not use old preparations.

Hygienic measures are of great importance both in prevention and in treatment.

Corneal scarring may require corneal transplantation. Entropion and trichiasis require plastic surgery to evert the lids. Dacryocystorhinostomy may be required in nasolacrimal duct obstruction.

B. Inclusion Keratoconjunctivitis: This is a sexually transmitted infection that causes subclinical cervicitis in the female and urethritis in the male. About 40% of cases of nongonorrheal urethritis in men are caused by chlamydiae. The agent is transmitted by intercourse, and the eye is occasionally infected by contact with genital secretions. The newborn contracts the disease by passage through the infected birth canal. In the past, the disease had been transmitted by exposure of the eyes to contaminated water in swimming pools, and for this reason it was referred to as "swimming pool conjunctivitis." Adequate chlorination of swimming pools has eliminated this mode of transmission.

Inclusion conjunctivitis (blennorrhea) of the newborn usually occurs about 5–12 days after birth. The disease is characterized by bilateral redness, a mucopurulent exudate, papillary hypertrophy, and, in some cases, a diffuse punctate keratitis. If pseudomembranes occur, the disease may result in fine conjunctival scars. Corneal scars occur rarely and never lead to blindness, as in trachoma.

In babies, treatment with tetracycline eye drops, 1% in oil instilled 5–6 times daily for 2–3 weeks, is very effective.

Adult inclusion conjunctivitis occurs most frequently in sexually active young adults. The disease starts with acute redness, discharge, and irritation. The eye findings consist of follicular conjunctivitis with mild keratitis. A nontender preauricular lymph node can often be palpated. Healing leaves no sequelae. The cytology of the conjunctival scrapings is similar to that of trachoma, but cytoplasmic inclusions are found more frequently.

In adults, the 1% tetracycline drops in oil should be supplemented by tetracycline, 1–1.5 g daily orally for 2–3 weeks. (See pp 881–883.)

Ophthalmia Neonatorum

Any infection of the newborn conjunctiva is referred to as ophthalmia neonatorum. The eyes of the newborn are usually inoculated with the offensive agent during passage through the birth canal. The causes of ophthalmia neonatorum include *Neisseria gonorrhoeae,* the agent of inclusion conjunctivitis, herpesvirus hominis type 2 (genital herpes), and certain opportunistic bacteria. The etiologic agent should be identified in Giemsa- and Gram-stained scrapings of the conjunctiva and smears of exudates and by conjunctival cultures for bacteria and viruses.

The Credé 1% silver nitrate prophylaxis is effective for the prevention of gonorrheal ophthalmia but does not protect against herpesvirus infection or inclusion blennorrhea. Appropriate topical antibiotics should be instilled to treat bacterial infections.

Allergic Conjunctivitis

Allergic conjunctivitis is a common disorder that is most often associated with hay fever. It causes bilateral tearing, itching, and redness and a minimal stringy discharge. It is usually chronic and recurrent.

Short-term local corticosteroid therapy is often effective. Allergy is the usual cause of the alarming sudden painless chemosis seen in children.

Fungal & Parasitic Conjunctivitis

Fungal and parasitic conjunctivitides are rare in most parts of the world and are usually unilateral. They often present with a localized inflammatory granuloma. A more common example is *Leptothrix* conjunctivitis, which occurs in persons in close contact with cats.

Darougar S et al: Clinical and epidemiological features of adenovirus keratoconjunctivitis in London. *Br J Ophthalmol* 1983;**67**:1.

Feducowicz HB: *External Infections of the Eye: Bacterial, Viral, and Mycotic,* 2nd ed. Appleton-Century-Crofts, 1978.

Pierce JM et al: Ophthalmia neonatorum in the 1980's. *Br J Ophthalmol* 1982;**66**:728.

Tabbara KF, Bobb AA: Lacrimal system complications of trachoma. *Ophthalmology* 1980;**87**;298.

Vaughan D, Asbury T: Conjunctiva. Chap 7, pp 58–84, in: *General Ophthalmology,* 10th ed. Lange, 1983.

PINGUECULA

Pinguecula is a yellow elevated nodule on either side of the cornea (more commonly on the nasal side) in the area of the palpebral fissure. Histologically, pinguecula is an elastoid degeneration of the conjunctival substantia propria. The nodules rarely grow, but inflammation (pingueculitis) may occur. No treatment is indicated. Pinguecula is common in persons over age 35.

PTERYGIUM

Pterygium is a fleshy, triangular encroachment of the conjunctiva onto the nasal side of the cornea and is usually associated with constant exposure to wind, sun, sand, and dust. Pterygium may be either unilateral or bilateral. There may be a genetic predisposition, but no hereditary pattern has been described. Excision is indicated if the growth threatens vision by approaching the pupillary area. Pterygium is fairly common in the southwestern USA. Treatment is surgical, but recurrences are frequent.

Paton D: Pterygium management based upon a theory of pathogenesis. *Trans Am Acad Ophthalmol Otolaryngol* 1975; **79**:603.

UVEITIS
(Iritis, Iridocyclitis)

Uveitis is any inflammation of the uveal tract (iris, ciliary body, and choroid). Inflammation primarily of the iris is called anterior uveitis, iridocyclitis, or iritis; inflammation of the choroid (and usually the retina as well) is called posterior uveitis or retinochoroiditis.

Uveitis may be either granulomatous (exogenous) or nongranulomatous (endogenous); the latter is more common. The disease is usually unilateral, and signs and symptoms are similar in both types, varying only in intensity. Early diagnosis and treatment are important to prevent the formation of posterior synechiae.

All patients with uveitis should have a thorough history, systems review, and physical examination. Pertinent laboratory studies should include at least an erythrocyte sedimentation rate, VDRL, and FTA-ABS. PPD and anergy skin tests should be performed. Obtain x-rays of the chest and (if symptomatic) the sacroiliac joint.

Uveitis must be differentiated from conjunctivitis, acute glaucoma, and corneal ulcer.

Nongranulomatous Uveitis (Endogenous)

Nongranulomatous uveitis is primarily an anterior noninfectious disease, and it is occasionally associated with ankylosing spondylitis or Crohn's disease. The iris and ciliary body are primarily affected, but occasional foci are found in the choroid.

The onset is acute, with marked pain, redness, photophobia, and blurred vision. A circumcorneal flush, caused by dilated limbal blood vessels, is present. Fine white keratic precipitates on the posterior surface of the cornea can be seen with the slit lamp or with a loupe. The pupil is small, and there may be a collection of fibrin with cells in the anterior chamber. If posterior synechiae are present, the pupil will be irregular and the light reflex will be absent.

Local corticosteroid therapy tends to shorten the course. Warm compresses will decrease pain. Atropine, 1%, 2 drops in the affected eye twice daily, will prevent posterior synechia formation and alleviate photophobia. Recurrences are common, but the prognosis is good.

Granulomatous Uveitis (Exogenous)

Granulomatous uveitis usually follows invasion by the causative organism, eg, *Mycobacterium tuberculosis* or *Toxoplasma gondii,* although these pathogens are rarely recovered. Other common causes are *Treponema pallidum* and *Mycobacterium leprae.* Any or all parts of the uveal tract may be affected, but there is a predilection for the choroid.

Granulomatous uveitis is more subtle than nongranulomatous uveitis in that there is usually less pain and redness, but the permanent eye damage is relatively devastating. The onset is usually slow, and the affected eye may be only slightly and diffusely red. Because of vitreous haze and retinal involvement, vision may be more blurred than would be expected in view of the apparent mildness of the process. Pain is minimal or absent, and photophobia is slight. The pupil may be normal or, if posterior synechiae are present, irregular and slightly smaller than normal. Large gray "mutton fat" keratic precipitates on the posterior surface of the cornea may be seen with the slit lamp or loupe. The anterior chamber may be cloudy. Iris nodules are commonly present, and there may be vitreous haze. Fresh lesions of the choroid appear yellow when viewed with the ophthalmoscope.

Treatment depends on the causative agent. The pupil should be kept dilated with atropine and associated systemic disease treated as indicated. Chronic long-standing refractory uveitis may require surgery to control specific complications of the disease. The visual prognosis is fair.

Lowder CY, Char DH: Uveitis: A review. *West J Med* 1984; **140**:421.

Mines JA, Coles RS: Surgical approaches to uveitis. *Med Times* (June) 1984;**112**:52.

O'Connor GR: Factors related to the initiation and recurrence of uveitis. XL Edward Jackson Memorial Lecture. *Am J Ophthalmol* 1983;**96**:577.

DISORDERS OF THE LIDS & LACRIMAL APPARATUS

Hordeolum

Hordeolum is a common staphylococcal abscess that is characterized by a localized red, swollen, acutely tender area on the upper or lower lid. Internal hordeolum is a meibomian gland abscess that points to the skin or to the conjunctival side of the lid; external hordeolum or sty (infection of the glands of Moll or Zeis) is smaller and on the margin.

The chief symptom is pain of an intensity directly related to the amount of swelling.

Warm compresses are helpful. Incision is indicated if resolution does not begin within 48 hours. An antibiotic or sulfonamide instilled into the conjunctival sac every 3 hours may be beneficial during the acute stage. Internal hordeolum may lead to generalized cellulitis of the lid.

Chalazion

Chalazion is a common granulomatous inflammation of a meibomian gland characterized by a hard, nontender swelling on the upper or lower lid. It may be preceded by a sty. Most chalazions point toward the conjunctival side.

If the chalazion is large enough to impress the cornea, vision will be distorted. The conjunctiva in the region of the chalazion is red and elevated.

Excision is done by an ophthalmologist.

Tumors

Verrucae and papillomas of the skin of the lids can often be excised by the general physician if they do not involve the lid margin. Cancer should be ruled out by microscopic examination of the excised material.

Blepharitis

Blepharitis is a common chronic, bilateral inflammation of the lid margins. It may be ulcerative (*Staphylococcus aureus*) or nonulcerative (seborrheic). The latter type may be caused by *Pityrosporum ovale*, although the relationship is not definite. Both types are usually present. Seborrhea of the scalp, brows, and frequently of the ears is almost always associated with seborrheic blepharitis.

Symptoms are irritation, burning, and itching. The eyes are "red-rimmed," and scales or "granulations" can be seen clinging to the lashes. In the staphylococcal type, the scales are dry, the lid margins are red and ulcerated, and the lashes tend to fall out; in the seborrheic type the scales are greasy, ulceration is absent, and the lid margins are less red. In the more common mixed type, both dry and greasy scales are present, and the lid margins are red and may be ulcerated.

Cleanliness of the scalp, eyebrows, and lid margins is essential to effective local therapy. Scales must be removed from the lids daily with a damp cotton applicator.

An antistaphylococcal antibiotic or sulfonamide eye ointment is applied with a cotton applicator 3 times daily to the lid margins. The treatment of both types is similar except that in severe staphylococcal blepharitis antibiotic sensitivity studies may be required.

Entropion & Ectropion

Entropion (inward turning of the lid, usually the lower) occurs occasionally in older people as a result of degeneration of the lid fascia and may follow extensive scarring of the conjunctiva and tarsus. Surgery is indicated if the lashes rub on the cornea.

Ectropion (outward turning of the lower lid) is fairly common in elderly people. Surgery is indicated if ectropion causes excessive tearing, exposure keratitis, or a cosmetic problem.

Dacryocystitis

Dacryocystitis is a common infection of the lacrimal sac. It may be acute or chronic and occurs most often in infants and in persons over 40. It is usually unilateral.

The cause of obstruction is usually unknown, but a history of trauma to the nose may be obtained. In acute dacryocystitis, the usual infectious organisms are *Staphylococcus aureus* and beta-hemolytic streptococci; in chronic dacryocystitis, *Streptococcus pneumoniae* (rarely, *Candida albicans*). Mixed infections do not occur.

Acute dacryocystitis is characterized by pain, swelling, tenderness, and redness in the tear sac area; purulent material may be expressed. In chronic dacryocystitis, tearing and discharge are the principal signs. Mucus or pus may be expressed from the tear sac.

Acute dacryocystitis responds well to systemic antibiotic therapy, but recurrences are common if the obstruction is not surgically removed. The chronic form may be kept latent by using antibiotic eye drops, but relief of the obstruction is the only cure.

OPEN-ANGLE (CHRONIC) GLAUCOMA

Essentials of Diagnosis

- Insidious onset in older age groups.
- No symptoms in early stages.
- Gradual loss of peripheral vision over a period of years, resulting in tunnel vision.
- Persistent elevation of intraocular pressure associated with pathologic cupping of the optic disks.
- *Note:* "Halos around lights" are not present unless the intraocular tension is markedly elevated.

General Considerations

In open-angle glaucoma, the intraocular pressure is consistently elevated. Over a period of months or years, this results in optic atrophy with loss of vision varying from a slight constriction of the upper nasal peripheral visual fields to complete blindness.

The cause of the decreased rate of aqueous outflow in open-angle glaucoma has not been clearly demonstrated. The disease is bilateral and is genetically determined, most likely as an autosomal recessive trait which is so common that it is easily confused with dominant inheritance (pseudodominant). Infantile glaucoma usually has an autosomal recessive mode of inheritance.

In the USA it is estimated that there are 2 million people with glaucoma; about 25% of these cases are undetected. About 90% of all cases of glaucoma are of the open-angle type.

Clinical Findings

Patients with open-angle glaucoma have no symptoms initially. On examination, there may be slight cupping of the optic disk. The visual fields gradually constrict, but central vision remains good until late in the disease.

Tonometry, ophthalmoscopic visualization of the optic nerve, and central visual field testing are the 3 prime tests for the diagnosis and continued clinical evaluation of glaucoma. The normal intraocular pressure is about 10–25 mm Hg. Except in acute glaucoma, however, the diagnosis is never made on the basis of one tonometric measurement, since various factors can influence the pressure (eg, diurnal variation). Transient elevations of intraocular pressure do not constitute glaucoma (for the same reason that periodic or intermittent elevations of blood pressure do not constitute hypertensive disease).

Prevention

All persons over age 20 should have tonometric and ophthalmoscopic examinations every 3–5 years. The examination may be performed by the general physician, internist, or ophthalmologist. If there is a family history of glaucoma, annual examination is indicated. Mydriatic and cycloplegic drugs should not be used in any patient with a narrow anterior chamber angle.

Treatment

Most patients can be controlled with miotics, eg, pilocarpine, 1–2%, 3–4 times daily. Pilocarpine increases the rate of outflow of aqueous. Carbonic anhydrase inhibitors—eg, acetazolamide—decrease the rate of aqueous production. Epinephrine eye drops, 0.5–2%, decrease aqueous production and increase outflow. (*Caution:* Epinephrine is contraindicated if the anterior chamber angle is narrow.) Timolol, a beta-adrenergic blocking agent, is a new and effective antiglaucoma agent. It is used alone (every 12 hours) or in combination with other intraocular pressure-lowering agents.

Prognosis

Untreated chronic glaucoma that begins at age 40–45 will probably cause complete blindness by age 60–65. Early diagnosis and treatment will preserve useful vision throughout life in most cases.

Glaucoma. *Ophthalmology* 1981;**88**:175. [Entire issue.]

Kolker AE, Hetherington J: *Becker-Shaffer's Diagnosis and Therapy of the Glaucomas,* 5th ed. Mosby, 1982.

Maumenee AE et al: Causes of optic nerve damage in glaucoma. *Ophthalmology* 1983;**7**:741.

Wise J: Long-term control of adult open-angle glaucoma by argon laser treatment. *Ophthalmology* 1981;**88**:197.

Yanoff M, Stone RA: A clinicopathologic study of four cases of primary open-angle glaucoma compared to normal eyes. *Am J Ophthalmol* 1981;**91**:88.

Zimmerman TJ et al: Timolol update. *Surv Ophthalmol* (Dec) 1983;**28(Suppl)**:227.

RETINAL DISORDERS ASSOCIATED WITH SYSTEMIC DISEASES

Many systemic diseases are associated with retinal manifestations. Some of the more common ones include essential hypertension, diabetes mellitus, preeclampsia-eclampsia of pregnancy, blood dyscrasias, sarcoidosis, syphilis, and toxoplasmosis. The retinal damage caused by these disorders can be easily observed with the aid of the ophthalmoscope.

One method of classifying hypertensive retinopathy (modified after Keith and Wagener) is shown in Table 5–2.

Diabetic retinopathy is the leading cause of new blindness among American adults aged 20–65. In recent years, it has been broadly classified as proliferative or nonproliferative.

Nonproliferative retinopathy is characterized by dilatation of veins, microaneurysms, and retinal hemorrhages plus retinal edema and hard and soft exudates. **Proliferative retinopathy** is more devastating and is characterized by neovascularization and hemorrhage that result in fibrovascular proliferation into the vitreous, a forerunner of virtually untreatable total retinal detachment. In general, the visual progno-

Table 5–2. A classification of hypertensive retinopathy. (Modified after Keith and Wagener.)

Stage	Ophthalmoscopic Appearance	Clinical Classification
I	Minimal narrowing or sclerosis of arterioles.	"Essential" hypertension (chronic, benign, "arteriosclerotic").
II	Thickening and dulling of vessel reflection (copper wire appearance). Localized and generalized narrowing of arterioles. Changes at arteriovenous crossings (A-V nicking). Scattered tiny round or flame-shaped hemorrhages. Vascular occlusion may be present.	
III	Sclerotic changes may not be marked. "Angiospastic retinopathy": localized arteriolar spasm, hemorrhages, exudates, "cotton wool patches," retinal edema.	Malignant hypertensive retinopathy.
IV	Same as III, plus papilledema.	

sis with proliferative retinopathy is much worse than with nonproliferative retinopathy.

It should be emphasized that if nonproliferative retinopathy is recognized early, laser photocoagulation treatment will prevent progression of the disease and preserve vision. Patients with insulin-dependent diabetes mellitus should have a careful yearly ophthalmoscopic examination through dilated pupils. Examination by an ophthalmologist is usually advisable if the diabetes is of more than 10 years' duration, or earlier if ocular symptoms are present or if there are suspicious findings of retinopathy on ophthalmoscopic examination. Failure to diagnose nonproliferative retinopathy by ophthalmoscopic examination is common (see Sussman reference below). Fluorescein angiography may be required when an ophthalmologist wishes to verify a clinical diagnosis of nonproliferative retinopathy. There is adequate evidence now to show that the risk of diabetic retinopathy can be lessened by careful control of blood glucose levels and of coexisting hypertension.

Senile macular degeneration is the leading cause of new cases of visual impairment and blindness in persons over age 65 in the USA. Initially there is irregular thickening of the choroid, drusen deposits, and associated sclerosis of the choroid capillaries. The overlying pigment epithelium is disturbed, especially in the macula and at the disk margin. In the early stages, which may continue for many years, there may be only a small loss of visual acuity. Later there may be neovascularization, bleeding, and serous detachment of the pigment epithelium. The later complications cause severe loss of central vision. In a small percentage of cases, if the macular degeneration is diagnosed early and neovascularization has not spread to the fovea, preliminary reports suggest that some patients may be treated successfully with argon laser photocoagulation.

Preeclampsia-eclampsia is manifested in the retina as rapidly progressive hypertensive retinopathy, and extensive permanent retinal damage may occur if the pregnancy is not terminated. Occasionally, the choroidal circulation is mainly affected, leading to infarction of the retinal pigment epithelium.

In **blood dyscrasias,** various types of hemorrhages are present in both the retina and choroid and may lead to blindness. If the underlying dyscrasia is successfully treated and macular hemorrhages have not occurred, it is possible to regain normal vision.

The chorioretinitis associated with **syphilis** is striking. There are many small yellow dots and pigment clumps in the peripheral fundus, giving a typical "salt and pepper" appearance.

Toxoplasmosis produces necrotizing lesions of retinochoroiditis that may involve the posterior pole and the macular area. The active lesion appears as a white elevated granuloma with inflammatory cells in the vitreous. The vitreous appears hazy and may sometimes obscure the lesion. In the healed stage, a punched-out pigmented chorioretinal lesion develops through which the sclera is clearly visible. Treatment consists of the administration of sulfadiazine and pyrimethamine.

Retinal Vasculitis

Inflammation of the retinal veins (retinal periphlebitis) may occur as an isolated phenomenon or as part of a multisystem disorder such as sarcoidosis or Behçet's disease. Fluffy white thickening of the vein wall with associated venous occlusion may occur.

Patients with retinal vasculitis may need systemic steroids or cytotoxic therapy. Recently, cyclosporine has been shown to be effective in Behçet's disease.

Acquired Immunodeficiency Syndrome (AIDS)

Patients with AIDS who develop retinal cotton wool spots and hemorrhages may be suffering from opportunistic invasion of the eye by normally harmless organisms such as *Pneumocystis carinii* or cytomegalovirus. Patients have low white cell counts and a marked reversal of normal helper/suppressor T lymphocyte ratios. Overwhelming opportunistic infection may be apparent on ocular examination before other clinical features of AIDS appear.

Constable IJ et al: Assessing the risk of diabetic retinopathy. *Am J Ophthalmol* 1984;**79**:53.

Dumonde D et al: Anti-renal autoimmunity and circulating immune complexes in patients with retinal vasculitis. *Lancet* 1982;**2**:787.

Freeman MK et al: The use of radionuclide retinal scintigraphy for the assessment of retinopathy in diabetes mellitus. *Ophthalmology* 1983;**90**:513.

Khadem M et al: Ophthalmological findings in acquired immune deficiency syndrome (AIDS). *Arch Ophthalmol* 1984;**102**:201.

Spalton D: Fundus changes in histologically confirmed sarcoidosis. *Br J Ophthalmol* 1981;**65**:348.

Sussman EJ, Tsiaras WG, Soper KA: Diagnosis of diabetic eye disease. *JAMA* 1982;**247**:3231.

RETINAL DETACHMENT

Essentials of Diagnosis

- Blurred vision in one eye becoming progressively worse. ("A curtain came down over my eye.")
- No pain or redness.
- Detachment seen by ophthalmoscopy.

General Considerations

Detachment of the retina is usually spontaneous but may be secondary to trauma. Spontaneous detachment occurs most frequently in persons over 50 years of age. Predisposing causes such as aphakia, myopia, and trauma are common.

Clinical Findings

As soon as the retina is torn, a transudate from the choroidal vessels, combines with abnormal vitreous traction on the retina and the force of gravity to strip the retina from the choroid. The superior temporal area is the most common site of detachment. The area of detachment rapidly increases, causing corresponding progressive visual loss. Central vision remains intact until the macula becomes detached.

On ophthalmoscopic examination, the retina is seen hanging in the vitreous like a gray cloud. One or more retinal tears, usually crescent-shaped and red or orange, are always present and can be seen by an experienced examiner.

Differential Diagnosis

Sudden partial loss of vision in one eye may also be due to retinal or vitreous hemorrhage and central retinal vessel (artery or vein) occlusion.

Treatment

All cases of retinal detachment should be referred immediately to an ophthalmologist. During transportation over a long distance, the patient's head should be positioned so that the detached portion of the retina will fall back with the aid of gravity. For example, a patient with a superior temporal retinal detachment in the right eye should lie supine, head turned to the right. Head position is less important during transportation for a short distance.

Treatment consists of drainage of the subretinal fluid and closure of the retinal tears by diathermy, with or without scleral buckling or the application of a Lincoff sponge. Diathermy produces an inflammatory reaction that causes the retina to adhere to the choroid. Photocoagulation is of value in a limited number of cases of minimal detachment. It consists of focusing a strong light ("burning glass") through the pupil to create an area of inflammation between the choroid and the retina. The laser is used in the same manner as the photocoagulator. The main use of both instruments is in the prevention of detachment by sealing small retinal tears before detachment occurs.

Cryosurgery is widely and effectively used in the treatment of retinal detachment. A supercooled probe is applied to the sclera to cause a chorioretinal scar with minimal scleral damage. In areas of the world where it is available, cryosurgery has replaced diathermy in the operative management of retinal detachment.

Prognosis

About 80% of uncomplicated cases can be cured with one operation; an additional 10% will need repeated operations; the remainder never reattach. The prognosis is worse if the macula is detached, if there are many vitreous strands, or if the detachment is of long duration. Without treatment, retinal detachment almost always becomes total in 1–6 months. Spontaneous detachments are ultimately bilateral in 20–25% of cases.

Chawla HB: A review of techniques employed in 1100 cases of retinal detachment. *Br J Ophthalmol* 1982;**66:**636.

Verdaguer J: Juvenile retinal detachment. *Am J Ophthalmol* 1982;**93:**145.

CATARACT

Essentials of Diagnosis

- Blurred vision, progressive over months or years.
- No pain or redness.
- Lens opacities (may be grossly visible).

General Considerations

A cataract is a lens opacity. Cataracts are usually bilateral. They may be congenital or may occur as a result of trauma or, less commonly, systemic disease. Senile cataract is by far the most common type; most persons over 60 have some degree of lens opacity.

Clinical Findings

Even in its early stages, a cataract can be seen through a dilated pupil with an ophthalmoscope, a slit lamp, or an ordinary hand illuminator. As the cataract matures, the retina will become increasingly more difficult to visualize, until finally the fundus reflection is absent. At this point, the pupil is white and the cataract is mature.

The degree of visual loss corresponds to the density of the cataract.

Treatment

Only a small percentage of senile cataracts require surgical removal. Degree of visual impairment is the prime surgical criterion; other factors include age, general health, and occupation. Treatment of senile cataract consists of removal of the entire lens followed by refractive correction with a spectacle cataract lens. Contact lenses are replacing the heavy cataract lenses mainly in younger patients and patients of any age requiring surgery in one eye only.

Implantation of **intraocular lenses** at the time of cataract removal has become increasingly popular within the past few years. The original intraocular lenses developed in London by Ridley in 1949 proved to be disastrous. However, greatly improved lens design has made the concept more attractive to patients, despite the increased risk as compared with the standard intracapsular operation. There are a number of pre-existing ocular diseases, including diabetes and uveitis, that cause intraocular lenses to be poorly tolerated.

An alternative to the intraocular lens is the continuous wear soft contact lens that can be worn day and night for weeks to months at a time. Considerable improvement in this device has also occurred within recent years.

Intraocular lenses are being inserted by an increasing number of cataract surgeons throughout the world.

Prognosis

If surgery is indicated, lens extraction improves visual acuity in 95% of cases. The remainder either have preexisting retinal damage or develop postoperative complications such as glaucoma, hemorrhage, retinal detachment, or infection.

Drews RC et al: Cataracts: Intraocular lens. *Ophthalmology* 1983;**4**:301.

Frayer WC: What's new in surgery? Ophthalmic surgery. *Bull Am Coll Surg* 1982;**67**:32.

Klein B et al: Cataracts and macular degeneration in older Americans. *Arch Ophthalmol* 1982;**100**:571.

Yanoff M: Cataract surgery: When and how. *Geriatrics* (Nov) 1982;**37**:71.

●   ●   ●

PRINCIPLES OF TREATMENT OF OCULAR INFECTIONS

Identification of Pathogen

Before one can determine the drug of choice, the causative organism must be identified. For example, a pneumococcal corneal ulcer will respond to treatment with a sulfonamide, penicillin, or any broad-spectrum antibiotic, but this is not true in the case of corneal ulcer due to *Pseudomonas aeruginosa,* which requires vigorous treatment with polymyxin or gentamicin. Another example is staphylococcal dacryocystitis, which, if it does not respond to penicillin, is most likely to respond to erythromycin.

Choice of Alternative Drugs

In the treatment of infectious eye disease, eg, conjunctivitis, one should always use the drug that is the most effective, the least likely to cause complications, and the least expensive. It is also preferable to use a drug that is not usually given systemically, eg, sulfacetamide or bacitracin. Of the available antibacterial agents, the sulfonamides come closest to meeting these specifications. Two reliable sulfonamides for ophthalmic use are sulfisoxazole and sodium sulfacetamide. The sulfonamides have the added advantages of low allergenicity and effectiveness against the chlamydial group of organisms. They are available in ointment or solution form.

Two of the most effective broad-spectrum antibiotics for ophthalmic use are gentamicin and neomycin. Both of these drugs have some effect against gram-negative as well as gram-positive organisms. Allergic reactions to neomycin are common. Other antibiotics frequently used are erythromycin, the tetracyclines, bacitracin, and polymyxin. Combined bacitracin-polymyxin ointment is often used prophylactically after corneal foreign body removal for the protection it affords against both gram-positive and gram-negative organisms.

Method of Administration

Most ocular anti-infective drugs are administered locally. Systemic administration as well is required for all intraocular infections, corneal ulcer, orbital cellulitis, dacryocystitis, and any severe external infection that does not respond to local treatment.

Ointment Versus Liquid Medications

Ointments have greater therapeutic effectiveness than solutions, since contact can be maintained longer. However, they do cause blurring of vision; if this must be avoided, solutions should be used.

Barza M, Baum J: Ocular infections. *Med Clin North Am* 1983; **67**:131.

Burns RP (editor): Symposium on drugs. *Ophthalmology* 1979; **86**:79.

Havener WH: *Ocular Pharmacology,* 5th ed. Mosby, 1983.

Robin JS, Ellis PP: Ophthalmic ointments. *Surv Ophthalmol* 1978;**22**:335.

Vaughan D, Asbury T: *General Ophthalmology,* 10th ed. Lange, 1983.

TECHNIQUES USED IN THE TREATMENT OF OCULAR DISORDERS

Instilling Medications

Place the patient in a chair with head tilted back, both eyes open, and looking up. Retract the lower lid slightly and instill 2 drops of liquid into the lower cul-de-sac. Have the patient look down while finger contact on the lower lid is maintained. Do not let the patient squeeze the eyes shut.

Ointments are instilled in the same general manner.

Self-Medication

The same techniques are used as described above, except that drops are usually better instilled with the patient lying down.

Eye Bandage

Most eye bandages should be applied firmly enough to hold the lid securely against the cornea. An ordinary patch consisting of gauze-covered cotton is usually sufficient. Tape is applied from the cheek to the forehead. If more pressure is desired, use 2 or 3 bandages. The black eye patch is difficult to sterilize and therefore is seldom used.

Warm Compresses

A clean towel or washcloth soaked in warm tap water is applied to the affected eye for 10–15 minutes 2–4 times a day.

Removal of a Superficial Corneal Foreign Body

Record the patient's visual acuity, if possible, and instill sterile local anesthetic drops. With the patient sitting or lying down, an assistant should direct a strong light into the eye so that the rays strike the cornea obliquely. Using either a loupe or a slit lamp, the physician locates the foreign body on the corneal surface. It may then be removed with a sterile wet cotton applicator or, if this fails, with a spud, with the lids held apart with the other hand to prevent blinking. An antibacterial ointment (gentamicin) is instilled after the foreign body has been removed. It is preferable not to patch the eye, but the patient must be seen on the following day to make certain healing is under way.

PRECAUTIONS IN MANAGEMENT OF OCULAR DISORDERS

Use of Local Anesthetics

Unsupervised self-administration of local anesthetics is dangerous because the patient may further injure an anesthetized eye without knowing it. The drug may also prevent the normal healing process. An abrasion expected to heal in 24 hours may still be present after a month or more of "treatment" with a local anesthetic.

Pupillary Dilation

Use cycloplegics and mydriatics with caution. Dilating the pupil can precipitate an acute glaucoma attack if the patient has a narrow anterior chamber angle.

Local Corticosteroid Therapy

Repeated use of local corticosteroids presents several serious hazards: herpes simplex (dendritic) keratitis, fungal overgrowth, open-angle glaucoma, and cataract formation. Furthermore, perforation of the cornea may occur when the corticosteroids are used for herpes simplex keratitis.

Contaminated Eye Medications

Ophthalmic solutions must be prepared with the same degree of care as fluids intended for intravenous administration.

Tetracaine, proparacaine, and fluorescein are most likely to become contaminated. The most dangerous is fluorescein, as this solution is frequently contaminated with *Pseudomonas aeruginosa*, an organism that can rapidly destroy the eye. Sterile fluorescein filter paper strips are now available and are recommended in place of fluorescein solutions.

The following rules should be observed in handling eye medications for use in the diagnostic examination of uninjured eyes: (1) Obtain solutions in small amounts from the pharmacy. (2) Be certain that the solution is sterile as prepared and that it contains an effective antibacterial agent. (3) Date the bottle at the time it is procured.

Plastic dropper bottles are in widespread use; solutions from these bottles are safe to use in uninjured eyes. Whether in plastic or glass containers, eye solutions should not remain in use for long periods after the bottle is opened. Two weeks after opening is a reasonable maximal time to use a solution before discarding.

If the eye has been injured accidentally or by surgical trauma, it is of the greatest importance to use sterile medications supplied in sterile disposable single-use eyedropper units.

Ocular Irritation

Patients receiving long-term topical therapy may develop local toxic reactions to preservatives, especially if there is inadequate tear secretion. Burning and soreness are exacerbated by drop instillation; occasionally, fibrosis and scarring of the conjunctiva and cornea may occur.

Fungal Overgrowth

Since antibiotics, like corticosteroids, when used over a prolonged period of time in bacterial corneal ulcers, favor the development of secondary fungal corneal infection, the sulfonamides should be used whenever they are adequate for the purpose.

Systemic Effects of Ocular Drugs

The systemic absorption of certain topical drugs (through the lacrimal drainage system) must be considered when there is a systemic medical contraindication to the use of the drug. Exercise caution, for example, when using ophthalmic solutions of the beta-blocker timolol (Timoptic) in patients with cardiac disease, asthma, or diabetes mellitus. Atropine ointment should be prescribed for children rather than the drops, since absorption of the 1% topical solution may be toxic. Phenylephrine eye drops can precipitate hypertensive crises. Also to be considered are adverse interactions between systemically administered and ocular drugs. Patients who have used echothiophate drops to manage glaucoma are at risk of prolonged apnea from succinylcholine used in anesthesia. On the other hand, oral levodopa administration has been shown to reduce the mydriasis following topical phenylephrine. A few minutes of nasolacrimal occlusion or eyelid closure improves efficacy and decreases systemic side effects of topical agents.

Sensitization

An antibiotic instilled into the eye can sensitize the patient to that drug and cause a hypersensitivity reaction upon subsequent systemic administration.

Table 5—3. Adverse ocular effects of systemic drugs.

Drug	Possible Side Effects
Respiratory agents	
Oxygen	Retrolental fibroplasia (in premature infants). Blurring of vision, constriction of visual fields.
Cardiovascular system drugs	
Cardiac glycosides (digitalis, etc)	Disturbances of color vision, blurring of vision, scotomas.
Quinidine	Toxic amblyopia.
Thiazides (Diuril, etc)	Xanthopsia (yellow vision), myopia.
Carbonic anhydrase inhibitors (acetazolamide)	Ocular hypotony, transient myopia.
Gastrointestinal drugs	
Anticholinergic agents (eg, atropine)	Risk of angle-closure glaucoma due to mydriasis. Blurring of vision due to cycloplegia (occasional).
Central nervous system drugs	
Barbiturates	Extraocular muscle palsies with diplopia, ptosis, cortical blindness.
Chloral hydrate	Diplopia, ptosis, miosis.
Phenothiazines (eg, chlorpromazine)	Toxic amblyopia, deposits of pigment in conjunctiva, cornea, lens, and retina. Oculogyric crises.
Amphetamines	Widening of palpebral fissure. Dilatation of pupil, paralysis of ciliary muscle with loss of accommodation.
Monoamine oxidase inhibitors	Nystagmus, extraocular muscle palsies, amblyopia (toxic).
Tricyclic agents	Dilatation of pupil (risk of angle-closure glaucoma), cycloplegia.
Phenytoin	Nystagmus, diplopia, ptosis, slight blurring of vision (rare).
Neostigmine	Nystagmus, miosis.
Morphine	Miosis.
Hormones	
Corticosteroids	Cataract (posterior subcapsular), local immunologic suppression causing susceptibility to viral (herpesvirus hominis), bacterial, and fungal infections; steroid-induced glaucoma.
Female sex hormones	Retinal artery thrombosis, retinal vein thrombosis, papilledema, ocular palsies with diplopia, nystagmus, optic neuritis and atrophy, retinal vasculitis, scotomas, migraine, and mydriasis and cycloplegia.
Antibiotics	
Chloramphenicol	Optic neuritis and atrophy. Toxic amblyopia (rare).
Streptomycin	Toxic amblyopia (rare).
Antimalarial agents	
Eg, chloroquine	Macular changes, central scotomas, pigmentary degeneration of the retina, chloroquine keratopathy, ocular palsies, ptosis, ERG depression.
Chemotherapeutic agents	
Sulfonamides	Conjunctivitis in Stevens-Johnson syndrome causing cicatrization of the conjunctiva. Toxic amblyopia (rare).
Ethambutol	Toxic amblyopia, optic neuritis and atrophy.
Isoniazid	Toxic amblyopia, optic neuritis and atrophy.
Aminosalicylic acid	Toxic amblyopia.
Heavy metals	
Gold salts	Deposits in the cornea and conjunctiva.
Lead compounds	Toxic amblyopia, papilledema, ocular palsies.
Oral hypoglycemic agents	
Chlorpropamide	Transient change in refractive error, toxic amblyopia, diplopia.
Vitamins	
Vitamin A	Papilledema, retinal hemorrhages, loss of eyebrows and eyelashes, nystagmus, diplopia, blurring of vision.
Vitamin D	Band-shaped keratopathy.
Antirheumatic agents	
Salicylates	Toxic amblyopia, cortical blindness (rare).
Indomethacin	Corneal deposits, toxic amblyopia, diplopia, retinal changes.
Phenylbutazone	Toxic amblyopia, retinal hemorrhages.

• • •

References

Abrahamson IA: Eye changes after forty. *Am Fam Physician* (April) 1984;**29**:171.

Adler AG et al: Systemic effects of eye drops. *Arch Intern Med* 1982;**142**:2293.

Beard C: *Ptosis*, 3rd ed. Mosby, 1981.

Chumbley LC: *Ophthalmology in Internal Medicine*. Saunders, 1981.

Cogan DG: *Ophthalmic Manifestations of Systemic Vascular Disease*. Saunders, 1974.

Ellis PP: *Ocular Therapeutics and Pharmacology*, 6th ed. Mosby, 1981.

Fraunfelder FT: *Drug-Induced Ocular Side Effects and Drug Interactions*, 2nd ed. Lea & Febiger, 1980.

Hansten PD: *Drug Interactions*, 4th ed. Lea & Febiger, 1979.

Harrington DO: *The Visual Fields: A Textbook and Atlas of Clinical Perimetry*, 5th ed. Mosby, 1981.

Havener WH: *Ocular Pharmacology*, 5th ed. Mosby, 1983.

Havener WH: *Synopsis of Ophthalmology*, 5th ed. Mosby, 1979.

Henkind P et al (editorial consultants): *Physicians' Desk Reference (PDR) for Ophthalmology*. Medical Economics, 1983.

Hughes WF (editor): *Year Book of Ophthalmology*. Year Book, 1982.

Kaufman HE, Zimmerman TJ (editors): *Current Concepts in Ophthalmology*. Vol 7. Mosby, 1981.

Kolker AE, Hetherington J: *Becker-Shaffer's Diagnosis and Therapy of the Glaucomas*, 5th ed. Mosby, 1982.

Melamed MA: A generalist's guide to eye emergencies. *Emergency Med* (Feb 15) 1984;**16**:99.

Miller NR: *Walsh & Hoyt's Clinical Neuro-Ophthalmology*, 4th ed. Vol 1. Williams & Wilkins, 1982.

Moses RA: *Adler's Physiology of the Eye: Clinical Application*, 7th ed. Mosby, 1981.

Newell FW: *Ophthalmology: Principles and Concepts*, 5th ed. Mosby, 1982.

Schachter J, Dawson CR: *Human Chlamydial Infections*. PSG Publishing Co, Inc., 1978.

Scheie HG, Albert DM: *Textbook of Ophthalmology*, 9th ed. Saunders, 1977.

Schoene RB et al: Effects of betaxolol, timolol and placebo on pulmonary function in asthmatic bronchitis. *Am J Ophthalmol* 1984;**97**:86.

Trevor-Roper PD: *Lecture Notes on Ophthalmology*, 6th ed. Blackwell, 1980.

Vaughan D, Asbury T: *General Ophthalmology*, 10th ed. Lange, 1983.

Von Noorden GK: *Von Noorden–Maumenee's Atlas of Strabismus*, 4th ed. Mosby, 1983.

Zimmerman TJ et al: Improving the therapeutic index of topically applied ocular drugs. *Arch Ophthalmol* 1984;**102**:55.

6 | Ear, Nose, & Throat

Wayne W. Deatsch, MD

DISEASES OF THE EAR

HEARING LOSS

Classification

A. Sensorineural (Nerve) Deafness:
1. Receptor end organ (cochlea).
2. Neural pathways.
3. Central. Auditory cortex lesions are bilateral.

B. Conductive Deafness: Disturbances of the external or middle ear preventing normal sound transmission.

C. Mixed Deafness: Combined sensorineural and conductive deafness.

D. Functional Deafness: No organic lesion can be detected.

General Considerations

Five to 10% of the population have a severe temporary or permanent hearing impairment.

Sensorineural hearing loss may be congenital, due to birth trauma, maternal rubella, erythroblastosis fetalis, or malformations of the inner ear; or it may be due to traumatic injury to the inner ear or eighth nerve, vascular disorders with hemorrhage or thrombosis in the inner ear, ototoxic agents (Table 6–1), bacterial and viral infections (meningitis, encephalitis, mumps, etc), severe febrile illnesses, Meniere's disease, posterior fossa tumors, multiple sclerosis, presbycusis (due to aging), tertiary syphilis, myxedema, or prolonged or repeated exposure to loud sound. Two or more of these causative factors may be synergistic (eg, noise may potentiate drug ototoxicity).

Conductive hearing loss may also be congenital, due to malformations of the external or middle ear. Trauma may produce perforation of the eardrum or disruption of the ossicular chain. Inflammatory middle ear disease may produce serous otitis media, acute or chronic purulent otitis media, or adhesive otitis media. Otosclerosis, a common familial conductive hearing loss with onset in middle life, produces ankylosis of the stapes by overgrowth of new spongy bone; the cause is not known.

Clinical Findings

The older patient will usually be aware of hearing loss of significant degree, and an accurate history is of importance to determine the cause. All of the causes of hearing loss listed above must be investigated. In particular, the age at onset, degree of loss, progression,

Table 6–1. Ototoxic agents.*

Drug	Auditory Disturbance	Vestibular Disturbance	Remarks
Antibiotics			
Capreomycin	+	+	Rare.
Gentamicin and all aminoglycoside antibiotics	+	++	Frequent.
Kanamycin	++	+	Occasional. Onset may be delayed.
Neomycin	++	±	Occasional. Any route of administration.
Paromomycin	++	±	Occasional.
Streptomycin	++	++	Frequent.
Vancomycin	++	+	Occasional.
Viomycin	++	++	Frequent.
Diuretics			
Ethacrynic acid	++	+	Occasional. Usually transient.
Furosemide	++	+	Following intravenous use. Usually transient.
Salicylates	+	++	Tinnitus. Tone decay. Usually reversible.
Antimalarials			
Chloroquine	++	+	Rare. Progressive, irreversible.
Quinine (and quinidine)	+	++	Tinnitus. Usually reversible, transitory deafness (rare).

*Ototoxicity of offending drugs may be enhanced by (1) impaired renal function due to renal damage, shock, dehydration, etc; (2) high dosages of drug, such as salicylates in rheumatoid arthritis; (3) use of 2 aminoglycosides simultaneously; and (4) perhaps by potentiation by other drugs (eg, diuretics, especially furosemide). Many other drugs and industrial, agricultural, and household chemicals are also reported to produce ototoxicity.

Table 6–2. Differentiation of sensorineural and conductive deafness.

	Conductive Deafness	Sensorineural Deafness
Patient's voice	Speaks softly	Speaks loudly
Effect of noisy environment	Hears best	Hears poorly
Speech discrimination	Good	Poor
Hearing on telephone	Good	Poor
Weber test lateralization	To diseased ear	To good ear
Rinne test	Negative (AC < BC)	Positive (AC > BC)

AC = Air conduction. BC = Bone conduction.

associated tinnitus or vertigo, exposure to head trauma, sound trauma, ototoxic drugs, previous infection, and severe febrile illnesses must be checked.

In infants and young children, the diagnosis is often suggested by failure of speech development, lack of cooperation, inability to concentrate, and slow progress in learning.

A complete ear, nose, and throat examination is essential for all patients with hearing loss. Most important is examination of the ear canal, eardrum, and middle ear with the magnifying otoscope to detect even slight abnormalities. Attention must be given to obstructing or infected adenoids and tonsils, nasal and sinus infection, and evidences of other cranial nerve disturbance. Alert parents and family physicians often can detect hearing loss in young infants (6–9 months) by their failure to respond to appropriate sounds. Special attention should be paid to "high-risk" newborns, those with Rh incompatibilities, premature infants, or infants delivered after prolonged or difficult labor or whose mothers had viral infections during pregnancy.

Special tests of value are as follows:

(1) Whispered and spoken voice test: In a quiet room, with the other ear covered, the tested normal ear should be able to accurately perceive the spoken voice at 6 m and the whispered voice at 4.5 m.

(2) Tuning fork tests: The 500-Hz and 1000-Hz forks are the most important. These tests detect lateralization of the sounds of the fork and comparative disturbances of air conduction and bone conduction (to distinguish conductive loss and nerve type loss).

(3) Audiometric tests (pure tone, speech tests, and other highly specialized audiometric tests) provide quantitative measurements of hearing loss. Audiometry is invaluable in following the progress of patients with ear disorders and hearing impairment and for the proper evaluation of hearing aids.

(4) Labyrinthine tests give valuable objective evidence of inner ear function. An absent or altered labyrinthine response is quite significant. The test is done by irrigating the ear canals with hot or cold water to produce nystagmus and vertigo. The response in each ear should be equal.

(5) The electronystagmogram (ENG) may be of value in the identification and interpretation of nystagmus, especially in response to labyrinthine tests.

Treatment

A. Hearing Loss in Children: Recurrent otitis media and serous otitis media are the commonest causes of conductive hearing loss in children and require prompt diagnosis and medical treatment (see pp 108–111). In persistent cases, investigation of nasal allergy or infection and adenoidectomy and insertion of ventilating tubes may be necessary. At about age 12 years, improved immune response and improved auditory tube function with growth result in a marked decrease in ear problems. Chronic otitis media with mastoiditis, cholesteatoma, or granulation tissue may require extensive tympanoplastic surgery.

Sensorineural hearing loss or uncorrectable conductive hearing loss in children usually requires aural rehabilitation. This includes early diagnosis, use of a hearing aid, and lip reading and speech training.

B. Hearing Loss in Adults:

1. Nerve deafness–Nerve loss due to acoustic trauma will sometimes improve over a period of 6 months if the patient can avoid exposure to loud noise. The best treatment is prevention of exposure to loud noise either by avoiding the sources of noise (industry, recreation, military) or by wearing suitable protective earplugs or other noise attenuators. Exposure to highly amplified "rock" music should be avoided.

Drugs known to be ototoxic (see p 106) should be used with caution; measurement of blood levels to control drug dosage may be required. Prompt evaluation of hearing and vestibular problems (decreased hearing, tinnitus, instability while walking) by careful history and physical examination and, when indicated, audiometry and electronystagmography may help prevent severe sensorineural hearing loss. Additional causes of sensorineural hearing loss in adults that require prompt, effective treatment include central nervous system infections (eg, meningitis, syphilis), diabetes mellitus, Meniere's disease, and vestibular nerve tumors.

The nerve loss of Meniere's disease often improves with treatment and between attacks. A fluctuating loss has a more favorable prognosis than a sudden severe loss. Medical management consists of a low-sodium diet, potassium substitution for sodium (KCl, 1 g 3 times daily for 1–2 weeks), antihistamines (eg, diphenhydramine, 4 times daily for 1–2 months), nicotinic acid in flushing doses 4 times daily, and reassurance. There is no medical or surgical treatment for actual nerve damage in other forms of sensorineural deafness except as mentioned above.

Acoustic neuroma or other cerebellopontine angle tumor will produce a unilateral sensorineural hearing loss. This is usually slowly progressive and associated with tinnitus and, later, unsteadiness. Diagnostic audiometry, impedance audiometry, and special diagnostic audiometry (site-of-lesion testing), combined with tests of labyrinthine function (electronystagmography) and x-ray studies of the temporal bone (plain films, polytomography, CT scanning, and posterior fossa myelography), distinguish this from other unilateral sensorineural hearing loss. Early diagnosis is essential for best surgical results, so any unilateral sensorineural hearing loss should be carefully studied.

2. Conductive deafness–Important advances have been made recently in the surgical treatment of middle ear deafness. Otosclerosis may be treated successfully by a direct operation on the fixed stapes through the ear canal and middle ear. Techniques involve removal of the stapes and replacement of the foot plate with a graft and replacement of the stapes crura with a prosthesis.

Perforations of the eardrum can be repaired by fascia or skin grafting (myringoplasty).

Mastoid and middle ear operations have been designed for the treatment of suppuration and the removal of cholesteatoma and to preserve or improve hearing by skin grafting and by replacing or realigning the ossicular chain (tympanoplasty).

For serous otitis media, see p 110.

3. Aural rehabilitation of adults–This should include provision for satisfactory amplification of sound. A hearing aid should neither be recommended for nor denied to a patient until feasibility of use is determined by careful audiometric testing (pure tone and speech). Total auditory abilities and deficits as well as the desires of the individual patient must be considered. Advanced age itself does not preclude satisfactory use of a hearing aid. Lip reading is of value to patients who have difficulty with speech discrimination or who require good speech reception at work.

Cochlear implantation is currently approved in the USA for selected profoundly deaf adults who have already developed speech.

Council on Scientific Affairs, American Medical Association: Cochlear implants. *JAMA* 1983;**250**:391.

D'Alonzo BJ, Cantor MB: Ototoxicity: Etiology and issues. *J Fam Pract* 1983;**16**:489.

Dobie RA: Hearing conservation in industry. *West J Med* 1982;**137**:499.

Guidotti TL, Novak RE: Hearing conservatism and occupational exposure to noise. *Am Fam Physician* (Oct) 1983;**28**:181.

Irvine PW: The hearing-impaired elderly patient. *Postgrad Med* (Oct) 1982;**72**:115.

Ludman H: ABC of ENT: Assessing deafness. *Br Med J* 1981;**282**:207.

Paparella MM: Differential diagnosis of hearing loss. *Laryngoscope* 1978;**88**:952.

Symposium on audiology. *Otolaryngol Clin North Am* 1978; **11**:597. [Entire issue.]

DISEASES OF THE EXTERNAL EAR

1. IMPACTED CERUMEN

Cerumen is the normal secretion of the cartilaginous part of the ear canal; it serves a protective function. Normally it dries and falls out of the ear canal, but it may accumulate within the canal because of dryness or scaling of the skin, narrowing or tortuos-

ity of the ear canal, or excess hair in the ear canal. It may be packed in deeper by repeated unskilled attempts to remove it. There are usually no symptoms until the canal becomes completely occluded, when a feeling of fullness, deafness or tinnitus, or a cough due to reflex stimulation of the vagus nerve may occur. Otoscopy reveals the mass of yellow, brown, or black wax that may be sticky and soft, waxy, or hard.

If the mass is firm and movable, it may be removed through the speculum with a dull ring curet or a cotton applicator. If this is painful, the impaction may be removed by irrigation with water at body temperature, directing the stream of water from a large syringe at the wall of the ear canal and catching the solution in a basin held beneath the ear. If the impaction is hard and adherent and cannot be readily removed by irrigation, it must be softened by repeated instillations of oily (baby oil) ear drops, glycerin (70% by volume), or hydrogen peroxide (3%) and irrigated again in 2–3 days.

2. EXTERNAL OTITIS

External otitis may vary in severity from a diffuse mild eczematoid dermatitis to cellulitis or even furunculosis of the ear canal. It is frequently referred to as a fungal infection of the ear, although in many cases there is no infection and the reaction is a contact dermatitis (earphones, earrings) or a variant of seborrheic dermatitis. Infections of the ear canal are usually bacterial (staphylococci and gram-negative rods), with occasional secondary infection by fungi (*Aspergillus, Mucor, Penicillium*). Predisposing factors are moisture in the ear canal resulting from a warm, moist climate or from swimming or bathing; trauma due to attempts to clean or scratch the itching ear; and seborrheic and allergic dermatitis.

Clinical Findings

A. Symptoms and Signs: Itching and pain in the dry, scaling ear canal are the chief symptoms. There may be a watery or purulent discharge and intermittent deafness. Pain may become extreme when the ear canal becomes completely occluded with edematous skin and debris. Preauricular, postauricular, or cervical adenopathy or fever indicates increasing severity of infection.

Examination shows crusting, scaling, erythema, edema, and pustule formation. Cerumen may be absent. There may be evidence of seborrhea elsewhere.

B. Laboratory Findings: The white count may be normal or elevated.

C. Special Examinations: After the canal is cleansed so that the eardrum is visible, otitis media can often be excluded if tuning fork tests indicate normal or nearly normal hearing.

Differential Diagnosis

Diffuse eczematoid dermatitis of the ear canal, diffuse infected dermatitis, and furuncle of the ear canal must be distinguished from dermatitis due to contact with foreign objects (eg, hearing aids) or infected material draining from the middle ear through a perforated eardrum or tumor of the external ear.

Treatment

A. Systemic Treatment: If there is evidence of extension of infection beyond the skin of the ear canal (lymphadenopathy or fever), systemic antibiotics may be necessary. Analgesics are required for pain.

B. Local Treatment: The objectives of local treatment are to keep the ear canal clean and dry and to protect it from trauma. Debris may be removed from the canal by gently wiping it with a cotton applicator or with suction or, occasionally, irrigation. The use of Debrox (carbamide peroxide in anhydrous glycerol) 3 times daily often helps to remove debris.

Topical antibiotic ointments and ear drops (eg, neomycin, polymyxin, bacitracin) applied to the ear canal with a cotton wick for 24 hours followed by the use of ear drops twice daily help to control infection. Topical corticosteroids aid in decreasing inflammatory edema and controlling the underlying dermatitis that is often present. Topical antifungal and antimicrobial agents must be used with caution because of the possibility of local sensitivity reactions. Compresses of Burow's solution or 0.5% acetic acid are sometimes effective against acute weeping infected eczema when other measures fail. Seventy percent alcohol frequently controls itching in the dry, scaling ear canal.

Malignant external otitis occurs in elderly diabetics or severely debilitated younger patients. Infection with *Pseudomonas aeruginosa* produces necrosis of external canal skin and bone and extends to deeper tissue and intracranially, producing paralysis of cranial nerves VII, X, XI, and XII. It is characterized by persistent granulations at the junction of the cartilaginous and bony canals. These patients must be hospitalized and treated vigorously, with control of the diabetes and the use of intravenous moxalactam and topical polymyxin B sulfate or colistimethate sodium. Even with the most vigorous treatment, the mortality rate is 30–50%.

Prognosis

Depending upon the cause, external otitis may be refractory to treatment, and recurrences are frequent.

Dehner LP, Chen KTK: Primary tumors of the external and middle ear. *Arch Otolaryngol* 1980;**106**:13.

Lucente FE: External otitis. In: *Current Therapy in Otolaryngology: Head and Neck Surgery 1982–1983*. Gates GA (editor). Mosby, 1982.

Madder JT, Love JT: Malignant external otitis. *Arch Otolaryngol* 1982;**108**:38.

3. FOREIGN BODY IN THE EAR CANAL

Foreign bodies in the ear canal are more common in children than in adults. When removing an object, care must be taken not to push it farther into the ear canal and thereby cause injury to the bony ear canal, tympanic membrane, or middle ear structures.

Small objects that do not occlude the ear canal can be removed with a dull curet or small blunt hook that can be maneuvered past the foreign body or by suction or irrigation. Vegetable foreign bodies that can absorb moisture and swell should be irrigated with care. Objects that completely occlude the ear canal may require removal by operation, with anesthesia, magnification, and even surgical enlargement of the ear canal.

Upchurch DT: Removing foreign bodies from ears, nose and throat. *Consultant* (March) 1982;**22**:283.

DISEASES OF THE MIDDLE EAR

1. ACUTE OTITIS MEDIA

Essentials of Diagnosis

- Ear pain, a sensation of fullness in the ear, and hearing loss; aural discharge.
- Onset following an upper respiratory tract infection.
- Fever and chills.

General Considerations

Acute otitis media most commonly occurs in infants and children, but it may occur at any age. Suppuration of the middle ear usually occurs following or accompanying disease of the upper respiratory tract. Beta-hemolytic streptococci, staphylococci, pneumococci, and *Haemophilus influenzae* are the usual infecting organisms. The acute inflammatory reaction that occurs in the middle ear mucosa is followed by acute suppuration and then a more severe suppuration with perforation of the tympanic membrane, occasionally with necrosis of the middle ear mucosa and eardrum.

Clinical Findings

A. Symptoms and Signs: The principal symptoms are ear pain, deafness, fever, chills, and a feeling of fullness and pressure in the ear. The eardrum at first shows dilatation of the blood vessels on the malleus and at the tympanic annulus; this is followed by diffuse dullness and hyperemia of the eardrum and loss of normal landmarks (short process of malleus) and bulging of the drum as the pressure of retained secretions increases in the middle ear. If the eardrum ruptures, discharge is found in the ear canal; the discharge may be pulsating. Fever is usually present.

B. Laboratory Findings: The white count is usually increased. Culture of the drainage will reveal the infecting organism.

C. Special Examinations: Hearing tests will show a conductive hearing loss.

Differential Diagnosis

Acute otitis media with bulging of the eardrum

must be distinguished from myringitis bullosa, usually by the presence of more than one bleb in the ear canal and the absence of marked hearing loss. Acute otitis media with drainage must be distinguished from acute external otitis. The history of a preceding upper respiratory tract infection and hearing loss confirm the diagnosis of otitis media. Acute exacerbation of chronic otitis media is diagnosed by a history of otorrhea and hearing loss and by finding scar tissue on the eardrum. Otalgia due to referred pain from such causes as pharyngitis, laryngitis, dental disease, and temporomandibular joint disease may be present if there are no acute inflammatory changes in the ear canal or eardrum and if there is no fever.

Complications

Acute mastoiditis, labyrinthitis, or meningitis may occur as complications.

Treatment

A. Systemic Treatment: Bed rest, analgesics, and systemic antibiotics are usually required. Penicillin or a broad-spectrum antibiotic is usually the drug of choice. Tetracycline should not be used in children or pregnant women because staining of the teeth of the child or fetus may occur. Ampicillin or amoxicillin is often used in children below age 6 or 8 years because of the higher incidence of *H influenzae* infection.

B. Local Treatment: Ear drops are of limited value except in the mildest cases. Local heat may hasten resolution. Local cold applications relieve pain occasionally. Oral decongestants may hasten resolution of edema of the auditory tube. The most important aspect of treatment is myringotomy when the infection does not resolve promptly or when bulging of the eardrum indicates that a discharge is present and is under pressure. Myringotomy should also be promptly performed if there is continued pain or fever, increasing hearing loss, or vertigo.

Prognosis

Acute otitis media adequately treated with antibiotics and myringotomy if indicated resolves with rare exceptions. Complicating mastoiditis occurs most commonly following inadequate or no treatment. Persistent conductive hearing loss with or without middle ear fluid may occur following incomplete resolution of the infection. It is imperative to examine the ears and to test the hearing after otitis media to prevent persistent conductive hearing loss with serous otitis media or "glue ear."

Bluestone CD: Otitis media in children: To treat or not to treat? *N Engl J Med* 1982;**306**:1399.

Feigin RD: Otitis media: Closing the information gap. (Editorial.) *N Engl J Med* 1982;**306**:1417.

Howie VM et al: Acute otitis media: One year in general pediatric practice. *Am J Dis Child* 1983;**137**:155.

2. CHRONIC OTITIS MEDIA

Chronic inflammation of the middle ear is nearly always associated with perforation of the eardrum. It is important to distinguish the relatively benign chronic otitis associated with auditory (eustachian) tube disease—characterized by central perforation of the eardrum and often mucoid otorrhea occurring with an upper respiratory tract infection—from the chronic otitis associated with mastoid disease that is potentially much more dangerous; the latter is characterized by perforation of Shrapnell's membrane or posterior marginal perforation of the eardrum, often with foulsmelling drainage and cholesteatoma formation. Drainage from the ear and impaired hearing are frequent symptoms.

Treatment of the chronic "tubal ear" should be directed at improving auditory tube function by correcting nasal or sinus infection or treating infected or hypertrophied tonsils or adenoids, nasal polyps, deviated nasal septum, and nasal allergy. Ear drops (antibiotic solutions) or dusting powders (iodine, boric acid, or antibiotics) and frequent cleansing of the ear are of value. Systemic antibiotics are often of value. If there is evidence of continued suppuration or if mastoiditis or other complications occur, radical or modified radical mastoidectomy should be done. In some cases of chronic otitis media where hearing loss has occurred—and if the middle ear infection is quiescent and auditory tube function is adequate—reconstructive middle ear operations (tympanoplasty) can be attempted to improve the hearing.

Duval AJ III, Lowell SH: The "chronic" ear: How to manage mild to severe otitis. *Postgrad Med* (Aug) 1979;**66**:94.

3. SEROUS OTITIS MEDIA

Serous otitis media is characterized by the accumulation of sterile fluid (serous or mucoid) in the middle ear, producing symptoms of hearing loss, a full, plugged feeling in the ear, and an unnatural reverberation of the patient's voice. It may be caused by (1) an obstruction of the auditory tube that prevents normal ventilation of the middle ear and subsequent transudation of serous fluid; (2) an incompletely resolved exudate of purulent otitis media; or (3) an allergic exudate of serous fluid into the middle ear.

Examination shows a conductive hearing loss and a retracted eardrum, often with a characteristic "ground glass" amber discoloration and impaired mobility of the eardrum with the pneumatic otoscope. Air-fluid bubbles or a fluid level can sometimes be seen through the eardrum.

The absence of fever, pain, and toxic symptoms distinguishes serous otitis media from acute otitis media. Cancer of the nasopharynx must be ruled out in persistent unilateral serous otitis media in an adult.

Local treatment consists of auditory tube inflations, paracentesis of the eardrum with aspiration of the middle ear contents, and nasal decongestants (0.25% phenylephrine nasal spray or phenylpropanolamine, 25–50 mg orally 3 times daily). Antihistamines should be given if there is any suggestion of contributing nasal allergy. Underlying factors must be corrected by control of nasal allergy and treatment of nasal or sinus infection. Tonsillectomy and adenoidectomy may sometimes be necessary. Indwelling plastic ventilating tubes after myringotomy and local or systemic use of corticosteroids may help in persistent cases.

Brenman AK, Meltzer CR, Milner RM: Myringotomy and tube ventilation in adults. *Am Fam Physician* (Oct) 1982;**26**:181.
Christiansen TA: When to consider the PE tube. *Postgrad Med* (Feb) 1984;**75**:195.

4. MASTOIDITIS

Acute mastoiditis is a complication of acute suppurative otitis media. Bony necrosis of the mastoid process and breakdown of the bony intercellular structures occur in the second to third week. When this occurs there is evidence of continued drainage from the middle ear, mastoid tenderness, systemic manifestations of sepsis (fever, headache), and x-ray evidence of bone destruction.

If suppurative mastoiditis develops in spite of antibiotic therapy, mastoidectomy must be done. Acute mastoiditis is rarely seen since antibiotic therapy has become available for the treatment of acute suppurative otitis media.

Chronic mastoiditis is a complication of chronic otitis media. If the disease occurs in infancy, the mastoid bone does not develop cellular structure but becomes dense and sclerotic. Infection is usually limited to the antral area. However, an x-ray finding of a sclerotic mastoid does not necessarily mean that a chronic infection is present, only that an infection was present in infancy and that as a result the mastoid air cells are not well developed. The presence of infection must be determined by clinical findings. In some cases of marginal perforation of the eardrum, cholesteatomas develop. Cholesteatoma is produced by the ingrowth of squamous epithelium from the skin of the external ear canal into the middle ear or mastoid, forming an epithelial cyst. Desquamation and laminated growth of the cyst may produce erosion of adjacent bone or soft tissue.

Antibiotic drugs are usually of limited usefulness in clearing the infection in chronic mastoiditis, but they may be effective in the treatment of complications. Some cases of chronic otitis media and mastoiditis can be managed by local cleansing of the ear and instillation of antibiotic powders or solutions. Other cases may require radical or modified radical mastoidectomy or tympanoplasty.

Shaffer HL: Acute mastoiditis and cholesteatoma. *Otolaryngology* 1978;**86**:394.
Wolferman A: Twenty-five years of tympanoplasty: A critical evaluation. *Ann Otol Rhinol Laryngol* 1977;**86(Suppl 37)**:3.

COMPLICATIONS OF MIDDLE EAR INFECTIONS

Following Acute Suppurative Otitis Media & Mastoiditis

A. Subperiosteal abscess following acute otitis media and mastoiditis is infrequent. Simple mastoidectomy is required.

B. Facial nerve paralysis developing in the first few hours or days after the onset of acute otitis media is due to edema of the nerve in the bony facial canal. Conservative treatment is usually indicated (antibiotics, myringotomy, supportive measures).

C. Meningitis, epidural, subdural, and brain abscess, and sigmoid sinus thrombosis are serious complications that may be masked by antibiotic drugs. Surgical treatment of the mastoid disease and its complications is required.

D. Conductive deafness: See p 108.

Following Chronic Otitis Media

A. Acute exacerbations of chronic otitis media and mastoiditis may lead to meningitis; epidural, subdural, and brain abscess; and sigmoid sinus thrombosis, requiring antibiotic therapy and surgery.

B. Facial nerve paralysis is usually the result of direct pressure on the nerve by cholesteatoma or granulation tissue. Mastoidectomy and decompression of the facial nerve are necessary.

C. Conductive deafness: See p 108.

Portmann M: Principles of management for sequelae of otitis. *J Laryngol Otol* 1983;**8(Suppl)**:70.

DISEASES OF THE INNER EAR

1. MENIERE'S DISEASE (Paroxysmal Labyrinthine Vertigo)

Essentials of Diagnosis

- Intermittent attacks of vertigo, nausea and vomiting, and profuse sweating.
- Progressive, often unilateral nerve type hearing loss and continuous tinnitus.

General Considerations

Meniere's disease is characterized by recurrent episodes of severe vertigo associated with deafness and tinnitus. It is encountered most often in men in the age group from 40 to 60. The cause is not known, but "endolymphatic hydrops" with marked dilatation of the cochlear duct is the pathologic finding. Meniere's disease may follow head trauma or middle ear infection, but many cases develop without apparent damage to the nervous system or ear.

Clinical Findings

Intermittent severe vertigo, which may cause the patient to fall, is the principal symptom. "Spinning" of surrounding objects is often noted. Nausea, vomiting, and profuse perspiration are often associated. The attacks may last from a few minutes to several hours. The frequency of attacks varies considerably, even in the same patient. Headache, nerve type hearing loss, and tinnitus occur during and persist between attacks. Hearing loss is apt to be progressive, and is unilateral in 90% of cases. Nystagmus may occur during attacks of vertigo. An altered labyrinthine response is often demonstrated by means of the caloric test. There is increased sensitivity to loud sounds. Audiometric tests show recruitment, decreased speech discrimination, and a nerve type hearing loss.

Differential Diagnosis (See Chapter 17.)

Distinguish the vertigo from that produced by posterior fossa tumors (other findings such as papilledema, increased cerebrospinal fluid pressure and protein, and brain stem signs) and the relatively common benign vestibular neuronitis that results from irritation of the vestibular portion of the eighth nerve. Differentiate dizziness and lightheadedness from those seen in some systemic diseases, brain stem vascular disease (vertebrobasilar artery syndrome), and psychiatric disorders. Special diagnostic audiometry, electronystagmography, and x-rays of the internal auditory canals are often necessary for differential diagnosis.

Treatment

Reassurance is important, since many of these patients have a marked psychic overlay. A salt-free diet and ammonium chloride, 1–2 g 4 times daily, may be helpful. Nicotinic acid, 50–150 mg orally 3–4 times daily, has been found useful. The antihistamines, especially diphenhydramine (Benadryl) and dimenhydrinate (Dramamine), in doses of 50–100 mg 3–4 times daily, appear to be of benefit to some patients. Parenteral diphenhydramine or dimenhydrinate—or atropine sulfate, 0.6 mg—may stop the acute attack.

Surgery on the labyrinth or vestibular nerve may be necessary in a few severe cases that do not respond to medical measures.

Prognosis

Meniere's disease is a chronic recurrent disease that persists for several years. Remission or improvement of vertigo, tinnitus, and hearing loss after treatment is often noted; however, tinnitus and deafness may be unaffected and permanent. Progression is slow and sometimes stops before complete deafness occurs.

Cessation of attacks of vertigo may follow complete loss of hearing.

Procedures that destroy or interrupt an affected vestibular portion of acoustic nerve (such as destruction of the labyrinth or section of the acoustic nerve) may prevent further attacks of vertigo.

Endolymphatic shunt or the "tack" operation of Cody attempts to relieve the vertigo and preserve hearing.

Schmidt PH, Brunsting RC, Antvelink JB: Meniere's disease: Etiology and natural history. *Acta Otolaryngol (Stockh)* 1979; **87**:410.

Snow JB Jr, Kimmelman CP: Assessment of surgical procedures for Meniere's disease. *Laryngoscope* 1979;**89**:737.

Wiet RJ: A holistic approach to Meniere's disease: Medical and surgical management. *Laryngoscope* 1981;**91**:1647.

2. TINNITUS

Tinnitus is a sensation of noise in the ears or head that may be objective (heard by the examiner) or subjective. Objective tinnitus is uncommon and is usually caused by transmitted vascular vibrations in the blood vessels of the head and neck or by rhythmic rapid contractions of the muscles of the soft palate or middle ear. The examiner can often hear the sound through a stethoscope placed over the ear or can see movements of the eardrum or palate.

Subjective tinnitus usually accompanies hearing loss or other disorders of the external, middle, or inner ear. Although the cause is unknown, tinnitus is presumed to be due to irritation of nerve endings in the cochlea by degenerative vascular or vasomotor disease. Most patients state that the noise is bearable during the day but is much louder and more disturbing at night when the masking effect of environmental sounds is not present.

If possible, treatment is directed at the underlying cause. If the cause cannot be determined, reassurance may be all that is necessary. An air conduction hearing aid during the day and a pillow speaker for music or other masking sound during the night may be necessary in severe cases. Sedation may be used sparingly. Difficult cases may require the close cooperation of an otolaryngologist, internist, neurologist, and psychiatrist.

Liebman EP: Tinnitus: Multiple causes, varying significance. *Consultant* (April) 1984;**26**:47.

Pulec JL, Hodell SF, Anthony PF: Tinnitus: Diagnosis and treatment. *Ann Otol Rhinol Laryngol* 1978;**87**:821.

3. ACUTE NONSUPPURATIVE LABYRINTHITIS

Acute inflammation of the inner ear characteristically follows respiratory tract infections and is manifested by intense vertigo, usually with marked tinnitus, nausea, a staggering gait, and nystagmus. Hearing is often unimpaired.

Bed rest, preferably in a darkened room, is indicated until severe symptoms subside. Antibiotics are of little value unless there is associated infection of the middle ear or mastoid bone. Antihistamine drugs (as for motion sickness) may be of value. Sedation with diazepam or phenobarbital is generally helpful. Chlorpromazine hydrochloride (Thorazine), 50 mg intramuscularly (or other phenothiazine derivative), is useful in the acute early phase.

Attacks of labyrinthitis may last for several days. Recovery is usually complete.

Maragos NE, Neel HB III, McDonald TJ: Dissection of dizziness: With emphasis on labyrinthine vertigo. *Postgrad Med* (May) 1981;**69**:109.

4. ACUTE SUPPURATIVE LABYRINTHITIS

Acute suppurative labyrinthitis is an infection of the intralabyrinthine structures. It may occur following acute otitis media and mastoiditis, acute exacerbations of chronic otitis media and mastoiditis, or meningitis unrelated to ear diseases. There is usually total destruction of labyrinthine function in the affected area and complete unilateral deafness.

Antibiotics and surgical drainage are indicated.

5. CHRONIC LABYRINTHITIS

Chronic labyrinthitis is secondary to erosion of the bony labyrinthine capsule (usually the lateral semicircular canal) by cholesteatoma. The patient has chronic episodes of vertigo, and attacks of vertigo can be reproduced by increasing the air pressure in the ear canal with a pneumatic otoscope (positive fistula test).

Mastoidectomy and removal of the cholesteatoma are required.

DISEASES OF THE NOSE

NASAL VESTIBULITIS

Inflammation of the nasal vestibule may occur as a dermatitis of the skin of the nose, often as a result of irritation from a nasal discharge; as a fissure resulting from chronic dermatitis or the trauma of picking or wiping the nose; or as a furuncle, usually after pulling hairs from the nose. Symptoms vary from scaling and weeping to edema, hyperemia, intense pain, and abscess formation. Fissures usually occur at the junction of the columella with the ala or with the floor of the nose. Careful cleansing of the nostrils, refraining from pulling out hairs, and protection with petrolatum or boric acid ointment may prevent these problems and the grave complications of cavernous sinus thrombosis.

The application of soothing, protective, and antimicrobial ointments (eg, 5% ammoniated mercury, 3% iodochlorhydroxyquin cream, neomycin, polymyxin, or bacitracin ointments) several times daily for several days after symptoms disappear is usually adequate treatment. For more severe infections, systemic antibiotics, local heat, and general supportive measures may be necessary.

If the infection localizes into a small furuncle, the furuncle can be incised and drained without squeezing or manipulation when the infection is pointing. Systemic antibiotics for staphylococcal infection (dicloxacillin or cephalosporin) will speed recovery and minimize the risk of retrograde infection into the cavernous sinus. This is an infrequent but life-threatening complication of any infection in the middle one-third of the face (see p 116).

NASAL SEPTAL HEMATOMA & ABSCESS

Septal hematoma occurs following trauma to the nose. The swollen septum produces nasal obstruction and frontal headache. Septal abscess usually is the result of an infected septal hematoma. It may occur following a furuncle in the vestibule and produces nasal obstruction, headache, fever, malaise, pain in the nose, and tenderness over the nasal dorsum.

A small septal hematoma may be treated conservatively by observation for possible infection; it should resolve in 4–6 weeks. It may also be relieved by aspiration with a large-bore needle or by incision and drainage, taking extreme precautions to prevent infection. Large hematomas should always be drained.

Septal abscess must be drained by wide incision of one side of the septum and suction. Necrotic pieces of cartilage may be cautiously removed. The incision must be wide enough to prevent early closure or must be spread open daily. Nasal packing may be necessary to control bleeding. Systemic antibiotic therapy is required.

Destruction of cartilage causes saddle deformity.

"COMMON COLD"
(Coryza)

This exceedingly common respiratory tract syndrome may be caused by a wide variety of viruses, including the rhinoviruses (30 different serologic types), adenovirus, echoviruses, coxsackievirus, influenza viruses, parainfluenza viruses, and mycoplasmal organisms. All of the viruses exist in multiple antigenic types, and recurrent infection is common. There is considerable individual variation in susceptibility. The contributory role of environmental exposure (eg, cold and dampness) is not known.

Clinical Findings

A. Symptoms and Signs: The patient complains of malaise, "feverishness," and headache. Nasal discomfort with watery discharge and sneezing is followed shortly by mucoid to purulent discharge and nasal obstruction. Throat symptoms include "dryness," "soreness" rather than actual pain, and hoarseness.

The nasal mucosa is reddened and edematous. The pharynx and tonsils show mild to moderate injection, usually without edema or exudate. Cervical lymph nodes may be enlarged and slightly tender. Herpes labialis is common.

B. Laboratory Findings: The white count may be slightly elevated, but in most cases this is due to secondary bacterial infection. Throat cultures are repeatedly negative for bacterial pathogens.

Differential Diagnosis

Many specific infectious diseases present initial manifestations indistinguishable from those of common respiratory disease (eg, streptococcal infection, meningococcal infection, diphtheria).

Influenza is recognized by its epidemic occurrence and by serologic confirmation.

Exanthematous diseases in their preeruptive phase (especially measles and chickenpox) may simulate common respiratory disease.

Complications

Complications result from secondary bacterial infections, often aided by the obstruction of respiratory passages (eg, sinus ostia, bronchioles). They include purulent sinusitis, otitis media, bacterial pneumonia, and tonsillitis. Serious bronchial obstruction may occur in patients with underlying bronchopulmonary disease.

Treatment

No specific treatment is available for this syndrome. Antibiotics are used only for treatment of complicating secondary infections.

General measures consist of rest, sufficient fluids to prevent dehydration, and a balanced diet as tolerated. Aspirin may be given for headache, sore throat, muscle soreness, and fever. Phenylephrine (Neo-Synephrine), 0.25%, several drops in each nostril every 2–3 hours, or phenylpropanolamine (Propadrine), 25–50 mg every 4–6 hours, gives temporary relief of nasal obstruction and rhinorrhea. Warm glucose or saline gargles may relieve throat discomfort. Cough may be reduced by inhaling steam or with cough suppressants as needed (see p 126). Application of heat to the area of the sinuses may relieve nasal obstruction.

The use of large doses of vitamin C (1 g or more daily) remains of unproved value.

Mills J: Viral URIs: How to fight back. *Mod Med* (Nov) 1983;**51**:88.
Reed SF: The aetiology and epidemiology of common colds, and the possibilities of prevention. *Clin Otolaryngol* 1981;**6**:379.

ALLERGIC RHINITIS
(Hay Fever)

Essentials of Diagnosis

- Watery nasal discharge, sneezing, itching eyes and nose.
- Pale, boggy mucous membranes.

- Eosinophilia of nasal secretions and blood.
- Onset usually in childhood.
- Occurrence pattern:
    Seasonal–Spring (pollens), summer (grasses and molds), autumn (ragweed).
    Perennial–Dusts and danders.
- Family history of allergic disease.
- Positive skin tests.

General Considerations

See discussion under Bronchial Asthma.

Clinical Findings

A. Symptoms and Signs: The principal symptoms are nasal congestion; a profuse, watery nasal discharge; itching of the nasal mucosa leading to paroxysms of violent sneezing; conjunctival itching and burning; and lacrimation. The nasal mucosa is pale blue and boggy. Polyps may be present. The conjunctiva is often reddened and swollen.

B. Laboratory Findings: A smear of the nasal secretions reveals increased numbers of eosinophils. (In infections, neutrophils predominate.) The peripheral blood may reveal mild (5–10%) or occasionally marked (30–40%) eosinophilia, even between clinical episodes.

Skin tests may be of aid in the detection of allergens but are significant only when the results are correlated with the clinical picture.

Differential Diagnosis

A history of an allergy aids in distinguishing allergic rhinitis from the common upper respiratory infections; hay fever should be suspected in young children as the real cause of repeated "colds."

Treatment

A. Specific Measures: There is no true specific treatment. Hyposensitization or desensitization is sometimes beneficial and consists of administering the allergen (usually pollen) in gradually increasing doses to induce an "immunity." For best results, therapy should be started 3–6 months before the beginning of the hay fever season.

B. General Measures:

1. Antihistamines give relief in 60–80% of patients, but their effectiveness often wanes as the season continues. (See p 17.)

2. Sympathomimetic drugs such as ephedrine and phenylpropanolamine are effective by themselves or in combination with the antihistamines.

3. Mild sedatives for short periods may be of value for tense or nervous patients.

4. The corticosteroids are useful in severe hay fever that cannot be controlled by the agents mentioned above. Prednisone, 20–40 mg by mouth daily in divided doses, may be used for several days until the symptoms are controlled. Dosage should then be reduced gradually (over 7–10 days) to the smallest daily dose that will serve to suppress symptoms. Discontinue corticosteroid therapy as soon as possible.

Topical sprays of beclomethasone dipropionate and flunisolide are very effective in relieving nasal congestion in about half of patients with nasal pollen allergy.

5. Maintenance of an allergen-free atmosphere and the use of dust-proof respirator masks and room air filters are often of value during the pollen season if the patient must remain in the area. When dust is the offending agent, prepare a dust-free bedroom as follows: Cover the mattress and pillow with an airtight nonantigenic material (plastic or sheet rubber). Remove all carpets, drapes, bedspreads, and other lint-producing materials and all ornate furniture or other objects which are not easily dusted. Blankets should be of synthetic material if possible.

Household pets must be considered possible sources of allergens.

Prognosis

Allergic rhinitis is a self-limited though recurrent disorder associated with mild morbidity.

Buesse WW: Chronic rhinitis: A systematic approach to diagnosis and treatment. *Postgrad Med* (Feb) 1983;**73**:325.

Jacobs RL: A practical classification of chronic rhinitis. *J Resp Dis* (May) 1981;**2**:20.

Soss TL: Allergy in otolaryngology. *Laryngoscope* 1983;**93**:408.

SINUS INFECTION

Essentials of Diagnosis

Acute:

- History of acute upper respiratory infection, dental infection, or nasal allergy.
- Pain, tenderness, redness, swelling over the involved sinus.
- Nasal congestion and purulent nasal discharge.
- Clouding of sinuses on x-ray or transillumination.
- Fever, chills, malaise, headache.
- Teeth hurt or feel "long" (maxillary sinusitis), or swelling occurs near the nasal canthus of the eye (ethmoid sinusitis).

Chronic:

- Nasal obstruction.
- Postnasal discharge.
- Sinus clouding on x-ray or transillumination.
- Pain is not a common finding.

General Considerations

Acute sinus infection usually follows an acute upper respiratory infection, swimming or diving, dental abscess or extractions, or nasal allergies, or occurs as an exacerbation of a chronic sinus infection. Isolated acute frontal sinus infection is rare. Acute ethmoiditis is most common in infants and children. Chronic pyogenic infections of single sinuses do occur, but this is less common than pansinusitis. The usual infecting organisms are *Staphylococcus, Streptococcus,* pneumococci, and *Haemophilus influenzae,* making ampicillin or a cephalosporin the antibiotics of choice. Many patients with bronchopulmonary disease (eg, asthma) have x-ray evidence of sinusitis even in the absence of nasal symptoms.

Clinical Findings

A. Symptoms and Signs:

1. Acute sinusitis–The symptoms resemble those of acute rhinitis but are more severe. There is headache and facial pain, tenderness and swelling with nasal obstruction, and a purulent nasal and postnasal discharge, sometimes causing sore throat and cough. The headache typically is worse during the day and subsides in the evening. Acute maxillary sinusitis may cause pain in the teeth and a feeling of "long teeth." Acute ethmoiditis causes headache between and behind the eyes, and eye motion increases the pain. Tenderness medially in the roof of the orbit occurs with frontal sinusitis. Fever and systemic symptoms vary with the severity of the infection.

2. Chronic sinusitis–Chronic sinus infection may produce no symptoms, or only a mild postnasal discharge and a musty odor or nonproductive cough. Nasal obstruction and profuse purulent nasal and postnasal discharge may occur.

B. Laboratory Findings: In acute sinusitis the white count may be elevated, and culture of nasal discharge usually shows the pyogenic organisms.

C. Other Examinations: X-ray and transillumination show clouding of the involved sinuses.

Differential Diagnosis

Acute dental infection usually produces greater facial swelling lower in the face, with more marked tenderness of the involved tooth, than does maxillary sinusitis. Tear sac infection is distinguished from ethmoiditis by the more localized swelling and tenderness and the greater involvement of the eyelids, with absence of nasal discharge. X-ray examination gives more definite evidence of sinus involvement.

An isolated chronic maxillary sinusitis without obvious cause suggests dental disease or neoplasm.

Complications

Chronic sinusitis is the commonest complication of acute sinusitis. Orbital cellulitis and abscess may follow ethmoiditis or frontal sinusitis. Frontal sinusitis may be complicated by meningitis or extradural, subdural, or brain abscess. Osteomyelitis of the facial or frontal bones may occur. Cavernous sinus thrombosis is an infrequent complication of any infection in the middle one-third of the face.

Treatment

A. Acute Sinusitis: Place the patient at bed rest and give sedatives, analgesics, a light diet, and fluids. Oral nasal decongestants (eg, phenylpropanolamine, 25–50 mg 3 times daily) and systemic antibiotics frequently produce prompt resolution of the infection. Ampicillin or erythromycin, 1–2 g/d, is most commonly used. Other antibiotics may be used as determined by culture and sensitivity testing.

Local heat, topical nasal decongestants (eg,

0.25% phenylephrine), and gentle spot suctioning of the nasal discharge are helpful.

The sinuses must not be manipulated during the acute infection. Antrum irrigation is of value after the acute inflammation has subsided. Acute frontal sinusitis is treated medically and conservatively; cannulation is rarely warranted. Trephining of the sinus floor may occasionally be indicated in acute fulminating infections. Acute ethmoid infections respond to medical management; if external fluctuation develops, incision and drainage are indicated.

B. Chronic Sinusitis: When the infecting organism has been identified, the most effective antibiotic can be chosen by antibiotic sensitivity tests. Irrigation of the antra or Proetz displacement may help drainage. Conservative surgery to promote drainage is of value (removal of polyps, submucous resection of an obstructing septum, intranasal antrotomy). If conservative treatment is not effective, more radical sinus surgery by the external approach may be considered.

C. Treatment of Complications:

1. Osteomyelitis, meningitis, abscess–Give supportive measures and antibiotics. Remove necrotic bone and drain abscesses as required.

2. Orbital fistulas–Treat the underlying sinus disease and close the tract surgically.

3. Oroantral fistula–Remove underlying sinus infection by the Caldwell-Luc operation and close the tract.

4. Mucoceles (mucopyoceles)–Surgical excision.

5. Cavernous sinus thrombosis is recognized by a high spiking fever; ophthalmoplegia with involvement of the third, fourth and sixth cranial nerves with absence of the pupillary reflex; visual field defects; and, at times, total blindness in the affected eye and swelling of the conjunctiva. Treatment is with high-dosage antibiotic therapy (nafcillin, chloramphenicol, or cephalosporins for staphylococcal infection), anticoagulation therapy, and surgical drainage of the infected sinuses.

Prognosis

Acute infections usually respond to medical management and irrigation.

Chronic infections often require surgical correction. Chronic frontal sinusitis is especially likely to persist or recur.

Fairbanks DNF: Effective treatment of ear, nose and throat infections. Parts 1 and 2. *Drug Ther* (Sept and Oct) 1981;**11**:49, 127.

Rhea JT, DeLuca SA: Acute sinusitis. *Am Fam Physician* (April) 1982;**25**:121.

Wald ER: Acute sinusitis and orbital complications in children. *Am J Otolaryngol* 1983;**4**:424.

Wald ER et al: Acute maxillary sinusitis in children. *N Engl J Med* 1981;**304**:749.

Yarington CT: Sinusitis as an emergency. *Otolaryngol Clin North Am* 1979;**12**:447.

NASAL TUMORS

Benign Tumors

Angioma, fibroma, papilloma, chondroma, and osteoma are the most common types of benign neoplasms of the nose and sinuses. Nasal tumors produce obstruction and nasal discharge when they become large enough. Severe epistaxis occurs with angioma. Secondary infection may occur. Pressure atrophy of surrounding structures, widening of the nasal bridge, and displacement of the eye may occur. X-rays and biopsy usually establish the diagnosis.

Treatment consists of complete removal with permanent intranasal drainage of involved sinuses.

Malignant Tumors

Many nasal cancers originate in the sinuses and extend into the nose. Sarcoma and carcinoma occur. Symptoms and signs may not occur until late; the most common are obstruction, discharge, epistaxis, pain, swelling of the face, and diplopia. X-ray shows clouding of the sinuses that may suggest infection; secondary infection is frequently present. Bony destruction may show on x-rays. Cytologic smears of antrum irrigation fluid and "cell buttons" may rarely show malignant cells. Biopsy is diagnostic.

Surgical excision is usually the treatment of choice. Some cases may be treated by biopsy followed by x-ray therapy or, occasionally, surgery plus irradiation or cautery.

Donald PJ: Recent advances in paranasal sinus surgery. *Head Neck Surg* (Nov/Dec) 1981;**4**:146.

Weymuller EA Jr, Reardon EJ: A comparison of treatment modalities in carcinoma of the maxillary antrum. *Arch Otolaryngol* 1980;**106**:625.

EPISTAXIS
(Nosebleed)

The most common sites of nasal bleeding are the mucosal vessels over the cartilaginous nasal septum (Kiesselbach's area) and the anterior tip of the inferior turbinate. Bleeding is usually due to external trauma, nose picking, nasal infection (especially with vigorous nose blowing), or drying of the nasal mucosa. Up to 5% of nosebleeds originate posteriorly in the nose, where the bleeding site cannot be seen; these can cause great problems in management. If the blood drains into the pharynx and is swallowed, bloody vomitus may be the first clue of nosebleed.

Underlying causes of nosebleed such as blood dyscrasias, hypertension, hemorrhagic disease, nasal tumors, and certain infectious diseases (measles or rheumatic fever) must be considered in any case of recurrent or profuse nosebleed without obvious cause.

Treatment

A. Specific Measures: Examine and treat for any contributing systemic disease. (See above.)

B. Local Measures: Have the patient sit up and forward, head tipped downward, to prevent swallowing and aspiration of blood. Good illumination is essential to proper examination and treatment.

1. Anterior epistaxis–Pressure over the area (pinching the nose) for 5 minutes is often sufficient to stop bleeding. This may be combined with packing the bleeding nostril with 0.25% phenylephrine or 1:1000 epinephrine solution.

After active bleeding has stopped (or if pressure fails to stop bleeding), a cotton pledget moistened with a topical anesthetic (1% tetracaine or 5% cocaine) applied to the bleeding area will provide anesthesia for cauterization with a chromic acid bead, trichloroacetic acid, or an electrocautery. After cauterization, lubrication with petrolatum helps prevent crusting. A second cauterization is infrequently necessary.

If the source of bleeding is not accessible to cauterization or is not controlled by cauterization, the nasal cavity must be packed. After maximum shrinkage of the mucosa has been achieved with a suitable decongestant (0.25% phenylephrine or 2% ephedrine) and topical anesthesia, the nasal cavity can be tightly packed with half-inch gauze lubricated with petrolatum or cod liver oil. Pack the gauze into the nose in layers, starting either in the vault or on the floor of the nasal cavity. The packing may be left in place as long as 5–6 days if necessary. The patient should be given analgesics for pain and antibiotic medication for suppurative otitis media and sinusitis as needed.

2. Posterior epistaxis–Posterior bleeding can sometimes be controlled only by means of a posterior nasal pack. This accomplishes 2 things: It compresses and controls bleeding sites in the nasopharynx or posterior choana, and it prevents very firm anterior packing from being dislodged into the pharynx.

The postnasal pack is prepared as follows: (1) Sew 3 strings (No. 1 braided silk) through and through the center of a rolled 10- × 10-cm gauze sponge. (2) Pass a soft rubber catheter through the bleeding nostril into the pharynx and out through the mouth. (3) Attach 2 of the strings to the catheter tip and draw them through the mouth and out through the bleeding nostril. (4) Guide the gauze pack with a finger into the nasopharynx and posterior choana, taking care not to roll the uvula upward beneath the pack. (5) Anchor the 2 strings over a gauze bolster at the anterior nares. (6) Allow the third string to remain in the mouth and tape it to the face, or cut it about 10 cm long and allow it to dangle in the pharynx; it is used later to remove the pack. Inserting a Foley catheter with a 30-mL bag in the nose with inflation of the bag in the nasopharynx is often an easier way to provide a posterior nasal pack.

The pack should not be left in place for more than 4 days. The patient's ears should be examined daily for evidence of acute otitis media. If bleeding recurs while the pack is in place or when it is removed, it must usually be changed or reinserted under general anesthesia.

If anterior and posterior packing fail to arrest the bleeding, ligation of specific arteries must be considered.

Prognosis

Most anterior nosebleeds are easily treated as an office procedure; complicated nosebleed or posterior nosebleed may require hospitalization for 2–3 weeks.

Johnson JT, Rood SR: Epistaxis management. *Postgrad Med* (Nov) 1981;**70**:231.

Kirchner JA: Current concepts in otolaryngology: Epistaxis. *N Engl J Med* 1982;**307**:1126.

DISEASES OF THE PHARYNX

SORE THROAT

Sore throat is a common presenting symptom of many illnesses ranging from simple catarrhal pharyngitis to severe streptococcal infection (see below). Diagnosis and treatment are aimed at establishing bacterial versus viral or other etiology. Treatment of bacterial sore throat (most often beta-streptococcal but also caused by *Staphylococcus, Pneumococcus, Haemophilus influenzae,* and *Neisseria gonorrheae*) is with systemic antibiotics as well as local and symptomatic measures such as rest, light diet, adequate fluids, warm saline gargles, and throat irrigations and analgesics. Viral, allergic, and other causes are treated symptomatically. Persistent sore throat requires careful study for sources of referred pain, such as cervical arthritis, hypopharyngeal and laryngeal neoplasm, or systemic illnesses with local manifestations (eg, chronic brucellosis, iron deficiency anemia). Not all patients with sore throat require throat culture. Bacterial infection, especially with streptococci, is suggested if there is a history of exposure to a similar infection, tender cervical lymphadenopathy, tonsillar or pharyngeal exudate, or fever over 38.3 °C (101 °F). Sore throat associated with respiratory symptoms (rhinitis and cough) suggests viral infection. For treatment, see below under pharyngitis and tonsillitis.

SIMPLE PHARYNGITIS

Acute simple (catarrhal) pharyngitis is an acute inflammation of the mucosa of the pharynx that to some extent involves the lymphatic structures also. It usually occurs as part of an upper respiratory tract disorder that may also affect the nose, sinuses, larynx, and trachea. The most common causes are bacterial or viral infection; rarely, it is due to inhalation of irritant gases or ingestion of irritant liquids. Pharyngitis may occur as part of the syndrome of an acute specific infection (eg, measles, scarlet fever, whooping cough).

The inflammation may be diffuse or localized (lateral pharyngitis). Drying of the mucosa occurs in pharyngitis sicca.

In acute pharyngitis, the throat is dry and sore. Systemic symptoms are fever and malaise. The pharyngeal mucosa is red and slightly swollen, with thick, sticky mucus. The disease lasts only a few days.

Chronic pharyngitis may produce few symptoms, eg, throat dryness with thick mucus and cough; or recurrent acute episodes of more severe throat pain, dull hyperemia and mild swelling of the mucosa (especially the tonsillar pillars), and thick tenacious mucus, often in the hypopharynx.

The treatment of acute pharyngitis is symptomatic: rest, light diet, analgesics, and warm, nonirritating gargles or throat irrigations. Antibiotics may be used for initial or complicating bacterial infection.

Chronic pharyngitis is treated by removing underlying causes such as infections of the nose, sinuses, or tonsils and by restricting irritants such as alcohol, spicy foods, and tobacco. Local removal of the tenacious secretion with suction or saline irrigation and application of 2% silver nitrate are helpful.

ACUTE TONSILLITIS
(See also Chapter 24.)

Acute tonsillitis is nearly always a bacterial infection, often due to streptococci. It is a contagious airborne or food-borne infection that can occur in any age group but is more common in children. Associated adenoidal infection in children is usual.

The onset is sudden, with sore throat, fever, chills, headache, anorexia, and malaise. The tonsils are swollen and red, and pus or exudate is present on the tonsils or in the crypts. The cervical lymph nodes frequently are tender and enlarged. The white count may be elevated, and throat cultures will show the infecting organism.

Other causes of sore throat and fever that must be distinguished from acute tonsillitis include simple pharyngitis, infectious mononucleosis, Vincent's angina, diphtheria, agranulocytosis, and mycotic infections. Smear and culture from the throat identify the bacterial and mycotic infections. The white count helps distinguish viral infections and blood dyscrasias. The white count and heterophil antibody titer will make the diagnosis of infectious mononucleosis.

The complications of local extension are chronic tonsillitis, acute otitis media, acute rhinitis and sinusitis, peritonsillar abscess or other deep neck abscess, and cervical lymph node abscess. Nephritis, osteomyelitis, rheumatic fever, or pneumonia may follow streptococcal tonsillitis.

Treatment consists of bed rest, fluids, a light diet, analgesics, and antibiotics as required. Streptococcal infection can be treated with penicillin G benzathine, 1.2 million units intramuscularly, or penicillin V, 500 mg 4 times daily orally for 10 days, or, in penicillin-sensitive patients, erythromycin, 0.5–1 g/d for 10 days. Tonsillitis and pharyngitis caused by other pathogens (*Haemophilus influenzae*, pneumococci, staphylococci) may require use of other antibiotics as

determined by culture and sensitivity tests. Local relief of pain may be obtained with frequent hot, nonirritating gargles or throat irrigations.

Spontaneous resolution usually occurs after 5–7 days. Vigorous treatment may shorten the course, prevent many complications, and make the patient more comfortable.

Schwartz RH et al: Penicillin V for group A streptococcal pharyngotonsillitis: A randomized trial of seven vs ten days' therapy. *JAMA* 1981;**246:**1790.
Wormser GP, Hewlett D: Strategy for streptococcal pharyngitis. *Hosp Med* (May) 1984;**20:**13.

CHRONIC TONSILLITIS

Chronic tonsillitis usually results from repeated or unresolved acute infection. It is manifested by persistent dull hyperemia. Mild edema and scarring of the tonsils and tonsillar pillars may occur, and the crypts may contain abnormal secretions. In children, chronic adenoiditis may occur, with findings of enlargement and exudate visible only with a mirror or endoscope. Other symptoms and signs may range from a mild scratching sensation in the throat to cough, fetid breath, and a pharyngeal exudate. An enlarged cervical lymph node is common. The size of the tonsils is of little significance in determining the presence of chronic infection. Chronic infection may predispose to recurrent acute infections.

The treatment of significant chronic tonsillar infection is surgical excision (see below). Intercurrent acute infections and chronic infections in people who are poor operative risks (because of advanced age or severe systemic or hemorrhagic diseases) are treated medically as outlined above for acute infections. Chronic infection can rarely be eradicated by conservative treatment.

Adenotonsillectomy

The value of adenotonsillectomy, the indications for and contraindications to the operation, and the optimal time for the operation when it is indicated have been the subject of much controversy. Most surgeons agree that there are occasions when the operation is of definite benefit to the patient and that there are circumstances in which it is definitely contraindicated. The recent trend is away from tonsil and adenoid surgery for chronic serous otitis media and recurrent acute otitis media in favor of treatment with ventilating tubes. Even when a strong indication for surgery is present, however, the decision to operate must not be made until all pertinent restraining factors (eg, medical, psychologic, social) have been evaluated. In some cases, after culture and antibiotic sensitivity tests, a prolonged course of appropriate antibiotic therapy (2–3 weeks) will eradicate the infection.

A. Strong Indications: Whenever the infected or hypertrophied tonsils and adenoids are almost certainly the underlying or only cause of the disease, or when the tonsils are malignant.

1. Recurrent acute infection or chronic infection of tonsils and adenoids despite adequate antibiotic treatment.

2. Recurrent acute ear infections.

3. Peritonsillar abscess.

B. Equivocal Indications: When the infected or hypertrophied tonsils are likely to be the cause of the disease or are aggravating the disease: (Other possible contributing factors must first be investigated and ruled out or treated.) The risk/benefit ratio of the complications of surgery and anesthesia to the expected improvement must be carefully considered.

1. Snoring and mouth breathing.

2. Allergic rhinitis and asthma.

3. Systemic disease, eg, nephritis, rheumatic or congenital heart disease, rheumatic fever.

C. Relative Contraindications: When the operation may do more harm than good unless special precautions are taken. Surgery is contraindicated during acute tonsillar infection. The mere enlargement of tonsils and adenoids is not an indication for surgery.

1. Cleft palate–Further speech impairment can occur following adenotonsillectomy. Only the lateral adenoidal masses should be removed.

2. Systemic disease, eg, intercurrent infection, uncontrolled diabetes, tuberculosis, heart disease.

3. Hemorrhagic disease (eg, hemophilia).

Neel HB III, McDonald TJ: Tonsillectomy and adenoidectomy: Are there any indications? *Postgrad Med* (Sept) 1981;**70**:107.

Sasaki CT, Koss N: Chronic bacterial tonsillitis. *Otolaryngology* 1978;**86**:858.

PERITONSILLAR ABSCESS
(Quinsy)

Peritonsillar abscess is a complication of acute tonsillitis that occurs when the infection spreads to the potential peritonsillar space deep to the tonsil between the tonsillar capsule and the constrictor pharyngis muscle. Mixed pyogenic organisms (streptococci, staphylococci, pneumococci) are usually obtained upon culture. The sore throat of tonsillitis suddenly becomes more severe on one side when the infection breaks through the tonsillar capsule; dysphagia increases, trismus may be present, and one-sided swelling pushes the tonsil and tonsillar pillar toward or across the midline. The swelling extends to the soft palate, and the uvula is displaced. Fluctuation develops between the third and fifth days.

Symptomatic care and antibiotic therapy are indicated. After the abscess becomes fluctuant, it must be incised and drained. The walls of the abscess should be spread daily to prevent re-formation of the abscess. After the infection subsides, tonsillectomy should be done to prevent recurrences.

Hora JF: Deep-neck infections. *Arch Otolaryngol* 1963;**77**:129.

LUDWIG'S ANGINA
(Cellulitis of the Floor of the Mouth)

Ludwig's angina is a severe pyogenic infection of the sublingual and submaxillary spaces of the floor of the mouth and the anterior neck. A rapidly spreading diffuse cellulitis or abscess formation pushes the tongue upward against the roof of the mouth, limiting its motion and causing pain. The airway may become obstructed, or the infection may spread downward in the neck.

Supportive treatment and large doses of antibiotics are necessary. If abscess occurs, external incision and drainage should be performed. Local anesthesia avoids the danger of immediate obstruction of the airway, which may occur if general anesthesia is used. Because of the diffuse nature of the infection, large quantities of free pus are seldom obtained. Incision must be adequate, and the fascial spaces above and below the hyoglossus muscle must be opened by blunt dissection. A tracheostomy may be necessary.

RETROPHARYNGEAL ABSCESS

Retropharyngeal abscess is a pyogenic infection that occurs most often in infants and children. Suppuration occurs in the fascial space between the posterior pharyngeal wall and the prevertebral fascia as a result of suppurative lymph node infection, usually following tonsillar, nasal, or sinus infection. The symptoms are fever and difficulty in swallowing and breathing. The posterior pharyngeal wall is tender and swollen.

Early treatment (antibiotics, hydration) may produce resolution. If fluctuation occurs, incision and drainage are required, with the patient in full Trendelenburg position, adequate lighting, and suction equipment at hand. General anesthesia is avoided because of the danger of laryngeal obstruction and aspiration. Tracheostomy may be necessary.

Johnson JT, Tucker HM: Recognizing and treating deep neck infection. *Postgrad Med* (June) 1976;**59**:95.

PARAPHARYNGEAL ABSCESS

Parapharyngeal abscess is a pyogenic infection that occurs as a complication of acute tonsillitis, peritonsillar abscess, dental infection, or acute pharyngitis. It is localized in the fascial space outside the constrictor pharyngis muscle and deep to the investing cervical fascia, in close relationship to the carotid sheath and the stylopharyngeus and stylohyoid muscles. Infection can spread along the carotid sheath into the mediastinum. There are signs and symptoms of sepsis, bulging of the lateral pharyngeal wall, and trismus. The veins of the neck and scalp may be distended as a consequence of pressure upon the jugular vein. Brawny swelling and redness may develop later in the neck below the angle of the mandible.

Early treatment consists of hydration and antibiotics in large doses. Intraoral incision and drainage should be done only by a surgeon familiar with this area because of the danger of hemorrhage from large blood vessels. External incision and drainage at the angle of the jaw and upper neck can be done if pus is sought deep in the neck by blunt dissection.

Caution is required in giving general anesthesia because of the hazard of airway obstruction. Local anesthesia or a tracheostomy for general anesthesia should be considered.

Eliacher I, Peleg H, Joachims HZ: Mediastinitis and bilateral pyopneumothorax complicating a parapharyngeal abscess. *Head Neck Surg* (May/June) 1981;**3**:438.

Kreutzer EW et al: Ultrasonography in the preoperative evaluation of neck abscesses. *Head Neck Surg* (March/April) 1982;**4**:290.

DISEASES OF THE LARYNX

ACUTE LARYNGITIS

Acute inflammation of the laryngeal mucosa due to bacterial or viral infection may occur alone or in association with acute rhinitis, pharyngitis, or tracheitis. It may also occur with influenza, measles, or diphtheria, or as a result of inhalation of irritants. Hoarseness is the chief symptom. Pain and cough are often present. Stridor and dyspnea may occur if edema is marked. Examination of the larynx shows redness of the mucosa and edema with or without exudate. The acute inflammation may extend into the bronchi and lungs, and slight hemoptysis may occur if coughing ruptures small blood vessels.

Treatment consists of voice rest; decreased smoking; control of underlying nasal, sinus, or throat infections; and control of cough. Steam inhalations and local cold or heat to the neck may provide relief. Systemic antibiotics should be given for bacterial infections. If marked edema produces dyspnea and stridor, parenteral steroids may sometimes decrease the edema sufficiently so that tracheostomy can be withheld.

ACUTE EPIGLOTTITIS

Acute epiglottitis is most common in preschool children but occurs also in older children and adults. It is a potentially lethal infection that typically starts with a sore throat which can progress rapidly in a few hours to extreme sepsis, airway obstruction, and death. The infecting organism in children is usually *Haemophilus influenzae* type B, which is recovered in blood cultures in 80% of cases. Symptoms of rapidly progressive sore throat and fever, pain on swallowing progressing to inability to swallow saliva, and the desire to sit up,

leaning forward, in order to ease the inspiratory effort should alert the physician to the diagnosis. If the pharynx is examined with a tongue depressor, a cherry-red, extremely edematous epiglottis may be seen. If the diagnosis is suspected, it is probably best not to attempt visualization of the epiglottis for fear of producing terminal airway obstruction. Lateral soft tissue x-ray examination of the pharynx and larynx will show the enlarged epiglottis. Throat cultures may be misleading, showing a variety of organisms (eg, *H influenzae*, streptococci, staphylococci, gram-negative diplococci) that may often be found in healthy individuals. Blood culture is more useful. Often no pathogen is found in either throat or blood cultures. If the diagnosis is suspected, the patient should be taken immediately to the hospital, where further diagnostic procedures, pharyngeal examination with tongue depressor and laryngeal mirror, x-ray examination, and laboratory tests can be conducted in an environment where immediate treatment of airway obstruction, sepsis, and shock is available. This is often done in the intensive care unit or operating room. In the case of children, in whom airway obstruction usually occurs more rapidly and is more severe, diagnostic maneuvers should be kept to a minimum until after the airway is secured, in order to prevent the sudden onset of airway obstruction caused by a struggling child.

Treatment is primarily aimed at maintaining the airway. In children, this means immediate tracheostomy or endotracheal intubation (oral or nasal). Medical treatment is with ampicillin or chloramphenicol with added nafcillin or cloxacillin for penicillinase-producing organisms. In adults, the obstructive symptoms may be less severe and the symptoms may subside with medical treatment alone, but very close observation in the hospital must be maintained and tracheostomy or endotracheal intubation done at the first sign of airway impairment. Good nursing care of the artificial airway is essential to prevent secretions from blocking the tube, with humidification of the air and frequent suctioning of the tube after instillation of saline. The infection usually subsides in a few days, and the artificial airway can usually be terminated in 2–8 days. Prior to nasotracheal extubation, the epiglottis is inspected, and if the patient is deemed sufficiently recovered, the tube is removed in an environment (the operating room) where if needed the tube or a bronchoscope can be immediately reinserted and tracheostomy performed. Tracheostomy tubes can be removed after a gradual reduction in size and after a trial of plugging the tube with an obturator.

Cantrell RW, Bell RA, Morioka WT: Acute epiglottitis: Intubation versus tracheostomy. *Laryngoscope* 1978;**88**:994.

Cohen EL: Epiglottitis in the adult: Recognizing and treating the acute case. *Postgrad Med* (May) 1984;**75**:309.

Johnson GK, Sullivan JL, Bishop LA: Acute epiglottitis. *Arch Otolaryngol* 1977;**100**:333.

Schoss MD, Hanallah R, Baxter JD: Acute epiglottitis: Twenty-six years of experience at the Montreal Children's Hospital. *J Otolaryngol* 1979;**8**:3.

CHRONIC LARYNGITIS

Chronic inflammation of the laryngeal mucosa may be due to many causes, including repeated acute laryngitis, chronic vocal abuse, chronic inhalation of irritants (including smoking), chronic sinus and throat infection, syphilis and tuberculosis (rare today), allergy, and hypometabolic states. Chronic hoarseness is the chief symptom. Cough, expectoration of tenacious secretions, and a feeling of dryness in the throat are often present. Examination shows signs of chronic inflammation; a thickened, dull, edematous mucosa of the vocal cords; and polypoid changes, whitish plaques, and thickened secretions. Ulceration is occasionally seen.

Chest x-ray and other tests for signs of tuberculosis, serologic tests for syphilis, and biopsy to rule out carcinoma may be required.

Treatment consists of correcting the underlying cause, if any; antibiotics for sinus and throat infections; antiallergenic measures when indicated; decreased smoking; and voice rest.

TUMORS OF THE LARYNX

Essentials of Diagnosis

- Hoarseness is the principal symptom.
- Respiratory obstruction.
- Sore throat, "sticking" sensation in throat, pain referred to the ear.
- Cough or hemoptysis.
- Dysphagia.

General Considerations

Tumors of the larynx may be benign or malignant. Both produce similar symptoms and may be considered together. The symptoms depend upon the size and location of the tumor.

Benign laryngeal tumors may be neoplastic (eg, papilloma, fibroma), may be due to allergy or metabolic disturbance (polyps), or may be due to extrinsic or intrinsic trauma (singer's nodules, intubation granuloma). Ninety-five percent of malignant laryngeal tumors are squamous cell carcinomas, but sarcoma, adenocarcinoma, and others occur.

Clinical Findings

Hoarseness is the earliest and principal manifestation of vocal cord tumor. As the tumor enlarges, stridor and dyspnea may occur, usually late. With tumors elsewhere in the larynx (false cord, epiglottis, arytenoepiglottic fold, piriform sinus), voice change may be a late symptom and minor throat discomfort (sometimes referred to the ear), dysphagia, or mild cough may be the only early symptoms. Laryngeal examination usually shows a mass or ulceration at the tumor site. Submucosal tumors may be manifested only as a fullness or swelling of the affected area. Biopsy examination establishes the diagnosis.

Differential Diagnosis

Tumors of the larynx must be distinguished from chronic laryngitis, tuberculosis, syphilis, contact ulcer, granulomas, and laryngeal paralysis. Laryngeal symptoms lasting longer than 2–3 weeks must be investigated. Direct or indirect laryngoscopy is often diagnostic. Chest x-ray and other tests for tuberculosis, serologic tests for syphilis, laryngeal biopsy, and bacteriologic cultures usually establish a firm diagnosis.

Treatment & Prognosis

Almost all of the techniques involved in intralaryngeal manipulation and surgery require the skills of an otolaryngologist.

Small, asymptomatic benign tumors may require no treatment other than diagnosis to rule out cancer. Vocal cord polyps or ulcers due to metabolic disturbances (allergy or hypothyroidism) or to vocal misuse or other trauma may improve when the underlying problem is treated. Small benign tumors of the vocal cord producing hoarseness may be locally excised under direct or indirect laryngoscopy. Direct laryngoscopy with use of the operating microscope with microlaryngeal instruments and the carbon dioxide laser has made possible greater precision in laryngeal surgery. Larger benign tumors—especially papillomas, which have a great tendency to recur—may require laryngotomy for adequate excision.

Malignant tumors are treated by external irradiation or surgical excision. Irradiation is suitable for superficial malignant tumors confined to the vocal cord that show no evidence of invasion of muscle or cartilage. More extensive tumors require surgical excision and often en bloc neck node dissection. At times, combined planned preoperative irradiation followed by surgical excision can provide better control of cancer.

Decker J, Goldstein JC: Risk factors in head and neck cancer. *N Engl J Med* 1982;**306**:1151.

DeSanto LW: The options in early laryngeal carcinoma. *N Engl J Med* 1982;**306**:910.

Nahum AM: The needle biopsy comes of age. *Head Neck Surg* (July/Aug) 1981;**3**:457.

Sessions DG: Recent advances in surgery of the larynx and trachea. *Head Neck Surg* (Sept/Oct) 1982;**5**:42.

TRACHEOSTOMY

There are 5 indications for tracheostomy: (1) respiratory obstruction at the level of the larynx or above; (2) inability to clear tracheobronchial secretions; (3) need for some way of administering anesthesia; (4) need to place the larynx at rest; and (5) need for prolonged tracheal intubation for ventilatory assistance.

The causes of airway obstruction at or above the larynx include infections (laryngotracheobronchitis, epiglottitis, and diphtheria), tumors, edema (allergic, infectious, postirradiation), trauma, and foreign bodies. Upper airway obstruction produces supra-sternal, intercostal, and epigastric retraction and signs of hypoxia, including restlessness, increasing pulse, and, as a late finding, cyanosis. Disorders that interfere with normal sphincter action of the larynx, permit aspiration of pharyngeal secretions, and prevent effective cough include loss of consciousness and organic muscular paresis due to poisoning, cerebrovascular accidents, postoperative state, poliomyelitis, and organic central nervous system disease. Obstructive sleep apnea syndrome relieved by tracheostomy has been reported. There are some surgical situations, especially in surgery of the head or neck, where an endotracheal tube cannot be introduced through the nose or mouth but can be introduced through a tracheostomy. Intralaryngeal disease rarely may require tracheostomy to place the larynx at rest.

Two kinds of tracheostomies are performed: emergency and elective. **Emergency tracheostomy** must be done immediately even if proper equipment and assistance are not available. In these circumstances, **cricothyrotomy** is a safe procedure that can be performed rapidly as follows: With a scissors or knife, the skin is cut vertically over the cricothyroid membrane (the part of the airway nearest the skin), a transverse incision is made in this membrane, and the wound is spread with the knife handle or other dilator. It is essential to stay in the midline and to promptly replace this emergency airway with a proper tracheostomy. If a laryngoscope and endotracheal tube or a bronchoscope are available, the airway may be established with one of these devices and a deliberate tracheostomy then performed.

Elective tracheostomy is done under general or local anesthesia while the patient's airway is still adequate or has been reestablished with an endotracheal tube or bronchoscope. The precise surgical technique may vary, eg, with midline or horizontal incision, blunt or sharp dissection, retraction or division of the thyroid isthmus; but the principles are the same in all: (1) avoid trauma to the cricoid cartilage, (2) stay in the midline to avoid trauma to lateral neck structures, and (3) do not close the incision tightly, thus minimizing subcutaneous emphysema.

Posttracheostomy care must include humidifying the inspired air to keep secretions loose and prevent the formation of plugs and crusts, frequent cleaning (every 2–4 hours) of the inner tube, avoidance of heavy sedation, and constant attention during the first 24–48 hours. Uninterrupted observation may not be necessary with some adults, but with small children it is absolutely necessary that a nurse, hospital attendant, or member of the family be in constant attendance as long as the tracheostomy is maintained.

The use of cuffed tracheostomy tubes facilitates positive pressure assisted or controlled respiration. The cuff must be deflated intermittently because prolonged inflation may result in tracheal mucosal ulceration and granuloma formation or tracheal stenosis.

Guilleminault C et al: Progressive improvement of apnea index and ventilatory response to CO_2 after tracheostomy in obstructive sleep apnea syndrome. *Am Rev Resp Dis* 1982;**126**:14.

Linscott MS, Horton WC: Management of upper airway obstruction. *Otolaryngol Clin North Am* 1979;**12**:351.

FOREIGN BODIES IN THE AIR & FOOD PASSAGES*

Foreign bodies may lodge in the larynx, bronchi, or esophagus, usually during eating; following sudden inspiration caused by surprise; as a result of simple carelessness while holding something in the mouth; or during unconsciousness. Eighty percent of cases of inhaled or swallowed foreign bodies occur in children under 15 years of age. In adults, most foreign bodies are large boluses of food or bones lodged in the esophagus as a result of hasty eating or full dentures that impair normal sensation in the mouth.

Esophageal foreign bodies are usually found at the level of the cricothyroid muscle; the inlet to the esophagus; or less commonly, at the cardia or mid esophagus. If laryngeal foreign bodies completely block the airway, asphyxia is imminent. A foreign body small enough to pass the glottis will seldom lodge in the trachea but will be found in the bronchi. The relatively sharp angle of the left bronchus and the straight right bronchus cause most bronchial foreign bodies to be found in the right side. Nearly all foreign bodies that enter food or air passages through the mouth and do not enter the stomach can be removed by the same route.

Laryngeal Foreign Bodies

Laryngeal foreign bodies may produce hoarseness, stridor, cough, and gagging; may obstruct the airway partially or completely and cause dyspnea, stridor, or asphyxia; and may produce inflammatory symptoms of fever, pain, tenderness, and swelling. They can be removed with a grasping forceps through a direct laryngoscope under topical or general anesthesia. The patient should be in the Trendelenburg position to prevent the foreign body from entering the trachea or esophagus, and a bronchoscope and esophagoscope of proper size should be available in case this happens.

A small laryngeal foreign body may become lodged in the bronchi (see below).

Bronchial Foreign Bodies

Bronchial foreign bodies usually produce an initial episode of coughing followed by an asymptomatic ("silent") period varying from a few hours (some vegetable foreign bodies) to months or years (less irritating nonvegetable foreign bodies) before obstructive and inflammatory symptoms occur (cough, wheezing, atelectasis, and pulmonary infection). If the

*See Appendix, p 1113.

foreign body lodges in such a way as to create a valve effect, obstructive emphysema of a pulmonary segment or lobe may be present. Recurrent episodes of cough and pulmonary infection, especially if unilateral, are suggestive of foreign body. X-rays will show a foreign body if it is radiopaque. Nonradiopaque foreign bodies will be revealed on x-ray only by the signs of bronchial obstruction and infection. Vegetable foreign bodies produce earlier and more severe inflammatory symptoms than nonvegetable objects.

In the differential diagnosis, it is necessary to consider pneumonia, bronchiectasis, lung abscess, and tuberculosis.

Bronchial foreign bodies are removed through a bronchoscope with suitable forceps by a skilled endoscopist. General anesthesia is usually employed. In the case of very small radiopaque foreign bodies (eg, straight pins) in the periphery of the lung that cannot be located with the bronchoscope alone, a biplane fluoroscope can sometimes be used. Thoracotomy is occasionally necessary to remove foreign bodies in the periphery of the lung.

Unrecognized bronchial foreign bodies may produce severe and progressive pulmonary infection, with pneumonia, abscess, and empyema. In children, bronchoscopic manipulation may produce laryngeal edema severe enough to require tracheostomy.

Esophageal Foreign Bodies

Esophageal foreign bodies usually produce immediate symptoms of coughing and gagging; pain in the neck at the level of the thyroid cartilage, with a sensation of something "stuck in the throat"; and difficulty in swallowing or inability to swallow food or saliva. Occasionally, however, especially in children, weeks or months may pass before symptoms of infection or obstruction occur. Pooling of saliva in the piriform sinuses is suggestive of esophageal obstruction. X-rays will show opaque objects but often will not show a bolus of meat or a bone. Fluoroscopic observation as the patient swallows a capsule filled with barium sulfate or a wisp of cotton impregnated with barium sulfate is a useful means of locating suspected foreign bodies, since the radiopaque test object will be delayed by the foreign body in its transit through the esophagus.

Esophageal foreign bodies near the cardia may produce pain in the interscapular area.

Esophageal foreign bodies should be removed through the esophagoscope by a skilled endoscopist. Only rarely does an esophageal foreign body constitute an emergency, and so the delay involved in referral is not usually hazardous. Blind probing in an effort to dislodge a foreign body is extremely hazardous.

Perforation of the esophagus by an esophageal foreign body or during endoscopic removal may lead to mediastinal infection (fatal in 50% of cases) or, rarely, severe hemorrhage.

Cohen SR, Lewis GB: Foreign bodies in the airway. *Ann Otol Rhinol Laryngol* 1980;**89**:437.

• • •

References

Ballenger JJ: *Diseases of the Nose, Throat, Ear, Head and Neck,* 13th ed. Lea & Febiger, 1984.
DeWeese DD, Saunders WH: *Textbook of Otolaryngology,* 6th ed. Mosby, 1982.
Levy ML, Ericsson CD, Pickering LK: Infections of the upper respiratory tract. *Med Clin North Am* 1983;**67**:153.
Paparella MM, Shumrick DA (editors): *Otolaryngology,* 2nd ed. 3 vols. Saunders, 1980.

7 | Respiratory Tract & Mediastinum

R. Morton Manson, MD, & James L. Rushing, MD

Commonly Used Abbreviations
(See also Table 7–1.)

ARDS	Adult respiratory distress syndrome
COPD	Chronic obstructive pulmonary disease
CPAP	Continuous positive airway pressure
CPPB	Continuous positive pressure breathing
D_LCO	Diffusion capacity of carbon monoxide by the lung
FEF	Forced expiratory flow
FEV	Forced expiratory volume
F_{IO_2}	Fraction of inspired oxygen
FRC	Functional residual capacity
FVC	Forced vital capacity
IMV	Intermittent mandatory ventilation
MBC	Maximum breathing capacity
MVV	Maximum voluntary ventilation
Pa_{CO_2}	Arterial carbon dioxide tension
Pa_{O_2}	Arterial oxygen tension
PEEP	Positive end-expiratory pressure
RV	Residual volume
TLC	Total lung capacity
VC	Vital capacity

NONSPECIFIC MANIFESTATIONS

Cough

Cough is the most common symptom of respiratory disease. It may be produced by disturbances located anywhere from the oropharynx to the terminal bronchioles. Cough may also occur in diseases not primarily respiratory in nature, eg, congestive heart failure, mitral valve disease, otitis media, or subdiaphragmatic irritation. Cough may be either dry or accompanied by sputum; paroxysmal cough suggests bronchial obstruction. Patients often overlook or minimize a chronic cough, but an explanation should always be sought for any persistent cough.

Dyspnea

Exertional dyspnea may be due to impaired ventilation (eg, restrictive or obstructive defects), inefficient mechanics of breathing, or diffusion defects.

Dyspnea at rest is more characteristic of congestive heart failure than of chronic pulmonary disease,

but it does appear in diffuse pulmonary diseases causing a diffusion defect and when secondary factors are superimposed on a low pulmonary reserve (eg, bronchitis in an emphysematous patient). Acute illnesses (pneumonia, spontaneous pneumothorax, asthma, atelectasis) can produce marked dyspnea at rest.

Orthopnea is usually considered to be presumptive evidence of congestive heart failure, but some pulmonary patients breathe more easily in a sitting position (eg, asthmatics).

Expectoration

The characteristics of the sputum must be noted. Mucoid sputum is seen in tracheobronchitis and asthma. A yellow or greenish sputum suggests bacterial infection. Foul-smelling sputum suggests anaerobic infection (eg, putrid lung abscess). Pink, frothy sputum is seen in pulmonary edema. "Rusty" sputum is typical of pneumococcal pneumonia. Copious sputum separating into layers is characteristic of bronchiectasis.

The production of large amounts of sputum upon a change of posture (eg, upon arising in the morning) occurs when dependent cavities or bronchiectatic spaces suddenly empty into the bronchial tree.

Wheezing

Wheezing is the characteristic manifestation of bronchial narrowing. It occurs during expiration. Forced expiration may elicit wheezing that is absent during normal breathing. In asthma, it is paroxysmal and diffuse. Acute left ventricular failure may produce diffuse wheezing that is differentiated from asthma and bronchitis by associated signs of congestive failure. A persistent localized wheeze is evidence of local bronchial obstruction (eg, carcinoma, inflammatory stenosis, foreign body).

Chest Pain

Pain due to lung disease is usually due to involvement of the parietal pleura (the visceral pleura is insensitive to pain) or the chest wall, including its bony and cartilaginous structures. Pleural pain is usually unilateral and aggravated by changes in intrathoracic pressure (eg, cough, sneeze, deep breathing). Diaphragmatic irritation may cause pain referred to the anterior shoulder (central irritation) or to the upper abdomen (peripheral irritation). Involvement of the chest wall structures is usually accompanied by tenderness, and pain from this location is more constant and less affected by breathing and coughing.

Localized swelling, pain, and tenderness of one or more costosternal cartilages, caused by nonspecific inflammation, occur occasionally (Tietze's syndrome) and may be mistaken for cardiac or pulmonary disease.

Cardiac pain is usually retrosternal and frequently radiates to the neck, jaw, left shoulder, or arm. Such pain produced by exercise and relieved by rest is almost always due to myocardial ischemia. Pericardial inflammation produces retrosternal or precordial pain that is aggravated by deep breathing. Pain from esophageal irritation or spasm is deep and central and is altered by swallowing. Deep, persistent, aching chest pain may be caused by localized neoplasms.

A careful history is essential to the identification of chest pain. Character, location, duration, aggravating factors (exercise, deep respiration, deglutition, etc), and radiation, if any, are important elements in determining the cause of the pain.

Hemoptysis

Spitting or coughing of blood may occur in many bronchopulmonary diseases. Bronchitis, tuberculosis, carcinoma, and bronchiectasis are the most common causes. Bleeding of more than a few ounces is uncommon. Fatal hemorrhage is rare. Bleeding from the nose or pharynx may lead to a history of blood spitting. Collateral circulation between the bronchial and pulmonary veins may cause hemoptysis in mitral stenosis. When associated with acute chest pain, hemoptysis suggests pulmonary infarction. The possibility of bleeding from the upper gastrointestinal tract must be considered. When in doubt, gastric irrigation will usually make the diagnosis.

Cyanosis

Cyanosis represents increased concentration of reduced hemoglobin in the blood (> 5 g/dL), which can result from a number of defects of function in pulmonary disease: (1) impaired diffusion of oxygen from alveoli to capillaries; (2) inadequate gross ventilation of alveoli; and (3) disturbed perfusion/ventilation relationships (increased intrapulmonary "shunts"). Cyanosis is less evident or does not occur in patients with hypoxia due to anemia or histotoxic hypoxia. It is more marked if the patient is cold.

Reduced hemoglobin in the blood may not be manifested as frank cyanosis even when present to a significant degree. The presence or absence of hypoxemia should be confirmed by measuring the oxygen tension of the arterial blood (Pa_{O_2}).

Polycythemia (See also Chapter 10.)

Increase in the total erythrocyte mass may be very striking as a compensatory response to the chronic hypoxemia of pulmonary insufficiency. Primary polycythemia (erythremia) is usually associated with a normal arterial oxygen saturation, but differentiation from the secondary variety is not always easy on this or any other basis.

Digital Clubbing & Hypertrophic Osteoarthropathy

Digital clubbing and the far less common secondary hypertrophic osteoarthropathy are apparently different manifestations of the same incompletely understood cause. Both conditions are found most often in association with bronchogenic carcinoma, but clubbing also occurs with other thoracic and gastrointestinal neoplasms and chronic inflammations and with a wide variety of congenital and acquired cardiac disorders. True clubbing is due to thickening of the soft tissues of the distal phalanges and should not be diagnosed unless the angle between the nail and skin is greater than 180 degrees. Marked curvature of the nails is sometimes mistaken for clubbing. Clubbing occurs occasionally as a benign hereditary trait. Hypertrophic osteoarthropathy is a proliferative periostitis occurring over the distal portions of the long bones. There is usually pain, tenderness, and swelling of the overlying soft tissue. Both conditions may disappear after removal of the primary lesion.

Irwin RS, Carrao WM, Pratter MR: Chronic persistent cough in the adult: The spectrum and frequency of causes and successful outcome of specific therapy. *Am Rev Respir Dis* 1981;**123**:413.

Shneerson JM: Digital clubbing and hypertrophic osteoarthropathy: The underlying mechanisms. *Br J Dis Chest* 1981;**75**:113.

PULMONARY FUNCTION TESTING
(See Table 7–1.)

Although the value of pulmonary function testing in screening asymptomatic patients remains a matter of controversy, there is general agreement that pulmonary function testing is valuable in the diagnosis of patients with symptoms referable to the cardiopulmonary system (eg, dyspnea, wheezing). There is also agreement that in patients known to have lung disease, serial pulmonary function tests are of value in assessing response to therapy and progression or improvement of physiologic impairment over time. In addition, a strong case can be made for preoperative pulmonary function screening (ie, FVC, FEV_1, FEF_{25-75}, and $FEF_{200-1200}$) in patients with known pulmonary risk factors such as smoking or obesity who are to undergo major abdominal or thoracic surgery. The above-mentioned tests can be obtained from a single spirometric maneuver and may be supplemented by measurement of arterial blood gases where needed.

Table 7–1 contains the definition and clinical significance of the more common pulmonary function measurements.

Tisi G: Preoperative evaluation of pulmonary function: Validity, indications, and benefits. *Am Rev Resp Dis* 1979;**119**:293.

Williams DO, Cugell DW: Current perspective on lung function testing. *Hosp Med* (Oct) 1983;**19**:31.

Table 7—1. Common pulmonary function tests and their clinical significance.

Test	Definition	Clinical Significance
Forced vital capacity (FVC)	Total volume of air (in liters) that can be exhaled from the lungs during a forced expiration following a maximal inhalation.	Nonspecific indicator of pulmonary disease; serial measurements are useful to measure deterioration or improvement in same patient.
Forced expiratory flow in 1 second (FEV_1)	Volume of air (in liters) exhaled during the first second of FVC.	Reduced volume suggests obstruction; improvement after bronchodilatation demonstrates reversibility. Most common screening method for detecting significant obstructive disease.
Forced expiratory flow 25–75% (FEF_{25-75})	Rate of air flow (in L/min) during the middle half (25–75%) of the FVC.	Most useful screening test for "small airway disease" (obstructive disease in airways $\leqslant 2$ mm in diameter).
Forced expiratory flow 200–1200 ($FEF_{200-1200}$)	Rate of air flow (in L/min) measured between 200 mL and 1200 mL of the FVC.	Best single measurement of ability to cough. Low value indicates high probability of postoperative pulmonary complications.

Arterial blood gas values while breathing room air		
Test	**Clinical Significance**	**Normal Values**
O_2 tension (Pa_{O_2})	Objective measurement of oxygenation of blood.	104 mm Hg minus (0.4 $\times$ age in years)
CO_2 tension (Pa_{CO_2})	Most reliable assessment of adequacy of ventilation.	38–42 mm Hg
pH	Measure of acidity or alkalinity of arterial blood. Necessary for diagnosis of acidosis or alkalosis.	7.38–7.42

TRACHEOBRONCHIAL DISEASES

ACUTE TRACHEOBRONCHITIS

Acute infection of the upper airway is characterized by cough, with or without sputum. Sputum may be mucoid or purulent. Tracheobronchial infection often follows acute pharyngitis or laryngitis. Fever may occur, and there may be some retrosternal discomfort. On examination, musical rhonchi and occasionally wheezing may be heard. Chest x-ray is negative. Acute tracheobronchitis is usually due to a viral infection, and symptoms may be prolonged by secondary bacterial infection. The disease is rarely serious in the healthy adult but may be life-threatening in patients with severe chronic obstructive pulmonary disease. Sputum cultures usually yield the common mouth organisms. Occasionally, specific pathogens such as pneumococci or *Haemophilus influenzae* are found.

Treatment

Rest and cessation of smoking are advisable. Sufficient fluids should be taken to prevent dehydration. Steam or cool mist inhalation may help relieve irritation. Severe cough may be controlled with a liquid antitussive preparation containing codeine or hydrocodone, given every 4 hours as needed. A nonnarcotic preparation containing dextromethorphan may be sufficient. Cough-suppressing drugs should be avoided in patients with chronic obstructive pulmonary disease. Oral theophylline preparations, eg, aminophylline 100–200 mg every 6 hours, may be helpful if wheezing is present.

Antibiotics are generally unnecessary or inadvisable in the treatment of acute tracheobronchitis. However, they may help prevent secondary infection in patients with impaired respiratory or cardiac function or in patients debilitated by other illnesses. Treatment is with one of the following given orally every 6 hours: tetracycline, 250–500 mg; ampicillin, 250–500 mg.

For a discussion of chronic bronchitis, see p 150.

ACUTE OBSTRUCTION OF THE UPPER AIRWAY

Acute obstruction of the upper airway produces dramatic life-threatening symptoms of suffocation and is usually due to an inhaled foreign body or to acute laryngeal edema (see pp 122–123). The obstruction must be relieved promptly by removal of the foreign body or by an emergency tracheostomy. The Heimlich procedure is especially applicable with obstruction due to an inhaled bolus of food (see p 1113).

CHRONIC OBSTRUCTION OF THE UPPER AIRWAY

Chronic upper airway disease producing either fixed or variable narrowing of the trachea is frequently mistaken for asthma, bronchitis, or emphysema. Causes include scarring from a previous tracheostomy, vocal cord paralysis, compression from an enlarged thyroid, tumors, enlarged lymph nodes, and tracheal malacia. An accurate diagnosis is important because the lesion is often surgically correctable.

Tracheal narrowing may be suspected in the presence of wheezing and dyspnea associated with a stridorous cough, especially if symptoms are aggravated when the patient is in the recumbent position. Inspiratory stridor is an indication that may be demonstrated by auscultation over the trachea.

Obstruction to air flow during both inspiratory and expiratory phases occurs in fixed tracheal obstruction. Predominant inspiratory obstruction occurs when the narrowing is not fixed (eg, vocal cord paralysis). Characteristic patterns of obstruction can be demonstrated in the pulmonary function laboratory by the study of flow-volume loops.

Treatment and prognosis depend on the cause of the obstructing lesion.

A sleep apnea syndrome due to partial upper airway obstruction occurring during sleep has been described. It is characterized by loud snoring punctuated by apneic periods and hypoxemia that may occasionally reach dangerous levels. Other symptoms include daytime somnolence, deterioration of intellectual capacity, personality changes, impotence, morning headache, and abnormal motor activity during sleep. The cause of the airway obstruction may be redundant mucosa that can be resected from the oropharynx and palate. Other patients with severe symptoms and with no demonstrated cause have been cured by permanent tracheostomy. Before consideration of such procedures, the presence of severe obstructive apnea should be documented by nighttime sleep monitoring.

Farmer W, Littner MR, Gee BL: Assessment of therapy of upper airway obstruction. *Arch Intern Med* 1977;**137**:309.
Kryger M et al: Diagnosis of obstruction of the upper and central airways. *Am J Med* 1976;**61**:85.
Simmons FB, Guilleminault C, Miles EM: A surgical treatment for snoring and obstructive sleep apnea. *West J Med* 1984;**140**:43.

PULMONARY DISEASES DUE TO IMMUNOLOGIC REACTIONS

Progress in immunology within the past 2 decades has resulted in greater understanding of the pathogenesis of a large group of lung diseases that were thought to be unrelated. Recent studies of enzymes and cellular elements in bronchopulmonary washings have helped to elucidate the immunopathogenesis of several pulmonary disorders. Some disorders are currently categorized as hypersensitivity manifestations of the immunologic reactions described and classified by Coombs and Gell (types 1–4). Examples are as follows:

Type I: Anaphylactic: Atopic asthma, immediate.
Type II: Cytotoxic: Pneumoconiosis, Goodpasture's syndrome, and certain drug reactions.

Type III: Immune complex disease: Pulmonary vasculitis (in systemic lupus erythematosus and other collagen disorders), serum sickness.
Type IV: Cell-mediated: Pulmonary eosinophilia due to parasites.

Danielle RP (editor): Symposium on immune complex injury of the lung. *Am Rev Respir Dis* 1981;**124**:738.
Reynolds HY: Immunologic lung disease. (2 parts.) *Chest* 1982; **81**:126, 745.
Schatz M, Patterson R, Fink J: Immunologic lung disease. *N Engl J Med* 1979;**300**:1310.

ASTHMA

Essentials of Diagnosis

- Recurrent acute attacks of dyspnea, cough, and mucoid sputum, usually accompanied by wheezing.
- Prolonged expiration with generalized wheezing and musical rales.
- Bronchial obstruction reversible by drugs.

General Considerations

Asthma is due to hyperreactive airways that constrict and secrete excessive mucus in response to a variety of stimuli (allergens, infections, noxious fumes, cold air, and other irritants). The airway obstruction is due to a combination of bronchoconstriction, mucosal edema, and inspissated mucus and is usually reversible.

Atopic, or "extrinsic," asthma has been thought to result from sensitization of the bronchial mucosa by tissue-specific antibodies. The antibodies produced are immunoglobulins of the IgE (type I) class, and the total serum IgE concentration is usually elevated. Exposure to the appropriate allergens by inhalation results in an antigen-antibody reaction that releases vasoactive bronchoconstrictive chemical mediators, causing the characteristic tissue changes. More recent work suggests that immunoglobulin G (IgG) may play a role similar to that of IgE in some cases.

Approximately 50% of asthmatics are of the nonatopic ("intrinsic") type in which the bronchial reaction occurs in response to nonimmunologic stimuli such as infection, irritating inhalants, cold air, exercise, and emotional upset. These patients do not demonstrate elevated IgE antibodies in their serum, and the history does not suggest hypersensitivity to specific allergens, although there may be other immunologic mechanisms that have not yet been demonstrated.

Certain chemicals such as isocyanates and metal dusts encountered in the workplace cause asthma by direct irritation, protein denaturation, and hypersensitization by mechanisms as yet unknown. Hypersensitization has been shown to occur in susceptible individuals after repeated exposure to very low concentrations of isocyanates and sulfites, well within the limits permitted by occupational safety laws. Occupational asthma should be suspected when symptoms occur repeatedly at work or within several hours thereafter and improve away from work. Improvement may require several days. Sulfites are widely used in the preservation of foods and even medicines and are considered to be the cause of some cases of "nonatopic" asthma.

Beta-adrenergic blocking agents such as propranolol cause intense bronchial constriction in patients with asthma, apparently due to parasympathetic nerve stimulation.

Aspirin and nonsteroidal anti-inflammatory agents may cause severe asthma in some patients.

Clinical Findings

A. Symptoms and Signs: Asthma is characterized by recurrent attacks of dyspnea, cough, and expectoration of tenacious mucoid sputum, and usually wheezing. Symptoms may be mild and may occur only in association with respiratory infection, or they may occur in various degrees of severity to the point of being life-threatening. Classic allergic (atopic) asthma usually begins in childhood and becomes progressively more severe throughout life, although spontaneous remissions may occur in adulthood. Hay fever often accompanies atopic asthma.

The acute attack is characterized by dyspnea usually associated with expiratory wheezing that may be heard without a stethoscope. Cough may be present but is usually not the predominant symptom. There is a small group of patients with asthma in whom paroxysmal cough may be the predominant symptom.

When asthma becomes prolonged, with severe intractable wheezing, it is known as status asthmaticus.

B. Laboratory Findings: The sputum is characteristically tenacious and mucoid, containing "plugs" and "spirals." Eosinophils are seen microscopically. The differential blood count may show eosinophilia. In severe, acute bronchospasm, arterial hypoxemia may be present as a result of disturbed perfusion/ventilation relationships, alveolar hypoventilation, or functional right-to-left shunts. An elevated P_{aCO_2} is unusual and, when present, is a cause for concern.

C. X-Ray Findings: Chest films usually show no abnormalities. Reversible hyperexpansion may occur in severe paroxysms, or hyperexpansion may persist in long-standing cases. Transient, migratory pulmonary infiltrations may be present. Severe attacks are sometimes complicated by pneumothorax.

Differential Diagnosis

Distinguish wheezing from that due to other disorders such as bronchitis, obstructive emphysema, and congestive heart failure.

Treatment

The treatment may be divided into 2 phases: (1) treatment of the acute attack and (2) interim therapy. Mild attacks may be relieved by nebulized bronchodilators. Subcutaneous epinephrine, with or without intravenous aminophylline, is more effective for moderate wheezing. (Epinephrine should not be used in patients with hypertension or angina or in elderly patients.) For status asthmaticus or for acute asthma in epinephrine-resistant patients, adrenal corticosteroids are usually necessary.

A. Acute Attack: Maintain adequate rest and relieve apprehension by reassurance. Treat respiratory infections vigorously with antibiotics. Give fluids orally or parenterally as necessary to prevent dehydration and liquefy secretions.

1. Drugs–

a. Nebulized adrenergic stimulators are effective agents for mild attacks. In the emergency department or office, isoetharine 1% (Bronkosol) or isoproterenol 1:200 (Isuprel), 0.5 mL in 2–3 mL of water or normal saline, is delivered by nebulizer using compressed air or oxygen as the pressure source. The patient is encouraged to take slow, deep inhalations. The treatment may be repeated in 20 minutes if necessary. In the absence of the above equipment, these agents can be administered by a pressurized, metered dose inhaler (Bronkometer, Medihaler-Iso). The usual dose is 2–3 inhalations initially, followed by 2 inhalations in 20 minutes, if necessary, then every 4 hours. Several minutes should be allowed after the first inhalation before repeating, to produce deeper bronchial penetration.

b. Epinephrine (1:1000), 0.2–0.5 mL subcutaneously, is the most effective drug for moderate and severe wheezing. It can be repeated in 20 minutes and then every 1–2 hours. (Note the above precautions.)

c. Aminophylline (a theophylline-ethylenediamine complex), 250 mg in 10–20 mL of normal saline *slowly* intravenously, can be used if epinephrine is not effective and the patient is not already receiving a theophylline preparation. Both epinephrine and aminophylline can be given initially.

d. Corticosteroid drugs–Most effective in severe attacks that do not respond to the above bronchodilators. Hydrocortisone sodium succinate (Solu-Cortef), 250 mg intravenously, can be given in a single dose together with prednisone, 40–60 mg orally in divided doses the first day. The daily dose of prednisone is gradually reduced to zero over the next 7–10 days.

e. Oxygen by nasal prongs or mask is indicated in moderate to severe wheezing.

f. Fluids–Patients with persistent symptoms who require hospitalization need supplemental intravenous fluids to help liquefy secretions.

2. Status asthmaticus–When severe wheezing persists after use of the measures listed above, hospitalization is required. A P_{aO_2} of less than 50 mm Hg is an indication for hospitalization. Elevation of the P_{aCO_2} signifies an urgent need for hospitalization.

The principal drugs for the treatment of the hospitalized patient are the following:

a. Aminophylline–Give an initial dose of 6 mg/kg intravenously in 100 mL 5% dextrose in water over 20 minutes. Reduce or eliminate the loading dose (see below) for patients who have been taking theophylline preparations. (In overweight patients, calculation of the dose should be based on ideal rather than actual body weight, because theophylline does not penetrate fatty tissue.)

The intravenous infusion should be continued according to the dosage schedule recommended by the FDA, which is lower than previously recommended by various authors: children and young adult smokers, 1 mg/kg/h for 12 hours, then reduce to 0.8 mg/kg/h; healthy nonsmoking adults, 0.7 mg/kg/h, reduced to 0.5 mg/kg/h after 12 hours; older patients and those with cor pulmonale, 0.6 mg/kg/h, reduced to 0.3 mg/kg/h after 12 hours; patients with congestive heart failure and liver failure, 0.5 mg/kg/h, reduced to 0.1–0.2 mg/kg/h after 12 hours.

The subsequent dosage schedule should be determined by the serum concentration; 10–20 μg/mL is the recognized therapeutic range.

For patients who have been taking theophylline drugs, determine (if possible) the amount and time of the last medication (1.2 mg aminophylline is equivalent to 1 mg theophylline) and reduce the loading dose accordingly. When this information is not available, give a reduced loading dose of aminophylline of 2.9 mg/kg, then continue with the maintenance schedule outlined above.

b. Corticosteroids–The drugs of choice are either hydrocortisone sodium succinate (Solu-Cortef), 250 mg, or methylprednisolone sodium succinate (Solu-Medrol), 125 mg given intravenously every 4 hours until improvement is established. Prednisone, 20 mg, or methylprednisolone (Medrol), 16 mg orally 4 times daily, can be started at the same time and continued in decreasing doses after the intravenous steroids are no longer needed.

B. Other Measures: Oxygen by nasal prongs or mask should be given in sufficient concentration to relieve hypoxemia.

Dehydration is frequently present and must be corrected by intravenous replacement. Use up to 4 liters of 5% dextrose in water in 24 hours for an average-sized adult. Electrolytes should be monitored during continued intravenous replacement.

Nebulized isoetharine (Bronkosol), 0.5 mL in 3 mL of 0.5 N saline, may be added every 3–4 hours. The use of intermittent positive pressure breathing has no clear advantage over a simple nebulizer driven by compressed air or oxygen. The addition of chest percussion and postural drainage every 2–4 hours will usually aid in clearing tenacious secretions.

Arterial blood gases should be monitored every 30–60 minutes initially. Unrelieved hypoxemia or a rising Pa_{CO_2} or, if blood gas measurements are not available, clinical deterioration of the patient is an indication for intubation and assisted or controlled respiration. After intubation, sedation with small doses of diazepam or morphine intravenously may be necessary to permit ventilatory control by the respirator.

When control of wheezing cannot be accomplished by the above measures, general anesthesia with halothane may be lifesaving. Cardiac rhythm and blood pressure must be monitored carefully.

C. Interim Therapy: Attempt to identify the offending allergens and protect the patient from further contact. Desensitization may be indicated occasionally. Emotional disturbances should be eliminated if possible. Patients with "intrinsic" asthma (usually associated with bronchitis) may be helped by antibiotic therapy.

Long-acting theophylline preparations (Theo-Dur, Theolair) in doses sufficient to produce therapeutic blood levels, usually 300 mg every 12 hours, are the bronchodilators of choice.

Various combinations of ephedrine with aminophylline and a barbiturate or hydroxyzine have been used for many years with benefit in mild asthma, but side effects (tachycardia and central nervous system stimulation) are frequent and may limit their usefulness. The newer beta-adrenergic stimulators have a relatively greater degree of beta$_2$ specificity and longer action; accordingly, they are somewhat more effective and have fewer side effects. Terbutaline (Brethine, Bricanyl) may be given orally (2.5–5 mg 3 times daily). Albuterol (Proventil, Ventolin) may be given orally (2–4 mg 3 or 4 times daily) or as a metered dose aerosol (1–2 inhalations every 4–6 hours). These agents cause an initial adrenergic response of anxiety and tremor, but this tends to decrease over a few days even while drug intake continues. Patients should be advised against excessive use.

The other nebulized drugs, isoproterenol (Isuprel), metaproterenol (Alupent, Metaprel), and isoetharine (Bronkosol) are useful in relieving or preventing mild wheezing when used in a hand bulb or pressurized nebulizer. Proper use of the nebulizer is important. Patients should be instructed to direct the nebulized spray into the back of the pharynx during inhalation with the mouth open. Two inhalations separated by a 5-minute interval will produce the maximum effect.

Patients who are not helped by other measures may be treated on a long-term basis with a corticosteroid. The dosage employed should be sufficient to keep the patient comfortable and relatively free of symptoms. Begin with 10 mg 3–4 times daily and reduce gradually to the lowest effective maintenance dose, preferably on an alternate-day schedule.

An aerosolized corticosteroid, beclomethasone dipropionate (Beclovent, Vanceril), has been found to be effective in many asthmatic patients who require corticosteroids. It is virtually unabsorbable and thus has no systemic side effects. Its action occurs in the bronchial mucosa. It is not effective during an acute attack, since its action depends on deposition deep in the bronchial tree. It is best introduced after wheezing has been controlled by a systemic corticosteroid, which can then be reduced or eliminated as the nebulized drug takes effect. In patients who have been receiving long-term treatment with a systemic corticosteroid, joint pains and other symptoms may appear as that drug is reduced. Prolonged gradual weaning may be necessary. Some patients will continue to require systemic corticosteroid drugs in smaller dosage. Some receive no benefit from the aerosolized form. In a recent report, no adverse effects were found in mothers or infants when inhaled beclomethasone was used during pregnancy in the recommended dosage.

Beclomethasone may be used after administration of a rapidly acting nebulized bronchodilator such as isoetharine or albuterol to achieve deeper deposition in the bronchial tree. The initial dose is 2 inhalations 4 times daily, with subsequent adjustment to the lowest effective dose. Doses as frequent as 8 times daily are acceptable if significant improvement results. (However, the isoetharine or albuterol should not be used more often than every 4 hours.) Some patients are well maintained on twice-daily treatments. Even patients who are well controlled with the nebulized drug may have occasional increased wheezing during colds or intense exposure to allergens. Short courses of prednisone may be required.

A troublesome side effect—oral candidiasis—can be avoided by rinsing the mouth thoroughly with water after each nebulizer treatment; rinsing with a liquid nystatin suspension, 2 mL 4 times daily, is usually effective if this side effect develops.

Atropine has long been known to be an effective bronchodilator but has uncomfortable side effects. An aerosolized form (not yet available in the USA) may produce the desired anticholinergic effect on the bronchi without systemic absorption and side effects.

Cromolyn sodium (Intal) is useful mainly in atopic asthma and asthma induced by exercise. It acts to specifically inhibit the liberation of mediators initiated by the antigen-antibody reaction. It is effective only during remissions to prevent recurrent attacks and to reduce the requirement for corticosteroids. It is administered as a micronized powder by inhalation. Occasional pharyngeal and tracheal irritation has been noted, but no systemic side effects have been reported.

Prognosis

Most patients with asthma adjust well to the necessity for continued medical treatment throughout life. Inadequate control or persistent aggravation by unmodified environmental conditions may lead to the development of incapacitating or even life-threatening complications.

Bukowskyj M, Nakatsu K, Munt PW: Theophylline reassessed. *Ann Intern Med* 1984;**101**:63.

Chodosh S: Rational management of bronchial asthma. *Arch Intern Med* 1978;**138**:1394.

Corrao WM, Braman SS, Irwin RS: Chronic cough as the sole presenting manifestation of bronchial asthma. *N Engl J Med* 1979;**300**:633.

Fatal asthma. (Editorial.) *Lancet* 1979;**2**:337.

Greenberger PA, Patterson R: Beclomethasone dipropionate for severe asthma during pregnancy. *Ann Intern Med* 1983;**98**:478.

Josephson GW et al: Emergency treatment of asthma. *JAMA* 1979;**242**:639.

Kass I, Nair SV, Patil KD: Beclomethasone dipropionate aerosol in the treatment of steroid-dependent asthma: An assessment of 18 months of therapy. *Chest* 1977;**71**:703.

Rossing TH, Fanta CH, McFadden ER Jr: Effect of outpatient treatment of asthma with beta agonists on the response to sympathomimetics in an emergency room. *Am J Med* 1983;**75**:781.

Schwartz SH: Treatment of status asthmaticus with halothane. *JAMA* 1984;**251**:2688.

Sheppard D: Occupational asthma. *West J Med* 1982;**137**:480.

Sogn D: The ubiquitous sulfites. (Editorial.) *JAMA* 1984; **251**:2986.

Van Arsdell PP Jr, Paul GH: Drug therapy in the management of asthma. *Ann Intern Med* 1977;**87**:68.

Webb-Johnson DC, Andrews JL Jr: Bronchodilator therapy. (2 parts.) *N Engl J Med* 1977;**297**:476, 758.

Williams MH Jr: Life-threatening asthma. *Arch Intern Med* 1980; **140**:1604.

PULMONARY INFILTRATIONS WITH EOSINOPHILIA

The most common cause of pulmonary infiltrations with eosinophilia is aspergillosis. It occurs in atopic individuals and may go unrecognized as a cause of asthma. Both type I and type III immune reactions appear to be operative.

The disease typically appears as an asthmatic syndrome in young adults, many of whom had ordinary childhood asthma. The additional clinical features include marked (up to 80%) eosinophilia of the peripheral blood and of the sputum, pulmonary infiltrates that are often migratory, dense pulmonary lesions secondary to impacted mucous plugs, and, occasionally, bronchiectasis.

Other diagnostic findings include positive skin tests, both immediate and delayed, to *Aspergillus* extracts, positive sputum cultures for *Aspergillus fumigatus,* and significant elevation of serum IgE levels.

Other causes of pulmonary eosinophilia without asthma include *Candida* infection, reaction to certain bacterial enzymes *(Bacillus subtilis),* systemic helminthic infections that have a pulmonary cycle (ascariasis, filariasis), and a number of common drugs. The pulmonary eosinophilia caused by most of these agents may be transient and migratory (Löffler's syndrome) or may be chronic and result in irreversible pulmonary fibrosis.

Treatment is largely symptomatic. Systemic corticosteroids are usually very effective for controlling symptoms and clearing pulmonary infiltrates. Anthelmintic agents should be used when indicated; antifungal agents are not effective. Mucoid impaction may result in permanent areas of fibrosis and bronchiectasis.

Schatz M, Wasserman S, Patterson R: The eosinophil and the lung. *Arch Intern Med* 1982;**142**:1515.

ASBESTOSIS

Exposure to asbestos is far more common than heretofore recognized. In addition to the obvious exposures of mining and manufacture of asbestos products, many opportunities for more subtle exposure to asbestos fibers occur in other settings, such as the use of products containing the substance, removal of insulation from buildings and plumbing, and even working and living near operations that discharge fibers into the air.

Pulmonary asbestosis usually requires prolonged exposure to asbestos fibers, although lung damage following exposure for a single day has been reported. There also appears to be a genetically determined susceptibility to the development of progressive pulmonary disease. A decrease in cell-mediated immunity and an increase in humoral immune factors have been observed, but the significance of these changes in the pathogenesis of the disease remains to be determined. Cigarette smokers and persons with preexisting chronic pulmonary disease are at greater risk.

Bronchogenic carcinoma occurs more frequently in the presence of asbestosis, especially in smokers, in whom the incidence is 100 times greater than that in smokers in the general population. Pleural mesothelioma—long associated with asbestosis—has been noted to occur more frequently following relatively trivial exposure, such as residing near asbestos plants.

Asbestos is a silicate of iron and magnesium that occurs in fibers thin enough to be inhaled to the level of the respiratory bronchioles. Chrysotile is the commonest form in nature. Crocidolite and amosite ores produce smaller but equally damaging fibers. Once deposited in the distal bronchioles, the fibers are coated with macrophages and ferritin granules, producing the characteristic ferruginous (asbestos) bodies. The resulting tissue reaction is usually a diffuse fibrosis beginning in the alveoli and extending to the interstitial tissue, predominantly in the lower lobes.

Pleural plaques are another common manifestation, and these frequently calcify. Progression of the process results in loss of lung volume and elasticity and eventual pulmonary failure. The presence of pleural plaques without pulmonary fibrosis may indicate asbestos exposure but may not indicate significant disease or disability. The determination of disability for compensation purposes requires a documented history of exposure, compatible x-ray findings, demonstration of ferruginous bodies in sputum or tissue, and significant alteration of pulmonary function tests (sometimes demonstrated only by exercise testing).

X-ray changes in asbestosis consist of diffuse infiltrates, predominantly in the lower lobes, and pleural thickening, which occasionally calcifies, especially the diaphragmatic pleura.

There is no effective treatment for asbestosis. Exposure must be prevented by dust control and the use of masks and other devices to guard against inhalation of asbestos fibers.

SILICOSIS

Essentials of Diagnosis

- History of exposure to dust containing silicon dioxide (eg, hard rock mining, sandblasting, foundry work).
- Characteristic x-ray changes: Bilateral nodules, fibrosis, hilar lymphadenopathy.
- Recurrent respiratory infections.
- *Note:* Tuberculosis is a common complication.

General Considerations

Silicosis is one of the chronic fibrotic pulmonary diseases caused by inhalation of inorganic occupational dusts (the pneumoconioses, Table 7–2). In the case of silicosis, free silica (silicon dioxide) is by far the most common offender. Prolonged exposure is usually required. Various immunoglobulins have been identified in silicotic tissue and in bronchoalveolar washings, but the exact role of immunologic factors in the pathogenesis of silicosis has yet to be demonstrated.

Clinical Findings

A. Symptoms and Signs: Symptoms may be absent or may consist only of unusual susceptibility to upper respiratory tract infections, "bronchitis," and pneumonia. Dyspnea on exertion is the most common complaint. It may progress slowly. Cough usually develops and is dry initially but later becomes productive, frequently with blood-streaked sputum. Severe, occasionally fatal hemoptysis may occur.

Physical findings may be absent in patients with advanced silicosis.

B. Laboratory Findings: Sputum studies for acid-fast bacilli are indicated to rule out silicotuberculosis or other mycobacterial infection. Pulmonary function tests characteristically show reduced lung volumes, decreased diffusion capacity, decreased compliance, and normal or increased flow rates. Lung biopsy is occasionally indicated to establish the diagnosis for compensation purposes.

C. X-Ray Findings: Chest x-rays are not diagnostic but often strongly suggest the diagnosis. Abnormalities are usually bilateral, symmetric, and predominant in the inner mid-lung fields. Small nodules tend to be of uniform size and density. Enlargement of hilar nodes is a relatively early finding. Peripheral calcification of the nodes, giving an "eggshell" appearance, may occur later. Interstitial fibrosis is manifested by fine linear markings and reticulation. Coalescence of nodules produces larger densities, sometimes quite large (progressive massive fibrosis), which may have the radiologic appearance of a neoplasm. Associated emphysema gives an x-ray picture of increased radiolucency, often quite striking at the lung bases.

Treatment

No specific treatment is available. Symptomatic treatment is indicated for chronic cough and wheezing.

Table 7—2. Pneumoconioses.*

Disease and Occupation	Causative Particle and Pathology	Clinical Features	X-Ray Findings
Silicosis† (mining, drilling, blasting, grinding, abrasive manufacture; various other processes exposing silica to high temperatures, such as iron molding or ceramic manufacture)	Free silica, cristobalite, and tridymite (toxic isomers produced by exposure of silica to high temperatures) cause immunologic tissue reactions producing nodules, fibrosis, lymphatic blockage, emphysema, and hilar adenopathy.	Required exposure is 2–20 years. May remain asymptomatic for years after lesions appear on x-ray. Then, dyspnea on exertion, dry cough, hemoptysis. Frequent infections, especially tuberculosis. Pulmonary insufficiency, chronic cor pulmonale.	Nodules (inner, midlung fields), interstitial fibrosis, hilar adenopathy; peripheral ("eggshell") calcification of hilar nodes. Signs of associated tuberculosis (inflammatory infiltrates, cavitation) may be present.
Asbestosis‡ (asbestos mining and processing, handling asbestos products)	Iron, calcium, and magnesium silicates; chrysotile, amosite, crocidolite. Causes diffuse pulmonary fibrosis, thickened alveolar walls, pleural plaques, ferruginous (asbestos) bodies in the tissue.	Exposure is usually prolonged but may be short. Lesions appear years after exposure. Increased incidence of bronchogenic carcinoma and malignant mesothelioma even after trivial exposure.	Fine, diffuse infiltrates in lower lobes, with late appearance of interstitial fibrosis. Thickening and sometimes calcification of pleura, which may occur without parenchymal changes.
Berylliosis (beryllium production, machining, and drilling; use of beryllium alloys and ceramics in the electronics and space vehicle industries)	Beryllium particles. **Acute:** Patchy infiltrations resembling bronchial pneumonia. **Chronic:** Alveolar septal granuloma causing fine nodules. Fibrosis not prominent. Elastic tissue damaged, causing emphysema. No hilar adenopathy.	**Acute:** After a few weeks of exposure, upper respiratory symptoms; "bronchitis," "pneumonia" later. **Chronic:** Required exposure 6–18 months. Dyspnea, cough, weight loss, cyanosis, skin lesions, pulmonary insufficiency, cor pulmonale.	**Acute:** Clear at first, then patchy infiltrations. **Chronic:** Scattered minute ("sandpaper") nodules. Later, larger nodules, diffuse reticular markings. No hilar adenopathy.
Bauxite pneumoconiosis (Shaver's disease; aluminosis)	May be due to other toxic contaminants rather than aluminum dust per se, causing fibrosis, hilar adenopathy, atelectasis.	Required exposure is several months to 2 years. Dyspnea (marked pulmonary insufficiency). Attacks of spontaneous pneumothorax.	Hilar and mediastinal adenopathy, irregularity of diaphragms, fibrosis, emphysema.
Anthracosis (rarely dissociated from silicosis) (mining, city dwellers)	Coal dust, causing black discoloration of lungs, nodes, distant organs (nodules rare).	Progressive disease (fibrosis, emphysema) reported in Welsh soft-coal workers. Silica may be an important factor.	"Reticulation," fine nodules. Coal dust may produce large densities by deposition without fibrosis.
Siderosis (iron ore processing, metal drilling, electric arc welding)	Iron oxides, metallic iron, causing "red" (oxides) and "black" (metallic) discoloration of lung. "Red" type leads to fibrosis. "Black" type associated with silicosis.	Findings are those of associated silicosis. (See above.)	Dependent mainly on associated silicosis.

*Actual exposure is rarely to one dust alone.
†Silicosis is discussed more fully on p 131.
‡Asbestosis is discussed more fully on p 131.

When tuberculosis occurs (a not uncommon complication), antituberculosis drugs must be given as for the treatment of advanced tuberculosis (Table 7–3). In the presence of a positive tuberculin skin test and no other evidence of active tuberculosis, isoniazid, 300 mg daily, should be given for 2 years.

Prognosis

Gradually progressive dyspnea may be present for years. The development of complications, especially tuberculosis, markedly worsens the prognosis.

Craighead JE, Mossman BT: The pathogenesis of asbestos-associated diseases. *N Engl J Med* 1982;**306:**1446.

De Shazo RD: Current concepts about the pathogenesis of silicosis and asbestosis. *J Allergy Clin Immunol* 1982;**70:**41.

Golden JA: Asbestos related lung disease: Medical Staff Conference, University of California School of Medicine, San Francisco. *West J Med* 1979;**131:**225.

Hassan FM, Nash G, Kazemi H: The significance of asbestos exposure in the diagnosis of mesothelioma. *Am Rev Respir Dis* 1977;**115**:761.

Parkes WR: *Occupational Lung Disorders*, 2nd ed. Butterworth, 1982.

Weill H: Occupational lung diseases. *Hosp Pract* (May) 1981; **16**:53.

OTHER PNEUMOCONIOSES
(See Table 7–2.)

The following substances, when inhaled, cause varying degrees of pulmonary inflammation, fibrosis, emphysema, and disability, usually to a lesser degree than silicon dioxide: coal dust, bauxite (aluminum and silicon), talc (hydrous magnesium silicate), graphite (crystallized carbon plus silicon dioxide), beryllium, and diatomaceous earth. The latter is almost pure silicon dioxide but produces effects essentially like those of silicosis only when heated (flux calcined) in the manufacture of abrasives.

Identification of these pulmonary dust diseases depends upon a careful inquiry into possible occupational or casual exposure.

Treatment is symptomatic.

SARCOIDOSIS
(Boeck's Sarcoid)

Essentials of Diagnosis

- Hilar adenopathy and nodular or fibrous infiltration of both lungs on the chest x-ray.
- Tuberculin reaction usually negative; no bacteriologic evidence of tuberculosis.
- Biopsy (most commonly the lymph nodes and skin) reveals noncaseating granuloma.
- Occasionally, the skin, bones, joints, salivary glands, and uvea are also involved.
- Black race more often affected.

General Considerations

Boeck's sarcoid is a chronic noncaseating epithelioid cell granuloma that may involve various organs but most commonly the lungs. More than one immunologic mechanism appears to be involved. Type IV cell-mediated immunity, which is associated with granuloma formation, was identified earlier. More recently, increased IgM and IgG immunoglobulins have been demonstrated in sarcoid lung tissue and airway secretions. It is now believed that granuloma formation is preceded by a mononuclear cell alveolitis made up primarily of T lymphocytes and alveolar macrophages. The immunogenic stimulus causing the alveolitis has not been identified. The alveolitis is transformed into a noncaseating epithelioid granuloma that usually resolves spontaneously but may persist and progress to pulmonary fibrosis. Distribution of sarcoidosis is worldwide, but the incidence is highest in the temperate zones, especially in the southeastern USA. The incidence in the black population is 14 times that in whites. The usual age range is 20–40.

Since the lungs and mediastinal nodes are most commonly involved, sarcoidosis is an important entity in the differential diagnosis of pulmonary and mediastinal diseases.

Clinical Findings

A. Symptoms and Signs: Pulmonary symptoms and signs are commonly absent in spite of marked x-ray abnormalities. Constitutional symptoms, such as night sweats, fever, and loss of weight, are often minimal or absent. Cough and dyspnea occur late in patients with progressive pulmonary lesions, although they may occasionally occur early in the presence of an acute onset.

Skin lesions consist of nodules and diffuse infiltrations, especially of the face, ears, nose, and extensor surfaces. Atrophic scars may follow healing. Erythema nodosum may occur.

Other clinical manifestations are very uncommon. Enlargement of the tracheobronchial nodes may produce cough and dyspnea owing to compression. Persistent painless enlargement of the parotid and other salivary glands may occur. There may also be lacrimal gland involvement; variable involvement of the eyes, with conjunctivitis, iritis, and corneal and vitreous opacities; and involvement of the retina.

Polyarthritis may occur.

Myocardial lesions may result in arrhythmias, conduction defects, and even cardiac failure.

Paralysis of the facial muscles, soft palate, and vocal cords and peripheral neuritis may be found.

B. Skin Tests: Type IV cell-mediated hypersensitivity reactions are known to be impaired in sarcoidosis, and tuberculin and various fungus antigen skin tests are usually negative even when these infections are present. Antigen prepared from sarcoid nodes and injected intracutaneously reproduces the sarcoid tubercle locally, usually after weeks or months, in most patients with sarcoidosis (Kveim reaction). The value of this test is limited because of the time required and also because positive reactions may occur in the presence of lymphadenopathy due to diverse causes.

C. Laboratory Findings: Routine laboratory tests are usually not helpful. Tissue biopsy is the most definitive diagnostic test. Lymph nodes are involved in 80% of sarcoid patients, and the most frequent sites are supraclavicular anterior to the scalenus anticus muscle and in the mediastinum. Other biopsy procedures include transbronchial lung biopsy through the flexible bronchoscope when there is x-ray evidence of pulmonary infiltration and blind-needle biopsy of the liver, where granulomas are found in 20–40% of asymptomatic sarcoidosis patients. Biopsy material should also be cultured for tubercle bacilli and fungi.

Recent studies of material obtained by bronchoalveolar lavage through the flexible bronchoscope have greatly expanded our understanding of the pathogenesis of pulmonary sarcoidosis. T lymphocytes and other mononuclear cells can be identified and quantified. Another procedure is based on the propensity of intravenously administered Gallium citrate Ga 67 to localize in the alveolar macrophages of active sarcoid alveolitis, permitting these cells to be quantified by a lung scan. As these 2 procedures become more available, diagnosis will be facilitated, and the course and outcome of the disease may be more predictable.

D. X-Ray Findings: Prominent bilateral hilar adenopathy is common. Interstitial nodular infiltration may occur with or without adenopathy and is usually bilateral. In later stages, the infiltrations are replaced by fibrosis that may eventually become extensive and cause bullous emphysema and bronchiectasis. Prior to the appearance of fibrosis, the process may be entirely reversible. Characteristic "punched-out" areas in the bones of the fingers and toes may be seen but are uncommon.

Differential Diagnosis

The most important diseases to be differentiated are tuberculosis, the malignant lymphomas (especially Hodgkin's disease), the collagen diseases, mycotic infections, and other diseases producing x-ray patterns of hilar lymphadenopathy or miliary pulmonary nodules. The relatively asymptomatic nature of sarcoidosis in the presence of obvious clinical disease is an important differential feature.

Treatment

There is no specific treatment. Absence of symptoms and spontaneous resolution are common. When extensive pulmonary disease is present that is symptomatic or progressive, corticosteroid treatment may be helpful. Prednisone, 40 mg orally daily, should be given for at least 1 month. If no symptomatic or x-ray improvement has occurred, discontinue the drug gradually. If there has been improvement, reduce the prednisone gradually to 20 mg daily and continue as long as further clearing occurs. When stability of symptoms or x-ray lesions has been achieved, continue the corticosteroid for another 4–6 weeks in gradually decreasing doses until the drug is eliminated. Exacerbations of symptoms or x-ray lesions may indicate the need for more prolonged treatment.

Prognosis

Sarcoidosis is a relatively benign disease. The overall mortality rate is about 5%. Hilar adenopathy usually resolves without treatment. Pulmonary lesions are more likely to persist and be replaced by fibrosis with or without treatment. Complications may include cardiac failure (due to actual myocardial involvement or cor pulmonale) and pulmonary insufficiency when pulmonary lesions are progressive. The altered diffusion capacity may persist even after other signs and symptoms have cleared.

Hanson RR et al: Transbronchial biopsy via fiberoptic bronchoscope: Results in 164 patients. *Am Rev Respir Dis* 1976; **114**:67.

Kaltreider HB, Caldwell JL, Ayoub EM: Pulmonary and cardiac diseases. Chap 28, pp 544–559, in: *Basic & Clinical Immunology*, 5th ed. Stites DP et al (editors). Lange, 1984.

Keogh BA et al: The alveolitis of pulmonary sarcoidosis: Evaluation of natural history and alveolitis-dependent changes in lung function. *Am Rev Respir Dis* 1983;**128**:256.

Mitchell DN, Scadding JG: Sarcoidosis. *Am Rev Respir Dis* 1974;**110**:774.

Rohatgi PK: Breakthroughs in understanding pulmonary sarcoidosis. *Drug Ther* (March) 1984;**14**:138.

GOODPASTURE'S SYNDROME

This disease consists of chronic, relapsing pulmonary hemosiderosis, often in association with fatal glomerulonephritis. The cause is unknown. Both type II and type III immunoglobulins have been identified in association with this disease, but their roles in pathogenesis have not been determined.

Clinical features include cough with recurrent hemoptysis, dyspnea, pulmonary infiltrates, and hypochromic iron deficiency anemia resulting from hemoptysis and the breakdown of large amounts of hemoglobin and its deposit as hemosiderin in the lungs. Transbronchial lung biopsy through a flexible fiberoptic bronchoscope is a valuable diagnostic procedure. It is necessary to demonstrate IgG deposits on the alveolocapillary membrane by immunofluorescence staining in order to distinguish this condition from idiopathic pulmonary hemosiderosis. An even more sensitive test is the demonstration of serum anti-glomerular basement membrane antibody by radioimmunoassay, a specific finding in Goodpasture's syndrome. Evidence of glomerulonephritis and progressive renal failure is common and usually occurs later than the pulmonary manifestations. Needle biopsy of the kidney may be necessary. The appearance of the glomeruli with immunofluorescence staining is diagnostic.

The prognosis is poor. Immunosuppressive treatment with prednisone and cyclophosphamide has apparently been effective in some patients. Increasingly, patients with progressive respiratory disease and renal failure are reported to be improved after multiple plasma exchanges (plasmapheresis).

When the principal manifestation of the disease is renal failure, hemodialysis may be indicated. Selected patients should be considered for bilateral nephrectomy and renal transplant.

Abboud RT et al: Goodpasture's syndrome: Diagnosis by transbronchial lung biopsy. *Ann Intern Med* 1978;**89**:635.

Levin M et al: Goodpasture's syndrome: Treatment with plasmapheresis, immunosuppression, and anticoagulation. *Arch Dis Child* 1983;**58**:697.

PULMONARY VASCULITIS

This is a group of hypersensitivity diseases in which pulmonary vasculitis is a manifestation of a systemic disease. The immunologic mechanism seems also to involve type III antibody formation in response to various antigens such as heterologous serum, RNA, DNA, streptococci, and certain drugs such as sulfonamides, hexamethonium, and nitrofurantoin. Serum sickness, polyarteritis nodosa, systemic lupus erythematosus, and interstitial pneumonitis are manifestations of this type of reaction. (See Chapter 14.)

Wegener's Granulomatosis

This is a necrotizing granuloma of unknown cause that involves the upper respiratory tract and the lungs and is associated with a diffuse vasculitis involving both arteries and veins. Deposition of IgG and complement in vessel walls and glomerular membrane has been demonstrated. Renal failure due to glomerulitis and pulmonary failure is the usual cause of death. A limited form of the disease has been described with pulmonary lesions, with or without upper respiratory disease, and no renal or other systemic involvement. Most patients with Wegener's disease do have renal involvement, and this is the determining factor in the prognosis. The disease occurs somewhat more frequently in males and usually appears in the fourth and fifth decades in previously healthy people. The condition may be a variant of disseminated polyarteritis.

Clinical manifestations include epistaxis, severe sinusitis, hemoptysis, pulmonary consolidation, hemorrhagic skin lesions, and progressive renal failure.

Treatment with cytotoxic agents, especially cyclophosphamide (Cytoxan) and azathioprine (Imuran), has definitely improved the prognosis in Wegener's disease, which formerly had a 2-year mortality rate of 80% when renal involvement was present. However, the incidence of serious side effects is significant, and treatment is indicated for multiple progressive lesions only. Kidney transplantation has proved to be successful for the treatment of patients in whom end-stage renal disease has developed. Corticosteroid treatment does not alter the prognosis but may be helpful in the presence of acute inflammatory manifestations.

Israel HL, Patchefsky AS, Saldama MJ: Wegener's granulomatosis, lymphoid granulomatosis, and benign lymphocytic angiitis and granulomatosis of lung. *Ann Intern Med* 1977; **87**:691.

Steinman TI et al: Recurrence of Wegener's granulomatosis after kidney transplantation: Successful re-induction of remission with cyclophosphamide. *Am J Med* 1980;**68**:458.

EXTRINSIC ALLERGIC ALVEOLITIS
(Hypersensitivity Pneumonitis)

Extrinsic allergic alveolitis is caused by exposure to dusts containing various fungi, molds, thermophilic actinomycetes, and pigeon serum proteins (in pigeon droppings). Type III and, more recently, type IV immune responses have been associated with the disease. The role of each in the pathogenesis is not yet defined.

Various environmental exposures have been identified as sources of offending antigens: thermophilic actinomycetes in moldy hay (farmer's lung), pressed sugar cane (bagassosis), mushroom compost (mushroom worker's disease), and contaminated air conditioning (humidifier lung); fungi in barley (malt worker's lung), maple bark (maple bark disease), wood pulp (wood pulp worker's disease); proteins in pigeon droppings (pigeon breeder's disease). Exposure in sensitized individuals causes interstitial and alveolar inflammatory processes. However, the fact that only a small percentage of those exposed develop the disease suggests hereditary or other host factors.

The clinical picture is that of an acute onset of fever, dry cough, dyspnea, and malaise that occurs 5–6 hours after substantial exposure to the offending antigen. Chest x-rays show a diffuse fine granular infiltration. Eosinophilia usually does not occur. A detailed history of exposure is important in the diagnosis. Continuous mild exposure to such an antigen may produce chronic pulmonary and systemic symptoms. Hypersensitivity to *Aspergillus* antigens produces a more chronic clinical picture. (See Pulmonary Infiltrations with Eosinophilia, p 130.)

Treatment consists of cessation of exposure and, if symptoms are severe, a course of corticosteroid treatment. Mild chronic exposure can sometimes be controlled by wearing a simple cloth or paper mask. Pulmonary fibrosis may result from severe or repeated episodes.

Cockcroft DW, Dosman JA: Respiratory health risks in farmers. *Ann Intern Med* 1981;**95**:380.

Fink JN et al: Interstitial lung disease due to contamination of forced air systems. *Ann Intern Med* 1976;**84**:406.

Reyes CN Et al: The pulmonary pathology of farmer's lung disease. *Chest* 1982;**81**:142.

Schlueter DP: Infiltrative lung disease: Hypersensitivity pneumonitis. *J Allergy Clin Immunol* 1982;**70**:50.

IDIOPATHIC INTERSTITIAL PNEUMONIA OR FIBROSIS

This disease entity is characterized by cellular infiltrates or fibrosis in the pulmonary interstitium. It was first described by Hamman and Rich in 1933. Their cases were rapidly progressive and fatal. Since then, many cases with similar pathologic findings and varying rates of progression have been described. It is now recognized that the disease is often chronic and may occasionally be reversible. Immunologic mechanisms may play a role in some instances, and rheumatoid factor is frequently present in the serum. Circulating immune complexes (type III) and deposition of immunoglobulin (IgG) and complement in the lungs have been demonstrated in some patients with interstitial fibrosis. All of the known causes of pulmonary fibrosis and interstitial pneumonitis, such as infection, exposure to toxic inhalants, systemic use of drugs and toxic substances, and various systemic diseases (eg, rheumatoid arthritis) must be excluded before this diagnosis can be made.

Symptoms include progressive dyspnea and nonproductive cough. Physical findings may be absent or minimal initially. Fine end-inspiratory rales eventually appear. Clubbing of the fingers is also common. Signs of pulmonary hypertension and right ventricular failure appear in the more advanced stages of the disease. Routine laboratory studies are not characteristic. Pulmonary function tests show primarily restriction and diminished diffusion capacity for carbon monoxide. Arterial blood gases show hypoxemia with hypocapnia (widened arterial-alveolar P_{aO_2} difference). The hypoxemia has been shown to be the result of ventilation/perfusion abnormalities rather than the thickened pulmonary interstitium ("alveolar-capillary block syndrome"). Chest x-rays may show coarse reticular infiltrates, reticulonodular infiltrates, a "ground glass" pattern with air bronchograms, or typical honeycombing. Lung biopsy is necessary for definitive diagnosis. This can be done transbronchially with the flexible fiberoptic bronchoscope. However, open biopsy may be necessary in order to obtain an adequate specimen in many cases.

Treatment with large doses of corticosteroids (prednisone, 1 mg/kg/d) for several weeks followed by gradual reduction to a lower maintenance dose may have a favorable effect in the early stages before pulmonary fibrosis is established, but the course is unpredictable.

Desquamative interstitial pneumonia is a pathologic entity believed by some to be distinct from other forms of interstitial lung disease. Other writers consider it to be an early inflammatory stage of idiopathic interstitial fibrosis. The clinical presentation is identical to that described above. However, it appears that when the characteristic alveolar desquamation pattern is present, the course is more favorable and the disease is more responsive to corticosteroid treatment. This may be correlated with lack of fibrosis rather than the desquamation per se. Corticosteroid dosage is as outlined above.

Carrington CB et al: Natural history and treated course of usual and desquamative interstitial pneumonia. *N Engl J Med* 1978; **298**:801.

Dreisin RB et al: Circulating immune complexes in the idiopathic interstitial pneumonias. *N Engl J Med* 1978;**298**:353.

Fulmer JD: The interstitial lung diseases. *Chest* 1982;**82**:172.

Keogh BA: Pulmonary function testing in interstitial pulmonary disease. *Chest* 1980;**78**:856.

Luce JM: Interstitial lung disease. *Hosp Pract* (July) 1983;**18**:173.

Poe RH et al: Sensitivity and specificity of non-specific transbronchial lung biopsy. *Am Rev Respir Dis* 1979;**119**:25.

INFECTIONS OF THE LUNG*

Acute pneumonia continues to be a major cause of death and disability; it is the fifth leading cause of death in the USA. A significant cause of the continued prevalence of these infections is the large number of compromised hosts resulting from alcohol and drug abuse, cancer therapy, and an aging population.

Approximately half of the acute pneumonias are of bacterial origin. The other principal causes are viruses, mycoplasma, and parasites. Early identification of the infectious agent is essential for the proper treatment of pneumonia.

A careful history will often help to differentiate bacterial from viral infections and also identify noninfectious diseases masquerading as pneumonia. A sudden onset of symptoms, including fever, chills, cough, and often chest pain, suggests bacterial infection. Viral pneumonia is more often gradual in onset, with malaise and low-grade fever without chills, and is more likely to follow an upper respiratory infection. Elderly patients, especially those with chronic obstructive pulmonary disease and other chronic illnesses, may have bacterial pneumonias without typical symptoms and usually require more aggressive management.

Tachycardia, tachypnea, and signs of pulmonary consolidation are more common with bacterial pneumonia. There is often a paucity of physical findings with nonbacterial pneumonias.

Leukocytosis may occur with either bacterial or viral infections, although significantly abnormal white counts are more common with the former. Examination of an adequate sputum sample by Gram's stain is mandatory and may help to suggest appropriate treatment. A sputum sample that contains many squamous epithelial cells is heavily contaminated with saliva and is not valid. A better sample has to be obtained by nasotracheal suction or transtracheal aspiration. In bacterial pneumonias, sputum usually shows abundant neutrophils and predominance of one bacterial organism. In nonbacterial pneumonias, there are few neutrophils, and the gram-stained smear contains a mixed respiratory flora. Culture of valid sputum may show a predominant bacterial pathogen.

Foul-smelling sputum usually indicates mixed bacterial infection, including anaerobes, and is suggestive of a lung abscess. Anaerobic cultures of such sputum are indicated.

Blood cultures may help identify the causative organisms and should always be done before starting antimicrobial drugs.

Radiologic findings may be nondiagnostic, but dense consolidations and pleural effusions are more common with bacterial pneumonias, and viral infections are more likely to be interstitial.

*By Ernest Jawetz, MD, PhD.

Fick RB, Reynolds HY: Changing spectrum of pneumonia. (Editorial.) *Am J Med* 1983;**74**:1.

Pulmonary complications of the acquired immunodeficiency syndrome: Report of a National Heart, Lung, and Blood Institute Workshop. *N Engl J Med* 1984;**310**:1682.

PNEUMOCOCCAL PNEUMONIA

Essentials of Diagnosis

- Sudden onset of shaking chills, fever, chest pain, and cough with rust-colored sputum.
- X-rays show infiltration, often lobar in distribution, but sometimes patchy.
- Pneumococci are present in the sputum and often in the blood.
- Leukocytosis.

General Considerations

Pneumonia is an inflammatory process in lung parenchyma most commonly caused by infection. The consolidation of pneumonia must be differentiated from pulmonary infarction, atelectasis with bronchial obstruction, and congestive heart failure, but it may coexist with any of these conditions. The pneumococcus accounts for 50–80% of community-acquired bacterial pneumonias; types 1–9 and 12 are most commonly found in adults, whereas types 6, 14, 19, and 23 are most common in children. These bacteria frequently are in the normal flora of the respiratory tract. The development of pneumonia must therefore usually be attributed to an impairment of natural resistance. Conditions leading to aspiration of secretions include suppression of the cough or epiglottic reflex, impairment of upward migration of mucous sheets (propelled by cilia), and impairment of alveolar phagocyte function. Among conditions that predispose to pneumonia are viral respiratory diseases, malnutrition, exposure to cold, noxious gases, alcohol intoxication, depression of cerebral functions by drugs, and cardiac failure. Pulmonary consolidation may be in one or more lobes or may be patchy in distribution.

Clinical Findings

A. Symptoms and Signs: The onset is usually sudden, with shaking chills, "stabbing" chest pain (exaggerated by respiration but sometimes referred to the shoulder, abdomen, or flank), high fever, cough and blood-tinged or "rusty" sputum, and occasionally vomiting. A history of recent upper respiratory illness can often be elicited.

The patient appears severely ill, with marked tachypnea (30–40/min) but no orthopnea. Respirations are grunting, nares flaring, and the patient often lies on the affected side in an attempt to splint the chest. Herpes simplex facial lesions are often present.

Initially, chest excursion is diminished on the involved side, breath sounds are suppressed, and fine inspiratory rales are heard. Later, the classic signs (absent breath sounds, dullness, etc) of consolidation appear. A pleural friction rub or abdominal distention may be present. During resolution of the pneumonia, the signs of consolidation are replaced by rales. Physical findings are often inconclusive, and repeated x-ray examination is helpful.

B. Laboratory Findings: Blood cultures are positive for pneumococci in 15–25% of cases early in the disease. In peripheral blood, leukocytosis (20–35 thousand/μL) is the rule, and a low white blood cell count carries a poorer prognosis.

Sputum must be examined by Gram's stain and by culture. In the smears, the presence of many squamous epithelial cells suggests heavy contamination with saliva, and such specimens are of no value. Typical sputum from pneumococcal pneumonia contains many red and white cells (PMNs) and many pneumococci. If good sputum specimens are not obtainable, a transtracheal aspirate may reveal the causative agent, but this procedure is not without risk. A microscopic "quellung" reaction with pooled antiserum rapidly identifies pneumococci in fresh sputum.

C. X-Ray Findings: Initially, there may be only a vague haziness across the involved part of the lung field. Later, typical consolidation is well defined either in lobar or in patchy distribution. Fluid shadows in the costophrenic angles may appear before pleural exudate can be detected by physical examination. During resolution of the consolidation, which may require 8–10 weeks, areas of radiolucency may appear, suggesting "pseudocavitation."

Treatment

A blood culture and a good sputum specimen for smear and culture should always be obtained before treatment is started. The dosage and route of administration of antimicrobial drugs are influenced to some extent by the clinical severity of the disease, the presence of unfavorable prognostic signs (see below), and the presence of complications.

A. Antibacterial Therapy: Penicillin G is the drug of choice. It is given initially in dosages ranging from 600,000 units of procaine penicillin every 12 hours intramuscularly for moderate illness to 1 million units of aqueous penicillin G given every 4 hours rapidly into an intravenous infusion in severe cases. Only after there has been a definite response to treatment should oral penicillin V (400,000 units every 4–6 hours) be considered. All pneumococci are susceptible to penicillin at present, although strains requiring 4 units/mL of penicillin G have occurred in South Africa and, rarely, elsewhere. Some strains resistant to tetracyclines, erythromycin, or lincomycin have been encountered. Therefore, these alternatives to penicillin (eg, in patients with documented hypersensitivity) may fail, but they (or cephalexin or cephradine, 0.5 g every 4–6 hours) can be tried orally in mildly ill patients. In more severely ill persons, cefazolin, 4 g intravenously daily, is a reasonable alternative. Treatment with an effective drug should be continued for 3 days after defervescence.

Sulfonamides are not in favor now because the therapeutic response is slower than with penicillin.

However, sodium sulfadiazine, 4–6 g intravenously, followed by maintenance doses intravenously or orally, is adequate (if not optimal) treatment for many cases of pneumococcal pneumonia. The precautions outlined in Chapter 29 must be observed when administering sulfonamides.

B. General Supportive Treatment:

1. Ventilation and oxygenation–An adequate airway must be maintained—if necessary, by tracheal suction, endotracheal tube, or tracheostomy. Oxygen must be supplied to any patient with severe pneumonia, cyanosis with P_{aO_2} below 60, or marked dyspnea; this will also help to prevent pulmonary edema. Oxygen may be supplied by nasal catheter, soft rubber mask, or oxygen tent. With masks, a 95% oxygen concentration can be maintained, whereas with nasal tubes or tents the concentration will reach only 40–50%. However, masks are difficult to tolerate because of cough and expectoration. Oxygen must be humidified to prevent drying of secretions.

2. Management of shock and pulmonary edema–These are the most frequent causes of death in pneumonia. Oxygen administration tends to prevent pulmonary edema; impending right heart failure must be managed, and digitalization is urgent. Treat shock as outlined in Chapter 1.

3. Management of toxic delirium–Toxic delirium occurs in any severe pneumonia and may be particularly difficult to manage in alcoholics. Delirium, anxiety, and restlessness during waking hours may be treated with diazepam, 5 mg, or chlordiazepoxide, 10 mg, or phenobarbital, 15–30 mg orally 4–6 times daily. Pentobarbital, 0.1 g, or flurazepam (Dalmane), 30 mg, at bedtime helps to ensure adequate rest. If sedatives or tranquilizers are given, it is helpful to check the patient's sensorium frequently for any change suggestive of meningitis, which requires a diagnostic lumbar puncture.

4. Fluids–Patients with pneumococcal pneumonia may perspire profusely and lose much fluid and salt. Sufficient fluid must be given to maintain a daily urinary output of at least 1500 mL. Electrolytes must be kept in balance.

5. Diet–Initially, the dyspneic patient is anorectic, and a liquid diet is preferred. With improvement, a normal diet will be tolerated. If complications suggest a long illness, a high-protein, high-calorie diet with vitamin supplementation is indicated.

6. Cough–If cough interferes with sleep and rest, it may be suppressed with codeine phosphate, 15–30 mg every 3–4 hours subcutaneously or orally; or by elixir of terpin hydrate with codeine, 4 mL every 3–4 hours as necessary.

7. Pleuritic pain–For mild pain, spray ethyl chloride over the area of greatest pain for about 1 minute or inject a local anesthetic to anesthetize the involved dermatomes to provide temporary relief. Codeine phosphate, 15–30 mg, may be given as necessary for pain. For very severe pain, use meperidine, 50–100 mg subcutaneously, or morphine sulfate, 10–15 mg subcutaneously.

8. Abdominal distention–Abdominal distention is usually due to air swallowing in severe dyspnea and is a frequent problem in patients with pneumonia. Neostigmine methylsulfate, 1:2000, 1 mL subcutaneously, and insertion of a rectal tube will usually produce rapid initial decompression. Gastric dilatation can be relieved by suction through a nasal tube passed into the stomach.

9. Congestive failure–(Distinguish from shock and pulmonary edema.) In elderly patients or patients with preexisting heart disease, congestive failure may be precipitated by pneumonia. Rapid digitalization is indicated.

10. Cardiac arrhythmias–Extrasystoles usually require no treatment. If atrial fibrillation or flutter develops, rapid heart failure may be precipitated. Rapid digitalization is usually indicated in these cases.

C. Evaluation of Treatment: With proper selection of antimicrobial drugs, there should be marked improvement and defervescence in 72 hours or less. If this fails to occur, one must consider 3 main possibilities: (1) the presence of a serious complication such as empyema, pulmonary suppuration associated with bronchial obstruction, endocarditis, or meningitis; (2) infection by an organism other than the pneumococcus and resistant to the drug used; and (3) possible drug fever or other associated disease. If there is much pleural fluid, it must be aspirated promptly, smeared, and cultured to detect infection or empyema that requires drainage. If an organism other than the pneumococcus is shown to be the probable agent, treatment must be directed against it.

Complications

Complications of pneumococcal pneumonia occur with the following approximate frequencies: sterile pleural effusion (4–8%), empyema (0.5–2%), endocarditis and meningitis (0.1–0.3%), and pericarditis (0.1%). Other complications such as pneumococcal arthritis or lung abscess are even more rare. Fibrous organization of the pneumonia (in place of resolution) occurs sometimes but rarely causes disability. Major pleural fluid collections must be aspirated and examined by smear and culture to permit early treatment of empyema.

Prognosis

Untreated pneumococcal pneumonia has a mortality rate of 20–40%. The following are unfavorable prognostic signs: age over 50 years, presence of underlying disease (eg, heart failure, cirrhosis), pregnancy, bacteremia, marked proteinuria, absence of leukocytosis, pulmonary edema, and shock.

With early and adequate antimicrobial treatment, the fatality rate is about 5–8% but in bacteremic pneumonia it is 17–25%. Most fatalities occur in the age groups under 2 years and over 50 years. In untreated, uncomplicated cases, resolution by crisis (or more gradual resolution) occurs 7–10 days after onset.

Prevention

A polyvalent vaccine containing polysaccharides from the 23 pneumococcus types encountered most commonly in bacteremic pneumonias in the USA is available. It has given significant protection against disease in persons at high risk: persons with sickle cell disease, splenectomized children, persons with chronic bronchopulmonary, cardiac, or renal disease, and elderly or debilitated persons. A single dose of 0.5 mL is given intramuscularly and may cause local erythema, soreness, or fever. It should not be given during pregnancy. Children at high risk can receive vaccine at age 6 months and again at 2 years. In addition, prophylactic penicillin may be required. Regrettably, some children under 2 years of age and some patients with myeloma or lymphoma have a poor antibody response to the vaccine. In adults, the need for revaccination is not established.

Boerner DF, Zwadyk P: The value of the sputum Gram's stain in community-acquired pneumonia. *JAMA* 1982;**247**:642.

George WL, Finegold SM: Bacterial infections of the lung. *Chest* 1982;**81**:502.

Kantor HG: The many radiologic facies of pneumococcal pneumonia. *Am J Roentgenol* 1981;**137**:1213.

Murray BE, Moellering RC: Antimicrobial agents in pulmonary infections. *Med Clin North Am* 1980;**64**:319.

OTHER BACTERIAL PNEUMONIAS

Primary bacterial pneumonias caused by single bacterial species other than the pneumococcus may account for up to 25% of community-acquired and 80% of hospital-acquired pneumonias. All of these pneumonias may have somewhat similar physical findings and x-ray evidence of pulmonary infiltration or consolidation. For proper treatment, it is crucial to identify the causative agent by blood culture and by sputum examination with stained smear and culture. Transtracheal aspiration, fiberoptic bronchoscopy, or even lung biopsy may be needed for specific diagnosis and treatment.

Klebsiella Pneumonia

Klebsiella pneumoniae occurs as a member of the normal bacterial flora in the respiratory tract or gut of 5–20% of the population. Primary pneumonia due to this organism occurs mainly in persons over 40 years of age with a history of alcoholism, malnutrition, or debilitating diseases. *Klebsiella* pneumonia also occurs as superinfection in persons hospitalized for serious disease, including other types of pneumonia treated with antimicrobial drugs.

The onset is usually sudden, with chills, fever, dyspnea, cyanosis, and profound toxicity. The sputum is often red ("currant jelly"), mucoid, sticky, and difficult to expectorate. Physical findings and white counts are variable. The disease may be fulminating and progress rapidly to a fatal outcome. In subacute

forms, there is a tendency toward necrosis of lung tissue and abscess formation.

The diagnosis is based on finding short, encapsulated gram-negative bacteria as the predominant organism in sputum smears (in poorly stained smears they may be mistaken for pneumococci) and klebsiellae in blood and sputum cultures. Immediate intensive antimicrobial treatment is essential. Cefotaxime, 1–2 g intravenously as a bolus every 4–6 hours (or a similar cephalosporin), is given, often in combination with an aminoglycoside (eg, tobramycin, 5–7 mg/kg/d intramuscularly). Antimicrobial treatment may have to be continued for more than 2 weeks to avoid relapses. General supportive treatment is the same as for pneumococcal pneumonia.

The fatality rate in untreated *Klebsiella* pneumonia is 40–60%. Even with apparently adequate treatment, the fatality rate may be near 30%.

Reyes MP: The aerobic gram-negative bacillary pneumonias. *Med Clin North Am* 1980;**64**:363.

Haemophilus influenzae Pneumonia

This is a rare form of primary bacterial pneumonia in adults. It has occurred in the presence of cardiac disease, hypogammaglobulinemia, and chronic lung disease. Symptoms and signs do not distinguish this from other bacterial pneumonias. The sputum may be bloody, but Gram-stained smears may be misinterpreted. The diagnosis ultimately rests on the results of cultures of blood and sputum.

Ampicillin, 12 g/d, or moxalactam, 150–200 mg/kg/d, is given intravenously. An alternative treatment is with chloramphenicol, 0.5 g orally or intravenously every 6 hours. Trimethoprim with sulfamethoxazole has been occasionally successful in pneumonia due to penicillinase-producing *Haemophilus influenzae*. General measures are the same as for pneumococcal pneumonia.

Stratton CW et al: *Hemophilus influenzae* pneumonia in adults: Report of five cases caused by ampicillin-resistant strains. *Am Rev Respir Dis* 1980;**121**:595.

Proteus, Pseudomonas, & Serratia Pneumonia

Pneumonias caused by various species of *Proteus, Pseudomonas,* and *Serratia* occur with increasing frequency in debilitated persons with chronic lung or heart disease and alcoholism, or as nosocomial infections in patients who have required inhalation therapy or tracheal suction and have received antimicrobial drugs. In fibrocystic disease, pulmonary infection with mucoid *Pseudomonas aeruginosa* is prominent. The hands of medical staff and contaminated equipment are important in transmission.

These pneumonias are associated with early delirium, massive consolidation often proceeding to necrosis and multiple abscess formation, and a high fatality rate. Treatment is with an aminoglycoside (eg, tobramycin, 5–7 mg/kg/d) plus ticarcillin, 10–18 g/d, or a new cephalosporin (eg, moxalactam, 12 g/d) given intravenously. With renal insufficiency, dosage has to be adjusted (see Chapter 29).

The prognosis in gram-negative bacterial pneumonias must be guarded.

Valdivieso M et al: Gram-negative bacillary pneumonia in the compromised host. *Medicine* 1977;**56**:241.

Streptococcal Pneumonia

Pneumonia due to hemolytic streptococci occurs usually as a sequela to viral infection of the respiratory tract, especially influenza or measles, or in persons with underlying pulmonary disease. The patients are usually in a severely toxic condition and cyanotic. Pleural effusion develops frequently and early and progresses to empyema in one-third of untreated patients. The diagnosis rests on finding large numbers of streptococci in smears of sputum and culturing hemolytic streptococci from blood and sputum.

The treatment of choice is with penicillin G in a dosage similar to that for pneumococcal pneumonia (see above). If treatment is started early, the prognosis is good.

Staphylococcal Pneumonia

Pneumonia caused by *Staphylococcus aureus* occurs as a sequela to viral infections of the respiratory tract (eg, influenza) and in debilitated (eg, postsurgical) patients or hospitalized infants, especially after antimicrobial drug administration. There is often a history of a mild illness with headache, cough, and generalized aches that abruptly changes to a very severe illness with high fever, chills, and exaggerated cough with purulent or blood-streaked sputum and deep cyanosis. There may be early signs of pleural effusion, empyema, or tension pneumothorax. X-ray examination reveals lung consolidation, pneumatoceles, abscesses, empyema, and pneumothorax. The demonstration of pyopneumothorax and of cavities with air-fluid levels by x-ray is highly suggestive of staphylococcal pneumonia. The diagnosis must be confirmed by stained smear of sputum (masses of white cells and gram-positive cocci, many intracellular) and culture (predominantly *S aureus*), and also by means of cultures of pleural fluid and blood. The white count is usually more than 20,000/μL.

Initial therapy (based on sputum smear) consists of nafcillin, 6–12 g/d, or vancomycin, 2 g/d, given intravenously in divided doses as a bolus. If the staphylococcus proves to be penicillin-sensitive by laboratory test, penicillin G, 20–60 million units/d intravenously, is the antibiotic of choice. Drugs should be continued for several weeks. If empyema develops, drainage must be established. If pneumothorax develops, it is treated as described on p 172.

The prognosis varies with the underlying condition of the patient and the drug susceptibility of the organism.

Musher DM, Franco M: Staphylococcal pneumonia: A new perspective. *Chest* 1981;**79**:172.

Bacteroides Pneumonia

Pneumonias caused by anaerobic *Bacteroides* species occur as complications of abdominal or pelvic *Bacteroides* infections in patients with chronic lung disease or in whom aspiration of secretions has occurred. Pleural effusions and empyema develop early and are a main feature of the disease, which is often subacute or chronic. The diagnosis is based on the foul odor of the empyema and the demonstration of pleomorphic gram-negative anaerobes. Drainage of empyema must be combined with intensive penicillin, cefoxitin, or clindamycin treatment.

Davidson M, Tempest B, Palmer DL: Bacteriologic diagnosis of acute pneumonia: Comparison of sputum, transtracheal aspirates and lung aspirates. *JAMA* 1976;**235**:158.

Melioidosis

Pseudomonas pseudomallei occurs in soil and water of many subtropical and tropical countries. Animals and humans commonly are infected via the respiratory route. Most infections are subclinical, but some result in glanderslike lesions, and others cause a pneumonitis that may range from subacute or chronic to fulminating and rapidly fatal. Among persons who have mild or subclinical pneumonitis, latent infection may persist for years and may be reactivated by immunosuppression, eg, in drug abusers.

Diagnosis rests on bacteriologic and serologic findings, particularly in chronic pulmonary consolidation, which resembles mycobacterial or fungal pneumonias. Blood cultures are positive in the fulminating forms seen in Southeast Asia.

The organism is susceptible to tetracyclines, chloramphenicol, and sulfonamides, and these drugs, singly or in combination, have been effective in controlling the pneumonic process if given for several weeks. Lung abscesses may have to be drained.

No preventive measures are known. Human-to-human transmission is very rare.

Patamasucon P, Schaad UB, Nelson JD: Melioidosis. *J Pediatr* 1982;**100**:175.

Legionella Pneumonia

The eponym legionnaires' disease has been given to a serious pneumonia that afflicted people attending the American Legion Convention in Philadelphia in 1976. Other outbreaks have been diagnosed retrospectively at least since 1965, and sporadic infections have occurred at least since 1947 in many places.

Legionella pneumophila is a poorly staining gram-negative bacterium that grows slowly on special media (eg, charcoal-yeast extract) at 35 °C. There are at least 8 species of *Legionella,* some with multiple serotypes. These organisms can be recovered in human disease from sputum, bronchial washings, pleural fluid, lung biopsies, or blood. *Legionella* species occur in the environment and are acquired by humans from aerosols, dust from air-conditioning systems, water, or soil. The infection is not usually communicable from patient to contacts. Asymptomatic infection is common at all ages, whereas symptomatic infection is most often an opportunistic pneumonia in immunocompromised individuals.

Asymptomatic infection is evident only by a rise in specific antibodies. Symptomatic infection is observed mainly in elderly persons, smokers, and patients undergoing hemodialysis or renal transplant.

The incubation period is estimated to be 2–10 days. Initial symptoms are malaise, diffuse myalgias, and headache, followed in 12–48 hours by high, nonremittent fever and chills. Nausea, vomiting, and diarrhea are frequent early in the illness. On the third day a dry cough begins that is nonproductive or produces scanty mucoid, sometimes blood-streaked sputum. Dyspnea and hypoxia become marked as signs of consolidation develop. Pleuritic chest pain occurs in one-third of patients. Severe confusion or delirium may occur.

There is leukocytosis (10,000–20,000/μL) with a shift to the left, hyponatremia, abnormal liver function tests, and, occasionally, microscopic hematuria. Chest x-rays reveal patchy, often multilobar pulmonary consolidation, and, occasionally, small pleural effusions. The illness usually worsens for 4–7 days before improvement begins in those who recover. During severe outbreaks, the mortality rate has been 10% in those with manifest disease. Death is attributed to respiratory or renal failure or shock, with disseminated intravascular coagulation.

The diagnosis is based on a clinical picture compatible with the specific features of the disease and on negative results of bacteriologic laboratory tests for other pneumonias. The organism can be identified by immunofluorescence in cultures, lung biopsy, and, rarely, sputum specimens. A retrospective diagnosis is based on a significant rise in specific serum antibodies detected by immunofluorescence.

The treatment of choice is erythromycin, 0.5–1 g every 6 hours intravenously or orally for 2–3 weeks. This usually results in improvement in 2–3 days. Rifampin, 10–20 mg/kg/d, and doxycycline, 100–200 mg/d, are alternative drugs. Assisted ventilation and management of shock are essential.

Edelstein PH, Meyer RD: Legionnaire's disease: A review. *Chest* 1984;**85**:114.

Kirby BD et al: Legionnaires' disease: Report of 65 nosocomially acquired cases and review of the literature. *Medicine* 1980; **59**:188.

Orenstein WA et al: The frequency of *Legionella* infection in children hospitalized with pneumonia. *J Pediatr* 1981; **99**:403.

Pneumocystis carinii Pneumonia

This parasitic infection occurs in debilitated children or immunodeficient adults. It has been a prominent opportunistic infection in AIDS patients (see Chapter 22). The diagnosis is made by bronchoalveolar lavage or open lung biopsy and the demonstration of typical cysts of *P carinii* in smears stained with methenamine-silver. Early treatment with sulfameth-

oxazole-trimethoprim can cure the pneumonia. The same drug has been effective in prophylaxis during immunosuppression. An alternative, more toxic drug is pentamidine isethionate (available through the Centers for Disease Control, Atlanta, GA 30333).

Hughes WT et al: Successful chemoprophylaxis for *Pneumocystis carinii* pneumonitis. *N Engl J Med* 1977;**297**:1419.

Winston DJ et al: Trimethoprim-sulfamethoxazole for the treatment of *Pneumocystis carinii* pneumonia. *Ann Intern Med* 1980;**92**:762.

"MIXED" BACTERIAL PNEUMONIAS
(Hypostatic Pneumonia, "Terminal" Pneumonia, Bronchopneumonia)

Essentials of Diagnosis

- Variable onset of fever, cough, dyspnea, expectoration.
- Symptoms and signs often masked by primary (debilitating) disease.
- Greenish-yellow sputum (purulent) with mixed flora.
- Leukocytosis (often absent in aged and debilitated patients).
- Patchy infiltration on chest x-ray.

General Considerations

Mixed bacterial pneumonias include those in which culture and smear reveal several organisms, not one of which can clearly be identified as the causative agent. These pneumonias usually appear as complications of anesthesia, surgery, aspiration, trauma, or various chronic illnesses (cardiac failure, advanced cancer, uremia). They are common complications of chronic pulmonary diseases such as bronchiectasis and emphysema. Old people are most commonly affected ("terminal" pneumonia). Patients treated with intermittent positive pressure breathing apparatus or immunosuppressive drugs may develop pneumonia caused by gram-negative rods.

The following findings in a debilitated, chronically ill, or aged person suggest a complicating pneumonia: (1) worsening of cough, dyspnea, cyanosis; (2) low-grade, irregular fever; (3) purulent sputum; and (4) patchy basal densities on a chest film (in addition to previously noted densities caused by a primary underlying disease, if any), sometimes with local necrosis and cavitation.

Clinical Findings

A. Symptoms and Signs: The onset is usually insidious, with low-grade fever, cough, expectoration, and dyspnea that may become marked and lead to cyanosis. Physical findings are extremely variable and may not be impressive against a background of cardiac or pulmonary disease. The signs listed under Other Bacterial Pneumonias may also be present.

B. Laboratory Findings: The appearance of a

greenish or yellowish (purulent) sputum should suggest a complicating pneumonia. Smears and cultures reveal a mixed flora, often including anaerobes. Predominant types should be noted. Leukocytosis is often absent in the aged and debilitated patient presenting with a mixed infection.

C. X-Ray Findings: X-ray shows patchy, irregular infiltrations, most commonly posterior and basal (in bedridden patients). Abscess formation may be observed. Careful interpretation will avoid confusion with shadows due to preexisting heart or lung disease.

Differential Diagnosis

Mixed bacterial pneumonias must be differentiated from tuberculosis, carcinoma, and other specific mycotic, bacterial, and viral pulmonary infections (to which they may be secondary).

Treatment

Clear the airway and correct hypoxia. Unless a probably significant etiologic agent can be identified, give one of the new cephalosporins (eg, cefotaxime, 12 g/d intravenously) as initial therapy. This will be modified according to clinical and laboratory results.

Prognosis

The prognosis depends upon the nature and severity of the underlying pulmonary disease and varies with the predominating organism.

Donowitz GR, Mandell GL: Empiric therapy for pneumonia. *Rev Infect Dis* 1983;**5:**S40.
Eickhoff TC: Pulmonary infections in surgical patients. *Surg Clin North Am* 1980;**60:**175.
Verghese A, Berk SL: Bacterial pneumonia in the elderly. *Medicine* 1983;**62:**271.

ASPIRATION PNEUMONIA

Aspiration pneumonia is an especially severe type of pneumonia, often with a high mortality rate. It results from the aspiration of gastric contents in addition to aspiration of upper respiratory flora in secretions. Important predisposing factors include impairment of the swallowing mechanism (eg, esophageal disease), inadequate cough reflex (eg, anesthesia, postoperative state, central nervous system disease, drug abuse), and impaired gastric emptying (eg, pyloric obstruction). Pulmonary injury is due in large part to the low pH (< 2.5) of gastric secretions.

Scattered areas of pulmonary edema and bronchospasm occur, and the x-ray appearance may be confused with that of pulmonary emboli, atelectasis, bronchopneumonia, and congestive heart failure.

Removal of aspirated material by catheter suction or bronchoscopy may be attempted, but this usually fails to remove all aspirate completely. Corticosteroids (eg, prednisone, 100 mg orally on the first or second day) may reduce the intensity of the inflammatory reaction to acidic gastric secretion, but the value of

corticosteroids in the treatment of aspiration pneumonia is not proved, and they increase the risk of superinfection. Some aspiration pneumonias have no bacterial component, but in many others a mixed bacterial flora is involved. Antimicrobial drugs directed against the latter (eg, penicillin G plus an aminoglycoside or the best available cephalosporin) are sometimes administered without waiting for evidence of progressive pulmonary infection. In doing so, however, there is a risk of favoring the development of resistant microorganisms. Therefore, administration of antimicrobials should not continue without laboratory and clinical evidence of microbial infection. Assisted ventilation and supplementary oxygen are beneficial.

Brook I, Finegold SM: Bacteriology of aspiration pneumonia in children. *Pediatrics* 1980;**65:**1115.
Wolfe JE et al: Effects of corticosteroids in the treatment of patients with gastric aspiration. *Am J Med* 1977;**63:**719.
Wynne JW, Modell JH: Respiratory aspiration of stomach contents. *Ann Intern Med* 1977;**87:**466.

LIPOID PNEUMONIA

This disease is an aspiration pneumonia associated with the use of oily medications. Fibrosis and the presence of macrophages containing oil droplets are the histologic features.

Symptoms and signs vary widely, at times resembling those of acute pneumonia (fever, productive cough) or chronic lung disease (weight loss, night sweats). There may be no symptoms but striking x-ray densities. Patients must be carefully questioned about the use of mineral oil, oily nose drops, or ointments used in the nose. Physical signs vary accordingly and are not diagnostic. Peribronchial infiltrations, diffuse lobar densities, scattered discrete densities, and even central cavitation have all been described on x-ray. Leukocytosis may occur with acute symptoms. Proper examination of the sputum for oil droplet-laden macrophages will often establish the diagnosis.

Treatment is nonspecific and symptomatic. Use of the oil-containing preparation must be discontinued. When this is done, further progression of the disease usually does not occur, and the prognosis is good. Large solitary masses may require resection.

Heckers H et al: Long-term course of mineral oil pneumonia. *Lung* 1978;**155:**101.

MYCOPLASMAL PNEUMONIA

Essentials of Diagnosis

- Cough of increasing intensity with scanty sputum.
- Minimal physical signs on chest examination.
- X-ray evidence of pulmonary infiltrate, sometimes extensive.
- White blood cell count in normal range.

General Considerations

Mycoplasmas are bacteria that lack a cell wall. Although many mycoplasmas cause diseases in animals, only one, *Mycoplasma pneumoniae,* clearly produces disease in humans. *Mycoplasma salivarium* and *Mycoplasma orale* are part of the normal flora of the oropharynx. *Mycoplasma hominis* and *Ureaplasma urealyticum* occur in the genital tract and may cause urethritis and salpingitis. *M pneumoniae* is a significant respiratory pathogen occurring endemically, with the main spread (by respiratory secretions) in the family, but also in outbreaks in military or school populations. Within a family the infection spreads slowly, beginning with school children and progressing to adults, often involving most of the susceptibles. Pneumonia occurs in about 30% of infected family members (mostly children and young adults) and in about 10% of infected military adults. Tracheobronchitis is more common than pneumonia, often with pharyngitis, and sometimes with bullous myringitis. In young children, mycoplasmal infection often presents as an upper respiratory infection.

Clinical Findings

A. Symptoms and Signs: There is a gradual onset of lassitude, respiratory symptoms, headache, myalgia with slowly rising fever, and increasing cough. Cough—sometimes paroxysmal—becomes more and more severe and may be accompanied by chest pains. Sputum is scanty and sometimes blood-flecked. Fever is regularly present with pneumonia and occasionally with tracheobronchitis, but there are no shaking chills. Patients usually do not appear seriously ill. Findings on chest examination are often minimal (rales, signs of consolidation), and the x-ray findings are disproportionately greater than expected from the physical findings. Segmental lower lobe consolidation on x-ray is sometimes accompanied by pleural fluid. The x-ray pattern is variable and not diagnostic.

B. Laboratory Findings: Leukocyte counts are usually within normal limits. The scanty sputum shows only normal flora by smear and culture. During the second week of illness, about 50% of patients develop "cold agglutinins," ie, their serum in a dilution of 1:32 or higher agglutinates human type O red cells at 4 °C. This is a nonspecific reaction. Specific antibodies to *M pneumoniae* can be demonstrated by growth inhibition or complement fixation tests in special laboratories. A 4-fold titer rise in paired sera is required for specific etiologic diagnosis. *M pneumoniae* can be grown from throat swabs or sputum after prolonged incubation on special media.

Differential Diagnosis

Mycoplasmal pneumonia is part of a "primary atypical pneumonia" complex that includes such non-bacterial pneumonias as Q fever *(Coxiella burnetii),* psittacosis *(Chlamydia psittaci),* and adenoviral and influenzal pneumonias. Other causes of pulmonary infiltrates must be considered, including mycobacteria and fungi, infarction, and neoplasms. Mycoplasmal

infection can also mimic many other types of viral and bacterial upper respiratory disease (eg, parainfluenza or respiratory syncytial virus).

Course

This is quite variable. Fever and cough may persist for 3 days to 4–6 weeks. Slow recovery is the rule. Radiologic signs resolve slowly and relapses occur, but deaths are very rare. Rarely, high-titer cold agglutinins are associated with intravascular hemolysis. Other rare complications include atelectasis, persistent pleural effusions, myocarditis, and secondary bacterial pneumonia.

Treatment

The general measures are as for pneumococcal pneumonia. In mild or moderate cases of mycoplasmal pneumonia, antimicrobial drugs are not indicated. Severe cases may be treated with a tetracycline or erythromycin, 0.5 g orally every 4–6 hours. No effective vaccine is available at present.

Levine DP, Lerner AM: The clinical spectrum of *Mycoplasma pneumoniae* infections. *Med Clin North Am* 1978;**62**:961.

PNEUMONIAS DUE TO SPECIFIC VIRUSES, RICKETTSIAE, & CHLAMYDIAE

The important specific viral, rickettsial, and chlamydial infections that may produce pneumonia include influenza, adenovirus infection, cytomegalovirus infection, Q fever, Rocky Mountain spotted fever, typhus, and chlamydial infections. The exanthematous viral diseases (rubeola, varicella) give rise occasionally to specific interstitial pneumonias.

These pneumonias were called "atypical" because they resemble mycoplasmal pneumonias and differ from classic bacterial pneumonias in physical and x-ray findings. Diagnosis depends upon recognition of the specific systemic disease by extrapulmonary features (eg, rash), a history of exposure to vectors (eg, parrots, ticks), exanthematous infections (especially varicella-herpes zoster), epidemiologic information, and isolation of the organism by special methods or demonstration of a significant rise in specific antibody titers. Bacterial superinfection in viral disease may be difficult to rule out.

Chlamydial pneumonitis in infants under 6 months of age is clinically recognizable by cough, pulmonary hyperinflation, eosinophilia, marked elevation of IgM antibodies, and little or no fever. This entity and psittacosis of adults are discussed in Chapter 24. The treatment of viral pneumonias is symptomatic. Treat rickettsial pneumonias as described in Chapter 23.

Murray HW, Tuazon C: Atypical pneumonias. *Med Clin North Am* 1980;**65**:507.

Ramsey PG et al: Herpes simplex virus pneumonia. *Ann Intern Med* 1982;**97**:813.

Schachter J, Grossman M: Chlamydial infections. *Annu Rev Med* 1981;**32**:45.

See also references under Pneumococcal Pneumonia.

LUNG ABSCESS

Essentials of Diagnosis

- Development of pulmonary symptoms about 1–2 weeks after possible aspiration, bronchial obstruction, or previous pneumonia.
- Septic fever and sweats, and periodic sudden expectoration of large amounts of purulent, foul-smelling, or "musty" sputum. Hemoptysis may occur.
- X-ray density with central radiolucency and fluid level.

General Considerations

Lung abscess develops when necrosis and liquefaction occur in an area where necrotizing pneumonia is present. Symptoms and signs occur 1–2 weeks after the following events: (1) massive aspiration of upper respiratory tract secretions and microbial flora, especially during profound suppression of cough reflex (eg, with alcohol, drugs, unconsciousness, anesthesia, brain trauma); (2) bronchial obstruction (eg, by atelectasis, foreign body, neoplasm); (3) presence of pneumonias, especially those caused by gram-negative bacteria or staphylococci; or (4) formation of septic emboli from other foci of infection, or, during bacteremia, with pulmonary infarcts. Abscess is more commonly in the lower dependent portions of the lung. The main etiologic organisms are related to the underlying condition, but a dense mixed anaerobic flora is often prominent, particularly when aspiration has occurred.

Clinical Findings

A. Symptoms and Signs: Onset may be abrupt or gradual. Symptoms include septic fever, sweats, cough, and chest pain. Cough is often nonproductive at onset. Expectoration of foul-smelling brown or gray sputum (anaerobic flora) or of purulent sputum without foul odor (pyogenic organism) may occur abruptly and in large quantity. Blood-streaked sputum is also common.

Pleural pain, especially with coughing, is common because the abscess is often subpleural.

Weight loss, anemia, and pulmonary osteoarthropathy may appear when the abscess becomes chronic (8–12 weeks after onset).

Physical findings may be minimal. Consolidation due to pneumonitis surrounding the abscess is the most frequent finding. Rupture into the pleural space produces signs of fluid or pneumothorax.

B. Laboratory Findings: Sputum cultures are usually inadequate in determining the bacterial cause of a lung abscess. Transtracheal aspirates should be obtained with the proper technique employed to culture anaerobic organisms in addition to the usual aerobic cultures. Special methods of transporting specimens are required for anaerobic organisms, and appropriate culture media and methods must be employed.

Smear and cultures for the tubercle bacilli are required, especially in lesions of the upper lobe and in chronic abscess.

C. X-Ray Findings: A dense shadow, usually located posteriorly in the lung, is the initial finding. A central radiolucency, often with a visible fluid level, appears as surrounding densities subside. Computerized tomography can supply the detailed localization of the abscess and may also reveal primary lesions (eg, bronchogenic carcinoma) and provide guidance for contemplated surgery. Various x-ray procedures also permit localization of pleural involvement to facilitate drainage.

D. Instrumental Examination: Fiberoptic bronchoscopy may help to diagnose location and nature of obstructions (foreign body, tumor), obtain specimens for microbiologic and pathologic examination. If secretions are copious, a rigid bronchoscope is preferred.

Differential Diagnosis

Differentiate from other causes of pulmonary cavitation: tuberculosis, bronchogenic carcinoma, mycotic infections, and staphylococcal or gram-negative bacterial pneumonia.

Treatment

Postural drainage and bronchoscopy are important to promote drainage of secretions.

A. Acute Abscess: Intensive antibacterial therapy is necessary to prevent further destruction of lung tissue. While cultures and sensitivity tests are pending, treatment should be started with penicillin G, 2–6 million units daily. In penicillin hypersensitivity, clindamycin and chloramphenicol are alternatives. If the patient improves on antimicrobial drugs (and postural drainage), the drugs should be continued for 4–8 weeks. If the patient fails to respond significantly to the initial treatment, sensitivity tests may suggest other antimicrobials, eg, nafcillin for staphylococci, cefotaxime for *Klebsiella*, cefoxitin or metronidazole for mixed anaerobes. Postural drainage is important adjunctive treatment. Percutaneous catheter drainage has been used successfully in selected cases. Surgical therapy is indicated mainly for severe hemoptysis and for the infrequent abscesses that fail to respond to antimicrobial management. Failure of fever to subside after 2 weeks of therapy, abscess diameter of more than 6 cm, and very thick cavity walls are all factors that lessen the likelihood of success with nonsurgical treatment alone.

B. Chronic Abscess: After acute systemic manifestations have subsided, the abscess may persist. Although many patients with chronic lung abscess can be cured with long-term treatment with antibacterial agents, surgery may occasionally be required.

Complications

Rupture of pus into the pleural space (empyema) causes severe symptoms: increase in fever, marked pleural pain, and sweating; the patient becomes "toxic" in appearance. Adequate drainage of empyema is mandatory. In chronic abscess, severe and even fatal hemorrhage may occur. Metastatic brain abscess is a well-recognized complication, and the infection may seed other organ sites. Bronchiectasis may occur as a sequela to lung abscess even when the abscess itself is cured.

Prognosis

The prognosis in acute abscess is excellent with prompt and intensive antibiotic therapy. About 80% of patients are healed within 7–8 weeks. The incidence of chronic abscess is consequently low. In chronic cases, surgery is curative.

Irwin RS et al: Sampling lower respiratory tract secretions in primary lung abscess: A comparison of the accuracy of four methods. *Chest* 1981;**79**:559.

Johanson WG, Harris GD: Aspiration pneumonia, anaerobic infections, and lung abscess. *Med Clin North Am* 1980;**64**:385.

Levison ME et al: Clindamycin compared with penicillin for the treatment of anaerobic lung abscess. *Ann Intern Med* 1983;**98**:466.

Vainrub B et al: Percutaneous drainage of lung abscess. *Am Rev Respir Dis* 1978;**117**:153.

PULMONARY TUBERCULOSIS

Essentials of Diagnosis

- Presenting signs and symptoms are usually minimal: malaise, lassitude, easy fatigability, anorexia, mild weight loss, afternoon fever, cough, apical rales, hemoptysis.
- Symptoms and signs may be entirely absent.
- Positive tuberculin skin test; especially a recent change from negative to positive.
- Apical or subapical infiltrates, often with cavities.
- *Mycobacterium tuberculosis* in sputum or in gastric or tracheal washings.

General Considerations

Pulmonary tuberculosis is a specific pulmonary infection caused by the acid-fast organism *M tuberculosis* and characterized by the formation of tubercles in the lung. Infection occurs almost exclusively by means of the inhalation of organisms carried on microscopic airborne droplets produced by the cough of a person with tubercle bacilli in the sputum. The danger of infection from contaminated surfaces is negligible. The first, or primary, infection is usually a self-limited disease in children that escapes detection. A few patients develop progressive primary tuberculosis. Another small percentage of patients, after a latency period of months to years, develop progressive pulmonary disease of the adult type. Primary infection occurring in adults may evolve into the adult kind of disease

without developing the characteristic changes of primary disease seen in children. Once primary infection has occurred, the individual's subsequent risk is from the primary infecting bacilli. Superinfection ("exogenous reinfection") occurs rarely if at all. Although most people who are infected at any age never develop the disease, it is not always possible to predict which ones are at risk. Malnutrition, diabetes, measles, chronic corticosteroid administration, silicosis, and general debility favor progression of infection to the stage of overt disease.

Refugees arriving in the USA from Southeast Asia since 1979 have been found to have a high incidence of tuberculosis. Continued operation of existing case-finding and treatment programs is essential to ensure that the disease remains controlled.

Clinical Findings

A. Symptoms and Signs: Symptoms may be absent—or mild and nonspecific—in the presence of active disease. When present, the most frequent symptoms are cough, malaise, easy fatigability, weight loss, low-grade afternoon fever, night sweats, and pleuritic pain. Cough, when present, has no specific characteristics. Blood in the sputum is strongly suggestive of tuberculosis. Patients with pulmonary tuberculosis occasionally present with symptoms due to extrapulmonary complications such as laryngeal, renal, or central nervous system involvement.

Pulmonary signs may be difficult to elicit even in the presence of active disease. Fine persistent rales over the upper lobes may be found. These are best heard during inspiration after a slight cough. Advanced disease may lead to retraction of the chest wall, deviation of the trachea, wheezes, rales, and signs of pulmonary consolidation. Signs of cavitation are unreliable.

Pulmonary tuberculosis cannot be ruled out by physical examination alone. A chest x-ray is the minimum diagnostic requirement.

B. Skin Testing: The **tuberculin skin test** is based on delayed skin hypersensitivity to a specific bacterial protein antigen. Tuberculin should be administered intracutaneously (Mantoux). The intracutaneous method employing purified protein derivative (PPD-S) in intermediate strength (5 tuberculin units) is most reliable. A standardized liquid PPD is the preferred preparation and is more stable than dissolved tablets, which quickly lose their potency in solution.

Multiple puncture methods (tine, Mono-Vacc) should be used for screening only and only when intradermal testing is not feasible. Positive tests must be confirmed by intradermal PPD.

1. A skin reaction of 10 mm or more of induration in 24–72 hours indicates past or present infection. The test becomes positive 2–8 weeks after infection with the tubercle bacillus. The incidence of positive reactions varies with population groups and is higher among disadvantaged segments in all countries. False-positive reactions may occur as a result of cross-sensitivity to atypical mycobacteria (see p 150)

or previous vaccination with BCG. When testing close contacts of active cases, a 5-mm induration should be considered significant.

2. A skin reaction of 5 mm or less in a person with no known recent exposure makes tuberculosis unlikely. Anergy (disappearance or marked decrease in the tuberculin reaction in the presence of a tuberculous infection) occasionally occurs with overwhelming tuberculosis, exanthematous diseases, corticosteroid treatment, sarcoidosis, debility, and increased age. The possibility of defective testing material must also be considered. When the clinical picture strongly suggests tuberculosis, further diagnostic measures are indicated.

3. A skin reaction of 5–9 mm may be due to recent infection, cross-sensitivity to nontuberculous mycobacteria, or partial anergy due to one of the causes listed above. Repeat the test within 1 week. If it is still doubtful and the chest x-ray is negative, repeat the test in 3 months. If the induration is still less than 10 mm, it can be considered negative.

4. A "conversion" reaction is one that has shown an increase of at least 6 mm of induration, from less than 10 mm to more than 10 mm in diameter. If this change has occurred within 2 years, the person is considered to be newly infected and should receive preventive treatment (see p 147, ¶ D).

C. Bacteriologic Studies: Recovery of the tubercle bacillus from sputum or gastric or tracheal washings is the only incontrovertible diagnostic finding. Tracheal wash with saline or sputum induction by inhalation of a heated aerosol (5% saline) produces a more reliable specimen for bacteriologic examination if there is no spontaneous sputum production. Pleural effusions or biopsy may yield the organisms on culture.

1. Sputum–Direct smears are positive by acid-fast stain when the bacterial count is high. Positive smears should always be confirmed by culture, although treatment is usually started before culture results are completed. Sensitivities to the major antituberculosis drugs of organisms obtained by culture should be determined.

Fresh sputum should be obtained for culture, although tubercle bacilli will usually survive several days in specimens transmitted by mail.

Culture is more sensitive than smear examination, but the time required for growth of organisms (4–6 weeks) is a disadvantage. Certain atypical acid-fast organisms may cause confusion. Bacteriologic methods usually permit the differentiation of *M tuberculosis* from atypical mycobacteria as well as differentiation of the several groups of the latter (see below).

2. Gastric washings–Gastric specimens should be obtained in the morning after the patient has fasted for 8–10 hours. Stained smears of gastric washings are of no value because of the occurrence of nontuberculous acid-fast organisms. Culture of gastric contents is especially useful for patients who cannot cooperate (eg, children, senile patients).

D. Biopsies: Enlarged lymph nodes in supraclavicular or cervical areas should be searched for carefully, since they may reveal an extension of the underlying pulmonary disease easily accessible by biopsy. In addition to histologic examination, excised nodes should always be cultured for tubercle bacilli and fungi. Pleural and pulmonary biopsy may also give valuable diagnostic information.

E. X-Ray Findings: Chest films disclose disease in almost all cases. Failures occur where lesions are hidden behind ribs, cardiovascular structures, and the diaphragm. A single film is usually insufficient for diagnosis. Although many features suggest the likelihood of tuberculosis (see below), there is no pathognomonic x-ray pattern.

Hilar lymph node enlargement associated with a small parenchymal lesion that heals with calcification is the usual picture of primary infection. Many "primaries" (proved by change of tuberculin skin test from negative to positive) do not present x-ray abnormalities. Very large nodes are unusual in adults, in whom primary infection cannot be distinguished from postprimary progression by x-ray findings.

Apical and subapical infiltrations are the usual presenting x-ray features of "adult" (postprimary progression) tuberculosis. Lordotic views may be required to reveal such lesions where uncertainty exists in the posteroanterior projection.

Cavitation is presumptive evidence of tuberculous activity. Tomograms are occasionally necessary for the demonstration of cavities. Cavitation may persist in some treated, sputum-negative patients.

Fibrotic disease, with dense, well-delineated strands, may dominate the picture. Without negative sputum cultures, the physician should not assume that these lesions are inactive.

Solitary nodules, miliary lesions, and lobar consolidation (acute caseous pneumonia) present difficult problems in differential diagnosis.

Lower lung field tuberculosis in the absence of upper lobe lesions is uncommon (about 3% of all cases).

Serial films are often crucial in the establishment of activity and are indispensable in the selection and evaluation of therapy.

Differential Diagnosis

Tuberculosis can mimic almost any pulmonary disease. Important diseases to be considered are bacterial and viral pneumonias, lung abscess, pulmonary mycoses, bronchogenic carcinoma, sarcoidosis, pneumoconioses, and nontuberculous mycobacterial infections.

Recovery of tubercle bacilli by culture establishes the diagnosis of tuberculosis. A negative tuberculin skin test makes the diagnosis of tuberculosis very unlikely. If carcinoma is suspected and cannot be promptly excluded, early tissue diagnosis by thoracotomy may be indicated without waiting for culture results.

Prevention

A. Isolation Precautions: Persons in contact with patients with tuberculosis who are newly diagnosed or suspected of having the disease should wear masks, although the protection afforded is questionable. Patients must be taught to effectively cover the mouth and nose with tissue during coughing. The patient should wear a mask when outside the isolation room and when hospital personnel are present.

Patients with previously untreated disease who are cooperative and not coughing (or who cover the mouth when coughing) and who have been on antituberculosis drug treatment for at least 2 weeks do not present a risk of contagion even without special precautions and even though tubercle bacilli may still be present in the sputum. Hospital personnel with negative tuberculin skin tests who are in contact with tuberculosis patients should repeat skin tests twice a year.

B. Examination of Contacts: Close contacts must be examined by skin test when a case of tuberculosis is discovered. Persons with positive tests should have chest x-rays. Those with negative skin tests should be retested 2 months after contact with the infectious case has been broken. Those with positive skin tests and negative x-rays should receive preventive treatment with isoniazid (see ¶ D, below). Some authorities recommend giving all close contacts (with negative x-rays) isoniazid for 1 year whether the skin test is positive or negative.

C. BCG Vaccination: Although it is generally agreed that BCG vaccination offers some protection to tuberculin-negative persons, several factors limit its usefulness. In most parts of the world, the risk of developing tuberculosis is slight among tuberculin-negative persons. Converting tuberculin-negative people to positive reactors by vaccination deprives the clinician of an important tuberculosis control measure, ie, the discovery of early infection by skin testing and treatment of converters with isoniazid. For these reasons, BCG vaccination is recommended only where exposure to tuberculosis is great and the usual tuberculosis control measures are not possible.

D. Treatment of Tuberculin Reactors (Without Other Evidence of Disease): Certain tuberculin reactors should be given preventive treatment with isoniazid. These include the following:

(1) Close contacts of recently diagnosed tuberculosis patients. Infants and children who have had such exposure should be given isoniazid even if the tuberculin test is negative. If they are still negative 3 months after exposure has been discontinued, treatment may be stopped. Adult contacts who are initially negative to tuberculin should be retested in 2 months and treated if the test has become positive.

(2) Persons with positive skin tests and x-ray findings compatible with nonprogressive tuberculosis.

(3) Those who have had a conversion from a negative to a positive skin test within 2 years.

(4) Persons with special risk factors such as prolonged corticosteroid treatment for other disease, immunosuppressive therapy, hematologic and reticuloendothelial system disorders (eg, Hodgkin's disease, leukemia), insulin-dependent diabetes mellitus, silicosis, and postgastrectomy.

(5) Preventive treatment should be given to children up to age 6 and should be strongly recommended for persons up to age 21.

(6) Positive reactors in the 21–35 age group who are otherwise healthy should be considered for preventive treatment on an individual basis.

Preventive treatment for the above groups consists of isoniazid, 300 mg daily (10 mg/kg, up to 300 mg, daily for children) for 1 year.

Prior to treatment, the presence of possible contraindications should be determined:

(1) A history of adverse reaction to isoniazid.

(2) Evidence or strong suspicion of progressive tuberculosis. (These patients should be treated as outlined below.)

(3) A previous course of adequate treatment with isoniazid.

(4) The presence of active liver disease.

(5) Pregnancy. Because of potential risk to the fetus, preventive treatment should be postponed until the postpartum period.

Because of the known—although low—incidence of isoniazid-induced liver damage, patients receiving preventive treatment should be cautioned regarding the symptoms of isoniazid toxicity (unexplained fever, rash, gastrointestinal symptoms) and advised to stop the drug and report to the physician if such symptoms appear. Routine liver function testing of patients without a history of liver disease is not useful. Patients with a history of liver disease for whom preventive treatment is strongly indicated should be investigated before treatment and monitored periodically during treatment.

When infection has been acquired from a patient with organisms known to be resistant to isoniazid, preventive treatment may be given with rifampin (see below). However, the efficacy of this drug for this purpose has not been established.

Treatment

A. Drug Therapy: (See Table 7–3.) Drug treatment is the most important single measure in the management of tuberculosis and is indicated in all cases.

Bed rest is advisable if there are symptoms such as fever, hemoptysis, or severe cough and usually is needed only for a few weeks. In general, return to normal physical activity is permitted following a brief period of observation after an effective drug regimen has been established. Patients with positive sputum must be isolated until effective treatment has been given for at least 2 weeks.

Extensive field trials in recent years have shown that the currently available drugs can be used in a number of different ways and achieve the same end result, ie, 95–100% cure of initially treated pulmonary tuberculosis. Also, it has been shown that the treatment period for pulmonary tuberculosis caused by susceptible organisms can be greatly shortened from

Table 7—3. Pulmonary tuberculosis drug therapy schedules.

Drug	Adult Dose	Remarks
A. Isoniazid Rifampin	300 mg daily 600 mg daily	Current preferred regimen for compliant patients with presumed susceptible organisms. Give each drug in a single dose daily for 9 months.

B. 1. Isoniazid
     Rifampin
     Ethambutol
B. 2. Isoniazid
     Rifampin
	300 mg daily
	600 mg daily
	15 mg/kg daily
	900 mg twice weekly
	600 mg twice weekly
		An alternate regimen for compliant patients. Use schedule B1 for the first month and schedule B2 for the next 8 months. Give each drug in a single dose.

C. Isoniazid
   Rifampin
   Streptomycin
	300 mg daily
	600 mg daily
	0.75–1 g daily
		This schedule should be used when resistant organisms may be present (previous treatment failure, recent arrival from another country). Continue daily streptomycin until organism sensitivity is determined. If sensitive, continue as above (A). If resistance is present, a longer treatment period with the appropriate drugs may be required.*

D. Isoniazid
   Rifampin
   Streptomycin
	900 mg twice weekly
	600 mg twice weekly
	1 g IM twice weekly
		This schedule may be used for noncompliant patients with susceptible organisms. The twice-weekly regimen is supervised and should be preceded by 2 months of daily treatment (C), usually in the hospital. The total duration of supervised treatment is 9 months or until sputum has been negative at least 6 months.

*Patients with organisms resistant to one or more of the major drugs need more intensive and carefully monitored treatment with a combination of 3 or 4 of the primary or secondary drugs to which the organisms have in vitro sensitivity. The reader is referred to the references on this subject.

the previously recommended 18 months. Additionally, by giving larger doses of the most effective drugs twice weekly, it is now feasible to provide supervised treatment for otherwise noncompliant patients and achieve the same excellent results.

It should be noted that these shortened treatment regimens are not yet recommended for extrapulmonary tuberculosis, drug-resistant disease, or tuberculosis complicated by other illness such as silicosis, diabetes, and immunosuppressed states.

The principal drugs currently used in the treatment of tuberculosis are isoniazid, rifampin, streptomycin, and ethambutol. A second-line drug, pyrazinamide, which is not widely used in the USA, has found new usefulness in the intermittent shorter term regimens. The choice of regimens may be modified by sensitivity tests, patient tolerance, and coexisting liver disease.

Toxicity of the major antituberculosis drugs, except streptomycin, is quite low, with side effects in 3–4% of patients. Both isoniazid and rifampin cause occasional gastrointestinal symptoms. About 10% of patients receiving isoniazid have elevated serum values of SGOT and SGPT. Significant hepatitis occurs in 1–2%, with a slightly higher incidence in those over age 50. Isoniazid interferes with the excretion of phenytoin and may result in phenytoin toxicity when given concurrently with this drug. Rifampin has less hepatotoxicity than isoniazid. Other minor side effects of rifampin include yellowish discoloration of the urine and sweat and interaction with various drugs. It accelerates the metabolism of birth control pills and oral anticoagulants, corticosteroids, methadone, oral hypoglycemic agents, and digitoxin. Ethambutol occasionally causes gastrointestinal disturbances, elevated uric acid, and a reversible optic neuropathy with loss of visual acuity, especially with prolonged treatment with more than 15 mg/kg/d. Pretreatment visual acuity determination with a Snellen chart and periodic

reexamination are advisable in patients who require prolonged treatment. Streptomycin's side effects include pain at injection sites, occasional hypersensitivity reactions, and, rarely, eighth nerve damage causing dysequilibrium or hearing loss, especially in elderly patients.

If treatment for active tuberculosis is required during pregnancy, isoniazid and ethambutol are the preferred drugs, and they appear to be well tolerated by the mother and fetus.

The corticosteroids are used occasionally in conjunction with antituberculosis drug treatment in certain extrapulmonary forms of tuberculosis. Their use in pulmonary tuberculosis is beneficial only in extensive disease with severe toxic symptoms.

Sensitivity tests on tubercle bacilli recovered by culture should be started, using the major drugs, before treatment is initiated. When the results of these studies are obtained (4–6 weeks later), it may be necessary to modify the drug regimen.

B. Collapse Therapy (Pneumothorax, Pneumoperitoneum): This type of treatment is no longer used in the treatment of tuberculosis.

C. Surgery:

1. Pulmonary resection–Resection is an important mode of treatment in selected cases, although very few patients now require surgery for pulmonary tuberculosis. Pulmonary resection is indicated in any of the following circumstances: (1) When there is a localized pulmonary nodule and the possibility of cancer cannot be excluded. (2) For bronchial stenosis. (3) For any localized chronic focus that has not improved substantially after 6 months of adequate drug therapy, and where tubercle bacilli persist in the sputum.

2. Thoracoplasty–This operation is no longer used as a primary treatment measure. It is occasionally used (1) to reduce the pleural "dead space" after a large pulmonary resection and thus minimize distention of the remaining lung, or (2) to close a chronic empyema space.

D. Diet: No special diets have been shown to be of benefit in tuberculosis. Normal weight should be maintained.

E. Climate: There is little evidence that climate is of any significance in the management of tuberculosis. The availability of good medical care is far more important.

F. Symptomatic Treatment: The patient should be reassured that symptoms will disappear as the illness is brought under control.

1. Cough–In general, cough in tuberculosis should not be abolished with drugs. Productive cough should be encouraged, and the patient should be taught to cover the mouth with disposable tissues and cough with minimal effort. If it becomes necessary to suppress exhausting cough, give codeine phosphate, 8–15 mg orally every 4–6 hours as necessary. Patients with large cavities who produce copious amounts of sputum may be helped by postural drainage. When secondary infection is present, appropriate antibiotics may be indicated.

2. Hemorrhage–The chief danger of hemorrhage in tuberculosis is not sudden death but aspiration of the infected blood and spread of the disease to other parts of the lungs. Observe the patient for shock (see Chapter 1). Reassurance is most important in allaying apprehension. Diazepam, 5–10 mg, may be of value in quieting the apprehensive patient. Use cough inhibitors carefully in the treatment of hemorrhage. Codeine phosphate, 8–15 mg every 4–6 hours, should be given to suppress (but not to abolish) cough. *Caution:* Do not give morphine.

Bed rest is essential during periods of hemorrhage. Instruct the patient in the proper method of coughing (see above).

G. Response to Treatment: A favorable symptomatic response to treatment is usually reported within 2–3 weeks; improvement can usually be observed within 4 weeks; and positive sputum usually becomes negative within 2 months. There is good evidence that most patients with previously untreated tuberculosis who are on a good drug regimen do not transmit the disease after 2–3 weeks of treatment even though tubercle bacilli may still be present in the sputum. Repeated x-ray examination and sputum tests, preferably cultures, should be done at monthly intervals during the first few months of treatment. When improvement is established, the interval between x-rays can be lengthened. When sputum becomes negative on culture and surgery is not indicated, a rapid return to normal activities can be permitted (see below). If there is no x-ray improvement or sputum conversion within 3 months, the treatment program should be reevaluated. Tuberculosis is no longer classified as "active" or "inactive." Instead, the patient's status is described in terms of whether exposure and infection have occurred and whether disease is present. Additional terms describe location of disease, bacteriologic status, status of chemotherapy, x-ray findings, and skin test results. It should be emphasized that patients who are on a good chemotherapy regimen and are asymptomatic may resume normal activities while receiving treatment. Of course, arrangements for continuation of treatment must be made and followed.

Patients who are noncompliant with the usual treatment schedules can be successfully treated with a supervised program adjusted to meet their special needs. This is accomplished by twice-weekly administration of larger doses of the principal drugs in a suitable location (ie, physician's office or clinic, or in the home or place of work by a public health nurse). The twice-weekly schedule should be preceded by 1–2 months of daily treatment with conventional doses of the drugs, usually in the hospital. Such supervised treatment can be completed in 9–12 months when the organisms are susceptible (Table 7–3). Patients treated on this schedule should be instructed to report symptoms of possible drug reaction (flu symptoms, gastrointestinal symptoms, petechiae, hematuria).

Prognosis

Very few people die of pulmonary tuberculosis when modern treatment methods are used before the disease reaches a very advanced stage. Most patients, including those with advanced disease, can be restored to a normal state of health within 12 months (although, as noted above, drug treatment may have to be continued for a longer period). Shorter periods of drug treatment are now possible with combinations that include rifampin.

A good treatment program should result in a 95% cure rate in all cases of initially treated disease. Of those who remain well 2 years after cessation of proper treatment, less than 1% can be expected to relapse. Prolonged follow-up of this group of patients is unnecessary. Inadequately treated patients should have regular follow-up examinations indefinitely.

American Thoracic Society: Treatment of tuberculosis and other mycobacterial diseases. *Am Rev Respir Dis* 1983;**127:**790.

American Thoracic Society: The tuberculin skin test. *Am Rev Respir Dis* 1981;**124:**356.

BCG vaccination. *Br Med J* 1975;**4:**603.

Coleman DL, Slutkin G: Chemoprophylaxis against tuberculosis. *West J Med* 1984;**140:**106.

Comstock GW, Woolpert SL: Tuberculin conversions: True or false? (Editorial.) *Am Rev Respir Dis* 1977;**118:**215.

Dutt AK, Stead WW: Short-course chemotherapy: The Arkansas experience. *Chest* 1982;**80:**724.

Farer LS: Chemoprophylaxis. *Am Rev Respir Dis* 1982;**125(pt 2):**102.

Glassroth J, Robins AG, Snider DE Jr: Tuberculosis in the 1980s. *N Engl J Med* 1980;**302:**1441.

Judson FN et al: Tuberculosis screening: Evaluation of a food handlers' program. *Chest* 1983;**83:**879.

Kopanoff DE, Snider DE Jr, Canas GJ: Isoniazid-related hepatitis: A US Public Health Service Cooperative Surveillance Study. *Am Rev Respir Dis* 1978;**117:**991.

McDonald RJ, Memon AM, Reichman LB: Successful supervised management of tuberculosis treatment failures. *Ann Intern Med* 1982;**96:**297.

Mitchell JR et al: Isoniazid liver injury: Clinical spectrum, pathology, and probable pathogenesis. *Ann Intern Med* 1976; **84**:181.

Powell KE et al: Tuberculosis among Indochinese refugees in the United States. *JAMA* 1983;**249**:1455.

Sbarbaro JA, Cotlin BJ, Iseman M: Long-term effectiveness of intermittent therapy for tuberculosis. *Am Rev Respir Dis* 1979; **119**:409.

Taylor WC et al: Should young adults with a positive tuberculin test take isoniazid? *Ann Intern Med* 1981;**94**:808.

Thompson NJ et al: The booster phenomenon in serial tuberculin testing. *Am Rev Respir Dis* 1979;**119**:587.

PULMONARY DISEASES DUE TO NONTUBERCULOUS MYCOBACTERIA

Certain mycobacteria other than the tubercle bacillus, which are ordinarily saprophytic and widely distributed in nature, may under certain circumstances produce chronic progressive pulmonary disease that is clinically similar to pulmonary tuberculosis. Cervical lymphadenitis is now more commonly due to these organisms (in the USA) than to tuberculosis and is very similar clinically.

These organisms are identical with tubercle bacilli microscopically and are differentiated by certain characteristics on bacterial culture.

Pulmonary disease is caused by 2 principal groups: photochromogens, the best known of which are *Mycobacterium kansasii* and *Mycobacterium marinum,* and the nonphotochromogens, which more closely resemble tubercle bacilli. *Mycobacterium avium* and *Mycobacterium intracellulare* (the Battey bacillus), the principal organisms in this group, cannot be distinguished by common laboratory examinations or by their behavior in human infection. Most authorities refer to them as *M avium-intracellulare* or the *M avium* complex. These mycobacteria cause pulmonary disease that is clinically similar to tuberculosis. Because these nontuberculous acid-fast bacilli usually exist as nonpathogenic saprophytes in humans, care must be taken to identify them as the true cause of disease.

Infection with nontuberculous mycobacteria and subsequent delayed hypersensitivity to them may result in cross-sensitivity to the tuberculin skin test antigen (PPD-S). The size of the reaction to PPD-S in these infections is considerably less than that due to tuberculosis.

Human-to-human transmission has not been reported, and isolation of patients is not required. Nontuberculous mycobacterial infection is more frequently seen in people with chronic pulmonary and systemic diseases in which natural immunity is compromised.

In spite of frequent in vitro drug resistance, patients with nontuberculous mycobacterial infection may show marked response to multiple drugs. This is especially true of *M kansasii;* more than 80% of patients with this infection may expect cure on the regi-mens used for *M tuberculosis,* especially when rifampin is included. Disease due to *M avium-intracellulare* responds less favorably, but with the use of additional drugs a good result may be achieved. In addition to the usual drugs, cycloserine, ethionamide, and pyrazinamide have been used. Simultaneous administration of combinations of as many as 5 of these drugs has been recommended. Surgical resection may be required for localized persistent disease.

Treatment with the chemotherapeutic agents that are effective in tuberculosis has been less predictable.

Ahn CH et al: Short course chemotherapy for pulmonary disease caused by *Mycobacterium kansasii. Am Rev Respir Dis* 1983;**128**:1048.

Bass JB Jr, Hawkins EL: Treatment of disease caused by nontuberculous mycobacteria. *Arch Intern Med* 1983;**143**:1439.

Rosenzweig DY: Pulmonary mycobacterial infections due to *M intracellulare-avium* complex: Clinical features and course in 100 consecutive cases. *Chest* 1979;**75**:115.

OBSTRUCTIVE DISEASES

CHRONIC OBSTRUCTIVE PULMONARY DISEASE (COPD)
(Chronic Bronchitis, Emphysema)

COPD is probably the most common cause of death and disability due to lung disease in the USA. The entity referred to as COPD may be subdivided into at least 2 categories: (1) chronic bronchitis (which may have varying degrees of centrilobular emphysema) and (2) predominant panacinar emphysema (alpha$_1$-antitrypsin deficiency). As the previous statement implies, there may be considerable overlapping of the 2 clinical entities.

1. CHRONIC BRONCHITIS

Chronic bronchitis is probably the most common debilitating respiratory disease in the USA. There is a strong association with inhalation of irritant substances, most commonly cigarette smoke and various forms of air pollution. The pathologic findings include hyperplasia and hypertrophy of the submucosal bronchial mucous glands, hyperplasia of bronchiolar goblet cells, squamous metaplasia of bronchial mucosal cells, chronic and acute inflammatory infiltrates in the bronchial submucosa, profuse inflammatory exudates in the lumens of bronchi and bronchioles, and denudation of bronchial mucosa. As mentioned previously, centrilobular emphysema consisting of dilatation of respiratory bronchioles of all orders, with subsequent communication between these distended air spaces, is not uncommonly found in patients with chronic bronchitis. (See following section on panacinar emphysema.)

Clinical Findings

A. Symptoms and Signs: The hallmark of chronic bronchitis is chronic cough and sputum production. Specifically, the definition of chronic bronchitis requires that productive cough be present on most days for a minimum of 3 months in the year in at least 2 consecutive years in order to make the diagnosis. The disease is most commonly seen in smokers over age 35. Initially, cough with sputum production, often in the morning, may be the only symptom. Gradually the cough and sputum production increase and symptoms of dyspnea on exertion develop.

As the disease progresses, the patient's course is usually marked by recurrent episodes of acute respiratory failure resulting from infectious exacerbations of the bronchitis. Clinically, these are marked by increased cough, change in sputum from clear and mucoid to purulent, fever, dyspnea, and varying degrees of respiratory distress. Respiratory failure often ensues, with both elevated Pa_{CO_2} and diminished Pa_{O_2}. These episodes are often reversible at first with appropriate antibiotics, bronchodilators, and respiratory therapy.

Signs and symptoms of cor pulmonale are frequent in chronic bronchitis and are exacerbated along with episodes of acute respiratory failure.

The course of the disease is one of gradual increase in frequency and severity of episodes of acute infection and respiratory failure, eventually resulting in intubation and the need for almost constant ventilatory assistance. Death usually occurs during an episode of respiratory failure.

Depending on the stage in which the patient is examined, the physical findings may vary. During relatively quiescent periods, the only finding may be increased anteroposterior diameter of the chest, hyperresonance to percussion, prolonged expiratory phase, scattered diffuse coarse to medium rhonchi and rales, and wheezing. Later, the patient may manifest the signs and symptoms of pulmonary hypertension and right ventricular failure, ie, increased second heart sound, pedal edema, hepatomegaly, and ascites. These patients commonly have a plethoric appearance resulting from secondary polycythemia.

If examined during an acute attack, the patient will be in respiratory distress, as evidenced by tachypnea and use of accessory muscles of respiration, in addition to the signs described above. Cough is often prominent, and cyanosis during acute attacks is not uncommon. For these reasons, patients with predominant bronchitis have been called "blue bloaters."

B. Laboratory Findings: Routine laboratory studies often demonstrate the presence of secondary polycythemia (eg, hematocrit greater than 55%). Also, if right ventricular failure and hepatic congestion are present, there may be aberrations in liver function tests (SGOT, alkaline phosphatase, bilirubin, etc). Culture of sputum often shows *H influenzae* and *Streptococcus pneumoniae*. Several studies have indicated that these organisms may colonize the upper and lower airways of patients with chronic bronchitis, and their

significance in the pathogenesis of acute exacerbations is unknown at present. Arterial blood gases show hypoxemia with either low, normal, or elevated Pa_{CO_2}.

If the patient has chronically retained CO_2, serum bicarbonate will also be elevated, and there will be only a modest degree of acidemia. If CO_2 retention is the result of an acute exacerbation, there will not be an elevation of bicarbonate, and respiratory acidosis with acidemia may be pronounced.

Pulmonary function studies uniformly show expiratory air flow obstruction (ie, reduced FEV_1, $FEF_{200-1200}$, FEF_{25-75}). Vital capacity may be normal or reduced, and there is often evidence of air trapping, with increased residual volume, total lung capacity, and ratio of RV to TLC. Expiratory reserve volume also is often diminished, and functional residual capacity is increased. Diffusion capacity for carbon monoxide may be normal or decreased.

More sophisticated pulmonary function studies show normal elastic recoil, increased airway resistance, and relatively normal compliance in pure bronchitis.

C. X-Ray Findings: Chest x-rays show evidence of pulmonary overinflation, with increased anteroposterior diameter, flattened diaphragms, and increased retrosternal air space (unless right ventricular hypertrophy has supervened). There are often prominent and increased bronchial markings at the lung bases, seen as parallel or tapering shadows ("tram lines"), which reflect the increased thickness of the bronchial wall. Bullae of varying sizes may be seen primarily in the upper lung fields rather than the lung bases (as in alpha$_1$-antitrypsin deficiency).

Treatment

There is no doubt that smoking hastens the progression of emphysema and shortens the life span of patients with the disease. Patients must be vigorously encouraged to discontinue cigarette smoking and avoid exposure to other toxic inhalants when possible. Since the risk of infection resulting in respiratory failure is great, these patients should be immunized against pneumococci and influenza. The efficacy of prophylactic or regular antibiotic treatment is unproved and controversial, and it is reasonable to reserve antibiotics for management of acute exacerbations, as manifested by change in sputum character, increased dyspnea, etc.

The preferred drug is ampicillin, 250–500 mg every 6 hours, or erythromycin, 500 mg every 6 hours, for 5–7 days. When exacerbations are associated with respiratory failure, appropriate treatment measures must be instituted (see pp 164 and 167). Since many of these patients display varying degrees of chronic bronchospasm, most authorities treat chronically with bronchodilators. Oral aminophylline in dosages sufficient to give serum theophylline levels of 10–20 μg/mL is the drug of choice (usual dosage 250–500 mg 4 times daily or 200 mg of sustained-release preparations twice daily). Inhaled bronchodilators (Bronkometer, Alupent Inhaler, etc) may also be useful in the chronic management of these patients. The usual dosage is 2–3 puffs 4 times daily. Sympathomimetic beta-agonists (terbutaline, 2.5–5 mg 3 times daily, or metaproterenol, 10–20 mg 3 times daily) are often useful in chronic management.

Many patients with chronic bronchitis develop right ventricular failure, and there is also a considerable body of evidence suggesting that left ventricular dysfunction is common as well. For this reason, signs and symptoms referable to cardiac dysfunction (either right- or left-sided) are managed with diuretics. The administration of digitalis is controversial; some authors prefer not to use it unless there is documented evidence of left ventricular failure (ie, increased pulmonary capillary wedge pressure) or a digitalis-responsive arrhythmia (eg, atrial flutter).

The use of corticosteroids in patients with COPD/bronchitis is controversial also. Many authorities feel that there is a significant subgroup of patients who respond favorably to the administration of corticosteroids (eg, prednisone, 20–50 mg daily). No clinical or laboratory markers for this group of patients have been definitely identified, and there are no well-documented studies proving the efficacy of corticosteroid therapy. Nonetheless, many authorities use corticosteroids as a last resort in patients with severe disease.

Other measures, such as low-flow home oxygen and patient education regarding coughing and postural drainage exercises, are often useful.

Course & Prognosis

The course of the disease in any one patient is quite variable. However, in general there is progressive deterioration of pulmonary function with increasing frequency of respiratory failure episodes until death. Once patients become severely symptomatic with clinically obvious disease, the prognosis for survival beyond 5–10 years is not good. Some authorities feel that cessation of smoking may interrupt or reverse the disease process if instituted early.

2. EMPHYSEMA

The term emphysema denotes a disease entity characterized pathologically by destruction of interalveolar septa, including blood vessels, and coalescence of air spaces to form abnormal cystic or bullous areas in the lungs that do not function in gas exchange. The underlying lesion is destruction of pulmonary elastic tissue, with resultant loss of elastic recoil and increased compliance. This has been associated with deficiencies in alpha$_1$-antitrypsin, a protein that inactivates the enzyme trypsin. The postulated pathogenesis is that trypsin and various other enzymes (eg, elastases) digest the elastic tissue in smaller airways and the pulmonary interstitium in the absence of the inhibitor alpha$_1$-antitrypsin. The disease is inherited, and signs and symptoms commonly become manifest

in the third and fourth decade in homozygotes. The risk of disease for heterozygotes is unclear at present.

Clinical Findings

A. Symptoms and Signs: Insidious onset of progressive dyspnea on exertion is the most common symptom. The patient may complain of chronic cough with sputum production, although this is not characteristic. In far-advanced disease, symptoms of cor pulmonale may become evident (eg, pedal edema, ascites). Findings on physical examination will vary depending upon the stage of disease at which the patient is examined. In general, they are associated with air trapping and hypoxemia and include increased anteroposterior diameter of the chest; hyperinflation of the lungs, with depressed diaphragm and very little diaphragmatic motion; hypertrophy of accessory muscles of respiration (eg, sternocleidomastoids); hyperresonance of the chest to percussion; decreased breath sounds with increased expiratory phase; and, in some patients, wheezing. In far-advanced disease, one may see clubbing of the digits and signs of pulmonary hypertension (increased second heart sound, pedal edema, hepatomegaly, and ascites).

Patients with pure emphysema tend not to have CO_2 retention until the disease is far advanced. Likewise, P_{aO_2} is often maintained in the high 60 or low 70 mm Hg range, which is sufficient to saturate hemoglobin to an extent obviating cyanosis. Therefore, these patients have been called "pink puffers."

B. X-Ray Findings: Chest x-rays characteristically show signs of lung hyperinflation, with increased anteroposterior diameter, lowered flattened diaphragms, and increased retrosternal air space. The cardiac silhouette appears small in most cases, and it has been suggested that a normal-sized cardiac silhouette in this setting is suggestive of left ventricular enlargement. There may be prominent bullous changes, especially at the lung bases.

C. Laboratory Findings: As mentioned previously, many patients will be found to be deficient in serum alpha$_1$-antitrypsin, which can be assayed directly. Pulmonary function studies show enlarged total lung capacity (TLC) and residual volume (RV) with normal or decreased vital capacity. The ratio of RV to TLC is increased, and there is usually marked diminution of all expiratory flow parameters (eg, FEV_1, $FEF_{200-1200}$, FEF_{25-75}). Also, the carbon monoxide diffusing capacity (D_LCO) is characteristically decreased in these patients. More sophisticated pulmonary function studies will demonstrate loss of elastic recoil and hence increased pulmonary compliance. Arterial blood gases characteristically show mild to moderate hypoxemia with reduced or normal P_{aCO_2}. There may be abnormalities in liver function tests owing to deposition of granules of alpha$_1$-antitrypsin in the hepatic parenchyma.

Treatment

Although there is no effective treatment for the underlying disease process per se, a number of symptomatic measures may improve the patient's quality of life, and appropriate treatment of episodes of respiratory failure may prolong life. Cigarette smoking must be discontinued and other toxic inhalants must be avoided. Since patients are at very high risk for developing respiratory failure with even minor pulmonary infection, they should be vaccinated against pneumonia and influenza on a regular basis. Administration of antibiotics early in the course of lower respiratory infection (eg, fever, purulent sputum) is often recommended. The antibiotic of choice is ampicillin, 250–500 mg 4 times daily, or erythromycin, 500 mg 4 times daily.

Treatment of episodes of acute respiratory failure is often necessary. (See Acute Respiratory Failure, p 164.) The long-term prognosis of the disease is poor, with progressive diminution of pulmonary function and the occurrence of respiratory failure, which accounts for most of the deaths.

Other supplemental measures that may be useful include home oxygen, usually low-flow, administered by nasal cannula with any one of a number of portable oxygen-containing devices.

Ayres SM: Chronic bronchitis: A clinical guide. *Hosp Med* (May) 1984;**20**:213.
Hodgkin JE (editor): *Chronic Obstructive Pulmonary Disease.* American College of Chest Physicians, 1979.
IPPB Trial Group: Intermittent positive pressure breathing therapy of chronic obstructive pulmonary disease: A clinical trial. *Ann Intern Med* 1983;**99**:612.
Morse JO: Alpha₁-antitrypsin deficiency. (2 parts.) *N Engl J Med* 1978;**299**:1045, 1099.
Petty TL, Zwillich C (editors): The 22nd Aspen Lung Conference: Chronic obstructive pulmonary disease. *Chest* 1980;**77** (**Suppl**):249.
Snider GL: The pathogenesis of emphysema: Twenty years of progress. *Am Rev Respir Dis* 1981;**124**:321.
Tobin MJ, Hutchison DCS: α_1-Antitrypsin deficiency: Current and future therapeutic strategies. *Drug Ther* (May) 1983;**13**:189.

ATELECTASIS

Essentials of Diagnosis

- Acute: tachycardia, dyspnea, fever, hypoxemia.
- Chronic: there may be no symptoms or signs other than x-ray abnormalities, even with lobar involvement.
- Radiologic findings consistent with atelectasis, eg, a lobar or segmental density, which is often homogeneous, and reduction in size of the involved lobe. Tracheal deviation, mediastinal shift, and elevation of the diaphragm may occur with massive atelectasis.

General Considerations

Atelectasis is the collapse of part or all of a lung. It is probably most commonly seen in the immediate postoperative period following major abdominal or thoracic surgery. In this circumstance it is secondary to poor inspiration and lack of coughing by the patient as a result of the painful incision. This leads to resorption of alveolar air and possibly loss of surfactant and other local mechanisms that are not well understood. In this instance, the major bronchi are not obstructed.

In patients with chronic bronchitis, the atelectasis may result from failure to clear respiratory secretions by coughing, with resultant partial or complete obstruction of bronchi.

The incidence of postoperative atelectasis varies from 3 to 5% in individuals with previously normal lungs to over 50% in patients with chronic obstructive pulmonary disease. Obese patients may also be at increased risk owing to closure of airways in the lung bases, which results from low lung volumes. The low lung volumes are caused by difficulty in expanding the massive chest wall.

The other principal cause of atelectasis is bronchial obstruction resulting from neoplasm or foreign body.

Clinical Findings

A. Symptoms and Signs: The severity of symptoms depends upon the site of collapse, the rate at which it develops, and the presence or absence of infection in the atelectatic area. The more acute the onset (eg, postoperative atelectasis), the more marked the symptoms. Massive acute atelectasis causes marked dyspnea, cyanosis, tachycardia, and fever. Lesser degrees of collapse produce variable symptoms, but atelectasis involving even a small segment of lung may produce symptoms.

The physical findings in acute atelectasis include tachycardia and decrease of chest motion on the affected side. There may be displacement of the mediastinum to the involved side, as shown by shift of the trachea and heart. Percussion dullness and decreased or absent vocal fremitus, breath sounds, and voice sounds may be apparent over the atelectatic area. Bronchial breath sounds are occasionally present over portions of collapsed lung.

In chronic atelectasis, displacement of the mediastinum may be modified by the slowness of compensatory changes, rigidity of the mediastinum due to the underlying disease, and changes of elasticity of surrounding diseased lung.

B. X-Ray Findings: The atelectatic lobe or segment is usually densely consolidated and smaller than normal. Fissure lines are displaced toward the area of density. Tracheal deviation to the affected side commonly occurs in upper lobe atelectasis but is a useful diagnostic sign only when the deviation is marked. Lower lobe atelectasis may cause elevation of the corresponding part of the diaphragm, but this may also result from other causes. Mediastinal shift to the involved side is seen with massive atelectasis. Compensatory overexpansion of lung adjacent to the atelectatic area is often present. The presence of air bronchograms in the area of density indicates that the central airways are clear and that any obstruction is in the segmental or subsegmental branches.

Differential Diagnosis

Atelectasis must be distinguished from pneumonia, pulmonary infarction, pleural effusion (in massive atelectasis), and chronic fibrotic changes.

Complications

The sequelae of unrelieved atelectasis are infection, destruction of lung tissue, and bronchiectasis.

Treatment

A. Postoperative Atelectasis: The prevention and treatment of postoperative atelectasis involve various measures to induce deep breathing and stimulate coughing. Incentive spirometers, blow bottles, and other similar devices are widely used and are as effective as intermittent positive pressure breathing (IPPB) in the prevention and treatment of postoperative atelectasis. In patients unable to perform or respond to the above measures, there may be a role for IPPB to expand partially collapsed segments. In patients who are unable to cough or breathe deeply despite the previously mentioned maneuvers, small catheters (Intracath) introduced transtracheally through the cricothyroid membrane and taped in place may be used to inject 2–3 mL of saline at regular intervals to stimulate coughing.

The key element in these procedures is probably the deep breathing and consequent expansion of lung produced by the maneuvers. Likewise, stimulation of cough facilitates removal of secretions and prevents partial or complete bronchial obstruction due to tenacious sputum. Appropriate preoperative instruction (eg, cessation of smoking, deep breathing exercises), voluntary deep breathing, and early ambulation after surgery are undoubtedly the most cost-effective methods for the prevention of atelectasis. In the case of the postoperative patient being maintained on a ventilator via an endotracheal tube, a sigh breath 1½ times the tidal volume should be delivered at least 4–6 times per hour.

Recent studies have indicated that removal of bronchial obstruction by fiberoptic bronchoscopy is of no greater effectiveness than aggressive physical and respiratory therapy in the reexpansion of acute lobar atelectasis, in both postoperative and nonoperative patients. Therefore, one should exhaust all means of conservative treatment (incentive spirometry, percussion, vibration, drainage, etc) before proceeding with fiberoptic bronchoscopy.

B. Spontaneous Atelectasis: Bronchoscopy is required to determine the cause of spontaneously occurring atelectasis, especially if it is chronic in nature. This is necessary in order to identify and possibly remove foreign bodies as well as to make the diagnosis of endobronchial neoplasm.

Prognosis

Although the outlook is usually good in postoperative atelectasis, unrelieved collapse may result in death (when massive) or in prolonged illness (when lobar or segmental). The prognosis in other types of atelectasis depends on the underlying lesion producing the bronchial obstruction.

Bartlett RH et al: Respiratory maneuvers to prevent postoperative pulmonary complications: A critical review. *JAMA* 1973; **224:**1017.

Iverson LI et al: A comparative study of IPPB, the incentive spirometer, and blow bottles: The prevention of atelectasis following cardiac surgery. *Ann Thorac Surg* 1978;**25:**197.

Marini JJ, Pierson DJ, Hudson LD: Acute lobar atelectasis: A prospective comparison of fiberoptic bronchoscopy and respiratory therapy. *Am Rev Respir Dis* 1979;**119:**971.

BRONCHIECTASIS

Essentials of Diagnosis

- Chronic cough with expectoration of large amounts of purulent sputum; hemoptysis.
- Rales and rhonchi over lower lobes.
- X-ray of chest reveals little; bronchograms show characteristic dilatations.

General Considerations

Bronchiectasis is a dilatation of small and medium-sized bronchi resulting from destruction of bronchial elastic and muscular elements. It may be caused by pulmonary infections (eg, pneumonia, pertussis, tuberculosis) or by a bronchial obstruction (eg, foreign bodies or extrinsic pressure). In many patients, a history of onset following one or more episodes of pulmonary infection, usually in early childhood, is obtained. However, since infection does not regularly produce significant bronchiectasis, unknown intrinsic host factors presumably are present. The incidence of the disease has been reduced by treating pulmonary infections with antibiotics.

Clinical Findings

A. Symptoms and Signs: Most patients with bronchiectasis have a history of chronic cough with expectoration of large volumes of sputum, especially upon awakening. The sputum has a characteristic quality of "layering out" into 3 layers upon standing, a frothy top layer, a middle clear layer, and a dense particulate bottom layer. It is usually purulent in appearance and foul-smelling.

Intermittent hemoptysis, occasionally in dangerous proportions, is often combined with intercurrent respiratory infections. Symptoms occur most often in patients with idiopathic bronchiectasis (ie, childhood respiratory infections). However, patients who have bronchiectasis secondary either to tuberculosis or chronic obstruction may not exhibit characteristic symptoms. Idiopathic bronchiectasis occurs most frequently in the middle and lower lobes and posttuberculous bronchiectasis in the upper lobes.

Hemoptysis is thought to result from erosion of bronchiolar mucosa with resultant destruction of underlying blood vessels. Pulmonary insufficiency may result from progressive destruction of pulmonary tissue.

Physical findings consist primarily of rales and rhonchi over the affected segments. If the condition is far-advanced, emaciation, cyanosis, and digital clubbing may appear.

B. Laboratory Findings: There are no characteristic laboratory findings. If hypoxemia is chronic and severe, secondary polycythemia may develop. There may be either restrictive or obstructive pulmonary function defects associated with bronchiectasis. Hypoxemia and hypocapnia or hypercapnia may also be associated with the disease, depending on the severity of the underlying condition.

C. X-Ray Findings: Plain films of the chest often show increased bronchopulmonary markings in affected segments; in severe cases, there may be areas of radiodensities surrounding portions of radiolucency. Early in the course of bronchiectasis, however, the chest x-ray may be normal.

Iodized contrast media instilled into the bronchial tree (a bronchogram) demonstrates saccular, cylindric, or fusiform dilatation of small and medium bronchi with consequent loss of the normal branching pattern. Cylindric changes of bronchiectasis that may result from acute pneumonia will revert to normal after 6–8 weeks, but saccular dilatations represent long-standing damage and permanent disease.

Differential Diagnosis

The differential diagnosis includes other disorders that lead to chronic cough, sputum production, and hemoptysis, ie, chronic bronchitis, tuberculosis, and bronchogenic carcinoma. The diagnosis of bronchiectasis is suggested by the patient's history and can be confirmed only by bronchographic examination or histopathologic examination of surgically removed tissue.

Complications

Recurrent infection in poorly drained pulmonary segments leads to chronic suppuration and may cause pulmonary insufficiency. Complications include hemoptysis, respiratory failure, chronic cor pulmonale, and amyloidosis. There is also an increased incidence of brain abscess, which is thought to be secondary to abnormal anastomoses between bronchial (systemic) and pulmonary venous circulation. These anastomoses produce right-to-left shunts and allow for the dissemination of septic emboli.

Treatment

A. General Measures and Medical Treatment:

1. Environmental changes–The patient should avoid exposure to all common pulmonary irritants such as smoke, fumes, and dust and should stop smoking cigarettes.

2. Control of bronchial secretions (improved drainage)–

a. Postural drainage often gives effective relief of symptoms and should be utilized in every case. The patient should assume the position that gives maximum drainage, usually lying on a bed in the prone, supine, or right or left lateral decubitus position with the hips elevated on several pillows and no pillow under the head. Any effective position should be maintained for 10 minutes, 2–4 times a day. The first drainage should be done upon awakening and the last drainage at bedtime. Family members can be trained in the art of chest percussion to facilitate drainage.

b. Liquefaction of thick sputum may be promoted by inhaling warm mists and, in some cases, mucolytic agents such as acetylcysteine or 5% sodium bicarbonate given by aerosol may also be helpful.

3. Control of respiratory infection–Exposure to respiratory infections should be minimized and the patient should be vaccinated against influenza and pneumococcal pneumonia. Antibiotic therapy is indicated for acute exacerbations (ie, increased production of purulent sputum, hemoptysis, etc). Long-term or prophylactic antibiotic therapy is controversial, since it has not been conclusively shown to be of lasting benefit. Therefore, it seems rational to treat acute exacerbations in order to control infection but minimize the emergence of resistant strains. Because the bacteria most commonly involved are *H influenzae* and *S pneumoniae,* the drug most commonly employed is ampicillin, 250–500 mg orally every 6 hours for 5 days. Alternative therapies for the penicillin-allergic patient are erythromycin, given in the same dosage schedule as ampicillin, or trimethoprim-sulfamethoxazole, 2 double-strength tablets twice a day for 5 days.

B. Surgical Treatment: Surgical treatment is most often employed when hemoptysis with bronchiectasis is recurrent and severe. Despite antibiotic therapy, localized bronchiectasis (eg, in a lower lobe or segment) with progressive uncontrolled infection and sputum production may be an indication for surgical removal of the affected segments.

Other Considerations

Bronchiectasis is also associated with mucoviscidosis. It is thought to be secondary to the thick viscid secretions that cannot be cleared by normal cough mechanisms and that lead to stasis of sputum and chronic infection. This disorder, usually associated with sinusitis, may be accompanied by other manifestations of mucoviscidosis. Its most common organisms are *S aureus* or *Pseudomonas aeruginosa.*

Bronchiectasis is also associated with certain abnormalities of cellular ciliary function, the most common of which is Kartagener's syndrome, a combination of sinusitis, situs inversus, and bronchiectasis. Patients with this disorder show immotile cilia secondary to ultrastructural abnormalities, stasis of sputum, failure to clear secretions, and chronic pulmonary infection that results in bronchiectasis.

Antibiotic treatment of mucoviscidosis and Kartagener's syndrome must be guided by sensitivity studies of organisms cultured from sputum.

Annest LS, Kratz JM, Crawford FA: Current results of treatment of bronchiectasis. *J Thorac Cardiovasc Surg* 1982;**83**:546.

Similä S et al: Chronic lung damage caused by adenovirus type 7: A ten-year follow-up study. *Chest* 1981;**80**:127.

Yarnal JR et al: The immotile cilia syndrome: Explanation for many a clinical mystery. *Postgrad Med* (Feb) 1982;**71**:195.

VASCULAR DISEASES

PULMONARY EMBOLISM

Essentials of Diagnosis

- Sudden onset of dyspnea and anxiety, with or without substernal pain, is characteristic of a large pulmonary embolus. Signs of acute right heart failure and circulatory collapse may follow shortly.
- Less severe dyspnea, pleuritic pain, cough, hemoptysis, and an x-ray density in the lung are characteristic of congestive atelectasis or pulmonary infarction.
- Gradually developing, unexplained dyspnea with or without pulmonary x-ray densities may indicate repeated minor embolization to the lungs.
- A history or clinical findings of thrombophlebitis are common in patients with pulmonary embolism.

General Considerations

In the past, pulmonary embolism was thought to be quite common and probably underdiagnosed, since autopsy studies showed thrombosis in the pulmonary arterial tree to be a common finding. Recent studies, however, suggest that at least in selected populations of patients, pulmonary embolism may be overdiagnosed. This is because until recently the diagnosis of pulmonary embolism was based on nuclear medicine scanning procedures, which have high sensitivity but relatively low specificity for pulmonary embolism.

Most pulmonary emboli appear to arise from silent thromboses in the pelvic veins or the deep venous system of the lower extremities. Therefore, patients at high risk for pulmonary embolism are the same as those at high risk for pelvic or venous thrombosis. These include the following: (1) Patients rendered immobile by illness or trauma (chronic bed rest, multiple fractures with casts, etc). (2) Patients with congestive heart failure. (3) Patients with a variety of neoplasms, especially adenocarcinomas of the gastrointestinal tract. (4) Postsurgical patients, especially following abdominal or orthopedic surgery. (5) Those with intrinsic venous disease. (6) Normal people who are relatively immobile for long periods. (7) Pregnant women or women in the immediate postpartum period. (8) Women taking oral contraceptives (perhaps). (See also Chapter 9, pp 292 ff.)

Clinical Findings

A. Symptoms and Signs: The symptoms of pulmonary embolism vary according to the size of the artery occluded and whether or not pulmonary infarction has occurred as a result of the embolus. If the embolus is small and lodges in a small pulmonary artery, the only symptom may be relatively sudden onset of dyspnea with or without pleuritic chest pain. With massive pulmonary embolism (eg, occlusion of a main pulmonary artery), one may see sudden onset of dyspnea, anxiety, substernal chest pain, and other manifestations of frank shock. Various combinations of symptoms between these 2 extremes are possible with emboli of intermediate size. The most common symptom of all forms of pulmonary emboli is sudden onset of dyspnea. Pleuritic chest pain is also a common finding, and if pulmonary infarction develops (which occurs 12–36 hours after embolization), hemoptysis may appear in roughly one-third of patients. Of all patients with pulmonary embolism, approximately 10% have pulmonary infarction as a result.

Physical examination will also vary depending upon the location and size of the embolus. Patients with massive emboli will show tachypnea, tachycardia, extreme anxiety, overt respiratory distress, hypotension, accentuated pulmonary second heart sound, and distended neck veins. Supraventricular and ventricular tachyarrhythmias are not uncommon in this setting. In patients with smaller emboli, findings may consist merely of tachycardia with or without tachycardia or pleural friction rub. Mild elevation of temperature (37.2–38.3 °C [99–101 °F]) may occur. Physical signs of pleural effusion may be evident (eg, dullness to percussion and decreased breath sounds).

Patients with pulmonary infarction commonly have pleural friction rub, dullness to percussion, decreased breath sounds, and rales over the area of infarction. Diffuse wheezing may also occur with both small and large pulmonary emboli.

There is a distinctive syndrome of multiple small recurrent pulmonary emboli occurring predominantly in young women and characterized by the insidious onset of dyspnea on exertion. There is often no underlying history of cardiopulmonary disease. Physical examination is usually unremarkable until relatively late in the course, when pulmonary hypertension supervenes and signs of cor pulmonale (accentuated pulmonary second heart sound, pedal edema, hepatomegaly, ascites, etc) become manifest. This syndrome often requires lung biopsy for definitive diagnosis, and the pathologic features are quite similar to those of primary pulmonary hypertension. Unlike other forms of pulmonary embolism, this type seems relatively refractory to anticoagulant therapy, and no effective form of treatment is currently available.

B. Laboratory Findings: Routine laboratory studies are not helpful in the diagnosis of pulmonary embolism. Arterial blood gases are also not helpful, since diminished P_{aO_2} (< 80 mm Hg) may occur in a variety of circumstances clinically similar to pulmonary embolism, and normal P_{aO_2} is not uncommon in the presence of pulmonary embolism. Serum LDH, bilirubin, fibrin degradation products, and leukocyte count may be elevated.

C. Electrocardiographic Findings: The ECG is not specifically helpful in diagnosis. The most common electrocardiographic finding is sinus tachycardia. Other findings observed with varying frequency in different series are prominent S in lead I, abnormal Q with inverted T in lead III, right axis deviation, right ventricular strain pattern, and incomplete right bundle branch block. It should be emphasized that all of these are nonspecific findings that may be present with many clinical entities and are not diagnostic of pulmonary embolism.

D. X-Ray Findings: Chest x-rays are of limited value in the diagnosis of pulmonary emboli. A large percentage of patients with documented emboli have completely normal chest x-rays. Common findings, however, may include subsegmental atelectasis, segmental infiltrates, and pleural effusion. None of these are specific for pulmonary embolism. However, a good-quality chest x-ray is important for the interpretation of perfusion lung scans.

E. Ventilation and Perfusion Lung Scanning: Although the role of lung scanning in the diagnosis of pulmonary embolism is highly controversial, it is generally agreed that a negative perfusion lung scan virtually rules out the diagnosis. Therefore, all patients suspected of having pulmonary embolism should first have a perfusion lung scan. If this is normal, no further studies are necessary. The contribution of an abnormal perfusion lung scan to the diagnosis of pulmonary embolism remains quite controversial, as does the question of whether or not adding a ventilation scan to the perfusion scan increases the accuracy of the former. There have been reports of patients with ventilation/perfusion matched defects (ie, lack of ventilation and perfusion to the same pulmonary segment) who have had angiographically demonstrated pulmonary emboli. This combination of scan findings was previously thought to be virtually diagnostic of nonembolic pulmonary disease (eg, COPD). Thus, the role of a positive perfusion scan and of ventilation scans in the diagnosis of pulmonary embolism remains unresolved.

F. Pulmonary Angiography: Pulmonary angiography is necessary for the definitive diagnosis of clinically significant pulmonary emboli. The morbidity and mortality rates of pulmonary angiography have been reported to be approximately 1% and 0.5%, respectively, in a large multicenter study. These centers, however, were highly skilled in the performance of angiography and performed large numbers of angiograms, and the relevance of these data to community hospitals is unclear at present. There is also evidence that thromboemboli in vessels less than 2.5 mm in diameter may not be detected by pulmonary angiography. Most authorities, however, feel that emboli this small are not clinically significant and should not be treated.

Approach to Diagnosis

Although the subject is controversial, the following diagnostic approach seems reasonable.

In otherwise healthy adults (including women taking oral contraceptives) who are not in high-risk categories for the occurrence of pulmonary embolism and in whom clinical findings suggest the diagnosis, a perfusion lung scan should be performed. If this is completely normal, the diagnosis of pulmonary embolism is excluded. If the lung scan is abnormal (regardless of "probability" of pulmonary embolism read on scan), pulmonary arteriography should be done to avoid the consequences of an unwarranted diagnosis of pulmonary embolism (difficulty in obtaining insurance, cessation of contraception, avoidance of pregnancy, etc). Pulmonary arteriography should be performed also if the patient has a relative contraindication to anticoagulant therapy (eg, bleeding diathesis, peptic ulcer disease) or if interruption of the vena cava is being considered.

Patients at high risk for pulmonary embolism (except otherwise healthy women taking oral contraceptives) who develop clinical signs and symptoms suggestive of pulmonary embolism may be presumptively diagnosed as having pulmonary embolism on the basis of positive perfusion scans, especially if the scans show lobar or multiple segmental defects in areas where the chest x-ray is normal. In such cases it is essential that the patient have no contraindications to anticoagulant therapy and that the physician realize the diagnosis is only a presumptive one.

There is also evidence that pulmonary angiography is indicated for the diagnosis of pulmonary embolism in another subgroup of patients—those in intensive care units with acute respiratory failure from a variety of causes (eg, diffuse pneumonia, ARDS). Patients in this setting should also have angiography unless the perfusion lung scan is completely normal.

Prevention

In the case of surgical patients, there are sufficient data to show that "minidose heparin" (5000 units subcutaneously every 8–12 hours) is effective in preventing perioperative thrombosis and pulmonary embolism in patients undergoing major abdominal or orthopedic procedures, with the exception of total hip replacement. Heparin is begun shortly before surgery and continued through the operative period and thereafter until the patient is ambulatory. Several studies have documented the effectiveness of this regimen, and there have been no reports of increased incidence of major bleeding complications. The efficacy of this regimen in treating other high-risk patients (eg, those who are bedridden or who have congestive heart failure) is not known, but it seems reasonable to expect comparable benefits. Once a documented embolism has occurred, prevention of further embolization on a long-term basis is best achieved with oral coumarin anticoagulants. (See section below on treatment.)

Treatment

A. Heparin: Adequate prolongation of the clotting time with heparin is the treatment of choice. This is best achieved with fewest side effects when heparin is administered by constant intravenous infusion via infusion pump. An initial loading dose of 5000–10,000 units is given intravenously, and approximately 1000 units of heparin per hour are then administered via constant infusion. The heparin dosage is titrated according to clotting studies. Either the partial thromboplastin time or the whole blood clotting time may be used to regulate heparin dosage. The partial thromboplastin time is maintained at 1.5–2 times baseline control levels; whole blood clotting time is maintained at 2–3 times the control value. It appears that the measurement of clotting activity is helpful in assuring a heparin dose sufficient to prevent further clotting and embolization, but such monitoring probably has no effect on the rate of bleeding complications.

If facilities for administration of continuous infusion are not available, therapy may be given with a loading dose of 5000–10,000 units intravenously followed by intermittent intravenous doses of 5000–10,000 units intravenously every 4–6 hours. This regimen is also titrated by the whole blood clotting time or partial thromboplastin time, as discussed above. Samples for these tests should be drawn approximately 1 hour before a heparin dose is given.

If angiography is indicated but is not immediately available, heparin therapy should be started if there is clinical suspicion of pulmonary embolism. It can then be discontinued briefly (half-life about 90 minutes) before angiography is done. One should never withhold heparin therapy if the clinical suspicion of pulmonary embolism is great unless there is a strong contraindication to anticoagulation (gastrointestinal bleeding, cerebrovascular accident, etc).

The principal complications of heparin therapy are bleeding and thrombocytopenia. Heparin is a hazardous drug, and its effects must be closely monitored.

Continue heparin therapy for at least 10 days. Oral anticoagulants are begun as discussed below.

B. Warfarin: Although the subject is controversial, most authorities feel that treatment with warfarin derivatives should be continued for at least 3–6 months following an episode of pulmonary embolism. This is most effective if drug therapy is begun several days before discontinuation of heparin therapy. No loading dose is necessary, and one can begin the patient on warfarin sodium, 10–15 mg/d. The dose is titrated by monitoring the prothrombin time, which is not significantly altered by concomitant heparin therapy. The aim is to achieve a one-stage prothrombin time of 2–2.5 times the control. In certain patients who have chronic underlying disorders that place them at high risk (eg, severe congestive heart failure, severe venous disease), it may be necessary to continue oral anticoagulation indefinitely.

C. Adjunctive Therapy: Patients with pulmonary embolism may be hypoxemic, and administration of supplemental oxygen to achieve a P_{aO_2} in the range of 60–70 mm Hg is helpful. If pleuritic chest pain is severe, it may be alleviated with morphine sulfate given intravenously, 1 mg at a time up to a total of 5–10 mg. In patients with major or massive pulmonary emboli and hypotension, administration of a pressor agent may be indicated. Dopamine in doses of 5–10 $\mu g/kg/min$ is currently the agent of choice. The patient's blood volume status should be closely monitored, and antiarrhythmic agents should be employed in appropriate circumstances.

D. Thrombolytic Agents: There is definite evidence that the exogenous plasminogen activators streptokinase and urokinase produce the following effects when used in therapy of acute pulmonary embolism: (1) lysis of clots; (2) improvement of abnormal hemodynamics of right heart and pulmonary circulation; and (3) more rapid reperfusion of the previously embolized area when compared with heparin therapy.

Although the value of thrombolytic therapy versus heparin therapy remains unsettled, some authorities feel that the long-term effect of thrombolytic therapy may be to improve the circulation in the pulmonary microvasculature by resolution of microemboli. Prompt thrombolytic therapy may therefore be useful in patients with massive or submassive pulmonary emboli (ie, who are hemodynamically unstable) in whom embolectomy is deemed impossible or inappropriate. Therapy must be started within 7 days of onset of symptoms, and no contraindications should be present.

Absolute contraindications to the use of thrombolytic therapy are active internal bleeding or cerebrovascular process, disease, or procedure within the preceding 2 months. Relative contraindications include recent major surgery, organ biopsy, or puncture of noncompressible blood vessels; the immediate postpartum period; cardiopulmonary resuscitation with presence of rib fractures; recent thoracentesis, paracentesis, or lumbar puncture; or other potentially serious bleeding diatheses such as uncontrolled coagulation defects, uncontrolled severe hypertension, or pregnancy. Many authorities feel that any history of cerebrovascular disease or surgical procedure within the past 2 months or even longer is a relative contraindication.

The following dosage regimens are recommended in the treatment of acute pulmonary embolism: Both streptokinase and urokinase should be given intravenously by means of continuous pump infusion. A loading dose should be administered. With streptokinase, the recommended dose is 250,000 units over a 30-minute period. With urokinase, the recommended dosage is 4400 units/kg over 10 minutes. The maintenance dose, also delivered by continuous pump infusion, is urokinase, 4400 units/kg/h for 12–24 hours, or streptokinase, 100,000 units/h for 24–72 hours.

Any of the following coagulation tests may be used for monitoring therapy: whole blood euglobulin lysis time, thrombin time, partial thromboplastin time, or prothrombin time. The test selected should be performed before therapy and then 3–4 hours after the beginning of therapy; the objective is significant prolongation of the test. If the test obtained 3–4 hours after therapy shows prolongation of greater than twice the baseline value, no further monitoring is necessary until infusion is stopped. If there is no significant prolongation of clotting parameters with streptokinase, another loading dose must be administered and the infusion continued. If clotting parameters are still not prolonged, the patient has a high titer of streptokinase antibodies from previous streptococcal infections, and the agent should be discontinued and urokinase begun.

When thrombolytic therapy is completed, partial thromboplastin time should be determined; when thromboplastin time is less than twice the baseline value, intravenous heparin therapy should be initiated in the conventional manner and continued for at least 10 days. Oral anticoagulants should be given as described above.

One side effect of thrombolytic agents is bleeding from venipuncture, cutdown, and arterial puncture sites. Mild bleeding is usually limited to oozing from skin sites and can be controlled with compression bandages. When bleeding is more severe, however, the thrombolytic agent should be stopped. If blood replacement is clinically indicated, fresh whole blood will best reverse the coagulation abnormalities. If it is unobtainable, give packed red blood cells with either fresh frozen plasma or cryoprecipitate.

Other complications include febrile and allergic reactions, especially to streptokinase. These can often be obviated by infusion of 100 mg of hydrocortisone before streptokinase therapy and repeat infusions of 100 mg every 12 hours during therapy.

E. Surgical Therapy:

1. Pulmonary embolectomy–Surgical removal of massive pulmonary emboli has been lifesaving in a few situations. The operation depends upon prior demonstration of an embolus by pulmonary angiography and the availability of cardiac surgeons and cardiopulmonary bypass equipment. It should be considered only for patients with documented massive emboli who are in shock and refractory to medical management and who would otherwise probably die.

2. Vena caval interruption–Many devices and procedures are available for interrupting the inferior vena cava. This procedure should be done in the following circumstances: recurrent pulmonary emboli during adequate anticoagulant therapy; a single massive pulmonary embolus in the face of adequate anticoagulant therapy; pulmonary embolism in a patient in whom anticoagulant drugs are strongly contraindicated; extreme sensitivity to heparin therapy, including the development of thrombocytopenia; in association with pulmonary embolectomy; in instances of paradoxic embolism to the arterial tree.

The procedure has a substantial operative mortality risk, and the postoperative complications include edema of the lower extremities, recurrent thrombophlebitis, leg ulcers, stasis dermatitis, acute massive venous thrombosis, venous claudication, and recurrent emboli occurring through collateral vessels. Because

of the risk of recurrent embolism and thrombophlebitis, patients should be maintained on long-term warfarin anticoagulation as soon as feasible following interruption of the inferior vena cava.

Griner PF et al: Application of principles of test selection and interpretation. *Ann Intern Med* 1981;**94:**571.

Hull RD et al: Pulmonary angiography, ventilation lung scanning, and venography for clinically suspected pulmonary embolism with abnormal perfusion lung scan. *Ann Intern Med* 1983;**98:**891.

Moser KM et al: Deep venous thrombosis and pulmonary embolism: Frequency in a respiratory intensive care unit. *JAMA* 1981;**246:**1422.

Murray JF: Pulmonary embolism: Solutions to the D_x and R_x puzzle. *Mod Med* (Feb) 1984;**52:**176.

Salzman EW et al: The management of heparin therapy: Controlled prospective trial. *N Engl J Med* 1975;**292:**1046.

Sasahara AA et al: Pulmonary thromboembolism. *JAMA* 1983; **249:**2945.

Sharma GVRK et al: Thrombolytic therapy. *N Engl J Med* 1982; **306:**1268.

PULMONARY ARTERIOVENOUS MALFORMATIONS

Pulmonary arteriovenous malformations are abnormal communications between the pulmonary arterial system and the pulmonary venous system whereby these 2 circulations connect directly without an intervening capillary bed. The incidence of the malformations is unknown, and they may be hereditary or acquired. Most hereditary arteriovenous malformations are associated with the hereditary hemorrhagic telangiectasia (Osler-Weber-Rendu) syndrome. Patients usually have other characteristics of the syndrome, eg, mucosal telangiectasia, gastrointestinal hemorrhage, or epistaxis. Hereditary hemorrhagic telangiectasia is an autosomal dominant disorder. Approximately 15% of affected patients also have pulmonary arteriovenous malformations, which may be multiple in as many as one-third of the patients.

Rarely, hereditary pulmonary arteriovenous malformations may occur without associated hereditary hemorrhagic telangiectasia.

Acquired arteriovenous malformations may result from (1) trauma, (2) pulmonary schistosomiasis, (3) hepatic cirrhosis, or (4) carcinoma. Although the incidence of these illnesses is unknown, the number of patients with chronic liver disease who also have pulmonary arterial "spiders" may be significant, especially if radionuclide scanning techniques are used to determine the presence of shunts.

The gross pathologic features consist of pulmonary arteries connected by aneurysmal saclike structures to pulmonary veins. Under a microscope, these saclike structures display varying amounts of muscle, fibrous tissue, and thrombosis and, occasionally, small amounts of calcium.

Clinical Findings

A. Signs and Symptoms: The symptoms associated with pulmonary arteriovenous malformations may be those of the Osler-Weber-Rendu syndrome (epistaxis, gastrointestinal bleeding, etc). If they result from the pulmonary arteriovenous malformations themselves, the most apparent symptom is dyspnea on exertion. This condition is often worse when the patient stands erect. Since the malformations constitute a true right-to-left shunt, either septic or bland emboli to the central nervous system may occur through the shunts. Such patients may present with findings of cerebrovascular accident.

The nature of the physical examination will depend on the underlying cause of the arteriovenous malformation. Patients with hereditary hemorrhagic telangiectasia will often have mucosal telangiectasia as well as other signs. Those who have pulmonary arteriovenous malformations with cirrhosis invariably have the hallmarks of severe chronic liver disease, especially arteriovenous cutaneous spiders. Patients with pulmonary arteriovenous malformations secondary to schistosomiasis may have signs of liver disease secondary to the parasite and other indications of schistosomiasis, eg, eggs in the stool. Pulmonary arteriovenous malformations resulting from trauma usually have obvious physical findings of the underlying trauma to the chest.

There are ordinarily no outstanding physical findings on chest examination. An occasional patient will have a continuous murmur that can be heard over the malformations. Other findings are nonspecific and related to the degree and severity of hypoxemia (eg, clubbing, cyanosis).

B. Laboratory Findings: Most patients with significant pulmonary arteriovenous malformations demonstrate hypoxemia refractory to oxygen in high concentrations. Since most arteriovenous malformations are located in the lower lobes, hypoxemia will often be aggravated by sitting or standing. Many patients with chronic hypoxemia also have secondary polycythemia, although those with hereditary hemorrhagic telangiectasia may present with anemia secondary to epistaxis or gastrointestinal blood loss. As previously mentioned, arterial blood gases usually show hypoxemia with chronic hyperventilation (hypocapnia). There are no characteristic abnormalities of pulmonary function.

C. X-Ray Findings: Pulmonary arteriovenous malformations usually appear on the chest x-ray as single or multiple nodules, most often in the lower lobes. Tomography will often demonstrate the artery and vein that "feed" the malformations, and pulmonary angiography will readily show the presence of the arteriovenous connections.

Complications

Hypoxemia and disabling dyspnea are the chief complications. Bland or septic central nervous system emboli can occur, and hemoptysis and hemothorax are found in approximately 10% of patients.

Treatment

Surgical removal of the malformation is the only effective treatment available. Indications for surgery include severe hypoxemia, severe hemoptysis, and lesions that are enlarging rapidly. Since as many as 33% of patients with pulmonary arteriovenous malformations have multiple lesions a significant number of which may not be visible on a plain chest film, pulmonary angiography is mandatory before surgical removal of a pulmonary arteriovenous malformation. Angiography delineates the vessels involved in the anomaly and identifies other malformations that may need to be resected.

Dines DE et al: Pulmonary arteriovenous fistulas. *Mayo Clin Proc* 1974;**49**:460.
Robin ED et al: Detection, quantitation and pathophysiology of lung "spiders." *Trans Assoc Am Physicians* 1975;**88**:202.
Robin ED et al: Platypnea related to orthodeoxia caused by true vascular lung shunts. *N Engl J Med* 1976;**294**:941.
Wolfe JD et al: Hypoxemia of cirrhosis: Detection of abnormal small pulmonary vascular channels by a quantitative radionuclide method. *Am J Med* 1977;**63**:746.

PULMONARY NEOPLASMS

BRONCHOGENIC CARCINOMA

Essentials of Diagnosis

- Insidious onset, with cough, localized wheeze, or hemoptysis; often asymptomatic.
- May present as an unresolved pneumonia, atelectasis, or pleurisy with effusion (often bloody), or as a pulmonary nodule seen on x-ray.
- Metastases to other organs may produce initial symptoms.
- Endocrine, biochemical, and neuromuscular disorders (see below) may be the presenting features of bronchogenic carcinoma.

General Considerations

Cancer arising in the mucosa of the bronchial tree is the most common intrathoracic cancer. Lung cancer now accounts for 25% of all cancer deaths. It is the most common cause of cancer deaths in men, and if present trends continue, it will soon be the leading cause in women.

The importance of genetic and environmental factors in the etiology of bronchogenic carcinoma is not known. However, more than 75% of all lung cancer cases are attributable to smoking; the disease is relatively rare in nonsmokers.

The principal histologic types of bronchogenic carcinoma according to the World Health Organization classification are as follows:

Epidermoid (squamous cell) carcinomas
Small cell anaplastic carcinomas
    Fusiform cell type

Polygonal cell type
Lymphocytelike ("oat cell") type
Others
Adenocarcinomas
   Bronchogenic
   Acinar
   Papillary
Bronchiolo-alveolar
Large cell carcinomas
   Solid tumors with mucinlike content
   Solid tumors without mucinlike content
   Giant cell carcinomas
   "Clear cell" carcinomas
Combined epidermoid and adenocarcinomas

The cell type, together with the staging of the disease, has important implications for treatment and prognosis. (See American Thoracic Society reference for staging system.)

The 5-year survival rate for all bronchogenic cancers is 8%. Epidermoid tumors have the most favorable prognosis, and small cell anaplastic ("oat cell") carcinomas have the worst. The prognosis for the other cell types is intermediate.

Small peripheral lesions, with the exception of the small cell anaplastic type, have a better prognosis following excision than centrally located lesions.

Bronchiolo-alveolar carcinoma (previously called alveolar cell or bronchiolar carcinoma) appears to be a peripherally located form of adenocarcinoma. It frequently takes the form of a diffuse infiltration mimicking a pneumonia.

Clinical Findings

A. Symptoms and Signs: Symptoms, when present, are caused by the effects of the primary growth, the metastatic lesions, or systemic manifestations of the tumor. Persistent nonproductive cough, hemoptysis, and localized persistent wheeze are the major symptoms produced by bronchial irritation, erosion, and partial obstruction, although there may be no symptoms. These are often attributed to "cigarette cough" or "chronic bronchitis."

Pulmonary infections (pneumonitis, lung abscess) occurring distal to a bronchial obstruction frequently dominate the clinical picture and mask an underlying neoplasm. Any atypical pulmonary infection (persisting, recurring, or responding incompletely to therapy) should suggest carcinoma.

Metastases frequently give rise to the first symptoms. Local metastases may invade the chest wall, ribs, and spine, causing deep persistent pain or pleural effusion. Mediastinal metastases may cause superior vena caval obstruction, esophageal obstruction, or recurrent laryngeal nerve involvement with vocal cord palsy. Bronchogenic carcinoma in the apex of the lung may produce Pancoast's syndrome (shoulder, arm, and chest wall pain and ipsilateral Horner's syndrome). Distant metastases most often involve bones, the central nervous system, or the liver.

In general, pulmonary signs result from the sequelae of bronchial erosion, bronchial obstruction, pleural involvement, and mediastinal invasion. When a solitary small lesion does not produce hemoptysis, significant bronchial obstruction, or pleural involvement, there are no clinical findings. If the lesion is large enough, there may be physical (and x-ray) signs of partial or complete bronchial obstruction with associated atelectasis and infection.

Local spread is characterized by pleural fluid (bloody effusion is commonly present), signs of mediastinal invasion (pericardial effusion, hoarseness and brassy cough, stridor, dysphagia), and signs of regional metastases. Bronchogenic carcinoma in the upper part of the lung may produce Pancoast's syndrome (ipsilateral Horner's syndrome and shoulder-arm pain).

A careful search should be made for enlarged cervical, supraclavicular, and axillary lymph nodes and for liver nodules, which are frequent sites of metastases.

Paraneoplastic syndromes are uncommon metabolic manifestations of bronchogenic carcinoma— symptoms resembling those of myasthenia gravis; peripheral neuritis involving both sensory and motor components; clubbing of the digits; Cushing's syndrome; carcinoid syndrome (hyperserotoninemia), even when the tissue is not carcinoid; hypercalcemia not due to osseous metastases; and hyponatremia due to inappropriate excessive secretion of antidiuretic hormone (ADH). These changes may disappear when the tumor is removed and do not necessarily signify a grave prognosis.

B. Laboratory Findings:

1. Sputum cytology–A positive diagnosis of bronchogenic carcinoma can be made in 40–60% of cases on the basis of sputum cytology in squamous cell carcinoma and less frequently with other cell types. At least 3 fresh specimens should be studied.

2. Bronchoscopy–Biopsy by forceps or brush is possible in 75–80% of cases of bronchial tumor by use of the flexible fiberscope under fluoroscopic guidance. This method also permits transbronchial biopsy of diffuse lesions.

3. Needle aspiration biopsy of localized lesions under careful fluoroscopic control appears to be a useful and safe procedure.

4. Biopsy of palpable nodes in the neck or axilla may yield the diagnosis.

5. Mediastinoscopy–In the absence of palpable lymph nodes, mediastinoscopy is a valuable procedure to obtain tissue for diagnosis and to determine operability. Its greatest value as a diagnostic procedure is in the investigation of centrally located tumors, especially those with mediastinal involvement.

6. Prior to thoracotomy, a search should be made for metastases that would contraindicate surgery. Radioisotope scans of liver and bone and a brain scan by computerized tomography (CT) are indicated when clinical findings suggest such involvement. CT scan is also effective in identifying mediastinal metastases. When effusion is present, the fluid should be examined

for tumor cells and the pleura should be biopsied.

7. Exploratory thoracotomy may be the only way to establish a diagnosis when other studies are negative.

C. X-Ray Findings: The chest film offers the greatest possibility of early diagnosis and cure. Solitary nodules that do not cause symptoms or signs can be detected only by this method. Thirty percent of these "coin" lesions have proved to be carcinomas at thoracotomy.

Bronchogenic carcinoma may also present on x-ray as a perihilar mass (34–36%), atelectasis (segmental or lobar) (21–23%), pleural effusion (5–15%), or mediastinal lymph node enlargement (5–15%).

Apparent pneumonias that do not clear as expected may be the first indication of carcinoma and should be investigated with the appropriate diagnostic procedures.

Treatment

Early detection and surgical removal before metastases occur offer the only hope of cure. For this reason, a routine chest x-ray once a year for all men over 40 who are smokers has been strongly recommended despite the small yield in terms of curable disease. Pulmonary function should be carefully evaluated prior to thoracotomy. A ventilation/perfusion lung scan may add valuable information in this assessment.

Symptoms due to inoperable lesions may be temporarily controlled by nonoperative means. The coordination of radiation therapy with the available chemotherapeutic agents used in combinations of smaller, less toxic doses administered over a longer period of time seems to offer some hope of improved palliation and, rarely, a cure except in squamous cell tumors, where excision is the only treatment available.

Prognosis

The survival rate is related to both the stage of the disease and the cell type. Resectable lesions without lymph node or mediastinal metastases have the best prognosis. In this group, squamous cell carcinoma has a more favorable prognosis (50% 5-year survival rate in some series) than adenocarcinoma. Undifferentiated tumors have a poor prognosis, and the small cell (oat cell) variant has the worst of all. Small cell bronchogenic carcinoma metastasizes early and widely and is not amenable to surgery. Some encouraging results in palliation and longer survival have been reported with the newer treatment regimens noted above.

American Thoracic Society: Clinical staging of primary lung cancer. *Am Rev Respir Dis* 1983;**127**:659.

Centers for Disease Control: Lung cancer among women— Canada. *MMWR* 1984;**33**:67.

Faling LJ et al: Computed tomographic scanning of the mediastinum in the staging of bronchogenic carcinoma. *Am Rev Respir Dis* 1981;**124**:690.

Gelb AF, Epstein JD: Nd-YAG laser in lung cancer. *West J Med* 1984;**140**:393.

Jett JR, Cortese DA, Fontana RS: Lung cancer: Current concepts and prospects. *CA* 1983;**33**:74.

Kessinger A, Foley JF, Lemon HM: Therapeutic management of small cell lung cancer. *JAMA* 1983;**250**:3188.

Lacquet L et al: Mediastinoscopy and bronchial carcinoma: Experience with 600 mediastinoscopies. *Thorax* 1975;**30**:141.

Shure D, Astarita RW: Bronchogenic carcinoma presenting as an endobronchial mass: Optimal number of specimens for diagnosis. *Chest* 1983;**83**:865.

Shure D, Fedullo P: Transbronchial needle aspiration of peripheral masses. *Am Rev Respir Dis* 1983;**128**:1090.

Strauss MJ: New developments in the treatment of advanced lung cancer. *Am Rev Respir Dis* 1979;**120**:967.

Symposium on lung cancer. *Chest* 1977;**71**:624. [9 papers.]

Weisenthal LM: Treatment of small cell lung cancer—1981. *Arch Intern Med* 1981;**141**:1499.

Williams DE et al: Survival of patients surgically treated for stage 1 lung cancer. *J Thoracic Cardiovasc Surg* 1981;**82**:70.

Woolner LW et al: Mayo Lung Project: Evaluation of lung cancer screening. *Mayo Clin Proc* 1981;**56**:544.

SOLITARY PULMONARY NODULE

The solitary nodule ("coin lesion") presents an important diagnostic challenge to the clinician. A significant number of these lesions, which are usually asymptomatic and found by incidental chest x-rays, are malignant. The percentage of malignancy varies from less than 10% in solitary nodules found in community-wide x-ray screening to 35% in preselected patients who are referred for surgery. Age and geographic location are modifying factors. (Nodules in persons under age 30 are almost always nonneoplastic. Pulmonary nodules due to coccidioidal infection are common in the southwestern USA.)

Important elements of diagnosis include a careful medical history of symptoms, travel to endemic areas, and other possible exposures. Most importantly, previous chest x-rays should be obtained for comparative purposes.

The physical examination should include a search for enlarged lymph nodes and evidence of other neoplasms that might cause pulmonary metastasis.

Skin tests for tuberculosis, histoplasmosis, and coccidioidomycosis are essential. When all are negative, neoplasm becomes a stronger consideration. A positive skin test obviously does not exclude cancer but indicates other diagnostic possibilities that should also be investigated. Sputum, if present, should be examined for tumor cells, and appropriate cultures should be started. Bronchoscopy to obtain biopsy and culture material is helpful in lesions accessible to the flexible fiberoptic scope and brush or forceps. Small peripheral lesions are not usually accessible. These can sometimes be reached by needle aspiration biopsy with fluoroscopic direction by someone experienced with this procedure. If available, this method might be considered in patients in whom the probability of cancer is low.

Special x-ray views, tomography, and CT scanning are often needed to define the character and location of the nodule and may also reveal additional nodules. The presence of calcification is strong evidence against cancer and will usually justify continued observation.

When it cannot be determined within 2 months that a pulmonary nodule is benign, it should be excised, especially when the patient has a higher risk of cancer (based on age, smoking history, family history, etc).

When, after appropriate examinations, observation of a solitary nodule is undertaken, careful follow-up x-ray examinations with comparable technique should be continued for at least 2 years. Monthly films should be done for the first 3–4 months. Any increase in size of the lesion should result in prompt excision.

When a solitary nodule is due to cancer, the 5-year survival rate after excision is approximately 40% regardless of the histologic features of the tumor.

Felson B: Calcification in pulmonary nodules. Pages 479–489 in: *Chest Roentgenology.* Felson B (editor). Saunders, 1973.
Higgins GA, Shields TW, Keehn RJ: Solitary pulmonary nodule: 10-year follow-up of Veterans Administration–Armed Forces Cooperative Study. *Arch Surg* 1975;**110**:570.
Ray JF et al: The coin lesion story: Update 1976. *Chest* 1976;**70**:332.

BRONCHIAL ADENOMA

Bronchial adenoma (neoplasm arising in the glandular structures of the bronchial mucous membranes) is the most common (80%) "benign" bronchopulmonary neoplasm. The sex distribution is equal; the age incidence is somewhat lower than that of bronchogenic carcinoma. Bronchial adenoma is locally invasive.

The great majority of bronchial adenomas arise in the proximal bronchi. The onset is insidious. Cough and localized wheeze are similar to those found in bronchogenic carcinoma. These tumors are quite vascular, and hemoptysis is common, occurring in 25–30% of cases.

Since bronchial adenoma does not tend to exfoliate, examination of the sputum is not helpful. Differentiation from bronchogenic carcinoma therefore depends upon bronchoscopic biopsy or exploratory thoracotomy.

In many cases, bronchial adenoma can be distinguished from bronchogenic carcinoma only by histologic and cytologic study. Distinguish also from other benign obstructions, eg, foreign body, tuberculous bronchial stenosis.

Treatment
It is usually necessary to remove the neoplasm by lobectomy. Occasionally, pedunculated noninvasive adenomas may be removed by bronchoscopy, but serious bleeding can occur in such cases (even with biopsy alone).

The prognosis is good. The tumor tends to be locally invasive, but 5–10% metastasize slowly. Fatalities are not usually due to metastases but are associated with bronchiectasis, pneumonitis, hemorrhages, the complications of surgery, or asphyxiation secondary to obstruction by the tumor.

DeLima R: Bronchial adenoma: Clinicopathologic study and results of treatment. *Chest* 1980;**77**:81.
Lawson RM et al: Bronchial adenoma: A review of an 18-year experience at Brompton Hospital. *Thorax* 1976;**31**:245.

BRONCHOALVEOLAR CARCINOMA
(Bronchiolar Carcinoma, Alveolar Cell Carcinoma, Pulmonary Adenomatosis)

Bronchoalveolar carcinoma is a relatively uncommon pulmonary cancer (3–5% of lung cancers) that grows slowly and metastasizes late. In contrast to bronchogenic carcinoma, it is often multicentric. The neoplastic cells line the alveoli and bronchioles. Sex distribution is equal. Most cases occur in the age group from 50 to 60 years.

This lesion develops in the bronchiolar or alveolar lining and does not involve the major bronchi. Lesions are solitary or multicentric and are made up of secretory, nonsecretory, or undifferentiated cells. The latter have a uniformly poor prognosis and usually metastasize. Multicentric lesions of any type also have a poor prognosis. Solitary lesions that are not the undifferentiated type have a favorable prognosis when resected.

Cytologic examination of the sputum is positive in only 25% of multicentric undifferentiated lesions, even though copious sputum production is common. Transbronchial biopsy through a flexible fiberscope may be necessary. Solitary lesions yield few cells in the sputum, and aspiration needle biopsy or resection is preferred.

There are usually no diagnostic features that distinguish this from other types of lung cancer. Bilateral lesions, either discrete or diffuse, are more common. Solitary lesions may partly calcify and resemble granulomas.

The tumor metastasizes by bronchogenic spread of exfoliated cells and also by lymphatic and hematogenous routes.

Treatment
If involvement is unilateral and localized and there is no evidence of extrapulmonary extension, surgical excision is warranted.

Prognosis
Widespread pulmonary involvement is the usual cause of death. Metastases occur in 50% of cases (25% are lymphatic or hematogenous). With resection of solitary lesions, 5-year survival rates of 25–35% have been reported.

Tao LC et al: Bronchioloalveolar carcinoma: A correlative clinical and cytologic study. *Cancer* 1978;**42**:2759.

MISCELLANEOUS PULMONARY DISEASES

ACUTE RESPIRATORY FAILURE

The function of the lungs and pulmonary vasculature is to provide adequate oxygenation for the tissues' metabolic needs and to eliminate carbon dioxide in order to maintain normal acid-base balance. The diagnosis of respiratory failure is made by obtaining arterial blood gas determinations while the patient is breathing room air (inspired oxygen concentration of 21%). Respiratory failure is defined as a P_{aO_2} of 55 mm Hg or less or a P_{aCO_2} equal to or greater than 45 mm Hg. The causes of respiratory failure are many, and they fall into 2 main categories: nonpulmonary and pulmonary.

The more common nonpulmonary causes of acute respiratory failure include the following:

(1) Central nervous system depression: Drugs causing depression (opiates, barbiturates, etc); intracranial hemorrhage or infarction, intracranial masses; head injury.

(2) Neuromuscular diseases: Muscular dystrophies; multiple sclerosis; drugs (aminoglycosides; curare, etc); poliomyelitis; Guillain-Barré syndrome; spinal cord injuries.

(3) Chest wall abnormalities: Congenital (kyphoscoliosis, severe pectus excavatum); flail chest.

(4) Cardiovascular: Left ventricular failure; right-to-left intracardiac shunt; pulmonary emboli.

(5) Trauma: Noncardiogenic pulmonary edema. (See Adult Respiratory Distress Syndrome, p 167.)

Primary pulmonary conditions that can lead to acute respiratory failure include the following:

(1) Emphysema.
(2) Chronic bronchitis.
(3) Asthma.
(4) Interstitial fibrosis.
(5) Massive pleural effusions.
(6) Severe pneumonias.

Symptoms & Signs

The initial manifestations of acute respiratory failure are those of hypoxemia or hypercapnia. The cardinal symptoms and signs of hypoxemia include disorientation, restlessness, agitation, hypertension, tachycardia, and cyanosis (late). Hypercapnia presents with somnolence, confusion, hypotension, and asterixis. If not corrected, these conditions often lead to coma, cardiovascular collapse with superimposed metabolic acidosis, arrhythmias, and death.

Laboratory Findings

The laboratory findings in acute respiratory failure are those outlined above in the definition of the syndrome. Not uncommonly, the clinician faces a situation of acute respiratory failure occurring in patients with chronic respiratory disease. Helpful diagnostic laboratory findings in this situation include elevation of serum bicarbonate concentration above normal and elevated hemoglobin and hematocrit in the presence of normal hydration.

Treatment

Acute respiratory failure often has many causes that require multiple concurrent treatments. However, *the chief aim of treatment is correction of hypoxemia.* Particular attention should also be directed toward correcting acidosis and normalizing arterial pH.

Specific treatment measures should include the following:

A. Oxygenation: The object of supplemental oxygen is to maintain P_{aO_2} at 55 mm Hg or more. Various means are available, including nasal cannulas, Venturi masks, nonrebreathing masks, etc. In patients with chronic obstructive pulmonary disease, adequate oxygenation must be maintained without increasing P_{aCO_2}, which would lead to respiratory acidosis. Oxygenation is often best achieved by using low-flow nasal prongs delivering a flow of oxygen at 1–2 L/min or a Venturi mask delivering oxygen concentrations of 24–28%. Arterial blood gases must be closely monitored.

B. Reversal of Bronchospasm: Bronchospasm is best treated with a variety of approaches, which may include the following:

1. Intravenous bronchodilators–The most commonly used intravenous bronchodilator is aminophylline. It is given intravenously in a loading dose of 5.6 mg/kg over a 30-minute period, followed by subsequent doses of 0.9 mg/kg/h. Serum levels should be determined about 12 hours after the start of treatment, and a serum concentration of 15–20 μg/mL should be maintained. Congestive heart failure, a history of previous treatment with theophylline, liver dysfunction, and severe illness will require appropriate reductions in dosage. Side effects in decreasing order of occurrence include tachycardia, nausea, agitation, arrhythmias, and seizures.

2. Aerosolized bronchodilators–Aerosolized bronchodilators may be given via nebulized mist (eg, Acorn or deVilbiss nebulizer, intermittent positive pressure device, etc) and include isoproterenol, isoetharine, and terbutaline. Isoproterenol and isoetharine, 1:200, are administered via nebulized mist, 0.5 mL in 2–2.5 mL of normal saline, given every 2–4 hours. The dose for terbutaline is 0.75–1.5 mg in 2 mL of normal saline, administered by nebulized mist every 2–4 hours. A new hand-held aerosolized medication, albuterol, has recently been introduced. Recommended dosage is 2 inhalations 4 times a day. Possible side effects include tachycardia, agitation, abdominal distention (particularly with intermittent positive pressure breathing), hyperthermia, and cardiac arrhythmias. These may often be avoided by alternating the above drugs at prescribed intervals.

3. Systemic beta-adrenergic drugs–Beta-adrenergic agents have additive effects when combined with xanthine derivatives or aerosolized bronchodilators. Included in this category are terbutaline and metaproterenol. Usual doses for terbutaline are 0.25–0.75 mg subcutaneously or 2.5–5 mg orally 3 times daily; metaproterenol is given in doses of 10–20 mg orally 3 times daily. The recommended dose for albuterol is 2–4 mg 3–4 times a day. Side effects include tremor, tachycardia, agitation, increased blood pressure, and cardiac arrhythmias.

4. Corticosteroids–The general effectiveness of corticosteroids in the treatment of acute respiratory failure is controversial. However, a specific subgroup of patients, those with eosinophilia and intermittent bronchospastic disease, has demonstrated improvement following administration of these drugs. The usual dosage is prednisone, 1 mg/kg/d orally, or, for severely ill patients, methylprednisolone, 20–100 mg intravenously every 6–8 hours. The onset of action of these compounds is delayed at least 6–12 hours; they have not proved to be helpful when immediate effects are required. The dosage should be adjusted so that total eosinophil counts are less than 50/mL. Possible side effects are few but include salt and water retention. Aerosolized corticosteroids appear to have no place in the treatment of acute respiratory failure.

C. Mobilization of Secretions: Patients in acute respiratory failure often have difficulty with increased or inspissated secretions. Vigorous attempts to mobilize secretions often result in rapid improvement in the patient's condition. The most useful methods include the following:

1. Nebulized mist–Nebulized water mist with or without supplemental oxygen is helpful in reducing viscosity of secretions and aiding in their removal.

2. Physical therapy–Physical therapy includes coughing, deep breathing, and postural drainage by trained personnel.

3. Mucolytic agents–Acetylcysteine or 5% sodium bicarbonate effectively liquefies sputum in some patients. The dosage is 2–5 mL of acetylcysteine 20% or 2–3 mL of bicarbonate via aerosol every 4 hours. In a small number of patients, bronchospasm has occurred following the administration of mucolytic agents, specifically acetylcysteine. This can most often be prevented by administering an inhaled bronchodilator first.

D. Treatment of Underlying Disease: Treatment must be directed toward correcting the underlying causes of acute respiratory failure. Antibiotics for pneumonia or bronchitis, stabilization of the chest wall in patients with flail chest, removal or reversal of factors depressing respiratory function, and diuretics for pulmonary edema are examples of specific measures that should be instituted in addition to the treatments described above.

E. Tracheal Intubation and Mechanical Ventilation: In spite of appropriate and timely administration of all measures outlined above, the condition of some patients will progressively deteriorate, and they will require mechanical ventilation. Some general indications for intubation and ventilation are as follows:

1. Inability to maintain Pa_{O_2} of 55 mm Hg or

more with $F_{I_{O_2}}$ of 50% or more over a period of 6–12 hours.

2. Unacceptable respiratory acidosis following oxygen administration, even at low flows. A pH of 7.25 or less is usually an indication for mechanical ventilation.

3. Obviously tiring, moribund, or potentially comatose patient.

4. Vital capacity of less than 10 mL/kg body weight.

5. Patient's inability to cough effectively and clear secretions requiring some means of facilitating suction and pulmonary toilet.

Intubation can be accomplished with either an orotracheal tube or a nasotracheal tube by someone skilled in this procedure. As large a tube as possible (preferably with an internal diameter of at least 8 mm) should be used. The use of a large tube helps to minimize upper airway resistance (which in the normal adult is approximately equal to an 8-mm tube), facilitate suctioning, and allow for fiberoptic bronchoscopy should this become necessary. After intubation, mechanical ventilation may be initiated. In general, volume-cycled ventilators are preferable to pressure-cycled devices, because they are generally easier to operate and deliver a set volume of gas even in situations where pulmonary compliance is decreased.

A physiologic method of delivering mechanical ventilation is intermittent mandatory ventilation (IMV). In this technique, the patient receives a predetermined number of breaths per minute from the ventilator, but by virtue of a one-way valve may breathe without the machine from an oxygen reservoir in between respirator breaths. This intermittent technique helps to obviate the development of dangerous alkalosis from overventilation and also allows the patient's respiratory muscles to remain in use while the patient is on the respirator. Although individual circumstances vary greatly, the following general guidelines for respiratory settings may be helpful.

(1) Patients with normal or increased pulmonary compliance (eg, chronic obstructive pulmonary disease, neuromuscular disease, etc): Begin with a tidal volume of approximately 10 mL/kg body weight at a rate of 10–12 breaths/min delivered by intermittent mandatory ventilation. In order to prevent atelectasis, sighs should be administered at a rate of 5–12/h and at a volume that is about 1.5 times the administered tidal volume.

(2) Patients with reduced pulmonary compliance (eg, diffuse alveolar filling disease: pulmonary edema, severe diffuse pneumonia, etc): These patients should receive a higher tidal volume than patients with normal compliance, eg, 15 mL/kg body weight at an initial rate of 10–12/min. Sighs are not mandatory.

Supplemental oxygen. The fraction of inspired oxygen ($F_{I_{O_2}}$) delivered through the respirator should be sufficient to maintain Pa_{O_2} at 55 mm Hg or more. All ventilator settings, eg, tidal volume, rate, and $F_{I_{O_2}}$ must be based on the patient's arterial blood gas values, which should be monitored frequently and which are the primary guide to determining when any change in ventilator settings is necessary. Following any adjustments in settings, arterial blood gases should be measured after a 20- to 30-minute wait.

Positive end-expiratory pressure (PEEP). Patients with diffuse alveolar filling disease (noncardiogenic pulmonary edema, diffuse pneumonia, etc) often have widespread microatelectasis, and oxygenation may be difficult. If adequate arterial oxygenation cannot be maintained with a nontoxic F_{IO_2} (ie, $\leqslant 50\%$) for a period of time exceeding 6–12 hours, then PEEP is indicated. PEEP functions by holding alveoli open during expiration, thereby reducing the intrapulmonary right-to-left shunt. If PEEP is used, insertion of a Swan-Ganz flow-directed catheter into the pulmonary artery is desirable in order to monitor pulmonary capillary wedge pressure. Attempts should be made to maintain pulmonary capillary wedge pressure between 6 and 12 mm Hg, utilizing intravenous diuretics if necessary. Measurement of cardiac output is useful for detecting left ventricular dysfunction that can be treated by diuresis and inotropic agents. Reduction in cardiac output is one of the most significant side effects of PEEP, and the optimal level of PEEP is the pressure just below that at which cardiac output becomes reduced.

Guidelines for using PEEP are as follows: Begin with pressures of 3–5 cm of water and increase by increments of 2–3 cm while monitoring arterial blood gases and cardiac output. Side effects of PEEP include pneumomediastinum, subcutaneous emphysema, and pneumothorax. The goal of PEEP is to achieve satisfactory arterial oxygenation with nontoxic levels of F_{IO_2} without compromising cardiac output.

F. Weaning From the Ventilator: After a satisfactory clinical response has been achieved, weaning from the ventilator must be considered. The patient's clinical condition will dictate how weaning can best be accomplished. For example, young patients with posttraumatic acute respiratory failure (adult respiratory distress syndrome) but otherwise normal lungs may often be weaned more easily than patients with severe chronic obstructive pulmonary disease and chronic CO_2 retention. The general method is to reduce the number of ventilator breaths provided per minute, thus allowing the patient to breathe spontaneously for a progressively longer period of time. When the rate of intermittent mandatory ventilation is 2–5 breaths/min and when other indices of pulmonary function are satisfactory (Table 7–4), the patient may be weaned from the ventilator by means of a T-tube. The patient is removed from the ventilator and breathes a fixed concentration of supplemental oxygen from a nebulizer through the endotracheal tube with no mechanical assistance. Most patients will develop some degree of hypoxemia when placed on a T-tube, and the F_{IO_2} should therefore be increased by a factor of one-third when the patient is being weaned from the ventilator to a T-tube. The F_{IO_2} need not be further increased when extubation is accomplished and mask oxygen is used.

Most methods of ascertaining a patient's readiness for weaning and use of a T-tube utilize certain common measurements (eg, vital capacity, P_{aO_2}, etc). One way of evaluating a patient's readiness for extubation is a scoring system, as outlined in Table 7–4. If the various measurements indicate that the patient is a suitable candidate for extubation, the patient is removed from the ventilator and placed on a T-tube for a period of 1–2 hours. A second set of measurements is then performed. If the second evaluation confirms the findings of the initial assessment, the endotracheal tube is removed, and the patient is observed very closely; arterial blood gas determinations must be

Table 7–4. Guidelines for extubation.
(Measured before and after 1-hour T-tube trial.)*

Physiologic Category	Score†			
	0	1	2	3
State of consciousness	Comatose	Disoriented, uncooperative	Awake, content	Awake, wants tube out
Circulation	Receiving pressor or antiarrhythmic drug	Use of pressor or antiarrhythmic drugs under consideration	Abnormal pulse or blood pressure but no drugs required or under consideration	Normal
Respiration‡				
Rate	50/min	40–50/min	40/min	40/min
Secretions	Thick or copious	Thick or copious	Modest	Negligible
Vital capacity (mL/kg)	< 8	8–13	14–20	≥ 21
Oxygenation ratio§	< 1.4	1.5–2.4	2.5–3.4	≥ 3.5
CO_2 elimination P_{aCO_2} (mm Hg)	≥ 50 and rising	≥ 50 and stable	≤ 49	≤ 49
Inspiratory force (cm water)	< 20	20–25	26–30	> 30

*Modified and reproduced, with permission, from: Lecky JH, Ominsky AJ: Postoperative respiratory management. *Chest* 1972;**62** (Suppl):50S.

†A zero score in any category usually precludes extubation; a pair of ones usually precludes extubation.

‡Place patient in lowest category consistent with rate and secretions.

§To calculate oxygenation ratio, divide P_{aO_2} in mm Hg by inspired oxygen in percent.

made within 1–2 hours after extubation and as needed thereafter.

Balk R, Bone RC: The adult respiratory distress syndrome. *Med Clin North Am* 1983;**67**:685.

Brehus B, Snider G: The bronchodilator effect of aerosolized terbutaline. *JAMA* 1977;**238**:2277.

Downs JB et al: Intermittent mandatory ventilation: A new approach to weaning patients from mechanical ventilators. *Chest* 1973;**64**:331.

Feeley TW, Hedley-White J: Weaning from controlled ventilation and oxygen. *N Engl J Med* 1975;**292**:903.

Horn BR et al: Total eosinophil counts in the management of bronchial asthma. *N Engl J Med* 1975;**292**:1152.

Petty TL, Newman JH: Adult respiratory distress syndrome. *West J Med* 1978;**128**:399.

Piafsky KM, Ogilvie RI: Dosage of theophylline in bronchial asthma. *N Engl J Med* 1975;**292**:1218.

Sahn SA, Lakshminarayan S, Petty TL: Weaning from mechanical ventilation. *JAMA* 1976;**235**:2208.

Sutter PM, Fairley BH, Isenberg MD: Optimum end-expiratory airway pressure in patients with acute pulmonary failure. *N Engl J Med* 1975;**292**:284.

Wilson RS, Rie MA: Management of mechanical ventilators. *Surg Clin North Am* 1975;**55**:591.

ACUTE PULMONARY EDEMA OF EXTRINSIC ORIGIN

Pulmonary edema in the absence of underlying cardiac disease and arising de novo in previously healthy lungs has been described after the use of some drugs (nitrofurantoin, heroin), the inhalation of smoke and other toxic substances (causing altered capillary permeability), fluid overload, and rapid ascent to altitudes exceeding 3000 m ("altitude pulmonary edema") (see p 996). Pulmonary edema also occurs in some patients after severe central nervous system trauma. This appears to be neurogenically mediated and has been shown to be due to adrenergic overactivity, causing a shift of blood from the systemic to the pulmonary circulation.

General measures that may be helpful in the treatment of pulmonary edema due to these causes include supplemental oxygen, bed rest, and mechanical ventilation when indicated. (See Adult Respiratory Distress Syndrome.)

Specific measures (depending on the cause) include intravenous diuretics and possibly corticosteroid therapy (advocated by some for pulmonary edema secondary to inhalation of toxic substances or due to drug reaction).

Wray NP, Nicotra MB: Pathogenesis of neurogenic pulmonary edema. *Am Rev Respir Dis* 1978;**118**:783.

ADULT RESPIRATORY DISTRESS SYNDROME

Essentials of Diagnosis

- Anxiety, dyspnea, and tachypnea in a patient being treated for trauma, shock, or sepsis.
- Arterial hypoxemia with hypocapnia.
- Diffuse alveolar and interstitial infiltrates (which may progress to consolidation) on chest x-ray.
- Decreased pulmonary compliance.

General Considerations

The term adult respiratory distress syndrome (ARDS) describes noncardiogenic pulmonary edema occurring in certain characteristic clinical situations. Although the exact incidence is uncertain, this condition may occur in as many as one-third of all patients in severe shock or trauma. It occurs in association with massive trauma, hypotension of any cause, cardiopulmonary bypass procedures, septicemia, viral pneumonia, aspiration pneumonitis, other severe infections, intravenous narcotic overdose, fat embolism, and pancreatitis. The pathogenesis is unclear, but the end result is damage to the pulmonary capillary endothelium, producing increased permeability and interstitial and alveolar hemorrhage and edema. Consequently, loss of surfactant occurs, causing widespread alveolar atelectasis with right-to-left shunting of capillary blood past collapsed alveolar units. The increased amount of extravascular water in the lung and diffuse alveolar atelectasis result in decreased compliance and diminished functional residual capacity, respectively.

Clinical Findings

A. Symptoms and Signs: Symptoms typically appear 12–24 hours after the initial injury. The predominant symptoms are those of hypoxemia, ie, anxiety, dyspnea, and altered sensorium. The physical examination typically shows tachypnea and tachycardia. Auscultation of the chest reveals few or no rales or rhonchi. If hypoxemia is severe, cyanosis may be present.

B. Laboratory Findings: Arterial blood gas determinations show progressively severe hypoxemia with hypocapnia. There is inability to oxygenate arterial blood even with increasingly high concentrations of inspired oxygen (F_{IO_2}). Normal or elevated Pa_{CO_2} occurs late in the course and is an ominous prognostic sign. The arterial pH is usually normal or elevated.

C. X-Ray Findings: Chest x-rays show interstitial and alveolar infiltrates that progress to areas of consolidation (in the absence of cardiomegaly).

Treatment

A. Respiratory Support: The patient should receive mechanical ventilation with large tidal volumes (15 mL/kg) delivered by a volume ventilator (because of the high pressures required as a result of decreased pulmonary compliance). If a Pa_{O_2} of 60 mm Hg cannot be maintained with a nontoxic F_{IO_2} (inhaled oxygen concentration less than 50%), positive end-expiratory pressure (PEEP) is indicated. Positive end-expiratory pressure reduces the magnitude of right-to-left shunting by preventing collapse of alveoli and allows adequate oxygenation of arterial blood with a lower

F_{IO_2}. However, the level of positive end-expiratory pressure must be closely monitored with regard to the patient's cardiac output, since reduction in cardiac output frequently occurs. Other frequent side effects of positive end-expiratory pressure are pneumothorax, pneumomediastinum, and subcutaneous emphysema.

B. Fluid Balance: The most accurate and dependable method of assessing fluid balance and administering intravenous fluid therapy in patients with adult respiratory distress syndrome is the Swan-Ganz pulmonary artery catheter. With this device, the pulmonary capillary wedge pressure can be maintained at an optimal pressure of between 5 and 10 mm Hg. (Higher pressures may predispose to pulmonary edema because of leakage through the injured capillary endothelium.) To maintain optimal pulmonary capillary wedge pressure, fluid administration should be restricted to 20–25 mL/kg body weight daily. Intravenous diuretics (eg, furosemide) should be administered when necessary in order to achieve optimal wedge pressure. If it is necessary to administer fluids intravenously to maintain cardiac output, crystalloid solutions (eg, saline, Ringer's lactate) are preferable to albumin or colloid solutions, since the latter leak into the pulmonary interstitium, thereby providing an osmotic stimulus favoring continued pulmonary edema. Packed red blood cells are also an acceptable form of intravenous volume replacement and should be given in quantities sufficient to maintain the hemoglobin concentration at a minimum of 10 g/dL.

C. Treatment of Underlying Conditions: Underlying conditions that result in adult respiratory distress syndrome (eg, continued hemorrhage, pancreatitis, persistent infection) must be corrected. Particular attention should be given to eradicating infection either within the thorax or at distant sites. Several studies have shown that the single worst prognostic factor is ongoing infection, even that occurring outside the thorax. In such infections, the bacteria may elaborate substances that circulate in the blood and further damage the pulmonary capillary endothelium. There is no evidence that prophylactic use of antibiotics to prevent infection in these patients is helpful; in fact, such usage may predispose to superinfection with organisms resistant to antimicrobials.

D. Corticosteroids: According to some experimental evidence, the alveolar capillary membrane may be damaged by activation of the complement system with neutrophil aggregation in the pulmonary microvasculature. However, there is clinical evidence that early use of high-dose intravenous corticosteroids may prevent this (eg, 1–2 g of methylprednisolone every 6 hours for the first 2–4 days of the illness).

E. Prognosis: Mechanical ventilation is sometimes necessary for several weeks. When changes in the mechanical ventilation regimen are contemplated, measurements of arterial blood gases, mixed venous P_{O_2} and cardiac output are the best indicators of the patient's status. The mortality rate is 50–80%. Most patients who survive regain their previous level of pulmonary function within 1 year.

Boggis CRM, Greene R: Adult respiratory distress syndrome. *Br J Hosp Med* 1983;**29**:167.

Eaton RJ, Taxman RM, Avioli LV: Cardiovascular evaluation of patients treated with PEEP. *Arch Intern Med* 1983;**143**:1958.

Flick MR, Murray JF: High-dose corticosteroid therapy in the adult respiratory distress syndrome. *JAMA* 1984;**251**:1054.

Hopewell PC: Adult respiratory distress syndrome. *Basics of RD* [Respiratory Distress] (March) 1979;**7**:1.

Keren A, Klein J, Stern S: Adult respiratory distress syndrome in the course of acute myocardial infarction. *Chest* 1980;**77**:161.

Rinaldo JE et al: Adult respiratory distress syndrome: Changing concepts of lung injury and repair. *N Engl J Med* 1982; **306**:900.

SILO-FILLER'S DISEASE

Silo-filler's disease is an agricultural pulmonary disease caused by inhalation of nitrogen dioxide and sulfur dioxide fumes emanating from silos that have been freshly filled (eg, with corn or alfalfa). The toxic inhalant causes increased capillary permeability resulting in a form of pulmonary edema. (See also Acute Pulmonary Edema of Extrinsic Origin, p 167.)

The initial phase, appearing promptly after exposure, consists of cough, dyspnea, and weakness. This may progress or be followed by a decrease in symptoms, which may then reappear and become progressively worse. Diffuse rales and rhonchi are heard, and the chest x-ray shows bilateral fluffy infiltrates that may coalesce into dense areas of pulmonary edema. The mortality rate is approximately 30%, with death usually occurring 1–3 weeks after onset. Most patients who recover have no residual pulmonary damage. A small number have permanently reduced pulmonary function and x-ray evidence of pulmonary fibrosis.

Corticosteroids are usually effective. Initial dosage should be the equivalent of hydrocortisone, 500–600 mg daily, with a gradual reduction as improvement occurs. Parenteral medication is replaced with prednisone as soon as improvement is established. The drug should be continued for 6–8 weeks. Supplementary oxygen and respiratory assistance are used to correct hypoxemia.

Preventive measures include avoiding entry into silos if fumes are present and assuring good ventilation of silos by any means necessary.

Horvath EP et al: Nitrogen dioxide–induced pulmonary disease. *J Occup Med* 1978;**20**:103.

OBESITY & HYPOVENTILATION

This syndrome consists of chronic hypercapnia and hypoxemia in morbidly obese individuals. There may be associated signs of right ventricular failure. Clinically, the patient presents with daytime somnolence. This symptom complex has been termed the "Pickwickian syndrome" because of its similarity to Dickens' description of the fat boy in *The Pickwick Papers*.

Weight reduction appears to reverse the abnormality (see p 812). Oral progesterone therapy has been reported to stimulate ventilation in some patients. Rarely, if weight reduction cannot be accomplished and episodes of nocturnal hypoxemia are severe in patients with mechanical upper airway obstruction, tracheostomy may be necessary.

Goldman AL, Morrison D, Foster LJ: Oral progesterone therapy: Oxygen in a pill. *Arch Intern Med* 1981;**141**:574.

ALVEOLAR PROTEINOSIS

Alveolar proteinosis is a chronic, progressive, often fatal disease of unknown cause (and unrecognized before 1958) characterized by progressive dyspnea, cough, intermittent fever, pulmonary infiltrations on x-ray, and pulmonary insufficiency due to impaired alveolar-capillary diffusion. Definitive diagnosis is based on the histologic findings (at biopsy or autopsy) of striking replacement of the alveolar air spaces with granular, amorphous material that stains characteristically with alcian blue–PAS stain. However, the clinical diagnosis can also be made, without biopsy, from material obtained by segmental saline lavage through a flexible bronchoscope. The aspirate is centrifuged, and the sediment button is processed in the same way as a biopsy specimen. The chemical similarity between this material, which appears to be a phospholipid (palmitoyl lecithin), and the surface-active agent normally secreted by the alveolar epithelium suggests the possibility of an abnormal hypersecretion of this substance. These patients seem prone to develop nocardiosis and fungal infections.

Methods have been described for irrigating the involved lung with saline or heparin solutions via endobronchial catheter. Large quantities of the proteinaceous material can thus be removed, and this results in clearing (as seen by x-ray) and temporary or prolonged improvement in pulmonary function.

Corticosteroids are of no value.

Claypool WD, Rogers RM, Matuschak GM: Update on the clinical diagnosis, management and pathogenesis of pulmonary alveolar proteinosis (phospholipidosis). *Chest* 1984;**85**:550.
Martin RJ et al: Pulmonary alveolar proteinosis: The diagnosis by segmental lavage. *Am Rev Respir Dis* 1980;**121**:819.

PULMONARY CONTUSION

Pulmonary contusion is the major contributing factor in 25% of deaths following high-speed deceleration automobile injuries and a factor (though not the major one) in 25–50% of the remainder. It is the major factor in respiratory insufficiency developing 12–24 hours after multiple injuries are sustained. Damage to pulmonary tissue may occur from blunt or sharp trauma with or without accompanying rib fracture.

Alveolar rupture due to trauma results in fluid transudation into the alveolar space and extravasation of blood. This fluid may or may not communicate with the endobronchial tree. The presence of hemoptysis is helpful in diagnosis.

Clinical Findings

A. Symptoms and Signs: Significant chest wall trauma, including adjacent rib fractures or chest wall hematoma, is usually obvious. Severe localized chest pain is present with or without physical evidence of injury. Paradoxic motion of the chest wall (inward with inspiration and outward with expiration) is present in 75% of cases.

B. Laboratory Findings: Arterial blood gas studies may show hypoxemia and hypocapnia or hypercapnia.

C. X-Ray Findings: The chest x-ray is normal or minimally abnormal initially. An area of consolidation or cavitation develops after 12–24 hours.

Treatment

At the scene, sandbags should be used to stabilize the area of paradoxic motion.

Fluid management as described by Trinkle (see references) consists of restriction of fluids to 1000 mL intravenously at resuscitation and 50 mL/h thereafter; methylprednisolone, 500 mg intravenously every 6 hours for 3 days; plasma, 50 mL/h; and replacement of blood loss by whole blood or plasma. General measures include vigorous pulmonary toilet, pain control with intercostal nerve blocks and narcotics, and supplemental oxygen to maintain a P_{aO_2} of more than 60 mm Hg. Intubation and mechanical ventilation are required for patients in whom the P_{aO_2} drops below 60 mm Hg, in those receiving supplemental oxygen therapy, and in those with severe ventilatory disturbances manifested by hypercapnia and acidemia. (See Acute Respiratory Failure, p 164.)

Prognosis

The prognosis depends on the extent of the accompanying injuries. Treatment as described above has resulted in decreased morbidity and mortality rates in this class of patients.

Kohn MS: Management of chest injuries. *Topics in Emergency Medicine* 1979;**1**:79.
Lucas C, Tintinalli JE: Flail chest. *JACEP* (Sept) 1979;**8**:380.
Trinkle JK: Flail chest: A new therapeutic approach. *Resident Staff Physician* (Jan) 1979;**102**:15.

DISEASES OF THE PLEURA

FIBRINOUS PLEURISY

Deposition of a fibrinous exudate on the pleural surface is the cardinal pathologic feature of fibrinous pleurisy. This is usually secondary to pulmonary disease: pneumonia, pulmonary infarction, and neoplasm are the most frequent causes. Fibrinous pleurisy may precede the development of pleural effusion.

Chest pain is typically "pleuritic," ie, it is greatest during inspiration. Pain is minimal or absent when the breath is held or when the ribs are splinted. Referred pain may occur from the diaphragmatic pleura to the shoulder and neck (central diaphragm) or upper abdomen (peripheral diaphragm).

Pleural friction rub ("to-and-fro," "squeaky-leather," or "grating" sounds) with respirations is pathognomonic. It may occur without pleuritic pain and vice versa. Splinting of the involved chest is characteristic, with decreased motion and shallow, "grunting" respirations. The patient lies on the painful side. Other findings reflect the underlying pulmonary disease.

Treatment is aimed at the underlying disease. The treatment of the pleurisy consists only of relieving pain. Analgesics may be used as necessary. Strapping the chest with adhesive tape may give relief by restricting movement. Lidocaine intercostal nerve block may be used in more severe cases.

Fibrinous pleurisy clears promptly with the resolution of the primary process. Pleural scars may remain and create minor diagnostic difficulties on future chest x-rays.

PLEURAL EFFUSION

Essentials of Diagnosis

- Dyspnea if effusion is large; may be asymptomatic.
- Pain of pleurisy often precedes the pleural effusion.
- Decreased breath sounds, flatness to percussion, egophony.
- The underlying cardiac or pulmonary disease may be the major source of symptoms and signs.
- X-ray evidence of pleural fluid.

General Considerations

Any fluid collection (transudate or exudate) in the pleural space constitutes a pleural effusion. Numerous disease processes of inflammatory, circulatory, and neoplastic origin can cause pleural effusion. Every effort should be directed toward the diagnosis of the primary disease. "Idiopathic" pleural effusion often proves to be of tuberculous origin.

Clinical Findings

A. Symptoms and Signs: There may be no symptoms. Chest or shoulder pain may be present at onset, especially when fibrinous pleuritis precedes the effusion. Dyspnea may be mild or, with large or rapidly forming effusions, severe. Cardiac failure may be associated with effusion. Fever, sweats, cough, and expectoration may occur, depending upon the underlying cause.

Physical findings include decreased motion of the chest and decreased to absent vocal fremitus on the side of the fluid, flat percussion note and decreased to absent breath sounds over the fluid, and egophony (e-to-a sound) at the upper level of the fluid. With large effusions, the mediastinum shifts away from the fluid (as shown by displacement of the trachea and the cardiac apex), although underlying atelectasis may result in a shift toward the fluid. Signs resembling those of consolidation (dullness, bronchial breath sounds, bronchophony) are occasionally elicited over the fluid, presumably as a result of compression of the underlying lung by large, rapidly forming effusions.

B. X-Ray Findings: Three hundred milliliters or more must be present before fluid can be demonstrated by x-ray. Obliteration of the costophrenic angle is the earliest sign. Later, a homogeneous triangular density with a concave medial border extends upward to the axilla; other borders are formed by the lateral chest wall and the diaphragm. The mediastinum shifts away from the fluid (displaced heart and tracheal air shadow). The mobility of the fluid shadow, which "pours" into dependent areas of pleural space when the patient is placed on the involved side, may aid in the demonstration of small effusions. An atypical distribution of fluid along the interlobar fissures or in loculated areas may be noted.

C. Thoracentesis: This is the definitive diagnostic procedure. It demonstrates conclusively the presence of fluid and provides samples for study of physical characteristics, protein content, cells, and infectious agents. Thoracentesis should be done carefully to avoid introducing infection and puncturing the visceral pleura.

1. Removal of fluid for examination–Remove 50–1000 mL. Use a 3-way stopcock to avoid introduction of air. Care must be exercised to avoid contaminating the pleural space.

2. Pleural fluid examination–(Specimen must be fresh.) A specific gravity of more than 1.015 or protein of more than 3 g/dL usually indicates an exudative fluid. More reliable indicators include a ratio of pleural fluid protein to serum protein greater than 0.5; a fluid LDH to serum LDH ratio of more than 0.6; or a pleural fluid LDH of more than 200 IU, especially if all 3 conditions are present.

A stained smear should be examined for the detection of organisms and the nature of the cellular content. Collect a specimen in a heparinized tube for cell count. Cultures on appropriate media are indicated for all fluids from unexplained pleural effusions to demonstrate the presence of tubercle bacilli, other bacteria, or fungi. Cytologic examination of the remaining fluid should be done if a neoplasm is suspected.

Lactic dehydrogenase (LDH) levels are frequently increased in effusions due to cancer. Chylous effusions usually signify interruption of the thoracic duct by cancer.

D. Pleural Biopsy: This procedure has become very simple and valuable as a result of the development of better biopsy needles (eg, Abrams' needle) that permit thoracentesis and removal of multiple tissue specimens with the same needle. Pleural biopsy is indicated whenever the diagnosis is in doubt. If the tissue is not diagnostic, several more specimens should be taken. If pleural fluid examination and needle biopsy do not yield a diagnosis, open pleural biopsy must be considered. A portion of the biopsy material should be cultured.

Treatment

A. Postpneumonic and Other Sterile Effusions: Remove readily obtainable fluid by multiple thoracentesis, at daily intervals if necessary. Removal of more than 1000 mL initially is not advisable. Reexamine subsequent fluid specimens to rule out empyema if the pleuritis does not respond to treatment.

B. Tuberculous Effusion: Uncomplicated pleural effusion due to tuberculosis is treated essentially as minimal pulmonary tuberculosis. A course of isoniazid plus one of the other major antituberculosis drugs (Table 7–3) is recommended. Many patients with untreated tuberculous effusions develop pulmonary tuberculosis later, usually within 5 years.

Removal of all readily available fluid by thoracentesis is advisable to minimize later pleural fibrosis. When high fever persists for longer than 2 weeks, hematogenous dissemination should be suspected.

C. Effusions Due to Malignant Tumors: These tend to reaccumulate rapidly and require frequent removal. An attempt should be made to control the re-formation of fluid by irradiation of the hemithorax or by the use of intrapleural tetracycline or cytotoxic agents.

Prognosis

The prognosis is that of the underlying disease.

Poe RH et al: Sensibility, specificity and predictive value of closed pleural biopsy. *Arch Intern Med* 1984;**144**:321.

Sahn SA: The differential diagnosis of pleural effusions. *West J Med* 1982;**137**:99.

HYDROTHORAX

The term hydrothorax generally denotes the presence of a collection of serous fluid having a specific gravity of less than 1.015 or a protein content of less than 3 g/dL (transudate). The most common cause is congestive heart failure, but lymphatic obstruction and obstruction of the superior vena cava or vena azygos may also cause hydrothorax. The not unusual finding of hydrothorax in hepatic cirrhosis with ascites (6%) is explained by observations of ready transfer of radio-iodine-labeled albumin from the peritoneal to the pleural spaces. The initial examination of the pleural fluid should be as described above.

The fluid should be removed by thoracentesis when it causes dyspnea.

The prognosis is that of the underlying disease.

HEMOTHORAX

Hemothorax (pooling of blood in a pleural space) is most commonly due to trauma but may also follow tumor, tuberculosis, and pulmonary infarction. The physical findings are the same as those of pleural effusion. Military experience has shown that early removal of all blood from the pleural space is desirable. If this cannot be accomplished by thoracentesis, an intercostal tube with water-seal drainage is indicated. If bleeding continues, thoracotomy is indicated. Great care must be taken during aspiration to avoid bacterial contamination of the pleural cavity. Surgical removal of residual blood clots may be necessary.

PLEURAL EMPYEMA
(Nontuberculous)

Acute infection of the pleural space may result from (1) direct spread from adjacent bacterial pneumonia, (2) postsurgical infection, (3) posttraumatic (including thoracentesis) infection. Underlying chronic obstructive pulmonary disease or bronchogenic carcinoma is frequently present. The availability of early and specific therapy for these conditions has made empyema an uncommon disease. However, the mortality rate remains high (30% in some series). Hospital-acquired infections have a more serious prognosis.

The clinical findings are often obscured by the primary underlying disease. Pleural pain, fever, and "toxicity" after clinical improvement of the primary disease, in association with physical and x-ray signs of pleural fluid, are characteristic. Thoracentesis reveals a frankly purulent exudate from which the causative organism may be cultured. Empyema, like lung abscess, may become chronic, with a prolonged course and little tendency to spontaneous resorption.

The key to nonsurgical treatment of acute empyema is early diagnosis. Any collection of fluid occurring in the course of pulmonary inflammatory disease should be removed at once. If pus is present, a specimen should be obtained for Gram staining and cultures, including cultures for anaerobic organisms. Specimens for anaerobic culture must be collected without exposure to air and must be placed into suitable transport media immediately. (Coagulase-positive *Staphylococcus aureus* and gram-negative bacilli are the most common aerobic bacteria causing empyema; *Bacteroides* and peptostreptococci are the most frequently encountered anaerobic organisms.) The empyema should be aspirated as completely as possible. Some early localized empyemas can be treated by thoracentesis and antibiotic therapy alone. Any large or loculated empyema should be drained immediately via an intercostal tube. Open thoracotomy is sometimes required to ensure adequate drainage.

As soon as specimens have been obtained for culture, parenteral antibiotic treatment should be started with penicillin, 600,000 units intramuscularly every 6 hours, or, alternatively, cephalothin, 8 g intravenously daily. When the pus has a foul odor or the empyema is thought to be secondary to an intra-abdominal infection, chloramphenicol, 50 mg/kg daily orally, should be added to the initial treatment. The object is to obliterate the empyema space as soon as possible. Irrigations with saline through the catheter may be necessary. Chronic empyema usually results from inadequately treated acute empyema or from a bronchopleural fistula. Surgical drainage with or without decortication is usually necessary.

Davis WC, Johnson LF: Adult thoracic empyema revisited. *Am Surg* 1978;**44**:362.

De la Rocha AG: Empyema thoracis. *Surg Gynecol Obstet* 1982; **155**:839.

Finland M, Barnes MW: Changing ecology of acute bacterial empyema: Occurrence and mortality at Boston City Hospital during 12 selected years from 1935 to 1972. *J Infect Dis* 1978; **137**:274.

Varkey B et al: Empyema thoracis during a ten-year period. *Arch Intern Med* 1981;**141**:1771.

SPONTANEOUS PNEUMOTHORAX

Essentials of Diagnosis

- Sudden onset of chest pain referred to the shoulder or arm on the involved side; associated dyspnea.
- Hyperresonance, decreased chest motion, decreased breath and voice sounds on involved side; mediastinal shift away from involved side.
- Chest x-ray revealing retraction of the lung from the parietal pleura is diagnostic.

General Considerations

The cause of spontaneous pneumothorax is unknown in 90% of cases, but it may be secondary to pulmonary disease. The idiopathic form typically occurs in healthy young males with no demonstrable pulmonary disease other than the subpleural blebs usually found on thoracotomy or (rarely) autopsy.

Entry of air into the pleural space from a rent in the visceral pleura causes partial to complete collapse of the underlying lung. Collapse usually is self-limited by rapid sealing of the tear. Occasionally a "valve effect" occurs, with progressive entry of air on inspiration and failure of exit on expiration, and with increasing intrapleural pressure (tension pneumothorax). This has a profound effect on cardiorespiratory dynamics and may be fatal if not treated promptly.

Clinical Findings

A. Symptoms and Signs: Symptoms are occasionally minimal (vague chest discomfort, dry cough) or may even be overlooked. Characteristically, however, the onset is sudden and not necessarily related to exertion, with chest pain referred to the shoulder and arm on the affected side. Pain is aggravated by physical activity and by breathing, producing dyspnea.

Fever is usually not present. Shock and cyanosis occur in tension pneumothorax, where high intrapleural pressure interferes with venous return to the heart.

Physical findings consist of decreased chest motion and decreased to absent vocal fremitus and breath sounds on the affected side. (Breath sounds may be abnormally loud and harsh on the normal side.) The percussion note is hyperresonant over the involved side. With large pneumothorax, the mediastinum shifts away from the affected side and a metallic "close to" sound can be heard with the stethoscope when one coin is tapped against another held to the chest ("coin sign"). "Tapping," roughly synchronous with the heartbeat, occasionally occurs in left-sided pneumothorax.

B. X-Ray Findings: Air in the pleural space with a visible border of retracted lung (difficult to see if the pneumothorax is small) is best seen over the apex and in films taken in expiration. Retraction may be confined to one area of the lung (pleural adhesions in other areas). Contralateral shift of the mediastinum is demonstrated by displacement of the tracheal air shadow and cardiac apex. (Great amounts of air are present with tension pneumothorax.) Pleural fluid (bleeding from a ruptured area or torn adhesion) is occasionally visible but is seldom present in large quantities.

Differential Diagnosis

Spontaneous pneumothorax may be secondary to pulmonary disease (eg, tuberculosis, abscess, bullous emphysema) but is most commonly due to unexplained rupture of small blebs on the visceral lung surface. The cause of bleb formation and the exact mechanism of rupture in idiopathic cases are not known. Fifty percent of cases occur in the age group from 20 to 24 years, and 85% occur in men. Onset may occur during exercise or at complete rest. Chest pain must be differentiated from that of myocardial infarction (especially when there is shoulder-arm radiation), pulmonary embolism, and acute fibrinous pleurisy.

Treatment

A. Emergency Measures for Tension Pneumothorax: *Note: This is a medical emergency!* Insert a trocar or large-bore, short-beveled needle into the anterior part of the affected chest (just into the pleural space to avoid trauma to the expanding lung). After tension has been relieved, a simple one-way valve made from a rubber glove finger, slit at the end, can be tied to the hub of the trocar or needle. As soon as possible, a No. 14 or No. 16 Foley catheter should be introduced into the pleural space via a trocar or by direct incision and attached to a water trap with the end of the tubing under 1–2 cm of water. (A plastic catheter mounted on a disposable aluminum stylet and packaged ready to use is available. It obviates the need for a trocar and is suitable for both emergency and definitive treatment.) A suction pump (with a maximum vacuum of −30 cm of water) may be attached to the water trap.

If pain is severe, give morphine sulfate, 8–15 mg

subcutaneously. Treat shock (see Chapter 1). Follow-up treatment is as for spontaneous pneumothorax.

B. Spontaneous Pneumothorax Without Increased Intrathoracic Pressure: Bed rest is essential until the air leak has stopped. Pleural pain should be treated with analgesics. If cough is annoying, codeine sulfate, 15–60 mg every 3–4 hours, should be used. Aspirate air if dyspnea is present or if the pneumothorax space is large enough to aspirate safely. If there is no apparent underlying lung disease or pleural effusion, the air can be aspirated via a small catheter introduced into the second anterior interspace through a No. 16-gauge needle with a 50 mL syringe and a 3-way stopcock. If pneumothorax does not recur after 48 hours, no further treatment is required for this episode. If air leakage continues, an intercostal catheter attached to a water trap and suction (see above) may be necessary. Continue suction until the lung has been reexpanded for 24 hours. Administer oxygen if dyspnea is present. In some cases of spontaneous pneumothorax where the lung does not expand or if there are repeated episodes of collapse, exploratory thoracotomy may be necessary.

Prognosis

The outlook is very good in "idiopathic" cases but is more serious in secondary cases because of the danger of infection of the pleural space. Recurrence occurs in 15–20%, usually on the same side. After 2 episodes, surgical correction should be considered. Patients with a history of spontaneous pneumothorax should be advised to avoid high altitudes and flying in unpressurized aircraft. Empyema may occur where underlying disease, especially tuberculosis, is present. Failure of lung to reexpand, with fibrothorax, is rare in the idiopathic type.

Tension pneumothorax is a true emergency.

Bevelaqua FA, Aranda C: Management of spontaneous pneumothorax with small lumen catheter manual aspiration. *Chest* 1982;**81**:693.

Pierce AK: Pneumothorax. Page 560 in: *Pulmonary Medicine,* 2nd ed. Guenter CA, Welch MH (editors). Lippincott, 1982.

TRAUMATIC PNEUMOTHORAX

Note: This is an emergency! Open chest wounds (sucking wounds) must be made airtight by any available means (eg, bandage, handkerchief, shirt, or other material) and closed surgically as soon as possible.

Traumatic pneumothorax due to lung puncture or laceration (fractured rib, bullet, etc) is managed like spontaneous pneumothorax (above). Surgery is frequently required.

DISEASES OF THE MEDIASTINUM

MEDIASTINAL TUMOR

Mediastinal masses are often clinically "silent" until they become large. They are frequently discovered on routine chest x-rays and fluoroscopy, where their position, density, and mobility are of aid in differential diagnosis. Biopsy is often the only way to make a differential diagnosis.

Because of their proximity to the heart, great vessels, esophagus, air passages, and surrounding nerves, even benign lesions are potentially serious.

The symptoms and signs are usually due to compression and distortion of surrounding structures. Pain is usually retrosternal. It originates in the afferent lower cervical and upper thoracic segments (may mimic "cardiac" pain) and occasionally radiates to the shoulder, neck, arms, or back. Cough suggests tracheal and bronchial involvement. Dyspnea is due to airway obstruction (which may lead to pulmonary infections). Respirations may be stertorous, with suprasternal retraction on inspiration. Hoarseness is associated with compression paralysis of the thoracic portion of the left recurrent laryngeal nerve. Mild to severe dysphagia is due to extrinsic compression of the esophagus with obstruction.

Compression of the heart or great vessels is an unusual cause of symptoms.

Tracheal shift is due to displacement by mass. Tracheal tug is associated with adjacent aortic aneurysms with transmitted pulsations.

The superior vena cava syndrome consists of dilated neck veins, fullness of the neck and face, and collateral veins on the thoracic wall. It is caused by compression of the superior vena cava.

Horner's syndrome (ipsilateral miosis, ptosis, and enophthalmos) is due to compression of sympathetic outflow pathways.

Chest x-rays after a swallow of barium will often delineate the mass and demonstrate any enlarged mediastinal nodes. A CT scan of the thorax is the most precise noninvasive method of detecting mediastinal tumors. Mediastinoscopy or mediastinotomy and, occasionally, thoracotomy are necessary to obtain tissue for diagnosis.

Treatment will depend upon the primary disease. The prognosis is variable depending upon the cause and the histologic characteristics of the mass.

Economou JS et al: Management of primary germ-cell tumors of the mediastinum. *J Thorac Cardiovasc Surg* 1982;**83**:643.

Hussain SA: Posterior mediastinal mass. *JAMA* 1976;**235**:849.

Silverman NA, Sabiston DC Jr: Mediastinal masses. *Surg Clin North Am* 1980;**60**:757.

PNEUMOMEDIASTINUM

Essentials of Diagnosis

- Sudden onset of severe retrosternal pain.
- Crepitus on palpation of neck and chest.
- Crunching sound simultaneous with heartbeat.
- X-ray is diagnostic.

General Considerations

Free air in the mediastinum may be secondary to perforation of the intrathoracic esophagus or respiratory tract or may be caused by spontaneous rupture of alveoli into the perivascular interstitial tissues of the lung. Air may also be sucked into the mediastinum through an open neck wound or from an area of emphysema in the neck resulting from a chest wound. Spontaneous pneumomediastinum is often associated with spontaneous pneumothorax, most often of the tension type.

Clinical Findings

A. Symptoms and Signs: Symptoms are often minimal. Typically, the air escapes into the subcutaneous tissues of the neck and then over the rest of the body and retroperitoneally. If pneumothorax (especially tension pneumothorax) is present also, there is usually a sudden onset of severe retrosternal pain radiating to the neck, shoulders, and anus (retroperitoneal dissection).

Dyspnea is not usually severe. Uncommonly, high intramediastinal pressure results in compression of the heart and blood vessels, with marked dyspnea, shock, and even death ("air block"); hemodynamics are similar to those of pericardial tamponade.

Subcutaneous emphysema with crepitus on palpation of the skin of the neck or upper chest is common. Air may cause grotesque puffing of the neck and face.

"Crackling" or "crunching" sounds (Hamman's sign) in the retrosternal and precordial areas synchronous with the heartbeat are characteristic but are occasionally due to left-sided pneumothorax.

B. X-Ray Findings: These are definitive, showing radiolucency surrounding the heart border and radiolucent streaking of the upper mediastinum; and radiolucency of the retrosternal area on a lateral film taken at full expiration and in the subcutaneous tissues of the neck and shoulder areas.

Differential Diagnosis

The pain of pneumomediastinum may simulate that of myocardial infarction.

Treatment

No treatment is usually required unless infection occurs, but a prompt search should be made for the underlying cause (eg, pneumothorax, ruptured bronchus, perforated esophagus).

Prognosis

Spontaneous recovery usually occurs if the underlying cause is corrected. If symptoms are progressive, the condition may be due to a ruptured esophagus, and emergency tracheostomy may be required.

ACUTE MEDIASTINITIS

Acute inflammation of the mediastinal space may be due to traumatic perforation of the esophagus or trachea (eg, during instrumentation or by lodged foreign bodies); spontaneous perforation of the esophagus (as in carcinoma); or lymphatic and direct spread from an infection of the neck or head, eg, retropharyngeal and cervical abscess.

Onset is usually within 24 hours after perforation. Findings include retrosternal and neck pain; progressive dysphagia, dyspnea, fever, chills, prostration, and "toxicity"; and signs of pneumomediastinum.

There may be no radiographic findings. Mediastinal widening is visible as a diffuse soft tissue density. Mediastinal mass (abscess), with or without a fluid level, may be visible.

Treatment

Treatment consists of large doses of penicillin plus chloramphenicol until organism sensitivities are determined. Surgical drainage in the cervical region is indicated when a collection of pus bulges in that area. Drainage by mediastinotomy is indicated when a widened mediastinal shadow is seen by x-ray.

Prognosis

Without treatment, the mortality rate is high; with treatment, the prognosis is markedly improved.

CHRONIC MEDIASTINITIS

Granulomatous and fibrous mediastinitis accounts for about 10% of the lesions presenting as a mediastinal mass by x-ray. The most common causes are histoplasmosis, tuberculosis, and sarcoidosis.

The clinical manifestations include widening of the mediastinum on x-ray, superior vena caval obstruction, and, occasionally, partial esophageal or tracheobronchial obstruction.

Scalene or mediastinal node biopsy may establish the cause, or exploration may be necessary.

Granulomatous disease may respond to specific treatment and corticosteroids. Obstruction due to fibrosis may be amenable to surgical resection.

James EC, Harris SS, Dillenburg CJ: Tracheal stenosis: An unusual presenting complication of idiopathic fibrosing mediastinitis. *J Thorac Cardiovasc Surg* 1980;**80**:410.

Rabinowitz JG et al: Mediastinal histoplasmosis. *Mt Sinai J Med (NY)* 1980;**47**:356.

Table 7–5. Differential diagnosis of mediastinal tumors.
Metastases may occur in any portion of the mediastinum. Among infrequent mediastinal masses are lipoma and meningocele.

Lesion	Density	Mobility (Fluoroscopy)	Clinical Features
Anterior			
Teratoma	Translucent upper area merging with denser underlying shadow. Presence of teeth or bone is pathognomonic. Tends to calcify.	May change in shape with respirations (fluid contents compressible).	Often clinically silent. Occasional rupture into bronchus with coughing up of hair and sebaceous material. May be associated with other congenital anomalies.
Hernia (Morgagni)	May contain gut (gas) or omentum (soft tissue density).	Barium studies may be diagnostic.	May be asymptomatic.
Lymphoma (Hodgkin's disease, lymphosarcoma)	Dense, rounded masses. Usually bilateral.	May show transmitted pulsations when close to vessels. Relatively fixed.	Prominent systemic symptoms (eg, fever, cachexia, anemia, pruritus). Lymphadenopathy in palpable areas.
Retrosternal thyroid	Merges with soft tissue of neck. May have hazy calcification.	Moves with swallowing. Usually displaces trachea.	Upper portion is often palpable in the neck. Signs of thyrotoxicosis may be present.
Thymus thymoma	Soft tissue density.	Usually fixed.	Physiologic in infants; usually malignant in adults. Benign enlargement is present in up to 15% of cases with myasthenia gravis.
Pericardial cysts	Soft tissue.	Usually solitary; move with heart.	Asymptomatic.
Middle			
Bronchogenic cyst	May contain air over fluid (communication with bronchus).	May be seen to rise with swallowing.	May become infected, simulating ordinary lung abscess.
Neurogenic tumors (phrenic, vagus)	Soft tissue density, circumscribed.	Phrenic tumor may move with heart.	Asymptomatic.
Sarcoidosis	Dense hilar masses, usually bilateral.	Fixed.	Asymptomatic.
Leiomyoma of the eosphagus	A single circumscribed mass.	Fixed. Outline with barium in the esophagus.	Usually a history of dysphagia.
Lymphoma: See above.			
Aneurysm, arch of aorta	Calcification of wall may occur.	May be expansile.	
Posterior			
Neurofibroma	Close relationship to thoracic spine.	Fixed.	Often "silent" when discovered. Radicular pain may be prominent. Usually not associated with generalized neurofibromatosis (Von Recklinghausen). May produce compression of spinal cord.
Ganglioneuroma	Close relationship to thoracic spine.	Usually in children.	Potentially malignant.
Neuroblastoma	Close relationship to thoracic spine.	Usually in children.	Malignant.
Hernia (Bochdalek)	Soft tissue density. May be fluid level.	May contain kidney, spleen, or bowel.	Usually asymptomatic.
Aneurysm of descending aorta		Expansile.	Erosion of vertebrae may produce back pain.
Lymphoma: See above.			

• • •

References

Bone RC (editor): Symposium on respiratory failure. *Med Clin North Am* 1983;**67**:549.

Guenter CA, Welch MH (editors): *Pulmonary Medicine*, 2nd ed. Lippincott, 1982.

Hinshaw HC, Murray JF: *Diseases of the Chest*, 4th ed. Saunders, 1981.

Pulmonary Disease Committee, American College of Physicians: Pulmonary disease: An annotated bibliography of recent literature. *Ann Intern Med* 1983;**98**:1033.

Rabin CB, Baron MG: *Radiology of the Chest*, 2nd ed. Williams & Wilkins, 1980.

Shields TW: *General Thoracic Surgery*, 2nd ed. Lea & Febiger, 1983.

West JB: *Pulmonary Pathophysiology*, 2nd ed. Williams & Wilkins, 1982.

Ziment I: *Respiratory Pharmacology and Therapeutics*. Saunders, 1978.

8 | Heart & Great Vessels

Maurice Sokolow, MD

The diagnosis of any cardiovascular disease consists of (1) determining the cause, (2) identifying the structural changes, (3) defining the physiologic abnormalities, and (4) assessing the remaining functional capacity of the heart. Treatment and the estimation of prognosis are both based upon a clear understanding of these 4 factors.

Investigation of the cause of heart disease requires consideration of the patient's age, the history, the specific abnormalities present, and appropriate laboratory studies. Abnormalities of cardiac structure and function are identified by careful physical examination combined with radiologic, echocardiographic, and electrocardiographic studies and isotopic imaging. Cardiac catheterization is needed to determine the extent of shunts and to measure the pressures in the heart chambers, aorta, or pulmonary artery. Dye dilution tests are useful in some otherwise undetectable right-to-left or left-to-right shunts. Biplane angiography and cineangiography are of great value in outlining the anatomy of congenital and acquired abnormalities, the degree of valvular insufficiencies, and intracardiac tumor masses and thrombi, as well as assessing left ventricular function by calculation of left ventricular volumes, left ventricular ejection fraction, and similar data.

Radioisotope scanning of the heart with technetium 99m pyrophosphate, technetium albumin, and thallium 201 is a noninvasive technique that has been shown to be reliable for the early detection of myocardial infarction and for serial determination of the size of the infarct. Regional wall motion and ejection fraction (global myocardial function) can be assessed by nuclear angiography. The anatomic area of the infarction correlates well with electrocardiographic and pathologic evidence of infarction. Regional myocardial perfusion and wall motion abnormalities, whether reversible or not, can be demonstrated by thallium imaging and by nuclear angiography at rest and during exercise.

Ultrasound (echocardiography), especially when combined with phonocardiography (echophonocardiography), is of considerable value in diagnosing pericardial effusion, valvular disease (especially mitral stenosis), abnormal motion of the anterior mitral leaflet in hypertrophic cardiomyopathy, mitral valve prolapse, and left atrial tumor. Ultrasound also allows estimation of the ejection fraction, the relative sizes of the septum and the atrial and ventricular muscle walls, and the dimensions and volume of the atria and ventricles and is helpful in the recognition of ventricular aneurysm, ventricular septal defect, and vegetations in infective endocarditis. Sector scans offer more detailed information than M mode echocardiograms.

Left ventricular function can be assessed indirectly by determining the ejection fraction by 2-dimensional echocardiography or left ventricular angiography or by estimating semiquantitatively the number and degree of contraction abnormalities revealed by left ventricular angiography or less reliably by 2-dimensional echocardiography. Newer techniques to evaluate cardiac function and metabolism that are now being investigated include digital angiography, x-ray tomography, positron-computed tomography, and nuclear magnetic resonance imaging.

Goldberg HL et al: Digital subtraction intravenous left ventricular angiography: Comparison with conventional intraventricular angiography. *J Am Coll Cardiol* 1983;**1**:858.

Hoffman JIE, Rudolph AM, Heymann MA: Pulmonary vascular disease with congenital heart lesions: Pathologic features and causes. *Circulation* 1981;**64**:873.

Pohost GM, Ratner AV: Nuclear magnetic resonance: Potential applications in clinical cardiology. *JAMA* 1984;**251**:1304.

Tavel ME: Phonocardiography: Clinical use with and without combined echocardiography. *Prog Cardiovasc Dis* 1983;**26**:145.

NONSPECIFIC MANIFESTATIONS

The most common symptoms resulting from heart disease are dyspnea, fatigue, chest pain, palpitations, and edema. However, because any of these symptoms may be due to noncardiac disorders (even in patients with known heart disease), the proper interpretation of their significance depends upon systematic inquiry and diagnostic studies. These symptoms are described in detail below.

Dyspnea

Dyspnea due to heart disease is almost always associated with cardiac enlargement and other structural or physiologic changes and is an indication of left ventricular failure (ie, elevated pulmonary wedge pressure). However, dyspnea in the absence of left ventricular failure may be due to pulmonary venous congestion in such conditions as mitral stenosis, intracardiac shunts, and atrial myxomas.

The most common type of dyspnea due to heart disease is **exertional dyspnea**—distinct shortness of breath upon moderate exertion that is relieved by rest.

Orthopnea is dyspnea in recumbency that is promptly relieved by sitting up.

Paroxysmal nocturnal dyspnea suddenly awakens the patient, who must then sit on the side of the bed or stand up for relief. It may be the first symptom of left ventricular failure or tight mitral stenosis.

Acute pulmonary edema is discussed on p 253.

Noncardiac causes of exertional dyspnea include poor physical condition, obesity, debility, advanced age, chronic lung disease, anemia, and obstruction of the nasal passages. Orthopnea occurs in extreme obesity, tense ascites due to any cause, abdominal distention due to gastrointestinal disease, and in the third trimester of pregnancy. Paroxysmal nocturnal dyspnea can be simulated by bronchial asthma appearing in adult life for the first time and by airway obstruction due to paratracheal tumors.

Anxiety states and cardiac neuroses can produce any form of dyspnea, but such patients often describe sighing respirations and complain of inability to take in a satisfying breath. Psychogenic dyspnea (hyperventilation) is also associated with acute respiratory alkalosis, which causes lightheadedness or mental clouding, paresthesias of the limbs or around the mouth, and at times frank tetany, tremulousness, and apprehension.

Fatigue

Easy fatigability that is relieved by rest is common in low-output states and heart failure. It may be the chief complaint (rather than dyspnea) in congenital heart disease, cor pulmonale, or mitral stenosis complicated by pulmonary hypertension. Asthenia—chronic exhaustion and lethargy not improved by rest—may be due to such psychologic disorders as depression, cardiac neuroses, and chronic anxiety or may be a component of effort syndrome ("neurocirculatory asthenia"). Noncardiac organic causes of fatigue include chronic infections, anemia, endocrine and metabolic disorders, chronic poisoning, habitual use of depressant or sedative drugs, cancer, connective tissue diseases, and any debilitating illness.

Chest Pain

Chest pain occurs in the following cardiovascular disorders: angina pectoris (in which the pain is due to intermittent ischemia of the myocardium), myocardial infarction, myopericarditis, pericardial effusion or tamponade, aortic dissection or aneurysm, hypertrophic cardiomyopathy, mitral valve prolapse, and pulmonary embolism or infarction.

Chest pain is one of the most common presenting complaints in medicine. Careful evaluation includes inquiry concerning its quality, location, radiation, and duration and the factors that precipitate, aggravate, or relieve it. Serial examinations are often required as well as laboratory tests. Exercise tests, radioisotope and metabolic studies, therapeutic tests, and selective coronary cineangiography are sometimes required.

The following noncardiac disorders are often associated with chest pain that resembles or is indistinguishable from that of heart disease: (1) Musculoskeletal arthritis or disk disease of the lower cervical and upper thoracic spine (dorsal or cervical nerve root pain); local chest wall pain, eg, costochondritis, strain or inflammation of the pectoral or intercostal muscles and ligaments; periarthritis of the left shoulder; neoplastic invasion of ribs or vertebrae. (2) Pulmonary and mediastinal disorders, eg, spontaneous pneumothorax, pleurisy, spinal cord disease, mediastinal tumor, mediastinal emphysema. (3) Gastrointestinal disease, eg, esophagitis secondary to hiatal hernia, acute or chronic cholecystitis, acute pancreatitis, cardiospasm, peptic ulcer. (4) Neurocirculatory asthenia and other emotional disorders with cardiac neurosis.

Palpitation

Consciousness of rapid, forceful, or irregular beating is the most common complaint referable to the heart. In the vast majority of instances, palpitation is due to cardiac arrhythmia or to increased awareness of normal heart action, either because of anxiety about the presence of heart disease or secondary to long-standing emotional disorders such as neurocirculatory asthenia. Organic causes are anemia, thyrotoxicosis, debility, and paroxysmal arrhythmias.

Two types of palpitation are most often described: **Sinus tachycardia**, a rapid, forceful pounding that may begin gradually or suddenly but invariably slows gradually, occurs normally on exertion or during excitement. **Premature ventricular systoles** cause a sensation of the heart "skipping a beat" or "stopping and turning over."

Patients with true paroxysmal tachycardia describe a rapid, regular palpitation or "fluttering" sensation that begins suddenly, lasts minutes or hours, and then ceases abruptly. In younger patients, there are no other symptoms unless the attacks are prolonged. In older patients, paroxysmal arrhythmias may produce angina pectoris, congestive heart failure, dizziness, or syncope. Paroxysmal atrial fibrillation is felt as a rapid irregular pounding that begins and ends suddenly. Chronic atrial fibrillation and flutter are often not perceived by the patient except after exercise or excitement, when the ventricular rate increases.

An ECG taken during an episode of palpitation establishes the diagnosis. However, clinical observation of the heart rate and rhythm and venous pulses and the effect of exercise and carotid sinus pressure, together with an assessment of the overall clinical picture (age of patient, associated heart and other diseases), permits diagnosis in the great majority of cases without ECGs.

SIGNS OF HEART DISEASE

Valuable information pertaining to the cause, nature, and extent of heart disease is often found on general physical examination, eg, Argyll Robertson pupils, splinter hemorrhages, splenomegaly, diffuse goiter, large kidneys, congenital anomalies, or epigastric bruit. Abnormal pulsations of the neck veins or precordium, height of the venous pressure, cyanosis, clubbing, and edema should be carefully noted. Careful palpation may disclose right or left ventricular hypertrophy, thrills, and diastolic movements as well as abnormal pulsations or a palpable gallop rhythm. An audible gallop should also be sought. Close attention should be paid to the character of the left ventricular impulse, whether heaving, hyperdynamic, or normal, and whether displaced to the left or not.

Edema

Edema caused by right heart failure appears first in the ankles and lower legs of ambulatory patients and over the sacrum, flanks, buttocks, and posterior thighs of bedridden patients.

The mere presence of edema does not establish a diagnosis of heart failure in a patient who also complains of dyspnea. Significant edema occurs often in obese patients and those with incompetent leg veins and healed thrombophlebitis. Garters, rolled or elastic-top stockings, tight girdles, prolonged sitting or standing, premenstrual fluid retention, and "idiopathic edema of women" are other common noncardiac causes. Nephrosis or terminal nephritis, cirrhosis with tense ascites, congenital or acquired lymphedema, hypoproteinemia, severe malnutrition or anemia, and obstruction of the inferior vena cava can produce dependent edema. If the edema is of cardiac origin, an elevated venous pressure will be evident on evaluation of the neck veins. (See p 253 for discussion of pulmonary edema.)

Cyanosis

Cyanosis is classified as central or peripheral. Central cyanosis results from low arterial oxygen saturation caused by intracardiac right-to-left shunts, pulmonary arteriovenous fistulas, certain chronic lung diseases, or pneumonia. It is differentiated from peripheral cyanosis by being present also on warm mucous membranes such as the insides of the lips and cheeks and on the tongue and conjunctiva, and is established by determining the arterial oxygen tension (P_{O_2}) and saturation. Polycythemia vera may produce central cyanosis despite normal oxygen saturation, since the larger numbers of red cells produce a proportionately greater increase in the amount of reduced hemoglobin. A useful means of differentiating cyanosis caused by a shunt in the heart or lung from that caused by primary lung disease is to administer 100% oxygen: cyanosis caused by shunt will be unaffected, whereas that due to parenchymal lung disease will disappear or decrease.

Peripheral cyanosis occurs in the presence of normal arterial oxygen saturation. It only occurs on cool portions of the body, such as the fingertips, nose, ears, and cheeks. It is caused by slowed circulation through peripheral vascular beds, which allows the capillary blood to give up more than normal amounts of oxygen. Reduced cardiac output due to mitral stenosis, pulmonary stenosis, or heart failure causes peripheral cyanosis. The most common causes, however, are nervous tension with cold, clammy hands and exposure to cold.

Murmurs, Sounds, & Clicks

Auscultation permits the examiner to determine the presence of structural or functional abnormalities by noting changes in the first or second heart sounds; by ascertaining the presence of additional heart sounds, extracardiac sounds, systolic pulmonary or aortic ejection clicks, or mid and late systolic clicks associated with mitral disease; and by analyzing murmurs. The examiner must also recognize the sounds that have no known pathologic significance: normally split first sound, normal third sound, cardiorespiratory murmurs, and the "innocent" heart murmurs. Accurate interpretation of murmurs is difficult in the presence of gross heart failure with very low cardiac output or rapid ventricular rates. In these situations, restoration of compensation or slowing of the ventricular rate may cause prominent murmurs to decrease in intensity; previously faint or inaudible murmurs may in turn become loud. Murmurs are graded on the basis of intensity into grades I (least intense) to VI (most intense). Experienced examiners rarely differ by more than one grade in evaluating a murmur.

A. Systolic Murmurs: A soft short systolic murmur at any valve area may be innocent if there are no other abnormalities and if it changes markedly with respiration and position. Exercise and tachycardia increase the intensity of any murmur. This so-called innocent or functional systolic murmur, usually present at the mitral or pulmonary area, is "ejection" in type (crescendo-decrescendo, ending before systole is complete, and related to the ejection of blood from the right or left ventricle into the pulmonary artery or aorta, respectively). It is most easily heard in recumbent, thin-chested individuals; full inspiration causes it to disappear or diminish markedly, whereas full expiration may accentuate it considerably. The louder a systolic murmur, the more likely it is to be organic in origin. Any systolic murmur associated with a thrill at that valve area is due to valvular or outflow tract disease unless there is gross anemia. An apical pansystolic murmur (a "regurgitant" murmur) which merges with and replaces the first sound and which is well transmitted into the left axilla or left infrascapular area is organic, ie, is due to deformity of the mitral valve or dilatation of the mitral valve ring with regurgitation. An aortic systolic murmur is "ejection" in type and midsystolic. It is transmitted into the carotids or upper interscapular area when due to organic disease of the aortic valve or to dilatation of the base of the aorta, and is often heard well at the apex of the heart.

B. Diastolic Murmurs: Diastolic murmurs may result from dilatation of the heart (acute myocarditis, severe anemia), dilatation of the aortic ring (marked hypertension), deformity of a valve, altered placement of a papillary muscle, rapid diastolic flow, or intracardiac shunts. When listening for diastolic murmurs, one should focus attention only on diastole, excluding from awareness as far as possible (once one has determined the timing) the first heart sound and any systolic murmurs. The position of the patient is often important in evaluation. Mitral diastolic murmurs are best heard in the left lateral position and may be quite well localized. Aortic diastolic murmurs are best heard by having the patient sit forward in expiration.

• • •

FUNCTIONAL & THERAPEUTIC CLASSIFICATION OF HEART DISEASE*

Functional Capacity Classification (Four classes.)
Class I: No limitation of physical activity. Ordinary physical activity does not cause undue fatigue, palpitation, dyspnea, or anginal pain.
Class II: Slight limitation of physical activity. Comfortable at rest, but ordinary physical activity results in fatigue, palpitation, dyspnea, or anginal pain.
Class III: Marked limitation of physical activity. Comfortable at rest, but less than ordinary activity causes fatigue, palpitation, dyspnea, or anginal pain.
Class IV: Unable to carry on any physical activity without discomfort. Symptoms of cardiac insufficiency or of the anginal syndrome may be present even at rest. If any physical activity is undertaken, discomfort is increased.

Therapeutic Classification (Five classes.)
Class A: Physical activity need not be restricted.
Class B: Ordinary physical activity need not be restricted, but unusually severe or competitive efforts should be avoided.
Class C: Ordinary physical activity should be moderately restricted, and more strenuous efforts should be discontinued.
Class D: Ordinary physical activity should be markedly restricted.
Class E: Patient should be at complete rest, confined to bed or chair.

CONGENITAL HEART DISEASES

Congenital lesions account for only about 2% of all heart disease in adults. For this reason, discussion

*Criteria Committee, New York Heart Association.

of these diseases here will be limited to the most common conditions seen by the physician in adult patients. It should be appreciated that the discussion in the various sections on prognosis refers to untreated patients. Following corrective surgery, even though patients show considerable clinical improvement and are often symptom-free, few are completely normal. They may develop cardiac arrhythmias or conduction defects, symptoms and signs of cardiac failure, and infective endocarditis and may show residual defects if thoroughly studied. Further long-term follow-up may reveal additional difficulties. The reader is referred to the references.

Engle MA, Diaz S: Long-term results of surgery for congenital heart disease. (2 parts.) *Circulation* 1982;**65:**415, 634.
McNamara DG, Latson LA: Long-term follow-up of patients with malformations for which definitive surgical repair has been available for 25 years or more. *Am J Cardiol* 1982; **50:**560.
Vetter VL, Horowitz LN: Electrophysiologic residua and sequelae of surgery for congenital heart defects. *Am J Cardiol* 1982;**50:**588.

PURE PULMONARY STENOSIS (WITH INTACT SEPTUM)

Stenosis of the pulmonary valve or infundibulum increases the resistance to outflow, raises the right ventricular pressure, and limits the amount of pulmonary blood flow. Since there is no shunt, arterial saturation is normal, but severe stenosis causes peripheral cyanosis by reducing cardiac output. Clubbing or polycythemia does not develop unless a patent foramen ovale or atrial septal defect is present, permitting shunting of blood from the right to the left atrium.

Clinical Findings
A. Symptoms and Signs: Mild cases (right ventricular–pulmonary artery gradient < 50 mm Hg) are asymptomatic. Moderate to severe stenosis (gradients exceeding 80 mm Hg) causes dyspnea on exertion (in the absence of heart failure), fainting, and chest pain. Right ventricular failure develops eventually in severe cases, producing edema, increased dyspnea, and fatigue.

There is a palpable right ventricular heave. A loud, harsh systolic murmur and a prominent thrill are present in the left second and third interspaces parasternally; the murmur is in the third and fourth interspaces in infundibular stenosis. The second sound is obscured by the murmur in severe cases; the pulmonary component is diminished, delayed, or absent. Both components are audible in mild cases. A presystolic gallop and a prominent *a* wave in the venous pulse are present in severe cases.
B. X-Ray Findings and Fluoroscopy: The heart size may be normal, or there may be a prominent right ventricle and atrium or gross cardiac enlargement, depending upon the severity. The pulmonary artery is dilated, with weak or absent pulsations, in valvular

stenosis; but it is normal in infundibular stenosis. Pulmonary vascularity is normal or (in severe cases with right-to-left shunts) diminished.

C. Electrocardiographic Findings: Right axis or right ventricular hypertrophy; peaked P waves as evidence of right atrial overload.

D. Special Studies: Cardiac catheterization permits estimation of the gradient across the pulmonary valve, determines whether the stenosis is valvular or infundibular, and, together with dye studies, demonstrates the presence or absence of associated shunts. Angiography delineates the anatomy of the defect, including the infundibulum of the right ventricle. Echocardiography is of little value except in excluding the diagnosis.

Treatment

Pure pulmonary stenosis with evidence of progressive hypertrophy and resting gradients of over 75–80 mm Hg is treated surgically, with an operative mortality rate of 3–4% and excellent results in most cases. All lesions are corrected under direct vision; those with associated outflow tract hypertrophy are often approached through a ventriculotomy. Percutaneous balloon valvuloplasty has been reported to have favorable results in a few cases; the same is true for dilatation of the coarctation site of the aorta (see below). Further experience for both lesions is awaited.

Prognosis

Patients with mild stenosis may have normal life expectancy unless infective endocarditis occurs. Severe stenosis causes refractory heart failure in the 20s and 30s. Moderate stenosis may be asymptomatic in childhood and adolescence, but cardiac symptoms and cardiac failure occur with increasing frequency as the patient becomes older. Only 12% of untreated patients live past age 50. In patients with pure pulmonary stenosis, the incidence of infective endocarditis is about 1% per year.

Rocchini AP et al: Percutaneous balloon valvuloplasty for treatment of congenital pulmonary valvular stenosis in children. *J Am Coll Cardiol* 1984;3:1005.

COARCTATION OF THE AORTA

The adult type of coarctation of the aorta consists of localized narrowing of the aortic arch just distal to the origin of the left subclavian artery in the region of the ligamentum arteriosum. A bicuspid aortic valve is present in 25% of cases. Blood pressure is elevated in the aorta and its branches proximal to the coarctation and decreased distally. Collateral circulation between the high- and low-pressure aortic segments develops through the intercostal arteries and branches of the subclavian arteries.

Clinical Findings

A. Symptoms and Signs: There are no symp-

toms until the hypertension produces left ventricular failure or cerebral hemorrhage. The latter can occur from hypertension or from associated cerebral aneurysms. Strong arterial pulsations are seen in the neck and suprasternal notch. Hypertension is present in the arms, but the pressure is normal or low in the legs. This difference is exaggerated by exercise, which is helpful in the diagnosis of doubtful cases. Femoral pulsations are absent or weak, and delayed in comparison with the brachial pulse. Visible or palpable collateral arteries are present in the intercostal spaces and along the borders of the scapulas. Patients with large collaterals may have relatively small gradients but still have severe coarctation. Late systolic ejection murmurs at the base are often heard better posteriorly, especially over the spinous processes. There may be an associated aortic insufficiency murmur due to a bicuspid aortic valve.

B. X-Ray Findings: X-ray shows scalloping of the ribs due to enlarged collateral intercostal arteries, dilatation of the left subclavian artery and poststenotic aortic dilatation ("3" sign), and left ventricular enlargement.

C. Electrocardiographic Findings: The ECG shows left ventricular hypertrophy; it may be normal in mild cases.

D. Invasive Studies: Left ventricular angiography or aortography is often employed, as well as cardiac catheterization, to determine the pressure difference across the stenosis of the aorta and the cardiac output and to exclude associated lesions.

Treatment

Resection of the coarcted site is a more difficult operative procedure than ligation of a patent ductus arteriosus, and the surgical mortality rate is in the neighborhood of 1–4%. The risks of the disease are such, however, that if a skilled heart surgeon is available, all coarctations in patients up to age 20 years should be resected, usually with patch angioplasty. In patients between ages 20 and 35, surgery is advisable if the patient is showing evidence of left ventricular strain. The mortality rate rises considerably in patients over age 50 years, and surgery in this age group is of doubtful value.

Prognosis

Cardiac failure is common in infancy and in older untreated patients; it is uncommon in late childhood and in young adult life. Most untreated patients with the adult form of coarctation die before age 40 from the complications of hypertension, rupture of the aorta, infective endocarditis of the aortic valve or endarteritis at the coarctation site, or cerebral hemorrhage (congenital aneurysms). About one-fourth of patients continue to be hypertensive years after surgery, and they may have all the complications associated with hypertension. However, 25% have a normal cardiovascular prognosis and die of causes unrelated to the coarctation.

ATRIAL SEPTAL DEFECT

The most common form of atrial septal defect is persistence of the ostium secundum in the mid septum; less commonly, the ostium primum (which is low in the septum, involving the endocardial cushion) persists, in which case mitral or tricuspid abnormalities may also be present. A third form involves a defect of the upper part of the septum known as the sinus venosus defect, which is often associated with partial anomalous drainage of the pulmonary veins into the superior vena cava. Rarely, the latter may occur alone. In any case, normally oxygenated blood from the left atrium passes into the right atrium, increasing the right ventricular output and the pulmonary blood flow. In the primum defect, mitral valve insufficiency produces, additionally, strain on the left ventricle.

Clinical Findings

A. Symptoms and Signs: Most patients with moderate secundum defects are asymptomatic. With large shunts, exertional dyspnea or cardiac failure may develop. Prominent right ventricular pulsations are readily visible and palpable. A moderately loud systolic ejection murmur can be heard in the second and third interspaces parasternally as a result of increased flow across the pulmonary valve, as well as an apical or xiphoid middiastolic soft murmur due to increased flow across the tricuspid valve, especially on inspiration. Thrills are uncommon. The second sound is widely split and does not vary with breathing.

B. X-Ray Findings: Large pulmonary arteries with vigorous pulsations, increased pulmonary vascularity, an enlarged right atrium and ventricle, and a small aortic knob.

C. Electrocardiographic Findings: Right axis or right ventricular hypertrophy may be present in ostium secundum defects. Incomplete or complete right bundle branch block is present in most cases, and left superior axis deviation with counterclockwise rotation in the frontal plane in ostium primum defect.

D. Special Studies: Cardiac catheterization permits calculation of the amount of blood shunted, the intracardiac and pulmonary pressures, and the pulmonary vascular resistance. Hemodynamic evidences of cardiac failure may be found, eg, raised pulmonary capillary wedge pressure and decreased cardiac output. Cardiac failure is usually associated with the late development of atrial fibrillation in older patients. If right heart failure has occurred because of the development of pulmonary hypertension, right ventricular diastolic pressure and right atrial pressure will be elevated. The catheter may pass through the defect into the left atrium. Contrast or nuclear angiocardiography may reveal primum defects or mitral insufficiency. Echocardiography can demonstrate right ventricular size, septal motion, and left-to-right shunt. Two-dimensional echocardiography may disclose a sinus venosus defect in the superior aspect of the atrial septum. Contrast echocardiography can cause a temporary shunt from right to left with the passage of bubbles

into the left heart, documenting an atrial septal defect. Radioisotope studies can often estimate the size of the shunt.

Treatment

Small atrial septal defects do not require surgery. Defects with a large left-to-right shunt (more than 2 or 3 times systemic flow) with slight or no increased pulmonary arterial resistance should be closed surgically even in older patients. The surgical risks are now sufficiently low so that patients with pulmonary to systemic flow ratios between 1.5 and 2.0 may be operated on if the total clinical picture warrants, according to the physician's judgment. Ratios exceeding 2:1 are an indication for surgical closure of the defect.

Surgery should be withheld from patients with pulmonary hypertension with reversed shunt because of the risk of acute right heart failure. Relocation of pulmonary veins is required in patients with partial anomalous venous drainage. In ostium primum defects, in addition to closure of the defect, suture of the valve clefts, especially those of the mitral valve, is advisable if mitral regurgitation of any significant degree is present.

Prognosis

Patients with small shunts may live a normal life span; with larger shunts, they survive to middle or late life before pulmonary hypertension or heart failure appears. The latter is precipitated most often by atrial fibrillation or raised pulmonary vascular resistance. Large shunts cause disability by age 40. Raised pulmonary vascular resistance secondary to pulmonary hypertension rarely occurs in childhood or young adult life in secundum defects but is more common in primum defects; after age 40, pulmonary hypertension, cardiac arrhythmia, and left ventricular failure may occur in secundum defects.

The surgical mortality rate with cardiac bypass is low (< 1%) in patients under age 45 who are not in cardiac failure and have pulmonary artery pressures < 60 mm Hg. It increases to 6–10% in patients over age 40 with cardiac failure or pulmonary artery pressures > 60 mm Hg. Most survivors show considerable improvement.

Hurwitz RA et al: Current value of radionuclide angiocardiography for shunt quantification and management in patients with secundum atrial septal defect. *Am Heart J* 1982;**103**:421.

St. John Sutton MG, Tajik AJ, McGoon DC: Atrial septal defect in patients ages 60 years or older: Operative results and long-term postoperative follow-up. *Circulation* 1981;**64**:402.

Smallhorn JF et al: Assessment of atrioventricular septal defects by two-dimensional echocardiography. *Br Heart J* 1982;**47**:109.

PATENT DUCTUS ARTERIOSUS

The embryonic ductus arteriosus fails to close normally and persists as a shunt connecting the left pulmonary artery and aorta, usually near the origin of the left subclavian artery. Blood flows from the aorta through the ductus into the pulmonary artery continuously in systole and diastole; it is a form of arteriovenous fistula, increasing the work of the left ventricle. In some patients, obliterative changes in the pulmonary arterioles cause pulmonary hypertension. Then the shunt is bidirectional or right-to-left (Eisenmenger's syndrome).

Clinical Findings
A. Symptoms and Signs: There are no symptoms until or unless left ventricular failure develops. The heart is of normal size or slightly enlarged, with a forceful apex beat. Pulse pressure is wide and diastolic pressure low. A continuous, rough "machinery" murmur, accentuated in late systole at the time of S_2, is heard best in the left first and second interspaces at the sternal border. Thrills are common. Paradoxic splitting of the second sound may be present if there is considerable left ventricular hypertrophy.

B. X-Ray Findings: The heart is normal in size and contour, or there may be left ventricular and left atrial enlargement. The pulmonary artery, aorta, and left atrium are prominent.

C. Electrocardiographic Findings: Normal pattern or left ventricular hypertrophy, depending upon the width of the ductus.

D. Special Studies: Cardiac catheterization establishes the presence of a left-to-right shunt. The catheter may be passed through the ductus into the aorta from the pulmonary artery, and, when combined with angiography, excludes other lesions that may cause a similar murmur.

Treatment
In premature infants with cardiac failure, a trial of indomethacin, an inhibitor of prostaglandin synthesis, may result in closure of the ductus and relief of the cardiac failure. Surgical correction is recommended for older infants 2–3 months of age and for premature infants with cardiac failure who fail to respond to indomethacin. Prostaglandin E_1 (alprostadil; Prostin VR Pediatric) may provide palliation for infants with ductus-dependent cyanotic congenital heart disease.

Asymptomatic older adults with no left ventricular hypertrophy are at low risk of developing infective endocarditis or endarteritis, and surgery may be unwise.

The indications for ligation or division of a patent ductus arteriosus in the presence of pulmonary hypertension are controversial. Current opinion favors ligation whenever the pulmonary vascular resistance is low or only moderately elevated and the flow through the ductus is permanently or intermittently from left to right, ie, when pulmonary blood flow is increased and the pulmonary artery pressure is < 100 mm Hg.

Prognosis
Large shunts cause a high mortality rate from cardiac failure early in life. Smaller shunts are compatible with long survival, congestive heart failure being

the most common complication. Infective endocarditis or endarteritis may also occur. A small percentage of patients develop pulmonary hypertension and reversal of shunt, such that the lower legs, especially the toes, appear cyanotic and clubbed in contrast to normally pink fingers. At this stage, the patient is inoperable.

Heymann MA: Pharmacologic use of prostaglandin E_1 in infants with congenital heart disease. *Am Heart J* 1981;**101**:837.

VENTRICULAR SEPTAL DEFECT

In this lesion, a persistent opening in the upper interventricular septum resulting from failure of fusion with the aortic septum permits blood to pass from the high-pressure left ventricle into the low-pressure right ventricle with small or moderately large ventricular septal defects; with large ventricular septal defects, the pressures in the 2 ventricles are equal, and the shunt depends on the relative pulmonary and systemic vascular resistance. In one-fourth to one-third of cases, the shunt is not large enough to overload the heart. With large shunts, both left and right ventricular overload may develop.

Clinical Findings
A. Symptoms and Signs: The clinical features are dependent upon the size of the defect and the presence or absence of a raised pulmonary vascular resistance. Cardiac failure is common in infancy and in the first months of life if the defect is large. If pulmonary vascular resistance is normal and the defect is small, the left-to-right shunt is small; if the defect is large, the resistance to flow between the ventricles is small and the left-to-right shunt is large; a rise in pulmonary vascular resistance decreases the left-to-right shunt and converts the pansystolic murmur into a "lopsided" diamond ejection murmur. A long, loud, harsh systolic murmur and thrill are found in the left third and fourth interspaces along the sternum and may be the only findings in small defects. About one-third of small or moderate defects and, infrequently, larger shunts may close spontaneously over a period of a few years. In large shunts a right ventricular heave is palpable and a middiastolic "flow murmur" and a third heart sound may be heard at the apex.

B. X-Ray Findings: With large shunts the right or left ventricle (or both), the left atrium, and the pulmonary arteries are enlarged, and pulmonary vascularity is increased.

C. Electrocardiographic Findings: May be normal or may show right, left, or biventricular hypertrophy, depending on the size of the defect and the pulmonary vascular resistance.

D. Special Studies: Cardiac catheterization permits a definitive diagnosis in all but the most trivial defects. Infants with cardiac failure should be studied to establish the diagnosis and determine the appropriate medical or surgical treatment.

Echocardiography, especially the 2-dimensional

type, can demonstrate chamber size and allow estimation of the magnitude of the pulmonary flow as well as of ejection fraction.

Treatment

Ventricular septal defects vary in severity from trivial asymptomatic lesions with normal cardiac hemodynamics to extensive lesions causing death from cardiac failure in infancy. The former do not require surgery. The ideal case for curative repair with cardiac bypass techniques is one with a large left-to-right shunt, left ventricular hypertrophy, and only moderate pulmonary hypertension. When severe pulmonary hypertension is present (pulmonary arterial pressures > 85 mm Hg) and the left-to-right shunt is small, the surgical mortality risk is at least 50%. If the shunt is reversed, surgery is contraindicated. If surgery is required because of unrelenting cardiac failure in infancy due to a large left-to-right shunt, pulmonary artery banding may decrease the shunt and tide the patient over until age 5 or 6, when definitive repair can be done. Early closure of the defect rather than banding is now the preferred procedure in most centers, with a surgical mortality rate of 2–3% for primary repair. It has become increasingly evident that some defects (perhaps as many as 30–50%) close spontaneously. Therefore, surgery should be deferred until late childhood unless the disability is severe or unless pulmonary hypertension is observed to progress or to develop.

Prognosis

Patients with the typical murmur as the only abnormality have a normal life expectancy except for the threat of infective endocarditis. With large shunts, congestive heart failure may develop early in life, and survival beyond age 40 is unusual. Shunt reversal occurs in an estimated 25%, producing Eisenmenger's syndrome. Postoperative studies show that surgery is of no benefit if the pulmonary vascular resistance exceeds one-third of the systemic vascular resistance.

Blake RS et al: Conduction defects, ventricular arrhythmias, and late death after surgical closure of ventricular septal defect. *Br Heart J* 1982;**47**:305.
Jablonsky G et al: Rest and exercise ventricular function in adults with congenital ventricular septal defects. *Am J Cardiol* 1983;**51**:293.

TETRALOGY OF FALLOT

Pulmonary stenosis (usually infundibular or pulmonary atresia), together with a high ventricular septal defect that allows the right ventricle to empty into the aorta, prevents venous blood from passing normally into the pulmonary artery. Instead, blood passes from the right ventricle into the aorta and into the left ventricle. Aortic blood is therefore markedly unsaturated, and cyanosis, polycythemia, and clubbing appear early. Exercise causes cyanosis to deepen.

Clinical Findings

A. Symptoms and Signs: Physical development is retarded in severe cases. Dyspnea is common, squatting relieves fatigue and dyspnea, and syncope occasionally occurs. Prominent signs are cyanosis and clubbing, a slight right ventricular heave and absent apical impulse, and a short, harsh systolic murmur and thrill along the left sternal border. The heart is not enlarged. A single loud second sound is heard unless the lesion is mild, when the second sound is split, with the pulmonary component decreased in amplitude.

B. X-Ray Findings: The lung fields are abnormally clear. The apex of the heart is blunted, with a concavity in the pulmonary artery segment (boot-shaped heart). A right aortic arch is present in 25% of cases.

C. Electrocardiographic Findings: Moderate right ventricular hypertrophy is usually present. Prominent right atrial P waves are occasionally present.

D. Special Studies: Cardiac catheterization and right ventricular angiocardiography together establish the diagnosis and define the anatomic defect. Aortography has been recommended as a routine procedure in patients who are being considered for "total" corrective surgery, to show the aortic branches and unexpected associated defects. Demonstration of shunting of blood across the ventricular septal defect on hemodynamic study is dependent on the relative resistance of the systemic and pulmonary circulations. Variation of the systemic vascular resistance varies the magnitude of right-to-left shunting.

E. Echocardiography: Echocardiography can determine the presence and extent of overriding of the aorta and demonstrate the break in continuity of echoes representing ventricular septal defect. It therefore can help distinguish between tetralogy of Fallot and pulmonary stenosis.

Treatment

Tetralogy of Fallot is treated surgically, using extracorporeal circulation, and the operative mortality rate is reasonably low. Patients with underdeveloped pulmonary arteries and those weighing less than 15 kg should be given a preliminary Blalock-Taussig type of shunt operation. The Potts anastomosis is obsolete.

Complete repair of the defect is always indicated in adult patients. If the patient has reached adult life without surgical treatment, the lesion is likely to be mild, and complete correction should be comparatively easy. The mortality rate of the operation is 3–5%. The operation may be more difficult in patients who have had prior palliative surgery of the Blalock-Taussig or Potts type. The late results of surgery in survivors is usually good; most patients are asymptomatic, but about one-third have residual obstruction of the right ventricular outflow tract, residual ventricular septal defect, or left-to-right shunt, as shown by postoperative hemodynamic studies.

Propranolol (Inderal) has been used with benefit for episodes of syncope due to infundibular contraction.

Prognosis

Tetralogy of Fallot is the commonest cause of cyanotic congenital heart disease in adults, although survival to adult life is not common. Severe hypoxemia is the commonest cause of death. Cerebral thromboses secondary to polycythemia are also common. The severity of the syndrome is dominated by the degree of stenosis; the greater the stenosis, the greater the right-to-left shunt and the smaller the pulmonary blood flow.

Brandenburg RO et al: Clinical follow-up study of paroxysmal supraventricular tachyarrhythmias after operative repair of a secundum type atrial septal defect in adults. *Am J Cardiol* 1983;**51**:273.

Katz NM et al: Late survival and symptoms after repair of tetralogy of Fallot. *Circulation* 1982;**65**:403.

Partridge JB, Fiddler GI: Cineangiocardiography in tetralogy of Fallot. *Br Heart J* 1981;**45**:112.

ACQUIRED HEART DISEASES

RHEUMATIC FEVER

Criteria for Diagnosis (Modified After Jones)
  A. Major Criteria:
  1. Carditis.
  2. Sydenham's chorea.
  3. Subcutaneous (fascial) nodules.
  4. Erythema marginatum.
  5. Polyarthritis.

  B. Minor Criteria:
  1. Fever.
  2. Polyarthralgia.
  3. Reversible prolongation of PR interval.
  4. Increased sedimentation rate.
  5. Evidence of antecedent beta-hemolytic streptococcal infection.
  6. Verified history of previous rheumatic fever or presence of rheumatic valvular disease.

The diagnosis of rheumatic fever is almost certain when 2 or more major criteria are present. Nevertheless, rheumatoid arthritis, neurocirculatory asthenia, infective endocarditis, connective tissue diseases, serum sickness, penicillin reaction, and chronic infectious disease can reproduce the early manifestations of rheumatic fever.

General Considerations

Rheumatic fever is an acute, subacute, or chronic systemic disease that is a sequela to hemolytic streptococcal infection. For unknown reasons it may either be self-limiting or lead to slowly progressive valvular deformity.

Rheumatic fever is the most common precursor of heart disease in people under age 50 years in less developed countries; it is now uncommon in the USA. In overall incidence, rheumatic valvular heart disease ranks third behind hypertension and atherosclerotic coronary disease. Rheumatic fever is somewhat more common in males than in females, but chorea is seen more frequently in females. The peak incidence occurs between ages 5 and 15; it is rare before age 4 and after 50.

Rheumatic fever is initiated by an infection with group A hemolytic streptococci, appearing usually 1–4 weeks after tonsillitis, nasopharyngitis, or otitis.

The acute phase of rheumatic fever may involve the endocardium, myocardium, pericardium, synovial joint linings, lungs, or pleura. The characteristic lesion is a perivascular granulomatous reaction and vasculitis. The mitral valve is attacked in 75–80% of cases, the aortic valve in 30%, the tricuspid and pulmonary valves in less than 5%. Small pink granules appear on the surface of the edematous valve. Healing may be complete, or a progressive scarring due to subacute or chronic inflammation may develop over months and years.

Clinical Findings
  A. Major Criteria:
  1. Carditis–The presence of carditis establishes the diagnosis of rheumatic fever whenever there is (1) a definite history of rheumatic fever, or (2) valvular disease clearly of rheumatic origin, or (3) a streptococcal infection of the upper respiratory tract known to have occurred within the preceding 4 weeks. Carditis is most apt to be evident in children and adolescents; in adults, it is often best detected by serial electrocardiographic study. Any of the following establishes the presence of carditis.

  a. Pericarditis–Either fibrinous or with effusion of any degree. It is uncommon in adults and is at times diagnosed by the progressive increase in "heart shadow" on serial chest x-rays or by echocardiography.

  b. Cardiac enlargement, detected by physical signs or x-ray, indicating dilatation of a weakened, inflamed myocardium. Serial x-rays are often needed to detect the change in size.

  c. Frank congestive failure, right- and left-sided–Right heart failure is more prominent in children, and painful liver engorgement is a valuable sign.

  d. Mitral or aortic diastolic murmurs, indicative of dilatation of a valve ring or the myocardium with or without associated valvulitis.

  In the absence of any of the above definite signs, the diagnosis of carditis depends upon the following less specific abnormalities considered in relation to the total clinical picture.

  (1) Electrocardiographic changes: PR prolongation greater than 0.04 s above the patient's normal that returns to normal as rheumatic activity subsides is the most significant abnormality; changing contour of P waves or inversion of T waves is less specific.

  (2) Changing quality of heart sounds.

(3) Pansystolic apical murmur that persists or becomes louder during the course of the disease and is transmitted into the axilla. The Carey-Coombs short middiastolic murmur should be carefully sought.

(4) Gallop rhythm: Difficult to differentiate from the physiologic third sound in children and adolescents.

(5) Sinus tachycardia out of proportion to the degree of fever, persisting during sleep and markedly increased by slight activity.

(6) Arrhythmias, shifting pacemaker, ectopic beats.

2. Erythema annulare and subcutaneous nodules–The former begin as rapidly enlarging macules that assume the shape of rings or crescents with clear centers. They may be slightly raised and confluent. The rash may be transient or may persist for long periods.

Subcutaneous nodules are uncommon except in children. The nodules may be few or many; are usually small (2 cm or less in diameter), firm, and nontender; and are attached to fascia or tendon sheaths over bony prominences. They persist for days or weeks, are usually recurrent, and are clinically indistinguishable from the nodules of rheumatoid arthritis.

3. Sydenham's chorea may appear suddenly as an isolated entity. Eventually, 50% of cases have other signs of rheumatic fever. Girls are more frequently affected, and occurrence in adults is rare. (See Chapter 17.)

4. Arthritis–The arthritis of rheumatic fever is characteristically a migratory polyarthritis that involves the large joints sequentially, one becoming hot, red, swollen, and tender as the inflammation in the previously involved joint subsides. In adults, only a single or a small joint may be affected. The acute arthritis lasts 1–5 weeks and subsides without residual deformity—except for the rare persistent arthritis known as Jaccoud's arthritis. Prompt response of arthritis to therapeutic doses of salicylates is characteristic (but not diagnostic) of rheumatic fever.

B. Minor Criteria: These are nonspecific manifestations and are of help only when considered in conjunction with major criteria. These consist of fever (which may be low-grade, continuous, or intermittent); malaise; asthenia; weight loss or anorexia; abdominal pain (from engorgement of the liver or rheumatic peritonitis), especially in children; recurrent epistaxis; or various arthralgias known as "growing pains."

C. Laboratory Findings: Laboratory findings include nonspecific evidence of inflammatory disease as shown by a raised sedimentation rate or white cell count; a high or increasing titer of antistreptolysin O demonstrating an antecedent beta-hemolytic streptococcal infection; and occasional proteinuria and microscopic hematuria.

Differential Diagnosis

Rheumatic fever may be confused with the following: rheumatoid arthritis, osteomyelitis, traumatic joint disease, neurocirculatory asthenia or cardiac neurosis, infective endocarditis, pulmonary tuberculosis, chronic meningococcemia, acute poliomyelitis, disseminated lupus erythematosus, serum sickness, drug sensitivity, leukemia, sickle cell anemia, inactive rheumatic heart disease, congenital heart disease, and "surgical abdomen."

Complications

Congestive heart failure occurs in severe cases. Other complications include cardiac arrhythmias, pericarditis with large effusion, rheumatic pneumonitis, pulmonary embolism and infarction, cardiac invalidism, and early or late development of permanent heart valve deformity.

Prevention of Recurrent Rheumatic Fever

The principles of prevention are to avoid beta-hemolytic streptococcal infections if possible and to treat streptococcal infections promptly and intensively with appropriate antibiotics.

A. Prevention of Infection: Two methods of prevention are now advocated.

1. Penicillin–The preferred method of prophylaxis is with benzathine penicillin G (Bicillin), 1.2 million units intramuscularly every 4 weeks. Oral penicillin (200–250 thousand units daily before breakfast) may be used instead but is less reliable. Prophylaxis is advocated especially for children who have had one or more acute attacks and should be given throughout the school years and continued until about age 25. Adults should receive preventive therapy for about 5 years after an attack or until about age 30 if they are exposed to children with recurrent streptococcal infections.

2. Sulfonamides–If the patient is sensitive to penicillin, give sulfadiazine, 1 g daily throughout the year. *Caution:* Patients receiving sulfonamides should have periodic blood counts and urinalyses. If there is any tendency toward leukopenia, the drug should be stopped immediately.

3. Erythromycin–If allergy to penicillin and sulfonamides is present, erythromycin, 250 mg orally 4 times a day, may be used.

B. Treatment of Streptococcal Sore Throat: It has been shown that prompt therapy of streptococcal infections initiated within 24 hours and continued for 10 days will prevent most attacks of acute rheumatic fever. (See Chapter 24.)

Treatment

A. Medical Measures:

1. The salicylates markedly reduce fever, relieve joint pain, and may reduce joint swelling. There is no evidence that they have any effect on the natural course of the disease.

a. Sodium salicylate or aspirin is the most widely used of this group of drugs; aspirin must be used if the patient has evidence of cardiac failure. The salicylates should be used with antacids after meals or with milk to reduce gastric irritation. A usually satisfactory dose for children is 15–25 mg/kg given every 4 hours during the day for a week, with the dose then decreased by half. Adults may require 0.6–0.9 g every 4 hours during the day to allay symptoms and fever. Early toxic reactions to the salicylates include tinnitus, vomiting, and hyperpnea. The antiplatelet action of aspirin must be kept in mind and evidences of bleeding searched for. These, however, are infrequent to rare. The doses recommended are arbitrary and can be varied depending upon response. Determination of blood salicylate levels is infrequently required unless the patient develops symptoms suggesting salicylate poisoning (see p 1016). *Caution:* Never use sodium salicylate or sodium bicarbonate in patients with acute rheumatic fever who have associated cardiac failure. Other antiinflammatory agents (eg, indomethacin) have not been used in large-scale studies.

b. Aspirin may be substituted for sodium salicylate, with the same dosages and precautions.

2. Penicillin should be employed in the treatment at any time during the course of the disease to eradicate any existing streptococcal infection.

3. Corticosteroids–There is no clear or consistent proof that cardiac damage is prevented or minimized by corticosteroids. Corticosteroids are effective anti-inflammatory agents for reversing the acute exudative phase of rheumatic fever and are probably more potent for this purpose than salicylates. A short course of corticosteroids usually causes rapid improvement in the acute manifestations of rheumatic fever and is indicated in severe cases.

A suggested schedule, to be started as soon as severe rheumatic fever is diagnosed, is as follows: Give prednisone, 5–10 mg orally every 6 hours for 3 weeks, and then gradually withdraw over a period of 3 weeks by reducing and then discontinuing first the nighttime, then the evening, and finally the daytime doses. In severe cases the dosage should be increased, if necessary, to levels adequate to control symptoms. (See the discussion of the methods, dangers, and precautions in the use of corticosteroids in Chapter 19.)

B. General Measures: Bed rest should be enforced until all signs of active rheumatic fever have disappeared. The criteria for this are as follows: return of the temperature to normal with the patient at bed rest and without medications; normal sedimentation rate; normal resting pulse rate (under 100 in adults); return of ECG to normal or fixation of abnormalities. The patient may then be allowed up slowly, but several months should elapse before return to full activity unless the rheumatic fever was exceedingly mild. Maintain good nutrition.

C. Treatment of Complications:

1. Congestive failure–Treat as for congestive failure, with the following variations:

a. A low-sodium diet and diuretics are of particular value in promoting diuresis and treating failure in acute rheumatic fever.

b. Digitalis is usually not as effective in acute rheumatic fever as in most cases of congestive failure and may accentuate the myocardial irritability, producing arrhythmias that further embarrass the heart. However, digitalis should be given a cautious trial because it may be helpful to the individual patient.

c. Many cases of congestive failure are due to acute myocarditis. These often respond dramatically to corticotropin or the corticosteroids. When sodium-retaining hormonal agents are employed, rigorous sodium restriction (< 200 mg daily) or thiazide drugs are imperative.

d. Other measures of treating cardiac failure, such as vasodilators and inotropic agents such as dopamine, may be tried in severe cases. (See under Cardiac Failure.)

2. Pericarditis–Treat as any acute nonpurulent pericarditis. The rheumatic effusion is sterile, and antibiotics are of no value. The general principles include relief of pain, by opiates if necessary, and removal of fluid by cardiac paracentesis if tamponade develops. This is rarely necessary. Nonsteroidal anti-inflammatory agents may be helpful, but their complications must be kept in mind. Corticotropin and the corticosteroids, as well as salicylates, should be continued or started, as they seem to have a specific favorable effect in aiding resorption of fluid. Serial echocardiograms are the most effective means of detecting pericardial effusion and early hemodynamic limitation. Serial assessment of the jugular venous pressure or measurement of the central venous pressure should be determined if pericardial effusion is present.

Prognosis

Initial episodes of rheumatic fever last months in children and weeks in adults. Twenty percent of children have recurrences within 5 years. Recurrences are uncommon after 5 years of well-being and rare after age 21. The immediate mortality rate is 1–2%. Persistent rheumatic activity with a greatly enlarged heart, heart failure, and pericarditis indicate a poor prognosis; 30% of children thus affected die within 10 years of the initial attack. Otherwise the prognosis for life is good. Eighty percent of all patients attain adult life, and half of these have little if any limitation of activity. Approximately one-third of young patients have detectable valvular damage after the initial episode, most commonly a combination of mitral stenosis and insufficiency. After 10 years, two-thirds of surviving patients will have detectable valvular disease. In adults, residual heart damage occurs in less than 20% and is generally less severe. Mitral insufficiency is the commonest residual effect, and aortic insufficiency is much more common than in children. Twenty percent of patients who have chorea develop valvular deformity even after a long latent period of apparent well-being.

Sanyal SK et al: Sequelae of the initial attack of acute rheumatic fever in children from North India: A prospective 5-year follow-up study. *Circulation* 1982;**65:**375.

Stollerman G et al: Jones Criteria (revised) for guidance in the diagnosis of rheumatic fever. *Circulation* 1984;**69:**203A.

RHEUMATIC HEART DISEASE
(Rheumatic Valvulitis, Inactive)

Chronic rheumatic heart disease results from single or repeated attacks of rheumatic fever that produce rigidity and deformity of the cusps, fusion of the commissures, or shortening and fusion of the chordae tendineae. Stenosis or insufficiency results, and both often coexist, although one or the other predominates. The mitral valve alone is affected in 50–60% of cases; combined lesions of the aortic and mitral valves occur in 20%; pure aortic lesions in 10%. Tricuspid involvement occurs only in association with mitral or aortic disease in about 10% of cases. The pulmonary valve is rarely affected.

Clinical Findings

A history of rheumatic fever is obtainable in only 60% of patients with rheumatic heart disease.

The earliest evidence of organic valvular disease is a significant murmur. The earliest evidence of hemodynamically significant valvular lesions is found on x-ray, fluoroscopy, and electrocardiographic study, since these will reveal the earliest stages of specific chamber enlargement. Careful physical examination also permits accurate diagnosis of advanced valve lesions.

The important findings in each of the major valve lesions are summarized in Table 8–1. Hemodynamic changes, symptoms, associated findings, and course are discussed below.

Management of Asymptomatic Valvular Heart Disease

A. Prevention:

1. Recurrences of acute rheumatic fever can be prevented (see p 185).

2. The patient should be given advice regarding dental extraction, urologic procedures, surgical procedures, etc, to prevent bacteremia and possible infective endocarditis.

B. General Measures:
Vocational guidance is necessary to anticipate possible reduced exercise tolerance in later life. Follow-up observations should emphasize early recognition of disturbances of thyroid function, anemia, and arrhythmias; maintenance of general health; and avoidance of obesity and excessive physical exertion.

1. MITRAL STENOSIS

Over 75% of patients with mitral stenosis are women below age 45. Relatively slight degrees of narrowing are sufficient to produce the auscultatory signs.

As indicated in Table 8–1, the characteristic finding of mitral stenosis is a localized, delayed diastolic murmur that is low in pitch and whose duration varies with the severity of the stenosis and the heart rate. Because it is thickened, the valve opens in early dias-

tole with a snap known as the opening snap. The sound is sharp, is widely distributed over the chest, and occurs early after A_2 in severe and later in milder varieties of mitral stenosis. If the patient has severe mitral stenosis with a poor cardiac output and slow flow across the mitral valve, the murmur may be absent or extremely difficult to find, but the opening snap can usually be heard unless the patient has a grossly calcified mitral valve, in which case neither an opening snap nor a murmur can be heard. It is in these cases that echocardiography is particularly valuable in demonstrating the presence of mitral stenosis in the patient with pulmonary venous congestion and with unsuspected mitral stenosis (see below) when the valve has narrowed. If the patient has both mitral stenosis and mitral insufficiency, the dominant features may be the systolic murmur of mitral regurgitation with or without a short diastolic murmur, a delayed opening snap, and a right ventricular lift from a large left atrium that forces the right ventricle anteriorly.

When the valve has narrowed to less than 1.5 cm², the left atrial pressure must rise to maintain normal flow across the valve and a normal cardiac output. This results in a pressure difference between the left atrium and left ventricle during diastole, which may be present in mild cases only during periods of rapid ventricular filling (in mid diastole or following atrial systole) and, in more severe cases, may persist all through diastole. The pressure gradient (and the length of the diastolic murmur) reflects the severity of the mitral stenosis; they persist throughout diastole when the lesion is severe or when the ventricular rate is rapid. The duration is shorter and confined to the middle of diastole when the lesion is slight or the ventricular rate is slow. Both the flow and the pressure gradient must be known in order to compute the valve area according to Gorlin's formula. When the left atrial pressure is raised, the pulmonary venous capillary "wedge" pressure is also raised. The latter increases further as a consequence of incomplete left atrial emptying, when the heart rate increases and the duration of diastole decreases with exercise or tachycardia. In mild cases, the left atrial pressure and the cardiac output may be essentially normal and the patients asymptomatic, but in moderate stenosis (valve area < 1 cm²) with tachycardia or exercise, dyspnea and fatigue appear as the left atrial pressure rises. With severe stenosis, the left atrial pressure is sufficiently high at rest to produce pulmonary venous congestion at rest, worsening rapidly with exercise.

Recumbency at night further increases the pulmonary blood volume, causing orthopnea, paroxysmal nocturnal dyspnea, or actual transudation of fluid into the alveoli, leading to acute pulmonary edema. Severe pulmonary congestion may also be initiated by acute bronchitis or any acute respiratory infection, by development of subacute infective endocarditis, or by recurrence of acute rheumatic carditis. As a result of long-standing pulmonary venous hypertension, anastomoses develop between the pulmonary and bronchial veins in the form of bronchial submucosal varices.

Table 8—1. Differential diagnosis of rheumatic heart disease.

	Mitral Stenosis	Mitral Insufficiency	Aortic Stenosis	Aortic Insufficiency	Tricuspid Stenosis	Tricuspid Insufficiency
Inspection	Malar flush. Precordial bulge and diffuse pulsation in young patients.	Usually forceful apical impulse to left of MCL.	Localized heaving PMI. Carotid pulsations weak, exhibiting slow rise.	Generalized pallor. Strong, abrupt carotid pulsations. Forceful PMI to left of MCL and down. Capillary pulsations.	Giant a wave in jugular pulse with sinus rhythm. Often olive-colored skin (mixed jaundice and local cyanosis).	Large v wave in jugular pulse.
Palpation	"Tapping" sensation over area of expected PMI. Middiastolic and/or presystolic thrill at apex. Right ventricular pulsation left third to fifth ICS parasternally when pulmonary hypertension is present.	Forceful, brisk PMI; systolic thrill over PMI. Pulse normal, small, or slightly collapsing.	Powerful, heaving localized PMI to left of MCL and slightly down. Systolic thrill over aortic area (best felt with patient leaning forward, breath held in maximum expiration). Plateau pulse, small and slowly rising; best appreciated in the carotid pulse.	Apical impulse forceful and displaced significantly to left and down. Water-hammer pulses.	Middiastolic thrill between lower left sternal border and PMI. Presystolic pulsation of liver (sinus rhythm only).	Right ventricular pulsation. Occasionally systolic thrill at lower left sternal edge. Systolic pulsation of liver.
Percussion	Dullness in left third ICS parasternally. ACD normal or slightly enlarged to left only.	ACD increased to left of MCL and slightly down.	ACD slightly enlarged to left and down.	Definite cardiac enlargement to left and down.		Usually cardiac enlargement to left and right.
Heart sounds, rhythm, and blood pressure	Loud snapping M_1. Opening snap along left sternal border or at apex. Atrial fibrillation common. Blood pressure normal.	M_1 normal or buried in murmur. Third heart sound. Delayed opening snap occasionally present. Atrial fibrillation common. Blood pressure normal.	A_2 normal, or delayed and weak; may be absent. Blood pressure normal or systolic pressure normal with high diastolic level. Ejection click occasionally present just preceding murmur.	Sounds normal or A_2 loud. Wide pulse pressure with diastolic pressure < 60 mm Hg.	M_1 often loud.	Atrial fibrillation usually present.
Murmurs: Location and transmission	Sharply localized at or near apex. Graham Steell murmur along lower left sternal border in severe pulmonary hypertension.	Loudest over PMI; transmitted to left axilla, left infrascapular area.	Right second ICS parasternally and/or at apex; heard in carotids and occasionally in upper interscapular area.	Loudest along left sternal border in third to fourth interspace. Heard over aortic area and apex.	Third to fifth ICS along left sternal border out to apex.	As for tricuspid stenosis.
Timing	Onset at opening snap ("middiastolic") with presystolic accentuation if in sinus rhythm. Graham Steell begins with P_2 (immediate diastolic).	Pansystolic: begins with M_1 and ends at or after A_2.	Midsystolic: begins after M_1, ends before A_2, reaches maximum intensity in mid systole.	Begins immediately after aortic second sound and ends before first sound.	As for mitral stenosis.	As for mitral insufficiency.
Character	Low-pitched, rumbling; presystolic murmur merges with loud M_1 in a "crescendo." Graham Steell high-pitched, blowing.	Blowing, high-pitched; occasionally harsh or musical.	Harsh, rough.	Blowing, often faint.	As for mitral stenosis.	Blowing, coarse, or musical.

Optimum auscultatory conditions	After exercise, left lateral recumbency. Bell chest piece lightly applied.	After exercise; diaphragm chest piece.	Patient resting, leaning forward, breath held in full expiration. Bell chest piece, lightly applied.	Slow heart rate; patient leaning forward, breath held in expiration. Diaphragm chest piece.	Murmur usually louder during and at peak of inspiration. Patient recumbent. Bell chest piece.
X-ray and fluoroscopy*	Straight left heart border. Large left atrium sharply indenting esophagus. Large right ventricle and pulmonary artery if pulmonary hypertension present. Elevation of left branches. Occasional calcification seen in mitral valve.	Enlarged left ventricle and left atrium; systolic expansion of left atrium if enlargement not extreme.	Concentric left ventricular hypertrophy. Prominent ascending aorta, small knob. Calcified valve common.	Moderate to great left ventricular hypertrophy. Prominent aortic knob. Strong aortic pulsation on fluoroscopy.	Enlarged right atrium only.
ECG	Broad P waves in standard leads; broad negative phase of diphasic P in V_1. Normal axis. If pulmonary hypertension is present, tall peaked P waves, right axis deviation or right ventricular hypertrophy appear.	Left axis deviation or frank left ventricular hypertrophy. P waves broad, tall, or notched in standard leads; broad negative phase of diphasic P in V_1.	Left ventricular hypertrophy.	Left ventricular hypertrophy.	Wide, tall peaked P waves. Normal axis.
Echocardiography† M mode	Slow early diastolic filling slope, left atrial enlargement, normal to small left ventricle.	Loss of the A wave with only minimal reduction of the early diastolic filling slope, hyperdynamic enlarged left ventricle.	Dense persistent echoes from the aortic valve with poor leaflet excursion, left ventricular hypertrophy (LVH) with preserved contractile function.	Low-frequency diastolic vibrations of the anterior leaflet of the mitral valve and septum, early closure of the mitral valve when condition is severe, dilated left ventricle with normal contractility.	Tricuspid valve thickening, decreased early diastolic filling slope of the tricuspid valve.
Two-dimensional	Maximum diastolic orifice size reduced, subvalvular apparatus foreshortened, variable thickening of other valves.	Portions of the mitral valve fail to collapse in systole.	Above plus poststenotic dilatation of the aorta, restricted opening of the aortic leaflets, bicuspid aortic valve in about 30%.		Above plus enlargement of the right atrium.

Murmur usually becomes louder during inspiration.	
Enlarged right atrium and ventricle.	
Right axis usual.	
Systolic reflux of intravenous contrast agent (saline) from the superior vena cava to the inferior vena cava.	
Same as above.	

*Technetium 99m pertechnetate radioisotope scans and echocardiography are being increasingly used to augment x-ray studies.
†With the assistance of Dr Nelson B Schiller.

A_2 = Aortic second sound   MCL = Midclavicular line
ACD = Area of cardiac disease P_2 = Pulmonary second sound
ICS = Intercostal space   PMI = Point of maximal impulse
M_1 = Mitral first sound

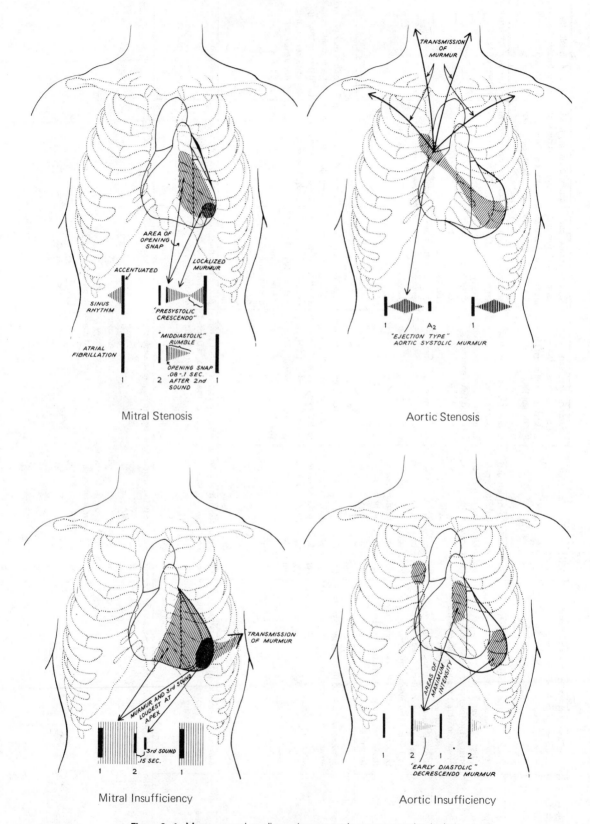

Figure 8–1. Murmurs and cardiac enlargement in common valve lesions.

These often rupture, producing mild or severe hemoptysis.

Fifty to 80% of patients develop paroxysmal or chronic atrial fibrillation that, until the ventricular rate is controlled, may precipitate dyspnea or pulmonary edema. Twenty to 30% of these patients in turn will later have major emboli in the cerebral, visceral, or peripheral arteries as a consequence of thrombus formation in the left atrium.

In a few patients, for unknown reasons, the pulmonary arterioles become narrowed or constricted; this greatly increases the pulmonary artery pressure and the pulmonary vascular resistance and accelerates the development of right ventricular hypertrophy and right ventricular failure. These patients have relatively little dyspnea but experience great fatigue and weakness on exertion because of the markedly reduced cardiac output.

Special diagnostic studies such as echocardiography, left ventricular angiocardiography, dye dilution, and pressure curves from the left ventricle and left atrium during left heart catheterization or left ventricular puncture may prove helpful in difficult cases. Echocardiography is particularly valuable in the diagnosis of mitral stenosis, showing a decreased closing slope of the anterior mitral valve leaflet in mid diastole. The anterior and posterior leaflets are fixed and move together, rather than in opposite directions as is normal. If the left ventricle fills rapidly in association with an increase in its diastolic size, mild and not severe disease is usually inferred. Left atrial size can be determined by echocardiography. Increased size denotes an increased chance of atrial fibrillation or systemic emboli. Mitral valve area can also be estimated. Serial studies are valuable in the postoperative period.

Treatment

Medical treatment for mild mitral stenosis may be feasible if it is thought that the stenosis does not warrant a valvotomy or mitral valve replacement. If the patient has episodic pulmonary venous congestion associated with high sodium intake or excessive physical exertion, therapy can be directed toward avoiding the precipitating factors, and diuretics can also be added. If the patient has paroxysmal atrial fibrillation, this can be treated by quinidine (see p 234), although if severe symptoms occur, there is usually a sufficiently severe stenosis of the mitral valve to warrant valve replacement or valvotomy. (See sections on arrhythmias and cardiac failure, pp 231 and 244.)

Closed mitral valvulotomy is advisable only if symptoms are due to mechanical obstruction of a noncalcific mitral valve and not due to mitral insufficiency or associated aortic valve disease. Most surgeons prefer to perform all mitral valvulotomies under "open bypass," believing that a better repair is possible under direct vision. If the signs of mitral stenosis are present but there is no systolic murmur, mitral regurgitation is exceedingly unlikely. If there is a loud pansystolic murmur at the apex in association with an accentuated,

often early third heart sound, a soft first sound, and no opening snap, the diagnosis of predominant mitral regurgitation is likely even if a short middiastolic murmur can be heard at the apex. Unless hypertension or an aortic valvular lesion is present, left ventricular hypertrophy shown on electrocardiography should make one very cautious in recommending closed operation for mitral stenosis because in this circumstance the mitral valve is probably regurgitant. If there is a moderate systolic murmur at the apex, the diagnosis depends upon a consideration of the total findings.

Replacement of the valve is indicated when combined stenosis and insufficiency are present, or if anatomically the mitral valve is so distorted and calcified that a satisfactory fracture is not possible, even if the operation is performed "open" under cardiopulmonary bypass (see Mitral Insufficiency). Systemic embolism, in the presence of other indications for surgery, probably is an indication for open operation. Systemic emboli in the presence of only mild to moderate disease is not an indication for surgery but should be treated with anticoagulants.

Because the course of mitral stenosis is highly variable and because of the significant mortality rate (3–5%) as well as morbidity associated with mitral surgery, operation is not advised in mild cases with slight exertional dyspnea and fatigue only. Indications for surgery include the following: (1) Signs of mitral stenosis with a pliable valve (opening snap, snapping first sound). (2) Uncontrollable pulmonary edema. (3) Disabling dyspnea and occasionally pulmonary edema. (4) Evidence of pulmonary hypertension with right ventricular hypertrophy and early congestive failure. (5) Increased pulmonary arteriolar resistance, with marked dyspnea and increased P_2. These patients are apt to develop right heart failure and emboli. (6) Right heart failure or tricuspid incompetence (or both) when secondary to marked mitral valve disease.

Problems associated with prosthetic valves are thrombosis, paravalvular leak, endocarditis, and degenerative changes in porcine valves. Continuous anticoagulant therapy is required for patients treated by valve replacement (see Thrombophlebitis, p 292), although such therapy is often discontinued after 3 months in patients with aortic porcine valves.

Cohn LH et al: The in-hospital risk of rereplacement of dysfunctional mitral and aortic valves. *Circulation* 1982;**66:**1153.

Gore JM, Dalen JE: Complications of prosthetic heart valves: When to reoperate. *J Cardiovasc Med* 1983;**8:**1153.

Kotler MN et al: Noninvasive evaluation of normal and abnormal prosthetic valve function. *J Am Coll Cardiol* 1983;**2:**151.

Rutledge R et al: Mitral valve replacement after closed mitral commissurotomy. *Circulation* 1982;**66(Suppl 1):**162.

2. MITRAL INSUFFICIENCY

During ventricular systole, the mitral leaflets do not close normally, and blood is forced back into the atrium as well as through the aortic valve. The net effect is an increased volume of work by the left ventricle. The left atrium enlarges progressively, but the pressure in pulmonary veins and capillaries rises only transiently during exertion. Patients have exertional dyspnea and fatigue that usually progress slowly over many years. Left ventricular failure eventually develops, and orthopnea and paroxysmal dyspnea may appear, followed rapidly by the symptoms of right heart failure.

The chronic course described here is for rheumatic mitral insufficiency; the course may be different and more acute when mitral insufficiency is due to causes other than rheumatic fever. (See Nonrheumatic Mitral Insufficiency, below.)

When heart failure is fully developed, the response to therapy is incomplete, and the patient remains incapacitated. Mitral insufficiency, like stenosis, predisposes to atrial fibrillation; but this arrhythmia is less likely to provoke acute pulmonary congestion, and fewer than 5% of patients have peripheral arterial emboli. Mitral insufficiency especially predisposes to infective endocarditis.

Clinically, mitral insufficiency is characterized by a pansystolic murmur maximal at the apex, radiating to the axilla and occasionally to the base; a hyperdynamic left ventricular impulse and a brisk carotid upstroke; and a prominent third heart sound. When there is slight associated mitral stenosis, a short middiastolic murmur and a late opening snap may be present. The first heart sound is often diminished, but care should be taken to exclude a prolonged PR interval to explain this finding. The magnitude of the left ventricular hypertrophy is usually moderate, both clinically and electrocardiographically, and most of the enlargement of the cardiac shadow seen on x-ray is due to considerable diffuse enlargement of the left atrium. Calcification of the mitral valve is common, though less common than in pure mitral stenosis. The same is true of enlargement of the main pulmonary artery on x-ray.

Hemodynamically, the most striking feature of severe rheumatic mitral insufficiency is an elevated left atrial pressure with a large v wave and a rapid y descent due to rapid filling of the left ventricle. Overwork of the left ventricle ultimately leads to left ventricular failure and reduced cardiac output, but for many years the left ventricular end-diastolic pressure and the cardiac output may be normal at rest, even with considerable increase in left ventricular volume.

Patients with rheumatic mitral insufficiency have systemic emboli and pulmonary hypertension less often—and atrial fibrillation more often—than do patients with mitral stenosis. Because of the frequency of combined mitral stenosis and insufficiency, and because of the difficulty in some patients with fixed valves to specify which is dominant, dogmatic differentiation is unwise.

When mitral insufficiency is combined with aortic stenosis or aortic insufficiency, patients may become symptomatic with lesser hemodynamic abnormalities of both valves than if the valves were diseased individually.

Nonrheumatic mitral insufficiency. Mitral insufficiency may be due to causes other than rheumatic fever and have different clinical findings and a different clinical course. The most common are those secondary to mitral valve prolapse or rupture of the chordae tendineae, usually secondary to infective endocarditis but occasionally occurring spontaneously or after trauma, and those secondary to infective endocarditis with perforation of a cusp.

Mitral valve prolapse is a genetic disorder of collagen, usually asymptomatic but sometimes associated with nonspecific chest pain, dyspnea, and fatigue. It is characterized by mitral insufficiency associated with a late systolic murmur, a nonejection midsystolic click, and a characteristic echocardiographic finding of scalloping of the posterior mitral valve leaflet in late systole. Its significance is in dispute because of the frequency (about 10%) with which it is diagnosed in healthy young men and women and the high frequency with which prolapse has been found in unselected cardiac patients who have had left ventriculograms. Although it is probable that mitral valve prolapse has been overdiagnosed when the diagnosis is based solely on echocardiographic findings, recent studies indicate that this lesion may not be as benign as previously thought. A spectrum of the disease exists, and one should distinguish between patients who have mitral insufficiency and those who have only a midsystolic click. Follow-up studies have shown that the latter is almost always benign but that patients with a late or pansystolic murmur may develop worsening of mitral insufficiency and infective endocarditis over a period of years in 3–10% of cases. Sudden death is uncommon and is usually related to supraventricular arrhythmias and ventricular tachycardias. The arrhythmias may be revealed by ambulatory echocardiographic monitoring. If they are of the complex variety, they should be treated vigorously (see p 237).

Papillary muscle dysfunction or necrosis following acute myocardial infarction is less common. When the mitral insufficiency is due to papillary dysfunction, it may subside as the infarction heals. Other causes include cardiac tumors, especially left atrial myxoma, and surgically acquired mitral insufficiency. In contrast to rheumatic mitral insufficiency, the other varieties usually develop cardiac failure more rapidly, are in sinus rhythm rather than atrial fibrillation, occur in males more often than females, have little or no enlargement of the left atrium, have no calcification of the mitral valve, have no associated mitral stenosis, and often present an angiographic appearance that may be helpful. The difference in the clinical picture may be due to the fact that nonrheumatic causes of mitral insufficiency are more acute and patients get into trouble within months or 1–2 years, whereas in rheumatic mitral insufficiency the course develops over a period of many years. Because the course of nonrheumatic mitral insufficiency may be more fulminant, surgical treatment with replacement of the valves is often a more urgent consideration.

Echocardiography is valuable in demonstrating

disruption of chordal support of the mitral valve with prolapse of either or both mitral valve leaflets; the diagnostic finding is posterior prolapse of the leaflet in systole, usually associated with early diastolic anterior motion of the posterior leaflet. Two-dimensional echocardiography (the long axis view is best) may show systolic "whipping" of the posterior leaflet into the left atrium in flail mitral valve with acute severe mitral incompetence. Such patients may have marked systolic expansion of the left atrium associated with left atrial volume overload. The magnitude of regurgitation can be estimated by cardiac gated pool imaging. Most patients with mitral valve prolapse have few or no symptoms unless they have severe mitral incompetence. This is to be contrasted with the echocardiographic findings of the midsystolic click, late systolic murmur syndrome (Barlow's syndrome), in which there is late systolic prolapse (notching of the posterior mitral valve leaflet) without the diagnostic early anterior motion seen in chordal rupture.

Treatment

Medical treatment can be used for minimal left ventricular failure or arrhythmias if the lesion is considered sufficiently mild not to warrant cardiac surgery (see references under Mitral Stenosis, p 191). Vasodilators may improve left ventricular function prior to valve replacement in urgent situations (see also p 249).

Reconstructive operations on the mitral valve are infrequent today and are usually performed for a perforated leaflet in infective endocarditis or, rarely, because of ruptured chordae. When the disability is great enough to warrant the surgical risk, open heart surgery using cardiopulmonary bypass is almost always required, with replacement of the diseased valve with a prosthetic device. The choice of valves is related to durability and the likelihood of obstruction and embolus formation—and also depends in part on the surgeon's preference. Porcine valves are valuable in patients in whom anticoagulant therapy is contraindicated or unwise, because thromboembolic phenomena may be less with these tissue valves. However, porcine valves may degenerate after 5 or 6 years, and one should hesitate to use them in patients under 30 years of age.

Late complications with all of the valves have included degenerative changes, endocarditis, and displacement of the valve. In addition to changes in the valve itself, late complications of valve replacement include systemic embolization, leaks of the valve, hemolytic anemia, and, occasionally, sudden death.

Prognosis

The early and late embolic complications of mitral insufficiency must be recognized, but the surgical mortality rate has declined with greater experience. The fate of the prosthesis over the long term is uncertain. Follow-up studies have shown considerable improvement in surviving patients, including reversal of pulmonary and left atrial hypertension. Usually, however, some hemodynamic abnormality persists.

Greenberg BH et al: Arterial dilators in mitral regurgitation: Effects on rest and exercise hemodynamics and long-term clinical follow-up. *Circulation* 1982;**65**:181.

McGoon MD et al: Aortic and mitral valve incompetence: Long-term follow-up (10 to 19 years) of patients treated with the Starr-Edwards prosthesis. *J Am Coll Cardiol* 1984;**3**:930.

Nestico PF et al: Mitral annular calcification: Clinical, pathophysiology, and echocardiographic review. *Am Heart J* 1984;**107**:989.

Oliveira DBG et al: Chordal rupture. 1. Aetiology and natural history. 2. Comparison between repair and replacement. *Br Heart J* 1983;**50**:312, 318.

Selzer A: Nonrheumatic mitral regurgitation: Clinical aspects. *Primary Cardiol* (March) 1982;**8**:119.

Waller BF et al: Etiology of clinically isolated, severe, chronic, pure mitral regurgitation: Analysis of 97 patients over 30 years of age having mitral valve replacement. *Am Heart J* 1982;**104(2–Part 1)**:276.

3. AORTIC STENOSIS

Aortic valvular stenosis may follow rheumatic fever, may be congenital and bicuspid, or may be degenerative and calcific, especially in older people. Progressive calcification may occur, leading rapidly to severe aortic stenosis. Valvular stenosis must be distinguished from supravalvular obstruction and from outflow obstruction of the left ventricular infundibulum (muscular subaortic obstruction; idiopathic hypertrophic subaortic stenosis; see p 266). The former is congenital and uncommon; surgical experience is limited, and results depend on the findings in the ascending aorta. In the latter variety, the obstruction may be intermittent, aggravated by digitalis or inotropic influences, and relieved by propranolol (Inderal) or sedation. If patients are symptomatic, have severe obstruction to left ventricular flow, and achieve no benefit from propranolol, surgery is advised. Myotomy and limited resection of the hypertrophied muscle have produced gratifying results.

Over 80% of patients with aortic stenosis are men. Slight narrowing, roughened valves, or aortic dilatation may produce the typical murmur and thrill without causing significant hemodynamic effects. In mild-to-moderate cases, the characteristic signs are a systolic ejection murmur at the aortic area transmitted to the neck and apex and a systolic ejection click at the aortic area; in severe cases, a palpable left ventricular heave, often reversed splitting of the second sound, and a weak to absent aortic second sound (see Table 8–1). The chest film reveals dilatation and, frequently, calcification of the ascending aorta in valvular stenosis. When the valve area is less than one-fifth of normal, ventricular systole becomes prolonged and the typical plateau pulse develops, characterized by a delayed upstroke (in the carotid artery). At this stage, exertional dyspnea, fatigue, and pounding of the heart are noted. Cardiac output is ultimately markedly reduced, so that patients have angina pectoris, great weakness or giddiness on exertion, or syncope. Survival beyond 3 years is uncommon if any of these appear. Many patients develop myocardial infarction, and 30% or more die suddenly. The stenosis may be valvular, subvalvular, or supravalvular, requiring identification and differential surgical procedures. Eighty-five percent of patients with significant aortic stenosis may be identified by the combination of (1) slow carotid upstroke, (2) left ventricular heave, and (3) left ventricular hypertrophy as shown on electrocardiography. Syncope may be due to arrhythmias as well as to decreased cerebral perfusion resulting from increased blood flow to the exercising muscles. There is an increased incidence of sudden death in patients with severe aortic stenosis.

Angina pectoris frequently occurs in aortic stenosis. One-third to one-half of patients with calcific aortic stenosis and angina have significant coronary disease, whereas coronary disease is noted at only half this rate in the absence of angina. The prognosis is worse with coexisting coronary disease. Coronary arteriograms should be obtained whenever angina is present, and some authorities believe that they should be performed in all cases of aortic stenosis being considered for surgery.

Most patients require complete preoperative study, including right and left heart catheterization and aortic, coronary, and left ventricular angiograms, to evaluate the presence and degree of associated valve regurgitation and coronary stenoses. Coronary angiography is probably not needed if angina pectoris is not a symptom, because of the low prevalence of coronary disease in this group of patients. Echocardiography is helpful in demonstrating impaired or absent aortic valve motion with increased reflectance of the valve structures, increased aortic root diameter, and increased septal and left ventricular posterior wall thickness. Ultrasound is less reliable in estimating the severity of the aortic stenosis.

Hemodynamically, the cardinal feature of valvular aortic stenosis is a systolic gradient across the aortic valve (systolic pressure difference between the left ventricle and the aorta). As the valve area narrows (size can be estimated if both gradient and flow across the valve are known), the gradient increases; the elevated left ventricular systolic pressure causes considerable concentric left ventricular hypertrophy, which allows a normal cardiac output until relatively late in the course of the disease. The left ventricular end-diastolic pressure may be elevated because of decreased compliance of the ventricle, even with normal cardiac output and no or minimal symptoms. Later, left atrial pressure rises with exercise, left ventricular volume increases and left ventricular failure may occur, and the cardiac output is reduced, especially with exercise. At this point, syncope on unaccustomed effort, left ventricular failure, and angina pectoris all may coexist as a triad, and a critical aortic valve area of 0.6–0.7 cm² is reached. Syncope, of course, can be due to other causes such as ventricular tachyarrhythmia, which may cause sudden death.

The arterial pulse characteristically is slow-rising, is of low amplitude, and has a well-defined anacrotic shoulder on the ascending limb—low in severe and high in mild aortic stenosis.

Echocardiography is less valuable in aortic stenosis than in mitral stenosis.

Treatment

Medical treatment for aortic stenosis is usually limited to serial observations of the patient, including yearly chest x-rays, ECGs, and echocardiograms, to facilitate early recognition of left ventricular hypertrophy, enlargement, or failure; arrhythmias; and progressive aortic valve calcification. When cardiac failure occurs, the usual medical measures for treatment of failure should not be continued; it is wise at this point to consider aortic valve replacement.

The indications for surgical correction of aortic stenosis are progressive left ventricular failure, attacks of syncope due to cerebral ischemia, angina pectoris when it is thought to be due to the decreased cardiac output of aortic stenosis and not to associated coronary artery disease, or hemodynamic (aortic valve area < 1 cm²) and clinical evidence of severe aortic stenosis even in patients with few symptoms. In contrast to dominant aortic insufficiency with a large left ventricle and depressed systolic function, valvular replacement probably should not be instituted before the onset of symptoms in aortic stenosis. When combined coronary bypass surgery and aortic valve replacement are necessary, the surgical mortality rate is at least double that occurring with aortic valve replacement alone. In the presence of both mitral and aortic stenosis, surgical correction or replacement of both valves can be performed at the same procedure.

Follow-up of patients who have had valve replacement reveals an early surgical mortality rate of 3% and a late mortality rate of 10–15%. Good results occur in 85% of the surviving patients. Striking hemodynamic improvement can be documented in those judged clinically to have a good result.

In the first month following surgery, arrhythmias are the most common cause of death, whereas during 5 years following surgery the most common causes of death are ventricular fibrillation and cardiac failure from coronary disease.

Lytle BW et al: Replacement of aortic valve combined with myocardial revascularization: Determinants of early and late risk for 500 patients, 1967–1981. *Circulation* 1983;**68**:1149.

Wagner S, Selzer A: Patterns of progression of aortic stenosis: A longitudinal hemodynamic study. *Circulation* 1982;**65**:709.

4. AORTIC INSUFFICIENCY

For many years the only sign may be a soft aortic diastolic murmur, ie, "auscultatory" aortic insufficiency, indicating regurgitation of a small amount of blood through the incompetent leaflets during diastole. As the valve deformity increases, larger and larger amounts regurgitate, diastolic blood pressure falls, the pulse wave assumes its characteristic contour, and the left ventricle progressively enlarges. This is the stage of "dynamic" aortic insufficiency. Many patients remain asymptomatic even at this point or experience exertional dyspnea. Left ventricular failure often begins abruptly with acute pulmonary edema or recurrent paroxysmal nocturnal dyspnea and orthopnea; fatigue, weakness, and exertional dyspnea are then incapacitating. The murmur of aortic insufficiency may be absent in the presence of severe heart failure and may reappear following treatment. A_2 is usually increased in intensity. Angina pectoris or protracted chest pain simulating angina appears in many. The heart failure is relatively refractory to treatment and is the chief cause of death. Ten to 15% of patients with aortic insufficiency die suddenly.

Hemodynamically, because of the large volume load upon the left ventricle, patients show a large stroke output but no abnormality of the minute cardiac output or left ventricular end-diastolic pressure until late in the course of the disease. The latter (unlike aortic stenosis) remains normal until late in the disease and may abruptly rise when failure occurs and be reflected in a rise in left atrial pressure. The left ventricular volume is increased, but compliance does not decrease until late, when the combination of decreased compliance and left ventricular failure raises the left ventricular end-diastolic pressure. Abnormal left ventricular systolic function, as manifested by ejection fraction and end-systolic left ventricular dimension, is a late sign of aortic regurgitation; it can assist in the timing of surgery and is predictive of survival after valvular replacement. The arterial pulse characteristically has a rapid rise and fall (Corrigan's pulse), with an elevated systolic and lowered diastolic pressure and thus a widened pulse pressure. A mid- or late-diastolic low-pitched murmur (Austin Flint murmur) may be heard in advanced aortic insufficiency as forward flow through the mitral valve and backward flow through the aortic valve meet and set up turbulence. Echocardiography is helpful in establishing the presence of aortic valve insufficiency by demonstrating fluttering of the mitral valve leaflet during diastole and in determining ejection fraction, left ventricular volume, and end-systolic dimension. The magnitude of the aortic insufficiency is best quantified by supra-aortic cineangiography, but it can be estimated semiquantitatively by cardiac gated pool imaging. This measurement is less valuable when aortic stenosis is also present. Early closure of the mitral valve by echocardiography is a valuable sign of severe aortic insufficiency.

Nonrheumatic aortic insufficiency. Although rheumatic aortic insufficiency is the most common variety, other causes must be considered such as congenital (bicuspid) aortic valve, dissection of the aorta, infective endocarditis, hypertension, rheumatoid arthritis, ankylosing spondylitis, syphilis, and ruptured aneurysm of the sinus of Valsalva. When aortic insufficiency develops acutely (as in dissecting aorta or perforated cusp during infective endocarditis), left ventricular failure may develop rapidly, and surgery may be urgently required. Differentiation of the clinical pictures of acute and chronic aortic insufficiency is as important as it is in acute and chronic mitral insufficiency. Patients with acute aortic insufficiency may not have the large dilated left ventricle that is so common in chronic aortic insufficiency, and acute left ventricular failure may occur in these individuals with great rapidity.

Treatment

Aortic insufficiency usually requires prosthetic replacement of the entire valve. The substantial surgical risk (3–5%) and the uncertain prognosis limit the indications to patients with class III or class IV lesions. The ideal time for replacement is uncertain because many patients survive for 5–10 years on medical treatment despite substantial insufficiency and left ventricular hypertrophy. However, the operative morbidity and mortality rates are significantly greater and the long-term benefits are fewer if surgery is delayed until there is considerable increase in left ventricular end-systolic volume and left ventricular dysfunction with decrease in the ejection fraction. Serial echocardiographic studies may document increasing left ventricular size and help to time aortic valve replacement.

When left ventricular failure develops, it is rarely wise to continue conventional medical measures for the treatment of cardiac failure except as a preliminary to surgical evaluation and treatment or when surgical treatment is not feasible. Undue prolongation of medical treatment may increase the risk and decrease the benefit of operation. Continuous anticoagulants are required unless a homograft or porcine heterograft has been used.

Aortic insufficiency that appears or worsens after infective endocarditis may lead to severe cardiac failure in weeks or months even though the infection is controlled. Surgical removal of the valve is indicated even during the infection if cardiac failure worsens despite medical treatment. Patients should be observed closely for many months after endocarditis.

Replacement of the valve may become a surgical emergency if perforation of a cusp or rupture of the sinus of Valsalva or of the subaortic valvular structure occurs, causing acute severe left ventricular failure. Great judgment is required to determine the timing of and need for physiologic studies.

Bonow RO et al: Timing of operation for chronic aortic regurgitation. Am J Cardiol 1982;**50**:325.

DePace NL et al: Comparison of echocardiography and angiography in determining the cause of severe aortic regurgitation. Br Heart J 1984;**51**:36.

5. TRICUSPID STENOSIS

Most patients with tricuspid stenosis are women, and mitral valve disease is usually present also. Tricuspid stenosis acts as a mechanical block to the return of blood to the heart, and the systemic venous engorgement is analogous to the pulmonary venous engorgement caused by mitral stenosis. Tricuspid stenosis should be suspected when "right heart failure" appears early in the course of mitral disease, marked by hepatomegaly, ascites, and dependent edema. These are more prominent when atrial fibrillation is present. Severe fatigue is usual. Cardiac cirrhosis develops early, and patients acquire a characteristic complexion that is a blend of peripheral cyanosis and slight jaundice. Careful examination is needed to differentiate the typical diastolic rumble along the lower left sternal border from the murmur of mitral stenosis. In the presence of sinus rhythm, a presystolic liver pulsation can be found in half of the patients. In atrial fibrillation, only the slow emptying of the jugular vein during diastole is noted. A giant right atrium on a chest film or angiogram is frequently found in tricuspid valve disease.

Hemodynamically, a diastolic pressure gradient of 5–15 mm Hg is found across the tricuspid valve between the right atrium and the right ventricle in conjunction with a raised pressure in the right atrium and jugular veins, with prominent a waves and a slow y descent because of slow right ventricular filling. Hepatic enlargement, ascites, and dependent edema develop when the mean right atrial pressure is about 15 mm Hg. The cardiac output is usually low, but it rises slightly with exercise.

Echocardiography may sometimes allow recognition of tricuspid stenosis by the decreased slope of tricuspid valve filling and emptying.

Treatment

Congenital tricuspid stenosis is associated with an underdeveloped right ventricle and does not lend itself to valvotomy. Diversion of the superior vena caval flow into the right lung is a relatively safe closed procedure that confers a sizable degree of palliation.

Acquired tricuspid stenosis may be amenable to valvotomy under direct vision, but it usually requires a prosthetic valve replacement.

Daniels SJ, Mintz GS, Kotler MN: Rheumatic tricuspid valve disease: 2-dimensional echocardiographic, hemodynamic, and angiographic correlations. *Am J Cardiol* 1983;**51**:492.

Guyer DE et al: Comparison of the echocardiographic and hemodynamic diagnosis of rheumatic tricuspid stenosis. *J Am Coll Cardiol* 1984;**3**:1135.

6. TRICUSPID INSUFFICIENCY

Tricuspid insufficiency affects the right ventricle just as mitral insufficiency affects the left ventricle. Tricuspid insufficiency may occur in a variety of situations other than disease of the tricuspid valve itself. The most common is right ventricular overload resulting from left ventricular failure due to any of several causes but chiefly to coronary heart disease, hypertensive heart failure, cardiomyopathy, and mitral or aortic valve disease. Tricuspid insufficiency occurs in association with right ventricular infarction due to stenosis or occlusion of the right coronary artery and inferior myocardial infarction. It is common in infective endocarditis in intravenous drug abusers, but in these situations it is due to disease on the tricuspid valve itself. The symptoms and signs of organic tricuspid valve disease due to rheumatic heart disease are identical with those resulting from right ventricular failure due to any cause. In the presence of mitral disease, the tricuspid valvular lesion can be suspected on the basis of a relatively early onset of right heart failure and a harsh systolic murmur along the lower left sternal border which is separate from the mitral murmur and which often increases in intensity during and just after inspiration.

Hemodynamically, tricuspid insufficiency is characterized by a prominent regurgitant systolic (v) wave in the right atrium and jugular venous pulse, with a rapid y descent and a small or absent x descent, and by regurgitation of blood from the right ventricle to the right atrium during systole as seen in right ventricular angiography. The regurgitant wave, like the systolic murmur, is increased with inspiration, and its size depends upon the size of the right atrium. When right ventricular hypertrophy and right ventricular failure occur, a right ventricular S_3 (also known as a right atrial gallop) may be present. The volume of regurgitation can be estimated by right ventricular angiography.

Treatment

Replacement of the tricuspid valve is being performed with decreasing frequency in recent years. Tricuspid insufficiency secondary to severe mitral valve disease may regress when only the mitral valve is replaced.

• • •

Prognosis of Rheumatic Heart Disease (Untreated)

Recurrent rheumatic fever may produce fatal heart failure at any time, and infective endocarditis is a constant threat. However, many patients may remain asymptomatic for years.

A. Mitral Stenosis: In general, patients with severe mitral stenosis die of intractable congestive failure in their 30s or 40s after a prolonged period of disability.

B. Mitral Insufficiency and Aortic Valve Lesions: These patients become symptomatic later in life, but death occurs within a few years after the onset of symptoms of congestive heart failure.

C. Aortic Stenosis: When angina, left ventricular failure, or syncope is present, death usually occurs within 3 years.

D. Tricuspid Lesions: These are usually associated with mitral valve disease. The prognosis is surprisingly good, with survival for up to 10 years after the onset of edema, but patients are incapacitated by fatigue.

INFECTIVE ENDOCARDITIS*

Essentials of Diagnosis

- Fever.
- Heart murmur.
- Embolic phenomena.
- Splenomegaly.
- Anemia.
- Blood culture positive.

General Considerations

Infective endocarditis implies the presence of microorganisms (bacteria, fungi, chlamydiae, etc) in lesions of the endocardium. Traditionally, endocarditis was called "acute" or "subacute," but it is more desirable to group endocarditis according to the causative microorganism. The traditional "subacute" infective endocarditis (SIE) has an insidious onset, with slow deterioration, anemia, valve damage leading to heart failure, cachexia, and death. It is superimposed mainly on preexisting congenital, rheumatic, or calcific abnormalities of the heart. Bacteremia occurs frequently with dental procedures and endoscopic or other manipulations of the respiratory, urinary, or gastrointestinal tracts. Viridans (50%) and fecal (10%) streptococci are among the commoner causative agents, but virtually any microorganism can cause endocarditis.

The initial event is an abnormality in blood flow resulting in endothelial damage. A thrombotic lesion develops, consisting of fibrin, platelets, and leukocytes. Any microorganisms circulating in the blood may be implanted into this lesion to form a vegetation, and pieces of vegetation may break off, sending emboli to various organs and sites. Immune complex nephritis often develops and may lead to renal failure. Mycotic aneurysms and septic infarcts result from dissemination of infected vegetation.

The traditional "acute" infective endocarditis (AIE) is a rapidly progressive, destructive infection of normal, abnormal, or prosthetic valves, usually developing in the course of intense bacteremia, intravenous narcotic abuse, surgery on infected tissues, urologic procedures, or insertion of a prosthesis. Staphylococci and gram-negative enteric bacteria are common pathogens. Among intravenous drug users, staphylococci, *Candida,* enterococci, and gram-negative bacteria are prominent causes of endocarditis.

Acute endocarditis may produce large, friable vegetations, severe embolic episodes with metastatic abscess formation, and rapid perforation, tearing, or destruction of the affected valves or rupture of chordae tendineae. Nonbacterial thrombotic endocarditis is found post mortem in some patients dying of chronic illness, notably cancer. It is often clinically silent during life.

Clinical Findings

A. Symptoms and Signs: Fever is present in most cases, but afebrile periods may occur, especially in the aged. Any or all of the following may occur also: night sweats, chills, malaise, fatigue, anorexia, weight loss; myalgias, arthralgia, or redness and swelling of joints; sudden visual disturbances, aphasia, or hemiplegia due to cerebral emboli; pain in the abdomen, chest, or flanks due to mesenteric, splenic, pulmonary, or renal emboli; nosebleeds, easy bruisability, and symptoms of heart failure. In AIE, the course is more fulminating, and the patient is very toxic.

In SIE, evidence of rheumatic, congenital, or calcific heart disease is often present. Findings include tachycardia; splenomegaly; petechiae of the skin, mucous membranes, and ocular fundi, or beneath the nails as "splinter hemorrhages"; clubbing of the fingers and toes; pallor or a yellowish-brown tint of the skin; neurologic residual effects of cerebral emboli; and tender red nodules of the finger or toe pads. Heart murmurs may be "insignificant" in infection of the tricuspid and pulmonary valve, where recurrent pulmonary infarction suggesting pneumonia may be prominent. The clinical picture is often atypical in older persons; fever, chills, and heart murmurs may be absent, but stroke or renal failure may be prominent.

AIE presents as a severe infection associated with chills, high fever, prostration, and multiple, serious embolic phenomena. These may be superimposed on the antecedent causative infection (eg, pneumonia) or may appear abruptly following instrumentation, surgery, or self-injection of narcotics. Heart murmurs may change rapidly, and heart failure occurs early.

Infective endocarditis may develop during "prophylactic" or inadequate therapeutic antibiotic administration. In these circumstances the onset is "masked," and a sudden embolic episode, the appearance of petechiae, unexplained heart failure, changing murmurs, or fever may be the first clue.

B. Laboratory Findings: In suspected infective endocarditis, take 2 blood cultures daily for 2–3 days. Within 2–7 days of incubation, 80–90% of these cultures will grow organisms and permit specific drug selection. In AIE, take 2 or 3 cultures during the emergency workup, then begin antibiotic treatment. In the presence of repeated negative blood cultures (eg, in uremic patients), bone marrow should be cultured.

The administration of an antimicrobial drug may interfere with positive blood cultures for 7–10 days.

Normochromic anemia, a markedly elevated sedimentation rate, variable leukocytosis, microscopic hematuria, proteinuria, and casts are commonly present in infective endocarditis. Nitrogen retention may be the first clue, especially in older patients. Rheumatoid factor is demonstrable in the serum of 50–60% of cases of infective endocarditis of more than 6 weeks' standing. Echocardiography may define large vegetations.

Complications

The complications of infective endocarditis include peripheral arterial emboli (producing hemiplegias or aphasia; infarction of the bowel, kidney,

---

*By Ernest Jawetz, MD, PhD.

lung, or spleen; or acute arterial insufficiency of an arm or leg), congestive heart failure, uremia, hemorrhagic tendency, anemia, and metastatic abscess formation. Abscesses may cause relapse or lack of response to therapy.

Differential Diagnosis

Infective endocarditis must be differentiated from various seemingly primary disease states. Hemiplegia, intractable heart failure, anemia, a bleeding tendency, or uremia may be caused by infective endocarditis. If a patient presenting with any of these illnesses has fever or a heart murmur, blood cultures should be taken.

Specific diseases that require differentiation are lymphomas, leukemias, acute rheumatic fever, disseminated lupus erythematosus, polyarteritis nodosa, chronic meningococcemia, brucellosis, septic thrombophlebitis, disseminated tuberculosis, mycoses, and nonbacterial thrombotic endocarditis or various chronic wasting diseases.

Infective endocarditis may present as an exacerbation of an existing infection. It can be recognized only by noting rapid clinical deterioration, bacteremia, the appearance or sudden change of heart murmurs, heart failure, and major embolic accidents, especially those affecting the central nervous system.

Prevention

A. Medical Measures: Some cases of endocarditis arise after dental procedures or surgery of the oropharynx or genitourinary tract. Patients with known cardiac anomalies who are to have any of these procedures should be prepared in one of the following ways, although failures sometimes occur.

1. For dental and upper respiratory tract procedures–

a. Oral–Penicillin V, 2 g 1 hour before procedure and 1 g 6 hours later. For penicillin allergy, give erythromycin, 1 g 1 hour before procedure and 0.5 g 6 hours later.

b. Parenteral–Ampicillin, 1 g, or penicillin G, 2 million units intramuscularly or intravenously, plus gentamicin, 1.5 mg/kg intramuscularly or intravenously, each given 1 hour before procedure and again 8 hours later. In penicillin allergy, give vancomycin, 1 g intravenously as a 1-hour infusion beginning 1 hour before procedure, and repeat once 8 hours later.

2. For gastrointestinal or genitourinary tract procedures–

a. Parenteral–Ampicillin, 2 g intravenously or intramuscularly, plus gentamicin, 1.5 mg/kg intravenously or intramuscularly, each given 1 hour before procedure and once 8 hours later. In penicillin allergy, give vancomycin as above, alone or with gentamicin as above.

b. Oral–Oral prophylaxis (amoxicillin, 3 g 1 hour before procedure and 1.5 g 6 hours later) is probably less desirable than parenteral prophylaxis.

Many alternative regimens have been proposed. For none of them is there absolute proof of efficacy. Any form of antimicrobial prophylaxis may favor the selection of resistant organisms in the normal flora, with subsequent implantation of such organisms in infective endocarditis.

B. Surgical Measures: Surgery is warranted for the prevention of infective endocarditis in selected patients with surgically correctable congenital lesions (patent ductus arteriosus) or acquired lesions (symptomatic aortic and mitral valvular disease). Preoperative antibiotics should be instituted as above. Mycotic aneurysms also must be treated surgically.

Treatment

A. Specific Measures: The most important consideration in the treatment of infective endocarditis is a bactericidal concentration of antibiotics in contact with the infecting organism, which is often localized in avascular tissues or in vegetations. Penicillins, because of their high degree of bactericidal activity against many bacteria that produce endocarditis and because of their low toxicity, are by far the most useful drugs. Synergistic combinations of antibiotics have proved valuable at times. Few cases have been cured by bacteriostatic drugs used alone.

Positive blood cultures are invaluable to confirm the diagnosis and to guide treatment with tests of susceptibility of the infecting organism to various antibiotics or combinations of antibiotics. See ¶ B, p 197, for blood culture directions.

Note: **Control of antimicrobial treatment.** Negative blood cultures are a minimal initial requirement of effective therapy. An assay of serum bactericidal activity is the best guide to support the selection of drugs and the daily dose after treatment has been started. During therapy, the patient's serum diluted 1:5 or 1:10 should (at least during part of the interval between drug doses) be rapidly bactericidal in vitro under standardized laboratory conditions for the organisms originally grown from the patient's bloodstream. Drugs are initially administered by the intravenous or intramuscular route. If clinical and laboratory response is good, drugs may later be given orally, under control of serum bactericidal tests.

Specific antimicrobial regimens are as follows:

1. Endocarditis due to *S viridans* (*Streptococcus salivarius*, *Streptococcus mutans*, *Streptococcus sanguis*, *Streptococcus bovis*)–Viridans streptococci (usually originating in the oropharynx) are the infecting organisms in over 60% of spontaneously arising cases of typical slow-onset endocarditis. Most such organisms are susceptible to 0.1–1 unit/mL penicillin G in vitro. Penicillin G, 5–10 million units daily (in divided doses given as a bolus every 4 hours into an intravenous infusion) continued for 3–4 weeks, is generally curative. Enhanced bactericidal action is obtained if an aminoglycoside (eg, gentamicin, 3–5 mg/kg/d intramuscularly) is added during the first 10–14 days of treatment. More resistant organisms may require daily doses of penicillin G of 20–50 million units. Probenecid, 0.5 g orally 3 times daily, further enhances blood levels of penicillin by interfering with its tubular excretion.

2. Endocarditis due to *Streptococcus faecalis* –This organism causes 5–10% of cases of spontaneously arising endocarditis and occasionally also follows abuse of intravenous drugs. Treatment requires the simultaneous use of penicillin and an aminoglycoside. Penicillin G, 20–40 million units daily, or ampicillin, 6–12 g daily, is given in divided doses as bolus injections every 2–4 hours into an intravenous infusion. An aminoglycoside (eg, gentamicin, 5 mg/kg/d) selected by appropriate laboratory test is injected intramuscularly 2–3 times daily in divided doses. The cell wall-inhibitory drug (eg, penicillin, vancomycin) enhances the entry of the aminoglycoside and permits killing of the enterococci. Treatment must be continued for 4–5 weeks; cephalosporins cannot be substituted for penicillins.

3. Endocarditis due to staphylococci *(Staphylococcus aureus, Staphylococcus epidermidis)* –If the infecting staphylococci are *not* penicillinase producers, penicillin G, 10–20 million units in divided doses, is the treatment of choice. If the staphylococci produce penicillinase, nafcillin, 8–12 g daily, given as a bolus every 2 hours into an intravenous infusion, is the drug of choice. In probable or established hypersensitivity to penicillin, the alternative drug is vancomycin, 2–3 g intravenously daily in divided doses every 4 hours. This treatment must be continued for 5–6 weeks, and a frequent careful check for metastatic lesions or abscesses must be conducted (and lesions drained) to avoid reseeding of cardiac sites from such reservoirs of infectious organisms.

4. Endocarditis due to gram-negative bacteria –The susceptibility of these organisms to antimicrobial drugs varies so greatly that effective treatment must be based on laboratory tests. An aminoglycoside (gentamicin, 5–7 mg/kg/d; amikacin, 15 mg/kg/d; or tobramycin, 5–7 mg/kg/d) is often combined with a cell wall-inhibitory drug (ticarcillin, 18 g/d; cefotaxime or cefoperazone, 12 g/d) to enhance penetration of the aminoglycoside. Laboratory guidance is essential not only for susceptibility tests but also to establish the presence of sufficient bactericidal activity in serum obtained during treatment. The dosage of aminoglycosides must be adjusted if renal function is impaired, as determined by serum creatinine levels. Suggested modifications in time-dose regimens for aminoglycosides and other nephrotoxic drugs are given in Chapter 29. Each of these drugs can also cause eighth nerve damage, and the patient should be monitored often for hearing loss and vestibular function.

Whenever large doses of penicillins or cephalosporins are given, the following must be considered: (a) Each million units of potassium penicillin G contains about 1.7 meq of potassium, which might give rise to toxicity, especially in the presence of renal failure. (b) At very high concentrations of penicillin, there is enough diffusion into the central nervous system to cause neurotoxicity. (c) With *any* intravenous infusions of long duration, there is a significant risk of superinfection; to minimize this possibility, injection sites must be changed every 48 hours and must be kept scrupulously clean. Prolonged high concentrations of antimicrobials are irritating and favor the development of thrombophlebitis. Therefore, bolus injection of a portion of the total daily dose over a 20- to 30-minute period (through a Volutron or similar device) every 2–6 hours into a continuous infusion (drip) of 5% glucose in water is preferable to a steady flow of antibiotic.

5. Endocarditis due to yeasts and fungi –This type rarely arises spontaneously but is seen with increasing frequency in abusers of intravenous drugs, after cardiac surgery, or in immunosuppressed individuals. *Candida albicans, Candida parapsilosis,* and *Torulopsis glabrata* are among the agents encountered commonly, but virtually any fungus, including *Aspergillus* and even *Histoplasma,* can be seen. Fungal endocarditis is often associated with bulky, friable vegetations that tend to produce massive emboli in large arteries. *Candida* endocarditis has occurred early after the insertion of prosthetic valves, and the diagnosis may be based on the finding of pseudohyphae in emboli surgically removed from large vessels. Blood cultures may require 1–3 weeks to grow these organisms.

The drugs most active against yeasts and fungi are amphotericin B (0.4–0.8 mg/kg/d) and flucytosine (150 mg/kg/d orally). However, these drugs rarely eradicate fungal endocarditis. Early surgical excision of the involved valve tissue during antifungal therapy and continuation of the latter for several weeks offer the best opportunity for cure.

6. Prosthetic valve endocarditis –This may occur early, within days after insertion of a valve, and then is usually caused by staphylococci, gram-negative enteric bacteria, or *Candida*. The most common organism may be *S epidermidis* resistant to lactamase-resistant penicillins (eg, nafcillin); it requires treatment with vancomycin plus rifampin.

Alternatively, prosthetic valve endocarditis may occur after insertion of the prosthesis, presumably as a consequence of spontaneous bacteremia. Antimicrobial treatment alone rarely succeeds in eradicating the infection. Drugs aimed at the infecting organisms are given before, during, and after removal of the infected prosthesis and its replacement. There is a substantial mortality rate (over 10%) involved in such a replacement.

7. Culture-negative endocarditis –With a clinical picture suggestive of infective endocarditis but with persistently negative blood cultures, empiric treatment with penicillin G, 20–50 million units/d intravenously, plus an aminoglycoside (eg, gentamicin, 5 mg/kg/d intramuscularly), can be given for 4 weeks. There should be significant clinical improvement within 7–10 days. If not, a therapeutic trial with other drugs may be warranted.

8. Bacteriostatic drugs –Tetracyclines, erythromycins, lincomycins, chloramphenicol, and similar drugs that are mainly bacteriostatic are not drugs of choice in most cases of infective endocarditis. If administered to patients with fever of unknown origin, these drugs suppress bacteremia temporarily and produce symptomatic improvement but fail to eradicate the infection. They interfere with specific diagnosis by blood culture and permit progression of the lesion, and they should therefore be avoided.

9. Follow-up and recurrences–At the end of the established treatment period of 3–6 weeks, all antimicrobial therapy should be stopped. After 3 days, blood cultures are taken once weekly for 4 weeks while the patient is observed carefully. Most bacteriologic relapses occur during this time, but some recurrences are delayed for several months. Embolic phenomena and fever may occur both during and after successful treatment and—by themselves—are not adequate grounds for retreatment. An initial adequate course of therapy in culture-positive infective endocarditis can result in up to 90% microbiologic cure. If relapse occurs, the organism must be isolated and tested again, and a second—and often longer—course of treatment administered with properly selected drugs.

In spite of microbiologic cure, 50% of patients treated for infective endocarditis progress to cardiac failure in 5–10 years. This mechanical failure can be attributed in part to valvular deformities (eg, perforation of cusp, tearing of chordae) caused by the infection and in part to the healing and scarring process. Therefore, surgical correction of abnormalities in cardiovascular dynamics or possible valvular protheses must be considered as part of the follow-up.

B. General Measures: Supportive treatment, as for any severe infection, must be given. Anemia, if severe, may require transfusion of blood or red cell mass. Anticoagulants (eg, heparin, dicumarol) are not indicated in uncomplicated infective endocarditis and may contribute to hemorrhagic complications. They might even be discontinued in prosthetic endocarditis.

C. Treatment of Complications:

1. Infarctions of organs in the systemic circulation usually result from emboli originating in vegetations in the left heart. Emboli derived from right heart lesions may produce pulmonary infarction. Treatment is symptomatic, and anticoagulants are sometimes helpful. Embolectomy can be attempted if an accessible site can be located. Fungal vegetations may produce massive arterial occlusions.

2. Cardiac failure–Myocarditis, which frequently accompanies infective endocarditis of long duration, and increasing deformity of heart valves may precipitate cardiac failure and require digitalization and sodium restriction. In such patients, the sodium salts of drugs are undesirable, and potassium salts are preferred. Early valve replacement must be considered during antimicrobial therapy if there is evidence of progressive severe heart failure. Because of the bad prognosis of progressive aortic insufficiency developing with endocarditis, insertion of an aortic valve prosthesis may be essential after only 1–2 weeks of effective antimicrobial drug therapy.

3. Renal failure–Infective endocarditis often leads to renal failure resulting from immune complex glomerulonephritis. Rising serum creatinine requires

adjustment of drug dosage and—rarely—temporary treatment of uremia until renal function improves during antimicrobial therapy.

Prognosis

Infective endocarditis is uniformly fatal unless the infection can be eradicated, but in some cases surgical removal of an infected arteriovenous fistula, patent ductus arteriosus, or infected prosthesis has been curative. The poorest prognosis for microbiologic cure exists in patients with consistently negative blood cultures and long delay in therapy, in those with very highly resistant organisms, and in those with an infected prosthesis. If microbiologic cure is accomplished, the prognosis depends on the adequacy of cardiovascular function as mechanical distortions and impairment of dynamics develop during infection and healing. Only about 60% of patients with microbiologically cured infective endocarditis are well 5 years after treatment. Among valve lesions, aortic insufficiency carries the worst outlook and merits the most prompt surgical consideration. Among embolic events, those to the brain have the poorest prognosis. Cerebral emboli and rupture of mycotic aneurysms may occur even after microbiologic cure. Renal functional impairment is generally reversible during early adequate antimicrobial therapy but requires dose adjustment of drugs.

Archer GL, Armstrong BC: Alteration of staphylococcal flora in cardiac surgery patients receiving antibiotic prophylaxis. *J Infect Dis* 1983;**147:**642.

Brandenburg RO et al: Infective endocarditis: A 25-year overview of diagnosis and therapy. *J Am Coll Cardiol* 1983;**1:**280.

Clemens JD et al: A controlled evaluation of the risk of bacterial endocarditis in persons with mitral valve prolapse. *N Engl J Med* 1982;**307:**276.

Cooper R, Mills J: *Serratia* endocarditis. *Arch Intern Med* 1980; **140:**199.

Jawetz E: The doctor's dilemma: Have I chosen the right drug? An adequate dose regimen? Can laboratory tests help in my decision? Pages 109–120 in: *Current Clinical Topics in Infectious Diseases*. Remington JS, Swartz MN (editors). McGraw-Hill, 1981.

Kaplan EL et al: Prevention of bacterial endocarditis. *Circulation* 1977;**56:**139A.

Karchmer AW, Archer GL, Dismukes WE: *Staphylococcus epidermidis* causing prosthetic valve endocarditis: Microbiologic and clinical observations as guides to therapy. *Ann Intern Med* 1983;**98:**447.

Korzeniowski O, Sande MA: The National Collaborative Endocarditis Study Group: Combination antimicrobial therapy for *Staphylococcus aureus* endocarditis in patients addicted to parenteral drugs and in nonaddicts. *Ann Intern Med* 1982;**97:**496.

Mayer KH, Schoenbaum SC: Evaluation and management of prosthetic valve endocarditis. *Prog Cardiovasc Dis* 1982;**25:**43.

Palmer SR, Young SEJ: Q-fever endocarditis in England and Wales, 1975–81. *Lancet* 1982;**2:**1448.

Pesanti EL, Smith IM: Infective endocarditis with negative blood cultures: An analysis of 52 cases. *Am J Med* 1979;**66:**43.

Pringle TH et al: Clinical, echocardiographic, and operative findings in active infective endocarditis. *Br Heart J* 1982;**48:**529.

Reisberg BE: Infective endocarditis in the narcotic addict. *Prog Cardiovasc Dis* 1979;**22**:193.

Rubenson DS et al: The use of echocardiography in diagnosing culture-negative endocarditis. *Circulation* 1981;**64**:641.

Simon GL: Transient bacteremia and endocarditis prophylaxis. *Arch Intern Med* 1984;**144**:34.

Stratton JR et al: Bacteremia and the heart: Serial echocardiographic findings in 80 patients. *Am J Med* 1982;**73**:851.

Wilson WR: Symposium on infective endocarditis. (2 parts.) *Mayo Clin Proc* 1982;**57**:3, 81.

Wilson WR, Geraci JE: Antibiotic treatment of infective endocarditis. *Annu Rev Med* 1983;**34**:413.

HYPERTENSIVE CARDIOVASCULAR DISEASE

The criteria for the diagnosis of hypertension are arbitrary, because the arterial pressure rises with age and varies from one occasion of measurement to another. Most authorities consider hypertension to be present when the diastolic pressure consistently exceeds 100 mm Hg in a person more than 60 years of age or 90 mm Hg in a person less than 50 years of age. WHO places upper limits of normal at 160/95 mm Hg. The vascular complications of hypertension are thought to be the consequence of the raised arterial pressure and associated atherosclerosis of major arterial circuits.

Hypertension is uncommon before age 20, although recent data suggest a higher frequency if one uses different criteria for children, such as pressure exceeding the 90th percentile for age. In young people it is commonly caused by chronic glomerulonephritis, renal artery stenosis, pyelonephritis, or coarctation of the aorta.

Hypertension that has not demonstrably affected the heart is called hypertensive vascular disease. When left ventricular hypertrophy, heart failure, or coronary artery disease is present, "hypertensive cardiovascular disease" is the appropriate term.

Transient elevation of blood pressure caused by excitement, apprehension, or exertion and the purely systolic elevation of blood pressure in elderly people caused by loss of elasticity in the major arteries do not constitute hypertensive disease if the mean blood pressure is less than 107 mm Hg. However, systolic elevation is a significant disease reflecting atherosclerosis of the aorta, and the prognosis is therefore correspondingly less good. Treatment with antihypertensive agents has not been established as effective in decreasing the mortality rate in this group, and they must be used cautiously and in small doses to prevent hypotension and decreased cardiac output.

Hypertension is an important preventable cause of cardiovascular disease; prospective studies have shown that without treatment, hypertension greatly increases the incidence of cardiac failure, coronary heart disease with angina pectoris and myocardial infarction, hemorrhagic and thrombotic stroke, and renal failure. Epidemiologic studies have shown that only a portion of the population is receiving effective antihypertensive therapy; education of the physician and the patient is necessary to identify the patient with hypertension, to ensure adequate treatment, and to reinforce the concept that treatment is a lifelong process and that compliance with the treatment program is essential to an effective result. The prevention—as well as the reversibility—of hypertensive complications by antihypertensive therapy is a major public health concern.

Etiology & Classification

A. Primary Hypertension: In about 90% of cases of hypertensive vascular or cardiovascular disease, no cause can be established. The condition is common and occurs in 10–15% of white adults and 20–30% of black adults in the USA. The onset of essential hypertension is usually between ages 25 and 55. The family history is usually suggestive of hypertension (stroke, "sudden death," heart failure). Women are affected more often than men.

Elevations in pressure are transient early in the course of the disease but eventually become permanent. Even in established cases, the blood pressure fluctuates widely in response to emotional stress, especially anger, resentment, and frustration. The resting blood pressure is lower than single casual office readings and can be determined after several hours' rest in bed. Blood pressures taken by the patient at home or during daily activities using a portable apparatus are lower than those recorded in the office, clinic, or hospital and are more reliable in estimating prognosis. *Note:* All of the foregoing may be true in other forms of hypertension also. A diagnosis of essential hypertension is warranted only after repeated, thorough search for specific causes has been unsuccessful, but such extensive, invasive, and expensive studies are warranted only in selected cases.

Primary hypertension does not always have uniform pathophysiologic features; there is evidence that subsets of patients can be identified in terms of factors that regulate the blood pressure and salt and water content of the blood in the normal population. These include baroreceptor activity, cardiac output, systemic vascular resistance, blood volume, activity of the sympathetic and central nervous systems, and the renin-angiotensin-aldosterone system. **Renin,** a proteolytic enzyme, is secreted by the juxtaglomerular cells surrounding the afferent arterioles in response to a signal that is related to stretch of the afferent arteriole or to decreased volume or sodium content. Renin exists in the plasma in an inactive (prorenin) and an active (renin) form. The latter acts on a substrate in the plasma, producing angiotensin I, which is then acted upon by a converting enzyme to form angiotensin II, which is the most potent pressor substance known. Angiotensin II, by an effect on the zona glomerulosa of the adrenal cortex, increases the secretion of aldosterone, which results in sodium and water retention by its characteristic action on the distal renal tubule, thus restoring blood volume; by negative feedback, the secretion of renin is then reduced until equilibrium results. Approximately 20% of hypertensive patients have low plasma renin but normal aldosterone production, and 15% have high plasma renin in the absence of the accelerated (malignant) phase. These subsets may have important prognostic and therapeutic implications. Patients with low-renin hypertension respond very well to drugs such as thiazides, spironolactone, and other diuretics that deplete plasma and extracellular volume. The effect of the diuretics is less dramatic in patients with high-renin hypertension; arteriolar vasoconstriction is thought to be the dominant physiologic abnormality raising the systemic vascular resistance. Propranolol and other beta-adrenergic blocking agents are more effective in reducing the plasma renin activity in the high-renin group than in low-renin hypertension. Measurement of renin in clinical practice outside of research centers has limited application.

The role of the renin-angiotensin system in the regulation of blood pressure is being studied with the use of inhibitors of components of the system. (See pp 208 and 250.)

Factors opposing a rise in blood pressure may also have physiologic significance in hypertension. These factors include poor baroreceptor reflex control and local vasodilator enzymes such as prostaglandins, kallikreins, adenosine, and perhaps other peptides, as well as hormones of the renal medulla.

The role of the sympathetic nervous system has been intensively studied. Although there is some evidence for increased sympathetic activity in borderline or mild hypertension (raised cardiac output, heart rate, and ejection fraction), circulating plasma norepinephrine usually is not significantly different between normotensive subjects and patients with established hypertension. Plasma norepinephrine is labile and varies with even minor stressful situations and procedures, such as venipuncture, posture, and exercise. The role of sodium has also been controversial, although some (but not most) individuals may be salt-sensitive and respond to increased sodium intake with increased blood pressure. The urinary excretion of sodium and potassium is not significantly different between normotensive and hypertensive subjects; salt intake and blood pressure are not closely related.

Prostaglandins are known to modulate blood flow within the kidney, but their possible etiologic role in hypertension is still unclear.

B. Secondary Hypertension:

1. Renal hypertension–(See also p 274.)

a. Vascular–Narrowing of one or both renal arteries due to atherosclerosis, fibromuscular hyperplasia, or other causes has come to be recognized as perhaps the most common cause of curable hypertension. It may present in the same manner as essential hypertension but may be suspected in the following circumstances: (1) if the onset is after age 50, especially if the course is severe and of short duration; (2) if there are epigastric or renal artery bruits; (3) if there is atherosclerosis elsewhere; (4) if there are variations in the size and appearance of the kidneys as shown by

x-ray, time of appearance of contrast media, or delayed hyperconcentration of contrast material in the involved kidney on the intravenous urogram; (5) if there are increased amounts (relative to the other kidney) of renin activity in renal vein blood; (6) if there is abnormal excretion of radioactive materials as shown by renal scan; or (7) if atherosclerosis or fibromuscular hyperplasia can be demonstrated by renal artery angiogram. Renal angiograms should be performed if anatomic stenosis is suggested strongly by the history, signs, abnormal intravenous urogram, and severity of hypertensive disease.

The functional significance of an established lesion is determined (1) by demonstrating increased renal vein renin on the involved side as compared to the opposite side, and (2) by means of the Howard-Stamey test, with decreased sodium concentration and increased osmolality in the urine on the involved side. When both tests are positive in the presence of a severely stenosed proximal renal artery lesion, reconstructive surgery or transluminal angioplasty (see p 219) offers a good prognosis.

b. Parenchymal–Chronic glomerulonephritis and pyelonephritis have in the past accounted for the largest group of known causes of hypertension. Unilateral pyelonephritis is rare but can often be cured by surgery. Polycystic kidney disease and congenital or acquired obstructive hydronephrosis are rare causes. The primary role of the kidney in causing hypertension (especially acute hypertension) has been documented in acute glomerulonephritis, scleroderma, Goodpasture's syndrome, and the acute vasculitis associated with lupus erythematosus and polyarteritis nodosa.

2. Endocrine–Pheochromocytoma (see Chapter 19).

3. Coarctation of the aorta–See p 180.

4. Miscellaneous–Hypertension of varying severity is present in preeclampsia-eclampsia, following use of oral contraceptive agents, with increased intracranial pressure due to tumor or hematoma, and with overdistention of a neurogenic bladder.

C. Malignant Hypertension: (See Acute Hypertensive Crises, p 209.) Any form of sustained hypertension, primary or secondary, may abruptly become accelerated, with diastolic pressure rising rapidly above 130 mm Hg and causing widespread arteriolar necroses and hyperplasia of the intima of the interlobular arteries of the kidney, in turn causing ischemic atrophy of the nephron. Without treatment, there is rapidly progressive renal failure, left ventricular failure, and stroke. The raised arterial pressure results in papilledema and hemorrhages and exudates in the retinas; these signs may precede clinical evidence of renal impairment and are the most reliable definitive clinical signs of malignant hypertension, although fibrinoid necrosis of the kidney may occur in the presence of soft exudates and hemorrhages alone. If no treatment is given, the mortality rate approaches 100% in 2 years, with an 80% mortality rate in 1 year. Examination of the retina for evidence of accelerated hypertension is necessary in all hypertensive patients because the early stages of the malignant phase may be essentially asymptomatic. Cardiac and renal failure may occur with great rapidity, and treatment to lower the blood pressure is urgent (see p 205).

Pathogenesis

Essential and renal hypertension are due to increased peripheral arteriolar resistance of unknown mechanism. Unless heart failure or edema is present, cardiac output and blood volume are not affected in well-established cases. In young hypertensives with hyperkinetic syndrome, however, cardiac output may be raised with normal systemic vascular resistance. Renal pressor substances may play a role in essential and renal hypertension, but their exact role and mechanisms are unknown.

In pheochromocytoma, hypertension is due to varying combinations of increased cardiac output and peripheral resistance caused by epinephrine and norepinephrine, respectively.

The mechanism of production of hypertension by changes in plasma volume, adrenal glucocorticoids, aldosterone, angiotensin, and deoxycorticosterone, as well as the factors leading to structural systemic vascular resistance, are not known. The hypertension of coarctation of the aorta is thought to result directly from the constriction, which causes the left ventricle to eject blood into a "short chamber," although the renal mechanism may be involved. Adrenergic impulses from the central nervous system may, by the mechanism of autoregulation, cause vasoconstriction of the arterioles and later structural changes.

Pathology

Sustained hypertension causes the initially reversible ("functional") arteriolar narrowing to become permanent ("structural") as a result of intimal thickening, hypertrophy of the muscular coats, and hyaline degeneration. In malignant hypertension, arteriolar necrosis (especially in the renal vessels) develops rapidly and is responsible for the acute onset of renal failure. The dominant manifestations of hypertension are secondary to left ventricular hypertrophy and failure and to the widespread arteriolar and arterial lesions. Hypertension accelerates the development of coronary and cerebral artery atherosclerosis; myocardial infarction and cerebral hemorrhage or thrombosis are common sequelae.

Clinical Findings

The clinical and laboratory findings are mainly referable to the degree of vascular deterioration and involvement of the "target organs": heart, brain, kidneys, eyes, and peripheral arteries.

A. Symptoms: Mild to moderate essential hypertension is compatible with normal health and well-being for many years. Vague symptoms usually appear after patients learn they have "high blood pressure." Suboccipital headaches, characteristically occurring early in the morning and subsiding during the day, are common, but any type of headache may occur (even simulating migraine). Other common complaints are lightheadedness, tinnitus, "fullness in the head," easy fatigability, loss of energy, and palpitations. These symptoms are caused by anxiety about hypertension or by associated psychologic disturbances.

Patients with pheochromocytoma that secretes predominantly norepinephrine usually have sustained hypertension but may have intermittent hypertension. Intermittent release of catecholamines causes attacks (lasting minutes to hours) of acute anxiety, palpitation, profuse perspiration, pallor, trembling, and nausea and vomiting; blood pressure is markedly elevated during the attack, and angina or acute pulmonary edema may occur. In primary aldosteronism, patients may have recurrent episodes of generalized muscular weakness or paralysis, as well as paresthesias, polyuria, and nocturia due to associated hypokalemia.

Cardiac involvement secondary to increased work of the left ventricle in overcoming the raised systemic vascular resistance often leads to paroxysmal nocturnal dyspnea or cardiac asthma with or without symptoms of chronic left ventricular failure. Angina pectoris or myocardial infarction may develop.

Progressive renal involvement may not produce striking symptoms, but nocturia or intermittent hematuria may ultimately occur.

Peripheral arterial disease most commonly causes intermittent claudication. When the terminal aorta is narrowed or occluded, pain in the buttocks and low back pain appear on walking, and men become impotent.

Cerebral involvement causes (1) hemiplegia or aphasia due to thrombosis or (2) sudden hemorrhage from rupture of small intracerebral aneurysms (Charcot), leading to death in hours or days. In malignant hypertension (and occasionally in its absence), severe headache, confusion, coma, convulsions, blurred vision, transient neurologic signs, and nausea and vomiting may occur ("hypertensive encephalopathy"). Their mechanism of production is probably acute capillary congestion and exudation with cerebral edema. The findings are usually reversible if adequate treatment is given.

B. Signs: Physical findings depend upon the cause of hypertension, its duration and severity, and the degree of effect on target organs.

1. Blood pressure–The diagnosis of hypertension is not warranted in patients under age 50 unless the blood pressure exceeds 140/90 mm Hg on at least 3 separate occasions after the patient has rested 20 or more minutes in familiar, quiet surroundings. Casual readings (ie, those taken in the usual fashion) may be much higher than this in the absence of hypertensive disease, since with rest the pressures return to normal; this condition is vascular hyperreactivity, not hypertension, although these transient rises may often represent a precursor to sustained hypertension.

2. Retinas–The Keith-Wagener (KW) classification of retinal changes in hypertension, although it has deficiencies, has prognostic significance and correlates well with the clinical course.

KW1 = Minimal arteriolar narrowing and irregularity.

KW2 = More marked narrowing and arteriovenous nicking. Implies arteriosclerotic as well as hypertensive changes.

KW3 = Flame-shaped or circular hemorrhages and fluffy "cotton wool" exudates.

KW4 = Any of the above plus papilledema, ie, elevation of the optic disk, obliteration of the physiologic cup, or blurring of the disk margins. By definition, malignant hypertension is always associated with papilledema.

3. Heart and arteries–A loud aortic second sound and an early systolic ejection click may occur. Evidence of left ventricular enlargement with a left ventricular heave indicates well-established disease. With onset of left ventricular failure, pulmonary basal rales, gallop rhythm, and pulsus alternans may be noted; a presystolic gallop alone may not imply failure but may be due to decreased compliance of the left ventricle.

4. Pulses–Direct bilateral comparison should be made of both carotid, radial, femoral, popliteal, and pedal pulses, and the presence or absence of bruits over major vessels, including the abdominal aorta and iliacs, should be determined. Blood pressure should be taken in both arms and legs.

5. Cerebrum–Neurologic residuals of cerebral thrombosis or hemorrhage may be present, ranging from only a positive Babinski or Hoffman reflex to frank hemiplegia or hemianopia.

C. Laboratory Findings: Routine urinalysis may disclose a low fixed specific gravity compatible with advanced renal parenchymal disease or hypokalemic nephropathy of primary aldosteronism. In both, blood urea nitrogen and serum creatinine are elevated, and anemia due to advanced azotemia may be present. In aldosteronism, however, the serum potassium is low and the serum sodium and HCO_3^- elevated; the reverse is true in uremia associated with primary renal disease.

Proteinuria, granular casts, and occasionally microhematuria occur in nephrosclerosis; differentiation from chronic nephritis on this basis is impossible.

Demonstrable bacilluria in a fresh clean specimen suggests chronic pyelonephritis; white cell casts are rarely found. Pyuria is frequently absent. Quantitative culture of a clean specimen must be performed on all patients and repeated at intervals, since bacilluria in chronic pyelonephritis may be intermittent.

See Chapter 19 for laboratory findings associated with endocrine abnormalities.

Appropriate laboratory tests should seek other elements known to be risk factors for the development of atherosclerosis, such as serum cholesterol and triglyceride level determinations, evidence of diabetes, or hyperuricemia.

D. Hemodynamics: The basic hemodynamic abnormality in established hypertension is a raised systemic vascular resistance with a normal cardiac output. The latter may be raised in the early phase of borderline or mild hypertension but is usually normal in established cases.

E. X-Ray Findings: Chest x-ray may disclose rib notching and the small aortic knob of coarctation and indicate the degree of cardiac enlargement caused by hypertension. Intravenous urograms yield valuable information on relative renal size, relative rate of appearance and disappearance of the contrast material, renal displacement, obstruction, and pyelonephritis and are diagnostic of polycystic disease.

F. Electrocardiographic Findings: Electrocardiography can estimate the degree of left ventricular hypertrophy and will show signs of coronary artery disease with conduction disturbances and significant Q waves. In aldosteronism and Cushing's disease, the QT interval is prolonged and the ST segment may be depressed (hypokalemia).

G. Echocardiography: Echocardiography is valuable in assessing the presence and degree of left ventricular hypertrophy because it demonstrates increased left ventricular septal and posterior free wall thickness and dimensions and increased left ventricular mass. These abnormalities may be found even in patients without cardiac symptoms; they appear earlier and are a more reliable index of left ventricular hypertrophy than electrocardiographic signs.

H. Special Studies: Selective renal angiography combined with intravenous urograms and tomography is useful in visualizing adrenal tumors. Computerized tomography (CT scans) and the newer nuclear magnetic resonance scans may help to define the location and size of an adrenal tumor and may replace invasive studies. If renal artery stenosis is suspected, intravenous urograms are indicated. It may also be necessary to perform aortography, differential radioisotope excretion studies, or renal vein renin determinations on the 2 kidneys, or differential urinary function studies on each kidney (differential water, electrolyte, inulin, aminohippurate sodium [PAH], and dye excretion measurements).

I. Physiologic and Biochemical Studies of Cardiac Output, Blood Volume, Systemic Vascular Resistance, Plasma Renin, Angiotensin, and Aldosterone: As indicated on p 201, subsets of patients with hypertension may have prognostic and therapeutic significance, and new technology allows determination of these factors with precision.

J. Follow-Up Studies: If specific causes have been excluded, periodic ophthalmoscopic study and evaluation of cardiac and renal status by electrocardiography, chest x-ray, creatinine clearance, blood urea nitrogen, urinary specific gravity, and urine protein determinations are advised to observe the progression of the disease.

Treatment With Hypotensive Drugs

Many patients with mild hypertension, especially middle-aged women, live years in comfort without treatment. Great care should therefore be exercised before subjecting these patients to the disagreeable side effects and potential dangers of a continuous program of drug therapy, especially if the diastolic pressure is less than 100 mm Hg.

Factors that unfavorably influence the prognosis in chronic arterial hypertension and that accordingly determine the nature of drug therapy to be recommended include the following: (1) high diastolic and systolic blood pressure levels, (2) male gender, (3) early age at onset, (4) black race, (5) retinal abnormalities (see p 203), (6) cardiac abnormalities (eg, electrocardiographic changes, cardiomegaly, angina), (7) cerebrovascular accidents, (8) renal abnormalities, and (9) family history of hypertension.

Large-scale Veterans Administration studies demonstrate convincingly that appropriate drug treatment of asymptomatic moderate degrees of chronic hypertension ($\geq$ 105 mm Hg diastolic) results in significantly lower morbidity and mortality rates from cardiovascular diseases (heart failure, hemorrhagic stroke, renal failure) than are reported in untreated control patients. Multicenter trials showed that in patients with diastolic pressures less than 105 mm Hg, the 5-year mortality rate from all causes was 20% lower in a stepped-care experimental group than in similar patients treated in the community. A review of the trials suggests that nonpharmacologic treatment (with observation at least every 6 months) may be started instead of drug therapy in patients whose blood pressure is consistently less than 100 mm Hg and in whom there are no other risk factors or vascular complications, in which case drug therapy can be begun at a lower diastolic pressure such as 95 mm Hg or even 90 mm Hg. If the blood pressure rises during the observation period, drug therapy should be begun. That treatment of hypertension decreases the incidence of clinical coronary disease is suggested but not established by data from both the Hypertension Detection Study and the multicenter Australian trial. Current insurance data have shown that even slight increases in blood pressure decrease survival, especially by causing premature atherosclerosis.

In mild to moderate hypertension, therapy is usually initiated with thiazides or (less frequently) other classes of diuretics (see below for details). Beta-adrenergic blocking drugs (see Table 8–3) such as propranolol, atenolol, metoprolol, pindolol, timolol, and nadolol have been recommended as initial therapy, especially in younger patients. Current data do not provide evidence clearly in favor of diuretics or beta-blockers; both are effective. Postsynaptic alpha-adrenergic blocking agents such as prazosin or its analogs have some advocates, especially if diuretics or beta-adrenergic blocking drugs produce side effects. If blood pressure is not controlled by the first drug alone after a period of 1–3 weeks, a second drug may be reserpine, hydralazine, methyldopa, a beta-adrenergic blocking drug, clonidine, prazosin, or guanabenz (see below). If a beta-blocker was the first drug used, a diuretic can be added as the second one. In moderate arterial hypertension (diastolic pressure of 110–130 mm Hg), it may be advisable to initiate treatment with

a combination of thiazides and one of the second group of drugs mentioned above. The combination of a vasodilator (hydralazine or prazosin) and a beta-blocking drug counteracts the increased sympathetic discharge resulting from vasodilators and has proved effective, with few side effects. If the combination fails to lower the pressure, prazosin can be added to hydralazine; even though both are vasodilators, they act by different mechanisms. Calcium entry-blocking agents are vasodilators, but they have not yet been approved by the FDA for treatment of hypertension. In severe cases or when patients fail to respond to the other agents, minoxidil, captopril, or guanethidine may be used. Analogs of captopril such as enalapril have been reported to be effective and to have a longer duration of action with fewer side effects than captopril. Preliminary reports are encouraging. In general, guanethidine should replace rather than be added to reserpine or methyldopa when these drugs are ineffective. If hypertension is complicated by renal failure, methyldopa and hydralazine have been the most effective agents, although drugs such as prazosin, clonidine, and minoxidil have distinct advantages. Minoxidil is the most powerful vasodilator of the oral antihypertensive agents. Treat malignant hypertension with rapidly acting drugs.

The monoamine oxidase inhibitors should not be used in combination with any of the antihypertensive drugs because of the possibility of provoking hypertensive crises. Amphetamines and tricyclic antidepressants block the effectiveness of guanethidine and may occasionally aggravate hypertension.

A. Indications for Antihypertensive Drugs:

1. Definite indications–Antihypertensive drug therapy is definitely indicated in malignant hypertension; in hypertensive cardiac failure (pulmonary edema); for rapidly increasing diastolic blood pressure with left ventricular hypertrophy and dilatation; for hypertensive encephalopathy; when there is evidence of deterioration in the heart and fundi (exudates and hemorrhages), especially in young (particularly male and black) patients; in dissecting aorta in hypertensive individuals; or when there are persistent diastolic pressures exceeding 100–105 mm Hg. In acute myocardial infarction, hypertension should be treated cautiously.

Antihypertensive drugs are indicated in recurrent mild cerebral thrombosis with neurologic sequelae and high diastolic pressure; in intractable coronary insufficiency with high diastolic pressure; when the diastolic pressure varies between 100 and 105 mm Hg without evidence of complications of hypertension, especially in patients under age 50; or for severe intractable hypertensive headaches (in the absence of obvious emotional stress). Younger patients, those with family histories of early death from cardiovascular disease, black males, and patients with evidence of target organ damage should be treated if they have consistent diastolic pressures exceeding 90–95 mm Hg.

2. Doubtful indications–Antihypertensive drug therapy is probably not indicated for mild benign essential hypertension (pressures approximating 160/90–95 mm Hg in the absence of vascular abnormalities) in elderly women or for early transient hypertension (slight rises above 140/90 mm Hg on some occasions but readings well below this on other occasions, especially if the rises occur in the setting of emotional stress) in young people with no objective evidence of vascular deterioration or complications.

B. Drugs Available: Antihypertensive agents, once begun for significant hypertension, should usually be continued indefinitely, especially in those with severe hypertension before treatment. If blood pressure is well-controlled for a year, attempts may be made to decrease the dose of one agent or to gradually stop a second drug if combined therapy is being used.

1. Oral diuretic agents–Diuretics are drugs that suppress renal tubular reabsorption of sodium. They are used in the treatment of diseases associated with excess sodium retention and consequent fluid accumulation and edema such as cardiac failure (see p 260) or in the treatment of hypertension to increase the excretion of sodium and water, to decrease plasma volume, and ultimately to decrease systemic vascular resistance. See Table 8–2 for useful oral diuretics. The marked sodium loss caused by diuretics is accompanied by potassium diuresis of a potentially serious degree, especially if digitalis is given concurrently.

Thiazides are ineffective in renal failure and must be used in smaller doses and with careful observation in patients with cirrhosis of the liver and in those receiving digitalis. Thiazides such as chlorothiazide reduce the required dose of blocking agents to about half and are additive with other agents. Give chlorothiazide, 0.5–1 g/d in divided doses, with due caution for electrolyte depletion, especially in elderly patients or those receiving digitalis; or hydrochlorothiazide, 50 mg 1–2 times daily. If patients respond well, the dose may be decreased to 25 mg. Other oral diuretic agents such as chlorthalidone and metolazone are as effective and are longer-lasting. The more potent diuretics (ethacrynic acid and furosemide) may lead to electrolyte and volume depletion more readily than the thiazides and therefore are not ordinarily used in hypertension, except in the presence of renal failure.

Hypovolemia, caused by any of the diuretics, leads to decreased renal blood flow with a rise in the serum creatinine, especially in older patients. The rise in serum creatinine is usually reversible, but the evidence is unclear about the long-term significance and reversibility of this rise in older persons. The so-called loop diuretics are more effective in renal failure. Hypokalemia can be avoided by a high-potassium diet with fresh fruit and green vegetables. Some authorities advise adding potassium-retaining drugs such as spironolactone, 25 mg 3 times daily, triamterene, or amiloride, 5–15 mg/d in divided doses when oral diuretics are used. If this is done, serum potassium must be checked frequently and potassium salts not used to avoid hyperkalemia. The potassium-retaining drugs should not be used in renal failure or oliguria. As indicated previously, diuretics (including spironolactone) are most effective in low-renin hypertension. Hyperuricemia and hyperglycemia may also occur with the use of thiazides, and probenecid, allopurinol, or oral hypoglycemic agents may be necessary. Other untoward effects are allergic reactions such as skin rashes, pruritus, and, rarely, bone marrow depression.

2. Beta-adrenergic blocking agents–(Table 8–3.) These drugs are effective in hypertension because they inhibit adrenergic mediators at their receptor sites in the heart and thus decrease the heart rate and cardiac output. Even after continued use for a number of years, cardiac output remains decreased and systemic vascular resistance does not increase. The drugs also decrease renin release and in larger doses have a quinidinelike effect. They neutralize the reflex tachycardia caused by vasodilators such as hydralazine and prazosin in the treatment of hypertension. Propranolol is begun in a dosage of 10–20 mg twice daily and increased to a total daily dose of 160–320 mg/d. Metoprolol is started in a dose of 50 mg twice daily and increased as necessary depending on response to 200 mg twice daily. Because it is cardioselective, it is

Table 8–2. Useful oral diuretics.

	Daily Dose
Amiloride (Moduretic)	5–15 mg
Bendroflumethiazide (Naturetin)	5–10 mg
Benzthiazide (Exna)	25–100 mg
Bumetanide (Bumex)	0.5–2 mg
Chlorothiazide (Diuril)	250–1000 mg
Chlorthalidone (Hygroton)	50–200 mg
Cyclothiazide (Anhydron, Fluidil)	1–2 mg
Ethacrynic acid (Edecrin)	100–200 mg
Flumethiazide (Ademol)	250–1000 mg
Furosemide (Lasix)	40–80 mg
Hydrochlorothiazide (Esidrix, HydroDiuril)	25–100 mg
Hydroflumethiazide (Di-Ademil, Saluron)	25–100 mg
Indapamide (Lozol)	2.5–5 mg
Methyclothiazide (Aquatensen, Enduron)	2.5–10 mg
Metolazone (Zaroxolyn)	2.5–10 mg
Polythiazide (Renese)	1–4 mg
Quinethazone (Hydromox)	50–100 mg
Spironolactone (Aldactone)	50–100 mg
Triamterene (Dyrenium)	100–200 mg
Trichlormethiazide (Metahydrin, Naqua)	2–8 mg

Table 8–3. Beta-adrenergic blocking drugs approved by FDA.

Agent	Cardio-selectivity	Half-Life (hours)	Average Daily Dose; Frequency
Propranolol	No	4–6	160–320 mg; 2–3 divided doses
Atenolol	Yes	6–9	50–100 mg; once daily
Metoprolol	Yes	3–6	50–200 mg; 2 divided doses
Pindolol	No	3–5	5–10 mg; 2 divided doses
Timolol	No	4–6	10–30 mg; 2 divided doses
Nadolol	No	20–24	40–200 mg; once daily

preferred to propranolol in patients with chronic lung disease. Nadolol is given in an initial dosage of 40 mg once daily. This may be gradually increased in 40- to 80-mg increments until an optimal effect is achieved. The usual maintenance dose is 80–320 mg once daily. Dosage adjustments are necessary in patients with renal impairment. Atenolol is begun with 25–50 mg daily in a single dose and may be gradually increased, usually to not more than 100 mg/d. Pindolol can be started in a dosage of 5 mg twice daily, with increments at 2- to 3-week intervals, to a maximum of about 40 mg/d. The average effective maintenance dose is about 20–25 mg/d. The beta-blocking drugs are all approximately equal in effectiveness but differ clinically with respect to their effect on the β_2-receptors of the bronchi (cardioselectivity), their duration, and whether they are lipid-soluble and enter the brain. Trial and error and experience lead to the physician's preference of one over another.

The side effects of all the beta-blockers, which can be either absolute or relative contraindications, are the development of bronchial asthma in patients who have had allergy in the past; severe bradycardia; atrioventricular conduction defects; left ventricular failure because of the negative inotropic action of the sympatholytic action of the drug; Raynaud's phenomenon, especially in women in cold weather; and, rarely, central nervous system symptoms with excitement and confusion.

3. Hydralazine hydrochloride–The initial dosage of this drug is 10–25 mg orally twice daily, progressively increasing to a total dosage of 200 mg/d. The results of the oral use of this drug as a sole method of therapy are often not impressive; however, because it is a vasodilator and does not decrease the renal blood flow, it is useful as an adjunct to oral postganglionic or ganglionic blocking agents as well as to the oral diuretics, especially if there is impaired renal function. (See p 209 for the parenteral use of hydralazine.)

Toxic side effects are common when large doses of hydralazine are used alone but uncommon when the drug is used in combination with chlorothiazide in doses not exceeding 200 mg/d or with rauwolfia or propranolol. The most important are headache and palpitations with tachycardia due to reflex baroreceptor response to the lowered pressure induced by vasodilatation. A syndrome resembling systemic lupus erythematosus has occurred, usually after large doses have been given for many months.

4. Prazosin (Minipress)–Prazosin relaxes smooth muscle by blocking alpha-adrenergic receptors and thereby decreasing afterload and systemic vascular resistance. Because prazosin causes dilatation of both arteries and veins, it is of particular value when hypertension is associated with cardiac failure. Give an initial dose of 0.5–1 mg twice a day increased as necessary to a usual total oral daily dose of 10–15 mg, with increments at least a week apart. Because the first dose may cause marked postural hypotension and syncope, it should be no greater than 0.5 mg and should be given at bedtime. Potency of the drug is approximately

equal to that of methyldopa or hydralazine. It does not increase the cardiac output as much as hydralazine and does not appreciably decrease the renal blood flow or glomerular filtration rate. Tachycardia and headache may occur.

5. Methyldopa (Aldomet)–Methyldopa decreases sympathetic peripheral outflow by a central sympatholytic action, thereby lowering blood pressure. An initial dose of 250 mg 2 or 3 times daily orally is gradually increased at intervals of 2–3 days to a total daily dose (divided into 2–4 doses) of 0.75–2.5 g. Both supine and standing pressures are reduced in about two-thirds of cases of moderate hypertension; the postural effect may predominate, especially in patients receiving reserpine. Concomitant thiazide therapy is desirable both to potentiate the hypotensive effects of the drug and to counteract the fluid retention that (with drowsiness) is its main side effect. Decreased vigor, impotence, and hepatitis may also occur with methyldopa and limit its applicability. A positive Coombs test and hemolytic anemia (uncommon) may occur. Fever is a rare toxic reaction. As with other hypotensive agents, methyldopa should be given under close supervision by the physician until a stable dose schedule is established. (The parenteral use of methyldopa is discussed on p 209.)

6. Clonidine (Catapres)–Clonidine stimulates alpha-adrenergic receptors in the depressor center of the medulla that decrease efferent sympathetic vasoconstrictor impulses to the heart, thus lowering systemic vascular resistance and blood pressure in hypertension. An initial dose of 0.1 mg is given once or twice daily. The average daily dose given once or twice a day in divided doses is 0.1–0.6 mg. Because the first dose may cause marked drowsiness, it should be no greater than 0.1 mg and should be given at bedtime. Careful observation is required during the first week. Increments can be given at 1-week intervals. The side effects include dry mouth, drowsiness, and, if the drug is stopped abruptly, a considerable rebound hypertension and symptoms of sympathetic overactivity. If the drug is to be stopped, dosage should be tapered rather than abruptly stopped. The rebound effect is not confined to clonidine and has been observed with other antihypertensive agents as well, but not as dramatically.

7. Guanabenz–Guanabenz is a centrally acting alpha$_2$-adrenergic agonist that decreases the blood pressure by a mechanism similar to that of clonidine. Its efficacy is similar to that of both clonidine and methyldopa; heart rate and cardiac output are not affected. Further data are required to compare the centrally acting drugs.

8. Rauwolfia drugs–Rauwolfia is a central nervous system depressant that has a relatively slight hypotensive action but may be useful because of its mild sedative effect and its value as an adjunct when combined with hydralazine or chlorothiazide. Nasal stuffiness, gastric hyperacidity, sodium retention, and severe depression may occur, in which case the drug should be withdrawn. Recent studies have not confirmed earlier reports of reserpine's association with breast cancer. Give either of the following: (1) Reserpine, 0.1–0.25 mg daily orally. *Caution:* Do not use if there is a history of previous mental depression. Reserpine may also be given intramuscularly, 1–2.5 mg every 8–12 hours, for a short time in hypertensive emergencies. (2) Rauwolfia, 100–200 mg daily.

9. Captopril–Agents that inhibit the formation of angiotensin II from angiotensin I, such as the converting enzyme inhibitor captopril (or its analog enalapril), decrease systemic vascular resistance by inhibiting the pressor action of angiotensin II, thereby lowering arterial pressure. Oral captopril has effectively lowered the blood pressure in hypertensive patients regardless of initial plasma renin levels, although it is more effective when plasma renin is high. Captopril has the advantage of increasing the glomerular filtration rate in some patients.

Caution must be exercised, because severe hypotension may occur in patients who are sodium-depleted. The optimum dose has not been clarified, and 5–10% of patients develop a rash that may represent a hypersensitivity reaction. Some patients have also developed proteinuria suggesting renal damage. The dose of captopril in different studies has varied considerably (from 25 to 600 mg daily). Even with larger doses, the blood pressure may not fall to normal, and other drugs, such as the diuretics, must be added. The specificity of captopril has been questioned because it not only blocks the formation of angiotensin II but also inactivates bradykinin and may inhibit prostaglandins, which are potent vasodilators. The approach to the treatment of hypertension using inhibitors of the renin-angiotensin system is of considerable interest, but further experience is required.

10. Guanethidine–Guanethidine acts by blocking the postganglionic adrenergic neurons; tolerance rarely occurs. The drug can be given in a single daily dose, is effective, and does not produce parasympathetic blockage. The initial dose is 10 mg orally, increasing gradually to tolerance at weekly intervals. Postural hypotension (especially in the morning on awakening and after exercise), diarrhea, muscle aching, and lack of ejaculation in men are the major symptoms of toxicity.

11. Combined alpha- and beta-adrenergic blocking agents (labetalol)–A combination blockade of the 2 adrenergic systems may offer significant advantages. Alpha-receptor blockade counteracts the reflex increase in heart rate and cardiac output produced by vasodilating drugs such as hydralazine. Postural hypotension may occur. Labetalol can be used either orally or intravenously. The intravenous dose is 50 mg; the oral dose may be considerably higher and must be titrated to the needs of the individual patient. Further data are required to establish its role in treatment.

12. Calcium entry-blocking drugs–These agents inhibit the entry of calcium into the cell, resulting in arterial vasodilation and decreased blood pressure in hypertension. They also (especially verapamil) have a variable negative inotropic action that

may lead to cardiac failure if beta-blocking agents are used concurrently or may worsen cardiac failure if it is already present. The most common agents are nifedipine, verapamil, and diltiazem. They all have been effective in the treatment of severe hypertension, but treatment must often be supplemented with diuretics or other antihypertensive agents (see also pp 214 and 233).

13. Minoxidil (Loniten)–This drug is a potent vasodilator that reflexly increases heart rate and cardiac output; sodium retention usually also occurs. It is most useful in the treatment of severe hypertension which has not responded to more moderate therapy and which usually requires associated diuretic therapy and beta-blocking drugs, if tachycardia and headache warrant. Furosemide rather than the thiazides is usually necessary, because sodium and water retention can be severe. A major side effect of the drug is the development of hirsutism, a considerable disadvantage for women.

Side Effects and Hazards of Antihypertensive Agents

(1) Acute hypotensive reactions are manifested by faintness, weakness, and nausea and vomiting. The patient should be instructed to lie down immediately with the feet higher than the head. Unless the hypotensive effect is too severe, the symptoms pass rapidly with this postural assistance. If the symptoms persist, give a vasopressor drug such as phenylephrine hydrochloride or methoxamine subcutaneously, or a slow, continuous intravenous infusion of levarterenol bitartrate, 4 mg/L, titrated carefully, because occasional patients are unusually sensitive to some vasopressors.

(2) Acute or progressive renal failure due to decreased renal blood flow or filtration pressure may necessitate discontinuing the drug.

(3) Vascular thromboses (especially cerebral) and renal failure are hazards in older patients who suffer severe and abrupt falls of blood pressure.

(4) A low-sodium diet potentiates the action of blocking compounds. If an individual receiving fixed doses of the drug is given a low-sodium diet, hypotensive symptoms may occur. It is usually wise to place the patient on a 2-g sodium diet at onset of therapy.

(5) Alcohol, hot climate, vasodilator drugs, vigorous exercise, and salt depletion potentiate the action of ganglionic and postganglionic compounds.

Determination of Adequate Treatment

Although determination of the proper drug dosage is difficult, it is usually considered satisfactory if standing diastolic pressures of 90–100 mm Hg or less are achieved (especially after exercise) or a systolic pressure of 150–160 mm Hg or less. Since the effectiveness of the drug cannot be determined by casual blood pressure readings in the physician's office, the following methods have been used to determine effective dosage: (1) Home blood pressure readings are recorded and shown to the physician at the regular visits. The physician may increase or decrease the dose, and the patient is instructed to decrease the dose whenever the blood pressure falls below 150/90 mm Hg, and not to take a dose if the blood pressure is below 130/80 mm Hg in the recumbent position. (2) "Near-basal" blood pressure levels can be obtained by having a nurse take repetitive blood pressures under quiet surroundings in the office in the physician's absence. Pressures are obtained every 1–5 minutes for 30–60 minutes, and the average of the 3 lowest readings is considered to be the basal pressure. These near-basal pressures correlate more closely with the development of vascular complications than do routine office pressure readings. (3) Ambulatory blood pressure recordings taken throughout the day give a more representative record of the patient's usual pressures and may predict clinical outcome more reliably than office pressures. The apparatus is commercially available. (4) Motionless standing for 1 minute before taking the drug is advocated to prevent excessive hypotension. Blood pressure will then be high enough that an additional quantity can be taken without harm. This only guards against excessive dosage; it does not indicate when the dose has been inadequate.

Acute Hypertensive Crises

Patients with acute severe hypertension (diastolic blood pressure > 140 mm Hg) or with pressures somewhat lower but with commanding symptoms of headache, visual disturbance, somnolence, or other "crises" noted below must be hospitalized and treated on an emergency basis with parenteral hypotensive drugs. The most important of the hypertensive "crises" are those of acute hypertensive encephalopathy, acute pulmonary edema associated with a marked rise in blood pressure in hypertensive patients with left ventricular failure, malignant hypertension, acute dissecting aorta with a high arterial pressure, and hemorrhagic stroke with marked elevation of blood pressure.

Constant monitoring of blood pressure, preferably in an intensive care unit, is required. The patient should sit up or the head of the bed should be elevated 30 degrees. Blood urea nitrogen and serum creatinine should be determined daily if blood urea nitrogen is > 50 mg/dL. Advance preparation should be made to treat excessive pressure drop (see Chapter 1).

Parenteral Antihypertensive Therapy

Several parenteral antihypertensive drugs are available, but no single agent can be classified as the drug of choice.

A. Rapidly Acting Agents:

1. Diazoxide (Hyperstat), 75–300 mg intravenously in a single dose, acts promptly as a vasodilator without decreasing cardiac output or renal blood flow. It has been used most often in preeclampsia-eclampsia, malignant hypertension, and acute hypertensive encephalopathy. Side effects include hypotension, which may be severe and which necessitates starting with a smaller dose in young or elderly patients, or, alternatively, a slow infusion over 30 min, which is usually as

effective and better tolerated. Hyperglycemia and sodium and water retention may occur. For these reasons, the drug should be used only for short periods and combined with a potent diuretic such as furosemide.

2. The ganglionic blocking agent trimethaphan (Arfonad), 1 ampule of 500 mg in 1 L of 5% dextrose in water, is given intravenously at a rate of 1–4 mL/min and titrated with the patient sitting so as to utilize gravity if the hypotensive effect is excessive. It takes effect within a few minutes and lasts for the duration of the infusion. The objective should be to reduce the diastolic blood pressure to about 110 mm Hg over a period of about 1 hour.

3. Sodium nitroprusside (8–50 μg/min) by controlled intravenous infusion titrated to the desired effect. It lowers the blood pressure within seconds by direct arteriolar and venous vasodilatation, decreasing preload as well as afterload. As with trimethaphan, close monitoring by nurse or physician is essential to avoid excessive fall in blood pressure.

B. Delayed Acting Agents: These agents do not require as close monitoring as the rapidly acting agents (above) and can be used in less urgent cases.

1. Reserpine, 1–2.5 mg intramuscularly every 8 hours; effect not predictable.

2. Hydralazine (Apresoline), 5–20 mg intramuscularly every 2–4 hours. Propranolol may be necessary to counteract tachycardia. The combination of reserpine and hydralazine parenterally has proved of considerable value in the acute hypertension associated with acute glomerular nephritis in children.

3. Methyldopa (Aldomet), 500 mg intravenously every 2–4 hours, takes effect more slowly than the ganglioplegics, and its effect lasts for 8–12 hours.

C. Subsequent Therapy: When the blood pressure has been brought under control, combinations of oral antihypertensive agents can be added as parenteral drugs are tapered off over a period of 2–3 days.

Other Methods of Treatment

A rigid low-sodium diet (350 mg of sodium or less per day) is unnecessary with the use of chlorothiazide; 2 g of sodium are usually allowed.

Attempts to treat hypertensive patients with psychotherapeutic methods have not been successful, although attention to the emotional needs of such patients is an important adjunct to treatment.

If the patient is anxious, attempt to treat the underlying cause with or without the help of a psychiatrist or a psychologist. If necessary, give phenobarbital, 15 mg 3 times daily, or similar mild sedatives (but not if the patient is receiving reserpine or methyldopa). Tricyclic antidepressants and phenothiazines should be avoided if guanethidine is used, because they compete with guanethidine uptake and the antihypertensive effect of the latter is diminished.

Hypertension in the Presence of Renal Failure

In the presence of renal failure, hypertension is dependent on blood volume. If the blood pressure is not reduced by vigorous use of antihypertensive drugs, including furosemide, beta-blocking drugs, and minoxidil, or by repeated injections of diazoxide, renal dialysis should be employed; in most instances, the blood pressure will be reduced as the patient achieves a dry weight state. Rarely—especially in those patients with high plasma renin levels—bilateral nephrectomy is necessary to control severe hypertension. The presence of renal failure is an adverse prognostic sign, but vigorous therapy often can reverse the malignant phase associated with renal failure and thus prolong life.

Treatment of Complications

The cardiac, cerebral, and renal complications of hypertension are discussed under congestive failure, angina pectoris, myocardial infarction, cerebral hemorrhage, cerebral thrombosis, and renal failure.

The mechanism of the headache in benign hypertension is unknown; the headache is often intermittent, with no apparent change in blood pressure, and it is thought to be caused at times by emotional tension. It may be relieved by antihypertensive therapy. Severe suboccipital headache is common in accelerated or malignant hypertension (see p 202); lowering the blood pressure is the most effective treatment.

Prognosis

Although many patients with slight elevation of blood pressure live a normal life span, most patients with untreated hypertensive cardiovascular disease die of complications within 20 years. Before effective antihypertensive drugs were available, 70% of patients died of heart failure or coronary artery disease, 15% of cerebral hemorrhage, and 10% of uremia.

Antihypertensive therapy has dramatically changed the prognosis of hypertensive patients. Within the past 10 years, the mortality rate has decreased 40%. Cardiac failure, renal failure, and malignant hypertension rarely occur in the well-treated patient, and the incidence of hemorrhagic stroke and dissecting aorta is greatly decreased. Furthermore, heart failure and malignant hypertension may be reversed by the introduction of antihypertensive drugs. It has been reported that treatment of hypertension with antihypertensive drugs may decrease the incidence of clinical coronary manifestations as contrasted with that in an untreated group. If this is confirmed, it may partially explain the recent epidemiologic finding that the mortality rate from coronary disease has decreased in recent years in the population at large.

The results of treatment are of course related to its adequacy; poor treatment has essentially the same result as no treatment. The response to treatment should therefore be monitored and the patient's compliance sought by education, prevention of long waiting times at visits, and persuasion to continue a lifelong program of drug treatment that often has some unpleasant side effects. The benefits of antihypertensive therapy are most obvious in younger patients, before atherosclerosis has occurred, and less obvious in older patients who have other risk factors of atherosclerosis (see p 211)

such as hypercholesterolemia, hypertriglyceridemia, diabetes, cigarette smoking, etc. Attention to multiple risk factors in the hypertensive patient should improve prognosis; various studies are under way throughout the world to test this hypothesis.

The Australian Therapeutic Trial in Mild Hypertension: Report by the Management Committee. *Lancet* 1980;**1**:1261.

Berglund G, Andersson O: Beta-blockers or diuretics in hypertension? A six-year follow-up of blood pressure and metabolic side effects. *Lancet* 1981;**1**:744.

Biglieri EG: Adrenocortical components in hypertension. *Cardiovasc Rev Rep* 1982;**3**:734.

Colucci WS: Alpha-adrenergic receptor blockage with prazosin: Consideration of hypertension, heart failure, and potential new applications. *Ann Intern Med* 1982;**97**:67.

Cressman MD, Gifford RW: Hypertension and stroke. *J Am Coll Cardiol* 1983;**1(2–Part 1)**:521.

Dean RH, Smith BM: How valuable is revascularization for hypertension and renal failure? *J Cardiovasc Med* 1983;**8**:84.

des Combes JB et al: Ambulatory blood pressure recordings: Reproducibility and unpredictability. *Hypertension* 1984;**6**:110.

Doroghazi RM et al: Long-term survival of patients with treated aortic dissection. *J Am Coll Cardiol* 1984;**3**:1026.

Dunn FG et al: Enalapril improves systemic and renal hemodynamics and allows regression of left ventricular mass in essential hypertension. *Am J Cardiol* 1984;**53**:105.

Helgeland A: Treatment of mild hypertension: A five-year controlled drug trial. The Oslo Study. *Am J Med* 1980;**69**:725.

Hollenberg NK: Medical therapy of renovascular hypertension: Efficacy and safety of captopril in 269 patients. *Cardiovasc Rev Rep* 1983;**4**:852.

Houston MC: Clonidine hydrochloride: Review of pharmacologic and clinical aspects. *Prog Cardiovasc Dis* 1981;**23**:337.

Hypertension Detection and Follow-Up Program Cooperative Group: The effect of treatment on mortality in "mild" hypertension. *N Engl J Med* 1982;**307**:976.

Hypertension Detection and Follow-Up Program Cooperative Group: Five-year findings of the hypertension detection and follow-up program. 3. Reduction in stroke incidence among persons with high blood pressure. *JAMA* 1982;**247**:633.

Kaplan NM, Lowenstein J (guest editors): First-line therapy for hypertension: Changing directions. (Symposium.) *Am J Cardiol* 1984;**53**:1A. [Entire issue.]

Linas SL, Nies AS: Minoxidil. *Ann Intern Med* 1981;**94**:61.

Lund-Johansen P: Haemodynamics in essential hypertension: State of the art review. *Clin Science* 1980;**59(Suppl 6)**:343s.

Mahler F et al: Lasting improvement of renovascular hypertension by transluminal dilatation of atherosclerotic and nonatherosclerotic renal artery stenosis: A follow-up study. *Circulation* 1982;**65**:611.

Okun R: Effectiveness of prazosin as initial antihypertensive therapy. *Am J Cardiol* 1983;**51**:645.

Oparil S: Hypertension and oral contraceptives. *J Cardiovasc Med* 1981;**6**:381.

Perloff D: Hypertensive emergencies. Chap 9, pp 181–201, in: *Cardiac Emergencies*. Scheinman MM (editor). Saunders, 1984.

Perloff D, Sokolow M, Cowan R: The prognostic value of ambulatory blood pressures. *JAMA* 1983;**249**:2792.

Rabkin SW, Mathewson FA, Tate RB: Relationship of blood pressure in 20- to 39-year-old men to subsequent blood pressure and incidence of hypertension over a 30-year observation period. *Circulation* 1982;**65**:291.

Reichek N et al: Anatomic validation of left ventricular mass estimates from clinical 2-dimensional echocardiography: Initial results. *Circulation* 1983;**67**:348.

Smuckler AL et al: Echocardiographic diagnosis of aortic root dissection by M-mode and two-dimensional techniques. *Am Heart J* 1982;**103**:897.

Tarazi RC, Zanchetti A (guest editors): Symposium of First European Meeting on Hypertension held in Milan: Response to antihypertensive treatment. *Hypertension* 1983;**5(pt II)**: 1.

Veterans Administration Cooperative Study Group on Antihypertensive Agents: Comparison of prazosin with hydralazine in patients receiving hydrochlorothiazide: A randomized, double-blind clinical trial. *Circulation* 1981;**64**:772.

Veterans Administration Cooperative Study Group on Antihypertensive Agents: Comparison of propranolol and hydrochlorothiazide for the initial treatment of hypertension. 1. Results of short-term titration with emphasis on racial differences in response. 2. Results of long-term therapy. *JAMA* 1982;**248**:1996, 2004.

Veterans Administration Cooperative Study Group on Antihypertensive Agents: Efficacy of nadolol alone and combined with bendroflumethiazide and hydralazine for systemic hypertension. *Am J Cardiol* 1983;**52**:1230.

CORONARY HEART DISEASE
(Arteriosclerotic Coronary Artery Disease; Ischemic Heart Disease)

Coronary heart disease, or obliterative atherosclerosis of the coronary arteries, is the commonest underlying cause of cardiovascular disability and death. Smooth muscle cell proliferation combined with a disorder of lipid metabolism is thought to be responsible for the localized subintimal accumulations of fatty and fibrous tissue that progressively obstruct the epicardial portions of the coronary arteries and their main branches. A deficiency or imbalance in certain tissue enzymes such as prostaglandins has been proposed as the mechanism that allows adherence of platelets and accelerates the atherosclerotic process. This subject is under intensive investigation.

Although it has been considered for years that total serum cholesterol and low-density lipoproteins are the most important components of lipids with respect to atherosclerosis, some recent data suggest that high-density lipoproteins may be equally important. There is an inverse relationship between the concentration of subclasses of high-density lipoproteins and the incidence of clinical coronary events, so a high concentration is protective.

Risk factors (established by prospective studies) that predispose to the development of ischemic heart disease include age, genetic predispositions, hypercholesterolemia, arterial hypertension, diabetes mellitus, hypertriglyceridemia, and cigarette smoking. Other factors of less importance include obesity and possibly physical fitness and personality type.

Prevention of Ischemic Heart Disease: Management of the Patient With High Risk Factors

Although it has been shown that individuals who have the risk factors listed above—especially if they are present in combination and if the patient is under age 50—have an increased risk of developing clinical disease, there is evidence that correcting them will prevent further progression of the disease once it has occurred. However, recent reports indicate that in men with type II hypercholesterolemia, lessening serum cholesterol by diet and cholestyramine decreases the incidence of initial clinical coronary events, decreases progression, and increases survival rates in persons with pre-existing coronary disease (see references on p 217). Emphasis should therefore be given to prevention. Hypertension, hypercholesterolemia, and diabetes should be adequately treated; cigarette smoking should be discouraged; and optimal weight and physical fitness should be encouraged.

The classification of hyperlipidemias has been a subject of "confusion and controversy." The Fredrickson classification (Table 20–7, p 788), while no longer completely adequate because of the emergence of new information regarding the genetic and metabolic aspects of hyperlipidemic states, is a useful approach to the evaluation and management of the hyperlipidemias.

For detailed discussion, see pp 787–792.

Pathophysiology

Men are more often affected than women by an overall ratio of 4:1; before age 40 the ratio is 8:1, and beyond age 70 it is 1:1. In men the peak incidence of clinical manifestations is at age 50–60; in women, at age 60–70. Advanced stages of atherosclerotic coronary artery disease, even complete occlusion, may remain clinically silent, being discovered incidentally after death due to other causes. At present, the only means of determining the location and extent of narrowing is coronary angiography, although the effect of coronary stenoses in different parts of the heart can be inferred from regional wall motion abnormalities detected by radionuclide angiography or 2-dimensional echocardiography. Myocardial ischemia can be induced by exercise, by cold, by atrial pacing to increase the heart rate, or by ergonovine in graduated doses to induce coronary vasoconstriction; the development of ischemia can be monitored by noninvasive techniques such as thallium 201 imaging, blood pool or first pass radionuclide angiography, or electrocardiography (see below). There is no correlation between the clinical symptoms and signs and the extent of disease.

1. ANGINA PECTORIS

Essentials of Diagnosis

- Squeezing or pressurelike pain, retrosternal or slightly to the left, that appears quickly during exertion, may radiate in a set pattern, and subsides with rest.
- Seventy percent have diagnostic electrocardiographic abnormalities after mild exercise; the re-

maining 30% have normal tracings or nondiagnostic abnormalities.

General Considerations

Angina pectoris is usually due to arteriosclerotic heart disease, but in rare instances it may occur in the absence of significant disease of the coronary arteries as a result of coronary spasm (see p 214), severe aortic stenosis or insufficiency, syphilitic aortitis, increased metabolic demands as in hyperthyroidism or after thyroid therapy, marked anemia, or paroxysmal tachycardias with rapid ventricular rates. The underlying mechanism is a discrepancy between the myocardial demands for oxygen and the amount delivered through the coronary arteries, either by increased demand (as in exercise) or decreased coronary flow (coronary spasm) or both (see p 214).

Clinical Findings

A. History: The diagnosis of angina pectoris depends almost entirely upon the history, and it is of the utmost importance that the patient be allowed sufficient time to describe the symptoms without help from the examiner, using gestures to characterize the location and quality of the symptom. (The patient often makes a fist.) The history should specifically include the following categories:

1. Circumstances that precipitate and relieve angina–Angina most commonly occurs during walking, especially up an incline or a flight of stairs. Exertion that involves straining, closing the glottis, and immobilizing the thorax precipitates an attack most rapidly. Regardless of the type of activity, angina occurs *during* exertion and subsides promptly if the patient stands or sits quietly. Patients prefer to remain upright rather than lie down. Some patients obtain relief by belching and for this reason may attribute their distress to "stomach trouble." The amount of activity required to produce angina varies with each patient, but it is always less after meals, during excitement, or on exposure to a cold wind. Heavy meals, hypoglycemia, or strong emotion can provoke an attack in the absence of exertion.

2. Characteristics of the discomfort–Patients often do not refer to angina as a "pain" but as a sensation of squeezing, burning, pressing, choking, aching, bursting, "gas," or tightness. It is commonly attributed to "indigestion." The distress of angina is never a sharply localized or darting pain that can be pointed to with a finger. It appears quickly during exertion and increases rapidly in intensity until the patient is compelled to stop and rest, even though the initial discomfort may not be severe. Discomfort may occur at rest or at night as a result of coronary spasm not preceded by changes in pulse or blood pressure (see p 214).

3. Location and radiation–The distribution of the distress may vary widely in different patients but is always the same for each individual patient. In 80–90% of cases the discomfort is felt behind or slightly to the left of the sternum. When it begins farther to the left or, uncommonly, on the right, it characteristically moves centrally and is felt deep in the chest. Although angina may radiate to any segment from C8 to T4, it radiates most often to the left shoulder and upper arm, frequently moving down the inner volar aspect of the arm to the elbow, forearm, wrist, or fourth and fifth fingers. Radiation to the right shoulder and distally is less common, but the characteristics are the same. Occasionally angina may be referred to or felt initially in the lower jaw, the base or back of the neck, the interscapular area, or high in the left back.

Angina may almost certainly be excluded when the patient designates the only site of pain by pointing to the area of the apical impulse with one finger.

4. Duration of attacks–Angina is of clearly defined short duration and subsides completely without residual discomfort. If the attack is precipitated by exertion and the patient promptly stops to rest, the distress of angina usually lasts less than 3 minutes (although most patients think it is longer). Attacks following a heavy meal or brought on by anger often last 15–20 minutes.

5. Effect of nitroglycerin–The diagnosis of angina pectoris is strongly supported (1) if 0.4 mg of nitroglycerin invariably shortens an attack and (2) if that amount taken immediately before exertion invariably permits greater exertion before the onset of angina or prevents angina entirely. However, this source of diagnostic information is less reliable than the characteristic history.

6. Unrelated disorders that intensify or mimic angina should be considered. Cholecystitis, reflux esophagitis, thyrotoxicosis, paroxysmal arrhythmias, orthostatic hypotension, acute increase in blood pressure, or left ventricular failure may account for unusual variants of angina pectoris.

B. Signs: Examination during a spontaneous or induced attack frequently reveals a significant elevation in systolic and diastolic blood pressure; occasionally, gallop rhythm is present during pain only. Carotid sinus massage often causes the pain to subside more quickly than usual if it slows the cardiac rate, and it is a helpful maneuver in instances of "atypical angina."

It is important to detect signs of diseases that may contribute to arteriosclerotic heart disease, eg, diabetes mellitus (retinopathy or neuropathy), xanthomatosis (tuberosa, plana, or tendinosa); or of disorders that intensify the angina, such as hypertension, thyrotoxicosis, orthostatic hypotension, and aortic stenosis or mitral stenosis.

The cardiovascular examination is normal in 25–40% of patients with angina. In the remainder, evidence of occlusive disease of the peripheral arteries, hypertensive retinopathy and cardiomegaly, significant murmurs, or signs of cardiac failure may be noted.

C. Laboratory Findings: Look for risk factors associated with the development of atherosclerosis, such as serum cholesterol, high-density lipoproteins, triglycerides, evidence of diabetes, hyperuricemia, and hypoglycemia. Contributing factors such as anemia, evidence of renal disease, myxedema, syphilis, or other cardiac disorders should be sought.

D. Electrocardiography: The resting ECG is normal in over one-fourth of patients with angina. In the remainder, abnormalities include atrioventricular or intraventricular conduction defects, patterns of left ventricular hypertrophy, old myocardial infarction, or nonspecific ST–T changes.

E. Exercise Stress Test: Exercise has been the most common noninvasive technique used for many years to provide objective evidence of myocardial ischemia by inducing the typical chest discomfort of which the patient complains. Most commonly, stress exercise employs serial graded exercise, using a bicycle ergometer or motorized treadmill, that the physician can stop at any time. Interpretation may be difficult if the patient is receiving digitalis, beta-adrenergic blocking drugs, or quinidine and if the pretest likelihood of disease is low (see below). The original criteria for a positive test in the past consisted of a horizontal down-sloping ST segment depression varying from 1 to 2 mm. Recent refinements of the test attempt to measure the degree of positivity and not merely to classify the test as either positive or negative. The factors considered in these refinements include the contour, depth, and area of ST segment change (depression or elevation), the time or stage of appearance of the abnormalities, their duration, the pulse rate achieved in relation to the maximum predicted for the age and sex of the patient, the coexistent development of anginal pain, and hypotension or complex ventricular beats during exercise. A strongly positive test consists of ST changes of 2 mm or more that appear early at a heart rate less than 85% of predicted maximum and are associated with angina, hypotension, or complex arrhythmias. The greater the abnormality, the more marked the positivity and the more likely the presence of multi-vessel disease, including left main coronary artery disease.

1. Precautions to be observed during exercise stress test–Exercise should not be performed if a recent myocardial infarction or unstable angina is suspected or if the patient has an acute illness, severe cardiac failure, or other conditions in which exercise would be unwise. Acute myocardial infarction may be precipitated if exercise testing is done in patients with acute or subacute myocardial ischemia and pain of recent origin. The test must be done under the supervision of a physician, who should observe and examine the patient during the exercise and be able to perform resuscitative measures in the event of ventricular fibrillation. The physician should also observe a continuous ECG obtained during the exercise in order to stop the test if the patient develops moderately severe angina, frequent or complex ventricular premature beats, significant hypotension or hypertension, marked dyspnea or fatigue, or if a satisfactory ECG is not being recorded.

2. Significance of a postive exercise stress electrocardiographic test–There is considerable controversy about the desirability of performing exercise tests in asymptomatic middle-aged individuals because of the likelihood of both false-positive and false-negative tests, especially in population groups in whom the presence or possibility of coronary disease is relatively low. Despite the rigorousness of the criteria one uses for a positive test and whether one uses a qualitative or quantitative treadmill score, one must consider the population from which the patient was drawn and the pretest probability of coronary disease in order to interpret the exercise stress test. The sensitivity, specificity, and predictive accuracy of the quantitative exercise electrocardiographic stress test are being correlated with the results of radioisotope studies and of coronary arteriography. All 3 tests correlate significantly, although thallium 201 testing is generally more sensitive to hypoperfusion at rest and gated blood pool cardiac imaging is more sensitive to wall motion abnormalities than are stress electrocardiographic tests, although the latter are perhaps more specific. All tests become more specific when they follow ischemia induced by exercise and reversed with redistribution after several hours (reversible ischemia).

F. Radioisotope Studies: Redistribution myocardial ischemia revealed by serial thallium 201 scans may be positive in patients with atypical chest pain who have negative exercise electrocardiographic studies. Reduced perfusion with thallium 201 on exercise, combined with the finding of abnormally contracting segments or hypokinesis on blood pool scans, is a reliable index of myocardial ischemia, although false-negative results occur in a small percentage of cases (see also p 222). Decreased ejection fraction may be demonstrated by 2-dimensional echocardiography.

G. Coronary Angiography: In the past few years, selective coronary cineangiocardiography has been performed with increased frequency in many centers, utilizing multiple views with either the Sones or the Judkins technique. Low mortality rates in the range of 0.2% have been described by experienced operators, but morbidity rates vary from 1 to 7%. Episodes of cardiac ischemia, arrhythmias, pulmonary edema, or thrombosis of arteries used in the study prevent its use in all patients with coronary disease. The procedure demands experienced physicians and facilities for monitoring of rhythm and other vital functions, as well as resuscitation equipment. Cost is a major concern. The procedure should not be used solely for the purpose of diagnosis of angina except infrequently. High-quality films are required, taken in multiple projections and interpreted by experienced physicians.

Coronary arteriography should be performed according to the following indications:

(1) In patients being considered for coronary bypass surgery because of disabling stable angina who have failed to improve on an adequate medical regimen.

(2) In patients in whom coronary bypass surgery is being considered because of myocardial infarctions in rapid succession or repeated admissions to the hospital because of unstable angina.

(3) In patients with aortic valve disease who also have angina pectoris, especially if the aortic valve gradient is only modest, in order to determine whether the angina is due to coronary disease or to aortic stenosis.

(4) In patients who have had coronary bypass surgery with initial improvement and subsequent relapse of symptoms, to determine whether the bypass graft is patent or occluded, or if there are new coronary stenoses in vessels previously patent or only slightly stenotic.

(5) In patients with coronary disease with ischemic cardiomyopathy and cardiac failure in whom a left ventricular aneurysm, mitral insufficiency, or perforated interventricular septum is suspected that can be treated surgically if bypassable lesions in the coronary arteries can be operated upon at the same time.

(6) For diagnostic purposes in patients with nonanginal chest pain of uncertain cause who will be benefited by knowing that the pain is not due to coronary disease, especially when important decisions regarding vocation or avocation depend upon the accuracy of the diagnosis.

Whereas the diagnosis of angina pectoris is made on the basis of the history, the degree and variety of coronary stenotic lesions and the presence and adequacy of collateral circulation—as well as impairment of left ventricular contractility—require anatomic visualization. There are good clinical data to indicate that the prognosis in patients with clinical coronary disease and angina pectoris is directly related to the extent of the coronary lesion (whether the stenoses affected one, 2, or all 3 coronary arteries, are proximal, or involve the main left coronary artery) and the left ventricular function and contractility; the 5-year mortality rate has been shown to be 3–6 times as great if 3 vessels—as opposed to one—are involved, if the ejection fraction is reduced, or if ventricular aneurysm or its lesser manifestations of dyskinesis or akinesis are present. Left ventricular function is more important prognostically than the number of stenotic arteries.

Most patients with abnormal coronary angiograms have ischemic exercise ECGs, but about one-third of patients with negative exercise tests have positive coronary angiograms.

Sones has shown that single-vessel disease occurs in 25% of patients with angina pectoris or myocardial infarction and that isolated disease of the left main or circumflex coronary artery is rare. Patients with cardiac failure, left ventricular asynergy, or decreased ejection fractions usually have 2- or 3-vessel disease.

H. Left Ventricular Angiography: Left ventricular angiography should be combined with coronary angiography in the evaluation of patients. Nitroglycerin, previously given prior to coronary angiography, is now withheld until the cine films have been obtained, because nitroglycerin may mask coronary spasm (see below). If invasive procedures are required, both are necessary to properly evaluate the anatomy of the coronary arteries, left ventricular function, the presence of ventricular aneurysm or mitral insufficiency, the degree of collateral circulation, and the volume and presence of abnormally contracting segments of the left ventricle.

I. Coronary Spasm (Prinzmetal's Variant Angina): Coronary artery spasm, formerly suggested as a possible cause of variant angina pectoris, has in recent years been found to contribute to a variety of manifestations of ischemic cardiac disease (see below, under Treatment).

Hemodynamic and radioisotopic studies have shown that spasm of the large coronary arteries with resulting decreased coronary blood flow may occur spontaneously or may be induced by mechanical irritation from a coronary catheter, by exposure to cold, or by ergot-derivative drugs. Spasm may occur both in normal and in stenosed coronary arteries. Angina pectoris and even myocardial infarction may occur as a result of spasm in the absence of visible obstructive coronary heart disease (normal coronary arteriogram), although most instances of coronary spasm occur in the presence of coronary stenosis. It is thus necessary to rule out spasm before diagnosing organic stenosis of a coronary artery during coronary arteriography. Multiple views should be obtained and sublingual nitroglycerin, isosorbide dinitrate, or verapamil or nifedipine should be administered in an attempt to reverse possible spasm. Verapamil, nitroglycerin, and propranolol (or other beta-blockers) may be given intravenously, or the nitroglycerin may be injected directly into the involved coronary artery.

Prinzmetal's variant angina is more apt to occur at rest than with effort, may occur at odd times during the day or night (even awakening patients from sleep), and is apt to be associated with arrhythmias or conduction defects; the ST segment is more commonly elevated rather than depressed, as during angina of effort. Both variant angina and angina of effort respond rapidly to sublingual nitrates or calcium entry-blocking agents (see p 208). Variant angina is more common in women under age 50; angina of effort is uncommon in women of this age in the absence of severe hypercholesterolemia, hypertension, or diabetes mellitus.

The occurrence of coronary spasm during coronary arteriography, perfusion defects on radioisotope studies during induced spasm, and the occurrence of angina pectoris at rest, myocardial infarction, and ventricular arrhythmias in the absence of stenosis of the coronary arteries have elucidated the role of coronary spasm in clinical disease.

Angina has been provoked by ergotamine used for the treatment of migraine, and it has been specifically induced by ergonovine for diagnosis during coronary arteriography. Because the resulting spasm may be intense and may induce angina, arrhythmias, or myocardial infarction, these drugs, if used at all, should be used with considerable caution, in small doses, and under close clinical observation and with resuscitation equipment at hand.

If patients with angina resulting from coronary spasm do not respond rapidly to nitrates, then nifedipine, diltiazem, or verapamil are usually effective. These drugs may also benefit the usual angina of effort, in which spasm may be superimposed. The negative inotropic action of verapamil, as well as its electrophysiologic action by decreasing conduction through the sinus and atrioventricular nodes, must be appreciated (see also p 233). Coronary artery spasm due to neurohumoral influences may occur in patients with or without coronary artery stenosis and may play a role in the frequent association of emotional events and angina pectoris.

J. Newer Diagnostic Studies: Subtraction coronary angiography, positron emission tomography, and nuclear magnetic resonance are in the process of being evaluated. They show promise because they are essentially noninvasive.

Differential Diagnosis

Psychophysiologic cardiovascular reactions are a loosely defined group of disorders having in common dull aching chest pains often described as "heart pain," lasting hours or days, often aggravated by exertion but not promptly relieved by rest. Darting, knifelike pains of momentary duration at the apex or over the precordium are often present also. Emotional tension and fatigue make the pain worse. Dyspnea of the hyperventilation variety, palpitation, fatigue, and headache, and continual exhaustion are common.

The "anterior chest wall syndrome" is characterized by sharply localized tenderness of intercostal muscles, pressure on which reproduces the chest pain. Sprain or inflammation of the chondrocostal junctions, which may be warm, swollen, and red (so-called Tietze's syndrome), may result in diffuse chest pain that is also reproduced by local pressure. Intercostal neuritis (herpes zoster, diabetes mellitus, etc) may confuse the diagnosis.

Cervical or thoracic spine disease (degenerative disk disease, postural strain, "arthritis") involving the dorsal roots produces sudden sharp, severe chest pain similar to angina in location and "radiation" but related to specific movements of the neck or spine, recumbency, and straining or lifting. Pain due to cervical thoracic disk disease involves the outer or dorsal aspect of the arm and the thumb and index fingers rather than the ring and little fingers.

Peptic ulcer, chronic cholecystitis, cardiospasm, and functional gastrointestinal disease are often suspected because some patients indisputably obtain relief from angina by belching. In these disorders, symptoms are related to food intake rather than physical exertion. X-ray and fluoroscopic study are helpful in diagnosis.

Reflux esophagitis is characterized by lower chest and upper abdominal pain after heavy meals, occurring in recumbency or upon bending over. The pain is relieved by bland diet, antacids, semi-Fowler position, and walking.

Degenerative and inflammatory lesions of the left shoulder or cervical rib and the scalenus anticus syndrome differ from angina in that the pain is precipitated by movement of the arm and shoulder, paresthesias are present in the left arm, and postural exercises and pillow support to the shoulders in bed give relief.

"Tight" mitral stenosis or pulmonary hypertension resulting from chronic pulmonary disease can produce chest pain indistinguishable from angina pectoris, including ST segment sagging or depression. The clinical findings of mitral stenosis or of the lung disease are evident, and the ECG invariably discloses right axis deviation or frank right ventricular hypertrophy.

Spontaneous pneumothorax may cause chest pain as well as dyspnea and may create confusion with angina as well as myocardial infarction.

Treatment

A. Treatment of Acute Attack:

1. Nitroglycerin is the drug of choice; it acts in about 1–2 minutes. This drug (and all nitrates) decreases arteriolar and venous tone, reduces preload and afterload, and lowers the oxygen demand of the heart. As soon as the attack begins, place one fresh 0.3-mg tablet under the tongue and allow it to dissolve. The dose may be increased to 0.4–0.6 mg if no relief is obtained from a smaller dose. Nitroglycerin may be used freely whenever an attack occurs or may be used in order to prevent an attack (see below). It may cause headache and hypotension, especially if larger doses are used.

2. Sublingual nifedipine, 10–20 mg, may rapidly relieve angina, especially if spasm is the cause.

3. Oral isosorbide dinitrate and nitroglycerin ointment do not act as rapidly as nitroglycerin but have a longer duration of action and can be used at 4- to 6-hour intervals during the day or at bedtime. Sublingual isosorbide dinitrate takes effect more rapidly than the oral form and may be used instead of sublingual nitroglycerin. Transdermal nitroglycerin provides slow continuous release of the drug over a 24-hour period and is more convenient than nitroglycerin ointment.

4. General measures–The patient should stand still, sit, or lie down as soon as the pain begins and remain quiet until the attack is over. Most patients do cease activity, but some try to "work the attack off," and patients should be warned against this.

B. Prevention of Further Attacks:

1. Angina may coexist with or be aggravated by left ventricular failure, obvious or incipient. Treatment of the cardiac failure with diuretics or digitalis or both, as well as with other methods such as prolonged rest, may be extremely helpful.

2. Nitroglycerin, 0.3–0.6 mg under the tongue just before activity.

3. Long-acting nitrates–Isosorbide dinitrate (Isordil, Sorbitrate), 2.5–10 mg sublingually 3 or more times daily or 10–40 mg orally 4 times daily. Transdermal nitroglycerin, an adhesive patch delivering nitroglycerin to the skin at a predetermined rate of usually 5 or 10 mg/24 h, may be used during the day and has a duration of action of 24 hours (see p 218). There is no convincing evidence that these agents prolong life, but they do relieve pain.

4. Beta-blocking agents–Propranolol (Inderal), 10–80 mg 3–4 times daily by mouth; metoprolol (Lopressor), 50 mg twice daily; nadolol (Corgard), 40 mg once daily; atenolol (Tenormin), 50–100 mg once daily; pindolol (Visken), 5–10 mg twice daily; or timolol (Blocadren), 10–20 mg twice daily (each drug then increased to tolerance) has been given with benefit to patients with angina who have never had left ventricular failure. Care must be exercised during use of these drugs, and the precautions noted on p 206 should be observed. Combination therapy with long-acting nitrates such as isosorbide dinitrate or with calcium-entry blocking agents (see below) has been shown to be significantly more effective than single-drug therapy.

5. Calcium entry-blocking agents–(See Table 8–4.) Nifedipine, verapamil, and diltiazem are valuable agents in the treatment of angina, whether or not coronary spasm coexists. They dilate the coronary epicardial arteries and decrease the blood pressure. Care must be taken in the presence of cardiac failure, especially if the drugs are combined with beta-blocking agents. New agents are being developed— analogs of the above 3 with both shorter and longer duration of action. Further experience is required.

6. General measures–The patient must avoid all habits and activities known to bring on an attack. Coexisting disorders (especially anemia or cardiac arrhythmias) that may lead to increased cardiac ischemia must be treated. Most patients with angina do not require prolonged bed rest, but rest and relaxation are beneficial. Adequate mental rest is also important. Obese patients should be placed on a reducing diet and their weight brought to normal or slightly subnormal levels. Use of tobacco should be stopped or avoided because it produces tachycardia and elevation in blood pressure and because cigarette smoking has been shown to be a risk factor in coronary heart disease. Smoking may precipitate ventricular arrhythmias and sudden death in patients with coronary disease. Physical fitness resulting from a regular exercise program has been thought to be helpful, but the benefits may be mainly psychologic, ie, an improved overall sense of well-being. Evidence that such a program prolongs life is inconclusive.

7. Sedatives or tranquilizers–These may reduce the frequency of attacks.

8. Oral vasodilator therapy, eg, hydralazine combined with diuretic therapy with or without oral nitroglycerin, long-acting nitrates, or calcium entry-blocking drugs are often helpful in decreasing left ventricular work.

9. Prevent arrhythmias–(See p 237.)

10. Control hyperlipidemia–(See pp 211 and 787.)

11. Control hypertension–(See p 201 and also Surgery for Coronary Heart Disease, p 218.)

12. Platelet-inhibiting agents–Recent work on the synthesis of prostaglandins and on the competitive roles of thromboxane (which causes aggregation of platelets) and prostacyclin (which decreases platelet aggregation and causes vasodilatation) has suggested the use of anti-platelet-aggregating drugs such as clofibrate, sulfinpyrazone, aspirin, dipyridamole, and possibly beta-adrenergic blocking agents in coronary disease. The clinical value of these agents (with the exception of beta-blocking drugs, which have been shown to decrease the likelihood of recurrent myocardial infarction and the incidence of sudden death and cardiac death) is still controversial, and the long-term benefits remain to be determined.

Prognosis

The average mortality rate of angina pectoris over a period of 5 years is approximately 3–4% per year. The percentage varies from 1 to 15% depending upon whether there is one-, 2-, or 3-vessel disease; whether the stenosis is proximal or distal; whether the collateral circulation is adequate; whether the ejection fraction is less than 50%; whether abnormal contraction patterns are present; and whether the patient has evidence of resting ischemic changes on the ECG, hypertension, or evidence of left ventricular failure at the time of the angina pectoris. The course is unpredictable in the individual patient, although groups with higher and lower risks can be identified. Hypertension increases the afterload of the left ventricle, leading to myocardial hypertrophy, which contributes to the increased requirement of coronary blood flow.

The course is prolonged, with variable frequency and severity of attacks punctuated by periods of complete remission and episodes of myocardial infarction, or terminated by sudden death. The last is often unpredictable and contributes to the great anxiety caused by

Table 8–4. Oral calcium entry–blocking drugs.

Agent	Inhibition of Atrioventricular Conduction	Coronary Vasodilatation	Decreased Inotropic Action	Hypotension, Edema	Dose (Initial; Daily)*
Verapamil (Calan, Isoptin)	+++	++	++	++	40–80 mg; 240–360 mg
Diltiazem (Cardizem)	+ to ++	++	+	+	30–60 mg; 180–240 mg
Nifedipine (Procardia)	0 to +	+++	0	+++	20 mg; 40–120 mg

*Give in divided doses.

the disease. Diabetes, hypertension, cardiac hypertrophy, congestive failure, myocardial infarction, arrhythmias, and conduction defects shorten life expectancy. Onset prior to age 40 or a family history of early cardiac death is prognostically unfavorable.

Half of all patients die suddenly, and an additional one-third die after myocardial infarction. Heart failure accounts for most of the remainder of deaths.

Brensike JF et al: Effects of therapy with cholestyramine on progression of coronary arteriosclerosis: Results of the NHLBI type II coronary intervention study. *Circulation* 1984;**69**:313.

Brown BG, Bolson EL, Dodge HT: Arteriographic assessment of coronary atherosclerosis: Review of current methods, their limitations, and clinical applications. *Arteriosclerosis* 1982;**2**:2.

Fozzard HA: Electrophysiology of the heart: The effects of ischemia. *Hosp Pract* (May) 1980;**15**:61.

Froelicher VF: Exercise testing and training: Clinical applications. *J Am Coll Cardiol* 1983;**1**:114.

Havel RJ, Kane JP: Therapy of hyperlipidemic states. *Annu Rev Med* 1982;**33**:417.

Herfkens RJ, Brundage BH, Lipton MJ: Cardiovascular applications of computed tomography. *Cardiovasc Rev Rep* 1983;**4**:979.

Kannel WB et al: Optimal resources for primary prevention of atherosclerotic diseases. *Circulation* 1984;**70**:157A.

Klocke FJ: Measurements of coronary blood flow and degree of stenosis: Current clinical implications and continuing uncertainties. *J Am Coll Cardiol* 1983;**1**:31.

Lipid Research Clinics Program: The lipid research clinics coronary primary prevention trial results. 1. Reduction in incidence of coronary heart disease. 2. The relationship of reduction in incidence of coronary heart disease to cholesterol lowering. *JAMA* 1984;**251**:351, 365.

Mark DB et al: Clinical characteristics and long-term survival of patients with variant angina. *Circulation* 1984;**69**:880.

Maseri A, Parodi O, Fox KM: Rational approach to the medical therapy of angina pectoris: The role of calcium antagonists. *Prog Cardiovasc Dis* 1983;**25**:269.

Moncada S: Prostacyclin and arterial wall biology. *Arteriosclerosis* 1982;**2**:193.

Packer M et al: Hemodynamic consequences of combined beta-adrenergic and slow calcium channel blockade in man. *Circulation* 1982;**65**:660.

Parmley WW: The combination of beta-adrenergic-blocking agents and nitrates in the treatment of stable angina pectoris. *Cardiovasc Rev Rep* 1982;**3**:1425.

Pitt B et al: Prostaglandins and prostaglandin inhibitors in ischemic heart disease. *Ann Intern Med* 1983;**99**:83.

Proceedings of a symposium on calcium-entry blockers in coronary artery disease. *Circulation* 1982;**65**(1–**Part 1**). [Entire issue.]

Proceedings of a symposium on new strategies in the management of ischemic heart disease. *Am Heart J* 1982;**103**(4–**Part 2**):583.

Proudfit WJ et al: Fifteen-year survival study of patients with obstructive coronary artery disease. *Circulation* 1983;**68**:986.

Reeder GS, Seward JB, Tajik AJ: The role of two-dimensional echocardiography in coronary artery disease: A critical appraisal. *Mayo Clin Proc* 1982;**57**:247.

Ross R: Atherosclerosis: A problem of the biology of arterial wall cells and their interactions with blood components. *Arteriosclerosis* 1981;**1**:293.

Ruderman NB, Haudenschild C: Diabetes as an atherogenic factor. *Prog Cardiovasc Dis* 1984;**26**:373.

Shub C et al: The unpredictable progression of symptomatic coronary artery disease: A serial clinical-angiographic analysis. *Mayo Clin Proc* 1981;**56**:155.

Stadel BV: Oral contraceptives and cardiovascular disease. (2 parts.) *N Engl J Med* 1981;**305**:612, 672.

Stamler J, Stamler R: Intervention for the prevention and control of hypertension and atherosclerotic diseases: United States and international experience. *Am J Med* 1984;**76**:13.

ten Kate LP et al: Familial aggregation of coronary heart disease and its relation to known genetic risk factors. *Am J Cardiol* 1982;**50**:945.

Thompson RH: The clinical use of transdermal delivery devices with nitroglycerin. *Cardiovasc Rev Rep* 1983;**4**:91.

Twelfth Bethesda Conference: Noninvasive technology in the assessment of ventricular function. *Am J Cardiol* 1982;**49**:1309.

Weksler BB et al: Differential inhibition by aspirin of vascular and platelet prostaglandin synthesis in atherosclerotic patients. *N Engl J Med* 1983;**308**:800.

Winniford MD, Huxley RL, Hillis LD: Randomized, double-blind comparison of propranolol alone and a propranolol-verapamil combination in patients with severe angina of effort. *J Am Coll Cardiol* 1983;**1**(2–**Part 1**):492.

2. UNSTABLE ANGINA
(Intermediate Coronary Syndrome)

This syndrome, called by some preinfarction angina, intermediate coronary syndrome, premature or impending myocardial infarction, or coronary insufficiency, refers to a syndrome intermediate between the angina pectoris of effort and acute myocardial infarction in the spectrum of clinical events that occur in coronary heart disease. It has received special attention because of the adverse prognosis and unpredictability of sudden onset of myocardial infarction in some of these patients. Since the mortality rate in acute myocardial infarction is greatest in the first few hours, recognition of a syndrome with increased likelihood of impending infarction requires hospitalization and monitoring in the coronary care unit to avert sudden arrhythmias and death.

The syndrome is recognized by the appearance of pain which has a different character, duration, radiation, and severity—or which over a period of hours or days has a crescendo quality of increased ease of production, or which occurs at rest or during the night. The ischemic nature of the pain should be documented by demonstrating transient ischemic electrocardiographic changes during the pain. Angina that appears for the first time usually indicates occlusion of a coronary branch and may progress to myocardial infarction or gradually subside, but the same close monitoring is required.

Patients who have the clinical features described but do not develop signs of myocardial infarction are considered to be in precarious balance between coronary supply and demand and should be treated as though they have had a small myocardial infarction.

Patients with rest angina, especially if the ST segment is elevated during pain, are likely to have coronary vasoconstriction resulting in decreased supply rather than increased demand and are usually benefited by calcium entry-blocking agents (see below and Table 8-4). Radioisotope studies with pyrophosphate (see under Acute Myocardial Infarction, p 222) have revealed areas with diffuse necrosis in 20–30% of such patients, but diffuse uptake is unreliable and may occur with fibrosis due to cardiomyopathy or other cause. Focal, well-defined uptake of isotope should be required before one diagnoses acute myocardial necrosis.

The prognosis following medical treatment of unstable angina has varied considerably in different reports; the consensus is that the mortality rate during hospitalization is low—on the order of 5%—but the mortality rate over the next 1–2 years is about 15%. A randomized study by the Veterans Administration has indicated a similar mortality rate over a 2- to 5-year period with either medical or surgical treatment of unstable angina after the first few days. Relief of anginal pain is a consistent finding in all of the studies, yet return to gainful employment is not greater in surgically treated patients.

Patients with unstable angina should be treated with bed rest; nitrates, including intravenous nitroglycerin; beta-blocking drugs such as propranolol, atenolol, metoprolol, pindolol, timolol, or nadolol; calcium antagonists such as verapamil, diltiazem, or nifedipine; and psychologic rest and reassurance. Nitrates can be given as isosorbide dinitrate (Isordil, Sorbitrate), 2.5–10 mg sublingually every 2 hours when awake, or transdermal nitroglycerin (see p 215), one 5-mg patch daily. If there is rest angina or ST elevation during pain, the calcium entry-blocking agents nifedipine, diltiazem, and verapamil should be used. If there is associated left ventricular failure, caution should be exercised before combining a beta-blocking and a calcium entry-blocking agent, especially verapamil.

If the symptoms do not subside with this therapy or if they become worse, intra-aortic balloon assist devices (see under Acute Myocardial Infarction, p 226) may temporarily improve the situation so that hemodynamic investigations combined with left ventricular angiography and coronary angiography may be performed with the intention of doing coronary bypass surgery if there are bypassable stenoses. Because of the lower surgical mortality rate, delaying surgery at least a month is desirable if possible.

Follow-up shows that patients who entered the coronary care unit because of acceleration of the clinical coronary syndrome suggesting infarction but in whom infarction was not demonstrated have a higher death rate over a 1- to 2-year period than ordinary angina pectoris patients and so need close supervision. (See also Surgery for Coronary Heart Disease, below.)

3. SURGERY FOR CORONARY HEART DISEASE

Aortocoronary Bypass

Considerable progress has been made in the indications for and modifications of bypass procedures for coronary artery stenosis. The procedure most commonly used is anastomosis of a graft of the saphenous vein or internal mammary artery from the aorta to the distal portion of the obstructed coronary artery, beyond the stenosis. One to 5 bypass grafts have been made in the same patient, and the data show that in some patients there is improvement of left ventricular function, increased cardiac output, improved cardiac contraction, and relief of angina pectoris. The grafts have remained patent in about 80–85% of patients, but it is still uncertain how long patency will be maintained. Apart from a surgical mortality rate of about 1–3% and an incidence of late closure of the bypass graft of about 10–20%, the major complication of coronary bypass surgery is the development of intraoperative myocardial infarction in 5–10% of patients. Further study of the incidence of postoperative myocardial infarction and late recurrence of angina or development of impaired left ventricular function will place the indications for the procedure into proper perspective.

The indications for bypass surgery include major stenosis (at least 50–70%) of the left main coronary artery, severe unacceptable angina pectoris, and 3-vessel coronary disease with only slightly impaired left ventricular function—especially if there is a high risk of reinfarction or sudden death associated with previous myocardial infarction, left ventricular failure, complex ventricular arrhythmias, or large segmental contraction abnormalities.

Left ventricular function must be efficient enough to enable the patient to survive surgery and accommodate the depressed left ventricular function that occurs postoperatively. A poor ejection fraction, a large left ventricular volume, and cardiac failure secondary to ischemic cardiomyopathy from coronary disease are contraindications to bypass surgery because the surgical mortality rate is high and the benefits small.

Randomized studies show that bypass surgery prolongs life when there is significant left main coronary artery stenosis or 3-vessel disease with slightly or moderately impaired left ventricular function and the patient is in a high-risk group, as indicated above. Evidence for prolongation of life by surgery in 3-vessel disease in this group has required a follow-up of 5–10 years. Relief of anginal pain occurs after surgery in 85% of cases.

The availability of this surgical procedure has sharpened and broadened the indications for **coronary angiography.** The most common indication is unacceptable angina pectoris unimproved by restricted activity, nitrates, beta-blocking, or calcium entry-blocking agents. Indications for coronary angiograms and possible bypass surgery have been extended to include unstable angina after the acute phase has subsided and residual angina that persists following a myocardial infarction. Because of the frequent coexistence of dyskinesia or aneurysm of the left ventricle, dysfunction of the papillary muscle, or ventricular septal defect, patients studied by coronary angiography should have concurrent left ventricular cineangiography and radionuclide studies to determine localized areas of dyskinesia or mitral insufficiency.

Ventricular aneurysms and areas of dyskinesia and akinesia have been found to occur more frequently than previously thought, primarily because they were not obvious on a plain film of the chest but could be seen in a left ventricular cineangiogram or by means of 2-dimensional echocardiograms or radioangiographic studies. (See p 223 for spectrum of abnormalities.) At present it is not considered wise to resect the aneurysm unless there is a well-demarcated, discrete akinesia and cardiac failure or ventricular ectopy that cannot be controlled by medical treatment. Repeated systemic emboli are a lesser indication and are controversial. Resection of the aneurysm is unwise unless at least 40–50% of regional myocardial contractility remains. In patients who have ventricular tachycardia resistant to conventional medical therapy, endocardial electrophysiologic mapping should be performed to determine the site of origin of the ectopic activity; surgical resection of this endocardial area can then be combined with resection of the aneurysm. Patients with left ventricular failure of undetermined cause should have a coronary angiogram and a left ventricular cineangiogram to exclude left ventricular aneurysm or localized areas of impaired contraction secondary to coronary heart disease that might be amenable to surgery.

Complications of acute myocardial infarction (see below) such as ventricular septal defect, papillary muscle rupture, or false ventricular aneurysm should be sought, because they usually require surgical intervention.

Percutaneous Transluminal Coronary Angioplasty (See also p 277.)

Percutaneous transluminal angioplasty is a new form of treatment developed by Grüntzig, in which a balloon catheter is passed percutaneously under local anesthesia through a systemic artery into the coronary artery and inflated to dilate the obstruction. This method can also be used for renal artery lesions causing hypertension. Single, proximal, localized noncalcified atheromas, especially of the left anterior descending artery (about 10% of all cases), are the lesions most suitable for treatment by physicians experienced in this method. As with coronary bypass surgery, patients should have disabling angina pectoris not responding adequately to medical teatment. About half of patients treated to date have shown clinical improvement, manifested by a reduced pressure gradient across the stenosis, improved exercise capacity, decreased ischemia with exercise (as shown by thallium scans and radionuclide angiography), and decreased angina. Ejection fraction, indicating improved left ventricular performance, has increased after exer-

cise in some patients. The procedure is investigational because of complications such as dissection of the coronary artery, thrombosis, lack of success in dilating the obstruction, and about a 20% rate of recurrent stenosis over a period of a few months. A backup surgical team is necessary. The procedure is being performed in many centers, and its proper role will be clarified in the near future.

Biagini A et al: Vasospastic ischemic mechanism of frequent asymptomatic transient ST–T changes during continuous electrocardiographic monitoring in selected unstable angina patients. *Am Heart J* 1982;**103**:13.

Coronary artery surgery study (CASS): A randomized trial of coronary artery bypass surgery: Survival data. *Circulation* 1983;**68**:939.

European Coronary Surgery Study Group: Prospective randomised study of coronary artery bypass surgery in stable angina pectoris: Second interim report by the European Coronary Surgery Study Group. *Lancet* 1980;**2**:491.

Gerstenblith G et al: Nifedipine in unstable angina: A double-blind, randomized trial. *N Engl J Med* 1982;**306**:885.

Hamby RI et al: Recurrent angina after bypass surgery: Evaluation by early and late arteriography. *Am Heart J* 1980;**99**:607.

Kaplan K et al: Intravenous nitroglycerin for the treatment of angina at rest unresponsive to standard nitrate therapy. *Am J Cardiol* 1983;**51**:694.

Krikler DM, Rowland E: Clinical value of calcium antagonists in treatment of cardiovascular disorders. *J Am Coll Cardiol* 1983;**1**:355.

Lawrie GM et al: Clinical results of coronary bypass in 500 patients at least 10 years after operation. *Circulation* 1982;**66(2–Part 2)**:11.

Mock MB et al: Survival of medically treated patients in the Coronary Artery Surgery Study (CASS) registry. *Circulation* 1982;**66**:562.

Mulcahy R et al: Unstable angina: Natural history and determinants of prognosis. *Am J Cardiol* 1981;**48**:525.

National Heart, Lung, and Blood Institute: Proceedings of the National Heart, Lung, and Blood Institute Workshop on the outcome of percutaneous transluminal coronary angioplasty. *Am J Cardiol* 1984;**53**:1C. [Entire issue.]

National Institutes of Health Consensus-Development Conference Statement: Coronary-artery bypass surgery: Scientific and clinical aspects. *N Engl J Med* 1981;**304**:680.

Norris RM et al: Coronary surgery after recurrent myocardial infarction: Progress of a trial comparing surgical with nonsurgical management for asymptomatic patients with advanced coronary disease. *Circulation* 1981;**63**:785.

Ott DA et al: Improved cardiac function following left ventricular aneurysm resection: Pre- and postoperative performance studies in 150 patients. *Tex Heart Inst J* 1982;**9**:267.

Roberts KB et al: The prognosis for patients with new onset angina who have undergone cardiac catheterization. *Circulation* 1983;**68**:970.

Victor MF et al: Unstable angina pectoris of new onset: A prospective clinical and arteriographic study of 75 patients. *Am J Cardiol* 1981;BR,**47**:228.

4. SUDDEN DEATH

Sudden death is the initial and only clinical manifestation of coronary heart disease in about one-fourth of all patients. Most sudden deaths are not totally unexplained or unexpected. In many cases, the patient is known to have had coronary or hypertensive heart disease, hypertrophic cardiomyopathy, fascicular blocks, or recurrent ventricular arrhythmias, or the patient may have recently sought medical care or noticed the onset of symptoms that were subsequently disregarded or misinterpreted. Sudden death during exercise is the most common cause of death in young athletes with hypertrophic cardiomyopathy. The recurrence rate of ventricular fibrillation—the mechanism of "sudden death syndrome"—is high: about 30% of patients experience recurrence in the first year, and 50% experience ventricular fibrillation again within 3 years. Survivors of out-of-hospital ventricular fibrillation who are subsequently studied by cardiac catheterization and coronary arteriography have demonstrated a high prevalence of advanced coronary atherosclerosis, and three-fourths have abnormalities of left ventricular wall motion, indicating the likelihood of previous myocardial infarction. Over a 2-year period, those who experienced recurrences of ventricular fibrillation or who died suddenly had a significantly higher prevalence of severe abnormalities of left ventricular wall motion. Of the patients who were resuscitated but who died in subsequent months, at least two-thirds had "recurrent sudden death," indicating that the final event was similar to the initial event, usually ventricular fibrillation. Vigorous antiarrhythmic drug therapy combined with management of adverse psychologic factors may reduce the recurrence rate of ventricular fibrillation and the likelihood of sudden death in this subset of patients (see p 225).

Differential Diagnosis

In deaths investigated by the coroner's office, sudden unexpected, unexplained deaths that occur within 1 hour after onset of symptoms are most always due to coronary heart disease. When death is delayed more than 2 hours, coronary disease is less commonly the cause but is still the cause in at least half of cases. Other causes are overwhelming sepsis; other cardiac disorders such as myocarditis, cardiomyopathy, or aortic stenosis; cerebral hemorrhage; shock due to any cause; bowel obstruction; and aortic dissection. The so-called café coronary, resulting from tracheal obstruction caused by food while the person is eating, may be confused with sudden death from coronary disease.

Prevention

Since most deaths from coronary heart disease occur suddenly, usually owing to ventricular fibrillation, successful resuscitation depends upon how quickly trained persons can institute appropriate measures to sustain the patient until defibrillation can be accomplished.

Data from multiple sources indicate that beta-adrenergic blocking agents decrease the incidence of cardiac death, sudden death, and re-infarction when begun about a week after acute myocardial infarction (see references on p 229).

A. Cigarette Smoking: The positive relationship between cigarette smoking and sudden death has been extensively documented.

B. Physical Activity: The high incidence of both coronary disease and coronary deaths in the lumberjacks of northeastern Finland indicates that hard physical activity does not protect against sudden death and coronary heart disease, although it has psychologic benefit and creates a sense of well-being.

Emergency Measures

The value of resuscitation in ventricular fibrillation has been demonstrated in a number of community studies in which the 1-year survival rate of those who were resuscitated with prompt defibrillation was about 70%. Resuscitated patients with primary ventricular fibrillation are often able to return to work with adequate left ventricular function. There is an increased likelihood of recurrence of ventricular fibrillation within the next year, and the long-term prognosis is guarded unless antiarrhythmic agents and attention to social, psychologic, and environmental factors are employed to reduce adrenergic impulses operating "through the mind" that may produce coronary vasoconstriction.

There is increasing evidence that implanted ventricular automatic pacemakers in patients who have recurrent ventricular tachycardia or ventricular fibrillation may sense the appearance of the arrhythmia and deliver an electric shock that may terminate it. Technical advances are still needed, because the pacemaker is not programmable and must be individually tailored to the anticipated rate of the arrhythmia. The value in some patients has been dramatic; further experience is awaited.

Greenberg HM, Dwyer EM Jr: Sudden coronary death. *Ann NY Acad Sci* 1982;**382**. [Entire issue.]

Lown B: Mental stress, arrhythmias and sudden death. *Am J Med* 1982;**72**:177.

Miller DD et al: Clinical characteristics associated with sudden death in patients with variant angina. *Circulation* 1982;**66**:588.

Mirowski M et al: The automatic implantable defibrillator: New modality for treatment of life-threatening ventricular arrhythmias. *PACE* 1982;**5**:384.

Morady F et al: Electrophysiologic testing in the management of survivors of out-of-hospital cardiac arrest. *Am J Cardiol* 1983;**51**:85.

Myerburg RJ et al: Survivors of prehospital cardiac arrest. *JAMA* 1982;**247**:1485.

Ruberman W et al: Ventricular premature complexes and sudden death after myocardial infarction. *Circulation* 1981;**64**:297.

Weaver WD, Cobb LA, Hallstrom AP: Ambulatory arrhythmias in resuscitated victims of cardiac arrest. *Circulation* 1982;**66**:212.

5. ACUTE MYOCARDIAL INFARCTION

Essentials of Diagnosis

- Sudden but not instantaneous development of

prolonged constricting anterior chest pain that may produce arrhythmias, hypotension, shock, or cardiac failure.

- Rarely painless, masquerading as acute congestive heart failure, syncope, cerebral thrombosis, or "unexplained" shock.
- Fever, leukocytosis, rising sedimentation rate, elevated serum enzymes such as myocardial band isoenzymes of CPK (CPK-MB), SGOT, or LDH, within 24–48 hours. CPK-MB is the most specific and appears earliest in the serum.
- Electrocardiography: Abnormal Q waves, elevated ST; later, symmetric inversion of T waves.
- Early findings of segmental, localized wall motion abnormalities by radioangiography or 2-dimensional echocardiography.

General Considerations

Myocardial infarction is ischemic necrosis due to occlusion of a coronary artery by thrombus or subintimal hemorrhage at the site of atheromatous narrowing. Less often, complete occlusion by intimal plaques or by hemorrhage into a plaque is responsible. Infarction may occur in the absence of complete occlusion if coronary blood flow is temporarily reduced, as in postoperative or traumatic shock, gastrointestinal bleeding or hypotension due to any cause, or dehydration. Coronary vasoconstriction or spasm may be intense and prolonged and has been proved to result in myocardial infarction in a small number of cases. Rarely, embolic occlusion, syphilitic aortitis, or acute vasculitis causes infarction.

The location and extent of infarction depend upon the anatomic distribution of the vessel, the site of current and previous occlusions, and the adequacy of collateral circulation. Thrombosis occurs most commonly in the anterior descending branch of the left coronary artery, resulting in infarction of the anterior left ventricle. Occlusion of the left circumflex artery produces anterolateral infarction. Right coronary thrombosis leads to infarction of the posteroinferior portion of the left ventricle and might involve the right ventricular myocardium (see below).

The hemodynamic findings are related directly to the extent of necrosis or scarring of the myocardium. In mild infarction, the hemodynamics may be normal (see p 224). With more severe disease, there may be a raised left ventricular end-diastolic pressure with associated increase in the pulmonary artery diastolic pressure, decreased cardiac output, and decreased ejection fraction. When the patient is hypotensive or in shock, the cardiac output is considerably reduced in conjunction with evidences of left ventricular failure and a high left ventricular filling pressure. The "wedge" and left ventricular diastolic pressure may be raised, with no abnormality in the right ventricular diastolic pressure or the right atrial pressure; thus, the superior vena cava or right atrial pressures are often misleading because they do not reflect left ventricular events. They are, however, valuable if the pressures are very low, indicating the possibility of hypovo-

lemia; the response to volume loads may be helpful in producing an increased cardiac output. The presence of a large V wave in the pulmonary wedge pressure pulse is helpful in diagnosing acute mitral insufficiency due to papillary muscle dysfunction in patients who abruptly worsen, with development of cardiac failure. Similarly, raised oxygen content in the right ventricle under similar circumstances helps in diagnosis of perforated ventricular septum.

Clinical Findings

A. Symptoms:

1. Premonitory pain–Over one-third of patients give a history of alteration in the pattern of angina, sudden onset of typical or atypical angina, or unusual "indigestion" felt in the chest.

2. Pain of infarction–This may begin during rest (even in sleep) or activity. It is similar to angina in location and radiation but is more severe, does not subside with rest, and builds up rapidly or in waves to maximum intensity in the space of a few minutes or longer. Nitroglycerin has little effect. The pain may last for hours if unrelieved by narcotics and is often unbearable. Patients break out in a cold sweat, feel weak and apprehensive, and move about, seeking a position of comfort. They prefer not to lie quietly. Lightheadedness, syncope, dyspnea, orthopnea, cough, wheezing, nausea and vomiting, or abdominal bloating may be present singly or in any combination.

3. Painless infarction–In 5–15% of cases, pain is absent or minor and is overshadowed by the immediate complications, notably acute pulmonary edema or rapidly developing heart failure, profound weakness, shock, syncope, or cerebral thrombosis.

B. Signs:
Physical findings are highly variable; the presence of rales, gallop rhythm, tachycardia, arrhythmia or bradycardia, and hypotension correlate well with hemodynamic and clinical evidences of the severity of the attack and the extent of the necrosed myocardium.

1. Shock–Shock may be described as a systolic blood pressure below 80 mm Hg (or slightly higher with prior hypertension) along with gray facial color, mental dullness, cold clammy skin, peripheral cyanosis, decreased urine output, tachycardia or bradycardia, and weak pulse. Shock is present only in severe attacks (incidence about 8–14%). Shock may be caused primarily by the pain rather than the hemodynamic effects of the infarction; if so, distinct improvement occurs within 30–60 minutes after relief of pain and administration of oxygen.

2. Cardiac effects–(See discussion of complications on p 223.) In the severe attack, the first and second heart sounds are faint, are often indistinguishable on auscultation, and assume the so-called tic-tac quality. Gallop rhythm (S_3), distended neck veins, and basal rales are often present. Acute pulmonary edema or rapidly progressive congestive failure may dominate the picture. In less severe attacks, examination is normal or there may be diminished intensity of the first sound or low systolic blood pressure; arrhythmia, hypoxemia, radiologic evidence of pulmonary venous congestion, and echocardiographic evidence of left ventricular distention may be present. Pericardial friction rub appears in 20% of cases between the second and fifth days; it is often transient or intermittent and is rarely of clinical significance unless the patient is taking anticoagulants, in which case a large hemorrhagic effusion may develop.

The presence of right ventricular failure with raised venous pressure disproportionate to left ventricular failure in the presence of an inferior myocardial infarction should make one consider right ventricular infarction (see below). In the usual case of severe left ventricular failure followed by right ventricular failure, the former dominates. When the reverse is true, right ventricular infarction associated with enlargement and hypokinesis of the right ventricle may be present. The ventricular septum and the posterior left and right ventricles are usually infarcted.

3. Fever–Fever is absent at the onset (in contrast to acute pericarditis) and during prolonged shock. It usually rises to 37.8–39.4 °C (100–103 °F)—rarely to 40.6 °C (105 °F)—within 24 hours and persists for 3–7 days (rarely longer).

C. Laboratory Findings: Leukocytosis of 10–20 thousand cells/μL usually develops on the second day and disappears in 1 week. The sedimentation rate is normal at onset, rises on the second or third day, and remains elevated for 1–3 weeks. SGOT activity increases in 6–12 hours, reaches a peak in 24–48 hours, and returns to normal in 3–5 days. Serum lactic acid dehydrogenase may remain elevated for 5–7 days. Serial determinations are helpful in equivocal instances. Creatine phosphokinase (CPK) isoenzyme activity may increase earliest (especially the MB isoenzyme, derived almost exclusively from the myocardium), and, when determined every 2 hours, gives an estimate of the magnitude of the infarction, although for diagnosis, CPK determination every 6–12 hours is adequate.

D. Electrocardiography: Electrocardiographic changes do not correlate well with the clinical severity of the infarction. The characteristic pattern consists of specific changes that undergo a stereotyped "evolution" over a matter of weeks in the average case. At the onset there are elevation of ST segment and T wave and abnormal Q waves; the ST segment progressively returns to the baselines as T waves become symmetrically inverted. An unequivocal electrocardiographic diagnosis of infarction can only be made in the presence of all 3 abnormalities. Serial ST–T changes alone are compatible with but not diagnostic of infarction. The characteristic changes are not seen in the presence of left bundle branch block or when a previous infarct has permanently altered the ECG. Even in these instances an ECG taken early in an attack often shows ST segment displacement.

E. Radioisotope Studies: Radioisotope imaging has been employed extensively in the study of acute myocardial infarction. The most commonly used radioisotope is technetium 99m pyrophosphate, which binds to calcium and accumulates in the mitochondria when cardiac cells necrose. It appears in the area of the infarction as an intense, well-localized "hot spot" that conforms to the area of the infarction in experimental animals. Wall-motion studies with the intravenous use of human serum albumin labeled with radioactive technetium (^{99m}Tc)—so-called gated blood pool scintigraphy or gated angiography—imaged with an Anger camera may demonstrate hypokinesis, dyskinesis, or a localized aneurysm in an area of the myocardium that is infarcted. The specificity of regional myocardial wall-motion hypokinesis revealed by these tests has been confirmed by comparison with left ventriculograms and has been shown to occur in the distribution of stenosed coronary arteries seen on coronary arteriography. Pyrophosphate imaging is valuable primarily in acute myocardial infarction during the first few days. Decreased perfusion, or "cold spots," obtained with thallium 201 when the patient is at rest suggest an old myocardial infarction or myocardial scar, but the findings are not specific. Serial radioisotope imaging may demonstrate shrinkage or increase in size of the myocardial infarction and may serve not only as a prognostic index but also as an aid to evaluating the effect of various therapeutic interventions. The magnitude of segmental wall motion abnormality is a determinant of the degree of functional disturbance of the left ventricle. The most important prognostic factor after acute myocardial infarction is the state of left ventricular function as determined by symptoms, by ejection fraction, and by the degree of hypokinesis, akinesis, or dyskinesis. Serial isotope imaging is also an indicator of survival during the acute phase of infarction. New methods of imaging with other radioactive materials have been used in various centers, but it is too soon to tell which will prove most specific and most sensitive.

Right ventricular infarction can be diagnosed by abnormal radionuclide uptake localized to the right ventricle or by localized hypokinesis of the right ventricle as shown on gated blood pool angiography. Infarction of the right ventricle may explain predominant right ventricular failure in patients with acute inferior myocardial infarction.

F. Hemodynamic Findings: These are discussed in detail along with Cardiac Failure and Shock, pp 224 and 225.

Differential Diagnosis

In acute pericarditis, fever often precedes the onset of pain, which may be predominantly pleuritic and is significantly relieved by breath-holding and leaning forward and made worse by swallowing. The friction rub appears earlier, is louder, is heard over a greater area, and is more persistent than in infarction, and a pleuropericardial rub is often present. There are no QRS changes, and ST elevation and T wave inversion are more widespread, without reciprocal changes (except in aVR). SGOT and LDH are rarely elevated.

Dissection of the aorta causes violent chest pain that is often of maximum severity at onset. It typically spreads up or down the chest and back over a period of hours. Changes in pulses, changing aortic murmurs, and left pleural effusion or cardiac tamponade are distinctive features. Blood pressure does not fall early. Syncope or neurologic abnormalities are common. Electrocardiographic changes are not diagnostic of infarction unless the coronary ostia are involved in the proximal dissection.

Acute pulmonary embolism may cause chest pain indistinguishable from myocardial infarction as well as hypotension, dyspnea, and distended neck veins, but the ECG, regardless of coronarylike changes, will often show right axis deviation or right ventricular conduction defect early in the course of the acute process. SGOT and LDH are often elevated, as in myocardial infarction. The myocardial band isoenzyme of CPK is not elevated in acute pulmonary embolism. If the attack is not fatal, pulmonary infarction may follow, frequently causing pleuritic pain, hemoptysis, and localized lung findings. Thrombophlebitis is often found when careful examination is made of the legs, the groins, and the lower abdomen.

Cervical or thoracic spine disease produces sudden, severe chest pain similar to myocardial infarction; but orthopedic measures give relief and the ECG is normal.

Reflux esophagitis may simulate the pain of infarction, and the T waves may be flat or even inverted during the attack, but there is no hypotension or subsequent fever, leukocytosis, or increase in sedimentation rate, SGOT, LDH, or CPK.

Acute pancreatitis and acute cholecystitis may superficially mimic infarction by causing ST–T changes; Q wave abnormalities are rare. A past history of gastrointestinal symptoms, present findings in the abdomen, jaundice, elevated serum amylase, and x-ray findings differentiate these. Most helpful is the absence of diagnostic serial electrocardiographic changes and absence of elevated CPK-MB.

Spontaneous pneumothorax, mediastinal emphysema, preeruptive herpes zoster, and severe psychophysiologic cardiovascular reactions may have to be differentiated from myocardial infarction.

Complications

Congestive heart failure and shock may be present at onset of infarction or may develop insidiously or abruptly following an arrhythmia or pulmonary embolization. Sedation and weakness may mask the presence of dyspnea and orthopnea. Distention of neck veins, persistent basal rales, gallop rhythm (S_3 not S_4), the appearance of the murmur of mitral insufficiency, abnormal cardiac pulsations, an enlarging tender liver, and peripheral edema should be sought daily. If increasing cardiac failure or evidence of poor cardiac output develops, a Swan-Ganz flow-directed balloon catheter should be inserted to determine precisely the hemodynamic abnormalities and to assist in treatment (see p 225). Portable chest x-ray films to recognize pulmonary venous congestion are desirable. If anticoagulants are not given, pulmonary embolism secondary to phlebitis of the leg or pelvic veins occurs in 5–10% of patients during the acute and convalescent stage.

Arrhythmias occur commonly after myocardial infarction and are thought to be the cause of death in about 40% of patients. The mechanism is either cardiac arrest or ventricular fibrillation; the former occurs following shock or heart failure, and the latter is more apt to be a primary event (although it can be secondary). Continuous monitoring has revealed a higher incidence of ventricular tachycardia, complete atrioventricular block, and other less serious arrhythmias than was formerly suspected. The *appearance* of left anterior hemiblock, especially combined with right bundle branch block, often precedes the development of complete atrioventricular block and requires insertion of a prophylactic pacemaker. Ventricular premature beats often precede more serious arrhythmias in late or secondary but may not in early or primary ventricular fibrillation. Atrial arrhythmias are less common and often transient, as is the case with atrial fibrillation. The prompt recognition of arrhythmias is essential in order to initiate treatment.

Cerebrovascular accident may result from a fall in blood pressure associated with myocardial infarction or from embolism secondary to a mural thrombus. It is advisable to take an ECG in all patients with "cerebrovascular accident."

Recurrent myocardial infarction or extension of the infarction occurs in about 5% of patients during recovery from the initial attack.

Rupture of the heart is uncommon. When it occurs, it is usually in the first week.

Perforation of the ventricular septum is rare, characterized by the sudden appearance of a loud, harsh systolic murmur and thrill over the lower left parasternal area or apex and acute heart failure. This must be distinguished from mitral insufficiency caused by papillary muscle infarction or dysfunction. The diagnosis may sometimes be made by passing (at the bedside) a pulmonary artery flow-directed catheter and noting the size of the *v* wave in the wedged position and the oxygen content in the right ventricle. Two-dimensional echocardiography may demonstrate the perforation of the ventricular septum and so obviate the need for catheterization. Both lesions may precipitate cardiac failure and require cardiac surgery when the patient's condition has stabilized in weeks or months and right and left heart catheterization reveals a significant hemodynamic lesion. Emergency surgical repair is sometimes required but has a high mortality rate. An effort should be made to delay surgery for at least a month.

Ventricular aneurysm and peripheral arterial embolism may occur early or not for months after recovery. The spectrum of ventricular aneurysm is now recognized to extend from frank outpocketing of an area of myocardium with well-demarcated paradoxic pulsations to localized poor contraction or irregular pulsation seen on cineangiography. Approximately 20% of patients develop some form of aneurysm or left ventricular hypokinesis, recognized clinically by abnormal paradoxic precordial pulsations and proved by gated pool scintigraphy, 2-dimensional echocardiography, cinefluoroscopy, or left ventricular cineangiography. Some of these patients develop refractory cardiac failure and benefit from surgical excision.

Oliguria, anuria, or, rarely, tubular necrosis may result if shock persists.

Treatment

A. Immediate Treatment: There is convincing evidence that patients are treated best in a special coronary care unit equipped with continuous monitoring, alarm, recording, pacemaker, and resuscitation equipment, and with specially trained nurses and physicians. The risk of ventricular fibrillation and sudden death is much greater in the first few hours after the onset of the myocardial infarction. Every effort should be made to admit these patients to the coronary care unit as soon as possible to decrease the incidence of death outside the hospital. Some cities are using specially equipped ambulances to minimize the fatalities by providing "pre-coronary unit care." Prophylactic antiarrhythmic programs and immediate intravenous beta-blocking drugs are also under study. Intracoronary thrombolysis is being used increasingly throughout the world, but the benefits and problems are still being identified. The procedure must be used within the first few hours after an acute infarction.

1. Sedation–Patients with acute myocardial infarction are apprehensive and anxious and often have a feeling of impending doom. Opiates, in addition to relieving pain, produce physical and mental rest by allaying anxiety; if they are ineffective, drugs such as diazepam, 5–10 mg orally every 6 hours, may be helpful. If pain is not present and patients are restless and unable to sleep, sedatives (including morphine) should be used as necessary, because adequate sleep is vital for physical and mental rest.

2. Analgesia–When pain is severe, give morphine sulfate, 2–5 mg slowly intravenously, repeated at 15-minute intervals unless the respirations fall below 12/min or the P_{CO_2} rises above 45 mm Hg. Subcutaneous morphine can be used (5–15 mg) if the pain is not severe and the patient is not in shock, but it takes longer to act, may be inadequately absorbed in patients with poor peripheral perfusion, and interferes with evaluation of SGOT and total CPK. When the pain is relieved and perfusion improved, further injections can be given subcutaneously. *Caution:* Do not give a second dose of morphine if respirations are below 12/min. Morphine may cause venous pooling and decreased cardiac output with fainting if the patient is allowed to sit or stand or is transported with the head elevated.

Meperidine and hydromorphone are preferred by some physicians because these agents are thought to produce less nausea and vomiting. The dosage of hydromorphone is 4 mg given intramuscularly or intravenously. The dosage of meperidine is 50–100 mg given intramuscularly as needed or smaller doses intravenously.

Aminophylline, 0.5 g intravenously very slowly (1–2 mL/min), may be helpful if the pain is not relieved by opiates or oxygen (see below). It may produce tachycardia and arrhythmias if given too rapidly.

3. Oxygen is often useful and sometimes necessary for the relief of dyspnea, cyanosis, pulmonary edema, shock, and chest pain. Positive pressure breathing often induces struggling and decreased venous return and may aggravate myocardial ischemia.

4. Anticoagulant therapy is a controversial matter in the milder cases (rapid relief of pain, minimal signs of myocardial necrosis, absence of shock or cardiac failure). In severe cases of myocardial infarction, coumarin anticoagulants may be recommended but are of marginal benefit. Prophylactic "low-dose" heparin is not advised.

5. Thrombolytic therapy of acute myocardial infarction– A more recent invasive procedure, which is still investigational but shows promise, is intracoronary thrombolysis, usually utilizing streptokinase. It has been shown that about 80% of patients with acute myocardial infarction have an acute thrombus that may be lysed by the infusion of streptokinase, resulting in improved coronary blood flow across the obstructed artery. The procedure is not simple and must be done within 3–6 hours of the onset of infarction, which usually means that diagnosis of myocardial infarction is uncertain and that the patient is hemodynamically unstable and is at risk of reperfusion hemorrhage. Following this procedure, some patients have shown increased flow of contrast media on repeat angiography and improved wall motion with radionuclide angiography. The subsequent benefits have not yet been determined. Risks and benefits are being studied in a multicenter trial conducted by the National Institutes of Health.

B. Observation and Activity: Alert clinical observation for evidence of extension of the infarction, new infarction, the appearance of complications, or symptoms requiring treatment is essential. Recurrent pain after the initial pain has subsided suggests extension of the myocardial necrosis; confirmation should be sought in the ECG, by serial measurement of serum enzymes, and in other clinical features. For activity, see p 228.

C. Treatment of Complications:

1. Cardiac failure and cardiogenic shock– (See also p 244.) Left ventricular performance suffers in all patients with acute myocardial infarction. The degree of failure depends upon the magnitude of the new infarction and the state of the myocardium as modified by previous episodes of myocardial ischemia, myocardial infarction, or left ventricular disease due to hypertension or to other cardiac diseases. A small first myocardial infarction in a patient with no underlying cardiac disease usually produces no or minimal evidence of impaired left ventricular performance as judged by symptoms and signs and by hemodynamic monitoring of cardiac output, left ventricular filling pressure, and arterial pressure. If the myocardial infarction is large and occurs in a patient who has had previous infarctions with large areas of scar and borderline compensation, the patient may rapidly go into severe cardiac failure. When hypotension and impaired perfusion of the vital organs are present, cardiogenic shock may occur. The range of possibilities is from no evidence of impaired cardiac function to gross cardiogenic shock with a high mortality rate. It is appropriate to discuss the subject as a continuum, with treatment adjusted according to the degree of severity.

a. Clinical findings of cardiac failure–Some degree of cardiac failure, usually left ventricular, can be detected in 20–50% of patients with acute myocardial infarction unless the attack is mild. The findings are usually not overt. The patient may or may not complain of dyspnea; clinical examination may reveal pulmonary rales, a third heart sound, an accentuated pulmonary second sound, pulsus alternans, and pulmonary venous congestion as shown by radiologic examination. The typical central congestion with bat wing densities does not occur unless the patient develops acute pulmonary edema. The development of Kerley B lines occurs later, with chronic failure, and may not be present even though the pulmonary venous wedge pressure is elevated. The increased pulmonary congestion in the upper lobes is usually part of a generalized pulmonary venous congestion at this phase, but if the process continues there may be reversal of the normal flow pattern, with upper lobe congestion and lower lobe oligemia as pulmonary arterial constriction occurs in the lower lobes. The radiologic findings may be out of phase with the clinical findings because they take somewhat longer to develop and to regress. It is valuable to obtain serial portable chest films to check for the presence of unsuspected pulmonary venous congestion. In patients who are being monitored by a bedside Swan-Ganz catheter, a raised pulmonary venous wedge pressure can be found in the absence of the radiologic findings.

b. Treatment of cardiac failure–If the evidence of left ventricular failure is minimal or subclinical, treatment can be conservative, consisting of oral diuretics such as hydrochlorothiazide, 50–100 mg; oxygen to relieve hypoxemia; and avoidance of sodium-containing fluids. A Swan-Ganz catheter need not be inserted, and hemodynamic measurements are not necessary.

If patients with **moderate left ventricular failure** require passage of a flow-directed balloon thermodilution catheter for monitoring wedge pressure, pulmonary pressure, and cardiac output, see below.

With more severe left ventricular failure that is not promptly relieved by diuretic therapy, more aggressive therapy (see ¶ e, below) should be considered—preceded by hemodynamic monitoring of the arterial pressure, of the pulmonary venous wedge pressure (left ventricular filling pressure), and of the cardiac output (usually by thermodilution technique).

Stroke work index is computed by the following formula: Stroke work volume × (mean systolic arterial pressure − mean pulmonary capillary wedge pressure) × 0.0136. The normal range is 40–80 g-m/m². *It is hazardous to continue to use potent therapeutic agents unless hemodynamic monitoring is available so that the results of the intervention can be observed and the dose of the various drugs adjusted.*

c. Interpretation and treatment of hypotension with volume repletion–Hypotension is often the first sign that cardiac failure may be more severe than is suggested by slight dyspnea and pulmonary rales, especially if it persists after pain is relieved. When monitoring reveals that the left ventricular filling pressure is low (< 12 mm Hg) and the cardiac output is normal, despite the low arterial pressure, hypovolemia is the most probable cause and should be treated by increments of volume replacement beginning with 100 mL of half-normal saline. Increments of volume repletion can be given every 5–10 minutes until left ventricular filling pressure rises. Other fluids, such as serum albumin, dextran 40, or lactated Ringer's injection, can be used so that fluid does not rapidly leave the intravascular space. If the cardiac output does not increase as the left ventricular filling pressure increases to 15–20 mm Hg, further volume replacement should be stopped to prevent pulmonary edema, which may occur quite abruptly. If the only hemodynamic abnormality is a raised left ventricular filling pressure, with blood pressure and output normally maintained, more vigorous diuresis can be attempted with larger doses of furosemide. Excessive diuresis must be avoided because the patient may then become dehydrated, and although the filling pressure may fall, the blood pressure may also fall, and the patient will need further volume repletion.

d. Treatment of hypotension with vasopressors–Some patients with acute myocardial infarction have hypotension with impaired tissue perfusion primarily from failure of compensatory peripheral vasoconstriction without a substantial change in filling pressure or cardiac output; these patients often respond with a rise in arterial pressure to sympathomimetic amines (norepinephrine and dopamine) that stimulate the beta-adrenergic receptors. Both drugs should be infused at a slow rate to avoid tachycardia, marked increases in blood pressure, and ventricular arrhythmias. The physician's aim is not only to maintain the blood pressure but also to prevent arrhythmias.

e. Vasodilator treatment of severe cardiac failure and cardiogenic shock–(See also p 249.) When the cardiac dysfunction is more severe, with reduced cardiac output, increased left ventricular filling pressure (above 20 mm Hg), and arterial blood pressure at or above 90 mm Hg, vasodilator therapy can be cautiously begun while the hemodynamic result is monitored. Drugs such as sodium nitroprusside, 15–400 µg/min given by intravenous drip and titrated to the patient's response, decrease the impedance to left ventricular ejection, reduce left ventricular volume and filling pressure, may improve the left ventricular stroke work index, decrease the myocardial oxygen consumption (MVO_2), and improve perfusion to the brain, kidney, and heart. Vasodilator therapy (intravenous nitroprusside, nitrates, hydralazine, calcium-blocking agents, or captopril) cannot be used if there is considerable reduction in arterial pressure, because further reduction by the vasodilator therapy may aggravate the situation. Efforts, therefore, must be made to raise the arterial pressure to about 100 mm Hg with inotropic agents such as dobutamine or dopamine (with caution regarding tachycardia) before vasodilator therapy can be used.

f. Treatment with inotropic agents–Digitalis, the time-honored inotropic agent, is infrequently used today in the treatment of cardiac failure in the setting of acute myocardial infarction, primarily because of its tendency to produce ventricular arrhythmias and its relative ineffectiveness in the setting of severe left ventricular pump failure. When cardiac failure is severe and inotropic agents are required, dopamine, dobutamine, or amrinone should be tried. The last drug is not yet approved in USA. In milder varieties of cardiac failure, digitalis should probably be withheld, primarily because the development of ventricular arrhythmias places the physician in the dilemma of deciding whether they are the result of the digitalis therapy or a natural consequence of the myocardial ischemia. Digitalis should still be used if the patient has atrial fibrillation with a rapid ventricular rate.

g. Treatment with aortic balloon counterpulsation–If the arterial pressure cannot be raised with vasopressors without worsening the left ventricular filling pressure and aggravating the cardiac failure, aortic balloon counterpulsation may be used as a dramatic temporary circulatory assist to raise the arterial pressure and to make vasodilator therapy possible. Counterpulsation decreases aortic pressure during systole and increases it during diastole. The decreased aortic pressure during systole decreases the impedance to left ventricular ejection, reduces afterload and the work of the left ventricle, and results in a fall in left ventricular filling pressure similar to that achieved by vasodilators. Raising the aortic pressure in diastole increases coronary perfusion and improves left ventricular function by decreasing myocardial ischemia.

The combination of counterpulsation followed by vasodilator therapy with infusion of nitroprusside, 60–200 μg/min, has reduced the mortality rate in cardiogenic shock and allowed patients to leave the hospital even though they continued to show some evidences of left ventricular failure. The long-term prognosis in patients who have been successfully treated by balloon assist for cardiogenic shock is still poor (approximately 10% survival in 1 year) because of extensive underlying disease.

Invasive balloon counterpulsation can be used as a temporary measure to tide the patient over acute "power failure" and gain time to consider the desirability of performing coronary angiograms as well as the feasibility of coronary bypass surgery if the lesions are shown to be amenable to surgery. The surgical

mortality rate in patients recovering from cardiogenic shock is high, and more data are required before a definite conclusion can be reached about the feasibility of bypass surgery in such cases.

h. Poor response to treatment of cardiac failure–The poor response to medical as well as surgical therapy in patients with cardiogenic shock following myocardial infarction can be appreciated when one considers that at least 50% of the left ventricle has been shown to be damaged or necrosed in autopsy studies of such patients. The left ventricular filling pressure is usually considerably more than 20 mm Hg. The left ventricular stroke work index is usually less than 20 gram-meters per square meter (g-m/m^2) and often less than 15 g-m/m^2, and a P_{O_2} of less than 40–50 mm Hg is frequently found. The high wedge pressure (left ventricular filling pressure) induces dyspnea; impaired peripheral perfusion resulting from the decreased cardiac output is recognized clinically by cold, pale, clammy skin, cerebral obtundation, low urine output, and evidence of venous constriction.

Monitoring of the hemodynamic parameters mentioned above is valuable in prognosis. Patients with left ventricular filling pressures less than 15 mm Hg and stroke work indices of more than 35 or 40 g-m/m^2 have a good prognosis, whereas if the filling pressure exceeds 20 mm Hg and the stroke work index is less than 20 g-m/m^2—or especially if it is 15 g-m/m^2—a poor outcome is likely. It is in patients with a poor prognosis that aggressive therapy is warranted before severe deterioration of the patient has occurred. The various drugs and forms of therapy discussed should be considered as therapeutic trials; the physician should tailor therapy depending upon the hemodynamic response. One cannot be dogmatic in advance about doses and preferences for certain drugs over others; adjustments are necessary as treatment proceeds.

2. Arrhythmias–Ventricular premature beats are common. They indicate increased irritability of the damaged myocardium and may presage ventricular tachycardia or fibrillation. Lidocaine (Xylocaine), 50–100 mg intravenously, followed by an intravenous infusion at a rate of 1–4 mg/min, is the drug of choice. There are data suggesting that prophylactic intravenous lidocaine infusion should be initiated early to prevent ventricular tachycardia or fibrillation. Alternatives are procainamide, quinidine sulfate, disopyramide (Norpace), or, if digitalis is thought to be responsible for the arrhythmia, potassium salts. Disopyramide is an effective antiarrhythmic agent; however, because of its negative inotropic action, it should be used with caution in patients who are in cardiac failure or who have a history of cardiac failure. Aggressive treatment of ventricular arrhythmias may prevent ventricular fibrillation and cardiac arrest. New antiarrhythmic drugs are being developed but are not yet available in the USA. One of the most promising new drugs is amiodarone.

Ventricular tachycardia is an emergency (see p 235). Ventricular fibrillation should be instantly recognized on the alarm system at the nursing station, and defibrillation should be accomplished within 30 seconds. Lidocaine should be given by intravenous infusion (1–4 mg/min) to prevent recurrence.

Recurrent ventricular arrhythmias, when they occur following myocardial infarction—especially if associated with ventricular aneurysm and cardiac failure—may respond to surgical resection of the aneurysm combined with endocardial resection of the area that is initiating the arrhythmia (ascertained by electrophysiologic mapping at surgery) and bypass surgery, which should be considered whenever the arrhythmias are life-threatening and difficult to control with drugs.

Atrial fibrillation is usually transient. If this persists, if the patient tolerates it poorly, or if congestive heart failure occurs, digitalize with care or treat by cardioversion.

3. Stokes-Adams attack with heart block – (See p 242.) *This is an emergency.* Complete heart block complicates acute myocardial infarction in 6–10% of cases. It has a high mortality rate, usually lasts less than a week, and often can be treated by artificial pacing through a transvenous catheter placed in the right ventricle. Pacing at a rate of 70–80 may greatly improve the cardiac output and tissue perfusion and prevent Stokes-Adams attacks. Stokes-Adams attacks with fatal syncope are rare in the presence of inferior myocardial infarction because the atrioventricular conduction damage is nodal and due to transient ischemia or edema from occlusion of a branch of the right coronary artery. When atrioventricular conduction defects occur in anterior infarction, they usually represent widespread necrosis of the septum and the conduction system, involving the bundle of His or the bundle branches, usually with decreased left ventricular function and ventricular asynergy. Complete heart block may occur rapidly, and a temporary artificial demand pacemaker should therefore be introduced if second- or third-degree atrioventricular block occurs or when right bundle branch block and left anterior hemiblock develop acutely in the presence of anterior infarction (see section on atrioventricular conduction system defects). Demand pacemakers are preferred over fixed rate pacemakers because the atrioventricular conduction defects are usually transient and subside within a week, and ventricular arrhythmias may result from competition between the artificial pacemaker and the patient's own natural pacemaker (see below). Temporary pacemakers are usually left in place for a week after the atrioventricular conduction becomes normal. Rarely, a permanent pacemaker may be required in anterior infarction, although some authorities recommend it even when sinus rhythm has been restored, because of the presumed higher mortality rate over the next 1–2 years in patients who are not permanently paced. This procedure is under study.

Second-degree atrioventricular block with Wenckebach pauses (see below) and narrow QRS complexes is not routinely paced if the patient has inferior infarction. His bundle recordings have demonstrated that if the conduction defect is in the atrioventricular node, above the bundle of His (as is the usual finding in inferior infarctions), Stokes-Adams attacks are uncommon even if complete block develops. This is in contrast to the atrioventricular conduction defect that occurs in anterior infarctions, in which His bundle recordings and pathologic data show that the block is usually distal to the atrioventricular node, within the bundle of His or in the bundle branches; Stokes-Adams attacks with fatalities occur if the patient is not protected by a pacemaker.

Sinus bradycardia (see p 231), especially in inferior infarction with hypotension, may precede atrioventricular block and provide a setting in which ventricular arrhythmias may occur. Further, with the decreased cardiac output seen in acute myocardial infarction, perfusion of the vital organs may be inadequate with a slow heart rate. Atropine, 0.25–1 mg intravenously, is desirable in such situations, with close observation to determine its effectiveness and side effects, since ventricular arrhythmias have resulted from atropine. If atropine is ineffective or if the bradycardia is marked or associated with block, a temporary prophylactic transvenous demand pacemaker should be inserted into the right ventricle. Asystole may occur unpredictably, so electrode catheters should be placed prophylactically in patients with anterior infarctions who have complete atrioventricular block or type II Mobitz atrioventricular block, in those with inferior infarctions with complete atrioventricular block, and in patients in whom left anterior hemiblock with or without left or right bundle branch block appears during the course of the infarction, even with a normal PR interval. Infusions of lidocaine should be given to prevent ventricular fibrillation if atrioventricular block subsides and competition with the patient's own pacemaker occurs. Demand rather than fixed rate pacemakers are preferable for this reason.

Ventricular fibrillation is the major hazard associated with pacing in acute myocardial infarction because of competition between the patient's own pacemaker and that of the artificial *fixed* pacemaker. For this reason, patients with first-degree atrioventricular block or with type I second-degree atrioventricular block with Wenckebach pauses and narrow QRS complexes in inferior infarction are not routinely paced. A demand pacemaker, activated by a delay in the appearance of the QRS complex, is always preferred, so that when atrioventricular conduction is unstable and intermittent, competition between the normal and artificial pacemaker will not occur.

4. Thromboembolic phenomena are relatively uncommon (5–10%) during the course of myocardial infarction. Anticoagulants should be administered promptly. For treatment of pulmonary embolism, see Chapter 7.

5. Oliguria, anuria, acute tubular necrosis – See Chapter 16.

6. Rupture, perforation of the interventricular septum, mitral insufficiency from papillary muscle dysfunction or rupture, and aneurysm – Surgical repair is indicated for perforated ventricular septum or mitral insufficiency after the lesion has stabilized (for 4–10 weeks, if possible), if cardiac failure has persisted. Patients with mitral insufficiency following myocardial infarction, when it is associated with left ventricular failure requiring surgery, have a high incidence of raised left ventricular end-diastolic pressure (more than 15 mm Hg) or a reduced cardiac index (less than 2.5 L/min/m²). The surgical mortality rate is higher than in replacement of the mitral valve in other varieties of mitral insufficiency, but the end results are often gratifying. Resection of aneurysm is recommended in the presence of unequivocal ventricular aneurysm with persistent cardiac failure but not for minor asymptomatic aneurysm or for diffuse, flabby, irregular hypokinesis and cardiac failure of ischemic cardiomyopathy. No treatment is available for cardiac rupture except in rare cases where the leak is slow and is diagnosed and surgery is available (pseudoaneurysm).

7. Rare post-myocardial infarction syndromes–

a. Dressler's syndrome–Pericarditis, pericardial friction rub, and fever, with or without pneumonitis, may occur weeks or months after acute myocardial infarction. Dressler's syndrome is considered to be a hypersensitivity reaction similar to postcardiotomy syndrome and must be differentiated from a new myocardial infarction, pulmonary infarction, or cardiac failure on the basis of appropriate clinical and laboratory tests. The syndrome subsides spontaneously in a few days or weeks, but improvement is more rapid if indomethacin or corticosteroids are given. Anticoagulants should not be used because of the hazards of hemorrhagic pericardial effusion.

b. Shoulder-hand syndrome–Shoulder-hand syndrome, consisting of stiffness, limitation of motion, and pain in the shoulder and arm (especially the left-hand side) is caused by prolonged immobilization. It may last days or weeks and is benefited by symptomatic treatment, including physical therapy.

D. Activity: Patients are encouraged to increase their activity in bed after the first 2 days, to sit up on the third day, and to walk on the fifth to seventh days, provided there have been no complications and the infarction has been mild. Cautious controlled ambulation allows the patient with mild myocardial infarction and a good home situation to leave the hospital between the tenth and 14th days. Early hospital discharge is unwise if, during the acute phase of infarction, the patient has had multiple ventricular premature beats, ventricular tachycardia or fibrillation, second- or third-degree atrioventricular block, cardiac failure with pulmonary edema or cardiogenic shock, sinus tachycardia, systemic hypotension, atrial arrhythmias, or evidence of extension of the infarction. These complications preclude early ambulation in at least half of patients with infarction.

During ambulation and before discharge, the response of the patient should be monitored so that pulse rate, blood pressure, and the presence of symptoms can be determined. If untoward developments occur, the process of rehabilitation can be slowed until a stable state is achieved. In uncomplicated cases, between 3 and 6 weeks after acute myocardial infarction, a limited electrocardiographic exercise stress test, not allowing the pulse rate to exceed 120/min, helps the physician to determine the patient's capacity for further activity, gives the patient confidence, and may be of prognostic value. Ischemic depression of the ST segment or complex ventricular arrhythmias at this time indicate a greater risk for subsequent recurrent clinical disease.

E. Treatment of Chronic Coronary Heart Disease: Antiplatelet Agents: Secondary prevention of myocardial infarction has utilized various drugs that affect platelet aggregation, as well as various rehabilitation programs. Sulfinpyrazone (Anturane) has been shown in 2 studies to reduce the incidence of sudden death and recurrent myocardial infarction. In the 1980 study, treatment reduced the rate of sudden death only up to the seventh month after infarction; no further benefit was found after this time. Further studies are required to settle the matter.

A large multicenter myocardial infarction study group found that aspirin, which interferes with platelet aggregation, did not reduce the number of deaths in patients with a history of myocardial infarction.

Beta-adrenergic blocking drugs have been shown in several studies to decrease the likelihood of sudden death and reinfarction in the months following acute myocardial infarction. All beta-blockers studied have been beneficial. Timolol, propranolol, alprenolol, and metoprolol may all be used.

Rehabilitation programs, with early ambulation under close surveillance and progressive activities that will restore patients to a normal or nearly normal life-style, have been shown to increase physical work ability and improve morale. There is much less evidence for improvement in ventricular function and little convincing evidence that these programs, with exercise, decrease the recurrence of myocardial infarction or the mortality rate. However, the safety of rehabilitation programs under good supervision seems well established.

Prognosis

The overall mortality rate (including the prehospital phase) during the first month after the infarction averages 30%. Most of the deaths occur in the first 12 hours. In the mild attack, clinical manifestations subside promptly, and the initial mortality rate is less than 5%. Clinically severe myocardial infarction may require 6–12 weeks for recovery. The mortality rate rises to 60–90% with prolonged shock, severe early heart failure, leukocytosis over 25,000/μL with eosinophilia, fever above 40 °C (104 °F), uncontrolled diabetes mellitus, old age, and previous definite infarction, especially if these occur in combination. Pulmonary embolism that is not treated with anticoagulants, persistent arrhythmias, and extension of the infarct superimpose a mortality rate of 15–20% during early convalescence.

The seemingly poorer late prognosis in non-transmural (subendocardial) infarction compared to transmural infarction may be because many patients with the former condition have an already damaged myocardium owing to previous infarction.

Long-term survival is related to the availability of medical care and the presence of other chronic diseases in addition to the residuals of infarction. Complete clinical and electrocardiographic recovery is compatible with survival of 10–20 years. Patients with residual heart failure usually die within 1–5 years.

Various prospective studies are under way to improve the clinician's ability to predict which patients surviving myocardial infarction are apt to die prematurely. Those with findings suggesting higher risks (frequent or complex ventricular arrhythmias, evidence of residual ischemia on the ECG, ischemia induced by submaximal stress electrocardiography, evidence of left ventricular dysfunction on history or physical examination, echocardiography or radioisotopic nucleotide studies documenting decreased ejection fraction and extensive segmental wall motion abnormalities, cardiac failure, conduction defects, and atherosclerosis elsewhere) may have a considerably higher mortality rate than patients with findings suggesting lowest risks. The extent of the anatomic stenosis and the left ventricular function are the major factors in prognosis.

Following recovery from an acute myocardial infarction, 30–40% of patients demonstrate advanced degrees of ventricular arrhythmia on monitoring and exercise stress tests. Efforts are under way to determine the value of antiarrhythmic therapy in preventing ventricular fibrillation and sudden death in these patients. Total abolition of ventricular arrhythmias may not be necessary; it may be sufficient to abolish complex and "malignant" arrhythmias. Control of coffee, alcohol, and tobacco intake and exercise conditioning have been disappointing in preventing premature beats.

Beta-blocking agents have been reported to decrease the incidence of reinfarction and sudden death when given continuously after recovery from acute myocardial infarction. Some reports indicate that these agents improve prognosis when given immediately after the onset of acute myocardial infarction.

β-Blocker Heart Attack Trial Research Group: A randomized trial of propranolol in patients with acute myocardial infarction. 1. Mortality results. *JAMA* 1982;**247**:1707.

Bigger JT et al: The relationships among ventricular arrhythmias, left ventricular dysfunction, and mortality in the 2 years after myocardial infarction. *Circulation* 1984;**69**:250.

Corbett JR et al: Left ventricular functional alterations at rest and during submaximal exercise in patients with recent myocardial infarction. *Am J Med* 1983;**74**:577.

Dewhurst NG, Muir AL: Comparative prognostic value of radionuclide ventriculography at rest and during exercise in 100 patients after first myocardial infarction. *Br Heart J* 1983;**49**:111.

Graham I et al: Natural history of coronary heart disease: A study of 586 men surviving an initial acute attack. *Am Heart J* 1983;**105**:249.

Gray RJ, Sethna D, Matloff JM: The role of cardiac surgery in acute myocardial infarction. 1. With mechanical complications. *Am Heart J* 1983;**106**:723.

Grüntzig A: Results from coronary angioplasty and implications for the future. *Am Heart J* 1982;**103**:779.

Hjalmarson A et al: Effect on mortality of metoprolol in acute myocardial infarction: A double-blind randomised trial. *Lancet* 1981;**2**:823.

Hutter AM et al: Nontransmural myocardial infarction: Hospital and late clinical course of patients with that of matched patients with transmural anterior and transmural inferior myocardial infarction. *Am J Cardiol* 1981;**48**:595.

May GS et al: Secondary prevention after myocardial infarction: A review of short-term acute phase trials. *Prog Cardiovasc Dis* 1983;**25**:335.

Mirowski M: Management of malignant ventricular tachyarrhythmias with automatic implanted cardioverter-defibrillators. *Mod Concepts Cardiovasc Dis* 1983;**52**:41.

The Multicenter Postinfarction Research Group: Risk stratification and survival after myocardial infarction. *N Engl J Med* 1983;**309**:331.

Murray GC, Beller GA: Cardiac rehabilitation following coronary artery bypass surgery. *Am Heart J* 1983;**105**:1009.

National Heart, Lung, and Blood Institute Coronary Artery Surgery Study. *Circulation* 1981;**63**(6–Part 2). [Entire issue.]

Norris RM et al: Prognosis after recovery from first acute myocardial infarction: Determinants of reinfarction and sudden death. *Am J Cardiol* 1984;**53**:408.

The Norwegian Multicenter Study Group: Timolol-induced reduction in mortality and reinfarction in patients surviving acute myocardial infarction. *N Engl J Med* 1981;**304**:801.

Pantridge JF, Webb SW, Adgey AAJ: Arrhythmias in the first hours of acute myocardial infarction. *Prog Cardiovasc Dis* 1981;**23**:265.

Rapaport E, Remedios P: The high risk patient after recovery from myocardial infarction: Recognition and management. *J Am Coll Cardiol* 1983;**1**(2–Part 1):391.

Rechnitzer PA et al: Relation of exercise to the recurrence rate of myocardial infarction in men: Ontario exercise-heart collaborative study. *Am J Cardiol* 1983;**51**:65.

Rentrop KP, Blanke H, Karsch KR: Effects of nonsurgical coronary reperfusion on the left ventricle in human subjects compared with conventional treatment: Study of 18 patients with acute myocardial infarction treated with intracoronary infusion of streptokinase. *Am J Cardiol* 1982;**49**:1.

Roberts WC (editor-in-chief): The Goteborg Metoprolol trial in acute myocardial infarction. (Symposium.) *Am J Cardiol* 1984;**53**:1D. [Entire issue.]

Schröder R et al: Intravenous short-term infusion of streptokinase in acute myocardial infarction. *Circulation* 1983;**67**:536.

Shaw LW: Effects of a prescribed supervised exercise program on mortality and cardiovascular morbidity in patients after a myocardial infarction. *Am J Cardiol* 1981;**48**:39.

Smalling RW et al: Sustained improvement in left ventricular function and mortality by intracoronary streptokinase administration during evolving myocardial infarction. *Circulation* 1983;**68**:131.

Sorensen SG et al: Noninvasive detection of ventricular aneurysm by combined two-dimensional echocardiography and equilibrium radionuclide angiography. *Am Heart J* 1982;**104**:145.

Tans AC, Lie KI, Durrer D: Clinical setting and prognostic significance of high degree atrioventricular block in acute inferior myocardial infarction: A study of 144 patients. *Am Heart J* 1980;**99**:4.

Van Reet RE et al: Comparison of two-dimensional echocardiography with gated radionuclide ventriculography in the evaluation of global and regional left ventricular function in acute myocardial infarction. *J Am Coll Cardiol* 1984;**3**:243.

Visser CA et al: Echocardiographic-cineangiographic correlation in detecting left ventricular aneurysm: A prospective study of 422 patients. *Am J Cardiol* 1982;**50**:337.

Weiner DA et al: Prognostic importance of a clinical profile and exercise test in medically treated patients with coronary artery disease. *J Am Coll Cardiol* 1984;**3**:772.

Wenger NK: Rehabilitation of the coronary patient: Scope of the problem and responsibility of the primary care physician. *Cardiovasc Rev Rep* 1981;**2**:1249.

DISTURBANCES OF RATE & RHYTHM

The presence of a significant arrhythmia should be suspected in any of the following circumstances: (1) when there is a history of sudden onset and sudden termination of palpitation or rapid heart action; (2) when the heart rhythm is grossly irregular; (3) when the heart rate is below 40 or above 140 per minute; (4) when the heart rate does not change with breath-holding or exercise; (5) when a rapid heart rate suddenly slows during carotid sinus massage; (6) when the first heart sound varies in intensity; or (7) when a patient develops sudden anginal pain, shock, congestive heart failure, or syncope.

The diagnosis of an arrhythmia consists of accurate identification of the site of origin of the abnormality and proper assessment of its significance. The most common arrhythmias are sinus arrhythmia, sinus tachycardia, sinus bradycardia, atrial and ventricular premature beats, and paroxysmal atrial tachycardia. These occur in normal and diseased hearts alike and have no significance except insofar as they alter circulatory dynamics. Atrial fibrillation and flutter occur most commonly in patients with arteriosclerotic or rheumatic heart disease, but thyrotoxicosis, acute infections, alcoholism, intravenous drug abuse, or trauma may precipitate them in the absence of heart disease. Ventricular tachycardia appears most often in the presence of advanced coronary artery disease. Partial or complete heart block also results from coronary heart disease but is most commonly due to fibrosis of the conduction system. Digitalis toxicity is a frequent cause of many types of arrhythmia.

From the physiologic standpoint, arrhythmias are harmful to the extent that they reduce cardiac output, lower blood pressure, and interfere with perfusion of the vital territories of the brain, heart, and kidney. Rapid heart rates may cause any or all of these changes and, in the presence of heart disease, may precipitate acute heart failure or pulmonary edema, angina pectoris or myocardial infarction, syncope, poor cerebration with confusion, or cerebral thrombosis. Patients with otherwise normal hearts may tolerate rapid rates with no symptoms other than palpitation or fluttering,

but prolonged attacks usually cause weakness, exertional dyspnea, and precordial aching. The rate at which slow heart rates produce symptoms at rest or on exertion depends upon the underlying state of the cardiac muscle and its ability to increase its stroke output. If the heart rate abruptly slows, as with the onset of complete heart block or transient standstill, syncope or convulsions may result.

If possible, elicit a history of previous attacks and precipitating factors, symptoms of heart failure, and anginal pain. Examine for cardiac enlargement, significant murmurs, signs of heart failure, and hypotension. Count the heart rate for 1 minute. If the rate is seemingly regular, repeat the count twice to determine if the rate is absolutely regular; if irregular, determine whether pulse deficit is present. If there is no severe failure, angina, or recent infarction, determine the effects of breath-holding, exercise, and change of position on the heart rate and rhythm. Massage the right and left carotid sinus successively for 30 seconds while listening to the heart; cease massage as soon as a change in rate occurs. Note whether the first heart sound varies in intensity. Examine the neck veins for abnormal pulsations or cannon waves.

The final diagnosis of arrhythmias depends upon the ECG. However, consideration of the patient's age, the type of associated heart disease, and the results of the examination permit a diagnosis in most cases before the ECG is taken.

His bundle recordings aid in the interpretation of complex arrhythmias, especially when there is a question about whether the rhythm is atrial or ventricular, by demonstrating the supraventricular or ventricular origin of wide QRS complexes. If the QRS complex follows the His bundle spike, ventricular aberrancy is present, and treatment is influenced accordingly. His bundle recordings also aid in the recognition of concealed premature depolarizations, especially of the His bundle with antegrade and retrograde atrioventicular block; His bundle depolarizations affect subsequent cycles by retrograde conduction to the atrioventricular node, producing a prolonged PR interval and nonconducted P waves (see below).

Dimarco JP et al: Intracardiac electrophysiologic techniques in recurrent syncope of unknown cause. *Ann Intern Med* 1981;**95**:542.

Fisher JD: Role of electrophysiologic testing in the diagnosis and treatment of patients with known and suspected bradycardias and tachycardias. *Prog Cardiovasc Dis* 1981;**24**:25.

Nademanee K, Singh BN: Advances in antiarrhythmic therapy: The role of newer antiarrhythmic drugs. *JAMA* 1982;**247**:217.

Scheinman MM, Morady F: Invasive cardiac electrophysiologic testing: The current state of the art. (Editorial.) *Circulation* 1983;**67**:1169.

Walker PR: Pacemakers: Techniques, indications, results and implications. Pages 367–379 in: *Scientific Foundations of Cardiology*. Sleight P, Jones JV (editors). Heinemann, 1983.

SINUS ARRHYTHMIA

Sinus arrhythmia is a cyclic increase in normal heart rate with inspiration and decrease with expiration. It results from reflex changes in vagal influence on the normal pacemaker and disappears with breath-holding or increase of heart rate due to any cause. The arrhythmia has no significance except in older persons, when it may be associated with coronary artery disease.

SINUS TACHYCARDIA

Sinus tachycardia is a heart rate faster than 100 beats/min that is caused by rapid impulse formation by the normal pacemaker secondary to fever, exercise, emotion, anemia, shock, thyrotoxicosis, or drug effect. The rate may reach 180/min in young persons but rarely exceeds 160/min. The rhythm is basically regular, but serial 1-minute counts of the heart rate indicate that it varies 5 or more beats per minute with changes in position, with breath-holding or sedation, or with correction of the underlying disorder. The rate slows gradually, but tachycardia may begin abruptly in response to sudden emotional stimuli.

SINUS BRADYCARDIA
(See also p 239.)

Sinus bradycardia is a heart rate slower than 55/min due to increased vagal influence on the normal pacemaker. The rate increases after exercise or administration of atropine. Slight degrees have no significance, especially in youth, unless there is underlying heart disease, especially coronary heart disease or acute myocardial infarction. Elderly patients may develop weakness, confusion, or even syncope with slow heart rates. Atrial and ventricular ectopic rhythms are more apt to occur with slow ventricular rates. It may be desirable to use ephedrine or atropine in some patients to speed the heart rate. Rarely, artificial pacemakers are necessary.

ATRIAL PREMATURE BEATS
(Atrial Extrasystoles)

Atrial premature beats occur when an ectopic focus in the atria fires off before the next expected impulse from the sinus node. Ventricular systole occurs prematurely, and the compensatory pause following this is only slightly longer than the normal interval between beats. Such premature beats occur with equal frequency in normal and diseased hearts and are never sufficient basis for a diagnosis of heart disease. Speeding of the heart rate by any means usually abolishes premature beats. Early atrial premature beats may cause aberrant QRS complexes or be nonconducted to the ventricle because the latter is still refractory.

PAROXYSMAL ATRIAL TACHYCARDIA

This is the commonest paroxysmal tachycardia. It occurs more often in young patients with normal hearts. Attacks begin and end abruptly and usually last several hours. The heart rate may be 140–240/min (usually 170–220/min) and is perfectly regular, ie, the rate will not vary more than 1–2 beats per minute. Exercise, change of position, breath-holding, carotid sinus massage, or induced gagging or vomiting either has no effect or promptly abolishes the attack. Patients are asymptomatic except for awareness of rapid heart action unless there is underlying heart disease, especially mitral stenosis and coronary heart disease. In prolonged attacks with rapid rates, dyspnea or tightness in the chest may be felt. Paroxysmal atrial tachycardia may result from digitalis toxicity, and then is associated with atrioventricular block so that only every second or, rarely, every third atrial impulse reaches the ventricles (so-called paroxysmal atrial tachycardia with block).

The most common mechanism of paroxysmal atrial tachycardia is reentry from an atrial premature beat through an atrioventricular node whose conduction has been slowed, combined with unidirectional block in a neighboring fiber. Alternative mechanisms are abnormal automaticity and, more rarely, triggered activity. In addition to the atrioventricular node, the reentry circuit may include the sinoatrial node, the atrium, or an accessory bypass tract. The depolarization wave front proceeds antegradely through the fiber whose conduction is slowed and returns retrogradely in a nearby fiber that had unidirectional antegrade block. When this returning echo reaches the site of its origin, it may then reexcite the fiber, which is now no longer refractory. Thus, repetitive reentry may result, precipitating paroxysmal tachycardia, if the atrial premature beat is appropriately timed and if the other conditions noted above are present. Similarly, a single atrial premature beat may terminate atrial tachycardia by making the reentry pathway refractory. Recent evidence indicates that about one-third of patients have aberrant pathways to the ventricles.

Prevention of Attacks

A. Specific Measures: Attempt to find and remove the cause, especially emotional stress, fatigue, or excessive use of alcohol or tobacco.

B. Drugs:

1. Quinidine is a valuable drug in the management of most cardiac arrhythmias. It increases the effective refractory period of cardiac muscle, slows the rate of atrial and ventricular conduction, decreases the excitability and contractility of the myocardium, reduces vagal tone, and has a general depressant action on smooth muscle, causing vasodilatation. It is useful both in the prevention and in the treatment of atrial and ventricular arrhythmias. Quinidine is rapidly absorbed following oral administration, reaches a peak level of effectiveness in about 2 hours, and is excreted slowly; about 30% of the peak level remains after 12 hours. Only 10–20% of orally administered quinidine is excreted in the urine; the remainder is metabolized in the body. If quinidine is used with digitalis, the digitalis blood level doubles. Quinidine idiosyncrasy with fever, purpura, thrombocytopenia, rash, or severe hypotension or the presence of advanced atrioventricular block are absolute contraindications to the use of quinidine. Relative contraindications are bundle branch block, thyrotoxicosis, acute rheumatic fever, and infective endocarditis. Quinidine sulfate may be used to prevent frequent and troublesome attacks. Begin with small doses and increase if the attacks are not prevented and toxic effects do not occur. Long-acting quinidine (quinaglute, 1 tablet every 12 hours) or procainamide SR (every 6–8 hours) may be used in patients who have gastrointestinal symptoms with quinidine sulfate or have difficulty complying with the 4-hourly schedule.

2. Digitalis–If quinidine is not effective or not tolerated, full digitalization and maintenance may prevent or decrease the frequency of attacks.

3. Verapamil–Verapamil is the drug of choice in the treatment of acute paroxysmal atrial tachycardia, but it prevents recurrent attacks in only about 50% of patients—although it does decrease the frequency and duration of attacks. Oral verapamil is given in a dosage of 80–160 mg 3 times daily after an initial trial of 40 mg. The major side effects are constipation and hypotension. Data on chronic use are sparse.

4. Beta-blocking agents–Propranolol (Inderal), 10–40 mg 3–4 times daily; metoprolol (Lopressor), 50 mg twice daily; nadolol; or atenolol (see p 206) prevents recurrent atrial arrhythmias even in patients refractory to quinidine and procainamide. Use *cautiously* (if at all) in patients with early heart failure, heart block, or bronchospasm.

5. Procainamide (Pronestyl) depresses ectopic pacemakers, prevents arrhythmias, and is primarily useful in the treatment of junctional and ventricular arrhythmias. It can also be used in atrial arrhythmias but is less effective. The drug is used in a maintenance dosage of 250–500 mg 3 times daily when quinidine and digitalis are not successful. Long-acting procainamide (Procan SR) given every 6–8 hours may result in better compliance.

6. New investigational drugs–The most promising is amiodarone (see p 238). This drug frequently produces side effects and should only be used in severe cases unresponsive to the conventional therapy described above.

7. His bundle ablation–In desperate cases with repeated attacks that are difficult to control, ablation of the atrioventricular node, His bundle, or accessory pathways has been accomplished by cryosurgery, surgical interruption, and catheter electrical ablation of the His bundle in order to prevent reentry. The number of cases treated has been small, but the results have been gratifying when the severity of the situation warrants this drastic therapy. A ventricular pacemaker is necessary because complete atrioventricular block is often produced.

Treatment of the Acute Attack

In the absence of heart disease, serious effects are rare. Most attacks subside spontaneously, and the physician should not use remedies that are more dangerous than the disease. Particular effort should be made to terminate the attack quickly if it persists for several days; if cardiac failure, syncope, or anginal pain develops; or if there is underlying cardiac disease. Because reentry is the most common mechanism for paroxysmal atrial tachycardia, effective therapy requires that conduction be interrupted at some point in the reentry circuit.

A. Mechanical Measures: A variety of methods have been used to interrupt attacks, and patients may learn to perform these themselves. These include Valsalva's maneuver (holding the breath and contracting the chest and abdominal muscles), stretching the arms and body, lowering the head between the knees, coughing, and breath-holding. These maneuvers, as is true also of carotid sinus pressure (see below), stimulate the vagus, delay atrioventricular conduction and thereby prolong the AH interval, and so block the reentry mechanism, terminating the arrhythmia.

B. Vagal Stimulation:

1. Carotid sinus pressure–*Caution:* Do *not* use this method if the patient has carotid bruits or a history of transient cerebral ischemic attacks. With the patient relaxed in the semirecumbent position, firm but gentle pressure and massage are applied first over one carotid sinus for 10–20 seconds and then over the other. Pressure should not be exerted on both carotid sinuses at the same time. Continuous auscultation of the heart is required so that carotid sinus pressure can be withdrawn as soon as the attack ceases. Carotid sinus pressure will interrupt about half of the attacks, especially if the patient has been digitalized or sedated. *Do not apply eyeball pressure.*

2. Induced vomiting (except in cases of syncope, anginal pain, or severe cardiac disease) is effective but rarely used today because drug therapy is so much more potent.

C. Drug Therapy: If mechanical measures fail and the attack continues (particularly if the above symptoms are present), one of the following drugs should be employed: (1) Verapamil, which slows conduction in the atrioventricular node, prolonging the AH interval, 40–80 mg every 6 hours. If the attack is symptomatic—especially if it induces angina, syncope, or left ventricular failure—calcium entry-blocking drugs can be given intravenously: verapamil, 5–10 mg, or diltiazem, 0.15 mg/kg (10–15 mg), over a 2-minute period. They can be repeated in 30 minutes at half the initial dose. (2) Parasympathetic stimulating drugs such as edrophonium (Tensilon), 5–10 mg intravenously, which result in enhancement of the atrioventricular conduction delay, breaking the reentry mechanism. (3) Pressor agents, which reflexly stimulate the baroceptors and cause vagal stimulation. (4)

Procainamide. (5) Beta-blockers. (6) Digitalis. (7) Quinidine.

D. Cardioversion: (See p 234.) Use if the clinical situation is severe enough to warrant anesthesia and electric precordial shock. If digitalis toxicity is present or strongly suspected, do not use DC shock but consider atrial pacing instead. If digitalis has been given but toxicity is doubtful, electric shock can be used in progressively increasing amounts beginning with 10 watt-seconds. If ventricular premature beats develop, use lidocaine (Xylocaine), 50–100 mg intravenously, and, if the premature beats disappear, one can repeat the shock. Cardioversion should be abandoned for the time being if the premature beats recur. Alternatively, rapid atrial pacing may terminate the attack and may be the preferred treatment if digitalis excess is present and Wolff-Parkinson-White syndrome is *not* present. External radio-frequency stimulation of an artificial ventricular or atrial pacemaker may stop the attack by interrupting the reentry cycle through the mechanism of a beat that fortuitously enters the atrioventricular node, making it refractory to the circus pathway. An implantable automatic pacemaker has been employed to sense the appearance of a supraventricular tachycardia and to deliver electric shocks that may interrupt the reentry circuit and stop the arrhythmia.

E. Stopping Any Offending Drug Therapy: Paroxysmal atrial tachycardia, usually with 2:1 block, may be due to digitalis toxicity (increased dosage or excessive potassium diuresis). Treatment consists of stopping digitalis and diuretics and treating the patient for digitalis toxicity with potassium, if necessary.

Betriu A et al: Beneficial effect of intravenous diltiazem in the acute management of paroxysmal supraventricular tachyarrhythmias. *Circulation* 1983;**67**:88.

Hartzler GO, Holmes DR Jr, Osborn MJ: Patient-activated transvenous cardiac stimulation for the treatment of supraventricular and ventricular tachycardia. *Am J Cardiol* 1981;**47**:903.

Klein GJ et al: Comparison of the electrophysiologic effects of intravenous and oral verapamil in patients with paroxysmal supraventricular tachycardia. *Am J Cardiol* 1982;**49**:117.

Luceri RM et al: The arrhythmias of dual-chamber cardiac pacemakers and their management. *Ann Intern Med* 1983;**99**:354.

Mauritson DR et al: Oral verapamil for paroxysmal supraventricular tachycardia: A long-term, double-blind randomized trial. *Ann Intern Med* 1982;**96**:409.

Morady F, Scheinman MM: Paroxysmal supraventricular tachycardia. 1. Diagnosis. 2. Treatment. *Mod Concepts Cardiovasc Dis* 1982;**51**:107, 113.

ATRIAL FIBRILLATION

Atrial fibrillation is the commonest chronic arrhythmia. It occurs most frequently in rheumatic heart disease, especially mitral stenosis, and arteriosclerotic heart disease. It may appear paroxysmally before becoming the established rhythm in thyrotoxicosis and other disorders. Infection, trauma, surgery, poisoning, or excessive alcohol intake may cause attacks of atrial fibrillation in patients with normal hearts. It is the only common arrhythmia in which the ventricular rate is rapid and the rhythm irregular. An ectopic atrial pacemaker fires 400–600 times per minute. The impulses pass through the atria at varying speeds and are mostly blocked at the atrioventricular node. The ventricular response is completely irregular, ranging from 80 to 160/min in the untreated state. Because of the varying stroke volumes induced by the varying periods of diastolic filling, not all ventricular beats result in a palpable peripheral pulse. The difference between the apical rate and pulse rate is the "pulse deficit"; this deficit is greater when the ventricular rate is high. Exercise intensifies the irregularity when the heart rate is slow. Carotid sinus massage usually slows the ventricular response but does not terminate the arrhythmia.

Prevention

Procainamide is relatively ineffective. If quinidine alone does not prevent the attacks, it may be added after the patient has been on maintenance doses of digitalis.

Treatment

A. Paroxysmal Atrial Fibrillation:

1. Verapamil–Verapamil selectively increases atrioventricular block at the atrioventricular node and slows the ventricular rate. Enough experience has now accumulated to indicate that verapamil has probably superseded digitalis as the drug of choice to slow the ventricular rate in atrial fibrillation, or it may be combined with digitalis to slow the excessive ventricular rate that frequently occurs during mild to moderate exercise. Verapamil increases the concentration of serum digoxin, and the dose of the latter should be decreased if the combination is used. Verapamil does not usually terminate atrial fibrillation. Caution should be exercised in the use of verapamil or other calcium entry-blocking agents, because they may produce sinus or atrioventricular block with cardiac arrest. Because of their negative inotropic action, they may cause cardiac failure or hypotension, especially when used in combination with beta-adrenergic blocking drugs or disopyramide. Particular caution should be used when beta-blockers and calcium entry blockers are given in combination intravenously. Verapamil should be avoided when atrial fibrillation complicates Wolff-Parkinson-White syndrome (see also pp 208 and 214).

2. Digitalis–Digitalis may be used instead of verapamil, especially when the symptoms or signs of cardiac failure have appeared. *Note:* Digitalis should not be used when atrial fibrillation occurs in Wolff-Parkinson-White syndrome; it may decrease atrioventricular conduction in the normal pathway and enhance it in the aberrant pathway, possibly resulting in very rapid ventricular rates (see p 243).

Digitalis inhibits atrioventricular conduction, thus slowing the ventricular rate, which is the immediate objective of treatment. Give full digitalizing doses, with the objective of slowing the ventricular rate to 70–80/min and avoiding toxic manifestations. In paroxysmal fibrillation there is no clear evidence that the use of digitalis will result in established fibrillation.

3. Cardioversion–Cardioversion should be used at once to convert the rhythm to sinus rhythm in patients with severe underlying heart disease or when the rapid ventricular rate with decreased cardiac output causes severe dyspnea, hypotension, or myocardial ischemia. It may also be used as the primary therapy in patients in whom atrial fibrillation persists. Quinidine is used rarely today to effect conversion to sinus rhythm.

B. Chronic Atrial Fibrillation: In general, conversion to sinus rhythm is attempted whenever it is thought that the patient will be better off with sinus rhythm than with atrial fibrillation: (1) Atrial fibrillation persisting after thyrotoxicosis has been treated surgically or by other means. (2) Atrial fibrillation of a few weeks' duration in an individual with no or only slight cardiac disease. (3) Atrial fibrillation associated with frequent embolic phenomena. (4) Refractory cardiac failure induced by the atrial fibrillation. (5) Severe palpitations resulting from inability to decrease the ventricular rate with digitalis, verapamil, or beta-blocking agents; this may be obvious only on exertion. (6) Atrial fibrillation appearing for the first time post-operatively in patients with a technically successful mitral valvulotomy. Opinion varies on whether anticoagulant therapy should be used in patients with atrial fibrillation in whom reversion to sinus rhythm is attempted. In general, anticoagulants are advised in patients with a recent history of systemic emboli and in patients with mitral valve disease, especially mitral stenosis, and in patients with hypertrophic cardiomyopathy, in whom atrial thrombi can be anticipated.

1. Digitalis–Digitalization is the first step in the absence of preexcitation. The patient is then usually placed on maintenance digitalis indefinitely if atrial fibrillation is not terminated by cardioversion or if it recurs and if preexcitation is not present. The object of digitalization is to slow the ventricular rate and to improve myocardial efficiency, but digitalis toxicity is to be avoided, and digitalis is stopped for 2 days before cardioversion.

2. Verapamil slows the ventricular rate and may produce symptomatic relief until countershock can be used. Infrequently, however, the drug may accelerate the ventricular response during atrial fibrillation, especially if preexcitation is present. Electrophysiologic testing should precede the use of verapamil in preexcitation, just as it should with digitalis. Neither drug should be given when atrial fibrillation complicates preexcitation. When the ventricular rate rises inordinately with mild exercise, the drug can be combined with digitalis as noted above.

3. Countershock–Synchronized DC countershock, 2.5 ms, 10–400 J, under intravenous or general anesthesia, has converted many patients to sinus rhythm even when quinidine has failed or was not tolerated in adequate dosage. It is now the procedure of choice in converting chronic atrial fibrillation (or flutter). DC shock should be avoided in the presence of digitalis toxicity. Relapses have been a problem but can be decreased by the long-term use of quinidine after countershock has produced sinus rhythm.

4. Quinidine is used to abolish the ectopic rhythm once the ventricular rate is controlled with digitalis if countershock is not available. It is potentially hazardous and should be used only in carefully selected cases by a physician thoroughly familiar with the drug and by a method that ensures close medical supervision (preferably in the hospital) while conversion to sinus rhythm is being attempted. Maintenance doses are used following conversion with countershock to maintain sinus rhythm by preventing reversion to atrial fibrillation. *Caution:* See p 231 for dangers of quinidine therapy.

5. Beta-blocking drugs–(See also p 206.) These drugs may be used alone or combined with digitalis to slow the ventricular rate when digitalis alone fails. Use *cautiously* (if at all) in the presence of cardiac failure, heart block, or bronchospasm.

Kannel WB et al: Epidemiologic features of chronic atrial fibrillation. *N Engl J Med* 1982;**306**:1018.

Mancini JGB, Goldberger AL: Cardioversion of atrial fibrillation: Consideration of embolization, anticoagulation, prophylactic pacemaker, and long-term success. *Am Heart J* 1982;**104**:617.

Schwartz J et al: Acute and chronic pharmacodynamic interaction of verapamil and digoxin in atrial fibrillation. *Circulation* 1982;**65**:1163.

ATRIAL FLUTTER

Atrial flutter is uncommon and usually occurs in patients with rheumatic or coronary heart disease, cor pulmonale, or atrial septal defect or as a result of quinidine effect on atrial fibrillation. Ectopic impulse formation occurs at rates of 250–350, with transmission of every second, third, or fourth impulse through the atrioventricular node to the ventricles. The ventricular rate is usually one-half the atrial rate (2:1 conduction), or 150/min. Carotid sinus massage causes sudden slowing or standstill, with rapid return of the rate to the original level on release of pressure. When the ventricular rate is 75 (4:1 block), exercise may cause sudden doubling of the rate to 150 (2:1 block). The first heart sound varies slightly in intensity from beat to beat (but not when the patient is in a constant 2:1 flutter).

Prevention
Similar to prevention of atrial fibrillation.

Treatment
A. Paroxysmal Atrial Flutter: Treatment is similar to that of paroxysmal atrial tachycardia except that digitalis is the drug of choice. The arrhythmia

tends to become established more often than does atrial or junctional tachycardia. If hemodynamic status is seriously compromised, DC shock should be used promptly without digitalis.

B. Chronic Atrial Flutter:

1. DC countershock as in atrial fibrillation (see above). This is the treatment of choice because of the ease and effectiveness of the procedure in restoring sinus rhythm and because the toxic effects of large doses of digitalis and quinidine can be avoided.

2. Digitalis is the drug of choice if countershock is not available or in the rare instances when it is ineffective, unless preexcitation is present. It increases the atrioventricular block and allows a 4:1 conduction with a ventricular rate of about 75/min. By decreasing conduction in the atrioventricular node, digitalis prevents a 2:1 or 1:1 conduction response. In about half of cases, atrial fibrillation or sinus rhythm results from full digitalization. Oral medication is usually sufficient, although the intravenous route may be used if the situation is critical and DC cardioversion is not available. Digitalis must often be given in larger doses than are usually required for cardiac failure. When a fixed 4:1 conduction is produced by digitalis, a slightly increased dose may convert the flutter to atrial fibrillation or sinus rhythm; or DC countershock may be used. Verapamil may be used to increase atrioventricular block and slow the ventricular rate.

3. Beta-adrenergic or calcium entry-blocking drugs may be used as in atrial fibrillation to slow the ventricular rate if this is difficult with digitalis. (See Atrial Fibrillation, above).

4. Quinidine should not be used to treat atrial flutter unless the patient is fully digitalized, with a slow ventricular rate, because of the danger of producing a 1:1 conduction. If digitalis results in only a 4:1 conduction or produces atrial fibrillation that does not spontaneously convert to sinus rhythm, quinidine may be given if DC cardioversion is not available.

ATRIOVENTRICULAR JUNCTIONAL RHYTHM

The atrial-nodal junction or the nodal–His bundle junction may assume pacemaker activity for the heart, usually at a rate of 40–60/min. This may occur in normal hearts, myocarditis, coronary artery disease, or as a result of digitalis or quinidine toxicity. The rate responds normally to exercise, and the diagnosis is often a surprise finding on electrocardiography. Careful examination of the jugular pulse may reveal the presence of cannon waves. Patients are often asymptomatic. Digitalis toxicity must always be considered.

Junctional rhythm is often an escape rhythm because of depressed sinus node function with sinoatrial block or impaired transmission of the impulse from the sinus node to the atrioventricular node. This is a passive rhythm and should be differentiated from junctional rhythm or tachycardia that results from increased automaticity of the junctional tissues from such conditions as digitalis toxicity, hypoxia, or ischemia. In these latter circumstances, the rhythm is often called nonparoxysmal junctional tachycardia and is associated with a narrow QRS and a rate usually less than 120–130/min. It is usually considered benign when it occurs in acute myocardial infarction, but the ischemia that induces it may also induce ventricular tachycardia and ventricular fibrillation.

ATRIOVENTRICULAR JUNCTIONAL TACHYCARDIA

This arrhythmia is due to rapid, regular impulse formation in the atrioventricular nodal junction or bundle of His, with regular transmission to the ventricles. The usual rates are 140–240/min. Junctional tachycardia may be a benign condition or may reflect serious myocardial disease; it is more common than other arrhythmias in cor pulmonale and may often be the result of digitalis toxicity, which increases the rate of impulse formation in subsidiary pacemaker cells.

Differentiation From Ventricular Tachycardia

The differentiation of ventricular tachycardia from supraventricular tachycardia with aberrant conduction is often difficult in patients with a QRS duration of 0.12 s or more. Utilizing His bundle recordings to establish the site of origin of the tachycardia, Wellens (1978) found that the following electrocardiographic changes favored (but did not establish) a ventricular origin: (1) a QRS duration exceeding 0.14 s; (2) left axis deviation; (3) atrioventricular dissociation; (4) capture or fusion beats (infrequent); (5) monophasic (R) or biphasic (qR, QR, or RS) complexes in V_1; and (6) a qR or QS complex in V_6. A supraventricular origin was favored by (1) a triphasic QRS complex, especially if there was initial negativity in leads I and V_6; (2) ventricular rates exceeding 170/min; (3) QRS duration longer than 0.12 s but not longer than 0.14 s; and (4) the presence of preexcitation syndrome.

The relationship of the P waves to the ventricular complex is helpful. A one-to-one relationship usually means a supraventricular origin except in the case of ventricular tachycardia with retrograde P waves. If the P waves are not clearly seen, Lewis leads may be employed, in which the right arm electrode is placed in the V_1 position 2 interspaces higher than usual and the left arm electrode is placed in the usual V_1 position. This accentuates the size of the P waves. Esophageal leads, in which the electrode is placed directly posterior to the left atrium, achieve the same effect and may also be helpful in differentiating supraventricular from ventricular arrhythmias by making it possible to note any disparity between atrial and ventricular rates. Right atrial electrograms may also help to clarify the diagnosis by accentuating the P waves.

His bundle recordings clarify the origin of the arrhythmia by noting the relationship of the A, H, and V spikes. His bundle electrograms may also be helpful. A bipolar or tripolar catheter can be inserted percutaneously via the femoral vein and positioned in the right ventricle in the region of the tricuspid valve. It is then possible to record impulses from the atria, bundle of His, and His-Purkinje-ventricular system. In any given arrhythmia, one can see whether the His bundle spikes precede each QRS complex, in which case the rhythm originates above the ventricles. If the ventricular complex is not preceded by a His spike or atrial activity, the ectopic focus arises distal to the bundle of His. One can determine the interval between the atrial spike and the His spike and between the His spike and the beginning of the QRS to determine where atrioventricular conduction delays occur. His bundle recordings are also valuable in atrial fibrillation to distinguish between aberrant conduction from a rapid ventricular rate and ventricular premature beats, or ventricular tachycardia. If the His spike precedes each ventricular complex in the ECG, ventricular tachycardia is excluded.

If the diagnosis can be made by clinical and routine electrocardiography, the cost and hazards of cardiac catheterization should be avoided.

Treatment is along the same lines as for atrial tachycardia. However, when tachycardia induces severe hemodynamic abnormalities, is recurrent, and is refractory to medical treatment, surgical ablation of the retrograde limb of the tachycardia circuit has successfully prevented recurrence of the tachycardia (Guarnieri, 1984). This procedure requires expertise in electrophysiology to study and manage the patient.

Guarnieri T et al: The nonpharmacologic management of the permanent form of junctional reciprocating tachycardia. *Circulation* 1984;**69**:269.

Wellens HJJ, Bär FWHM, Lie KI: The value of the electrocardiogram in the differential diagnosis of a tachycardia with a widened QRS complex. *Am J Med* 1978;**64**:27.

VENTRICULAR PREMATURE BEATS*

Ventricular premature beats are similar to atrial premature beats in mechanism and manifestations but are much more common. Together, they are the commonest causes of a grossly irregular rhythm with a normal heart rate. Ectopic impulse formation causes ventricular contraction to occur sooner than the next expected beat. The sound of this contraction is audible. The pause between the ectopic ventricular beat and the next normally occurring ventricular beat is longer than the usual interval between 2 regular beats. When this pause, combined with the coupling interval (the interval between the *preceding* regular ventricular beat and the ectopic beat), equals twice the cycle length of regularly occurring ventricular beats, the pause is compensatory, whereas the pause is not compensatory in atrial premature beats because the sinus node is

*See also Arrhythmias under Myocardial Infarction, p 226.

depolarized and must start a new basic rhythm. Single premature beats that occur after every normal beat produce bigeminy. Exercise generally abolishes premature beats in normal hearts, and the rhythm becomes regular.

Premature beats have no definite significance in the absence of coronary disease, hypertrophic cardiomyopathy, or prolapse of the mitral valve unless they arise early in diastole, are frequent, occur from multiple foci, occur with rapid ventricular rates or in runs, interrupt the T wave (R-on-T phenomenon), or are due to digitalis toxicity. The importance of the R-on-T phenomenon in predicting the likelihood of ventricular fibrillation is still being debated (see also p 243). Sudden death occurs more frequently (presumably as a result of ventricular fibrillation) when ventricular premature beats occur in the presence of known coronary disease, hypertension, cardiomyopathy, and possibly prolapsed mitral valve, but not in individuals with no known cardiac disease even in the middle-aged normal population.

Ambulatory electrocardiographic monitoring or continuous electrocardiography during graded exercise reveals more frequent and complex ventricular premature beats than occur in a single routine ECG. Although it is felt that these exercise-induced premature beats have a worse prognosis than those which occur spontaneously, the benefit and safety of long-term antiarrhythmia therapy are not yet established.

Treatment

If no associated cardiac disease is present and if the ectopic beats are infrequent, occur late in diastole, and produce no palpitations, no specific therapy is indicated. If the patient has known coronary disease and the ventricular premature beats are frequent or complex (multiform, paired, in salvos, or early on the T wave), antiarrhythmic agents such as quinidine, procainamide, beta-adrenergic blocking drugs, disopyramide, or (especially if heart failure exists) digitalis may be used (see also p 226). In the presence of coronary disease, if hemodynamic deterioration results, if the patient has symptoms of angina or dyspnea, or if the palpitations are very troublesome, then antiarrhythmic therapy should be given. Conventional drugs such as those just listed may be ineffective in patients with advanced heart disease. Complex ventricular premature beats may lead to ventricular tachycardia and fibrillation; new investigational agents are now being given extensive trial for treatment of these disorders. There is evidence that by suppressing complex ventricular arrhythmias, ventricular fibrillation and sudden death may be prevented. Further data on this point are being accumulated. Some of these newer drugs include amiodarone, aprindine, encainide, flecainide, mexiletine, and tocainide (see references).

If ventricular premature beats are due to digitalis toxicity, withdraw digitalis and diuretics for 3–5 days or until the arrhythmia disappears and then resume medication in smaller dosage. Phenytoin may be of value (see below). At times, however, patients with cardiac failure who are receiving digitalis may develop ventricular premature beats that are due not to digitalis toxicity but to inadequate digitalization and cardiac failure. If in doubt as to the cause, withdraw digitalis for several days and treat the cardiac failure with other available methods (see p 253). In these circumstances, the ventricular premature beats often disappear as the cardiac failure improves.

Horan MJ, Kennedy HL: Ventricular ectopy: History, epidemiology, and clinical implications. *JAMA* 1984;**251**:380.

Kostis JB et al: Premature ventricular complexes in the absence of identifiable heart disease. *Circulation* 1981;**63**:1351.

PAROXYSMAL VENTRICULAR TACHYCARDIA

This is an uncommon serious arrhythmia due to rapid ectopic impulse formation in the ventricles. The rate may be 160–240. It usually lasts hours but may persist for days if untreated. The rhythm is almost completely regular but is less regular than in atrial tachycardia, and the first sound may vary slightly in intensity from beat to beat. Carotid sinus massage has no effect.

Paroxysmal ventricular tachycardia usually occurs after myocardial infarction, dilated cardiomyopathy, hypertrophic cardiomyopathy, or mitral valve prolapse or as a result of digitalis or quinidine toxicity. It infrequently occurs in the absence of known cardiac disease. Pain due to myocardial ischemia, fall in blood pressure, and shock are common.

Prevention

The drugs of choice are quinidine, procainamide, and disopyramide, or, if ventricular premature beats occur during acute myocardial infarction, a constant infusion of lidocaine at a rate of 1–4 mg/min. If severe ventricular tachycardia recurs following these drugs, electrophysiologic studies should be done to guide therapy with the investigational drugs discussed under Treatment, above, and below.

Treatment

A. Average Case:

1. DC countershock has replaced pharmacologic methods of treatment of ventricular tachycardia in all but the mildest cases.

2. Lidocaine (Xylocaine), 50–100 mg intravenously followed by 1–4 mg/min intravenously, has largely replaced quinidine and procainamide because of its short duration of action and infrequent hypotensive effect (see below).

3. Procainamide (Pronestyl), 0.5–1.5 g orally every 4–6 hours, may be substituted for quinidine if quinidine is ineffective or produces toxicity. Long-acting procainamide sustained release (Procan SR), every 6–8 hours, may also be used.

4. Quinidine, 0.4 g orally every 2 hours for 3 doses, if the attack is well tolerated and the patient is not in shock and if DC cardioversion is not available. If the attack continues and there is no toxicity from the quinidine, increase the dose to 0.6 g orally every 2 hours for 3 doses or use DC countershock. If countershock is not available and the larger oral dosage of quinidine is not successful, change to procainamide.

5. Disopyramide (Norpace), 100–200 mg 4 times daily, often preceded by a loading dose of 300 mg; it can also be given as a dose of 2 mg/kg intravenously. Side effects are due to the anticholinergic activity of the drug and include dry mouth, urinary retention, and aggravation of sick sinus syndrome. Cardiac failure has occurred (because of the negative inotropic action of the drug) in patients who previously had cardiac failure. Disopyramide should be used with caution or not at all in these instances.

6. Phenytoin (Dilantin), 5 mg/kg intravenously or 100–500 mg intravenously very slowly, has been used with success in ventricular arrhythmias, especially when they are due to digitalis. Sinus rhythm may be induced, and digitalis-induced ventricular arrhythmias may be prevented when DC shock is given. Slow administration and careful electrocardiographic and blood pressure monitoring are necessary.

B. Urgent Case:

1. DC countershock, depolarizing the entire heart, has proved of great value in patients not responding to lidocaine or procainamide, even in acute myocardial infarction. Under general anesthesia or intravenous diazepam, a DC shock, synchronized to the downstroke of the R wave of the ECG, 2.5 ms in duration, 50–400 J, can be given.

2. Lidocaine (Xylocaine), 1 mg/kg in 1 or 2% solution (50–100 mg for an adult) given intravenously, has proved effective. If the arrhythmia recurs, one may give an intravenous infusion of 60–240 mg/h (1 g diluted to 1 L of 5% glucose) (about 1–4 mg/min) or repeat the intravenous injection twice at 20-minute intervals.

3. Procainamide hydrochloride (Pronestyl), 1 g *slowly* intravenously (at a rate not to exceed 100 mg/min). During the infusion, continuous electrocardiography and repeated blood pressure determinations are essential. Severe hypotension may result from the medication.

4. Quinidine may be given intravenously as quinidine gluconate, 0.8 g diluted with 50 mL of 5% glucose *slowly* (1 mL/min), with continuous electrocardiographic and blood pressure determinations. When giving intravenous quinidine in severe cases, the physician should be alert to the possibility of precipitating ventricular fibrillation or asystole. (See Heart-Lung Resuscitation, p 1109.) Complete atrioventricular block is a contraindication to the use of quinidine.

5. Propranolol (Inderal) or its equivalent may be given slowly intravenously in 0.5-mg doses under constant clinical electrocardiographic monitoring. The precautions noted under the atrial arrhythmias should be observed. Propranolol is rarely used in ventricular tachycardia unless cardioversion is not available.

6. Vasopressor drugs for shock–If shock is present as a result of ventricular tachycardia or results from the drugs given intravenously, it can be treated with vasopressor drugs as described under the treatment of shock (see Chapter 1).

7. Digitalis is usually contraindicated in ventricular tachycardia; however, in some patients with cardiac failure in whom the above-mentioned drugs have failed to restore sinus rhythm, full digitalization, performed carefully, has been successful.

8. Temporary transvenous cardiac pacing may capture the rhythm from the ectopic ventricular tachycardia and has been used when antiarrhythmic drugs have failed. Implantable programmable pacemakers are being used on an investigational basis to permit salvos of rapid ventricular pacing during supraventricular and ventricular tachycardia in order to interrupt the reentry circuit. Preliminary results are promising but seem more suitable for patients with chronic recurrent tachycardia (see below).

9. Investigational drugs–One of the most effective and best-studied of these drugs is **amiodarone.** It can be given either as a continuous infusion of 200–1400 mg/d or as an acute injection of 5 mg/kg over 15–20 minutes. Side effects have been few in the relatively small number of patients in which intravenous amiodarone has been used, but one should be prepared for hypotension and worsening of hemodynamic status, especially if the patient had cardiac failure prior to the use of the drug. Close monitoring with Swan-Ganz catheters in place should be used in these circumstances. Hemodynamic deterioration may occur rapidly in patients with ventricular tachycardia, and if conventional drugs are ineffective, the newer investigational ones should be used. These drugs may be used in urgent cases also.

Chronic Recurrent Ventricular Tachycardia

Chronic recurrent ventricular tachycardia is an arrhythmia that is often life-threatening and difficult to treat. It has increased in frequency in recent years because of the greater numbers of patients who have been resuscitated after ventricular fibrillation or who have been shown to have unsuspected left ventricular aneurysm after recovery from acute myocardial infarction. Treatment in the past has been largely empiric, with antiarrhythmic drugs used alone or in combination. A new approach is the initiation and termination of ventricular tachycardia in the laboratory with intracardiac programmed stimulation. Various antiarrhythmic drugs can then be given in sequence to determine which agents prevent the induction of ventricular tachycardia. Drugs that prevent the electrical induction of ventricular tachycardia in the laboratory are likely to be effective in vivo for long-term therapy; long-term use of a particular drug may still be effective even if the arrhythmia is not prevented in the laboratory.

Endocardial catheter mapping should be employed in patients who have frequent recurrences of ventricular tachycardia with life-threatening symptoms that fail to respond to drugs approved by the FDA or to the newer investigational drugs not yet approved, such as amiodarone, aprindine, encainide, flecamide, mexiletine, tocainide, and others. The origin and sequence of activation can be determined; this is essential if surgical treatment or cryotherapy is being considered. The indications for surgical treatment and the various approaches are still in a state of flux, but the results have often been dramatic when all else has failed. Surgery should be performed only in specialized electrophysiologic laboratories and centers experienced in the techniques and only when long-term medical treatment of recurrent ventricular tachycardia is unsatisfactory despite the use of the newer potent investigational drugs or if their use induces intolerable side effects. Because of the extensive myocardial damage in these patients, drug therapy is often not the long-term answer, and earlier aggressive therapy should be considered.

The automatic implantable ventricular pacemaker is being used more frequently in experienced electrophysiologic centers, with encouraging results. Further improvement of the pacemaker so that it both senses the arrhythmia and delivers electric shocks to terminate it will increase its usefulness. In successful cases of previously severe recurrent ventricular tachycardia or fibrillation, the implantable pacemaker sometimes obviated the need for repeated defibrillations and cardioversions and for surgical treatment. Further experience is awaited.

The importance of the precipitating role of acute psychologic reactions in ventricular arrhythmias has been reemphasized recently; the central nervous system should always be considered and treated.

Chesnie B et al: Encainide for refractory ventricular tachyarrhythmia. *Am J Cardiol* 1983;**52:**495.

Graboys TB et al: Long-term survival of patients with malignant ventricular arrhythmia treated with antiarrhythmic drugs. *Am J Cardiol* 1982;**50:**437.

Josephson ME, Harken AH, Horowitz LN: Long-term results of endocardial resection for sustained ventricular tachycardia in coronary disease patients. *Am Heart J* 1982;**104:**51.

Kienzle MG et al: Subendocardial resection for refractory ventricular tachycardia: Effects on ambulatory electrocardiogram, programmed stimulation and ejection fraction, and relation to outcome. *J Am Coll Cardiol* 1983;**2:**853.

Lerman BB et al: Disopyramide: Evaluation of electrophysiologic effects and clinical efficacy in patients with sustained ventricular tachycardia or ventricular fibrillation. *Am J Cardiol* 1983;**51:**759.

Lown B: Mental stress, arrhythmias and sudden death. *Am J Med* 1982;**72:**177.

Mirowski M: Management of malignant ventricular tachyarrhythmias with automatic implanted cardioverter-defibrillators. *Mod Concepts Cardiovasc Dis* 1983;**52:**41.

Podrid P, Ruskin J (editors): The role of oral mexiletine in the management of ventricular arrhythmias. (Symposium.) *Am Heart J* 1984;**107:**1053. [Entire issue.]

Roy D et al: Clinical characteristics and long-term follow-up in 119 survivors of cardiac arrest: Relation to inducibility at electrophysiologic testing. *Am J Cardiol* 1983;**52:**969.

Singh BN, Nademanee K: New agents in antiarrhythmia therapy. (2 parts.) *Primary Cardiol* (Feb) 1982;**8**:16 and (March) 1982;**8**:16.

Spurrell R: Use of cardiac pacemakers in the management of tachycardia. *Cardiovasc Rev Rep* 1982;**3**:123.

Wellens HJJ et al: Medical treatment of ventricular tachycardia: Considerations in the selection of patients for surgical treatment. *Am J Cardiol* 1982;**49**:186.

Zipes DP, Prystowsky EM, Heger JJ: Amiodarone: Electrophysiologic actions, pharmacokinetics and clinical effects. *J Am Coll Cardiol* 1984;**3**:1059.

ACCELERATED IDIOVENTRICULAR RHYTHM

Accelerated idioventricular rhythms are ventricular rhythms that simulate ventricular tachycardia but occur in selected situations and at a relatively slow rate. Two mechanisms have been invoked: (1) an escape rhythm due to suppression of higher pacemakers resulting from sinoatrial and atrioventricular block or from depressed sinus node function; and (2) a slow ventricular tachycardia due to reentry or increased automaticity due to ischemia, as in acute myocardial infarction. In the latter instance, the attacks of tachycardia consist of paroxysms of relatively short duration that are relatively slow (less than 100/min). It is uncertain whether the idioventricular rhythm, if not associated with escape rhythms, has the same or a better prognosis than ventricular tachycardia in general. The incidence of ventricular fibrillation is considerably less than that of ventricular tachycardia with a rapid rate. Ventricular fibrillation must be distinguished from the idioventricular or junctional rhythm with rates less than 40–45/min that occurs in the presence of complete atrioventricular block. Atrioventricular dissociation but not atrioventricular block occurs in most cases of accelerated idioventricular rhythm.

VENTRICULAR FLUTTER & FIBRILLATION

These arrhythmias represent more advanced stages of ventricular tachycardia in which the rate of impulse formation is more rapid and transmission becomes irregular, resulting in ineffective ventricular contractions. Diagnosis can be established only by electrocardiography. Ventricular flutter-fibrillation is rapidly fatal unless terminated by defibrillation. It is usually associated with severe myocardial damage but may be precipitated by epinephrine, quinidine, or digitalis.

Treatment

A. Surgical and Mechanical Measures: External cardiac massage and prompt ventilation until electric defibrillation is the treatment of choice (see Appendix). Continuous monitoring of patients with acute myocardial infarction has shown at least half of sudden cardiac deaths to be due to ventricular fibrillation.

Prompt treatment may be lifesaving. Surgical exposure of the heart with direct cardiac massage is infrequently performed today except during cardiac operations.

B. Medical Measures: Usually ineffective. In paroxysmal episodes, try to prevent (as in ventricular tachycardia).

DISTURBANCES OF CONDUCTION

SICK SINUS SYNDROME; BRADYCARDIA-TACHYCARDIA

In recent years a syndrome known as the "sick sinus" syndrome, or tachycardia-bradycardia syndrome, has become increasingly noted, but its significance has been disputed, especially since low heart rates are frequent in elderly patients, in whom escape rhythms may occur. Pathologic causes of the syndrome include coronary disease, degenerative fibrotic lesions of the cardiac conduction system, and other conditions in which sclerotic or granulomatous lesions may occur, including scleroderma, Chagas' disease, and various cardiomyopathies. The diagnosis should not be made in the absence of significant symptoms of syncope or near-syncope during the bradycardia phase and palpitations or dyspnea during the tachycardia phase, and it should be documented by Holter monitoring. The syndrome consists of abnormalities of the pacemaker function of the sinus node or abnormalities in conduction from the sinus node to the atrioventricular node. The patients may have sinus bradycardia, sinus standstill, or sinoatrial block. In conjunction with a slow atrial rate resulting from these abnormalities, paroxysmal atrial or junctional arrhythmias and perfusion abnormalities may occur. The patient may have alternately a slow rate (which may not be adequate to perfuse the vital organs) and a rapid atrial or junctional tachycardia or atrial fibrillation that may produce symptoms as a result of the rapid ventricular rate. Treatment of the atrial arrhythmias with drugs such as quinidine or digitalis may enhance the conduction difficulties of the sinus node or the sinoatrial transmission; treatment is best effected by inserting an artificial demand pacemaker into the right ventricle to prevent sinus slowing and then using various antiarrhythmic agents to prevent the paroxysmal atrial arrhythmias.

In some patients, the increased heart rate resulting from the implanted artificial pacemaker may improve left ventricular function over a period of weeks or months, so that the recurrent atrial arrhythmias become less frequent and the pharmacologic treatment becomes less urgent; the patient may become asymptomatic with the use of the implanted pacemaker alone.

SINOATRIAL BLOCK
(See p 239.)

In sinoatrial block the normal pacemaker fails to initiate the depolarizing impulse at irregular or regular intervals or, rarely, in a fixed 2:1 ratio, or the sinus node discharges but there is exit block. This failure is apparently due to heightened vagal tone and is not usually related to the presence of heart disease but may be due to digitalis. Exercise and atropine may therefore abolish sinoatrial block. This arrhythmia can be recognized by the fact that no sound is audible during the prolonged interval between beats (in contrast to ventricular premature beats). There are no symptoms unless the period of standstill extends over the span of several beats, in which case momentary faintness or even syncope may occur. In susceptible individuals, carotid sinus massage induces sinoatrial block. The sick sinus syndrome, in which sinoatrial block is combined with sinus arrest, sinus bradycardia, and paroxysmal atrial arrhythmia, is discussed under sinus bradycardia, above (see p 231).

Beta-adrenergic blocking agents slow the heart rate by decreasing adrenergic impulses in the sinus node. Vagal stimuli slow the sinus rate by cholinergic effects and can be reversed by atropine.

Any fibrotic, ischemic, or inflammatory lesion can produce conduction defects involving the sinoatrial or atrioventricular conduction pathways.

Treatment

In most cases no treatment is required. The causative factors, especially digitalis, should be eliminated if possible. The following drugs may be tried: (1) atropine sulfate, 0.6 mg 4 times daily orally; (2) ephedrine sulfate, 25 mg orally 4 times daily. In more prolonged cases, give atropine, 0.5–1 mg intravenously. When sinoatrial block is associated with the sick sinus syndrome with paroxysmal atrial arrhythmias, therapy requires a combination of a transvenous artificial pacemaker and an antiarrhythmic drug as described under sinus bradycardia.

Chung EK: Sick sinus syndrome: Current views. (2 parts.) *Mod Concepts Cardiovasc Dis* 1980;**49**:61, 67.

Ferrer MI: Sick sinus syndrome. *J Cardiovasc Med* 1981;**6**:743.

Gillette PC: Recent advances in mechanisms, evaluation, and pacemaker treatment of chronic bradydysrhythmias in children. *Am Heart J* 1981;**102**:920.

Mazuz M, Friedman HS: Significance of prolonged electrocardiographic pauses in sinoatrial disease: Sick sinus syndrome. *Am J Cardiol* 1983;**52**:485.

ATRIOVENTRICULAR CONDUCTION SYSTEM

Bundle Branch Block

Conduction of the cardiac impulse from the atria to the ventricles should be considered as a continuous system: the impulse originates normally in the sinoatrial node and passes via various internodal tracts to the atrioventricular node. From here, the impulse spreads via the bundle of His and a "septal" fascicle into a trifascicular branching system consisting of a right bundle and the left anterior superior and left posterior inferior branches of the left bundle. Conduction then continues via the Purkinje system to the ventricular myocardium. Atrioventricular block may occur anywhere from the atrioventricular node to involvement of both bundle branches. Block need not be due to disease in the atrioventricular node itself; His bundle recordings have demonstrated that the site of the block or blocks can be single or multiple and may be localized in the atrioventricular node, the bundle of His, or anywhere in the conduction system distal to the bundle of His. Types of bilateral bundle branch block involving both bundles, the common bundle, or the right bundle and one of the left branches have all been shown to be involved in some cases of atrioventricular block. Stressing the conduction system by increasing the heart rate by atrial pacing can produce atrioventricular block, usually proximal to the bundle of His. Newly acquired bundle branch block in the absence of acute myocardial infarction is relatively uncommon; only 125 cases were noted during an 18-year follow-up of the Framingham group. Organic heart disease is more frequent and mortality rates are greater in left than in right bundle branch block.

Conduction defects may be due to drugs (such as digitalis), coronary heart disease, acute inflammatory myocarditis, rheumatic fever, fibrosis of the conduction system of the cardiac skeleton, or infiltrative diseases such as sarcoidosis, amyloidosis, or Chagas' disease.

Prognosis and treatment may vary depending on whether the block is proximal or distal to the bundle of His and whether it is chronic or developed during acute myocardial infarction (see p 227). The prognosis is better when the block is proximal. His bundle recordings—in conjunction with clinical studies—have demonstrated that block is almost always in the atrioventricular node when there is only partial atrioventricular block with prolonged PR interval or when the second-degree atrioventricular block (see below) is characterized by the Wenckebach phenomenon, with partial progressive PR delay with dropped beats, and when QRS complexes are narrow. This is the usual situation in congenital atrioventricular block and in inferior myocardial infarction. Syncope and Stokes-Adams attacks are uncommon. In contrast, the conduction defect is almost always distal to the atrioventricular node, with a greater likelihood of the development of complete atrioventricular block, syncope, and sudden death, when there is Mobitz type II or second-degree atrioventricular conduction defect with dropped beats not preceded by progressive delay of previous PR intervals when the QRS complex is widened; and when the atrioventricular conduction defects occur in the setting of anterior myocardial infarction.

Bifascicular Block

Bifascicular block discovered during routine electrocardiography or mass screening or in asymptomatic persons only infrequently progresses to complete atrioventricular block. Neither His bundle conduction studies nor insertion of pacemakers is justified unless symptoms documented as being due to second- or third-degree atrioventricular block are clearly established. When clinical heart disease is present, as is often the case when bifascicular block is discovered on electrocardiography in patients with cardiac symptoms, the degree of the underlying cardiac disease rather than the presence of any abnormal conduction intervals determines the prognosis. Although these patients have an increased cardiovascular mortality rate because of the presence of associated cardiac disease, complete atrioventricular block (documented by Holter monitoring) or sudden death is uncommon. Insertion of a pacemaker is indicated only if second- or third-degree block is present or if transient neurologic symptoms are proved to be due to intermittent atrioventricular block. Such symptoms may be due to relative bradycardia and not to atrioventricular block and can sometimes be improved by a pacemaker. The overall mortality rate and the incidence of sudden death have not been significantly decreased in these patients by the use of a pacemaker. Ambulatory electrocardiographic monitoring, with careful correlation between symptoms and electrocardiographic evidence of block or arrhythmia, is essential before resorting to pacemaker therapy.

If one studies patients with right or left bundle branch blocks with His bundle techniques, atrioventricular conduction defects are occasionally found when not seen in the ordinary ECG; in others, they may appear with the passage of time. A combination that is more likely to develop atrioventricular block is right bundle branch block and left anterior hemiblock, with a frontal plane axis of approximately −45 to −60 degrees. This bifascicular block may be present for months or years without symptoms or atrioventricular conduction delay. The incidence of subsequent atrioventricular block is on the order of perhaps 1–2% over a period of years.

Atrioventricular Block

A. Partial (or First-Degree) Atrioventricular Block: Partial atrioventricular block consists of prolongation of the conduction time of the normal impulse from the atria to the ventricles; as indicated above, this can occur distal as well as proximal to the bundle of His. Atrioventricular block is classified by the degree of block: In partial atrioventricular block, the PR interval is prolonged to 0.21 s or more (at normal heart rates), but every atrial impulse reaches the ventricles. Its presence can be suspected clinically when the first heart sound is faint in the presence of a vigorous apical impulse. There may be a presystolic gallop rhythm caused by audible atrial contraction.

B. Second-Degree Atrioventricular Block: In second-degree atrioventricular block the delay in conduction increases to the point where every sinus impulse does not reach the ventricles, resulting in failure of a ventricular contraction, ie, every so often a beat is dropped. After a beat is dropped, the atrioventricular conduction system recovers, and in 2:1 block the next PR interval is usually normal. The cycle may be repeated regularly or irregularly, producing a 2:1, 3:1, or other interval of rhythm. Dropped beats are distinguished from premature beats by the fact that during the interval between peripheral pulses there is no sound at the apex as well as no beat felt at the wrist, whereas in premature beats there may be no beat felt at the wrist but one can hear a faint premature beat at the apex.

Second-degree atrioventricular block is divided into (1) Mobitz type I, with partial progressive atrioventricular block and dropped beats (Wenckebach pauses), and (2) Mobitz type II, with intermittent dropped beats not preceded by a prolonged PR interval. As indicated in the section on myocardial infarction, Mobitz type I usually occurs when the conduction defect is in the atrioventricular node—as during an inferior myocardial infarction—and infrequently leads to Stokes-Adams attacks. Type II is due to a block in or distal to the bundle of His. It is more apt to occur in anterior myocardial infarction and frequently leads to Stokes-Adams attacks with complete atrioventricular block and, therefore, requires artificial pacing.

The classification as Mobitz type I and Mobitz type II is only partially reliable, because patients may have both types in the same lead, and one cannot predict the site of origin of the 2:1 atrioventricular block from the ECG. In most cases with Mobitz type II the block is distal to the bundle of His, but it may be in the atrioventricular node. Rare exceptions occur in which the Mobitz type I block is *distal* to the atrioventricular node, but it is more likely to be *in* the atrioventricular node. The width of the QRS complexes assists in differentiating whether the block is nodal or infranodal. When they are narrow, the block is usually nodal; when they are wide, the block is usually infranodal.

C. Complete (Third-Degree) Heart Block: This is a more advanced form of block. Complete atrioventricular block is usually due to a lesion distal to the His bundle and associated with bilateral bundle branch block; occasionally, the block is proximal to the bundle of His. In the latter case, the QRS is usually (but not always) normal in width (less than 0.12 s), and the ventricular rate is faster—usually greater than 50/min. In the former case, the QRS is wide and the ventricular rate is slower, usually less than 50/min. Inferior infarction causes ischemia of the atrioventricular node due to a compromised nodal artery from the right coronary, whereas anterior infarction results in destruction of the ventricular septum with bilateral bundle branch block. Transmission of atrial impulses through the atrioventricular node is completely blocked, and a ventricular pacemaker maintains a slow, regular ventricular rate, usually less than 45/min. Exercise does not increase the rate. The first heart sound varies greatly in loudness; wide pulse pressure, changing systolic blood pressure level, and cannon venous pulsations in the neck are also present. Patients may be asymptomatic or complain of weakness or dyspnea if the rate is less than 35/min—at times at even higher rates if the left ventricle cannot increase its stroke output. During periods of transition from partial to complete heart block, certain patients have ventricular asystole that lasts several seconds to minutes. Syncope occurs abruptly, and if the asystole is prolonged beyond a few seconds, convulsive movements appear (Stokes-Adams syndrome). Asystole of 2–3 minutes is usually fatal.

Treatment

A. Prolonged Conduction and Incomplete Heart Block: In the absence of Stokes-Adams syndrome with syncope (see below), treatment of atrioventricular conduction defects is rarely successful except by elimination of drugs, if they are causative, or by the subsidence of acute myocarditis, acute myocardial infarction, or ischemia. Prolongation of the atrioventricular conduction itself usually needs no treatment (except careful observation) unless there is complete heart block (see below) or anterior infarction, especially if the atrioventricular conduction defect is associated with left anterior hemiblock or bundle branch block. Cardiac failure or weakness may occur with slow ventricular rates, in which instance a demand pacemaker should be inserted to increase the ventricular rate.

See above for a discussion of the danger of complete atrioventricular block in patients with partial atrioventricular block and bundle branch block.

B. Complete Heart Block and Stokes-Adams Syndrome: Try to eliminate or treat the cause. The objective of treatment is to obtain a ventricular rate of 70/min or more.

Artificial transvenous or epicardial pacemaker. Dramatic improvement in cardiac failure, cerebral symptoms, and syncopal attacks has resulted in earlier use of transvenous right ventricular pacing in many patients. When syncopal attacks due to bradyarrhythmia have occurred, a catheter pacemaker may be lifesaving.

Pacemakers are now introduced following a single proved Stokes-Adams attack and are used with increasing frequency when slow ventricular rates induce cerebral or cardiac insufficiency. Follow-up of patients with pacemakers is essential to establish early the presence of faulty functioning.

When atrioventricular block is intermittent but causing syncope, a demand pacemaker is preferable because it is activated only during bradycardia, thus decreasing the likelihood of ventricular fibrillation caused by stimulation of the heart during the vulnerable period and resulting from competition between the natural and artificial pacemakers.

Syncope of Undetermined Origin

This represents a troublesome clinical dilemma.

Electrophysiologic studies have been performed to determine if a cardiovascular cause could be found in patients in whom clinical and noninvasive tests were not diagnostic. About half of cases remain unexplained; about one-fifth are due to noncardiac causes, but about one-third have a treatable cardiovascular cause, usually episodic ventricular arrhythmias, but occasionally sinonodal and atrioventricular nodal block. It seems worthwhile to recommend electrophysiologic studies in patients in whom the cause of syncope could not be determined otherwise.

Dancy M, Leech G, Leatham A: Significance of complete right bundle-branch block when an isolated finding: An echocardiographic study. *Br Heart J* 1982;**48**:217.

Harthorne JW: Indications for pacemaker insertion: Types and modes of pacing. *Prog Cardiovasc Dis* 1981;**23**:393.

Hess DS, Morady F, Scheinman MM: Electrophysiologic testing in the evaluation of patients with syncope of undetermined origin. *Am J Cardiol* 1982;**50**:1309.

McAnulty JH, Rahimtoola SH: Bundle branch block. *Prog Cardiovasc Dis* 1984;**26**:333.

Pacemaker Study Group: Optimal resources for implantable cardiac pacemakers. *Circulation* 1983;**68**:227A.

Reid JM, Coleman EN, Doig W: Complete congenital heart block: Report of 35 cases. *Br Heart J* 1982;**48**:236.

Scheinman MM et al: Value of the H–Q interval in patients with bundle branch block and the role of prophylactic permanent pacing. *Am J Cardiol* 1982;**50**:1316.

See also references for Paroxysmal Ventricular Tachycardia, p 238.

IDIOPATHIC LONG QT SYNDROME

Idiopathic long QT syndrome is an uncommon disease that was first described in deaf siblings, although deafness is not essential to the disease. The syndrome is characterized by recurrent syncope, a long QT interval (usually 0.5–0.7 s), documented ventricular arrhythmias, and sudden and unexpected death. Patients with the disease demonstrate neural degeneration of the conduction system. Acquired prolongation of the QT interval secondary to use of antiarrhythmic agents or antidepressant drugs, electrolyte abnormalities, myocardial ischemia, or significant bradycardia may result in ventricular tachycardia. The role of a prolonged QT interval is difficult to evaluate, because antiarrhythmic agents such as quinidine, encainide, and others increase the QT interval and yet are effective in treating the ventricular tachyarrhythmias. The importance of acquired QT interval prolongation requires further study.

Recent research emphasizes the role that the sympathetic nervous system (especially the left stelloid ganglion) plays in the pathogenesis of the syndrome. Acute arrhythmic episodes are treated by local anesthetic block of the left stelloid ganglion, and recurrent episodes are treated by resection of this ganglion as well as of the first 3 or 4 thoracic ganglia. Before resection of the left stelloid ganglion is considered, patients should be treated with propranolol or other beta-adrenergic blocking drugs or with phenytoin, which has proved beneficial in some patients.

Milne JR et al: The long QT syndrome: Effects of drugs and left stellate ganglion block. *Am Heart J* 1982;**104(2–Part 1)**:194.

Moss AJ, Schwartz PJ: Delayed repolarization (QT or QTU prolongation) and malignant ventricular arrhythmias. *Mod Concepts Cardiovasc Dis* 1982;**51**:85.

Pryor R: The long Q–T syndrome. *Primary Cardiol* (Feb) 1981; **7**:52.

VENTRICULAR PREEXCITATION
(Wolff-Parkinson-White Syndrome; Accelerated Conduction Syndrome)

Preexcitation occurs in 2 major forms: the Lown-Ganong-Levine syndrome and the more common Wolff-Parkinson-White syndrome. In the Lown-Ganong-Levine syndrome (partial atrioventricular nodal bypass), the upper part of the atrioventricular node is bypassed by the James accessory tract. The impulse that spreads through the atria reaches the lower part of the atrioventricular node by the posterior intra-atrial tract and the James fibers and excites the ventricles prematurely. Atrial arrhythmias occur in this syndrome as they do in the Wolff-Parkinson-White syndrome, in which the cardiac impulse is initiated in the normal way in the sinus node but then short-circuits the atrioventricular node in an anomalous fashion, usually via the bundle of Kent, but also by the Mahaim fibers, which spread from the bundle of His to the ventricular septum.

Preexcitation of the Wolff-Parkinson-White variety has been characterized into different types depending upon the location of the accessory bypass tracks, but this classification is incomplete, and there are subclassifications more complex than the conventional types A and B. Type A is from a left accessory bypass, producing an electrocardiographic pattern in V_1 of right ventricular hypertrophy or right bundle branch block; type B preexcitation results from early activation via a right lateral accessory pathway, producing an electrocardiographic pattern similar to that of left bundle branch block. In addition to the characteristic electrocardiographic changes (see below), Wolff-Parkinson-White syndrome is associated with frequent atrial paroxysmal arrhythmias, usually atrial tachycardia but occasionally atrial flutter or fibrillation. The mechanism of the atrial arrhythmia is thought to be reentry in which impulses from the atria pass through the normal atrioventricular conduction system to the ventricle and then return in retrograde fashion to the atria via the anomalous pathway. When the atria, the atrioventricular junction, or the atrioventricular node is no longer refractory, the retrograde impulse may reexcite portions of the specialized normal atrioventricular pathway that conducts to the ventricles and so set up a self-perpetuating circuit. Recent electrophysiologic studies have shown that the circuit is antegrade through the normal atrioventricular pathway and retrograde

through the anomalous pathway because the refractory period of the latter is shorter, but the circuit may be in reverse fashion.

Determination of the refractory period of the accessory pathway and of the atrioventricular node is desirable in patients with Wolff-Parkinson-White syndrome with atrial arrhythmias, especially if atrial fibrillation or flutter is the mechanism of the atrial arrhythmia. In the latter instance, any drug that decreases the refractory period of the accessory pathway is dangerous and may lead to ventricular tachycardia or fibrillation. A substantial number of patients with paroxysmal supraventricular tachycardia may have a concealed accessory retrograde conduction pathway that is revealed only by electrophysiologic studies. Antegrade conduction is normal.

Clinical Findings

The diagnosis is usually made electrocardiographically, even in patients who do not have a history of paroxysmal arrhythmia. During the arrhythmia it may be difficult to see the characteristic pattern, especially if there is a rapid atrial rate. The typical findings include a short PR interval, a wide QRS complex, and a slurred delta wave at the onset of the QRS, representing the bypass through the accessory pathway. The total PR plus the QRS interval is essentially normal; it has been called "falsely long" bundle branch block. The delta wave is usually short—about 0.05 s—and the PR interval in some cases may be essentially normal. Rarely, the delta wave may be negative, especially in leads II, III, and aVF, and may simulate inferior myocardial infarction. Negative delta waves occur elsewhere, and careful scrutiny of the cardiogram usually demonstrates a positive slurred delta wave elsewhere in the ECG. About half of patients have no symptoms, while the other half have episodes of paroxysmal atrial arrhythmia that may only be noted by 12- to 24-hour Holter monitoring. The arrhythmia may be the precipitating symptom in many patients, may last a few seconds and produce trivial or no symptoms, or may last hours and be disabling. It was formerly thought that death was rare during an attack of arrhythmia; this opinion has changed, possibly because of the very rapid ventricular rates that may occur if the patient has atrial fibrillation and the refractory period of the anomalous pathway is decreased by drugs such as digitalis.

One way of estimating the likelihood that ventricular fibrillation will develop after digitalis therapy is to determine the RR cycle interval (the ventricular rate) during spontaneous atrial fibrillation. When this interval is 220 ms or less (a rapid ventricular rate) during spontaneous atrial fibrillation, a short refractory period of the accessory pathway is probably present, and the hazard of ventricular fibrillation following the administration of digitalis is substantial.

If there is any question that paroxysmal tachycardia is in fact paroxysmal atrial fibrillation, electrophysiologic studies should be performed and atrial fibrillation induced to determine the refractory period of the accessory pathway, to determine the RR interval, and to test the effect on the refractory period of the accessory pathway of various antiarrhythmic agents that might be used clinically (see below under Treatment).

In the Lown-Ganong-Levine syndrome, the characteristic findings are a short PR interval (less than 0.11 s in adults) but a normal QRS complex and no delta wave. The ECG may appear normal except for the short PR interval. As indicated previously, these patients may have paroxysmal atrial arrhythmias.

Treatment

Asymptomatic patients in whom the condition is discovered by chance during a routine ECG should be alerted to the possibility of the development of atrial arrhythmias, especially if the arrhythmia is atrial fibrillation, for which digitalis should not be used because it increases the block in the atrioventricular node while decreasing the refractory period of the anomalous pathway. The rapid atrial impulses may then be transmitted directly to the ventricle, and rapid ventricular rates or even ventricular fibrillation may ensue. During acute atrial arrhythmias—especially atrial fibrillation—DC cardioversion is the procedure of choice.

Patients who have episodes of paroxysmal atrial arrhythmias require a different approach; it is wise to determine electrophysiologically the refractory period of both the normal and the anomalous pathways to the ventricle so as to select drugs that do not decrease the refractory period of the anomalous pathway. Newer studies using His bundle recording and induced premature beats make this possible. Most cases of paroxysmal atrial tachycardia can be treated in the usual fashion by interrupting the reentry circuit by increasing the block in the atrioventricular node through maneuvers such as carotid sinus massage, drugs that stimulate the vagus, or digitalis if the rhythm is paroxysmal atrial tachycardia and not atrial fibrillation or flutter (see Paroxysmal Atrial Tachycardia, p 231). Drugs that increase the block or prolong the refractory period in the anomalous pathway may be helpful; of these, procainamide, quinidine, disopyramide, and amiodarone are the most effective. Beta-blocking drugs and verapamil are less desirable because they increase the block in the atrioventricular node without appreciably affecting the refractory period of the accessory pathway, thereby decreasing the refractory period of the accessory pathway relative to that of the normal pathway and sometimes increasing the ventricular rate in atrial fibrillation. Atrial pacing has been used because a random beat might by chance excite a portion of the reentrant pathway, making it refractory to the oncoming circus wave; there is a risk that atrial pacing may increase the impulses to the ventricles via the anomalous pathway and so raise the ventricular rate. DC shock (cardioversion) or procainamide or propranolol intravenously should be considered in emergency situations or in atrial fibrillation. If the attacks of atrial arrhythmia are frequent and difficult to control, surgical treatment (see below) or efforts to prevent the arrhythmia are indicated and constitute some of the recent developments in the field.

Prevention of Atrial Arrhythmias

Drugs that prevent the reentry phenomena by slowing conduction or increasing the refractory period of the atrioventricular node may all be helpful, as in paroxysmal atrial tachycardia in the absence of Wolff-Parkinson-White syndrome. Quinidine, propranolol, procainamide, disopyramide, encainide, and amiodarone are valuable. Drugs used in combination may sometimes be effective when one used singly is not. Side effects from one may prevent it from being used to maximum effect, such as when bradycardia complicates the use of propranolol. A ventricular pacemaker with a radio-frequency transmitter may be inserted and may be activated externally by a radio-frequency signal in the hope that a chance premature beat may interrupt the reentry cycle.

Surgical resection or cryoablation of the anomalous pathway is being performed with increasing frequency in a few specialized centers; the procedure is preceded by electrophysiologic studies and endocardial and epicardial mapping to determine the area of earliest ventricular excitation. When the anomalous pathway is clearly mapped, resection or cryoablation may interrupt the pathway and prevent both the delta wave and the subsequent arrhythmias.

Benson DW Jr et al: Localization of the site of ventricular preexcitation with body surface maps in patients with Wolff-Parkinson-White syndrome. *Circulation* 1982;**65**:1259.

Morady F et al: Electrophysiologic testing in the management of patients with the Wolff-Parkinson-White syndrome and atrial fibrillation. *Am J Cardiol* 1983;**51**:1623.

Prystowsky EN et al: Clinical efficacy and electrophysiologic effects of encainide in patients with Wolff-Parkinson-White syndrome. *Circulation* 1984;**69**:278.

Wellens HJJ: Wolff-Parkinson-White syndrome. 1. Diagnosis, arrhythmias, and identification of the high risk patient. 2. Treatment. *Mod Concepts Cardiovasc Dis* 1983;**52**:53, 57.

CARDIAC FAILURE

Essentials of Diagnosis

Left ventricular failure:
- Exertional dyspnea, cough, fatigue, orthopnea, paroxysmal nocturnal dyspnea, cardiac enlargement, rales, gallop rhythm, and pulmonary venous congestion.

Right ventricular failure:
- Elevated venous pressure, hepatomegaly, dependent edema.

Both:
- Combination of above.

General Considerations

The function of the heart is to pump an adequate volume of blood (which it receives from the veins) to the various tissues of the body as required by their metabolic needs. Left ventricular performance is a function of preload, afterload, contractility, and heart rate. Various compensatory mechanisms such as increased sympathetic activity resulting in raised systemic vascular resistance, increased contractility, and salt and water retention due to activation of the renin-angiotensin-aldosterone system (see below) are brought into play when the heart is diseased, when the work load is increased, or when the tissue demands are enhanced. When these compensatory methods fail or are inappropriate, a clinical syndrome develops which may only be obvious when the demands on the heart are increased, as with exercise or emotion, but which may be absent at rest. Heart failure may be present, therefore, when the cardiac output is elevated, normal, or decreased with respect to the average; but regardless of the absolute level, the cardiac output in cardiac failure is reduced relative to the metabolic demands of the body, assuming an adequate venous return. Markedly reduced venous return (as in hemorrhage) constitutes peripheral vascular failure, not cardiac failure. In thyrotoxicosis with heart failure, the cardiac output may be greater than usual and yet insufficient for the increased metabolic needs occasioned by the increased secretion of thyroxine.

The left or right ventricle alone may fail initially—usually the former—but ultimately, especially after salt and water retention occurs (see below), combined failure is the rule.

Left ventricular failure is most commonly due to cardiomyopathy, hypertension, coronary heart disease, or valvular heart disease, usually aortic valvular disease. Less commonly, mitral valvular disease, hypertrophic cardiomyopathy, left-to-right shunts, congenital heart lesions, and drugs are responsible. Infective endocarditis may occur de novo or may complicate other valvular diseases and aggravate left ventricular failure. Cardiac failure may also occur in various connective tissue disorders, thyrotoxicosis, severe anemia, arteriovenous fistulas, myocarditis, beriberi, and myocardial involvement by tumors or granulomas.

Right ventricular failure is most commonly due to mitral stenosis with raised pulmonary vascular resistance, pulmonary parenchymal or vascular disease (the latter may be primary or secondary to ventricular or atrial septal defects or patent ductus arteriosus), pulmonary valvular stenosis, right ventricular infarction (in association with inferior myocardial infarction), or, less commonly, tricuspid valvular disease or infective endocarditis involving the right side of the heart. Carcinoid involving the pulmonary valve or tricuspid valve is a rare cause.

In at least half of cases, demonstrable precipitating diseases or factors that increase the work load of the heart may be present, and these factors should be sought in every patient with cardiac failure. They include omission of therapy, arrhythmias, respiratory infection, myocardial infarction, pulmonary embolism, rheumatic carditis, thyrotoxicosis, anemia, excessive salt intake, corticosteroid administration, pregnancy, and excessive or rapid administration of parenteral fluids.

Etiology

The basic causes of ventricular failure are as follows:

A. Myocardial Weakness or Inflammation: Coronary artery disease, myocarditis, congestive cardiomyopathies, and drugs.

B. Excess Work Load:

1. Increased resistance to ejection–Hypertension, stenosis of aortic or pulmonary valves, hypertrophic cardiomyopathy.

2. Increased stroke volume–Aortic insufficiency, mitral insufficiency, tricuspid insufficiency, congenital left-to-right shunts.

3. Increased body demands–Thyrotoxicosis, anemia, pregnancy, arteriovenous fistula.

Hemodynamics & Pathophysiology

The compensatory mechanisms by which the heart responds to an increased load include the following: (1) concentric hypertrophy, which provides larger contractile cells; (2) increased fiber length or dilatation, which increases the force of contraction in accordance with the Frank-Starling law; and (3) increased sympathetic nervous system activity, which increases the force of contraction at any fiber length without increasing the filling pressure.

Concentric hypertrophy is most apt to occur when the load placed on the heart is due to increased resistance to ejection with increased impedance, characteristically seen in aortic stenosis and hypertension. The increased thickness of the left ventricle decreases its distensibility, or compliance, so that the left ventricular end-diastolic pressure is raised with a normal left ventricular volume; the raised filling pressure is required to augment left ventricular output according to the Starling principle. Left ventricular systolic function becomes impaired with increased end-systolic volume. Later, left ventricular volume increases (because cardiac hypertrophy alone is insufficient to compensate), the left ventricular end-diastolic pressure rises even further, and left ventricular failure occurs.

When the increased cardiac load is due to increased stroke volume, typically represented by aortic insufficiency, the increased stretch increases fiber length and so increases the force of left ventricular contraction according to the Frank-Starling principle. As the stretch increases, left ventricular volume increases, as can be demonstrated by the enlargement of the heart seen on the plain film of the chest, by echocardiography, or by left ventricular angiography. In these circumstances, distensibility is not decreased, and it is common to find an increased left ventricular volume with a normal or increased cardiac output and left ventricular filling pressure. When left ventricular performance falls in the latter stages of this type of lesion (as well as in the various types of secondary cardiomyopathies, known as congestive cardiomyopathy), the ejection fraction (the difference between left ventricular diastolic and systolic volume) becomes decreased from its normal value of 60–70% as left ventricular failure occurs and may be as low as 10–20% in very severe failure. Patients tolerate increased volume load better than increased resistance load.

Increased sympathetic stimulation can be demonstrated in patients with cardiac failure by increased concentration of catecholamines in the blood and urine and by depletion of norepinephrine in cardiac tissue; cardiac contractility is thus improved. Beta-adrenergic blocking drugs such as propranolol, by decreasing the sympathetic drive to the heart, may worsen or precipitate left ventricular failure.

Early in the course of various cardiac diseases, the compensatory mechanisms are adequate to maintain a normal cardiac output and normal intracardiac pressures at rest and after exercise. Hypertrophy can be recognized on the ECG, echocardiogram, or plain chest film. This stage of compensated heart disease becomes "decompensated" as volumes and filling pressures of the respective ventricles increase. As the filling pressure increases, pulmonary venous congestion occurs as the raised left atrial pressure is transmitted backward. This leads to interstitial and then alveolar edema of the lungs, resulting in a continuum of symptoms of left ventricular failure. Cardiac output may be normal at this phase—especially at rest—but may be decreased on exercise; as the cardiac output on exercise diminishes, tachycardia occurs and thus increases the minute cardiac output when the stroke volume cannot increase adequately. The atrioventricular oxygen difference widens so that the tissues can extract more oxygen to compensate for the decreased cardiac output. When the ventricular filling pressure is increased—especially when compliance is decreased—atrial hypertrophy increases the force of atrial systole and so aids filling; the loss of this so-called atrial kick can be devastating when atrial fibrillation occurs.

Apart from the changes in pressure, volume, compliance, and contractility just described, secondary retention of salt and water due to increased aldosterone secretion secondary to enhanced sympathetic activity is responsible for many of the symptoms and signs of cardiac failure. The increased sodium and water retention leads to an increase in blood volume, which, by raising the hydrostatic pressure in the capillaries, leads first to interstitial edema and then to transudation of fluid into tissues that have decreased tissue pressure, such as the subcutaneous tissues. As a result, edema of the ankles and lower extremities occurs when the patient is ambulatory and edema of the sacral area when the patient is recumbent. Symptoms such as dyspnea and edema are aggravated by salt and water retention and are reversed by the use of diuretics and low-sodium diets.

The precise point at which "cardiac failure" occurs in the course of cardiac disease is difficult to determine, although in the overt stage cardiac failure is quite obvious.

Clinical Findings

These vary depending on the nature of the cardiac failure (acute or chronic), the location of the increased load (on the left ventricle, right ventricle, or both), and the cause.

A. Symptoms and Signs:

1. Left ventricular failure–Left ventricular failure is characterized predominantly by symptoms: exertional dyspnea, cough, fatigue, weakness, and nocturia. **Exertional dyspnea,** which is caused by pulmonary venous engorgement and increased stiffness of the lungs, resembles the normal ventilatory response to exercise but is associated with increased awareness of breathlessness and difficulty in breathing. In heart failure, the patient regularly becomes short of breath during an amount of exertion that previously caused no difficulty. As the pulmonary engorgement progresses, less and less activity brings on dyspnea until it is present even when the patient is at rest (rest dyspnea). **Orthopnea,** or shortness of breath occurring in recumbency that is promptly relieved by propping up the head or trunk, is precipitated by the further increase in pulmonary engorgement on recumbency. **Paroxysmal nocturnal dyspnea** or **cough** may appear at any time and is often the first indication of left ventricular failure caused by severe hypertension, aortic stenosis or insufficiency, or myocardial infarction. Paroxysmal nocturnal dyspnea also occurs in patients with tight mitral stenosis in advanced stages. It is an exaggerated form of orthopnea, the patient awakening from sleep gasping for breath and compelled to sit or stand up for relief. Cough is frequently present. With bronchospasm, patients may have inspiratory and expiratory wheezing (so-called cardiac asthma). The paroxysmal cough and dyspnea may pass in a few minutes to several hours or may progress to acute pulmonary edema. Patients become pale or frankly cyanotic, sweat profusely, and complain of great air hunger. Cough productive of frothy white or pink sputum is characteristic. The attack may subside in 1 to several hours, or the left ventricle may progressively weaken, leading to shock and death.

These forms of dyspnea must be distinguished from those occurring in many other conditions. Advanced age, debility, poor physical condition, obesity, chronic pulmonary disease, and severe anemia commonly produce exertional dyspnea. Extreme obesity (Pickwickian syndrome), ascites from any cause, abdominal distention from gastrointestinal disease, or advanced stages of pregnancy may produce orthopnea in the absence of preexisting heart disease. Bronchial asthma appearing in middle life may be symptomatically difficult to distinguish from the paroxysmal nocturnal dyspnea of left ventricular failure. Patients with neurocirculatory asthenia or anxiety states with psychophysiologic cardiovascular reactions may suffer from sighing respirations simulating dyspnea.

Exertional fatigue and weakness due to reduced cardiac output are late symptoms and disappear promptly on resting. Severe fatigue, rather than dyspnea, is the chief complaint of patients with mitral stenosis who have developed pulmonary hypertension and low cardiac output.

Nocturia occurs as a result of the excretion of edema fluid accumulated during the day and the increased renal perfusion in the recumbent position; it reflects the decreased work of the heart at rest and often the effects of diuretics given during the day.

Signs of left ventricular failure are seen on examination, which should disclose the following: (1) the basic cause of the left ventricular failure (hypertension, aortic or mitral valve disease, myocardial infarction); (2) left ventricular hypertrophy, in which the apical impulse is forceful or heaving and displaced to the left and downward, confirmed by electrocardiography, echocardiography, and chest x-ray; and (3) radiologic evidence of pulmonary venous distention such as redistribution of blood to the upper lobes, Kerley B lines, or, in acute left ventricular failure, butterfly pattern hilar congestion. Hydrothorax may be present.

The following may or may not be present and are not necessary for diagnosis: basilar parenchymal rales that do not clear on coughing, gallop rhythm, pulsus alternans, and an accentuated pulmonary component of the second sound (P$_2$). The chest x-ray may reveal pulmonary venous congestion and left atrial enlargement in the case of mitral stenosis and shows unquestioned left ventricular enlargement in the usual case, except with acute myocardial infarction or cardiac arrhythmia. The symptoms and signs of left ventricular failure may not correlate with noninvasive and invasive tests of left ventricular performance, perhaps because prolonged raised left ventricular filling pressure may cause increased pulmonary interstitial pressure (which counteracts hydrostatic pressure), and patients therefore may not develop alveolar fluid accumulation and dyspnea. Exercise tolerance may be better than that expected from the degree of left ventricular dysfunction inferred from the decreased ejection fraction.

2. Right ventricular failure–Right ventricular failure is characterized predominantly by signs. **Anorexia, bloating,** or **exertional right upper abdominal pains** are common, reflecting hepatic and visceral engorgement secondary to elevated venous pressure. **Oliguria** is present in the daytime; **polyuria** at night. Weakness and mental aberration are present in severe cases.

The jugular venous pressure is raised and has an abnormal systolic pulsation; the pressure can be estimated by noting the extent of jugular filling (during normal expiration) above the level of the clavicles when the patient's torso is propped up to make a 30-degree angle with the bed. A simple water manometer allows serial determinations of the peripheral venous pressure at the bedside (zero level junction of lower and middle thirds of the anteroposterior diameter of the chest is a commonly used reference point). Normal pressure is 6–10 cm of water.

Right ventricular hypertrophy is demonstrated by a lower sternal or left parasternal palpable systolic heave independent of the apical impulse. The liver is enlarged, tender, and pulsating. Ascites is rarely prominent; when it appears early and in massive amounts, cardiac tamponade, constrictive pericarditis, or tricuspid stenosis should be considered. Dependent edema caused by heart failure usually subsides overnight initially but eventually persists and increases in extent. Pleural effusion is more common on the right side. Coolness of the extremities and peripheral cyanosis of the nail beds are due to reduced peripheral blood flow. Sinus tachycardia is present. A right ventricular S$_3$ may be present.

The electrocardiographic and echocardiographic findings indicate pure right ventricular hypertrophy in pure right-sided failure and, usually, evidence of left ventricular hypertrophy or coronary artery disease when left-sided failure is also present and is predominant.

Right atrial and ventricular enlargement is noted on the chest film in pure right heart failure, but specific chamber enlargement is difficult to define when right heart failure is secondary to left heart failure.

Echocardiography may provide an indirect means of assessing impaired left ventricular function prior to the development of cardiac failure. Left ventricular cineangiograms or nuclide scans quantitate the left ventricular contraction and ejection fraction.

B. Laboratory Findings: Red and white cell counts, hemoglobin, packed cell volume, and sedimentation rate are normal in uncomplicated left heart failure. Polycythemia and right-to-left shunt may occur in chronic cor pulmonale. Urinalysis often discloses significant proteinuria and granular casts. The blood urea nitrogen may be elevated because of reduced renal blood flow, but the urine specific gravity is high in the absence of primary renal disease. The serum sodium, potassium, CO$_2$, and chloride are within normal limits in ordinary congestive heart failure before diuretics are used. Serum norepinephrine and plasma renin levels are usually increased in advanced cardiac failure; plasma renin levels may also be raised because of diuretic therapy.

C. Echocardiography: Echocardiography may reveal separation of the septum from the E point of the mitral valve. It can also be used to demonstrate left ventricular mass and volume and ejection fraction.

D. Nuclear Scans: Electrocardiography-gated (synchronized) nucleotide angiography may quantify ventricular dimensions, segmental abnormalities of contraction, and (regional and global) ejection fraction and thus contribute to the understanding of left ventricular function.

Echocardiography and nuclear scans help to exclude the presence of aortic and mitral stenosis, cardiac tumors, pericardial effusion, left ventricular aneurysm, ventricular septal defect, and vegetations from infective endocarditis.

Differential Diagnosis

Congestive heart failure must be differentiated from cardiac tumors, pericardial effusion, constrictive pericarditis, pulmonary venous congestion due to mitral stenosis, neurocirculatory asthenia, acute and chronic pulmonary disease, bronchial asthma, cirrhosis, carcinoma of the lung, nephrosis or nephritis, mediastinal tumor, repeated pulmonary emboli, obstruction of the vena cava, anemia, and idiopathic "edema"; the last has been attributed to rebound salt and water retention following the use of diuretics and should be considered in patients who present with edema, fatigue, and rapid weight gain.

Consideration of the history, together with physical findings of organic cardiovascular disease, enlarged heart with ventricular heaves, character of the arterial pulse, gallop rhythm, pulsus alternans, and elevated venous pressure and increased systolic pulsations of the jugular veins in the absence of collateral venous circulation, differentiates congestive heart failure from these conditions.

Treatment

The objectives of treatment are to remove the cause, increase the force and efficiency of myocardial contraction, and reduce the abnormal retention of sodium and water. The patient shares a large responsibility in the management of the disease because treatment is long-term and involves restrictions in diet and activity and the reliable use of cardiac drugs.

Potentially curable causes of congestive heart failure must be specifically considered: valvular heart disease, constrictive pericarditis, congenital heart lesions, infective endocarditis, ruptured chordae tendineae, thyrotoxicosis, myxedema heart, peripheral arteriovenous fistula, beriberi, and recurrent arrhythmias.

Specific search should be made for reversible noncardiac causes of failure originating outside the heart, eg, thyrotoxicosis, anemia, myxedema, nutritional disturbances (especially vitamin B deficiency), arteriovenous fistulas, polycythemia vera, and Paget's disease.

Determine, treat, and eliminate, if possible, the factor precipitating the cardiac failure, eg, infection (especially respiratory); pulmonary infarction; overexertion; increased sodium intake; discontinuation of medication; the onset of arrhythmia, particularly with rapid ventricular rates (eg, atrial fibrillation); myocardial infarction; and anemia.

A. Rest: Rest in bed or sitting in a chair decreases the work of the heart and promotes sodium diuresis. Morphine- or barbiturate-induced sleep comes as a welcome relief to a patient who has spent many sleepless, dyspneic nights with the disease. Adequate rest should be maintained until compensation has occurred and then should be replaced by progressive ambulation. Most patients can use a bedside toilet with no more effort than is required for a bedpan.

Rest should be continued as long as necessary to permit the heart to regain reserve strength but should not be so prolonged as to cause generalized debility of the patient.

Patients are usually more comfortable in a cool room.

Cardiac patients at bed rest are prone to develop phlebitis. They should be given passive or active leg exercises and an elastic stocking to prevent phlebothrombosis.

B. Diet: At the onset of therapy, give frequent (4–6) small, bland, low-calorie, low-residue meals with vitamin supplements. The degree of sodium restriction depends upon the severity of the failure and the ease with which it can be controlled by other means. Even with the use of diuretics, unlimited sodium intake is unwise. Evaluation of the previous intake of sodium will provide a baseline upon which to gauge the degree of restriction required. The use of sodium-containing substances other than salt in the diet should be curtailed, and the patient should be warned regarding the use of bicarbonate of soda, Alka-Seltzer, or water softeners, all of which increase the sodium intake. Before drastic sodium restriction is instituted, the renal function should be evaluated to determine if the kidneys can conserve sodium. Because cardiac failure is a long-term illness, dietary and other restrictions should be modified according to the habits and preferences of the patient. The availability of potent oral diuretics usually allows the patient to have at least a 2-g sodium diet, which usually means no added salt at the table and avoidance of highly salted foods such as ham, bacon, and potato chips. It is often helpful early in the course of treatment to see whether cardiac failure can be treated by rest and sodium restriction alone so as to avoid the side effects of diuretic therapy. Most patients, however, find a low-sodium diet difficult to maintain, and total reliance on a strict low-sodium intake is usually inadvisable. Vitamin supplements may be indicated. Restricted diets and anorexia may lead to malnutrition and avitaminosis, with a superimposed beriberi type of failure.

C. Digitalis: (See pp 226 and 250.)

D. Removal of Sodium and Water:

1. Thiazide diuretics–(See also p 206.) Sodium diuresis is most conveniently accomplished by the use of an orally active agent such as chlorothiazide or any of its analogs. The diuretics can be given daily or, preferably, intermittently depending on the need. Some authorities prefer diuretics to digitalis when salt and water retention is excessive, but the primary problem concerns the heart. Patients may require both a diuretic and digitalis. Dietary or supplementary potassium must be adequate to prevent potassium depletion and digitalis toxicity.

2. Furosemide (Lasix), 40–80 mg orally; **ethacrynic acid (Edecrin),** 25–100 mg orally; and **bumetanide (Bumex),** 0.5–2 mg once daily orally, are potent diuretics with a short duration of action. They cause nausea and diarrhea more often than the thiazides, especially with regular dosage. The considerable diuresis may cause hypokalemia and a significant fall in glomerular filtration rate, and these drugs must therefore be used with considerable caution. The rapid onset of action (within 30 minutes) makes them valuable on occasion for treatment of acute pulmonary edema, but their potency increases the hazards, and the thiazides are probably preferable for the average patient with congestive failure unless there is associated renal failure. They are effective even in the presence of low glomerular filtration rates or in disturbances in acid-base balance or electrolyte metabolism.

3. Aldosterone antagonists and other potassium-conserving drugs –Spironolactone antagonizes aldosterone, the adrenal steroid that controls renal tubular reabsorption of sodium, thereby causing sodium diuresis without potassium loss, and can be combined with a thiazide to neutralize the potassium-wasting effect of thiazides. The onset of clinical effect may be delayed for 1 week. Response is variable but may be striking. The initial dosage is 25 mg 4 times daily. Drowsiness, hyperkalemia, hypovolemia, hypotension, and breast tenderness may occur. Similar potassium sparing may occur with either triamterene or amiloride, which inhibit potassium secretion in the distal portion of the distal tubule. Triamterene or amiloride may be used in combination with thiazides, ethacrynic acid, or furosemide (see below). *Caution:* Check serum potassium, avoid potassium supplements, and use with particular care in the presence of impaired renal function.

4. Mercurial diuretics –The mercurial diuretics are slightly more potent than the thiazide diuretics but are infrequently used today because they must be given parenterally. Mercurials in doses of 0.1–1 mL reveal their effect in about 2 hours and last 10–12 hours.

E. Oxygen Therapy: Useful when respiratory distress with hypoxemia is present.

F. Vasodilators: (See also p 225.) These drugs may either have a predominant effect on the arterial or venous system or an equal effect on both. Drugs that decrease preload by dilating the venous vessels are particularly valuable when patients have severe dyspnea and a high wedge pressure but normal or near-normal cardiac output and arterial pressure. Intravenous nitroglycerin, for example, may be valuable under these circumstances. When patients have only slightly raised left ventricular filling pressure but decreased cardiac output, drugs that dilate the arterial system are preferred (hydralazine, captopril, or nifedipine). When both preload and afterload are increased with raised wedge pressure and reduced cardiac output, drugs that affect both systems such as sodium nitroprusside or prazosin are preferred. Intravenous nitroglycerin is given by controlled infusion at a rate of 10 μg/min, gradually increasing every 10 minutes until a satisfactory fall in wedge pressure is obtained. (See below for use of sodium nitroprusside.) Hemodynamic studies in coronary care units showed that patients with left ventricular failure and cardiogenic shock who have low cardiac output and a high left ventricular filling pressure (LVFP) (more than 20 mm Hg) often improve when impedance to left ventricular output (afterload) is reduced by vasodilator therapy. Vasodilator therapy was then used to *decrease afterload* in patients with other types of severe chronic cardiac failure (especially left ventricular failure) who did not respond adequately to the usual

therapy discussed above. The results of sodium nitroprusside treatment are often impressive. There is a prompt reduction in left ventricular filling pressure and an increase in cardiac output; the heart rate is slowed; and there may be a marked increase in the ejection fraction and stroke volume. Diuresis and clinical improvement accompany the hemodynamic changes. Sodium nitroprusside (Nipride) is begun at a rate of 5–15 μg/min and the drip is increased by 5 μg/min at intervals of 3–5 minutes to be certain that the arterial pressure remains above 95–100 mm Hg. Other intravenous agents besides nitrates can be used —eg, alpha-adrenergic blocking agents such as phentolamine (Regitine) can be infused intravenously at a rate of 10–40 mg/kg/min. Intravenous vasodilator therapy should be used only when patients can be monitored closely (as in the coronary care unit), when hypotension can be avoided, and when serum thiocyanate levels can be monitored (if nitroprusside is infused over a period of days) to avoid toxicity. Once clinical improvement has occurred following the intravenous infusions, it is possible to maintain improvement with oral vasodilator agents. Oral hydralazine, 75 mg, which decreases afterload and systemic vascular resistance, alone or in combination with nitrates such as isosorbide dinitrate (Isordil), 10–20 mg orally 3–4 times a day, which decreases the venous return and reduces the filling pressure of the left ventricle **(preload reduction),** have proved helpful, but the beneficial effects often decrease over a period of months. The combination of nitrates and hydralazine is more effective than either alone. The effect can be enhanced with the use of transdermal nitroglycerin in a 5-mg patch, which provides nitrate absorption over a 24-hour period.

Other vasodilators such as captopril (see below), prazosin, minoxidil, verapamil, diltiazem, or nifedipine have also been used with at least temporary good results. The long-term benefits are controversial, because of the high 1- and 2-year mortality rates in patients receiving vasodilators. Care must be exercised with minoxidil because of its sodium- and water-retaining properties. As little as 2.5 mg twice a day may result in massive pleural and pericardial fluid and peripheral edema in 1 week. Potent diuretics must be used whenever minoxidil is prescribed. The magnitude of the salt and water retention varies in different patients, and some patients with cardiac failure have received as much as 20 mg without this untoward effect.

These drugs produce arterial or venous dilatation (or both) by different mechanisms, such as direct action on vascular muscle, inhibition of postsynaptic alpha-adrenergic receptors, inhibition of the conversion of angiotensin I to angiotensin II, and other mechanisms. The appropriate drug can be selected depending on whether one wishes to decrease preload or afterload or both.

Intravenous vasodilators with nitroprusside or nitroglycerin can be combined with inotropic agents (see below) in appropriate amounts in order to achieve the greatest hemodynamic benefit without inducing significant hypotension. If nitroprusside is continued for more than a few days, thiocyanide levels should be monitored. Calcium entry-blocking agents are valuable adjuncts, but caution should be exercised, particularly with verapamil, because its negative inotropic action may worsen cardiac failure. Nifedipine does not have this side effect and is preferred in cardiac failure. Newer vasodilators have been undergoing preliminary trials; their ultimate place has not been determined.

G. Sympathetic and Other Inotropic Agents: Isoproterenol, beta-adrenergic agonists, dopamine, and dobutamine may have a place in therapy if digitalis is contraindicated, especially in the postoperative period after open heart surgery or following acute myocardial infarction.

A synthetic positive inotropic drug, amrinone, has been reported to be effective when used intravenously in the treatment of chronic cardiac failure unresponsive to diuretics and digitalis; it has also been shown to be a vasodilator. There have been reports of thrombocytopenia, but the frequency of this toxic effect is not known, and further data are required. Analogs of amrinone (eg, milrinone) show promise, because their effects are longer-lasting, they appear to be more potent, and thrombocytopenia has not been a problem. Further data are required.

H. Inhibitors of the Renin-Angiotensin System: The oral converting enzyme inhibitor captopril and its analog enalapril have been shown to be beneficial in patients with chronic cardiac failure. Following their use, vasodilation occurs, cardiac output rises, the right atrial and left ventricular filling pressures fall, and systemic vascular resistance decreases. Clinical use is increasing; benefits appear greater in patients whose control plasma renin activity is normal or high. Hypotension, hypersensitivity reactions, rash, proteinuria, and renal glomerular membrane changes have occurred following captopril administration, and the long-term safety remains to be determined. The beneficial effects produced by inhibitors of the system suggest that the renin-angiotensin system plays an important role in the compensatory rise in systemic vascular resistance that occurs in chronic cardiac failure.

I. Mechanical Measures: Paracentesis of fluid in the chest and abdomen should be undertaken if respiration is embarrassed. Since sodium retention may occur as a result of fluid collection in the chest, abdomen, and legs, diuresis may occur following the procedure. Phlebotomy (in low-output failure in the absence of anemia), rotating tourniquets, Southey tubes, and acupuncture may be beneficial if the more conventional forms of treatment fail or are not available. Southey tubes and acupuncture are especially valuable in severe right heart failure with obstinate dependent edema. Take care to avoid a severe low-sodium syndrome with hyperkalemia or hypokalemia.

J. Peritoneal Dialysis: Hypertonic peritoneal dialysis is an effective method reserved for patients with severe heart failure, dilutional hyponatremia, and renal failure. Some remissions have been dramatic,

and the method should be given a greater trial.

K. Observation During Treatment of Cardiac Failure: Record the following at every visit:
1. Status of original symptoms.
2. New symptoms or signs.
3. Morning weight or weight with same clothes.
4. Presence of the signs of congestive failure (venous engorgement and pulsations, pulmonary rales, pleural fluid, engorgement of the liver, presence of edema).
5. Examination of the heart and blood vessels (cardiac sounds, gallop rhythm, friction rub, cardiac rhythm and apical rate, cardiac size, peripheral arterial pulsations, and status of the veins).
6. Blood pressure and presence of pulsus alternans.
7. Evidence of phlebothrombosis.

Treatment With Digitalis (See also p 226.)

Digitalis increases the speed and force of cardiac contraction. Increased cardiac output, decreased cardiac volume and ventricular diastolic pressure, and a fall in right atrial and peripheral venous pressure frequently follow digitalization in patients with cardiac failure. The beneficial effect of decreasing conduction through the atrioventricular node and thus slowing the ventricular rate is more striking in patients with atrial fibrillation and a rapid ventricular rate. Cardiac failure associated with sinus rhythm may improve with digitalis, especially when the failure is severe and chronic. The drug may increase the left ventricular obstruction and should probably not be used in hypertrophic states such as hypertrophic cardiomyopathy and in right heart failure secondary to pulmonary disease (cor pulmonale). Digitalis is less effective in acute myocardial infarction with severe cardiac failure, when other more potent inotropic agents such as dopamine or dobutamine should be used. The glycosides available are qualitatively similar. They differ in speed of action, dosage, and rate of excretion. It is advisable to become familiar with a rapid intravenous and a rapid oral method of digitalization. Rapid digitalization is indicated in atrial flutter and fibrillation with fast ventricular rates and in acute pulmonary edema; otherwise, slow digitalization is preferred.

Caution must be exercised when quinidine is added to the regimens of patients receiving digitalis. Serum digoxin levels also rise when calcium entry-blocking drugs are given to patients receiving digitalis.

Digitalis produces characteristic changes in the ECG; the most typical of which are sagging of the ST segment and displacement of the T waves in a direction opposite to that of the main deflection. Later the PR interval may be prolonged. ST-T changes cannot be used as criteria of toxicity, for the effects appear before saturation occurs and persist for 2–3 weeks after digitalis has been stopped. However, ECGs are often of value in determining whether digitalis has been given in the previous 2–3 weeks and may give an idea of the amount.

A. Indications for Administration of Digitalis:

Table 8–5. Digitalis and digitalislike preparations.*†

Glycoside and Preparations Available	Adult Dose		Rapid Method of Administration	Speed; Maximum Action and Duration
	Digitalizing	Maintenance		
Parenteral preparations				
Ouabain, 1- and 2-mL ampules, 0.25 mg	0.25–0.5 mg	Not used for maintenance	0.25–0.5 mg (1–2 mL) diluted in 10 mL saline slowly IV; follow with another drug (see below).	½–1½ hours; duration, 2–4 days.
Deslanoside (Cedilanid-D), 2- and 4-mL ampules, 0.4 and 0.8 mg	8 mL (1.6 mg)	0.2–0.4 mg (1–2 mL)	1.2 mg (6 mL) IV or IM and follow with 0.2–0.4 mg (1–2 mL) IV or IM every 3–4 hours until effect is obtained.	1–2 hours; duration, 3–6 days.
Digitoxin (dilute before use), 1- and 2-mL ampules, 0.2 and 0.4 mg	1.2 mg (6 mL)	0.05–0.2 mg	0.6 mg (3 mL) IV or IM followed by 0.2–0.4 mg every 4–6 hours until 1.2 mg has been given.	3–8 hours; duration, 14–21 days.
Digoxin (Lanoxin), 2-mL ampules, 0.25 mg/mL	1.5 mg (6 mL)	0.25–0.75 mg (1–3 mL)	0.5–1 mg (2–4 mL) IV and 0.25–0.5 mg (1–2 mL) in 3–4 hours; then 0.25 mg (1 mL) every 3–4 hours until effect is obtained.	1–2 hours; duration, 3–6 days.
Oral preparations				
Digitalis, 0.03-, 0.06-, and 0.1-g tablets	1–1.5 g	0.05–0.2 g	0.6 g at once; 0.4 g in 6–8 hours; 0.2 g every 6 hours for 2–3 doses; then 0.1 g twice daily until effect is obtained.	6–8 hours; duration, 18–21 days.
Digitoxin, 0.1-, 0.15-, and 0.2-mg tablets	1.2 mg	0.05–0.2 mg	0.6 mg at once and repeat in 12 hours and then 0.2 mg twice daily until effect is obtained.	6–8 hours; duration, 14–21 days.
Digoxin, 0.25- and 0.5-mg tablets	1.5–3 mg	0.15–0.5 mg	1 mg at once, and then 0.25–0.5 mg every 6 hours. Total, 1.5–3 mg.	4–6 hours; duration, 2–6 days.
Deslanoside (Cedilanid-D), 0.5-mg tablets	7.5 mg	0.5–1.5 mg	2 mg at once, and then 0.5–0.75 mg every 6 hours until effect is obtained.	

*Check manufacturer's descriptive literature. Dosage sizes of tablets and ampules change from time to time.
†It must be recognized that the signs of digitalis toxicity may occur with any of the above drugs in doses below the averages or maximums stated.

(1) Cardiac failure (left, right, or combined) with sinus rhythm (controversial) or atrial fibrillation.

(2) Atrial fibrillation or flutter with a rapid ventricular rate.

(3) Supraventricular paroxysmal tachycardia.

(4) Prevention of paroxysmal atrial arrhythmias when quinidine has failed or cannot be tolerated, or in combination with quinidine.

B. Choice of Digitalis Preparation: (See Table 8–5.) All of the cardiac glycosides have similar pharmacologic properties, differing only in dose, absorption, speed of onset of action, and duration of action. With digitalis leaf and digitoxin there is a long latent period before maximal effect is achieved (half-life, 4–6 days), and the duration of effect is long. Digoxin (Lanoxin) and deslanoside (Cedilanid-D) have a much more rapid onset of action and briefer duration of effect (half-life, 36 hours). Ouabain exerts its effect within a few minutes, but it is infrequently used in the USA because other parenteral glycosides are available.

C. Routes of Administration of Digitalis:

1. Parenteral administration–

a. Emergency digitalization–(1) Acute pulmonary edema or other severe failure. Caution should be used in giving the full digitalizing dose in a single injection intravenously under these circumstances. The drug should be given slowly, in divided doses. (2) Treatment of atrial arrhythmias when the need for control of the ventricular rate is urgent.

b. Inability to take digitalis orally, eg, in nausea and vomiting due to any cause, in coma, and postoperatively.

2. Oral administration–Oral administration is used unless parenteral administration is indicated (Table 8–6).

D. Methods of Digitalization:

1. Untreated cases–(When the patient has received no digitalis in the preceding 2 weeks.)

a. Parenteral digitalization–*Caution:* Never administer a full digitalizing dose intravenously unless it is certain that no digitalis has been given in the

Table 8–6. Oral administration of the digitalis drugs for the average-sized adult.

Urgency	Drug	Dosage
Moderate	Digitalis	0.4 g every 8 hours for 3 doses
	Digitoxin	0.4 mg every 8 hours for 3 doses
	Digoxin	0.5 mg every 8 hours for 3 doses
Intermediate	Digitalis	0.2 g 3 times daily for 2 days, or 0.1 g 4 times daily for 3 days
	Digitoxin	0.2 mg 3 times daily for 2 days
	Digoxin	0.5 mg twice daily for 2 days, or 0.25 mg 3 times daily for 3 days
Least	Digitalis	0.1 g 3 times daily for 4–5 days
	Digitoxin	0.1 mg 3 times daily for 4–6 days
	Digoxin	0.25 mg daily

preceding 2 weeks. Always give intravenous preparations slowly.

Select the drug on the basis of the rapidity of effect needed. Except in extreme emergencies do not give the entire average digitalizing dose in a single dose. A good general rule if it is desired to digitalize rapidly (within a day) is to give one-half to two-thirds of the average digitalizing dose immediately and then give increments of one-fourth at intervals of 2–4 hours until the desired effect occurs. Observe carefully for digitalis toxicity. When the initial dose is given parenterally, it is advisable to give also an average oral maintenance dose of a digitalis preparation if the patient is able to swallow. Optimal digitalization can thus be achieved and maintained from the start. It is not necessary to give the same glycoside orally that was used for the initial medication; for example, the physician may digitalize with intravenous deslanoside (Cedilanid-D) and give digoxin for maintenance. Optimal digitalization may be quite difficult to determine in a patient with sinus rhythm.

A history of digitalis therapy is often difficult to obtain, and digitalis toxicity has occurred in patients who have denied or were unaware of having received the drug. This is another reason for not giving a full digitalizing dose in a single injection as well as for determining digitalis blood levels.

Individualize the dosage for each patient.

b. Rapid oral digitalization (within 24 hours)–It is usually unwise to attempt to digitalize with a single oral dose, since nausea and vomiting are common and make it very difficult to estimate the degree of digitalization. Multiple oral doses are usually adequate for initial digitalization. Close medical observation is required before each dose is given, and further doses should be withdrawn at the first sign or symptom of toxicity.

c. Slow digitalization–At times it is desirable to digitalize slowly over the course of a week, especially if the patient cannot be closely observed during this period. Any of the digitalis preparations can be given in daily doses 2 or 3 times the average maintenance dose for 2–4 days. If rapid digitalization is not indicated, one can slowly digitalize over the course of a week by giving a maintenance dose of digoxin, 0.25 mg once or twice daily for 2 or 3 days and then daily; or one can give this dose daily, so that digitalization occurs in 7–10 days. The total digitalizing dose may be somewhat greater than when digitalization is rapid. As soon as toxic symptoms appear the drug should be stopped for 1 day and then the patient given the average maintenance dose.

2. Partially treated cases–If a digitalis preparation has been taken within 2 weeks, give one-fourth of the estimated digitalizing dose and then give additional digitalis cautiously, observing the response at intervals of 6–12 hours.

3. Adjustment of average doses–The ''average'' doses of digoxin or other digitalis preparations must be decreased in cases of renal failure, hepatic failure, hypothyroidism, or elderly or small patients,

or if quinidine or calcium entry–blocking agents are added to the regimen of a patient receiving digitalis. Digoxin blood levels may double, and toxicity may occur. Correct hypokalemia before giving digitalis.

E. Maintenance Doses and Methods: The oral route is preferred in maintaining digitalization. The exact maintenance dose must be determined clinically for each patient.

F. Toxic Effects of Digitalis: There are no nontoxic digitalis preparations, and the difference between the therapeutic and toxic level is very small.

1. Slight toxicity–Anorexia, occasional ventricular ectopic beats, sinus bradycardia.

2. Moderate toxicity–Nausea and vomiting, headache, malaise, frequent or complex ventricular premature beats.

3. Severe toxicity–Diarrhea, blurring of vision, confusion, disorientation, junctional tachycardia, atrioventricular dissociation, paroxysmal atrial tachycardia with block, atrial fibrillation, ventricular tachycardia, sinoatrial or atrioventricular block.

4. Extreme toxicity–High-degree conduction blocks and ventricular fibrillation.

Because many arrhythmias occur in the absence as well as in the presence of digitalis toxicity, it is often difficult for the physician to know whether the drug has caused the arrhythmia. A high degree of probability exists with respect to multifocal ventricular beats, junctional atrioventricular nodal tachycardia, atrioventricular dissociation not associated with atrioventricular block, and paroxysmal atrial tachycardia with block. Ventricular tachycardia is common in acute myocardial infarction but may be due to digitalis toxicity. When digitalis is continued despite the presence of the above arrhythmias (thought likely as an index of digitalis toxicity), the mortality rate is high.

Although there is an overlap in the serum concentrations of digoxin as determined by radioimmunoassay, Smith found that the serum levels in patients considered to be digitalis toxic averaged 2 (± 1.5) ng/mL, as compared to 1 (± 0.7) in patients judged to be nontoxic. Serum levels may prove helpful in the case of doubtful digitalis toxicity but must be interpreted in the light of factors other than toxicity that influence serum levels.

G. Relationship of Digitalis to Potassium Ion: There is an antagonism between potassium and digitalis, and digitalis toxicity is more likely to occur in any clinical situation in which potassium is decreased in the cells or serum, eg, as a result of potassium diuresis due to certain diuretics (thiazide, furosemide, or ethacrynic acid), gastrointestinal losses, or following corticosteroid therapy. In these circumstances, potassium ion should be given.

H. Relationship of Digitalis to Quinidine: When quinidine is given to a patient receiving digoxin, the serum concentration of digoxin will approximately double, and toxicity may ensue. If the dose of digoxin is reduced by half and the serum digoxin level is monitored, the risk of toxicity will be lower, and the digoxin dosage can then be adjusted appropriately.

When adjustment is made, the serum digoxin concentration must be assayed to determine the effect of the quinidine.

I. Treatment of Severe Digitalis Toxicity: Withhold digitalis and diuretics until the manifestations of toxicity have subsided, and treat the cardiac failure, if present, with other means such as bed rest, low-sodium diet, and vasodilators when failure is more severe. Give potassium salts, 4–8 g orally per day in divided doses, or, depending upon the clinical urgency, well-diluted intravenous potassium salts slowly (not more than 20–30 meq/h). In emergency circumstances, potassium may be given more rapidly under electrocardiographic control. Do not give potassium salts intravenously in the presence of high-grade atrioventricular block or renal failure. One can treat premonitory ventricular arrhythmias with lidocaine, phenytoin, propranolol, or procainamide. Life-threatening digitalis intoxication has been treated safely and effectively with antibodies to purified digoxin-specific Fab fragments. *Caution:* Cardioversion should be used with great caution if digitalis toxicity is suspected. It may precipitate digitalis-induced arrhythmias or be followed by more serious arrhythmias such as ventricular tachycardia. If essential, administer electrical cardioversion in small graded increments or use atrial pacing.

The differentiation of digitalis toxicity and inadequate digitalization is sometimes quite difficult, but serum digitalis levels may be helpful. The only safe procedure, if one is uncertain, is to withhold digitalis and diuretics and treat the cardiac failure with restriction of sodium and other means to improve cardiac function. Nausea, vomiting, and arrhythmias that are in fact due to digitalis toxicity will subside in 2–3 days. *Caution:* Do not give rapid-acting intravenous digitalis preparations to a patient taking digitalis who is apparently in failure unless it is certain that the manifestations observed are not due to digitalis toxicity.

Prognosis

The availability of potent diuretics, effective antihypertensive therapy, newer vasodilator and inotropic drugs, surgical replacement of stenotic and regurgitant cardiac valves, and correction of some congenital lesions have considerably improved the outlook for patients with these conditions. However, the prognosis is still unsatisfactory in severe congestive cardiomyopathy with failure, myocardial infarction with failure, and any condition not remediable by surgery or correction of the underlying pathogenetic factor. Less than half of these patients survive 2 years, especially if they fail to respond to digitalis, diuretics, and oral vasodilators. Pulmonary embolization secondary to venous thrombosis in the leg veins is common, as are pulmonary infections, cardiac cirrhosis, and peripheral arterial embolization from mural thrombi on the endocardium. In general, the speed and adequacy of response to therapy are the most reliable guides to prognosis. Detection and removal of a precipitating condition prolong survival. The age of the patient, the degree of cardiac enlargement, the extent of myocardial damage, and the severity of underlying cardiac and associated diseases must all be considered. Survival is longer in failure precipitated by atrial fibrillation or due to mitral insufficiency, unless it is due to "acute" mitral regurgitation (see Nonrheumatic Mitral Insufficiency, p 192). Survival is shorter when failure is due to dilated cardiomyopathy, mitral stenosis, syphilitic aortic insufficiency, calcific aortic stenosis, myocardial infarction, chronic pulmonary disease, and severe hypertension.

SPECIAL PROBLEMS IN THE MANAGEMENT OF CONGESTIVE HEART FAILURE

Acute Pulmonary Edema

Acute pulmonary edema is a grave emergency. Treatment may vary depending upon the cause (cardiac, or noncardiac as in heroin toxicity) and severity. For example, in a mild attack, morphine and rest in bed alone may suffice; in an attack due to atrial fibrillation with rapid ventricular rate, lanatoside D or digoxin given intravenously or cardioversion may be required.

The patient should be elevated to the semi-Fowler position or placed in a chair; this decreases the venous return to the heart. Morphine sulfate, 3–5 mg intravenously or 5–10 mg intramuscularly, relieves anxiety, increases venous compliance and decreases preload, depresses pulmonary reflexes, and induces sleep. Relief from forceful respiration decreases the negative intrathoracic pressure and the venous return to the heart.

Sublingual nitroglycerin, 0.4–0.6 mg, repeated every 10 minutes for several doses, if necessary, may be immediately effective in acute pulmonary edema. The blood pressure should be monitored to avoid hypotension, and if the pressure begins to fall, the next dose should be smaller. Nifedipine inhibits the effect of calcium in excitation-contraction coupling and induces vascular smooth muscle relaxation. It has rapidly relieved acute pulmonary edema when given in doses of 10 mg sublingually.

Oxygen should be administered in high concentrations by mask or (for children) by hood or tent. Moderate concentrations (40–60%) can be achieved with an oxygen tent or nasal catheter. Oxygen relieves hypoxia and dyspnea and decreases pulmonary capillary permeability.

Furosemide (Lasix; see p 248), 40–80 mg intravenously, or ethacrynic acid (Edecrin), 25–100 mg orally or 25–50 mg intravenously, is useful because of the potent and prompt vasodilatory and diuretic action of these drugs; they also decrease preload, which precedes diuresis.

Vasodilator therapy should be employed (see ¶ F, p 249), including sublingual nitrates and nifedipine as indicated above. Intravenous infusion of sodium nitroprusside or nitroglycerin may be valuable in acute pulmonary edema in hypertensive patients requiring hospitalization. Oral therapy with hydralazine and long-acting nitrates may be valuable in left ventricular failure associated with mild pulmonary edema, or if the patient has only orthopnea or nocturnal dyspnea quickly relieved by sitting up.

Rapid digitalization is of value. Extreme care should be taken in giving digitalis intravenously to a previously digitalized patient.

Aminophylline, 0.25–0.5 g slowly intravenously, is often helpful. It increases cardiac output, renal blood flow, glomerular filtration rate, and urine output of water and sodium. Rectal aminophylline suppositories, 0.25–0.5 g, are often helpful and are more convenient for the patient.

Soft rubber tourniquets or blood pressure cuffs, applied with sufficient pressure to obstruct venous but not arterial flow and rotated every 15 minutes, will effectively reduce the venous return to the heart. The tourniquets should be removed gradually as the attack subsides. About 700 mL of blood may be trapped in the extremities by this method. Venesection (300–700 mL) is the most direct way of reducing the venous return to the heart and may strikingly increase cardiac output and decrease right atrial and peripheral venous pressure in low-output cardiac failure. It is contraindicated if anemia is present.

In the acute recurrent pulmonary edema of hypertensive heart disease and in the presence of severe hypertension, vasodilator therapy as outlined above (in addition to other measures outlined for acute hypertensive emergencies on p 209) may be helpful. Care must be taken not to produce hypotension.

Refractory Cardiac Failure

When the treatment measures outlined above do not result in clinical improvement, reevaluate the total situation with particular attention to the following questions:

(1) Is the diagnosis correct?

(2) Has bed rest been adequate? Is the patient receiving more sodium than ordered? Have treatment measures been carefully and properly administered? A review of the patient's activities, diet, and medications is essential.

(3) Are any of the following present or to be considered: unrecognized recurrent pulmonary infarction, anemia, masked hyperthyroidism, vitamin deficiency, infective endocarditis, abrupt worsening or production of valvular insufficiencies, silent myocardial infarction, arrhythmias, malfunction of prosthetic valve, ventricular aneurysm, arteriovenous fistulas, use of corticosteroids, or uncontrolled hypertension?

(4) Have complications such as acute rheumatic myocarditis or infective endocarditis been superimposed upon a rheumatic heart?

(5) Are there electrolyte abnormalities that may have resulted from diet or diuretics? Electrolyte disturbances produce a low-sodium syndrome or, in the case of low potassium, enhance digitalis intoxication.

(6) Is the renal function adequate for the use of thiazides? If not, furosemide should be used.

(7) Has the patient been taking the prescribed medication regularly? If so, has there been a change in the preparation of digitalis? (See p 250 regarding digitalis administration.)

(8) If questions 1–7 noted above have all been answered, if conventional therapy has not controlled the cardiac failure, and if symptoms of left ventricular or congestive failure persist or recur, oral vasodilator agents should be used alone or combined with inotropic agents, as discussed in ¶ F, p 249.

Management of Convalescence

Provide adequate rest and exercise within tolerance. Careful attention should be paid to the treatment of noncardiac causes of cardiac failure and to the avoidance of precipitating factors.

A. Digitalization: Once digitalis is started for cardiac failure, it is usually necessary to continue it for life, unless the diagnosis is faulty or the failure is acute and secondary to paroxysmal arrhythmias, overwhelming systemic disorders, or shock due to acute myocardial infarction or surgically corrected disease.

B. Low-Sodium Diet: Allow 1.5 g of sodium chloride (600 mg of sodium) per day. It is advisable to check serum sodium frequently to be certain that hyponatremia and hypovolemia are not occurring. An inadequate sodium intake in the presence of severe renal impairment can precipitate hyperkalemia or fatal renal failure. If thiazide compounds are used, it is wise ·to allow the ambulatory patient at least 2 g of sodium a day in the diet.

A high-sodium diet is particularly apt to maintain cardiac failure if the patient concurrently is up and about, stimulating aldosterone secretion. Dietary review often reveals that the patient is not restricting sodium adequately.

C. Diuretics: The adequately digitalized (short of toxicity) patient on a sodium-restricted diet may still accumulate edema fluid. Diuretic drugs should be added to the regimen in the amounts necessary to prevent this accumulation. There are some who recommend the use of diuretics prior to the use of digitalis in cardiac failure. Salt and water depletion are ancillary to improving the contractile power of the heart. Intensive diuretic therapy may produce hypovolemia, hypokalemia, and weakness.

The thiazide diuretics, because of the greater convenience of oral administration, are most widely used. Any one of the agents listed in Table 8–6 can be given (preferably intermittently) several times each week but can be given daily if necessary. Because potassium depletion is a hazard in the use of the thiazide diuretics, potassium must be added, either as potassium chloride, 1 g 3 times daily, or by the use of fruit juices, fruits (dried apricots, dates, prunes, bananas), and vegetables. Potassium-sparing diuretics (spironolactone or triamterene) can be added instead. Do not use spironolactone or triamterene if renal failure or oliguria is present.

D. Oral Vasodilators and Inotropic Agents:
(See pp 249 and 250.)

Electrolyte Disturbances in Cardiac Failure

During treatment of cardiac failure, several types of electrolyte disturbance may be seen.

A. Hypochloremic Alkalosis: This is due to chloride excretion out of proportion to sodium loss following diuresis, resulting in low serum chloride and high serum bicarbonate. Serum sodium and potassium levels may be normal or low. Symptoms of dehydration may be present.

Almost always there is associated potassium deficit. Correction of the hypochloremia is usually accomplished by use of potassium chloride.

Low serum sodium may be dilutional and may occur in association with hypokalemic alkalosis; restriction of fluids and administration of potassium salts such as potassium chloride may be helpful.

B. Low-Sodium Syndrome: In the absence of edema, the onset of weakness, oliguria, sweating, and azotemia heralds the "low-salt syndrome." Excessive diuresis, hot weather, fever, and vomiting are additional predisposing factors. Low serum sodium may be present without alkalosis or acidosis, or it may be complicated by dehydration and acidosis. It may follow severe sodium restriction accompanied by diuresis.

In mild cases treatment consists merely of increasing the sodium intake. For severe cases, treat very cautiously with intravenous hypertonic saline.

The total body sodium is usually increased when edema is present in spite of hyponatremia. In such cases, do not give sodium but restrict water to counteract the dilutional hyponatremias.

C. Hypokalemia: This may result from excessive potassium excretion due to the administration of thiazide or the more potent diuretics if the patient is taking a high-sodium diet. Hypokalemia may induce digitalis intoxication.

Treatment consists of giving potassium chloride, 3–6 g daily orally, provided renal function is adequate. Parenteral administration of potassium salts may be tried with caution in the presence of acidosis or mild renal failure if the need for potassium requires it. Monitor effects by noting changes on the ECG (tall T waves) and by determining serum potassium levels.

D. Hyperkalemia: This may result from spironolactone treatment and renal failure and may occur with severely restricted sodium intake (even with normal renal function) owing to lack of sodium ion in the distal tubule to exchange with potassium ion (see Chapter 3).

High-Output Failure

The term "high-output failure" means that in the presence of fully developed congestive heart failure, the cardiac output is greater than normal but still insufficient for the needs of the body. It occurs characteristically when preexisting heart disease is complicated by thyrotoxicosis, severe anemia (hemoglobin < 8 g/dL), pregnancy, arteriovenous fistula, beriberi, and occasionally Paget's disease of bone or chronic pulmonary disease or liver disease with arterial oxygen unsaturation.

The clinical picture of congestive heart failure is present except for more marked tachycardia, overactive heart, bounding pulses, and warm hands and skin generally. The circulation time may be short or normal in the face of elevated venous pressure. This is never seen in uncomplicated heart failure unless fever or one of the disorders listed above is present.

Treatment is directed at the failure as well as at the associated illness, eg, anemia, thyrotoxicosis.

See also sections on digitalis and diuretics (pp 206 and 250).

Arnold SB et al: Long-term digitalis therapy improves left ventricular function in heart failure. *N Engl J Med* 1980; **303:**1443.

Baim DS et al: Evaluation of a new bipyridine inotropic agent—milrinone—in patients with severe congestive heart failure. *N Engl J Med* 1983;**309:**748.

Captopril Multicenter Research Group: A placebo-controlled trial of captopril in refractory chronic congestive heart failure. *J Am Coll Cardiol* 1983;**2:**755.

Chatterjee K, Parmley WW: Vasodilator therapy for acute myocardial infarction and chronic congestive heart failure. *J Am Coll Cardiol* 1983;**1:**133.

DiCarlo L et al: Enalapril: A new angiotensin-converting enzyme inhibitor in chronic heart failure: Acute and chronic hemodynamic evaluations. *J Am Coll Cardiol* 1983;**2:**865.

Franciosa JA et al: Survival in men with severe chronic left ventricular failure due to either coronary heart disease or idiopathic dilated cardiomyopathy. *Am J Cardiol* 1983;**51:**831.

Lee DC et al: Heart failure in outpatients: A randomized trial of digoxin versus placebo. *N Engl J Med* 1983;**306:**699.

Maskin CS et al: Inotropic therapy in the management of congestive heart failure. *Cardiovas Rev Rep* 1982;**3:**837.

Miller RR et al: Differential systemic arterial and venous actions and consequent cardiac effects of vasodilator drugs. *Prog Cardiovasc Dis* 1982;**24:**353.

Packer M: Vasodilator and inotropic therapy for severe chronic heart failure: Passion and skepticism. *J Am Coll Cardiol* 1983;**2:**841.

Popp RL: M mode echocardiographic assessment of left ventricular function. *Am J Cardiol* 1982;**49:**1312.

Ports TA et al: Trimazosin in chronic congestive heart failure: Improved left ventricular function at rest and during exercise. *Am Heart J* 1983;**106:**1036.

Smith TW et al: Digitalis glycosides: Mechanisms and manifestations of toxicity. (2 parts.) *Prog Cardiovasc Dis* 1984;**26:**413, 495.

Wilson JR et al: Prognosis in severe heart failure: Relation to hemodynamic measurements and ventricular ectopic activity. *J Am Coll Cardiol* 1983;**2:**403.

See references for Cardiac Failure on p 255.

DISEASES OF THE PERICARDIUM

ACUTE INFLAMMATORY PERICARDITIS
(For Pericarditis With Effusion, see p 257.)

Essentials of Diagnosis

- Pleuritic or persisting substernal or precordial pain referred to the left neck, shoulder, or back.
- Pericardial friction rub.
- Electrocardiography: Early, concordant ST elevation; late, general symmetric T wave inversion without Q waves or reciprocal changes except in aVR.

General Considerations

In approximate order of frequency, infectious pericarditis is caused by viruses, pyogenic bacteria associated with bacteremia or septicemia (pneumococcus, hemolytic *Streptococcus, Staphylococcus aureus,* meningococcus, gonococcus), *Mycobacterium tuberculosis,* and *Brucella*. Inflammatory pericarditis includes all diseases associated with acute vasculitis, most commonly disseminated lupus erythematosus, acute rheumatic fever, rheumatoid arthritis, and serum sickness. A miscellaneous group includes pericarditis that occurs after pericardiotomy, myocardial infarction, or trauma; pericarditis associated with uremia, metastatic tumors, and the lymphomas; and hemorrhagic pericarditis due to dissecting aorta.

Acute pericarditis is traditionally classified as fibrinous pericarditis or pericarditis with effusion, in which the pericardial cavity contains significant amounts of transudate, blood, exudate, or pus. Varying degrees of myocarditis accompany pericarditis and are responsible for the electrocardiographic changes in ST–T contours.

Pericarditis is a spectrum of diseases ranging from acute fibrinous pericarditis through pericardial effusion with or without cardiac tamponade to subacute seroconstrictive or typical chronic constrictive pericarditis.

Clinical Findings

A. Symptoms and Signs: Acute viral pericarditis is more common in men age 20–50 years and often follows a "viral" respiratory infection. The onset of pain is usually sudden; pain is precordial or substernal, pleuritic or steady (or both), and radiates to the left neck, shoulder, back, or epigastrium. It is worse in the supine position and may be accentuated by swallowing. Tachycardia and a pericardial (often pleuropericardial) friction rub are present.

Fever is 37.8–39.4 °C (100–103 °F) or higher in infectious pericarditis and is determined by the febrile pattern of the underlying disease in the other varieties.

B. Laboratory Findings: Leukocytosis of 10–20 thousand/μL is usually present in acute viral pericarditis; leukopenia may be noted in pericarditis associated with disseminated lupus erythematosus. LE cells should be sought in isolated acute pericarditis.

C. X-Ray Findings: An enlarged cardiac silhouette, pneumonitis, and pleural effusion may be seen.

D. Electrocardiography: Initially, electrocardiographic changes consist only of ST–T segment elevation in all leads, with preservation of normal upward concavity. Return to the baseline in a few days is followed by T wave inversion. Reciprocal changes are absent except in aVR, and Q waves do not appear.

E. Echocardiography: Echocardiography is most valuable in the diagnosis of pericardial effusion. The fluid occupies an echo-free space separating the anterior wall of the right ventricle from the chest and the posterior wall of the left ventricle from the lung. The procedure is valuable in the differentiation between cardiac dilatation and pericardial effusion, especially in the presence of what may be cardiac tamponade.

Differential Diagnosis

A. Acute Myocardial Infarction: Acute viral pericarditis usually follows a respiratory infection, occurs in the age group from 20 to 50 years, and characteristically presents with pleuritic pain. Fever, friction rub, leukocytosis, and an elevated sedimentation rate are found at the onset rather than 24–72 hours later. Electrocardiographic changes are usually distinctive. SGOT, CPK, and LDH are only rarely elevated even in severe pericarditis. In severe cases, the diagnosis of acute myocardial infarction can be established by endomyocardial biopsy.

B. Acute Pleurisy: Pericardial friction rub is differentiated from pleural friction rub by its persistence when the breath is held, although there may also be a pleuropericardial friction sound that is related to respiration and is also heard when the breath is held. Electrocardiographic changes may be diagnostic of pericarditis in the absence of a rub.

C. Confusion of Rub With Murmurs: Pericardial friction rubs are differentiated by their pressure with the breath held, changing character, lack of association with the usual areas of murmurs, highpitched or "scratchy" quality, asynchrony with heart sounds, and often triple character.

Complications

Pericardial effusion is the most noteworthy complication, but if myocarditis is present there may be cardiac dilatation as well as pericardial effusion, resulting in a poorer prognosis. Arrhythmias are frequent, especially if myocarditis is present. The pericarditis may be recurrent for weeks or months, perhaps as a result of immunologic mechanisms.

Treatment

Treat the underlying condition and give analgesics as necessary for relief of pain. Salicylates and corticotropin or the corticosteroids are useful in rheumatic pericarditis. In severe acute myocarditis or if cardiac failure develops rapidly, corticosteroids combined with immunosuppressive drugs have been shown to reverse the myocardial infiltrate with resultant clinical benefit. See below for pericardial effusion and tamponade.

Prognosis

The prognosis of viral pericarditis is usually excellent. Recovery occurs in 2 weeks to 3 months; recurrences, however, are relatively common (due to an autoimmune mechanism or an unsuspected infection). The effusion may recur at intervals of weeks or months and may persist for 1 or 2 years. Residual pericardial thickening or persistent electrocardiographic abnormalities are rare. Constrictive pericarditis has been reported following viral pericarditis but is rare. Similarly, dilated cardiomyopathy has been described, but it is also rare following an acute infection. The promptness and adequacy of antibiotic and surgical treatment determine the outcome in tuberculous and purulent pericarditis. Other manifestations of disseminated lupus erythematosus may become apparent after an attack of presumed "viral" pericarditis. In the miscellaneous group, the basic disorder determines the prognosis.

Hancock EW: Management of pericardial disease. *Primary Cardiol* (May) 1980;**6**:19.

Spodick DH: The normal and diseased pericardium: Current concepts of pericardial physiology, diagnosis, and treatment. *J Am Coll Cardiol* 1983;**1**:240.

Thompson ME, Rault RM, Reddy PS: Uremic pericarditis. *Cardiovasc Rev Rep* 1981;**2**:755.

PERICARDITIS WITH EFFUSION

The most common causes of pericardial effusion are uremia, cancer, lymphoma, connective tissue disorders, viral pericarditis, radiation of the mediastinum, myxedema, tuberculosis, rheumatoid arthritis, and purulent pericarditis. Infrequent causes include sarcoidosis and chylous and "chronic idiopathic" pericarditis.

The speed of accumulation determines the physiologic importance of the effusion. Massive pericardial effusions (over 1000 mL), if they accumulate slowly, may produce no symptoms. However, sudden hemorrhage into the pericardium or sudden accumulation of relatively small effusions (about 200 mL) may raise the intrapericardial pressure to the point of cardiac tamponade, in which the fluid limits venous inflow and diastolic filling of the heart. In tamponade the cardiac output falls, the pulse pressure narrows, and tachycardia and elevation of the central venous pressure appear as compensatory mechanisms. Shock and death may result if tamponade is not relieved.

Clinical Findings

A. Symptoms and Signs: Pain is often absent but may be present as in acute pericarditis and as a dull, diffuse, oppressive precordial or substernal distress. Dyspnea and cough cause the patient to sit up and lean forward for relief. Dysphagia is prominent. Fever and other symptoms depend upon the primary disease (eg, septicemia, empyema, cancer).

The area of "cardiac" dullness is enlarged and the apex beat is often not palpable or is well within the lateral border of dullness. Friction rub may persist despite a large effusion. In tamponade, distended neck veins, inspiratory distention of the neck veins, narrow pulse pressure, and paradoxic pulse are present. Paradoxic pulse is a decrease in the volume of the arterial pulse and blood pressure with inspiration, due to decreased dimensions of the left ventricular cavity and decreased stroke output, and increase of those of the right ventricular cavity and increased stroke output. This is an exaggerated form of the normal respiratory response and can be demonstrated by echocardiography. Paradoxic pulse is absent when pericardial effusion complicates atrial septal defect, presumably because of the equilibration of pressures and volumes in the 2 atria and therefore the absence of a disproportionate decrease in left ventricular volume during inspiration. Liver enlargement, ascites, and leg edema depend upon the degree and duration of tamponade. Acute cardiac tamponade produces the clinical picture of shock.

B. Laboratory Findings: The cause of acute effusion is determined by bacteriologic and cytologic study of aspirated fluid and by the presence of primary disease elsewhere (tuberculosis, lupus erythematosus, cancer, myxedema, sarcoidosis, septicemia, lymphoma, etc). The cause of chronic effusion is determined by pericardial biopsy. Leukocytosis and a rapid sedimentation rate are present when the effusion is infectious or inflammatory. The arm-to-tongue circulation time is normal in the presence of large effusion without tamponade: this is often a clue to the correct interpretation of a "large heart shadow" on chest x-ray. In myxedema, pericardial effusion and prolongation of the circulation time are present without tamponade.

C. X-Ray Findings: A rapidly enlarging "cardiac" silhouette with sharply defined margins, an acute right cardiophrenic angle, clear lung fields, and pleural effusion are common. Cardiac pulsations are feeble or absent.

D. Electrocardiographic Findings: The T waves are low, flat, diphasic, or inverted in all leads; the QRS voltage is uniformly low. Electrical alternans may be present.

E. Echocardiography: Echocardiography has replaced the invasive procedures and is the best and simplest method of diagnosis (see p 256).

Differential Diagnosis

Cardiac dilatation with congestive heart failure may be impossible to differentiate from pericarditis with effusion if pleural effusion is also present. Pulmonary rales, gallop rhythm, and raised jugular venous pressure may be of clinical value in assessing cardiac failure. Rapid changes in heart size as seen by x-ray, clear lung fields with normal hilar vessels, definite paradoxic pulse, and absent cardiac pulsations on fluoroscopy are rare in congestive failure. Echocardiography is often definitive in the diagnosis of pericardial effusion. In a patient with "heart failure," the absence of significant murmurs, arrhythmia, and hypertension should suggest pericarditis with effusion.

Complications

Cardiac tamponade is a serious complication. Rapidly developing pericardial effusions or hemorrhage into the pericardial sac may so impede venous return and cardiac filling that cardiac output falls and irreversible shock occurs. Anticoagulant therapy creates a serious hazard of hemorrhage.

Purulent pericarditis is usually secondary to other infection elsewhere but is at times caused by contamination of a previous pericardial tap.

Pericardial effusion may be recurrent over a period of weeks to months, possibly because of immunologic mechanisms.

Treatment

A. Emergency Treatment (Paracentesis): The indications for pericardial paracentesis are the symptoms and signs of cardiac tamponade. As the pericardial fluid increases in amount, and particularly when it increases rapidly, the venous pressure may rise toward its limit of 22–24 cm of water, and the cardiac output may progressively fall. When this occurs, the patient becomes weak, pale, and dyspneic, and the pulse pressure becomes very narrow and the pulse rapid and thready, ie, the patient goes into shock. Under these circumstances, removal of pericardial fluid may be lifesaving; fluid should be removed slowly to avoid cardiac dilatation or sudden reflex changes in rate and rhythm. Fluid should be removed in the catheterization laboratory, with resuscitation equipment available.

B. Specific Measures:

1. Tuberculous pericarditis–Treat the systemic infection with bed rest, attention to nutrition and other general factors, and intensive antituberculosis chemotherapy. If fever and signs of pericardial effusion do not rapidly subside and are still obvious in 1 month, surgical decortication of the pericardium should be considered in order to prevent chronic constrictive pericarditis. Good judgment is required to determine when the disease is progressing despite medical treatment and when signs of constriction are appearing.

2. Rheumatic pericarditis with effusion–Treat as for rheumatic fever. The salicylates may help in causing fluid resorption. Paracentesis is usually unnecessary but should be performed if tamponade occurs.

3. Hydropericardium due to heart failure– Treatment of the congestive failure is usually sufficient.

4. Hemopericardium due to rupture of adjacent structure (usually posttraumatic)–If fluid accumulation is excessive, remove fluid *at once*.

5. Infection–Treat infection with appropriate chemotherapeutic agents and perform paracentesis as needed to relieve pressure. When fluid is being removed instill 50–150 thousand units of penicillin or the equivalent topical amount of streptomycin or other indicated antibiotic into the pericardial sac, and repeat whenever a tap is performed. Chemotherapeutic agents should be continued as long as purulent effusion is present. If fluid is encapsulated or the patient is not responding to therapy, surgical drainage via pericardiotomy may be necessary.

6. Uremic pericarditis often clears clinically after dialysis therapy is started. Severe tamponade may require pericardiotomy.

7. Myxedema–Treat cautiously, beginning with small doses of T_3 or T_4. Some prefer to begin with T_3, because its short half-life is protective in case angina or arrhythmia occurs, and then change to T_4 after 1–2 weeks.

8. Connective tissue disorders–Treat with corticosteroids.

9. Others–Treat sarcoidosis with corticosteroids (see p 134). Lymphoma and tumors may be treated with radiotherapy or chemotherapy.

Prognosis

Tuberculous pericarditis causes death in the majority of untreated cases and results in chronic constrictive pericarditis in many who survive. The mortality rate is very low with early and adequate treatment; the long-term effect on the incidence of constrictive pericarditis is not known.

Acute benign pericarditis is only rarely fatal. Increase in central venous pressure may precede other significant hemodynamic changes. Venous pressure should be measured serially in pericardial effusion, especially when tamponade is suspected.

Rheumatic pericarditis, if severe and protracted, is associated with myocarditis, and this determines the immediate prognosis. Residual pericardial disease of clinical significance does not occur.

Purulent pericarditis, since it is usually associated with a bloodstream infection or infection elsewhere, is usually fatal if not treated; however, it responds satisfactorily to antibiotics and pericardial drainage when necessary.

Grose R et al: Cardiac tamponade in medical patients. *Circulation* 1981;**64**:1981.

Shabetai R: Diagnosis and treatment of pericardial effusion. *J Cardiovasc Med* 1981;**6**:125.

CHRONIC CONSTRICTIVE PERICARDITIS

Essentials of Diagnosis

- Markedly elevated venous pressure.
- Slight to moderate cardiac enlargement and quiet heart action.
- Paradoxic pulse.

- Ascites out of proportion to degree of ankle edema.

General Considerations

In the past, tuberculosis was overwhelmingly the most common cause of constriction of the pericardium, and this is still true in areas of the world where tuberculosis remains a public health problem. Constriction, especially the subacute variety, can occur following viral pericarditis but is uncommon. Trauma, radiation therapy of the mediastinum (especially for Hodgkin's disease), cardiac surgery, and malignant involvement of the pericardium may lead to subacute constriction, which with time will become fibrous and perhaps calcified. In many cases the cause is not determined, possibly because the inciting incident occurred years previously.

Encasement of the myocardium by an adherent, dense fibrous pericardium may be asymptomatic or may prevent ventricular expansion during diastole. If this happens, the stroke volume is low and fixed, and cardiac output can be increased only by tachycardia. Venous pressure rises as in congestive heart failure; together with renal retention of sodium and water, this produces the peripheral signs of right heart failure.

Clinical Findings

A. Symptoms and Signs: The principal symptoms are slowly progressive dyspnea, fatigue, and weakness on exertion; abdominal distention; and leg edema. Examination shows markedly distended neck veins with weak or absent systolic pulsations but prominent diastolic retraction, a moderately enlarged heart with a quiet precordium in the presence of tachycardia, faint heart sounds, a palpable and audible pericardial knock in early diastole, a low pulse pressure with a high diastolic level, paradoxic pulse, enlarged liver, ascites, and edema of both legs and the scrotum. Atrial fibrillation is frequently present.

B. Laboratory Findings: Rarely, tuberculous infection of the lungs or other organ is noted.

C. X-Ray and Fluoroscopic Findings: The "heart" is usually moderately enlarged. Its shape is not consistent with valvular or hypertensive heart disease. Pulsations are weak or absent. Lung fields are clear. Pericardial calcification is common but is not diagnostic of constrictive pericarditis. Diagnostic ultrasound may be of assistance.

D. Electrocardiographic Findings: T waves are flat or inverted; low voltage of QRS complexes is variable. Atrial fibrillation is common.

E. Echocardiography: The abrupt cessation of ventricular filling and decreased excursion of the left ventricular endocardium occurring in chronic constrictive pericarditis can be seen on 2-dimensional echocardiography and contrasts with the ventricular dilatation and slow ejection rate associated with cardiomyopathy, which is the major disease to be considered in the differential diagnosis. Thickening of the pericardium may be seen.

F. Computerized Tomography: CT scans of the chest may show pericardial thickening or fluid and may demonstrate tumors. Demonstration of a thickened pericardium in patients with constriction can thus differentiate patients with restrictive cardiomyopathy and a normal pericardium.

Differential Diagnosis

Marked venous engorgement in the neck without systolic pulsation, slight to moderate cardiac enlargement, absence of significant murmurs or hypertension, paradoxic pulse, and electrocardiographic changes distinguish chronic constrictive pericarditis from tricuspid stenosis and congestive heart failure from any cause, especially cardiomyopathy. Restrictive or dilated cardiomyopathy often causes confusion. CT scans of the chest may be diagnostic by demonstrating a thickened pericardium. Cirrhosis of the liver, mediastinal tumor, nephrosis, and obstruction of the vena cava must also be considered. Diagnosis may be difficult and require cardiac catheterization.

Complications

In tuberculous cases, a miliary spread or acute flare-up of the intrapericardial infection may occur.

Thrombophlebitis of the leg veins may occur secondary to elevated venous pressure, venous stasis, and inactivity. Nephrotic syndrome has been described.

Treatment

Give a low-sodium diet and diuretics as in cardiac failure to combat ascites and congestive failure. Excessive diuresis may be dangerous. Digitalis is usually of little value unless the patient has atrial fibrillation.

Surgical removal of the constricting pericardium can frequently restore a patient to normal health. If congestive phenomena are chronic or the pericarditis is progressive, surgical intervention is the only method offering possible cure. The recent surgical mortality rate is 3–5%, and most patients benefit greatly from the procedure.

Prognosis

Constrictive pericarditis known to be due to tuberculosis is usually fatal without antituberculosis drugs and surgery. Most patients with constrictive pericarditis due to any cause have increasing disability because of ascites and edema and die of mechanical "heart failure." A few patients show no progression of symptoms or signs for years. Spontaneous regression is rare.

Fowler NO: Constrictive pericarditis: New aspects. *Am J Cardiol* 1982;**50:**1014.

Gottdiener JS et al: Late cardiac effects of therapeutic mediastinal irradiation: Assessment by echocardiography and radionuclide angiography. *N Engl J Med* 1983;**308:**569.

Hancock EW: Constrictive pericarditis: Modern view of diagnosis and management. *J Cardiovasc Med* 1980;**5:**367.

Isner JM et al: Computed tomography in the diagnosis of pericardial heart disease. *Ann Intern Med* 1982;**97:**473.

DISEASES OF
THE MYOCARDIUM

PRIMARY PULMONARY
HYPERTENSION

Primary pulmonary hypertension is a condition of pulmonary hypertension and raised pulmonary vascular resistance in the absence of any other disease of the lungs or heart. Its cause is unknown. Pathologically, it is characterized by diffuse narrowing of the pulmonary arterioles without obvious reason. Late in the course of the disease, thrombi may develop in the areas of the pulmonary arterioles, and there may be evidence of pulmonary embolism as a result of the chronic low-output failure. Pulmonary embolism contributes to the downhill course. Primary pulmonary hypertension must be distinguished from chronic pulmonary heart disease and from mitral stenosis. The condition is infrequent and seems to have become less common in recent years, perhaps because infrequent causes of pulmonary heart disease formerly overlooked—such as left-to-right shunt, left ventricular failure, sarcoidosis, recurrent pulmonary emboli, and idiopathic pulmonary fibrosis—have been recognized with more regularity. The main differential steps are to exclude primary lung or pulmonary thromboembolic disease by appropriate clinical and pulmonary function studies and to exclude aortic and mitral valvular disease by clinical findings, cardiac catheterization, echocardiography, and other techniques.

The clinical picture is similar to that of pulmonary hypertension from any other cause. Patients present themselves with evidence of right heart failure that is usually progressive, leading to death in 2–8 years. Patients have the manifestations of low cardiac output, with weakness and fatigue, as well as edema and ascites as right heart failure advances. Peripheral cyanosis is present, and syncope on effort may occur.

Previously, there was no effective treatment for primary pulmonary hypertension, but recent studies with oral phentolamine (a drug that dilates the pulmonary artery) have been promising. The drug, 5 mg intravenously, causes a fall in peak pulmonary artery pressure; after oral therapy the effects are sustained for a number of months. Hydralazine, 75–100 mg, verapamil, and nifedipine have been reported to be effective with some patients, but more information is needed.

Bell WR, Simon TL: Current status of pulmonary thromboembolic disease: Pathophysiology, diagnosis, prevention, and treatment. *Am Heart J* 1982;**103**:239.

Haworth SG: Primary pulmonary hypertension. *Br Heart J* 1983;**49**:517.

Hermiller JB et al: Vasodilators and prostaglandin inhibitors in primary pulmonary hypertension. *Ann Intern Med* 1982;**97**:480.

CHRONIC OR SUBACUTE
PULMONARY HEART DISEASE
(Chronic or Subacute Cor Pulmonale)

Essentials of Diagnosis
- Symptoms and signs of chronic bronchitis and pulmonary emphysema.
- No significant murmurs or hypertension.
- Electrocardiography: Tall, peaked P waves; right axis deviation; and right ventricular hypertrophy.
- Chest x-ray: Enlarged right ventricle and pulmonary artery.

General Considerations
Cor pulmonale refers to the right ventricular hypertrophy and eventual failure resulting from pulmonary parenchymal or vascular disease. It may be acute, subacute, or, most commonly, chronic, and its clinical features depend upon both the primary disease and its effects on the heart.

Chronic cor pulmonale is most commonly caused by chronic obstructive pulmonary emphysema, often referred to as "chronic asthmatic bronchitis." Less common or rare causes include pneumoconiosis, pulmonary fibrosis or schistosomiasis, kyphoscoliosis, primary pulmonary hypertension, repeated episodes of subclinical or clinical pulmonary embolization, Pickwickian syndrome, and obliterative pulmonary capillary or lymphangitic infiltration from metastatic carcinoma. Emphysema and associated fibrosis result in obliteration of capillaries and disturbance of pulmonary function, with resultant hypoxia. Compensatory polycythemia and increased cardiac output also appear. The combined effect of these changes is increased pulmonary artery pressure, leading to right ventricular hypertrophy and eventual failure of the "high-output" variety.

Clinical Findings
A. Symptoms and Signs: The dominant symptoms of compensated cor pulmonale are respiratory in origin: chronic productive cough, exertional dyspnea, wheezing respirations, undue fatigability, and weakness. When the pulmonary disease has advanced sufficiently to cause right ventricular failure, these symptoms are intensified. Dependent edema, right upper quadrant pain, and digestive disturbances may also appear. The signs of cor pulmonale include cyanosis, clubbing, distended neck veins, right ventricular heave or gallop (or both), prominent lower sternal or epigastric pulsations, an enlarged tender liver, and dependent edema. The heart size cannot be determined because of emphysema, but there is no evidence of valvular disease. Pulses are full and the extremities warm unless the patient is terminal or in shock.

B. Laboratory Findings: Polycythemia is usually present in cor pulmonale secondary to emphysema. The arterial oxygen saturation is below 85%; P_{CO_2} is often elevated. Venous pressure is significantly elevated in right ventricular failure, but the circulation time may be normal or only slightly prolonged. Pulmonary function studies define the nature of the pulmonary disease.

C. X-Ray Findings: Chest x-ray discloses the presence or absence of parenchymal disease and a prominent or enlarged right ventricle, pulmonary conus, and artery.

D. Electrocardiographic Findings: The ECG shows right axis deviation and peaked P waves. Deep S waves are present in lead V_6. Left axis deviation and low voltage may be noted in patients with pulmonary emphysema. Frank right ventricular hypertrophy is uncommon except in "primary pulmonary hypertension." The ECG often mimics myocardial infarction because of the loss of anterior forces in the precordial leads, resulting from right ventricular hypertrophy. Q waves may be present in II, III, and aVF because of the vertically placed heart, but they are rarely deep or wide, as in inferior myocardial infarction. Arrhythmias are frequent and nonspecific.

E. Other Studies: Cardiac catheterization and right ventricular angiograms reveal pulmonary artery pressures and right ventricular anatomy. Perfusion pulmonary scans are rarely of value in chronic pulmonary heart disease. If they are negative in the presence of an acute episode, they are valuable in excluding pulmonary emboli; when positive, they lack specificity. The diagnosis of pulmonary emboli is improved when combined perfusion and ventilation scans are positive and can be confirmed by pulmonary angiography, which is the most specific method of diagnosis. In chronic pulmonary hypertension, echocardiography may show right ventricular enlargement and hypertrophy.

Differential Diagnosis

In its early stages, cor pulmonale can be diagnosed only on x-ray or electrocardiographic evidence. When frank congestive signs appear, differentiation from primary left ventricular failure is possible by considering the predominant history of respiratory complaints, the absence of orthopnea, the degree of cyanosis, bounding pulses, and warm extremities in the presence of edema. Electrocardiographic demonstration of right axis deviation, normal or only moderately prolonged circulation time, and absence of demonstrable factors pointing to left failure are helpful. Catheterization of the right heart, angiography, and pulmonary function studies will establish a definitive diagnosis.

Complications

Intercurrent respiratory infections increase dyspnea, cough, and cyanosis and further increase the pulmonary artery pressure. This may precipitate a dangerous degree of respiratory acidosis in advanced emphysema. Neurologic manifestations of CO_2 narcosis may appear: disorientation, somnolence, papilledema, coma, and occasionally convulsions.

Treatment

A. Specific Measures: Give appropriate antibi-

otic therapy for the respiratory infection that so commonly precedes failure in this type of case. The patient may be afebrile.

B. General Measures: The details of the treatment of chronic pulmonary disease (chronic respiratory failure) are discussed in Chapter 7.

Prognosis

Compensated cor pulmonale has the same outlook as the underlying pulmonary disease. Once congestive signs appear, the average life expectancy is 2–5 years, but survival is significantly longer when uncomplicated emphysema is the cause. Left ventricular failure secondary to coronary artery disease, hypertension, or aortic valve lesions may develop and shorten expectancy accordingly.

Kereiakes DJ et al: Computerized tomography in chronic thromboembolic pulmonary hypertension. *Am Heart J* 1983;**106:**1432.

Wood LDH, Prewitt RM: Cardiovascular management in acute hypoxemic respiratory failure. *Am J Cardiol* 1981;**47:**963.

SYPHILITIC CARDIOVASCULAR DISEASE
(See also Chapter 25.)

Essentials of Diagnosis

- Linear calcification or localized dilatation of the ascending aorta on x-ray.
- Aortic valvular insufficiency without stenosis or mitral valve disease.
- Aneurysm of the aorta.
- Coronary ostial stenosis.
- Evidence of syphilitic origin: history of infection, positive serologic test for syphilis, or presence of other forms of late syphilis.

General Considerations

Syphilitic "heart disease" may consist of aortic valvular insufficiency (most common), aortic dilatation or aneurysm, or narrowing of the coronary ostia. It comprises less than 5% of all heart disease in population groups that have ready access to effective treatment of syphilis. It is more common in men (3:1) and is usually diagnosed between ages 35 and 55 (10–20 years after the primary infection). Serologic tests for syphilis are positive in about 85% (and almost 100% with the fluorescent treponemal antibody absorption test [FTA-ABS]; see p 885) of untreated cases. The ascending aorta, arch, and descending aorta are most commonly affected; the abdominal aorta is rarely involved. Aortic valve insufficiency occurs in about 10% of cases of untreated syphilitic aortitis. One or both of the coronary ostia may be partially occluded.

Clinical Findings

A. Aortitis: There are no symptoms, and physical signs are absent unless dilatation has occurred. In a patient under age 40 without hypertension or demonstrable arteriosclerosis, a ringing or accentuated second aortic sound with or without a soft aortic systolic murmur is "suggestive" of syphilitic aortitis. Fluoroscopic evidence of increased width and pulsation of the ascending aorta, best seen in the left anterior oblique view, in the absence of elongation, is also suggestive. Linear calcification that is limited to the root of the aorta and arch is almost a sure diagnostic sign. There is echocardiographic evidence of aortic root dilatation.

B. Aortic Insufficiency: Clinical, x-ray, and electrocardiographic manifestations are as for rheumatic aortic insufficiency. Ten percent of cases are associated with saccular aneurysm of the aorta. Aortic insufficiency may produce no symptoms for long periods; once heart failure develops, however, it soon becomes refractory to treatment. In most cases death from aortic insufficiency occurs within 2–5 years if not treated surgically (prosthetic valves).

C. Aortic Aneurysm: Symptoms and signs are dependent upon the site and size of the aneurysm. Aneurysm of the ascending aorta is characterized by visible pulsation or dullness on palpation at the manubrium and in the first to third interspaces parasternally, lowered blood pressure in the right arm, and an aortic systolic murmur and thrill without peripheral signs of aortic stenosis. Aneurysm of the aortic arch is characterized by cough, dyspnea, and recurrent pulmonary infections (compression of trachea or right main stem bronchus); hoarseness (compression of recurrent laryngeal nerve); tracheal tug, edema of the face and neck, distended neck veins, and prominent veins over upper chest (compression of superior vena cava); and dysphagia (compression of the esophagus). Aneurysm of the descending aorta is usually asymptomatic; when it is large it may erode the ribs or spine, producing pain that is worse in recumbency and visible or palpable pulsations medial to the left scapula.

X-ray findings consist of saccular or sharply defined fusiform bulging of the thoracic aorta with increased pulsation. Clot formation or periaortic fibrosis may dampen the pulsations and simulate a solid tumor. Aortography demonstrates continuity of the aorta with the lumen of the aneurysm.

D. Narrowing of the Coronary Artery Ostia: Angina pectoris is identical to that seen in coronary heart disease. Its syphilitic origin can only be inferred in the presence of one of the other manifestations of syphilitic aortitis.

Differential Diagnosis

The clinical picture can mimic rheumatic and arteriosclerotic heart disease, ankylosing spondylitis, Reiter's disease, and rheumatoid arthritis. Syphilitic aneurysms are indistinguishable clinically from those caused by arteriosclerosis.

Treatment

A. Specific Measures: Treat syphilis as outlined in Chapter 25 if the patient has not had a full course of treatment.

B. General Measures: Bed rest may be desirable during treatment with penicillin because of the possibility of Herxheimer's reaction.

C. Surgical Measures: Surgical repair of the aneurysm has been attempted but is hazardous. Successful surgical aortocoronary bypass for coronary ostia stenosis has been accomplished. Surgical correction of aortic insufficiency may be necessary.

Complications

A. Aortic Insufficiency: Left ventricular hypertrophy, which may progress to failure.

B. Aortic Aneurysm: Recurrent pulmonary infection, bronchiectasis, atelectasis, bronchial hemorrhage, and rupture of the aneurysm.

Prognosis

A. Aortitis: Ten to 20% of patients develop aortic insufficiency and other manifestations of syphilitic cardiovascular disease; in the remainder, life expectancy is not affected.

B. Aortic Insufficiency: If penicillin is given when the signs of aortic insufficiency are purely auscultatory, the progress of the lesion may be slowed or even arrested; this significantly improves the prognosis for survival.

C. Aortic Aneurysm: Once aneurysms have reached sufficient size to produce symptoms by compression of adjacent structures, life expectancy is measured in months. Longer survival is possible when the aneurysm is small and effective therapy for syphilis has been given. Death is usually due to rupture of the aneurysm.

D. Narrowing of the Coronary Artery Ostia: This condition tends to aggravate the heart failure due to syphilitic aortic insufficiency and predisposes to sudden death. Surgical correction (aortocoronary bypass) has been successfully accomplished.

CARDIOMYOPATHIES

Diseases of the myocardium are a complex and heterogeneous group of disorders that are diagnostically confusing. There are various causes, not all of which are known; some are associated with general systemic disorders, and the disease is not confined to the heart. The clinical manifestations vary from a trivial illness recognizable only by nonspecific electrocardiographic abnormalities, mild chest pain, or slight enlargement of the heart to fulminant cardiac failure, recurrent ventricular arrhythmias, and death. Myocarditis may be acute or chronic, and the acute form may be benign or fulminant. The terms chronic myocarditis and chronic cardiomyopathy are often used interchangeably, since the cause of the disease is often unknown and because the inflammatory infiltrate suggests infection ("-itis"). "Chronic idiopathic cardiomyopathy" goes by a variety of names; the term "dilated cardiomyopathy" was preferred by a group of individuals trying to devise a uniform nomenclature. Myocarditis may be a primary disease of the heart or may be secondary to such systemic diseases as the connective tissue disorders.

Myocarditis is often associated with pericarditis (myopericarditis), especially in viral infections. The endocardium and the valves are less often involved except in the case of acute rheumatic fever or endocardial fibrosis. Myocardial disease due to drug toxicity is becoming increasingly more common with use of cardiotoxic drugs (see below).

ACUTE MYOCARDITIS

Acute myocarditis is a focal or diffuse inflammation of the myocardium occurring during or after many viral, bacterial, rickettsial, spirochetal, fungal, and parasitic diseases or after administration of various drugs. Mild forms are common and recognizable only by serial electrocardiographic changes. Severe myocarditis producing symptoms and signs occurs most commonly in acute rheumatic fever, diphtheria, scrub typhus, and Chagas' disease (*Trypanosoma cruzi* infection). Bacteremia, viral pneumonia and encephalitis, and trichinosis may be associated with myocarditis of varying severity.

The most common cause of acute viral myocarditis is coxsackie B virus, usually type B3 or B5. The disease is diagnosed by isolating the virus from throat washings, feces, or blood; by detecting a 4-fold increase in serum antibody titers from paired sera; or, in fatal cases, by isolating the virus from the myocardium.

Clinical Findings

A. Symptoms and Signs: In acute myocarditis, the patient usually presents with an acute febrile illness associated with fever, malaise, arthralgias, chest pain, dyspnea, and palpitations. The patient may have associated pericarditis, with chest pain characteristic of pericardial involvement. The chest pain is frequently vague and nondiagnostic. An acute febrile illness with symptoms suggesting cardiac involvement should provoke a meticulous search for signs of heart disease. The patient may experience syncope (Stokes-Adams attacks) if conduction defects are present.

1. Cardiac signs–Tachycardia out of proportion to the fever suggests the diagnosis of acute myocarditis. There are usually no abnormalities on inspection or palpation except for displacement of the cardiac impulse to the left. The blood pressure is usually normal. Auscultation may reveal a tic tac rhythm, a "functional" systolic murmur, and a gallop rhythm with S_3. In the presence of cardiac failure, the patient may have a raised pulmonary venous or jugular venous pressure. Various types of ventricular arrhythmias or atrioventricular conduction defects may be found.

Acute circulatory collapse, with hypotension, cold and clammy extremities, oliguria, and obtundation, may occur when myocardial damage is severe. Emboli and sudden death may occur.

2. Signs of associated disease–Signs of associated disease may be present in the lungs, skin, liver, kidneys, or elsewhere in patients with secondary myocardial disorders.

B. Electrocardiographic Findings: Findings on the ECG are usually nonspecific. ST–T changes, often in the inferior leads, are the most common abnormalities. If the inflammatory or infiltrative process affects the conduction system, the patient may have conduction defects.

C. X-Ray Findings: The radiologic findings are also nonspecific. The chest film may show an enlarged and globular heart and pericardial or pleural effusion or pulmonary venous congestion. If the patient has sarcoidosis, there may be hilar adenopathy and pulmonary infiltration. In lymphomatous and malignant disease, the radiologic examination may show evidence of tumor in various parts of the body.

D. Noninvasive Tests: Echocardiography may reveal enlargement of the left ventricle, E point separation in severe cardiac failure, and pericardial effusion. It is a means of ruling out other diseases (eg, hypertrophic cardiomyopathy and mitral stenosis).

E. Cardiac Catheterization: Cardiac catheterization is rarely performed in acute myocarditis unless the diagnosis is in doubt.

F. Endomyocardial Biopsy: Right ventricular endomyocardial biopsy is being used with increasing frequency. It occasionally establishes the specific cause of the myocarditis but more commonly shows a nonspecific inflammatory infiltrate that establishes a diagnosis of myocarditis but not its cause. Serial biopsies may prove the value of treatment with corticosteroids or immunosuppressive drugs but are not recommended for routine use.

Differential Diagnosis

Acute myocarditis resulting from infection with viruses (eg, coxsackieviruses), protozoa (eg, trypanosomes), or bacteria (eg, pneumococci) must be distinguished from acute toxic myocarditis due to drugs or diphtheria and from myocarditis associated with acute rheumatic fever, connective tissue disorders, and acute glomerulonephritis.

Nonviral myocarditis is recognized on the basis of the manifestations of the underlying disease. In acute myocardial toxicity due to drugs, awareness of the use of drugs for treatment of an underlying disease, their dosage, and the nature of the disease being treated help differentiate myocardial toxicity from acute myocarditis. The differentiation may be quite difficult in patients with acute lupus erythematosus with fever, pericarditis, and vasculitis, and specific diagnostic procedures such as LE cell preparations and serial neutralizing antibody determinations for viral infections may be required.

Treatment

In the absence of effective specific antiviral therapy, treatment consists of general supportive care, avoidance of vigorous exercise, and management of cardiac failure, arrhythmias, or conduction defects if they occur. Immunosuppressive drugs combined with corticosteroids may be used in severe cases in patients with rapidly developing cardiac failure.

In nonviral acute myocarditis, treatment is directed toward the underlying cause if known, as it is with diphtheria or pneumococcal infections. Some patients with *Candida* infections respond to amphotericin B or flucytosine. Anti-*Toxoplasma* chemotherapy (pyrimethamine and sulfonamide) results in marked clinical improvement or complete remission in patients with toxoplasmosis. Most cases of disseminated toxoplasmosis and myocarditis occur in immunosuppressed individuals or those who have defects in cellular immunity. Particular inquiry should be made regarding drugs that have a toxic effect on the myocardium such as drugs used in the treatment of leukemia and drugs used in depressed states, among others (see below).

Prognosis

Depending upon the cause, the cardiac failure of myocardial disease may differ from that due to ischemic cardiomyopathy or severe valvular disease. In acute viral myocarditis or peripartum cardiomyopathy, for example, cardiac failure may be completely reversible over a period of 1–2 months. In the case of viral myocarditis, cardiac failure may be recurrent; follow-up of patients with coxsackie B acute myocarditis indicates that most patients have no definite symptoms or signs of myocarditis, but chronic cardiac failure may result infrequently.

Daly K et al: Acute myocarditis: Role of histological and virological examination in the diagnosis and assessment of immunosuppressive treatment. *Br Heart J* 1984;**51**:30.

Fenoglio JJ et al: Diagnosis and classification of myocarditis by endomyocardial biopsy. *N Engl J Med* 1983;**308**:12.

Heikkila J, Karjalainen J: Evaluation of mild acute infectious myocarditis. *Br Heart J* 1982;**47**:381.

Mason JW, Billingham ME, Ricci DR: Treatment of acute inflammatory myocarditis assisted by endomyocardial biopsy. *Am J Cardiol* 1980;**45**:1037.

ACUTE MYOCARDIAL DAMAGE DUE TO DRUG TOXICITY

Acute myocardial damage has been noted in the past after use of a variety of drugs, notably emetine, digitalis, sympathomimetic drugs, corticosteroids, arsenic, antimony, amphetamines, and tricyclic antidepressants (amitriptyline and imipramine, among others). The decreased inotropic action of beta-adrenergic blocking drugs, verapamil, and disopyramide (Norpace) has also caused cardiac failure, especially when there have been previous episodes of cardiac failure. Myocardial toxicity is occurring with greater frequency as a result of the use of high doses of multiple cytotoxic drugs in the treatment of serious diseases. Recent observations indicate that about one-fourth of patients receiving high-dose multiple chemotherapy may die of acute myopericardial failure during treat-

ment as a result of endothelial injury, pericardial effusion, cardiac failure, and cardiac arrhythmias.

The toxic effects of cytotoxic agents are dose-related and more apt to occur when such drugs are used in combination. The total dose of doxorubicin in adults should not exceed 500 mg/m^2 body surface—less in children or if the patient has received radiation therapy to the mediastinum or is receiving concomitant therapy with other potentially cardiotoxic agents. Doxorubicin cardiotoxicity is decreased when the drug is given by continuous infusion as compared to the more usual route of slow intravenous injection (see Legha reference). Endomyocardial biopsy may show degenerative changes in the myocardium at doses lower than this.

As in any other variety of acute myocardial disease or toxicity, the patient may present with cardiac failure, arrhythmias, conduction defects, postural hypotension, or electrocardiographic T wave abnormalities. Patients receiving emetine (for amebiasis) or antimony (for schistosomiasis) may demonstrate electrocardiographic abnormalities without clinical symptoms or signs; it is then desirable to use alternative drugs or proceed with smaller dosages and close observation. Onset of failure may be rapid or delayed.

Serial ECGs, chest films, and echocardiograms, cautious restriction of total dosage, and close clinical observation for early evidence of cardiac involvement are advised. Decrease in the height of the R wave is an early sign of cardiac toxicity, and the risk/benefit ratio of continued therapy must be assessed.

Treatment

Withdraw cardiotoxic drugs and treat cardiac failure and arrhythmias.

Prognosis

The prognosis is good if appropriate measures are taken before severe cardiac failure occurs; poor if the offending drug is continued after early cardiac toxicity is manifest. Mild to moderate cardiac failure subsides gradually after the cardiotoxic drug is stopped.

Legha SS et al: Reduction of doxorubicin cardiotoxicity by prolonged continuous intravenous infusion. *Ann Intern Med* 1982;**96**:133.

Marshall JB, Forker AD: Cardiovascular effects of tricyclic antidepressant drugs: Therapeutic usage, overdose, and management of complications. *Am Heart J* 1982;**103**:401.

Saltiel E, McGuire W: Doxorubicin (Adriamycin) cardiomyopathy: A critical review. *West J Med* 1983;**139**:332.

CHRONIC CARDIOMYOPATHIES

This is a miscellaneous group of heart muscle diseases of unknown cause, divided on the basis of the clinical and hemodynamic features into 3 types: (1) congestive cardiomyopathy, with clinical features of cardiac enlargement, increased cardiac volume, and symptoms and signs of congestive failure with poor pump function; (2) hypertrophic cardiomyopathy (see p 266); and (3) restrictive cardiomyopathy, with infiltrative myocardial disease associated with endomyocardial fibrosis, amyloid disease, scleroderma, hemochromatosis, and other disorders that interfere with left ventricular filling and emptying (decreased distensibility). Restrictive cardiomyopathy is uncommon, and no further discussion will be presented. See the references for further information.

In cases of myocardial disease, the damage may include the ventricular conduction system and may cause destruction of the sinoatrial or atrioventricular node or large portions of the Purkinje system. Stokes-Adams attacks, arrhythmias, and sudden death are common in such disorders as scleroderma, sarcoidosis, and Chagas' disease, in which fibrosis dominantly involving the conduction system may occur.

1. CONGESTIVE (IDIOPATHIC) DILATED OR PRIMARY CARDIOMYOPATHY

Idiopathic dilated congestive cardiomyopathy is a nonspecific diagnosis, and there are no characteristics that distinguish it from congestive cardiomyopathy caused by a variety of myocardial diseases that have a similar end point: congestive failure. Excessive alcohol intake over a period of many years is a possible cause in many cases, as is ischemic coronary disease.

Clinical Findings

A. Symptoms: The disease is suspected early in patients who have dyspnea, chest pain, or palpitations. When right heart failure supervenes, peripheral edema may be a prominent symptom.

The chest pain is nondescript and not typical of angina pectoris. It may be related to pulmonary congestion or, if pleuritic, to pulmonary embolism. Pericardial pain is rare.

Patients who complain of palpitations may have chronic atrial fibrillation or paroxysmal atrial or ventricular arrhythmia. The arrhythmias may be incidental or may dominate the clinical picture. Ventricular premature beats occur in about half of cases; ventricular tachycardia or fibrillation usually occurs late.

Dizziness or syncope may occur from bradyarrhythmia or ventricular conduction defects secondary to fibrosis.

Symptoms of pulmonary or systemic emboli may occur, sometimes dominating the clinical features.

B. Signs: The signs are those of cardiac hypertrophy or cardiac failure (see p 244), and they do not differ from those seen in congestive heart failure resulting from other causes. The blood pressure is usually normal. A history of hypertension or intermittently raised pressure is present in 30–40% of patients with cardiomyopathy, but hypertension is not usually present in patients presenting with cardiac failure.

Signs of pulmonary emboli or systemic emboli may be found when these complications occur.

C. Laboratory Findings: There are no specific laboratory findings unless the congestive cardiomyopathy is due to a specific disease.

D. Electrocardiographic Findings: Changes evident on the ECG include left ventricular hypertrophy, conduction defects, and nonspecific ST–T abnormalities.

E. X-Ray Findings: The x-ray changes are those of cardiac enlargement, chiefly left ventricular, with a large cardiac volume and with pulmonary congestion but without disproportionate left atrial enlargement, calcified valves, or abnormalities of the aorta.

F. Echocardiography: Echocardiography is helpful in ruling out pericardial effusion, aortic stenosis (when the murmur is not heard because of a severely decreased cardiac output), and mitral valve disease, as well as in estimating left ventricular volume and ejection fraction. Massive increases in diastolic volume or decreases in ejection fraction (less than 20%) are poor prognostic signs.

G. Hemodynamic Findings and Angiography: The findings in advanced cases are those of a heart with large volume, poor contractions and generalized hypokinesis, decreased ejection fraction (usually 30–40% or less), increased left ventricular filling pressure, and possibly increased right atrial and right ventricular pressure. The left ventricular filling pressure may be raised out of proportion to right ventricular filling pressure, which helps to differentiate congestive or hypertrophic cardiomyopathy from constrictive pericarditis. This sign is not completely reliable, because if right ventricular failure occurs secondary to the left ventricular failure, the filling pressure may be approximately equal in the 2 ventricles.

Differential Diagnosis

A. Ischemic Cardiomyopathy: Increased left ventricular volume with decreased ejection fraction and generalized hypokinesis are seen on left ventricular angiography in both idiopathic cardiomyopathy and ischemic cardiomyopathy. The latter, however, may have segmental defects in contraction rather than symmetric hypokinesis. A history of myocardial infarction may be elicited, and myocardial ischemia may be induced by exercise.

B. Other Disorders: Other forms of cardiac disease (eg, valvular heart disease), hypertension, and secondary cardiomyopathies are discussed elsewhere.

Treatment

There are no specific measures for idiopathic dilated cardiomyopathy or endomyocardial fibrosis. Treat cardiac failure. Anticoagulant and antiarrhythmic treatment may be valuable in some cases.

Cardiac failure may be severe and unrelenting in idiopathic congestive cardiomyopathy, and the use of intravenous and oral vasodilators should be considered if the usual therapeutic agents fail.

Prognosis

The prognosis of advanced idiopathic cardiomyopathy is poor. Even with the best of care, survival for only 2–3 years is the rule, although some patients have survived 5–6 years. Prolonged bed rest and intensive treatment of cardiac failure may improve the prognosis. There are no data on whether vasodilator therapy to decrease the impedance against which the left ventricle contracts may prolong life, but this should be attempted if conventional therapy fails and cardiac failure persists.

Acquatella H et al: M mode and two-dimensional echocardiography in chronic Chagas' heart disease: A clinical and pathologic study. *Circulation* 1980;**62**:787.

Botstein GR, LeRoy EC: Primary heart disease in systemic sclerosis (scleroderma): Advances in clinical and pathologic features, pathogenesis, and new therapeutic approaches. *Am Heart J* 1981;**102**:913.

Fauci AS et al (moderators): NIH conference: The idiopathic hypereosinophilic syndrome: Clinical, pathophysiologic, and therapeutic considerations. *Ann Intern Med* 1982;**97**:78.

Feller ER et al: Familial hemochromatosis: Physiologic studies in the precirrhotic stage of the disease. *N Engl J Med* 1977; **296**:1422.

Goodwin JF: The frontiers of cardiomyopathy. *Br Heart J* 1982;**48**:1.

Johnson RA, Palacios I: Dilated cardiomyopathies of the adult. (2 parts.) *N Engl J Med* 1982;**307**:1051, 1119.

Kyle RA, Greipp PR: Amyloidosis (AL): Clinical and laboratory features in 229 cases. *Mayo Clin Proc* 1983;**58**:665.

Morkin E, Flink IL, Goldman S: Biochemical and physiologic effects of thyroid hormone on cardiac performance. *Prog Cardiovasc Dis* 1983;**25**:435.

Parrillo JE et al: The results of transvenous endomyocardial biopsy can frequently be used to diagnose myocardial diseases in patients with idiopathic heart failure. *Circulation* 1984;**69**:93.

Wahr DW, Schiller NB: Evaluating myopericardial disease with echocardiography. *J Cardiovasc Dis* 1982;**7**:799.

Weatherall DJ, Pippard MJ, Callender ST: Iron loading in thalassemia: Five years with the pump. (Editorial.) *N Engl J Med* 1983;**308**:456.

2. HYPERTROPHIC (OBSTRUCTIVE) CARDIOMYOPATHY
(Idiopathic Hypertrophic Subaortic Stenosis, IHSS; Asymmetric Septal Hypertrophy)

Hypertrophic cardiomyopathy, a genetic disease of unknown cause, is more common than was formerly thought. It is due essentially to asymmetric hypertrophy of the septum and free wall of the left ventricle in association with variable obstruction of the left ventricular outflow tract. Hypertrophy of the right ventricle with obstruction of the right ventricular outflow tract may coexist. The degree of obstruction is highly variable and is related to the contractile force of the left ventricle, the systemic vascular resistance (the "afterload"), and the left ventricular diastolic volume. Factors that increase the force of left ventricular contraction, such as inotropic agents (digitalis, isoproterenol) or the first beat following a postextrasystolic pause, cause or increase obstruction and result in a pressure difference, or gradient, across the left ventricular cavity below the aortic valve. Similarly, decrease in the systemic vascular resistance (such as occurs with amyl nitrite) decreases the impedance to left ventricular outflow, and the pressure gradient becomes increased as obstruction develops.

Clinical Findings
A. Symptoms: Dyspnea on exertion and chest pain are the commonest presenting symptoms. The pain is similar but not identical to angina pectoris and is not relieved by nitroglycerin. Fatigue and dizziness are often present. The dizziness is not related to unaccustomed exertion, as in aortic stenosis. Hypertrophic cardiomyopathy has been reported to be the most common cause of sudden death in young athletes. The symptoms are often related to the degree of obstruction in the infundibulum of the left ventricle. Anything that reduces systemic vascular resistance, such as a hot environment, pregnancy, exercise, or suddenly assuming the erect position, may induce symptoms. Left ventricular failure is a late manifestation, sometimes following atrial fibrillation.

B. Signs: The obstruction to left ventricular outflow is thought by some to be due to decreased volume of the left ventricular cavity resulting from forceful contraction of the thick left ventricle; others believe it is caused by impingement of the anterior leaflet of the mitral valve against the hypertrophied septum, which can be recognized clearly on echocardiography. The abnormal position of the anterior leaflet also results in mitral insufficiency with its characteristic pansystolic murmur; patients have as well a late crescendo systolic ejection murmur resulting from the left ventricular outflow tract obstruction. The carotid pulse and the left ventricular pressure pulse have a rapid upstroke time, since the forceful contraction of the hypertrophied left ventricle ejects most of the blood during the initial part of systole. When the increased force of contraction results in obstruction of the outflow tract, the ejection of blood is abruptly slowed, and a slower (double-humped) secondary wave then appears in both the left ventricular pressure pulse and the carotid artery as ejection continues. The palpable fourth heart sound due to decreased compliance of the left ventricle causes a "triple-humped" pressure pulse that can be demonstrated by palpation and by the apexcardiogram.

C. Laboratory Findings and Special Studies: Patients with hypertrophic cardiomyopathy demonstrate left ventricular hypertrophy electrocardiographically and radiologically. Left ventricular catheterization and angiography demonstrate the variable pressure gradient (which can be induced during the study; see above) across the ventricular outflow tract; the narrow systolic left ventricular outflow tract with marked, irregular septal hypertrophy; delayed left ventricular diastolic filling and relaxation; and abnormalities of systolic contraction that differ from those seen in valvular aortic stenosis. Amyl nitrite inhalation and isoproterenol induce or exaggerate the outflow obstruction murmur by reducing systemic vascular resistance and exaggerating the outflow obstruction.

Phenylephrine increases the systemic vascular resistance, decreases the outflow obstruction, and reduces the pressure gradient across the outflow track. The left ventricular end-diastolic pressure is almost always raised, especially after exercise, owing to the considerably decreased diastolic compliance of the hypertrophied left ventricle. A characteristic feature is impaired diastolic function with general and regional abnormalities of relaxation (see Goodwin reference, above). Inflow obstruction from decreased distensibility causes slow filling of the left ventricle, a large *a* wave, a slow *y* descent, and a small *v* wave in the left atrium. Decreased left ventricular filling due to decreased diastolic compliance is in contrast to the "pump failure" of dilated idiopathic cardiomyopathy. Coronary arteriograms are usually normal.

Echocardiographic findings are rapidly becoming the most practical and satisfactory means of making the diagnosis, obviating the need for cardiac catheterization in asymptomatic or mild cases. The 2 diagnostic features are asymmetric hypertrophy of the ventricular septum (the width of the septum is at least 1.3 times as great as the width of the posterior myocardium) and systolic anterior motion of the anterior cusp of the mitral valve, which approaches or impinges on the ventricular septum. The aortic valve is normal on echocardiography. The echocardiographic signs may be too sensitive and may occur in other conditions.

Course of the Disease

The course of the disease is variable. It may be first recognized by the symptoms of dyspnea, angina, or dizziness, which indicate a more advanced stage of the disease; by the pansystolic murmur of mitral insufficiency; by the presence of left ventricular hypertrophy; or by the demonstration of echocardiographic abnormalities. The inflow obstruction ultimately worsens, and as the left ventricular end-diastolic pressure and left atrial pressure rise, dyspnea may occur; later, cardiac output falls. Holter monitoring has shown that about half of patients have multiform or complex ventricular premature beats, including ventricular tachycardia, which may explain the frequency of syncope and sudden death in this syndrome. Sudden death, which occurs in about one-third of patients with this disease, unfortunately cannot be clearly related to the severity of symptoms or obstruction or to the degree of left ventricular hypertrophy. Sudden death can sometimes be associated with a family history of the disease where sudden death occurred, with rapidly worsening symptoms and signs, or with complex arrhythmias and ventricular tachycardia, but it may also occur in apparently healthy individuals, especially during vigorous exercise. Frequent ambulatory electrocardiographic monitoring and appropriate antiarrhythmic drugs may prove helpful.

Atrial fibrillation may, by further interfering with left ventricular filling, precipitate congestive heart failure. Systemic embolism, angina pectoris, syncope, and sudden death may also terminate the disease. Infective endocarditis may involve the mitral valve.

Treatment

Treatment is often not satisfactory, because it may not prevent progression of the disease or increase survival rates. Treatment begins with beta-adrenergic blocking agents such as propranolol to reduce the left ventricular end-diastolic pressure induced by exercise and sympathetic stimulation; compliance is increased and left ventricular contractility is decreased, lessening the obstruction to left ventricular outflow. Verapamil may be beneficial by improving left ventricular diastolic function. The effects have not been dramatic. In some patients, sinus bradycardia and sinus arrest may occur. Vasodilatation induced by the drug may increase left ventricular obstruction and induce symptoms. Care must be used in the presence of severe obstruction, left ventricular failure, or sinus node abnormalities. Because of the frequency of ventricular tachycardia and other ventricular arrhythmias shown by ambulatory monitoring, antiarrhythmic therapy should be considered in order to prevent sudden death. Amiodarone has been used with some success in these patients. If the patient remains symptomatic and receives no benefit from propranolol, surgery may be advised. Myotomy and limited resection of the hypertrophied muscle have occasionally produced gratifying results.

Chatterjee K et al: Hypertrophic cardiomyopathy: Therapy with slow channel inhibiting agents. *Prog Cardiovasc Dis* 1982;**25**:193.

Jones M, Barnhart GR, Morrow AG: Late results after operations for left ventricular outflow tract obstruction. *Am J Cardiol* 1982;**50**:569.

Maron BJ, Roberts WC, Epstein SE: Sudden death in hypertrophic cardiomyopathy: A profile of 78 patients. *Circulation* 1982;**65**:1388.

Nishimura RA, Giuliani ER, Brandenburg RO: Hypertrophic cardiomyopathy. *Cardiovasc Rev Rep* 1983;**4**:931.

PRIMARY CARDIAC TUMORS

Primary cardiac tumors are rare and constitute only a small fraction of all tumors that involve the heart or pericardium. Metastases may appear in the myocardium or the pericardium and infrequently affect left ventricular function, although when pericardial effusion occurs, the patient may show manifestations of pericardial tamponade. The most common primary cancers of the heart are sarcomas of various types.

A cardiac tumor may obstruct the venous or arterial vessels in the region of the heart, may obstruct the superior or inferior vena cava, or may interfere with left ventricular filling or left ventricular output.

The diagnosis is suggested by bizarre outlines of the cardiac shadow on plain films; by a clinical picture of cancer elsewhere; by the relationship of posture to symptoms of syncope or vertigo as well as to murmurs; and, in the case of pericardial effusion, by the finding of malignant cells in the fluid. Definitive diagnosis is by cineangiocardiography, which may demonstrate obstruction of any chamber. A recent patient presented with evidences of tricuspid stenosis due to angiosarcoma of the right atrium.

The most common benign tumor of the heart is myxoma—usually left atrial myxoma—although the right atrium may be involved and, more rarely, either ventricle. The patient usually presents in one of 3 ways: (1) With intermittent symptoms of syncope, vertigo, and dyspnea as well as signs suggesting mitral valve disease. There may be changing murmurs and differences of opinion among examiners. The tumor is usually on a stalk and is mobile, and the degree of mitral valve obstruction varies depending upon its position, the position of the patient, and varying hemodynamic events. (2) Systemic emboli (common in about one-third of cases). In some patients, the diagnosis can be made by histologic recognition of myxoma in the embolic tissue removed at surgery. (3) Systemic symptoms and signs that are thought to be immunologic in origin, consisting of fever, tachycardia, raised sedimentation rate, anemia, clubbed fingers, protein abnormalities, raised serum globulin, etc.

The diagnosis of left atrial myxoma is made by echocardiography, which shows multiple dense echoes representing a mass with its stalk posterior to the anterior mitral valve leaflet in diastole, and by cineangiocardiography, in which a filling defect is demonstrated. In carcinoid disease, echocardiography shows right ventricular volume overload and a thickened, shortened tricuspid valve with decreased mobility.

Treatment of myxoma consists of surgical excision, including removal of the base of the stalk to prevent recurrences. Surgical treatment of carcinoid valves has been of limited value but is being considered more often recently.

Gutman JM, Schiller NB: Carcinoid heart disease: Diagnostic usefulness of echocardiography. *Primary Cardiol* 1983; **9**:130.

Sutton MGSJ et al: Atrial myxomas: A review of clinical experience in 40 patients. *Mayo Clin Proc* 1980;**55**:371.

THE CARDIAC PATIENT & SURGERY

Major surgery in the cardiac patient is inevitably more hazardous than in patients with normal hearts. When shock, hemorrhage, hypoxia, struggling during induction of anesthesia, thromboembolism, and hypoventilation occur in a patient with heart disease, the danger of coronary occlusion, myocardial infarction, cardiac failure, and arrhythmias is increased.

The major cardiac lesions that increase the risks of surgery are rheumatic heart disease (especially aortic stenosis); coronary heart disease (about 5% additional hazard); and syphilitic cardiovascular disease, especially if there is involvement of the coronary ostia

(as suggested by associated angina). Hypertension without cardiac or renal involvement does not usually add to the surgical risk.

If possible, surgery of important magnitude and duration in patients with recent congestive failure should be delayed until 3 weeks after recovery; in patients with recent myocardial infarction a delay of 3–6 months is advisable. The patient should be brought into the best cardiac state possible before surgery, with medications, diet, and vitamin supplements. Anemia should be corrected. Presurgical electrolyte management is also very important in the cardiac patient.

In inducing and maintaining anesthesia in a cardiac patient, adequate ventilation, oxygenation, and smooth induction without struggling are important.

During surgery, hypotension should be treated promptly if it occurs, anemia avoided, and fluid therapy given to maintain optimal cardiac reserve.

Improvements in anesthesia and surgical skill have reduced the risk of major surgery in recent years. The presence of cardiac disease increases the risk but should not per se deny patients the benefits of elective but necessary surgery.

Gazes PC: Noncardiac surgery and dentistry and cardiac patients. Parts 1 and 2. *Primary Cardiol* 1983;**9**:139.

Goldman L: Cardiac risks and complications of non-cardiac surgery. *Ann Intern Med* 1983;**98**:504.

Rogers MC: Anesthetic management of patients with heart disease. *Mod Concepts Cardiovasc Dis* 1983;**52**:29.

Thibault GE et al: Medical intensive care: Indications, interventions, and outcomes. *N Engl J Med* 1980;**302**:938.

Tinker JH et al: Management of patients with heart disease for noncardiac surgery. *JAMA* 1981;**246**:1348.

Wells PH, Kaplan JA: Optimal management of patients with ischemic heart disease for noncardiac surgery by complementary anesthesiologist and cardiologist interaction. *Am Heart J* 1981;**102**:1029.

THE CARDIAC PATIENT & PREGNANCY*

The following information will assist in estimating the likelihood of cardiac failure in a pregnant woman: (1) functional class before pregnancy, (2) the age of the patient, (3) the size of the heart, (4) the structural lesion of the heart, (5) the presence of arrhythmias, (6) the patient's socioeconomic status (eg, if children are at home or if the patient must work), (7) the intelligence and cooperation of the patient, and (8) the presence of associated disease.

Assessment of Risk of Heart Disease in Pregnancy

A. Little or No Functional Incapacity: Almost all patients who are asymptomatic or who have only

*See also Chapter 13 for discussion of hypertension of pregnancy and other obstetric subjects.

mild symptoms with ordinary activities can continue to term under close medical supervision. If the patient develops more severe symptoms with activity, she should be hospitalized, treated for cardiac failure, and kept in bed until term.

B. Moderate or Marked Functional Incapacity: If the patient has pure mitral stenosis and develops acute pulmonary edema or has moderate to marked symptoms with activity, mitral valvulotomy should be considered. This has been successfully accomplished up to the eighth month. If the patient does not have an operable lesion, she should be hospitalized, treated for cardiac failure, and kept in bed until term.

C. Severe Functional Incapacity: All patients seen during the first trimester who have symptoms on little or no activity and who do not have an operable cardiac lesion should be aborted because of the high incidence of recurrent failure and death in this group of patients. Tubal ligation should be considered.

Physiologic Load That Pregnancy Imposes on the Heart

The work of the heart increases by about 50% at the beginning of about the third month, when the blood volume and cardiac output increase. In a normal pregnant woman, these physiologic factors can produce systolic "flow" murmurs. This, together with a normal physiologic S_3, can lead the physician to a false diagnosis of heart disease. The placenta acts as an arteriovenous fistula. Cardiac failure may occur at any time from the end of the first trimester up to 2–3 weeks before term, at which time the load for some unaccountable reason decreases. Cardiac arrhythmias, not uncommon (as in any variety of heart disease), may occur especially in patients with mitral valve or congenital heart disease.

Sodium should be restricted after the second month. Anticoagulants should be avoided and care taken with the use of any drugs in pregnancy.

Management of Labor

Current opinion holds that vaginal delivery is to be preferred except when there is an obstetric indication for cesarean section. Coarctation of the aorta may be the only cardiac disease that contraindicates vaginal delivery, because of the danger of aortic rupture.

The second stage should be made as short as possible, using forceps when possible. Ergonovine maleate (Ergotrate) should probably not be used because of the increased work of the heart that it causes.

Postpartum Cardiac Failure

Cardiac failure occurring in days or weeks after delivery in an apparently normal woman has been observed particularly in the tropics, where physicians believe it to be a distinct disease entity. Hemodynamic and echocardiographic studies indicate that left ventricular function is relatively normal despite edema and dyspnea. Clinical findings are not characteristic of congestive cardiomyopathy. The combination of fluid retention from high salt intake and increased cardiac output resulting from lying in heated beds (a tribal custom) may be the basic cause of the disease. Many patients promptly improve when they are hospitalized under normal environmental circumstances. Late follow-up indicates a good prognosis.

Cockburn J et al: Final report of study on hypertension during pregnancy: The effects of specific treatment on the growth and development of the children. *Lancet* 1982;**1**:647.

Elliot DL et al: Medical illness and pregnancy: An annotated bibliography of recent literature. *Ann Intern Med* 1983;**99**:83.

Lindheimer MD, Katz AI: Pathophysiology of pre-eclampsia. *Annu Rev Med* 1981;**32**:273.

Rotmensch HH, Elkayam U, Frishman W: Antiarrhythmic drug therapy during pregnancy. *Ann Intern Med* 1983;**98**:487.

Rubin PC et al: Placebo-controlled trial of atenolol in treatment of pregnancy-associated hypertension. *Lancet* 1983;**1**:431.

Selzer A: Management of pregnant patients with valvular heart disease. *Primary Cardiol* (Feb) 1981;**7**:127.

Tamari I et al: Medical treatment of cardiovascular disorders during pregnancy. *Am Heart J* 1982;**104**:1357.

• • •

References

Artman M, Parrish MD, Graham TP: Congestive heart failure in childhood and adolescence: Recognition and management. *Am Heart J* 1983;**105**:471.

Bennett WM et al: Drug therapy in renal failure: Dosing guidelines for adults. (2 parts.) *Ann Intern Med* 1980;**93**:62, 286.

Braunwald E (editor): *Heart Disease: A Textbook of Cardiovascular Medicine*, 2nd ed. Saunders, 1984.

Braunwald E, Mock MM, Watson JT (editors): *Congestive Heart Failure: Current Research and Clinical Application*. Grune & Stratton, 1982.

Cardiovascular diseases: An annotated bibliography of recent literature. *Ann Intern Med* 1983;**98**:679.

Gibson GS, Gibbons A: Hypertension among Blacks: An annotated bibliography. *Hypertension* 1982;**4**(1-Part 2):I1.

Goldman MJ: *Principles of Clinical Electrocardiography*, 11th ed. Lange, 1982.

Grossman W (editor): *Cardiac Catheterization and Angiography*, 2nd ed. Lea & Febiger, 1980.

Hagan AD et al: *Two-Dimensional Echocardiography*. Little, Brown, 1983.

Hatle L, Angelsen B: *Doppler Ultrasound in Cardiology*. Lea & Febiger, 1982.

Hurst JW, Logue RB: *The Heart, Arteries and Veins*, 5th ed. McGraw-Hill, 1982.

Johnson RA, Haber E, Austen WG (editors): *The Practice of Cardiology*. Little, Brown, 1980.

Marcus HL: *The Coronary Circulation in Health and Disease*. McGraw-Hill, 1983.

Morganroth J, Parisi AF, Pohost GM: *Noninvasive Cardiac Imaging*. Year Book, 1983.

Nadel JN (editor): *Physiology and Pharmacology of the Airways*. Marcel Dekker, 1980.

The National Conference on Cardiopulmonary Resuscitation and Emergency Cardiac Care: Standards and guidelines for cardiopulmonary resuscitation (CPR) and emergency cardiac care (ECC). *JAMA* 1980;**244:**453.

Scheinman MM (editor): *Cardiac Emergencies*. Saunders, 1984.

Selzer A: *Principles of Clinical Cardiology: An Analytical Approach*, 2nd ed. Saunders, 1983.

Shabetai R: *The Pericardium*. Grune & Stratton, 1981.

Sleight P, Jones JV (editors): *Scientific Foundations of Cardiology*. Heinemann, 1983.

Sokolow M, McIlroy MB: *Clinical Cardiology*, 3rd ed. Lange, 1981.

•   •   •

Key References

Borer JS: Key references: Obstructive and nonobstructive asymmetric septal hypertrophy. *Circulation* 1980;**62:**662.

Cardiovascular Diseases: An annotated bibliography of recent literature. *Ann Intern Med* 1983;**98:**679.

Cheitlin MD: Key references: Cardiovascular trauma. (2 parts.) *Circulation* 1982;**65:**1529 and **66:**244.

Cohn JN: Key references: Vasodilators in congestive heart failure. *Circulation* 1980;**61:**661.

Conti CR: Key references: Coronary artery spasm. *Circulation* 1980;**61:**862.

Fowler NO: Key references: Pericardial diseases. *Circulation* 1981;**63:**1429.

Gibson GS, Gibbons A: Hypertension among Blacks: An annotated bibliography. *Hypertension* 1982;**4(1-Part 2):**1.

Higgins CB: Key references: Coronary arteriography. *Circulation* 1980;**62:**439.

Karliner JS: Key references: Calcium-channel blockers in heart disease. *Circulation* 1982;**66:**675.

Kloster FE, Morris CD: Key references: Natural history of valvular heart disease. *Circulation* 1982;**65:**1283.

Mehta J: Key references: Prostaglandin and cardiovascular disease. *Circulation* 1982;**66:**474.

Nies AS: Key references: Beta blockers. *Circulation* 1982;**66:**1342.

Perloff JK: Key references: The cardiomyopathies: Dilated and restrictive. *Circulation* 1981;**63:**1189.

Roberts R: Key references: Modification of infarct size. *Circulation* 1980;**61:**458.

Rosen KM: Key references: Clinical cardiac electrophysiology. *Circulation* 1980;**61:**1262.

Sheffield LT: Key references: Clinical exercise stress testing. *Circulation* 1980;**61:**1053.

Spielman FJ, Popio KA: Key references: Pregnancy and heart disease. *Circulation* 1982;**65:**831.

Weisfeldt ML, Chandra N: Key references: Cardiopulmonary resuscitation. (2 parts.) *Circulation* 1982;**66:**898, 1133.

Blood Vessels & Lymphatics | 9

John M. Erskine, MD

DEGENERATIVE & INFLAMMATORY ARTERIAL DISEASES

Arteriosclerosis accounts for most forms of degenerative arterial disease. Its incidence increases with age; although manifestations of the disease may appear in the fourth decade, people over 40 (particularly men) are most commonly affected. Diseases that predispose to arteriosclerosis include the hyperlipidemic states, diabetes mellitus, and hypertension. Smoking apparently contributes to its development. Arteriosclerosis tends to be a generalized disease, with some degree of involvement of all major arteries, but it generally produces its major clinical manifestations by critical involvement of a limited number of arteries at a time. Gradual narrowing and ultimate occlusion of the artery are the most common manifestations of the disease, but weakening of the arterial wall, with aneurysmal dilatation of the arterial segment, also occurs, and both forms may be present in the same individual.

Less common forms of degenerative and inflammatory arterial disease that must be considered are cystic medial necrosis of the aorta, arteritis of both large and small arteries of undetermined cause, thromboangiitis obliterans (Buerger's disease), fibrodysplasia of visceral arteries, and syphilitic aortitis and arteritis. Radiation therapy will also result in a form of arteritis. The hemodynamic disturbances produced by these diseases may be very similar to those of arteriosclerosis.

DISEASES OF THE AORTA

ACUTE AORTIC DISSECTION

Essentials of Diagnosis
- Sudden severe chest pain with radiation to the back, abdomen, and hips.
- Shock may be present, though often not until the later stages.
- Central nervous system changes may occur.

- A history of hypertension is usually present.
- Dissection occurs most frequently in males.

General Considerations

Extravasation of blood into and along the wall of the aorta may occur, resulting in aortic dissection. Dissection generally begins either in the proximal aorta just above the aortic valve (types I and II, or proximal dissections) or at a site just beyond the origin of the left subclavian artery (type III, or distal dissections). The initial intimal tear probably results from the constant movement of the ascending and proximal descending aorta that occurs at these 2 points as a result of the pulsatile blood flow from the heart. Dissection can occur in a diseased aorta even without an intimal tear. Proximal dissections are more often in aortas involved with changes such as cystic medial necrosis or other forms of degeneration of the smooth muscle, elastic tissue, or collagen; distal dissections are more often associated with arteriosclerotic changes, they occur in a somewhat older age group, and hypertension is generally present prior to the dissection. When dissection occurs before age 40, Marfan's syndrome, pregnancy, or congenital heart disease is usually present, and hypertension may not be present in this group of patients. Both hypertension and a forceful pulse are important in the progression, which may extend from the ascending aorta distally to the abdominal aorta or beyond (type I). It may remain limited to the ascending aorta and the aortic valve area (type II), especially if hypertension is not present or is controlled early, and the distal (type III) dissections may progress not only distally but also proximally. Death may occur after hours, days, or weeks and is usually due to rupture of the aorta into the pericardial sac (cardiac tamponade) or into the left pleural cavity or the retroperitoneal area. The dissections may rupture back into the true lumen of the aorta (recanalization) with blood flow through both the true and false lumens; long-term survival can thus occur.

Clinical Findings

A. Symptoms and Signs: Severe, persistent pain of sudden onset is almost always present, most often in the anterior and posterior chest, although it may be limited to one or the other, and may later progress to the abdominal and hip areas. (Consider dissection in all adults with the abrupt onset of pain in those areas.) Radiation down the arms (so frequent in myocardial infarction) generally does not occur. Usually there is only a mild decrease in the prerupture hypertensive levels; if shock is present, it may respond to relatively small amounts of transfused blood. Partial or complete occlusion of the arteries arising from the aortic arch or of the intercostal and lumbar arteries may lead to such central nervous system findings as convulsions, hemiplegia, or paralysis of the lower extremities. Peripheral pulses and blood pressures may be diminished or unequal. Murmurs may appear over arteries along with signs of acute arterial insufficiency. An aortic diastolic murmur may develop as a result of dissection close to the aortic valve, resulting in secondary valvular insufficiency and heart failure. Fever is often present.

B. Laboratory Findings: Leukocytosis and LDH elevation are usually present. Electrocardiographic changes indicating left ventricular hypertrophy are often present; acute changes may not develop unless the dissection involves the coronary ostium or unless cardiac failure develops from acute aortic valvular insufficiency or from cardiac tamponade as a result of leakage into the pericardial sac.

C. X-Ray Findings: Chest x-rays often reveal an abnormal aortic contour or a wide superior mediastinum, with changes in the configuration and thickness of the aortic wall in successive films. There may be findings of pleural or pericardial effusion. CT scan with contrast enhancement, digital subtraction angiography, and radionuclide angiocardiographic studies are helpful diagnostic procedures and may be repeated to follow the clinical course. Aortography, when positive, may demonstrate an aortic wall greater than 1 cm in thickness, deformity of the true lumen, and a false channel with or without an open intimal tear.

Differential Diagnosis

Dissecting aneurysm is most commonly confused with myocardial infarction (see pp 220–230). Patients with dissecting aneurysm may also have heart disease, with old or recent electrocardiographic changes.

Treatment

A. Medical Measures: A combined and detailed program of intensive medical and surgical monitoring should be established promptly in an individual with severe spontaneous truncal pain; and, if hypertension is present, aggressive measures to lower the pressure should probably be initiated even before diagnostic studies have been completed. Treatment generally includes the simultaneous reduction of the systolic blood pressure to 100–120 mm Hg and reduction of the pulsatile aortic flow by means of the following:

(1) Start a rapid-acting antihypertensive agent as an intravenous infusion at a flow rate regulated by very frequent blood pressure determinations. Nitroprusside and trimethaphan (Arfonad) are the most commonly used drugs and may be given as follows: (a) Nitroprusside (50 mg in 1000 mL of 5% dextrose in water

and shielded from light by foil) is started at a rate of 0.5 mL/min, and the infusion rate may be increased by 0.5 mL every 5 minutes until adequate control of the pressure has been achieved. Daily serum thiocyanate levels should be obtained, and the infusion should be stopped if the drug level reaches 10 mg/dL. (b) Trimethaphan (1 or 2 mg/mL) may be infused at a flow rate determined by the blood pressure response and the possible side effects of the drug.

(2) The constant infusion of one of these 2 drugs is generally maintained for 24–48 hours, by which time the longer-acting agents, started shortly after the infusion, have become effective, and the infused drugs can then gradually be discontinued. A combination of propranolol and methyldopa may be indicated: (a) Propranolol, 1 mg intravenously over 20 minutes or 20 mg orally every 6 hours (or less if the pulse rate drops below 60/min). (b) Methyldopa, 250 mg intramuscularly or orally every 4–6 hours. If these drugs are not well tolerated or are contraindicated, reserpine, 0.25 mg orally every 12 hours (used in place of propranolol), and guanethidine, 25–50 mg orally every 12 hours (used in place of methyldopa), are other choices. A thiazide diuretic may also be used. (See p 206.)

Elevate the head of the bed 30–45 degrees and follow the ECG, blood pressure, central venous pressure, and hourly recording of urine output. If the state of consciousness worsens or urine output decreases significantly, allow the blood pressure to rise somewhat; if the chest and back pain does not diminish promptly, consider lowering the blood pressure to 70–80 mm Hg. Maintain urine output at 25–30 mL/h. Follow with daily chest films. An aortogram or one of the other x-ray studies that offers a full and detailed examination of the entire aorta should be obtained within hours of admission. If hypertension is not present, the pulsatile flow should still be reduced with oral reserpine (at least 0.5 mg/d) or propranolol (60–120 mg/d), and the drug should be continued for long-term therapy. If the patient's status becomes stabilized, oral intake may start in 3 days and ambulation in 2 weeks. Failure of this pharmacologic approach is suggested if (a) chest pain is not relieved or reappears; (b) a saccular aneurysm appears; (c) significant compromise or occlusion of a major branch of the aorta develops; or (d) progressive enlargement with impending rupture or leakage from the aneurysm occurs.

B. Surgical Measures: The emphasis in treatment has shifted toward surgery, as a result of increased proficiency in handling these very difficult technical problems. If a skilled cardiovascular team is available, all acute dissections involving the ascending aorta (types I and II) should probably be treated surgically to relieve or to prevent aortic valve insufficiency and to prevent rupture. Using total body hypothermia and circulatory arrest, the ascending aorta and, if necessary, the aortic valve and arch may be replaced with reattachment of the coronaries and brachiocephalic vessels.

Combined medical and surgical treatment is increasingly popular for the dissections arising in the descending thoracic aorta (type III); surgery is used after the hypertension and dissection have been stabilized by medical means. The origin of the dissection is then removed; the false lumen is closed; and a graft is inserted to deliver all blood flow through the normal lumen, thus relieving the occlusive pressure on the aortic branches.

Prognosis

Without treatment, the mortality rate at 3 months is 90%, but only 3% die immediately; 21% are dead in 24 hours, and 60% in 2 weeks. Survival without treatment, usually due to recanalization, does occasionally occur, and intensive pharmacologic methods to lower the pulse wave and blood pressure have led to healing of the dissected aorta in 50–80% of patients with an acute dissection and will convert others to a subacute or chronic form, which may then be treated by surgery. After 3 years, only 30% of the medically treated patients are alive as compared to 60% of those treated surgically. With the significant improvement in operative mortality rate, surgery by a skilled team now appears to be the treatment of choice.

Cachera JP et al: Surgical management of acute dissections involving the ascenda aorta: Early and late results in 38 patients. *J Thorac Cardiovasc Surg* 1981;**82**:576.

Ergin MA et al: Experience with profound hypothermia and circulatory arrest in the treatment of aneurysms of the aortic arch. *J Thorac Cardiovasc Surg* 1982;**84**:649.

Lemole GM et al: Improved results for dissecting aneurysms: Intraluminal sutureless prosthesis. *J Thorac Cardiovasc Surg* 1982;**83**:249.

Roberts WC: Aortic dissection: Anatomy, consequences, and cause. *Am Heart J* 1981;**101**:195.

Slater EE, DeSanctis RW: The clinical recognition of dissecting aortic aneurysm. *Am J Med* 1976;**60**:625.

ANEURYSMS OF THE THORACIC AORTA

The aneurysms of the ascending aorta are most commonly secondary to connective tissue disease, whereas those of the descending aorta are generally arteriosclerotic. Syphilitic aneurysms are now rare. Traumatic aneurysms may occur just beyond the origin of the left subclavian artery when the wall of the aorta is incompletely torn as a result of a rapid deceleration accident. Only one-sixth of aortic aneurysms are thoracic.

Clinical Findings

Manifestations depend largely on the size and position of the aneurysm and its rate of growth.

A. Symptoms and Signs: There may be no symptoms. Substernal, back, or neck pain may occur, as well as symptoms and signs due to pressure on (1) the trachea (dyspnea, stridor, a brassy cough), (2) the esophagus (dysphagia), (3) the left recurrent laryngeal nerve (hoarseness), or (4) the superior vena cava

(edema in the neck and arms, distended neck veins). The findings of regurgitation at the aortic valve may be present, together with manifestations of coronary or myocardial insufficiency.

B. X-Ray Findings: In addition to routine chest x-rays, aortography may be necessary to substantiate the diagnosis and to delineate the precise location and extent of the aneurysm and its relation to the vessels arising from the arch. CT scan is of more use than ultrasound in scanning thoracic aneurysms. Digital subtraction angiography, if available, is another means of evaluation. The coronary vessels and the aortic valve should also be studied if the ascending aorta is involved. An esophagogram may be of value.

Differential Diagnosis

It may be difficult to determine whether a mass in the mediastinum is an aneurysm, a neoplasm, or a cyst. The x-ray studies mentioned above (B) will distinguish an aneurysm. Radioactive isotope studies may be helpful in diagnosing a substernal goiter (^{125}I) or certain malignant tumors (gallium). Radionuclide angiocardiography may be helpful as a screening procedure before contrast angiography.

Treatment

Aneurysms of the thoracic aorta often progress, with increasing symptoms, and finally rupture. Resection of aneurysms is now considered the treatment of choice if a skilled surgical team is available and if the patient's general condition is such that the major surgical procedure usually required can be done with an acceptable risk. This is especially true if an aneurysm is large, associated with symptoms and signs, and limited to the ascending or descending aorta. Small asymptomatic aneurysms, especially in poor-risk patients, are perhaps better followed by x-ray and ultrasonography and treated only if progressive enlargement occurs. Hypertension—if present—should be controlled.

Saccular aneurysms with narrow necks can often be excised without occluding the aorta. Fusiform aortic aneurysms require resection and grafting of the aortic defect, often with the patient on partial or complete cardiac bypass. If the aortic valve is involved, an aortic valve replacement may be necessary, and reattachment of the coronary arteries or aortocoronary bypass grafts may also be indicated. Paraplegia is a dreaded complication of excision and graft replacement of aneurysms involving the descending thoracic aorta (3% of cases).

Prognosis

Small aneurysms may change very little over a period of years, and death may result from causes other than rupture. If the aneurysm is large, symptomatic, and associated with hypertension or arteriosclerotic cardiovascular disease, the prognosis is poor. In general, one-half will be dead in 3 years, one-half of survivors in 5 years, and two-thirds of those remaining in 10 years, but only about one-third of all deaths will result from rupture. Saccular aneurysms, those distal to the left subclavian artery, and even those limited to the ascending aorta can now be removed with an acceptable mortality rate. Resection of aneurysms of the transverse aortic arch involves major technical problems that can be dealt with by skilled surgical teams using hypothermia to protect the nervous system.

Crawford ES, Snyder DM: Aneurysms of the thoracic aorta: Basic principles of surgical treatment. *Contemp Surg* 1982; **21**:35.
Culliford AT et al: Aneurysms of the ascending aorta and transverse arch. *J Thorac Cardiovasc Surg* 1982;**701**:83.

ANEURYSMS OF THE ABDOMINAL AORTA

The vast majority of aneurysms of the abdominal aorta are below the origin of the renal arteries and generally involve the bifurcation of the aorta and thus the proximal end of the common iliac arteries. Aneurysms of the upper abdominal aorta are rare. Most aneurysms of the distal aorta are arteriosclerotic in origin and fusiform in shape. Eighty percent of aortic aneurysms are in the distal aorta.

Clinical Findings

A. Symptoms and Signs: Three phases can be recognized:

1. Asymptomatic–A pulsating mid and upper abdominal mass may be discovered on a routine physical examination, most frequently in men over 50. The calcification that frequently exists in the wall of the aneurysm may be discovered at the time of an abdominal x-ray examination. As a general rule, surgical resection should be advised even for an asymptomatic aneurysm, particularly if it is large. Although small aneurysms (< 6 cm) also rupture, surgery may occasionally be withheld if the patient is a poor operative risk and especially if there is significant cardiac, renal, pulmonary, or distal peripheral obliterative vascular disease. In such an individual, if hypertension is present, it should be controlled by medication. If the aneurysm later increases in size as determined by repeated physical and ultrasonic examinations or if it becomes symptomatic, operative treatment should be reconsidered.

2. Symptomatic–Pain is present in some form in one-fourth to one-third of cases and varies from mild midabdominal or lumbar discomfort to more severe constant or intermittent abdominal and back pain requiring narcotics for relief. Intermittent pain may be associated with a phase of enlargement or intramural dissection. Pain is an unfavorable prognostic sign that usually indicates the need for immediate surgery. Peripheral emboli may occur, even from small and unsuspected aneurysms, and symptomatic arterial insufficiency may result.

3. Rupture–Rupture of an aneurysm almost always causes death in a few hours and is therefore an indication for immediate surgical intervention without any of the delays associated with x-ray and laboratory studies. Pain is usually severe and sudden in onset. Because the hemorrhage is most often into the retroperitoneal tissues, which offer some resistance, shock and other manifestations of blood loss may at first be mild or absent; but free uncontrolled bleeding inevitably follows, resulting in death. There is an expanding, pulsating abdominal and flank mass, and subcutaneous ecchymosis is occasionally present in the flank or groin. About half of such patients can be saved by emergency surgery.

B. Laboratory Findings: Cardiac and renal function should be evaluated by means of electrocardiography, urinalysis, and blood urea nitrogen determination. Ultrasonic studies are of value and can be used to follow extension of aneurysms that are not removed following diagnosis.

C. X-Ray Findings: Curvilinear calcifications outlining portions of the aneurysm wall may be visible on plain films of the aortic area in approximately three-fourths of those with an aneurysm. In some cases the position of the aneurysm in relation to the renal arteries can be identified by intravenous urograms, but more often the examination is inconclusive. If distal occlusive disease or renovascular hypertension is suspected, an aortogram may be indicated to study the extent of the distal disease or the condition of the renal, carotid, and coronary arteries. CT scanning coupled with contrast-enhanced scanning or digital subtraction angiography can define the mass and its vascularity and may make arteriography unnecessary.

Treatment

Surgical excision and grafting of the defect is indicated for all aneurysms of the distal abdominal aorta in good-risk patients regardless of the size of the aneurysm. It is also advisable in all symptomatic aneurysms. Opinions differ as to whether asymptomatic small aneurysms in poor-risk patients with significant cardiovascular, pulmonary, or renal disease should be removed or should be followed closely by means of ultrasound measurements to detect any signs of growth. Patients with significant coronary or carotid artery disease are at risk during and following aneurysm resection, and surgery to lessen the chance of myocardial infarction or stroke prior to elective aneurysm surgery is sometimes advisable. If surgery is not performed, hypertension, if present, should be controlled. Individuals over age 80 with good preoperative risk factors can undergo elective surgery with an acceptable mortality rate; those with significant associated disease generally should not undergo operation without compelling indications.

Complications

Irreversible renal injury can occur if hemodynamic instability is allowed to develop through inadequate monitoring. The rather high incidence of early and late myocardial infarction in this group of patients may be diminished by preoperative coronary angiography in those with evidence of coronary disease and preoperative bypass grafting or angioplasty if indicated. Ischemia of the distal colon and of one or both legs occasionally occurs following this surgery; in most cases, it can be prevented by meticulous attention to detail before and during surgery.

Prognosis

The mortality rate following elective surgical resection is 3–8%, though in certain clinics it has recently approached 1%. Of those who survive surgery, approximately 60% are alive 5 years later, and of those who died, myocardial infarction was the leading cause of death. Among unoperated patients, less than 20% survive 5 years, and aneurysm rupture is the cause of 60% of the deaths. In general, a patient with an aortic aneurysm has a 3-fold greater chance of dying as a consequence of rupture of the aneurysm than of dying from surgical resection.

Crawford ES et al: Infrarenal abdominal aortic aneurysm: Factors influencing survival after operation performed over a 25-year period. *Ann Surg* 1983;**193**:699.

Crawford ES et al: Symposium: Prevention of complication of abdominal aortic reconstruction. *Surgery* 1983;**91**:93.

Szilagyi DE, Elliott JP, Smith RF: Clinical fate of the patient with asymptomatic abdominal aortic aneurysm and unfit for surgical treatment. *Arch Surg* 1972;**104**:600.

Whittemore AD et al: Aortic aneurysm repair: Reduced operative mortality associated with maintenance of optimal cardiac performance. *Ann Surg* 1980;**192**:414.

*   *   *

PERIPHERAL ARTERY ANEURYSMS
(Popliteal & Femoral)

Popliteal artery aneurysms rank third in frequency among aneurysmal lesions; most of the other peripheral aneurysms are femoral. Almost all are arteriosclerotic and occur in men. They are often multiple and bilateral, and aneurysmal disease of the aortoiliac vessels is commonly associated with the more peripheral aneurysms.

Popliteal Aneurysms

Almost half are asymptomatic when diagnosed, and they are generally discovered in the popliteal fossa as a pulsating mass 2 cm or more in diameter. Most aneurysms present with symptoms generally related to varying degrees of arterial insufficiency to the lower leg and foot, ie, intermittent claudication if insufficiency develops slowly, or severe ischemic manifestations with rest pain, pregangrene, or gangrene if sudden thrombosis of the aneurysm has developed or, less commonly, if distal embolization has occurred. (See pp 277–281.) When complete thrombosis has occurred, a nonpulsatile popliteal mass is noted. The large aneurysms may be associated with a degree of venous obstructive manifestations or pain from pressure on the nerves; thrombophlebitis is infrequent, and rupture is rare.

Angiography may be helpful in defining the aneurysm if it is not partly filled with clot and is certainly of value in defining the distal arterial tree and the collateral vessels. The actual size of the aneurysm is more clearly determined by ultrasound examination.

Popliteal aneurysms rank second to abdominal aortic aneurysms in the incidence of potentially serious complications. Even small aneurysms (2 cm in size) can become thrombosed or give rise to emboli, particularly if laminated clot is demonstrated within the lumen of the aneurysm. When thrombosis occurs, over 40% will require amputation. No amputation should be necessary when the aneurysm is treated surgically in the asymptomatic stage. Thus, surgery is usually advisable, and a reversed saphenous vein bypass graft with proximal and distal ligation of the aneurysm is generally employed. In large aneurysms with manifestations of vein or nerve compression, resection of the aneurysm with grafting of the arterial defect may be necessary.

Femoral Aneurysms

Femoral aneurysms, as manifested by a pulsatile mass in the femoral area on one or both sides, have the potential for the same complications as popliteal aneurysms, although rupture is a more frequent complication and limb-threatening episodes are less frequent in femoral aneurysms. Because the incidence of serious complications in the asymptomatic group seems to be considerably less than for popliteal aneurysms, there is more reason to follow rather than operate on smaller, asymptomatic femoral aneurysms and to deal first with aortoiliac and then popliteal aneurysms in preference to femoral aneurysms when aneurysmal disease exists in all of these areas.

Graham LM et al: Clinical significance of arteriosclerotic femoral artery aneurysms. *Arch Surg* 1980;**115**:502.

Szilagyi DE, Schwartz RL, Reddy DJ: Popliteal arterial aneurysms: Their natural history and management. *Arch Surg* 1981;**116**:724.

Whitehouse WM et al: Limb-threatening potential of arteriosclerotic popliteal artery aneurysms. *Surgery* 1983;**93**:694.

ARTERIOSCLEROTIC OCCLUSIVE DISEASE

OCCLUSIVE DISEASE OF THE AORTA & ILIAC ARTERIES
(The Leriche Syndrome)

Occlusive disease of the aorta and the iliac arteries begins most frequently just proximal to the bifurcation of the common iliac arteries and at or just distal to the bifurcation of the aorta. Atherosclerotic changes occur in the intima and media, often with associated perivascular inflammation and calcified plaques in the media. Progression involves the complete occlusion of one or both common iliac arteries and then the abdominal aorta up to the segment just below the renal vessels. Although atherosclerosis is a generalized disease, occlusion tends to be segmental in distribution, and when the involvement is in the aortoiliac vessels there may be minimal atherosclerosis in the more distal external iliac and femoral arteries. The best candidates for direct arterial surgery are those with localized occlusions at or just beyond the aortic bifurcation with relatively normal vessels proximally and distally.

Clinical Findings

Intermittent claudication is almost always present in the calf muscles and is usually present in the thighs and buttocks. It is most often bilateral and progressive, so that by the time the patient seeks help the pain may be produced by walking a block or less. Some complain only of weakness in the legs when walking or a feeling of "tiredness" in the buttocks. Difficulty in having or sustaining an erection is a common complaint in men. Coldness of the feet may be present; rest pain is infrequent.

Femoral pulses are absent or very weak. Pulses distal to the femoral area are usually absent. A pulsation in the abdominal aorta is usually present. A bruit may be heard over the aorta or the iliac or femoral arteries. Atrophic changes of the skin, subcutaneous tissues, and muscles of the distal leg are usually minimal or absent, and dependent rubor and coolness of the skin of the foot are minimal unless distal arterial disease is also present.

If surgery is being seriously considered, a translumbar aortogram will usually give valuable information regarding the level and extent of the occlusion and the condition of the vessels distal to the block. If coronary heart disease or carotid murmurs are present, arteriography should probably also include those vessels, for half of postoperative and later deaths are related to coronary artery disease. If significant disease is present, direct myocardial revascularization may be considered before aortic surgery.

Treatment

Surgical treatment is indicated if claudication interferes appreciably with the patient's essential activities or work. It is generally not advisable if the condition alters the individual's usual activities in only minor ways. The objective of treatment is reestablishment of blood flow through the narrowed or occluded aortoiliac segment to relieve claudication. If significant occlusive disease exists in the thigh and leg as well, relief of ischemic problems may also be necessary and can generally be achieved by means of surgery in the proximal aorto-iliac-femoral area.

A. Arterial Graft (Prosthesis): An arterial prosthesis bypassing the occluded segment is the treatment of choice in the more extensive aortoiliac occlusions. In general, the bifurcation graft extends from the infra-

renal abdominal aorta, usually by means of an end-to-end anastomosis, to the distal external iliac or common femoral arteries as end-to-side anastomoses. A patient with leg ischemia who is considered to be too poor a risk for the major surgical procedure in the aortoiliac area can be treated with little risk and generally good results by means of a graft from the axillary artery to one or both femoral arteries or, in the case of iliac unilateral disease, from the femoral artery with normal blood flow to the femoral artery distal to the stenotic iliac vessel. (See above for complications of aortic surgery.)

B. Thromboendarterectomy: This procedure, which avoids the use of a prosthesis, is generally used when the occlusion is limited to the common iliac arteries and when the external iliac and common femoral arteries are free of significant occlusive disease.

C. Percutaneous Transluminal Angioplasty: This is a very effective means of dealing with symptomatic iliac artery stenoses by the transfemoral artery approach. A major operation is avoided. It should not be used in complete common iliac artery occlusion because of the danger of embolization down the contralateral iliac artery. Postsurgical sexual problems in men are avoided by this technique, and in those already affected with impotence, relief of the problem may occur. See below for further details of this technique.

D. Sympathectomy: A bilateral lumbar sympathectomy should be added to the direct arterial procedure if there is occlusive disease in the arteries of the thighs or legs. Aortoiliac surgery, especially when combined with bilateral sympathectomies, may result in sexual dysfunction in men who are still sexually active, so sympathectomy should probably be avoided in these patients.

Prognosis

The operative mortality rate is 2–6%, and the immediate and long-term benefits are often impressive, particularly if there is no significant distal occlusive disease. In those with no distal occlusive disease, improvement is both subjective and objective, with relief of all or most of the claudication and, usually, return of all of the pulses in the extremities. Late occlusions in this group of patients are infrequent, and if proper judgment is used in patient selection, results are comparable for angioplasty, endarterectomy, and arterial grafting techniques.

Crawford ES et al: Aortoiliac occlusive disease: Factors influencing survival and function following reconstructive operation over a 25-year period. *Surgery* 1981;**90**:1055.

Darling RC et al: Aorto-iliac reconstruction. *Surg Clin North Am* 1979;**59**:565.

Ray LI et al: Axillofemoral bypass: Critical reappraisal of its role in the management of aortoiliac disease. *Am J Surg* 1979; **138**:117.

OCCLUSIVE DISEASE
OF THE FEMORAL
& POPLITEAL ARTERIES

In the region of the thigh and knee, the vessels most frequently blocked by occlusive disease are the superficial femoral artery and the popliteal artery. Atherosclerotic changes usually appear first at the most distal point of the superficial femoral artery, where it passes through the adductor magnus tendon into the popliteal space. In time, the whole superficial femoral artery may become occluded; the disease progresses into the popliteal artery less frequently. The common femoral and deep femoral arteries are usually patent and relatively free of disease, although the origin of the profunda femoris is sometimes narrowed. The distal popliteal and its 3 terminal branches may also be relatively free of occlusive disease.

Clinical Findings

As a rule, the changes are initially more advanced in one extremity than the other, although similar changes often appear later in the opposite extremity.

A. Symptoms and Signs: (See also p 278.) Intermittent claudication, which may appear after walking one-half to one block, is confined to the calf and foot. Atrophic changes in the lower leg and foot may be quite definite, with loss of hair, thinning of the skin and subcutaneous tissues, and diminution in the size of the muscles. Dependent rubor and blanching on elevation of the foot are usually present. When the leg is lowered after elevation, venous filling on the dorsal aspect of the foot may be slowed to 15–20 seconds or more. The foot is usually cool or cold. If these findings are marked or if rest pain is present, significant occlusive disease in the aortoiliac or lower leg vessels should also be suspected. The common femoral pulsations are usually of fair or good quality, although a bruit may be heard. No popliteal or pedal pulses can be felt. Pressure measurements in the distal leg, using ultrasound, will supply an objective functional assessment of the circulation and will aid in the decision whether to follow the patient or to go on to x-ray studies and possibly surgery.

B. X-Ray Findings: X-rays of the thigh and leg may show calcification of superficial femoral and popliteal vessels. A femoral arteriogram will show the location and extent of the block as well as the status of the distal vessels, and lateral or oblique views will reveal whether the origin of the profunda femoris is narrow. It is important to know the condition of the aortoiliac vessels also, since a relatively normal inflow as well as an adequate distal "run-off" is important in determining the likelihood of success of an arterial procedure. A translumbar aortogram or a retrograde transfemoral Seldinger catheter study with added oblique and leg and foot views will supply important information.

Treatment

Surgery is indicated (1) if intermittent claudication is progressive or incapacitating and thus interferes significantly with the patient's essential physical activities such as ability to work or (2) if there is rest pain or if there are pregangrenous or gangrenous lesions on the foot and it is hoped that a major amputation can be avoided. Procedures to improve blood flow to an extremity should not be employed if studies reveal that they have little or no chance of success.

A. Arterial Graft: An autogenous vein graft using a reversed segment of the great saphenous vein can be placed, bypassing the occluded segment. The distal anastomosis is usually to the popliteal artery, below the site of major occlusive disease. When the entire popliteal artery is occluded and gangrene or advanced ischemic changes are present in the foot, it is generally better to perform an amputation below the knee rather than an anastomosis to one of the leg arteries, though in very carefully selected patients anastomosis to a tibial or peroneal artery may save the extremity. Synthetic arterial prostheses, with the possible exception of the new PTFE (polytetrafluoroethylene; Gore-Tex) grafts, have not proved to be very successful in this area because of the relatively high incidence of early or late thrombosis.

B. Thromboendarterectomy: Thromboendarterectomy with removal of the central occluding core may be successful if the occluded and stenotic segment is very short.

When significant aortoiliac or common femoral occlusive disease exists as well as superficial femoral and popliteal occlusions, it is usually better to relieve the obstructions in the larger, proximal arteries and deliver more blood flow to the profunda femoris than to operate on the smaller distal vessels, where the chances of success are less. If the origin of the profunda femoris is narrowed as demonstrated by arteriography of the area, including oblique views, a limited procedure at that site—a profundoplasty—may be successful in improving blood flow to the leg and foot and may be used, especially in poor-risk patients with rest pain.

C. Percutaneous Transluminal Angioplasty: An advance in the treatment of arterial stenoses, either arteriosclerotic or fibromuscular, involves the introduction of a double-lumen catheter with a balloon near the tip through the skin into the artery. Under radiographic control, the Gruntzig balloon can be placed across a stenosis that can then be disrupted by dilating the balloon, which is calibrated to expand only to the size of that normal vessel segment. In the process, the intima is split, the media overstretched, and the stenosis generally eliminated. Fibrous healing results in a normal-sized lumen that persists for months or years. Although recurrent stenosis may occur, it may again be dilated, and failure of the procedure does not generally result in significant complications, nor does it interfere with early or late surgical bypass procedures to deal with the arterial insufficiency should such procedures become necessary.

1. Most favorable lesions–Single, short, discrete stenosis in medium-sized arteries such as the iliac-femoral-popliteal vessels.

2. Less favorable lesions–Multiple stenosis in series, those longer than 5 cm, complete occlusions less than 5 cm long, small arteries, recent acute occlusions (in conjunction with local intra-arterial streptokinase infusion).

3. Poor-risk surgical patients or those with stenosis in inaccessible areas such as the renal or coronary arteries are particularly suitable for treatment with this technique (see pp 202 and 218).

4. Stenotic arterial anastomoses or grafts may sometimes be dilated.

5. The technique is not suitable for carotid artery stenosis, because of the serious nature of even small emboli to the brain. Complications, though infrequent, include embolism, thrombosis of the dilated stenosis, and arterial perforation or rupture; a surgical team should generally be available to deal with such problems on an emergency basis. In the femoral-popliteal area, where arterial spasm following the dilatation may be a problem, heparin is often used. Antiplatelet therapy is usually employed for several months following the procedure.

Immediate and long-term success rates in properly selected cases are comparable to those achieved by surgical means, and the expense of this form of therapy is considerably less. Results in diabetics and in those who continue to smoke are less good.

D. Sympathectomy: Lumbar sympathectomy may be used as an adjunct to grafting or endarterectomy or as the only operation if an arterial procedure is thought inadvisable. The vasodilator effect of sympathectomy may improve the circulation to the skin of the lower leg and foot.

Prognosis

Thrombosis of the ''bypass'' graft or of the endarterectomized vessel either in the immediate postoperative period or months or years later is relatively frequent in the superficial femoral-popliteal area. This is particularly true if one or more of the 3 terminal branches of the distal popliteal artery are occluded or badly diseased or if endarterectomy or a synthetic prosthesis is used. For this reason, operation is usually not recommended for mild or moderate claudication, and approximately 80% of these patients will have relatively stable symptoms and will go for years without much progression of their symptoms or the development of ischemia or gangrene. Some may improve as collateral circulation develops. The chances of improvement after surgery are less in patients with ischemia or early gangrene, but the procedure is often justified because some limbs can be saved from amputation. Failure of the graft or the endarterectomy may make the condition of the limb worse than it was before the procedure and may complicate a subsequent amputation, particularly if the distal anastomosis is to a lower leg artery. The 5-year overall patency rate for the

saphenous vein bypass grafts—the procedure of choice in most cases—is in the range of 60–80%, or less if the bypass is to a tibial artery. The two-year patency rate after transluminal angioplasty is over 80% and thus compares favorably with the venous bypass results over that period, although the long-term results may not be as good. Only about 50% of these patients survive 5 years; most deaths are due to complications of arteriosclerosis, usually of the coronary arteries. After 5 years, the yearly mortality rate exceeds the rate of loss of patency of the graft.

Athanasoulis CA: Percutaneous transluminal angioplasty: General principles. *Am J Rad* 1980;**135**:893.
Bergan JJ et al: Symposium on transluminal angioplasty. *Arch Surg* 1981;**116**:804.
Mannick JA: Femoro-popliteal and femoro-tibial reconstructions. *Surg Clin North Am* 1979;**59**:581.
Roberts B, Ring EJ: Current status of percutaneous transluminal angioplasty. *Surg Clin North Am* 1982;**62**:357.
Szilagyi DE et al: Autogenous vein grafting in femoropopliteal atherosclerosis: The limits of its effectiveness. *Surgery* 1979; **86**:836.
Wilson AR, Fuchs JCA: Percutaneous transluminal angioplasty. *Surg Clin North Am* 1984;**64**:121.

OCCLUSIVE DISEASE OF THE ARTERIES IN THE LOWER LEG & FOOT

Occlusive processes in the lower leg and foot may involve, in order of incidence, the tibial and common peroneal arteries and their branches to the muscles, the pedal vessels, and occasionally the small digital vessels. Symptoms depend upon the vessels that are narrowed or thrombosed, the suddenness and extent of the occlusion, and the status of the proximal and collateral vessels. The clinical picture may thus vary from a rather stable or a slowly progressive form of vascular insufficiency that over months or years may ultimately result in atrophy, ischemic pain, and, occasionally, gangrene. A rapidly progressive and extensive thrombosis will result in acute ischemia and often gangrene.

Clinical Findings

Although all of the possible manifestations of vascular disease in the lower leg and foot cannot be described here, there are certain significant clinical aspects that enter into the evaluation of these patients.

A. Symptoms:

1. **Claudication**–Intermittent claudication is the commonest presenting symptom. Aching fatigue during exertion usually appears first in the calf muscles; in more severe cases a constant or cramping pain may be brought on by walking only a short distance. Less commonly, the feet are the site of most of the pain. Pain that lasts longer than 10 minutes after rest suggests some other disease, such as arthritis. The distance that the patient can walk before pain becomes severe enough to necessitate a few minutes' rest gives a

rough estimate of circulatory inadequacy: 2 blocks (360–460 m) or more is mild, 1 block is moderate, and one-half block or less is severe.

2. Rest pain–Rest pain may be due to sepsis or ischemia. The former is usually throbbing, whereas ischemia usually produces a persistent, gnawing ache with occasional spasms of sharp pain. Rest pain often comes on in bed at night, when the cardiac output is less. A degree of relief can often be obtained by uncovering the foot and letting it hang over the side of the bed. In more advanced stages, the pain may be constant and so severe that even narcotics may not relieve it. Ischemic neuropathy is an important factor in this condition. The patient may request amputation.

3. Muscle cramps–Sudden painful contractions that last only a few minutes but leave a feeling of soreness for minutes or days in a pulseless leg are usually related to the arterial disease.

B. Signs:

1. Absence of pulsations–Careful palpation over the femoral, popliteal, dorsalis pedis, and posterior tibial arteries should be done to determine which pulsations are present. Although the popliteal pulse may be present, both pedal pulses are usually absent. Exercise may make pedal pulses disappear in certain patients with arterial disease. If a strong popliteal pulse is present, a direct surgical approach on the vessels of the lower extremity is not likely to be of value unless emboli to the distal vessels are the cause of the ischemic changes.

2. Color changes in the feet–Defective blood supply causes anoxic paralysis of the capillaries and a bluish-red skin (rubor). The rate of return of color following blanching induced by local pressure is an inaccurate index of circulatory adequacy because the blood that returns on release of the pressure does not necessarily represent true circulation.

a. Pallor upon elevation–If pallor appears rapidly upon elevation of the foot from the horizontal—or if it appears when the leg is only slightly raised—the circulatory status is poor.

b. Flushing time–Color normally returns in a few seconds to a foot placed in a dependent position after 1–2 minutes of elevation of the entire lower extremity. The poorer the collateral circulation, the longer the interval before flushing begins to appear in the toes. If flushing time is over 20 seconds—and especially if it appears only after 45–60 seconds—the arterial disease is extensive.

c. Dependent rubor–Beefy redness of the toes or foot on dependency is frequently present in occlusive disease, but it may not reach its full extent until a minute or more after the leg has been placed in the dependent position. Dependent rubor implies moderate or severe arterial occlusive disease.

d. Rubor of stasis–When almost complete stasis in the distal vessels occurs, with venous as well as arterial thrombosis and extravasation of red blood cells, redness of the toes and forefoot may develop that may not completely disappear on elevation of the leg. Usually, however, there is pallor of the skin surround-

ing the red area in the elevated leg. This disorder is often associated with severe pain and is more commonly noted in thromboangiitis obliterans than in atherosclerosis.

e. Patchy cyanosis and pallor indicate severe ischemia; they are seen frequently following acute thrombosis or recent embolism.

3. Venous filling time–If the valves in the saphenous system are competent, venous filling is a valuable gauge of collateral circulation of the foot. If it takes the veins on the dorsum of the foot more than 30 seconds to fill when the leg is placed in a dependent position after having been elevated for a minute, the circulatory impairment in the leg is severe.

4. Local tissue changes–Diminished arterial flow causes wasting of the subcutaneous tissues of the foot and lower leg. Hair is lost over these areas, the skin becomes smooth and shiny, and the nails may become thickened and deformed. Infections are common following minor injuries or even without injury at the edge of a nail or under a thick callus. Once established, infection may become indolent and chronic, with the formation of an ischemic ulcer that is often located over a pressure point of the foot; or the infection may lead to localized or progressive gangrene. Local heat should not be used in the treatment of such an infection.

5. Skin temperature–If arterial circulation is inadequate, the leg will feel quite cool.

6. Sweating–The feet are often dry, but if a patient with occlusive disease still notes sweating of the feet, some degree of sympathetic activity is present and lumbar sympathectomy may be of benefit.

C. X-Ray Findings: Films of the lower leg and foot may show calcification of the vessels. If there is a draining sinus or an ulcer close to a bone or a joint, osteomyelitis may be apparent on the film. If fairly strong popliteal pulses can be felt, arteriography is not likely to be of much value as a guide to surgical treatment; sometimes, however, the status of the femoral or popliteal arteries must be evaluated in this way.

D. Physiologic Testing: Pressure and blood flow measurements may be done in an extremity distal to occlusive disease by utilizing ultrasonic Doppler measurements, radioactive isotope clearance, and plethysmography. These are useful in the initial evaluation and in following the progress of the vascular disease or evaluating the results of treatment.

E. Arterial Disease in Diabetic Patients: Atherosclerosis develops more often and earlier in patients with diabetes mellitus, especially if the disease has been poorly controlled over a period of years. Either the large or small vessels may be involved, but occlusion of the smaller vessels is relatively more frequent than in the nondiabetic, and diabetics thus more often have the form of the disease that may not be suitable for arterial surgery. Cigarette smoking, vascular impairment, and inadequate patient education and understanding of specific problems increase risk. The resistance to infection is less. Anesthesia of the toes and distal foot (due to diabetic neuropathy) develops in some and predisposes to injury and secondary ulcers. In patients with such neurogenic ulcers, pain may be minimal and the peripheral circulation may be adequate, so that local healing may take place at a relatively normal rate. Recurrent trouble is frequent, however, and because of the sensory deficit, injury and secondary infection may be advanced before the condition is noted. Poor vision due to diabetic retinopathy makes care of the feet more difficult and injuries more likely (see p 773).

Ulcers, when present, are more likely to be moist and infected, and healing, if it occurs at all, may be very slow. Gangrene may advance rapidly.

Treatment

A. Intermittent Claudication: The patient should be instructed to walk slowly, take short steps, avoid stairs and hills, and stop for brief rests to avoid pain. Walking, however, is the most effective way to develop collateral circulation, and walking up to the point of claudication, followed by a 3-minute rest, should be done at least 8 times a day.

B. Circulatory Insufficiency in the Foot and Toes: Lumbar sympathectomy may be indicated when ischemic or pregangrenous changes are present in the distal foot, when small ulcers are present in a foot with diminished circulation, and in patients who have mild to moderate rest pain. Sympathectomy reduces vasoconstrictive reflexes involving the vessels to the skin, often resulting in a dry, warm foot. There is usually no change in the circulation to the muscles and thus no relief from claudication or change in the level of an inevitable amputation. Predictive tests to calibrate the vasospastic activity and thus the possible benefit of the procedure are unreliable. Patients who cannot tolerate the surgical procedure may be considered for chemical sympathectomy with 6% phenol. Vasodilator drugs are of little or no value and may be harmful, but encouraging results are reported with prostaglandins E_2 and I_2 used intra-arterially or intravenously in critical situations (see Jacobsen reference, p 271). The general care of the feet is most important (see p 773).

C. Infections, Ulcers, and Gangrene of the Toes or Foot:

1. Early treatment of acute infections–Place the patient at complete bed rest with the leg in a horizontal or slightly depressed position. An open or discharging lesion should be covered with a light gauze dressing, but tape should not be used on the skin. Culture and sensitivity studies should be obtained if there is any purulent discharge, but if advancing infection is present an appropriate antibiotic should be started immediately. Drain purulent pockets.

Ulcerations covered with necrotic tissue can often be prepared for spontaneous healing or grafting with wet dressings of sterile saline changed 3–4 times a day. Petrolatum or Xeroform gauze and a bacitracin-neomycin ointment may also help soften crusted infected areas and aid drainage.

Treat diabetes and anemia, if present.

2. Early management of established gangrene–In most instances an area of gangrene will progress to a point where the circulation provided by the inflammatory reaction is sufficient to prevent progressive tissue death. The process will at least temporarily demarcate at that level. This can be encouraged by measures similar to those outlined in the preceding section on the treatment of acute infection. If the skin is intact and the gangrene is dry and due only to arterial occlusion, antibiotics should be withheld. If infection is present or if the gangrene is moist, antibiotics should be used in an effort to limit the process and prevent septicemia.

If the gangrene involves only a segment of skin and the underlying superficial tissue, sympathectomy and, if possible, an artery graft may reverse the process (see p 278). The necrotic tissue can then be removed and the ulcer grafted or allowed to heal as outlined above in the section on ulcers. If the hoped-for healing does not occur and amputation is required, it can sometimes be carried out at a more distal level because of those procedures.

3. Amputations for gangrene–

a. A toe that is gangrenous to its base can sometimes be amputated through the necrotic tissue and left open; this procedure may be employed to establish adequate drainage when there is active infection with undrained pus in addition to the gangrene.

b. When the distal part of the toe is gangrenous and there is sufficient circulation in the proximal toe, a closed amputation can be carried out after the area has become well demarcated and inflammation has subsided.

c. Transmetatarsal amputation can be considered if the gangrene involves one or more toes down to but not into the foot and if the circulation in the distal foot seems adequate to support healing.

d. Below the knee is the amputation level of choice when gangrene or ischemia in the foot is so distributed that local amputation (as outlined above) is not possible. The preservation of the knee and proximal part of the lower leg is most important in that a more useful prosthesis can be applied and the patient can walk. Even when the circulation below the knee is quite poor, successful healing of the stump is often achieved by the use of a meticulous and gentle technique and often a rigid cast to support a well-padded stump dressing. Amputation below the knee should be attempted if there is a chance of success. Amputation through the knee joint will sometimes succeed when a below-knee amputation would fail and provides a much more useful stump than the above-knee amputation.

e. Amputation above the knee (through the distal thigh in the supracondylar area) is indicated in patients with very advanced peripheral vascular disease requiring amputation because of gangrene, particularly if the leg as well as the foot is extensively involved with gangrene and infection. It is also employed if an attempted below-knee amputation has failed to heal.

Even if the femoral artery is obliterated, there will be sufficient collateral circulation to allow healing provided gentle technique with good hemostasis is used. Few of these patients have the strength and coordination to walk with a prosthesis; most are limited to wheelchair and bed.

    f. **Guillotine amputation**–Infection with bacteremia or septicemia occasionally develops secondary to gangrene of the lower extremity. This usually requires emergency amputation, and the mortality rate is 30%. In such a situation, it is often wise to leave the stump open so that it can heal by second intention or be revised or reamputated when the infection has been controlled. The mortality rate of a major amputation in this group of poor-risk patients is approximately 10%.

Delbridge L: Factors associated with development of foot lesions in the diabetic. *Surgery* 1983;**93**:78.

Imparato AM: Lumbar sympathectomy. *Surg Clin North Am* 1979;**59**:719.

Imparato AM et al: Intermittent claudication: Its natural course. *Surgery* 1975;**78**:795.

Stoney RJ: Ultimate salvage for the patient with limb-threatening ischemia: Realistic goals and surgical considerations. *Am J Surg* 1978;**136**:228.

Wheelock FC: Management of the diabetic foot. In: *Vascular Surgery.* Najarian JS, Delaney JP (editors). Year Book, 1978.

OCCLUSIVE CEREBROVASCULAR DISEASE

Although gradual mental deterioration, episodes of weakness or dizziness, blurred vision, or sudden complete hemiplegia may be due to a variety of causes, arteriosclerotic occlusive or ulcerative disease accounts for many of these problems (see Chapter 17). Single or multiple segmental lesions are often located in the extracranial arteries and account for approximately 40% of ischemic stroke syndromes. The extracranial areas most often involved are (1) the common carotid bifurcation, including the origins of the internal and external carotid arteries (approximately 90%); (2) the origin of the vertebral artery; and (3) the intrathoracic segments of the aortic arch branches (although these vessels may occasionally be occluded as a result of a nonspecific arteritis; see p 287). Because more than one vessel may be involved, complete evaluation of symptoms thought to be due to cerebral or brain stem ischemia on the basis of reduction of total blood flow to the brain below a critical point should include studies of the entire brachiocephalic system.

Clinical Findings

    A. Symptoms: The correlation between the clinical manifestations and the location and degree of the occlusive arterial disease is often imprecise. When the symptoms are secondary to carotid artery disease, they are generally contralateral to the dominant lesions and may consist of transient neurologic manifestations or permanent motor or sensory losses.

    Transient ischemic attacks (TIAs) may be the earliest manifestation of carotid arterial stenosis or ulceration, and the episode may last minutes or hours and be completely resolved within 24 hours. Significant carotid artery stenosis with temporary diminished blood flow to the brain or ulcerations with microemboli from the ulcer to the brain or the ipsilateral retinal artery are responsible for approximately half of TIAs and may precede a complete stroke within 5 years in one-third of these patients. The classic manifestations include unilateral weakness or sensory changes, speech alterations, and visual disturbance (usual temporary partial or complete loss of vision in one eye, known as amaurosis fugax).

    Dizziness and unsteadiness, particularly when associated with a quick change in position, are usually the result of postural hypotension or vertebrobasilar problems, and atypical neurologic symptoms or personality changes may require noninvasive carotid tests. Cardiac monitoring to eliminate arrhythmias as a cause of weakness or dizziness may also be necessary.

    B. Signs: Bruits, diminished or absent pulsations, and a blood pressure difference in the 2 arms of more than 10 mm Hg are indications of occlusive disease in the brachiocephalic arteries. The most significant bruit is one that is sharply localized high in the lateral neck close to the angle of the jaw (overlying the common carotid bifurcation), but a major stenosis sufficient to reduce the blood flow through the vessel is present in only a fourth of these arteries. The murmur of aortic stenosis may be heard as a bruit over the subclavian and carotid arteries; when there is no such heart murmur, the bruit generally denotes disease in these arteries. Bruits are often present without central nervous system symptoms, and the absence of a bruit does not exclude the possibility of carotid artery stenosis. Microemboli can arise from ulcerations of arteries without stenosis or bruit, particularly if the ulcer is large. Only the common carotid and superficial temporal pulses can be felt with accuracy; the internal carotid pulses cannot usually be palpated.

    A reduction in the retinal artery pressure as determined by oculoplethysmography may be present on the side of the significant carotid stenosis. The Doppler ultrasound devices are useful in determining information about the collateral flow to the brain by recording the direction of flow in the supraorbital artery with and without compression of the superficial temporal artery. Ultrasonic arteriography, sometimes used with Doppler spectral analysis, may yield a good image of the stenosis provided it is significant in degree. The noninvasive tests presently available are accurate in about 90% of cases and can be helpful in determining which patients need the more definitive x-ray studies.

    C. X-Ray Findings: Arteriographic visualization of the brachiocephalic arteries is of great value in defining the location and degree of stenoses, the presence of symptomatic or asymptomatic arterial occlusions, and the nature of the collateral flow to the brain in the presence of significant stenoses or thromboses. The study may also help to differentiate an arterial lesion from other central nervous system problems such as brain tumor or hematoma. The ideal study includes the carotid vessels with their intracranial branches and the vertebral-basilar system, usually by means of transfemoral percutaneous catheterization of the aortic arch and its branches (Seldinger technique). Selective arterial injections are safer than aortic arch studies, particularly if digital subtraction angiography equipment is also employed. Digital subtraction angiography by intravenous injection will provide much of the same information in about 60% of patients, and it is a valuable screening procedure; it is now also being used in carefully selected cases as the definitive preoperative examination in place of arteriography, because it is safer, is less expensive, does not require hospitalization, and is more easily tolerated by the patient. CT scan may be helpful in the overall evaluation of the patient.

Treatment

A. Medical Measures: Acute strokes, most progressive or evolving strokes, and those with major neurologic deficits are treated by medical means as discussed in the section on cerebrovascular accidents in Chapter 17. Patients with transient ischemic attacks may be treated with antiplatelet drugs (aspirin, 150 mg, dipyridamole, 100–150 mg, each day) or with oral anticoagulants (see p 294), though there is now some evidence that the former are both safer and more effective than the latter, particularly in men. If transient ischemic attacks continue despite treatment with antiplatelet drugs and if an operable carotid lesion has been demonstrated, surgery should be seriously considered. There is considerable evidence that carotid endarterectomy when expertly performed is the preferred treatment for properly evaluated transient ischemic attacks. There are those who recommend the same treatment for individuals with asymptomatic bruits in the neck who, on further investigation, prove to have carotid stenosis greater than 60–75% of the diameter of the internal carotid. Others recommend antiplatelet medication and periodic neurologic evaluation supplemented by noninvasive studies such as high-resolution ultrasound or digital subtraction angiography to determine if the carotid stenosis is static or progressing.

B. Surgical Measures: Endarterectomy is the procedure employed to treat those with transient cerebral ischemic attacks with significant occlusive or ulcerative lesions of the bifurcation of the common carotid, and it may be indicated in certain carefully selected individuals with asymptomatic bruits, chronic cerebral ischemia with personality changes, and stable strokes. Some think that it may be indicated as an emergency procedure in those with very early and fluctuating neurologic deficits and significant carotid stenosis. It is not indicated in those with acute strokes or progressing strokes or when there is also severe intracranial disease. The surgical technique is important in achieving good results, and many advocate the use of a temporary inlying bypass shunt to support cerebral circulation during the endarterectomy. Great

care should be taken to avoid hypotension in these patients; general anesthesia is usually used.

Occlusions at or close to the aortic arch can generally be treated using extrathoracic bypass grafts in the neck connecting a subclavian artery to the ipsilateral carotid artery. If both carotid and vertebral artery stenoses exist, the carotid lesion should be selected for treatment. When the internal carotid artery is completely occluded, microsurgical technique may be used to anastomose the superficial temporal artery to the middle cerebral artery on the surface of the brain.

Prognosis

The prognosis and results of therapy are related to the number of vessels involved, the degree of stenosis in each, the collateral flow in the circle of Willis, and the specific effects of the occlusive disease on the function of the brain. Expertly performed surgery can be done in carefully selected patients with an acceptable mortality rate of 1–2% or less and with 1–4% permanent major or minor neurologic complications. Transient ischemic attacks known to be secondary to significant carotid artery stenosis or ulceration can usually be eliminated by surgery, and although future strokes can occur in such patients, other arterial lesions, such as a contralateral carotid stenosis or intracranial arterial lesions, are usually responsible. The coronary vessels are generally responsible for a mortality rate that is rather similar in operated and unoperated groups. The operative procedure in patients with transient ischemic attacks is thought to reduce the chance of developing a permanent neurologic deficit within 5 years from 15–35% to 3–5%. The incidence of a later stroke after an uncomplicated endarterectomy is around 5–10%. Significant carotid artery stenosis without symptoms entails no more than a 6–18% stroke risk over 3–5 years, so a surgeon who advises operation for a patient with asymptomatic carotid artery stenosis must be technically skillful.

Machleder HI: Strokes, transient ischemic attacks and asymptomatic bruits. *West J Med* 1979;**130**:205.

Thompson JE, Talkington CM: Carotid surgery for cerebral ischemia. *Surg Clin North Am* 1979;**59**:539.

Whisnant JP et al: Carotid endarterectomy for unilateral carotid system transient cerebral ischemia. *Mayo Clin Proc* 1983;**58**:171.

RENOVASCULAR HYPERTENSION
(See Chapter 8 and p 277, ¶ C.)

VISCERAL ARTERY INSUFFICIENCY

Chronic intestinal ischemia generally results from atherosclerotic occlusive lesions at or close to the origins of the superior mesenteric, celiac, and inferior mesenteric arteries, leading to a significant reduction of blood flow to the intestines. Symptoms may be mild initially, more severe later, and typically consist of epigastric or periumbilical postprandial pains that last for 1–3 hours. To avoid pain, the patient limits oral intake, and weight loss results. Such a history in a person over 45 years of age who appears chronically ill and who may have epigastric bruit or findings of peripheral arterial disease is probably an indication for arteriography or digital subtraction angiography to determine the presence of significant occlusive lesions that can be treated by percutaneous transluminal angioplasty (see p 277), bypass surgery, or endarterectomy. If such studies reveal extrinsic compression of the celiac axis by the diaphragmatic ligamentous attachments, cutting the arcuate ligament and freeing and dilating the constricted celiac artery is sufficient.

Acute intestinal ischemia results from (1) embolic occlusions of the visceral branches of the abdominal aorta, generally in patients with heart disease (see pp 211 ff); (2) thrombosis of one or more of the visceral vessels involved with arteriosclerotic occlusive changes, sometimes in patients with a history of abdominal angina as described on p 382; (3) nonocclusive mesenteric vascular insufficiency, generally in patients with congestive heart failure and receiving digitalis therapy or patients in shock. The acute onset of crampy or steady epigastric and periumbilical abdominal pain combined with minimal or no findings on examination and often a high leukocyte count should suggest one of these 3 diagnoses. Emergency angiography of the superior mesenteric artery is essential for the early diagnosis and treatment of both occlusive and nonocclusive intestinal ischemia and should be performed, if possible, before physical findings develop. If vasospasm with or without occlusion is demonstrated, a constant infusion of papaverine should be started into the artery (30–60 mg/h), antibiotics should be started, digitalis should be stopped, and laparotomy usually should then be performed to reestablish blood flow to the bowel if possible and to remove necrotic bowel if present. Hyperbaric oxygen, continuous intravenous infusion of dextran, and possibly intraarterial infusion of streptokinase are also therapeutic considerations.

Through early diagnosis and aggressive treatment, the very poor prognosis of the past should yield to somewhat lower morbidity and mortality rates (see pp 382, 383, and 395).

Cooperman M: *Intestinal Ischemia.* Futura, 1983.

Orringer LW: The surgical management of acute occlusion of the superior mesenteric artery. *Ann Surg* 1978;**188**:721.

Stoney RJ, Olcott C: Visceral artery syndromes and reconstructions. *Surg Clin North Am* 1979;**59**:637.

ACUTE ARTERIAL OCCLUSION

Essentials of Diagnosis

- Symptoms and signs depend on the artery occluded, the organ or region supplied by the artery, and the adequacy of the collateral circulation to the area primarily involved.
- Occlusion in an extremity usually results in pain, numbness, tingling, weakness, and coldness. There is pallor or mottling; motor, reflex, and sensory alteration; and collapsed superficial veins. Pulsations are absent in arteries distal to the occlusion.
- Occlusions in other areas result in such conditions as cerebrovascular accidents, intestinal ischemia and gangrene, and renal or splenic infarcts.

Differential Diagnosis

The primary differentiation is between arterial embolism and thrombosis. In an older individual with both arteriosclerotic vascular disease and cardiac disease, the differentiation may be very difficult, and in 10–20% a definite diagnosis either cannot be made or turns out to be incorrect. Arterial trauma may result in either occlusion or spasm.

1. ARTERIAL EMBOLISM

Arterial embolism is generally a complication of heart disease; 22% of those with embolism have rheumatic heart disease, and 60% have arteriosclerotic heart disease, either with or without myocardial infarction. Atrial fibrillation is often present. Other forms of heart disease account for 6%, and miscellaneous causes, including those arising from arteriosclerotic ulcerations or aneurysms or those of undetermined origin, account for 13%. In 12%, there is more than one embolism, and recurrent emboli after initial successful treatment may occur.

Emboli tend to lodge at the bifurcation of major arteries, with over half going to the aortic bifurcation or the vessels in the lower extremities; the carotid system is involved in 20%, the upper extremity in 16%, and the mesenteric arteries in 5%. Emboli from arterial ulcerations are usually small, giving rise to transient symptoms in the toes or brain.

Clinical Findings

In an extremity, the initial symptoms are usually pain (sudden or gradual in onset), numbness, coldness, and tingling. Signs include absence of pulsations in the arteries distal to the block, coldness, pallor or mottling, hypesthesia or anesthesia, and weakness, rigidity, or muscle paralysis. The superficial veins are collapsed. Later, blebs and skin necrosis may appear, and gangrene may occur.

Emboli going to the carotid system and resulting in stroke are seldom treated surgically. See preceding section on Visceral Artery Insufficiency for management of visceral emboli.

Treatment

Immediate embolectomy is the treatment of choice in almost all early cases of emboli in extremities. It should be done within 4–6 hours of the embolic episode if possible. If a longer delay has occurred or if there is clinical evidence of tissue necrosis (particularly in muscle, noted as an area of rigidity), embolectomy may be associated with an unacceptably high mortality rate related to the release of substances from the revascularized but previously ischemic limb; in such circumstances, nonoperative measures (as outlined below) should be employed, and the possibility of amputation at a later date must be accepted in some of these cases. Embolectomy many days after the initial episode may occasionally be successful.

A. Emergency Preoperative Care:

1. Heparin–Heparin sodium, 5000 units intravenously, should be given as soon as the diagnosis is made or suspected in an effort to prevent distal thrombosis. The effect of this dose will usually be dissipated by the time the patient has been moved to surgery. If a delay is anticipated, intravenous heparin should be started (see p 294).

2. Cardiorenal support–Emergency measures to improve cardiac output (if inadequate) will help local tissue perfusion by means of the collateral circulation. If the status of renal function is uncertain or if there is likely to be edema in the ischemic tissue, mannitol may be of value.

3. Protect the part–Keep the extremity at or below the horizontal plane. Do not apply heat or cold to the involved extremity (but heat to an uninvolved extremity may help produce reflex vasodilatation). Protect from hard surfaces and overlying bedclothes.

4. Vasodilators–Papaverine, 60 mg intravenously every 2 hours, may be given. Whiskey, 45 mL 4 times daily, or nicotinic acid, 50 mg 4 times daily, may also be tried if surgery is not considered possible.

5. Analgesics–Pain may be severe and should be relieved with an appropriate analgesic.

6. Arteriography–Arteriography is often of value either before or during surgery. There may be more than one embolus in an extremity; x-ray studies may help locate a distal embolus or determine the extent of the thrombosis.

B. Surgical Measures: Local anesthesia is generally used if the occlusion is in an artery to an extremity. After removing the embolus through the arteriotomy, the proximal and distal artery should be explored for additional emboli or secondary thrombi by means of a specially designed catheter with a small inflatable balloon at the tip (Fogarty catheter). An embolus at the aortic bifurcation or in the iliac artery can often be removed under local anesthesia through common femoral arteriotomies with the use of these same catheters. Heparinization for a week or more postoperatively is indicated, and prolonged anticoagulation with warfarin is often desirable after that.

Delayed embolectomy carried out more than 12 hours following the embolism and when there is also evidence of a considerable degree of ischemia, as shown by mottled cyanosis, muscle paralysis and rigidity, anesthesia, or early evidence of tissue necrosis, involves a high risk of acute respiratory distress syndrome or acute renal shutdown; rapid deterioration

and death may result. Anticoagulation in liberal doses rather than surgery is the safer approach under such circumstances even though amputation may become necessary later. Where it appears that significant tissue necrosis has already taken place, a guillotine amputation at the appropriate level should be considered.

Prognosis

Arterial embolism is a threat not only to the limb (5–25% amputation rate) but also to the life of the patient (25–30% hospital mortality rate, with the underlying heart disease responsible for over half of these deaths). Emergency surgery, even under local anesthesia, is poorly tolerated by patients with advanced cardiopulmonary disease.

Emboli in the aortoiliac area are more dangerous than more peripheral emboli, and the mortality rate rises if there are multiple peripheral emboli or carotid or visceral emboli; the mortality rate is essentially 100% if all 3 areas are involved. Emboli associated with hypertensive or arteriosclerotic heart disease have a poorer prognosis than those arising from rheumatic valvular disease, and congestive heart failure significantly increases the mortality rate.

In patients with atrial fibrillation an attempt may be made to restore normal rhythm with quinidine or cardioversion, although restoration of normal rhythm tends to be permanent only in patients with recent or transitory fibrillation (see p 233). Long-term anticoagulant therapy definitely diminishes the danger of further emboli and in the majority of patients is the only long-term prophylactic measure that can be instituted (see p 347). Correction of mitral stenosis is indicated in selected individuals. Heart surgery done in the earlier stages of mitral stenosis diminishes the chance of later embolic complications (see p 191).

If no heart disease exists, arteriography may reveal an arteriosclerotic ulcer or small aneurysm to be the origin of the embolus; such a defect should be removed.

2. ACUTE ARTERIAL THROMBOSIS

Acute arterial thrombosis generally occurs in an artery extensively involved with arteriosclerosis, resulting in almost complete obliteration of the channel. Blood flowing through such a narrow, irregular, or ulcerated lumen may clot, leading to a sudden, complete occlusion of the narrow segment. The thrombosis may then propagate either up or down the artery to a point where the blood is flowing rapidly through a somewhat less diseased artery (usually to a significant arterial branch proximally or one or more functioning collateral vessels distally). Occasionally, the thrombosis is precipitated when the bloodstream dissects and displaces an arteriosclerotic plaque, blocking the lumen; trauma to the artery may precipitate a similar event. Inflammatory involvement of the arterial wall, with narrowing of the channel as in thromboangiitis obliterans, will also lead to acute thrombosis. Chronic mechanical irritation of the subclavian artery compressed by a cervical rib may also lead to a complete occlusion. Thrombosis in a diseased artery may be secondary to an episode of hypotension or cardiac failure. Polycythemia and dehydration also increase the chance of thrombosis.

Chronic, incomplete arterial obstruction usually results in the establishment of some collateral flow, and further flow will develop relatively rapidly through the collaterals once complete occlusion has developed. The extremity may go through an extremely critical period of hours or days, however, while the additional collateral circulation develops around the block. The survival of the tissue distal to the block depends on the development of adequate collateral circulation, which in turn depends on the location and length of the arterial thrombosis and whether conditions such as shock, heart failure, anemia, or hemoconcentration can be corrected promptly.

Clinical Findings

The local findings in the extremity are usually very similar to those described in the section on arterial embolism. The following differential points should be checked: (1) Are there manifestations of advanced occlusive arterial disease in other areas, especially the opposite extremity (bruit, absent pulses, secondary change as described on p 275)? Is there a history of intermittent claudication? These clinical manifestations are suggestive but not diagnostic of thrombosis. (2) Is there a history or are there findings of rheumatic heart disease or of a recent episode of atrial fibrillation or myocardial infarction? If so, an embolism is more likely than a thrombosis. (3) Electrocardiography and serum enzyme studies may give added information regarding the presence of a silent myocardial infarction and its likelihood as a source of an embolus (see pp 221 and 222). (4) An emergency arteriogram may be of value in making a more accurate differential diagnosis and in planning the therapy.

Treatment

Whereas emergency embolectomy is the usual approach in the case of an early occlusion from an embolus, a nonoperative approach is generally used in the case of thrombosis for 2 reasons: (1) The segment of thrombosed artery may be quite long, requiring rather extensive and difficult surgery (thromboendarterectomy or artery graft). The removal of a single embolus in a normal or nearly normal artery is, by comparison, relatively easy and quick. (2) The extremity is more likely to survive without development of gangrene because some collateral circulation has usually formed during the stenotic phase before acute thrombosis. With an embolism, this is not usually the case; the block is most often at a major arterial bifurcation, occluding both branches, and the associated arterial spasm is usually more acute.

Treatment is therefore as outlined under emergency preoperative care for arterial embolism (see above). Gradual improvement in the circulation of the distal areas of the extremity is usually noted. If this does not occur or if muscle tenderness and swelling are prominent, early angiography and surgery may be considered, but attempts at revascularization of an ischemic extremity often result in death of the patient owing to release of toxins and thrombotic material from ischemic tissues into the circulation when blood flow is reestablished. In most cases it is best not to risk the patient's life for the sake of an extremity and to accept the loss of the limb if tissue necrosis is present.

Prognosis

Limb survival usually occurs with acute thrombosis of the iliac or superficial femoral arteries; gangrene is more likely if the popliteal is suddenly occluded, especially if the period between occlusion and treatment is long or if there is considerable arterial spasm or proximal arterial occlusive disease. If the limb does survive the acute occlusion, a period of observation and evaluation is usually advisable, for significant functional recovery may occur gradually over a number of weeks. The later treatment and prognosis are outlined above in the section on occlusive disease of the iliac, femoral, and popliteal arteries. (See pp 275–281.)

Blaisdell FW et al: Management of acute lower extremity arterial ischemia due to embolism and thrombosis. *Surgery* 1978; **84:**822.

Elliott JP et al: Arterial embolization: Problems of source, multiplicity, recurrence and delayed treatment. *Surgery* 1980; **88:**833.

Gregg RO et al: Embolectomy or heparin therapy for arterial emboli? *Surgery* 1983;**93:**377.

McPhair NV et al: Management of acute thromboembolic limb ischemia. *Surgery* 1983;**93:**381.

• • •

THROMBOANGIITIS OBLITERANS (TAO)
(Buerger's Disease)

Essentials of Diagnosis

- Almost always in young men who smoke.
- Extremities involved with inflammatory occlusions of the more distal arteries, resulting in circulatory insufficiency of the toes or fingers.
- Thromboses of superficial veins may also occur.
- Course is intermittent and amputation may be necessary, especially if smoking is not stopped.

General Considerations

Buerger's disease is an episodic and segmental inflammatory and thrombotic process of the arteries and veins, principally in the limbs. It is seen most commonly in men between ages 25 and 40 who smoke. The effects of the disease are almost solely due to occlusion of the arteries. The symptoms are primarily due to ischemia, complicated in the later stages by infection and tissue necrosis. The inflammatory process is intermittent, with quiescent periods lasting weeks, months, or years.

The arteries most commonly affected are the plantar and digital vessels in the foot and those in the lower leg. The arteries in the hands and wrists may also become involved. Different arterial segments may become occluded in successive episodes; a certain amount of recanalization occurs during quiescent periods.

Superficial migratory thrombophlebitis is a common early indication of the disease.

The cause is not known, but alteration in the collagen in the vessels suggests that it may be a collagen disorder.

Clinical Findings

The signs and symptoms are primarily those of arterial insufficiency, and the differentiation from arteriosclerotic peripheral vascular disease may be difficult; however, the following findings suggest Buerger's disease:

(1) The patient is a man between ages 20 and 40 who smokes.

(2) There is a history or finding of small, red, tender cords resulting from migratory superficial segmental thrombophlebitis, usually in the saphenous tributaries rather than the main vessel. A biopsy of such a vein often gives microscopic proof of Buerger's disease.

(3) Intermittent claudication is common and is frequently noted in the palm of the hand or arch of the foot. Rest pain is common and, when present, is persistent. It tends to be more pronounced than in the patient with atherosclerosis. Numbness, diminished sensation, and pricking and burning pains may be present as a result of ischemic neuropathy.

(4) The digit or the entire distal portion of the foot may be pale and cold, or there may be rubor that may remain relatively unchanged by posture; the skin may not blanch on elevation, and on dependency the intensity of the rubor is often more pronounced than that seen in the atherosclerotic group. The distal vascular changes are often asymmetric, so that not all of the toes are affected to the same degree. Absence or impairment of pulsations in the dorsalis pedis, posterior tibial, ulnar, or radial artery is frequent.

(5) Trophic changes may be present, often with painful indolent ulcerations along the nail margins.

(6) There is usually evidence of disease in both legs and possibly also in the hands and lower arms. There may be a history or findings of Raynaud's phenomenon in the finger or distal foot. (See pp 287 and 288.)

(7) The course is usually intermittent, with acute and often dramatic episodes followed by rather definite remissions. When the collateral vessels as well as the main channels have become occluded, an exacerbation is more likely to lead to gangrene and amputation. The course in the patient with atherosclerosis tends to be less dramatic and more persistent (see pp 278–281).

Differential Diagnosis

Differences between thromboangiitis obliterans and arteriosclerosis obliterans are discussed above.

Scleroderma causes characteristic skin changes prior to definite vascular findings.

Raynaud's disease causes symmetric bilateral color changes, primarily in young women. There is no impairment of arterial pulsations.

Livedo reticularis and acrocyanosis are vasospastic diseases that do not affect peripheral pulsations (see p 288).

Treatment

The principles of therapy are the same as those outlined for atherosclerotic peripheral vascular disease, but the long-range outlook is better in patients with Buerger's disease, so that when possible the approach should be more conservative and tissue loss kept to a minimum.

A. General Measures: Smoking must be stopped; the physician must insist on it. The disease is almost sure to progress if this advice is not heeded.

See the discussion of instructions in the care of the feet on p 773.

B. Surgical Measures:

1. Sympathectomy–Sympathectomy is useful in eliminating the vasospastic manifestations of the disease and aiding in the establishment of collateral circulation to the skin. It may also relieve the mild or moderate forms of rest pain. If amputation of a digit is necessary, sympathectomy may aid in healing of the surgical wound.

2. Arterial grafts–Arterial grafting procedures are seldom indicated in patients with Buerger's disease because they do not usually have significant occlusive disease in the iliofemoral region.

3. Amputation–The indications for amputation are similar in many respects to those outlined for the atherosclerotic group (see p 280), although the approach should be more conservative from the point of view of preservation of tissue. Most patients with Buerger's disease who are managed carefully and stop smoking do not require amputation of the fingers or toes. It is almost never necessary to amputate the entire hand, but amputation below the knee is occasionally necessary because of gangrene or severe pain in the foot.

Prognosis

Except in the case of the rapidly progressive form of the disease—and provided the patient stops smoking and takes good care of his feet—the prognosis for survival of the extremities is good. Buerger's disease rarely results in death.

Shionoya S et al: Diagnosis, pathology, and treatment of Buerger's disease. *Surgery* 1974;**75:**695.

IDIOPATHIC ARTERITIS OF TAKAYASU
("Pulseless Disease")

Pulseless disease, most frequent in young women, is an occlusive polyarteritis of unknown cause with a special predilection for the branches of the aortic arch. It occurs most commonly in Orientals. Manifestations, depending upon the vessel or vessels involved, may include evidence of cerebrovascular insufficiency, with dizzy spells and visual disturbances; and absent pulses in the arms, with a rich collateral flow in the shoulder, chest, and neck areas.

Pulseless disease must be differentiated from vascular lesions of the aortic arch due to atherosclerosis (see p 278). Unless this disease is treated by bypass grafts ensuring adequate blood flow beyond the arterial occlusions, blindness and hemiplegia can result.

Lupiherrera E et al: Takayasu's arteritis: Clinical study of 107 cases. *Am Heart J* 1977;**93**:94.
Shumacker HB Jr et al: The management of stenotic and obstructive lesions of the aortic arch branches. *Am J Surg* 1977; **133**:351.

TEMPORAL ARTERITIS
(Giant Cell Arteritis)

This disorder is discussed in Chapter 14 (p 511).

VASOMOTOR DISORDERS

RAYNAUD'S DISEASE & RAYNAUD'S PHENOMENON

Essentials of Diagnosis
- Paroxysmal bilateral symmetric pallor and cyanosis followed by rubor of the skin of the digits.
- Precipitated by cold or emotional upset; relieved by warmth.
- Primarily a disorder of young women.

General Considerations
Raynaud's disease is the primary, or idiopathic, form of paroxysmal digital cyanosis. Raynaud's phenomenon, which is more common than Raynaud's disease, may be due to a number of regional or systemic disorders.

In Raynaud's disease the digital arteries respond excessively to vasospastic stimuli. The cause is not known, but some abnormality of the sympathetic nervous system seems to be active in this entity. The disease occurs primarily in females between puberty and age 40, and a family history of a vasospastic phenomenon can often be obtained. Immunologic abnormalities such as autoantibodies are present in many.

Clinical Findings
Raynaud's disease and Raynaud's phenomenon are characterized by intermittent attacks of pallor or cyanosis—or pallor followed by cyanosis—in the fingers (and rarely the toes), precipitated by cold or occasionally by emotional upsets. Early in the course of the disease, only 1–2 fingertips may be affected; as the disease progresses, all the fingers down to the distal palm may be involved. The thumbs are rarely affected. General as well as local body cooling is usually necessary to cause such attacks. Recovery usually begins near the base of the fingers as a bright red return of color to the cyanotic or pale digit. During recovery there may be intense rubor, throbbing, paresthesia, and slight swelling. Attacks usually terminate spontaneously or upon returning to a warm room or putting the extremity in warm water. Between attacks there may be no abnormal findings. Sensory changes that often accompany vasomotor manifestations include numbness, stiffness, diminished sensation, and aching pain. The condition may progress to atrophy of the terminal fat pads and the digital skin, and gangrenous ulcers, which may heal during warm weather, may appear near the fingertips. Although the radial and ulnar pulses are present, these arteries as well as the palmar and particularly the digital vessels may be involved with significant organic obstructive disease. Other patients may have only increased vasomotor tone without organic arterial disease.

Raynaud's disease appears first between ages 15 and 45, almost always in women. It tends to be progressive, and, unlike Raynaud's phenomenon (which may be unilateral and may involve only 1–2 fingers), symmetric involvement of the fingers of both hands is ultimately the rule. Spasm gradually becomes more frequent and prolonged, but the severe changes that may develop in those with Raynaud's phenomenon generally do not occur.

Differential Diagnosis
Raynaud's disease must be differentiated from the numerous disorders that may be associated with Raynaud's phenomenon. Arteriography, isotope scan, plethysmometry, or thermography may be helpful studies, and specific laboratory tests are also of value. A rapid sedimentation rate is an indicator of temporal cell arteritis (see p 511). The latex fixation test and rheumatoid factor help in identifying rheumatoid vasculitis. Extractable nuclear antigen and speckled ANA pattern help identify collagen vascular disease.

The differentiation from thromboangiitis obliterans is usually not difficult, since thromboangiitis obliterans is generally a disease of men; peripheral pulses are often diminished or absent; and, when Raynaud's phenomenon occurs in association with thromboangiitis obliterans, it is usually in only one or 2 digits (see p 285).

Raynaud's phenomenon may occur in patients with the thoracic outlet syndromes (including cervical rib and scalenus anticus problems). In these disorders involvement is generally unilateral, and symptoms referable to brachial plexus compression tend to dominate the clinical picture. The various maneuvers and tests helpful in diagnosing these conditions should be performed on any patient with unilateral Raynaud's phenomenon. Carpal tunnel syndrome should also be considered, and nerve conduction tests may be appropriate.

It may be difficult to differentiate the skin thickening in Raynaud's disease from the early stages of scleroderma with Raynaud's phenomenon. (See p 507.)

Raynaud's phenomenon is occasionally the presenting complaint in systemic lupus erythematosus, and this disease should be ruled out by appropriate tests, particularly the antinuclear antibody pattern. (See p 505.)

Because many patients with Raynaud's phenomenon have serum protein and serologic abnormalities, including a variety of autoantibodies, thorough evaluation is necessary, including tests for antinuclear antibodies and for antiglobulins. Involvement of the immune mechanism may be evidenced by depression of the serum level of the third component of complement. (See p 1105.)

In acrocyanosis, cyanosis of the hands is permanent and diffuse (see p 289).

Frostbite may lead to chronic changes with Raynaud's phenomenon. Ergot poisoning, particularly the prolonged or excessive use of ergotamine, must also be considered.

Treatment

A. General Measures: The body should be kept warm, and the hands especially should be protected from exposure to cold; gloves should be worn when out in the cold. The hands should be protected from injury at all times; wounds heal slowly, and infections are consequently hard to control. Softening and lubricating lotion to control the fissured dry skin should be applied to the hands frequently. Smoking should be stopped.

B. Vasodilators: Vasodilator drugs are of limited value but may be of some benefit in those patients who are not adequately controlled by general measures when there is peripheral vasoconstriction without significant organic vascular disease. With the relatively large doses used, side effects are troublesome. Shortening of temperature recovery time may occur with the use of reserpine, methyldopa, topical nitroglycerin (or a longer-acting nitrate orally), nicotinic acid, papaverine, guanethidine, and phenoxybenzamine. Regional medical sympathectomy can be achieved by intravenous injection of reserpine (0.5 mg in 50 mL of saline) into a hand vein after the venous blood has been drained from the extremity and a tourniquet has been inflated to hold the drug in the distal extremity for 20 minutes. If vasospasm is present, a good response will be achieved for about 2 weeks and will often get the patient through an acute exacerbation. The procedure can be easily repeated at intervals as necessary for symptomatic relief. Prostaglandin E intravenous infusion seems to be beneficial during acute vasospastic episodes, and its effect may last for weeks.

C. Surgical Measures: Sympathectomy may be indicated when attacks have become frequent and severe, interfering with work and well-being—and particularly if trophic changes have developed and medical measures have failed. In the lower extremities, complete and permanent relief usually results, whereas dorsal sympathectomies generally result in only temporary improvement in approximately 80% of patients treated with operation. Although vascular tone of the vessels in the hands usually ultimately reappears, the symptoms in the fingers that may thus recur in 1–5 years are usually milder and less frequent. When the symptoms do recur, carefully selected drugs may be of help. If the process is due to collagen vascular disease, sympathectomy may be used as adjuvant to vigorous systemic immunosuppressive therapy. Sympathectomies are of very limited value in far-advanced cases, and particularly if significant digital artery obstructive disease or scleroderma is present.

Prognosis

Raynaud's disease is usually benign, causing mild discomfort on exposure to cold and progressing very slightly over the years. In a few cases rapid progression does occur, so that the slightest change in temperature may precipitate color changes. It is in this situation that sclerodactylia and small areas of gangrene may be noted, and such patients may become quite disabled by severe pain, limitation of motion, and secondary fixation of distal joints.

LIVEDO RETICULARIS

Livedo reticularis is a vasospastic disorder of unknown cause that results in constant mottled discoloration on large areas of the extremities, generally in a fishnet pattern with reticulated cyanotic areas surrounding a paler central core. It occurs primarily in young women. It may be associated with occult cancer.

Livedo reticularis is most apparent on the thighs and forearms and occasionally on the lower abdomen and is most pronounced in cold weather. The color may change to a reddish hue in warm weather but never entirely disappears spontaneously. A few patients complain of paresthesias, coldness, or numbness in the involved areas. In severe cases there may be recurrent ulcerations in the lower extremities.

Bluish mottling of the extremities is diagnostic. The peripheral pulses are normal. The extremity may be cold, with increased perspiration.

Treatment consists of protection from exposure to cold, and use of vasodilators (see p 288) in more severe cases. In most instances, livedo reticularis is entirely benign. The rare patient who develops ulcerations or gangrene should be studied for underlying systemic disease.

ACROCYANOSIS

Acrocyanosis is an uncommon symmetric condition that involves the skin of the hands and feet and, to a lesser degree, the forearms and legs. It is associated with arteriolar vasoconstriction combined with dilatation of the subpapillary venous plexus of the skin, through which deoxygenated blood slowly circulates. It is worse in cold weather but does not completely disappear during the warm season. It occurs in either sex, is most common in the teens and 20s, and usually improves with advancing age or during pregnancy. It is characterized by coldness, sweating, slight edema, and cyanotic discoloration of the involved areas. Pain, trophic lesions, and disability do not occur, and the peripheral pulses are present. The individual may thus be reassured and encouraged to dress warmly in cold weather.

ERYTHROMELALGIA
(Erythermalgia)

Erythromelalgia is a paroxysmal bilateral vasodilative disorder of unknown cause. Idiopathic (primary) erythromelalgia occurs in otherwise healthy persons, rarely in children, and affects men and women equally. A secondary type is occasionally seen in patients with polycythemia vera, hypertension, gout, and organic neurologic diseases.

The chief symptom is bilateral burning distress that lasts minutes to hours, involving circumscribed areas on the soles or palms first and, as the disease progresses, the entire extremity. The attack occurs in response to stimuli producing vasodilatation (eg, exercise, warm environment), especially at night when the extremities are warmed under bedclothes. Reddening or cyanosis as well as heat may be noted. Relief may be obtained by cooling the affected part and by elevation.

No findings are generally present between attacks. With onset of an attack, heat and redness are noted in association with the typical pain. Skin temperature and arterial pulsations are increased, and the involved areas may sweat profusely.

Erythromelalgia must be differentiated from peripheral neuritis and organic occlusive diseases as well as from acrocyanosis.

In primary erythromelalgia, aspirin may give excellent relief. The patient should avoid warm environments. In severe cases, if medical measures fail, section or crushing of peripheral nerves may be necessary to relieve pain.

Primary idiopathic erythromelalgia is uniformly benign.

Machleder HL et al: Treatment of upper extremity ischemia by cervico-dorsal sympathectomy. *Vasc Surg* 1979;**13**:399.

Spittel JA Jr: Raynaud's phenomenon and allied vasospastic disorders. In: *Allen-Barker-Hines Peripheral Vascular Disease,* 5th ed. Juergens JJ, Spittel JA Jr, Fairbairn JF II (editors). Saunders, 1980.

Taylor LM et al: Treatment of finger ischemia with Bier block reserpine. *Surg Gynecol Obstet* 1982;**154**:39.

POSTTRAUMATIC SYMPATHETIC DYSTROPHY
(Causalgia)

Essentials of Diagnosis

- Burning or aching pain following trauma to an extremity of a severity greater than that expected from the initiating injury.
- Manifestations of vasomotor instability are generally present and include temperature, color, and texture alterations of the skin of the involved extremity.

General Considerations

Pain—usually burning or aching—in an injured extremity is the single most common finding, and the disparity between the severity of the inciting injury and the degree of pain experienced is the most characteristic feature. Crushing injuries with lacerations and soft tissue destruction are the most common causes, but closed fractures, simple lacerations, burns (especially electric), and elective operative procedures are also responsible for this syndrome. It is rare in children. The manifestations of pain and the associated objective changes may be relatively mild or quite severe, and the initial manifestations often change if the condition proceeds to a chronic stage.

Clinical Findings

In the early stages, the pain, tenderness, and hyperesthesia may be strictly localized to the injured area, and the extremity may be warm, dry, swollen, and red or slightly cyanotic. The involved extremity is held in a splinted position by the muscles, and the nails may become ridged and the hair long. In advanced stages, the pain is more diffuse and worse at night; the extremity becomes cool and clammy and intolerant of temperature changes (particularly cold); and the skin becomes glossy and atrophic. The joints become stiff, generally in a position that makes the extremity useless. The bones become osteoporotic. The dominant concern of the patient may be to avoid the slightest stimuli to the extremity and especially to the trigger points that may develop.

Prevention

During operations on an extremity, peripheral nerves should be handled only when absolutely necessary and then with utmost gentleness. Splinting of an injured extremity for an adequate period during the early, painful phase of recovery, together with adequate analgesics, may help prevent this condition.

Treatment & Prognosis

A. Conservative Measures: It is most important that the condition be recognized and treated in the early stages, when the manifestations are most easily reversed and major secondary changes have not yet developed. In mild, early cases with minimal skin and joint changes, physical therapy involving active and passive exercises combined with trifluoperazine, 1 or 2 mg twice daily, or diazepam, 2 mg twice daily, may relieve symptoms. Protecting the extremity from irritating stimuli is important, and the use of nonaddicting analgesics may be necessary.

B. Surgical Measures: If the condition fails to respond to conservative treatment or if there are more severe or advanced objective findings, sympathetic blocks (stellate ganglion or lumbar) are indicated, usually in a series on consecutive days. Intensive physical therapy may be used during the pain-free periods following effective blocks. Patients who achieve significant temporary relief of symptoms after sympathetic blocks but fail to obtain permanent relief by the blocks may be cured by sympathectomy. In the advanced forms—particularly in association with major local changes and emotional reactions—the prognosis for a useful life is poor. The newer neurosurgical approaches using implantable electronic biostimulator devices to block pain impulses in the cervical spinal cord have met with some success.

REFLEX SYMPATHETIC DYSTROPHY

Local sympathetic nervous system overactivity may be responsible for the changes in an extremity that occasionally occur in association with diseases involving the central nervous system, the spine, the heart, or other organs, as well as in association with trauma (in which case the syndrome may be referred to as Sudeck's atrophy). It is bilateral in one-third to one-half of cases, and the early acute manifestations include evidence of vasomotor instability, pain of a burning nature made worse by movement of the distal joints (or even the ipsilateral shoulder, as in shoulder-hand syndrome), swelling, and sweating. Later, atrophic changes in the skin, nails, bones, and joints may develop, with wasting of the soft tissues and stiffness of the joints. Patchy osteoporosis of the bones of the hands or feet develops, as well as proliferative changes of the joint capsules and around the joints.

Local and supportive measures include those as outlined for posttraumatic sympathetic dystrophy (see above). Prednisone may be beneficial.

Kleinert HE et al: Post-traumatic sympathetic dystrophy. *Orthop Clin North Am* 1973;**4**:917.
Kozin F et al: The reflex sympathetic dystrophy syndrome. *Am J Med* 1976;**60**:321.

DEGENERATIVE & INFLAMMATORY VENOUS DISEASE

VARICOSE VEINS

Essentials of Diagnosis
- Dilated, tortuous superficial veins in the lower extremities.
- May be asymptomatic or may be associated with fatigue, aching discomfort, or pain.
- Edema, pigmentation, and ulceration of the skin of the distal leg may develop.

General Considerations
Varicose veins develop predominantly in the lower extremities. They consist of abnormally dilated, elongated, and tortuous alterations in the saphenous veins and their tributaries. These vessels lie immediately beneath the skin and superficial to the deep fascia; they therefore do not have as adequate support as the veins deep in the leg, which are surrounded by muscles. An inherited defect seems to play a major role in the development of varicosities in many instances, but it is not known whether the basic valvular incompetence that exists is secondary to defective valves in the saphenofemoral veins or to a fundamental weakness of the walls of the vein, resulting in dilatation of the vessel. Periods of high venous pressure related to prolonged standing or heavy lifting are contributing factors, and the highest incidence is in women who have been pregnant. Fifteen percent of adults develop varicosities, and a family history is common.

Secondary varicosities can develop as a result of obstructive changes and valve damage in the deep venous system following thrombophlebitis, or occasionally as a result of proximal venous occlusion due to neoplasm. Congenital or acquired arteriovenous fistulas are also associated with varicosities.

The long saphenous vein and its tributaries are most commonly involved, but the short saphenous vein may also be affected. There may be one or many incompetent perforating veins in the thigh and lower leg, so that blood can reflux into the varicosities not only from above, by way of the saphenofemoral junction, but also from the deep system of veins through the incompetent perforators in the mid thigh or lower leg. Largely because of these valvular defects in the most proximal valve of the long saphenous vein or in the distal communicating veins, venous pressure in the superficial veins does not fall appreciably on walking; over the years, the veins progressively enlarge, and the surrounding tissue and skin develop secondary changes such as fibrosis, chronic edema, and skin pigmentation and atrophy.

Clinical Findings
A. Symptoms: The severity of the symptoms caused by varicose veins is not necessarily correlated

with the number and size of the varicosities; extensive varicose veins may produce no subjective symptoms, whereas minimal varicosities may produce many symptoms, especially in women. Dull, aching heaviness or a feeling of fatigue brought on by periods of standing is the most common complaint. Cramps may occur, often at night, and elevation of the legs typically relieves symptoms. One must be careful to distinguish between the symptoms of arteriosclerotic peripheral vascular disease, such as intermittent claudication and coldness of the feet, and symptoms of venous disease, since occlusive arterial disease usually contraindicates the operative treatment of varicosities distal to the knee. Itching from an associated eczematoid dermatitis may occur in the region of the veins.

B. Signs: Dilated, tortuous, elongated veins beneath the skin in the thigh and leg are generally readily visible in the standing individual, although in very obese patients palpation and percussion may be necessary to detect their presence and location. Secondary tissue changes may be absent even in extensive varicosities; but if the varicosities are of long duration, brownish pigmentation and thinning of the skin above the ankle are often present. Swelling may occur, but signs of severe chronic venous stasis such as extensive swelling, fibrosis, pigmentation, and ulceration of the distal lower leg usually denote the postphlebitic state (see p 298).

C. Trendelenburg's Test: Of use in determining competence at the proximal end of the long saphenous vein close to the saphenofemoral junction, in the long saphenous vein in thigh and leg, and in the communicating veins between superficial and deep vessels.

1. With the patient supine, elevate the leg. If there is no organic venous obstruction, varicosities will empty immediately.

2. Place a rubber tourniquet around the upper thigh and ask the patient to stand.

a. If the long saphenous vein remains empty for 30 seconds or more and then fills very slowly from below over a period of 1–2 minutes, the valves close to the saphenofemoral junction are incompetent, the valves in the communicating veins are competent, and the blood is flowing through them in the normal direction (superficial to deep). On release of the tourniquet, if the veins fill rapidly from above, the incompetence of the proximal valves is confirmed.

b. If the varicosities fill rapidly, the communicating veins between the deep and the superficial vessels are incompetent and blood is refluxing into the varicosed vessels. If, on release of the tourniquet, no additional filling of the varicosities occurs, the valves in the saphenous vein close to the saphenofemoral junction are competent; if, on the other hand, further distention of the varicosities occurs when the tourniquet is released, the valves at the upper end of the long saphenous vein are also incompetent. The precise site of these defective perforating veins can often be determined by repetition of this maneuver while placing the tourniquet at successively lower levels or using 2 or 3 tourniquets at different levels. If varices in the posterior leg fill within less than 30 seconds with the tourniquet at the level of the mid thigh but remain relatively empty with the tourniquet at the level of the knee, an incompetent short saphenous vein should be suspected.

Differential Diagnosis

Primary varicose veins should be differentiated from those secondary to (1) chronic venous insufficiency of the deep system of veins (the postphlebitic syndrome; see p 298); (2) retroperitoneal vein obstruction from extrinsic pressure or fibrosis; (3) arteriovenous fistula (congenital or acquired)—a bruit is present and a thrill is often palpable; and (4) congenital venous malformation. Venography may be of value in the investigation of some of these problems. Pain or discomfort secondary to arthritis, nerve root pressure, or arterial insufficiency should be distinguished from symptoms associated with coexistent varicose veins.

Complications

If thin, atrophic, pigmented skin has developed at or above the ankle, secondary ulcerations may occur—often as a result of little or no trauma. An ulcer will occasionally extend into the varix, and the resulting fistula will be associated with profuse hemorrhage unless the leg is elevated and local pressure is applied to the bleeding point.

Chronic stasis dermatitis with fungal and bacterial infection may be a problem (see pp 78 and 298).

Thrombophlebitis may develop in the varicosities, particularly in postoperative patients and pregnant or postpartum women or those taking oral contraceptives. Local trauma or prolonged periods of sitting may also lead to superficial venous thrombosis (see p 297). Extension of the thrombosis into the deep venous system by way of the perforating veins or through the saphenofemoral junction may occur. (See Thrombophlebitis, p 292.)

Prevention

Individuals with early or minimal varicosities, particularly if there is a family history of varicosities and their activities involve a great deal of standing, should use elastic stockings to protect their veins from the chronic venous hypertension that is not reduced by walking. Elastic stockings are particularly important in these individuals if pregnancy occurs.

Treatment

A. Nonsurgical Measures: The use of elastic stockings (medium or heavy weight) to give external support to the veins of the proximal foot and leg up to but not including the knee is the best nonoperative approach to the management of varicose veins. When elastic stockings are worn during the hours that involve much standing and when this is combined with the habit of elevation of the legs when possible, reasonably good control can be maintained and progression of the condition and the development of complications can often be avoided. This approach may be used in elderly patients, in those who refuse or wish to defer surgery, sometimes in women with mild or moderate varicosities who plan to have more children, and in those with mild asymptomatic varicosities.

B. Surgical Measures: The surgical treatment of varicose veins consists of interruption or removal of the varicosities and the incompetent perforating veins. Accurate delineation and division of the latter are required to prevent recurrence in the varicosities that are not to be removed. The most important phase of the procedure is transection and ligation of the incompetent long saphenous vein precisely at its junction with the common femoral vein, combined with ligation and division of the 5 or 6 tributaries joining the terminal 3–10 cm of this vein. The previously marked incompetent perforating veins and the large varicosed tributaries of the saphenous system can then be ligated and the long saphenous vein removed by the stripping method. The same technique may be applied to the short saphenous vein if varicosed, as it occasionally is. If the stripping procedure is not considered necessary or desirable, as in older individuals or those with minimal varicosities, the entire operation can be done under local anesthesia. Venous segments that are not demonstrated to be incompetent and varicosed should not be ligated or removed; they may be needed as artery grafts later in the patient's life.

Varicose ulcers that are small generally heal with local care, frequent periods of elevation of the extremity, and compression bandages or some form of compression boot dressing for the ambulatory patient (see p 298). It is best to defer a stripping procedure until healing has been achieved and stasis dermatitis has been controlled. Some ulcers require skin grafting.

C. Compression Sclerotherapy: Sclerotherapy to obliterate and produce permanent fibrosis of the collapsed veins is generally reserved for the treatment of residual small varicosities following definitive varicose vein surgery, although it is used by some who have become very competent in this technique as a primary form of treatment. With the patient reclining and following the aspiration of all blood from an isolated segment of vein, an injection of 0.5 mL sclerosing solution into the vein is made (3% sodium tetradecyl sulfate [Sotradecol] is often used), and this is followed by ambulation with continuous pressure to that segment of vein for 1–4 weeks. Complications such as phlebitis, tissue necrosis, or infection may occur.

Prognosis

Patients should be informed that even extensive and carefully performed surgery may not prevent the development of additional varicosities and that further (though usually more limited) surgery or scleropathy may be necessary in later years. Good results with relief of symptoms are usually obtained in most patients. If extensive varicosities reappear after surgery, the completeness of the high ligation should be questioned, and reexploration of the saphenofemoral area

may be necessary. Even after adequate treatment, secondary tissue changes may not regress.

Bernard KG et al: Relative importance of incompetent communicating veins in the production of varicose veins and venous ulcer. *Surgery* 1977;**82**:9.

Crane C: The surgery of varicose veins. *Surg Clin North Am* 1979;**59**:737.

Hobbs JT: Surgery and sclerotherapy in the treatment of varicose veins: A random trial. *Arch Surg* 1974;**109**:793.

Larson HL et al: Long-term results after vein surgery: Study of 1000 cases after 10 years. *Mayo Clin Proc* 1974;**49**:114.

THROMBOPHLEBITIS

Thrombophlebitis is partial or complete occlusion of a vein by a thrombus with secondary inflammatory reaction in the wall of the vein. The thrombotic process, once established, is generally quite similar in all cases no matter what the cause, although the initiating factors may be quite variable. Trauma to the endothelium of the vein wall resulting in exposure of subendothelial tissue to platelets in the venous blood may initiate thrombosis, especially if a degree of venous stasis also exists. Intravascular stimuli affecting the blood, such as antigen-antibody complexes, viruses, bacteria, endotoxins, or autonomic and adrenal reactions, may also result in the release of platelet constituents. Platelet aggregates form on the vein wall followed by the deposition of fibrin, leukocytes, and finally erythrocytes; a thrombus results that can then propagate along the veins as a free-floating clot. Within 7–10 days, this thrombus becomes adherent to the vein wall, and secondary inflammatory changes develop, although a free-floating tail may persist. The thrombus is ultimately invaded by fibroblasts, resulting in scarring of the vein wall and destruction of the valves. Central recanalization may occur later, with restoration of flow through the vein; however, because the valves do not recover function, directional flow is not reestablished, leading in turn to secondary functional and anatomic problems.

1. THROMBOPHLEBITIS OF THE DEEP VEINS

The deep veins of the lower extremities and pelvis are most frequently involved. The process arises approximately 80% of the time in the deep veins of the calf, although it can arise in the femoral or iliac veins. Radioisotope fibrinogen uptake studies on postoperative or posttrauma patients reveal the development of small thrombi in the deep calf veins within 24 hours in 27% of patients studied, and propagation of the thrombosis into the popliteal and femoral veins takes place in approximately 10% of these cases. The process may become clinically detectable 4–14 days following major surgery or trauma or the end of pregnancy. Approximately 3% of patients undergoing major general surgical procedures will develop clinical manifestations of thrombophlebitis; many others with the process will have no detectable findings. Twelve percent of patients undergoing total hip replacement develop evidence of thromboembolic complications. Illnesses that involve periods of bed rest, such as cardiac failure, stroke, sepsis, or cancer, are associated with a high incidence of thrombophlebitis, especially if shock, anemia, obesity, or dehydration is also present. Use of oral contraceptive drugs, especially by women over 30 and by those who smoke, is associated with coagulation abnormalities, resulting in thrombophlebitis in some women. These drugs should not be prescribed for women with a history of phlebitis or who are to have elective surgery, and they should be discontinued if there is any clinical suspicion of thrombophlebitis.

Clinical Findings

Approximately half of patients with thrombophlebitis have no symptoms or signs in the extremity in the early stages. The patient often suffers a pulmonary embolism, presumably from the leg veins, without symptoms or demonstrable abnormalities in the extremities.

A. Symptoms: The patient may complain of a dull ache, a tight feeling, or frank pain in the calf or, in more extensive cases, the whole leg, especially when walking. A feeling of anxiety is not uncommon.

B. Signs: Typical findings, though variable and unreliable and in about half of cases absent, are as follows: slight swelling in the involved calf, as noted by careful measurements; distention of the superficial venous collaterals; tenderness and induration or spasm in the calf muscles, with or without pain in the calf, produced by dorsiflexion of the foot (Homans' sign); warmth of the affected leg when both legs are exposed to room temperature for a few minutes; and slight fever and tachycardia. Any of these signs may occur without deep vein thrombosis. When the femoral and iliac veins are also involved, there may be tenderness over these veins, and the swelling in the extremity may be marked (phlegmasia alba dolens). The skin may be cyanotic if venous obstruction is severe (phlegmasia cerulea dolens), or pale and cool if a reflex arterial spasm is superimposed.

C. Diagnostic Techniques: Because of the difficulty in making a precise diagnosis by history and examination and because as accurate a diagnosis as possible is desirable before relatively prolonged and expensive therapy is initiated, diagnostic studies are being used with increasing frequency.

1. Ascending contrast venography, the most accurate and complete method of diagnosis thus far available, will define by x-ray means the location, extent, and degree of attachment of the thrombosis (thrombi in the profunda femoris and internal iliac veins will not be demonstrated). Bilateral studies are of importance in planning therapy. Because of the time, expense, and discomfort involved, this test is not used as a screening study and is unsuitable for repeated monitoring. It is particularly useful when the clinical picture strongly suggests calf vein thromboses but noninvasive tests are equivocal. It may on occasion produce or exacerbate a thrombotic process. A chest x-ray should be obtained on admission to the hospital and a pulmonary arteriogram may be necessary to determine if embolization has occurred.

2. The radioactive (^{125}I) fibrinogen uptake test defines the presence of small thrombi in the calf and allows observation of the thrombotic process over several days. It is the most sensitive test for deep venous thrombosis developing in the calf, popliteal, and femoral veins, and the process can be followed by daily testing. A perfusion and ventilation lung scan is often helpful in determining the presence of pulmonary emboli.

3. The Doppler ultrasound blood flow detector allows the major veins in an extremity to be examined for thrombosis. This test is of value as a rapid screening procedure for the detection of thrombosis in large veins in high-risk patients, and it may be particularly helpful in detecting an extension of small thrombi in the calf veins (see ¶ 2 above) into the popliteal and femoral veins. Venous plethysmography may also be used to detect the alteration of venous flow by obstruction of thrombi. Small thrombi in calf veins when collateral channels are patent or even large thrombi in the main channel if not fully obstructing may be missed. The combination of a Doppler examination and plethysmography is more sensitive and specific than either test alone. Because the accuracy of these methods in detecting main channel deep venous obstruction is approaching 85–95%, the decision to start anticoagulation therapy can be based in most cases on one of these tests. If available, these tests should be employed rather than starting anticoagulant therapy on the basis of clinical impression only.

Differential Diagnosis

Calf muscle strain or contusion may be difficult to differentiate from thrombophlebitis; phlebography may be required to determine the correct diagnosis.

Cellulitis may be confused with thrombophlebitis; with infection, there is usually an associated wound, and inflammation of the skin is more marked.

Obstruction of the lymphatics or the iliac vein in the retroperitoneal area from tumor or irradiation may lead to unilateral swelling, but it is usually more chronic and painless. An acute arterial occlusion is more painful, the distal pulses are absent, there is usually no swelling, and the superficial veins in the foot fill slowly when emptied.

Bilateral leg edema is more likely to be due to heart or kidney disease.

Complications

A. Pulmonary Embolism: See Chapter 7, p 156.

B. Chronic Venous Insufficiency: Chronic venous insufficiency with or without secondary varicosities is a late complication of deep thrombophlebitis. (See Chronic Venous Insufficiency, p 297.)

Prevention

Prophylactic measures may diminish the incidence of venous thrombosis in hospitalized patients.

A. Venous Stasis: Venous stasis may be avoided by the following measures–

1. Elevation of the foot of the bed 15–20 degrees will encourage venous flow from the legs, particularly if the head of the bed is kept low or horizontal. Slight flexion of the knees is desirable. This position is also maintained on the operating table and in the recovery room.

2. Leg exercises, carried out by the surgical team immediately following major surgery and during the early postoperative period and practiced by the patient when in bed, are important. A few minutes every hour of leg exercises against a footboard are helpful. The importance of frequent leg movements and exercises as well as ambulation and very limited chair sitting should be explained to patients so as to secure their cooperation.

3. Elastic antiphlebitic stockings may be employed, particularly in patients with varicose veins or a history of phlebitis who will require bed rest for a number of days.

4. Walking for brief but regular periods postoperatively and during long airplane and automobile trips should be encouraged, because active, healthy travelers may sometimes develop thrombotic problems.

B. Hypercoagulable Tendencies: Hypercoagulable tendencies may be modified by the following measures–

1. Avoiding or treating promptly predisposing conditions such as dehydration, anemia, shock, infection, or congestive heart failure and minimizing tissue trauma during surgery.

2. Anticoagulants may be used in patients considered high risk for venous thrombosis.

a. Low-dose heparin, 5000 units every 12 hours subcutaneously 2 hours preoperatively and during the postoperative period of bed rest and limited ambulation, appears to be effective in reducing the incidence of thromboembolic complications in high-risk patients, although its effectiveness in major pelvic and hip procedures has been disappointing. Significant postoperative or posttrauma bleeding is not generally a problem, but heparin should not be taken by patients who are also taking aspirin or those (10% of patients) who are unusually sensitive to the drug (consider preoperative drug response evaluation). It should not be used whenever limited bleeding would be dangerous, such as in brain and eye surgery.

b. Dextran, 500 mL of 10% low-molecular-weight solution started intravenously at the onset of surgery and repeated in the early postoperative period and the day following surgery, may be of value, although allergic reaction, bleeding, or congestive failure may complicate its use.

c. Aspirin, 150 mg daily, may have a prophylactic value in men when used both pre- and postoperatively.

Treatment of Acute Thrombophlebitis

A. Local Measures: The legs should be elevated 15–20 degrees, the trunk should be kept horizontal, and the head and shoulders may be supported with pillows. The legs should be slightly flexed at the knees. Bed rest should be maintained until local tenderness and swelling have disappeared, by which time the thrombus has generally become adherent to the vein wall; a week may be adequate for calf thrombosis and 10–14 days for thigh or pelvic thrombosis. Walking but not standing or sitting is then permitted; the time out of bed and walking is increased each day.

Below-the-knee elastic support may be started soon after diagnosis and should be used when ambulation is started and continued for a number of months, or years if the process has been extensive (see p 297). Intermittent elevation of the legs is also important.

B. Medical Measures (Anticoagulants): Therapy with anticoagulants is considered to be the preferred treatment in most cases of deep thrombophlebitis with or without pulmonary embolism. There is evidence that the relatively high incidence of fatal pulmonary embolism secondary to venous thrombosis is significantly reduced by adequate anticoagulant therapy, and the incidence of death from additional emboli following an initial embolism is apparently reduced from approximately 20% to 1–2%. Progressive thrombosis with its associated morbidity is also reduced considerably, and the chronic secondary changes in the involved leg are probably also less severe. When embolic fatalities do occur during well-established and adequate heparin therapy, it is likely that the thrombus responsible has already developed to the point of insensitivity to heparin. Heparin acts rapidly and must be considered the anticoagulant of choice for short-term therapy; it can only be given parenterally, so hospitalization is necessary. After the initial phase of therapy with heparin, and if a prolonged period of anticoagulation is advisable, an oral drug can be used. (See p 295; also see ¶ 4 on p 296 for contraindications to anticoagulants.)

The rate of subsidence of symptoms is variable, and occasional cases are quite refractory to therapy. A developing thrombus generally becomes more firmly adherent to the vessel wall in 7–10 days; thus, therapy should probably be continued for at least 9–12 days for venous thrombosis and 14–21 days for pulmonary embolism. It may have to be continued for a longer period if signs and symptoms of active or unresolved thrombosis persist or if the patient has a marked thrombotic tendency, with a history of recurrent acute episodes. In the patients who were not ill or postoperative at the time the thrombophlebitis developed (ie, those with a significant thrombotic tendency), long-term anticoagulant therapy over a period of 6 or more months is probably advisable. This is particularly true if there has been an associated pulmonary embolism.

1. Heparin–Before starting heparin therapy, baseline coagulation studies should be obtained that should include not only the clotting time study to be

used in following the heparin therapy but also a prothrombin time, a partial thromboplastin time, a bleeding time, a blood urea nitrogen measurement, and a
platelet count. The therapeutic range of the commonly
used clotting time studies is considered to be 1½–2
times the baseline pretreatment value, although there is
evidence that high doses resulting in greater prolongation of the clotting time should be used in the first 48
hours, when bleeding complications are least likely to
occur and when it is most difficult to reverse the
thrombotic process and associated symptoms such as
vasospasm and inflammation. The normal activated
clotting time (ACT) at 37 °C is 80–130 seconds, and
this is probably the most useful of the various clotting
time determinations in following heparin therapy. Because the test can be done at the bedside, any necessary
adjustment in the heparin dose can be made immediately. The desired therapeutic range is usually
140–170 seconds. The plasma activated partial thromboplastin time (APTT) is another available test. Serious bleeding complications, such as bleeding into the
brain or retroperitoneum, are more likely to occur in
patients with other serious concomitant illnesses; in
patients over age 60 (especially women); in patients
with hypertension, uremia, hemostatic defects, or
duodenal ulcer; or in patients who have had recent
trauma or surgery. Heparin should be used with great
care in such patients.

The patient's response to heparin must be observed closely by laboratory determinations, for the
dose of heparin required to maintain the clotting time at
a therapeutic level may vary considerably with individuals or even in the same patient at different times
during the course of treatment. Bleeding complications generally occur after the second day of treatment,
and the dose of heparin required can often be reduced
after the first 2–4 days. Platelet counts should be
performed every 2–3 days, and if thrombocytopenia
develops, heparin should be discontinued. A hematocrit and a test on urine and stool for occult blood every
2–3 days may help detect bleeding. Aspirin and similar anti-inflammatory drugs and intramuscular medication should be avoided during heparin therapy. Several
methods of administration are available.

Continuous intravenous infusion of heparin by
means of a reliable infusion pump is favored over
intermittent intravenous or subcutaneous therapy with
a total dose per 24 hours in a range of 480 units/kg ideal
weight. Before starting the constant infusion, an initial
loading dose of heparin should be given intravenously
as a bolus (100 units/kg is often used). The constant
infusion may then be started so that the average-sized
adult receives 1500 units of heparin per hour (250–500
mL of 5% dextrose solution containing 100 units/mL is
a convenient concentration), and the hourly dose is
subsequently adjusted depending on laboratory determinations performed every 2–3 hours on blood drawn
from the arm not being infused. A heparin algorithm
combined with an easily interpreted flowchart giving
specific instructions with respect to the volume per
hour required to deliver the desired dose of heparin is a
great help to personnel who administer this potentially
dangerous drug. Precautionary measures during treatment include tests for blood in stool, vomitus, and
urine and an automatic stop order in the event of
suspicious developments. After a stable infusion rate
has been achieved, as determined by at least 2 successive clotting times in the therapeutic range (140–170
seconds for the ACT), subsequent laboratory control
may be repeated every 8–12 hours or possibly less
often if a stable state develops. The therapeutic dose of
heparin usually becomes less within 2–4 days.

If reliable continuous infusion equipment with
skilled supervision is not available, intermittent intravenous heparin injected through a special needle retained in a vein for that purpose may be started using a
4- or 6-hour schedule, and the subsequent dose during
the initial regulatory period is based on the clotting
times as determined just before the next scheduled
injection, based on an ACT or APTT close to but not
more than one and one-half times the baseline pretreatment value. This method is apparently associated
with a higher incidence of bleeding complications but a
lower incidence of recurrent thrombosis.

2. Thrombolytic agents–The use of a plasminogen activator, eg, streptokinase or urokinase, requires
close monitoring and experience. (See p 158.)

3. Oral anticoagulants–Many prefer to use only
heparin for anticoagulation; those who shift to the
prothrombin depressant drugs usually do so after the
symptoms and signs of thrombosis have largely or
completely subsided and after the patient becomes
ambulatory. Heparin may thus be used for the first
7–14 days (sometimes even longer) and withdrawn
only when the prothrombin time has been depressed to
the therapeutic range for 3–4 days, by which time all
the anticoagulant effects of the drug will be in effect.

Prothrombin depressant drugs include coumarin
and indandione derivatives; of these, warfarin sodium
(Coumadin) is most commonly used now. The dose
during the first 48 hours of therapy is usually 10–15
mg/d. The usual maintenance dose is 2.5–7.5 mg daily
and must be determined for each individual patient.
The approximate duration of effect of the drug is 2–3
days. A pretreatment prothrombin time should be determined, and if it is prolonged as compared with the
control value, less drug should be used. Smaller doses
should be used in the elderly, in patients with kidney or
liver disease, and in those with congestive heart failure
or chronic illness. These drugs are contraindicated
during pregnancy. Interaction with many other drugs
does occur, and the anticoagulant effect may be either
potentiated or reduced; this possibility must be considered if the individual is already receiving other drugs at
the time the anticoagulant is started. Careful attention
to the maintenance dose is also required when a new
drug which enhances or inhibits the anticoagulant effect is added or one which was in use is withdrawn.
Interacting drugs should be avoided if possible. Many
of the drugs that increase and decrease the sensitivity to
coumarins are listed in Table 2 of the Appendix (p
1091).

A good therapeutic effect can usually be achieved in 3–5 days and exists when the prothrombin time is around 2 times the control value or 20–25% of the normal value. Further prolongation of the prothrombin time may result in bleeding complications (ie, hematuria, ecchymosis, epistaxis, gastrointestinal bleeding). At the beginning of treatment, daily prothrombin activities should be determined and the subsequent dose withheld until the report is received. In well-stabilized patients, weekly to monthly determination may be adequate.

4. Treatment of bleeding and overdosage–Any new development that occurs in a patient receiving anticoagulant therapy should be considered to be a complication of the anticoagulant until proved otherwise. Whereas bleeding complications will occur in at least 3% and death will result in 0.3% of patients receiving anticoagulants, the incidence of complications is considerably higher with heparin therapy and may be as high as 25–35% in some groups (older patients, especially women; patients with other serious concurrent disease or a history of bleeding problems or duodenal ulcer; and patients receiving other medication with anticoagulant properties or intramuscular medication). Complications appear most frequently after the first 3 days of heparin; they are infrequent when heparin is being given while diagnostic studies are in progress to determine whether thrombophlebitis is present, but hypotension can result, and in most cases, the heparin activity will disappear rapidly enough to make its use unnecessary. Protamine sulfate administered slowly intravenously will neutralize any previously administered heparin. In most clinical situations, heparin activity will disappear rapidly enough to obviate the need for protamine; the maximum dose is 100 mg intravenously. Phytonadione (Mephyton [oral] or AquaMephyton [intravenous]) will counteract the effect of prothrombin depressant drugs, and if transfusion is necessary, fresh blood or fresh frozen plasma should be used.

5. Thrombolytic therapy–The ideal treatment for thrombophlebitis involving the iliac, femoral, or popliteal veins or for a major pulmonary embolism would involve removal of the thrombus and restoration of blood flow through vessels that have been cleaned of the thrombus with little or no damage to their walls or valves. Heparin will not remove a thrombus and only serves to halt an ongoing thrombotic process. Streptokinase and urokinase, potent and expensive thrombolytic agents, will clear the vessels of fresh clots and may restore them to normal function, but such therapy involves a risk of bleeding that is definitely greater than that associated with the use of heparin. Such agents should be used only when the benefits outweigh the risks, when there is no known vessel defect that might be a source of bleeding (superficial or deep), and when extreme care and careful monitoring is employed during the course of therapy.

C. Surgical Measures:

1. Vein ligation–Ligation or plication of the inferior vena cava with a partially occluding plastic clip or, less commonly, of one or both common femoral veins is recommended when anticoagulant therapy is undesirable or contraindicated. Examples are patients with peptic ulcer, significant liver or kidney disease, or known clotting defect; those with malignant hypertension with retinopathy; those with a history of cerebrovascular hemorrhage or recent head trauma; or those who are 1–3 days postoperative, especially if the operation has involved extensive dissection or surgery on the brain or spinal cord. Vein ligation is also indicated if there are signs of propagation of the thrombus or if emboli continue to occur during adequate anticoagulant therapy (3–16% of patients), if pulmonary hypertension has developed from multiple small emboli, after pulmonary artery embolectomy, or if septic phlebitis is present. Simultaneous ligation of the ovarian veins is advocated if septic phlebitis is present.

The chance of a second, possibly fatal pulmonary embolism is appreciably reduced after ligation or plication of the inferior vena cava, but recurrent emboli may still occur (6–36%), and the surgical mortality rate is about 7–20%. Although some degree of chronic edema of the legs may develop as a result of ligation (15–30%), it can usually be minimized if anticoagulant therapy is resumed 1–2 days following surgery and if follow-up care, consisting of elastic supports to the lower legs and elevation of the legs at intervals, is continued for at least 1 year (see next section).

Inferior vena caval filter devices may be inserted under local anesthesia through the right internal jugular vein to the third lumbar level, using radiologic control. This approach is considerably safer than surgical ligation, is quite effective in trapping further emboli, generally does not result in later caval occlusion, and may be the preferred means of preventing embolism in those who require mechanical protection.

2. Femoral vein thrombectomy–In the rare case of massive venous occlusion (phlegmasia cerulea dolens) that has not responded to elevation of the leg, heparin, and fluid and electrolyte replacement, thrombectomy to remove the iliofemoral thrombosis may be considered if the condition is of recent onset (1–2 days) and venous gangrene is considered a possibility.

Prognosis

With adequate treatment the patient usually returns to normal health and activity within 3–6 weeks. The prognosis in most cases is good once the period of danger of pulmonary embolism has passed, but for the first 2–3 weeks it is guarded. Occasionally, recurrent episodes of phlebitis will occur in spite of good local and anticoagulant management. Such cases may even have recurrent pulmonary emboli as well. Chronic venous insufficiency may result, with its associated complications (see p 297).

Donaldson MC, Wirthlin LS, Donaldson GA: Thirty-year experience with surgical interruption of the inferior vena cava for prevention of pulmonary embolism. *Ann Surg* 1980;**191**:367.

Dosick SM, Blakemore WS: The role of Doppler ultrasound in acute deep vein thrombosis. *Am J Surg* 1978;**136**:265.

Greenfield LJ et al: Greenfield vena caval filter experience: Late results in 156 patients. *Arch Surg* 1981;**116**:1451.

Hull R et al: Warfarin sodium versus low-dose heparin in the long-term treatment of venous thrombosis. *N Engl J Med* 1979;**301**:855.

Kakkar VV: Deep vein thrombosis: Detection and prevention. *Circulation* 1975;**51**:8.

Madden JL, Hume M (editors): *Venous Thromboembolism: Prevention and Treatment.* Appleton-Century-Crofts, 1977.

Marder JM: The use of thrombolytic agents: Choice of patient, drug administration, laboratory monitoring. *Ann Intern Med* 1979;**90**:802.

O'Donnell TF et al: Diagnosis of deep venous thrombosis in the outpatient by venography. *Surg Gynecol Obstet* 1980;**150**:69.

Renney JTG, O'Sullivan EF, Burke PF: Prevention of postoperative deep vein thrombosis with dipyridamole and aspirin. *Br Med J* 1976;**1**:992.

Salzman EW, Davies GC: Prophylaxis of venous thromboembolism. *Ann Surg* 1980;**191**:207.

Sherry S: Low-dose heparin prophylaxis for postoperative venous thromboembolism. *N Engl J Med* 1975;**293**:300.

Skillman JJ: Postoperative deep vein thrombosis and pulmonary embolism: A selective review and personal viewpoint. *Surgery* 1974;**75**:114.

Wilson JE III et al: Heparin therapy in venous thromboembolism. *Am J Med* 1981;**70**:808.

2. THROMBOPHLEBITIS OF THE SUPERFICIAL VEINS

Essentials of Diagnosis

- Induration, redness, and tenderness along a superficial vein.
- No significant swelling of the extremity.

General Considerations

Superficial thrombophlebitis may occur spontaneously, as in pregnant or postpartum women or in individuals with varicose veins or thromboangiitis obliterans; or it may be associated with trauma, as in the case of a blow to the leg or following intravenous therapy with irritating solutions. In the migratory or recurrent form, thromboangiitis should be suspected. It may also be a manifestation of abdominal malignancy such as carcinoma of the pancreas and may be the earliest sign. The long saphenous vein is most often involved. Superficial thrombophlebitis may be associated with occult deep vein thrombosis in about 20% of cases. Pulmonary emboli are infrequent but do occur.

Short-term plastic venous catheterization of superficial arm veins is now in routine use. The catheter should be observed daily for signs of local inflammation. It should be removed if a local reaction develops in the vein, and in any case it should be removed in 48 hours. If further intravenous therapy is necessary, a new catheter may be inserted in a different vein. Serious septic complications can occur if this policy is not followed. The steel intravenous needle with the anchoring flange (butterfly needle) is less likely to be associated with phlebitis and infection than the plastic catheter.

Clinical Findings

The patient usually experiences a dull pain in the region of the involved vein. Local findings consist of induration, redness, and tenderness along the course of a vein. The process may be localized, or it may involve most of the long saphenous vein and its tributaries. The inflammatory reaction generally subsides in 1–2 weeks; a firm cord may remain for a much longer period. Edema of the extremity and deep calf tenderness are absent unless deep thrombophlebitis has also developed. If chills and high fever develop, septic thrombophlebitis exists.

Differential Diagnosis

The linear rather than circular nature of the lesion and the distribution along the course of a superficial vein serve to differentiate superficial phlebitis from cellulitis, erythema nodosum, erythema induratum, panniculitis, and fibromyositis. Lymphangitis and deep thrombophlebitis must also be considered.

Treatment

If the process is well localized and not near the saphenofemoral junction, local heat and bed rest with the leg elevated are usually effective in limiting the thrombosis. Phenylbutazone (Butazolidin), 100 mg orally 3 times daily for 5 days, may aid in the resolution of the inflammatory process but is contraindicated in individuals with peptic ulcer.

If the process is very extensive or is progressing upward toward the saphenofemoral junction, or if it is in the proximity of the saphenofemoral junction initially, ligation and division of the saphenous vein at the saphenofemoral junction are indicated. The inflammatory process usually regresses following this procedure, though removal of the involved segment of vein (stripping) may result in a more rapid recovery.

Anticoagulation therapy is usually not indicated unless the disease is rapidly progressing. It is indicated if there is extension into the deep system.

Septic thrombophlebitis requires excision of the involved vein up to its junction with an uninvolved vein in order to control bacteremia.

Prognosis

The course is generally benign and brief, and the prognosis depends on the underlying pathologic process. Phlebitis of a saphenous vein occasionally extends to the deep veins, in which case pulmonary embolism may occur.

Lofgren EP, Lofgren KA: The surgical treatment of superficial thrombophlebitis. *Surgery* 1981;**90**:49.

CHRONIC VENOUS INSUFFICIENCY

Essentials of Diagnosis

- A history is often obtained of phlebitis or leg injury.

- Ankle edema is the earliest sign.
- Stasis pigmentation, dermatitis, subcutaneous induration, and often varicosities occur later.
- Ulceration at or above the ankle is common (stasis ulcer).

General Considerations

Chronic venous insufficiency generally results from changes secondary to deep thrombophlebitis, although a definite history of phlebitis is not obtainable in about 25% of these patients. There is often a history of leg trauma. It can also occur in association with varicose veins (see p 290) and as a result of neoplastic obstruction of the pelvic veins or congenital or acquired arteriovenous fistula.

When insufficiency is secondary to deep thrombophlebitis (the postphlebitic syndrome), the valves in the deep venous channels and often in the perforating veins have been damaged or destroyed by the thrombotic process. The recanalized, nonelastic deep veins are functionally inadequate because of the damaged valves in the deep and communicating veins. The pumping action of the contracting calf muscles on the veins forcing blood upward out of the extremity is inefficient because the damaged valves do not prevent the retrograde flow of venous blood as they normally do, and the venous pressure, particularly in the superficial veins, is not lowered during walking, as is the case in the normal extremity. The venous pressure in the superficial veins, therefore, remains high at all times (ambulatory venous hypertension). This constant transmission of high venous pressure through the damaged perforating veins leads to secondary changes, including edema, fibrosis of subcutaneous tissue and skin, pigmentation of skin, and, later, dermatitis, cellulitis, and ulceration. Dilatation of the superficial veins may occur, leading to varicosities. Primary varicose veins with no abnormalities of the deep venous system may also result in changes characteristic of chronic venous stasis (see p 291), but edema is more pronounced in the postphlebitic extremities, and the secondary changes are more extensive and encircling.

Clinical Findings

Chronic venous insufficiency is characterized first by progressive edema of the leg (particularly the lower leg) and later also by secondary changes in the skin and subcutaneous tissues. The usual symptoms are itching, a dull discomfort made worse by periods of standing, and pain if an ulceration is present. The skin is usually thin, shiny, atrophic, and cyanotic; and a brownish pigmentation often develops. Eczema may be present, with superficial weeping dermatitis (see p 49). The subcutaneous tissues become thick and fibrous. Recurrent ulcerations are common, usually just above the ankle, on the medial or anterior aspect of the leg; healing results in a thin scar on a fibrotic base that breaks down with minor trauma. Varicosities often appear that are associated with incompetent perforating veins.

Differential Diagnosis

Congestive heart failure and chronic renal disease may result in bilateral edema of the lower extremities, but generally there are other clinical or laboratory findings of heart or kidney disease.

Lymphedema is associated with a brawny thickening in the subcutaneous tissue that does not respond readily to elevation; varicosities are absent, and there is often a history of recurrent episodes of cellulitis (see p 301).

Primary varicose veins may be difficult to differentiate from the secondary varicosities that often develop in this condition, as discussed above. Phlebography may occasionally be necessary to determine if the deep system is completely obstructed.

Other conditions associated with chronic ulcers of the leg include collagen diseases, arterial insufficiency (often very painful), sickle cell anemia (positive sickle cell test), erythema induratum (bilateral and usually on the posterior aspect of the lower part of the leg), and fungal infections (cultures specific; no chronic swelling or varicosities).

Prevention

Irreversible tissue changes and associated complications in the lower legs can be minimized through early and energetic treatment of actual thrombophlebitis with anticoagulants (see p 294) and specific measures to avoid chronic edema in subsequent years as described in section A, below.

Treatment

A. General Measures: Bed rest, with the legs elevated to diminish chronic edema, is fundamental in the treatment of the acute complications of chronic venous insufficiency. Measures to control the tendency toward edema include (1) intermittent elevation of the legs during the day and elevation of the legs at night (kept above the level of the heart with pillows under the mattress); (2) avoidance of long periods of sitting or standing; and (3) the use of well-fitting, heavy-duty elastic supports worn from the mid foot to just below the knee during the day and evening if there is any tendency for swelling to develop.

B. Stasis Dermatitis: Eczematous eruption may be acute or chronic; treatment varies accordingly. (See also pp 47, 77, and 79.)

1. Acute weeping dermatitis–

a. Wet compresses for 1 hour 4 times daily of solutions containing boric acid, potassium permanganate, buffered aluminum acetate (Burow's), or isotonic saline.

b. Compresses are followed with a local corticosteroid such as 0.5% hydrocortisone cream in a water-soluble base. (Neomycin and nystatin may be incorporated into this cream.)

c. Systemic antibiotics may be indicated if active infection is present.

2. Subsiding or chronic dermatitis–

a. Continue the hydrocortisone cream for 1–2 weeks or until no further improvement is noted. Cordran tape, a plastic tape impregnated with flurandrenolide, is a convenient way to apply both medication and dressing.

b. Zinc oxide ointment with ichthammol (Ichthyol), 3%, 1–2 times a day, cleaned off as desired with mineral oil.

c. Carbolfuchsin (Castellani's) paint to the toes and nails 1–2 times a week may help control dermatophytosis and onychomycosis. Miconazole cream (2%) may also be used.

3. Energetic treatment of chronic edema, as outlined in sections A and C, with almost complete bed rest is important during the acute phase of stasis dermatitis.

C. Ulceration: Ulcerations are preferably treated with compresses of isotonic saline solution, which aid the healing of the ulcer or may help prepare the base for a skin graft. A lesion can often be treated on an ambulatory basis by means of a semirigid boot applied to the leg after much of the swelling has been reduced by a period of elevation. The pumping action of the calf muscles on the blood flow out of the lower extremity is enhanced by a circumferential nonelastic bandage on the ankle and lower leg. The boot must be changed every 1–2 weeks, depending to some extent on the amount of drainage from the ulcer. The ulcer, tendons, and bony prominences must be adequately padded. Special ointments on the ulcer are not necessary. The semirigid boot may be made with Unna's paste (Gelocast, Medicopaste) or Gauztex bandage (impregnated with a nonallergenic self-adhering compound). After the ulcer has healed, heavy below-the-knee elastic stockings are used in an effort to prevent recurrent edema and ulceration. Occasionally, the ulcer is so large and chronic that total excision of the ulcer, with skin graft of the defect, is the best approach. This is often combined with ligation of all incompetent perforating veins.

D. Secondary Varicosities: Varicosities secondary to damage to the deep system of veins may in turn contribute to undesirable changes in the tissues of the lower leg. Varicosities should occasionally be removed and the incompetent veins connecting the superficial and deep system ligated, but the tendency toward edema will persist, because the chronic high venous pressure is usually not very effectively lowered during walking by the procedure, and thus the measures outlined above (¶ A) will be required for life. Varicosities can often be treated along with edema by elastic stockings and other nonoperative measures, and only about 15–20% require surgery. If the obstructive element in the deep system appears to be severe, phlebography may be of value in mapping out the areas of venous obstruction or incompetence in the deep system as well as the number and location of the damaged perforating veins. A decision about whether to treat with surgery may be influenced by such a study; if the varicosities furnish the chief route of venous return, they should not be removed. Venous valvular reconstructive surgery is now in a developmental stage.

Prognosis

Individuals with chronic venous insufficiency often have recurrent problems, particularly if measures to counteract persistent venous hypertension, edema, and secondary tissue changes are not conscientiously adhered to throughout life. Additional episodes of acute thrombophlebitis may occur.

Dale WA: Surgery for chronic peripheral venous hypertension. *Contemp Surg* (March) 1980;**16**:28.

Huse JF et al: Direct venous surgery for venous valvular insufficiency of the lower extremity. *Arch Surg* 1983;**118**:719.

SUPERIOR VENA CAVA OBSTRUCTION

Obstruction of the superior vena cava is a relatively rare condition that is usually secondary to the neoplastic or inflammatory process in the superior mediastinum. The most frequent causes are (1) neoplasms, such as lymphomas, primary malignant mediastinal tumors, or carcinoma of the lung with direct extension (over 80%); (2) chronic fibrotic mediastinitis, either of unknown origin or secondary to tuberculosis or pyogenic infection; (3) thrombophlebitis, often by extension of the process from the axillary or subclavian vein into the innominate vein and vena cava and often associated with catheterization of these veins for central venous pressure measurements or for hyperalimentation; (4) aneurysm of the aortic arch; and (5) constrictive pericarditis.

Clinical Findings

A. Symptoms and Signs: There usually is an insidious onset as progressive obstruction of the venous drainage of the head, neck, and upper extremities develops. The cutaneous veins of the upper chest and lower neck become dilated, and edema develops around the eyes. Later, edema of the face, neck, and arms develops, and cyanosis of these areas then appears. Cerebral and laryngeal edema ultimately results in impaired function of the brain as well as respiratory insufficiency. Bending over or lying down accentuates the symptoms; sitting quietly is generally preferred. The manifestations are more severe if the obstruction develops rapidly and if the azygos junction or the vena cava between that vein and the heart is obstructed.

B. Laboratory Findings: The venous pressure is elevated (often over 20 cm of water) in the arm and is normal in the leg. A supraclavicular lymph node biopsy may supply a tissue diagnosis.

C. X-Ray Findings: Chest x-rays and a CT scan will define the location and often the nature of the obstructive process, and phlebography will map out the extent and degree of the venous obstruction and the collateral circulation. Estimation of blood flow around the occlusion, as well as serial evaluation of the response to therapy, may be obtained by means of radionuclear scans using intravenous injection of technetium Tc 99m pertechnetate.

Treatment

If the primary problem is due to a malignant neoplasm, radiation therapy or chemotherapy may relieve the pressure on the superior vena cava. Surgery may be necessary in order to arrive at a diagnosis. When the caval obstruction is severe, urgent operation to bypass the obstruction using a large autogenous venous graft constructed from saphenous vein and placed between one internal jugular vein and the right atrium will provide immediate venous decompression that can be followed by radiation therapy or chemotherapy or both. Some consider radiation without surgery the preferred treatment for the obstructive problems secondary to cancer. If the process results from tuberculosis, antituberculosis chemotherapy is indicated. In cases secondary to mediastinal fibrosis, excision of the fibrous tissue around the great vessels may reestablish flow.

Prognosis

The prognosis depends upon the nature and degree of obstruction and its speed of onset. Slowly developing forms secondary to fibrosis may be tolerated for years. A high degree of obstruction of rapid onset secondary to cancer is often fatal in a few days or weeks, but bypass surgery followed by treatment of the tumor with radiation and drugs may result in significant palliation.

Lockridge SK et al: Obstruction of the superior vena cava. *Surgery* 1979;**85**:14.

Parish JM et al: Etiologic considerations in superior vena cava syndrome. *Mayo Clin Proc* 1981;**56**:407.

DISEASES OF THE LYMPHATIC CHANNELS

LYMPHANGITIS & LYMPHADENITIS

Essentials of Diagnosis

- Red streak from wound or area of cellulitis toward regional lymph nodes, which are usually enlarged and tender.
- Chills, fever, and malaise may be present.

General Considerations

Lymphangitis and lymphadenitis are common manifestations of a bacterial infection that is usually caused by hemolytic streptococci and usually arises from an area of cellulitis, generally at the site of an infected wound. The wound may be very small or superficial, or an established abscess may be present, feeding bacteria into the lymphatics. The involvement of the lymphatics is often manifested by a red streak in the skin extending in the direction of the regional lymph nodes, which are, in turn, generally tender and enlarged. Systemic manifestations include fever, chills, and malaise. The infection may progress rapidly, often in a matter of hours, and may lead to bacteremia or septicemia and even death.

Clinical Findings

A. Symptoms and Signs: Throbbing pain is usually present in the area of cellulitis at the site of bacterial invasion. Malaise, anorexia, sweating, chills, and fever of 37.8–40 °C (100–104 °F) develop rapidly. The red streak, when present, may be definite or may be very faint and easily missed. It is not usually tender or indurated, as is the area of cellulitis. The involved regional lymph nodes may be significantly enlarged and are usually quite tender. The pulse is often rapid.

B. Laboratory Findings: Leukocytosis with an increase in immature cells is usually present. Later, a blood culture may be positive. Culture and sensitivity studies on the wound exudate or pus may be helpful in treatment of the more severe or refractory infections.

Differential Diagnosis

Lymphangitis may be confused with superficial thrombophlebitis (see p 297), but the erythematous reaction associated with thrombosis overlies the induration of the inflammatory reaction in and around the thrombosed vein. Venous thrombosis is not associated with lymphadenitis, and a wound of entrance with the secondary cellulitis is generally absent. Superficial thrombophlebitis frequently arises as a result of intravenous therapy, particularly when the needle or catheter is left in place for more than 2 days; if bacteria have also been introduced, suppurative thrombophlebitis may develop.

Cat-scratch fever should be considered when multiple superficial cat scratches are noted on the extremities and lymphadenitis is present in which the nodes, though often very large, are relatively nontender.

Neither of these conditions is accompanied by the systemic manifestations that often occur with acute cellulitis with lymphangitis and lymphadenitis.

Treatment

A. General Measures: Prompt treatment should include heat (hot, moist compresses or heating pad), elevation when feasible, and immobilization of the infected area. Analgesics may be prescribed for pain.

B. Specific Measures: Antibiotic therapy should always be instituted when local infection becomes invasive, as manifested by cellulitis and lymphangitis. A culture of any purulent discharge available should be obtained (often there is nothing to culture), and antibiotic therapy should be started in full doses at once. The initial drug may have to be replaced by a second antibiotic if a clinical response is not apparent in 36–48 hours or if the culture and sensitivity studies indicate that it is not effective. Because the causative organism is so frequently the streptococcus, penicillin is usually the drug of choice. If the patient is allergic to penicillin, erythromycin or a cephalosporin may be used. (See Chapter 29.)

C. Wound Care: Drainage of pus from an infected wound should be carried out, generally after the above measures have been instituted and only when it is clear that there is an abscess associated with the site of initial infection. An area of cellulitis should not be incised, because the infection may be spread by attempted drainage when pus is not present. It is extremely important to differentiate cellulitis from soft tissue infections that require early and aggressive incision and often resection of necrotic infected tissue, eg, acute streptococcal hemolytic gangrene, necrotizing fasciitis, gram-negative anaerobic cutaneous gangrene, and progressive bacterial synergistic gangrene.

Prognosis

With proper therapy and particularly with the use of an antibiotic effective against the invading bacteria, control of the infection can usually be achieved in a few days. Delayed or inadequate therapy can still lead to overwhelming infection with septicemia and death.

Baxter CR: Surgical management of soft tissue infections. *Surg Clin North Am* 1972;**52**:1483.

LYMPHEDEMA

Essentials of Diagnosis

- Painless edema of one or both lower extremities, primarily in young women.
- Initially, pitting edema, which becomes brawny and often nonpitting with time.
- Ulceration, varicosities, and stasis pigmentation do not occur.
- There may be episodes of lymphangitis and cellulitis.

General Considerations

The underlying mechanism in lymphedema is impairment of the flow of lymph from an extremity. When due to congenital developmental abnormalities consisting of hypo- or hyperplastic involvement of the proximal or distal lymphatics, it is referred to as the primary form. The obstruction may be in the pelvic or lumbar lymph channels and nodes when the disease is extensive and progressive. The secondary form results when an inflammatory or mechanical obstruction of the lymphatics occurs from trauma, regional lymph node resection or irradiation, or extensive involvement of regional nodes by malignant disease or filariasis. Secondary dilatation of the lymphatics that occurs in both forms leads to incompetence of the valve system,

disrupting the orderly flow along the lymph vessels, and results in progressive stasis of a protein-rich fluid, with secondary fibrosis. Episodes of acute and chronic inflammation may be superimposed, with further stasis and fibrosis. Hypertrophy of the limb results, with markedly thickened and fibrotic skin and subcutaneous tissue and diminution in the fatty tissue.

Lymphangiography and radioactive isotope studies are often useful in defining the specific lymphatic defect.

Treatment

The treatment of lymphedema is often not very satisfactory. The majority of patients can be treated conservatively with some of the following measures. (1) The flow of lymph out of the extremity, with a consequent decrease in the degree of stasis, can be aided through intermittent elevation of the extremity, especially during the sleeping hours (foot of bed elevated 15–20 degrees, achieved by placing pillows beneath the mattress); the constant use of elastic bandages or carefully fitted heavy-duty elastic stockings; and massage toward the trunk—either by hand or by means of pneumatic pressure devices designed to milk edema out of an extremity. (The Wright linear pump delivers sequential pressure cycles that effectively milk fluid out of the foot and leg and then out of the thigh.) (2) Secondary cellulitis in the extremity should be avoided by means of good hygiene and treatment of any trichophytosis of the toes (see p 77). Once an infection starts, it should be treated by very adequate periods of rest, elevation, and antibiotics. Infection can be a serious and recurring problem and is often difficult to control. Intermittent prophylactic antibiotics may occasionally be necessary. (3) Intermittent courses of diuretic therapy, especially in those with premenstrual or seasonal exacerbations. (4) In carefully selected cases, there are operative procedures that may give satisfactory functional results. Lymphaticovenous anastomosis using microsurgery has yielded some satisfactory cosmetic and functional results, particularly in those with primary lymphedema. This technique may replace the more deforming procedures and those aimed at introducing lymphatic bridges or lymphatic venous connections. Amputation is used as a last resort in very severe forms or when lymphangiosarcoma develops in the extremity.

Montorsi M et al: Microsurgical treatment of lymphedemas of the limbs. *Int Surg* 1981;**66**:53.

Wolfe JHN, Kinmonth JB: The prognosis of primary lymphedema of the lower limbs. *Arch Surg* 1981;**116**:1157.

● ● ●

References

Bernstein EF (editor): *Noninvasive Diagnostic Techniques in Vascular Disease,* 3rd ed. Mosby, 1983.

Caspar M, Barker WF: *Peripheral Arterial Disease,* 3rd ed. Saunders, 1981.

Connolly JE (editor): Venous and arterial disease. *Surg Clin North Am* 1982;**62**:3. [Entire issue.]

Haimovici H (editor): *Vascular Surgery: Principles and Techniques,* 2nd ed. McGraw-Hill, 1984.

Hirsch J, Genton E, Hull R: *Venous Thromboembolism.* Grune & Stratton, 1981.

Juergens JL, Spittel JA Jr, Fairbairn JF II (editors): *Allen-Barker-Hines Peripheral Vascular Disease,* 5th ed. Saunders, 1980.

Moore WS: *Vascular Surgery: A Comprehensive Review.* Grune & Stratton, 1983.

Rutherford RB (editor): *Vascular Surgery.* 2nd ed. Saunders, 1983.

Wolfe WG, Sabiston DC Jr: *Pulmonary Embolism.* Saunders, 1980.

Blood | 10

Ralph O. Wallerstein, MD

ANEMIAS

Diagnosis of Anemia

Anemia is a common clinical finding, and an explanation must always be sought. Extensive investigations are sometimes required to determine the cause. The answers to the following 4 fundamental questions are always relevant to a complete evaluation of the anemia patient: (1) Is there evidence of iron deficiency? (2) Is the anemia megaloblastic? (3) Is there evidence of hemolysis? (4) Is the bone marrow hypoactive?

Iron deficiency must be considered in all anemias of obscure origin—regardless of red cell morphology. Serum ferritin levels below 12 ng/mL are diagnostic of iron deficiency anemia. The combination of low serum iron and elevated total iron-binding capacity (TIBC) is equally diagnostic, but serum iron measurements are useless in a febrile patient because they are always low.

The diagnosis of moderately severe megaloblastic anemia (fewer than 3 million red cells/μL) can always be made by examination of the blood and bone marrow. The blood shows oval macrocytes and hypersegmented granulocytes; the bone marrow contains megaloblasts.

The major hemolytic disorders, regardless of type, have in common reticulocytosis, slightly increased serum bilirubin (indirect), and an increased number of nucleated red cells in the marrow.

Table 10–1. The anemias.

Type	Characteristic Findings
Iron deficiency	Serum ferritin below 12 ng/mL, low serum iron, high TIBC.
Megaloblastic	Characteristic red cell, white cell, and marrow morphology.
Hemolytic	High reticulocyte count, low or absent haptoglobin, high indirect bilirubin.
Marrow failure Absolute (eg, aplastic anemia)	Pancytopenia; normal marrow tissue replaced by fat.
Relative (eg, infection, azotemia, cancer, liver disease, myxedema)	Red cell, white cell, and serum factors often have no distinguishing characteristics. The marrow picture is not striking.

In hypoplastic anemia, the bone marrow is fatty and contains relatively few nucleated red cells.

In any case of undiagnosed normocytic normochromic anemia that does not fall into the above 4 groups, the following causes must be considered: infection, azotemia, cancer, myxedema, and liver disease.

Wallerstein RO: Role of the laboratory in the diagnosis of anemia. *JAMA* 1976;**236**:490.

IRON DEFICIENCY ANEMIA

Essentials of Diagnosis

- Pallor, lassitude.
- Hypochromia, microcytosis. Red cell count less reduced than hemoglobin.
- Serum ferritin below 12 ng/mL.
- Serum iron low, total iron-binding capacity increased.
- Blood loss usually chronic and occult.

General Considerations

Iron deficiency anemia in the adult is almost always due to blood loss. Excessive menstrual flow and gastrointestinal bleeding (due to esophagitis, gastritis, peptic ulcer, previous gastrectomy, polyps, cancer, hemorrhoids, or excessive salicylate intake) are the principal causes. Gastrointestinal bleeding is usually chronic and occult. Rare causes include colonic vascular ectasias, hemosiderinuria, pulmonary hemosiderosis, excessive blood donation, faulty diet, and habitual starch eating.

A normal daily diet contains 12–15 mg of iron, or approximately 6 mg of iron per 1000 kcal, of which 5–10% (0.6–1.5 mg) is absorbed. (More iron is absorbed in iron deficiency anemia.) Normally, less than 1 mg of iron is excreted per day; iron metabolism is almost a closed system. Chronic bleeding of as little as 2–4 mL of blood per day may lead to a negative iron balance and iron deficiency anemia.

Clinical Findings

A. Symptoms and Signs: In addition to symptoms of the primary disease (if any), symptoms due to anemia may be present: easy fatigability, dyspnea, palpitation, angina, and tachycardia. Waxy pallor, brittle hair and nails, smooth tongue, cheilosis, and dysphagia are late findings. Pica—compulsive eating of anything—is probably more common than patients will admit.

B. Laboratory Findings: The hemoglobin may fall to as low as 3 g/dL, but the red cell count is rarely below 2.5 million/μL; the red cells are usually microcytic and hypochromic (although in approximately 20% of adults with iron deficiency, indices are normal). Reticulocytes and platelets are normal or increased. The white blood cell count is normal. Serum iron is usually below 30 μg/dL (normal is 90–150 μg/dL); total iron-binding capacity is elevated to 350–500 μg/dL (normal is 250–350 μg/dL). Iron saturation is 10% or less. The bone marrow aspirate contains increased numbers of nucleated red cells; the normoblasts have only scanty cytoplasm. Stainable iron is always absent.

Serum ferritin is below 12 ng/mL. Only iron deficiency can lower serum ferritin values. (Normal is 12–300 ng/mL; the mean value for men is 120 ng/mL and for women, 56 ng/mL; 1 ng/mL is equivalent to approximately 10 mg of storage iron.) Elevated serum ferritin values without increase in storage iron may occur with hepatitis, Hodgkin's disease, and acute leukemia. Serum ferritin levels of approximately 25 ng/mL may be seen in patients who have iron deficiency anemia complicated by inflammation or infection.

Differential Diagnosis

Iron deficiency anemia is the only anemia in which hemosiderin is absent in bone marrow; in all other types of anemia, iron is present in bone marrow in normal or increased amounts. In thalassemia minor (which also manifests as a hypochromic, microcytic anemia), the red cells are smaller and have a more abnormal appearance (for a given degree of anemia); the red cell count may be above normal and the hemoglobin is rarely below 9 g/dL; and the bone marrow hemosiderin, serum iron, and total iron-binding capacity are normal. Hemoglobin A_2 is usually increased.

Iron deficiency anemia must be differentiated from other hypochromic anemias.

A. Anemia of Infection: (See p 323.) Red cells are normocytic and mildly hypochromic. Serum iron is low, but total iron-binding capacity is also decreased. Serum ferritin levels are normal. Bone marrow hemosiderin is present.

B. Sideroblastic Anemias: See p 315.

C. Some Hemoglobinopathies: All hemoglobin abnormalities involving the thalassemia gene are microcytic and hypochromic, eg, thalassemia minor, sickle thalassemia, hemoglobin C-thalassemia, and hemoglobin H disease; the red cells in hemoglobin E disease may be quite small. The diagnosis is made by hemoglobin electrophoresis.

Complications

Severe dysphagia (Plummer-Vinson syndrome)

develops in some patients. Iron deficiency anemia may be the presenting finding in gastrointestinal cancer. In patients with heart disease, severe anemia may precipitate angina pectoris or congestive heart failure.

Treatment

The sources of blood loss must be identified and corrected. Iron is specific for this type of anemia. It should be started as soon as diagnosis is made. Transfusions are rarely needed. A satisfactory response to iron therapy, whether oral or parenteral, is a rise in hemoglobin of at least 2 g/dL in 3 weeks. Failure of hemoglobin levels to rise in a week or 2 does not necessarily mean failure of therapy. Reticulocytes often do not rise measurably when the baseline hemoglobin was over 7.5 g/dL.

A. Oral Preparations and Dosages: The maximum absorption of iron is about 25 mg/d. Give one of the following: (1) ferrous sulfate, 0.3 g 3 times daily after meals; or (2) ferrous gluconate, 0.3 g 3 times daily after meals. Oral iron administration should be continued for 3 months after hemoglobin values return to normal, in order to replenish iron stores.

Many other iron salts and chelates, often mixed with other metals or vitamins, are promoted, but none are more useful in iron deficiency anemia than ferrous sulfate. The degree of gastrointestinal irritation and the amount absorbed are functions of the iron content of the salt or complex.

B. Parenteral Iron: The indications are intolerance to oral iron, refractoriness to oral iron (poor absorption), gastrointestinal disease precluding the use of oral iron, continued blood loss, and replacement of depleted iron stores when oral iron fails. Parenteral iron should be given only in the amounts necessary to correct the deficiency. Calculate the total dosage as follows: 250 mg for each g of hemoglobin below normal. (Normal: men, 14 g; women, 12 g.)

Iron dextran injection (Imferon) for intramuscular use contains 5% metallic iron (50 mg/mL). Give 50 mg (1 mL) at first and then 100–250 mg intramuscularly daily or every other day until the total dose has been given. Inject deeply with a 5-cm needle into the upper outer quadrant of the buttock, using the "Z" technique (pulling the skin to one side before inserting the needle) to prevent leakage of the solution and discoloration of the skin. This preparation may also be given intravenously; it is best administered in doses of 250–500 mg. A test dose of 0.5 mL should be given first; if the patient experiences no unusual reaction, the entire amount may be given over 3–5 minutes. The intravenous route is preferred if repeated injections must be given, eg, in hereditary telangiectasia.

Prognosis

Following iron therapy, all the signs and symptoms of iron deficiency anemia are reversible unless blood loss continues. Bleeding in excess of 500 mL/wk over a period of weeks or months probably cannot be treated successfully by iron medication alone.

Clinical aspects of iron deficiency and excess. *Semin Hematol* 1982;**19**:1. [Entire issue.]

Cook JD, Finch CA: Assessing iron status of a population. *Am J Clin Nutr* 1979;**32**:2115.

Hamstra RD et al: Intravenous iron dextran in clinical medicine. *JAMA* 1980;**243**:1726.

PERNICIOUS ANEMIA
(Addisonian Anemia)

Essentials of Diagnosis

- Anorexia, dyspepsia; smooth, sore tongue.
- Constant, symmetric numbness and tingling of the feet.
- Pallor and a trace of jaundice.
- Oval macrocytes, pancytopenia, hypersegmented neutrophils.
- Megaloblastic bone marrow.

General Considerations

Pernicious anemia is a conditioned vitamin B_{12} deficiency due to an absorption defect, not dietary lack. Intrinsic factor is absent. The defect is rare before age 35; it is more common in individuals of Scandinavian, English, and Irish extraction and is very rare in Orientals. Predisposition to pernicious anemia is probably inherited as a single, dominant, autosomal factor. About 40% of patients have a 7S gamma "autoantibody" with activity against intrinsic factor in their serum; approximately twice that many have antibody against parietal cells. A precipitable antibody to intrinsic factor may also be present in their gastric juice.

Intrinsic factor is secreted by the gastric mucosa. It makes possible absorption of vitamin B_{12}, mostly at the distal ileum, in the presence of calcium and at a pH of 5–7. It is probably a mucopolypeptide or mucopolysaccharide with a molecular weight of 50,000.

Total body vitamin B_{12} content is estimated to be 5 mg; daily loss is approximately 2.5 μg. Clinical and hematologic evidence of pernicious anemia appears when the body vitamin B_{12} pool has been reduced to 10% of normal.

Clinical vitamin B_{12} deficiency may also be caused by gastrectomy, regional ileitis, certain intestinal malformations involving the ileum, resection of the ileum, and fish tapeworm disease.

Clinical Findings

A. Symptoms and Signs: Patients with pernicious anemia may tolerate their disease well and have few symptoms. Anemia may cause easy fatigability, dyspnea, palpitation, angina, and tachycardia. Vitamin B_{12} deficiency may lead to glossitis and gastrointestinal symptoms such as belching, indigestion, anorexia, and diarrhea; central nervous system symptoms occur in approximately 10% of patients and include constant symmetric numbness and tingling of the lower extremities, ataxia, mental disturbances, and loss of vibration sense and deep reflexes; sensory symptoms usually appear before motor symptoms and signs.

B. Laboratory Findings:

1. Blood–In addition to the characteristic large oval red cells there are a few small, misshapen red cells. This poikilocytosis is a reflection of the ineffective erythropoiesis in the marrow. The white blood cell count is usually under 5000/μL. The granulocytes, which constitute less than 50% of white cells, tend to be hypersegmented. Platelets usually are reduced (40–100 thousand/μL). Reticulocytes range from less than 1% to 3%. The unconjugated bilirubin is increased, but rarely above 2 mg/dL.

2. Bone marrow–The bone marrow is hyperactive. The characteristic megaloblastic abnormalities are particularly evident in the more mature forms of red blood cells. Giant metamyelocytes are prominent. Megakaryocytes are hypersegmented and reduced in number. Hemosiderin is increased and in the form of fine granules.

3. Other laboratory tests–Patients secrete no free gastric acid and very little gastric juice. Even after injection of pentagastrin, 0.6 mg/kg, a powerful physiologic acid secretagogue, the pH remains above 7. Serum LDH (lactate dehydrogenase) activity is excessively elevated. Haptoglobin is usually absent. Serum vitamin B_{12} concentration (normally 300–400 pg/mL) is usually less than 100 pg/mL. Routinely used radiodilution methods may yield inappropriately high values for cobalamin; readings of serum vitamin B_{12} are reliable when true intrinsic factor is used as binder or *Euglena gracilis* is used as assay method. Readings of falsely low serum vitamin B_{12} may occur with multiple myeloma or other gammopathies. Absorption of ^{57}Co-labeled vitamin B_{12} is greatly impaired. This is demonstrated by the Schilling test, which involves the oral administration of a small (0.5 μg) dose of radiocobalt-labeled vitamin B_{12} followed 2 hours later by the parenteral administration of 1000 μg of unlabeled vitamin B_{12}. Less than 5% of the radioactive vitamin B_{12} is excreted in the urine in 24 hours (normal: 15–40%); however, simultaneous administration of intrinsic factor increases the excretion of vitamin B_{12} 5-fold or more. The Schilling test is useful only in (1) differentiating addisonian pernicious anemia from megaloblastic anemias due to folic acid deficiency; (2) diagnosing addisonian pernicious anemia in remission; and (3) diagnosing defective vitamin B_{12} absorption in patients with combined system diseases before the onset of anemia. The Schilling test may give a falsely low value (decreased urinary radioactivity) in the following situations: inadequate urine collection, impaired kidney function, diarrhea, and occasionally hypothyroidism. Low values that are not improved by simultaneous administration of intrinsic factor are characteristically seen with malabsorption involving disease of the ileum and with fish tapeworm disease (even in asymptomatic carriers).

Some patients with pernicious anemia in relapse may have intestinal malabsorption as well; their Schilling tests are not improved by intrinsic factor until after several months of vitamin B_{12} therapy.

Differential Diagnosis

Pernicious anemia must be differentiated from folic acid deficiency (see below) by means of vitamin B_{12} absorption tests or serum levels of vitamin B_{12} and folic acid.

Large red cells are not seen exclusively in the megaloblastic anemias, but their oval appearance is characteristic, as are the hypersegmented white cells and the megaloblasts of the marrow.

In the various hemolytic anemias, some young nucleated red cells in the marrow may resemble megaloblasts; however, there are no oval macrocytes and no hypersegmented polymorphonuclear neutrophils, and the reticulocytes are above 3%.

Treatment

Pernicious anemia in relapse is treated with vitamin B_{12} (cyanocobalamin), 100 μg intramuscularly 1–3 times per week until blood values return to normal. Thereafter, 100 μg intramuscularly monthly are given. It must be impressed upon the patient that the need for vitamin B_{12} injections will continue for life.

Patients who have undergone total gastrectomy should receive maintenance doses of vitamin B_{12} (100 μg intramuscularly monthly).

Prognosis

Untreated pernicious anemia is fatal. With parenteral vitamin B_{12} therapy the reticulocytes begin to increase on the fourth day and reach a peak between the sixth and tenth days. The magnitude of the reticulocyte peak correlates well with the degree of anemia; with an initial red cell count of 1 million/μL, a maximum reticulocyte count of 40% may be anticipated. Normal hemoglobin values are obtained in about 6 weeks. Central nervous system symptoms are reversible if they are of relatively short duration (less than 6 months), but may be permanent if they have existed longer. Histamine-fast achlorhydria persists; the Schilling test remains abnormal. Hypokalemia may occur during initial therapy.

Carmel R: The laboratory diagnosis of megaloblastic anemias. *West J Med* 1978;**128**:294.

Chanarin I: Investigation and management of megaloblastic anemias. *Clin Haematol* 1976;**5**:747.

Lindenbaum J: Status of laboratory testing in the diagnosis of megaloblastic anemia. *Blood* 1983;**61**:624.

FOLIC ACID DEFICIENCY

Folic acid deficiency produces the same hematologic findings as pernicious anemia, but blood changes occur sooner, because folate storage lasts for only 1–2 months. The most common cause is malnutrition ("nutritional megaloblastic anemia"), especially in association with alcoholism. Folic acid deficiency may develop in sprue and may complicate certain chronic hemolytic anemias (eg, sickle cell anemia). It is occasionally seen in epileptics receiving primidone, pheny-toin, or phenobarbital, which interfere with absorption of folate; in patients following treatment with methotrexate, pyrimethamine, or triamterene, all of which block the reduction of folic acid to its metabolically active form, folinic acid; and in pregnancy. In megaloblastic anemias due to folic acid deficiency, central nervous system symptoms are lacking, free gastric acid may be present, and the vitamin B_{12} absorption test (Schilling) is normal. Serum folate activity is less than 3 ng/mL (normal is 7 ng/mL or more); red cell folic acid is less than 150 ng/mL (normal, 165–600). The presence of serum folate binders in patients with liver disease, uremia, or cancer can produce falsely low readings of serum folate. Associated iron deficiency may give falsely normal red cell folate levels.

"Pernicious," or megaloblastic, anemia of pregnancy is caused by folic acid, not vitamin B_{12}, deficiency. Poor nutrition is the major factor in its development. The requirement for folic acid increases markedly during pregnancy. Low serum folate levels are found in approximately 20% of pregnancies; the incidence of deficiency is much higher with twins, toxemia, or abruptio placentae. However, only a small percentage of women with low serum levels of folic acid have megaloblastic anemia.

The diagnosis is made by finding hypersegmented polymorphonuclear leukocytes in the blood and megaloblastic maturation in the marrow. Oval macrocytes are found less consistently than in other megaloblastic anemias; the red cell mean corpuscular volume is not as consistently elevated as in pernicious anemia.

In megaloblastic anemia of infancy and in megaloblastic anemia due to malnutrition or antiepileptic therapy, folic acid is given only until a hematologic remission is obtained. No maintenance therapy is necessary.

A patient with sprue or malabsorption syndrome may require initial therapy with parenteral folic acid and maintenance with oral folic acid. Some of these patients have an associated vitamin B_{12} or iron deficiency and have to be treated accordingly. Others require corticosteroids to relieve symptoms.

Folic acid is available in 1-mg tablets for oral administration and as solution (5 and 15 mg/mL) for intramuscular use. The oral dosage is 1 mg daily.

Beard MEJ et al: Acute onset of folate deficiency in patients under intensive care. *Crit Care Med* 1980;**8**:500.

Hillman RS, Steinberg SE: The effects of alcohol on folate metabolism. *Annu Rev Med* 1982;**33**:345.

Streiff RR: Folic acid deficiency anemia. *Semin Hematol* 1970; 7:23.

APLASTIC ANEMIA

Essentials of Diagnosis

- Lassitude, pallor, purpura, bleeding.
- Pancytopenia, fatty bone marrow.

- History of exposure to an offending drug or x-ray radiation.

General Considerations

Aplastic anemia may occur at any age. Its incidence is approximately 4 per million population per year. It is characterized by pancytopenia or a selective depression of red cells, white cells, or platelets. A number of toxins have been implicated, including therapeutic agents, especially chloramphenicol, phenylbutazone, and mephenytoin; cytotoxic agents; irradiation; hepatitis virus; benzene; and some insecticides. In over half of cases, the cause is not known. Absent or defective stem cells, immune-mediated suppression of blood formation, and abnormalities of the microenvironment of the marrow are among the factors thought to be responsible.

Clinical Findings

A. Symptoms and Signs: Anemia may cause lassitude, pallor, fatigue, tachycardia, thrombocytopenia, purpura, bleeding, neutropenia, and infections with high fever.

B. Laboratory Findings: The red cell count may be below 1 million/μL. The cells are usually slightly macrocytic. The reticulocyte count is often low but may be normal or even slightly elevated. The white blood cell count may be less than 2000/μL and the platelet count less than 30,000/μL. The serum bilirubin is usually low normal. The standard chemical analyses, including serum protein, GOT, and LDH and blood urea nitrogen, are normal. Bone marrow is fatty, with very few red and white cells and megakaryocytes. Hemosiderin is present.

Fixed tissue section made from the marrow aspirate or biopsy and stained with hematoxylin and eosin is best for demonstrating the characteristic architecture of an aplastic bone marrow; smears of the aspirate stained with Wright's stain are not adequate for diagnosis.

Differential Diagnosis

In hypersplenism, the marrow is hyperactive and the spleen is large.

In myelofibrosis, the spleen and liver are enlarged; red cells vary in size and shape; bizarre and tear-shaped cells may be seen; leukocytosis is common; the platelet count may be low, normal, or even elevated, and giant platelets are common; the marrow is fibrotic rather than fatty; extramedullary hematopoiesis may be seen in the liver and spleen.

Aleukemic leukemia, malignant lymphoma, and Hodgkin's disease may cause pancytopenia; the correct diagnosis is made by marrow biopsy.

Complications

Long-term transfusion therapy may lead to development of leukoagglutinins and hemosiderosis. Overwhelming infection secondary to leukopenia and bleeding secondary to thrombocytopenia are frequently terminal events.

Some patients make a partial recovery and develop a syndrome resembling paroxysmal nocturnal hemoglobinuria.

Treatment

A. General Measures: A very thorough search for possible toxic agents must be made. All unnecessary medications must be discontinued. A detailed history of the patient's personal and work habits is essential. Patients should be specifically asked whether they have taken any agents for infection, arthritis, or convulsions and whether they have been exposed to radiation. Even after a careful search, no cause can be found in approximately half of patients.

B. Marrow Transplant: This is the treatment of choice for young patients (under 50) with severe aplastic anemia (hemoglobin below 7 g/dL) who have an HLA-compatible donor. Graft-versus-host disease remains a major problem. Bacterial and fungal infections are common complications. Patients who have never been transfused do better (90% survival compared to 50% survival in the previously transfused group).

C. Androgenic Steroids: When marrow transplant is not feasible, a trial of these agents is warranted, although their efficacy in acute aplastic anemia is in some doubt. It usually takes 2–3 months to see an effect, if any. The most commonly used agents are as follows: (1) Fluoxymesterone, 40–100 mg daily orally (tablets, 2, 5, and 10 mg). (2) Oxymetholone, 2.5 mg/kg/d orally (tablets, 2.5, 5, 10, and 50 mg). (3) Nandrolone decanoate, 1.5–3 mg/kg/wk intramuscularly (50 mg/mL or 100 mg/mL). Adverse effects include virilization, amenorrhea, aspermia, sodium and water retention, and muscle cramps. The oral agents may cause cholestatic jaundice. All of these effects are reversible when the agents are withdrawn or the dose is reduced.

D. Other Agents: Corticosteroids are of little value; they are sometimes used for their stabilizing effect on capillary fragility in patients with severe thrombocytopenia.

Lithium carbonate, 300 mg 3 times daily, may be tried in an effort to raise the granulocyte count.

E. Transfusion: Transfusions are given in the form of packed red cells.

When platelets are needed, platelet concentrates can be given (see p 349).

Complications of transfusion therapy include development of leukoagglutinins (see p 350).

F. Treatment of Complications (Infections): Antibiotics should not be given prophylactically even when leukopenia is severe, but fever in a patient with granulocytopenia is probably caused by bacteremia, and intravenous antimicrobial agents should be started pending results of cultures. A semisynthetic penicillin (eg, ticarcillin, 3 g every 4 hours) plus an aminoglycoside (eg, tobramycin, 1.7 mg/kg every 8 hours) are currently the treatment of choice. Prevalent organisms and antimicrobial susceptibility in individual hospitals may modify the choice of agent somewhat. Patients must pay meticulous attention to personal hygiene and avoid exposure to infections.

Prognosis

The mortality rate with severe bone marrow depression is over 50%; hemorrhage and overwhelming infection are the main causes of death. The course—from onset of anemia to death—is usually only a few months. Some patients can be maintained on transfusions for years. Partial or complete spontaneous remission may occur.

Bortin MM, Gale RP, Rimm AA: Allogeneic bone marrow transplantation for 144 patients with severe aplastic anemia. *JAMA* 1981;**245**:1132.

Camitta BM, Storb R, Thomas ED: Aplastic anemia: Pathogenesis, diagnosis, treatment, and prognosis. (2 parts.) *N Engl J Med* 1982;**306**:645, 712.

Reilly RJ: Allogeneic bone marrow transplantation: Current status and future directions. *Blood* 1983;**62**:941.

Storb R et al: Marrow transplantation with or without donor buffy coat cells for 65 transfused aplastic anemia patients. *Blood* 1982;**59**:236.

ANEMIA OF LEAD POISONING

Coarse basophilic stippling is characteristic. The red cell indices in lead poisoning are usually normal but may show some hypochromia. Marked stippling in patients with normal or nearly normal hemoglobin levels is seen only in lead poisoning and thalassemia minor. It appears to be related to an acquired erythrocyte nucleotidase deficiency. Blood collected in double oxalate or calcium disodium edetate may inhibit formation of stippling. White cells and platelets are normal. Stippling is more striking in the bone marrow, but the marrow is otherwise not remarkable. Red cell ^{51}Cr survival shows moderately diminished red cell life spans (half-life, 18–28 days). Free red cell protoporphyrin is greatly increased and is a good screening test. Whole blood levels of lead are above 70 μg/dL (normal, 20–30 μg/dL); urinary delta-aminolevulinic acid levels are greater than 8 mg/24 h (normal, 3–5 mg); and urinary coproporphyrin levels are 1 mg/24 h or more (normal, 0.1–0.3 mg).

When lead poisoning is suspected but the above values are borderline, one should measure the 24-hour urinary lead after a provocative injection of calcium disodium edetate, 0.5 g dissolved in 10 mL of saline and given intramuscularly or intravenously. The test is positive when more than 0.8 mg of lead are excreted in 24 hours.

Sources of lead poisoning are paint chips ingested by children, industrial fumes inhaled by adults (eg, battery workers), radiators decorated with lead paint, and improperly glazed earthenware used as drinking vessels.

If symptoms are mild, no treatment is necessary. With fairly severe symptoms (eg, abdominal cramps), one may consider calcium disodium edetate, 0.5–1 g intravenously daily; if symptoms are less severe, give

penicillamine (Cuprimine), 250 mg orally 4 times daily.

Albahary C: Lead poisoning and hemopoiesis. *Am J Med* 1972; **52**:367.

Valentine WN et al: Lead poisoning: Association with hemolytic anemia, basophilic stippling, erythrocyte pyrimidine 5′-nucleotidase deficiency, and intraerythrocytic accumulation of pyrimidines. *J Clin Invest* 1976;**58**:926.

ANEMIA OF MYXEDEMA

Some patients with very low thyroid function have a moderately severe anemia either primary or secondary to hypopituitarism. The red blood cell count is rarely below 3 million/μL and the hemoglobin is rarely less than 9 g/dL. The anemia tends to be macrocytic and normochromic. However, iron deficiency, a frequent complication, especially in women with menorrhagia, will produce hypochromic microcytic anemia. Bone marrow cellularity is decreased, with increase in fat spaces. Erythropoiesis is normoblastic. White cells and platelets are normal.

Thyroid medication induces a gradual return to normal hemoglobin levels and red blood cell count in 3–4 months.

Tudhope GR, Wilson GM: *The Thyroid and the Blood.* Thomas, 1969.

PURE RED CELL APLASIA

This is a relatively rare condition (less common than aplastic anemia) characterized by moderate to severe anemia, very low reticulocyte counts, aplasia of red cell precursors, and normal white blood cells and platelets. It may occur as a congenital disorder, presenting as profound anemia in the first 3 months of life (Blackfan-Diamond syndrome).

The adult form may be secondary to several causes. Preleukemic leukemia must always be considered and the granulocytic series carefully scrutinized for abnormalities. Selective red cell hypoplasia develops in most patients with renal failure. Some cases are associated with thymoma. Some degree of red cell aplasia occasionally accompanies infections. Acute red cell aplasia may develop during the course of hemolytic anemia, eg, in hereditary spherocytosis or sickle cell anemia ("aplastic crisis"). Rarely, autoimmune hemolytic anemia may have an aplastic phase. A form of this disorder occurs in severe protein malnutrition (kwashiorkor). Under experimental conditions, riboflavin (vitamin B$_2$) deficiency has led to selective red cell aplasia. These disorders do not usually show the degree of red cell aplasia seen in the idiopathic cases and those that result from the toxic effects of drugs. Drugs that have been implicated on occasion as the causative agent in this anemia are chloramphenicol, phenytoin, quinacrine, sulfathiazole, benzol, and antituberculosis agents. These drugs usually produce pancytopenia and total marrow aplasia but occasionally cause only selected red cell aplasia.

The only signs and symptoms are those of anemia. The red cell count may be as low as 1 million/μL, but the red cells appear normal and have no inclusions. Reticulocytes are reduced to 0.1% or even less. White cells and platelets are normal in number and appearance. Serum iron may be elevated.

The marrow has a normal architecture and normal or increased iron stores. Nucleated red cells usually total less than 100 per 1000 white cells. They are normoblastic. White cells, megakaryocytes, and stromal cells are unremarkable. Erythropoietin is usually greatly increased. A serum creatinine below 2 mg/dL rules out azotemia as the cause. A normal chest x-ray and a negative test for antimuscle antibody rule out thymoma.

Underlying conditions must be corrected; if a thymoma is present, anemia will not respond to medication until the tumor has been removed.

Corticosteroids are very effective in children but are less consistently beneficial in adults. Prednisone, 10–20 mg 3–4 times daily, may be tried. Immunotherapy with cyclophosphamide and prednisone shows some promise. Testosterone may be helpful.

Sieff C: Pure red cell anemia. *Br J Haematol* 1983;**54**:331.

HEMOLYTIC ANEMIAS

1. ACQUIRED AUTOIMMUNE HEMOLYTIC ANEMIA

Essentials of Diagnosis

- Fatigue, malaise, pallor, jaundice.
- Splenomegaly.
- Persistent anemia and reticulocytosis.
- Coombs test usually positive.

General Considerations

A positive direct Coombs test (Table 10–2) means that a plasma protein, usually either IgG or complement, has become fixed abnormally and relatively irreversibly to the red cell surface. The protein is detected by the Coombs serum, which is prepared by immunizing certain laboratory animals against human immunoglobulins and complement.

When done with the usual "broad-spectrum" antiglobulin serum, a positive Coombs test indicates attachment to the red cell membrane of gamma globulin, components of complement, transferrin, a complex of certain drugs and gamma globulin, or possibly other globulins. A "weak" positive direct Coombs test without clinical hemolysis may be found occasionally in a variety of unrelated conditions, eg, rheumatoid arthritis, ulcerative colitis, and leukemia. Appropriate clinical information and a few serologic tests usually lead to the correct diagnosis. As routinely performed, a positive direct Coombs test requires more than 500

Table 10–2. Positive Coombs test.
(Most common examples of specific causes.)

Neoplastic	
Chronic lymphatic leukemia	G
Lymphosarcoma	G
Reticulum cell sarcoma	G and C
Hodgkin's disease	G
Collagen diseases	
Lupus erythematosus	G and C
Rheumatoid arthritis	G and C
Infectious diseases	
Cytomegalic virus disease	G
Viral pneumonia	C
Infectious mononucleosis	C
Drugs	
Penicillin	G
Methyldopa	G

Legend: G = anti-IgG
C = anticomplement

molecules of IgG per red cell (normal: < 35 per red cell). Approximately 5% of patients with autoimmune hemolytic anemia have only 50–500 molecules per red cell and hence a false-negative Coombs test.

Two major types of red cell coating with protein exist—the IgG type ("gamma Coombs") and the complement type ("nongamma Coombs"), often associated with a cold antibody. The former is found in lymphoma, systemic lupus erythematosus, and certain drug reactions, but in two-thirds of cases no specific cause is found. In the nongamma type, a component of complement rather than of gamma globulin is fixed to the red cell surface; the concentration of complement in the patient's serum is correspondingly low.

Frequently, warm autoantibodies have Rh specificity, eg, some patients with autoimmune hemolytic anemia or a positive direct Coombs test have antibodies against a specific antigen present on their own red cells; this situation usually involves anti-E, anti-c, or anti-e antibodies.

Cold autoantibodies with hemolytic anemia may develop after some infections, eg, mycoplasmal pneumonia, mononucleosis, and with lymphoreticular neoplasms. They usually bind complement, have anti-I specificity (anti-i in mononucleosis), and may show diffuse hypergammaglobulinemia or a narrow band in the gamma or beta region on electrophoresis. Cold antibodies sometimes occur also without apparent underlying disease. A monoclonal cold agglutinin indicates cancer.

Red cell coating in vivo as described above is always referred to as the "direct" Coombs test. In approximately half of these, the indirect Coombs test is also positive; this test measures circulating antibody in patients' serum. In autoimmune hemolytic anemias, the indirect Coombs test is, of course, only positive when the direct Coombs test is positive. The positive indirect test merely indicates an excess of antibody.

Autoimmune hemolytic anemia may occur following exposure to certain agents. Three different mechanisms are recognized:

(1) Penicillin in large doses can produce this type of hemolytic anemia; it may act as a hapten to stimulate antibody formation. The antigen-antibody combination "coats" red cells, and a positive direct Coombs test with hemolytic anemia may develop.

(2) Several drugs can bring some immune injury to red cells, platelets, and white cells without first attaching to the cell surface. These agents stimulate antibody formtion; the drug and its appropriate antibody then combine, attach to red cells, and damage them. The role of the red cells has been referred to as that of an "innocent bystander." The antibody is usually of the anticomplement or IgM type. Stibophen, quinidine, and quinine are among the drugs implicated in this type of reaction.

(3) A third mechanism for the development of a positive Coombs test has been observed with the use of the antihypertensive agent methyldopa. Approximately 20% of patients who take this drug develop a positive Coombs test, but only 1% develop hemolytic anemia. The drug, while of prime etiologic importance, does not itself participate in the ultimate reaction. It perhaps produces some subtle changes on the red cell surface, possibly by interfering with normal biosynthesis of membrane components, causing alterations that result in "new" antigens. Alternatively, it may involve an abnormality of immunoregulatory T cells.

A positive Coombs test in a patient who has been transfused recently (within a few weeks) must be interpreted with great caution. The "coated" cells may be incompatible donor cells in a patient who has antibodies from a prior transfusion. The incompatibility occasionally leads to delayed (by 4–14 days) transfusion reactions that may simulate "autoimmune" hemolytic anemia.

Hemolysis without antibody (negative Coombs test) may develop in uremia, cirrhosis, diffuse vasculitis, cancer, and some bacterial infections.

Clinical Findings

A. Symptoms and Signs: Manifestations of anemia (weakness, pallor, dyspnea, palpitation, dizziness) or hemolysis (fever, jaundice, splenomegaly, hepatomegaly) may be present.

B. Laboratory Findings: Acquired hemolytic anemia is usually normocytic and normochromic. Spherocytes and nucleated red cells may be seen. White cell and platelet counts are frequently elevated, but leukopenia and thrombocytopenia may occur. The reticulocyte count is usually over 10%, often very high (50% or even more), but occasionally low. The bone marrow shows marked erythroid hyperplasia and ample hemosiderin. Indirect bilirubin may be elevated to 4 mg/dL. There is no bile in the urine. Haptoglobin may be low or absent. Normal donor blood has short survival.

Differential Diagnosis

The hemoglobinopathies are differentiated by electrophoresis. In hemolytic anemia associated with cirrhosis, the primary disease is usually evident. In hereditary spherocytosis and in congenital nonspherocytic hemolytic anemia, the Coombs test is negative. In refractory normoblastic anemia with intramedullary hemolysis, the reticulocyte count is not elevated, bone marrow shows many sideroblasts, and donor blood survives normally.

Complications

The hemolytic anemia may become acute, with shock, upper abdominal pain, and prostration. Thrombocytopenic purpura and thromboembolic phenomena may develop.

Treatment

A. Transfusions: Treatment must often be directed against the underlying disease. Transfusions are only palliative, and their effects are dissipated rapidly, since donor cells are also destroyed at an accelerated rate. These patients frequently cannot be cross-matched, because they have a positive indirect—as well as direct—Coombs test. Nevertheless, they must be transfused to combat shock or severe anoxia. Type-specific red cells are given and may have to be repeated daily until the disease remits. Rarely is it necessary or desirable to raise hemoglobin levels above 8 g/dL with transfusions.

B. Medical Measures: Prednisone, 1 mg/kg/d or more, is the initial treatment of choice. A rise in hematocrit and a fall in reticulocyte count are the best indicators of response and may occur within a few days. Reduction of the dose or change to alternate-day dosage is desirable when a good response has occurred. A small maintenance dose may have to be continued for months.

Patients with cold agglutinin disease usually do not respond to prednisone and may present a serious problem of management; immunosuppressive therapy or plasmapheresis has been used.

C. Surgical Measures: When corticosteroids fail or when large doses are required for maintenance, splenectomy must be considered.

Prognosis

In the idiopathic form, permanent remissions may occur; other patients relapse or may stabilize at a clinically acceptable level. A positive Coombs test may persist for years, even in patients who appear clinically well. Hemolytic anemia refractory to all measurements may be fatal.

Conley CL et al: Autoimmune hemolytic anemia with reticulocytopenia and erythroid marrow. *N Engl J Med* 1982;**306**:281.

Crisp D, Pruzanski W: B-cell neoplasms with homogeneous cold-reacting antibodies (cold agglutinins). *Am J Med* 1982;**72**:915.

Garratty G, Petz LD: Drug-induced immune hemolytic anemia. *Am J Med* 1975;**58**:398.

Petz LD: Red cell transfusion problems in immunohematologic disease. *Annu Rev Med* 1982;**33**:355.

Pruzanski W, Shumak KH: Biologic activity of cold-reacting

antibodies. (2 parts.) *N Engl J Med* 1977;**297:**538, 583.
Zweiman B: Immunohematologic disease. *JAMA* 1982;**248:** 2677.

2. HEREDITARY SPHEROCYTOSIS
(Congenital Hemolytic Anemia; Congenital Hemolytic Jaundice)

Essentials of Diagnosis
- Malaise, abdominal discomfort.
- Jaundice, anemia, splenomegaly.
- Spherocytosis, increased osmotic fragility of red cells, negative Coombs test.

General Considerations
In hereditary spherocytosis, the red cells have a defective membrane that is abnormally permeable to sodium. The basic defect appears to be an abnormality of spectrin, a membrane protein. To prevent excessive intracellular sodium accumulation, which in turn would lead to influx of water and cell rupture, increased metabolic work must be done by the cells. The necessary energy is derived from increased glycolysis. Glucose deprivation, as it occurs in the spleen—and in vitro during the performance of the autohemolysis or incubated osmotic fragility tests—leads to red cell destruction. When red cells from a patient with hereditary spherocytosis are transfused to a normal recipient, they are destroyed in the (normal) spleen. On the other hand, normal donor blood survives almost normally in a patient with hereditary spherocytosis. The disease is chronic, hereditary, and transmitted as a dominant autosomal trait, and it is seen in all races. In 25% of cases no family involvement can be demonstrated. It may be first manifested in the newborn period, and may resemble hemolytic disease due to ABO incompatibility; in some patients, the disease is not discovered until after age 80.

Clinical Findings
A. Symptoms and Signs: There may be easy fatigability and moderate and constant jaundice; the spleen is almost always enlarged and may cause left upper quadrant fullness and discomfort. Splenic infarction may cause acute pain. The anemia may be intensified during infections, following trauma, and during pregnancy.

On rare occasions an acute "aplastic" crisis develops, with profound anemia and, in some cases, fever, headache, abdominal pain, and pancytopenia with hypoactive marrow. In occasional instances there may be no clinical findings; the diagnosis is made only because the discovery of the disease in a more severely afflicted relative has led to an intensive search and laboratory testing of the blood.

B. Laboratory Findings: The red blood cell count is moderately decreased (3–4 million/μL). The red cells are small (mean corpuscular volume = 70–80 fL) and hyperchromic (mean corpuscular hemoglobin concentration = 36–40%). Spherocytes in varying

numbers are seen on the smear. The reticulocyte count is usually increased; the white cell and platelet counts may be only moderately increased.

In the bone marrow there is marked erythroid hyperplasia; hemosiderin is present in only moderate amounts, since the spleen is the main reservoir of iron in this disorder.

Indirect serum bilirubin is usually elevated, haptoglobins often decreased or even absent. The Coombs test is negative.

Osmotic fragility is characteristically increased; hemolysis of 5–10% of cells may be observed at saline concentrations of 0.6% or even higher. The response may be normal in some patients, but a sample of defibrinated blood incubated at 37 °C for 24 hours ("incubated fragility test") will show increased hemolysis when compared to a sample of normal blood similarly treated.

Autohemolysis of defibrinated blood incubated under sterile conditions for 48 hours is usually greatly increased (10–20% compared to a normal value of less than 5%).

The addition of 10% glucose prior to incubation will decrease the amount of autohemolysis.

Red cell survival studies, using the patient's own blood labeled with ^{51}Cr, will show a greatly shortened red cell life span and sequestration in the spleen.

Differential Diagnosis
Spherocytes in large numbers occur in many patients with autoimmune hemolytic anemia. Osmotic fragility and autohemolysis are similarly increased but are less consistently improved by glucose. The positive Coombs test, negative family history, and sharply reduced survival of normal donor blood in these patients establish the diagnosis.

Spherocytes are also seen in hemoglobin C disease, in some cases of drug-induced hemolytic anemias, in some alcoholic patients, and in patients with extensive burns.

Complications
Gallstones composed principally of bile pigments (reflecting increased metabolism of hemoglobin) occur in up to 85% of adults and may develop even in children. Leg ulcers are occasionally seen. During febrile illnesses, aplastic crises may occur with profound anemia and decreased white cell and platelet counts but little jaundice.

Treatment
There is no medical treatment for this disorder.
A. Surgical Measures: Splenectomy should be done in patients with an enlarged spleen, anemia, or jaundice. Patients should be immunized with pneumococcal vaccine at the time of splenectomy. Preoperative transfusion is rarely necessary. When there is associated cholelithiasis, splenectomy should precede cholecystectomy unless both procedures are done at the same time. Splenectomy is usually deferred until after the first few years of life, but it

should be done before school age so growth is not stunted.

B. Treatment of Aplastic Crisis: Prompt and adequate transfusion therapy is necessary to prevent cardiovascular collapse. Antibiotics may be necessary to treat precipitating infections.

Prognosis

Splenectomy eliminates anemia, jaundice, and gallstone formation, but abnormal red cell morphology and abnormal osmotic fragility persist. Red cell life span is almost normal after splenectomy.

Lusher JM, Barnhart MI: The role of the spleen in the pathophysi-ology of hereditary spherocytosis and hereditary elliptocyto-sis. *Am J Pediatr Hematol Oncol* 1980;**2**:31.
Valentine WN: Hereditary spherocytosis revisited. *West J Med* 1978;**128**:35.

3. OVALOCYTOSIS
(Hereditary Elliptocytosis)

Ovalocytosis is inherited as an autosomal domi-nant trait with variable clinical expression. It is equally common in males and females and occurs in all ethnic groups. The determining gene is on the same chromo-some that carries the Rh blood group gene. Twenty-five to 90% of the red cells may be oval. It is thought to occur in 4 out of 10,000 individuals in the USA. About 12% of subjects have moderate anemia, a palpable spleen, slight jaundice, and elevated reticulocyte counts. Patients may have marked poikilocytosis and some spherocytes. Incubated osmotic fragility and au-tohemolysis may be increased but are restored to nor-mal by glucose. Splenectomy is usually beneficial in patients with overt hemolysis.

The disorder is usually asymptomatic, without anemia and with normal red cell indices, but red cell survival is often shortened. In some patients the red cells are more oval than elliptical; a few spherocytes may be seen.

Torlontano G et al: Hereditary elliptocytosis: Haematological and metabolic findings. *Acta Haematol* 1972;**48**:1.

4. ACUTE HEMOLYTIC ANEMIA

Essentials of Diagnosis

- Sudden onset with chills, fever, nausea and vom-iting, or pain in abdomen or back.
- Pallor, slight jaundice, splenomegaly.
- Red or dark urine.

General Considerations

Acute hemolytic anemia may be drug-induced, especially in sensitive individuals (see Glucose-6-Phosphate Dehydrogenase Deficiency); it may be due to certain infections, eg, *Escherichia coli* infections, hemolytic streptococcal septicemia, *Clostridium wel-chii* infections, and malaria; it may be seen in some

forms of cancer and malignant lymphomas and in certain other diseases, eg, lupus erythematosus and infectious mononucleosis. It is seen during the course of paroxysmal nocturnal hemoglobinuria, thrombotic thrombocytopenic purpura, and paroxysmal cold he-moglobinuria and when cold agglutinins of high titer develop during convalescence from viral pneumonia. Sometimes the cause is not known.

Clinical Findings

A. Symptoms and Signs: The onset is fulminat-ing, with chills, fever, abdominal pain, pallor, jaun-dice, weakness, and tachycardia.

B. Laboratory Findings: The anemia is usually normocytic and normochromic, but spherocytes, burr cells, microspherocytes, and nucleated red cells may be seen. The red cell count and hemoglobin are lowest several days after the onset of symptoms. The white cell count may reach $50,000/\mu L$ and the platelet count 1 million/μL, but occasionally both are decreased. A blood smear stained with methyl violet may show Heinz bodies (large remnants of denatured hemoglobin in red cells), which are not visible with Wright's stain. Reticulocytes may be greatly increased. The Coombs test is usually negative.

The bone marrow is hyperplastic, with a pre-dominance of nucleated red cells. There may be hemo-globinemia lasting a few hours, followed by methem-albuminemia (manifested by a brown discoloration of the serum) for a few days and usually a moderately elevated indirect bilirubin value. Haptoglobin, which can normally bind 50–150 mg/dL of free hemoglobin, disappears from the serum.

The urine may contain hemoglobin and hemosiderin; urobilinogen may be elevated, but the urine does not contain bile. Red cell enzyme studies may show a deficiency of glucose-6-phosphate dehy-drogenase; cold agglutinins may be found in myco-plasmal pneumonia; slightly acid serum may hemolyze the cells in paroxysmal nocturnal hemoglobinuria (Ham test); and a circulating hemolysin may be found in paroxysmal cold hemoglobinuria (Donath-Land-steiner test).

Differential Diagnosis

The fulminant onset of acute hemolytic anemia, with chills and fever, may simulate an infection. The abdominal pain may suggest surgical illness; the profound anemia may suggest blood loss. In acute hemolytic anemia, however, the serum is invari-ably pigmented as a result of the products of hemoly-sis. A pink serum indicates free hemoglobin; a brown serum, methemalbumin; and a yellow serum, bilirubin.

Complications

Shock may occur if the development of anemia is sufficiently abrupt or severe. Acute tubular necrosis secondary to profound ischemia and precipitated he-moglobin in the renal tubules may lead to acute renal failure.

Treatment

Acute hemolytic anemia may be an emergency. The patient should be hospitalized, all medications discontinued, and the possible causes investigated.

Spontaneous remission frequently occurs. Even patients who are not critically ill are observed for a few days for a gradual decline of reticulocytosis, followed by a hemoglobin rise of 1–2 g/dL/wk. Under these circumstances only supportive therapy need be given.

A. General Measures: Since acute renal failure is a potential hazard, serum electrolytes and blood urea nitrogen are determined and strict attention is paid to fluid intake and output and electrolyte administration.

B. Transfusions: Transfusions are used only to combat shock or anoxia; packed red cells are preferable to whole blood. Rarely is it necessary or desirable to raise the hemoglobin level above 8 g/dL with transfusions.

C. Corticosteroids: If reticulocytosis persists and hemoglobin levels do not rise, if there is a continuous drop in hemoglobin, or if the patient is severely ill, give prednisone (or equivalent), 10–20 mg 4 times daily. Corticosteroids are continued until serum and urine are clear of hemolytic products and the hemoglobin level is normal. The dose may be reduced rapidly at first to 20 mg/d and then decreased by 5 mg each week. Splenectomy is rarely (if ever) indicated in acute hemolytic anemia.

Prognosis

Acute hemolytic anemia usually remits spontaneously, either because the offending agent is removed or because only a portion of the patient's red cells, usually the older ones, are sensitive to the toxin. Hemolytic anemias secondary to serious underlying disorders such as metastatic cancer, thrombotic thrombocytopenic purpura, or *Clostridium welchii* infection (as seen with induced abortion) are often rapidly fatal.

Turtzo DF, Ghatak PK: Acute hemolytic anemia with *Mycoplasma pneumoniae* pneumonia. *JAMA* 1976;**236**:1140.

5. PAROXYSMAL NOCTURNAL HEMOGLOBINURIA

Paroxysmal nocturnal hemoglobinuria is a rare chronic hemolytic anemia of variable severity, characterized by rather constant hemoglobinemia and hemosiderinuria and recurrent episodes of acute hemolysis with chills, fever, pain, and hemoglobinuria.

The basic disorder is a membrane defect; hemolysis is produced by interaction between the abnormal cells and several factors present in normal serum: magnesium, properdin, and complementlike components.

The onset is usually in adult life; the disease is not familial. Spleen and liver may be slightly enlarged. White cell and platelet counts are often decreased; the reticulocyte count is increased. The bone marrow is usually hyperactive but may be hypoplastic; aplastic anemia occasionally precedes the clinical development of this disorder.

The indirect serum bilirubin is elevated. Hemoglobinemia and methemalbuminemia are often present. Haptoglobins are absent, LDH is markedly elevated, and the red cell acetylcholinesterase level is low. The intrinsic red cell defect is demonstrated by finding hemolysis on incubation of the patient's red cells in acidified normal serum (Ham test). The sucrose hemolysis ("sugar water") test can be used for screening. Hemoglobin electrophoresis and osmotic fragility are normal, and the Coombs test is negative.

Complications consist of overwhelming infection, aplastic crises, and thromboses. After years of hemosiderinuria, iron deficiency may develop.

Transfusion reactions may occur when the donor blood (plasma) hemolyzes the patient's red cells.

Blood transfusions are given for severe anemia or complications such as trauma, infections, thromboses, or leg ulcers. The administration of 1 L of 6% dextran solution, preferably of relatively high molecular weight (150,000), before transfusion may prevent hemolysis of the patient's own cells by donor serum. Patients may benefit from the administration of prednisone, 40 mg every other day. Prednisone apparently deactivates the alternative pathway of complement.

Clark DA et al: The kidneys in paroxysmal nocturnal hemoglobinuria. *Blood* 1981;**57**:83.

Rosse WF: Paroxysmal nocturnal hemoglobinuria: Present status and future prospects. *West J Med* 1980;**132**:219.

Rosse WF: Treatment of paroxysmal nocturnal hemoglobinuria. *Blood* 1982;**60**:20.

6. HEREDITARY NONSPHEROCYTIC HEMOLYTIC ANEMIA

Essentials of Diagnosis

- Moderate anemia.
- Familial and congenital.
- Spleen slightly enlarged.
- No spherocytes; osmotic fragility normal.
- High reticulocyte count.

General Considerations

This is a heterogeneous group of congenital hemolytic anemias caused by intrinsic red cell defects. Specific enzyme deficiencies have been found for most of them. These disorders are usually inherited as autosomal recessive traits. Some involve the Embden-Meyerhof (anaerobic) pathway. Pyruvate kinase deficiency, which is usually found in northern Europeans, is the most common in this group; the rest are rare. Others involve the hexose monophosphate (pentose phosphate) shunt, but, with the exception of glucose-6-phosphate dehydrogenase (G6PD) deficiency, which is described in more detail below, they are rare.

Clinical Findings

A. Symptoms and Signs: Anemia and jaundice are usually discovered in early childhood. The spectrum of clinical findings in pyruvate kinase deficiency varies from severe neonatal jaundice that requires exchange transfusions to fully compensated hemolysis; in general, it is more severe than hereditary spherocytosis.

B. Laboratory Findings: Hemoglobin levels vary from 6 to 12 g/dL. The red cells may be slightly large, and spiculed, contracted, and oval cells may be seen; reticulocyte counts are relatively high, especially after splenectomy. In all of these conditions, Howell-Jolly bodies (nuclear remnants in red cells) and Pappenheimer bodies (iron particle inclusions visible with Wright's stain) may be prominent, especially after splenectomy. White cells and platelets are normal. The marrow shows marked erythroid hyperplasia. Osmotic fragility is normal. In general, autohemolysis is increased after 48 hours and not reduced by glucose (Dacie type II).

A fluorescent spot test for pyruvate kinase deficiency is available for screening. The other rare abnormalities can be discovered only by sophisticated biochemical techniques.

Differential Diagnosis

In hereditary spherocytosis the red cells are small and round, osmotic fragility is increased, and jaundice is often prominent.

In acquired autoimmune hemolytic anemia the Coombs test is positive. In refractory normoblastic anemia the reticulocyte count is low and the spleen is not palpable. In the hemoglobinopathies the diagnosis is made by hemoglobin electrophoresis.

In the newborn this condition may be very difficult to differentiate from hemolytic anemia due to ABO incompatibility.

Complications

There may be associated cholelithiasis.

Treatment

Whole blood transfusions may be necessary. Splenectomy is not curative but may ameliorate some conditions, especially pyruvate kinase deficiency.

Beutler E et al: Hemolytic anemia due to pyrimidine-5'-nucleotidase deficiency: Report of eight cases in six families. *Blood* 1980;**56**:251.
Brewer GJ: Inherited erythrocyte metabolic and membrane disorder. *Med Clin North Am* 1980;**64**:579.

7. GLUCOSE-6-PHOSPHATE DEHYDROGENASE (G6PD) DEFICIENCY

This X-linked red cell enzyme is deficient in about 13% of American black males (hemizygous); 25% of American black women are carriers, and 1% are homozygous for the deficiency. Carriers (female heterozygotes) may be susceptible to hemolysis; because of X chromosome inactivation (Lyon phenomenon), they have 2 populations of red cells—one with normal enzyme levels and one with deficient red cells.

Enzyme levels reflect susceptibility to hemolysis; in general, one out of 4 carriers is subject to hemolysis. Red cell values are normal for all of these individuals with the African (A–) variant of the disorder until they are exposed to certain (oxidant) drugs such as primaquine, nitrofurantoin, and sulfonamides; then they develop an acute, moderately severe but self-limited hemolytic anemia. Hemolysis may also be precipitated by certain viral or bacterial infections and by diabetic acidosis. The Mediterranean variant (B–), which is found especially in Sardinians, Sicilians, Greeks, Sephardic Jews, Iranians, and Arabs, produces more severe disease than the African variant; some of these individuals have chronic hemolytic anemia, and their white cells also lack the enzyme. Following infections or upon exposure to drugs or (in some cases) fava beans, a profound hemolytic anemia may develop. Other variants of the enzyme defect have been observed in northern Europeans and Chinese.

Several laboratory methods have been devised for identifying susceptible individuals. There is a glutathione stability test, a dye reduction test using cresyl blue, a methemoglobin reduction test, and a commercially available dye reduction spot test. These tests may give a falsely normal reading in patients with young cells, ie, with high reticulocyte counts after acute hemolysis; one must wait a couple of weeks after the reticulocytosis for reliable measurements.

Treat the infection or discontine exposure to the offending drug or toxic substance. Recovery from the acute episode is the rule.

Beutler E: Glucose-6-phosphate dehydrogenase deficiency. Pages 1629–1653 in: *The Metabolic Basis of Inherited Disease*, 5th ed. Stanbury JB et al (editors): McGraw-Hill, 1983.
Desforges JF: Genetic implications of G6PD deficiency. *N Engl J Med* 1976;**294**:1438.
Schrier SL: Human erythrocyte G6PD deficiency: Pathophysiology, prevalence, diagnosis, and management. *Compr Ther* 1980;**6**:41.

8. MICROANGIOPATHIC HEMOLYTIC ANEMIA

This term describes a group of acquired hemolytic anemias due to various causes that are characterized by fragmented or helmet-shaped red cells, burr cells, or microspherocytes. Associated thrombocytopenia is common; normal donor cells are destroyed rapidly. This form of red cell distortion may be seen in association with the following conditions: preeclampsia-eclampsia, thrombotic thrombocytopenic purpura (discussed elsewhere in this chapter), metastatic cancer, post-cardiotomy, drug toxicity (perhaps in association with glucose-6-phosphate dehydrogenase deficiency), the hemolytic-uremic syndrome of infancy and pregnancy, postpartum malignant nephrosclerosis, malignant hypertension (rare), acute nephritis (rare), and uremia.

In some of these, small thrombi in arterioles and capillaries, especially in the kidney, may be found.

Some degree of disseminated intravascular coagulation may be present.

Except for those that are drug-induced, these anemias carry a very poor prognosis.

Spero JA et al: Disseminated intravascular coagulation: Findings in 346 patients. *Thromb Haemostas* 1980;**43**:28.

ANEMIAS WITH INTRAMEDULLARY HEMOLYSIS*
(Ineffective Erythropoiesis)

An important pathologic process in several anemias is the destruction of immature, nucleated red cells while they are still in the marrow. The erythroblasts apparently are defective in some way and are sequestered by reticuloendothelial cells. Some of these disorders (eg, pernicious anemia) may be associated with frank megaloblastosis; others (eg, refractory normoblastic anemias) show erythroblasts that resemble megaloblasts.

These disorders are characterized by marked erythroid hyperplasia in the marrow without elevation of reticulocyte counts and by ringed sideroblasts. Radioiron studies show greatly increased iron turnover and uptake, delayed release from the marrow, and poor incorporation into circulating red cells, with secondary accumulation in the liver. Red cell survival as measured with ^{51}Cr is moderately shortened; the peripheral erythrocytes made by the disordered marrow somehow survive.

Examples of anemia with intramedullary hemolysis are the following:

Refractory Normoblastic Anemia

This is a heterogeneous group of chronic, moderate to severe anemias. Patients may have symptoms of anemia and sometimes have slight splenic enlargement, but no other abnormal physical findings are present. Ringed sideroblasts, when present, are commonly caused by acute alcoholism. Red cells are mostly normocytic and normochromic, but a few hypochromic microcytic cells may be seen. Stippled hypochromic macrocytes are characteristic. White cells and platelets may be decreased. The bone marrow shows considerable erythroid hyperplasia and some erythrophagocytosis. Some of these patients are diabetic. Ten percent develop acute myeloblastic leukemia (see below).

Sideroblastic Anemias

In this often familial group, most of the red cells are hypochromic and microcytic, serum iron is high, and iron deposits in the marrow, liver, and spleen are excessive. Ringed sideroblasts are frequently seen. The spleen is usually enlarged. Some of these patients respond to pyridoxine (see below).

*Pernicious anemia, folic acid deficiency, and thalassemia are discussed elsewhere in this chapter.

Pyridoxine-Responsive Anemias

In some of the above groups of anemias, hemoglobin may be restored to normal by large doses (50–200 mg intramuscularly daily) of pyridoxine; the microcytosis and hypochromia may persist. The patients have no other signs of pyridoxine deficiency such as central nervous system and skin involvement. A few patients have macrocytic anemia and megaloblastic bone marrow that do not respond to vitamin B_{12} or folic acid.

Bateman CJ: Sideroblastic anemia. (Editorial.) *Arch Intern Med* 1980;**140**:1278.
Cheng DS, Kushner JP, Wintrobe MM: Idiopathic refractory sideroblastic anemia. *Cancer* 1979;**44**:724.
Pierce HI et al: Clinical studies in alcoholic sideroblastosis. *Arch Intern Med* 1976;**136**:283.
Refractory anemia. (Editorial.) *Br Med J* 1980;**2**:258.

ABNORMAL HEMOGLOBINS

The human red cell contains 200–300 million molecules of hemoglobin. Each molecule contains 4 heme groups and one globin molecule. The globin molecule is composed of 2 dissimilar pairs of polypeptide chains. The globin chains are designated alpha through delta, each chain being unique in amino acid composition. The members of each pair are identical. Each chain is made up of 141–146 amino acids. The production of the different globin chains is under the control of independent genetic loci.

The sequence of structural genes involved in globin synthesis and the distance between them can now be determined by sophisticated techniques. The alpha chains have 2 structural loci on chromosome 16. The nonalpha chains are encoded on chromosome 11. Gamma chains have 2 structural loci—beta and delta—but only one each. Within the regions that encode for specific chains are located DNA segments that are not translated (intervening DNA, or "introns").

Three different types of hemoglobin are normally present in adults. About 97% is hemoglobin A, with 2 alpha and 2 beta chains; the other 2 normal hemoglobins (A₂ and F) are present in trace amounts (1–3%). Hemoglobin A_2 possesses 2 alpha chains but in place of the beta chains has a pair of delta chains, which probably differ from the beta chain in fewer than 10 amino acids. Fetal hemoglobin (hemoglobin F) also contains 2 alpha chains but 2 gamma chains instead of beta chains; gamma chains differ from beta chains in numerous amino acid substitutions.

Hemoglobinopathies involve abnormalities in the hemoglobin chains. These are due to changes in the DNA template, a different order of bases in the one locus resulting in the production of different amino acids and therefore a structurally and functionally altered protein. Differences between normal and abnormal hemoglobins are relatively minute. For example, sickle (S) hemoglobin differs from normal hemoglobin in a single amino acid substitution in the beta chains (composed of 146 amino acids). Valine instead of glutamic acid is the sixth amino acid from the amino terminal position. Yet this small difference has far-reaching clinical effects that produce sickle cell disease. Most of the well-known hemoglobinopathies involve abnormalities of the beta chains. A few alpha chain abnormalities are known, eg, hemoglobin H disease.

Bank A et al: Disorders of human hemoglobin. *Science* 1980; **207**:486.

Weatherall DJ (editor): Haemoglobin: Structure, function, and synthesis. *Br Med Bull* 1976;**32**:193. [Entire issue.]

Winslow RM, Anderson WF: The hemoglobinopathies. Pages 1666–1710 in: *The Metabolic Basis of Inherited Disease*, 5th ed. Stanbury JB et al (editors). McGraw-Hill, 1983.

1. HEREDITARY HEMOGLOBINOPATHIES

Certain hereditary hemolytic anemias seen almost exclusively in blacks are characterized by the genetically determined presence of an abnormal type of hemoglobin in the red cells.

The heterozygous hemoglobin trait syndromes usually represent asymptomatic carriers, eg, in sickle cell trait, which occurs in about 9% of American blacks, there is no anemia. With hemoglobin C trait, which occurs in about 3% of American blacks, there is no anemia but target cells are common. The relative frequency of some hemoglobinopathies (per 1000 blacks) is as follows: A/S, 90; S/S, 2; A/F, 10; S/C, 0.66; A/C, 30; C/C, 0.166.

The homozygous hemoglobin disorders usually cause some anemia. The most common and the most serious is sickle cell anemia, which occurs in 1 in 500 American blacks. Homozygous hemoglobin C disease occurs only in 1 in 6000 and is a relatively mild disease. Double heterozygous diseases, eg, combinations of hemoglobin S and C, occur with an incidence of 1 in 1500. In addition, sickle thalassemia or C-thalassemia may occur, but it is much less severe than sickle cell anemia. Target cells are prominent in all, especially when the C trait is present.

In general, all of the homozygous disorders with the exception of sickle cell anemia and all of the double heterozygous disorders are characterized by splenomegaly. Fetal hemoglobin is increased in double heterozygous disorders when one of the genes is a thalassemia gene. Some fetal hemoglobin is also present in sickle cell anemia.

2. SICKLE CELL ANEMIA

Essentials of Diagnosis

- Recurrent attacks of fever, and pain in the arms, legs, or abdomen since early childhood in a black patient.
- Anemia, jaundice, reticulocytosis, positive sickle cell test, and demonstration of abnormal (S) hemoglobin.

General Considerations

Sickling occurs at low oxygen tension, especially at a low pH. The S (sickle) hemoglobin is less soluble in deoxygenated (reduced) form, the viscosity of the whole blood consequently increases, and the result is stasis and obstruction of blood flow in the capillaries, terminal arterioles, and veins. Localized sickling, vascular occlusion, and perivascular edema cause pain and swelling in the involved organs.

Sickle cell anemia (S/S) is a hereditary disorder, essentially confined to blacks; the abnormal hemoglobin is transmitted as a dominant trait. Heterozygous carriers have mixtures of normal and sickle hemoglobin in all of their red blood cells.

Clinical Findings

A. Symptoms and Signs: Most patients with sickle cell anemia have moderately severe anemia. Concurrent alpha thalassemia lessens the degree of severity of hemolytic anemia. The anemia usually is not the major problem, because a good oxygen supply to tissues is preserved by a shift of the oxygen dissociation curve to the right and an increased cardiac output. The disease is disabling, primarily because of the recurrent painful crises.

The diagnosis is usually made in childhood, but occasionally a patient will reach adult life before a well-documented crisis develops. Patients with sickle cell anemia tend to be of asthenic build with long spindly legs. Constant scleral icterus of moderate degree is common. The painful clinical crisis consists of attacks of bone and joint pain or abdominal pain, sometimes with fever, lasting hours or days. The tender, rigid abdomen may resemble surgical illness. Cerebral thrombosis may occur, producing headaches, paralysis, and convulsions.

B. Laboratory Findings: Hemoglobin values average about 8 g/dL and change only slightly during painful crises. The red cell indices are usually normal. In addition to the sickled cells, some target cells are commonly seen on the blood film. The reticulocyte count may be 15–20%. Serum iron is normal or slightly elevated. Serum LDH is often greatly elevated, and haptoglobin is usually absent. Serum bilirubin values usually vary between 2 and 4 mg/dL. Plasma hemoglobin is slightly elevated, and ^{51}Cr red cell survival is approximately 10 days.

Two screening tests are in common use: (1) The sodium metabisulfite test uses a drop of fresh 2% reagent mixed on a slide with 1 drop of patient's blood; sickling of most red cells will occur in a few minutes. Sodium metabisulfite is a strong reducing agent, and the deoxygenated red cells become distorted as their hemoglobin becomes insoluble. (2) "Sickledex" is a simple solubility test that does not require a microscope; sodium dithionite is used as a reducing agent, and saponin and phosphate buffer make up the precipitating agents. When 0.02 mL of blood is mixed

Table 10–3. Hematologic findings in some of the hemoglobinopathies.*

Hemoglobin Disorders	Erythrocytes (mill/μL)	Hemoglobin (g/dL)	RBC		Reticulocytes (%)	Target Cells (%)	Hemoglobins (%)	Fetal Hemoglobins (%)
			MCV	MCHC				
Normal (adult men and women A/A)	4.2–6.2	12–18	82–92 fL	32–36 %	0.5–1.5	0	A 97 A₂ 2–3	0–2
A/S (sickle trait)	N	N	N	N	N	0	A₂ 3–4 S 22–48	0–2
S/S (sickle cell anemia)	1.5–4.0	2–11	N	N	5–30	Some	A₂ 3–4 S 80–100	0–20
Sickle thalassemia	2.0–5.0	6–14	Small	Decr	4–20	Many	A₂ 3–8 S 50–90 A 2–3	1–26
S/C	2.5–5.5	8.1–15.1	N	N	0.2–10	5–85	C 37–67 S 30–60	0–8
S/D	2.5–4.0	7–12	N	N	7–13	2–Some	D 23–75 S 25–77	Trace
S-Persistent F	3.5–5.0	11–15	N	N	N	0	S 75 A₂ 0–1	25
A/C	N	N	N	N	N	0–40	A 50–70 C 30–50	0–2
C/C	3.1–5.0	7–14.5	N	Incr	1–12	20–100	C 97–100	0–3
A/D	N	N	N	N	N	0	D <50	0–2
D/D	5.5–7.1	12–13	Small	N	1–1.5	50–80	D 100	0–2
H-Thalassemia	1.6–6.4	8–11	Small	Decr	2–22	1–30	A 60–85 H 15–40 A₂ 0–1	Trace–4
Thalassemia minor	4.0–7.5	8.3–13.2	Small	Decr	0.5–9.0	0–10	A 90+ A₂ 2–9	0–10
Thalassemia major	1.0–4.0	2–8	Small	Decr	1.5–38	0–50	A 10–30 A₂ 2–3	70–90
Hereditary persistence of fetal hemoglobin (A/F)	N	N	N	N	N	0	A 70–90 A₂ 0–1	10–30

*Modified from Dacie JV: *The Hemolytic Anemias, Congenital and Acquired,* 2nd ed. Part I. Grune & Stratton, 1960.

with 2 mL of the reagent, normal blood will give a clear tube and S hemoglobin will produce a cloudy tube.

Differential Diagnosis

Sickle cell anemia is differentiated from other hemoglobinopathies by hemoglobin electrophoresis, the sickle cell test, and fetal hemoglobin determination. Hematuria may simulate genitourinary tumor, tuberculosis, or vascular disease. Bone and joint pain may resemble rheumatic fever. The abdominal pain may simulate surgical abdominal conditions; persistence of normal bowel sounds in sickle cell crisis may be a helpful differential diagnostic finding.

The spleen is not enlarged in adult sickle cell anemia. An anemic black patient with an enlarged spleen and a positive sickle cell preparation probably has a double heterozygous disorder (eg, "sickle thalassemia") rather than sickle cell anemia. The sickle cell test does not differentiate between sickle cell anemia (the homozygous disorder) and sickle cell trait (the heterozygous carrier state). In sickle cell anemia the red count is always low; the finding of a low hemoglobin with a normal red count in a black patient with a positive sickle cell preparation is not compatible with the diagnosis of sickle cell anemia but suggests iron deficiency anemia plus sickle cell trait.

An electrophoretic pattern indistinguishable from that of sickle cell anemia may be found in the following: (1) Sickle cell–hemoglobin D disease: Hemoglobin D has the same electrophoretic mobility as hemoglobin S, but electrophoresis on agar gel at pH 6.0 differentiates these 2 hemoglobins. Hemoglobins A and D migrate together and ahead of hemoglobin S. (2) Some instances of sickle thalassemia: Hemoglobin A is sometimes absent in sickle thalassemia because the formation of normal beta chains is prevented by the sickle cell gene and is suppressed by the thalassemia gene. Family studies may distinguish sickle thalassemia from sickle cell anemia. Hemoglobin A₂ is usually elevated in sickle thalassemia but normal in sickle cell disease. (3) Sickle cell–persistent fetal hemoglobin syndrome.

Complications

Complications of sickle cell anemia include leg ulcers, bone infarction, aseptic necrosis of the femoral head, osteomyelitis (especially due to *Salmonella*), cardiac enlargement with auscultatory findings similar to those of mitral stenosis, recurrent gross hematuria, focal hepatic necrosis or cirrhosis, and cholelithiasis. Infection may cause an aplastic crisis, with more severe anemia without jaundice or reticulocytosis.

Sickle cell lung disease is manifested by fever, pleuritic pain, lung infiltrates, and hypoxemia, usually due to pneumonia in children and pulmonary infarcts in adults.

Right upper quadrant syndrome shows right upper quadrant pain, fever, and deepening jaundice; it may be caused by sickling in the liver, gallbladder disease, or even hepatitis.

Treatment

Treatment is symptomatic. The frequency and severity of clinical manifestations vary greatly.

Adults with sickle cell anemia should be immunized against pneumococcal infection with Pneumovax.

A. Treatment of Painful Clinical Crisis: Adequate hydration and analgesics should be provided. Oxygen therapy, local measures, alkalinizing measures, vasodilators, and urea have all been tried but have failed to give beneficial results.

Partial exchange transfusions, consisting usually of removing 2 units of 500 mL and replacing them first with 500 mL of saline and then with 5 units of packed red cells, may be useful with clinical exacerbation of crises, strokes, and surgery.

B. Treatment of Hemolytic and Aplastic Crisis: Transfusions are mandatory. The hemoglobin level should be raised to 12–14 g/dL. Adequate hydration is necessary. A careful search for infections should be made and appropriate antibiotic therapy instituted.

C. Treatment of Complications:

1. Leg ulcers–The legs are immobilized and elevated. The ulcer area is cleansed and debrided. The patient is given sufficient blood to raise the hemoglobin level to 12–14 g/dL.

2. Cholelithiasis or orthopedic disorders requiring surgery–Give sufficient preoperative blood to raise the hemoglobin level to 12–14 g/dL.

3. Sickle cell anemia appearing during pregnancy–Transfuse to maintain a hemoglobin level of 10–12 g/dL in the third trimester.

4. Fever–Because pneumococcal septicemia is a common problem, especially in children, prompt institution of antibiotic therapy with penicillin is indicated.

Prognosis

Many patients die in childhood of cerebral hemorrhage or shock. Others live beyond age 50 years. There is a tendency to progressive renal damage, and death from uremia may occur.

Chang JC, Kan YW: A sensitive new prenatal test for sickle cell anemia. *N Engl J Med* 1982;**307**:30.

Charache S: Treatment of sickle cell anemia. *Annu Rev Med* 1981;**32**:195.

Maugh TH II: Sickle cell. 2. Many agents near trials: A better understanding of the molecular basis of sickle disease leads to new approaches to therapy. *Science* 1981;**211**:468.

Mears JG et al: Alpha thalassemia is related to prolonged survival in sickle cell anemia. *Blood* 1983;**62**:286.

Sheehy TW, Plumb VJ: Treatment of sickle cell disease. *Arch Intern Med* 1977;**137**:779.

Steinberg MH, Hebbel RP: Clinical diversity of sickle cell anemia: Genetic and cellular modulation of disease severity. *Am J Hematol* 1983;**14**:405.

Vichinsky EP, Lubin BH: Sickle cell anemia and related hemoglobinopathies. *Pediatr Clin North Am* 1980;**27**:429.

3. SICKLE CELL TRAIT

Sickle cell trait (A/S) rarely causes symptoms or signs. Blood counts, red cell morphology, and red cell life span are normal. Gross hematuria occurs in 3–4% of cases; renal concentrating capacity is usually impaired; and pregnant women with the trait have an increased susceptibility to pyelonephritis. Splenic infarcts on high altitude flying as well as pulmonary infarcts develop occasionally. Under the stress of anoxia, as in congestive heart failure, acute alcoholism, or shock due to any cause, massive, fatal infarct may occur.

Sears DA: The morbidity of sickle cell trait. *Am J Med* 1978;**64**:1021.

4. S/C HEMOGLOBIN DISEASE

Essentials of Diagnosis

- Recurrent attacks of abdominal, joint, or bone pain.
- Enlarged spleen.
- Minimal anemia.
- Positive sickle cell test; many target cells.

General Considerations

The racial incidence and mode of inheritance of hemoglobin S/C disease are similar to those of sickle cell anemia. It represents a double heterozygous state, ie, the patient must receive the gene for S from one parent and the gene for C from the other. The incidence of the disease is 1 in 1500 in the American black population.

Clinical Findings

A. Symptoms and Signs: The average age at time of diagnosis is 11 years. In addition to abdominal, bone, joint, or chest pain, there may be painless hematuria, vitreous hemorrhages, and pulmonary thromboses. Jaundice is minimal. The liver is slightly enlarged and the spleen is large in two-thirds of patients. Heart murmurs are uncommon.

B. Laboratory Findings: Red blood count and hemoglobin values are nearly normal unless a complication is present. Target cells are very prominent, but red cell indices are normal; a few sickled cells may be seen. The sickle cell test is positive. Red cell survival is slightly shortened. White cell and platelet counts are normal. The marrow shows increased erythropoiesis. On electrophoresis the percentages of hemoglobin S and hemoglobin C are nearly equal. Hemoglobin F is normal.

Differential Diagnosis

S/C hemoglobin disease is differentiated from sickle cell anemia by its more benign clinical picture and splenic enlargement and by its characteristic migration on hemoglobin electrophoresis. Sickle thalassemia is also more severe than S/C hemoglobin disease and is identified by hemoglobin electrophoresis. Other conditions with target cell formation include hemoglobin C disease and C trait, thalassemia minor, and jaundice, especially when due to cirrhosis and in patients who have undergone splenectomy.

Complications

Eye manifestations (eg, vitreous hemorrhages, retinal detachment), splenic infarcts, gross hematuria, aseptic necrosis of femoral heads, complications of pregnancy, or pulmonary thromboses may occur.

Treatment

Management is similar to that given for sickle cell anemia. Most patients require no therapy.

Prognosis

The outlook for these patients is considerably better than in sickle cell anemia. Some patients live into their 70s.

Serjeant GR et al: The clinical features of haemoglobin S-C in Jamaica. *Br J Haematol* 1973;**24:**491.

5. SICKLE THALASSEMIA

Some patients with this disease may have frequent episodes of jaundice, enlargement of the liver and spleen, recurrent bouts of fever, joint pain, and occasional abdominal pain. Others may have no symptoms and no splenic enlargement. The blood shows hypochromic, microcytic red cells varying in size and shape, with target and sickle forms. Different electrophoretic patterns are recognized. Patients may have relatively large amounts of hemoglobin S and increased amounts of hemoglobin A_2 (up to 6%) and F (up to 15%), and hemoglobin A varies from none to 40%; these probably represent hemoglobin S/beta thalassemia disease. Others have more hemoglobin A than S, and normal or low fractions of A_2 and F; they are classified as hemoglobin S/alpha thalassemia and are clinically much milder. The severity of anemia

varies from patient to patient and even may fluctuate in a given patient; hemoglobin levels may be normal.

Higgs DR et al: The genetics and molecular basis of alpha thalassaemia in association with Hb S in Jamaican Negroes. *Br J Haematol* 1981;**47:**43.

Serjeant GR et al: The clinical features of sickle-cell/β thalassaemia in Jamaica. *Br J Haematol* 1973;**24:**19.

6. HEREDITARY PERSISTENCE OF FETAL HEMOGLOBIN

Individuals with this condition have no clinical abnormalities and are not anemic. Their erythrocytes are characterized by the presence, throughout life, of large amounts of fetal hemoglobin. The trait is transmitted as a single factor allelic with the gene for hemoglobins S and C. The defect is DNA deletion. The heterozygous (hemoglobin A/F) form occurs in 1 in 1000 American blacks.

The red cells appear normal, and the reticulocytes and serum bilirubin are not elevated. Fetal hemoglobin is uniformly distributed among the erythrocytes. Hemoglobin A_2 is decreased.

Heterozygotes carry 10–30% hemoglobin F and have no hematologic abnormalities. In individuals heterozygous for hereditary persistence of fetal hemoglobin and hemoglobin S or C, the hemoglobin pattern consists of 20–35% hemoglobin F and the remainder is hemoglobin S or C; no hemoglobin A is present. Individuals heterozygous for hereditary persistence of fetal hemoglobin and hemoglobin S are healthy.

Conditions with lesser elevation of hemoglobin F include occasional cases of thalassemia minor and rare cases of aplastic anemia. Fetal hemoglobin values in this group may reach 20%.

Wood WG, Weatherall DJ, Clegg JB: Annotation. *Br J Haematol* 1979;**43:**509.

7. THALASSEMIA MINOR

Essentials of Diagnosis

- Mild but persistent anemia.
- Red blood count normal or elevated.
- Similar blood findings in one of the parents.
- Patient usually has a Mediterranean, Negro, or southern Chinese racial background.

General Considerations

In thalassemia, an insufficient amount of hemoglobin is made to fill the red cells. In beta thalassemia, the beta chains are defective and the alpha chains are normal; in alpha chain thalassemia (see hemoglobin H disease), the reverse is true. This defect can be caused by a variety of mutations in the gene controlling beta chain synthesis, and reduced amounts of globulin are formed. Beta thalassemia is the more common type seen in the USA, in individuals of southern Italian extraction, other Mediterraneans, southern Chinese, and some blacks. The greater the imbalance between beta chain production and alpha chain production, the more severe the disorder. The discrepancy is least in blacks, which is why the clinical disorder is milder in this racial group. The unbalanced synthesis leads to precipitation of the normal chains, which are in relative excess; the precipitated hemoglobin causes premature red cell death, either in the marrow (intramedullary hemolysis, ineffective erythropoiesis) or in the bloodstream (shortened survival of red cells). In beta thalassemia, the other "nonalpha" chains, ie, the gamma chains and the delta chains, compensate to some extent for the lack of beta chains, producing increase in hemoglobin F or hemoglobin A_2, respectively. Thalassemia minor is the heterozygous form of the disorder; thalassemia major is the homozygous state.

Clinical Findings
A. Symptoms and Signs: There are usually no symptoms. The spleen may be slightly enlarged. Occasionally there is upper left quadrant pain.

B. Laboratory Findings: The red cell count may exceed 6 million/μL. The hemoglobin does not fall below 9 g/dL in uncomplicated cases. The red cells are very small (mean corpuscular volume = 50–70 fL). Target cells and stippled cells are common. Red cells vary considerably in size and shape—more than in iron deficiency anemia of a comparable hemoglobin level. Some hypochromic macrocytes may be seen. Red cell patterns vary from one family to another. One group may have many target cells; another group may have stippled cells. Reticulocytes vary from 1 to 9%; platelets and white cells are not remarkable.

The bone marrow shows increased numbers of nucleated red cells. White cells and megakaryocytes are normal. Hemosiderin is present. In patients of Mediterranean ancestry, hemoglobin A_2 (a slow-moving normal hemoglobin component demonstrated on starch, cellulose acetate, or agar gel electrophoresis) is usually increased 2- to 3-fold. Fetal hemoglobin may be increased up to 6% in about half of patients; it is unevenly distributed among the red blood cells. In a much less common form of beta thalassemia, hemoglobin F levels are increased to 10–20%, but A_2 levels are normal. Clinically, patients with this form of beta thalassemia are similar to those with A_2 variant. Thalassemia minor with normal A_2 and F components probably is an alpha chain abnormality. (See Hemoglobin H Disease.)

Differential Diagnosis
Thalassemia minor must be differentiated principally from iron deficiency anemia. It is not a severe anemia; the hemoglobin level is almost always above 9 g/dL, and serum iron, total iron-binding capacity, and marrow hemosiderin are normal.

Other hypochromic, microcytic anemias with normal or even increased serum iron and marrow hemosiderin are as follows.

A. Certain hemoglobinopathies, especially he-moglobin H and hemoglobin E disease and the so-called Lepore trait, are diagnosed by hemoglobin electrophoresis.

B. Sideroblastic anemia, characterized by increased iron values, many sideroblasts, and biochemical evidence of disordered heme synthesis. Hemoglobin electrophoresis is normal.

Complications
Thalassemia does not respond to iron therapy, and prolonged treatment with parenteral iron could lead to excess iron storage.

Treatment & Prognosis
No treatment is required, and iron therapy must be avoided. During pregnancy, transfusions may be necessary to maintain hemoglobin above 9 g/dL. Patients with thalassemia minor have normal life spans.

Benz EJ Jr, Forget BG: The thalassemia syndromes. *Annu Rev Med* 1982;**33**:363.

Weatherall DJ: Molecular pathology of the thalassemia disorders. *West J Med* 1976;**124**:388.

8. THALASSEMIA MAJOR

Essentials of Diagnosis
- Severe anemia starting in infancy.
- Very large liver and spleen.
- Hypochromic, microcytic red cells with many erythroblasts.
- Greatly elevated fetal hemoglobin.

General Considerations
See discussion in previous section.

Clinical Findings
A. Symptoms and Signs: Severe anemia and a large liver and spleen are recognized in early childhood. Jaundice may be present.

B. Laboratory Findings: Severe microcytic, hypochromic anemia, target cells, and bizarrely shaped red cells are seen. Nucleated red cells are numerous. The reticulocyte count is moderately elevated. The platelet count and white cell count are normal or increased. Serum bilirubin is elevated. Haptoglobins are absent. Fetal hemoglobin may be increased to 90%. The bone marrow shows tremendous erythroid hyperplasia and ample stainable iron.

C. X-Ray Findings: Skeletal lesions are most prominent in the skull and long bones and consist of increase of the medullary portion and thinning of the cortex, the so-called hair-on-end appearance.

Differential Diagnosis
Other hemoglobinopathies involving varying mixtures of hemoglobin S, hemoglobin C, and others with thalassemia may give similar but less severe clinical pictures. Congenital nonspherocytic hemolytic anemia may resemble this disorder. Hemoglobin elec-

trophoresis, determination of fetal hemoglobin, and family studies make the correct diagnosis. Family studies show that both parents have the thalassemia trait.

Treatment

Regularly spaced transfusions are often necessary to maintain life. Rarely, folic acid may be helpful for associated folic acid deficiency. When secondary hemolytic anemia develops, with evidence of accelerated splenic sequestration of transfused red cells, splenectomy may be helpful. Reduction of the iron load by deferoxamine administered continuously by pump is showing considerable promise.

Complications

There may be cardiorespiratory symptoms due to the chronic anemia. Leg ulcers and cholelithiasis may develop. Transfusion-induced iron overload, with myocardial hemosiderosis, may lead to cardiac arrhythmia; intractable heart failure is a fairly common cause of death. Few patients survive into adult life.

Forget BS, Nathan DG: Molecular pathology of the thalassemias. *Adv Intern Med* 1978;**21**:97.
Kattamis C et al: Oral desferrioxamine in young patients with thalassaemia. *Lancet* 1981;**1**:51.

9. ALPHA THALASSEMIA; HEMOGLOBIN H DISEASE

Normally, 2 alpha chains are present on each of the chromosome-16 pairs. Alpha chain thalassemia is due to deletion of one or both of these structural genes. Deletion of 2 alpha genes is referred to as alpha thalassemia 1 and produces a red cell picture similar to that of beta thalassemia minor. In Asians, the 2 deletions are often on the same chromosome; in blacks, both chromosomes have a single deletion. Single deletion in Asians or blacks is clinically silent and is called alpha thalassemia 2. Alpha thalassemia 1 and 2 are relatively common in blacks. In hemoglobin H disease, one chromosome has 2 deletions, the other only one; it therefore is seen in Asians and not in blacks. Double deletion in both chromosomes is not compatible with life and leads to hydrops fetalis.

These disorders are found in Filipinos, Chinese, Thais, and sometimes blacks, Greeks, and other Mediterraneans. The silent carrier state is common in blacks. In hemoglobin H disease one of the parents has alpha thalassemia minor and the other is a silent carrier; it is thus a doubly heterozygous disorder. In the alpha thalassemias, hemoglobin F is not elevated; hemoglobin A_2 is lower than normal; and, at birth, hemoglobin Barts (4 gamma chains) is found in the cord blood.

Hemoglobin H disease is a hypochromic microcytic anemia that resembles thalassemia minor of the beta chain type. However, the morphologic abnormalities of the red cells are more striking, and at times the anemia becomes more severe, eg, with infections. Hemoglobin H has a very high affinity for oxygen, which means that it does not deliver oxygen well to the tissues. Acute hemolysis may follow the use of oxidant drugs.

The spleen is enlarged, a moderate degree of anemia is present, and the reticulocyte count is elevated. Hemoglobin H differs from normal hemoglobin by its more rapid electrophoretic mobility and by its instability. When blood from a patient with hemoglobin H disease is incubated for 30 minutes at room temperature with 1% brilliant cresyl blue, precipitates form in the red cells. Hemoglobin H, unlike hemoglobin I, the other "faster than normal" hemoglobin, migrates to the anode even at pH 6.5. Its isoelectric point is pH 5.6. Osmotic fragility is decreased, red cell life span is shortened to a half-life of 12–24 days, marrow erythropoiesis is effective, and glycolytic enzyme levels are normal. Hemoglobin H varies from a few percent up to 40% of the patient's hemoglobin. (It is composed of 4 beta chains.) A_2 hemoglobin is decreased.

Splenectomy may be helpful if anemia is severe.

Higgs DR: Detection of alpha thalassaemia in Negro infants. *Br J Haematol* 1980;**46**:39.
Higgs DR et al: The interaction of alpha thalassemia and homozygous sickle cell disease. *N Engl J Med* 1982;**306**:1441.
Pressley L et al: A new genetic basis for hemoglobin H disease. *N Engl J Med* 1980;**303**:1303.

HYPERSPLENISM

Essentials of Diagnosis

- Large spleen.
- Pancytopenia; active marrow.

General Considerations

The most common form of hypersplenism is congestive splenomegaly, often due to portal hypertension secondary to cirrhosis. Other causes are thrombosis, stenosis, atresia, or angiomatous deformity of the portal or splenic vein, external pressure due to cysts, and aneurysm of the splenic artery.

The spleen may be enlarged because of a specific infiltrate, as in Gaucher's disease, Niemann-Pick disease, Letterer-Siwe disease, tuberculosis, or Boeck's sarcoid. Nonspecific enlargement may occur, as in rheumatoid arthritis (Felty's syndrome).

In hypersplenism the platelet count, white cell count, and to some extent the red cell count are reduced because of pooling in or sequestration by the enlarged spleen.

Clinical Findings

A. Symptoms and Signs: Patients affected with hypersplenism due to congestive splenomegaly are usually under age 35 years. Some have little difficulty; others have sudden hematemesis due to esophageal varices. Gastrointestinal bleeding occurs in about half.

The large spleen may cause abdominal fullness. Sometimes the spleen is found accidentally during a routine examination. Some patients have purpura. In primary splenic neutropenia, fever and pain over the splenic region occur.

B. Laboratory Findings: The anemia is often mild, normocytic and normochromic; the reticulocyte count may be elevated. The ^{51}Cr red cell life span is decreased, with evidence of increased splenic sequestration. Platelets and white cells, particularly granulocytes, are greatly decreased, with a shift to the left.

The bone marrow shows varying degrees of generalized hyperactivity.

Differential Diagnosis

Hypersplenism is characterized by "empty blood, full marrow" and a large spleen.

Leukemia and lymphoma are diagnosed by marrow or lymph node biopsy and examination of the peripheral blood (white cell count and differential). In hereditary spherocytosis there are spherocytes, osmotic fragility is increased, and platelets and white cells are normal. The hemoglobinopathies with splenomegaly are differentiated on the basis of hemoglobin electrophoresis. Thalassemia major becomes apparent in early childhood, and the blood smear morphology is characteristic. In myelofibrosis, marrow biopsy shows proliferation of fibroblasts and replacement of normal elements. In idiopathic thrombocytopenic purpura, the spleen is not enlarged. In aplastic anemia, the spleen is not enlarged, and the marrow is fatty.

Complications

Gastrointestinal hemorrhage due to bleeding from esophageal varices may be fatal. Granulocytopenia may cause persistent leg ulcers or induce overwhelming infection.

Treatment

Therapy is usually that of the underlying condition. When the hematologic abnormalities are not severe, no treatment is required.

Splenectomy may be advisable for congestive splenomegaly due to a splenic vein abnormality alone and when leukopenia with recurrent infections or thrombocytopenic purpura is associated with the splenomegaly of tuberculosis, Gaucher's disease, Felty's syndrome, or sarcoidosis.

If congestive splenomegaly is due to liver or portal vein disease, splenectomy should be done only in conjunction with a splenorenal, splenocaval, or portacaval shunt.

Patients who have had a splenectomy should be immunized against pneumococcal sepsis with Pneumovax.

Prognosis

The prognosis is that of the underlying disorder. The course in congestive splenomegaly due to portal hypertension depends upon the degree of venous obstruction and liver damage. Without hematemesis, the course may be relatively benign, and splenectomy may not be necessary.

Clinicopathologic Conference: Rheumatoid arthritis with Felty's syndrome, hyperviscosity and immunologic hyperactivity. *Am J Med* 1981;**70**:89.

Eichner ER: Splenic function: Normal, too much and too little. *Am J Med* 1979;**66**:311.

Spivack JL: Felty's syndrome: An analytical review. *Johns Hopkins Med J* 1977;**141**:156.

ANEMIA OF CHRONIC DISEASE

In this category are included several diseases often associated with moderate anemia. Shortened red cell survival, suboptimal marrow compensation ("relative marrow failure"), defective reutilization of iron, and, at times, reduced production of erythropoietin are some of the causes.

The red cells appear normal, the reticulocyte count is not particularly elevated, white cells are normal, and platelets are at times elevated. Serum ferritin is normal; serum iron and total iron-binding capacity are low. A low serum ferritin (12–25 μg/mL) implies an element of iron deficiency complicating the anemia of chronic disease. Some of these disorders have their own characteristics, which are described below. It is important to recognize and treat complicating iron or folic acid deficiency.

Finch CA: Anemia of chronic disease. *Postgrad Med* (Oct) 1978; **64**:107.

1. ANEMIA OF CIRRHOSIS

Some degree of anemia is almost invariably seen in the patient with cirrhosis.

(1) Iron deficiency due to blood loss may occur (though not commonly) with gastritis, esophageal varices, hemorrhoids, or associated peptic ulcer.

(2) Folic acid deficiency and the characteristic megaloblastic picture are seen in only 5% of cirrhotic patients with anemia, but some degree of folic acid deficiency can be demonstrated in most patients by serum folate levels.

(3) A moderately severe hemolytic anemia is seen most frequently. The red cells are thin, flat, macrocytic, and slightly hypochromic and vary greatly in size but not in shape. Target cells are common, and the reticulocyte count is moderately elevated. The white count is normal or elevated, and the platelet count is usually increased. In some patients, particularly when the spleen is enlarged, white cell and platelet counts are decreased. ^{51}Cr red cell survival studies show a half-life of 15–25 days. The Coombs test is negative. The bone marrow is hyperplastic and contains many erythroblasts, frequent plasma cells, and increased numbers of megakaryocytes. With acute exacerbation

of chronic hepatitis, histiocytes filled with fat may be seen. In the more severe cases, spur cells and acanthocytes may be seen, bile salts apparently inhibit serum transesterase, cholesterol is not esterified, and free cholesterol accumulates in the membrane and deforms it.

The hemolytic anemia of cirrhosis does not respond to any specific measures or to corticosteroid therapy. The treatment is that of the underlying disorder.

(4) Acute hemolytic anemia develops occasionally after excessive alcohol intake. Jaundice, hyperlipemia, hypercholesterolemia, and spherocytosis are associated findings. Liver biopsy shows fatty infiltration and only minimal fibrosis. The syndrome improves rapidly with abstinence from alcohol.

Chanarin I: Alcohol and the blood. *Br J Haematol* 1979;**42**:333.
Cooper RD: Hemolytic syndromes: Red cell membrane abnormalities in liver disease. *Semin Hematol* 1980;**17**:103.
Eichner ER: The hematologic disorders of alcoholism. *Am J Med* 1973;**54**:521.

2. ANEMIA OF CANCER

Anemia of cancer may be due to any of the following:

(1) Chronic blood loss with subsequent development of iron deficiency anemia.

(2) Hemolysis, usually moderate and demonstrable only by ^{51}Cr red cell survival studies. Occasionally, hemolysis is severe and acute and features schistocytes.

(3) Replacement of functional marrow by the malignant tissue ("myelophthisic anemia").

Alexanian R, Alfrey CP Jr: Erythrokinetics and androgens in bone marrow cancer. *Cancer* 1976;**38**:833.
Laszlo J: Hematologic effects of cancer. Section 18-2, pp 1077–1082, in: *Cancer Medicine*, 2nd ed. Holland JF, Frei E (editors). Lea & Febiger, 1982.

3. ANEMIA OF INFECTION

Anemia usually develops only in chronic infections that are clinically obvious, eg, in patients with lung abscess, empyema, pelvic inflammatory disease, tuberculosis, or rheumatoid arthritis. The anemia in these cases is only moderately severe, and the hemoglobin rarely falls below 9 g/dL. The cells are normocytic and may be slightly hypochromic. The reticulocyte count is normal, low, or slightly elevated. Platelets and white cells are not remarkable, although there may be toxic granulation of polymorphonuclear cells. The serum iron is low, but (in contrast to iron deficiency anemia) the total iron-binding capacity is also low. The red cell life span is moderately shortened and there is an insufficient increase in erythropoiesis. Red cell protoporphyrin levels are high. Erythropoietin activity is decreased. Iron reutilization is

decreased. The bone marrow contains decreased, normal, or increased numbers of cells. Hemosiderin appears fuzzy and diffuse. No sideroblasts are seen. Severe anemia with a marked degree of hemolysis may develop during the course of subacute infective endocarditis, *Escherichia coli* infection, hemolytic streptococcal infection, or *Clostridium welchii* infection.

4. ANEMIA OF AZOTEMIA

Anemia commonly develops during the course of renal insufficiency from any cause. The red cells are normocytic and normochromic, and there is little variation from normal in size and shape. "Acanthocytes" (cells with thorny outpocketings) and schistocytes (contracted cells) are occasionally seen. The reticulocyte count is normal, low, or slightly elevated. The bone marrow usually shows a striking decrease in the number of nucleated red cells. Erythropoietin levels are very low. Ferrokinetic measurements show decreased red cell life span and an inadequate increase in bone marrow erythropoiesis. Hemolysis is occasionally severe, with greatly shortened red cell survival time. Renal failure may cause anemia if the blood urea nitrogen is above 50 mg/dL or the serum creatinine is above 2 mg/dL. Androgens may help to increase erythropoiesis. Iron and folic acid may be needed to repair associated specific deficiencies.

Fried W: Hematologic complications of chronic renal failure. *Med Clin North Am* 1978;**62**:1363.
Ho-Yen DO et al: Bone marrow cellularity and iron stores in chronic renal failure. *Acta Haematol* 1980;**64**:265.
Wallner SF, Vautrin RM: Anemia of chronic renal failure: Studies of iron transport in vitro. *J Lab Clin Med* 1980;**96**:67.

• • •

LEUKEMIAS

1. ACUTE LEUKEMIA

Essentials of Diagnosis
- Weakness, malaise, anorexia, bone and joint pain.
- Pallor, fever, petechiae, lymph node swelling, splenomegaly.
- Leukocytosis; immature, abnormal white cells in peripheral blood and bone marrow.
- Anemia, thrombocytopenia.

General Considerations
Acute leukemia is a disorder of the blood-forming tissue characterized by proliferation of abnormal white cells. It is a neoplasm that occurs in all races and may develop at any age.

Clinical Findings
A. Symptoms and Signs: Presenting complaints

are often general, consisting of weakness, malaise, anorexia, fever, and petechiae. Pain in the joints, lymph node swelling, or excessive bleeding after dental extraction may also be initial complaints. Spleen, liver, and lymph nodes are usually enlarged in acute lymphatic leukemia but in less than half of patients with acute myeloblastic leukemia. Sternal tenderness is common. Any organ may be involved.

B. Laboratory Findings: Normochromic, normocytic anemia occurs early. The platelet count is usually below 100,000/μL, while the white count varies from less than 10,000 to over 100,000/μL. One-third are leukopenic. On the blood smear immature and abnormal cells may be seen; on a thick or overstained smear they may be mistaken for lymphocytes.

Auer bodies, red-staining rods in the cytoplasm of myeloblasts or monoblasts, occur in 10–20% and are pathognomonic of acute nonlymphatic leukemia. Acute myelocytic leukemia may be differentiated from acute lymphocytic leukemia by the presence of peroxidase-staining cytoplasmic granules in the former. A new form, adult T cell leukemia, has recently been recognized. It is an acute, aggressive leukemia, with frequent dermal involvement, lymphadenopathy and splenomegaly, characteristic cell morphology, and hypercalcemia.

There is massive proliferation of primitive malignant cells in the bone marrow even when leukopenia exists.

Skeletal involvement can be seen radiologically in almost all of the children and in half of the adults. Diffuse osteoporosis, periosteal elevation, osteolytic lesions, and radiolucent metaphyseal bands are the most common lesions.

Complications

Fatal gastrointestinal tract hemorrhage, symptoms from pressure on the brain stem, brain hemorrhage, and overwhelming infection are the chief causes of death. Intracerebral hemorrhage occurs more frequently in patients with very high white cell counts (over 300,000/μL).

Differential Diagnosis

The combination of anemia, thrombocytopenia, and bone marrow proliferation of primitive white cells is found only in leukemia. Leukocytosis may or may not be present. Among the other features, petechiae may be seen in idiopathic thrombocytopenic purpura or in aplastic anemia, but the bone marrow is diagnostic. Enlarged lymph nodes and splenomegaly may be found in infectious mononucleosis, Hodgkin's disease, or lymphosarcoma, but the bone marrow and peripheral red cells and platelets are usually normal. Marked lymphocytosis is often seen in whooping cough and infectious lymphocytosis, but the white cells are mature and red cell and platelet counts are normal. Malignant tumors, eg, neuroblastoma, osteosarcoma, and metastatic cancer, may cause bone pain, anemia, and leukocytosis; if there is marrow invasion, these conditions may resemble leukemia. On occasion, mononucleosis may resemble acute leukemia clinically and even on the blood film. A marrow aspirate will clearly differentiate the 2 conditions; it is relatively normal in mononucleosis, with only a few abnormal lymphocytes and rarely a granuloma. The Monospot test may also help.

Treatment

Patients should be on a bacteria-free diet—no fresh fruit, salads, or uncooked vegetables; no spices added after cooking.

Allopurinol, 300 mg daily orally, should be given to all patients with large spleens, prominent lymph nodes, or high white blood cell counts.

Venous access by a tunneled silicone elastomer catheter (eg, Hickman) into the right atrium should be considered for most patients.

A. Acute Lymphatic Leukemia: Because it is generally believed that unless every leukemic cell in the body is destroyed the residual cells will multiply and cause a relapse, attempts are now being made to cure this disease by using multiple agents in an effort to kill all leukemic cells. It is estimated that the total burden of malignant cells when leukemia first presents clinically is in the neighborhood of 10^{12}–10^{13} cells. Initial therapy will reduce that to 10^9 cells, which results in an apparent clinical and hematologic remission, ie, the marrow will appear normal. Consolidation therapy will reduce the total number of leukemic cells to 10^6 or fewer. As the total burden of cells decreases, it becomes more difficult to treat the leukemic cells without damaging normal cells. It is not clear whether the body's own immunologic defenses can cope with this residue or whether additional aggressive chemotherapy is required. Multiple drug therapy attacks the leukemic cells in different phases of the mitotic cycle—eg, vincristine arrests cells in mitosis, prednisone lyses lymphoblasts in their resting phases or prevents their entry into DNA synthesis, mercaptopurine inhibits DNA synthesis, and methotrexate inhibits DNA, RNA, and protein synthesis. Use of these drugs sequentially or in combination also avoids drug resistance to a large extent and improves the chances of destroying cells that are in a "resting phase" (ie, nondividing) and are usually relatively insensitive to chemotherapy. Prophylactic therapy to the central nervous system eradicates foci of malignant cells in "sanctuaries" not reached by systemic therapy.

The current schemes of multiple drug therapy and prophylactic central nervous system treatment as compared to single drug treatment have a considerably higher morbidity, are more costly, and often remove patients from their home environment for longer periods of time. In deciding which approach to use, the physician must weigh these problems against the chance of prolonging survival. The following factors make a favorable response to chemotherapy considerably less likely: age greater than 70, secondary acute leukemia, and previous treatment for other neoplastic diseases, erythroleukemia, or myelodysplastic syndromes.

The following regimen incorporates most of the above considerations:

1. For rapid initial remission–

a. Vincristine, 0.05 mg/kg (usually maximum of 2 mg/m^2) intravenously once a week for 4 weeks, plus—

b. Prednisone, 1 mg/kg (40 mg/m^2) orally daily.

2. For consolidation and further distribution of drug–Methotrexate, 15 mg/m^2 orally twice a week.

3. To destroy residual leukemic blood in central nervous system–Radiation to cerebrospinal axis, 2400 rads. Intrathecal methotrexate, 5 mg dissolved in 10 mL of spinal fluid, administered every 3 days until the spinal fluid is clear, may be a valuable adjunct to oral or intramuscular methotrexate.

4. Prolonged maintenance–Mercaptopurine, 2.5 mg/kg daily orally, or methotrexate, 15 mg/m^2 twice a week orally, or cyclophosphamide, 200 mg/m^2 weekly orally.

5. Management of relapses–Acute relapses may be treated with vincristine and prednisone, as above, or cytarabine, 50–100 mg daily intravenously for 4 days, or daunomycin, 1 mg/kg intravenously daily for 4 days.

B. Acute Myelogenous Leukemia: This is usually a disease of adults. Six different types are recognized: M_1 myeloblastic without maturation (stem cell); M_2 myeloblastic with maturation; M_3 promyelocytic; M_4 myelomonocytic; M_5 monocytic; and M_6 erythroleukemia. Multiple drug therapy is used for the same reasons as in acute lymphatic leukemia, but the effective agents are different. Many schemes have been used. Intermittent therapy appears to minimize toxic suppression of normal cells. The following 3 regimens are most widely used in current practice:

1. Daunomycin and cytarabine–Daunomycin, 45 mg/m^2 (or doxorubicin, 30 mg/m^2) daily for 3 days by intravenous push, plus cytarabine, 100 mg/m^2 by intravenous infusion daily for 7 days.

2. DAT–A common form of induction is the DAT protocol: Daunomycin, 60 mg/m^2 by intravenous bolus infusion on days 1, 2, and 3; cytosine arabinoside, 100 mg/m^2 by intravenous infusion over one-half hour every 12 hours on days 1–7; 6-thioguanine, 100 mg/m^2 orally every 12 hours for 5 days.

3. Cytarabine and thioguanine–Cytarabine, 100 mg/m^2 by intravenous infusion daily for 7 days, plus thioguanine, 100 mg/m^2 orally every 12 hours daily for 7 days. Repeat at 4 weeks.

4. Consolidation and maintenance–The value of these additional therapies in prolonging remission is controversial. The possible benefits must be weighed against the possible complications of therapy, especially when anthracyclines are used. Some form of maintenance for a year or 2 seems reasonable. A good, fairly well tolerated regimen is cytarabine, 100 mg/m^2 intramuscularly daily for 5 days, plus thioguanine, 100 mg/m^2 daily in 2 divided doses 12 hours apart for 5 days; repeat every month.

5. Marrow transplant–This has become the procedure of choice for young adults in first remission, if they have a histocompatible sibling donor.

C. Treatment of Complications:

1. Local manifestations–Severe bone pain, massive lymph node enlargement interfering with respirations and swallowing, and central nervous system involvement with signs of increased intracranial pressure may be treated successfully with local irradiation.

2. Fever–In adult patients with leukemia, bacterial infection is ultimately proved in 75% of cases to be the cause of febrile episodes. Septicemia and infections of the throat, lungs, skin, urinary tract, and anorectal area are the usual causes. Gram-negative organisms—especially *Pseudomonas,* but also *Escherichia coli, Klebsiella, Proteus,* and *Bacteroides*—are frequently identified. New fever in a patient with granulocytopenia should be managed with a semisynthetic penicillin plus an aminoglycoside, as noted on p 307. Fungal infections, viral hepatitis, herpes zoster, cytomegalovirus, and infections with *Pneumocystis carinii* may also occur in the compromised host. These conditions require appropriate specific management.

3. Bleeding–For patients with severe thrombocytopenia and bleeding, platelet concentrates should be given to raise the platelet count to at least 60,000/μL. To estimate dosage, assume that 1 unit will raise the count of a 70-kg subject by 10,000/μL.

Prognosis

A. Acute Lymphatic Leukemia: Over 90% of patients under age 20 years treated as above can be brought into a state of remission. The mean duration of remissions is 1–3 years. By using the above approach or some variation of it, apparent cure can be achieved in one-third of patients who are treated for 2½ years.

B. Acute Myeloblastic Leukemia: Approximately two-thirds of patients with acute myeloblastic leukemia will achieve remissions on the above 2 regimens. The median duration of remissions is approximately 1 year, but survivals of several years occur occasionally.

Arlin ZA, Clarkson BD: The treatment of acute nonlymphoblastic leukemia in adults. *Adv Intern Med* 1983;**28**:303.

Blayney DW et al: The human T-cell leukemia/lymphoma virus, lymphoma, lytic bone lesions, and hypercalcemia. *Ann Intern Med* 1983;**98**:144.

Burns CP et al: Analysis of the presenting features of adult acute leukemia: The French-American-British Classification. *Cancer* 1981;**47**:2460.

Degnan T et al: Dysmyelopoietic syndrome: Current concepts. *Am J Med* 1984;**76**:122.

Geary CG: The diagnosis of preleukemia. *Br J Haematol* 1983;**55**:1.

Mauer AM: Review: Therapy of acute lymphoblastic leukemia in childhood. *Blood* 1980;**56**:1.

Powles R, McElvain T (editors): Leukemia and lymphoma. *Semin Hematol* 1982;**19** (Nos. 3 and 4); 1983;**20** (No. 1). [Entire issues.]

Weinstein HJ et al: Treatment of acute myelogenous leukemia in children and adults. *N Engl J Med* 1980;**303**:473.

Whittaker JA: Regular review: Advances in the management of adult acute myelogenous leukaemia. Br Med J 1980;281:960.

2. CHRONIC MYELOCYTIC LEUKEMIA

Essentials of Diagnosis

- Weakness, lassitude, fever, abdominal discomfort.
- Painless enlargement of spleen.
- Unexplained leukocytosis, immature white cells in peripheral blood and bone marrow.
- Anemia.

General Considerations

Chronic leukemia is characterized by proliferation of abnormal white cells, which invade the bloodstream and may infiltrate any part of the body to cause local symptoms. It is inevitably fatal. The abnormal cells carry the Philadelphia chromosome (Ph[1]). The Ph[1] abnormality is seen in 90% of patients with chronic myelocytic leukemia and involves a deletion of chromosome 22 and a translocation of that segment to chromosome 9. The chromosomal abnormality is acquired and of clonal origin and also occurs in erythroid cells and megakaryocytes but not in lymphocytes and fibroblasts.

In addition to their immaturity, leukemic neutrophilic cells have less alkaline phosphatase than normal white cells.

Chronic myelocytic leukemia is primarily a disease of young adults, but it may be found at any age. It accounts for approximately 25% of cases of leukemia; the incidence is one case per 100,000 population per year.

Clinical Findings

A. Symptoms and Signs: Pallor, weakness, sternal tenderness, fever, purpura, skin nodules, and retinal hemorrhages or exudate may be seen. There may be abdominal discomfort secondary to splenomegaly. Gum bleeding after dental extraction, or large ecchymoses or muscle bleeding after trauma—presumably manifestations of thrombasthenia—may be the presenting sign.

Some cases are diagnosed accidentally before the onset of symptoms when a high white cell count is found during a routine examination.

B. Laboratory Findings: The white cell count may exceed 500,000/μL, but fewer than 5% of the cells are "blasts." Nonfilamented neutrophils, metamyelocytes, and myelocytes predominate; the neutrophils are alkaline phosphatase negative; basophils, eosinophils, and platelets are increased; and a few normoblasts may be seen. Some degree of anemia is common. The marrow shows complete replacement of fat by cellular elements, mostly granulocytes, but few blasts.

Differential Diagnosis

In leukemoid reactions due to infection or meta-static cancer, eosinophils and basophils are decreased rather than increased, the leukocyte alkaline phosphatase is strongly positive, and the marrow is only moderately hyperplastic. In myelofibrosis, the spleen may be quite large but leukocytosis only moderate, the marrow is fibrotic, the granulocytes are usually alkaline phosphatase-positive, and the Philadelphia chromosome is not seen.

Complications

Probably no part of the body is exempt from leukemic infiltration. Complications depend on the area infiltrated, eg, pressure symptoms or hemorrhage if the central nervous system is infiltrated. The spleen may become large and painful. Half of patients die in a "blastic" crisis.

Treatment

A. General Measures: The aim of therapy is palliation of symptoms and correction of anemia. Initial manifestations and each exacerbation should be treated promptly. Specific treatment of the anemia is unnecessary, as it is usually corrected by treatment directed at the leukemic process. Blood counts are checked weekly at first and then once or twice a month until a satisfactory remission is obtained. During remission, patients are encouraged to resume normal activity, but follow-up visits are necessary every 1–3 months. The nature of the disease should be explained to the patient, and the necessity for periodic observation and lifelong treatment should be stressed.

B. Chemotherapy: Busulfan (Myleran), an alkylating agent, is the drug of choice. Initial dosage is 2 mg 2–4 times daily, continued until the white cell count is less than 10,000/μL. As a rule, the white cell count begins to drop within 2 weeks and normal values are reached in 2 months. When the white cell count reaches about 10,000/μL, the drug may be discontinued until relapse and then administered intermittently. Remissions may last for several months to more than a year. Overtreatment results in general depression of myelopoiesis; irreversible thrombocytopenia may develop. Since thrombocytopenia may occur before any significant drop in hemoglobin, platelet counts should always be done as part of the routine count. The drug should be withheld if platelet values are below normal.

Melphalan (Alkeran) is also effective. For blastic crisis, one may use either mercaptopurine, 2.5 mg daily orally alone, or the combination of prednisone, 40 mg/m² orally daily, plus vincristine, 2 mg intravenously once a week.

Hydroxyurea (Hydrea) is achieving a certain popularity because, unlike busulfan, it is not mutagenic and does not cause pulmonary fibrosis. The usual dose is 30 mg/kg/d. Its disadvantage is the brevity of its therapeutic effect, necessitating daily maintenance dosage.

C. Irradiation: X-ray therapy consists of total body irradiation or local therapy to the spleen, liver, or local infiltrates. (X-ray therapy localized to the spleen has a beneficial general effect on the hematopoietic system by mechanisms that are still unknown. Localized high-voltage x-ray over the spleen in doses of 50–100 R daily until a total of 600 R has been given is usually sufficient for clinical hematologic remission.) X-ray therapy (by a radiologist) is given over a period of a few weeks. X-ray is most effective in the treatment of local manifestations.

The results of treatment with radiophosphorus (^{32}P) are comparable to those of total body irradiation; it is less effective in the treatment of local manifestations. There is no radiation sickness. The dosage of ^{32}P depends upon the degree of leukocytosis. One millicurie (mCi) is equivalent to 15 R. If the white cell count is above 50,000/μL, the initial dosage of ^{32}P is 1–2.5 mCi intravenously; 2 weeks later, 1–1.5 mCi are given. Similar doses are given every 2 weeks until the white cell count is less than 20,000. During remission, patients are seen every 1–3 months. When the white cell count rises above 25,000, an additional 1–1.5 mCi are given.

Prognosis

The average life expectancy is 3–4 years. As the disease progresses, some degree of myelofibrosis may appear in the marrow; it is thought that a platelet-derived growth factor stimulates proliferation of fibroblasts. The terminal blast phase is thought to be the evolution of an altered clone of neoplastic cells derived from the Ph^1 cells; this is manifested by fever, splenomegaly, severe anemia, thrombocytopenia, and, sometimes, a marked increase in the number of basophils. In some cases the blasts may be lymphoblasts containing the enzyme terminal transferase; some patients temporarily respond to the combination of prednisone and vincristine. Terminal transferase–negative blasts respond even less well.

Koffler HP, Golde DW: Chronic myelocytic leukemia: New concepts. (2 parts.) *N Engl J Med* 1981;**304**:1201, 1269.

Spiers AS: The treatment of chronic granulocytic leukaemia. *Br J Haematol* 1976;**32**:291.

3. CHRONIC LYMPHATIC LEUKEMIA

Essentials of Diagnosis

- Pallor.
- Superficial lymph node enlargement.
- Absolute lymphocytosis in adults.

General Considerations

This disorder involves progressive accumulation of small lymphocytes that have lost the capacity to divide. The life span of these metabolically abnormal cells may be lengthened to several years; the total body lymphocyte mass expands considerably and may reach enormous proportions. The cells, which originate in lymph nodes, aggregate chiefly in the lymph nodes, spleen, blood, and marrow. The decline in levels of immunoglobulins commonly observed during the course of the disease may represent the replacement of normal, immunologically competent cells by cells that are functionally inert and have lost the ability to react to antigenic stimuli. These lymphocytes have a strikingly low mitotic rate.

The disorder may remain relatively quiescent for several years, free of symptoms and signs and with relatively stable lymphocyte counts; or it may become progressive, with various clinical manifestations and a rising blood count.

Chronic lymphatic leukemia is rare under age 30 and extremely rare in Orientals.

Clinical Findings

A. Symptoms and Signs: The onset is insidious, and the diagnosis is usually made accidentally during routine examination. Weakness and symptoms of hypermetabolism may be present. Enlarged lymph nodes may cause pressure symptoms (eg, tracheal compression with respiratory difficulty). The spleen, liver, and lymph nodes are not tender.

B. Laboratory Findings: At the time of diagnosis, the hemoglobin may be normal. Anemia and thrombocytopenia develop as the disease progresses. Lymphocytosis usually precedes the rise in total white cell count. Eventually, the white cell count rises and may reach 100–500 thousand/μL. Over 90% of the cells are mature lymphocytes; "smudge" cells are common. The platelet count tends to be low as the disease progresses. The initial marrow specimen may show normal architecture and diffuse or nodular involvement; with more aggressive disease, the normal architecture is destroyed and the marrow is diffusely invaded by lymphocytes.

Differential Diagnosis

Diffuse, nontender lymphadenopathy with increased numbers of mature lymphocytes on the blood film is seen almost exclusively in chronic lymphatic leukemias. Inflammatory conditions such as infectious mononucleosis, AIDS, toxoplasmosis, and cytomegalic inclusion disease may cause lymphadenopathy but are seen in a younger age group and associated with atypical lymphocytes on the blood film.

Lymphocyte counts of 50–100 thousand/μL may be seen in children with whooping cough or infectious lymphocytosis. Moderate lymphatic leukemoid reactions (with white cell counts of 20–30 thousand/μL) are occasionally seen with tuberculosis. Diffuse lymph gland enlargement may be found in lymphosarcoma and infectious mononucleosis and, rarely, in tuberculosis, syphilis, carcinomatosis, hyperthyroidism, brucellosis, lupus erythematosus, and toxoplasmosis. In Hodgkin's disease, lymph node enlargement is usually asymmetric or only in a single site.

Complications

Anemia, sometimes hemolytic with a positive Coombs test, may become a serious problem as the disease progresses. Some patients develop severe thrombocytopenia and purpura. Hypogammaglobulinemia is common.

Treatment

A. General Measures: It may be desirable to withhold therapy until clinical manifestations appear or until hematologic complications develop. Many older patients with this disorder remain relatively asymptomatic despite high leukocyte levels. All symptomatic patients and all patients with anemia or thrombocytopenia should be treated.

B. Irradiation: As for chronic myelocytic leukemia, but systemic control with splenic radiation is less frequent.

C. Chemotherapy:

1. Chlorambucil is widely used. The dosage is 0.1–0.2 mg/kg daily, or 0.4–0.6 mg/kg as a single dose once every 4 weeks or, if necessary, every 2 weeks. Clinical and hematologic improvement may not be evident for 3–4 weeks and maximum improvement may not be achieved for 2–4 months. The drug should be discontinued when the white cell count falls to 5000–10,000/μL. Side effects are relatively uncommon, although gastrointestinal irritation occurs. Pancytopenia may develop, but recovery usually occurs when the drug is discontinued.

2. Cyclophosphamide, 50–100 mg orally 1–3 times daily, may be used.

D. Corticosteroids: Some patients respond well to relatively small doses of corticosteroids. Initially one may give prednisone (or equivalent), 40 mg daily until a response occurs; maintenance may be as little as 10–20 mg every 48 hours.

E. Treatment of Complications:

1. Anemia–Anemia is caused by a combination of 2 factors: increased rate of red cell destruction and inadequate bone marrow compensation. It often fails to respond to antileukemic therapy, and transfusions may have to be given. Prednisone (or equivalent), 10–20 mg 4 times daily, is usually required. With remission of the anemia, corticosteroids may be gradually withdrawn. With severe hemolytic anemia and splenic sequestration of the red cells, splenectomy may have to be considered. Intercurrent anemia due to blood loss and iron deficiency is treated with iron.

2. Bleeding–Abnormal bleeding in leukemia is usually due to thrombocytopenia, which may be secondary to either the leukemic process or therapy. If due to the leukemia, it may be improved by appropriate chemotherapy; if due to chemotherapy, the marrow-depressing drugs must be discontinued and corticosteroid therapy instituted until the marrow has had a chance to recover.

3. Infections–Infections are treated with specific antibiotics. Prophylactic use of antibiotics is not recommended. Some patients develop low levels of gamma globulin. With gamma globulin levels of 0.7 g/dL or less, prophylactic gamma globulin may be needed. Initially, 0.66 mL/kg (0.3 mL/lb) is given in divided doses of 5 mL each; a maintenance dose of half this amount is administered once or twice a month.

Prognosis

The course depends on the stage of the disease.

With lymphocytosis but no enlargement of lymph nodes and spleen, no anemia, and no thrombocytopenia, survival is in excess of 12 years. When in addition to the above the spleen is enlarged, survival is about 6 years. When anemia is also present, the median survival is less than 2 years.

Binet JL et al: A new prognostic classification of chronic lymphocytic leukemia derived from a multivariate analysis. *Cancer* 1981;**48**:198.

Rozman C et al: Prognostic significance of bone marrow patterns in chronic lymphatic leukemia. *Br J Haematol* 1981;**47**:529.

Theml M, Love R, Begemann H: Factors in the pathomechanism of chronic lymphatic leukemia. *Annu Rev Med* 1977;**28**:131.

MYELOFIBROSIS
(Myelosclerosis, Agnogenic Myeloid Metaplasia)

Essentials of Diagnosis

- Weakness and fatigue.
- Large spleen.
- "Leukoerythroblastic" blood picture with poikilocytosis.
- "Dry tap" on bone marrow aspiration.

General Considerations

Myelofibrosis is a proliferative disorder of the mesenchymal tissue and is probably related to other myeloproliferative disorders such as chronic myelocytic leukemia and polycythemia vera. There are progressive fibrosis of the marrow and myeloid metaplasia in the liver and spleen. The disease is usually seen in adults beyond middle age. In about 10% of cases it is preceded by polycythemia vera. Fibrosis of the marrow is occasionally associated with tuberculosis, metastatic cancer, or Hodgkin's disease; a hairy cell leukemia invariably features some degree of myelofibrosis.

Clinical Findings

A. Symptoms and Signs: Patients may complain of fatigue, weakness, weight loss, occasionally bone pain, abdominal discomfort, and symptoms of anemia. The spleen is almost always enlarged, usually markedly so. The liver may be enlarged. The lymph nodes are not affected.

B. Laboratory Findings: Anemia may be severe. The red cells vary greatly in size and shape; teardrop-shaped, distorted red cells and nucleated and stippled cells may be seen. The reticulocyte count is often slightly elevated. The white cell count may be high (20–50 thousand/μL), with a marked shift to the left and many basophils. The white cell alkaline phosphatase reaction is usually strongly positive, but it may be negative in 10% of patients. The platelet count may be greatly increased initially, and giant platelets and megakaryocyte fragments may be seen. Bone marrow aspiration is usually unsuccessful, yielding only sheets of platelet and megakaryocyte fragments and a few erythroblasts and granulocytes. Bone marrow biopsy shows fibrous tissue replacing normal marrow spaces.

Complications

Rapid splenic enlargement may be painful. The patient may develop symptoms of hypermetabolism with fever, sweating, and weight loss.

Secondary hypersplenism may lead to thrombocytopenia and bleeding and to hemolytic anemia with splenic sequestration of red cells. Some patients die in an acute "blastic" crisis.

Differential Diagnosis

In chronic myelocytic leukemia the white cell alkaline phosphatase reaction is negative. Hemolytic anemias are readily differentiated by the great number of reticulocytes, hypercellularity, and red cell hyperplasia of the bone marrow. Lymphoma and metastatic cancer with "dry tap" are differentiated by marrow biopsy.

Treatment

If the spleen is not painful and the anemia only moderate, no treatment may be required. For severe anemia, an androgenic steroid may be used (see p 307). Many patients have to be maintained on multiple transfusions. For painful enlargement of the spleen one may try busulfan, 2 mg 1–3 times daily, or x-ray radiation. For hemolytic anemia with splenic sequestration give prednisolone (or equivalent), 10–20 mg 4 times daily orally, or consider splenectomy. For "blastic crisis," mercaptopurine, 2.5 mg/kg/d, may be tried.

Prognosis

The average survival from the time of diagnosis is 2–3 years. In some patients the disease remains quiescent for several years even without transfusions. Death is due to hemorrhage, secondary infection, or acute blastic crisis.

Groopman JE: Pathogenesis of myelofibrosis in myeloproliferative disorders. (Editorial.) *Ann Intern Med* 1980;**92**:857.

Lazlo J: Myeloproliferative disorders (MPD): Myelofibrosis, myelosclerosis, extramedullary hematopoiesis, undifferentiated MPD and hemorrhagic thrombocythemia. *Semin Hematol* 1975;**12**:409.

Lubin J, Rosen S, Rywlin AM: Malignant myelosclerosis. *Arch Intern Med* 1976;**136**:141.

Myelofibrosis. (Editorial.) *Lancet* 1980;**1**:127.

HODGKIN'S DISEASE

Essentials of Diagnosis

- Regional lymph nodes enlarged, firm, nontender, painless.
- Fever, weight loss, excessive sweating, pruritus, fatigue.
- Exacerbations and remissions.

General Considerations

Hodgkin's disease is seen in all races and occurs most commonly in young adults. It is characterized by abnormal proliferation, in one or several lymph nodes, of lymphocytes, histiocytes, eosinophils, and Reed-Sternberg giant cells. It starts most likely as a regionally localized process that tends to spread to contiguous lymphatic structures. Determination of the histologic pattern and accurate measurement of the extent, or clinical staging, of the disease when first diagnosed are essential for proper management and prognosis.

Clinical Findings

A. Symptoms and Signs: Regional unilateral lymphadenopathy (especially swelling of cervical nodes) is usually the presenting sign. The nodes are firm, nontender, and of various sizes. They may adhere to the deeper tissues, but the skin remains freely movable. If the mediastinum is involved early, respiratory difficulty may be the initial complaint. Hepatosplenomegaly and constitutional complaints—fever, excessive sweating, fatigue, and pruritus—usually appear late.

B. Laboratory and X-Ray Findings: The blood count may show an absolute lymphocytopenia, especially in the histologic types showing lymphocytic depletion. Occasionally some eosinophilia is seen. Anemia is a late finding. Diagnosis is made by lymph node biopsy, but the extent of the disease must be well established prior to therapy. This is done by chest x-ray

Table 10—4. Staging of Hodgkin's disease (Ann Arbor Symposium).*

Stage	Definition
I	Involvement of a single lymph node region (I) or of a single extralymphatic organ or site (I_E).
II	Involvement of 2 or more lymph node regions on the same side of the diaphragm (II) or localized involvement of extralymphatic organ or site and of one or more lymph node regions on the same side of the diaphragm (II_E). An optional recommendation is that the numbers of node regions involved be indicated by a subscript (eg, II_3).
III	Involvement of lymph node regions on both sides of the diaphragm (III), which may also be accompanied by localized involvement of extralymphatic organ or site (III_E) or by involvement of the spleen (III_S) or both (III_{SE}).
IV	Diffuse or disseminated involvement of one or more extralymphatic organs or tissues with or without associated lymph node enlargement. The reason for classifying the patient as stage IV should be identified further by defining site by symbols.

Symptoms: A = Free of general symptoms. B = (1) Unexplained weight loss of more than 10% body weight; (2) unexplained fever. Tissue involved: N = lymph node; H = liver; S = spleen; L = lung; M = marrow; P = pleura; O = bone; D = skin.

*Modified and reproduced, with permission, from Carbone PT et al: Report of the Committee on Hodgkin's disease staging classification. *Cancer Res* 1971;**31**:1860.

(if mediastinal or hilar nodes are involved, chest tomograms and CT scans should be added), lower extremity lymphangiogram or inferior venacavogram, scintiscan of the liver and spleen, bone marrow biopsy, and liver function tests. With clinical evidence of disease in the upper abdomen—ie, a large spleen or radiographically demonstrable involvement of upper lumbar lymph nodes—exploratory laparotomy and splenectomy are indicated. The extensive pretherapy diagnostic workup is important because many patients with apparent stage I or II disease actually have more extensive involvement than is apparent, and this greatly influences the plan of therapy. In general, patients with lymphocytic predominance and nodular sclerosis do better than patients with a mixed pattern (histiocytes and lymphocytes) or lymphocytic depletion.

Differential Diagnosis

Hodgkin's disease must be distinguished from other diseases that involve lymph tissue. Anticonvulsive agents may produce lymph node changes similar to those seen in Hodgkin's disease. Differential diagnosis is made by biopsy, blood smear, or serologic tests.

Complications

Hemolytic anemia, intractable itching, superior vena cava obstruction, and pleural effusion occur. Painful and tender Hodgkin's sarcoma may develop. Paraplegia from extradural cord compression may occur.

Radiation toxicity occurs in less than 5% of patients treated; it includes pericarditis, sterility, pneumonitis, hypothyroidism, and myelopathy (Lhermitte's sign of radiation-induced myelopathy with electrical paresthesias).

Treatment

Radiation is used for stages I, II, and IIIA in an effort to eradicate the disease. Chemotherapy is used for patients with stage IIIB or IV disease. Occasionally, the 2 methods are combined.

A. Irradiation: The treatment of choice for regionally localized disease (IA, IIA, IIIA) is wide-field megavoltage radiotherapy to 3500–4000 rads in 4 weeks. Depending on the site and extent of the disease, one ("extended field") or both ("total nodal") of the following fields will have to be irradiated: The "mantle" field covers the cervical, supraclavicular, infraclavicular, axillary, hilar, and mediastinal nodes to the level of the diaphragm; the "inverted Y" covers the splenic pedicle, celiac, para-aortic, iliac, inguinal, and femoral nodes.

B. Antitumor Chemotherapy (Used for Class III$_2$ A, Class IV, and all Class B Disease):

1. Combination chemotherapy–This is the treatment of choice. To obtain maximal antitumor effect with minimal damage to healthy tissue, combinations of drugs with different mechanisms of action and various dose-limiting toxicities have been employed in preference to a large dose of a single drug. The following scheme ("MOPP")* has been used: mechlorethamine, 6 mg/m^2 intravenously on days 1 and 8; vincristine, 1.4 mg/m^2 intravenously on days 1 and 8; procarbazine, 100 mg/m^2 orally daily for 14 days in each cycle; and prednisone, 40 mg/m^2 orally daily for 14 days during cycles 1 and 4 only. A complete cycle consists of these 2 weeks of therapy followed by a rest period of 2 weeks without any treatment. Cyclophosphamide, 650 mg/m^2 intravenously, may be substituted for mechlorethamine. Three to 6 cycles are normally given.

2. Resistant cases–In resistant cases, "ABVD" may be tried: Adriamycin (doxorubicin), 25 mg/mg^2 on days 1 and 14; bleomycin, 10 units/mg^2 on days 1 and 14; vinblastine, 6 mg/mg^2 on days 1 and 14; and dacarbazine, 150 mg/mg^2 on days 1 through 14.

Alternating MOPP with ABVD has gained favor recently.

C. Treatment of Complications:

1. Acquired autoimmune hemolytic anemia–See p 309.

2. Fever–(See p 5.) For fever that does not respond to antibiotics, one may try indomethacin, 25 mg orally 4 times daily, or colchicine, 3 mg in 20 mL of saline solution given slowly intravenously.

3. Mediastinal or spinal cord compression is treated with mechlorethamine, 0.4 mg/kg intravenously, followed 24 hours later by x-ray therapy.

Prognosis

Patients with true stage I or II disease who receive intensive radiotherapy and who have no new manifestations for 5 years (about 50% of patients so treated) have at least a 95% chance of being cured. New manifestations, usually by extension of disease from the original site, occur in the other 50% but usually within 2 years after initial therapy. Attempts are now being made to reduce the incidence of extension by prophylactically irradiating apparently uninvolved contiguous areas. The overall 5-year survival rate in Hodgkin's disease appears to be about 30% at the present time. Long-term complications from MOPP therapy are sterility in virtually all of the men and half of the women and the risk of acute myelogenous leukemia.

Desforges JF, Rutherford CR, Piro A: Hodgkin's disease. *N Engl J Med* 1979;**301**:1212.

DeVita VT Jr, Hubbard SM, Moxley JH III: The cure of Hodgkin's disease with drugs. *Adv Intern Med* 1983;**28**:277.

Golomb HM et al: Importance of substaging of stage III Hodgkin's disease. *Semin Oncol* 1980;**7**:136.

Hoppe RT: Stage I-II Hodgkin's disease: Current therapeutic options and recommendations. *Blood* 1983;**62**:32.

Kaplan HS: Hodgkin's disease: Biology, treatment, prognosis. *Blood* 1981;**57**:813.

---

*Acronym for *mechlorethamine, *O*ncovin (vincristine), *procarbazine, and *prednisone.

NON-HODGKIN'S LYMPHOMA

This group of disorders usually presents with painless lymphadenopathy, most frequently in the cervical region. While lymph node involvement is more frequently regional, it may be diffuse—spleen and liver may be involved. Some patients present with systemic symptoms such as fever or weight loss. Malignant lymphoma may present at an extranodal site and may suggest a primary tumor of the involved organ, eg, the stomach.

Pathologic classification determines the approach to staging and therapy.

Current classifications take into account (1) pathologic patterns—follicular or diffuse; (2) cell type—small cells, large cells, cleaved cells, noncleaved cells, blast forms; (3) immunologic markers—B cell or T cell origin; and (4) kinetics—low-grade, intermediate-grade, and high-grade malignancy. Two schemes for classification of these lymphomas are based on cell classes of the immune system (Table 10–5) and on prognostic criteria (Table 10–6).

The favorable lymphomas are all of B cell origin; they include the small lymphocytic diffuse type, and small cleaved cell, mixed small, or large cell and follicular type. In patients with these types, treatment is best deferred.

The intermediate-grade malignancies are also of B cell origin and include follicular large cell lymphoma, diffuse small cleaved cell, and diffuse cleaved and noncleaved large cell lymphomas. This group frequently but not always requires therapy.

The high-grade malignancies include diffuse large cell (diffuse ''histiocytic'') lymphoma, Burkitt's lymphoma, and lymphoblastic lymphoma (a T cell lymphoma). They always require intensive chemotherapy.

Table 10–5. Lymphomas as neoplasms of specific cell classes of the immune system.*

B Cell	
Pre-B cell	ALL (rare)
Medullary B cell	CLL, small lymphocytic lymphoma
Follicular B cell	Follicular lymphomas, large cell lymphoma, Burkitt's lymphoma
B immunoblast	Large cell lymphoma
T Cell	
Pre-T cell	ALL (common)
Thymic T cell	ALL (uncommon), lymphoblastic lymphoma
T cell	CLL (rare), Sézary—mycosis fungoides
T immunoblast	Large cell lymphoma (rare)
Histocytic	
Histocyte	Malignant histiocytosis, Hodgkin's disease (?)

ALL = acute lymphoblastic leukemia; CLL = chronic lymphocytic leukemia.

*Reproduced, with permission, from Strauchen JA: Malignant lymphomas: Cell surface markers and advances in classification. (Medical Progress.) *West J Med* 1981;**135**:276.

Table 10–6. A working formulation of non-Hodgkin's lymphomas for clinical usage—recommendations of an expert international panel.*

Low Grade
  Malignant lymphoma, small lymphocytic
  Malignant lymphoma, follicular, predominantly small cleaved cell
  Malignant lymphoma, follicular, mixed small cleaved and large cell
Intermediate Grade
  Malignant lymphoma, follicular, predominantly large cell
  Malignant lymphoma, diffuse, small cleaved cell
  Malignant lymphoma, diffuse, mixed small and large cell
  Malignant lymphoma, diffuse, large cell
High Grade
  Malignant lymphoma, large cell, immunoblastic
  Malignant lymphoma, lymphoblastic
  Malignant lymphoma, small noncleaved cell (Burkitt's and non-Burkitt's)
Miscellaneous
  Composite malignant lymphoma
  Mycosis fungoides
  Extramedullary plasmacytoma
  Unclassifiable
  Other

*Reproduced, with permission, from Berard CW et al: A multidisciplinary approach to non-Hodgkin's lymphomas. (NIH Conference.) *Ann Intern Med* 1981;**94**:218.

Treatment

A. For the rare patient with localized disease only (stage I or II), radiotherapy with curative intent is the proper treatment.

B. For palliative care of intermediate-grade malignancies, regimens are the following:

1. CVP–Cyclophosphamide, 15 mg/kg intravenously on day 1; vincristine, 0.25 mg/kg intravenously on day 1; and prednisone, 0.6 mg/kg orally daily for 5 days. No therapy is given on days 6–21. Repeat cyclophosphamide and vincristine on day 22. On day 42, start a new cycle. Repeat for 4–6 cycles.

2. CHOP–Cyclophosphamide, 750 mg/kg; [hydroxy]doxorubicin, 50 mg/m²; Oncovin (vincristine), 2 mg intravenously; and prednisone, 100 mg orally daily for 5 days. This regimen is repeated every 4 weeks for 6 courses.

C. In some patients with high-grade malignancy, especially with large cell (diffuse histiocytic lymphoma) disease, complete remission can be achieved. Regimens are the following:

1. CHOP–See above.

2. BACOP–Cyclophosphamide, 650 mg/m² intravenously on days 1 and 8; Adriamycin (doxorubicin), 25 mg/m² intravenously on days 1 and 8; Oncovin (vincristine), 1.4 mg/m² intravenously on days 1 and 8; and bleomycin, 5 unit*/m² intravenously on days 15 and 22; prednisone, 60 mg/m² orally on days 15–28 inclusive. This regimen is repeated every 4 weeks for 6 courses.

*1 unit = 1 mg.

3. M-BACOD–Bleomycin, 4 unit*/m² intravenously on day 1; Adriamycin (doxorubicin), 45 mg/m² intravenously on day 1; cyclophosphamide, 600 mg/m² intravenously on day 1; Oncovin (vincristine), 1 mg/m² intravenously on day 1; dexamethasone, 60 mg/m² orally every day for 5 days; methotrexate, 200 mg/m² intravenously on days 8 and 15; leucovorin, 15 mg/m² orally every 6 hours for 8 doses starting on days 9 and 16.

Berard CW et al: A multidisciplinary approach to non-Hodgkin's lymphomas. (NIH Conference.) *Ann Intern Med* 1981; **94**:218.

Cabanillas F et al: Sequential chemotherapy and late intensification for malignant lymphoma of aggressive histologic type. *Am J Med* 1983;**74**:382.

Golomb HM: Non-Hodgkin lymphoma. *Semin Oncol* 1980; **7**:221.

Rosenberg SA: Non-Hodgkin's lymphoma: Selection of treatment on the basis of histologic type. *N Engl J Med* 1979; **301**:924.

Skarin AT et al: Improved prognosis of diffuse histiocytic and undifferentiated lymphoma by use of high dose methotrexate alternating with standard agents (M-BACOD). *J Clin Oncol* 1983;**1**:91.

Strauchen JA: Malignant lymphomas: Cell surface markers and advances in classification. *West J Med* 1981;**135**:276.

HAIRY CELL LEUKEMIA
(Leukemic Reticuloendotheliosis)

This variant of malignant lymphoma is characterized by splenomegaly without lymphadenopathy, pancytopenia, and the typical "hairy" cells, ie, lymphoid cells with cytoplasmic projection on a freshly made peripheral blood film; these cells contain tartrate-resistant acid phosphatase. On biopsy, the marrow shows mononuclear cells with striking fibrosis; occasionally the marrow is hypoplastic.

The clinical course is usually chronic. The most frequent complications are infection and purpura. Splenectomy is indicated in cases of frank hypersplenism. Over half of the patients survive longer than 4 years, and many long survivals have occurred. Chemotherapy is usually reserved for patients who have life-threatening disease with extensive infiltration of the marrow.

Bouroncle BA: Leukemic reticuloendotheliosis (hair cell leukemia). *Blood* 1979;**53**:412.

Golomb HM: Hairy cell leukemia. *Adv Intern Med* 1984;**29**:245.

IMMUNOBLASTIC LYMPHADENOPATHY

This recently described entity resembles Hodgkin's disease but differs from it pathologically in several important ways. Patients have fever, sweats,

weight loss, in some cases a rash, and diffuse, striking lymphadenopathy. Polyclonal hyperglobulinemia and hemolytic anemia with a positive Coombs test and lymphopenia are frequent findings. Lymph nodes show proliferation of arborizing blood vessels, interstitial amorphous acidophilic material, but no Reed-Sternberg cells. The disorder is thought to represent a nonneoplastic hyperimmune proliferation of B lymphocytes. It is frequently fatal in a year or so. Occasional cases have been reported to respond to combination treatment with cyclophosphamide, vincristine, and prednisone.

Cullen MK et al: Angioimmunoblastic lymphadenopathy. *Am J Med* 1979;**48**:151.

Pangalis A, Moran EM, Rappaport H: Blood and bone marrow findings in angioblastic lymphadenopathy. *Blood* 1978; **51**:71.

MYCOSIS FUNGOIDES

Mycosis fungoides is a malignant, progressive, proliferative disease, primarily of the skin. Initially, the lesions may resemble eczema, seborrheic dermatitis, psoriasis, or erythroderma; eventually they may become elevated and form tumors. Lymph nodes, liver, and spleen may become involved. Pathologically, the disease probably belongs to the lymphoma group; the malignant growth arises in the lymphoreticular system. The early histopathologic features are usually nonspecific. In the later stages, the characteristic findings are pleomorphic cellular infiltrates in the skin, with focal collections of mononuclear cells in the epidermis. When the cellular aggregates form tumors, they may break through the epidermis and ulcerate. At this stage, histologic distinction from reticulum cell sarcoma and Hodgkin's disease may be impossible. Generalized itching and lymph node enlargement are frequent systemic manifestations. Mycosis fungoides also resembles Sézary's syndrome (erythroderma with atypical lymphocytes).

The interval between the first appearance of a seemingly benign chronic skin eruption and the definite diagnosis of mycosis fungoides may be several years. Most patients die within 3–4 years after the tissue diagnosis is made.

Treatment is palliative, but good results may be obtained with electron beam radiation to give very little skin penetration and permit total body irradiation without visceral damage. Chemotherapy with mechlorethamine, cyclophosphamide, or methotrexate is the alternative. Weekly topical application of mechlorethamine (10 mg in 50 mL of water) may be helpful in the early stages.

Bunn PA Jr et al: Prospective staging evaluation of patients with cutaneous T-cell lymphomas. *Ann Intern Med* 1980;**93**:223.

Levi JA, Wiernik PH: Management of mycosis fungoides: Current status and future prospects. *Medicine* 1975;**54**:73.

*1 unit = 1 mg.

SÉZARY'S SYNDROME

This syndrome is characterized by chronic skin lesions, chiefly intensely pruritic erythroderma with mononuclear infiltration of the dermis and many abnormal lymphoid cells in the blood; they are thought to be of thymic origin (T cells). The cells may contain periodic acid–Schiff-positive cytoplasmic granules that are resistant to diastase. The disorder resembles mycosis fungoides in several ways and is treated similarly.

Bunn PA Jr et al: Patterns of cell proliferation and cell migration in the Sézary syndrome. *Blood* 1981;**57**:452.

HISTIOCYTOSIS

The histiocytic cell series includes monoblasts, monocytes, and immature and mature tissue macrophages. Each of these cells may undergo malignant transformation. These entities are not familial and may occur in all races.

Acute monocytic leukemia results from malignant transformation of the monoblast. Malignant lymphoma, histiocytic type (reticulum cell sarcoma), arises from poorly differentiated macrophages.

Histiocytic medullary reticulosis, which clinically resembles acute leukemia and is characterized by striking phagocytosis of red cells, white cells, and platelets, also arises from immature macrophages.

Histiocytosis X is a term that has been applied to a group of disorders including eosinophilic granuloma of bone, Hand-Schüller-Christian disease, and Letterer-Siwe disease. These conditions are of unknown cause. They are characterized by proliferation of well-differentiated histiocytes and reticulum cells, and they may be closely related, perhaps differing only in individual host resistance.

Eosinophilic granuloma of bone is a relatively benign, usually solitary osteolytic lesion. It is frequently asymptomatic and is discovered only on x-ray. It may cause pain, tenderness, swelling, and pathologic fracture. Biopsy shows histiocytic proliferation with eosinophilic infiltration. It can be treated successfully by curettage, excision, or radiation; it may also recur at another site. It is most frequently seen in children and adolescents; the commonest sites are the pelvis, skull, ribs, and vertebrae. The blood is usually not involved.

Hand-Schüller-Christian disease is a disseminated disorder involving many bones, especially the flat bones, with multiple osteolytic lesions. It is a disease of childhood. Clinically, it frequently causes diabetes insipidus. Other manifestations may be exophthalmos, eczema or eczematoid dermatitis, otitis media, and upper respiratory infections. The lymph nodes, liver, and spleen may be enlarged. The diagnosis is established by biopsy. The blood is usually not involved. Treatment may include radiation or chemotherapy with prednisone or vincristine.

Letterer-Siwe disease is characterized by proliferation of histiocytes in the skin, liver, spleen, lymph nodes, and sometimes the bones and lungs. Patients are often wasted; they have marked enlargement of the spleen and liver, maculopapular skin lesions, and recurrent infections. Pancytopenia is common, and the marrow may be replaced by histiocytes. It is most commonly seen in children under age 3 years, but it occurs also in older children, usually with a better prognosis. Prednisone and several antimetabolites may be used in therapy.

Groopman JE, Golde DW: The histocytic disorders: A pathophysiologic analysis. *Ann Intern Med* 1981;**94**:95.

Nezelof C et al: Disseminated histiocytosis X. *Cancer* 1979; **44**:1824.

Osband ME et al: Histiocytosis X. *N Engl J Med* 1981;**304**:146.

MASTOCYTOSIS
(Systemic Mast Cell Disease)

Mastocytosis is a systemic disorder of unknown cause, usually of adults, associated with hyperplasia of mast cells. There is often a complicating or underlying hematologic disease (eg, leukemia, myeloid metaplasia, or myelosclerosis). It has been suggested that manifestations are nonspecific and are due to release of histamine in the various body tissues. Urticaria pigmentosa, which consists of generalized small to medium-sized brownish macules or papules with urticaria and dermographia, is the most common clinical characteristic, although the systemic disorder has been reported to exist in the absence of skin lesions. Other clinical findings are variable and may include episodic flushing, headache, rhinitis, weakness, fever, tachycardia, gastrointestinal disturbances, lymphadenopathy, hepatosplenomegaly, bone pain, and weight loss. Laboratory findings may include anemia, x-ray evidence of lytic bone lesions, generalized cystic osteoporosis or bone sclerosis, and elevation of tissue, blood, and urine histamine levels. A definitive diagnosis can only be made by histologic demonstration of mast cell infiltration of skin, bone marrow, liver, and other body tissues.

There is no known effective treatment. Antihistamines, corticosteroids, anti-infectives, and other drugs are of no value. Urticaria pigmentosa of childhood frequently disappears, without recurrence. Patients with systemic mastocytosis often live fairly comfortably for many years, although the disease may terminate fatally within a few months of onset.

Clinicopathologic Conference: Systemic mastocytosis. *Am J Med* 1976;**61**:671.

Webb TA et al: Systemic mast cell disease: A clinical and hematopathologic study of 26 cases. *Cancer* 1982;**49**:927.

MULTIPLE MYELOMA

Essentials of Diagnosis

- Weakness, weight loss, recurrent pneumonia.
- Constant, severe bone pain aggravated by motion, often associated with pathologic fractures.
- Anemia, rapid sedimentation rate, and elevated serum globulin.
- Immature, atypical plasma cells in bone marrow.

General Considerations

Malignant plasma cells synthesize one of the immunoglobulins to excess, usually IgG or IgA. This accounts for the monoclonal spike on protein electrophoresis. Synthesis of normal immunoglobulins is usually decreased. The immunoglobulin consists of 2 pairs of polypeptide chains: a pair of "heavy" chains (molecular weight approximately 55,000 each) whose subunits determine whether the whole molecule belongs to the IgG, IgA, or IgM class; and a pair of "light" chains (molecular weight 20,000 each) that is the same for all 3 molecules. Dimers of light chains form Bence Jones protein, which has no heavy chains. Synthesis of heavy and light chains may be unbalanced, eg, an excess of light chain production leads to Bence Jones proteinuria. The malignant cells may also synthesize only part of an immunoglobulin molecule, eg, in Bence Jones myeloma, which is characterized by generalized hypogammaglobulinemia in the serum and excretion of large amounts of Bence Jones proteins in the urine, giving a paraprotein spike on urine electrophoresis. Much less commonly, only heavy chains—or portions of heavy chains—are synthesized. These "heavy chain diseases," which may involve excessive production of part of the IgG, IgA, or IgM molecule, clinically resemble lymphosarcoma more than they do multiple myeloma.

Myeloma usually appears in later life. It is seen in all races and is twice as common in men as in women. The lytic bone lesions in multiple myeloma are probably caused by an osteoclast-activating factor.

Amyloidosis, whether primary or secondary, is probably always associated with plasma cell neoplasia; abnormal gamma globulin products, particularly those of the Bence Jones type, are directly involved in these tissue ("amyloid") infiltrates.

Clinical Findings

A. Symptoms and Signs: Symptoms of anemia may be the only complaint, or there may be constant bone pain, especially on motion, and tenderness (especially of the back) and spontaneous fractures. Weight loss is common. Lymph nodes, spleen, and liver are not enlarged. Extramedullary plasma cell tumors are occasionally found in the oropharynx, on the skin, or near the spinal cord.

B. Laboratory Findings: Anemia is moderate and normocytic or slightly macrocytic. Rouleau formation may be marked and interfere with the technique of the red cell count, blood smear, typing, and crossmatching. The sedimentation rate is greatly elevated; white cell count, platelet count, and morphology are usually normal. The bone marrow may show sheets of plasma cells with large nuclei and nucleoli.

Serum globulin may exceed 10 g/dL. The electrophoretic pattern is characterized by a tall, sharp peak in contrast to the broad gamma peaks seen in other illnesses with hyperglobulinemia. The "paraprotein" globulin peak represents more than 3 g of globulin per 100 mL. It is usually associated with reduction of the other globulin. Exact identification into IgG, IgA, or IgM is made by immunoelectrophoresis. Cryoglobulin, a serum protein that precipitates in the cold, may be found. Serum calcium levels are often elevated, but phosphorus and alkaline phosphatase values remain normal. Nitrogen retention, proteinuria, and renal casts also occur. Bence Jones proteinuria is found in about 40% of myeloma patients. The abnormal globulins may interfere with thrombin formation and lengthen the PT and PTT.

The bony lesions appear on x-rays as rounded, punched-out, or mottled areas. New bone formation is lacking. Sometimes there is merely diffuse osteoporosis. In about 10% of cases x-rays are normal early in the disease. Bone scans are usually normal.

Differential Diagnosis

Pathologic fractures and osteolytic lesions are also found in reticulum cell sarcoma and lymphosarcoma, and in metastatic cancer, particularly if the origin is the breast, kidney, prostate, or thyroid. In most of these lesions some attempt at new bone formation is evident. Lymphosarcoma is particularly difficult to differentiate from multiple myeloma when there are bony tumors, oral cavity tumors, cord compression with paraplegia, or invasion of the bone marrow by atypical cells. Electrophoresis usually provides the answer.

Hyperparathyroidism is differentiated by low serum phosphorus, high parathyroid hormone level, and high alkaline phosphatase values. In primary macroglobulinemia (Waldenström), the electrophoretic pattern is similar to that of multiple myeloma, but the diagnosis is made by demonstration of "specific" macroglobulin paraprotein by immunoelectrophoresis. Hemorrhagic phenomena are prominent, and the spleen is usually enlarged. Bone lesions are rare, and the pathologic cells resemble lymphocytes rather than plasma cells. In the "heavy chain diseases," no light chains are demonstrable by immunoelectrophoresis.

In cirrhosis of the liver, cancer, infections, AIDS, and hypersensitivity reactions, up to 25% of mature plasma cells may be seen in the bone marrow, but they tend to aggregate near histiocytes and blood vessels and do not form sheets of cells. Hyperglobulinemia may be seen in sarcoidosis, lupus erythematosus, cirrhosis, lymphogranuloma venereum, and kala-azar infections. In most of these disorders, however, the basic disorder is obvious, the plasma cells are adult, and the electrophoretic pattern shows a broad gamma elevation rather than a sharp peak.

A monoclonal "spike" on serum electrophoresis may be observed occasionally in patients who have no other clinical or laboratory stigmas of myeloma or macroglobulinemia. Lymphoma, leukemia, and cancer may be associated disorders. Transient "spikes" may be seen in some infections. In some cases, no disease is found.

Complications

Complications include paraplegia due to cord compression, hemorrhage due to thrombocytopenia or interference with the normal coagulation mechanism, recurrent infections due to disturbance of antibody formation, renal failure, and liver disease.

Treatment

A. General Measures: Good urine output must be maintained to prevent protein precipitation in the renal tubules. Ambulation is encouraged to combat negative calcium balance, but patients must avoid exposure to trauma because of their susceptibility to fractures. Frequent blood transfusions may be necessary to combat the anemia. Analgesics may be needed to control pain.

B. Irradiation: Radiation therapy is best for localized bone pain and pathologic fractures.

C. Chemotherapy: The usual treatment is melphalan (Alkeran), 0.25 mg/kg orally daily for 4 days, plus prednisone, 1 mg/kg orally daily for 4 days, given together, every 4–6 weeks. The addition of vincristine, 1 mg intravenously every 4 weeks, may be valuable. For resistant cases, prednisone, 60 mg/m² for 5 days every 3 weeks, may be tried. The combination of cyclophosphamide, melphalan, vincristine, prednisone, and carmustine may be more effective, but it is less well tolerated.

D. Treatment of Complications:

1. Hypercalcemia–Hypercalcemia may be treated by giving intravenous fluids, including saline, 3–4 L daily, plus furosemide; or prednisone, 60–80 mg/d; or mithramycin, 25 μg/kg intravenously every other day for 2–4 doses.

2. Cord compression–Laminectomy may be necessary for emergency decompression.

Prognosis

The average survival time after diagnosis is 1½–2 years. Occasionally a patient may live for many years in apparent remission.

Bloch KJ: Plasma cell dyscrasias and cryoglobulin. *JAMA* 1982;**248**:2670.

Hoogstraten B: Multiple myeloma: A therapeutic enigma. *Am J Clin Oncol* 1982;**5**:13.

Kyle RA: Monoclonal gammopathy of undetermined significance: Natural history of 241 cases. *Am J Med* 1978;**64**:814.

Kyle RA: Treatment of multiple myeloma. *N Engl J Med* 1984;**310**:1382.

Solomon A: Bence-Jones proteins: Malignant or benign? (Editorial.) *N Engl J Med* 1982;**306**:605.

Stone MJ, Frenkel EP: The clinical spectrum of light chain myeloma. *Am J Med* 1975;**58**:601.

MACROGLOBULINEMIA OF WALDENSTRÖM

Macroglobulinemia is a chronic neoplastic disease of the bone marrow that bears some clinical resemblance to both multiple myeloma and chronic lymphocytic leukemia. It is characterized by excessive production of gamma M (IgM) globulin. The disorder usually develops after age 50. Symptoms of anemia (weakness, easy fatigability), hemorrhagic phenomena (petechiae and ecchymoses, mucous membrane bleeding), signs of hypermetabolism (fever and weight loss), or peripheral neuropathy may be the presenting findings. Increased serum viscosity may cause headache, dizziness, drowsiness, and even coma; on physical examination the most noteworthy finding is an abnormality of the veins in the optic fundi, which show alternating bulges and constrictions.

Some patients have a moderately enlarged spleen or diffuse lymphadenopathy. The blood may show some degree of pancytopenia; rarely, abnormal white cells; and often some rouleau formation. The marrow may be difficult to aspirate; the biopsy demonstrates a diffuse infiltrate with lymphoid elements and some plasma cells. Precipitated protein may be seen on the marrow smear. Total serum globulin may exceed 7 g/dL. Most sera with a concentration of macroglobulins greater than 2 g/dL and with an electrophoretic mobility in the gamma region will give a positive Sia water (euglobulin) test. Serum protein electrophoresis shows a sharp peak and is indistinguishable from multiple myeloma. Differentiation from multiple myeloma is made by immunoelectrophoresis. About 10% of patients have Bence Jones protein in their urine. Renal and osteolytic lesions are rare. Many patients have greatly increased blood volumes; an increase in serum viscosity is common. Smaller amounts of macroglobulin, usually less than 15% of the total globulin, may be seen in malignant lymphomas, collagen diseases, sarcoidosis, cirrhosis, and nephrosis.

In some patients the course is benign over several years. The average survival is about 4 years.

Treatment is with chlorambucil, 0.1–0.2 mg/kg daily, as described on p 328; or melphalan as described above.

The manifestations of hyperviscosity may require repeated plasmapheresis for control. Two to 4 units of plasma may have to be removed each week until alkylating agents become effective in slowing down production of the abnormal proteins.

Krajny M, Purzanski W: Waldenström's macroglobulinemia: Review of 45 cases. *Can Med Assoc* 1978;**114**:899.

CRYOGLOBULINEMIA

Serum globulins that precipitate on cooling and redissolve on warming may occur in a variety of disorders (eg, myeloma, macroglobulinemia, malignant lymphoma, collagen diseases, glomerulonephritis, infectious mononucleosis, syphilis, and cytomegalovirus disease). They may represent homogeneous proteins that have become physically altered (myeloma), mixtures of immunoglobulins (eg, IgG and IgM), or immune complexes (ie, antigen and antibody), possibly with complement (eg, lupus erythematosus). The finding of cryoglobulinemia is often without any apparent significance. It is assumed that when symptoms do occur as a result of cryoglobulinemia, the abnormal protein, on cooling, precipitates in smaller vessels and causes increased viscosity, stasis, thrombosis, or hemorrhage.

Clinical manifestations may include a Raynaud-like phenomenon on exposure to cold, oronasal bleeding, purpura, petechiae, retinal vascular constriction and hemorrhage, urticaria, and mottling, ulcerations, necrosis, and gangrene, especially in dependent areas. In mixed cryoglobulinemia, there may also be arthralgia and hepatic and renal involvement. Cryoglobulins in significant concentrations (30 mg/dL) may be demonstrated in the blood.

Treatment consists of preventing exposure to cold and, when possible, treatment of the underlying disease. Penicillamine and immunosuppressive agents have been tried. In general, treatment is unsatisfactory.

Gorevic PD et al: Mixed cryoglobulinemia: Clinical aspects and long-term follow-up of 40 patients. *Am J Med* 1980;**69**:287.

Invernizzi F et al: Secondary and essential cryoglobulinemias: Frequency, nosological classification, and long-term follow-up. *Acta Haematol (Basel)* 1983;**70**:73.

POLYCYTHEMIA VERA

Essentials of Diagnosis

- Malaise, fatigue, weakness.
- Florid facies, dusky redness of mucosa.
- Greatly increased red cell values and increase in total red cell mass.

General Considerations

Polycythemia vera is a myeloproliferative disorder that often involves one or several formed elements, such as red cells, white cells, or platelets, in varying degrees. Symptoms are probably due to increased blood viscosity and hypermetabolism. Although the disease may occur at any age, it is usually a disorder of middle age. It is more common in men than in women. Erythropoietin production is greatly depressed.

Clinical Findings

A. Symptoms and Signs: Patients may complain of headache, inability to concentrate, some hearing loss, itching (especially after bathing), pain in the fingers and toes, and redness of the conjunctiva. They may have a decreased feeling of well-being and a loss of efficiency and energy. A dusky redness is particularly noticeable on the lips, fingernails, and mucous membranes. The retinal veins are frequently tortuous and black. There is no clubbing of the fingers. The spleen is palpable in about half of cases at initial examination.

B. Laboratory Findings: The red cell count is 6–10 million/μL; the hemoglobin is above 18 g/dL in men and above 16 g/dL in women; and the hematocrit is over 52%. The white cell count may be normal or as high as 20,000/μL, and there may be an increase in basophils. The leukocyte alkaline phosphatase content is increased; platelets often are elevated and may be above 1 million/μL, but may be normal. Some patients with greatly elevated platelet counts (over 1 million/μL) but hemoglobin concentrations in the normal range may have "masked polycythemia vera." In these cases the increased red cell volume may be obscured by a simultaneous rise in plasma volume. In others, chronic gastrointestinal bleeding may keep the red cell volume within the normal range.

The bone marrow shows hyperactivity of all elements, with a corresponding decrease in marrow fat; the increase in megakaryocytes may be striking.

The arterial oxygen saturation is normal or slightly low but always above 91%. The uric acid is frequently elevated to 5–10 mg/dL. The red cell volume is increased above the upper normal limit of 36 mL/kg (32 mL/kg in women).

Differential Diagnosis

Polycythemia vera must be differentiated from high normal values (see below), which remain relatively stable and do not increase; and from stress erythrocytosis, a state of decreased plasma volume, normal red cell volume, and rapid fluctuations in blood values seen occasionally in tense individuals. A transient rise in hematocrit, with no increase of red cell volume but reduced plasma volume, may occur with use of diuretics.

The upper limits of normal for men are as follows: hemoglobin, 18 g/dL; red blood cell count, 6.2 million; hematocrit, 54%. For women, the upper limits of normal are hemoglobin, 16 g/dL; red blood cell count, 5.4 million; hematocrit, 47%.

In secondary polycythemia the basic pulmonary or cardiac disorder is usually obvious, as in cyanotic heart disease and pulmonary fibrosis. Smoking in excess of 1½ packs a day may cause erythrocytosis. In marked obesity (Pickwickian syndrome), which may also result in hypoventilation, the arterial oxygen saturation is distinctly decreased, leukocytosis and thrombocytosis are absent, and bone marrow hyperplasia is limited to the erythroid series. (Emphysema rarely raises the hemoglobin more than 1–2 g/dL above normal.)

Occasionally, a structural hemoglobin abnormality is responsible for tight oxygen binding. The oxygen tension at which 50% saturation occurs—the so-called P_{50}—is markedly reduced, and dissociation at the tissue level is below normal.

Polycythemia may occur in association with renal tumors or cysts, pyelonephritis, renal obstructive disease, cerebellar hemangioblastoma, uterine myomas, and hepatoma. Some of these disorders may be responsible for excessive erythropoietin production. The spleen usually is not enlarged, and the white cells and platelets are not affected.

Complications

Hemorrhage (particularly gastrointestinal bleeding) and thrombosis (cerebral, pulmonary, or deep vein) may occur in uncontrolled polycythemia vera. Excessive bleeding at surgery is common. Secondary gout occurs in about 10% of patients.

Treatment

A. Radiophosphorus (^{32}P): The initial dosage varies from 3 to 5 mCi intravenously. If ^{32}P is given orally, the dose is increased by 25%.

After therapy, the patient should be seen at intervals of 3–4 weeks until a remission has occurred. Platelets begin to fall at 2 weeks and reach a low point in 3–5 weeks. Red cells begin to decrease at 1 month and reach a low point at 3–4 months. At 2 months, if there has been no effect on platelets or red cells, patients are re-treated with an additional 2–3 mCi of ^{32}P. If necessary, another 2–3 mCi dose is given at 6 months. When blood counts have returned to normal, patients are reexamined every 3 months.

Remissions may last 6 months to 2 years and occasionally longer. Relapse is treated by the total initial effective dose but should not exceed 5 mCi.

B. Venesection (Phlebotomy): Remove 500–2000 mL of blood per week until the hematocrit reaches 45%, and repeat phlebotomy whenever the hematocrit rises 4–5%. The average maintenance is 500 mL every 2–3 months. When phlebotomy is the only therapy, medicinal iron must not be given. A low-iron diet is not practical, but certain foods of very high iron content should be avoided (clams, oysters, liver, legumes).

C. Chemotherapy: Alkylating agents are no longer recommended, because they are associated with an increased incidence of acute leukemia. Hydroxyurea, 15 mg/kg/d, may produce remission; initial doses may have to be slightly larger. Intermittent maintenance therapy is usually required.

D. Treatment of Complications: Surgery in patients with polycythemia vera is frequently complicated by hemorrhage. Patients should be in hematologic remission before operation. Blood loss at surgery is replaced by whole blood transfusions. Fibrinogen (human), 4–6 g, is given if the bleeding is due to fibrinogen deficiency. Gout is treated the same as primary gout.

Prognosis

In properly treated patients, survival averages approximately 13 years. Three stages of the disease can be recognized: (1) the "florid" stage, with a high red cell count and hemoglobin, may last many years; (2) compensated myelofibrosis, not requiring treatment, may continue for several more years; (3) the anemic phase, with severe myelofibrosis, megakaryocytic hyperplasia, and a very large spleen, lasts for a few months up to 2 years. About 5% of patients die of acute leukemia.

Berk PD et al: Increased incidence of acute leukemia in polycythemia vera associated with chlorambucil therapy. *N Engl J Med* 1981;**304**:441.

Berlin NI (editor): Symposium on polycythemia. (2 parts.) *Semin Hematol* 1975;**12**:335; 1976;**13**:1.

Golde DW et al: Polycythemia: Mechanism and management. *Ann Intern Med* 1981;**95**:71.

AGRANULOCYTOSIS

Essentials of Diagnosis

- Chills, fever, sore throat, prostration.
- Ulceration of oral mucosa and throat.
- Granulocytopenia with relative lymphocytosis.
- Increased sedimentation rate.

General Considerations

Agranulocytosis is usually secondary to the use of certain drugs and chemicals, eg, chemotherapeutic agents, antithyroid drugs, sulfonamides, phenothiazines, phenylbutazone, and aminopyrine. Some of these agents lead to the production of circulating agglutinins against granulocytes; in other cases the cause of agranulocytosis is not known. Some drugs, eg, aminopyrine, cause an explosive onset of symptoms and leukopenia; others, eg, the antithyroid drugs and the phenothiazines, produce leukopenia only gradually after several days or weeks, even on readministration. Transient neutropenia may be seen in disorders that elaborate an endotoxin and in viral disease. In patients undergoing hemodialysis, transient neutropenia is caused by reversible intravascular margination of neutrophils.

Clinical Findings

A. Symptoms and Signs: Onset is often sudden, with chills, fever, and extreme weakness. There may be a brownish-gray exudate of the throat and greenish-black membranous ulcers of the oral mucosa, respiratory tract, vagina, and rectum. Regional adenopathy is common. Macules and papules developing into bullae may appear. The spleen and liver are not enlarged, and there is no bone tenderness.

B. Laboratory Findings: Granulocytes disappear from the blood, and monocytes and lymphocytes may also be reduced in absolute numbers. Red cells and platelets are not affected. The bone marrow appears hypoplastic; only a few early myeloid cells are seen, but red cell series and megakaryocytes are normal. After the offending drug is removed, recovery takes place in 8–10 days; lymphocytes and monocytes reappear before the granulocytes. During recovery, a transient excess of lymphocytes followed by a phase of primitive granulocyte proliferation may be observed in the marrow.

Differential Diagnosis

Differentiate from aplastic anemia (thrombocytopenia and anemia) and from acute aleukemic leukemia (hyperplastic marrow, predominance of malignant cells).

Complications

Complications include sepsis, pneumonia, hemorrhagic necrosis of mucous membrane lesions, perirectal abscess, and parenchymal liver damage with jaundice.

Treatment

A. General Measures: Discontinue suspected chemical agents or drugs. Obtain a blood sample for bacterial culture and antibiotic sensitivity testing. Supportive measures include good oral hygiene, adequate fluid intake, and reduction of fever. Patients should be isolated if possible to reduce exposure to infection.

B. Management of Fever: Fever in a patient with granulocytopenia is probably caused by bacteremia, and intravenous antimicrobial agents should be used pending results of cultures. The current treatment of choice is to give a semisynthetic penicillin (eg, ticarcillin, 3 g every 4 hours) plus an aminoglycoside (eg, tobramycin, 1.7 mg/kg every 8 hours). Prevalent organisms and antimicrobial susceptibility in individual hospitals may modify the choice of agent.

Prognosis

The mortality rate may approach 80% in untreated cases. With antibiotic therapy, the mortality rate is much lower, and when recovery occurs it is complete. Patients must be cautioned against reexposure to offending agents.

Arneborn P, Palmblad J: Drug-induced neutropenia. *Adv Sci* 1983;**212**:289.

Price TH, Dale DC: Selective neutropenias. *Clin Haematol* 1978; **7**:501.

HEMORRHAGIC DISORDERS

Coagulation Mechanisms (Fig 10–1.)

Blood clots when its fibrinogen is converted to fibrin by the action of thrombin. Prothrombin can be converted to thrombin either by a series of reactions involving factors VIII and IX (generally referred to as the intrinsic clotting reaction) or by tissue damage and the action of factor VII (extrinsic clotting reaction). One should note that in both reactions a complex of activated factors X and V, phospholipid ("platelet factor 3"), and calcium acts on prothrombin to yield thrombin. Both intrinsic and extrinsic clotting reactions must be intact for normal hemostasis.

One can visualize the clotting factors as falling into 3 groups:

(1) Factors XII and XI concern surface control.

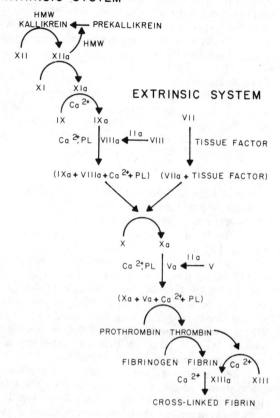

Figure 10–1. Cascade mechanism of blood coagulation. PL, phospholipid; Ca^{2+}, calcium ion; HMW, high-molecular-weight kininogen. (Adapted from Davie and Ratnoff. Reproduced, with permission, from Baugh RF, Hougie C: The chemistry of blood coagulation. *Clin Haematol* 1979;**8**:3.)

(2) Factors II, VII, IX, and X all depend on vitamin K for their synthesis. They are relatively small, are stable in bank blood, can be adsorbed by barium sulfate, and require calcium for their activation.

(3) Factors V, VIII, and fibrinogen are consumed or altered by the action of thrombin. Factors V and VIII are relatively large and are unstable.

Diagnosis of Coagulation Problems

In the study of a coagulation problem, the history is of utmost importance. The following questions must be answered:

(1) How long is the history of bleeding? Has bleeding been noted since early childhood, or is onset relatively recent? How many previous episodes have there been?

(2) What are the circumstances of the bleeding? Has it occurred after minor surgery, such as tonsillectomy or tooth extraction? Has it occurred after falls or participation in contact sports?

(3) What is the duration of the bleeding episode? (Prolonged oozing is more significant than massive hemorrhage.)

Table 10–7. Blood clotting factors.

I	Fibrinogen
I'	Fibrin monomer
I''	Fibrin polymer
II	Prothrombin
III	Tissue thromboplastin
IV	Calcium (Ca^{2+})
V	Labile factor
VII	Proconvertin
VIII	Antihemophilic globulin (AHG)
IX	Christmas factor, PTC
X	Stuart factor
XI	Plasma thromboplastin antecedent (PTA)
XII	Hageman factor
XIII	Fibrin-stabilizing factor
HMW-K	High-molecular-weight kininogen, Fitzgerald factor
Pre-K	Prekallikrein, Fletcher factor
Ka	Kallikrein
PL	Platelet phospholipid

(4) Is there a family history of bleeding?

(5) What is the type or character of the bleeding? Purpuric spots suggest a capillary or platelet defect; they are not characteristic of hemophilia. Hematomas, hemarthroses, or large ecchymoses at the site of trauma suggest hemophilia. Sudden, severe bleeding from multiple sites after prolonged surgery or during obstetric procedures suggests acquired fibrinogen deficiency. Massive bleeding from a single site without a history of purpura or previous bleeding suggests a surgical or anatomic defect rather than a coagulation defect.

Baugh RF, Hougie C: The chemistry of blood coagulation. *Clin Haematol* 1979;**8**:3.

Lewis JH, Spero JA, Hasiba U: Coagulopathies. *Disease-A-Month* (June) 1977;**23(9)**:3. [Entire issue.]

Rapaport SI: Preoperative hemostatic evaluation: Which tests, if any? *Blood* 1983;**6**:228.

HEMOPHILIA

Essentials of Diagnosis

- Lifelong history of bleeding in a male; usually congenital and familial.
- Slow, prolonged bleeding after minor injury.
- Recurrent hemarthroses and hematomas.
- Prolonged coagulation time and PTT.

General Considerations

Classic hemophilia (hemophilia A) is due to a deficiency of antihemophilic factor (AHF) activity, a constituent of normal plasma that is essential for thromboplastin formation. Patients with classic hemophilia (hemophilia A) lack part of the factor VIII molecule, the so-called VIII:C, a relatively small coagulant protein, which is usually measured by standard coagulation tests such as the PTT. Hemophiliacs have normal amounts of the larger VIII complex, a glyco-

protein usually referred to as VIII:R. When measured antigenically, this is referred to as VIIIR:Ag; when measured functionally, in tests for von Willebrand activity (see below), it is referred to as VIIIR:vW. The synthesis of VIII:R is under autosomal control. Factor VIII:C, which has a molecular weight of only 20,000, is rendered stable in plasma by VIII:R, which has a molecular weight over 1,000,000. Hemophilia A is transmitted as an X-linked recessive trait by clinically unaffected female carriers to male offspring. Female carriers can usually be identified by low or low normal levels of VIII:C with normal levels of VIIIR:Ag. About 85% of congenital bleeders have classic hemophilia. In one-third of these cases the occurrence is sporadic, ie, there is no family history of bleeding.

Plasma thromboplastin component (factor IX) deficiency (Christmas disease or hemophilia B), which accounts for about 2–3% of congenital bleeders (15% of hemophiliacs), has the same clinical manifestations and hereditary transmission as classic hemophilia. Differentiation is by specific factor assay and is essential for appropriate therapy. Several molecular types of this X-linked deficiency of factor IX have been defined. Ten percent are associated with abnormal antigen and 80% with reduced amounts of antigen.

Plasma thromboplastin antecedent (PTA) deficiency accounts for 1% of hemophiliacs. It is an autosomal recessive trait, therefore affecting both males and females. It occurs almost exclusively in Jews. Patients have only mild bleeding tendencies. Spontaneous bleeding is unusual, though some patients bruise easily. Bleeding usually only occurs after injury and some surgical procedures; hemarthroses do not occur. The differentiation from factor VIII and IX deficiency is made by specific factor assay. Fresh frozen plasma is used for treatment; no therapeutic concentrate exists as yet.

Clinical Findings

A. Symptoms and Signs: Patients with hemophilia rarely have massive hemorrhages. Bleeding is usually a delayed and prolonged oozing or trickling, occurring after minor trauma or surgery, eg, tonsillectomy or tooth extraction. With extravasation of blood, hematomas form in the deep subcutaneous or intramuscular tissue. Joint deformity results from repeated hemorrhage into joint spaces. Gastrointestinal bleeding and hematuria are also prominent.

The frequency of bleeding episodes is variable. There may be periods of spontaneous bleeding from multiple sites followed by a phase during which there is neither spontaneous bleeding nor bleeding following minor trauma.

In mild cases, a history of spontaneous bleeding may be lacking; problems occur only after dental or surgical procedures.

B. Laboratory Findings: In patients with severe hemophilia, the coagulation time may range from 30 minutes to several hours. Partial thromboplastin time (PTT) is greatly prolonged. Antihemophilic factor

(AHF) is virtually absent from the plasma. During clinically silent periods these laboratory tests remain abnormal. Capillary fragility, bleeding time (except after ingestion of aspirin), prothrombin time, fibrinogen content, and platelet values are normal.

In mild cases, the coagulation time is normal but the PTT is prolonged. The plasma contains only 5–40% of antihemophilic factor (normal: 50–150%).

Differential Diagnosis

Abnormal bleeding with long PTT occurs in several conditions. Patients with von Willebrand's disease have no joint bleeding; bleeding time is prolonged. In prothrombin complex disorders, the prothrombin time is prolonged.

Prolonged PTT but normal prothrombin time with clinical bleeding is seen in disseminated intravascular coagulation, the hemophilias, fibrinogen deficiency, and dysfibrinogenemia and in patients on heparin. Long PTT without bleeding is seen in congenital deficiency of factor XII, prekallikrein, or high-molecular-weight kininogen.

In fibrinogen deficiency, the blood does not clot at all in the test tube, or a clot may form at a normal rate and then contract to a tiny residue.

Complications

Repeated hemarthroses may lead to ankylosis. Hematoma formation around the peripheral nerves may cause permanent damage with pain, anesthesia, or muscle atrophy. Retroperitoneal bleeding may be fatal. Autoimmune anticoagulants (anti-AHF) following repeated transfusions develop in approximately 5% of patients. Receiving plasma from multiple donors exposes hemophiliacs to several risks. Many hemophiliacs have positive tests for hepatitis B antibody. Between 2% and 3% of hemophiliacs develop jaundice at some time. Abnormal liver function tests are common. Acquired immunodeficiency syndrome (AIDS) may become a hazard.

Prevention

Patients should be warned against contact sports and physically hazardous occupations. Before surgical procedures, including tooth extractions, they should receive appropriate infusions of prophylactic concentrate.

Treatment

A. General Measures: Aspirin-containing medication must not be given. Substitute acetaminophen, pentazocine, propoxyphene, or plain codeine to alleviate pain.

Treatment is based on raising the level of AHF in the patient's blood and maintaining it at this level until hemostasis is obtained. The half-disappearance time of AHF in vivo is about 12 hours. Treatment is evaluated by the clinical response. Correction of abnormal PTT is not a useful indicator.

The management of factor IX deficiency is similar; however, since factor IX is stable at blood bank conditions for long periods, plasma need not be fresh.

B. AHF Concentrates: Cryoprecipitate has some disadvantages. It must be started in the fibrinogen state; its factor VIII content varies more than that of commercial concentrates; and when a large number of units are given, it must be type-specific. It also has some important advantages. It is much less likely to lead to acquired immunodeficiency syndrome, and unlike commercial concentrates, it can be used in von Willebrand's disease. Several companies process fresh plasma to produce AHF concentrate. Labels of vials from each batch are imprinted with the content of AHF.

C. Plasma: (Fresh frozen plasma, 140 units/200 mL.) Just prior to infusion, the plasma is thawed at 37 °C until all solid material is liquefied. For maximum response it is administered as an initial dose of 15–20 mL/kg over a period of 1–2 hours.

For both concentrates and plasma, half the initial dose is repeated every 12 hours until bleeding stops.

D. Factor IX Complex: Proplex (Hyland) or Konyne (Cutter) contains factors II, VII, IX, and X. The 30-mL bottle contains approximately 500 units of factor IX in a dried form. For common bleeding (eg, hemarthroses), give 1 bottle or approximately 10 units/kg. For severe bleeding and surgical procedures, give 20 units/kg.

Fresh frozen plasma—or any kind of plasma—may be used for factor IX deficiency. The dosage considerations are similar to those for factor VIII deficiency. None of the factor VIII concentrates are effective for factor IX deficiency.

E. Desmopressin–Desmopressin can cause a quick rise in plasma levels of the factor VIII complex components, presumably by releasing them from vascular endothelial cells; it can be used effectively in the management of acute hemorrhages and minor surgery, requiring only one dose of 0.3 mg/kg in patients with mild hemophilia and in classic von Willebrand's disease. It is given by slow intravenous drip over 15–30 minutes.

F. Special Problems:

1. Bleeding–For the simpler bleeding episodes, the VIII:C level should be raised to 30%. For more severe bleeding and for surgical operations, levels of above 50% should be maintained. To calculate the proper dosage, infuse one unit of VIII:C per kilogram for every 2 percentage points increase desired. Cryoprecipitate contains on the average about 80 units per bag; commercial concentrates contain about 500 units per vial. For maintenance, infusions every 8–12 hours are needed. After dental work, one may give aminocaproic acid (Amicar) syrup, 15 mL (3.75 g) 4 times daily for 8 days, starting 24 hours before surgery.

2. Surgical procedures–Patients are prepared by infusing, just prior to surgery, enough concentrate to reach 75% AHF levels (eg, one bag of cryoprecipitate/3 kg, or AHF, 30 units/kg; one bag/6 kg at 6 hours and again at 12 hours; and then one bag/6 kg every 12 hours until the wound has healed, which may be 1–2 weeks after surgery). To assess efficacy of therapy, the AHF level must be determined; the PTT cannot be used for this.

Aminocaproic acid (Amicar, EACA) may be a valuable adjunct to therapy. Give 5 g intravenously 24 hours before surgery and then 6 g 4 times daily intravenously for 1 week. (Do not use with factor IX concentrate.) Plasma factor levels should be maintained at no less than 50% during the phase of primary wound healing (minimum of 2 weeks).

3. Hemarthroses–During the bleeding phase, the joint must be put at rest, in the position of comfort, and possibly packed with ice or put into a protective case. If pain is severe, aspiration may be necessary.

As soon as pain and bleeding have been controlled, usually within 3–5 days, muscle-stretching exercises are begun. When swelling subsides, active motion of the joint is encouraged. Weight bearing is not permitted until the periarticular soft tissues have returned to nearly normal and motion and muscle power of the joint are normal.

4. Hematuria–Give oral prednisone (2 mg/kg/d) for 2 days; the dose is then tapered and stopped after 5 days.

5. Inhibitors of anticoagulants–Five to 10% of hemophiliacs develop inhibitors. Initial manifestations are uncontrolled bleeding and failure of PTT and factor VIII levels to normalize after appropriate therapy with concentrate. Addition of normal plasma to patient's plasma in vitro does not correct the PTT. (With low level inhibitor, an incubation period may be necessary to demonstrate binding of the antigen.)

Large amounts of concentrate are usually ineffective in overcoming the inhibitor. Immunosuppressive therapy with prednisone, 1–2 mg/kg/d, and cyclophosphamide, 2.5 mg/kg/d, is occasionally successful. Success has been reported with the use of anti-inhibitor coagulation complex (Autoplex; Hyland) and, on occasion, with plasmapheresis.

Prognosis

Spontaneous hemorrhages into joints and bleeding from minor injuries or surgery are rarely dangerous. Major trauma and bleeding into loose tissues, eg, the retroperitoneal space, may be fatal despite therapy with plasma. Intracranial bleeding is the most common cause of death. Fatal, uncontrollable hemorrhage may also occur if inhibitors (anti-AHF factor) develop.

Abildgaard CF et al: Anti-inhibitor coagulant complex (Autoplex) for treatment of factor VIII inhibitors in hemophilia. *Blood* 1980;**56**:978.

Buchanan GR: Hemophilia. *Pediatr Clin North Am* 1980;**27**:309.

Kasper CK: Desmopressin acetate (DDAVP): Good news. (Editorial.) *JAMA* 1984;**251**:2564.

Kasper CK et al: Hemophilia B: Characterization of genetic variants and detection of carriers. *Blood* 1977;**50**:351.

Lusher JM et al: Efficacy of prothrombin-complex concentrates in hemophiliacs with antibodies to factor VIII. *N Engl J Med* 1980;**303**:421.

VON WILLEBRAND'S DISEASE
(Vascular Hemophilia, Pseudohemophilia)

Essentials of Diagnosis

- History of excessive bruising and frequent nosebleeds since childhood.
- Prolonged bleeding time, normal platelet count.
- Slightly prolonged PTT.

General Considerations

This relatively common disorder resembles hemophilia in that it causes prolonged bleeding, particularly after oropharyngeal surgery or trauma; however, it occurs in both sexes, and the bleeding time is prolonged.

In classic von Willebrand's disease, factor VIII/Willebrand factor-related clotting elements are all reduced. These include factor VIII procoagulant (VIII:C), factor VIII–related antigen (VIIIR:Ag), and factor VIII–related ristocetin cofactor (VIIIR:WF). VIIIR:WF in normal plasma causes platelets to adhere to glass surfaces and to agglutinate in the presence of the antibiotic ristocetin.

Clinical Findings

A. Symptoms and Signs: There is a history of frequent nosebleeds in childhood, prolonged bleeding from small cuts (eg, kitchen knife, razor cuts while shaving), excessive menstrual flow, prolonged oozing following oropharyngeal or minor gynecologic surgery, and easy bruisability. Other family members are usually affected. Skin bleeding is ecchymotic rather than petechial.

B. Laboratory Findings: A prolonged bleeding time (Ivy) is essential for diagnosis; it is greatly prolonged following the ingestion of as little as 0.6 g of aspirin. The PTT is usually slightly prolonged, reflecting low factor VIII in the range of 15–50%. The platelets are not aggregated by the antibiotic ristocetin in vitro. Platelet adhesiveness, as measured by the Salzman test, in which blood is passed through a tube with fine glass beads, is characteristically decreased (ie, more platelets than normal pass through the tube without adhering). Platelet count, platelet aggregation, prothrombin time, and clot retraction are all normal.

Differential Diagnosis

Vascular hemophilia must be differentiated from conditions with qualitative platelet defects. Glanzmann's syndrome is also characterized by a prolonged bleeding time and a normal platelet count; platelet morphology is abnormal; bleeding is often severe and may even be fatal. In macroglobulinemic purpura, ecchymoses and prolonged bleeding time may occur. In the recently described platelet-collagen interaction defect, platelet aggregation is faulty. A common aspect of all of these conditions is that factor VIII levels are normal.

Treatment

For serious bleeding episodes, the low factor VIII

level should be corrected by cryoprecipitate only; purified factor VIII concentrates may contain little Willebrand factor. If the bleeding site is accessible, bleeding can be controlled by local pressure with thrombin-soaked Gelfoam.

Prognosis

Bleeding is usually self-limited, although it may be prolonged. Fatal bleeding may occur, especially after minor surgical procedures. Childbirth and major abdominal procedures are less likely to be complicated by excessive bleeding. Bleeding tends to become less severe with increasing age.

Abildgaard CF et al: Serial studies in von Willebrand's disease: Variability versus "variants." *Blood* 1980;**56**:712.

Nachman RL: Von Willebrand's disease: A clinical and molecular enigma. *West J Med* 1982;**136**:318.

PURPURA

Petechiae, ecchymoses, and easy bruisability may be caused by thrombocytopenia, qualitative platelet disorders, or vascular defects. Qualitative platelet defects are either inherited or accompany certain diseases, eg, uremia, multiple myeloma, macroglobulinemia; they may also be drug-induced, especially by aspirin. Vascular defects may involve some hereditary disorders, autoimmune phenomena, or infections. A form of vascular purpura, characteristically confined to the upper torso, may be seen with trauma and fat embolism.

1. IDIOPATHIC (PRIMARY) THROMBOCYTOPENIC PURPURA

Essentials of Diagnosis

- Petechiae, ecchymoses, epistaxis, easy bruising.
- No splenomegaly.
- Decreased platelet count, prolonged bleeding time, poor clot retraction.

General Considerations

The thrombocytopenia is the result of increased platelet destruction; the platelet count is closely related to the rate of destruction. Normal platelet survival is 8–10 days. Survival is usually only 1–3 days in chronic idiopathic thrombocytopenic purpura and even less in the acute form. Most patients have increased levels of IgG on their platelets. Despite an apparent increase in the number of megakaryocytes in the marrow, platelet production is usually not increased; antibodies may disturb megakaryocytic development and lead to ineffective production. The disorder may be postinfectious, eg, following infectious mononucleosis or rubella; may be caused by isoimmunity, eg, following transfusions or in the neonatal period; may develop in diseases with autoimmune manifestations, eg, lupus erythematosus or lymphoproliferative

disorders; or may follow the use of certain drugs, eg, quinidine, quinine, thiazides, sulfonamides, phenylbutazone, acetazolamide, aminosalicylic acid, gold, heparin, and others.

The spleen, while not large, contributes to the thrombocytopenia in 2 ways: (1) it sequesters the subtly damaged platelets and (2) it manufactures some antibody.

Acute thrombocytopenic purpura is more common in children; 85% of patients are less than 8 years old. It usually remits spontaneously in 2 weeks to a few months. Chronic thrombocytopenic purpura may start at any age and is more common in females. At onset it cannot be distinguished from the acute form by laboratory test. There may be clinical remissions and exacerbations, but the platelet count is always low.

Clinical Findings

A. Symptoms and Signs: The onset may be sudden, with petechiae, epistaxis, bleeding gums, vaginal bleeding, gastrointestinal bleeding, or hematuria. In the chronic form, there may be a history of easy bruising and recurrent showers of petechiae, particularly in pressure areas. The spleen is not palpable.

B. Laboratory Findings: The platelet count is below $100,000/\mu L$ and may be below $10,000/\mu L$. Platelets may be absent on the peripheral blood smear. White cells are not affected; anemia, if present, is secondary to blood loss.

The bone marrow megakaryocytes are increased in number but not surrounded by platelets; they are abnormal, with single nuclei, scant cytoplasm, and often vacuoles. The chief value of the marrow examination is to rule out leukemia and aplastic anemia.

The bleeding time is prolonged, but PTT and PT are normal. Clot retraction is poor. Prothrombin consumption is decreased in severe cases. Capillary fragility (Rumpel-Leede test) is greatly increased. An antinuclear antibody (ANA) test and a prothrombin time and PTT should be done to look for lupus erythematosus, which may present as purpura.

Differential Diagnosis

Purpura may be the first sign of acute leukemia or macroglobulinemia. The diagnosis is made by finding the characteristic malignant cells in the blood or bone marrow. In thrombocytopenia accompanying aplastic anemia, the marrow fat is increased and megakaryocytes are decreased or absent. Thrombotic thrombocytopenic purpura is associated with hemolytic anemia, jaundice, central nervous system symptoms, fever, and schistocytes.

Thrombocytopenic purpura may also be seen in association with a variety of disorders causing splenomegaly and hypersplenism: congestive splenomegaly, Felty's syndrome, Gaucher's disease, tuberculosis, sarcoidosis, and myelofibrosis. Lupus erythematosus may be associated with thrombocytopenic purpura with or without splenomegaly. Other conditions that may have to be ruled out before making the diagnosis of idiopathic thrombocytopenic purpura include septicemia (especially with gram-negative organisms) and disseminated intravascular coagulation (often associated with schistocytes). Thrombocytopenia is relatively common in acute severe alcoholism.

In the newborn, thrombocytopenic purpura may also be caused by septicemia, congenital syphilis, cytomegalic inclusion disease, hemolytic disease of the newborn, a congenital lack of megakaryocytes, or a congenital giant hemangioma. In Wiskott-Aldrich syndrome, an X-linked recessive disorder, thrombocytopenic purpura is associated with eczema; increased susceptibility to infection; and deficiency of isoagglutinins, immunoglobulins, and lymphocytes.

Scurvy may cause purpura and massive skin and muscle hemorrhage, especially into hair follicles of the legs and extensor surfaces of the arms. Coagulation tests are normal.

Complications

Fatal cerebral hemorrhage occurs in 1–5% of cases; hemorrhage from the nose and gastrointestinal and urinary tracts may be dangerously severe. Pressure of a hematoma on nerve tissue may cause pain, anesthesia, or paralysis. Children born to mothers with idiopathic thrombocytopenic purpura may have transient neonatal purpura.

Treatment

A. General Measures: Patients should avoid trauma, contact sports, elective surgery, and tooth extraction. All unnecessary medications and exposure to potential toxins must be discontinued.

Children with mild purpura following viral infections do not require any therapy. They should be observed until petechiae disappear and the platelet count returns to normal.

B. Corticosteroids: Corticosteroids are warranted in patients with moderately severe purpura of short duration, especially when there is bleeding from the gastrointestinal or genitourinary tract. Corticosteroids are also given to patients with purpura who have complications contraindicating surgery. Prednisolone (or equivalent), 10–20 mg 4 times daily, is usually required to control bleeding. The dosage is continued until the platelet count returns to normal, and then it is gradually decreased.

C. Splenectomy: Splenectomy is indicated for all patients with well-documented thrombocytopenic purpura of more than 1 year's duration, for all patients with moderately severe purpura who have relapsed 2–3 times after corticosteroid therapy, and for all patients with severe idiopathic thrombocytopenic purpura who do not respond to corticosteroids.

If splenectomy must be performed on a patient who has been on corticosteroids, full doses of corticosteroids should be maintained for 3 days after surgery and then decreased gradually.

The platelet count rises promptly following splenectomy and often doubles within the first 24 hours. Maximum values are reached 1–2 weeks postoperatively. Sometimes the platelet count will exceed 1 million/μL before leveling off. Anticoagulant therapy is not necessary with even higher platelet counts. Splenectomy may be considered successful only when counts stay normal for at least 2 months.

D. Immunosuppressive Therapy: In patients who do not respond to corticosteroids and in whom splenectomy has failed to raise the platelet count, either vincristine, 1.4 mg/m^2, or vinblastine, 7.5 mg/m^2, once weekly intravenously for 4–6 weeks, may raise the platelet count to acceptable levels without further maintenance therapy.

E. Therapy for Refractory Cases: In desperate cases, intravenous immunoglobulin, 400 mg/kg given intravenously for 5 consecutive days, has been used. Another possible agent is danazol, an impeded androgen with reduced masculinizing capacity; the dose is 200 mg 2–4 times a day for 2 months or more.

Prognosis

Spontaneous and permanent recovery occurs in 75% of all cases of childhood idiopathic thrombocytopenic purpura and in 25% of all adult cases. Splenectomy is curative in 70–90% of all patients.

In thrombocytopenia caused by drugs, the platelet count may rise promptly (within a few days) when the drug is discontinued and return to normal within a few weeks. Occasionally, this return to normal is delayed, and the initial rise may not take place for several weeks.

Bussel JB, Hilgartner MW: The use and mechanism of action of intravenous immunoglobulin in the treatment of immune hematologic disease. *Br J Haematol* 1984;**56**:1.

Harrington WJ et al: Treatment of thrombocytopenic purpura. *Hosp Pract* (Sept) 1983;**18**:205.

Karpatkin S: Autoimmune thrombocytopenic purpura. *Blood* 1980;**56**:329.

McMillan R: Chronic idiopathic thrombocytopenic purpura. *N Engl J Med* 1981;**304**:1135.

Mueller-Eckhardt C et al: The clinical significance of platelet-associated IgG: A study on 298 patients with various disorders. *Br J Haematol* 1980;**46**:123.

2. DISORDERS WITH QUALITATIVE PLATELET DEFECTS

Skin purpura after minor trauma, dependent petechiae, and mucocutaneous bleeding may be seen. Some patients have abnormal bleeding after surgery. Platelet counts are usually normal but may be slightly low. Platelets may look abnormal on the blood smear; depending on the disorders, they may be small (eg, Wiskott-Aldrich syndrome) or large (eg, May-Hegglin anomaly), or they may fail to aggregate (Glanzmann's disease). The Ivy bleeding time is prolonged in all of these disorders, especially after a test dose of 0.6 g of aspirin. All of these patients should avoid the therapeutic use of aspirin. Other tests helpful in classifying the various entities in this group are clot retraction; platelet aggregation in response to collagen, adenosine diphosphate (ADP), epinephrine, and thrombin; and platelet factor 3 availability.

Aspirin may cause a defect in aggregation of platelets and prevent the release reaction; bleeding time is slightly prolonged. Aspirin irreversibly acetylates cyclooxygenase, an enzyme active in synthesis of prostaglandins.

Thrombasthenia (Glanzmann's Disease)

This is an autosomal recessive disorder. The platelet count is normal, but the platelets appear isolated on the blood smear. Bleeding time is prolonged, clot retraction is absent or decreased, and platelets do not aggregate with ADP as measured on the aggregometer. Platelet fibrinogen content is low. Platelet factor 3 availability is impaired.

Bernard-Soulier Syndrome

This is a rare congenital disorder characterized by mild to severe thrombocytopenia, large platelets on peripheral blood smear, prolonged bleeding time, normal platelet aggregation except with ristocetin, and defective platelet adhesion. The defect is thought to be a decreased concentration of platelet membrane glycoprotein Ib.

Primary Familial Platelet-ADP Release Dysfunction

This is a milder disorder than thrombasthenia, but the symptoms are similar. Easy bruising is a common finding. The bleeding time is less prolonged than in thrombasthenia, and the clot retraction is normal. The platelets look normal on the blood smear. Platelet aggregation is impaired or absent following exposure to collagen and epinephrine, and abnormal aggregation is seen following exposure to ADP.

Von Willebrand's Disease

This disorder (see p 341) may present with purpura.

Acquired Platelet Defects

Many drugs may cause defective aggregation of platelets or prevent the release reaction. Aspirin is the most important such agent, but the nonsteroidal antiinflammatory agents have similar action. Purpura and bleeding may also occur in patients who receive large parenteral doses of penicillin, carbenicillin, and similar agents. The bleeding tendency in uremia is also caused by a functional platelet defect that can be reversed by dialysis or administration of cryoprecipitate.

In macroglobulinemia and some cases of multiple myeloma, abnormal globulin may coat platelets and impair aggregation and platelet factor 3 availability.

Hochman R et al: Bleeding in patients with infections. *Arch Intern Med* 1982;**142**:1440.

Huebsch LB, Harker LA: Disorders of platelet function: Mechanisms, diagnosis and management. *West J Med* 1981; **134**:109.

Jason PA et al: Treatment of the bleeding tendency in uremia with cryoprecipitate. *N Engl J Med* 1980;**303**:1318.

Shattil SJ, Bennett JS: Platelets and their membranes in hemostasis: Physiology and pathophysiology. *Ann Intern Med* 1981; **94**:108.

3. HENOCH-SCHÖNLEIN SYNDROME
(Anaphylactoid Purpura)

This is an acquired hemorrhagic disorder characterized by general vasculitis involving multiple organ systems. It is much more common in children than in adults. Purpura may be associated with abdominal pain, gastrointestinal bleeding, hemoptysis, hematuria, proteinuria, glomerulonephritis, and arthralgia. The disorder is thought to be of immunologic origin. The purpura may be urticarial at first, followed by red macular lesions, often involving the palms and soles. All tests of coagulation, including bleeding time, are normal.

Henoch-Schönlein purpura. (Editorial.) *Br Med J* 1977;**1**:190.

HEREDITARY HEMORRHAGIC TELANGIECTASIA
(Rendu-Osler-Weber Disease)

Essentials of Diagnosis

- Telangiectatic lesions on face, mouth, nose, hands.
- Epistaxis or gastrointestinal bleeding.
- Familial involvement.

General Considerations

This is a vascular abnormality involving primarily the veins; vessels are dilated and their walls are thin. The disorder is inherited as a dominant trait. Males and females are involved equally. A positive family history can be obtained in 80% of cases.

Skin and mucous membrane lesions may be asymptomatic for many years; the diagnosis is established by inference when telangiectases and angiomas are noted in patients with a history of otherwise inexplicable attacks of epistaxis or gastrointestinal bleeding.

Clinical Findings

A. Symptoms and Signs: Multiple bright-red lesions 1–4 mm in diameter that blanch on pressure are seen on the face, oral or nasopharyngeal membranes, and upper extremities in over 90% of patients. The lesions are often first noticed in childhood, but severe bleeding is unusual before age 30; the peak incidence of severity occurs in the sixth decade. Approximately 5% of patients have pulmonary arteriovenous fistulas.

Epistaxis is the most common form of bleeding. Gastrointestinal bleeding occurs in about 15% of cases; it may be severe enough to require surgery, but the actual gastrointestinal lesions may be difficult to demonstrate at operation and too widespread to resect.

B. Laboratory Findings: Laboratory tests are helpful only in ruling out other causes of bleeding;

bleeding and clotting times, prothrombin time, platelet count, clot retraction, and tourniquet tests are normal. Secondary iron deficiency anemia is common.

Differential Diagnosis

Petechiae do not blanch on pressure, are more purple, and are not particularly common on the lips and tongue. Spider angiomas are arteriolar, can be shown to pulsate on pressure, and have several fine channels extending from their centers.

Complications

Severe bleeding may cause chronic iron deficiency anemia. Bleeding may exceed 1000 mL per week from the gastrointestinal tract.

Treatment

There is no cure. Asymptomatic lesions require no therapy. Local pressure and topical hemostatic agents may be tried in accessible bleeding areas. Cauterization of the nasal mucous membranes may be necessary.

For uncontrollable gastrointestinal bleeding unsuitable for surgery, iron therapy is indicated. If bleeding is severe (50–100 mL/d), give iron dextran injection, 5–10 mL intravenously once weekly. For more severe bleeding, transfusions are necessary.

Halpern M et al: Hereditary hemorrhagic telangiectasia. *Radiology* 1968;**90**:1143.

THROMBOTIC THROMBOCYTOPENIC PURPURA

This is a severe, acute illness with a poor prognosis. The major clinical manifestations are fever, jaundice, purpura, drowsiness with fluctuating neurologic signs, thrombocytopenia, hemolytic anemia with characteristically fragmented red blood cells, and renal abnormalities. Any one of these features may be absent, especially initially. The Coombs test is negative, red cell enzymes are not decreased, and Heinz bodies are absent.

The pathologic diagnosis depends upon vascular lesions located at arteriolocapillary junctions, with widespread distribution in many organs. The lesions consist of subintimal deposition of periodic acid–Schiff–positive material, hyaline thrombi, and vessel wall weakening, leading to aneurysmal dilatations. The thrombotic phenomena are thought to be secondary reactions to the damaged vascular walls. Circulating immune complexes may be responsible.

Infusion of fresh-frozen plasma should be started immediately after the diagnosis is made; 6–8 units a day may have to be used. In patients not responding, plasmapheresis should be instituted. Improvement in neurologic status, decrease in serum LDH, and rise in platelet count indicate improvement.

Cuttner J: Thrombotic thrombocytopenic purpura: A ten-year experience. *Blood* 1980;**56**:302.

MacHin SJ: Thrombotic thrombocytopenic purpura. *Br J Haematol* 1984;**56**:191.

Myers TJ et al: Thrombotic thrombocytopenic purpura: Combined treatment with plasmapheresis and antiplatelet agents. *Ann Intern Med* 1980;**92**:149.

Ridolfi RL, Bell WR: Thrombotic thrombocytopenic purpura: Report of 25 cases and review of the literature. *Medicine* 1981; **60**:413.

DISSEMINATED INTRAVASCULAR COAGULATION
(Defibrination Syndrome, DIC)

Essentials of Diagnosis

- Diffuse bleeding from the skin and mucous membranes.
- Poor, small clot.
- Reduced platelets on smear.
- Prolonged prothrombin time.

General Considerations

This is a pathologic form of coagulation that differs from normal clotting in 3 principal ways: (1) it is diffuse rather than localized; (2) it damages the site of clotting instead of protecting it; and (3) it consumes several clotting factors to such a degree that their concentration in the plasma becomes so low that diffuse bleeding may occur. It is seen in certain obstetric catastrophes and following some types of surgery, particularly involving the lung, brain, or prostate. In some of these conditions and in malignant tumors (especially of the prostate), septicemia, hemolytic transfusion reaction, and hemolytic uremic syndrome in infancy, deposition of fibrin in small blood vessels may lead to serious and even fatal tissue necrosis. Examples are (1) glomerular capillary thrombosis leading to cortical necrosis or a pattern similar to that of acute tubular necrosis, (2) adrenal sinusoidal thrombosis with resultant hemorrhagic necrosis of the adrenals (Waterhouse-Friderichsen syndrome), and (3) hemorrhagic skin necrosis in purpura fulminans. These conditions are caused in part by a failure to clear fibrin. Some relationship may exist between irreversible endotoxin shock and disseminated intravascular clotting.

Unexpected, profuse, or uncontrollable bleeding in certain surgical or obstetric situations suggests acute defibrination. Multiple coagulation factors are involved.

Clinical Findings

A. Symptoms and Signs: The most common manifestation is diffuse bleeding from many sites at surgery and from needle puncture. Minimal trauma may cause severe bleeding, or there may be spontaneous ecchymoses, epistaxis, or gastrointestinal hemorrhage. Uncontrollable postpartum hemorrhage may be a manifestation of intravascular coagulation.

B. Laboratory Findings: The combination of a poor, small clot, reduced platelets on the blood smear, and a prolonged prothrombin time is very suggestive of this disorder. With marked fibrinogen depletion (fibrinogen < 75 mg/dL), the clot that forms in a test tube may be quite flimsy and friable. It may be so small and retracted that it may not even be visible, thus simulating findings of fibrinolysis. The contents of the test tube should be poured into a Petri dish or onto a piece of filter paper for closer examination. If a blood clot can be demonstrated, it suggests that fibrinogen depletion, and not fibrinolysis, is the primary process.

A form of hemolytic anemia associated with fragmentation of the red blood cells (microangiopathic hemolytic anemia) may accompany some of these conditions.

Platelet counts usually vary from 30 to 120 thousand/μL. Screening tests for fibrinogen (Hyland Laboratories Fi test) usually indicate values of less than 100 mg/dL. The activated PTT (normal: < 35 seconds) is prolonged to as much as 100 seconds. The thrombin time is prolonged, and the prothrombin time is moderately prolonged.

Abnormalities in the metabolism of fibrinogen are first documented by finding the presence of fibrin monomers in the plasma by the protamine sulfate test or the ethanol gelation test. The best diagnostic confirmation of disseminated intravascular coagulation is the demonstration, by immunologic techniques, of markedly increased fibrin fragments (FDP) by the latex agglutination test or the staphylococcus clumping test.

Differential Diagnosis

Prolonged prothrombin time and a long PTT may be due to vitamin K deficiency, especially postoperatively, and a trial of vitamin K should be given. Disseminated intravascular coagulation—which, like all clotting, is associated with secondary fibrinolysis—must be distinguished from primary fibrinolysis, a much rarer clinical phenomenon requiring very different management. This latter syndrome may occur with disseminated carcinoma (especially of the prostate), with septicemia, and with very severe liver disease. Diffuse bleeding similar to that encountered in intravascular coagulation does not occur, and platelets, factor V, and factor VIII are less strikingly decreased; a clot may form initially but dissolves completely in less than 2 hours. As in secondary fibrinolysis, fibrinogen is low or absent; consequently, prothrombin and thrombin times are prolonged, plasminogen is low, and plasmin levels are increased.

Other conditions where clots fail to form in vitro are circulating anticoagulant and heparin administration. In vitro clotting may be prolonged to 1 hour or more in the hemophilias and in factor XII deficiency.

Treatment

If possible, treat the underlying disorder, eg, shock or sepsis. Heparin may be effective to stop pathologic clotting, and it may also control bleeding. In adults, the usual dose of heparin is 100 USP units/kg every 4–6 hours intravenously; in children, 50 units/kg every 4 hours after an initial dose of 100 units. If the

diagnosis of intravascular coagulation was correct and therapy is effective, fibrin degradation products should fall and fibrinogen levels, PTT, and PT should improve within 24 hours and platelet count within a few days. Whole blood may be necessary to combat shock. With severe fibrinogen deficiency, cryoprecipitate may have to be given. The average bag of cryoprecipitate contains at least 250 mg of fibrinogen. Platelet concentrates may be used in severe platelet deficiency.

Prognosis

In fibrinogen deficiency due to liver disease or cancer, the prognosis is usually that of the underlying disorder. Excessive bleeding during brain or lung surgery or at delivery may be completely and permanently corrected by heparin and possibly fibrinogen.

Feinstein DI: Diagnosis and management of disseminated intravascular coagulation: The role of heparin therapy. *Blood* 1982;**60:**284.

Spero JA et al: Disseminated intravascular coagulation: Findings in 346 patients. *Thromb Haemostas* 1980;**43:**28.

DISORDERS INVOLVING FIBRINOGEN

Increased synthesis of fibrinogen is seen in many inflammatory diseases, but decreased synthesis is rare. It can occur in congenital afibrinogenemia and after treatment with asparaginase for leukemia. The low levels of fibrinogen observed in diseases of the liver and in disseminated intravascular coagulation are caused by accelerated catabolism of fibrinogen. Several functionally defective molecular variants of fibrinogen have been described—the dysfibrinogenemias—many of them are clinically inert, but some cause bleeding or abnormal wound healing. On rare occasions, thrombotic episodes have been described.

Laboratory findings include prolonged thrombin time, prolonged reptilase time, and low values of fibrinogen as measured by clotting assays, but normal ones as measured by immunologic or chemical assay. In severe liver disease, dysfibrinogenemia may develop as an acquired disorder.

Treatment is with cryoprecipitate. Human fibrinogen is no longer recommended because of the high incidence of hepatitis associated with its use.

Gralnick HR et al: Dysfibrinogenemia associated with hepatoma. *N Engl J Med* 1978;**299:**221.

Ratnoff OD: Criteria for the differentiation of dysfibrinogenemic states. *Semin Hematol* 1976;V**13:**141.

ACQUIRED PROTHROMBIN COMPLEX DISORDERS
(Factors V, VII, & X & Prothrombin)

Essentials of Diagnosis

- Ecchymoses and epistaxis, spontaneously or after minimal trauma.

- Postoperative wound hemorrhage.
- Bleeding from venipuncture.

General Considerations

In all of these disorders an underlying process is usually evident, eg, liver disease or anticoagulant therapy. Regardless of which member of the prothrombin complex is deficient—prothrombin (factor II), factors V, VII, or X—the prothrombin time is prolonged.

There are 3 forms of prothrombin complex deficiency.

A. Vitamin K Deficiency: Factors VII, IX, X, and prothrombin are synthesized in the liver and resemble the protein trypsin. They are functionally inert until vitamin K adds gamma-carboxyl groups to glutamyl residues at the amino-terminal end of the molecule. This enables prothrombin and factors VII, IX, and X to bind calcium and bind to phospholipids. In the presence of vitamin K antagonists, such as coumadin, or in vitamin K deficiency, this carboxylation does not occur, and antigenically detectable but functionally inactive factors circulate. Vitamin K is derived from the diet and from bacterial synthesis in the bowel. Malnutrition, malabsorption, and antibiotics that sterilize the bowel can produce vitamin K deficiency. This can develop quite rapidly after surgery, especially if there is an element of renal failure.

B. Severe Liver Disease: There is primarily a deficiency of factor V, but factors II, VII, IX, and X may also be low.

C. Excessive Utilization: (See Intravascular Coagulation.) A severe bleeding disorder may accompany systemic amyloidosis. It is caused by acquired deficiency of factor X, which apparently is rapidly absorbed by the amyloid deposits in tissues.

Clinical Findings

A. Symptoms and Signs: There is no previous history of hemorrhagic manifestations. Ecchymoses and epistaxis may occur spontaneously or after minimal trauma. Gastrointestinal bleeding, hematuria, and postoperative wound hemorrhage are common. Bleeding into joints does not occur.

B. Laboratory Findings: The prothrombin time measures deficiencies in any member of the prothrombin complex, ie, if there is a deficiency in prothrombin (factor II), factor V, factor VII, or factor X, or if the fibrinogen levels are less than 125 mg/dL, the prothrombin time will be prolonged. Conversely, if the prothrombin time is normal, one can assume that all prothrombin complex components are adequate. Specific tests for these factors are of value when a congenital defect is suspected or when the underlying cause of the prolonged prothrombin time is not evident.

In these acquired prothrombin complex disorders the prothrombin time is usually below 40–50%; surgical bleeding may occur below 50%; spontaneous bleeding, at 10–15%. Prothrombin consumption, coagulation time, bleeding time, capillary fragility,

and clot retraction are normal unless there is associated thromboplastin deficiency.

Treatment

A. General Measures: Deficiency due to vitamin K lack or warfarin excess is successfully treated by administration of vitamin K. The deficiency of liver disease, however, does not respond to vitamin K. Replacement therapy with whole blood or plasma is generally unsatisfactory because of the lability of factor V in vitro and the very rapid disappearance rate of factor VII in vivo.

B. Vitamin K:

1. Phytonadione (Mephyton) for the treatment of warfarin excess–To restore prolonged prothrombin time to normal, give 5 mg orally. For major bleeding, 10–15 mg of Aqua-Mephyton given slowly intravenously at a rate not exceeding 10 mg/min will shorten the prothrombin time in 2 hours and produce safe therapeutic levels in 4–6 hours. Very severe bleeding may call for transfusions of whole blood and prothrombin concentrate (Proplex).

2. Synthetic, water-soluble vitamin K (menadione sodium bisulfite [Hykinone], menadiol [Synkayvite]) is sufficient for the treatment of vitamin K deficiency due to malabsorption. The dosage is 5 mg daily.

Prognosis

Vitamin K deficiency and the effect of warfarin excess can be corrected by parenteral or oral administration of vitamin K. The prognosis in other conditions depends upon the underlying disorder.

Friedman PA: Vitamin K–dependent proteins. *N Engl J Med* 1984;**310**:1458
O'Reilly RA: Vitamin K and the anticoagulant drugs. *Annu Rev Med* 1976;**27**:245.
Vansell JE, Kumar R, Deykin D: The spectrum of vitamin K deficiency. *JAMA* 1977;**238**:40.

CIRCULATING ANTICOAGULANTS

Essentials of Diagnosis

- Ecchymoses.
- Gastrointestinal bleeding.
- Hemarthroses.
- Prolonged PTT.

General Considerations

A circulating anticoagulant is an abnormal blood component that inhibits the coagulation of normal blood. Circulating anticoagulants may appear at any age and in either sex. Most circulatory anticoagulants interfere with thromboplastin formation, probably by immune alloantibody production; the majority are directed against AHF and occur either in patients with hemophilia after many transfusions or spontaneously and transiently 8–10 weeks after obstetric delivery. Circulating anticoagulants may be clinically silent and manifested only by an otherwise unexplained prolonged PTT as an isolated abnormality. The so-called lupus inhibitor is not associated with abnormal bleeding; the inhibitor is probably directed against the phospholipid used in the usual PTT procedure.

Clinical Findings
A. Symptoms and Signs: Patients develop sudden spontaneous hemorrhages characterized by ecchymoses, subcutaneous and intramuscular hematomas, hematuria, hemarthroses, gastrointestinal bleeding, and bleeding into the tongue and pharynx. Abnormal uterine bleeding may occur in women.

B. Laboratory Findings: In all patients the coagulation time is prolonged (30 minutes to several hours), but once a clot forms, it is of good quality and contracts normally. PTT is prolonged. Prothrombin time is normal in the hemophilialike group but is prolonged with the type of circulating anticoagulants seen in lupus erythematosus. Bleeding time and platelet counts are normal. The existence of circulatory anticoagulants can be proved if relatively small amounts (20–40%) of patient's blood or plasma inhibit coagulation of normal blood or plasma. Inhibitors of factor VIII may become apparent only after prolonged incubation of patient plasma and normal plasma. If circulating anticoagulants are present only in small amounts, however, more refined methods of demonstrating the inhibitory effect are necessary.

Differential Diagnosis
Another group of inhibitors of coagulation causing hemorrhagic phenomena (chiefly petechiae, epistaxis, and abnormal uterine bleeding) are the abnormal proteins, macroglobulins, myelomas, and cryoglobulins.

Treatment
The treatment of a bleeding hemophiliac with a circulating anticoagulant to AHF may require massive doses of AHF concentrate (Hyland Antihemophilic Factor-Method Four) to overload the inhibitor.

Prednisolone orally in relatively large doses (15–20 mg 4 times daily) with cyclophosphamide (Cytoxan), 2.5 mg/kg/d, may be tried.

Occasionally, success has been reported after the administration of factor IX concentrate (eg, Proplex).

Prognosis
The presence of circulating anticoagulants in the blood is a serious disorder. If anticoagulants develop in the course of hemophilia, the outcome is often fatal. Circulating anticoagulants that develop after pregnancy disappear spontaneously after several months.

Cosgriff TM, Martin BA: Low functional and high antigenic antithrombin III level in a patient with the lupus anticoagulant and recurrent thrombosis. *Arthritis Rheum* 1981;**24**:94.

Lupus anticoagulant. (Editorial.) *Lancet* 1984;**1**:1157.

Shapiro SS: Antibodies to blood coagulation factors. *Clin Haematol* 1979;**8**:207.

BLOOD TRANSFUSIONS

Blood transfusions are used to restore blood volume after hemorrhage; to improve the oxygen-carrying capacity of the blood in severe anemia; and to combat shock in acute hemolytic anemia. Blood volume or red cell mass should be restored to approximately 70% of normal after hemorrhage. Adequate oxygen-carrying capacity can usually be maintained in chronic anemia by raising the hemoglobin value to 50–70% of normal. Shock in acute hemolytic or acute aplastic anemia can be prevented by maintaining hemoglobin values at 50–70% of normal.

Rate of Transfusion
Except in the case of emergencies, blood should be given at a rate of 80–100 drops/min, or 500 mL in 1½–2 hours. For rapid transfusions, it is best to use a 15-gauge needle and allow the blood to run freely. The use of pressure is dangerous unless it can be applied by gentle compression of collapsible plastic blood containers.

Serologic Considerations
The antigens for which routine testing are always performed in donors and recipients are A, B, and D (Rh$_0$). Pretransfusion compatibility tests use the serum of the recipient and the cells of the donor (major cross-match). To ensure a maximal margin of safety, each transfusion should be preceded by a 3-part compatibility procedure: (1) at room temperature in saline; (2) at 37 °C fortified by the addition of albumin; and (3) at 37 °C followed by an antiglobulin test.

Miscellaneous Considerations
The age of the blood (within the expiration period) is relatively unimportant in restoring volume deficits or repairing oxygen-carrying capacity defects. Fresh blood is required only if functioning platelets are needed. Red cell mass (hematocrit about 70%), infused through 17- to 18-gauge needles, is the treatment of choice in chronic anemias. Precipitates of platelets, leukocytes, and fibrinogen or fibrin in some bank bloods may clog the filters in administration sets and cause the infusion rate to slow down; when this happens, the filters should be replaced.

Barton JC: Nonhemolytic noninfectious transfusion reaction. *Semin Hematol* 1981;**18**:95.

Boral LI et al: The type and antibody screen, revisited. *Am J Clin Pathol* 1979;**71**:578.

Mollison PL: *Blood Transfusion in Clinical Medicine,* 6th ed. Davis, 1979.

Tibor JG: Pathogenesis and management of hemolytic transfusion reaction. *Semin Hematol* 1981;**18**:84.

FRESH BLOOD

Concern about the freshness of blood has to do with 4 considerations: **(1) Platelets:** Platelets are in adequate supply in whole blood up to about 24 hours after collection. **(2) Factors V and VIII:** All coagulation factors except V and VIII are stable in banked blood for at least 21 days; factors V and VIII decline fairly rapidly within a few days after collection. **(3) Levels of 2,3-diphosphoglycerate (2,3-DPG):** As red cells age—usually after a week or so—levels of 2,3-diphosphoglycerate decline, which causes increased affinity of hemoglobin for oxygen and results in less supply to the tissues. Although normal affinity is restored in a few hours after transfusion, massive infusions of older blood may make a critically ill patient worse. The problem of declining 2,3-diphosphoglycerate levels may be largely solved when citrate-phosphate-dextrose (CPD) replaces acid-citrate-dextrose (ACD) as the standard anticoagulant in blood banking. **(4) Levels of plasma potassium, lactic acid, and ammonia:** Plasma levels rise very little above baseline for the first 4–5 days of storage and become potentially important only after 2 weeks. Most transfusions are given for acute blood loss—either post-traumatic, during surgery where blood loss is inevitable, or in patients with acute hemorrhage from the gastrointestinal tract. In none of these 3 categories is the age of blood particularly important, and fresh blood should not be ordered.

The recognized occasions when the age of the blood may be specified are the following:

(1) Open heart surgery, where heparinized blood is needed. Heparinized blood cannot be used later than 24 hours after procurement.

(2) Massive transfusions, ie, more than 10 units in a few hours. Platelets may become a problem (see next section).

(3) In renal dialysis and in patients with liver failure, blood can be given within a week after procurement.

PLATELET TRANSFUSIONS

Platelet transfusions may be indicated in patients with aplastic anemia or whose platelet counts have fallen below 10,000/μL after chemotherapy for acute leukemia. Platelets do not have to be ABO type-specific; concentrates do not contain enough red cells to cause a reaction. These transfusions raise the platelet count by 10,000 platelets per μL per platelet unit given; survival is usually about 2 days. After repeated transfusions of platelets, recipients may become immunized to random platelets; HLA-matched platelets should then be given. Platelet transfusions are of little value in conditions associated with rapid destruction of platelets such as idiopathic thrombocytopenic purpura.

WHITE CELL TRANSFUSIONS

Granulocyte concentrates can now be transfused. They are obtained by leukapheresis from a single donor who must be ABO compatible but need not be matched for HLA or granulocyte-specific antigens. If the patient has been alloimmunized, granulocyte transfusions may induce severe chill and fever reactions and will fail to have a clinical effect. In such cases, HLA typing of family members may yield a compatible match. Indications for granulocyte transfusions are a granulocyte count of less than 500/μL, with fever and infection that have failed to respond to antibiotics administered for 48 hours, and a marrow that shows no sign of imminent recovery.

TRANSFUSIONS IN BLEEDING PROBLEMS

Fresh frozen plasma, which contains all the clotting factors except platelets, may be used in a patient who continues to ooze postoperatively for several days if the suspicion of some type of hemophilia is strong and diagnostic results are not immediately available. Plasma is not a clinically useful source of fibrinogen because its fibrinogen concentration is too low.

When over 10 units of bank blood have to be given in a few hours, the levels of factors V and VIII may decrease sufficiently to cause prolongation of the PTT, but they usually do not fall below hemostatically adequate levels. Thrombocytopenic bleeding may become a problem. Platelet concentrates may have to be given. Central venous pressure should be monitored to protect against overtransfusion.

Higby DJ, Burnett D: Granulocyte transfusions: Current status. *Blood* 1980;**55**:2.

HEMOLYTIC TRANSFUSION REACTIONS

Essentials of Diagnosis
- Chills and fever during blood transfusion.
- Pain in the back, chest, or abdomen.
- Hemoglobinemia and hemoglobinuria.

General Considerations
In all significant hemolytic transfusion reactions there is immediate, easily visible hemoglobinemia with pinkish or red plasma. A normal serum color during or immediately after a transfusion rules out hemolysis as the cause of even severe symptoms.

In transfusion reaction due to ABO incompatibility the donor cells are hemolyzed instantaneously in the general circulation. Reactions caused by some of the other blood groups (such as Rh), have more gradual hemolysis and may last hours, most of the destruction occurring in the reticuloendothelial tissues.

Serious transfusion reactions are often caused by clerical errors such as improper labeling of specimens or improper identification of patients.

Clinical Findings

A. Symptoms and Signs: There may be chills and fever, and pain in the vein at the local injection site or in the back, chest, or abdomen. Anxiety, apprehension, and headache are common. In the anesthetized patient, spontaneous bleeding from different areas may be the only sign of a transfusion reaction.

B. Laboratory Findings: Posttransfusion blood counts fail to show the anticipated rise in hemoglobin; spherocytes may be present on the blood smear; and initial leukopenia at 1–2 hours is followed by a slight leukocytosis. Free hemoglobin can be detected within a few minutes. Methemalbumin, an acid hematin-albumin complex giving a brown color to the serum, may appear after a few hours and persist for several days. Elevated bilirubin levels, when present, are usually greatest 3–6 hours after the transfusion. Haptoglobin disappears from the serum. Hemoglobinuria and oliguria may occur.

After the reaction occurs it is essential to draw a fresh specimen from the patient, perform a direct Coombs test, and check it against the blood in the transfusion bottle (not the pilot tube) by the indirect Coombs test. If the indirect Coombs test is positive, exact identification of the offending antibody may be made by matching the patient's serum against a panel of known test cells. Unusual antibodies found in transfusion reactions are anti-c, anti-K (Kell), anti-E, anti-Fy^a (Duffy), anti-Le^a (Lewis), anti-Jk^a (Kidd), anti-C, and anti-P.

Differential Diagnosis

Transfusion in the presence of leukoagglutinins, which usually develop after 5 or more transfusions or after previous pregnancy, may cause severe chills and high fever and pulmonary infiltrates. There is no fall in hematocrit, a cross-match is compatible, and there are no pigmentary changes in the serum; leukoagglutinins can be demonstrated by cytotoxicity studies. All subsequent transfusions must be in the form of packed red cells, "white cell poor," ie, with the buffy coat removed.

In allergic transfusion reactions, the above tests also are negative, and no leukoagglutinins are present; recipients who lack IgA develop hives on the basis of anti-IgA.

Complications

Acute tubular necrosis and azotemia may follow a hemolytic transfusion reaction.

Treatment

Hives, chills, and fever following the transfusion of blood are not necessarily due to hemolysis; if the patient's serum remains clear, the transfusion may be continued. However, once the diagnosis of hemolysis is established by appropriate tests, the main problems are to combat shock and treat possible renal damage.

A. Treatment of Shock: After antibody screening of the patient's serum, transfusions with properly matched blood may be advisable. If no satisfactory answer can be found to account for the transfusion reaction, plasma expanders, such as dextran, and plasma may have to be used instead of whole blood. Pressor agents may be necessary.

B. Treatment of Renal Failure: Some studies suggest that osmotic diuretics such as mannitol can prevent renal failure following a hemolytic transfusion reaction. After an apparent reaction and in oliguric patients, a test dose of 12.5 g of mannitol (supplied as 25% solution in 50-mL ampules) is administered intravenously over a period of 3–5 minutes; this dose may be repeated if no signs of circulatory overload develop. A satisfactory urinary output following the use of mannitol is 60 mL/h or more. Mannitol can be safely administered as a continuous intravenous infusion; each liter of 5–10% mannitol should be alternated with 1 liter of normal saline to which 40 meq of KCl have been added to prevent serious potassium depletion. If oliguria develops, treat as for acute renal failure.

Prognosis

The hemolysis is self-limited. Renal involvement is comparatively infrequent. The death rate from hemolytic transfusion reactions is about 10%.

Goldfinger D: Acute hemolytic transfusion reactions: A fresh look at pathogenesis and considerations regarding therapy. *Transfusion* 1977;**17**:85.

POSTTRANSFUSION HEPATITIS

The risk of contracting hepatitis from a unit of whole blood is approximately 0.3%. It is only one-third as high when blood from donors negative for hepatitis B antigen (HBsAg) is used. Approximately 0.1–1% of potential donors are positive; it is thought that only one-third of hepatitis-transmitting donors can be detected by current methods, but severe cases may be entirely eliminated by screening for positive donors. Many cases of hepatitis following transfusion are of the non-A, non-B variety.

The incidence of hepatitis with blood from positive donors is 50–75%. The risk of hepatitis from fibrinogen may approach 25%; the risk from pooled plasma is about 10%.

Miller DJ: Seroepidemiology of viral hepatitis: Correlation with clinical findings. *Postgrad Med* (Sept) 1980;**68**:137.

Ratey GG: Transfusions and hepatitis, update 1978. (Editorial.) *N Engl J Med* 1978;**298**:1413. [This editorial reviews the status of hepatitis and transfusions and points out the role of non-A, non-B transfusional hepatitis.]

Sugg U et al: Clotting factors and non-A, non-B hepatitis. (Letter.) *N Engl J Med* 1980;**303**:943.

•   •   •

References

Biggs R, Rizza CR (editors): *Human Blood Coagulation, Haemostasis and Thrombosis,* 3rd ed. Mosby, 1983.

Carter SK, Bakowski MT, Hellman K: *Chemotherapy of Cancer,* 2nd ed. Wiley, 1981.

Chanarin I: *The Megaloblastic Anemias,* 2nd ed. Blackwell, 1979.

Colman RW et al: *Hemostasis and Thrombosis: Basic Principles and Clinical Practice.* Lippincott, 1982.

Mollison PL: *Blood Transfusion in Clinical Medicine,* 7th ed. Mosby, 1983.

Sandberg AA et al: Chromosome analysis in hematologic disorders: The leukemias. *Am J Med* 1984;**76:**971.

Stites DP et al (editors): *Basic & Clinical Immunology,* 5th ed. Lange, 1984.

Williams WJ et al: *Hematology,* 3rd ed. McGraw-Hill, 1983.

Wintrobe MM et al: *Clinical Hematology,* 8th ed. Lea & Febiger, 1981.

11 | Alimentary Tract & Liver

C. Michael Knauer, MD, John V. Carbone, MD,
Lloyd L. Brandborg, MD, & Sol Silverman, Jr., DDS

NAUSEA & VOMITING

These intensely disagreeable symptoms may occur singly or concurrently and may be due to a wide variety of factors (see below). The pathophysiology of vomiting is not completely understood. Vomiting appears to involve 2 functionally distinct medullary centers: the vomiting center, which initiates and controls the act of emesis; and the chemoreceptor trigger zone, which is activated by many drugs and endogenous and exogenous toxins. The vomiting center may receive stimuli from the alimentary tract and other organs, from the cerebral cortex, from the vestibular apparatus, and from the chemoreceptor trigger zone. Two or more stimuli may coexist.

An oversimplified classification of causes of vomiting is as follows:

(1) Alimentary disorders: Irritation, inflammation, or mechanical disturbance at any level of the gastrointestinal tract.

(2) Hepatobiliary and pancreatic disorders.

(3) Acute systemic infection.

(4) Central nervous system disorders: Increased intracranial pressure, stroke, migraine, infection, toxins, radiation sickness.

(5) Labyrinthine disorders: Motion sickness, infection, Meniere's syndrome.

(6) Endocrine disorders: Diabetic acidosis, adrenocortical crisis, pregnancy, starvation, lactic acidosis.

(7) Genitourinary disorders: Uremia, infection, obstruction.

(8) Cardiovascular disorders: Acute myocardial infarction, congestive heart failure.

(9) Drugs: Morphine, meperidine, codeine, excess alcohol, anesthetics, anticancer drugs, many others.

(10) Psychologic disorders: Reaction to pain, fear, or displeasure, chronic anxiety reaction, anorexia nervosa, psychosis.

Complications of vomiting include fluid and electrolyte disturbances, pulmonary aspiration of vomitus, gastroesophageal mucosal tear (Mallory-Weiss syndrome), malnutrition, and postemetic rupture of the esophagus (Boerhaave's syndrome).

Treatment

Simple acute vomiting such as occurs following dietary or alcoholic indiscretion or during morning sickness of early pregnancy (see p 480) may require little or no treatment. Avoiding known aggravating factors and taking simple corrective dietary measures usually suffice.

Severe or prolonged nausea and vomiting usually require careful medical management in the hospital. Attempt to determine and correct the causes of the vomiting as soon as possible. The vomiting patient should be checked to see if aspiration has occurred. The following general measures may be used as adjuncts to specific medical or surgical treatment:

A. Fluids and Nutrition: Maintain adequate hydration and nutrition, and correct any electrolyte imbalance that may occur. Hypokalemia and metabolic alkalosis are common in patients with severe vomiting. Withhold food temporarily and give intravenously 5% dextrose in saline with appropriate KCl supplementation (see pp 36 and 37). If vomiting continues, employ a nasogastric tube to intermittent suction for gastric decompression. When oral feedings are resumed, begin with dry foods in small quantities, eg, salted crackers, graham crackers. With "morning sickness," these foods may best be taken before arising. Later, change to frequent small feedings of simple palatable foods. Hot beverages (tea and clear broths) and cold beverages (iced tea and carbonated liquids, especially ginger ale) are tolerated quite early. Avoid lukewarm beverages. Always consider the patient's food preferences.

B. Medical Measures: *Note:* All unnecessary medication should be withheld from pregnant women during the critical early phase of fetal development. Unless nausea and vomiting of pregnancy are severe or progressive, avoid using medication for this purpose. The possible teratogenic effects of many classes of drugs are now being investigated.

Antiemetic drugs are usually better for preventing vomiting, but they may be employed selectively if the cause of vomiting cannot be treated effectively. The drugs should be used cautiously to avoid masking the development of serious illness. The choice of drug treatment depends on the reasons for the vomiting, the needs of the patient, and the known pharmacology of the available drugs:

(1) Sedatives, alone or with anticholinergics, may be helpful in patients with psychogenic vomiting.

(2) Antihistamines, eg, dimenhydrinate, 50 mg orally or intramuscularly every 4 hours or 100 mg by

suppository twice daily, may be useful for patients with vestibular disorders (eg, Meniere's syndrome, motion sickness).

(3) Phenothiazines, eg, prochlorperazine, 5–10 mg orally or intramuscularly 3 times daily or 25 mg by suppository twice daily, may be preferred for vomiting caused by drugs, radiation sickness, or surgery.

(4) Metoclopramide, 10 mg orally or intravenously, is particularly helpful for the nausea and vomiting of diabetic gastroparesis and for the prevention of the nausea and vomiting of cancer chemotherapy.

(5) Tetrahydrocannabinol (from marihuana) is currently under investigation as treatment for refractory vomiting induced by cancer chemotherapy.

C. Psychotherapy: Attempt to determine the possible psychic basis of prolonged nausea and vomiting, but avoid aggressive psychotherapy during the acute phase of the illness. Hospitalization and restricted visiting may be necessary. Avoid unpleasant psychic stimuli such as strange odors, foul-smelling or foul-tasting medication, unattractive objects, and foods that are improperly prepared or served.

DiPalma JR: Drugs for nausea and vomiting of pregnancy. *Am Fam Physician* (Oct) 1983;**28**:272.

Malagelada J-R, Camilleri M: Unexplained vomiting: A diagnostic challenge. *Ann Intern Med* 1984;**101**:211.

Stoudemire A, Cotanch P, Laszlo J: Recent advances in the pharmacologic and behaviorial management of chemotherapy-induced emesis. *Arch Intern Med* 1984;**144**:1029.

HICCUP
(Singultus)

Hiccup, although usually transient and benign, may be caused by or associated with a wide range of disorders. Of importance are disease processes just above and below the diaphragm, such as (1) inflammation (pneumonia, esophagitis, subphrenic abscess, pancreatitis); (2) gastric distention; (3) neoplasms; (4) myocardial infarction or pericardial disease; (5) metabolic derangements (azotemia); (6) central nervous system disorders (infection, tumors); and (7) idiopathic disorders. Correction of potentially remediable causes will be most effective in the management of hiccup.

Treatment

Countless measures have been suggested for interrupting the rhythmic reflex that produces hiccup. At times, however, none of these may be successful, and the symptom may be so prolonged and severe as to jeopardize the patient's life.

A. Simple Home Remedies: These measures probably act by diverting the patient's attention; they consist of distracting conversation, fright, painful or unpleasant stimuli, or of having the patient perform such apparently purposeless procedures as breath-holding, sipping ice water, or inhaling strong fumes.

B. Medical Measures:

1. Sedation–Any of the common sedative drugs may be effective, eg, pentobarbital sodium, 0.1 g orally or 0.13 g by rectal suppository.

2. Stimulation of nasopharynx–A soft catheter introduced nasally to stimulate the nasopharynx and pharynx is often successful.

3. Local anesthetics–Viscous lidocaine, 15 mL orally, may be of some use. General anesthesia may be tried in intractable cases.

4. Antispasmodics–Atropine sulfate, 0.3–0.6 mg, may be given subcutaneously.

5. Amyl nitrite inhalations may be effective.

6. CO_2 inhalations–Have the patient rebreathe into a paper bag for 3–5 minutes, or give 10–15% CO_2 mixture by face mask for 3–5 minutes.

7. Tranquilizers–Phenothiazine drugs have been used successfully for prolonged hiccup.

8. Antacids.

C. Surgical Measures: Various phrenic nerve operations, including bilateral phrenicotomy, may be indicated in extreme cases that fail to respond to all other measures and are considered to be a threat to life.

CONSTIPATION

The frequency of defecation and the consistency and volume of stools vary so greatly from individual to individual that it is often difficult to determine what is "normal." Familial, social, and dietary customs may help determine individual differences in bowel habits. Normal bowel movements may range in frequency from 3 to 12 stools per week, and the weights may range from 35 to 235 g of stool per day. The complaint of constipation often reflects the attitude of the patient with respect to the expected pattern of bowel movements. The patient should be considered to be constipated only if defecation is unexplainably delayed for days or if the stools are unusually hard, dry, and difficult to express. Constipation may result from repeatedly ignoring the urge to defecate because of unwillingness to interrupt social, recreational, or occupational activities.

Because there are many specific organic causes of constipation (see below), it is essential to explore such possibilities in patients with unexplained constipation. Be especially suspicious of organic causes when there have been sudden and unaccountable changes in bowel habits, or blood in the stools.

Causes of Constipation

(1) Dietary factors: Highly refined and low-fiber foods, inadequate fluids.

(2) Physical inactivity: Inadequate exercise, prolonged bed rest.

(3) Pregnancy.

(4) Advanced age (often multifactorial).

(5) Drugs: Anesthetics, antacids (aluminum and calcium salts), anticholinergics, anticonvulsants, antidepressants (tricyclics, monoamine oxidase inhibitors), antihypertensives (ganglionic blocking agents), antiparkinsonism drugs, antipsychotic drugs (pheno-

thiazines), beta-adrenergic blocking agents, bismuth salts, diuretics, iron salts, laxatives and cathartics (chronic use), metallic intoxications (arsenic, lead, mercury), muscle relaxants, opiates.

(6) Metabolic abnormalities: Hypokalemia, hyperglycemia, uremia, porphyria, amyloidosis.

(7) Endocrine abnormalities: Hypothyroidism, hypercalcemia, panhypopituitarism, pheochromocytoma, glucagonoma.

(8) Structural abnormalities of the colon, rectum, and anus or functional disorders such as prediverticular disease of the sigmoid colon and diverticulosis coli. Intrinsic or extrinsic inflammation or neoplastic lesions may also be associated with constipation.

(9) Neurogenic abnormalities: Innervation disorders of the bowel wall (aganglionosis, autonomic neuropathy), spinal cord disorders (trauma, multiple sclerosis, tabes dorsalis), disorders of the splanchnic nerves (tumors, trauma), cerebral disorders (strokes, parkinsonism, neoplasm).

(10) Psychogenic disorders.

(11) Enemas (chronic use).

Treatment

The patient should be told that a daily bowel movement is not essential to health or well-being and that many symptoms (eg, lack of "pep") attributed to constipation have no such relationship.

A. Reestablishment of Regular Evacuation: A regular period should be set aside after a meal for a bowel movement, even when the urge to defecate is not present. Cathartics and enemas should not be used for simple constipation, since they interfere with the normal bowel reflexes. If it seems inadvisable to withdraw such measures suddenly from a patient who has employed them for a long time, the milder laxatives and enemas (see below) can be used temporarily. Cathartic and enema "addicts" often defy all medical measures, and treatment is especially difficult when there is a serious underlying psychiatric disturbance.

B. Diet: The diet may be modified to satisfy the following requirements:

1. Adequate volume–Often "constipation" is merely due to inadequate food intake.

2. Adequate bulk or residue–Foods with high fiber content such as bran and raw fruits and vegetables may be helpful.

3. Vegetable irritants–Unless there is a specific contraindication (eg, intolerance), stewed or raw fruits (particularly prunes and figs) or vegetables may be of value, especially in the "atonic" type of constipation.

4. Adequate fluids–The patient should be encouraged to drink adequate quantities of fluids to permit passage of intestinal contents. Six to 8 glasses of fluid per day, in addition to the fluid content of foods, are ordinarily sufficient. A glass of hot water taken one-half hour before breakfast seems to exert a mild laxative effect.

C. Exercise: Moderate physical exercise is essential. Bed patients may require active and passive exercises. Good tone of the external abdominal mus-

cles is important. Corrective physical therapy may be employed in patients with protuberant abdomens.

D. Laxatives: Laxatives may be classified as (1) stimulants (irritants), (2) bulk-forming agents, (3) saline laxatives, (4) wetting agents, and (5) lubricants. They are intended for temporary use on a selective basis by patients with simple constipation. Laxatives should *never* be given to patients with undiagnosed abdominal pain or when there is a possibility of intestinal obstruction or fecal impaction. Prolonged use of laxatives is seldom justified unless definitive therapy for specific disease is not possible. Chronic laxative use interferes with normal bowel motility and reflexes, thereby setting up a pattern for persistent constipation. Habitual use may also result in damage to the myenteric plexus of the colon and rectum. Melanosis coli may occur with certain laxatives but is probably not functionally important. Compulsive laxative use often defies all medical measures, and treatment is especially difficult when there are serious underlying psychiatric disturbances. There are no advantages—and there may be serious disadvantages—to mixing various laxatives.

1. Stimulant (irritant) laxatives–

a. Docusate sodium (eg, Colace, Doxinate), 50–350 mg/d. This agent interferes with sodium resorption in the colon, leading to increased water content in stool. Docusate sodium is also an "irritant" that produces mucosal changes in the small bowel, but the effect of this action on stool character or frequency is unclear.

b. Cascara sagrada aromatic fluid extract, a mild agent; 4–8 mL acts within 6–12 hours.

c. Bisacodyl (Dulcolax, etc), a mild to moderate laxative that stimulates sensory nerve endings of the colon to produce parasympathetic reflexes; 10–15 mg acts within 6 hours. Efficacious in suppository form as well; particularly useful in patients with spinal cord injury.

d. Phenolphthalein, a potent over-the-counter laxative; 30–240 mg acts within 4–6 hours.

e. Glycerin suppository, an agent for lubricating hard fecal material and stimulating the rectocolic reflex; 3 g acts within 30 minutes.

2. Bulk-forming agents–

a. Psyllium hydrophilic mucilloid (Metamucil), more than 14 g (1–2 rounded teaspoonfuls), 2–3 times daily after meals in a full glass of water, is probably one of the least harmful mild laxatives when administered with an adequate or high fluid intake. It is particularly useful in elderly patients and in those with irritable colon syndrome.

b. Unprocessed bran, one-fourth cup daily with cereal or in unsweetened applesauce.

3. Osmotic laxatives–

a. Milk of magnesia (magnesium hydroxide), 15–30 mL at bedtime, is a common mild-to-moderate generically available laxative. It should not be used by patients with impaired renal function.

b. Citrate of magnesia, 120–240 mL. Avoid use for patients with renal impairment.

c. Sodium phosphate, 4–8 g in hot water before breakfast.

d. Lactulose syrup, 15–60 mL daily.

4. Wetting agents–Docusate sodium is a detergent; see ¶ 1(a) above.

5. Lubricants–Liquid petrolatum (mineral oil), 15–30 mL per rectum, may help soften stool. Administration orally should be avoided because of risk of aspiration with resulting lipid pneumonia, and because petrolatum may interfere with intestinal absorption of fat-soluble vitamins.

E. Enemas: Because they interfere with restoration of a normal bowel reflex, enemas should ordinarily be used only as a temporary expedient in chronic constipation or fecal impaction. Infrequently, it may be necessary to administer enemas for prolonged periods.

1. Saline enema (nonirritating)–Warm physiologic saline solution, 500–2000 mL.

2. Warm tap water (irritating)–500–1000 mL.

3. Soapsuds (SS) enema (irritating)–75 mL of soap solution per liter of water.

4. Oil retention enema–180 mL of mineral oil or vegetable oil instilled in the rectum in the evening, retained overnight, and evacuated the next morning.

Elliot DL, Watts WJ, Girard DE: Constipation: Mechanisms and management of a common clinical problem. *Postgrad Med* (Aug) 1983;**74**:143.

Graham DY, Moser SE, Estes MK: The effect of bran on bowel function in constipation. *Am J Gastroenterol* 1982;**77**:599.

FECAL IMPACTION

Hardened or puttylike stools in the rectum or colon may interfere with the normal passage of feces; if the impaction is not removed manually, by enemas, or by surgery, it can cause partial or complete intestinal obstruction. The impaction may be due to organic causes (painful anorectal disease, tumor, or neurogenic disease of the colon) or to functional causes (bulk laxatives, antacids, residual barium from x-ray study, low-residue diet, starvation, drug-induced colonic stasis, or prolonged bed rest and debility). The patient may give a history of obstipation, but more frequently there is a history of watery diarrhea. There may be blood or mucus in the stool. Physical examination may reveal a distended abdomen, palpable "tumors" in the abdomen, and a firm stool in the rectum. The impaction may be broken up digitally or dislodged with a sigmoidoscope. Cleansing enemas (preferably in the knee-chest position) or, in the case of impaction higher in the colon, colonic irrigations may be of value. Daily oil retention enemas followed by digital fragmentation of the impaction and saline enemas may be necessary.

Bustin MP, Iber F: Management of common nonmalignant GI problems in the elderly. *Geriatrics* (March) 1983;**38**:69.

GASTROINTESTINAL GAS

The amount of gastrointestinal gas varies considerably from individual to individual. Subjective estimates by patients may be at considerable variance from observed findings. Five gases—nitrogen and oxygen from swallowed air, and carbon dioxide, hydrogen, and methane produced in the gut—constitute more than 99% of gastrointestinal gas. Excessive belching or eructation is usually due to air swallowed during eating or drinking, or it may be due to a nervous habit of sucking in air; the latter may be severe.

Excessive passage of flatus per rectum is due largely to gases formed by bacterial fermentation of malabsorbed carbohydrates and cellulose in the intestine. Rectal gas consists predominantly of H_2, CO_2, CH_4—all odorless; there is little objective information on the malodorous gases. Many problems of abdominal bloating or distention with pain appear to be caused by disordered bowel motility rather than by excessive gas. Since excessive gastrointestinal gas may be due to both functional and organic disease, complaints of unusual belching, bloating, and flatulence may require search for specific causes.

Treatment

A. Specific Treatment: Eliminate specific causes, if known.

B. Correction of Aerophagia: Anxiety states are often associated with deep breathing and sighing and consequent swallowing of considerable quantities of air. When possible, treat underlying anxiety.

C. Correction of Physical Defects: These sometimes interfere with normal swallowing or breathing: (1) Structural deformities of the nose and nasopharynx, eg, nasal obstruction and adenoids. (2) Spatial defects of the teeth or ill-fitting dentures.

D. Good Hygiene and Eating Habits: Instruct the patient to avoid dietary indiscretions, eating too rapidly and too much, eating while under emotional strain, drinking large quantities of liquids with meals, taking laxatives, and chewing gum.

E. Diet: The diet should be nutritious as tolerated and enjoyed by the patient, but eliminate foods that may lead to excessive flatulence in susceptible individuals. (See p 803.)

F. Medications: Drugs (including charcoal, simethicone, and antiflatulence tablets) are generally unsatisfactory and at times are only of placebo value. Anticholinergic-sedative drugs serve to diminish the flow of saliva (which is often excessive in some patients), thereby reducing the aerophagia that accompanies swallowing; bowel motility is reduced.

Levitt MD: Gastrointestinal gas and abdominal symptoms. (Part 2.) *Practical Gastroenterol* (Jan/Feb) 1984;**8**:6.

Levitt MD: Intestinal gas production: Recent advances in flatology. *N Engl J Med* 1980;**302**:1474.

DIARRHEA

Diarrhea is defined as an increase in the frequency, fluidity, and volume of bowel movements. Normal bowel function varies from individual to individual, and the definition of diarrhea must take this variation into account. Factors influencing stool consistency are poorly understood; water content is not the sole determinant. Thus, the definition of diarrhea in a clinical sense is an increase in frequency or increased fluidity of bowel movements in a given individual. In pathophysiologic terms, diarrhea results from the passage of stools containing excess water, ie, from malabsorption or secretion of water. Although daily stool weight or water is probably the best single index to diarrhea, "small-volume diarrhea" with frequent evacuations of blood, mucus, or exudate is a syndrome often signifying disease of the distal colon.

Pathophysiology

A. Types of Diarrhea:

1. With excess fecal water–

a. Osmotic diarrhea–Excess water-soluble molecules in the bowel lumen cause osmotic retention of intraluminal water.

b. Secretory diarrhea–Excessive active ion secretion by the mucosal cells of the intestine.

c. Deletion or interference with normal ion absorption–This is usually a congenital problem.

d. Exudative disease–Abnormal mucosal permeability, with intestinal loss of serum proteins, blood, mucus, or pus.

e. Impaired contact between intestinal chyme and absorbing surface–Rapid transit, short bowel syndromes.

2. Without excess fecal water–Frequent small, painful evacuations are usually a result of disease of the left colon or rectum.

B. Causes of Diarrhea: Most diarrheal states are self-limited and pose no special diagnostic problem. They are often due to dietary indiscretions or mild gastrointestinal infections. The following list of the causes of diarrhea is indicative of the extensive diagnostic evaluation that may be required in patients with unexplained, profound, or chronic diarrhea.

1. Psychogenic disorders–"Nervous" diarrhea.

2. Intestinal infections:

a. Viral infections–Enterovirus, rotavirus.

b. Bacterial infections–Most common are *Campylobacter jejuni, Shigella, Salmonella,* and *Yersinia enterocolitica.*

c. Bacterial toxins–*Clostridium difficile,* pathogenic *Escherichia coli, Staphylococcus, Vibrio parahaemolyticus,* and *Vibrio cholerae.*

3. Parasitic infections–*Giardia lamblia, Entamoeba histolytica, Cryptosporidium,* and *Isospora* are the most common.

4. Other intestinal factors–Fecal impaction, antibiotic therapy, inflammatory bowel disease, catharsis habituation, vagotomy, carcinoma, heavy metal poisoning, and gastrocolic fistula (see Table 24–1).

5. Cholestatic syndromes–Hepatitis and bile duct obstruction may result in steatorrhea and mild diarrhea.

6. Malabsorption states–Primary small bowel mucosal diseases (eg, celiac sprue), short small bowel states, and intestinal blind loop syndrome (eg, diverticula, afferent loop).

7. Pancreatic disease–Pancreatic insufficiency, pancreatic endocrine tumors.

8. Reflex from other viscera–Pelvic disease (extrinsic to gastrointestinal tract).

9. Neurologic disease–Tabes dorsalis, diabetic neuropathy.

10. Metabolic disease–Hyperthyroidism.

11. Immunodeficiency disease–IgA deficiency.

12. Malnutrition–Marasmus, kwashiorkor.

13. Food allergy.

14. Dietary factors–Excessive fresh fruit intake.

15. Factitious–Surreptitious laxative ingestion.

16. Unknown.

Diagnosis

Specific diagnosis is based on careful examination of diarrheal material for polymorphonuclear cells and bacteria and, if indicated, for parasites. This is best accomplished at sigmoidoscopy prior to preparation with a cleansing enema. Cotton swabs should not be used in making slides, as both polymorphonuclear cells and parasites cling to cotton. The presence of polymorphonuclear cells indicates an inflammatory process. Rectal biopsy may prove helpful, particularly when *Entamoeba histolytica* is being considered and there is colitis. These studies should be performed prior to barium studies and treatment.

Treatment

Culture for bacterial pathogens and examination of several stools for polymorphonuclear cells and parasites must be done before barium studies or treatment is begun. Treat specific diseases whenever possible.

A. Correct Physiologic Changes Induced by Diarrhea:

1. Acid-base disturbance, fluid loss.

2. Electrolyte depletion (hyponatremia, hypokalemia, hypocalcemia, hypomagnesemia).

3. Malnutrition, vitamin deficiencies.

4. Psychogenic disturbances (eg, fixation on gastrointestinal tract or anxiety regarding incontinence in cases of long-standing diarrhea).

B. Diet:

1. Acute severe–Food should be withheld for the first 24 hours or restricted to clear liquids—a physiologic glucose and salt solution, sipped slowly as needed to replace large fluid and electrolyte losses, may be especially useful in patients with severe watery diarrhea. Frequent small soft feedings are added as tolerated. Milk and milk products are the last foods to be added, since lactase deficiency frequently is present after an "insult" to the small intestine.

2. Convalescent–Food should be incorporated into the diets of patients convalescing from acute diarrhea as tolerated. Nutritious food, preferably all cooked, in small frequent meals, is usually well tolerated. *Avoid* raw vegetables and fruits, fried foods, bran, whole grain cereals, preserves, syrups, candies, pickles, relishes, spices, coffee, and alcoholic beverages.

A diet free of milk and milk products and with no uncooked foods is a restricted diet. These patients may require vitamin supplements if the diet is prolonged.

3. Chronic diarrhea–Chronic diarrhea is due to many causes. Nutritional disturbances range from none to marked depletion of electrolytes, water, protein, fat, and vitamins. Treat specific disease when known (eg, gluten-free diet in celiac sprue and enzyme replacement in pancreatic insufficiency). Give fat-soluble vitamins (vitamins A, D, E, K) when steatorrhea is present. Some patients are so ill that they require parenteral hyperalimentation, sometimes at home.

C. Antidiarrheal Agents:

1. Pepto-Bismol–Give 30 mL 3–6 times per day for symptomatic treatment of diarrhea.

2. Narcotic analogs–Avoid with possible acute infectious diarrhea, as they may worsen and prolong the course.

a. Lomotil (diphenoxylate with atropine), 2.5 mg 3–4 times daily as needed. It must be used cautiously in patients with advanced liver disease and in those who are addiction-prone or who are taking sedatives.

b. Loperamide (Imodium), 2 mg 2–4 times daily, is effective in acute and chronic diarrhea.

3. Narcotics–Narcotics must be avoided in chronic diarrheas and are preferably avoided in acute diarrheas unless there is intractable diarrhea, vomiting, and colic. Always exclude the possibility of acute surgical abdominal disease before administering opiates. Give any of the following:

a. Paregoric, 4–8 mL after liquid movements as needed or with bismuth.

b. Codeine phosphate, 15–65 mg subcutaneously, if the patient is vomiting, after liquid bowel movements as needed.

c. Strong opiates–Morphine should be reserved for selected patients with severe acute diarrhea who fail to respond to more conservative measures.

4. Anticholinergic drugs, particularly when used in combination with sedatives, exert a mild antiperistaltic action in acute and chronic diarrheas associated with anxiety tension states. It may be necessary to administer the various drugs to a point near toxicity in order to achieve the desired effect.

Antidiarrheal drugs must be used with great caution in inflammatory bowel disease and amebiasis because of the risk of "toxic" dilatation of the colon. Unless diarrhea is severe, they should be avoided in bacillary dysentery, since they prolong the carrier state.

D. Psychotherapy: Many cases of chronic diar-

rhea are of psychogenic origin. A survey of anxiety-producing mechanisms should be made in all patients with this complaint. Antidepressant drug therapy may be useful, particularly since many of these agents have an anticholinergic effect.

Blaser MJ et al: *Campylobacter* enteritis in the United States: A multicenter study. *Ann Intern Med* 1983;**98:**360.

Fordtran JS: Diarrhea. In: *Gastrointestinal Disease,* 3rd ed. Sleisinger MH, Fordtran JS (editors). Saunders, 1983.

Gorbach SL: Traveler's diarrhea. (Editorial.) *N Engl J Med* 1982;**307:**881.

Kaplan JE et al: Epidemiology of Norwalk gastroenteritis and the role of Norwalk virus in outbreaks of acute nonbacterial gastroenteritis. *Ann Intern Med* 1982;**96:**756.

Read NW et al: Chronic diarrhea of unknown origin. *Gastroenterology* 1980;**78:**264.

MASSIVE UPPER GASTROINTESTINAL HEMORRHAGE

Massive upper gastrointestinal hemorrhage is a common emergency. It may be defined as rapid loss of sufficient blood to cause hypovolemic shock. The actual volume of blood loss required to produce shock varies with the size, age, and general condition of the patient and with the rapidity of bleeding. Sudden loss of 20% or more of blood volume (blood volume is approximately 75 mL/kg of body weight) produces hypotension, tachycardia, and other signs of shock. For example, a previously well 70-kg man who develops shock as a result of gastrointestinal hemorrhage will have lost at least 1000–1500 mL of blood. The immediate objectives of management are (1) to restore an effective blood volume and (2) to establish a diagnosis on which definitive treatment can be based.

The major causes of upper gastrointestinal bleeding are peptic ulceration of the duodenum, stomach, or esophagus, esophageal varices, and gastritis. In addition, bleeding may be due to Mallory-Weiss syndrome, hemorrhagic gastritis due to ulcerogenic drugs such as aspirin, or alcohol.

Clinical Findings

A. Symptoms and Signs: There is usually a history of sudden weakness or fainting associated with or followed by tarry stools or vomiting of blood. Melena occurs in all patients and hematemesis in over half. Hematemesis is especially common in esophageal varices (90%), gastritis, and gastric ulcer. The patient may or may not be in shock when first seen but will at least be pale and weak if major blood loss has occurred. If the patient is not vomiting, a stomach tube will often help determine if the bleeding is in the upper gastrointestinal tract. There may be a history of peptic ulcer, chronic liver disease, other predisposing disease, alcoholic excess, or severe vomiting.

There is usually no pain, and the pain of peptic ulcer disease often stops with the onset of bleeding.

Abdominal findings are not remarkable except when hepatomegaly, splenomegaly, or a mass (neoplasm) is present. Bowel sounds may be increased due to blood in the gut.

The cause of bleeding should be established as promptly as possible, since management will in part be dependent on the findings. This is particularly true if emergency surgery is anticipated, so that surgical approach and type of procedure can be determined.

A history of peptic ulcer or of antacid ingestion suggests duodenal ulcer. Ingestion of aspirin or other nonsteroidal anti-inflammatory agents on a regular or intermittent basis suggests gastric ulcer or hemorrhagic erosive gastritis. A history of alcoholism or evidence of chronic liver disease, such as jaundice, hepatosplenomegaly, spider angioma, liver palms, ascites, or encephalopathy, indicates probable portal hypertension with variceal bleeding. Aspiration of gastric contents by nasogastric tube is diagnostically useful and permits estimation of the continued rate of bleeding.

The principal diagnostic procedures that should be carried out after necessary emergency treatment has been given are outlined below.

B. Laboratory Findings: In addition to the baseline studies of a complete blood count, urinalysis, and serum electrolyte and creatinine measurements, the following may prove helpful in selected patients.

1. Liver tests–Serum bilirubin, transaminase, albumin/globulin, alkaline phosphatase, and prothrombin time may help support a diagnosis of chronic liver disease (portal hypertension).

2. Coagulation studies–In addition to the prothrombin time, other tests may sometimes be indicated. Determine bleeding time in cases of suspected ingestion of aspirin or nonsteroidal anti-inflammatory agents or of azotemia; a platelet count when platelets are low on the complete blood count; and a partial thromboplastin time when there is a history of excessive dental, gynecologic, or other bleeding.

C. Endoscopy: Fiberoptic oral panendoscopy should be the first definitive examination performed if an experienced endoscopist is available. This procedure permits visualization of the upper gastrointestinal tract from the cricopharyngeus to the second or third portion of the duodenum and can identify mucosal lesions not readily seen by other techniques. Sometimes, sclerosis of bleeding esophageal varices or other treatment can be accomplished during panendoscopy. When it is unclear that bleeding is from the upper gastrointestinal tract, sigmoidoscopy should be the first diagnostic procedure.

D. X-Ray Findings: The cause of upper gastrointestinal bleeding can be demonstrated on x-ray in up to 75% of cases. If upper gastrointestinal endoscopy does not reveal the bleeding site, selective angiography should be considered if the bleeding persists. Arteriography may not be successful if the bleeding is less than 1 mL/min.

If angiography fails to demonstrate the site of bleeding, then an upper gastrointestinal series is done.

The patient's vital signs should be monitored during the procedure.

Treatment

A. General Measures: The patient should be under the observation of both the primary care physician and a surgeon from the outset. Bed rest and charting of fluid intake, urine output, and temperature are ordered. Insert a large-bore nasogastric tube to verify the source of hemorrhage and to remove gastric contents (see below). If bleeding continues or if tachycardia or hypotension is present, monitor and treat the patient for shock (see Chapter 1). Insert a Foley catheter and a central venous pressure or pulmonary artery wedge pressure line. Blood is obtained immediately for complete blood count, hematocrit, and cross-matching of at least 3 or 4 units of packed red blood cells. In interpreting the hematocrit, it should be kept in mind that after acute blood loss, a period of 24–36 hours may be required for reequilibration of body fluids. Meanwhile, the hematocrit poorly reflects extent of blood loss. Frequent determination of vital signs, especially those associated with postural changes, is helpful in estimating acute blood loss. Replacement therapy through a large-bore intravenous needle (18-gauge minimum) or catheter is started immediately with normal saline. If shock is severe or if the patient has portal hypertension, fresh frozen plasma is given while a blood transfusion is being prepared.

Aqueous vasopressin (Pitressin), 20 units in 200–250 mL of 5% glucose in water intravenously over a 30- to 40-minute period, may cause temporary arteriolar vasoconstriction and lowering of the portal venous pressure for variceal bleeding. Infusion of vasopressin through the angiographic catheter may be effective in controlling hemorrhage, if the bleeding is from small vessels. The entire matter of using vasopressin therapy to control hemorrhage is unclear at present. (See Fogel reference below.)

Water-soluble vitamin K (menadiol sodium diphosphate [Synkayvite]), 5–10 mg intramuscularly, is given empirically if hepatobiliary disease is suspected. Restlessness may be due to continued hemorrhage, shock, or hypoxia.

B. Blood Replacement: Treatment of shock by transfusion with blood cells or fresh frozen plasma (or both) is begun without delay. Hematocrit determinations are done every few hours until they are stabilized. The objective of blood replacement is to relieve shock and restore blood volume. The amount of blood required is estimated on the basis of vital signs, measured loss, central venous pressure, and renal perfusion as measured by urine output, usually with the aim of a minimum hematocrit of 30%. While a patient is actively bleeding, at least 6 units of packed red blood cells and fresh frozen plasma should be available for emergency transfusion; rapid administration will control shock. When blood pressure and pulse have been restored to relatively normal levels and clinical signs of hypovolemia are no longer present, the rate of transfusion can be slowed. The total volume of blood given is determined by the course of the disease. A poor response usually means continued bleeding (see below) or inadequate replacement. Venous pressure or pulmonary artery wedge pressure is useful in gauging adequacy of blood replacement and detecting overtransfusion and congestive heart failure in the clinically fragile patient.

C. Medical Measures: Acid peptic digestion is a causative or aggravating factor in many cases of massive upper gastrointestinal hemorrhage, perhaps including varices. Feedings and oral medications for ulcer are begun as soon as shock and nausea have subsided. Continued slight bleeding is not a contraindication for the following regimen:

1. Diet–Liquid diet for the first 24 hours, followed by a soft or regular diet, depending on the clinical situation.

2. Acid reduction–While a nasogastric tube is still in place, antacids such as aluminum hydroxide-magnesium hydroxide mixtures can be administered hourly by mouth in a dose of 30 mL to protect the distal esophagus from reflux and to help neutralize gastric contents not suctioned by the tube. In the fasting patient, cimetidine, 300 mg intravenously every 6 hours, reduces acid output, although it does not affect the rate of recurrent bleeding. For the nonfasting patient with ulcer disease, the H_2 receptor antagonists (cimetidine, ranitidine), antacids, and sucralfate are equally efficacious in inducing healing. Therapeutic doses of antacids, 1 and 3 hours after meals and at bedtime, may cause diarrhea.

3. Mild sedation.

4. A nasogastric tube may be useful to permit continued decompression of the stomach and evacuation of blood by lavage with saline. The tube is also useful to monitor the rate of continued bleeding. Whenever the tube is placed, the patient should be in a moderate reversed Trendelenberg position, if possible, to minimize reflux around the tube. See above concerning antacid use.

D. Management of Bleeding Esophageal Varices: When varices are the cause of bleeding, special measures are indicated (see p 414).

E. Indications for Emergency Operation: Emergency surgery to stop active bleeding should be considered under any of the following circumstances: (1) When the patient has received 3 L or more of blood but shock is not controlled or recurs promptly. (2) When acceptable blood pressure and hematocrit cannot be maintained with a maximum of 500 mL of blood every 8 hours. (3) When bleeding is slow but persists more than 2–3 days. (4) When bleeding stops initially but recurs while the patient is receiving adequate medical treatment. (5) When the patient is over age 50. The death rate from exsanguination in spite of conservative measures is greater in the older age group.

Some patients have visible vessels on endoscopy. About half of these patients will have uncontrolled or recurrent bleeding and are therefore candidates for urgent surgery.

Prognosis

The overall mortality rate of about 14% indicates the seriousness of massive upper gastrointestinal hemorrhage. Fatality rates vary greatly, depending upon the cause of bleeding and the presence of other serious systemic disease. The overall operative mortality rate for emergency surgery to stop bleeding is high, and best results are obtained when bleeding can be controlled medically and surgery deferred until the patient has recovered from the effects of bleeding. Hemorrhage from duodenal ulcer causes death in about 3% of treated cases, whereas in bleeding varices the mortality rate may be as high as 50%.

Baker D et al: Cimetidine and tranexamic acid in the treatment of acute upper-gastrointestinal tract bleeding. *N Engl J Med* 1983;**308:**1571.

Fogel MR et al: Continuous intravenous vasopressin in active upper gastrointestinal bleeding. *Ann Intern Med* 1982;**95:**565.

Roth HP: Proceedings of the NIH consensus workshop. 1. Potential benefits of diagnostic endoscopy. 2. Potential benefits of therapeutic endoscopy. 3. Risks and complications of gastrointestinal endoscopy. 4. Other diagnostic approaches to the bleeding patient. 5. Epidemiology, cost effectiveness, future studies. *Dig Dis Sci* 1981;**26(Suppl).** [Entire issue.]

Zucherman G et al: Controlled trial of medical therapy for active upper gastrointestinal bleeding and prevention of rebleeding. *Am J Med* 1984;**76:**361.

MASSIVE LOWER GASTROINTESTINAL HEMORRHAGE

Massive lower gastrointestinal bleeding occurs most frequently in older, poor-risk patients and is always a *medical emergency*. Colonic diverticulosis and angiodysplasia (acquired arteriovenous malformation) are the most common causes of hemodynamically significant lower gastrointestinal bleeding, but other possibilities—including massive upper gastrointestinal hemorrhage—must be considered (see below).

Causes of Massive Lower Abdominal Hemorrhage

A. Colonic Disorders:

1. Inflammatory–Ulcerative colitis, regional enteritis, infectious diarrhea (eg, shigellosis), radiation colitis.

2. Diverticular–Diverticulosis.

3. Vascular–Hemorrhoids, angiodysplasia (vascular ectasia), bowel ischemia, colonic varices, aortic aneurysm.

4. Neoplastic–Benign and malignant disorders.

5. Hereditary–Telangiectasias, arteriovenous malformations.

6. Coagulopathies–Anticoagulant drugs, blood dyscrasias.

B. Upper Gastrointestinal Disorders:

1. Vascular–Esophageal varices, telangiectasias.

2. Ulcerative–Peptic ulceration.

3. Neoplastic–Benign and malignant disorders.

Management of Hemorrhage

The patient usually has a sudden onset of weakness and fainting, combined with or followed by passage of grossly bloody stools (which may be either bright red or dark red according to the time elapsed since the beginning of the hemorrhage). There may be a history and physical findings of one or more of the disorders listed above. The patient may appear pale and weak and may rapidly develop signs of shock.

If rectal bleeding is copious or if there is evidence of shock, the patient should be resuscitated with intravenous fluids and blood products before and during the diagnostic evaluation. Colonic bleeding stops spontaneously in about 75% of patients treated with bed rest and simple resuscitative measures.

A nasogastric tube should be inserted to rule out upper gastrointestinal bleeding (see above). However, unless bile is aspirated via this tube, one cannot be certain that bleeding is not duodenal in origin. Rectal examination and anosigmoidoscopy may identify bleeding lesions of the anorectal region as well as of the sigmoid mucosa. Lesions may require biopsy so that appropriate therapy can be instituted.

If several blood transfusions are necessary, further definitive diagnostic study is warranted. Radionuclide localization of shed technetium Tc 99m–labeled red cells is proving to be helpful in localizing lower gastrointestinal bleeding. Colonoscopy may sometimes be useful for identifying and fulgurating bleeding sites. Selective mesenteric angiography can often demonstrate and localize the site of hemorrhage in patients who are actively bleeding. Once the bleeding site is identified, selective intra-arterial infusion of vasopressin into the affected portion may control the bleeding, at least temporarily, in 75–80% of cases. If no bleeding site can be determined, laparotomy and appropriate surgical treatment are required.

Bar AH et al: Angiography in the management of massive lower gastrointestinal tract hemorrhage. *Surg Gynecol Obstet* 1980; **150**:226.

Richter JM et al: Angiodysplasia: Clinical presentation and colonoscopic diagnosis. *Dig Dis Sci* 1984;**29**:481.

Smith GW: Lower GI bleeding in the elderly. *Postgrad Med* (March) 1981;**69**:36.

Winzelberg GG et al: Radionuclide localization of lower gastrointestinal hemorrhage. *Radiology* 1981;**139**:465.

DISEASES
OF THE MOUTH

DISCOLORED TEETH

The most common causes of discolored teeth are food stains, bacteria, tobacco use, and drugs. These can be managed by altering habits and by dental prophylaxis. There may be pulpal hemorrhage induced by trauma, resulting in a deposition of hemosiderin on the internal crown surface. This causes a darkening of the tooth, which usually remains sterile and asymptomatic but nonvital. These teeth can be effectively bleached for aesthetic reasons. Occasionally, however, discoloration is due to changes in tooth structure caused by tetracyclines, congenital defects of enamel or dentin, fluorosis, and erythroblastosis fetalis.

Tetracycline discoloration occurs in some patients when these antibiotics (tetracycline, oxytetracycline, chlortetracycline, and demeclocycline) are given by mouth during the period of tooth development (infancy and childhood). Since an entire layer of dentin may be calcified in a few days, a small dosage over a short period may be incorporated into and appear to involve an entire tooth. The discoloration is gray-brown or yellow-brown. A typical yellow fluorescence is seen under ultraviolet light in undecalcified sections.

Dental fluorosis occurs most frequently when the fluoride in the water supply exceeds 2 ppm (1 ppm is the recommended concentration). Fluorosis can also be caused when the daily ingestion of fluoride-vitamin combinations exceeds the recommended levels (maximum of 1 mg of fluoride). The frequency and intensity of the discoloration are proportionate to the concentration in the water and the amount consumed during tooth development. The discoloration can vary from chalky-white to yellow-brown stains, often irregular in appearance. These teeth can be effectively bleached as required with 30% hydrogen peroxide (Superoxol).

Rare hereditary congenital defects may cause brownish discoloration of the teeth. Treatment is primarily for aesthetic reasons.

Black JB: Esthetic restoration of tetracycline-stained teeth. *J Am Dent Assoc* 1982;**104**:846.

ABSCESSES OF THE TEETH
(Periapical Abscess)

Dental decay is not self-limiting; unless it is removed, it will lead to infection of the pulp and subsequent periapical abscess. Death of the pulp and periapical infection may also result from physical and chemical trauma. The only treatment is root canal therapy (cleansing and filling of the entire canal) or extraction.

In the early stage of pulp infection, the symptoms may not be localized to the infected tooth. Intermittent throbbing pain is usually present and is intensified by local temperature change. In the later putrescent stage, the pain is extreme and continuous and may be accentuated by heat but is often relieved by cold. After the infection reaches the bone, the typical syndrome is localization, pain upon pressure, and looseness of the tooth. Symptoms may then disappear completely, and, if drainage occurs, a parulis (gumboil) may be the only finding. When drainage is inadequate, swelling, pain, lymphadenopathy, and fever are often present. At this stage, antibiotics are advisable before local therapy is undertaken. Diagnosis depends upon symptoms, pulp testing (hot, cold, electricity), percussion, x-rays (may not show the diagnostic periapical radiolucency), looseness, deep decay or fillings, parulis, and swelling. Rule out sinusitis, neuralgia, and diseases affecting the cervical lymph nodes.

Incision and drainage are indicated whenever possible. Antibiotics and analgesics may be given as necessary. Unless contraindicated from a history of hypersensitivity, penicillin is the antibiotic of choice. Do not use antibiotic troches.

If not eventually treated by root canal therapy or extraction, the abscess may develop into a more extensive osteomyelitis or cellulitis (or both) or may eventually become cystic, expand, and slowly destroy bone without causing pain.

VINCENT'S INFECTION
(Necrotizing Ulcerating Gingivitis, Trench Mouth)

Vincent's infection is an acute inflammatory disease of the gums that may be accompanied by pain, bleeding, fever, and lymphadenopathy. The cause is not known, and it is doubtful if the disease is communicable. It may occur as a response to many factors, such as poor mouth hygiene, inadequate diet and sleep, alcoholism, and various other diseases such as infectious mononucleosis, nonspecific viral infections, bacterial infections, thrush, blood dyscrasias, and diabetes mellitus. The presence of fusiform and spiral organisms is of no importance, since they occur in about one-third of clinically normal mouths and are absent in some cases of Vincent's infection.

Management depends upon ruling out underlying systemic factors and treating the signs and symptoms as indicated with systemic antibiotics, oxygenating mouth rinses (3% hydrogen peroxide in an equal volume of warm water), analgesics, rest, and appropriate dietary measures. Refer the patient to a dentist for further treatment (eg, curettage).

PERIODONTAL DISEASE

Periodontal disease is related to accumulations of microorganisms and substrate (plaque) on tooth surfaces. These may calcify and be recognized as calculus. Food, bacteria, and calculi that are present between the gums and teeth in areas called "dental pockets" may cause an inflammatory process and the formation of pus (pyorrhea) with or without discomfort or other symptoms. If this continues unchecked, the involved teeth will become loose and eventually will be lost as a result of resorption of supporting alveolar bone. If there is no drainage, accumulation of pus will lead to acute swelling and pain (lateral abscess).

The diagnosis depends upon a combination of findings, including localized pain, loose teeth, dental pockets, erythema, and swelling or suppuration. X-ray may reveal destruction of alveolar bone.

As in periapical abscess, the severity of signs and symptoms will determine the advisability of antibiotics. Local drainage and oxygenating mouth rinses (3% hydrogen peroxide in an equal volume of warm water) will usually reverse the acute symptoms and allow for routine follow-up procedures. Curettage or gingivectomy (or both) to reduce excess gum tissue helps prevent formation of the "dental pockets" that predispose to acute periodontal infections. In some cases, because of the advanced nature of the lesion (bone loss) or the position of the tooth (third molars in particular), extraction is indicated.

In some cases, periodontal disease occurs even in the presence of good hygiene and without obvious cause. Programs of regular dental care (periodic curettage and gingival or bone procedures) and home care (brushing, flossing, and rinsing) to remove dental plaque will at least slow alveolar bone destruction.

Murphy NC, Newman MG: Update and commentary on periodontics: Applying recent discoveries to your practice. *J Calif Dent Assoc* 1981;**9**:41.

Weeks DB: Tetracycline in the treatment of periodontal disease: Review of current literature. *J Am Dent Assoc* 1980;**101**:935.

APHTHOUS ULCER
(Canker Sore, Ulcerative Stomatitis)

An aphthous ulcer is a shallow mucosal ulcer with flat, fairly even borders surrounded by erythema. The ulcer is often covered with a pseudomembrane. It has never been adequately demonstrated that this lesion is due to a virus or any other specific chemical, physical, or microbial agent. One or more ulcers may be present, and they tend to be recurrent. They are often painful. Nuts, chocolates, and irritants such as citrus fruits often cause flare-ups of aphthous ulceration, but abstinence will not prevent recurrence. Aphthous ulcers may be associated with inflammatory bowel disease, Behçet's syndrome, infectious mononucleosis, and prolonged fever. The diagnosis depends mainly upon ruling out similar but more readily identifiable disease, a history of recurrence, and inspection of the ulcer.

Bland mouth rinses and hydrocortisone-antibiotic ointments reduce pain and encourage healing. Hydrocortisone in an adhesive base (Orabase) has been particularly useful. Sedatives and analgesics may be of help. Vaccines and gamma globulins have not proved significantly beneficial. Although caustics relieve pain by cauterizing the fine nerve endings, they also cause necrosis and scar tissue. Systemic antibiotics are contraindicated. Systemic corticosteroids in high doses for a short period of time may be very helpful for severe debilitating recurrent attacks.

Healing, which usually occurs in 1–3 weeks, may be only slightly accelerated by treatment. Occasionally, aphthous ulcers take the form of periadenitis, in which they are larger, persist sometimes for months, and may leave a scar. This form can be confused with carcinoma.

Ulcerative stomatitis is a general term for multiple ulcerations on an inflamed oral mucosa. It may be secondary to blood dyscrasias, erythema multiforme (allergies), bullous lichen planus, acute herpes simplex infection, pemphigoid, pemphigus, and drug reactions. If the lesions cannot be classified, they are referred to as aphthae.

Olson JA, Greenspan JS, Silverman S Jr: Recurrent aphthous ulcerations. *J Calif Dent Assoc* 1982;**10**:53.

HERPETIC STOMATITIS

Herpetic infections of the mouth can be primary (one episode) or secondary (recurrent attacks).

Primary gingivostomatitis due to herpesvirus hominis type 1 occurs in about 90% of the population before age 10. The disease has diverse manifestations, ranging from mild, almost unrecognizable signs and symptoms to multiple intraoral and lip ulcerations, erythema, edema, fever, cervical lymphadenopathy, and malaise. The course of the illness usually entails an increase in signs and symptoms for 1 week and then 1 week of progressive improvement as antibodies are produced (serum antibody titers will increase at least 4-fold). Adults who have never been infected or who have not developed adequate immunity may develop similar disease. Increasing susceptibility is seen in patients on immunosuppressive drugs. Infection with herpesvirus confers permanent immunity.

Herpetic gingivostomatitis must be differentiated from aphthous stomatitis, which is not due to a virus. The diagnosis is established by the history (no prior attack and short duration), characteristic signs and symptoms, and a confirmatory cytologic smear (pathognomonic pseudogiant cells). Direct cultures for herpes simplex virus are positive but impractical.

There is no evidence that the disease is contagious; however, this might be explained by existing immunologic resistance among the contacts.

Treatment is palliative (analgesics, bland mouth rinses, fluids, soft diet, and rest). In the differential diagnosis, erythema multiforme, infectious mononucleosis, and pemphigus must be considered.

Recurrent intraoral herpetic infections are extremely rare and only occur on the mucosa covering bone (gingiva and palate). The ulcers are small, shallow, and irregular in size and shape. They can be mistaken for traumatic abrasions. There is no effective therapy; the infection is self-limiting within 2 weeks.

Herpes labialis (cold sore) is due to recurrent herpesvirus infections. These lesions usually have a burning premonitory stage and are first manifested by small vesicles that soon rupture and scab. Factors that trigger herpesvirus migration by nerve pathways to the lip range from unidentifiable stimuli to temperature changes, chemical and physical irritants, or "stress."

The diagnosis is based on the history and appearance of the lesions. The differential diagnosis includes carcinoma, syphilitic chancre, and erythema multiforme. No method of treatment has been uniformly successful. Improvement has been claimed with the use of idoxuridine and acyclovir ointments, chloroform, or ether applications.

There is no firm evidence that type 1 herpesvirus is associated with oral carcinoma.

Hirsch MS, Schooley RT: Treatment of herpesvirus infections. (2 parts.) *N Engl J Med* 1983;**309**:963, 1034.

CANDIDIASIS
(Moniliasis, Thrush)

Thrush is due to overgrowth of *Candida albicans*. It is characterized by creamy-white curdlike patches anywhere in the mouth. The adjacent mucosa is usually erythematous, and scraping the lesions often uncovers a raw, bleeding surface. Quite commonly, a candidal lesion may appear as a slightly granular or irregularly eroded erythematous patch. Pain is commonly present; fever and lymphadenopathy are uncommon. Although this fungus appears in about one-third of normal-appearing mouths, overgrowth does not occur unless the "balance" of the oral flora is disturbed, so that the fungi can compete more favorably for glucose substrate.

Candidiasis is most commonly seen in denture wearers, with the appliances serving as a nutrient reservoir to foster fungal growth. It is also frequently seen in patients with debilitating or acute illness or in those being treated with antibiotics. Candidal growth also is favored by xerostomia (most commonly induced by drugs or head and neck irradiation), diabetes mellitus, iron deficiency anemia, and immunosuppressed status. Concomitant candidiasis of the gastrointestinal tract (including the pharynx and the esophagus) may occur.

The diagnosis is based upon the varied clinical picture of surface white patches or erythematous changes and may be confirmed by culture. A smear frequently will reveal characteristic spores and sometimes the more suggestive hyphae. In patients with active candidiasis, a biopsy from the lesion will often reveal pseudomycelia of *Candida* invading surface epithelium (periodic acid–Schiff stain).

Treatment is usually successful; however, the infection will often return in spite of treatment as long as causative factors are present. Therefore, treatment often should be prolonged well beyond the period of signs or symptoms. The patient should have a nutritious diet with vitamin supplementation and should get adequate rest. Mouth rinses made up of equal parts of peroxide and saline solution every 2 hours provide local relief and promote healing. Specific antifungal therapy consists of nystatin mouth rinses, 500,000 units 3 times daily (100,000 units/mL in a flavored vehicle), held in the mouth and then swallowed; nystatin vaginal troches (100,000 units) to be dissolved orally 4 times daily; clotrimazole troches (Mycelex) (10 mg) to be dissolved orally 5 times a day; and ketoconazole tablets (Nizoral), 200–400 mg with breakfast for 7–14 days. In denture wearers, nystatin powder (100,000 units/g) applied to the dentures 3–4 times daily for several weeks, can be helpful in reversing signs and symptoms.

Chronic angular cheilitis is often a manifestation of candidiasis. It is best treated with nystatin powder or Mycolog (nystatin-neomycin-gramicidin-triamcinolone) cream. Mucocutaneous candidiasis is rare and frequently does not respond well to any form of treatment, including immunostimulation.

Budtz-Jorgensen E: Clinical aspects of *Candida* infection in denture wearers. *J Am Dent Assoc* 1978;**96**:474.
Kirkpatrick CH, Alling DW: Treatment of chronic oral candidiasis with clotrimazole troches. *N Engl J Med* 1978;**299**:1201.

LEUKOPLAKIA

Leukoplakia (a white patch) of the oral mucous membranes is occasionally a sign of carcinoma; it is important to rule out cancer.

The most common cause of leukoplakia is epithelial hyperplasia and hyperkeratosis, usually in response to an irritant. In many cases the cause cannot be determined.

Leukoplakia is usually asymptomatic. It is often discovered upon routine examination or by patients feeling roughness in their mouths. Because there is no reliable correlation between clinical features and microscopic findings, a definitive diagnosis may be established only by histopathologic examination. However, because of the extensiveness of some intraoral leukoplakias, cytologic smears from the surface are helpful in supplementing both clinical and biopsy information.

Treatment consists of removing all irritants (eg, tobacco, ill-fitting dentures). If the leukoplakia is not reversible, excision should be performed when feasible. However, since some leukoplakias occur so diffusely that complete excision is often impractical, careful clinical examination and follow-up are essential. It must be remembered that the diagnosis must be reaffirmed periodically, since a leukoplakia may unpredictably be transformed into a malignant tumor. Electrodesiccation, cryosurgery, vitamin A, and proteolytic enzymes have not given predictably favorable results.

Silverman S Jr et al: Oral leukoplakia and malignant transformation: A follow-up study of 257 patients. *Cancer* 1984;**53**:563.

SIALADENITIS

Acute inflammation of a parotid or submandibular salivary gland is usually due to viral or bacterial infection or, less commonly, blockage of the duct. The gland is swollen and tender. Observation of Wharton's and Stensen's ducts may show absent or scanty secretion, with fluctuation of swelling, especially during meals, which indicates blockage; or a turbid secretion, which suggests infection. Clinical examination and x-ray may disclose ductal or glandular calcific deposits. Sialograms are of help in differentiating normal and diseased glands. Probing the ducts may reveal an inorganic plug or organic stenosis.

Dryness of the mouth (xerostomia) may be due to inflammation of the salivary glands, mouth breathing, dehydration, anticholinergic and psychotropic drugs, Sjögren's syndrome, and radiation injury. Mouth dryness is a common complaint in the elderly. Correct specific causes when possible. Frequent mouth rinsing and local troches may help.

Tumors may be confused with nonneoplastic inflammation. In these situations, biopsy (usually excisional) should be performed, but only after other diagnostic and therapeutic procedures have failed to yield a diagnosis. Neoplasms are usually not associated with an acute onset and, at least in the early phases, are not painful. The lymph nodes are intimately associated with the salivary glands, and consideration must be given to diseases in which lymphadenopathy is a prominent finding, eg, lymphomas and metastatic cancer.

In the acute stage, antibiotics, heat, and analgesics are indicated. Ductal stones that are too large for removal by massage and manipulation must be removed surgically (when the acute phase has subsided). If calcification or infection of the gland recurs often, extirpation of the gland must be considered. Radiation therapy may be effective in curing acute or recurrent sialadenitis that does not respond to other types of therapy.

McKenna RJ: Tumors of the major and minor salivary glands. *CA* 1984;**34**:24.
Rice DH: Advances in the management of salivary gland disease. *West J Med* 1984;**140**:238.

GLOSSITIS

Inflammation of the tongue (usually associated with partial or complete loss of the filiform papillae, which creates a red, smooth appearance) may be secondary to a variety of diseases such as anemia, nutritional deficiency, drug reactions, systemic infection, and physical or chemical irritations. Treatment is based on identifying and correcting the primary cause if possible and palliating the tongue symptoms as required. Many obscure cases are due to such conditions as geographic tongue and median rhomboid glossitis.

The diagnosis is usually based on the history and laboratory studies, including cultures as indicated. Empiric therapy may be of diagnostic value in obscure cases.

When the cause cannot be determined and there are no symptoms, therapy is not indicated.

Dreizen S: The telltale tongue. *Postgrad Med* (March) 1984;**75**:150.

GLOSSODYNIA, GLOSSOPYROSIS
(Chronic Lingual Papillitis)

Burning and pain, which may involve the entire tongue or isolated areas and may occur with or without glossitis, may be associated findings in hypochromic or pernicious anemia, nutritional disturbances, or diabetes mellitus and may be the presenting symptoms. Xerostomia, drugs (frequently diuretics), and candidiasis may be responsible. Smoking can be a causative irritant. Allergens (eg, in dentifrices) are rare causes of tongue pain. Certain foods may cause flare-ups but are not the primary causes. Dental prostheses, caries, and periodontal disease are usually of no causative significance.

Although most cases occur in postmenopausal women, these disorders are neither restricted to this group nor indicative of hypoestrogenemia.

In most cases a primary cause cannot be identified. Cultures are of no value, since the offending organisms are usually present also in normal mouths. Many clinicians believe that these symptoms occur on a primarily functional basis.

Treatment is mainly empiric, since causative factors usually are not identified. Important approaches include ruling out systemic conditions sometimes associated with these symptoms, changing the drugs being given for other disorders, and reassuring patients that there is no evidence of infection or neoplasia. Antihistamines, sedatives and tranquilizers, and vitamins are occasionally of value. Ointments and mouth rinses are of no value.

Partial xerostomia may be remedied by sucking on nonmedicated troches or by the administration of pilocarpine, 10–20 mg daily in divided doses.

Basker RM et al: Patients with burning mouths. *Br Dent J* 1978; **145**:9.

PIGMENTATION OF GINGIVAE

Abnormal pigmentation of the gingiva is most commonly a racially controlled melanin deposition in the epithelial cytoplasm. It is most prevalent in non-white peoples. The color varies from brown to black, and the involvement may be in isolated patches or a diffuse speckling. Nongenetic causes include epithelial or dermal nevi (rare), drugs (eg, bismuth, arsenic, mercury, or lead), and amalgam fragments that become embedded in the gums during dental work. (Mercury from this source has not been determined to be a health hazard.) Similar lesions may also appear during the menopause or in Addison's disease, intestinal polyposis, neurofibromatosis, and several other disorders associated with generalized pigmentations.

The most important consideration is to rule out malignant melanoma (extremely rare in the mouth), which is suggested by rapid growth and slight elevation.

Buchner A, Hansen LS: Pigmented nevi of the oral mucosa: A clinicopathologic study of 32 new cases and review of 75 cases from the literature. *Oral Surg* 1980;**49**:55.

Lockhart PB: Gingival pigmentation as the sole presenting sign of chronic lead poisoning in a mentally retarded adult. *Oral Surg* 1981;**52**:143.

ORAL CANCER

Cancers of the lips, tongue, floor of the mouth, buccal mucosa, palate, gingivae, and oropharynx account for about 4% of all cancers. Estimates from various surveys indicate that the average 5-year survival rate for all patients with oral cancer is less than 30%. However, with early detection, the 5-year survival rates are almost doubled. (By definition, detection is "early" when lesions are less than 3 cm in size, without evidence of metastases.) Therefore, early diagnosis followed by adequate treatment appears to be the most effective means of controlling oral cancer.

The lips and tongue are the most frequent sites of involvement. Squamous cell carcinoma is the most common type, accounting for over 90% of all oral cancers. Oral cancer is a disease of older people; over 90% of cases occur after age 45, and the average age is about 60. The male/female ratio is about 2:1.

The cause of oral cancer is not known. A genetic factor is not apparent. There is a definite increased risk with the use of tobacco and alcohol. Oral leukoplakia is an important precancerous lesion.

There are no reliable signs or symptoms in early oral carcinoma, although pain is the most frequent first complaint. An early cancer may appear as a small white patch (leukoplakia), an aphthouslike or traumatic ulcer, an erythematous plaque, or a small swelling. Biopsy is the only method of definitely diagnosing a carcinoma. However, immediate biopsy of every ill-defined or innocuous-appearing lesion is impractical and not indicated. Exfoliative cytology is a simple, reliable, and acceptable means of differentiating benign and early malignant neoplasms. In the case of small lesions whose gross appearance would be altered by biopsy, the clinician who will give the treatment should see the lesion before the biopsy is taken in order to determine the extent of resection or radiation required. Lymph nodes should not be incised for biopsy for fear of causing dissemination of tumor cells.

Curative treatment consists of surgery and radiation, alone or in combination. An attempt should be made to save the teeth necessary to support prostheses. Many teeth exposed to irradiation remain relatively free of disease and functional for long periods. The periodontium is maintained in optimal condition by periodic routine dental procedures. When areas that have been directly in the beam of irradiation are treated, extreme care is exercised and antibiotics may be selectively administered. Frequent fluoride applications appear to aid in minimizing tooth decalcification and caries. Daily mouth rinses containing 1 mg fluoride per 5 mL are a practical source of fluoride. Alterations of taste and saliva formation are usually not permanent, but there is no effective remedy if these changes do not reverse spontaneously. Pilocarpine solution, 5 mg 2–4 times daily, will often selectively increase salivation and contribute to the patient's comfort.

Decker J, Goldstein JC: Current concepts in otolaryngology: Risk factors in head and neck cancer. *N Engl J Med* 1982;**306:** 1151.

Silverman S, Gorsky M, Greenspan D: 1. Current trends in the occurrence of oral cancer. 2. Early detection of oral cancer. *J Dermatol Allergy* 1983;**6:**26.

DISEASES OF THE ESOPHAGUS

REFLUX ESOPHAGITIS
(Peptic Esophagitis)

Essentials of Diagnosis
- Substernal burning, cramping, severe pain, or pressure (any or all).
- Symptoms aggravated by recumbency or increase of abdominal pressure; relieved by upright position.
- Nocturnal regurgitation, cough, dyspnea, aspiration may be present.

General Considerations
Reflux esophagitis results from regurgitation of gastric contents into the esophagus. Acid, pepsins, or bile reflux is essential in pathogenesis. Hyperemia or exudates with erosions may be seen at endoscopy. The pathophysiology includes a permanently or intermittently incompetent lower esophageal sphincter, frequency and duration of reflux, and the inability of the esophagus to generate secondary peristaltic waves that normally prevent prolonged contact of the mucosa with acid and pepsin. A hiatal hernia may or may not be present. The presence of a hiatal hernia is of no consequence unless it is associated with reflux.

Clinical Findings
A. Symptoms and Signs: Pyrosis ("heartburn") is the most common symptom and is inconstantly indicative of the degree of esophagitis that is secondary to reflux. It is frequently severe, occurring 30–60 minutes after eating, and is initiated or accentuated by recumbency and relieved by sitting upright. Pain at the lower sternal level or xiphoid frequently radiates into the interscapular area, neck, jaw, or down the arms and may closely mimic angina pectoris.

The symptoms are the result of reflux of acid or alkaline gastric contents into the esophagus because of an incompetent lower esophageal sphincter. The conditions associated with an incompetent esophageal sphincter are hiatal hernia, pregnancy, obesity, recurring or persistent vomiting, and nasogastric tubes. Other symptoms include water brash (combination of regurgitation and increased salivation), dysphagia, and odynophagia due to diffuse spasm, stricture, or ulceration; hematemesis; and melena. Iron deficiency anemia may occur with chronic occult bleeding. Aspiration may cause cough, dyspnea, or pneumonitis.

B. X-Ray Findings: Esophageal reflux may be seen on x-ray. Unless stricture, ulcer, or motor abnormalities are present, esophagitis usually cannot be diagnosed by x-ray. In some patients, reflux may be impossible to document by radiographic techniques.

C. Special Examinations: The most objective means of demonstrating esophageal reflux is with the esophageal pH probe. Esophageal manometry is useful in determining lower esophageal sphincter pressure and esophageal motility disorders. All patients with esophageal dysfunction should undergo esophagoscopy. The gross features of esophagitis—hyperemia, friability, erosions, exudates, ulcerations, and strictures—are seen to some degree in 70% of those diagnosed as having esophagitis, on the basis of histologic criteria or a positive acid perfusion test. Multiple biopsies and cytologic examination of specimens obtained by brush biopsy or lavage will help in excluding the possibility of Barrett's esophagus or cancer. The acid perfusion (Bernstein) test usually reproduces the patient's symptoms if they are due to peptic esophagitis. Suction biopsy of the esophageal mucosa in the area 3–6 cm above the esophagogastric junction has a characteristic histopathologic picture even in the absence of gross esophagitis.

Differential Diagnosis
The differentiation of the retrosternal chest pain of esophagitis from that of angina pectoris or myocardial infarction requires sequential ECGs, enzyme determinations, and close clinical observation. Gastroduodenal ulcer disease, presenting with similar symptoms, can usually be distinguished by radiographic study.

Complications
Esophagitis, stricture, and esophageal ulcer are the most common complications. However, significant gastritis in the herniated portion of the stomach is sometimes a cause of occult bleeding and anemia.

Treatment
A. General Measures: Since obesity is often an associated or precipitating factor in esophagitis, weight reduction is essential. Other conditions that predispose to increased intra-abdominal pressure, eg, tight belts or corsets, should be avoided. The patient should also be advised to avoid lying down immediately after meals and to sleep with the head of the bed elevated 20–25 cm with wooden blocks. Medication should be taken with an ample amount of water,

preferably when the patient is in an upright position. Foods that decrease lower esophageal sphincter pressure should be avoided as much as possible, eg, dietary fat, chocolate, and peppermint. Tobacco and alcohol also decrease lower esophageal sphincter pressure and are best avoided. Many patients become symptomatic when they ingest citrus or tomato products and should avoid these foods.

B. Medical Measures:

1. Antacids–Thirty milliliters taken 1 and 3 hours after meals and at bedtime is effective in neutralizing residual acidic peptic gastric contents. Combination antacids containing aluminum hydroxide and magnesium carbonate (eg, Gaviscon), 1 or 2 tablets chewed thoroughly after meals and at bedtime, may be effective in preventing reflux.

2. Histamine H$_2$ receptor blockers–Cimetidine (Tagamet), 400 mg, or ranitidine (Zantac), 150 mg, at bedtime will suppress gastric secretions and thereby minimize nocturnal reflux.

3. Cholinergic agents–Bethanechol chloride, 10–20 mg at mealtime, may increase esophageal and gastric motility and speed gastric emptying, thereby decreasing reflux.

4. Gastrointestinal stimulants–Metoclopramide (Reglan), 10–20 mg/d, will increase the rate of gastric and esophageal emptying by stimulating the smooth muscle of the intestine. Its exact role in treatment has not been defined.

C. Surgical Measures: Antireflux operations may be indicated in a small number of patients who have persistent or recurrent symptoms despite adequate medical therapy. The most commonly performed antireflux procedure is Nissen fundoplication, which produces good results though with some recurrences reported after 5 years. Placement of an Angelchik ring around the distal esophagus in the infradiaphragmatic region is occasionally done. The long-term results of this procedure are unknown.

Prognosis

Most patients (85–90%) with esophagitis respond to management of weight reduction, antacids, elevation of the head of the bed, and other nonsurgical measures. Even those with strictures (see below) can usually be managed successfully with these measures plus bougienage. For those who cannot be managed medically, fundoplication produces good results in most instances.

Cooper JD, Jeejeebhoy KN: Gastroesophageal reflux: Medical and surgical management. *Ann Thorac Surg* 1981;**31**:557.
Corazziari E et al: Motor activity of the distal esophagus and gastroesophageal reflux. *Gut* 1984;**25**:1.
Dodds WJ et al: Mechanisms of gastroesophageal reflux in patients with reflux esophagitis. *N Engl J Med* 1982;**307**:1547.
Dodds WJ et al: Pathogenesis of reflux esophagitis. *Gastroenterology* 1981;**81**:376.
Richter JE, Castell DO: Gastroesophageal reflux: Pathogenesis, diagnosis and therapy. *Ann Intern Med* 1982;**97**:93.

BARRETT'S ESOPHAGUS

Barrett's esophagus is a disorder in which the esophagus is lined with columnar epithelium for varying lengths. It probably represents healing of esophagitis by replacement of the normal squamous epithelium with columnar cells. The symptoms are pyrosis or dysphagia. The incidence of this condition is 3 times greater in males than in females. The entity should be thought of when there is radiographic evidence of a high, benign stricture or a discrete "peptic ulcer" of the lower gullet. Esophagoscopy and biopsy are required to establish the histologic characteristics.

Treatment is the same as for esophagitis. These patients have about a 10% risk of developing adenocarcinoma in this abnormal epithelium. They should be followed closely with esophagoscopy, cytologic tests, and x-ray examination. The columnar epithelium may regress after successful antireflux surgery, possibly decreasing the chance of malignant degeneration.

Herlihy KJ et al: Barrett's esophagus: Clinical, endoscopic, histologic, manometric, and electrical potential difference characteristics. *Gastroenterology* 1984;**86**:436.

BENIGN STRICTURE OF THE ESOPHAGUS

Healing of any inflammatory lesion of the esophagus may result in stricture formation. Common causes are peptic esophagitis secondary to gastroesophageal reflux, indwelling nasogastric tube, Barrett's epithelium and ulcer formation, ingestion of corrosive substances, acute viral or bacterial infectious diseases, and, rarely, injuries caused by endoscopes.

The principal symptom is dysphagia, which may not appear for years after the initial insult. In patients who have swallowed caustics, the initial difficulty with swallowing caused by edema may be short-lived. However, it may be followed weeks or months later by stricture formation. Ability to swallow liquids is maintained the longest.

Odynophagia (painful swallowing) occurs not infrequently in association with dysphagia (difficult swallowing). The patient's description of the point at which the "hang-up" of food is perceived conforms with amazing accuracy to the level of the obstruction.

X-ray demonstration of smooth narrowing with no evidence of mucosal irregularity is usually diagnostic. However, esophagoscopy, biopsy, and cytologic examination are mandatory in all cases to rule out the possibility of cancer.

Dilatation is the definitive form of treatment, using Puestow dilators or mercury-filled (Maloney or Hurst) bougies to attain a lumen size of 44–60F. However, both patient and physician must be prepared for continuing bougienage, since recurrence of stenosis may occur if dilatation is terminated once swallowing again becomes normal. Monthly passage of the largest bougie the patient can tolerate usually prevents regression. If dilatation is unsuccessful, surgical replacement of the esophagus with a segment of stomach, jejunum, or colon will be indicated.

Patterson DJ et al: Natural history of benign esophageal stricture treated by dilatation. *Gastroenterology* 1983;**85**:346.

LOWER ESOPHAGEAL RING
(Schatzki's Ring)

The finding of a static but distensible lower esophageal ring signifies the presence of a sliding hiatal hernia that may or may not be symptomatic. Most rings histologically represent the esophagogastric junction. Manometric studies have also confirmed that the lower esophageal ring physiologically represents the point at which the esophagus and stomach meet. However, biopsies from both sides of the ring have rarely revealed esophageal mucosa. Some rings can be purely esophageal in origin.

The classic ring is 4 mm or less in thickness, is composed of a connective tissue core with muscularis mucosae, and is covered on the upper side by squamous epithelium and on the lower side by columnar epithelium. Submucosal fibrosis is present, but esophagitis is usually absent. Significant gastroesophageal reflux is not present.

Not all lower esophageal rings are mucosal in nature. Some are due to muscular contractions of the esophagus. Distention of the lower esophagus with barium does not obliterate a mucosal ring but accentuates it. Dysphagia is usually present when the ring reduces the internal esophageal lumen to a diameter of 13 mm or less and is often present with a diameter of 18 mm or less.

Most rings can be seen at endoscopy with fiberoptic instruments and can frequently be successfully treated simply by passing an esophagoscope through the ring, thereby dilating it. With a tight ring, one or 2 biopsies can be taken around its circumference, followed either by endoscopic bougienage or bougienage with mercury-filled dilators.

Hill M et al: The management of symptomatic Schatzki ring: A report of 7 cases. *Gastrointest Endosc* 1975;**21**:116.

Ott DJ et al: Review: Esophagogastric region and its rings. *AJR* 1984;**142**:281.

ACHALASIA OF THE ESOPHAGUS

Achalasia is a motor disorder of the esophagus characterized by loss of primary peristalsis, presence of a hypertonic lower esophageal sphincter that does not relax in response to a swallow, and evidence of denervation of the esophagus as shown by an exaggerated esophageal response to cholinergic agents. It is, in part, the result of impaired integration of parasympathetic stimulation. There is difficulty in swallowing both liquids and solids, at first of variable frequency and degree but later usually persistent and severe and characterized by dysphagia, occasional odynophagia, frequent regurgitation of food, and dilatation of the esophagus, as shown by radiography. Although achalasia may appear in infancy or old age, it most commonly afflicts patients in the third to fifth decades. It may predispose to esophageal carcinoma.

Two types of achalasia of the esophagus can be defined by differences in pathologic anatomy, symptoms, and radiographic findings. The first type (about 75% of cases) is characterized by a beaklike narrowing of the distal 2–4 cm of the esophagus. The more proximal portion is markedly dilated and tortuous, with the ultimate appearance of an elongated sigmoid configuration. Stasis of intraluminal contents is responsible for varying degrees of esophagitis. Patients with this form of achalasia characteristically experience dysphagia without chest pain. However, regurgitation may cause aspiration, with resultant pneumonitis, bronchiectasis, lung abscess, or pulmonary fibrosis.

The second form, vigorous achalasia, is characterized by recurring esophageal spasm, which may result in retrosternal and subxiphoid pain with frequent associated dysphagia or hypersalivation. The circular muscle of the esophagus appears hypertrophied, and the dilatation proximal to the lower esophageal sphincter is not as marked as with the first type.

Dysphagia may initially be intermittent, with food apparently sticking at the level of the xiphoid cartilage, and is associated with variable discomfort in the retrosternal or subxiphoid areas. Precipitation or accentuation of difficult swallowing may inconstantly follow the ingestion of solids or cold beverages and may be related to emotionally stressful situations. Continued esophageal dilatation with retention of food and liquids results in a sensation of fullness behind the sternum. Pain (when present) may also radiate to the back, neck, and arms and may occur independently of swallowing. Increased hydrostatic pressure within the esophagus will overcome the high resting pressure of the lower esophageal sphincter, and patients should therefore drink extra water and perform the Valsalva maneuver so that the esophageal contents will more readily enter the stomach. However, prolonged impairment of alimentation may cause varying degrees of malnutrition.

Radiographic diagnosis is based on the characteristic tapering of the distal esophagus in a conical fashion to a markedly narrowed distal segment, 1–3 cm long, which usually lies above the diaphragm. Fluoroscopy, cinefluorography, and films of the proximal esophagus reveal purposeless and ineffectual contractions as well as varying degrees of dilatation. Esophageal motility and manometric studies provide characteristic findings and may be required to establish a diagnosis of achalasia.

After a clear liquid diet for 24–36 hours and preendoscopic aspiration and lavage, esophagoscopy should be performed at least once in every case of achalasia to ascertain the severity of esophagitis and to eliminate the possibility of occult carcinoma.

Passage of a pneumatic dilator under fluoroscopic guidance—designed to split muscle fibers of the lower esophageal sphincter—has been recommended as nonsurgical treatment. Passage of mercury-filled bougies is only palliative at best but may be employed in a preparatory way to enable easier emptying of esophageal contents prior to pneumatic dilatation. Treatment of achalasia with long-acting nitrates (eg, isosorbide dinitrate) or calcium channel blockers (eg, nifedipine), which lower the resting pressure of the lower esophageal sphincter, has met with modest success. Esophagocardiomyotomy is required in approximately 20–25% of patients.

Richter JE, Castell DO: Diffuse esophageal spasm: A reappraisal. *Ann Intern Med* 1984;**100**:242.

Traube M et al: Effects of nifedipine in achalasia and in patients with high-amplitude peristaltic esophageal contractions. *JAMA* 1984;**152**:1733.

Vantrappen G, Hellmans J: Treatment of achalasia and related motor disorders. *Gastroenterology* 1980;**79**:144.

Winters C et al: Esophageal bougienage in symptomatic patients with the nutcracker esophagus. *JAMA* 1984;**252**:363.

CARCINOMA OF THE ESOPHAGUS

In the USA, carcinoma of the esophagus is predominantly a disease of men in the fifth to eighth decades. It usually arises from squamous epithelium. There is increased incidence of squamous cell carcinoma of the esophagus among smokers and in association with other otolaryngologic neoplasms. Stasis-induced inflammation such as is seen in achalasia or esophageal stricture and chronic irritation induced by excessive use of alcohol seemingly are etiologically important in the development of this neoplasm. Malignant tumors of the distal esophagus are frequently adenocarcinomas that originate in the stomach and spread cephalad to the gullet. Conversely, squamous cell carcinoma of the esophagus rarely invades the stomach. Primary adenocarcinoma of the esophagus is rare and probably arises in Barrett's epithelium. Regardless of cell type, the prognosis for cancer of the esophagus is usually poor.

Clinical Findings

A. Symptoms and Signs: Dysphagia, which is progressive and ultimately prevents swallowing of even liquids, is the principal symptom. Anterior or posterior chest pain that is unrelated to eating implies local extension of the tumor, whereas significant weight loss over a short period is an ominous sign.

B. X-Ray Findings: Barium swallow is positive for an irregular, frequently annular space-occupying lesion. CT scan of the esophagus can delineate extraesophageal involvement (eg, mediastinum, lymph nodes).

C. Special Examinations: Esophagoscopy, biopsy, and cytologic examination are confirmatory.

Differential Diagnosis

Achalasia can be differentiated by endoscopy, esophageal manometry, and cinefluorography. Since there is a significant association of stricture with malignant neoplasms, any narrowing of the lumen should be evaluated by esophagoscopy and biopsy.

Treatment & Prognosis

Although it was once considered a hopeless disease, improvements during the last 2–3 decades in anesthesia, surgical techniques, and radiation therapy have improved survival of patients with esophageal carcinoma. Irradiation generally is the best form of therapy, particularly for lesions in the proximal half of the gullet. When there is no evidence of metastases, tumors of the lower half of the esophagus may be treated by resection and esophagogastrostomy or jejunal or colonic interpositions. After dilatation of tumor-bearing portions of the esophagus, effective palliation and improved survival can often be accomplished by the use of prosthetic tubes that are inserted through the mouth to facilitate swallowing. Cure rates are still dismal, however, and do not exceed 5–10%.

Gastrostomy may improve nutrition but does not prolong survival, and the inability of completely obstructed patients to swallow even saliva makes the operation of questionable value for palliation. Anticancer drugs have not proved to be of value.

Ogilvie AL et al: Palliative intubation of oesophagogastric neoplasms at fibreoptic endoscopy. *Gut* 1982;**23**:1060.

Picus D et al: Computed tomography in the staging of esophageal carcinoma. *Radiology* 1983;**146**:433.

BENIGN NEOPLASMS OF THE ESOPHAGUS

Benign tumors of the esophagus are quite rare and are generally found accidentally by either the radiologist or prosector in the lower half of the esophagus. The most common of the benign neoplasms is the leiomyoma, which arises from one of the smooth muscle coats of the esophagus. This lesion may be circumferential or multiple, gradually increases in size (up to 2–2.5 cm), and may ultimately compromise the esophageal lumen or normal peristalsis, producing dysphagia. Other uncommon benign tumors are fibromas, lipomas, lymphangiomas, hemangiomas, and schwannomas. The diagnosis is made by barium swallow and esophagoscopy. Cytologic examination is not definitive, and biopsy may be inadequate or technically not feasible. Surgical removal is curative.

ESOPHAGEAL DIVERTICULA

Essentials of Diagnosis

- Dysphagia progressing as more is eaten; bad breath, foul taste in mouth.
- Regurgitation of undigested or partially digested food representing first portion of a meal.
- X-ray (barium) confirms diagnosis.

General Considerations

The clinical picture and pathologic effects of an esophageal diverticulum are to a large extent dictated by the location of the lesion. It is therefore convenient to distinguish pharyngoesophageal (pulsion or Zenker's), midesophageal (traction), and epiphrenic (traction-pulsion) diverticula by their locations. The first (pharyngoesophageal) develops through the space at the junction of the hypopharynx and esophagus just proximal to the cricopharyngeal sphincter, occurs chiefly in middle-aged men, and may attain large size. The second (midesophageal) type rarely is larger than 2 cm, may be multiple, frequently arises opposite the pulmonary hilar region, occurs with equal frequency in men and women, and usually causes no symptoms. The third and least common (epiphrenic) type occurs primarily in men in the esophageal segment immediately proximal to the hiatus, may be congenital in origin, and progressively enlarges, so that symptoms develop in middle age. Pharyngoesophageal and epiphrenic diverticula frequently produce nocturnal regurgitation and aspiration, with resultant bronchitis, bronchiectasis, and lung abscess.

Clinical Findings

A. Symptoms and Signs: The main symptoms of pharyngoesophageal (Zenker's) diverticula are dysphagia, regurgitation, gurgling sounds in the neck, nocturnal coughing, halitosis, and weight loss. Enlargement of the pouch results in its downward dissection between the postesophageal septum of the deep cervical fascia and the prevertebral fascia. When filled with food, the pouch may appear as a swelling at the side of the neck and internally may cause compression and obstruction of the proximal esophagus. There is occasionally so much compression of the esophagus that its entrance becomes slitlike, making it difficult to find endoscopically, and this readily explains the difficulty in swallowing and impaired nutrition.

Epiphrenic diverticula, which are occasionally associated with peptic strictures, usually cause no symptoms at first but ultimately may produce dysphagia, pain, and pulmonary complications.

Although midesophageal diverticula may rarely be responsible for mediastinal abscess or esophagobronchial fistulas and inconstantly may cause dysphagia, these lesions generally produce no symptoms.

B. X-Ray Findings: Barium swallow will usually demonstrate the 3 types of diverticula.

Differential Diagnosis

Regurgitation and difficult swallowing associated with diverticula must be distinguished from that caused by neoplasm, vascular anomalies, strictures, or motility dysfunction of the esophagus. Epiphrenic diverticula must also be differentiated from esophageal ulcer. Physical examination, radiography, and endoscopy will clarify the diagnosis.

Treatment & Prognosis

Large and symptom-producing pharyngoesophageal and epiphrenic diverticula should be treated surgically by amputation. Although recurrence or postoperative dysphagia is occasionally seen following operation for the former, long-term results are usually excellent. Cricopharyngeal sphincter myotomy has been advocated for pharyngoesophageal diverticula secondary to an abnormal sphincter. Since midesophageal pouches rarely produce complications or significant symptoms, therapy is usually not required.

Knuff TE, Benjamin SB, Castell DO: Pharyngeoesophageal (Zenker's) diverticulum: A reappraisal. *Gastroenterology* 1982;**82**:734.

ESOPHAGEAL WEBS

Esophageal webs are thin membranous structures that include in their substance only mucosal and submucosal coats. They are occasionally congenital but more commonly appear to be the sequelae of ulceration, local infection, hemorrhage, or mechanical trauma. Cervical vertebral exostoses are sometimes mentioned as a common cause. Most webs are found in the proximal portion of the esophagus and produce significant dysphagia with occasional laryngospasm secondary to aspiration. Difficult swallowing secondary to a web—when combined with iron deficiency anemia, splenomegaly, glossitis, and spooning of the nails and occurring almost invariably in premenopausal women—is called Plummer-Vinson syndrome. In this condition, a diaphanous web is usually located immediately below the cricopharyngeus and is associated with an atrophic pharyngoesophagitis. Esophagoscopy, (essential to rule out carcinoma) ameliorates dysphagia by disrupting the web. Bougienage with Maloney or Hurst dilators may occasionally be necessary.

ESOPHAGEAL CYSTS

Esophageal cysts probably result from buds of the primitive foregut or tracheobronchial branches. They may be asymptomatic but can cause dysphagia, dyspnea, cough, cyanosis, or chest pain, either because of their location or because they tend to contain acid-secreting epithelium that may produce peptic ulceration. The cysts are in the lower half of the esophagus between the muscle layers of the esophageal wall. Diagnosis is made by demonstration of a mediastinal mass on x-ray or at surgery. Surgical excision may be necessary.

Heithoff K et al: Bronchopulmonary foregut malformations: A unifying etiological concept. *Am J Roentgenol* 1976;**126**:46.

MALLORY-WEISS SYNDROME
(Mucosal Lacerations of the Esophagus or Cardioesophageal Junction)

Forceful or prolonged vomiting followed by the vomiting of bright-red blood suggests Mallory-Weiss syndrome. The bleeding is due to a vertical tear involving the mucosa of the cardioesophageal junction or, more commonly, the most proximal portion of the stomach. A hiatal hernia is frequently present. The diagnosis is based on the history of vomiting followed by hematemesis. The diagnosis is confirmed by the endoscopic demonstration of the mucosal tear. The treatment is conservative. The majority of lesions stop bleeding spontaneously.

Todd G, Zikria BA: Mallory-Weiss syndrome: A changing clinical picture. *Ann Surg* 1977;**186**:146.

DISEASES OF THE STOMACH

ACUTE GASTRITIS

Acute gastritis, probably the most common disturbance of the stomach, is frequently accompanied by generalized enteritis. It occurs in all age groups. The causes are as follows: (1) chemical irritants, eg, alcohol, salicylates; (2) bacterial infections or toxins, eg, staphylococcal food poisoning, scarlet fever, pneumonia; (3) viral infections, eg, "viral gastroenteritis," measles, hepatitis, influenza; and (4) allergy, eg, to shellfish.

Clinical Findings
A. Symptoms and Signs: Anorexia is usually the only symptom. There may be epigastric fullness and pressure and nausea and vomiting. Hemorrhage is frequent with chemical irritants (eg, salicylates, alcohol). Diarrhea, colic, malaise, fever, chills, headache, and muscle cramps are common with toxins or infections. The patient may be prostrated and dehydrated. Examination shows mild epigastric tenderness.

B. Laboratory Findings: Mild leukocytosis may be present. Leukopenia may be present with viral infections.

C. Special Examinations: Upper gastrointestinal endoscopy for hemorrhage may differentiate acute simple gastritis from erosive gastritis, peptic ulcer, or a mucosal laceration (Mallory-Weiss syndrome).

Treatment & Prognosis
Treat specific infections. Correct water and electrolyte disturbances. Give nothing by mouth until acute symptoms of pain and nausea have subsided. Then give clear liquid and progress to a soft diet as tolerated. Sedatives, phenothiazine tranquilizers, or opiates may be used as indicated. Symptoms last 1–7 days.

Strickland RG: Acute and chronic gastritis. *Hosp Med* (June) 1983;**19**:148.

ACUTE CORROSIVE ESOPHAGITIS & GASTRITIS

Ingestion of corrosive substances is most common in children but may occur in cases of attempted suicide. The substances most commonly swallowed are strong acids (sulfuric, nitric), alkalies (lye, potash), oxalic acid, iodine, bichloride of mercury, arsenic, silver nitrate, and carbolic acid. The esophagus is most severely injured. Gastric changes vary from superficial edema and hyperemia to deep necrosis and sloughing or even perforation.

Corrosion of the lips, tongue, mouth, and pharynx, along with pain and dysphagia due to esophageal lesions, is usually present. Nitric acid causes brown discoloration; oxalic acid causes white discoloration of mucous membranes. There is severe epigastric burning and cramping pain, nausea and vomiting, and diarrhea. The vomitus is often blood-tinged. Severe prostration with a shocklike picture and thirst may occur. Palpation of the abdomen may show epigastric tenderness or extreme rigidity. Leukocytosis and proteinuria are present.

Immediate treatment is supportive, including analgesics, intravenous fluids and electrolytes, sedatives, and antacids. Although the specific antidote (see Chapter 31) should be administered immediately, supportive measures must not be neglected. The benefit to be expected from the antidote appears miniscule if a large amount of corrosive has been ingested, and the benefit is doubtful considering that tissue damage occurs almost immediately. Avoid emetics and lavage if corrosion is severe, because of the danger of perforation.

The outcome depends upon the extent of tissue damage. Careful fiberoptic endoscopy may serve to determine the extent of injury. Emergency laparotomy may be indicated to resect the area of gangrene and potential perforation. If alkali has been ingested, prednisone, 20 mg every 8 hours started immediately, may prevent esophageal stricture. This dose should be tapered slowly over several weeks.

After the acute phase has passed, place the patient on a peptic ulcer regimen. If perforation has not occurred, recovery is the rule. However, pyloric stenosis may occur early or late, requiring gastric aspiration, parenteral fluid therapy, and surgical repair.

The amount of the corrosive substance, its local and general effects, and the speed with which it is removed or neutralized determine the outcome. If the patient survives the acute phase, gastric effects are usually overshadowed by esophageal strictures, although chronic gastritis or stricture formation at the pylorus may follow.

Maull KI: Surgical implications of acid ingestion. *Surg Gynecol Obstet* 1979;**148**:893.

Rumack BH, Burrington JD: Caustic ingestion: A rational look at diluents. *Clin Toxicol* 1977;**11**:27.

CHRONIC GASTRITIS

Essentials of Diagnosis

- Symptoms, if present, consist of vague, nondescript upper abdominal distress.
- Mild epigastric tenderness or no physical findings whatever.
- Gastric biopsy is the definitive diagnostic technique.

General Considerations

At best, a very poor correlation exists between the gastroscopic appearance considered to be gastritis and the histopathologic features.

Symptoms should not be attributed to chronic gastritis until all other possibilities have been excluded. Although the disorder is seen in association with gastric ulcer and gastric carcinoma, a cause and effect relationship has not been established. Patients with pernicious anemia have mucosal atrophy with varying amounts of gastritis.

Clinical Findings

A. Symptoms and Signs: The vast majority of persons with chronic gastritis do not have symptoms. Gastrointestinal symptoms, if they occur, may include anorexia, epigastric pressure and fullness, heartburn, nausea, vomiting, specific food intolerance, a peptic ulcer-like syndrome, and anemia or gross hemorrhage.

Physical findings are often absent or consist only of mild epigastric tenderness.

B. Laboratory Findings: The laboratory findings may be entirely normal. Hematologic studies may reveal evidence of macrocytic anemia. The Schilling test may be abnormal. Gastric analysis, although not diagnostic, frequently shows achlorhydria.

C. X-Ray Findings: The gastric folds are commonly thin or absent. Sometimes, however, the x-ray in chronic hypertrophic gastritis may show heavy folds.

D. Endoscopy and Biopsy: Endoscopy may show atrophy, as evidenced by blood vessels visible through the mucosa. Large folds that do not flatten with air inflation may be seen. Superficial erosions may be present. Pathologic examination shows varying degrees of atrophy and infiltration of the lamina propria with lymphocytes and plasma cells.

Differential Diagnosis

The disorders that must be differentiated include peptic ulcer, gastric tumor, cholecystitis, atypical angina pectoris, psychologic gastrointestinal disorders, and pancreatic disease.

Treatment & Prognosis

The treatment of chronic gastritis, except in those cases associated with pernicious anemia or iron deficiency anemia, is not very successful. A judicious diet—elimination of possible aggravating factors such as alcohol, salicylates and other nonsteroidal anti-inflammatory drugs, and caffeine—anticholinergic drugs, and mild sedatives may give symptomatic relief.

PEPTIC ULCER

A peptic ulcer is an acute or chronic benign ulceration occurring in a portion of the digestive tract that is accessible to gastric secretions. An active peptic ulcer does not occur in the absence of acid-peptic gastric secretions. Other than the requirement for acid and pepsin, the cause of peptic ulcer at any level of the gut remains obscure.

Other factors in peptic ulceration (besides the presence of gastric acid) include hypersecretion of hydrochloric acid and decreased tissue resistance.

Peptic ulcer may occur during the course of drug therapy (salicylates and other nonsteroidal anti-inflammatory drugs, reserpine). It may occur as a result of critical illness or severe tissue injury such as extensive burns or intracranial surgery (stress ulcer), and may be associated with endocrine tumors producing gastrin, which stimulates hypersecretion of hydrochloric acid and results in a very refractory peptic ulcer diathesis (Zollinger-Ellison syndrome, gastrinoma).

Grossman MI et al: Peptic ulcer: New therapies, new diseases. *Ann Intern Med* 1981;**95**:609.

1. DUODENAL ULCER

Essentials of Diagnosis

- Epigastric distress 45–60 minutes after meals, or nocturnal pain, both relieved by food, antacids, or vomiting.
- Epigastric tenderness and guarding.
- Chronic and periodic symptoms.
- Gastric analysis shows acid in all cases and hypersecretion in some.
- Ulcer crater or deformity of duodenal bulb on x-ray or with oral endoscopy.

General Considerations

The incidence of duodenal ulcer has been declining at a rate of about 8% per year for the past decade. It still remains a major health problem. Although the average age at onset is 33 years, duodenal ulcer may occur at any time from infancy to the later years. It is 4 times as common in males as in females. Occurrence during pregnancy is unusual.

Duodenal ulcer is 4 or 5 times as common as benign gastric ulcer. Illness due to peptic ulcer is a major public health problem.

About 95% of duodenal ulcers occur in the duodenal bulb or cap. The remainder are between this area and the ampulla. Ulcers below the ampulla are rare. The ulceration varies from a few mm to 1–2 cm in diameter and extends at least through the muscularis mucosae, often through to the serosa and into the pancreas. The margins are sharp, but the surrounding mucosa is often inflamed and edematous. The base consists of granulation tissue and fibrous tissue, representing healing and continuing digestion.

Clinical Findings

A. Symptoms and Signs: Symptoms may be absent, or vague and atypical. In the typical case, pain is described as gnawing, burning, cramplike, or aching, or as ''heartburn''; it is usually mild to moderate, located over a small area near the midline in the epigastrium near the xiphoid. The pain may radiate below the costal margins, into the back, or, rarely, to the right shoulder. Nausea may be present, and vomiting of small quantities of highly acid gastric juice with little or no retained food may occur. The distress usually occurs 45–60 minutes after a meal; is usually absent before breakfast; worsens as the day progresses; and may be most severe between 12 midnight and 2:00 AM. It is relieved by food, milk, alkalies, and vomiting, generally within 5–30 minutes.

Spontaneous remissions and exacerbations are common. Precipitating factors are often unknown but may include trauma, infections, or physical or emotional distress.

Signs include superficial and deep epigastric tenderness, voluntary muscle guarding, and unilateral (rectus) spasm over the duodenal bulb.

B. Laboratory Findings: Bleeding, hypochromic anemia, and occult blood in the stools occur in chronic ulcers. Gastric analysis shows acid in all cases and a basal and maximal gastric hypersecretion of hydrochloric acid in some.

C. X-Ray Findings: An ulcer crater is demonstrable by x-ray in 50–70% of cases but may be obscured by deformity of the duodenal bulb. When no ulcer is demonstrated, the following are suggestive of ulceration: (1) irritability of the bulb, with difficulty in retaining barium there, (2) point tenderness over the bulb, (3) pylorospasm, (4) gastric hyperperistalsis, and (5) hypersecretion or retained secretions.

D. Special Examinations: Duodenoscopy has proved to be a valuable adjunct in the diagnosis of duodenal ulcer not demonstrated radiographically. Duodenoscopy may also demonstrate duodenitis, a disorder that may have a pathogenetic mechanism in common with duodenal ulcer.

Differential Diagnosis

When symptoms are typical, the diagnosis of peptic ulceration can be made with assurance; when symptoms are atypical, duodenal ulcer may be confused clinically with functional gastrointestinal disease, gastritis, gastric carcinoma, and irritable colon syndrome. The final diagnosis often depends upon x-ray or endoscopic observation.

Complications

A. Intractability to Treatment: Most cases of apparently intractable ulcer are probably due to an inadequate medical regimen or failure of cooperation on the part of the patient. The designation ''intractable'' should be reserved for patients who have received an adequate supervised trial of therapy. The possibility of gastrinoma as well as complications of the ulcer must always be considered.

B. Hemorrhage Due to Peptic Ulcer: Hemorrhage is caused either by erosion of an ulcer into an artery or vein or, more commonly, by bleeding from granulation tissue. Most bleeding ulcers are on the posterior wall. The sudden onset of weakness, faintness, dizziness, chills, thirst, cold moist skin, desire to defecate, and the passage of loose tarry or even red stools with or without coffee-ground vomitus is characteristic of acute duodenal ulcer hemorrhage.

The blood findings (hemoglobin, red cell count, and hematocrit) lag behind the blood loss by several hours and may give a false impression of the quantity of blood lost. Postural hypotension and tachycardia and central venous pressure are more reliable indicators of hypovolemia than the hematocrit (see p 357).

C. Perforation: Perforation occurs almost exclusively in men 25–40 years of age. The symptoms and signs are those of peritoneal irritation and peritonitis; ulcers that perforate into the lesser peritoneal cavity cause less dramatic symptoms and signs. A typical description of perforated peptic ulcer is an acute onset of epigastric pain, often radiating to the shoulder or right lower quadrant and sometimes associated with nausea and vomiting, followed by a lessening of pain for a few hours and then by boardlike rigidity of the abdomen, fever, rebound tenderness, absent bowel sounds, leukocytosis, tachycardia, and even signs of marked prostration. X-ray demonstration of free air in the peritoneal cavity confirms the diagnosis.

D. Penetration: Extension of the crater beyond the duodenal wall into contiguous structures but not into the free peritoneal space occurs fairly frequently with duodenal ulcer and is one of the important causes of failure of medical treatment. Penetration usually occurs in ulcers on the posterior wall, and extension is usually into the pancreas; but the liver, biliary tract, or gastrohepatic omentum may be involved.

Radiation of pain into the back, night distress, inadequate or no relief from eating food or taking alkalies, and, in occasional cases, relief upon spinal flexion and aggravation upon hyperextension—any or all of these findings in a patient with a long history of duodenal ulcer usually signify penetration.

E. Obstruction: Minor degrees of pyloric obstruction are present in about 20–25% of patients with duodenal ulcer, but clinically significant obstruction is much less common. The obstruction is generally caused by edema and spasm associated with an active ulcer, but it may occur as a result of scar tissue contraction even in the presence of a healed ulcer.

The occurrence of epigastric fullness or heaviness and, finally, copious vomiting after meals—with the vomitus containing undigested food from a previous meal—suggests obstruction. The diagnosis is confirmed by the presence of an overnight gastric residual exceeding 50 mL containing undigested food, and x-ray evidence of obstruction, gastric dilatation, and hyperperistalsis. A succussion splash on pressure in the left upper quadrant may be present, and gastric peristalsis may be visible.

Treatment

Currently, antacids, histamine H_2 receptor antagonists, and sucralfate have all been shown to be equally effective in the treatment of duodenal ulcers when compared with placebos. These regimens provide symptomatic relief in the vast majority of patients. Less clear has been the therapeutic efficacy of various dietary measures. The limiting factor with existing therapies is that although the ulcers heal, the ulcer diathesis remains and recurrence rates are high.

A. Acute Phase:

1. General measures–The patient should be encouraged to have adequate rest and sleep, and it may sometimes be necessary to recommend 2 or 3 weeks' rest from work if that can be managed. In some instances, if the home situation is unsuitable or if the patient is unable to cooperate, hospitalization is recommended. The patient who must continue to work should be given careful instructions about the medical program. Arrangements should be made for rest periods and sufficient sleep. Anxiety should be relieved whenever possible.

Alcohol, a gastric secretagogue and irritant, should be strictly forbidden. The patient should also quit smoking, since smoking has been shown to markedly decrease the healing rate of duodenal ulcer even when optimal treatment is being given.

The following drugs may aggravate peptic ulcer or may even cause perforation and hemorrhage: rauwolfia, salicylates, phenylbutazone, indomethacin, and other nonsteroidal anti-inflammatory analgesics. They should be discontinued if possible.

2. Diet–All controlled clinical studies have documented that neither the type nor the consistency of diet will affect the healing of ulcers. The important principles of dietary management of peptic ulcer are as follows: (1) nutritious diet; (2) regular meals; (3) restriction of coffee, tea, cola beverages, decaffeinated beverages, and alcohol; and (4) avoidance of foods that are clearly known to produce unpleasant symptoms in a given individual.

In the acute phase, when there is partial gastric outlet obstruction, it is often useful to begin with a full liquid diet, provided that 1-hour postprandial gastric residuals are less than 100 mL. Milk, because of its secretagogue effect, should be avoided. Large amounts of milk and cream in the diet are associated with a striking increase in deaths from myocardial infarction in ulcer patients. Interval feedings should be avoided. Food of any type or consistency has been shown to markedly stimulate gastric acid secretion and to be ineffective as a buffer against acid in the stomach.

It is doubtful that any dietary measures other than elimination of known aggravating factors play a significant role in preventing ulcer recurrence.

3. Antacids–Antacids usually relieve ulcer pain promptly. Antacid dosage should be selected on the basis of neutralizing capacity. The response to antacids varies widely according to the preparation, the dosage, and the individual patient. Most tablet preparations are relatively ineffective and should not be given.

In order to be effective, antacids must be taken frequently. During the acute phase, a full dose 1 and 3 hours after meals and at bedtime should be sufficient. If pain relief is not achieved on this regimen, the stomach is emptying too rapidly or the patient is secreting more acid than the antacid can neutralize. (Suspect Zollinger-Ellison syndrome.)

Magnesium hydroxide-aluminum hydroxide mixtures (many preparations available) are effective and widely used antacids. The usual dose is 30 mL. When full therapeutic doses are given, the magnesium in the mixtures may produce diarrhea; it may be necessary to alternate with a straight aluminum hydroxide gel preparation (eg, Alternagel), which tends to be constipating. Prolonged ingestion of aluminum hydroxide gels may lead to phosphate depletion and osteoporosis. Magnesium salts should be used cautiously in patients with renal insufficiency.

Calcium carbonate has an excellent neutralizing action and may be used at times when the magnesium-aluminum gel antacids are inadequate. Antacid mixtures containing aluminum hydroxide, calcium carbonate, and magnesium hydroxide are available (Camalox), and the usual dose is 15–30 mL. A paradoxic calcium-induced gastric hypersecretion has been reported but probably has no clinical significance with this combination agent. However, when calcium carbonate alone is used, there may be hypercalcemia and its attendant complications.

4. Sucralfate (Carafate)–This nonabsorbable aluminum salt of sucrose octasulfate is a mucosal protective agent that has antipepsin activity and tends to adhere to areas of gastric and duodenal mucosal injuries, eg, ulcers. It is as effective with duodenal ulcer as antacids or H_2 receptor blockers and has the advantage of being nonsystemic. The only side effect reported to date is mild constipation in about 5% of patients. Dosage is 1 g 30–60 minutes before meals and at bedtime. Acid must be present for therapeutic effect, and, therefore, H_2 receptor blockers should not be used concomitantly. Antacids may be used when necessary but not within 1 hour of sucralfate.

5. Histamine H_2 receptor antagonists–

a. Cimetidine (Tagamet)–This drug markedly inhibits gastric secretion stimulated by food, gastrin, histamine, and caffeine. Cimetidine is approved in the USA for short-term treatment of duodenal ulcer and gastric ulcer, for use in preventing recurrence of duodenal ulcer (up to 1 year), for management of Zollinger-Ellison syndrome, and for treatment of other hypersecretory states such as systemic mastocytosis. The dosage is 300 mg 4 times daily before meals and at bedtime. The dose must be reduced by half in patients with renal insufficiency.

Rare side effects have included gynecomastia, galactorrhea, impotence, skin rashes, leukopenia, agranulocytosis, hepatitis, elevated serum creatinine, and decreased IgA and IgM. Of more concern are interactions between cimetidine and warfarin, theophylline, lidocaine, phenytoin, and other drugs, which occur via the P-450 cytochrome system of the liver.

b. Ranitidine (Zantac)–This H₂ receptor antagonist is more potent than cimetidine and does not interfere with the metabolism of drugs that use the P-450 cytochrome system of the liver. Ranitidine has been reported to be of value in treatment of duodenal ulcer, benign gastric ulcer, and Zollinger-Ellison syndrome. It is approved in the USA for treatment of active duodenal ulcer disease and Zollinger-Ellison syndrome. The dosage is 150 mg every 12 hours.

Rare side effects have included mild serum transaminase elevation, decreases in white blood cell and platelet counts, false-positive tests for proteinuria with Multistix, and some increase in headaches. Gynecomastia and impotence secondary to cimetidine have reversed when ranitidine is substituted. There have been no reports of galactorrhea or definite drug interactions.

6. Sedatives–Tense and apprehensive patients will usually benefit greatly from sedation. Hypnotic doses of the drugs may be necessary to ensure sleep.

7. Parasympatholytic (anticholinergic) drugs– Although the parasympatholytic drugs have been widely used over a long period of time for treatment of peptic ulcer, their effectiveness is questionable. Their usefulness is limited largely to the relief of refractory pain. The dosage necessary to produce significant gastric antisecretory effect may cause blurring of vision, constipation, urinary retention, and tachycardia. If patients have gastric retention, these drugs are contraindicated.

Note: Belladonna and other anticholinergic drugs should be avoided in patients with glaucoma, esophageal reflux, gastric ulcer, pyloric obstruction, cardiospasm, gastrointestinal hemorrhage, bladder neck obstruction, or serious myocardial disease.

a. Belladonna extract, 8–24 mg, or atropine, 0.25–0.5 mg, 20–30 minutes before meals and at bedtime with or without sedatives.

b. Synthetic parasympatholytics–Numerous proprietary tertiary and quaternary amines are available as belladonna or atropine substitutes. Although they do not have central nervous system side effects, it is difficult to substantiate other therapeutic advantages. They are also more expensive.

B. Convalescent Phase:

1. Reexamination–Once the diagnosis is established, it is unnecessary to repeat the gastrointestinal series unless complications develop. Anticholinergic therapy, if used, should be discontinued 72 hours prior to x-ray examination for duodenal ulcer.

2. Education of patient regarding recurrences–The patient should be informed about the chronic and recurrent nature of the illness and warned about the complications of careless or improper treatment. Although the cause of ulcer recurrence is not known, it may be associated with irregular eating habits, irregular living habits (long or irregular hours), use of alcohol or tobacco, emotional stress, and infections, particularly of the upper respiratory tract. The patient should be instructed to return to the ulcer regimen if symptoms recur or if conditions known to aggravate the ulcer cannot be avoided. Antacids or other medications should be readily available.

3. Rest and recreation–Provisions should be made for rest and recreation to promote physical and mental relaxation.

C. Treatment of Complications:

1. Hemorrhage–Institute immediate emergency measures for treatment of hemorrhage and shock (see p 357).

2. Perforation–Acute perforation constitutes a medical emergency. Immediate surgical repair, preferably by simple surgical closure, is indicated. More extensive operations may be unwise at the time of the acute episode because of the increased operative hazard due to the patient's poor physical condition. If the patient has had no previous therapy or if previous therapy has been inadequate, conservative medical treatment should be instituted.

The morbidity and mortality rates depend upon the amount of spillage and especially the time lapse between perforation and surgery. Surgical closure of the perforation is indicated as soon as possible. If surgery is delayed beyond 24 hours, gastric suction, antibiotics, and intravenous fluids are the treatment of choice.

3. Obstruction–Obstruction due to spasm and edema can usually be treated adequately by gastric decompression and ulcer therapy; obstruction due to scar formation requires surgery. It must be remembered that the obstruction may not represent a complication of an ulcer but may be due to a primary neoplastic disease, especially in those patients with no history or only a short history of peptic ulcer.

a. Medical measures (for obstruction due to spasm or edema) consist of bed rest, preferably in a hospital; continuous gastric suction for 48 hours; and parenteral administration of electrolytes and fluids. After 72 hours, begin liquid feedings. If continued obstruction is suspected, aspirate gastric juice to measure gastric residual. Do not use anticholinergic drugs, since they delay gastric emptying. Give sedative-tranquilizer drugs and a progressive diet as tolerated. Use antacids as with uncomplicated ulcer.

b. Surgical measures (for obstruction due to scarring) are indicated only after a thorough trial of conservative measures.

Prognosis

Duodenal ulcer tends to have a chronic course with remissions and exacerbations. Many patients can be adequately controlled by medical management. About 25% develop complications, and 5–10% ultimately require surgery. H_2 receptor blocking agents given at bedtime or sulcralfate given twice a day substantially reduces the recurrence rate.

Clinical trials of sucralfate. (Symposium.) *J Clin Gastroenterol* 1981;**147(Suppl 3)**:358.

Collen MJ et al: Comparison of ranitidine and cimetidine in the treatment of gastric hypersecretion. *Ann Intern Med* 1984;**100**:52.

Danilewitz M, Tim LO, Hirschowitz B: Ranitidine suppression of gastric hypersecretion resistant to cimetidine. *N Engl J Med* 1982;**306**:20.

Drake D, Hollander D: Neutralizing capacity and cost effectiveness of antacids. *Ann Intern Med* 1981;**94**:215.

Grossman MJ: New medical and surgical treatments for peptic ulcer disease. *Am J Med* 1980;**69**:647.

Hasan M, Sircus W: The factors determining success or failure of cimetidine treatment of peptic ulcer. *J Clin Gastroenterol* 1981;**3**:225.

Korman MG et al: Influence of smoking on healing rate of duodenal ulcer in response to cimetidine or high-dose antacid. *Gastroenterology* 1981;**80**:1451.

Martin F et al: Comparison of the healing capacities of sucralfate and cimetidine in the short-term treatment of duodenal ulcer: A double-blind randomized trial. *Gastroenterology* 1982; **82**:401.

Rawls DE, Dyck WP: Peptic ulcer: Previewing new drugs, reviewing current therapy. *Consultant* (Feb) 1984;**28**:85.

Sedman AJ: Cimetidine-drug interactions. (Review.) *Am J Med* 1984;**76**:109.

2. ZOLLINGER-ELLISON SYNDROME
(Gastrinoma)

Essentials of Diagnosis

- Severe peptic ulcer disease.
- Gastric hypersecretion.
- Elevated serum gastrin.
- Gastrinoma of pancreas, duodenum, or other ectopic site.

General Considerations

Zollinger-Ellison peptic ulceration syndrome, although uncommon, is not rare. Sixty percent of patients are males. Onset may be at any age from early childhood on but is most common in persons 20–50 years old. Most patients have the gastrin-secreting tumor in the pancreas; a few have tumors in the submucosa of the duodenum and stomach, the hilum of the spleen, and the regional lymph nodes. They may be either single or multiple. Approximately two-thirds of Zollinger-Ellison tumors are malignant with respect either to their biologic behavior or to their histologic appearance.

Clinical Findings

A. Symptoms and Signs: Pain is of the typical peptic ulcer variety but is more difficult to control by medical means. Diarrhea may occur as a result of the small bowel intraluminal pH dropping below 6.5, causing inactivation of lipase with fat maldigestion. Hemorrhage, perforation, and obstruction occur commonly.

B. Laboratory Findings: The most reliable means of establishing the diagnosis of Zollinger-Ellison syndrome is measurement of serum gastrin by radioimmunoassay. Patients with Zollinger-Ellison syndrome usually have serum gastrin levels > 300 pg/mL. Serum calcium levels are useful in revealing hypercalcemia to evaluate the possibility of hyperparathyroidism and multiple endocrine adenomatosis. Gastric analysis reveals basal gastric hypersecretion (> 15 meq/h). Maximal acid output following stimulation with histamine or betazole (Histalog) does not show the increased rate of gastric acid secretion as much as in normal people or in patients with peptic ulcer disease not of the Zollinger-Ellison type. In the Zollinger-Ellison patient, the basal acid output is greater than 60% of the maximal output, while in ordinary peptic ulcer disease the basal output is usually substantially less than 60% of the maximal. Intravenous secretin causes a marked elevation of serum gastrin in patients with gastrinomas and is of use in diagnosis.

C. X-Ray Findings: Gastrointestinal series reveal that 75% of the ulcers are in the first part of the duodenum and stomach and that the ulcers are usually not multiple. Ulcers occurring in the second, third, or fourth portion of the duodenum or in the jejunum are strongly suggestive of Zollinger-Ellison syndrome. Coarseness of the proximal jejunal folds and radiographic evidence of gastric hypersecretion also suggest Zollinger-Ellison syndrome.

Treatment

Total gastrectomy was the treatment of choice until recently. H_2 receptor blockers have been shown to markedly inhibit gastric acid secretion in patients with gastrinoma and have brought about healing of ulcers, and these drugs are now probably the treatment of choice. In patients poorly controlled with H_2 receptor blockers alone, vagotomy and pyloroplasty may also be necessary.

Jensen RT: Zollinger-Ellison syndrome: Current concepts and management. *Ann Intern Med* 1983;**98**:59.

3. GASTRIC ULCER

Essentials of Diagnosis

- Epigastric distress on an empty stomach, relieved by food, antacids, or vomiting.
- Epigastric tenderness and voluntary muscle guarding.
- Anemia, occult blood in stool, gastric acid.
- Ulcer demonstrated by x-ray or gastroscopy.
- Acid present on gastric analysis.

General Considerations

Benign gastric ulcer is in many respects similar to duodenal ulcer. Acid gastric juice is necessary for its production, but decreased tissue resistance appears to play a more important role than hypersecretion. Most patients have a history of aspirin or other nonsteroidal anti-inflammatory drug use.

About 60% of benign gastric ulcers are found within 6 cm of the pylorus. The ulcers are generally located at or near the lesser curvature and most frequently on the posterior wall. Another 25% of the ulcers are located higher on the lesser curvature.

If the radiographic appearance of the ulcer is benign, the occurrence of carcinoma is about 3.3%. If it is indeterminate (features of both benignancy and malignancy), it is approximately 9.5%. With evidence of associated duodenal ulcer, it is about 1%.

Clinical Findings

A. Symptoms and Signs: There may be no symptoms, or only vague and atypical symptoms. The epigastric distress is typically described as gnawing, burning, aching, or "hunger pangs," referred at times to the left subcostal area. Episodes occur usually 45–60 minutes after a meal and are relieved by food, alkalies, or vomiting. Nausea and vomiting are frequent complaints. There may be a history of remissions and exacerbations, especially if patients are taking aspirin or other nonsteroidal analgesics. Weight loss and fatigue are common.

Epigastric tenderness or voluntary muscle guarding is usually the only finding.

B. Laboratory Findings: If bleeding has occurred, there may be hypochromic anemia or occult blood in the stool. The gastric analysis always shows an acid pH after pentagastrin and usually the presence of low normal to normal secretion.

C. Other Examinations: An upper gastrointestinal series is the usual initial diagnostic procedure for the non-actively bleeding patient suspected of having a gastric ulcer. When the radiographic appearance of the ulcer is not clearly benign or when an ulcer is not 75% healed by 8 weeks or completely healed by 12 weeks, peroral endoscopy with multiple biopsies (6–10) of the ulcer margin and base is indicated to confirm cancer.

Differential Diagnosis

The symptoms of gastric ulcer, especially if atypical, must be differentiated from those of gastritis and functional gastrointestinal distress.

Most important is the differentiation of benign from malignant gastric ulcer. A favorable response to hospital management is presumptive evidence that the lesion is not malignant. Malignant ulcers may respond initially, but residual changes at the site usually demonstrate the nature of the process.

Complications

Hemorrhage, perforation, and obstruction may occur. (See Complications of Duodenal Ulcer, p 371.)

Treatment

Ulcer treatment (as for duodenal ulcer) should be intensive. Aspirin and other nonsteroidal anti-inflammatory agents must be avoided. Repeat x-rays should be obtained to document the rate of healing at 4- to 8-week intervals. Failure to respond in 8–12 weeks with significant healing may be an indication for surgical resection in the patient who has no contraindication to surgery. Gastroscopy and biopsy should be repeated. Histamine H_2 receptor antagonists are as effective as antacids in healing gastric ulcer. However, even a carcinoma may show improvement on an ulcer regimen, and clinical relief does not necessarily mean that the ulcer is benign. Follow-up at 3 and 6 months after apparently complete healing is therefore indicated. In the event of recurrence under intensive medical management, perforation, obstruction, or massive uncontrollable hemorrhage, surgery is mandatory.

Prognosis

Gastric ulcers tend to be recurrent. There is no evidence that malignant degeneration of gastric peptic ulceration ever occurs. Recurrent uncomplicated ulcer is not a serious event, and, in fact, it may heal more readily than the previous ulcer.

Isenberg JI et al: Healing of benign gastric ulcer with low-dose antacid or cimetidine: A double-blind, randomized, placebo-controlled trial. *N Engl J Med* 1983;**308:**1319.

Miller LJ et al: Dysfunction of the stomach with gastric ulceration. *Dig Dis Sci* 1980;**25:**857.

Rotter JI: Gastric and duodenal ulcer are each many different diseases. *Dig Dis Sci* 1981;**26:**154.

4. STOMAL (MARGINAL) ULCER (Jejunal Ulcer)

Marginal ulcer should be suspected when there is a history of operation for an ulcer followed by recurrence of abdominal symptoms after a symptom-free interval of months to years. The marginal ulcer incidence after simple gastroenterostomy is 15–20%; after subtotal gastrectomy or vagotomy and antrectomy, about 2%. Nearly all of the ulcers are jejunal, and the others are located on the gastric side of the anastomosis. The abdominal pain is burning or gnawing, often more severe than the preoperative ulcer pain, and is located lower in the epigastrium, even below the umbilicus and often to the left. The pain often covers a wider area and may radiate to the back.

The "food-pain rhythm" of peptic ulcer distress frequently occurs earlier (within an hour) in marginal ulcer as a result of more rapid emptying time; and relief with antacids, food, and milk may be incomplete and of short duration. Nausea, vomiting, and weight loss are common. Hematemesis occurs frequently. Low epigastric tenderness with voluntary muscle guarding is usually present. An inflammatory mass may be palpated. Anemia and occult blood in the stool are common. On x-ray, the ulcer niche at the stoma is often difficult to demonstrate or differentiate from postsurgical defects, despite use of compression films. Gastroscopy is the most effective means of diagnosing stomal ulcer.

Stomal ulcer must be differentiated from functional gastrointestinal distress, especially in a patient concerned about the possibility of recurrence of an ulcer after surgery. Atypical symptoms must be differentiated from "bile" gastritis and from biliary tract or pancreatic disease. Consider the possibility of Zollinger-Ellison syndrome.

Complications include gross hemorrhage, perforation, stenosis of the stoma, and gastrojejunocolic fistula.

Stomal ulcers are often resistant to medical therapy; vagotomy or a more extensive gastrectomy is usually necessary to decrease the acid secretion of the stomach.

Histamine H_2 receptor antagonists as used in treatment of duodenal and gastric ulcer often lead to healing.

X-ray therapy to the stomach will substantially reduce the gastric secretion of hydrochloric acid and in some instances may induce achlorhydria for varying periods of time. Since the advent of cimetidine, the use of x-ray therapy has been restricted to a few instances of complicating disease leading to increased surgical risk and to elderly patients.

Kennedy T, Green WER: Stomal and recurrent ulceration: Medical or surgical management? *Am J Surg* 1980;**139**:18.

POSTGASTRECTOMY SYNDROMES

Dumping Syndrome

Postgastrectomy dumping syndrome probably occurs in about 10% of patients after partial gastrectomy. The pathogenesis is complex and incompletely understood. The disorder is provoked mainly by soluble hypertonic carbohydrates, which, when present in the small intestine, have an osmotic effect resulting in rapid flow of fluid into the small intestine; increase in free plasma kinins; increase in peripheral blood flow; and a modest drop in plasma volume with a corresponding increase in hematocrit and a mild decrease in serum potassium. Whether sympathetic vasomotor responses contribute to the syndrome is uncertain.

One or more of the following symptoms occur within 20 minutes after meals: sweating, tachycardia, pallor, epigastric fullness and grumbling, warmth, nausea, abdominal cramps, weakness, and, in severe cases, syncope, vomiting, or diarrhea. Nonspecific electrocardiographic changes may be noted. Plasma glucose is not low during an attack.

It is important to distinguish this syndrome from the reactive hypoglycemia that occurs in some postgastrectomy patients. This latter syndrome occurs much later after the meal (1–3 hours) and is relieved by the ingestion of food.

Changing the diet to frequent (6) small, equal feedings high in protein, moderately high in fat, and low in simple carbohydrates usually lessens the severity of symptoms. Fluids should not be taken with meals. Sedative and anticholinergic drugs may be of value.

Meyer JH: Chronic morbidity after ulcer surgery. Pages 757–779 in: *Gastrointestinal Disease*, 3rd ed. Sleisenger MH, Fordtran JS (editors). Saunders, 1983.

Miranda R et al: Surgical treatment of the postgastrectomy dumping syndrome. *Am J Surg* 1980;**139**:40.

Afferent (Blind) Loop Syndrome

The afferent loop syndrome occurs after Billroth II gastrectomy or gastrojejunostomy. The syndrome may occur acutely early in the postoperative period or months to years following operation. An acute abdominal catastrophe (rare) may require emergency operation to release the obstruction and follow-up measures to prevent recurrence. More commonly, afferent loop syndrome is caused by chronic or recurring partial obstruction, although the exact etiologic mechanisms are not clear. The symptoms are caused by distention of and stasis within the afferent loop of the gastrojejunostomy. Typically, abdominal pain occurs 15–30 minutes after eating and is relieved by vomiting of bile fluid that does not contain food.

Poor emptying of the afferent loop may result in stasis of contents, leading to bacterial overgrowth. This in turn may lead to deficiency of vitamin B_{12} because of bacterial uptake of vitamin B_{12}. Deconjugation of bile salts may also occur, with subsequent impairment of micelle formation, leading to steatorrhea and its attendant complications.

Avoidance of the Billroth II procedure will prevent the afferent loop from occurring. Surgical reconstruction of the afferent loop to produce better emptying is the treatment of choice. Bacterial overgrowth can be temporarily controlled with repeated 7- to 10-day courses of a broad-spectrum antibiotic, such as tetracycline, 250 mg 4 times daily. With vitamin B_{12} deficiency, vitamin B_{12} should be administered.

Cooperman AM: Postgastrectomy syndromes. *Surg Annu* 1981;**13**:139.

Bile Reflux

Bile reflux is one of the most debilitating complications following gastric surgery. Bile reflux may occur after cholecystectomy and occasionally with no prior surgery. Typically, the patient experiences nausea, substernal distress, and anorexia. Vomiting or reflux of clear bile-stained fluid may occur.

Medical management is unsatisfactory. The surgical approach is a diversion of bile from the stomach. The Roux-en-Y gastrojejunostomy procedure serves this end.

Buxbaum KL: Bile gastritis occurring after cholecystectomy. *Am J Gastroenterol* 1982;**77**:305.

Goldstein F, Thorton JJ III, Abramson J: Bile reflux gastritis and esophagitis in patients without prior gastric surgery, with pilot study of the therapeutic effects of metoclopramide. *Am J Gastroenterol* 1981;**76**:407.

Miscellaneous

Other complications that may follow gastric surgery include reflux esophagitis, gastric retention, postvagotomy diarrhea, and the development of carcinoma in the gastric stump many years after surgery. Iron deficiency anemia occurs in 50% of patients 5 years or longer after a Billroth II gastrectomy, because of the bypassing of the duodenum, the major locus for iron absorption. The incidence of pulmonary tuberculosis is thought to be increased after gastrectomy.

CARCINOMA OF THE STOMACH

Essentials of Diagnosis

- Upper gastrointestinal symptoms with weight loss in patients over age 40.
- Palpable abdominal mass (very late).
- Anemia, occult blood in stools, positive cytologic examination.
- Gastroscopic and x-ray abnormality.

General Considerations

Carcinoma of the stomach is a common cancer of the digestive tract. It occurs predominantly in males over 40 years of age. Delay of diagnosis is caused by absence of definite early symptoms and by the fact that patients treat themselves instead of seeking early medical advice. Further delays are due to the equivocal nature of early findings and to temporary improvement with symptomatic therapy.

A history of the following possibly precancerous conditions should alert the physician to the danger of stomach cancer:

(1) Atrophic gastritis of pernicious anemia: The incidence of adenomas and carcinomas is *significantly increased.*

(2) Chronic gastritis, particularly atrophic gastritis: There is a wide variation in the reported incidence of gastritis with cancer, and a definite relationship has not been proved.

(3) Gastric ulcer: The major problem is in the differentiation between benign and malignant ulcer.

(4) Achlorhydria: The incidence of lowered secretory potential in early life is higher in those patients who later develop carcinoma.

(5) Patients who have had a partial gastrectomy for peptic ulcer 10–15 years previously have an increased risk of gastric cancer.

Carcinoma may originate anywhere in the stomach. Grossly, lesions tend to be of 4 types (Borrman):

Type I: Polypoid, intraluminal mass.
Type II: Noninfiltrating ulcer.
Type III: Infiltrating ulcer.

Type IV: Diffuse infiltrating process (to linitis plastica).

Gross typing generally correlates better with prognosis than the histologic grading of malignancy, ie, type I has a better prognosis than type II, etc.

Clinical Findings

A. Symptoms and Signs: Early gastric carcinoma, such as is detected in the mass surveys in Japan, causes no symptoms. The appearance of symptoms implies relatively advanced disease. The patient may complain of vague fullness, nausea, a sensation of pressure, belching, and heartburn after meals, with or without anorexia (especially for meat). These symptoms in association with weight loss and a decline in general health and strength in a man over age 40 years should suggest the possibility of stomach cancer. Diarrhea, hematemesis, and melena may be present.

Specific symptoms may be determined in part by the location of the tumor. A peptic ulcer-like syndrome generally occurs with ulcerated lesions (types II and III) and in the presence of acid secretion but may occur with complete achlorhydria. Unfortunately, symptomatic relief from antacids tends to delay diagnosis. Symptoms of pyloric obstruction are progressive postprandial fullness to retention type vomiting of almost all foods. Lower esophageal obstruction causes progressive dysphagia and regurgitation. Early satiety usually occurs with linitis plastica but may be seen with other cancers.

Physical findings are usually limited to weight loss and, if anemia is present, pallor. In about 20% of cases, a palpable abdominal mass is present; this does not necessarily mean that the lesion is inoperable. Liver or peripheral metastases may also be present.

B. Laboratory Findings: Achlorhydria (gastric pH > 6) after stimulation with pentagastrin, 6 μg/kg intramuscularly or subcutaneously, in the presence of a gastric ulcer is virtually pathognomonic of cancer; but this finding is present in only about 20% of patients with gastric cancer. The presence of acid does not exclude cancer. If bleeding occurs, there will be occult blood in the stool and mild to severe anemia. With bone marrow invasion, the anemia rarely may be normochromic and normocytic.

C. Other Examinations: Endoscopic biopsy and directed cytology and expert lavage cytology with chymotrypsin will provide the correct diagnosis in almost every case. These methods will also establish the important differential diagnosis between adenocarcinoma and the malignant lymphomas.

Differential Diagnosis

The symptoms of carcinoma of the stomach are often mistaken for those of benign gastric ulcer, chronic gastritis, irritable colon syndrome, or functional gastrointestinal disturbance; x-ray and gastroscopic findings must be differentiated from those of benign gastric ulcer or tumor. Nonhealing ulcers or ulcers that are enlarging with a strict ulcer regimen require surgery. Most of these will still be benign.

The clinical history of gastric leiomyosarcoma may be indistinguishable from that of carcinoma. Bleeding, particularly massive, is more common. These tumors account for approximately 1.5% of gastric cancers. A palpable mass is more frequent than in gastric carcinoma, and the x-ray picture is characteristically that of a well-circumscribed intramural mass with, frequently, a central crater.

With the decreasing incidence of carcinoma of the stomach in the USA, gastric lymphoma now accounts for about 10% of gastric malignant disease. Treatment consists of resection, if possible, followed by irradiation. The prognosis is much more favorable than in patients with carcinoma; cure may be anticipated in over half of patients if the tumor is confined to the stomach.

Treatment

Surgical resection is the only curative treatment. Signs of metastatic disease include a hard, nodular liver, enlarged left supraclavicular (Virchow's) nodes, skin nodules, ascites, rectal shelf, and x-ray evidence of osseous or pulmonary metastasis. If none of these are present and there is no other contraindication to operation, exploration is indicated. The presence of an abdominal mass is not a contraindication to laparotomy, since bulky lesions can often be totally excised. Palliative resection or gastroenterostomy is occasionally helpful. High-voltage x-ray therapy may be of some value. Multiple drug regimens are under study. Mitomycin C, 5-fluorouracil, adriamycin, and cytarabine (cytosine arabinoside) in various combinations have been reported to be beneficial.

Prognosis

There is wide variation in the biologic malignancy of gastric carcinomas. In many, the disease is widespread before symptoms are apparent; in a fortunate few, slow growth may progress over years and be resectable even at a late date. Approximately 10% of all patients with gastric carcinoma will be cured by surgical resection.

Ekbom GA, Gleysteen JJ: Gastric malignancy: Resection for palliation. *Surgery* 1980;**88**:476.

Green PHR, O'Toole KM: Early gastric cancer. (Editorial.) *Ann Intern Med* 1982;**97**:272.

LYMPHOMA OF THE STOMACH

Primary gastric lymphoma is an uncommon cancer of the stomach. It is an important consideration in patients presenting with enlarged gastric folds, masses, or ulcerations. Biopsy and cytology are essential in establishing the diagnosis. The treatment is surgical excision, radiation, or a combination of the 2.

Dworkin B et al: Primary gastric lymphoma: A review of 50 cases. *Dig Dis Sci* 1982;**27**:986.

BENIGN TUMORS OF THE STOMACH

Most benign tumors do not cause symptoms and often are so small that they are overlooked on x-ray examination. Their importance lies in the problem of differentiation from malignant lesions, their precancerous possibilities, and the fact that they occasionally cause symptoms.

These tumors may be of epithelial origin (eg, adenomas, papillomas) or mesenchymal origin (eg, leiomyomas, fibromas, hemofibromas, lipomas, hemangiomas). The mesenchymal tumors, which are intramural, rarely undergo malignant change. Most polyps of the stomach are hyperplastic ones with no malignant potential. Adenomas have a small but unknown potential for malignant change.

Clinical Findings

A. Symptoms and Signs: Large tumors may cause a vague feeling of epigastric fullness or heaviness; tumors located near the cardia or pylorus may produce symptoms of obstruction. If bleeding occurs, it will cause symptoms and signs of acute gastrointestinal hemorrhage (eg, tarry stools, syncope, sweating, vomiting of blood). Chronic blood loss will cause symptoms of anemia (fatigue, dyspnea). If the tumor is large, a movable epigastric mass may be palpable.

B. Laboratory Findings: The usual laboratory findings may be present.

C. X-Ray Findings: The x-ray is characterized by a smooth filling defect, clearly circumscribed, which does not interfere with normal pliability or peristalsis. Larger tumors may show a small central crater, especially leiomyomas.

Treatment & Prognosis

If symptoms occur (particularly hemorrhage), surgical resection is necessary. If there are no symptoms, the patient does not require surgery. These tumors may even regress spontaneously. Polyps may be excised by endoscopic electroresection.

DISEASES OF THE INTESTINES

REGIONAL ENTERITIS
(Regional Ileitis, Regional Enterocolitis, Granulomatous Ileocolitis, Crohn's Disease)
(See also Granulomatous Colitis, p 395.)

Essentials of Diagnosis

- Insidious onset.
- Intermittent bouts of diarrhea, low-grade fever, and right lower quadrant pain.
- Fistula formation or right lower quadrant mass and tenderness.

- X-ray evidence of abnormality of the terminal ileum.

General Considerations

Regional enteritis is a chronic inflammatory disease that may involve the alimentary tract anywhere from the mouth to the anus. The ileum is the principal site of the disease, either alone or in conjunction with the colon and jejunum. It generally occurs in young adults and runs an intermittent clinical course with mild to severe disability and frequent complications.

There is marked thickening of the submucosa with lymphedema, lymphoid hyperplasia, nonspecific granulomas, and often ulceration of the overlying mucosa. A marked lymphadenitis occurs in the mesenteric nodes.

The cause is unknown. Genetic factors appear to play a role. There is a higher than normal incidence in monozygotic twins and a greater than random familial incidence. The most common familial pattern involves 2 or more affected siblings. Regional enteritis and chronic ulcerative colitis occur in the same families. The possibility of an infectious origin for regional enteritis has been raised by studies demonstrating transmission of an agent from tissues with regional enteritis into immunologically deficient mice and rabbits. Viral agents, cell-wall-defective *Pseudomonas*-like bacteria, and *Mycobacterium kansasii* have been isolated by different investigators from patients with regional enteritis. The significance of these observations remains unknown.

Clinical Findings

A. Symptoms and Signs: The disease is characterized by exacerbations and remissions. Colicky or steady abdominal pain is present in the right lower quadrant or periumbilical area at some time during the course of the disease and varies from mild to severe. Diarrhea may occur, usually with intervening periods of normal bowel function or constipation. Patients with these symptoms are often diagnosed as having irritable or functional bowel disease. Fever may be low-grade or, rarely, spiking with chills. Anorexia, flatulence, malaise, and weight loss are present. Milk products and chemically or mechanically irritating foods may aggravate symptoms.

Abdominal tenderness is usually present, especially in the right lower quadrant, with signs of peritoneal irritation and an abdominal or pelvic mass in the same area. The mass is tender and varies from a sausagelike thickened intestine to matted loops of intestine.

Regional enteritis may pursue various clinical patterns. In certain instances, the course is indolent and the symptomatology mild. In other instances, the course is toxic, with fever, toxic erythema, arthralgia, anemia, etc. Still other patients pursue courses complicated by stricture or perforations of the bowel and suppurative complications of intra-abdominal perforation.

B. Laboratory Findings: There is usually a hypochromic (occasionally macrocytic) anemia and occult blood in the stool. The small bowel x-ray may show mucosal irregularity, ulceration, stiffening of the bowel wall, and luminal narrowing. Barium enema may show fissures or deep ulcers. Eccentric involvement, skipped areas of involvement, and strictures suggest Crohn's disease of the colon. Sigmoidoscopic examination may show an edematous hyperemic mucosa or a discrete ulcer when the colon is involved.

Differential Diagnosis

Acute regional enteritis may simulate acute appendicitis. Location in the terminal ileum requires differentiation from intestinal tuberculosis, *Yersinia enterocolitica* infection, and lymphomas. Regional enteritis involving the colon must be distinguished from idiopathic ulcerative colitis, amebic colitis, ischemic colitis, and infectious disease of the colon. The sigmoidoscopic and x-ray criteria distinguishing these various entities may not be absolute, and definitive diagnosis may require cultures, examinations of the stool for parasites, and biopsy in selected instances.

Complications

Ischiorectal and perianal fistulas occur frequently. Fistulas may occur to the bladder or vagina and even to the skin in the area of a previous scar. Mechanical intestinal obstruction may occur. Nutritional deficiency caused by malabsorption and maldigestion (the latter caused by a decreased bile salt pool) may produce a spruelike syndrome. Generalized peritonitis is rare because perforation occurs slowly. The incidence of colon or rectal cancer in regional enteritis patients is greater than in a control population. Migratory peripheral synovitis and axial arthropathy indistinguishable from sporadic ankylosing spondylitis may occur.

Treatment & Prognosis

A. General Measures: The diet should be high in calories and vitamins and adequate in protein. Raw fruits and vegetables should be avoided in patients who have obstructive symptoms. These patients may benefit from a nonresidue, well-balanced diet to maintain nutrition until obstructive symptoms subside. Anemia, dehydration, diarrhea, and avitaminosis should be treated as indicated.

B. Antimicrobial Agents: In our present state of knowledge about this disease, antimicrobials are indicated only for specific infectious problems, ie, abscess, fistulas.

1. Sulfasalazine –Sulfasalazine (Azulfidine), 2–8 g/d orally, has been shown to be effective.

2. Antibiotics –In cases of acute suppuration (manifested by tender mass, fever, leukocytosis), ampicillin, 4–8 g/d intravenously or 2–4 g/d orally, may be useful. Clindamycin and aminoglycosides are also effective. In cases where internal fistulization has led to a defunctionalized loop with bacterial overgrowth or where stricture formation has led to small bowel stasis with malabsorption, tetracycline, 1–2 g/d orally, may be valuable in combating bacterial overgrowth in the bowel and correcting absorptive malfunction.

3. Metronidazole–Metronidazole, 20 mg/kg/d, has been advocated for enterocutaneous fistulas.

C. Adrenocortical Hormones: These agents are often of use in the diffuse form of the disease and are particularly helpful in the toxic forms (arthritis, anemia, toxic erythemas). The complications of long-term therapy can be minimized by administering the drug on an alternate-day schedule (eg, prednisone, 15–40 mg every other day) once the patient's clinical symptoms have been brought under control. The National Cooperative Crohn's Disease Study conducted a randomized double-blind study comparing prednisone, sulfasalazine, and azathioprine in the treatment of regional enteritis. These data indicated that sulfasalazine and prednisone are effective in the acute phase of the disease but do not exert a prophylactic effect. Azathioprine proved to be of no value.

D. Other Medical Measures: When terminal ileal disease is present, vitamin B_{12} supplementation is often necessary. Calcium supplementation in the form of calcium gluconate or Os-Cal will alleviate the frequent calcium deficiency seen in these patients and is also helpful in decreasing excessive oxalate absorption, resulting in lowered incidence of oxalate urinary tract stones.

E. Surgical Measures: Surgical treatment of this disease is best limited to the management of its complications. Resection of the small bowel, particularly the extensive resection often necessary in regional enteritis, leads to a "short bowel" syndrome (diminished absorptive surface), ie, malabsorption of vitamin B_{12} to varying degrees (loss of terminal ileum), hyperoxaluria, steatorrhea, osteomalacia, and macrocytic anemia (due to folic acid and vitamin B_{12} deficiency). Short-circuiting operations may lead to blind loops (intestinal defunctionalization with bacterial overgrowth) with similar difficulties in absorption. When surgery is necessary in this disease, study of postsurgical bowel function is indicated to detect the possibility of impaired bowel function. If defects in absorption are present, appropriate therapy may prevent serious complications.

Dworken HJ: Crohn disease. (Editorial.) *Ann Intern Med* 1984; **101:**258.

Kirsner JB, Shorter RG: Recent developments in "nonspecific" inflammatory bowel disease. (2 parts.) *N Engl J Med* 1982; **306:**775, 837.

Korelitz BI: Current treatment of Crohn's disease. *Curr Concepts Gastroenterology* 1981;**6:**3.

Lee ECG: Aim of surgical treatment of Crohn's disease. *Gut* 1984;**25:**217.

Prior P et al: Mortality in Crohn's disease. *Gastroenterology* 1981;**80:**307.

Puntis J, McNeish AS, Allan RN: Long-term prognosis of Crohn's disease with onset in childhood and adolescence. *Gut* 1984;**25:**329.

Singleton JW (editor): The National Cooperative Crohn's Disease Study. *Gastroenterology* 1979;**74:**825.

Ursing B et al: A comparative study of metronidazole and sul-

fasalazine for active Crohn's disease: The cooperative Crohn's disease study in Sweden. 2. Result. *Gastroenterology* 1982; **83:**550.

Van Hees PA et al: Effect of sulphasalazine in patients with active Crohn's disease: A controlled double-blind study. *Gut* 1981; **22:**404.

TUMORS OF THE SMALL INTESTINE

Benign and malignant tumors of the small intestine are rare. There may be no symptoms or signs, but bleeding or obstruction (or both) may occur. The obstruction consists of either an intussusception with the tumor in the lead or a partial or complete occlusion in the lumen by growth of the tumor. Bleeding may cause weakness, fatigability, lightheadedness, syncope, pallor, sweating, tachycardia, and tarry stools. Obstruction causes nausea, vomiting, and abdominal pains. The abdomen is tender and distended, and bowel sounds are high-pitched and active. Malignant lesions produce weight loss and extraintestinal manifestations (eg, pain due to stretching of the liver capsule, flushing due to carcinoid). In the case of a duodenal carcinoma, a peptic ulcer syndrome may be present. A palpable mass is rarely found.

If there is bleeding, melena and hypochromic anemia occur. X-ray (small bowel series) may show the tumor mass or dilatation of the small bowel if obstruction is present; in the absence of obstruction, it is extremely difficult to demonstrate the mass.

Benign Tumors

Benign tumors may be symptomatic or may be incidental findings at operation or autopsy. Treatment consists of surgical removal.

Benign **adenomas** constitute 25% of all benign bowel tumors. **Lipomas** occur most frequently in the ileum; the presenting symptom is usually obstruction due to intussusception. **Leiomyomas** are usually associated with bleeding and may also cause intussusception. **Angiomas** behave like other small bowel tumors but have a greater tendency to bleed.

Multiple intestinal polyposis of the gastrointestinal tract (any level) associated with mucocutaneous pigmentation (Peutz-Jeghers syndrome) is a benign condition. Malignant change has been reported but is rare, and the entity becomes a problem only with complications such as obstruction or bleeding. The polyps are hamartomas, and the pigment is melanin. The pigment is most prominent over the lips and buccal mucosa.

Malignant Tumors

The treatment of malignant tumors and their complications is usually surgical.

Adenocarcinoma is the most common cancer of the small bowel, occurring most frequently in the duodenum and jejunum. Symptoms are due to obstructions or hemorrhage. The prognosis is very poor.

Lymphomas are also first manifested by obstruction or bleeding. Perforation or malabsorption may also occur. Postoperative radiation therapy may occasionally be of value. **Sarcomas** occur most commonly in the mid small bowel and may first be manifested by mass, obstruction, or bleeding. The prognosis is guarded.

     Carcinoid tumors arise from the argentaffin cells of the gastrointestinal tract. Ninety percent of these tumors occur in the appendix, and 75% of the remainder occur in the small intestine (usually the distal ileum). Carcinoids may arise in other sites, including the stomach, colon, bronchus, pancreas, and ovary. Most small bowel carcinoids do not produce carcinoid syndrome. The main problem is metastases. In general, carcinoid syndrome occurs only with malignant tumors that have metastasized. The tumor may secrete serotinin and bradykinin. The systemic manifestations may consist of (1) paroxysmal flushing and other vasomotor symptoms, (2) dyspnea and wheezing, (3) recurrent episodes of abdominal pain and diarrhea, and (4) symptoms and signs of right-sided valvular disease of the heart. The diagnosis is confirmed by finding elevated levels of 5-hydroxyindoleacetic acid in the urine. The primary tumor is usually small, and obstruction is unusual. The metastases are usually voluminous and surprisingly benign. Treatment is symptomatic and supportive; surgical excision may be indicated if the condition is recognized before widespread metastases have occurred. Response to treatment with serotonin antagonists has been irregular. Repeated administration of corticotropin or the corticosteroids may occasionally be of value. The prognosis for cure is poor, but long-term survival is not unusual.

Herbsman H et al: Tumors of the small bowel. *Curr Probl Surg* 1980;**17**:127.

MECKEL'S DIVERTICULITIS

     Meckel's diverticulum, a remnant of the omphalomesenteric duct, is found in about 2% of persons, more frequently in males. It arises from the ileum 60–90 cm from the ileocecal valve and may or may not have an umbilical attachment. Most are silent, but various abdominal symptoms may occur. The blind pouch may be involved by an inflammatory process similar to appendicitis; its congenital bands or inflammatory adhesions may cause acute intestinal obstruction; it may induce intussusception; or, in the 16% that contain heterotopic islands of gastric mucosa, it may form a peptic ulcer.

     The symptoms and signs of the acute appendicitis-like disease and the acute intestinal obstruction caused by Meckel's diverticulitis cannot be differentiated from other primary processes except by exploration. Ulcer type distress, if present, is localized near the umbilicus or lower and, more importantly, is not relieved by alkalies or food. If ulceration

has occurred, blood will be present in the stool. Other laboratory findings often cannot be differentiated from those of appendicitis or other causes of obstruction. Massive gastrointestinal bleeding and perforation may occur.

     Meckel's diverticulitis should be resected, either for relief or for differentiation from acute appendicitis. Surgery is curative.

Mackey WC, Dineen P: A fifty year experience with Meckel's diverticulum. *Surg Gynecol Obstet* 1983;**156**:56.

MESENTERIC VASCULAR INSUFFICIENCY

1. CHRONIC MESENTERIC VASCULAR INSUFFICIENCY (Abdominal Angina)

     The syndrome of intestinal angina has received increasing attention of late. Progress in angiographic techniques and vascular surgery has led to effective diagnostic and therapeutic approaches. The entity may be secondary to atherosclerosis and may precede vascular occlusion (see below). In some instances it is secondary to compression of the vessels either by the crura of the diaphragm or by anomalous bands.

     Localized or generalized postprandial pain is the classic picture. The intensity of pain may be related to the size of the meal; the relationship to eating leads to a diminution in food intake and, eventually, weight loss. An epigastric bruit may be heard. Laboratory evidence of malabsorption may be present. The small bowel series may reveal a motility disorder. Visceral angiograms are necessary to confirm narrowing of the celiac and mesenteric arteries. It is generally believed that 2 of the 3 main vessels must be involved in order for symptoms to occur.

     Surgical revascularization of the bowel is the treatment of choice if the patient's condition permits. Small, frequent feedings may prove helpful.

2. ACUTE MESENTERIC VASCULAR INSUFFICIENCY

Essentials of Diagnosis
- Severe abdominal pain with nausea, fecal vomiting, and bloody diarrhea.
- Severe prostration and shock.
- Abdominal distention, tenderness, rigidity.
- Leukocytosis, hemoconcentration.

General Considerations
     Mesenteric arterial or venous occlusion is a catastrophic abdominal disorder. Arterial occlusion is occasionally embolic but is more frequently thrombotic. Both occur more frequently in men and in the older age groups. Acute mesenteric vascular occlusion may also be a small vessel phenomenon, particularly in patients

with vasculitis in association with a variety of collagen diseases.

Involvement of the superior mesenteric artery or its branches is common. The affected bowel becomes congested, hemorrhagic, and edematous, and may cease to function, producing intestinal obstruction. True ischemic necrosis then develops.

Intestinal infarction may occur in the absence of mesenteric vascular thrombosis; nonocclusive disease may in fact be a more common cause of infarction than is occlusion. Most patients have been in severe congestive heart failure or shock or in a state of hypoxia. Although many patients with this syndrome have been receiving digitalis glycosides, the relationship of this agent to the bowel problem is unclear. Occlusive vascular disease may also play a role in reducing perfusion of the bowel in these patients.

Clinical Findings

A. Symptoms and Signs: Generalized abdominal pain often comes on abruptly and is usually steady and severe, but it may begin gradually and may be intermittent, with colicky exacerbations. Nausea and vomiting occur; the vomitus is rarely bloody. Bloody diarrhea and marked prostration, sweating, and anxiety may occur. For a period following the occlusion, symptoms are severe but the physical findings meager.

Shock may be evident. Abdominal distention occurs early, and audible peristalsis (evident early) may later disappear. As peritoneal irritation develops, diffuse tenderness, rigidity, and rebound tenderness appear.

B. Laboratory Findings: Hemoconcentration, leukocytosis (over $15,000/\mu L$ with a shift to the left), and blood in the stool may be present.

C. X-Ray Findings: A plain film of the abdomen shows moderate gaseous distention of the small and large intestines and evidence of peritoneal fluid.

Differential Diagnosis

Differentiate from acute pancreatitis and a perforated viscus. The elevated amylase in pancreatitis and free peritoneal air in perforation may help to differentiate these conditions. Amylase may be elevated in intestinal infarction.

Treatment & Prognosis

The treatment of acute mesenteric arterial thrombosis consists of the measures necessary to (1) restore fluid, colloid, and electrolyte balance; (2) decompress the bowel; and (3) prevent sepsis by administration of antimicrobial drugs. Unless there are absolute contraindications to surgery, laparotomy should be done as soon as possible and gangrenous bowel resected. If the infarction is due to an isolated thrombus or embolus of the superior mesenteric artery, embolectomy or thrombectomy may be possible. Anticoagulants are not indicated. The mortality rate is extremely high in the acute disease. The treatment of nonthrombotic intestinal infarction poses a therapeutic dilemma. Basically the principles are the same, ie, maintenance of

fluid, electrolyte, and colloid balance. However, in the face of congestive failure, this can be most difficult. Careful hemodynamic monitoring provides useful information but is not the solution to this problem. Surgical resection of gangrenous bowel in a patient with congestive failure is a formidable undertaking but should be tried if at all possible. The prognosis in either event is grave; survival is unusual.

Boley SJ, Brandt LJ, Veith FJ: Ischemic disorders of the intestines. *Curr Probl Surg* (April) 1978;**15**:1. [Entire issue.]

Camilleri M et al: Gastrointestinal manifestation of systemic vasculitis. *Q J Med* 1983;**52**:141.

Grendell JH, Ockner RK: Mesenteric venous thrombosis. *Gastroenterology* 1982;**82**:358.

ACUTE ORGANIC SMALL INTESTINAL OBSTRUCTION

Essentials of Diagnosis

- Colicky abdominal pain, vomiting, constipation, borborygmus.
- Tender distended abdomen without peritoneal irritation.
- Audible high-pitched tinkling peristalsis or peristaltic rushes.
- X-ray evidence of gas or gas and fluid levels without movement of gas.
- Little or no leukocytosis.

General Considerations

Acute organic intestinal obstruction usually involves the small intestine, particularly the ileum. Major inciting causes are external hernia and postoperative adhesions. Less common causes are gallstones, neoplasms, granulomatous processes, intussusception, volvulus, internal hernia, and foreign bodies.

Clinical Findings

A. Symptoms and Signs: Colicky abdominal pain in the periumbilical area becomes more constant and diffuse as distention develops. Vomiting, at first of a reflex nature associated with the waves of pain, later becomes fecal in obstruction of the distal bowel. Borborygmus and consciousness of intestinal movement, obstipation, weakness, perspiration, and anxiety are often present. The patient is restless, changing position frequently with pain, and is often in a shocklike state, with sweating, tachycardia, and dehydration. Abdominal distention may be localized, with an isolated loop, but usually is generalized. The higher the obstruction, the less the distention; the longer the time of obstruction, the greater the distention. Audible peristalsis, peristaltic rushes with pain paroxysms, high-pitched tinkles, and visible peristalsis may be present. Moderate generalized abdominal tenderness may be present, and there are no signs of peritoneal irritation. Fever is absent or low-grade. A tender hernia may be present.

B. Laboratory Findings: Hemoconcentration

may occur with true dehydration or may reflect sequestration of fluid in the obstructed loop or third space. Leukocytosis is absent or mild. Vomiting may cause electrolyte disturbances.

C. X-Ray Findings: Abdominal x-ray reveals gas- and fluid-filled loops of bowel, and the gas does not progress downward on serial x-rays. Fluid levels may be visible.

Differential Diagnosis

Differentiate from other acute abdominal conditions such as inflammation and perforation of a viscus or renal or gallbladder colic. The absence of peritoneal signs, ie, rigidity and rebound tenderness, should aid in differentiating small bowel obstruction from ileus secondary to peritonitis. The absence of leukocytosis and the presence of high-pitched bowel sounds or intestinal rushes are also helpful. Differentiate also from mesenteric vascular disease and torsion of an organ (eg, ovarian cyst). In the late stages of obstruction it may be impossible to distinguish acute organic intestinal obstruction from the late stage of peritonitis with ileus.

Complications

Strangulation (necrosis of the bowel wall) occurs with impairment of the blood supply to the gut. Strangulation is difficult to determine clinically, but fever, marked leukocytosis, and signs of peritoneal irritation should alert the clinician to this possibility. Strangulation may lead to perforation, peritonitis, and sepsis. Strangulation increases the mortality rate of intestinal obstruction to about 25%.

Treatment

A. Supportive Measures:

1. Decompression of the intestinal tract by nasogastric suction should relieve vomiting, reduce intestinal distention, and prevent aspiration. Tube decompression may be successful in relieving partial small bowel obstruction.

2. Correct fluid, electrolyte, and colloid deficits.

3. Give broad-spectrum antibiotics (gentamicin, ampicillin, or clindamycin) if strangulation is suspected.

4. The level of obstruction must be delineated; this is often best achieved initially by a barium enema.

B. Surgical Measures: Complete obstruction of the intestine is treated surgically after appropriate supportive therapy. Strangulation is always a danger as long as obstruction persists, and fever, leukocytosis, peritoneal signs, or blood in the feces mean that strangulation may have occurred and that immediate surgery is required.

If the bowel is successfully decompressed during the preoperative preparation period, with cessation of pain and passage of flatus and feces, surgery may be delayed. Otherwise, surgical relief of the obstruction is indicated. Surgery consists of relieving the obstruction and removing gangrenous bowel with reanastomosis.

Prognosis

Prognosis varies with the causative factor and the presence of strangulation.

Sarr MG, Bulkley GB, Zuidema GD: Preoperative recognition of intestinal strangulation obstruction: Prospective evaluation of diagnostic capability. *Am J Surg* 1983;**145**:176.

FUNCTIONAL OBSTRUCTION
(Adynamic Ileus, Paralytic Ileus, Pseudo-obstruction, Ogilvie's Syndrome)

Essentials of Diagnosis

- Continuous abdominal pain, distention, vomiting, and obstipation.
- History of a precipitating factor (surgery, peritonitis, pain).
- Minimal abdominal tenderness; decreased to absent bowel sounds.
- X-ray evidence of gas and fluid in bowel.

General Considerations

Adynamic ileus is a neurogenic impairment of peristalsis that may lead to intestinal obstruction. It is a common disorder that may be due to a variety of intra-abdominal causes, eg, gastrointestinal surgery, peritoneal irritation (hemorrhage, ruptured viscus, pancreatitis, peritonitis), or anoxic organic obstruction. Drugs with anticholinergic properties, renal colic, vertebral fractures, spinal cord injuries, severe infections, uremia, diabetic coma, and electrolyte abnormalities also may cause adynamic ileus.

Clinical Findings

A. Symptoms and Signs: There is mild to moderate abdominal pain, continuous rather than colicky, associated with vomiting (which may later become fecal) and obstipation. Borborygmus is absent. Symptoms of the initiating condition may also be present (eg, fever; prostration due to ruptured viscus).

Abdominal distention is generalized and may be massive, with nonlocalized minimal abdominal tenderness and no signs of peritoneal irritation unless due to the primary disease. Bowel sounds are decreased to absent. Dehydration may occur after prolonged vomiting or from sequestration of fluid in bowel loops. Other signs of the initiating disorder may be present.

B. Laboratory Findings: With prolonged vomiting, hemoconcentration and electrolyte imbalance may occur. Leukocytosis, anemia, and elevated serum amylase may be present, depending upon the initiating condition.

C. X-Ray Findings: X-ray of the abdomen shows distended gas-filled loops of bowel in the small and large intestines and even in the rectum. There may be evidence of air-fluid levels in the distended bowel. When the clinical problem is unclear, a barium enema and subsequent small bowel x-ray will rule out organic obstruction.

Differential Diagnosis

The symptoms and signs of obstruction with absent bowel sounds and a history of a precipitating condition leave little doubt about the diagnosis. It is important to make certain that the adynamic ileus is not secondary to an organic obstruction, especially anoxic, where conservative management is harmful and immediate surgery may be lifesaving.

Treatment

Most cases of adynamic ileus are postoperative and respond to restriction of oral intake with gradual liberalization of the diet as the bowel function returns. Severe and prolonged ileus may require gastrointestinal suction and complete restriction of oral intake. Parenteral restoration of fluids and electrolytes is essential in such instances. When conservative therapy fails, it may be necessary to operate for the purpose of decompressing the bowel by enterostomy or cecostomy and to rule out mechanical obstruction.

Those cases of adynamic ileus secondary to other diseases (eg, electrolyte imbalance, severe infection, intra-abdominal or back injury, pneumonitis) are managed as above plus treatment of the primary disease.

Prognosis

The prognosis varies with that of the initiating disorder. Adynamic ileus may resolve without specific therapy when the cause is removed. Intubation with decompression is usually successful in causing return of function.

Ellis H: *Intestinal Obstruction.* Appleton-Century-Crofts, 1981.

INTESTINAL PSEUDO-OBSTRUCTION

This idiopathic disorder, usually seen in teenagers or young adults, is characterized by recurring symptoms of small bowel obstruction but no evidence of organic obstruction on x-ray or with surgical exploration. All previously mentioned causes of functional obstruction are absent. The clinical course is progressively downhill unless the patient is treated with nasogastric suction, intravenous fluids, and parenteral nutrition as required.

Hirsh EH et al: Chronic intestinal pseudo-obstruction. *J Clin Gastroenterol* 1981;**3**:247.

Strodel WE et al: Therapeutic and diagnostic colonoscopy in nonobstructive colonic dilatation. *Ann Surg* 1983;**197**:416.

MALABSORPTION SYNDROMES
(Primary Mucosal Disease)

Malabsorption syndromes may be associated with a wide variety of small intestine mucosal disease processes that have in common the malabsorption of nutrients by the gastrointestinal tract. These syndromes should be contrasted to states of maldigestion where intraluminal abnormalities result in failure to absorb nutrients, such as pancreatic insufficiency, bile salt deficiency, and a variety of postsurgical abnormalities. The clinical and laboratory manifestations are summarized in Table 11-1.

Sleisenger MH et al: Malabsorption and nutritional support. *Clin Gastroenterol* 1983;**12**:323.

Table 11–1. Clinical and laboratory manifestations of malabsorption.*

Manifestation	Laboratory Findings	Malabsorbed Nutrient
Steatorrhea (bulky, light-colored)	Increased fecal fat; decreased serum cholesterol	Fat
Diarrhea (increased fecal water)	Increased fecal fat and/or positive bile salt breath test	Fatty acids and/or bile salts
Weight loss; malnutrition (muscle wasting); weakness, fatigue	Increased fecal fat and nitrogen; decreased glucose and xylose absorption	Calories (fat, protein, carbohydrates)
Abdominal distention		
Iron deficiency anemia	Hypochromic anemia; low serum iron	Iron
Megaloblastic anemia	Macrocytosis; decreased vitamin B_{12} absorption ([67]Co-labeled B_{12}); decreased serum vitamin B_{12} and folic acid activity (microbiologic assay)	Vitamin B_{12} and/or folic acid
Paresthesia; tetany; positive Trousseau and Chvostek signs	Decreased serum calcium, magnesium, and potassium	Calcium, vitamin D, magnesium, potassium
Bone pain; pathologic fractures; skeletal deformities	Osteoporosis; osteomalacia on x-ray	Calcium, protein
Bleeding tendency (ecchymoses, melena, hematuria)	Prolonged prothrombin time	Vitamin K
Edema	Decreased serum albumin; increased fecal loss of ^{51}Cr-labeled albumin	Protein (and/or protein-losing enteropathy)
Nocturia; abdominal distention	Increased small bowel fluid on x-ray	Water
Milk intolerance (cramps, bloating, diarrhea)	Flat lactose tolerance test; decreased mucosal lactase levels	Lactose

*Modified from Bayless TM: Malabsorption in the elderly. *Hosp Pract* (Aug) 1979;**14**:57.

CELIAC SPRUE
& TROPICAL SPRUE

Essentials of Diagnosis

- Bulky, pale, frothy, foul-smelling, greasy stools with increased fecal fat on chemical analysis of the stool.
- Weight loss and signs of multiple vitamin deficiencies.
- Impaired intestinal absorption of vitamins, fat; large amounts of fat in the stool.
- Hypochromic or megaloblastic anemia; small bowel x-ray pattern that of small bowel dilatation and dilution of barium.

General Considerations

Sprue syndromes are diseases of disturbed small intestine function characterized by impaired absorption, particularly of fats, and motor abnormalities. Celiac sprue responds to a gluten-free diet, whereas tropical sprue does not. The polypeptide gliadin is the offending substance in gluten. Although an infectious cause has not been conclusively demonstrated, tropical sprue behaves clinically like an infectious disease. It responds to folic acid and broad-spectrum antibiotics.

The clinical severity of sprue syndrome varies depending upon the extent of the lesion in the small intestine and the duration of the disease. Severe wasting, gastrointestinal protein loss, multiple vitamin deficiencies, and adrenal and pituitary deficiency may be associated with the severe forms of the disease. A flat intestinal mucosa without villi in the small intestine is noted, and some observers have described degenerative changes in the myenteric nerve plexuses.

Rare secondary varieties of sprue syndrome in which the cause of the small intestine dysfunction is known include gastrocolic fistulas, obstruction of intestinal lacteals by lymphoma, Whipple's disease, extensive regional enteritis, and parasitic infections such as giardiasis, cryptosporidiasis, strongyloidiasis, and coccidiosis.

Clinical Findings

A. Tropical Sprue: Patients with tropical sprue are either residents of, or have had prolonged visits in, tropical regions. The main symptom is diarrhea; at first it is explosive and watery; later, stools are fewer and more solid and characteristically pale, frothy, foul-smelling, and greasy, with exacerbations on high-fat diet. Indigestion, flatulence, abdominal cramps, weight loss (often marked), pallor, asthenia, irritability, paresthesias, and muscle cramps may occur. Quiescent periods with or without mild symptoms may occur especially on leaving the tropics. Symptoms may appear years after the patient has left endemic areas.

Vitamin deficiencies cause glossitis, cheilosis, angular stomatitis, cutaneous hyperpigmentation, and dry, rough skin. Abdominal distention and mild tenderness are present. Edema occurs late.

Anemia is usually macrocytic, and, with blood loss or malabsorption of iron, may be hypochromic, microcytic, or mixed. The fecal fat is increased. Serum proteins, calcium, phosphorus, cholesterol, and prothrombin are low. Gastric hypochlorhydria is frequent. The pancreatic enzymes are normal.

X-rays using nonflocculating barium show dilatation of the intestine and occasionally excess fluid and gas.

B. Celiac Sprue: This disorder is characterized by defective absorption of fat, protein, carbohydrates, iron, and water. Absorption of fat-soluble vitamins A, D, and K is impaired. Osteomalacia may ensue. Protein loss from the intestine may occur. Elimination of gluten from the diet causes dramatic improvement. The polypeptide gliadin is the offending substance in gluten. Gluten is found in wheat, barley, oats, and rye and is used as a filler in many prepared foods. Diligent elimination of this substance from the diet is important in achieving remission.

In one-third of patients with celiac sprue, symptoms begin in early childhood. Symptoms may persist into adult life, but there is usually a latent phase of apparent good health. The anemia is usually hypochromic and microcytic. The complications of impaired absorption are more severe: infantilism, dwarfism, tetany, vitamin deficiency signs, and even rickets may be seen. The definitive diagnosis of steatorrhea requires quantitative measurement of fecal fat, preferably on a known fat intake, and a characteristic small bowel biopsy.

A small group of patients with apparent celiac sprue are nonresponsive to a gluten-free diet. On closer inspection of the small bowel mucosal biopsy, a collagenous layer is found between the surface absorptive cells and the lamina propria. No consistently helpful medical therapy has yet been found.

Differential Diagnosis

It is necessary to differentiate between the various causes of malabsorption to permit selection of specific therapy, if any. Anatomic abnormalities such as fistulas, blind loops, and jejunal diverticulosis may be found on x-ray. Regional enteritis usually has a characteristic appearance but must be distinguished from intestinal tuberculosis and lymphoma. The small bowel x-ray appearance in Whipple's disease, nodular lymphoid hyperplasia, intestinal lymphoma, and amyloidosis is abnormal but not specific or diagnostic. In primary diseases of the small intestine, mucosal suction biopsy is the most effective way of making the diagnosis. The pathologic response in some diseases is patchy, and multiple specimens may be required. Pancreatic insufficiency due to obstruction may be diagnosed by a low water and bicarbonate secretion in response to intravenous administration of secretin.

Treatment

A. Tropical Sprue: Folic acid, 10–20 mg daily orally or intramuscularly for a few weeks, corrects diarrhea, anorexia, weight loss, glossitis, and anemia.

Tetracycline, 250 mg orally 4 times daily, is given at the outset of treatment. When complete remission occurs, the patient may be maintained on 5 mg of folic acid daily. If the patient has achlorhydria, giving vitamin B_{12} intramuscularly should also be considered. Hypochromic anemia can be treated with oral iron. A high-calorie, high-protein, low-fat diet can be given.

B. Celiac Sprue: Strict elimination of gluten from the diet will lead to clinical recovery. If there is no response, another diagnosis must be sought. The diet should be high in calories and protein, low in fat, and gluten-free. Prothrombin deficiency is treated by means of water-soluble vitamin K orally or, if urgent, parenterally. Treat hypocalcemia or tetany with calcium phosphate or gluconate, 2 g orally or intravenously 3 times daily, and vitamin D, 5–20 thousand units. Multiple vitamin supplements may also be advisable. Macrocytic anemia usually responds to vitamin B_{12}, 100 μg intramuscularly every month until the disease is in clinical remission.

The corticosteroids may be advantageous in certain patients with sprue, particularly the severely ill, since they increase the absorption of nitrogen, fats, and other nutrients from the gastrointestinal tract. They have a nonspecific effect in increasing appetite and inducing mild euphoria. Cortisol is best given in dosages of 100–300 mg/24 h intravenously and tapered off according to the patient's response.

Prognosis

With proper treatment, the response is good. Patients with celiac sprue have a late increased incidence of abdominal lymphoma and carcinomas. Patients who develop gastrointestinal symptoms while in remission on a gluten-free diet should be carefully evaluated for cancer.

Klipstein FA: Tropical sprue in travelers and expatriates living abroad. *Gastroenterology* 1981;**80**:590.

Ross IN et al: Immunologic changes in tropical sprue. *Q J Med* 1981;**50**:435.

Swinson CM et al: Coeliac disease and malignancy. *Lancet* 1983; **1**:111.

Trier JS: Celiac sprue. Pages 1050–1067 in: *Gastrointestinal Disease*, 3rd ed. Sleisenger MH, Fordtran JS (editors). Saunders, 1983.

DISACCHARIDASE DEFICIENCY

Lactase deficiency may occur in a congenital or adult-onset form. With the congenital form, the absence of lactase leads to acidic diarrhea (fecal pH 4.5–6). There are large amounts of lactic acid in the stool secondary to bacterial breakdown of lactose. The infant fails to thrive until lactose-containing foods are eliminated from the diet.

Lactase deficiency in the adult is common worldwide. It has been estimated from many studies that the incidence of lactase deficiency is 70–90% in Orientals, blacks, American Indians, and Mediterranean populations. The incidence of lactase deficiency in northern and western Europeans is 10–15%. Symptoms may vary from minor abdominal bloating, distension, and discomfort to markedly severe diarrhea in response to even small amounts of lactose. The diagnosis is confirmed by a lactose tolerance test; marked diarrhea usually occurs with this test. Onset in the adult may follow gastroduodenal surgery and may be associated with regional enteritis. The primary mucosal diseases of the small intestine usually have associated lactase deficiency.

Intercurrent acute illnesses, such as viral and bacterial enteritis, particularly in children, will frequently injure the microvilli of the mucosal cells of the small intestine, resulting in temporary lactase deficiency.

Other congenital defects described thus far are sucrose-isomaltose and glucose-galactose intolerance. Secondary disaccharidase deficiencies have been described in patients with giardiasis, celiac disease, ulcerative colitis, short bowel syndrome, and cystic fibrosis and postgastrectomy. Removal of the offending sugar from the diet will often result in remission (see p 801).

Ferguson A, Macdonald DM, Brydon WG: Prevalence of lactase deficiency in British adults. *Gut* 1984;**25**:163.

WHIPPLE'S DISEASE

Whipple's disease is an uncommon malabsorption disorder of unknown cause with widespread systemic manifestations. Histologic examination of a small bowel mucosal biopsy specimen reveals characteristic large, foamy mononuclear cells filled with cytoplasmic material that gives a positive periodic acid–Schiff staining reaction. Electron microscopic studies reveal bacterial bodies in the epithelium and lamina propria. The disease occurs primarily in middle-aged men and is of insidious onset; without treatment, it is usually fatal. The clinical manifestations include abdominal pain, diarrhea, steatorrhea, gastrointestinal bleeding, fever, lymphadenopathy, polyarthritis, edema, gray to brown skin pigmentation, and severe neurologic manifestations. Anemia and hypoproteinemia are common.

Treatment consists of tetracycline, 250 mg 4 times daily, or oral penicillin G, 600,000 units twice daily. The duration of treatment should be at least 6 months. Reappearance of symptoms after or during therapy suggests emergence of resistant organisms, and the antibiotic should be changed.

Bayless TM, Knox DL: Whipple's disease: A multisystem infection. (Editorial.) *N Engl J Med* 1979;**300**:920.

PROTEIN-LOSING ENTEROPATHY

Leakage of plasma proteins into the intestinal lumen is an integral phase of the metabolism of plasma proteins. In certain intestinal disease states, excessive protein loss into the intestinal lumen may be responsible for the hypoproteinemia that occurs. Excessive loss of plasma protein may be due to increased mucosal permeability to protein, inflammatory exudation, excessive cell desquamation, or direct leakage of lymph from obstructed lacteals. Gastrointestinal diseases associated with protein-losing enteropathy include all of the primary mucosal diseases of the small bowel, as well as gastric carcinoma, lymphoma, gastric rugal hypertrophy, sprue, and others.

Treatment consists of management of the primary disorder.

Sleisinger MH, Kim YS: Protein digestion and absorption. *N Engl J Med* 1979;**300:**659.

APPENDICITIS

Essentials of Diagnosis

- Right lower quadrant abdominal pain and tenderness with signs of peritoneal irritation.
- Anorexia, nausea, vomiting, and constipation.
- Low-grade fever and mild polymorphonuclear leukocytosis.

General Considerations

Appendicitis is initiated by obstruction of the appendiceal lumen by a fecalith, inflammation, foreign body, or neoplasm. Obstruction is followed by infection, edema, and, frequently, infarction of the appendiceal wall. Intraluminal tension develops rapidly and tends to cause early mural necrosis and perforation. All ages and both sexes are affected, but appendicitis is more common in males between 10 and 30 years of age.

Appendicitis is one of the most frequent causes of acute surgical abdomen. The symptoms and signs usually follow a fairly stereotyped pattern, but appendicitis is capable of such protean manifestations that it should be considered in the differential diagnosis of every obscure case of intra-abdominal sepsis and pain.

Clinical Findings

A. Symptoms and Signs: An attack of appendicitis usually begins with epigastric or periumbilical pain associated with 1–2 episodes of vomiting. Within 2–12 hours, the pain shifts to the right lower quadrant, where it persists as a steady soreness that is aggravated by walking or coughing. There is anorexia, moderate malaise, and slight fever. Constipation is usual, but diarrhea occurs occasionally.

At onset there are no localized abdominal findings. Within a few hours, however, progressive right lower quadrant tenderness can be demonstrated; careful examination will usually identify a single point of maximal tenderness. The patient can often place a finger precisely on this area, especially if asked to accentuate the soreness by coughing. Light percussion over the right lower quadrant is helpful in localizing tenderness. Rebound tenderness and spasm of the overlying abdominal muscles are usually present. Psoas and obturator signs, when positive, are strongly suggestive of appendicitis. Rectal tenderness is common and, in pelvic appendicitis, may be more definite than abdominal tenderness. Peristalsis is diminished or absent. Slight to moderate fever is present.

B. Laboratory Findings: Moderate leukocytosis (10–20 thousand/μL) with an increase in neutrophils is usually present. It is not uncommon to find microscopic hematuria and pyuria.

C. X-Ray Findings: There are no characteristic changes on plain films of the abdomen. However, visualization in the right lower quadrant of a radiopaque shadow consistent with fecalith in the appendix may heighten the suspicion of appendicitis. In uncertain cases, barium enemas are being used, as visualization of the entire appendix rules out acute appendicitis.

Factors That Cause Variations From the "Classic" Clinical Picture

A. Anatomic Location of Appendix: Abdominal findings are most definite when the appendix is in the iliac fossa or superficially located. When the appendix extends over the pelvic brim, abdominal signs may be minimal, greatest tenderness being elicited on rectal examination. Right lower quadrant tenderness may be poorly localized and slow to develop in retrocecal or retroileal appendicitis. Inflammation of a high-lying lateral appendix may produce maximal tenderness in the flank, and in the left lower quadrant in situs inversus. Bizarre locations of the appendix may rarely occur in association with a mobile or undescended cecum; in such cases, symptoms and signs may localize in the right upper or left lower quadrant.

B. Age:

1. Infancy and childhood–In infancy, appendicitis is relatively rare. When it does occur, history and physical findings are difficult to interpret. The disease tends to progress rapidly, and rupture results in generalized peritonitis.

2. Old age–Elderly patients frequently have few or no prodromal symptoms. Abdominal findings may be unimpressive, with slight tenderness and negligible muscle guarding, until perforation occurs. Fever and leukocytosis may also be minimal or absent. When the white count is not elevated, a shift to the left is significant evidence of inflammation.

3. Obesity–Obesity frequently increases the difficulty of evaluation by delaying the appearance of abdominal signs and by preventing sharp localization.

4. Pregnancy–See discussion in Chapter 13.

Differential Diagnosis

Acute gastroenteritis is the disorder most commonly confused with appendicitis. In rare cases it either precedes or is coincident with appendicitis. Vomiting and diarrhea are more common. Fever and the white blood count may rise sharply and may be out of proportion to abdominal findings. Localization of pain and tenderness is usually indefinite and shifting. Hyperactive peristalsis is characteristic. Gastroenteritis frequently runs an acute course. A period of observation usually serves to clarify the diagnosis.

Mesenteric adenitis may cause signs and symptoms identical with appendicitis. Usually, however, there are some clues to the true diagnosis. Mesenteric adenitis is more likely to occur in children or adolescents; respiratory infection is a common antecedent; localization of right lower quadrant tenderness is less precise and constant; and true muscle guarding is infrequent. In spite of a strong suspicion of mesenteric adenitis, it is often safer to advise appendectomy than to risk a complication of appendicitis by delay.

Meckel's diverticulitis may mimic appendicitis. The localization of tenderness may be more medial, but this is not a reliable diagnostic criterion. Because operation is required in both diseases, the differentiation is not critical. When a preoperative diagnosis of appendicitis proves on exploration to be erroneous, it is essential to examine the terminal 150 cm of ileum for Meckel's diverticulitis and mesenteric adenitis.

Regional enteritis, amebiasis, perforated duodenal ulcer, ureteral colic, acute salpingitis, mittelschmerz, ruptured ectopic pregnancy, and twisted ovarian cyst may also be confused with appendicitis.

Complications

A. Perforation: Appendicitis may rarely subside spontaneously, but it is an unpredictable disease with a marked tendency (about 95%) to progression and perforation. Because perforation rarely occurs within the first 8 hours, diagnostic observation during this period is relatively safe. Signs of perforation include increasing severity of pain, tenderness, and spasm in the right lower quadrant followed by evidence of generalized peritonitis or of a localized abscess. Ileus, fever, malaise, and leukocytosis become more marked. If perforation with abscess formation or generalized peritonitis has already occurred when the patient is first seen, the diagnosis may be quite obscure.

The treatment of perforated appendicitis is appendectomy unless a well-localized right lower quadrant or pelvic abscess has already walled off the appendix. Supportive measures are as for acute peritonitis.

1. Generalized peritonitis–This is a common sequela to perforation. Clinical findings and treatment are discussed elsewhere in this chapter.

2. Appendiceal abscess–This is one of the possible complications of untreated appendicitis. Malaise, toxicity, fever, and leukocytosis vary from minimal to marked. Examination discloses a tender mass in the right lower quadrant or pelvis. Pelvic abscesses tend to bulge into the rectum or vagina.

Abscesses usually become noticeable 2–6 days after onset, but antibiotic therapy may delay their ap-

pearance. Appendiceal abscess is occasionally the first and only sign of appendicitis and may be confused with neoplasm of the cecum, particularly in older persons, who may have little or no systemic reaction to the infection.

Treatment of early abscess is by intensive combined antibiotic therapy (eg, penicillin and gentamicin or clindamycin). On this regimen, the abscess will frequently resolve. Appendectomy should be performed 6–12 weeks later. A well-established progressive abscess in the right lower quadrant should be drained without delay. Pelvic abscess requires drainage when it bulges into the rectum or vagina and has become fluctuant.

B. Pylephlebitis: Suppurative thrombophlebitis of the portal system with liver abscess is a rare but highly lethal complication. It should be suspected when septic fever, chills, hepatomegaly, and jaundice develop after appendiceal perforation. Intensive combined antibiotic therapy with surgical drainage of the abscesses is indicated.

C. Other Complications: These include subphrenic abscess and other foci of intra-abdominal sepsis. Intestinal obstruction may be caused by adhesions.

Treatment

A. Preoperative Care:

1. Observation for diagnosis–Within the first 8–12 hours after onset, the symptoms and signs of appendicitis are frequently indefinite. Under these circumstances a period of close observation is essential. The patient is placed at bed rest and given nothing by mouth. *Note:* Laxatives should not be prescribed when appendicitis or any form of peritonitis is suspected. Parenteral fluid therapy is begun as indicated. Narcotic medications are avoided if possible, but sedation with tranquilizing agents is not contraindicated. Abdominal and rectal examinations, white blood count, and differential count are repeated periodically. Abdominal films and an upright chest film must be obtained as part of the investigation of all difficult diagnostic problems. In most cases of appendicitis, the diagnosis is clarified by localization of signs to the right lower quadrant within 12 hours after onset of symptoms.

2. Intubation–Preoperatively, a nasogastric tube is inserted if there is sufficient peritonitis or toxicity to indicate that postoperative ileus may be troublesome. In such patients the stomach is aspirated and lavaged if necessary, and the patient is sent to the operating room with the tube in place.

3. Antibiotics–In the presence of a marked systemic reaction with severe toxicity and high fever, preoperative administration of antibiotics (eg, penicillin and cephalothin or gentamicin) is advisable.

B. Surgical Treatment: In uncomplicated appendicitis, appendectomy is performed as soon as fluid imbalance and other significant systemic disturbances are controlled. Little preparation is usually required. Early surgery has a mortality rate of a fraction of 1%. The morbidity and mortality rates associated with this disease reflect the occurrence of gangrene and perforation that occur when operation is delayed.

C. Postoperative Care: In uncomplicated appendicitis, postoperative gastric suction is usually not necessary. Ambulation is begun on the first postoperative day. The diet is advanced from clear liquids to soft solids during the second to fifth postoperative days depending upon the rapidity with which peristalsis and gastrointestinal function return. Parenteral fluid supplements are administered as required. Enemas are contraindicated. Milk of magnesia or a similar mild laxative may be given orally at bedtime daily from about the third day onward if necessary. Antibiotic therapy (eg, penicillin and gentamicin or clindamycin) is advisable for 5–7 days, or longer if abdominal fluid at operation was purulent or malodorous, if culture was positive, or if the appendix was gangrenous. Primary wound healing is the rule, and the period of hospitalization is usually 1 week or less. Normal activity can usually be resumed in 2–3 weeks after surgery in uncomplicated cases.

D. Emergency Nonsurgical Treatment: When surgical facilities are not available, treat as for acute peritonitis. On such a regimen, acute appendicitis may subside, and complications will be minimized.

Prognosis

With accurate diagnosis and early surgical removal, mortality and morbidity rates are minimal. Delay of diagnosis produces significant mortality and morbidity rates if complications occur.

Recurrent acute attacks may occur if the appendix is not removed. "Chronic appendicitis" does not exist.

Buchman TG, Zuidema GD: Reasons for delay of the diagnosis of acute appendicitis. *Surg Gynecol Obstet* 1984;**158**:260.

Murray HW: Is the appendix boring? *Arch Intern Med* 1981; **141**:571.

ACUTE MESENTERIC LYMPHADENITIS

Essentials of Diagnosis

- Acute right lower quadrant or periumbilical pain in a child.
- Anorexia, nausea, vomiting, fever to 39.5 °C (103.1 °F).
- Right lower quadrant tenderness with minimal or no peritoneal irritation.
- Leukocytosis generally over $15,000/\mu L$.
- History of recent or current upper respiratory infection.

General Considerations

Mesenteric lymphadenitis is an acute benign inflammation of the mesenteric lymph nodes causing fever and abdominal pain. It is usually a disease of children, may be recurrent, and presents a major problem in differentiation from acute appendicitis,

Meckel's diverticulitis, renal infection or colic, and right lower lobe pulmonary infections in children with pain referred to the right lower quadrant. Episodes are often preceded or accompanied by upper respiratory infections. Bacteria (staphylococci, streptococci, yersiniae) and viruses have been implicated.

Clinical Findings

A. Symptoms and Signs: There is an acute onset of abdominal pain in the right lower quadrant or periumbilical area, generally steady from the onset rather than colicky, and associated with nausea, vomiting, and anorexia. Diarrhea often occurs. Abdominal tenderness is mild to severe and usually greatest in the right lower quadrant; point localization of pain is unusual. Peritoneal irritation and right vault rectal tenderness are mild or absent. Fever to 37.8–39.5 °C (100–103.1 °F) is usually present.

B. Laboratory Findings: There is polymorphonuclear leukocytosis with a shift to the left, generally over $15,000/\mu L$ and higher than would be expected from the findings.

Treatment & Prognosis

Exploration may be warranted to be certain that the patient does not have appendicitis. Complete resolution is the rule. *Yersinia* infection will usually respond to tetracyclines, kanamycin, or streptomycin.

Pai CH, Gillis F, Marks MI: Infection due to *Yersinia enterocolitica* in children with abdominal pain. *J Infect Dis* 1982; **146**:705.

INTESTINAL TUBERCULOSIS
(Tuberculous Enterocolitis)

Gastrointestinal tuberculosis may occur anywhere along the gastrointestinal tract. Involvement of the intestine frequently complicates pulmonary tuberculosis. Ingestion of milk containing tubercle bacilli is another means of infection.

The mode of infection is by ingestion of tubercle bacilli, with the formation of ulcerating lesions in the intestine, particularly the ileocecal region, and involvement of the mesenteric lymph nodes.

Symptoms may be absent or minimal even with extensive disease. When present, they usually consist of fever, anorexia, nausea, flatulence, distention after eating, and food intolerance. There may be abdominal pain and mild to severe cramps, usually in the right lower quadrant and often after meals. Constipation may be present, but mild to severe diarrhea is more characteristic. Tuberculosis may involve the peritoneum. It may appear as a primary infection, and the disease course is chronic.

Findings on abdominal examination are not characteristic, although there may be mild right lower quadrant tenderness. Fistula in ano may be evident. Weight loss occurs.

There are no characteristic laboratory findings.

The presence of tubercle bacilli in the feces does not correlate with intestinal involvement.

X-ray examination of the involved bowel reveals irritability and spasm, particularly in the cecal region; irregular hypermotility of the intestinal tract; ulcerated lesions and irregular filling defects, particularly in the right colon and ileocecal region; and usually pulmonary tuberculosis.

The prognosis varies with that of the pulmonary disease. The intestinal lesions usually respond to chemotherapy and rest when reexposure to infecting material is prevented. Operation may be required for intestinal obstruction or for diagnosis.

Kasulke RJ et al: Primary tuberculous enterocolitis: Report of 3 cases and review of literature. *Arch Surg* 1981;**116**:110.

DISEASES OF THE COLON & RECTUM

IRRITABLE BOWEL SYNDROME

Irritable bowel syndrome is a term denoting a clinical entity characterized by some combination of (1) abdominal pain; (2) altered bowel function, constipation, or diarrhea; (3) hypersecretion of colonic mucus; (4) dyspeptic symptoms (flatulence, nausea, anorexia); and (5) varying degrees of anxiety or depression. This common group of disorders has many names, eg, nervous indigestion, functional dyspepsia, pylorospasm, irritable colon, spastic "colitis," functional "colitis," mucous "colitis," intestinal neurosis, and laxative or cathartic "colitis."

Three main factors appear significant in the pathogenesis of irritable bowel syndrome.

(1) Colonic motor activity: There is no abnormality of either motility or electrical activity of the colon specific to the irritable bowel syndrome. However, prediverticular disease can be frequently demonstrated and is characterized by increased width of the sigmoid circular muscles, increased segmentation, and nonpropulsive intraluminal pressures. Colonic motor activity is abnormally increased in patients with colonic pain, eg, after meals, after administration of cholecystokinin or cholinergic drugs, or after emotional stress.

(2) Psychologic stress: Many patients with irritable bowel syndrome exhibit colonic symptoms at times of stress. The disturbances of colonic function are the usual bodily manifestations of emotional tension. The reaction, however, may be more severe in patients with irritable bowel.

(3) Diet: A low-residue diet in some patients may be a prominent predisposing factor. Intolerance of lactose and other sugars may account for irritable bowel syndrome in certain patients.

It is essential to eliminate the possibility of organic gastrointestinal disease. A history of "nervousness," neuropathic traits, and emotional disturbances can usually be obtained. Bowel consciousness and cathartic and enema habits are prominent features. There is a highly variable complex of gastrointestinal symptoms: nausea and vomiting, anorexia, foul breath, sour stomach, flatulence, cramps, and constipation or diarrhea; hysteria and depression are the most prevalent syndromes.

Nocturnal diarrhea, awakening the patient from a sound sleep, is frequently a result of organic disease of the bowel.

Examination discloses variable abdominal tenderness, particularly along the course of the colon. Sigmoidoscopy often reveals marked spasm and mucus in the colonic lumen and will frequently provoke the patient's spontaneously occurring symptoms. Laboratory studies should include a complete blood count and stool examination to rule out the presence of occult blood, ova, parasites, and pathogenic bacteria. Gastrointestinal x-rays may show altered gastrointestinal motility without other evidence of abnormalities.

Treatment

A. Diet: No single diet is applicable to all patients with irritable bowel syndrome. Some patients may respond to an increase in dietary fiber. Exclusion of milk and milk products may prove helpful. Irrational fear of foods must be dispelled.

B. Personal Habits: Regular hours and meals and adequate sleep, exercise, and recreation are important. Restriction of alcohol and tobacco may be indicated.

C. Psychotherapy: Reassurance is important. Once the diagnosis has been established, the patient should be reassured that the symptoms are not due to an organic disease. Anxiety states or depression should be treated appropriately.

D. Symptomatic Treatment: Sedative-antispasmodic medication may be of value.

E. Vegetable Mucilages: Psyllium hydrophilic mucilloid (Metamucil) may be useful.

Jones VA et al: Food intolerance: A major factor in the pathogenesis of irritable bowel syndrome. *Lancet* 1982;**2**:1115.

Schuster MM: Irritable bowel syndrome. Pages 880–895 in: *Gastrointestinal Disease*, 3rd ed. Sleisenger MH, Fordtran JS (editors). Saunders, 1983.

Thompson WG: Progress report: The irritable bowel. *Gut* 1984;**25**:305.

INFECTIOUS COLITIS

Bacterial infections are common causes of acute colitis and are usually associated with fever, cramps, and diarrhea with tenesmus and often with blood in the stool. The most common causes are *Campylobacter jejuni*, *Shigella*, *Salmonella*, and *Yersinia enterocolitica*. (See Chapter 24.) Anal intercourse may be responsible for additional infectious diseases of the rectum, including gonorrhea, syphilis, lymphogranuloma venereum, condyloma latum, and herpes simplex. Sigmoidoscopy will usually reveal acute colitis with small ulcerations; a mucus smear will reveal polyps; and cultures should reveal the organism. Tuberculosis is an uncommon cause.

Acute and chronic colitis caused by parasites such as the protozoon *Entamoeba histolytica* is common worldwide and not uncommon in the USA. It may be clinically indistinguishable from other types of acute and chronic colitis; differentiation can often be made by smears of aspirates at sigmoidoscopy, multiple stool examinations, and, in patients with sigmoidoscopic abnormalities, mucosal biopsy. In chronic forms, the areas of involvement are most commonly the cecum, sigmoid colon, or rectum. The chronic form may mimic granulomatous colitis or neoplasm. Complications include local abscess, liver abscess, and fistula formation. For treatment, see p 896.

Quinn TC et al: The etiology of anorectal infections in homosexual men. *Am J Med* 1981;**71**:395.

ANTIBIOTIC-ASSOCIATED COLITIS

Antibiotic-associated colitis may occur during antibiotic usage or up to 2 weeks subsequent to usage. The disease usually subsides when the offending antibiotic is withdrawn, but it is potentially lethal and diagnosis should be pursued.

Pseudomembranous colitis is characterized by profuse watery diarrhea with cramps, tenesmus, low-grade fever, and, rarely, blood per rectum. Current or recent antibiotic therapy is the usual cause. Almost all antibiotics have been implicated; clindamycin, ampicillin, and the cephalosporins are most common. Metronidazole has been reported to be effective in treatment of pseudomembranous enterocolitis, but it has also been reported to be a cause of this disease. Uncommonly, the disease occurs without antibiotic usage.

Diarrhea occurs secondary to selective overgrowth of the bacterium *Clostridium difficile,* which produces a toxin that causes the lesion of pseudomembranous colitis. Laboratory assays for detecting this toxin in stool are now available and are important in establishing the diagnosis.

Physical findings may be minimal but can include a distended, tender abdomen with a dilated bowel. Sigmoidoscopy may reveal a pseudomembrane characterized by adherent plaques (mushroom caps) of exudate with intervening normal mucosa. Occasionally the exudate is confluent. When the pseudomembrane is stripped away, capillary type bleeding will occur from the denuded mucosa. In a few patients, routine sigmoidoscopy is normal but colonoscopy shows involvement of the sigmoid colon or more proximal areas. Sometimes only the right colon is involved.

Vancomycin, 500–1000 mg/d orally for 7–10 days, is the drug of choice; it is very expensive but about 90% effective. Metronidazole, 1.5–2 g/d orally 3 times a day for 7–14 days, has recently been shown to be effective and is less expensive. Cholestyramine, 4 g orally 4 times daily has also been reported as useful.

Complications include dehydration with electrolyte imbalance, perforation, toxic megacolon, and death.

A similar colitis without pseudomembrane is clinically indistinguishable from pseudomembranous colitis and may be more common. It is usually (not always) *Clostridium difficile* toxin-related. Sigmoidoscopy and occasionally colonoscopy will show evidence of acute colitis, usually right-sided. Ampicillin is often associated. All antibiotics should be withdrawn, and treatment should proceed as with pseudomembranous colitis if the toxin is demonstrated. Otherwise, treat expectantly.

Cherry RD et al: Metronidazole: An alternate therapy for antibiotic-associated colitis. *Gastroenterology* 1982;**82**:849.
Daly JJ, Chowdary KVS: Pseudomembranous colitis secondary to metronidazole. *Dig Dis Sci* 1983;**28**:573.
Silva J Jr: Treatment of *Clostridium difficile* colitis and diarrhea with vancomycin. *Am J Med* 1981;**71**:815.

NONSPECIFIC ULCERATIVE COLITIS

Essentials of Diagnosis
- Bloody diarrhea with lower abdominal cramps.
- Mild abdominal tenderness, weight loss, fever.
- Anemia; no stool pathogens.
- Specific x-ray and sigmoidoscopic abnormalities.

General Considerations
Ulcerative colitis is a chronic inflammatory disease of the colon of unknown cause characterized by bloody diarrhea, a tendency to remissions and exacerbations, and involvement mainly of the left colon. It is primarily a disease of adolescents and young adults but may have its onset in any age group.

The pathologic process is that of acute nonspecific inflammation in the colon, particularly the rectosigmoid area, with multiple irregular superficial ulcerations. Repeated episodes lead to thickening of the wall with scar tissue, and the proliferative changes in the epithelium may lead to polypoid structures. Pseudopolyps are usually indicative of severe ulceration. The cause is not known; it may be multiple.

Clinical Findings
A. Symptoms and Signs: This disease may vary from mild cases with relatively minimal symptoms to acute and fulminating, with severe diarrhea and prostration. Diarrhea is characteristic; there may be up to 30 or 40 discharges daily, with blood and mucus in the stools, or blood and mucus may occur without feces. Blood in the stool is the cardinal manifestation of

ulcerative colitis. Constipation may occur instead of diarrhea.

Nocturnal diarrhea is usually present when daytime diarrhea is severe. Rectal tenesmus may be severe, and anal incontinence may be present. Cramping lower abdominal pain often occurs but is generally mild. Anorexia, malaise, weakness, and fatigability may also be present. A history of intolerance to dairy products can often be obtained, and there is a tendency toward remissions and exacerbations.

Fever, weight loss, and evidence of toxemia vary with the severity of the disease. Abdominal tenderness is generally mild and occurs without signs of peritoneal irritation. Abdominal distention may be present in the fulminating form and is a poor prognostic sign. Rectal examination may show perianal irritation, fissures, hemorrhoids, fistulas, and abscesses.

B. Laboratory Findings: Hypochromic microcytic anemia due to blood loss is usually present. In acute disease, a polymorphonuclear leukocytosis may also be present. The sedimentation rate is usually elevated. Stools contain blood, pus, and mucus but no pathogenic organisms. Hypoproteinemia may occur. In the fulminating disease, electrolyte disturbances may be evident.

C. X-Ray Findings: As shown by x-ray, the involvement may be regional to generalized and may vary from irritability and fuzzy margins to pseudopolyps, decreased size of colon, shortening and narrowing of the lumen, and loss of haustral markings. When the disease is limited to the rectosigmoid area, the barium enema may even be normal.

D. Special Examinations: Sigmoidoscopic changes are present in over 95% of cases and vary from mucosal hyperemia, petechiae, and minimal granularity in mild cases to ulceration and polypoid changes in severe cases. The mucosa, even when it appears grossly normal, is almost invariably friable when wiped with a cotton sponge. Colonoscopic examination may prove useful in defining the extent of ulcerative colitis and in permitting biopsy of radiographically suspect regions.

Differential Diagnosis

Differentiate from bacillary dysentery and amebic dysentery on the basis of specific stool pathogens and (for amebiasis) the indirect hemagglutination test. When rectal strictures have developed, differentiate from lymphogranuloma venereum by history and complement fixation test. Other entities that must be distinguished are functional diarrhea, granulomatous colitis, intestinal neoplasm, and diverticulitis. It is imperative that any cultures and parasitology specimens be obtained before barium examinations are performed or before therapy is begun. Rectal abscesses and fistulas are considerably less frequent than in granulomatous colitis.

Complications

A. Local Complications: Local complications in and around the large bowel include ischiorectal abscess, fistula in ano, rectovaginal fistula, rectal prolapse, fibrous stricture of the rectum or colon, colonic perforation, toxic dilatation of the colon, carcinoma, and massive colonic hemorrhage.

The incidence of carcinoma is significantly greater in patients with ulcerative colitis. It appears to be related to 2 factors. The first is the extent of involvement. Involvement of the entire colon carries a greater risk than minimal disease. The second factor is duration of the disease. The risk rises from approximately 2% at 10 years to 10–15% at 20 years.

B. Systemic Complications: Systemic complications include pyoderma gangrenosum, erythema nodosum, polyarthritis, ankylosing spondylitis, ocular lesions (episcleritis, iritis, uveitis), liver disease (fatty liver, pericholangitis, sclerosing cholangitis), anemia, pleuropericarditis, thrombophlebitis, and impaired growth and sexual development in children.

Treatment

Ulcerative colitis is characterized by recurrent exacerbations, varying degrees of damage to the colonic mucosa, and complications both intestinal and extraintestinal. The treatment programs should attempt to (1) terminate the acute attack, (2) prevent recurrent attacks, and (3) promote healing of the damaged mucosa. Long-term therapy may be modified by considerations relating to complications, eg, carcinoma and ocular disease. Symptomatic remission should not be the only index of therapeutic response.

The choice and intensity of therapy should be determined by the clinical severity of the disease.

A. Severe (Fulminant) Disease:

1. Hospitalization–Hospitalization is indicated. Patients with severe disease may deteriorate rapidly, with hemorrhage, perforation, toxic megacolon, and sepsis developing over a short period of time.

2. General measures–

a. Restore circulating blood volume with fluids, plasma, and blood as indicated.

b. Discontinue opiates and anticholinergics.

c. Correct electrolyte abnormalities.

d. Discontinue all oral intake. Institute nasogastric suction if the colon has become dilated.

3. Antimicrobial therapy–The clinical course of fulminant ulcerative colitis is associated with extensive necrosis of colonic mucosa, and perforation with sepsis is not uncommon in this form of the disease. Intravenous antibiotics are given these patients for presumed or potential sepsis. Ampicillin, cephalothin, cephapirin, chloramphenicol, and gentamicin have been used singly or in combination.

4. Adrenocorticosteroids–Give intravenous hydrocortisone, 300 mg daily, or prednisone, 60 mg daily, in divided doses at 6- to 8-hour intervals.

5. Surgery–If the patient with toxic colonic dilatation does not improve within 8–12 hours, colonic resection is usually indicated. In those patients who have fulminant disease but are not toxic, intravenous therapy is continued for 5–7 days. If improvement occurs, oral therapy can be substituted. If the patient fails to respond or deteriorates, colectomy should be considered. Malnourished patients may be benefited by total parenteral nutrition during this phase.

B. Moderate Disease: This group of patients has substantial evidence of activity, ie, diarrhea, abdominal cramping, weight loss, and anemia, and hospitalization should be advised. However, they are not in a toxic condition, ie, they do not have severe hypoproteinemia, fever, or leukocytosis.

1. Diet—Food served should be appealing and nutritious and contain adequate protein. Avoid foods known to exacerbate the individual patient's diarrhea or cramping. Some patients appear to be lactase-deficient and should avoid milk and milk products.

2. Adrenocorticosteroids—Give prednisone, 20–60 mg orally daily, and reduce by 5 mg per day per week when there is clinical and sigmoidoscopic evidence of improvement. Hydrocortisone enemas, 100 mg each night, may provide additional benefit.

3. Sulfasalazine—Sulfasalazine, 2–4 g daily in divided doses, has been shown to be beneficial in reducing inflammation and in decreasing the frequency of recurrent attacks in this form of the disease. It has been suggested that 5-aminosalicylic acid is the active moiety of sulfasalazine. Sulfasalazine has been shown to decrease fertility during the treatment period.

C. Mild Disease: These patients have minimal evidence of inflammatory bowel disease, ie, asymptomatic rectal bleeding, minimal involvement by sigmoidoscopic examination, and no systemic signs.

1. Diet—See ¶ 1 above.

2. Sulfasalazine—Sulfasalazine, 2–4 g daily in divided doses, as prolonged maintenance therapy.

3. Adrenocorticosteroids—Hydrocortisone enemas or suppositories, 100 mg each night until lesion heals or treatment proves ineffective.

D. Surgical Measures: Surgical excision of the colon is required for patients with refractory disease, severe extracolonic complications (growth suppression), prolonged widespread colon disease, massive hemorrhage, or extensive perirectal disease. The usual procedure is total colectomy with a permanent ileostomy. In some instance, the rectum may be preserved (stripped of its mucosa) and an ileoproctostomy performed with ileal mucosa replacing the stripped rectal mucosa. This allows intestinal continuity and avoids an ileostomy, but most of these patients will have 4–7 liquid stools per day.

Prognosis

The course may be characterized by remissions and exacerbations over a period of many years, or it may be fulminant. Permanent and complete cure on medical therapy is unusual, and life expectancy is shortened. The incidence of bowel cancer in patients with active disease rises with each decade after the diagnosis. Medical measures control the majority of cases, but colectomy is often necessary for fulminant, refractory disease and for complications. Because of potential complications with chronic ulcerative colitis,

close follow-up is indicated, particularly after the disease has been present for 8–10 years. Colonoscopy should be performed annually, and mucosal biopsies should be examined for dysplasia. Dysplasia is considered a precancerous lesion and is frequently thought to be an indication for colectomy.

Albrechtsen D et al: Elective surgery for ulcerative colitis: Colectomy in 158 patients. *Scand J Gastroenterol* 1981;**16**:825.

Bailar JC III: Cigarettes, ulcerative colitis, and inferences from uncontrolled data. (Editorial.) *N Engl J Med* 1983;**308**:275.

Kirsner JB: Observations on the medical treatment of inflammatory bowel disease. *JAMA* 1980;**243**:557.

Lennard-Jones JE et al: Cancer surveillance in ulcerative colitis. *Gastroenterology* 1984;**86**:770.

Peppercorn MA: Sulfasalazine: Pharmacology, clinical use, toxicity and related new drug development. *Ann Intern Med* 1984;**101**:377.

Prior P et al: Cancer morbidity in ulcerative colitis. *Gut* 1982;**23**:490.

Riddell RH et al: Dysplasia in inflammatory bowel disease: Standardized classifications with provisional clinical applications. *Hum Pathol* 1983;**14**:931.

Sales DJ, Kirsner JB: The prognosis of inflammatory bowel disease. (Review.) *Arch Intern Med* 1983;**143**:294.

Waterhouse JAH et al: Survival of patients with colorectal cancer complicating ulcerative colitis. *Gut* 1984;**25**:228.

TOXIC DILATATION OF THE COLON
(Toxic Megacolon)

Toxic megacolon is a life-threatening complication of idiopathic ulcerative colitis or Crohn's disease of the colon. The disease has also been observed in amebiasis, typhoid fever, cholera, and bacillary dysentery. It results from extensive damage to the mucosa, with areas of mucosal denudation and inflammation of the submucosal layers. Contributing factors include cathartics, opiates, anticholinergics, and hypokalemia. It is manifested clinically by evidence of systemic toxicity, fever, leukocytosis, tachycardia, and abdominal distention. Radiographically, the colon is seen to be dilated. Colonic dilatation per se without signs of systemic toxicity may be the result of potassium deficiency or anticholinergic or opiate therapy. The mortality rate of this fulminant complication is high, and treatment, both medical and surgical, should be instituted as soon as possible.

Treatment consists of the following urgent measures: (1) Decompress the bowel and pass an intestinal tube to prevent swallowed air from further distending the colon. (2) Replace lost fluids and electrolytes and restore colloid and blood volume. Remember that diarrhea and adrenal steroid therapy significantly reduce total body potassium and that this has an adverse effect on colonic function. (3) Suppress the inflammatory reaction with hydrocortisone, 100 mg intravenously every 8 hours. (4) Prevent sepsis with broad-spectrum antibiotics (tobramycin, clindamycin).

Careful observation with frequent abdominal

films during the period of 8–12 hours while the above therapy is being given determines whether or not the patient will require surgical treatment. If the colon decompresses, medical therapy is continued; if not, colectomy should be considered. These patients are desperately ill, and if surgery is necessary the procedure of choice is subtotal colectomy. This reduces operating time and the extent of operative trauma. Most of the patients who develop toxic dilatation of the colon but do not require emergency colectomy will require colectomy at a later time because of continuing disease.

Caprilli R et al: Risk factors in toxic megacolon. *Dig Dis Sci* 1980;**25**:817.

Grant CS et al: Toxic megacolon: Ultimate fate of patients after successful medical management. *Am J Surg* 1984;**147**:106.

Mungas JE, Moossa AR, Block GE: Treatment of toxic megacolon. *Surg Clin North Am* 1976;**56**:95.

GRANULOMATOUS COLITIS
(Crohn's Disease of the Colon)

Transmural colitis (Crohn's granulomatosis) may be difficult or impossible to distinguish from the mucosal form of colitis (idiopathic ulcerative colitis) by clinical criteria alone. The most distinguishing feature is transmural involvement in Crohn's colitis. Table 11–2 briefly summarizes the features of these 2 entities. However, the differential diagnostic criteria, when tested against the pathologic findings following colectomy, show a substantial overlap in clinical, radiographic, and histologic criteria.

The most common clinical manifestations are abdominal cramping, diarrhea, and weight loss. Extracolonic manifestations such as erythema nodosum, spondylitis, polyarthritis, and perirectal disease may antedate the colonic manifestations of the disease.

The treatment of granulomatous colitis is essentially the same as for idiopathic ulcerative colitis.

Korelitz BI: Carcinoma of the intestinal tract in Crohn's disease: Results of a survey conducted by the National Foundation for Ileitis and Colitis. *Am J Gastroenterol* 1983;**78**:44.

Lock MR et al: Recurrence and reoperation for Crohn's disease: The role of disease location in prognosis. *N Engl J Med* 1981; **304**:1586.

Tedesco FJ, Volpicelli NA, Moore FS: Estrogen- and progesterone-associated colitis: A disorder with the clinical and endoscopic features mimicking Crohn's colitis. *Gastrointest Endosc* 1982;**28**:247.

ISCHEMIC PROCTOCOLITIS

Interference with blood flow to the colon causes ischemic colitis. The rectum is usually spared because of its dual blood supply from the inferior mesenteric artery and, via the hemorrhoidal vessels, from the internal iliac artery. Most patients are 50–70 years old. Younger women taking oral contraceptives are also at risk.

Presenting symptoms are lower abdominal pain of sudden onset, fever, vomiting, and the passage of bright red blood and clots per rectum. A neutrophil leukocytosis is usual. The sigmoidoscopic examination is often normal, since involvement is usually of the more proximal portions of the colon, particularly the cecum, splenic flexure, and sigmoid colon. When the sigmoid colon is involved, a demarcation in mucosal color can often be seen at the rectosigmoid junction. Involvement of the sigmoid colon or the rectum (rare) may have the appearance on sigmoidoscopy of nonspecific proctocolitis or multiple ulcers, polypoid or nodular lesions, or, in some instances, hemorrhagic or necrotic membrane formation.

Plain films of the abdomen may show generalized dilatation of the colon. Barium enema normally shows a segmental area of involvement occurring, in descending order of frequency, in the splenic flexure, sigmoid colon, and ascending colon. Rectal involvement is rare because of its dual blood supply. The involved area is characterized by a variable combination of thumbprinting (edematous mucosal folds), saw-toothed mucosal irregularity, tubular narrowing, and sacculation. Angiograms may be helpful in showing vascular occlusions, particularly in patients who may have embolic potential. Most ischemic disease is nonocclusive, and angiograms will not be helpful. Inflammatory bowel involvement by Crohn's disease, idiopathic ulcerative colitis, and infection and stricture due to carcinoma must be ruled out.

Severe ischemia leading to gangrene is treated by replacement of blood volume, antibiotics (chloramphenicol, kanamycin, gentamicin), and excision of necrotic bowel. Less severe ischemia leading to stricture formation is treated by resection of the stricture. Transient ischemia requires no specific treatment.

Table 11–2. Differential features of ulcerative colitis and granulomatous colitis.*

	Ulcerative Colitis	Granulomatous Colitis
Clinical		
Toxicity	Common	Rare
Bleeding	Common	Rare
Perianal disease	Rare	Common
Fistula	Rare	Common
Perforation	Rare	Common
Sigmoidoscopy	Diffuse, friable superficial ulceration	Discrete, occasionally diffuse
X-ray		
Distribution	Continuous	Segmental
Mucosa	Serrated	Fissures to deep ulcers
Stricture	Rare	Common
Pathology	Mucosal micro-abscesses	Transmural involvement, granulomas

*Reference: Margulis AR et al: The overlapping spectrum of ulcerative and granulomatous colitis: A roentgenographic-pathologic study. *Am J Roentgenol* 1971;**113**:325.

The prognosis is good in transient proctocolitis. The mortality rate is high when gangrene occurs.

O'Connell TX, Kadell B, Tompkins RK: Ischemia of the colon. *Surg Gynecol Obstet* 1976;**142**:337.

DIVERTICULAR DISEASE OF THE COLON

Essentials of Diagnosis

- Intermittent, cramping left lower abdominal pain.
- Constipation or alternating constipation and diarrhea.
- Tenderness in the left lower quadrant.
- X-ray evidence of diverticula, thickened interhaustral folds, narrowed lumen.

General Considerations

Diverticula of the colon occur with increasing frequency after age 40. Although diverticula may occur throughout the gut, excluding the rectum, they are most common in the high-pressure areas of the colon (eg, sigmoid). They tend to dissect along the course of the nutrient vessels, and they consist of a mucosal coat and a serosa. The inflammatory complication, diverticulitis, probably affects 20–25% of patients at some time.

Inflammatory changes in diverticulitis vary from mild infiltration in the wall of the sac to extensive inflammatory change in the surrounding area (peridiverticulitis), with perforation or abscess formation. The changes are comparable to those that occur in appendicitis.

Clinical Findings

A. Symptoms and Signs: Left lower quadrant pain may be steady and severe and last for days or may be cramping and intermittent and relieved by a bowel movement. Constipation is usual, but diarrhea may occur. Occult blood is found in the stool in about 20% of cases. Diverticulosis coli is the most common cause of colonic hemorrhage; lower gastrointestinal hemorrhage is uncommon in diverticulitis.

B. Laboratory Findings: Noncontributory in uncomplicated diverticular disease.

C. X-Ray Findings: X-ray examination reveals diverticula and in some cases spasm, interhaustral thickening, or narrowing of the colonic lumen.

Complications

Diverticulitis is a complication of diverticular disease in which gross or microscopic perforation of the diverticulum has occurred. The clinical manifestations vary with the extent of the inflammatory process and may include pain, signs of peritoneal irritation, chills, fever, sepsis, ileus, and partial or complete colonic obstruction. Peritonitis and abscess formation may also occur. Urinary frequency and dysuria are associated with bladder involvement in the inflammatory process. Fistula formation usually involves the

bladder (usually vesicosigmoid) but may also be to the skin, perianal area, or small bowel. The white blood count shows polymorphonuclear leukocytosis. Red and white blood cells may be seen in the urine. Blood cultures may be positive.

Differential Diagnosis

The constrictive lesion of the colon seen on x-ray or at sigmoidoscopy must be differentiated from carcinoma of the colon. The appearance of a short lesion with abrupt transition to normal bowel suggests carcinoma. Colonoscopy with biopsy can be very useful in these instances.

Treatment

The treatment of uncomplicated diverticular disease consists primarily of increasing bulk in the diet by means of the following: (1) high-residue diet; (2) unprocessed bran, ¼ cup daily in fruit juice or muffins; or (3) bulk additives such as psyllium hydrophilic mucilloid (Konsyl, Metamucil, and others). Other measures that may be helpful are (1) stool softeners such as docusate sodium (Colace and others), 240 mg per day; and (2) anticholinergic drugs to decrease "spasm" in the sigmoid colon.

The treatment of acute diverticulitis requires antibiotic therapy. The antibiotic of choice is ampicillin. Other useful antibiotic drugs include cephalothin and combined treatment with penicillin and tobramycin.

Recurrent attacks of diverticulitis or the presence of perforation, fistula formation, or abscess formation requires surgical resection of the involved portion of the colon.

Massive diverticular hemorrhage usually stops spontaneously. Adequate blood replacement and careful endoscopic and barium studies are indicated to rule out other causes of bleeding. In certain instances, selective arteriography may localize the site of the bleeding and make it possible to control the bleeding with vasopressin. Operation may be required for uncontrolled bleeding.

Prognosis

The usual case is mild and responds well to dietary measures and antibiotics.

Almy TP, Howell DA: Diverticular disease of the colon. *N Engl J Med* 1980;**302**:324.
Hyland JMP et al: Does a high fibre diet prevent the complication of diverticular disease? *Br J Surg* 1980;**67**:77.
Larson DM: Medical and surgical therapy in diverticular disease: A comparative study. *Gastroenterology* 1976;**71**:734.

POLYPS OF THE COLON & RECTUM
(Intestinal Polyps)

Adenomatous polyps of the colon and rectum are common benign neoplasms that are usually asymptomatic but may cause painless rectal bleeding. They may be single or multiple, occur most frequently in the sigmoid and rectum, and are found incidentally in about 9% of autopsies. The incidence of polyps increases with age. The diagnosis is established by sigmoidoscopy, double contrast barium enema, and colonoscopy. When a polyp is found in the rectum, the colon should be studied by x-ray.

Whether polyps are precancerous is an important question. Pedunculated, adenomatous polyps probably have negligible malignant potential and may usually be treated by simple polypectomy through the sigmoidoscope or colonoscope. In most patients, more aggressive operation is not indicated unless the polyp grows on repeated observation or causes symptoms such as bleeding. Papillary (villous) adenomas are sessile lesions that are known to become metastasizing carcinomas and should be removed. The overwhelming majority of cancers of the colon and rectum arise de novo.

Familial intestinal polyposis is a rare hereditary disease characterized by innumerable adenomatous polyps of the colon and rectum. Gardner's syndrome involves colonic polyposis associated with sebaceous cysts, lipomas, fibromas, and leiomyomas of soft tissue and osteomas of bone (mandible, sphenoid, and maxilla). The colonic polyps in both situations are premalignant. Colectomy with ileoproctostomy is the treatment of choice and may be followed by spontaneous regression of the rectal polyps. The rectum should be examined regularly and residual polyps removed through the sigmoidoscope. If this is not possible, the rectum should also be excised.

Boland CR: Familiar Colonic Cancer Syndromes. (Medical Staff Conference.) *West J Med* 1983;**139**:351.

Sherlock P, Winawer SJ: Are there markers for the risk of colorectal cancer? *N Engl J Med* 1984;**311**: 118.

COLONIC OBSTRUCTION

Colonic obstruction may be acute or chronic. It may be simple, strangulating, paralytic, or closed loop. The most common cause of subacute and chronic obstruction of the colon is carcinoma. Other causes include drugs (phenothiazine, tricyclic antidepressants, morphine derivatives), fecal impaction, scleroderma, strictures caused by granulomatous colitis, and diverticular disease of the colon. Acute obstruction is usually due to volvulus, intussusception, or inguinal herniation of the colon.

Clinical Findings

A. Symptoms and Signs: Simple obstruction with constipation or obstipation may lead to the insidious development of pain. Severe continuous pain suggests strangulation. Borborygmus may be prominent. Nausea and vomiting are late signs. Physical examination discloses abdominal distention and tympany. High-pitched tinkles may be heard on auscultation. A localized mass suggests carcinoma, intussus-

ception, or strangulated closed loop. Peritoneal signs suggest perforation. Blood in the rectum suggests intussusception or carcinoma.

B. Laboratory Findings: Noncontributory unless strangulation has occurred.

C. X-Ray Findings: Colonic distention can be demonstrated by plain abdominal films. The barium enema will demonstrate the site of obstruction, but this procedure is contraindicated if there is ischemia with necrosis of the bowel wall. Barium by upper gastrointestinal series should never be given if there is any possibility of colonic obstruction.

Differential Diagnosis

In paralytic ileus the abdomen is silent, and cramping does not occur. Signs of peritonitis are present, or there is a history of drug ingestion or trauma to the back or pelvis.

In small bowel obstruction, vomiting is more common and occurs earlier. The abdominal pain is usually more severe, and x-ray may reveal the ladder configuration of distended small bowel with little or no colonic distention.

Complications

Delay in treatment may lead to strangulation with perforation, peritonitis, and sepsis.

Treatment

The treatment of colonic obstruction is usually surgical. However, sigmoid volvulus often can be decompressed with sigmoidoscopy or colonoscopy and intussusception by barium enema. The baseline medical treatment is to decompress the patient from above with nasogastric suction and to stabilize fluid, electrolyte, cardiac, and pulmonary status. Even patients acutely decompressed by nonsurgical means usually require surgery for definitive care.

Ballantyne GH: Review of sigmoid volvulus: History and results of treatment. *Dis Colon Rectum* 1982;**25**:494.

Kelley WE Jr et al: Penetrating, obstructing, and perforating carcinomas of the colon and rectum. *Arch Surg* 1981;**116**:381.

CANCER OF THE COLON & RECTUM

Essentials of Diagnosis

- Altered bowel function (constipation or diarrhea).
- Blood in the feces, unexplained anemia, weight loss.
- Palpable mass involving colon or rectum.
- Sigmoidoscopic or x-ray evidence of neoplasm.

General Considerations

Carcinoma is the only common cancer of the colon and rectum. Lymphoma, carcinoid, melanoma, fibrosarcoma, and other types of sarcoma occur rarely. The treatment of all is essentially the same.

Carcinoma of the colon and rectum causes more deaths than any other form of cancer. The only known predisposing causes are familial multiple polyposis, chronic ulcerative colitis, chronic lymphogranuloma venereum, chronic granuloma inguinale, and perhaps adenoma. Males are affected more commonly than females in a ratio of 3:2. The highest incidence is in patients about 50 years of age, but occasional cases have been reported in younger persons and even in children. The anatomic distribution of cancer of the large bowel is approximately 16% in the cecum and ascending colon, 5% in the transverse colon, 9% in the descending colon, 20% in the sigmoid, and 50% in the rectum.

Of all lesions of the colon and rectum, half to two-thirds lie within reach of the examining finger or sigmoidoscope and therefore can be biopsied on the first visit.

Clinical Findings

Symptoms vary depending upon whether the lesion is in the right or the left side of the colon. In either case, a persistent change in the customary bowel habits almost always occurs and should invariably alert the physician to investigate the colon. Bleeding is a cardinal diagnostic point. An acute abdominal emergency may be precipitated by perforation or colonic obstruction (due to circumferential narrowing, not intussusception). The diagnosis of colonic and rectal cancer is established by sigmoidoscopy and colonoscopy with biopsy and barium enema. Polyps and carcinoma not detected by barium enema may be detected by colonoscopy.

A. Carcinoma of the Right Colon: Because the fecal stream is fluid and the bowel lumen large in the right half of the colon, symptoms of obstruction occur less frequently than in left-sided tumors. Vague abdominal discomfort is often the only initial complaint. This may progress to cramplike pain, occasionally simulating cholecystitis or appendicitis. Secondary anemia with associated weakness and weight loss is found in half of patients with right colon lesions. The stools are usually positive for occult blood but rarely show gross blood. The patient is likely to have diarrhea. The first indication of cancer may be the discovery of a palpable mass in the right lower quadrant.

B. Carcinoma of the Left Colon: Obstructive symptoms predominate, particularly increasing constipation. There may be short bouts of diarrhea. Occasionally the first sign is acute colonic obstruction. A small amount of bright red blood with bowel movements is common, and anemia is found in about 20% of cases. At times a mass is palpable. About half of patients give a history of weight loss.

Differential Diagnosis

Diverticulitis is usually associated with fever and has a different x-ray appearance. Functional bowel distress may also simulate cancer of the colon symptomatically.

Treatment

The only curative treatment in cancer of the large bowel is wide surgical resection of the lesion and its regional lymphatics after adequate bowel preparation and appropriate supportive measures. When a significant degree of mechanical obstruction is present, a preliminary transverse colostomy or cecostomy is necessary. Even in the presence of metastatic disease, palliative resection may be of value to relieve obstruction, bleeding, or the symptoms of local invasion. Preoperative irradiation, 2000–2500 R in 10 fractions given over 12 days, has been shown to increase resectability and improve survival in patients undergoing abdominoperineal resection.

Prognosis

Over 90% of patients with carcinoma of the colon and rectum are suitable for either curative or palliative resection, with an operative mortality rate of 3–6%. The overall 5-year survival rate after resection is about 50%. If the lesion is confined to the bowel and there is no evidence of lymphatic or blood vessel invasion, the 5-year survival rate is 60–70%. Local recurrence of carcinoma in the anastomotic suture line or wound area occurs in 10–15% of cases. The incidence of local recurrence can be decreased if special precautions are taken at operation to avoid implantation of malignant cells. About 5% of patients develop multiple primary colon cancers. Early identification of resectable local recurrence or a new neoplasm depends upon careful follow-up with sigmoidoscopy and barium enema every 6 months for 2 years and yearly thereafter.

Burkitt DP: Etiology and prevention of colorectal cancer. *Hosp Pract* (Feb) 1984;**19**:67.

Hardcastle JD et al: Controlled trial of faecal occult blood testing in the detection of colorectal cancer. *Lancet* 1983; **2**:1.

Moore JRL, LaMont JT: Colorectal cancer: Risk factors and screening strategies. *Arch Intern Med* 1984;**144**:1819.

Nivatvongs S et al: Distribution of large-bowel cancers detected by occult blood test in asymptomatic patients. *Dis Colon Rectum* 1982;**25**:420.

Third International Symposium on Colorectal Cancer. *CA* 1984;**34**:130.

DISEASES OF THE ANUS

HEMORRHOIDS

Essentials of Diagnosis

- Rectal bleeding, protrusion, and vague discomfort.
- Mucoid discharge from rectum.
- Characteristic findings on external anal inspection or anoscopic examination.

General Considerations

Internal hemorrhoids are varices of the portion of the venous hemorrhoidal plexus that lies submucosally just proximal to the dentate margin. External hemorrhoids arise from the same plexus but are located subcutaneously immediately distal to the dentate margin. There are 3 primary internal hemorrhoidal masses: right anterior, right posterior, and left lateral. Three to 5 secondary hemorrhoids may be present between the 3 primaries. Straining at stool, constipation, prolonged sitting, and anal infection are contributing factors and may precipitate complications such as thrombosis. The diagnosis is suspected on the history of protrusion, anal pain, or bleeding and is confirmed by proctologic examination.

Carcinoma of the colon or rectum not infrequently aggravates hemorrhoids or produces similar complaints. Polyps may be present as a cause of bleeding that is wrongly attributed to hemorrhoids. For these reasons, the treatment of hemorrhoids is always preceded by sigmoidoscopy and barium enema. When portal hypertension is suspected as a causative factor, investigations for liver disease should be carried out. Hemorrhoids that develop during pregnancy or parturition tend to subside thereafter and should be treated conservatively unless persistent.

Clinical Findings

The symptoms of hemorrhoids are usually mild and remittent, but a number of disturbing complications may develop and call for active medical or surgical treatment. These complications include pruritus; incontinence; recurrent protrusion requiring manual replacement by the patient; fissure, infection, or ulceration; prolapse and strangulation; and secondary anemia due to chronic blood loss. Carcinoma has been reported to develop very rarely in hemorrhoids.

Treatment

Conservative treatment suffices in most instances of mild hemorrhoids, which may improve spontaneously or in response to a high-roughage diet, psyllium seed preparation, or nonirritating laxatives to produce soft stools. Local pain and infection are managed with warm sitz baths and insertion of a soothing anal suppository 2 or 3 times daily. Benzocaine and similar types of anal ointments should be avoided so as not to sensitize the patient to these agents. Prolapsed or strangulated hemorrhoids may be treated conservatively by gentle reduction with a lubricated gloved finger; by rubber band ligation or cryosurgery, or both; or by immediate surgical resection.

For severe symptoms or complications, complete internal and external hemorrhoidectomy is advisable and is a highly satisfactory procedure when properly done. Excision of a single external hemorrhoid, evacuation of a thrombosed pile, and the injection treatment of internal hemorrhoids fall within the scope of office practice. Injection therapy is effective, but there is a recurrence rate of more than 50%.

Evacuation of Thrombosed
External Hemorrhoid

This condition is caused by the rupture of a vein at the anal margin, forming a clot in the subcutaneous tissue. The patient complains of a painful lump, and examination shows a tense, tender, bluish mass covered with skin. If the patient is seen after 24–48 hours when the pain is subsiding—or if symptoms are minimal—hot sitz baths are prescribed. If discomfort is marked, removal of the clot is indicated. With the patient in the lateral position, the area is prepared with antiseptic, and 1% procaine or lidocaine is injected intracutaneously around and over the lump. A radial ellipse of skin is then excised and the clot evacuated. A dry gauze dressing is held in place for 12–24 hours by taping the buttocks together, and daily sitz baths are then begun.

Hooks VH: The diagnosis and treatment of common anorectal problems. *Cont Educ Fam Physician* (Jan) 1982;**16**:29.

Smith LE: Symptomatic internal hemorrhoids: What are your options? *Postgrad Med* (June) 1983;**73**:323.

CRYPTITIS & PAPILLITIS

Anal pain and burning of brief duration with defecation is suggestive of cryptitis and papillitis. Digital and anoscopic examination reveals hypertrophied papillae and indurated or inflamed crypts. Treatment consists of adding bulk agents, such as psyllium seed preparations, to the diet; sitz baths; and anal suppositories containing hydrocortisone after each bowel movement. Some recommend local application of 5% phenol in oil or carbolfuchsin compound to the crypts. If these measures fail, surgical excision of involved crypts and papillae should be considered.

FISSURA IN ANO
(Anal Fissure)

Acute fissures represent linear disruption of the anal epithelium due to various causes. They usually clear if bowel movements are kept regular and soft (eg, with a bulk agent, bran, or psyllium seed preparation). The local application of a mild styptic such as 1–2% silver nitrate or 1% gentian violet solution may be of value.

Chronic fissure is characterized by (1) acute pain during and after defecation; (2) spotting of bright red blood at stool, with occasional more abundant bleeding; (3) tendency to constipation through fear of pain; and (4) the late occurrence of a sentinel pile, a hypertrophied papilla, and spasm of the anal canal (usually very painful on digital examination). Regulation of bowel habits with use of bran or psyllium seed preparation in the diet or use of stool softeners, sitz baths, or anal suppositories (eg, Anusol) twice daily should be tried. If these measures fail, the fissure, sentinel pile, or papilla and the adjacent crypt must be excised surgically. Postoperative care is along the lines of the preoperative treatment.

Abcarian H: Surgical correction of chronic anal fissure. *Dis Colon Rectum* 1980;**23**:31.
Mazier W, Demoraes R, Dignan R: Anal fissure and anal ulcers. *Surg Clin North Am* 1978;**58**:479.

ANAL ABSCESS

Perianal abscess should be considered the acute stage of an anal fistula until proved otherwise. The abscess should be adequately drained as soon as localized. Hot sitz baths may hasten the process of localization. The patient should be warned that the fistula may persist after drainage of the abscess. It is painful and fruitless to search for the internal opening of a fistula in the presence of acute infection. The presence of an anal abscess should alert the clinician to the possibility of inflammatory bowel disease.

FISTULA IN ANO

About 95% of all anal fistulas arise in an anal crypt, and they are often preceded by an anal abscess. If an anal fistula enters the rectum above the pectinate line and there is no associated disease in the crypts, ulcerative colitis, regional ileitis, rectal tuberculosis, lymphogranuloma venereum, cancer, or foreign body should be considered in the differential diagnosis.

Acute fistula is associated with a purulent discharge from the fistulous opening. There is usually local itching, tenderness, or pain aggravated by bowel movements. Recurrent anal abscess may develop. The involved crypt can occasionally be located anoscopically with a crypt hook. Probing the fistula should be gentle because false passages can be made with ease, and in any case demonstration of the internal opening by probing is not essential to the diagnosis.

Treatment is by surgical incision or excision of the fistula under general anesthesia. If a fistula passes deep to the entire anorectal ring, so that all the muscles must be divided in order to extirpate the tract, a 2-stage operation must be done to prevent incontinence.

Adams D, Kovalcik PJ: Fistula in ano. *Surg Gynecol Obstet* 1981;**153**:731.
Hanley PH: Anorectal abscess fistula. *Surg Clin North Am* 1978; **58**:487.

ANAL CONDYLOMAS
(Genital Warts)

These wartlike papillomas of the perianal skin and anal canal flourish on moist, macerated surfaces, particularly in the presence of purulent discharge. They are not true tumors but are infectious and autoinoculable, probably owing to a sexually transmitted papovavirus. They must be distinguished from condylomata lata caused by syphilis. The diagnosis of the latter rests on a positive serologic test for syphilis or discovery of *Treponema pallidum* on darkfield examination.

Treatment consists of *cautious* accurate application of 25% podophyllum resin in tincture of benzoin to the lesion (with bare wooden or cotton-tipped applicator sticks to avoid contact with uninvolved skin). The compound should be washed off after 2–4 hours. Condylomas in the anal canal are treated through the anoscope and the painted site dusted with powder to localize the application and minimize discomfort. Electrofulguration under local anesthesia is useful if there are numerous lesions. Local cleanliness and the frequent use of a talc dusting powder are essential.

Condylomas tend to recur. The patient should be observed for several months and advised to report promptly if new lesions appear.

Owen WF: Sexually transmitted diseases and traumatic problems in homosexual men. *Ann Intern Med* 1982;**92**:805.
Quinn TC et al: The etiology of anorectal infections in homosexual men. *Am J Med* 1981;**71**:395.

BENIGN ANORECTAL STRICTURES

Traumatic

Acquired stenosis is usually the result of surgery or trauma that denudes the epithelium of the anal canal. Hemorrhoid operations in which too much skin is removed or which are followed by infection are the commonest cause. Constipation, ribbon stools, and pain on defecation are the most frequent complaints. Stenosis predisposes to fissure, low-grade infection, and, occasionally, fistula.

Prevention of stenosis after radical anal surgery is best accomplished by local cleanliness, hot sitz baths, and gentle insertion of the well-lubricated finger twice weekly for 2–3 weeks beginning 2 weeks after surgery. When stenosis is chronic but mild, graduated anal dilators of increasing size may be inserted daily by the patient. For marked stenosis, a plastic operation on the anal canal is advisable.

Inflammatory

A. Lymphogranuloma Venereum: This infectious disease is the commonest cause of inflammatory stricture of the anorectal region. It is most common in females and in male homosexuals. Acute proctitis due to lymphatic spread of the organism occurs early and may be followed by perirectal infections, sinuses, and formation of scar tissue (resulting in stricture). Frei and complement fixation tests are positive.

The tetracycline drugs are curative in the initial phase of the disease. When extensive chronic secondary infection is present or when a stricture has formed, repeated biopsies are essential because epidermoid carcinoma develops in about 4% of strictures. Local operation on a stricture may be feasible, but a colostomy or an abdominoperineal resection is often required.

B. Granuloma Inguinale: This disease may

cause anorectal fistulas, infections, and strictures. The Donovan body is best identified in tissue biopsy when there is rectal involvement. Epidermoid carcinoma develops in about 4% of cases with chronic anorectal granuloma.

The early lesions respond to tetracyclines. Destructive or constricting processes may require colostomy or resection.

Arko FR: Anorectal disorders. *Am Fam Physician* (Oct) 1980; **22**:121.

ANAL INCONTINENCE

Obstetric tears, anorectal operations (particularly fistulotomy), and neurologic disturbances are the most frequent causes of anal incontinence. When incontinence is due to surgery or trauma, surgical repair of the divided or torn sphincter is indicated. Repair of anterior childbirth lacerations should be delayed for 6 months or more.

Keighley MRB, Matheson DM: Results of treatment for rectal prolapse and incontinence. *Dis Colon Rectum* 1981;**24**:449.

SQUAMOUS CELL CARCINOMA OF THE ANUS

These tumors are relatively rare, comprising only 1–2% of all cancers of the anus and large intestine. Bleeding, pain, and local tumor are the commonest symptoms. Because the lesion is often confused with hemorrhoids or other common anal disorders, immediate biopsy of any suspicious lesion or mass in the anal area is essential. These tumors tend to become annular, invade the sphincter, and spread upward into the rectum.

Except for very small lesions (which can be adequately excised locally), treatment is by combined abdominoperineal resection. Radiation therapy is reserved for palliation and for patients who refuse or cannot withstand operation. Metastases to the inguinal nodes are treated by radical groin dissection when clinically evident. The 5-year survival rate after resection is about 50%.

Salmon RJ et al: Treatment of epidermoid anal canal cancer. *Am J Surg* 1984;**147**:43.

Schneider TC et al: Management of carcinoma of the anal canal. *Surgery* 1981;**90**:729.

Svenson EW et al: Results of treatment in transitional cloacogenic carcinoma. *Cancer* 1980;**46**:828.

DISEASES OF THE LIVER & BILIARY TRACT

JAUNDICE
(Icterus)

Since antiquity, a yellowish appearance of the skin and scleras has been recognized as a manifestation of liver disease. Jaundice is evidence of accumulation of bilirubin—a red pigment product of heme metabolism—in the body tissues; it has extrahepatic as well as hepatic causes. Hyperbilirubinemia may be due to abnormalities in the formation, transport, metabolism, and excretion of bilirubin. Total serum bilirubin is normally 0.2–1.2 mg/dL, and jaundice may not be clinically recognizable until levels are about 3 mg/dL.

From an anatomic standpoint, elevation of serum bilirubin levels is prehepatic, hepatic, or posthepatic. Prehepatic jaundice is due to excess production of bilirubin (eg, hemolysis). In hepatic jaundice, elevated serum bilirubin may be caused by qualitative or quantitative dysfunction of liver cells (eg, faulty uptake, metabolism, or excretion of bilirubin). Posthepatic jaundice results from interference with the physiologic removal of bilirubin from the hepatobiliary system (eg, obstruction of the common bile duct).

Because of the great diversity of causes of jaundice, no classification is entirely satisfactory; one that includes anatomy, biochemistry, and etiology is presented in Table 11–3.

Manifestations of Diseases Associated With Jaundice

A. Prehepatic: Weakness, abdominal or back pain may occur with acute hemolytic crises. Normal stool and urine color. Jaundice. Indirect unconjugated hyperbilirubinemia. Splenomegaly, except in sickle cell anemia. Hepatomegaly is variable. Hemolysis and indirect unconjugated hyperbilirubinemia.

B. Hepatic: ·

1. Acquired–Malaise, anorexia, low-grade fever, right upper quadrant discomfort. Dark urine, jaundice, amenorrhea. Enlarged, tender liver; vascular spiders; palmar erythema; ascites; gynecomastia; sparse body hair; fetor hepaticus; asterixis.

2. Congenital–May be asymptomatic; the intermittent cholestasis is often accompanied by pruritus, light-colored stools, and, occasionally, malaise.

C. Posthepatic: Colicky right upper quadrant pain, weight loss (carcinoma), jaundice, dark urine, light-colored stools. Fluctuating jaundice and intermittently colored stools indicate intermittent obstruction owing to stone or to carcinoma of the ampulla or junction of the intrahepatic ducts. Blood in the stools suggests cancer. Hepatomegaly, visible and palpable gallbladder (Courvoisier's sign), ascites, rectal (Blumer's) shelf, and weight loss also indicate cancer. Chills and fever suggest stone with cholangitis.

Table 11–3. Classification of jaundice.

Type of Hyperbilirubinemia	Location and Cause
Unconjugated hyperbilirubinemia (predominant indirect-acting bilirubin)	**PREHEPATIC** Increased bilirubin production (eg, hemolytic anemias, hemolytic reactions, hematoma, infarction). **HEPATIC** Impaired bilirubin uptake and storage (eg, posthepatitis hyperbilirubinemia, Gilbert's syndrome, drug reactions). Impaired glucuronyl transferase activity (eg, Crigler-Najjar syndrome, Gilbert's syndrome).
Conjugated hyperbilirubinemia (predominant direct-acting bilirubin)	Faulty excretion of bilirubin conjugates (eg, Dubin-Johnson syndrome, Rotor's syndrome). Biliary epithelial damage (eg, hepatitis, hepatic cirrhosis). Intrahepatic cholestasis (eg, viral hepatitis, alcoholic hepatitis, certain drugs, biliary cirrhosis). Hepatocellular damage or intrahepatic cholestasis resulting from miscellaneous causes (eg, viral hepatitis, spirochetal infections, infectious mononucleosis, cholangitis, sarcoidosis, lymphomas, industrial toxins). **POSTHEPATIC** Gallstones, biliary atresia, carcinoma of biliary duct, sclerosing cholangitis, choledochal cyst, external pressure on common duct, pancreatitis, pancreatic neoplasms.

Diagnostic Methods for Evaluation of Jaundice

A. Laboratory Studies: SGOT (AST) is valuable in the assessment of liver disease. Diagnostic usefulness is enhanced when the test is combined with complementary studies such as alkaline phosphatase and serum bilirubin. SGPT (ALT) may be useful in differentiating alcoholic from viral hepatitis, because SGPT levels are disproportionately low in alcoholic hepatitis.

B. Liver Biopsy: Percutaneous liver biopsy is a safe and accurate way of diagnosing diffuse hepatic disease. It is of less value in differentiating intrahepatic from extrahepatic cholestasis and is moderately successful in defining liver metastases.

C. Radiologic Studies: When the cause of jaundice cannot be determined on the basis of the patient's history and clinical and laboratory findings, it may be possible to differentiate hepatocellular and obstructive jaundice in 80–90% of cases by ultrasonography, CT scan, or radionuclide imaging, all of which are noninvasive. Dilated bile ducts demonstrated by these techniques indicate biliary obstruction, which helps distinguish between obstructive and hepatocellular disease. These methods do not depend on the presence of normal hepatic function—an important point, since conventional oral cholecystography is unsatisfactory when total bilirubin levels are greater than 3 mg/dL. Ultrasonography and CT scan can be used to demonstrate both hepatomegaly and intrahepatic tumors. Ultrasonography can also identify gallbladders and detect even 2-mm gallstones.

If surgical (obstructive) jaundice is initially suspected, some clinicians proceed directly from clinical and laboratory findings to percutaneous transhepatic cholangiography; this fine-needle technique often pinpoints the cause, location, and extent of the biliary obstruction. Unusual complications may include fever, bacteremia, bile peritonitis, and intraperitoneal hemorrhage. Endoscopic retrograde cholangiopancreatography, which requires a skilled endoscopist, is a fiberoptic technique comparable in accuracy to percutaneous cholangiography. It may also be utilized to demonstrate pancreatic causes of jaundice. Complications of the endoscopic procedure include pancreatitis and cholangitis, which occur in less than 3% of cases.

Ultrasonic examination is useful in demonstrating dilated hepatic ducts, an enlarged gallbladder, space-consuming hepatic lesions, and hepatosplenomegaly.

Liver scans using ^{99m}Tc sulfur colloid may be of value in detecting space-occupying lesions of the liver (tumors, abscesses, or cysts) and for assessing portal hypertension.

Corless JK, Middleton HM III: Normal liver function: A basis for understanding hepatic disease. *Arch Intern Med* 1983; **143**:2291.

Ferrucci JT et al: Advances in the radiology of jaundice. *Am J Radiol* 1983;**141**:1.

Fischer MG, Gelb AM, Weingarten LA: Cholestatic jaundice in adults: Algorithms for diagnosis. *JAMA* 1981;**245**:1945.

Richter JM, Silverstein MD, Schapiro R: Suspected obstructive jaundice. *Ann Intern Med* 1983;**99**:46.

Scharschmidt BF, Goldberg HI, Schmid R: Current concepts in diagnosis: Approach to the patient with cholestatic jaundice. *N Engl J Med* 1983;**308**:1515.

Venu RP et al: Endoscopic retrograde cholangiopancreatography: Diagnosis of cholelithiasis in patients with normal gallbladder x-ray and ultrasound studies. *JAMA* 1983;**249**:758.

Wolkoff AW et al: Bilirubin metabolism and hyperbilirubinemia. *Semin Liver Dis* 1983;**3**:1.

VIRAL HEPATITIS
(Hepatitis A, "Infectious," Short Incubation Period; Hepatitis B, "Serum," Long Incubation Period)

Essentials of Diagnosis

- Anorexia, nausea, vomiting, malaise, symptoms of upper respiratory throat infection or "flu"-like syndrome, aversion to smoking.
- Fever; enlarged, tender liver; jaundice.
- Normal to low white cell count; abnormal liver tests and liver function.

Table 11–4. Liver function tests: Normal values and changes in 2 types of jaundice.

Tests	Normal Values	Hepatocellular Jaundice	Uncomplicated Obstructive Jaundice
Bilirubin			
Direct	0.1–0.3 mg/dL	Increased	Increased
Indirect	0.2–0.7 mg/dL	Increased	Increased
Urine bilirubin	None	Increased	Increased
Serum albumin/ total protein	Albumin, 3.5–5.5 Total protein, 6.5–8.4	Albumin decreased	Unchanged
Alkaline phosphatase	30–115 IU	Increased (++)	Increased (++++)
Cholesterol			
Total	100–250 mg/dL	Decreased if damage severe	Increased
Esters	60–70% of total	Decreased if damage severe	Normal
Prothrombin time	60–100%. After vitamin K, 15% increase in 24 hours.	Prolonged if damage severe and does not respond to parenteral vitamin K	Prolonged if obstruction marked but responds to parenteral vitamin K
SGPT (ALT) SGOT (AST)	SGPT, 5–35 IU SGOT, 5–40 IU	Increased in hepatocellular damage, viral hepatitis	Minimally increased

- Liver biopsy shows characteristic hepatocellular necrosis and mononuclear infiltrate.

General Considerations

Hepatitis A is a viral infection of the liver that may occur sporadically or in epidemics. The liver involvement is part of a generalized infection but dominates the clinical picture. Although transmission of the virus may occur by contaminated needles, it is usually by the fecal-oral route. The excretion of hepatitis A virus (HAV) as determined by immune electron microscopy of stool occurs up to 2 weeks prior to illness. HAV is rarely demonstrated in feces after the third week of illness. There is no known carrier state with HAV. Blood and stools are infectious during the incubation period (2–6 weeks) and early illness until peak transaminase levels are achieved. Although theoretically possible, the short duration of viremia makes posttransfusion hepatitis unlikely. In fact, posttransfusion hepatitis due to HAV has not been documented. Although the mortality rate with hepatitis A is low, it may cause fulminant disease. The mortality rate (as with hepatitis B) appears to be age-related.

An unequivocal diagnosis of HAV is established by demonstrating the hepatitis A virus antigen (HAAg) in the stool or the IgM antibody to hepatitis A in serum. The absence of HAAg in the stool does not rule out HAV infection.

Antibodies to type A hepatitis appear early in the course of the illness and tend to persist in the serum. Immune electron microscopy and radioimmunoassay detect both IgM and IgG antibodies and are positive soon after the onset of the illness. Immune adherence hemagglutination reflects an IgG response and is positive later in the course of the disease. Peak titers of IgG antibodies occur after 1 month of disease and may persist for years. Peak titers of IgM antibodies occur during the first week of clinical disease and disappear within an 8-week period; therefore, measurement of these antibodies is an excellent test for demonstrating

acute hepatitis A infection. The presence of anti-HAV activity indicates (1) previous exposure to HAV, (2) noninfectivity, and (3) immunity to recurring HAV infection. It does not imply previous clinically apparent hepatitis, nor does it establish a relationship to ongoing liver disease unless seroconversion has been demonstrated.

The viral agent of hepatitis A is a small, 27-nm RNA virus that belongs to the picornavirus group, which also includes poliomyelitis virus and coxsackievirus. The agent is inactivated by ultraviolet light, by heating to 100 °C for 5 minutes, and by exposure to 1:4000 formalin solution.

Hepatitis B is a viral infection of the liver usually transmitted by inoculation of infected blood or blood products. However, the antigen has been found in most body secretions, and it is known that the disease can be

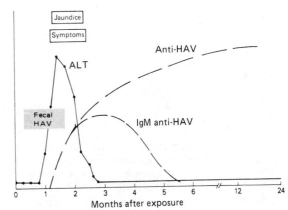

Figure 11–1. The typical course of acute type A hepatitis. HAV = hepatitis A antigen; anti-HAV = antibody to hepatitis A virus; ALT = alanine aminotransferase. (Reproduced, with permission, from Schafer DF, Hoofnagel JH: *Viewpoints on Digestive Diseases* 1982;**14**:5.)

spread by oral or sexual contact. Hepatitis B virus (HBV) is highly prevalent in homosexuals and intravenous drug abusers. Other groups at high risk include patients and staff at hemodialysis centers, physicians, dentists, nurses, and personnel working in clinical and pathology laboratories and blood banks. Approximately 5–10% of infected individuals become carriers, providing a substantial reservoir of infection. Forty to 70% of infants born to HBsAg-positive mothers will develop antigens to hepatitis B in the bloodstream. Fecal-oral transmission of virus B has also been documented. The incubation period of hepatitis B is 6 weeks to 6 months but may be prolonged by the administration of hyperimmune globulin. Clinical features of hepatitis A and B are similar; however, the onset in hepatitis B tends to be more insidious.

Hepatitis B virus is pleomorphic and occurs in spherical and tubular forms of different sizes. The largest of these, the Dane particle, is thought to be the complete infectious virus. The 42-nm Dane particle is composed of a core (27-nm particle) found in the nucleus of infected liver cells, and a double-shelled surface particle found in the cytoplasm. The other particles form an excess coating of the virus and contain no nucleic acid.

There are 3 distinct antigen-antibody systems that relate to HBV infection. In addition, DNA polymerase activity can be measured as a sensitive index of viral replication and infectivity.

The surface antigen (HBsAg) is the antigen routinely measured in blood. HBsAg is unaffected by repeated freezing and thawing or by heating at 56 °C overnight or at 60 °C for 1 hour. It is inactivated by heating between 85 and 100 °C for 15–30 minutes. HBsAg can exist in serum as 3 antigenically identical forms: (1) the outer coat of the intact Dane particle, (2) a spherical 22-nm particle, and (3) elongated tubular particles. The spherical and tubular particles do not contain nucleic acid and are not infectious. Four major antigenic subtypes of HBsAg have been recognized. Subtyping of HBsAg is primarily of epidemiologic importance. The presence of HBsAg is the first manifestation of HBV infection occurring before biochemical evidence of liver disease. HBsAg persists throughout the clinical illness. Persistence of HBsAg is usually associated with clinical and laboratory evidence of chronic hepatitis. The presence of HBsAg establishes infection with HBV and implies infectivity. Specific antibody to HBsAg (anti-HBs) occurs in most individuals after clearance of HBsAg. Anti-HBs is usually delayed after clearance of HBsAg. During this serologic gap, infectivity has been demonstrated. Development of anti-HBs signals recovery from HBV, noninfectivity, and protection from HBV infection.

Disruption of the Dane particle releases an antigenically distinct inner core structure (HBcAg). Antibodies against core antigen (anti-HBc) localize the core antigen primarily to the nucleus of infected human and primate liver cells. The core particles are not found in the serum. Core particles may be present in liver

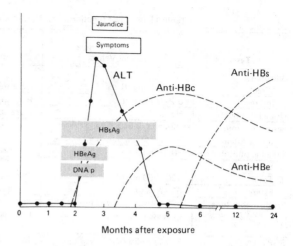

Figure 11–2. The typical course of acute type B hepatitis. HBsAg = hepatitis B surface antigen; anti-HBs = antibody to HBsAg; HBeAg = hepatitis Be antigen; anti-HBe = antibody to HBeAg; anti-HBc = antibody to hepatitis B core antigen; DNA p = DNA polymerase; ALT = alanine aminotransferase. (Reproduced, with permission, from Schafer DF, Hoofnagel JH: *Viewpoints on Digestive Diseases* 1982;**14**:5.)

tissue in the absence of H̊BsAg, and recovery from HBV is complete only when core particles are no longer detected in the liver. Anti-HBc appears shortly after HBsAg is detected and persists throughout the period of HBs antigenemia. It fills the serologic gap in patients who have cleared the HBsAg but have not demonstrated detectable amounts of anti-HBs. Anti-HBc can be found alone or in any combination with HBsAg or anti-HBs. Anti-HBc has been shown in all instances of acute HBV infection and appears simultaneously with the onset of clinical illness. Infectivity has been demonstrated in instances where donors are HBsAg-negative and positive for anti-HBc.

HBeAg is distinct from HBsAg. It is a soluble protein found only in HBsAg-positive sera. All patients with HBV infection demonstrate HBe antigenemia. HBeAg appears during the incubation period shortly after the detection of HBsAg and only during HBsAg reactivity. HBeAg may be a sensitive index of viral replication and infectivity. Anti-HBe is detected as early as the fourth week of illness. The clinical usefulness of this antigen-antibody system lies in its predictive value of infectivity.

DNA polymerase activity is first detectable at the time of peak HBsAg titer, suggesting that this enzyme is a manifestation of viremia and viral replication. DNA polymerase activity is usually transient but may persist for years in chronic carriers and is an indication of continued infectivity.

Clinical Findings

The clinical picture is extremely variable, ranging from asymptomatic infection without jaundice to a fulminating disease and death in a few days.

A. Symptoms:

1. Prodromal phase–The speed of onset varies from abrupt to insidious, with general malaise, myalgia, arthralgia and occasionally arthritis, easy fatigability, upper respiratory symptoms (nasal discharge, pharyngitis), and severe anorexia out of proportion to the degree of illness. Nausea and vomiting are frequent, and diarrhea or constipation may occur. Fever is generally present but is rarely over 39.5 °C (103.1 °F). Defervescence often coincides with the onset of jaundice. Chills or chilliness may mark an acute onset.

Abdominal pain is usually mild and constant in the upper right quadrant or right epigastrium and is often aggravated by jarring or exertion. (On rare occasions, upper abdominal pain may be severe enough to simulate cholecystitis or cholelithiasis.) A distaste for smoking, paralleling anorexia, may occur early.

2. Icteric phase–Clinical jaundice occurs after 5–10 days but may appear at the same time as the initial symptomatology. Some patients never develop clinical icterus. With the onset of jaundice, there is often an intensification of the prodromal symptoms, followed by progressive clinical improvement.

3. Convalescent phase–There is an increasing sense of well-being, return of appetite, and disappearance of jaundice, abdominal pain and tenderness, and fatigability.

B. Signs: Hepatomegaly—rarely marked—is present in over half of cases. Liver tenderness is usually present. Splenomegaly is reported in 15% of patients, and soft, enlarged lymph nodes—especially in the cervical or epitrochlear areas—may occur. Signs of general toxemia vary from minimal to severe.

C. Laboratory Findings: The white cell count is normal to low, especially in the preicteric phase. Large atypical lymphocytes, such as are found in infectious mononucleosis, may occasionally be seen. Mild proteinuria is common, and bilirubinuria often precedes the appearance of jaundice. Acholic stools are often present during the initial icteric phase. Blood and urine studies tend to reflect hepatocellular damage, with abnormal SGOT (AST) or SGPT (ALT) values, increased gamma globulin, and urobilinogenuria. In the cholangiolitic variety, alkaline phosphatase is elevated. HBsAg is usually positive in hepatitis B.

Delta Agent & Hepatitis B

The delta agent has an RNA genome, smaller than all known RNA animal viruses. The delta agent appears to be defective and depends upon external help to initiate and maintain replication. To date, it has been identified only in association with hepatitis B infection and specifically only in the presence of HBsAg; it is cleared when the latter is cleared. The distribution of the delta agent is global.

Clinically, the delta agent appears to be invariably pathogenic and may increase the severity of an acute HBV infection, aggravate previously existing HBV liver disease, or cause new disease in asymptomatic HBsAg carriers. When the delta agent is coincident with an acute HBV infection, the infection appears to be more severe, and the delta agent has recently been found in up to 50% of fulminant HBV infections. In chronic active hepatitis B, presence of the delta agent appears to carry a more severe prognosis. Vertical transmission of this agent appears to be much less frequent than that of HBV.

At present, there are no unique preventive or therapeutic measures for delta agent infections.

Hepatitis Non-A, Non-B

Although it has been generally accepted that virus A and virus B accounted for most instances of viral hepatitis, recent evidence provided by specific immunologic tests for virus types A and B, epidemiologic analysis of posttransfusion hepatitis, and response to prophylactic gamma globulin offers substantial evidence for the existence of one or more additional types of viral hepatitis (non-A, non-B hepatitis). These observations are of major importance in the problem of posttransfusion hepatitis. Although routine screening of HBsAg has appreciably reduced the incidence of posttransfusion type B hepatitis, its overall incidence has not changed. The incidence of posttransfusion hepatitis is approximately 7–10%. About 90% of the posttransfusion cases are caused by non-A, non-B hepatitis. The chronic carrier state of non-A, non-B hepatitis has been identified. The usual incubation period is 7–8 weeks, but it may vary from 2 to 20 weeks. Epidemiologic studies suggest that there are at least 2 non-A, non-B viruses. Aside from the exclusive use of volunteer blood donors, further reduction in the incidence of posttransfusion hepatitis will require development of serologic techniques to detect the agent or agents of non-A, non-B viral hepatitis.

The histologic findings in hepatitis A, B, and non-A, non-B are those of varying degrees of necrosis of the liver parenchymal cells and variable numbers of lymphocytes and monocytes in the portal areas and in areas of hepatocellular necrosis. The reticulum framework is well preserved, although there may be varying degrees of collapse if the insult is severe. In severe hepatitis, strands of collapsed reticulum may bridge from portal to portal, portal to central vein, or central vein to central vein; this is known as **bridging necrosis.** Healing occurs by regeneration from surviving cells—usually without distortion of the normal architecture.

Differential Diagnosis

The differential diagnosis of viral hepatitis should include, in addition to viruses A, B, and non-A, non-B, other viral diseases such as infectious mononucleosis and cytomegalic inclusion disease; spirochetal diseases such as leptospirosis and secondary syphilis; brucellosis; rickettsial diseases such as Q fever; and drug-induced liver disease.

The prodromal phase or the nonicteric form of the disease must be distinguished from other infectious diseases such as influenza, upper respiratory infections, and the prodromal stages of the exanthematous diseases. In the obstructive phase of viral hepatitis, it is necessary to rule out other obstructive lesions such as choledocholithiasis, chlorpromazine toxicity, and carcinoma of the head of the pancreas.

Prevention

Strict isolation of patients is not necessary, but hand washing after bowel movements is required. Thorough hand washing by medical attendants who come into contact with contaminated utensils, bedding, or clothing is essential. Disinfection of feces is not necessary when water-borne sewage disposal is available. Hepatitis B is for the most part transmitted by the parenteral route, but the possibility of fecal-oral infection as well as venereal transmission must be considered. Screening by means of HBsAg and SGOT determinations can remove potentially infectious individuals from blood donor lists. Unfortunately, there is increasing evidence that other viruses are responsible for similar clinical states. In blood donors, routine screening for HBsAg has reduced the incidence of posttransfusion hepatitis. In the USA, the avoidance of unnecessary transfusions and the exclusion of commercially obtained blood, along with clinical studies of the donor as well as the HBsAg and serum transaminase determinations, may be helpful in excluding potential sources of infectious blood. It may make possible the detection of one-third of infected donors. The use of disposable needles and syringes protects medical attendants as well as other patients.

Gamma globulin should be routinely given to all close personal contacts of patients with infectious hepatitis. An arbitrary dose of 5 mL for an adult has been found to be protective for hepatitis A if administered during the incubation period. It is also desirable that individuals traveling to or residing in endemic regions receive gamma globulin within 2 weeks after arrival. In the event of prolonged residence, a second dose should be given after 5–6 months.

Hepatitis B hyperimmune globulin may be protective if given in large doses within 7 days of exposure and again at 30 days. At present, this preparation is recommended for individuals exposed to hepatitis B surface antigen–contaminated material via the mucous membranes or through breaks in the skin. Persons who have had sexual contact with patients with acute hepatitis B surface antigen–positive disease should also receive hepatitis B hyperimmune globulin. Hepatitis B hyperimmune globulin is also indicated for newborn infants of HBsAg-positive mothers; give 0.5 mL very soon after birth and at ages 3 and 6 months. Hepatitis B hyperimmune globulin does not seem to be indicated in the prevention of transfusion-associated hepatitis.

A vaccine for the prevention of hepatitis B has been developed, extensively tested, and found safe. It reduces the incidence of hepatitis B by approximately 92% in highly exposed persons. The vaccine consists of highly purified, formalin-inactivated HBsAg particles derived from plasma of chronic antigen carriers. Recipients must have a negative serologic test for HBsAg and HBcAb. Potential candidates are persons at high risk, including renal dialysis patients and attending personnel, patients requiring repeated transfusions, spouses of HBsAg-positive individuals, male homosexuals, and newborns of HBsAg-positive mothers.

Treatment

A. General Measures: Bed rest should be at the patient's option during the acute initial phase of the disease, when symptoms are most severe. Bed rest beyond the most acute phase is not warranted. However, return to normal activity during the convalescent period should be gradual. If nausea and vomiting are significant problems, or if oral intake is substantially decreased, the intravenous administration of 10% glucose solution is indicated. If the patient shows signs of impending coma, protein should be temporarily interdicted and gradually reintroduced and increased as clinical improvement takes place. In general, dietary management consists of giving palatable meals as tolerated, without overfeeding. Patients with acute hepatitis should avoid strenuous physical exertion, alcohol, and hepatotoxic agents. While the administration of small doses of oxazepam or phenobarbital is safe (since they are not metabolized by the liver), it is recommended that morphine sulfate be avoided.

B. Corticotropin and Corticosteroids: Although these agents have been recommended by some authors for the treatment of fulminant hepatitis, controlled studies have demonstrated no benefit in patients with severe viral hepatitis treated relatively early in the course of the disease.

Prognosis

In most cases of viral hepatitis, clinical recovery is complete in 3–16 weeks. Laboratory evidence of disturbed liver function may persist for a longer period, but most of such patients usually go on to complete recovery. The overall mortality rate is less than 1%, but the rate is reportedly higher in older people (particularly postmenopausal women). Cirrhosis of the postnecrotic or macronodular type and chronic active (aggressive) hepatitis are infrequent.

Hepatitis tends to be more severe and potentially has a poorer prognosis in the elderly or in those with other complicating illnesses. Posttransfusion hepatitis occurs as a complication in 0.25–3% of blood transfusions and as many as 12% of pooled blood products. The asymptomatic carrier state and persistent viremia after acute disease make control of contamination in donor blood extremely difficult.

Aach RD, Kahn RA: Post-transfusion hepatitis: Current perspectives. *Ann Intern Med* 1980;**92**:539.

Alter HJ: The evolution, implications and applications of the hepatitis B vaccine. *JAMA* 1982;**247**:2272.

Dienstag JL: Non-A, non-B hepatitis. 1. Recognition, epidemiology and clinical features. 2. Experimental transmission, putative virus agents and markers, and prevention. *Gastroenterology* 1983;**85**:743.

Dienstag JL, Isselbacher KJ: Therapy for acute and chronic hepatitis. *Ann Intern Med* 1981;**141**:1419.

Feinstone SM, Hoofnagle JH: Non-A, maybe-B hepatitis. *N Engl J Med* 1984;**311**:185.

Hadler SC et al: Delta virus infection and severe hepatitis. *Ann Intern Med* 1984;**100**:339.

Health and Public Policy Committee, American College of Physicians: Hepatitis B vaccine. (Position Paper.) *Ann Intern Med* 1984;**100**:149.

Rinker J, Galambos JT: Prospective study of hepatitis B in thirty-two inadvertently infected people. *Gastroenterology* 1981; **81**:686.

Rizzetto M: The delta agent. *Hepatology* 1983;**3**:729.

Schafer DF, Hoofnagel JH: Serological diagnosis of viral hepatitis. *Viewpoints on Digestive Diseases* 1982;**14**:5.

Szmuness W et al: Hepatitis B vaccine: Demonstration of efficacy in a controlled clinical trial in a high-risk population in the United States. *N Engl J Med* 1980;**303**:833.

VARIANTS OF INFECTIOUS HEPATITIS

Cholangiolitic Hepatitis

There is usually a cholestatic phase in the initial icteric phase of viral hepatitis, but in occasional cases, this is the dominant manifestation of the disease. The course tends to be more prolonged than that of ordinary hepatitis. The symptoms are often extremely mild, but jaundice is deeper, and pruritus is often present. Laboratory tests of liver function indicate cholestasis with hyperbilirubinemia, biliuria, and elevated alkaline phosphatase and cholesterol.

Differentiation of this type of hepatitis from extrahepatic obstruction may be difficult. Percutaneous transhepatic cholangiography or endoscopic retrograde cholangiography may be necessary to make the distinction.

Boyer JL: The diagnosis and pathogenesis of clinical variants in viral hepatitis. *Am J Clin Pathol* 1976;**65**:898.

Fulminant Hepatitis

Hepatitis may take a rapidly progressive course terminating in less than 10 days. Extensive necrosis of large areas of the liver gives the typical pathologic picture of acute liver atrophy. Toxemia and gastrointestinal symptoms are more severe, and hemorrhagic phenomena are common. Neurologic symptoms of hepatic coma develop (see Cirrhosis, p 412). Jaundice may be absent or minimal, but laboratory tests show extreme hepatocellular damage.

The treatment of fulminant hepatitis is directed toward those metabolic abnormalities associated with severe liver cell dysfunction. They include coagulation defects; disordered fluid, electrolyte, and acid-base balance; hypoglycemia; and nitrogenous intoxication. Careful monitoring of the patient, with vigorous correction of the deficits noted, provides the hope that some patients will survive who might otherwise succumb before liver regeneration can occur.

Adrenocorticosteroids, exchange transfusions, and perfusions through pig and baboon livers have not proved effective.

Blitzer BL: Fulminant hepatic failure: A rare but often lethal syndrome. *Postgrad Med* (Sept) 1980;**68**:153.

Tygstrup N et al: Fulminant hepatic failure. *Clin Gastroenterol* 1981;**10**:191.

CHRONIC HEPATITIS

Chronic hepatitis is defined as a chronic inflammatory reaction of the liver of more than 6 months' duration, as demonstrated by persistently abnormal liver tests. For proper treatment, it is crucial to determine whether the disease will resolve, remain static, or progress to cirrhosis. The causes of chronic hepatitis are only partially defined. It may be a sequela of infection resulting from hepatitis B virus. Chronic hepatitis has also been seen as a sequela of non-A, non-B hepatitis. Hepatitis A virus has not yet been shown to lead to chronic hepatitis. Additionally, identical clinical entities may be associated with drug reactions, including oxyphenisatin, methyldopa, and isoniazid. Wilson's disease can also present as chronic liver disease, and α_1-antitrypsin deficiency is also associated with chronic liver disease.

1. CHRONIC PERSISTENT HEPATITIS

This form of chronic hepatitis represents an essentially benign condition with a good prognosis. The diagnosis is confirmed by liver biopsy. The biopsy may show portal tract infiltration with primarily mononuclear cells and occasional areas of focal inflammation in the parenchyma. The boundary between portal tracts and parenchyma remains sharp, and there is little or no "piecemeal necrosis" (a process in which the liver cells are gradually destroyed and replaced by fibrous tissue septa). In essence, the architecture of the hepatic lobule remains intact. The symptomatology varies from the asymptomatic state to various vague manifestations including fatigability, anorexia, malaise, and lassitude. Physical examination is usually normal.

Liver biopsy helps establish the diagnosis of persistent hepatitis. The treatment is mostly reassurance of the patient. Corticosteroids and immunosuppressive drugs should not be given. Dietary restrictions, excessive vitamin supplementation, and prolonged bed rest are not necessary. The prognosis is excellent. Rarely does the disease progress to chronic active hepatitis.

2. CHRONIC ACTIVE HEPATITIS

This form of chronic hepatitis is usually characterized by progression to cirrhosis, although milder cases may resolve spontaneously. The histologic changes include chronic inflammatory infiltration involving portal zones and extending into the parenchyma, with piecemeal necrosis and the formation of intralobular septa. **Piecemeal necrosis,** a process of inflammatory cells and hepatocyte necrosis occurring at the interface of the portal area and the liver lobule, may extend well into the lobule and across zonal boundaries. In severe cases, piecemeal necrosis may be associated with considerable hepatic failure or fibrosis and ultimately with cirrhosis. In very mild cases, it may be difficult to distinguish this entity from chronic persistent hepatitis. Liver biopsies repeated at varying intervals may be necessary to make the distinction as well as to monitor therapy.

Clinical Findings

A. Symptoms and Signs:

1. Chronic active hepatitis (lupoid type) –This is generally a disease of young people, particularly young women. However, the disease can occur at any age. The onset is usually insidious, but about 25% of cases present as an acute attack of hepatitis. Although the serum bilirubin is usually increased, 20% of these patients have anicteric disease. Examination often reveals a healthy-appearing young woman with multiple spider nevi, cutaneous striae, acne, and hirsutism. Amenorrhea may be a feature of this disease. Multisystem involvement, including kidneys, joints, lungs, and bowel, and Coombs-positive hemolytic anemia are associated with this clinical entity.

2. Chronic active hepatitis (HBsAg-positive type) –This type of hepatitis clinically resembles the lupoid type of disease. The histologic pictures of these 2 types of chronic active hepatitis are indistinguishable. The HBsAg form of chronic active hepatitis appears to affect males predominantly. It may be noted as a continuum of acute hepatitis or may be manifested only by biochemical abnormalities of liver function.

3. Delta agent in hepatitis B –(See p 405.) Acute delta infection superimposed on chronic HBV infection may be subclinical and manifested only by a transient transaminase rise; in this setting, chronic delta infection ensues. Delta infection among HBsAg carriers is common and is associated with the presence of liver damage, usually due to chronic active hepatitis with or without cirrhosis.

B. Laboratory Findings: The serum bilirubin is usually normal or only modestly increased (4.5–7 mg/dL); SGOT (AST), IgG, IgM, and gamma globulin levels are higher than normal. Late in the disease, serum albumin levels are usually decreased and prothrombin time may be significantly prolonged and will not respond to vitamin K therapy. Antinuclear and smooth muscle antibodies are positive 15–50% of the time but are nonspecific. Latex fixation tests for rheumatoid arthritis and anticytoplasmic and immunofluorescent antimitochondrial antibodies are positive in 28–50% of patients. Hepatitis B antigen is not found in the blood of patients with classic "lupoid" hepatitis.

The activity of chronic active hepatitis can be defined practically and accurately in terms of objective criteria. Thus, the magnitude of transaminase and gamma globulin elevations and the degree of hepatocellular necrosis are suitable means of defining activity and judging the response to treatment. Activity in chronic liver disease can be defined quantitatively quite readily by establishing arbitrary biochemical standards. For example, either a 10-fold increase in serum transaminase level or a 5-fold elevation of SGOT with a 2-fold increase in gamma globulin concentration constitutes "high-grade" activity.

Differential Diagnosis

Chronic active hepatitis can be confused with 5 other chronic liver conditions: cholestatic viral hepatitis, chronic persistent hepatitis, subacute hepatic necrosis, postnecrotic cirrhosis, and Wilson's disease. The differentiation is made on the basis of the clinical course, sequential laboratory testing, and liver biopsy.

Treatment

Prolonged or enforced bed rest has not been shown to be beneficial. Activity should be modified according to the patient's symptoms. The diet should be well balanced, without specific limitations other than sodium or protein restrictions as dictated by water retention or encephalopathy.

Prednisone has been shown to decrease the serum bilirubin, SGOT, and gamma globulin levels and reduce the piecemeal necrosis in patients with chronic active hepatitis. Data from controlled clinical trials indicate that the mortality rate in the group of patients treated with corticosteroids is significantly reduced. However, relapse after discontinuation of prednisone therapy occurs frequently. In assessing the necessity for corticosteroid therapy, the benefit of the therapy should outweigh its potential risk. For patients with chronic active hepatitis due to HBV infection, the risks of increasing viral replication and infectiousness with the use of corticosteroids are considerable and are a relative contraindication to their use. Patients with chronic active hepatitis who are symptomatic, those who are HBsAg-negative, and those who have severe histologic abnormalities appear at this time to be the most suitable candidates for corticosteroid therapy.

Prednisone or an equivalent drug is given initially in doses of 30 mg orally daily, with gradual reduction to the lowest maintenance level (usually 15–20 mg/d) that will control the symptomatology and reduce the abnormal liver function. If symptoms are not controlled, azathioprine (Imuran), 50–150 mg/d orally, is added, with the primary benefit being that doses of corticosteroids can be much lower. Azathioprine imposes a significant hazard of bone marrow depression, and complete blood counts should be obtained at least weekly until the dose has been stabilized for 6–8 weeks, and then at less frequent intervals as dictated by the maintenance dose and hematologic picture. In general, the combination of prednisone, 10–15 mg/d, and azathioprine, 25–50 mg/d, gives therapeutic efficacy with few significant side effects of both drugs.

Prognosis

The course of chronic active hepatitis is variable and unpredictable. The sequelae of chronic active hepatitis secondary to hepatitis B include cirrhosis, liver cell failure, and hepatocellular carcinoma. It has been stated that 40–50% of patients with chronic active hepatitis die within 5 years of the onset of symptoms. Most patients die of hepatocellular failure and associated complications of portal hypertension.

Czaja AJ et al: Clinical features and prognosis of severe chronic active liver disease (CALD) after corticosteroid-induced remission. *Gastroenterology* 1980;**78**:518.

Czaja AJ et al: Corticosteroid-treated chronic active hepatitis in remission. *N Engl J Med* 1981;**304**:5.

Gitnick GL: The long term course of non-A, non-B posttransfusion hepatitis. *Gastroenterology* 1980;**79**:893.

Redeker AG: Delta agent and hepatitis B. *Ann Intern Med* 1983; **98**:542.

Sherlock S: Chronic hepatitis. *Postgrad Med* (June) 1979;**65**:81.

Vyas GN, Blum HE: Hepatitis B virus infections: Current concepts of chronicity and immunity. *West J Med* 1984;**140**:754.

ALCOHOLIC HEPATITIS

Alcoholic hepatitis is an acute or chronic inflammation of the liver that occurs as a result of parenchymal necrosis induced by alcohol abuse. Although a variety of terms were used in the past to describe this type of hepatitis in chronic alcoholics, the term alcoholic hepatitis is now regarded as the most appropriate one to describe this injury, which is currently accepted as the precursor of alcoholic cirrhosis.

While alcoholic hepatitis is often a reversible disease, it is the most common cause of cirrhosis in the USA. This is especially significant, since cirrhosis ranks among the most common causes of death of adults in this country. Alcoholic hepatitis does not develop in all chronic heavy drinkers; the exact prevalence and incidence are not known but have been estimated to be about one-third. Women appear to be more susceptible than men.

Alcoholic hepatitis usually occurs after years of excessive drinking. Although it may not develop in many patients even after several decades of alcohol abuse, it appears in a few individuals within a year of excessive drinking. Over 80% of patients with alcoholic hepatitis were drinking 5 years or more before developing any symptoms that could be attributed to liver disease. In general, the longer the duration of drinking (10–15 or more years) and the larger the alcoholic consumption (usually more than 120 g of alcohol per day, which is equal to 8 oz of 100-proof whiskey, 30 oz of wine, or 100 oz of beer [eight 12-oz cans]), the greater the probability of developing alcoholic hepatitis and cirrhosis. It is also important to realize that while drinking large amounts of alcoholic beverages is essential for the development of alcoholic hepatitis, drunkenness is not. In drinking individuals, the rate of ethanol metabolism can be sufficiently high to permit the consumption of large quantities of spirits without raising the blood alcohol level over 80 mg/dL, the concentration at which the conventional breath analyzer begins to detect ethanol.

The roles of proteins, vitamins, and calories in the development of alcoholic hepatitis or in the progression of this lesion to cirrhosis are not understood.

Only liver biopsy can establish the diagnosis with certainty, since any of the manifestations of alcoholic hepatitis can be seen in other types of alcoholic liver disease such as fatty liver or cirrhosis.

Clinical Findings

A. Symptoms and Signs: Alcoholic hepatitis is usually seen after a recent period of heavy drinking. That history in addition to complaints of anorexia and nausea and the objective demonstration of hepatomegaly and jaundice strongly suggest the diagnosis. Abdominal pain and tenderness, splenomegaly, ascites, fever, and encephalopathy support the diagnosis. The clinical presentation of alcoholic hepatitis can vary from an asymptomatic patient with an enlarged liver to a critically ill individual who dies quickly.

B. Laboratory Findings: Anemia is variable and usually macrocytic and may in part reflect the socioeconomic status of the patient. Leukocytosis with shift to the left is common and is seen more frequently in patients with severe disease. Leukopenia is occasionally seen and disappears after cessation of drinking. About 10% of patients have thrombocytopenia that appears related to a direct toxic effect of alcohol on megakaryocytes.

SGOT (AST) is normal in 15–25% of patients; when increased, it is usually under 300 IU/mL. Values over 300 IU/mL imply increasing severity of the disease and correlate well with biopsy findings. Serum alkaline phosphatase is generally elevated, but rarely more than 3 times the normal value. Serum bilirubin is increased in 60–90% of patients, and when levels greater than 6 mg/dL are demonstrated it can be assumed that the process is severe. The serum albumin is depressed, and the gamma globulin is elevated in 50–75% of individuals with alcoholic hepatitis even in the absence of cirrhosis.

Liver biopsy is diagnostic and may reveal both cirrhosis and alcoholic hepatitis.

C. Special Procedures: Scintiphotographic evaluation (liver scanning) using ^{99m}Tc sulfur colloid will reveal patchy hepatic uptake of the isotope; marked bone marrow uptake, which is indicative of portal hypertension; and splenomegaly. Liver scanning is nonspecific and rarely indicated.

Differential Diagnosis

Nausea, vomiting, abdominal pain, jaundice, fever, right upper abdominal tenderness, leukocytosis, and elevated serum alkaline phosphatase with concomitantly minimal to moderate elevation of SGOT occur in both alcoholic hepatitis and diseases of the hepatobiliary tree such as cholecystitis and cholelithiasis. A history of chronic insobriety and recent debauch is helpful but far from conclusive. Percutaneous liver biopsy, if there is no contraindication, is the only reliable means of differentiation.

Complications

Clinical deterioration and worsening abdominal pain and tenderness may result in the unfortunate decision to perform celiotomy. The postoperative mortality rate of acutely ill patients with alcoholic hepatitis is far greater than that of those who are operated on for intra- or extrahepatic cholestasis.

Treatment

A. General Measures: Discontinue all alcoholic beverages. During periods of anorexia, every effort should be made to provide sufficient amounts of carbohydrate and calories to reduce endogenous protein catabolism and gluconeogenesis and to prevent hypoglycemia. Although the clinical value of intravenous hyperalimentation has not been established, the judicious administration of parenteral fluids is most important. Caloric intake is gratifyingly improved by the use of palatable liquid formulas during the transition period between totally intravenous alimentation and normal feeding. The administration of vitamins, particularly folic acid, is an important part of treatment and is frequently associated with dramatic clinical improvement in patients with alcoholic liver disease.

B. Steroids: The use of corticosteroids in this disorder has been evaluated over a period of more than 20 years, with reports of sporadic success. Anabolic steroids are not beneficial.

Prognosis

A. Short-Term: The severity of liver injury, which can be ascertained clinically, biochemically,

and histologically, enables valid speculation about prognosis. The presence of asterixis seems to be associated with an increased likelihood of death. Biochemically, it has been shown that when the prothrombin time is short enough to permit performance of liver biopsy without risk, the 1-year mortality rate is 7.1%, rising to 18% if there is progressive prolongation of that parameter during hospitalization. Individuals in whom the prothrombin time is so prolonged that liver biopsy cannot be attempted have a 42% mortality rate.

B. Long-Term: In the USA, the mortality rate over a 3-year period of persons who recover from acute alcoholic hepatitis is 10 times greater than that of average individuals of comparable age. The histologically severe form of the disease is associated with continued excessive mortality rates after 3 years, whereas the death rate is not increased after the same period in those whose liver biopsies show only mild alcoholic hepatitis.

The most important prognostic consideration is the indisputable fact that continued excessive drinking is associated with reduction of life expectancy in these individuals. The prognosis is indeed poor if the patient is unwilling to abstain from drinking.

Lieber CS: Alcohol, protein metabolism, and liver injury. *Gastroenterology* 1980;**79**:373.

Monroe PS, Baker AL: Alcoholic hepatitis: Update on recognition and management. *Postgrad Med* (April) 1981;**69**:32.

Zetterman RK, Sorrell MF: Immunologic aspects of alcoholic liver disease. *Gastroenterology* 1981;**81**:616.

Table 11–5. Uncommon hyperbilirubinemic disorders.

	Nature of Defect	Type of Hyper-bilirubinemia	Clinical and Pathologic Characteristics
Constitutional hepatic dysfunction (Gilbert's syndrome)	Glucuronyl transferase deficiency	Unconjugated (indirect) bilirubin	Benign, asymptomatic hereditary jaundice. Hyperbilirubinemia increased by 24- to 36-hour fast. No treatment required. Prognosis excellent.
Crigler-Najjar syndrome			Severe, nonhemolytic hereditary jaundice of neonates. Type I cases sustain CNS damage (kernicterus). Milder cases (type II) may persist into adult life and may benefit from treatment with phenobarbital.
Familial chronic idiopathic jaundice (Dubin-Johnson syndrome)	Faulty excretory function of liver cells (hepatocytes)	Conjugated (direct) bilirubin	Benign, asymptomatic hereditary jaundice. BSP excretion impaired. Gallbladder does not visualize on oral cholecystography. Liver darkly pigmented on gross examination. Biopsy shows centrilobular brown pigment. Prognosis excellent.
Rotor's syndrome			Similar to Dubin-Johnson syndrome but liver is not pigmented and the gallbladder is visualized on oral cholecystography. Prognosis excellent.
Benign intermittent cholestasis	Cholestatic liver dysfunction	Unconjugated plus conjugated (total) bilirubin	Benign intermittent idiopathic jaundice, itching, and malaise. Onset in early life and may persist for lifetime. Alkaline phosphatase and BSP retention are increased. Cholestasis found on liver biopsy. (Biopsy is normal during remission.) Prognosis excellent.
Recurrent jaundice of pregnancy			Benign cholestatic jaundice of unknown cause, usually occurring in the third trimester of pregnancy. Itching, gastrointestinal symptoms, and abnormal liver excretory function tests. Cholestasis noted on liver biopsy. Prognosis excellent, but recurrence with subsequent pregnancies or use of birth control pills is characteristic.

UNCOMMON HYPERBILIRUBINEMIA STATES

There are about a half-dozen hyperbilirubinemic states that must be distinguished from hemolytic disease, hepatitis, and surgical jaundice (see Table 11–5). The disorders are benign, with the notable exception of the rare type I Crigler-Najjar syndrome, for which there is no known effective treatment. These hyperbilirubinemic states are very uncommon, with the exception of Gilbert's syndrome, which may occur in up to 5% of the population.

Wolkoff AW et al: Bilirubin metabolism and hyperbilirubinemia. *Semin Liver Dis* 1983;**8**:1.

DRUG- & TOXIN-INDUCED LIVER DISEASE

The continuing synthesis, testing, and introduction of new drugs into clinical practice has resulted in an increase in toxic reactions of many types. Many widely used therapeutic agents may cause hepatic injury. The diagnosis of drug-induced liver injury is not always easy. Drug-induced liver disease can mimic viral hepatitis or biliary tract obstruction. The clinician must be aware of drug-induced liver disease and must question the patient carefully about the use of various drugs before dismissing this possibility.

Direct Hepatotoxic Group

The liver lesion caused by this group of drugs is characterized by (1) dose-related severity, (2) reproducibility in experimental animals, (3) a latent period following exposure, and (4) susceptibility in all individuals:

Acetaminophen	Phosphorus
Alcohol	Stilbamidine
Carbon tetrachloride	Tetracyclines
Chloroform	Valproic acid
Heavy metals	Vitamin A
Mercaptopurine	

Viral Hepatitis-Like Reactions

Reactions of this type are sporadic, suggesting host idiosyncrasy:

Aspirin	Methyldopa
Chloramphenicol	Oxacillin
Chlortetracycline	Phenylbutazone
Cinchophen	Pyrazinamide
Dantrolene	Streptomycin
Halothane	Sulfamethoxypyridazine
Isoniazid	Zoxazolamine
Methoxyflurane	

Cholestatic Reactions

There are 2 general categories that differ in clinical presentation and histopathologic features. These reactions are dose-dependent, but marked differences in individual susceptibility exist:

A. Noninflammatory: Probable direct effect of agent on bile secretory mechanisms and no inflammatory reactions:

Mestranol	Norethandrolone
Methyltestosterone	

B. Inflammatory: Inflammation of portal areas, with allergic features, eg, eosinophilia:

Chlorothiazide	Prochlorperazine
Chlorpromazine	Promazine
Chlorpropamide	Sulfadiazine
Erythromycin estolate	Thiouracils

Chronic Active Hepatitis

Clinically and histologically indistinguishable from chronic viral hepatitis:

Acetaminophen	Isoniazid
Aspirin	Methyldopa
Chlorpromazine	Nitrofurantoin
Halothane	Oxyphenisatin

Miscellaneous Reactions

A. Fatty Liver:
1. Large fatty inclusions–Alcohol, corticosteroids
2. Small cytoplasmic droplets–Tetracyclines

B. Granulomas:

Allopurinol	Phenytoin
Phenylbutazone	

C. Cirrhosis:
Methotrexate

Sherlock S: Hepatic reactions to drugs. *Gut* 1979;**20**:634.
Timbrell JA: Drug hepatotoxicity. (Review.) *Br J Clin Pharmacol* 1983;**15**:3.
Zafrani ES, Pinaudeau Y, Dhumeaux D: Drug-induced vascular lesions of the liver. *Arch Intern Med* 1983;**143**:495.

FATTY LIVER

It was formerly believed that malnutrition rather than ethanol was responsible for steatosis (fatty metamorphosis) of the liver in the alcoholic. More recently, it has come to be agreed that the role of deficient nutrition in such individuals has been overemphasized. However, it cannot be ignored that inadequate diets—specifically, those deficient in choline, methionine, and dietary protein—can produce fatty liver (kwashiorkor) in children.

Other nonalcoholic causes of steatosis are obesity (the commonest cause), starvation, diabetes mellitus, corticosteroids, poisons (carbon tetrachloride and yellow phosphorus), endocrinopathies such as Cushing's syndrome, tetracycline toxicity, Reye's syndrome, TPN, and, rarely, pregnancy.

Regardless of the cause, there are apparently at least 5 factors, acting in varying combinations, that are responsible for the accumulation of fat in the liver: (1) increased mobilization of fatty acids from peripheral adipose depots; (2) decreased utilization or oxidation of fatty acids by the liver; (3) increased hepatic fatty acid synthesis; (4) increased esterification of fatty acids into triglycerides; and (5) decreased secretion or liberation of fat from the liver.

Percutaneous liver biopsy is diagnostic.

Treatment consists of removing or modifying the offending factor.

Adler M, Schaffner F: Fatty liver hepatitis and cirrhosis in obese patients. *Am J Med* 1979;**67**:811.

Consensus Conference: Diagnosis and treatment of Reye's syndrome. *JAMA* 1981;**246**:2441.

Sherlock S: Acute fatty liver of pregnancy and the microvesicular fat diseases. *Gut* 1983;**24**:265.

CIRRHOSIS

The concept of cirrhosis that evolved during the past few decades includes only those cases in which hepatocellular injury leads to both fibrosis and nodular regeneration throughout the liver. These features delineate cirrhosis as a serious and irreversible disease that is characterized not only by variable degrees of hepatic cell dysfunction but also by portosystemic shunting and portal hypertension. Fibrosis alone, regardless of its severity, is excluded by the previous definition. Also excluded by definition are the earlier stages of chronic biliary obstruction and hemochromatosis, neither of which forms regenerating nodules until late.

An important part of this concept is the realization that the type of cirrhosis changes with the passage of time in any one patient. Terms such as "portal" and "postnecrotic" refer not so much to separate disease states with different causes as to stages in the evolution of cirrhosis.

Attempts to classify cirrhosis on the basis of cause or pathogenesis are usually unsuccessful when applied to individual patients. Such persons often represent end-stage cirrhosis, enabling only speculation about the evolutionary process. The use of a purely anatomic and descriptive categorization facilitates easier and more practical classification. One such classification that is currently employed divides cirrhosis into micronodular, mixed, and macronodular forms. It is important, however, to remember that these are stages of development rather than separate diseases.

(1) Micronodular cirrhosis is the form in which the regenerating nodules are no larger than the original lobules, ie, approximately 1 mm in diameter or less. It has been suggested that this feature results from the persistence of the offending agent (alcohol), a substance that prevents regenerative growth.

(2) Macronodular cirrhosis is characterized by larger nodules, which can measure several centimeters in diameter. This form corresponds more or less to

postnecrotic cirrhosis but does not necessarily follow episodes of massive necrosis and stromal collapse.

(3) Mixed macro- and micronodular cirrhosis points up the fact that the features of cirrhosis are highly variable and not always easy to classify. In any case, the configuration of the liver is determined by the mixture of liver cell death and regeneration as well as the deposition of fat, iron, and fibrosis.

Finally, it should be emphasized that there does exist a limited relationship between anatomic types and etiology as well as between anatomic types and prognosis. For example, alcoholics who continue to drink tend to have that form of cirrhosis that remains micronodular for long periods. The presence of fatty micronodular cirrhosis, although not an infallible criterion, is strongly suggestive of chronic alcoholism. On the other hand, liver cell carcinoma not uncommonly arises in macronodular rather than micronodular cirrhosis. Although speculative and subject to dispute, it is possible that this propensity to malignancy is related either to the increased regeneration in macronodular cirrhosis or to the longer period required for the process to develop.

Clinical Findings

A. Symptoms and Signs: Micronodular (Laennec's) cirrhosis may cause no symptoms for long periods, both at onset and later in the course (compensated phase). The onset of symptoms may be insidious or, less often, abrupt. Weakness, fatigability, and weight loss are common. In advanced cirrhosis, anorexia is usually present and may be extreme, with associated nausea and occasional vomiting. Abdominal pain may be present and is related either to hepatic enlargement and stretching of Glisson's capsule or to the presence of ascites. Diarrhea is frequently present, but some patients are constipated. Menstrual abnormalities (usually amenorrhea), impotence, loss of libido, sterility, and painfully enlarged breasts in men (rare) may occur. Hematemesis is the presenting symptom in 15–25%.

In 70% of cases, the liver is enlarged, palpable, firm if not hard, and has a blunt edge. Skin manifestations consist of spider nevi (usually only on the upper half of the body), palmar erythema (mottled redness of the thenar and hypothenar eminences), telangiectases of exposed areas, and evidence of vitamin deficiencies (glossitis and cheilosis). Weight loss, wasting, and the appearance of chronic illness are present. Jaundice— usually not an initial sign—is mild at first, increasing in severity during the later stages of the disease. Ascites, pleural effusion, peripheral edema, and purpuric lesions are late findings. The precoma state (asterixis, tremor, dysarthrias, delirium, and drowsiness) and encephalopathy or coma also occur very late. Gynecomastia, pectoral and axillary alopecia, and testicular atrophy may be present. Fever is present in 35% of cases and may reflect the presence of alcoholic hepatitis. (Infection with pneumococci or *Escherichia coli* and peritonitis secondary to tuberculosis should also be considered in any cirrhotic patient with ascites who is febrile for a prolonged period without a readily demonstrable cause.) Splenomegaly is present in 35–50% of cases. The superficial veins of the abdomen and thorax are dilated and reflect the intrahepatic obstruction to portal blood flow.

B. Laboratory Findings: Laboratory abnormalities are either absent or minimal in latent or quiescent cirrhosis. Anemia, a frequent finding, is usually macrocytic and represents, in the heavy drinker, direct suppression of erythropoiesis by alcohol as well as folate deficiency, hemolysis, and insidious or overt blood loss from the gastrointestinal tract. The white cell count may be low, elevated, or normal, reflecting hypersplenism or infection. Coagulation abnormalities may be a result of failure of synthesis of clotting constituents in the liver. Proteinuria may be present, and oliguria is frequent in active or decompensated disease with ascites.

Blood chemical studies show primarily hepatocellular injury and dysfunction, reflected by elevations of SGOT (AST), alkaline phosphatase, and bilirubin. Serum albumin is low; gamma globulin is increased.

Liver biopsy shows cirrhosis.

C. X-Ray Findings: Radiographic examinations may reveal the presence of esophageal or gastric varices if these vessels are sufficiently large. Plain films of the abdomen may reveal hepatic or splenic enlargement.

D. Special Examinations: Esophagogastroscopy demonstrates or confirms the presence of varices and detects specific causes of bleeding in the esophagus, stomach, and proximal duodenum. Splenoportography and arteriography are useful for evaluating the patency of the portal vein and splenic vein. Hepatic scanning using ^{99m}Tc sulfur colloid may occasionally be helpful in documenting splenomegaly; however, diffuse patchy uptake of the isotope in the liver makes this test useless in the evaluation of hepatoma. Peritoneoscopy is helpful in judging the type of cirrhosis present.

Differential Diagnosis

As previously noted, differentiation of one type of cirrhosis from another can be difficult. Actual visualization of the liver by peritoneoscopy, when correlated with biopsy results and the history, facilitates classification. Hemochromatosis may be associated with "bronzing" of the skin and diabetes mellitus. Special staining of liver biopsies will be positive for increased iron deposition in the hepatic parenchyma. Primary biliary cirrhosis tends to occur more frequently in women and is associated with marked pruritus, significant elevation of alkaline phosphatase, and positive antimitochondrial antibodies.

Complications

Upper gastrointestinal tract bleeding may occur from varices, hemorrhagic gastritis, or gastroduodenal ulcers. Hemorrhage may be massive, resulting in fatal exsanguination or portosystemic encephalopathy. Liver failure may also be precipitated by alcoholism, surgery, and infection. Carcinoma of the liver and portal vein thrombosis occur more frequently in patients with cirrhosis but are still uncommon. Lowered resistance often leads to serious infections, particularly of the lungs and peritoneum.

Treatment

A. General Measures: The principles of treatment include abstinence from alcohol and adequate rest, especially during the acute phase. The diet should be palatable, with adequate calories and protein (75–100 g/d) and, in the stage of fluid retention, sodium and fluid restriction. In the presence of hepatic precoma or coma, protein intake should be low or drastically reduced. Vitamin supplementation is desirable.

B. Special Problems:

1. Ascites and edema due to sodium retention, hypoproteinemia, and portal hypertension–Removal of ascites by paracentesis is usually not indicated unless it is critically important to relieve respiratory distress or patient discomfort or is essential for diagnosis of tumor or spontaneous bacterial peritonitis. Abdominal paracentesis can be associated with serious illness and even death. Hemorrhage, perforation of the bowel, and abscess may occur.

In many patients, there is a rapid diminution of ascites on dietary sodium and fluid restriction alone. In individuals who pose more significant problems of fluid retention and who are considered to have "intractable" ascites, the urinary excretion of sodium is less than 10 meq/L. Mechanisms that have been postulated to explain sodium retention in cirrhosis include impaired liver inactivation of aldosterone and increased aldosterone secretion secondary to increased renin production, which is associated with decreased renal cortical blood flow of uncertain cause. If such persons are permitted unrestricted fluids, serum sodium progressively falls, representing dilution. With a 200-mg sodium diet and 500-mL allowance of oral fluids per day, ascites production ceases and the patient's abdominal discomfort abates; however, this regimen is unrealistic in most clinical situations.

a. Restoration of plasma proteins–This is dependent upon improving liver function and serves as a practical index of recovery. The use of albumin intravenously is of doubtful value.

b. Diuretics–Spironolactone should be used after documentation of secondary aldosteronism, as evidenced by markedly low urinary sodium. Starting with spironolactone, 50 mg twice daily, and monitoring the aldosterone antagonist effect, reflected by the urinary sodium concentration and the fact that sodium excretion exceeds sodium intake, the dose of spironolactone is increased 100 mg every 3 days (up to a daily dosage of 1000 mg) until the urinary sodium excretion exceeds 60 meq/L. Diuresis commonly occurs at this point and may be augmented by the addition of a potent agent such as furosemide. This potent diuretic, however, will maintain its effect even with a falling glomerular filtration rate, with resultant severe renal damage. The dose of furosemide ranges from 40 to 120 mg/d, and the drug should be administered with careful monitoring of serum electrolytes.

The goal of weight loss in the nonedematous ascitic patient should be no more than 1–1½ lbs/d.

2. Hepatic encephalopathy–Hepatic encephalopathy is the result of biochemical abnormalities associated with hepatocellular deficit or hepatic bypass of portal vein blood into the systemic circulation. Although disturbed ammonia metabolism is inherent in the clinical entity of hepatic encephalopathy, it is not clear that ammonia per se is responsible for the disturbed mental status. The amount of ammonia produced is dependent upon the protein content, the bacterial flora, the pH, and the motility of the colon. Hepatic encephalopathy may be aggravated by sepsis. Bleeding into the intestinal tract from varices or ulcerations may significantly increase the amount of protein in the bowel and may precipitate rapid development of liver coma. Other factors that may precipitate hepatic encephalopathy include alkalosis, potassium deficiency induced by most diuretics, narcotics, hypnotics, and sedatives; medications containing ammonium or amino compounds; paracentesis with attendant hypovolemia; and hepatic or systemic infection.

Dietary protein may be drastically curtailed or completely withheld for short periods during acute episodes. Parenteral nutrition is usually indicated.

Gastrointestinal bleeding should be treated by all necessary medical and surgical means to prevent further bleeding and to remove blood. Give milk of magnesia, 30 mL 4 times daily, or magnesium sulfate, 10–15 g by indwelling nasogastric tube.

Lactulose (Cephulac), a nonabsorbable synthetic disaccharide, acidifies the colon contents, resulting in retention of ammonium ion and decreased ammonia absorption. When given orally, the initial dose of lactulose for acute hepatic encephalopathy is 30 mL 3 or 4 times daily, or a dose that will produce no more than 2–3 soft stools per day. When rectal use is indicated because of the patient's inability to take medicines orally, the dose is 300 mL of lactulose in 700 mL of saline as a retention enema for 30–60 minutes; it may be repeated every 4–6 hours. One liter of nonfat milk may be used instead.

The intestinal flora may also be controlled with neomycin sulfate, 0.5–1 g orally every 6 hours for 5–7 days. Side effects of neomycin include diarrhea, malabsorption, superinfection, phototoxicity, ototoxicity, and nephrotoxicity, usually only after prolonged use.

Treat shock as outlined in Chapter 1.

Treat infection with antibiotic agents chosen on the basis of culture and sensitivity studies. In some cases, broad-spectrum antimicrobials are indicated if the patient's condition is deteriorating.

If agitation is marked, give oxazepam, 10–30 mg orally, or sodium phenobarbital, 15–30 mg intramuscularly, cautiously as indicated. Avoid narcotics, tranquilizers, and sedatives excreted by the liver.

3. Anemia–For hypochromic anemia, give ferrous sulfate, 0.3-g enteric-coated tablets, one tablet 3 times daily after meals. Folic acid, 1 mg/d orally, is

indicated in the treatment of macrocytic anemia.

4. Hemorrhagic tendency–A bleeding tendency due to hypoprothrombinemia may be treated with vitamin K preparations. This treatment is ineffective in the presence of severe hepatic disease when other coagulation factors are deficient. Transfusions with packed red blood cells or fresh frozen plasma (or both) may be necessary to control bleeding tendencies. Give menadione, 1–3 mg orally 3 times daily after meals; or menadione sodium bisulfite, 2 mg subcutaneously every other day for a few days.

5. Hemorrhage from esophageal varices–When active variceal bleeding is evident, attempts should be made to sclerose the bleeding varices transendoscopically if a physician with skill in the technique is available. If this procedure cannot be performed or is not successful, bleeding can often be controlled by use of the quadruple lumen (Minnesota) tube. Unfortunately, there is a high incidence of recurrent variceal bleeding after balloon tamponade has been discontinued. Injection sclerotherapy has proved to be quite effective in stopping variceal bleeding. The advantages of this technique are simplicity and avoidance of a major surgical procedure in a poor-risk patient. Repeated injections may be necessary. Intravariceal injection sclerotherapy will achieve temporary control of variceal bleeding in about 80% of patients. If bleeding cannot be controlled by sclerotherapy, emergency surgical decompression of portal hypertension may be considered in selected patients. Morbidity and mortality rates are substantially lower when surgical shunting procedures are performed electively than when performed on an urgent basis. After the patient has been stabilized for 3–5 days, the beta-blocker propranolol can be given to lower the portal pressure. The dosage is usually 20–40 mg twice daily until the resting pulse rate has decreased by 25%.

6. Hemochromatosis–See p 415.

7. Spontaneous bacterial peritonitis–This occurs in cirrhotic patients with ascites. Abdominal pain, increasing ascites, fever, and progressive encephalopathy suggest the possibility, although symptoms may be very mild. Liver function is grossly abnormal in these patients. The mortality rate is high.

Prognosis

The prognosis in advanced cirrhosis has shown little change over the years. A major factor for survival is the patient's ability to discontinue the use of alcohol. In established cases with severe hepatic dysfunction, only 50% survive 2 years and only about 35% survive 5 years. Hematemesis, jaundice, and ascites are unfavorable signs.

Many latent cases are discovered only at autopsy.

Clearfield H: Drug therapy of ascites. *Am Fam Physician* (Jan) 1981;**23**:204.

Crossley IR, Wardle EN, Williams R: Biochemical mechanisms of hepatic encephalopathy. *Clin Sci* 1983;**63**:247.

Fogel MR et al: Continuous intravenous vasopressin in active upper gastrointestinal bleeding. *Ann Intern Med* 1982;**96**: 565.

Lebrec D et al: Propranolol for prevention of recurrent gastrointestinal bleeding in patients with cirrhosis: A controlled study. *N Engl J Med* 1981;**305**:1371.

Lindsay KL et al: Ascites. *West J Med* 1981;**134**:414.

Malt RA: Portasystemic venous shunts. (2 parts.) *N Engl J Med* 1976;**295**:24, 80.

Rogers EL, Rogers MC: Fulminant hepatic failure and hepatic encephalopathy. *Pediatr Clin·North Am* 1980;**27**:701.

Smith JL, Graham DY: Variceal hemorrhage: Problems of selecting therapy that reduces risk of death. *Consultant* (Oct) 1983; **27**:86.

Terblanche J et al: Acute bleeding varices: A five-year prospective evaluation of tamponade and sclerotherapy. *Ann Surg* 1981;**194**:521.

Weber FL: Therapy of portal-systemic encephalopathy: The practical and the promising. *Gastroenterology* 1981;**81**:174.

BILIARY CIRRHOSIS

1. PRIMARY BILIARY CIRRHOSIS

Primary biliary cirrhosis (chronic nonsuppurative destructive cholangitis) is a chronic disease of the liver manifested by cholestasis. It is insidious in onset, occurs usually in women aged 40–60, and is often detected by chance finding of elevated alkaline phosphatase levels. The disease is progressive and complicated often by steatorrhea, xanthomatous neuropathy, osteomalacia, and portal hypertension.

Clinical Findings

A. Symptoms and Signs: The onset is insidious and is heralded by pruritus. Jaundice usually occurs within 2 years of onset of pruritus. Physical examination reveals hepatosplenomegaly. Xanthomatous lesions may occur in the skin and tendons and around the eyelids.

B. Laboratory Findings: Hemograms are normal early in the disease. Serologic tests reflect cholestasis with elevation of alkaline phosphatase, cholesterol, and bilirubin. Mitochondrial antibodies are present in an incidence reported to be 83–98% in different series.

Differential Diagnosis

The disease must be differentiated from chronic biliary tract obstruction (stone or stricture), carcinoma of the bile ducts, and cholestatic liver disease associated with inflammatory bowel disease.

Treatment

Treatment is symptomatic. Cholestyramine may be beneficial for the pruritus. Vitamins A, K, and D should be administered parenterally if steatorrhea is present. Calcium supplementation may be helpful for osteomalacia. Two major clinical trials with penicillamine have shown some benefit. Corticosteroids and azathioprine have not proved to be of benefit.

Herlong HF, Recker RR, Maddery WC: Bone disease in primary biliary cirrhosis: Histologic features and response to 25-

hydroxy vitamin D. *Gastroenterology* 1982;**83**:103.

Matloff DS et al: A prospective trial of D-penicillamine in primary biliary cirrhosis. *N Engl J Med* 1982;**306**:319.

Roll J et al: The prognostic importance of clinical and histological features in asymptomatic and symptomatic primary biliary cirrhosis. *N Engl J Med* 1983;**308**:1.

Schaffner F: Primary biliary cirrhosis. *Curr Concepts Gastroenterol* (July/Aug) 1983;**8**:14.

2. SECONDARY BILIARY CIRRHOSIS

Secondary biliary cirrhosis follows chronic obstruction to bile flow. Superimposed infection may hasten the process. Bile flow is most commonly impaired in an extrahepatic site by calculus, neoplasm, stricture, or biliary atresia.

Clinical Findings

A. Symptoms and Signs: The clinical presentation is usually that of the underlying cause of the cholestasis (eg, carcinoma of the pancreas, choledocholithiasis, choledochal cysts).

B. Laboratory Findings: Hemograms are normal except insofar as they reflect the inciting lesion (eg, cholangitis associated with choledocholithiasis). Serologic tests reflect cholestasis with elevated alkaline phosphatase. The mitochondrial antibody is present in less than 1% of patients with secondary biliary cirrhosis.

C. X-Ray Findings and Ultrasonography: The most direct radiologic means of demonstrating the level and nature of the obstructing lesion is percutaneous transhepatic cholangiography, which has an accuracy rate of 95%. This procedure also allows for external drainage in the obstructed patient until a more definitive procedure is carried out. CT scan and ultrasound may reveal dilated ducts, cholelithiasis, or a mass. Endoscopic retrograde cholangiography may demonstrate the obstructing lesion when other methods prove unsuccessful.

Levitt RG et al: Accuracy of computed tomography of the liver and biliary tract. *Radiology* 1977;**124**:123.

Malini S, Sabel S: Ultrasonography in obstructive jaundice. *Radiology* 1977;**123**:429.

HEMOCHROMATOSIS

Primary or idiopathic hemochromatosis is considered to be a genetically determined disorder of iron metabolism characterized by increased accumulation of dietary iron. This iron is deposited as hemosiderin in the liver, pancreas, heart, adrenals, testes, pituitary, and kidneys. Eventually the patient may develop hepatic, pancreatic, and cardiac insufficiency. The disease usually occurs in males and is rarely recognized before the fifth decade. Clinical manifestations include arthropathy, hepatomegaly and evidence of hepatic insufficiency (late finding), occasional skin pigmentation (slate gray due to iron and brown due to melanin), cardiac enlargement and insufficiency, and diabetes mellitus with its complications. Bleeding from esophageal varices may occur, and in patients who develop cirrhosis, there is a 10% incidence of hepatic carcinoma.

Laboratory findings include elevated plasma iron, increased percentage saturation of transferrin, elevated serum ferritin, and the characteristic liver biopsy that stains positive for iron.

Early diagnosis and treatment in the precirrhotic phase of hemochromatosis is of great importance. Treatment consists initially of weekly phlebotomies (500 mL of blood for months—occasionally up to 2 or 3 years) until plasma iron and hematocrit determinations indicate depletion of iron stores. The chelating agent, deferoxamine, administered intramuscularly to patients with hemochromatosis, has been shown to produce urinary excretion of up to 5–18 g of iron per year. This rate of urinary excretion compares favorably with the rate of 10–20 g of iron removed annually by weekly or biweekly phlebotomies. The treatment, however, is painful and not always practical. Symptomatic and supportive treatment of diabetic, hepatic, and cardiac complications may be necessary.

Although the long-term benefits of iron depletion therapy have not been completely established, available data indicate that the course of the disease may be favorably altered by chelation or bleeding. There appear to be fewer cardiac conduction defects and lower insulin requirements with these treatments.

Rudy DR, Levin DM: Idiopathic hemochromatosis. *Am Fam Physician* (Nov) 1983;**28**:176.

Simon M et al: Idiopathic hemochromatosis: A study of biochemical expression in 247 heterozygous members of 63 families: Evidence for a single major HLA-linked gene. *Gastroenterology* 1980;**78**:703.

WILSON'S DISEASE

Wilson's disease (hepatolenticular degeneration) is a rare familial disorder that is inherited in an autosomally recessive manner and occurs in both males and females between the first and third decades. The condition is characterized by excessive deposition of copper in the liver and brain.

Awareness of the entity is important, since it may masquerade as chronic active hepatitis, psychiatric disorder, or neurologic disease. It is potentially reversible, and appropriate therapy will prevent neurologic and hepatic damage.

The major physiologic aberration in Wilson's disease is excessive absorption of copper from the small intestine and decreased excretion of copper by the liver, resulting in increased tissue deposition, especially in the liver, brain, cornea, and kidney. Ceruloplasmin, the plasma copper-carrying protein, is low. Urinary excretion of copper is high.

Wilson's disease can present primarily as a neuro-logic abnormality, with liver involvement appearing later; or the reverse may be true, with hepatic disease being the initial manifestation. It may first be clinically recognized when jaundice appears in the first few years of life. The diagnosis should always be considered in any child with manifestations of atypical hepatitis, splenomegaly with hypersplenism, hemolytic anemia, portal hypertension, and neurologic or psychiatric abnormalities. Wilson's disease should also be considered in young adults (under 30 years of age) with chronic active hepatitis.

The neurologic manifestations are related to basal ganglia dysfunction and are characterized by rigidity or parkinsonian tremor. Hepatic involvement is evidenced by signs of cirrhosis, portal hypertension, and biochemical confirmation of hepatocellular insufficiency. The almost pathognomonic sign of the condition is the Kayser-Fleischer ring, which represents fine pigmented granular deposits in Descemet's membrane in the cornea close to the endothelial surface. Scattering and reflection of light by these deposits give rise to the typically brownish or gray-green appearance of the ring. The ring itself is not always complete and is usually most marked at the superior and inferior poles of the cornea. It can frequently be seen with the naked eye and almost invariably by slit lamp examination.

The diagnosis is based on demonstration of increased urinary copper excretion ($> 100 \ \mu g/24$ h) or low serum ceruloplasmin levels (< 20 mg/dL), elevated hepatic copper concentration ($> 100 \ \mu g/g$ of dry liver). Histologically, the disease may present as an acute viral hepatitis. In other patients, it may present clinically and histologically as chronic active hepatitis. Cirrhosis ultimately occurs.

Early treatment is essential for removal of copper before it can produce neurologic or hepatic damage. Oral penicillamine (0.75–2 g/d in divided doses) is the drug of choice, making possible urinary excretion of chelated copper. Penicillamine therapy has to be supplemented with pyridoxine, 50 mg per week. Penicillamine is an antimetabolite of this vitamin. Triethylenetetramine may have an important place in the treatment of patients with Wilson's disease who have developed intolerance to penicillamine. The use of copper-restricted diets has not been beneficial and is superfluous when penicillamine is employed. The prognosis is excellent in patients who are effectively treated before liver or brain damage has occurred. Treatment should continue indefinitely.

McCullough AJ et al: Diagnosis of Wilson's disease presenting as fulminant hepatic failure. *Gastroenterology* 1983;**84**:161.

Sternlieb I: Copper and the liver. *Gastroenterology* 1980;**78**: 1615.

HEPATIC VEIN OBSTRUCTION
(Budd-Chiari Syndrome)

This uncommon disorder is due to occlusion of the hepatic veins from a variety of causes. Hepatovenous obstructions may be associated with caval webs, right-sided heart failure, polycythemia, use of birth control pills, pyrrolizidine alkaloids ("bush teas"), neoplasms causing hepatic vein occlusions, and pregnancy. Approximately 30% are idiopathic.

Clinical manifestations may include tender, painful hepatic enlargement; jaundice; splenomegaly; and ascites. With advanced disease, bleeding varices and hepatic coma may be evident. Isotopic liver scan may show prominent caudate lobes. Caval venogram can delineate caval webs and occluded hepatic veins. Percutaneous liver biopsy frequently shows a characteristic central lobular congestion.

Treatment consists of correcting the offending cause, when possible. Ascites should be treated with fluid and salt restriction and diuretics. Surgical decompression of the congested liver may be required. Mean survival is about 12–18 months, with a range of a few weeks to more than 20 years.

Mitchell MC et al: Budd-Chiari syndrome: Etiology, diagnosis and management. *Medicine* 1982;**61**:199.

HEPATIC ABSCESS

1. PYOGENIC ABSCESS

Single or multiple local collections of pus in the liver that are large enough to be seen with the naked eye are presently quite rare, principally because of the use of antibiotics and improved methods of diagnosis of appendicitis, which was formerly the most common precursor of liver abscess. Although the actual clinical incidence cannot be determined because the condition is aborted or modified by antimicrobial treatment, hepatic abscess is still reported in 0.5–1.5% of autopsy specimens. It is equally distributed between men and women, usually in the sixth or seventh decade.

There are apparently 5 ways in which the liver can be invaded by bacteria: (1) by way of the portal vein; (2) by way of ascending cholangitis in the common duct; (3) by way of the hepatic artery, secondary to bacteremia; (4) by direct extension from an infectious process; and (5) by traumatic implantation of bacteria through the abdominal wall.

Despite the use of antimicrobial drugs, 10% of cases of liver abscess are secondary to appendicitis. Another 10% have no demonstrable cause and are classified as idiopathic. At present, ascending cholangitis is the most common cause of hepatic abscess in the USA. Bacterial infection of the hepatobiliary tree is more likely to accompany obstruction by stone than obstruction by carcinoma of the head of the pancreas and is probably attributable to dissemination of bacteria from an acutely inflamed gallbladder. The most frequently encountered organisms are *Escherichia coli, Proteus vulgaris, Enterobacter aerogenes,* and multiple anaerobic species.

Clinically, fever is almost always present and may antedate other symptoms or signs. Pain is promi-

nent and is localized to the right hypochondrium or epigastric area. Jaundice, tenderness in the right upper abdomen, and either steady or swinging fever are the chief physical findings.

Laboratory examination reveals leukocytosis with a shift to the left. Chest roentgenograms will usually reveal elevation of the diaphragm if the abscess is on the right side. Left-sided abscess does not produce significant diaphragmatic elevation. Liver scanning, using ^{99m}Tc sulfur colloid, may reveal the presence of intrahepatic defects.

Treatment should consist of antimicrobial agents that are effective against coliform organisms. If adequate response to therapy is not rapid, surgical drainage should be undertaken. Failure to recognize and treat the condition is attended by mortality rates of about 60% in patients with multiple abscesses.

2. AMEBIC LIVER ABSCESS

Amebic abscess is more common as a primary presentation than is pyogenic abscess. Usual symptoms and signs, which may have been present for 1–30 days, are right upper quadrant pain, often with associated fever, and right pleuritic chest pain. Associated dysentery is uncommon, but 20% of patients will have had a significant recent diarrheal episode. Usually there is a history of travel to endemic areas.

Physical examination discloses fever in most cases, toxic appearance of varying degree, and a tender palpable liver with marked "punch" tenderness. Right lung base abnormalities and localized intercostal tenderness are common.

Laboratory findings usually consist of mild to moderate anemia, moderate leukocytosis with a shift to the left, and slightly abnormal liver tests. Serologic amebic gel diffusion test or indirect hemagglutination tests for *Entamoeba histolytica* are positive in 95% of patients.

An elevated right hemidiaphragm is frequently seen on chest x-ray. Ultrasonography, liver scan with ^{99m}Tc sulfur colloid, or CT scan is helpful in delineating the location and number of abscesses. Most are in the right lobe.

Metronidazole, 750 mg 3 times per day orally for 5–10 days, is the drug of choice. Occasionally, a second course is necessary. In the acutely toxic patient, percutaneous needle aspiration and decompression of the abscess bring about a greater feeling of well-being and also allow for demonstration of the ameba in over 50% of cases. Following completion of treatment for the abscess, the patient needs to take iodoquinol (Yodoxin), 650 mg 3 times a day for 20 days (for adults), to eradicate the intestinal cyst phase of amebiasis.

Fever usually subsides rapidly once treatment is initiated. The hepatic defect may persist for as long as 6 months.

Complications include rupture of the abscess transcutaneously, into the peritoneal cavity, pleural space, lungs, or pericardium, with a significant associated mortality rate if undiagnosed. Rarely, distal embolization has been reported.

Patterson M et al: The presentation of amebiasis. *Med Clin North Am* 1982;**66**:689.

NEOPLASMS OF THE LIVER

Neoplasms of the liver arise either in the hepatic parenchymal cells or biliary ductules. A tumor that arises from parenchymal cells is called a hepatoma; one that originates in the ductular cells is called a cholangioma.

Although hepatoma was formerly thought to occur only in underdeveloped parts of the world where hepatitis B, malnutrition, and parasitism are prevalent, its incidence is now increasing in the USA. This neoplasm occurs in up to 20% of cases of macronodular cirrhosis. In the Orient, hepatitis B and *Clonorchis sinensis,* the liver fluke, are etiologically significant.

Histologically, the tumor may be made up of cords or sheets of cells that roughly resemble the hepatic parenchyma. In the case of a cholangioma, a fibrous stroma or tissue containing structures that simulate bile ducts will be seen. Blood vessels such as portal or hepatic veins are commonly involved by tumor.

The presence of a hepatoma may be unsuspected until there is deterioration in the condition of a cirrhotic patient who was formerly stable. Cachexia, weakness, and weight loss are associated symptoms. The sudden appearance of ascites, which may be bloody, suggests portal or hepatic vein thrombosis by tumor or bleeding from the necrotic tumor.

Physical examination is positive for tender enlargement of the liver, with an occasionally palpable mass. Auscultation may reveal a bruit over the tumor, or a friction rub may be heard when the process has extended to the surface of the liver.

Laboratory tests may reveal leukocytosis, as opposed to the leukopenia that is frequently encountered in cirrhotic patients. Sudden and sustained elevation of the serum alkaline phosphatase in a patient who was formerly stable is a common finding. Hepatitis B surface antigen is present in more than 50% of cases. Alpha$_1$-fetoprotein—not usually found in adults—is demonstrable in 30–50% of patients with hepatoma. Cytologic study of ascitic fluid may reveal malignant cells.

Arteriography is frequently diagnostic, revealing a tumor "blush" that reflects the highly vascular nature of the tumor. Liver scanning with ^{99m}Tc sulfur colloid is occasionally helpful, but with diffuse liver disease, evaluation of findings is difficult. Liver biopsy is diagnostic.

No therapy, including hepatic perfusion with cytotoxic agents, has proved effective. Attempts at surgical resection are usually fruitless because of the presence of cirrhosis and the frequent multifocal characteristics of the tumor. On rare occasions, surgical resection of "solitary" hepatomas has resulted in 5-year "cures."

Benign and malignant neoplasms have been encountered in women taking oral contraceptives. Two distinct entities with characteristic clinical, radiologic, and histopathologic features have been described. Focal nodular hyperplasia occurs at all ages. It is usually asymptomatic and hypervascular and shows a normal uptake on liver scan. As shown microscopically, focal nodular hyperplasia consists of hyperplastic units of hepatocytes with centrally placed proliferating bile ducts. Liver cell adenoma occurs most commonly in the third and fourth decades of life; the clinical presentation is one of acute abdominal disease due to necrosis of the tumor with hemorrhage. The tumor is hypovascular and reveals a cold defect on liver scan. Grossly, the cut surface appears structureless. As seen microscopically, the liver cell adenoma consists of sheets of hepatocytes without portal tracts or central veins. The only physical finding in focal nodular hyperplasia or liver cell adenoma is an abdominal mass. Liver function is usually normal. Treatment of focal nodular hyperplasia is resection in the symptomatic patient. The prognosis is excellent. Liver cell adenoma often undergoes necrosis and rupture; resection is advised. Regression of benign hepatic tumors may follow cessation of oral contraceptives.

Beasley RF et al: Hepatocellular carcinoma and hepatitis B virus. *Lancet* 1981;**2**:1129.

Chuong JJH et al: The histopathologic and clinical indicators of prognosis in hepatoma. *J Clin Gastroenterol* 1982;**4**:547.

Hodgson HJF: Primary hepatocellular carcinoma. *Br J Hosp Med* 1983;**29**:240.

Neuberger J et al: Oral-contraceptive-associated liver tumours: Occurrence of malignancy and difficulties in diagnosis. *Lancet* 1980;**1**:273.

ACUTE CHOLECYSTITIS

Essentials of Diagnosis

- Steady, severe pain and tenderness in the right hypochondrium or epigastrium.
- Nausea and vomiting.
- Jaundice.
- Fever and leukocytosis.

General Considerations

Cholecystitis is associated with gallstones in over 90% of cases. It occurs when a calculus becomes impacted in the cystic duct and inflammation develops behind the obstruction. Vascular abnormalities of the bile duct or pancreatitis may rarely produce cholecystitis in the absence of gallstones. If the obstruction is not relieved, pressure builds up within the gallbladder as a result of continued secretion. Primarily as a result of ischemic changes secondary to distention, gangrene may develop, with resulting perforation. Although generalized peritonitis is possible, the leak usually remains localized and forms a chronic, well-circum-scribed abscess cavity.

Clinical Findings

A. Symptoms and Signs: The acute attack is often precipitated by a large or fatty meal and is characterized by the relatively sudden appearance of severe, minimally fluctuating pain which is localized to the epigastrium or right hypochondrium and which in the uncomplicated case may gradually subside over a period of 12–18 hours. Vomiting occurs in about 75% of patients and in half of instances affords variable relief. Right upper quadrant abdominal tenderness is almost always present and is usually associated with muscle guarding and rebound pain. A palpable gallbladder is present in about 15% of cases. Jaundice is present in about 25% of cases and, when persistent or severe, suggests the possibility of choledocholithiasis. Fever is usually present.

B. Laboratory Findings: The white count is usually high (12–15 thousand/μL). Total serum bilirubin values of 1–4 mg/dL may be reported even in the absence of common duct obstruction. Serum transaminase and alkaline phosphatase are often elevated—the former as high as 300 mU/mL and even higher when associated with ascending cholangitis. Serum amylase may also be moderately elevated.

C. X-Ray Findings: Films of the abdomen may show gallstones in 15% of cases. ^{99m}Tc hepatobiliary imaging agents (iminodiacetic acid compounds), also known as HIDA scan, are useful in demonstrating an obstructed cystic duct, which is the cause of acute cholecystitis in most patients. This test is reliable if the bilirubin is under 5 mg/dL.

Differential Diagnosis

The disorders most likely to be confused with acute cholecystitis are perforated peptic ulcer, acute pancreatitis, appendicitis in a high-lying appendix, perforated carcinoma or diverticulum of the hepatic flexure, liver abscess, hepatitis, and pneumonia with pleurisy on the right side. The definite localization of pain and tenderness in the right hypochondrium, with frequent radiation to the infrascapular area, strongly favors the diagnosis of acute cholecystitis.

Complications

A. Gangrene of the Gallbladder: Continuation or progression of right upper quadrant abdominal pain, tenderness, muscle guarding, fever, and leukocytosis after 24–48 hours suggests severe inflammation and possible gangrene of the gallbladder. Necrosis may occasionally develop without definite signs in either the obese or the elderly.

B. Cholangitis: Intermittently high fever and chills strongly suggest choledocholithiasis.

Treatment

Acute cholecystitis will usually subside on a conservative regimen (withholding of oral feedings, intravenous alimentation, analgesics and antibiotics if indi-cated). Cholecystectomy can be performed a few days after institution of hospitalization or can be scheduled for 2–3 months later, depending on the surgeon's preference and the clinical aspects of the individual case. If, as occasionally happens, recurrent acute symptoms develop during this waiting period, cholecystectomy is indicated without delay. If conservative treatment has been elected, the patient (especially if diabetic or elderly) should be watched carefully for evidence of gangrene of the gallbladder or cholangitis.

Operation is mandatory when there is evidence of gangrene or perforation. Operation during the first 24 hours can be justified as a means of reducing overall morbidity in good-risk patients in whom the diagnosis is unequivocal. It is usually best to defer surgery, if possible, in the presence of acute pancreatitis, unless choledocholithiasis is suspected.

A. Medical Treatment: During the acute period, the patient should be observed frequently, with careful abdominal examination and sequential determination of the white cell count several times a day. Analgesics such as pentazocine or meperidine should be used for pain control. Morphine derivatives in effective doses are known to produce spasm of the sphincter of Oddi and may cause spurious elevations of serum amylase. Meperidine may have the same effects but to a much lesser degree. Anticholinergic agents are rarely indicated for these patients, in part because they may mask the development of paralytic ileus or prolong its duration. Appropriate antimicrobial agents should be employed in all but the most mild and rapidly subsiding cases.

B. Surgical Treatment: When surgery is elected for acute cholecystitis, cholecystectomy is the procedure of choice. Cholangiography should be performed at the time of operation to ascertain the need for common duct exploration. In the poor-risk patient or when technical difficulties preclude cholecystectomy, cholecystostomy can be performed under local anesthesia.

Prognosis

Mild acute cholecystitis usually subsides, but recurrences are common. Symptomatic cholecystitis is a definite indication for surgery. Persistence of symptoms after removal of the gallbladder implies either mistaken diagnosis, functional bowel disorder, or technical error, since cholecystectomy is curative.

Detwiler RP, Kim DS, Longerbeam JD: Ultrasonography and oral cholecystography: A comparison of their use in the diagnosis of gallbladder disease. *Arch Surg* 1980;**115**:1096.

Fox MS et al: Acute acalculous cholecystitis. *Surg Gynecol Obstet* 1984;**159**:13.

Gupta SM: The role of nuclear scanning in evaluating hepatobiliary disease. *Med Times* (May) 1982;**110**:31.

Norrby S et al: Early or delayed cholecystectomy in acute cholecystitis: A clinical trial. *Br J Surg* 1983;**70**:163.

CHOLELITHIASIS

Gallstones are more common in women than in men and increase in incidence in both sexes and all races with aging. Data are available which indicate that in the USA 10% of men and 20% of women between the ages of 55 and 65 have gallstones and that the total exceeds 15 million people. Although it is less common in black people, cholelithiasis attributable to hemolysis has been encountered in over a third of individuals with sickle cell disease. American Indians have a high rate of cholesterol cholelithiasis. As many as 70% of Pima Indian women over age 25 have cholelithiasis. The incidence of gallstones is also high in individuals with certain diseases such as regional enteritis. Approximately one-third of individuals with inflammatory involvement of the terminal ileum have cholesterol gallstones due to disruption of bile salt resorption that results in decreased solubility of the bile. The incidence of cholelithiasis is also increased in patients with diabetes mellitus. Pregnancy as a significant cause of gallstones has been overemphasized.

The simplest classification of gallstones is according to chemical composition: stones containing predominantly cholesterol and stones containing predominantly calcium bilirubinate. The latter comprise less than 5% of the stones found in Europe or the USA but 30–40% of stones found in Japan.

Three compounds comprise 80–95% of the total solids dissolved in bile: conjugated bile salts, lecithin, and cholesterol. Cholesterol is a neutral sterol; lecithin is a phospholipid; and both are almost completely insoluble in water. However, bile salts are able to form multimolecular aggregates (micelles) that solubilize lecithin and cholesterol in an aqueous solution. Bile salts alone are relatively inefficient in solubilizing cholesterol (approximately 50 molecules of bile salt are necessary to solubilize 1 molecule of cholesterol), but the solubilization of lecithin in bile salt solutions results in a mixed micelle that is 7 times more efficient in the solubilization of cholesterol. Precipitation of cholesterol microcrystals may come about through a simultaneous change in all 3 major components.

Cholelithiasis is frequently asymptomatic and is discovered fortuitously in the course of routine radiographic study, operation, or autopsy. Although there is disagreement about the desirability of cholecystectomy in patients with "silent" gallstones, it is generally agreed that diabetic patients should undergo gallbladder removal to avoid complications. Operation is mandatory for symptomatic cholelithiasis.

Chenodeoxycholic acid (Chenix) is a bile salt that on oral administration is able to cause dissolution of some cholesterol stones. Although relatively safe, it may cause diarrhea or minor liver function test abnormalities. It is most effective in patients with a functioning gallbladder and an unobstructed biliary tract. Dissolution of gallstones may require 2 years or longer. Gallstones may recur when treatment stops. Obesity may induce resistance to therapy. Intermittent therapy is ineffective.

Bouchier IAD: Gallstone dissolving agents. (Review.) *Br Med J* 1983;**286:**778.
Heiss FW et al: Common bile duct calculi. 1. Surgical therapy. 2. Nonsurgical therapy. *Postgrad Med* (Feb 15) 1984;**75:**88, 109. [Special issue.]
Thistle JL et al: The natural history of cholelithiasis: The National Cooperative Gallstone Study. *Ann Intern Med* 1984;**101:**171.

CYSTIC DUCT SYNDROMES

Precholecystectomy

A small group of patients (mostly women) has been reported in whom right upper quadrant abdominal pain occurred frequently following meals. Conventional radiographic study of the upper gastrointestinal tract and gallbladder—including intravenous cholangiography—was unremarkable. Using cholecystokinin (CCK) as a gallbladder stimulant, contraction and evacuation of the viscus did not take place, as usually occurs in the 3- to 5-minute period after injection of the hormone. However, the gallbladder assumed a "golf ball" configuration, and biliary type pain was reproduced. At the time of cholecystectomy, the gallbladders were found to be enlarged and could not be emptied by manual compression. Anatomic and histologic examination of the operative specimens revealed obstruction of the cystic ducts either because of fibrotic stenosis at their proximal ends or because of adhesions and kinking.

Postcholecystectomy

Following cholecystectomy, a variable group of patients complain of continuing symptoms, ie, right upper quadrant pain, flatulence, and fatty food intolerance. The persistence of symptoms in this group of patients suggests the possibility of an incorrect diagnosis prior to cholecystectomy, eg, esophagitis, pancreatitis, radiculitis, or functional bowel disease. It is important to rule out the possibility of choledocholithiasis or common duct stricture as a cause for persistent symptoms in the postoperative period.

Pain has been associated with dilatation of the cystic duct remnant, neuroma formation in the ductal wall, foreign body granuloma, or traction on the common duct by a long cystic duct. The clinical presentation of colicky pain, chills, fever, or jaundice should suggest biliary tract disease. Liver tests for cholestasis, intravenous urography, abdominal ultrasonography, or percutaneous cholangiography may be necessary to rule out biliary tract disease. Surgery, with common duct exploration for stones and removal of the cystic duct remnant, may be necessary.

Hopkins SF et al: The problem of the cystic duct remnant. *Surg Gynecol Obstet* 1979;**148:**531.

CHRONIC CHOLECYSTITIS

The most common disability that results from cholelithiasis is chronic cholecystitis. It is characterized pathologically by varying degrees of chronic inflammation on gross inspection or microscopic examination of the gallbladder. In about 4–5% of cases, the villi of the gallbladder undergo polypoid enlargement due to deposition of cholesterol that may be visible to the naked eye ("strawberry gallbladder," cholesterolosis). In other instances, adenomatous hyperplasia of all or part of the gallbladder wall may be so marked as to give the appearance of a myoma (pseudotumor). Calculi are usually present, but the gallbladder may or may not be visualized on cholecystography. The diagnosis is often erroneously applied to collections of symptoms that are only vaguely or indirectly related to gallbladder dysfunction.

Clinical Findings

Chronic cholecystitis is associated with discrete bouts of right hypochondriac and epigastric pain that is either steady or intermittent. Discomfort is usually persistent, but, if intermittent, the height of pain may be separated by 15- to 60-minute intervals.

The onset of pain is usually abrupt, with maximum intensity and plateau reached within 15 minutes to 1 hour. Attacks of biliary colic may persist for as long as several hours or be as brief as 15–20 minutes, the average duration being about 1 hour. Pain referral to the interscapular area is occasionally noted.

Chronic indigestion is considered by many to be commonly due to gallbladder disease. Fatty food intolerance, belching, flatulence, a sense of epigastric heaviness, upper abdominal pain of varying intensity, and pyrosis are some of the symptoms that have been erroneously considered to be suggestive of cholelithiasis and cholecystitis. Efforts have therefore been made to evaluate "dyspeptic" symptomatology in relationship to objective evidence of gallbladder disease. In one prospective study of 142 women who experienced "chronic indigestion," only 24 had either gallstones or nonvisualization of the gallbladder on oral cholecystograms. Sixty-three (53%) of the 118 who had normal cholecystograms complained of "dyspepsia." Accordingly, it can be assumed that the association of chronic indigestion and gallstones is fortuitous. If cholecystectomy is performed in patients with calculi who have complained of a constellation of "dyspeptic" symptoms, the results of operation may be unpredictable and frequently unsatisfactory.

Physical examination is nonspecific, revealing abdominal tenderness which may be localized to the right hypochondrium and epigastric area but which may also be diffuse. Hydrops of the gallbladder results when subsidence of acute cholecystitis occurs but cystic duct obstruction persists, producing distention of the gallbladder with a clear mucoid fluid. The gallbladder in that circumstance is palpable in the right upper abdomen. The presence of jaundice obviously supports the diagnosis of cholecystitis with choledocholithiasis.

Laboratory studies are usually not diagnostic.

Films of the abdomen taken prior to oral cholecystography may reveal opacification of the gallbladder caused by high concentrations of calcium carbonate (limy bile) or radiopaque stones. Nonvisualization of the gallbladder implies cholecystitis provided there is radiologic evidence that the oral contrast material has been absorbed and excreted. It is important to remember the following technical reasons for nonvisualization: failure to ingest the dye, vomiting or diarrhea, gastric outlet obstruction or esophageal stricture, intestinal malabsorption, abnormal location of the gallbladder, liver disease (including preicteric hepatitis), Dubin-Johnson-Sprinz-Nelson syndrome, fat-free diet prior to cholecystography, and previous cholecystectomy.

Ultrasound examination of the gallbladder is a useful diagnostic examination. The accuracy of diagnosis of cholelithiasis in some centers is high (96%) and the incidence of false-positive results low (2%).

Differential Diagnosis

When nonspecific symptoms are present, it is necessary to consider the possibilities of gastroduodenal ulcer disease, chronic relapsing pancreatitis, irritable colon syndrome, and malignant neoplasms of the stomach, pancreas, hepatic flexure, or gallbladder. Barium enema and upper gastrointestinal series complement cholecystography. Microscopic examination of bile obtained by biliary drainage is occasionally helpful in demonstrating calculous disease of the gallbladder. (The test is valid only in the absence of hepatic disease.)

Complications

The presence of cholelithiasis with chronic cholecystitis can result in acute exacerbation of gallbladder inflammation, common duct stone, cholecystenteric fistulization, pancreatitis, and, rarely, carcinoma of the gallbladder.

Treatment

Although proved cholelithiasis and cholecystitis ideally should be managed surgically, significant metabolic and cardiovascular disease or other factors may preclude operation. Nonspecific "dyspeptic" symptoms (eg, heartburn, belching, abdominal pain, bloating, flatulence, constipation) frequently are ameliorated by careful use of low-fat diets and weight reduction. Anticholinergics and sedatives, along with antacids and hydrophilic agents, may prove helpful.

Surgical treatment is the same as for acute cholecystitis, with transhepatic and operative cholangiography employed if there is a possibility of choledocholithiasis.

Prognosis

The overall mortality rate of cholecystectomy is less than 1%, but hepatobiliary tract surgery is a more formidable procedure in the elderly and has a mortality rate of 5–10%. A technically successful surgical procedure in an appropriately selected patient is generally followed by complete cessation of symptoms.

Aranha GV et al: Cholecystectomy in cirrhotic patients: A formidable operation. *Am J Surg* 1982;**143:**55.

Berk RN et al: The radiological diagnosis of gallbladder disease: An imaging symposium. *Radiology* 1981;**141:**49.

Burnstein MJ et al: Results of combined biliary drainage and cholecystokinin cholecystography in 81 patients with normal oral cholecystogram. *Ann Surg* 1982;**196:**627.

See also references on pp 402 and 419.

CHOLEDOCHOLITHIASIS

Essentials of Diagnosis

- Often a history of biliary colic or jaundice.
- Sudden onset of severe right upper quadrant or epigastric pain, which may radiate to the right scapula or shoulder.
- Nausea and vomiting.
- Fever, often followed by hypothermia and gram-negative shock.
- Jaundice.
- Leukocytosis.
- Abdominal films may reveal gallstones.

General Considerations

About 15% of patients with gallstones have choledocholithiasis. The percentage rises with age, and the incidence in elderly people may be as high as 50%. Common duct stones usually originate in the gallbladder but may also form spontaneously in the common duct postcholecystectomy. The stones are frequently "silent," as no symptoms result unless there is obstruction.

Clinical Findings

A. Symptoms and Signs: A history suggestive of biliary colic or prior jaundice can usually be obtained. The additional features that suggest the presence of a common duct stone are (1) frequently recurring attacks of right upper abdominal pain that is severe and persists for hours; (2) chills and fever associated with severe colic; and (3) a history of jaundice that was chronologically associated with abdominal pain. The combination of pain, fever (and chills), and jaundice represents Charcot's triad and denotes the classic picture of cholangitis. The presence of altered sensorium, lethargy, and septic shock connotes acute suppurative cholangitis accompanied by pus in the obstructed duct and represents a surgical emergency.

Biliary colic in choledocholithiasis is apparently caused by rapidly increasing biliary pressure that is secondary to sudden obstruction to the flow of bile. Radiation of pain into the interscapular area may be helpful in differentiating choledocholithiasis from cholecystolithiasis. Hepatomegaly may be present in calculous biliary obstruction, and tenderness is usually present in the right hypochondrium and epigastrium. Usually, there are no specific physical findings.

B. Laboratory Findings: Bilirubinuria and elevation of serum bilirubin are present if the common duct is obstructed. Serum alkaline phosphatase elevation is especially suggestive of obstructive jaundice.

Because prolonged obstruction of the common duct results in hepatocellular dysfunction, SGOT (AST) will be abnormal. Prolongation of the prothrombin time occurs when there is disturbance of the normal enterohepatic circulation of bile, with its exclusion from the intestinal tract. When extrahepatic obstruction persists for more than a few weeks, differentiation of obstruction from primarily inflammatory disease becomes progressively more difficult.

C. X-Ray Findings: Although ultrasonography, CT scan, and radionuclide imaging may help to differentiate hepatocellular and obstructive jaundice, percutaneous transhepatic cholangiography provides the most direct and accurate nonsurgical means of determining the cause, location, and extent of obstruction.

Differential Diagnosis

The most common cause of obstructive jaundice is common duct stone. Next in frequency is carcinoma of the pancreas, ampulla of Vater, or common duct. Metastatic carcinoma (usually from the gastrointestinal tract) and direct extension of gallbladder cancer are other important causes of obstructive jaundice. Hepatocellular jaundice can usually be differentiated by the history, clinical findings, and liver tests, but liver biopsy is necessary on occasion.

Complications

A. Biliary Cirrhosis: Common duct obstruction lasting longer than 30 days results in severe liver damage. Hepatic failure with portal hypertension occurs in untreated cases.

B. Cholangitis: If bacteria enter the duct proximal to the obstruction and inoculation of these organisms into the bloodstream occurs as the result of elevated biliary pressure in the ductal system, fever (and chills), jaundice, and pain will appear (Charcot's triad). Cholangitis may be nonsuppurative or suppurative. The former usually responds well to antimicrobial therapy, whereas the latter is a surgical emergency. Untreated cholangitis is the most common cause of multiple pyogenic hepatic abscesses, resulting in a progressively downhill course and septic death.

C. Hypoprothrombinemia: Patients with obstructive jaundice or liver disease may bleed excessively as a result of prolonged prothrombin times. If the hypoprothrombinemia is due to faulty vitamin K absorption, the following preparations are of value. When prothrombin response to parenteral versus oral administration of these agents is compared, the nature of the underlying lesion (hepatocellular versus obstructive) can be determined; obstructive jaundice will respond to parenteral vitamin K or water-soluble oral vitamin K.

1. Subcutaneously–Phytonadione, 10 mg daily, is the preparation of choice. Menadione sodium bisulfite, 10 mg daily, may be used if phytonadione is not available.

2. Orally–Menadiol sodium diphosphate, 5 mg twice daily, is the preferred oral agent. It is water-soluble and is absorbed from the intestinal tract in the absence of bile.

Treatment

Common duct stone is usually treated by cholecystectomy and choledochostomy.

A. Preoperative Preparation: Emergency operation is rarely necessary unless severe ascending cholangitis is present. A few days devoted to careful evaluation and preparation will be well spent.

Liver function should be evaluated thoroughly. Prothrombin time should be restored to normal by parenteral administration of vitamin K preparations (see above). Nutrition should be restored by a high-carbohydrate, high-protein diet and vitamin supplementation. Cholangitis, if present, should be controlled with antimicrobials, but may necessitate more urgent surgical decompression.

B. Indications for Common Duct Exploration: At every operation for cholelithiasis, the advisability of exploring the common duct must be considered. Operative cholangiography via the cystic duct is a very useful procedure for demonstrating common duct stone.

1. Preoperative findings suggestive of choledocholithiasis include a history (or the presence) of obstructive jaundice; frequent attacks of biliary colic; cholangitis; a history of pancreatitis; and a percutaneous transhepatic cholangiogram showing stone, obstruction, or dilatation of the duct.

2. Operative findings of choledocholithiasis are palpable stones in the common duct; dilatation or thickening of the wall of the common duct; gallbladder stones small enough to pass through the cystic duct; and pancreatitis.

3. Alternative management of the patient with common duct stone, especially after cholecystectomy, includes endoscopic papillotomy. For the patient with a T tube and a common duct stone, manipulation with various special instruments via the T tube or T tube sinus tract is often successful in extracting the stone.

C. Postoperative Care:

1. Antibiotics–Postoperative antibiotics are not administered routinely after biliary tract surgery. Cultures of the bile are always taken at operation. If biliary tract infection was present preoperatively or is apparent at operation, penicillin or ampicillin is administered postoperatively until the results of sensitivity tests on culture specimens are available.

2. Management of the T tube–Following choledochostomy, a simple catheter or T tube is placed in the common duct for decompression. It must be attached securely to the skin or dressing because accidental removal of the tube may be disastrous. A properly placed tube should drain bile at the operating table and continuously thereafter; otherwise, it should be considered blocked or dislocated. The volume of bile drainage varies from 100 to 1000 mL daily (average, 200–400 mL). Above-average drainage may be due to obstruction at the ampulla (usually by edema), increased bile output, low resistance or siphonage ef-

fect in the drainage system, or a combination of these factors.

3. Cholangiography–A cholangiogram should be taken through the T tube on about the seventh or eighth postoperative day. Under fluoroscopic control, a radiopaque medium is aseptically and gently injected until the duct system is outlined and the medium begins to enter the duodenum. The injection of air bubbles must be avoided, since on x-ray they resemble stones in the duct system. Spot films are always taken. If the cholangiogram shows no stones in the common duct and the opaque medium flows freely into the duodenum, the tube is clamped overnight and removed by simple traction on the following day. A small amount of bile frequently leaks from the tube site for a few days. A rubber tissue drain is usually placed alongside the T tube at operation. This drain is partially withdrawn on the fifth day and shortened daily until it is removed completely on about the seventh day.

In poor-risk patients with common duct stones, an endoscopic sphincterotomy should be considered if a skilled endoscopist is available.

Allen B, Way LW et al: Management of recurrent and residual common duct stones. *Am J Surg* 1981;**142**:41.

Gordon P et al: Presence of gallstones is a poor indicator of the cause of obstructive jaundice. *Surg Gynecol Obstet* 1980; **151**:635.

Kozarek RA, Sandowski RA: Nonsurgical management of extrahepatic obstructive jaundice. *Ann Intern Med* 1982;**96**:743.

Roesch W et al: Long term follow-up after endoscopic sphincterotomy. *Endoscopy* 1981;**13**:152.

BILIARY STRICTURE

Benign biliary strictures are the result of surgical trauma in about 95% of cases. The remainder are caused by blunt external injury to the abdomen, pancreatitis, or erosion of the duct by a gallstone.

Signs of injury to the duct may or may not be recognized in the immediate postoperative period. If complete occlusion has occurred, jaundice will develop rapidly; but more often a tear has been accidentally made in the duct, and the earliest manifestation of injury may be excessive or prolonged loss of bile from the surgical drains. Bile leakage contributes to the production of localized infection, which in turn accentuates scar formation and the ultimate development of a fibrous stricture.

Cholangitis is the most common syndrome produced by stricture. Typically, the patient notices episodes of pain, fever, chills, and jaundice within a few weeks to months after cholecystectomy. With the exception of jaundice during an attack of cholangitis and right upper quadrant abdominal tenderness, physical findings are usually not significant.

Serum alkaline phosphatase is usually elevated. Hyperbilirubinemia is variable, fluctuating during exacerbations and usually remaining in the range of 5–10 mg/dL. Blood cultures may be positive during an episode of cholangitis. Percutaneous transhepatic cholangiography or endoscopic retrograde cholangiopancreatography can be valuable in demonstrating the stricture.

Differentiation from choledocholithiasis may require surgical exploration. Operative treatment of a stricture frequently necessitates performance of choledochojejunostomy or hepaticojejunostomy to reestablish bile flow into the intestine.

Biliary stricture is not a benign condition, since significant hepatocellular disease will inevitably occur if it is allowed to continue uncorrected. The death rate for untreated stricture ranges from 10 to 15%.

Bolton JS et al: Management of benign biliary stricture. *Surg Clin North Am* 1980;**60**:313.

PRIMARY SCLEROSING CHOLANGITIS

Primary sclerosing cholangitis is a rare nonspecific inflammatory reaction of unknown cause involving both the intra- and extrahepatic biliary ducts. It is characterized by a diffuse inflammation of the biliary tract leading to fibrosis and strictures of the biliary system. The disease is closely associated with ulcerative colitis, which is present in approximately two-thirds of patients with primary sclerosing cholangitis. Primary sclerosing cholangitis appears to be often associated with increased HLA-B8 histocompatibility antigen. Primary sclerosing cholangitis may occur at any period of life and may initially simulate a slowly growing bile duct carcinoma. However, the chronicity of the process militates against neoplasm. The criteria for making the diagnosis of primary sclerosing cholangitis are as follows: (1) progressive obstructive jaundice; (2) absence of calculi in the gallbladder or biliary ducts; (3) absence of prior surgical injury to the biliary tract; (4) absence of diseases causing cholangitis; (5) absence of congenital biliary anomalies; (6) thickening and narrowing of the biliary ductal system, demonstrated by palpation at surgery, biopsy, or x-ray techniques; (7) absence of biliary cirrhosis; and (8) exclusion of cholangiocarcinoma by long-term follow-up and multiple liver biopsies. Endoscopic retrograde cholangiography is the best means of establishing the diagnosis of primary sclerosing cholangitis other than surgical exploration.

Clinically, the disease presents as progressively obstructive jaundice, frequently preceded by malaise, pruritus, anorexia, and indigestion. Treatment consists of surgical bypass such as cholecystoduodenostomy. Corticosteroids and broad-spectrum antimicrobial agents have been employed with rare success, but generally the results have been inconstant and unpredictable. The prognosis is regarded as poor, with few individuals living more than a few years after the appearance of symptoms.

Chapman RW et al: Association of primary sclerosing cholangitis with HLA-B8. *Gut* 1983;**24**:38.

LaRusso NF et al: Primary sclerosing cholangitis. (Current concepts.) *N Engl J Med* 1984;**310**:899.

CARCINOMA OF THE BILIARY TRACT

Carcinoma of the gallbladder occurs in approximately 2% of all people operated on for biliary tract disease. It is notoriously insidious, and the diagnosis is usually made unexpectedly at surgery. Spread of the cancer—by direct extension into the liver or to the peritoneal surface—may be the initial manifestation.

Carcinoma of the extrahepatic bile ducts accounts for 3% of all cancer deaths in the USA. It affects both sexes equally but is more prevalent in individuals age 50–70. There is a questionable increased incidence in patients with chronic nonspecific ulcerative colitis.

Progressive jaundice is the most common and is usually the first sign of obstruction of the extrahepatic biliary system. Pain is usually present in the right upper abdomen and radiates into the back. Anorexia and weight loss are common and are frequently associated with fever and chills. Rarely, hematemesis may be a confusing presentation that results from erosion of tumor into a blood vessel. Fistula formation between the biliary system and adjacent organs may also occur. The course is usually one of rapid deterioration, with death occurring within a few months.

Physical examination will reveal profound jaundice. A palpable gallbladder with obstructive jaundice usually signifies malignant disease. Courvoisier's law states that the most frequent cause of obstructive jaundice distal to the cystic duct with a normal gallbladder wall is neoplasm. This clinical generalization has been proved to be accurate about 90% of the time. Hepatomegaly is usually present and is associated with liver tenderness. Ascites may occur with peritoneal implants. Pruritus and skin excoriations are common.

Laboratory examinations reveal hyperbilirubinemia, predominantly of the conjugated variety. Total serum bilirubin values range from 5 to 30 mg/dL. There is usually concomitant elevation of the alkaline phosphatase and serum cholesterol. SGOT (AST) is normal or minimally elevated.

The most helpful radiographic study prior to surgery is the percutaneous transhepatic cholangiogram. This procedure should be done to define the pathologic anatomy (ductal obstruction). Differentiation of benign strictures of the ductal system from progressive sclerosing cholangitis is suggested by a history of prior exploration of the hepatobiliary tree with resultant injury that was unrecognized at the time of the initial celiotomy.

Unless there are overwhelming contraindications, palliative surgery is indicated to decompress the hepatobiliary system and relieve jaundice. This can be accomplished by cholecystoduodenostomy or by T tube drainage of the common duct. The prognosis is poor, few patients surviving for more than 6 months after surgery.

Alexander F et al: Biliary carcinoma: A review of 109 cases. *Am J Surg* 1984;**147**:503.

Lees CD et al: Carcinoma of the bile ducts. *Surg Gynecol Obstet* 1980;**151**:193.

DISEASES OF THE PANCREAS

ACUTE PANCREATITIS

Essentials of Diagnosis

- Abrupt onset of dull epigastric pain, often with radiation to the back.
- Nausea, vomiting, sweating, weakness.
- Abdominal tenderness and distention, fever.
- Leukocytosis, elevated serum and urinary amylase, elevated serum lipase.
- History of previous episodes, often related to alcohol intake.

General Considerations

Acute pancreatitis is a severe intra-abdominal disease due to acute inflammation of the pancreas and associated "escape" of pancreatic enzymes from acinar cells into surrounding tissues. Most cases are related to biliary tract disease or heavy alcohol intake. Among the more than 80 other causes or associations are hypercalcemia, hyperlipidemias (types I, IV, and V), abdominal trauma (including surgery), total parenteral nutrition, drugs (including prednisone and thiazides), vasculitis, and viral infections. The exact pathogenesis is not known but may include edema or obstruction of the ampulla of Vater with resultant reflux of bile into pancreatic ducts, stenosis of the accessory pancreatic duct (duct of Santorini), and direct injury to the acinar cells.

Pathologic changes vary from acute edema and cellular infiltration to necrosis of the acinar cells, hemorrhage from necrotic blood vessels, and intra- and extrapancreatic fat necrosis. All or part of the pancreas may be involved.

Clinical Findings

A. Symptoms and Signs: Epigastric abdominal pain, generally abrupt in onset, is steady and severe and is often made worse by walking and lying supine and better by sitting and leaning forward. The pain usually radiates into the back but may radiate to the right or left. Nausea and vomiting are usually present. Severe weakness, sweating, and anxiety are noted in severe attacks. There may be a history of alcohol intake or a heavy meal immediately preceding the attack, or a history of milder but otherwise similar episodes in the past, even suggestive of biliary colic.

The abdomen is tender mainly in the upper abdomen, most often without guarding, rigidity, or rebound. The abdomen may be distended, and bowel sounds may be absent in associated paralytic ileus.

Fever of 38.4–39 °C (101.1–102.2 °F), tachycardia, hypotension (even true shock), pallor, and a cool clammy skin are often present. Mild jaundice is common. An upper abdominal mass may be present but is not characteristic. Acute renal failure may occur early in the course of acute pancreatitis.

B. Laboratory Findings: Findings of leukocytosis (10,000–30,000/μL), proteinuria, casts (25% of cases), glycosuria (10–20% of cases), hyperglycemia, and elevated serum bilirubin may be present. Blood urea nitrogen and serum alkaline phosphatase may be elevated and coagulation tests abnormal. Decrease in serum calcium may reflect a decreased serum albumin and correlates well with severity of disease; it is lowest on about the sixth day. Levels lower than 7 mg/dL are associated with tetany and an unfavorable prognosis.

Serum amylase and lipase are elevated within 24 hours in 90% of cases, and return to normal is variable depending on the severity of disease. Urine amylase and amylase activity in the peritoneal fluid, which may be very high, remain elevated longer than serum amylase. An amylase/creatinine clearance ratio of more than 5.5% usually indicates acute pancreatitis and is of some use in the differential diagnosis of hyperamylasemia. The only values needed are the concentrations of amylase and creatinine in simultaneously collected serum and urine. In some patients with acute pancreatitis, the ratio is not elevated. False-positive elevations of the clearance ratio may occur in patients with burns or ketoacidosis.

C. X-Ray Findings: A 2-way view of the abdomen may show gallstones, a "sentinel loop" (a segment of air-filled small intestine most commonly in the left upper quadrant), the "colon cutoff sign" (a gas-filled segment of transverse colon abruptly ending at the area of pancreatic inflammation), or linear focal atelectasis of the left lower lobe of the lungs with or without pleural effusion. These findings suggest acute pancreatitis but are not diagnostic. CT scan is useful in demonstrating an enlarged pancreas, in detecting pseudocysts, and in determining the extent of phlegmons. Ultrasonography is less reliable, because the echoes are deflected by the gas-distended small intestine frequently associated with acute pancreatitis.

D. Electrocardiographic Findings: ST–T wave changes may occur, but they usually differ from those of myocardial infarction. Abnormal Q waves do not occur as a result of pancreatitis.

Differential Diagnosis

Acute pancreatitis may be difficult to differentiate from an acutely perforated duodenal ulcer. One must keep in mind that pancreatitis may be the presenting clinical picture of choledocholithiasis with or without cholangitis, as well as of a penetrating duodenal ulcer. It may occur owing to infection by mumps virus or postoperatively owing to surgical manipulation in the area of the pancreas. Serum amylase may also be elevated in high intestinal obstruction, in mumps not involving the pancreas, in ectopic pregnancy, after administration of narcotics, and after abdominal surgery. Other conditions to be differentiated are acute cholecystitis, acute intestinal obstruction, dissecting aortic aneurysm, renal colic, and acute mesenteric vascular insufficiency or thrombosis.

Complications

Intravascular volume depletion secondary to leakage of fluids in the pancreatic bed and ileus with fluid-filled loops of bowel may result in prerenal azotemia and even acute tubular necrosis without overt shock. This usually occurs within 24 hours of the onset of acute pancreatitis and lasts 8–9 days. Some patients require peritoneal dialysis or hemodialysis.

One of the most serious complications of acute pancreatitis is pulmonary edema with or without cardiac failure ("shock lung"). It usually occurs 3–7 days after the onset of pancreatitis in patients who have required large volumes of fluid and colloid to maintain blood pressure and urine output. Most require assisted respiration with positive end-expiratory pressure for 1–2 weeks.

Pancreatic abscess is a suppurative process in necrotic tissue, with rising fever, leukocytosis, and localized tenderness and epigastric mass. This may be associated with a left-sided pleural effusion or an enlarging spleen secondary to splenic vein thrombosis.

Pseudocysts, encapsulated fluid collections with high enzyme content, commonly appear in pancreatitis when CT scans are used to monitor the evolution of an acute attack. Although the natural history of pseudocysts is not well delineated, it appears that most resolve spontaneously. Pseudocysts most commonly are within or adjacent to the pancreas but can present most anywhere (eg, mediastinal, retrorectal), having extended along anatomic planes. They may become secondarily infected, necessitating drainage as for an abscess. Erosion of the inflammatory process into a blood vessel can result in a major hemorrhage into the cyst.

Chronic pancreatitis develops in about 10% of cases.

Permanent diabetes mellitus and exocrine pancreatic insufficiency occur uncommonly after a single acute episode.

Prevention

Potential causative factors should be removed or corrected, eg, biliary tract disease, alcohol intake, hypercalcemia, duodenal ulcer, or certain offending drugs. The patient should be warned not to eat large meals or foods that are high in fat content and not to drink alcohol. The most common precipitating factor in acute pancreatitis is alcohol intake.

Treatment

A. Management of Acute Disease: The pancreatic rest program includes withholding food and liquids by mouth, bed rest, and in those with moderately severe pain or ileus, nasogastric suction. Pain is controlled with meperidine (Demerol), 100–150 mg intramuscularly every 3–4 hours as necessary. Other narcotics may be used if pain control is not achieved, but they may cause smooth muscle contractions (spasm of the ampulla of Vater). Atropine sulfate, 0.4–0.6 mg subcutaneously, may be given as an antispasmodic and to decrease pancreatic exocrine secretions but may complicate the picture in respect to possible ileus.

In more severe pancreatitis, there may be considerable leakage of fluids, necessitating more than the normal amount of intravenous fluids to maintain intravascular volume. Saline is chiefly used, but fresh-frozen plasma or serum albumin may be necessary. With colloid solutions, there may be an increased risk of developing adult respiratory distress syndrome. If shock persists after adequate volume replacement (including packed red cells), norepinephrine or dopamine may be required. For the severe pancreatitis patient requiring a large volume of parenteral fluids, central venous pressure and blood gases should be monitored at regular intervals.

Calcium gluconate must be given intravenously if there is evidence of hypocalcemia with tetany. Antibiotics should be reserved for specific infections. If fever exceeds 39 °C (102.2 °F) and blood, urine, sputum, and effusions (if present) have been obtained for culture, institution of antibiotic therapy has been recommended.

The patient with severe pancreatitis requires attention in an intensive care unit. Close follow-up of blood count, hematocrit, serum electrolytes, and creatinine is required.

B. Follow-Up Care: After the patient has recovered from shock (or if shock does not develop), it is necessary to choose between expectant medical management and exploratory surgery. Medical management is preferred. Observe the patient closely for evidence of continued inflammation of the pancreas or related structures. A surgeon should be consulted in all cases of suspected acute pancreatitis. If the diagnosis is in doubt and there is a strong possibility of a serious surgically correctable lesion (eg, perforated peptic ulcer, common duct stone), exploration is indicated.

Aggressive surgery and enteral or parenteral hyperalimentation may increase survival in patients with hemorrhagic or suppurative pancreatitis. Initially, enterostomy tubes and drainage are established. Subsequent surgery is performed to debride necrotic pancreas and surrounding tissue.

When acute pancreatitis is unexpectedly found on exploratory laparotomy, it is usually wise to close without intervention of any kind. If the pancreatitis appears mild and cholelithiasis is present, cholecystostomy or cholecystectomy may be justified. Patients with unsuspected pancreatitis who receive the least intra-abdominal manipulation have the lowest morbidity and mortality rates after laparotomy, except as noted above. Peritoneal lavage improves early survival in severe acute pancreatitis. Late septic complications are unaffected.

The development of a pancreatic abscess is an indication for prompt drainage, usually through the flank. If a pseudocyst develops and persists, surgical treatment may be required, although most subside over a period of 3–6 months. Pseudocysts may require drainage when associated with persisting pain, pancreatitis, or common duct obstruction.

The patient should be examined frequently. Periodic blood counts, blood glucose determinations, and serum and urine enzyme determinations should be carried out as indicated. Antibiotic therapy should be reserved for patients with septic complications.

No fluid or foods should be given orally until the patient is largely free of pain and has bowel sounds. Clear liquids are then given, and a gradual progression to a regular low-fat diet is pursued, guided by the patient's tolerance and by the absence of pain. Pancreatitis complicated by prolonged ileus (24 hours or more), abdominal distention, or vomiting require nasogastric suction until they subside, along with parenteral nutrition. Intravenous fluids are given as needed to replace lost fluids, electrolytes, and blood.

C. Convalescent Care: When clinical evidence of pancreatic inflammation has cleared, institute a low-fat diet.

Prognosis

Recurrences are common. The mortality rate for acute hemorrhagic pancreatitis is high, especially when hepatic, cardiovascular, or renal impairment is present. Surgery is indicated only when the diagnosis is in doubt, when the patient is desperately ill despite conservative therapy, or in the presence of an associated disorder such as stones in the biliary tract.

Barkin JS et al: Diagnosis of pancreatic abscess via percutaneous aspiration. *Dig Dis Sci* 1982;**27**:1011.

Fuller RK, Lovelorn JP, Frankel MH: An evaluation of the efficacy of nasogastric suction treatment in alcoholic pancreatitis. *Am J Gastroenterol* 1981;**75**:349.

Jasak EM et al: Pancreatitis in association with hypercalcemia in patients receiving total parenteral nutrition. *Gastroenterology* 1980;**79**:555.

Lankisch PD, Rahlf G, Koop H: Pulmonary complications in fatal acute hemorrhagic pancreatitis. *Dig Dis Sci* 1983;**28**:111.

Levitt MD, Johnson SG: Is the Cam/Ccr ratio of value for the diagnosis of pancreatitis? *Gastroenterology* 1978;**75**:118.

Mallory A, Kern F Jr: Drug-induced pancreatitis: A critical review. *Gastroenterology* 1980;**78**:813.

McCarthy MC, Dickerman RM: Surgical management of severe acute pancreatitis. *Arch Surg* 1982;**117**:476.

McConnell DB et al: Pancreatic pseudocyst. *Am J Surg* 1982;**143**:599.

Moossa AR: Current concepts: Diagnostic tests and procedures in acute pancreatitis. *N Engl J Med* 1984;**311**:639.

Stone HH, Fabian TC, Dunlop WE: Gallstone pancreatitis: Biliary tract pathology in relation to time of operation. *Ann Surg* 1981;**194**:305.

CHRONIC PANCREATITIS
(Chronic Relapsing Pancreatitis)

Chronic pancreatitis occurs most often in patients with alcoholism, hereditary pancreatitis, hypercalce-mia, and hyperlipoproteinemias (types I, IV, and V). Progressive fibrosis and destruction of functioning glandular tissue occur as a result. Pancreaticolithiasis and obstruction of the duodenal end of the pancreatic duct are often present. Pancreatitis recurring after cholecystectomy for cholelithiasis should raise the suspicion of a retained or newly developed common duct stone.

Differentiation of chronic from recurrent pancreatitis is important in that recurrent pancreatitis is initiated by a specific event (eg, alcoholic binge, passage of a stone), whereas chronic pancreatitis is a self-perpetuating disease characterized by pain and pancreatic exocrine or endocrine insufficiency.

Clinical Findings

A. Symptoms and Signs: Persistent or recurrent episodes of epigastric and left upper quadrant pain with referral to the upper left lumbar region are typical. Anorexia, nausea, vomiting, constipation, and flatulence are common. Abdominal signs during attacks consist chiefly of tenderness over the pancreas, mild muscle guarding, and paralytic ileus. Attacks may last only a few hours or as long as 2 weeks; pain may eventually be almost continuous. Steatorrhea (as indicated by bulky, foul, fatty stools) and other types of intestinal malabsorption may occur.

B. Laboratory Findings: Serum amylase and bilirubin may be elevated during acute attacks. Glycosuria may be present. Excess fecal fat may be demonstrated on chemical analysis of the stool.

C. X-Ray Findings: Plain films often show pancreaticolithiasis and mild ileus. A cholecystogram may reveal biliary tract disease, and upper gastrointestinal series may demonstrate a widened duodenal loop. Endoscopic retrograde cholangiopancreatography is a technique that has been widely used. It may show dilated ducts, strictures, or tumor. Failure to cannulate the duct occurs in about 20% of cases.

Complications

Narcotic addiction is common. Other frequent complications include diabetes mellitus, pancreatic pseudocyst or abscess, cholestatic liver disease with or without jaundice, steatorrhea, malnutrition, and peptic ulcer.

Treatment

Correctable coexistent biliary tract disease should be treated surgically.

A. Medical Measures: A low-fat diet should be prescribed. Alcohol is forbidden because it frequently precipitates attacks. Mild sedatives or anticholinergics may be helpful. Narcotics should be avoided if possible. Steatorrhea is treated with pancreatic supplements that are selected on the basis of their lipase activity. Cotazym, Festal, Ilozyme, Ku-Zyme HP, Pancrease, and Viokase have high lipase activity. The usual dose is 2 capsules before, during, and after meals. Concurrent administration of H_2 receptor antagonists decreases the inactivation of lipase by acid and may thereby decrease steatorrhea further; however, the drugs are expensive. It is not necessary to reduce fat excretion to normal to have a good clinical response. Treat associated diabetes as for any other patient. Every effort is made to manage the disease medically.

B. Surgical Treatment: The only indication for surgery in chronic pancreatitis, other than internal drainage of persistent pseudocysts or to treat other complications, is to attempt to relieve pain. The objectives of surgical intervention are to eradicate biliary tract disease, ensure a free flow of bile into the duodenum, and eliminate obstruction of the pancreatic duct. When obstruction of the duodenal end of the duct can be demonstrated by endoscopic retrograde cholangiopancreatography, dilatation of the duct or resection of the tail of the pancreas with implantation of the distal end of the duct by pancreaticojejunostomy may be successful. Anastomosis between the longitudinally split duct and a defunctionalized limb of jejunum without pancreatectomy may be in order. In advanced cases it may be necessary, as a last resort, to do subtotal or total pancreatectomy.

Prognosis

This is a serious disease and often leads to chronic invalidism. The prognosis is best when patients with acute pancreatitis are carefully investigated with their first attack and are found to have some remediable condition such as chronic cholecystitis and cholelithiasis, choledocholithiasis, stenosis of the sphincter of Oddi, or hyperparathyroidism. Medical management of the hyperlipidemias frequently associated with the condition may also prevent recurrent attacks. Surgical relief of these aggravating conditions may prevent recurrent pancreatic disease.

Dutta SK, Rubin J, Harvey J: Comparative evaluations of the therapeutic efficacy of a pH-sensitive enteric coated pancreatic enzyme preparation with conventional pancreatic enzyme therapy in the treatment of exocrine pancreatic insufficiency. *Gastroenterology* 1983;**84:**426.

Gowland M et al: Relative efficiency and predictive value of ultrasonography and endoscopic retrograde pancreatography in diagnosis of pancreatic disease. *Lancet* 1981;**2:**190.

Nagata A et al: A study of chronic pancreatitis by serial endoscopic pancreatography. *Gastroenterology* 1981;**81:**884.

CARCINOMA OF THE HEAD OF THE PANCREAS & THE PERIAMPULLARY AREA

Essentials of Diagnosis

- Obstructive jaundice (may be painless).
- Enlarged gallbladder may be painful.
- Upper abdominal pain with radiation to back, weight loss, and thrombophlebitis are usually late manifestations.

General Considerations

Carcinoma is the commonest neoplasm of the pancreas. About 75% are in the head and 25% in the body and tail of the organ. Carcinomas involving the head of the pancreas, the ampulla of Vater, the common bile duct, and the duodenum are considered together, because they are usually indistinguishable clinically.

Clinical Findings

A. Symptoms and Signs: Epigastric pain, jaundice, and weight loss are the most frequent findings in these tumors. Pain, which is present in over 70%, is often vague and diffuse in the epigastrium and is rarely comparable to biliary colic. Later, more persistent, severe pain develops and often radiates to the back. This usually indicates that the lesion has spread beyond the pancreas and is inoperable. The jaundice is obstructive and must be differentiated from the hepatocellular type. Unfortunately, it is often not possible to make the diagnosis before jaundice occurs. Diarrhea is seen occasionally. Migratory thrombophlebitis is a rare sign. It is a useful clinical rule (Courvoisier's law) that jaundice associated with a palpable gallbladder is indicative of obstruction by neoplasm. The gallbladder is usually not palpable. In addition, a hard, fixed, occasionally tender mass may be present.

B. Laboratory Findings: There may be mild anemia. Glycosuria, hyperglycemia, and impaired glucose tolerance or true diabetes mellitus are found in 10–20% of cases. The serum amylase or lipase level is occasionally elevated. Liver function tests are those of obstructive jaundice. Steatorrhea in the absence of jaundice is uncommon. The secretin test of exocrine secretion usually has a low volume with normal bicarbonate concentration. In about 60% of cases, duodenal cytology has shown malignant cells. Occult blood in the stool is suggestive of carcinoma of the ampulla of Vater. Carcinoembryonic antigen is elevated in most patients but is nonspecific.

C. X-Ray Findings: X-ray examination is usually noncontributory in involvement of the body and tail of the pancreas. With carcinoma of the head of the pancreas, the gastrointestinal series may show a widening of the duodenal loop, mucosal abnormalities in the duodenum ranging from edema to invasion or ulceration, or spasm or compression. Hypotonic duodenography and selective celiac and superior mesenteric arteriography may be most helpful by demonstrating either the encroachment of the duodenum or abnormal vessels in the region of the pancreas. Endoscopic retrograde cholangiopancreatography may delineate the pancreatic duct system and suggest carcinoma. Data are not available on how often this procedure leads to a therapeutic decision. CT scan is most helpful in delineating the extent of the pancreatic mass and allows for percutaneous aspiration of the mass for cytology.

Treatment

Abdominal exploration is usually necessary when cytologic diagnosis cannot be made or if resection is to be attempted, which includes about 30% of patients.

Radical pancreaticoduodenal resection is indicated for lesions strictly limited to the head of the pancreas, periampullary zone, and duodenum. When resection is not feasible, cholecystojejunostomy is performed to relieve the jaundice. A gastrojejunostomy is also done if duodenal obstruction is expected to develop later. High-voltage irradiation and combination drug chemotherapy should be considered.

Prognosis

Carcinoma of the head of the pancreas has a very poor prognosis. Reported 5-year survival rates range from 2.3 to 5.2%. Lesions of the ampulla, common duct, and duodenum have a better prognosis, with reported 5-year survival rates of 20–40% after resection. The reported operative mortality rate of radical pancreaticoduodenectomy is 10–15%.

Moossa AR: Pancreatic cancer: Approach to diagnosis, selection for surgery and choice of operation. *Cancer* 1982;**50**:2689.

CARCINOMA OF THE BODY & TAIL OF THE PANCREAS

About 25% of pancreatic cancers arise in the body or tail. Islet cell tumors arise in the pancreas, as do the non-B cell gastrin-secreting tumors associated with Zollinger-Ellison syndrome. There are no characteristic findings in the early stages. The initial symptoms are vague epigastric or left upper quadrant distress. Anorexia and weight loss usually occur. Later, pain becomes more severe and frequently radiates through to the left lumbar region. A mass in the mid or left epigastrium may be palpable. The spontaneous development of thrombophlebitis is suggestive. If suspected, the diagnosis can often be supported by CT scanning and confirmed by percutaneous aspiration of the mass for cytologic analysis. Sometimes, surgical exploration is necessary for diagnosis. Resection is rarely feasible, and cure is rarer still. The response to fluorouracil (5-FU) has been disappointing. Studies are under way to evaluate multiple-drug therapy.

Nix GA et al: Carcinoma of the head of the pancreas: Therapeutic implications of endoscopic retrograde cholangiopancreatography findings. *Am J Surg* 1984;**87**:37.

ACUTE PERITONITIS

Essentials of Diagnosis

- History of abdominal illness.
- Abdominal pain, vomiting, fever, and prostration.
- Abdominal rigidity and diffuse or local tenderness (often rebound).
- Later, abdominal distention and paralytic ileus.
- Leukocytosis.

General Considerations

Localized or generalized peritonitis is the most important complication of a wide variety of acute abdominal disorders. Peritonitis may be caused by infection or chemical irritation. Perforation or necrosis of the gastrointestinal tract is the usual source of infection. Chemical peritonitis occurs in acute pancreatitis and in the early stages of gastroduodenal perforation. Spontaneous bacterial peritonitis may occur in decompensated cirrhotics with ascites. Sclerosing peritonitis may be associated with neoplastic disease and certain drugs (eg, beta-blockers, methysergide).

Clinical Findings

A. Systemic Reaction: Malaise, prostration, nausea, vomiting, septic fever, leukocytosis, and electrolyte imbalance are usually seen in proportion to the severity of the process. If infection is not controlled, toxemia is progressive, and toxic shock may develop.

B. Abdominal Signs:

1. Pain and tenderness–Depending upon the extent of involvement, pain and tenderness may be localized or generalized. Abdominal pain on coughing, rebound tenderness referred to the area of peritonitis, and tenderness to light percussion over the inflamed peritoneum are characteristic. Pelvic peritonitis is associated with rectal and vaginal tenderness.

2. Muscle rigidity–The muscles overlying the area of inflammation usually become spastic. When peritonitis is generalized (eg, after perforation of a peptic ulcer), marked rigidity of the entire abdominal wall may develop immediately. Rigidity is frequently diminished or absent in the late stages of peritonitis, in severe toxemia, and when the abdominal wall is weak.

3. Paralytic ileus–Intestinal motility is markedly inhibited by peritoneal inflammation. Diminished to absent peristalsis and progressive abdominal distention are the cardinal signs. Vomiting occurs as a result of pooling of gastrointestinal secretions and gas, 70% of which is swallowed air.

C. X-Ray Findings: Abdominal films show gas and fluid collections in both large and small bowel, usually with generalized rather than localized dilatation. The bowel walls, when thrown into relief by the gas patterns, may appear to be thickened, indicating the presence of edema or peritoneal fluid. A gentle barium enema will determine whether large bowel obstruction is present or not.

D. Diagnostic Abdominal Tap: Recovery of ascitic fluid for amylase and protein measurements, culture and cytologic examination may be useful.

Differential Diagnosis

Peritonitis, which may present a highly variable clinical picture, must be differentiated from acute intestinal obstruction, acute cholecystitis with or without choledocholithiasis, pancreatitis, renal colic, gastrointestinal hemorrhage, lower lobe pneumonias, porphyria, periodic fever, hysteria, black widow spider bite, and central nervous system disorders (eg, tabes dorsalis).

Complications

The most frequent sequela of peritonitis is abscess formation in the pelvis, in the subphrenic space, between the leaves of the mesentery, or elsewhere in the abdomen. Antibiotic therapy may mask or delay the appearance of localizing signs of abscess. When fever, leukocytosis, toxemia, or ileus fails to respond to the general measures outlined for the management of peritonitis, a collection of pus should be suspected. This will usually require surgical drainage. Liver abscess and pylephlebitis are rare complications. Adhesions may cause early or, more frequently, late intestinal obstruction.

Treatment

The measures employed in peritonitis as outlined below are generally applicable as supportive therapy in most acute abdominal disorders. The objectives are (1) to control infection, (2) to minimize the effects of paralytic ileus, and (3) to correct fluid, electrolyte, and nutritional disorders.

A. Specific Measures: Operative procedures to close perforations, to remove sources of infection such as gangrenous bowel or an inflamed appendix, or to drain abscesses are frequently required. The cause of the peritonitis should always be identified and treated promptly.

B. General Measures: No matter what specific operative procedures are employed, their ultimate success will often depend upon the care with which the following general measures are performed:

1. Bed rest in the medium Fowler (semi-sitting) position is preferred.

2. Nasogastric suction is started as soon as peritonitis is suspected, to prevent gastrointestinal distention. Suction is continued until peristaltic activity returns and the patient begins passing flatus. A self-tending sump tube should be used, but it must be checked frequently for patency. In persistent paralytic ileus, the intestinal tract may be more adequately decompressed by means of a long intestinal tube (eg, Miller-Abbott), although passage of such a tube into the small bowel is frequently difficult because of poor intestinal motility. In rare cases, combined gastric and long intestinal tube suction may be necessary to relieve or prevent distention.

3. Give nothing by mouth. Oral intake can be resumed slowly after nasogastric suction is discontinued.

4. Fluid and electrolyte therapy and parenteral feeding are required.

5. Narcotics and sedatives should be used liberally to ensure comfort and rest.

6. Antibiotic therapy–Initial antibiotic therapy should be broad spectrum, eg, cephalothin, kanamycin, clindamycin-gentamicin. When cultures are available, antibiotics are chosen according to sensitivity studies.

7. Blood transfusions are used as needed to control anemia.

8. Septic shock, if it develops, requires intensive treatment.

Prognosis

If the cause of peritonitis can be corrected, the infection, accompanying ileus, and metabolic derangement can usually be managed successfully.

Clark C, Terris R: Sclerosing peritonitis associated with metoprolol. *Lancet* 1983;**1**:937.

Levy M: Intraperitoneal drainage. *Am J Surg* 1984;**147**:309.

PERIODIC DISEASE
(Benign Paroxysmal Peritonitis, Familial Mediterranean Fever, Periodic Fever, Recurrent Polyserositis)

Periodic disease is a heredofamilial disorder of unknown pathogenesis, probably metabolic, characterized by recurrent episodes of abdominal or chest pain, fever, and leukocytosis. It is usually restricted to people of Mediterranean ancestry, primarily Armenians, Sephardic Jews, and Arabs and to some extent people of Egypto-Arabic origin living in Turkey, Greece, and Italy. The disease suggests surgical peritonitis, but the acute attacks are recurrent, self-limited, and not fatal. Amyloidosis of the primary type occurs in some cases, and death may result from renal or cardiac failure. Acute episodes may be precipitated by emotional upsets, alcohol, or dietary indiscretion. Treatment is symptomatic and supportive. A low-fat diet may reduce the number and severity of attacks. Daily administration of colchicine, 0.5–1.8 mg, strikingly reduces the number of attacks.

Pras M et al: Variable incidence of Mediterranean fever among different ethnic groups. *Johns Hopkins Med J* 1982;**150**:22.

•   •   •

References

Buchanan KD (editor): Gastrointestinal hormones. *Clin Endocrinol Metabol* 1979;**8:**247. [Entire issue.]

Crane RK (editor): *Gastrointestinal Physiology III.* University Park Press, 1979.

Dooley CP et al: Double-contrast barium meal and upper gastrointestinal endoscopy. *Ann Intern Med* 1984;**101:**538.

Gastroenterology Committee, American College of Physicians: Gastroenterology: An annotated bibliography of recent literature. *Ann Intern Med* 1982;**97:**287.

Haaga J, Reich NE: *Computed Tomography of Abdominal Abnormalities.* Mosby, 1978.

Kirsner JB, Shorter RG: *Inflammatory Bowel Diseases,* 2nd ed. Lea & Febiger, 1980.

Lennard-Jones JE: Current concepts: Functional gastrointestinal disorders. *N Engl J Med* 1983;**308:**431.

Margulis AR, Burhenne HJ: *Alimentary Tract Roentgenology,* 3rd ed. Vols 1 and 2, 1983; Vol 3, 1979. Mosby.

Schiff L: *Diseases of the Liver,* 4th ed. Lippincott, 1975.

Sherlock S: *Diseases of the Liver and Biliary System,* 6th ed. Lippincott/Blackwell, 1981.

Silen W: *Cope's Early Diagnosis of the Acute Abdomen.* Oxford Univ Press, 1979.

Sleisenger MH (editor): Symposium on malabsorption. *Am J Med* 1979;**67:**979.

Sleisenger MH, Fordtran JS (editors): *Gastrointestinal Disease: Pathophysiology, Diagnosis, Management,* 3rd ed. Saunders, 1983.

Spiro HM: *Clinical Gastroenterology,* 3rd ed. Macmillan, 1983.

Taylor KB, Thomas HC: Gastrointestinal and liver diseases. Pages 520–543 in: *Basic & Clinical Immunology,* 5th ed. Stites DP et al (editors). Lange, 1984.

Welch CE, Malt RA: Abdominal surgery. (3 parts.) *N Engl J Med* 1983;**308:**624, 685, 753.

12 | Breast

Armando E. Giuliano, MD

CARCINOMA OF THE FEMALE BREAST

Essentials of Diagnosis

- Higher incidence in women who have delayed child bearing, those with a family history of breast cancer, and those with a personal history of breast cancer or some types of mammary dysplasia.
- Early findings: Single, nontender, firm to hard mass with ill-defined margins; mammographic abnormalities and no palpable mass.
- Later findings: Skin or nipple retraction; axillary lymphadenopathy; breast enlargement, redness, edema, pain, fixation of mass to skin or chest wall.
- Late findings: Ulceration; supraclavicular lymphadenopathy; edema of arm; bone, lung, liver, brain, or other distant metastases.

General Considerations

The breast is the most common site of cancer in women, and cancer of the breast is the leading cause of death from cancer among women in the USA. Breast cancer is the leading cause of death from all causes in women age 40–44 and is frequent in women of all ages over 30. The probability of developing the disease increases throughout life. The mean and the median age of women with breast cancer is 60–61.

There were about 115,000 new cases of breast cancer and about 35,000 deaths from this disease in women in the USA in 1983. At the present rate of incidence, one of every 11 American women will develop breast cancer during her lifetime. Women whose mothers or sisters had breast cancer are more likely to develop the disease than controls. Risk is increased when breast cancer has occurred before menopause, was bilateral, or was present in 2 or more first-degree relatives. However, there is no history of breast cancer among female relatives in over 90% of patients with breast cancer. Nulliparous women and women whose first full-term pregnancy was after age 35 have a slightly higher incidence of breast cancer than multiparous women. Late menarche and artificial menopause are associated with a lower incidence of breast cancer, whereas early menarche (under age 12) and late natural menopause (after age 50) are as-

sociated with a slight increase in risk of developing breast cancer. Mammary dysplasia (cystic disease of the breast), when accompanied by proliferative changes, papillomatosis, or atypical epithelial hyperplasia, is associated with an increased incidence of cancer. A woman who has had cancer in one breast is at increased risk of developing cancer in the opposite breast. Women with cancer of the uterine corpus have a breast cancer risk significantly higher than that of the general population, and women with breast cancer have a comparably increased endometrial cancer risk. In the USA, breast cancer is more common in whites than in nonwhites. The incidence of the disease among nonwhites (mostly blacks), however, is increasing, especially in younger women. In general, rates reported from developing countries are low, whereas rates are high in developed countries, with the notable exception of Japan. Some of the variability may be due to underreporting in the developing countries, but a real difference probably exists. There is some evidence that administration of estrogens to postmenopausal women may result in an increased risk of breast cancer. This increase is slight and may be seen only with higher, continuous doses of estrogens.

Women who are at greater than normal risk of developing breast cancer (Table 12–1) should be identified by their physicians and followed carefully. Screening programs involving periodic physical examination and mammography of asymptomatic high-risk women increase the detection rate of breast cancer and may improve the survival rate. Unfortunately, most women who develop breast cancer do not have signifi-

Table 12–1. Factors associated with increased risk of breast cancer.*

Race	White
Age	Older
Family history	Breast cancer in mother or sister (especially bilateral or premenopausal)
Previous medical history	Endometrial cancer
	Some forms of mammary dysplasia
	Cancer in other breast
Menstrual history	Early menarche (under age 12)
	Late menopause (after age 50)
Pregnancy	Late first pregnancy

*Normal lifetime risk in white women = 1 in 11.

cant identifiable risk factors, and analysis of epidemiologic data has failed to identify women who are not at significant risk and would not benefit from screening. Therefore, the cost-benefit ratio of screening programs to society as a whole is unclear. New, less expensive screening techniques, such as single-view mammography, are being investigated in an attempt to reduce the cost of widespread screenings.

Growth potential of tumor and resistance of host vary over a wide range from patient to patient and may be altered during the course of the disease. The doubling time of breast cancer cells ranges from several weeks in a rapidly growing lesion to nearly a year in a slowly growing one. Assuming that the rate of doubling is constant and that the neoplasm originates in one cell, a carcinoma with a doubling time of 100 days may not reach clinically detectable size (1 cm) for 8 years. On the other hand, rapidly growing cancers have a much shorter preclinical course and a greater tendency to metastasize to regional nodes or more distant sites by the time a breast mass is discovered.

The relatively long preclinical growth phase and the tendency of breast cancers to metastasize have led many clinicians to believe that breast cancer is a systemic disease at the time of diagnosis. Although it may be true that breast cancer cells are released from the tumor prior to diagnosis, variations in the host-tumor relationship may prohibit the growth of disseminated disease in many patients. For this reason, a pessimistic attitude concerning the management of localized breast cancer is not warranted, and many patients can be cured with proper treatment.

Staging (Table 12–2)

The extent of disease evident from physical findings and special preoperative studies is used to determine the clinical stage of the lesion. Histologic staging is performed after examination of the axillary specimen. The results of clinical staging are used in designing the treatment plan (Table 12–2). Both clinical and histologic staging are of prognostic significance.

Clinical Findings

The patient with breast cancer usually presents with a lump in the breast. Clinical evaluation should include assessment of the local lesion and a search for evidence of metastases in regional nodes or distant sites. After the diagnosis of breast cancer has been confirmed by biopsy, additional studies are often needed to complete the search for distant metastases or an occult primary in the other breast. Then, before any decision is made about treatment, all the available clinical data are used to determine the extent or "stage" of the patient's disease.

A. Symptoms: In taking the history, special note should be made of menarche, pregnancies, parity, artificial or natural menopause, date of last menstrual period, previous breast lesions, and a family history of breast cancer. Back or other bone pain may be the result of osseous metastases. Systemic complaints or weight loss should raise the question of metastases,

Table 12–2. Clinical and histologic staging of breast carcinoma and relation to survival.

Clinical Staging (American Joint Committee)	Crude 5-Year Survival (%)
Stage I	85
Tumor < 2 cm in diameter	
Nodes, if present, not felt to contain metastases	
Without distant metastases	
Stage II	66
Tumor < 5 cm in diameter	
Nodes, if palpable, not fixed	
Without distant metastases	
Stage III	41
Tumor > 5 cm or—	
Tumor any size with invasion of skin or attached to chest wall	
Nodes in supraclavicular area	
Without distant metastases	
Stage IV	10
With distant metastases	

Histologic Staging	Crude Survival (%)	
	5 Years	10 Years
All patients	63	46
Negative axillary lymph nodes	78	65
Positive axillary lymph nodes	46	25
1–3 positive axillary lymph nodes	62	38
> 4 positive axillary lymph nodes	32	13

which may involve any organ but most frequently the bones, liver, and lungs. The more advanced the cancer in terms of size of primary, local invasion, and extent of regional node involvement, the higher the incidence of metastatic spread to distant sites.

The presenting complaint in about 70% of patients with breast cancer is a lump (usually painless) in the breast (Table 12–3). About 90% of breast masses are discovered by the patient herself. Less frequent symptoms are breast pain; nipple discharge; erosion, retraction, enlargement, or itching of the nipple; and redness, generalized hardness, enlargement, or shrink-

Table 12–3. Initial symptoms of mammary carcinoma.*

Symptom	Percentage of All Cases
Painless breast mass	66
Painful breast mass	11
Nipple discharge	9
Local edema	4
Nipple retraction	3
Nipple crusting	2
Miscellaneous symptoms	5

*Adapted from report of initial symptoms in 774 patients treated for breast cancer at Ellis Fischel State Cancer Hospital, Columbia, Missouri. Reproduced, with permission, from Spratt JS Jr, Donegan WL: *Cancer of the Breast.* Saunders, 1967.

ing of the breast. Rarely, an axillary mass, swelling of the arm, or bone pain (from metastases) may be the first symptom. Thirty-five to 50% of women involved in organized screening programs have cancers detected by mammography only.

B. Signs: The relative frequency of carcinoma in various anatomic sites in the breast is shown in Fig 12–1. Almost half of cancers of the breast begin in the upper outer quadrant, probably because this quadrant contains the largest volume of breast tissue. The high percentage in the central portion is due to the inclusion of cancers that spread to the subareolar region from neighboring quadrants. Cancer is slightly more common in the left breast than in the right.

Inspection of the breast is the first step in physical examination and should be carried out with the patient sitting, arms at sides and then overhead. Abnormal variations in breast size and contour, minimal nipple retraction, and slight edema, redness, or retraction of the skin are best identified by careful observation in good light. Asymmetry of the breasts and retraction or dimpling of the skin can often be accentuated by having the patient raise her arms overhead or press her hands on her hips in order to contract the pectoralis muscles. Axillary and supraclavicular areas should be thoroughly palpated for enlarged nodes with the patient sitting (Fig 12–2). Palpation of the breast for masses or other changes should be performed with the patient both seated and supine with the arm abducted (Fig 12–3).

Breast cancer usually consists of a nontender, firm or hard lump with poorly delineated margins (caused by local infiltration). Slight skin or nipple retraction is an important sign. Minimal asymmetry of the breast may be noted. Very small (1–2 mm) erosions of the nipple epithelium may be the only manifestation of Paget's carcinoma. Watery, serous, or bloody

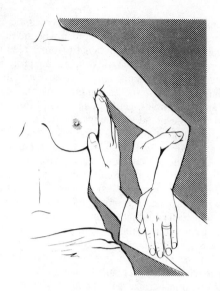

Figure 12–2. Palpation of axillary region for enlarged lymph nodes.

discharge from the nipple is an occasional early sign but is more often associated with benign disease.

A lesion smaller than 1 cm in diameter may be difficult or impossible for the examiner to feel and yet may be discovered by the patient. She should always be asked to demonstrate the location of the mass; if the physician fails to confirm the patient's suspicions, the examination should be repeated in 1 month. During the premenstrual phase of the cycle, increased innocuous nodularity may suggest neoplasm or may obscure an underlying lesion. If there is any question regarding the nature of an abnormality under these circumstances, the patient should be asked to return after her period.

The following are characteristic of advanced carcinoma: edema, redness, nodularity, or ulceration of the skin; the presence of a large primary tumor; fixation to the chest wall; enlargement, shrinkage, or re-

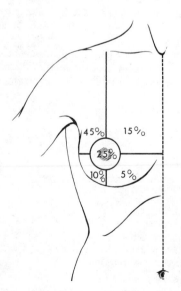

Figure 12–1. Frequency of breast carcinoma at various anatomic sites.

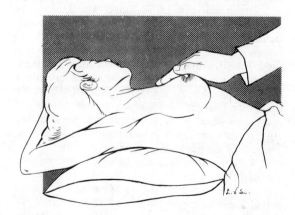

Figure 12–3. Palpation of breasts. Palpation is performed with the patient supine and arm abducted.

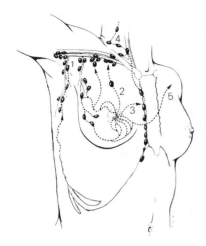

Figure 12–4. Lymphatic drainage of the breast to regional node groups. *1.* Main axillary group. *2.* Interpectoral node leading to apex of axilla. *3.* Internal mammary group. *4.* Supraclavicular group. *5.* Lymphatic channels to opposite axilla.

traction of the breast; marked axillary lymphadenopathy; supraclavicular lymphadenopathy; edema of the ipsilateral arm; and distant metastases.

Metastases tend to involve regional lymph nodes (Fig 12–4), which may be clinically palpable. With regard to the axilla, one or 2 movable, nontender, not particularly firm lymph nodes 5 mm or less in diameter are frequently present and are generally of no significance. Firm or hard nodes larger than 5 mm in diameter usually contain metastases. Axillary nodes that are matted or fixed to skin or deep structures indicate advanced disease (at least stage III). Histologic studies show that microscopic metastases are present in about 30% of patients with clinically negative nodes. On the other hand, if the examiner thinks that the axillary nodes are involved, this will prove on histologic section to be correct in about 85% of cases. The incidence of positive axillary nodes increases with the size of the primary tumor and with the local invasiveness of the neoplasm.

Usually no nodes are palpable in the supraclavicular fossa. Firm or hard nodes of any size in this location or just beneath the clavicle (infraclavicular nodes) are suggestive of metastatic cancer and should be biopsied. Ipsilateral supraclavicular or infraclavicular nodes containing cancer indicate that the patient is in an advanced stage of the disease (stage IV). Edema of the ipsilateral arm, commonly caused by metastatic infiltration of regional lymphatics, is also a sign of advanced (stage IV) cancer.

C. Special Clinical Forms of Breast Carcinoma:

1. Paget's carcinoma–The basic lesion is an infiltrating intraductal carcinoma, usually well differentiated and multicentric in the nipple and breast ducts. The nipple epithelium is infiltrated, but gross nipple changes are often minimal, and a tumor mass may not be palpable. The first symptom is often itching or burning of the nipple, with a superficial erosion or ulceration. The diagnosis is established by biopsy of the erosion.

Paget's carcinoma is not common (about 1–3% of all breast cancers), but it is important because it appears innocuous. It is frequently diagnosed and treated as dermatitis or bacterial infection, leading to unfortunate delay in detection. When the lesion consists of nipple changes only, the incidence of axillary metastases is about 5%. When a breast tumor is also present, the incidence of axillary metastases rises to about 67%, with an associated marked decrease in prospects for cure by surgical or other treatment.

2. Inflammatory carcinoma–This is the most malignant form of breast cancer and constitutes less than 3% of all cases. The clinical findings consist of a rapidly growing, sometimes painful mass that enlarges the breast. The overlying skin becomes erythematous, edematous, and warm. The diagnosis should be made when the redness involves more than one-third of the skin over the breast and biopsy shows invasion of the subdermal lymphatics. The inflammatory changes, often mistaken for an infectious process, are caused by carcinomatous invasion of the dermal lymphatics, with resulting edema and hyperemia. If the physician suspects infection but the lesion does not respond rapidly (1–2 weeks) to antibiotics, a biopsy must be performed. Metastases tend to occur early and widely, and for this reason inflammatory carcinoma is rarely curable. Mastectomy is seldom, if ever, indicated. Radiation, hormone therapy, and anticancer chemotherapy are the measures most likely to be of value.

3. Occurrence during pregnancy or lactation–Only 1–2% of breast cancers occur during pregnancy or lactation. Breast cancer complicates approximately one in 3000 pregnancies. The diagnosis is frequently delayed, because physiologic changes in the breast may obscure the true nature of the lesion. This results in a tendency of both patients and physicians to misinterpret the findings and to procrastinate in deciding on biopsy. When the neoplasm is confined to the breast, the 5-year survival rate after mastectomy is about 70%. On the other hand, axillary metastases are already present in 60–70% of patients, and for them the 5-year survival rate after mastectomy is only 30–40%. Pregnancy (or lactation) is not a contraindication to modified radical mastectomy, and treatment should be based on the stage of the disease as in the nonpregnant (or nonlactating) woman. Overall survival rates have improved as cancers are diagnosed earlier in pregnant women.

4. Bilateral breast cancer–Clinically evident simultaneous bilateral breast cancer occurs in less than 1% of cases, but there is a 5–8% incidence of later occurrence of cancer in the second breast. Bilaterality occurs more often in women under age 50 and is more frequent when the tumor in the primary breast is of the lobular type. The incidence of second breast cancers increases directly with the length of time the patient is alive after her first cancer.

In patients with breast cancer, mammography should be performed before primary treatment and at regular intervals thereafter, to search for occult cancer in the opposite breast. Routine biopsy of the opposite breast is usually not warranted.

D. Laboratory Findings: A consistently elevated sedimentation rate may be the result of disseminated cancer. Liver or bone metastases may be associated with elevation of serum alkaline phosphatase. Hypercalcemia is an occasional important finding in advanced cancer of the breast.

E. X-Ray Findings: Chest x-rays may show pulmonary metastases. CT scan of liver and brain is of value only when metastases are suspected in these areas.

F. Radionuclide Scanning: Bone scans utilizing technetium Tc 99m-labeled phosphates or phosphonates are more sensitive than skeletal x-rays in detecting metastatic breast cancer. Bone scanning has not proved to be of clinical value as a routine preoperative test in the absence of symptoms, physical findings, or abnormal alkaline phosphatase levels. The frequency of abnormal findings on bone scan parallels the status of the axillary lymph nodes on pathologic examination.

G. Biopsy: The diagnosis of breast cancer depends ultimately upon examination of tissue removed by biopsy. Treatment should never be undertaken without an unequivocal histologic diagnosis of cancer. The safest course is biopsy examination of all suspicious masses found on physical examination and, in the absence of a mass, of suspicious lesions demonstrated by mammography. About 30% of lesions thought to be definitely cancer prove on biopsy to be benign, and about 15% of lesions believed to be benign are found to be malignant. These findings demonstrate the fallibility of clinical judgment and the necessity for biopsy.

The simplest method is needle biopsy, either by aspiration of tumor cells or, preferably, by obtaining a small core of tissue with a Vim-Silverman or other special needle. This is an office procedure especially suitable for easily accessible lesions larger than a few centimeters in diameter. A negative needle biopsy should be followed by open biopsy, because false-negative needle biopsies may occur in 15–20% of cancers.

The preferred method is open biopsy under local anesthesia as a separate procedure prior to deciding upon definitive treatment. The lesion should be completely excised. The patient need not be admitted to the hospital. Decisions on additional workup for metastatic disease and on definitive therapy can be made and discussed with the patient after the histologic diagnosis of cancer has been established. This approach has the advantage of avoiding unnecessary hospitalization and diagnostic procedures in many patients, since cancer is found in only about 35% of patients who require biopsy for differential diagnosis of a breast lump.

As an alternative in patients for whom mastec-

tomy is considered to be the treatment of choice in highly suspicious circumstances, the patient may be admitted directly to the hospital, where the diagnosis is made on frozen section of tissue obtained by open biopsy under general anesthesia. If the frozen section is positive, the surgeon could proceed immediately with mastectomy.

In general, the 2-step approach—that is, outpatient biopsy followed by definitive operation at a later date—is preferred in the diagnosis and treatment of breast cancer, because patients can be given time to adjust to the diagnosis of cancer, can carefully consider alternative forms of therapy, and can seek a second opinion should they feel it important. Studies have shown no adverse effect from the short (1–2 weeks) delay of the 2-step procedure, and this is the current recommendation of the National Cancer Institute.

At the time of the initial biopsy of breast cancer, it is important for the physician to preserve a portion of the specimen for determination of estrogen receptors.

H. Cytology: Cytologic examination of nipple discharge or cyst fluid may be helpful on rare occasions. As a rule, mammography and breast biopsy are required when nipple discharge or cyst fluid is bloody or cytologically questionable.

I. Mammography: The 2 methods of mammography in common use are ordinary film radiography and xeroradiography. From the standpoint of diagnosing breast cancer, they give comparable results. It is now possible to perform a high-quality mammogram while delivering less than 1 rad to the mid breast.

Mammography is the only reliable means of detecting breast cancer before a mass can be palpated in the breast. Some breast cancers can be identified by mammography as long as 2 years before reaching a size detectable by palpation.

Although false-positive and false-negative results are occasionally obtained with mammography, the experienced radiologist can interpret mammograms correctly in about 90% of cases. Where mammography is employed proficiently, the yield of malignant lesions on biopsy remains around 35%. This is in spite of the fact that more biopsies are done.

Indications for mammography are as follows: (1) to evaluate the opposite breast when a diagnosis of potentially curable breast cancer has been made, and at intervals of 1–3 years thereafter; (2) to evaluate a questionable or ill-defined breast mass or other suspicious change in the breast, but only if mammographic findings will assist in determining whether or where a biopsy is to be performed; (3) to search for an occult breast cancer in a woman with metastatic disease in axillary nodes or elsewhere from an unknown primary; and (4) to screen at regular intervals a selected group of women who are at high risk for developing breast cancer (see below).

Patients with a dominant or suspicious mass must undergo biopsy despite mammographic findings. The mammogram should be obtained prior to biopsy so that other suspicious areas can be noted and the contralateral breast can be checked. Mammography is never a substitute for biopsy, because it may not reveal clinical cancer in a very dense breast, as may be seen in young women with mammary dysplasia, and often does not reveal medullary type cancer.

Early Detection

A. Screening Programs: A number of mass screening programs consisting of physical and mammographic examination of the breasts of asymptomatic women have been conducted. They are identifying more than 6 cancers per 1000 women. About 80% of these women have negative axillary lymph nodes at the time of surgery whereas, by contrast, only 45% of patients found in the course of usual medical practice have uninvolved axillary nodes. Detecting breast cancer before it has spread to the axillary nodes greatly increases the chance of survival, and about 84% of such women will survive at least 5 years.

Both physical examination and mammography are necessary for maximum yield in screening programs, since about 40% of early breast cancers can be discovered only by mammography and another 40% can be detected only by palpation. Women 20–40 years of age should have a breast examination as part of routine medical care every 2–3 years. Women over age 40 should have yearly breast examinations.

The American College of Radiology and the American Cancer Society have recently revised their recommendations regarding use of mammography in asymptomatic women. A baseline mammogram should be performed on all women between ages 35 and 40 years. Women aged 40–49 years should have a mammogram every 1–2 years. Annual mammograms are indicated for women age 50 years or older. High-risk women—those whose mothers or sisters had bilateral or premenopausal breast cancer, those who have had cancer of one breast, and those with histologic abnormalities associated with subsequent cancer (eg, atypical epithelial hyperplasia, papillomatosis, lobular carcinoma in situ)—should have an annual mammogram and biannual examinations. The usefulness of screening mammography in young women without identifiable risk factors is not yet of proved value. However, in a recent large study of women under age 50, nearly half of all cancers were detected by mammography alone. Mammographic patterns are not a reliable predictor of the risk of developing breast cancer.

Other modalities of breast imagery have been investigated. Automated breast ultrasonography is very useful in distinguishing cystic from solid lesions but should be used only as a supplement to physical examination and mammography in screening for breast cancer. Diaphanography (transillumination of the breasts) and thermography are of no proved screening value.

B. Self-Examination: All women over age 20 should be advised to examine their breasts monthly. Premenopausal women should perform the examination immediately after the menstrual period, and high-risk patients may be asked to perform a second examination in midcycle. The breasts should be inspected initially while standing before a mirror with the hands at the sides, overhead, and pressed firmly on the hips to contract the pectoralis muscles. Masses, asymmetry of breasts, and slight dimpling of the skin may become apparent as a result of these maneuvers. Next, in a supine position, each breast should be carefully palpated with the fingers of the opposite hand. Physicians should instruct their women patients in the technique of self-examination and advise them to report at once for medical evaluation if a mass or other abnormality is noted. Some women discover small breast lumps more readily when their skin is moist while bathing or showering.

Differential Diagnosis

The lesions most often to be considered in the differential diagnosis of breast cancer are the following, in order of frequency: mammary dysplasia (cystic disease of the breast), fibroadenoma, intraductal papilloma, duct ectasia, and fat necrosis. The differential diagnosis of a breast lump should be established without delay by biopsy, by aspiration of a cyst, or by observing the patient until disappearance of the lump within a period of a few weeks.

Pathologic Types

Numerous pathologic subtypes of breast cancer can be identified histologically (see Table 12–4). These pathologic types are distinguished by the histologic appearance and growth pattern of the tumor. In general, breast cancer arises either from the epithelial lining of the large or intermediate-sized ducts (ductal) or from the epithelium of the terminal ducts of the lobules (lobular). The cancer may be invasive or in situ. Most breast cancers arise from the intermediate ducts and are invasive (invasive ductal, infiltrating ductal), and most histologic types are merely subtypes of invasive ductal cancer with unusual growth patterns (colloid, medullary, scirrhous, etc). Ductal carcinoma that has not invaded the extraductal tissue is intraductal or in situ ductal. Lobular carcinoma may be either invasive or in situ.

The histologic subtypes have little bearing on prognosis when patients are compared after accurate staging. Various histologic parameters, such as invasion of blood vessels, tumor differentiation, invasion of breast lymphatics, and tumor necrosis have been examined, but they too seem to have little prognostic value.

The noninvasive cancers by definition lack the ability to spread. However, in patients whose biopsies show noninvasive intraductal cancer, associated invasive ductal cancers are present in about 1–3% of cases. Lobular carcinoma in situ is considered by some to be a premalignant lesion that by itself is not a true cancer. It lacks the ability to spread but is associated with the subsequent development of invasive cancer in at least 30% of cases.

Table 12-4. Histologic types of breast cancer.

	Percent Occurrence
Infiltrating ductal (not otherwise specified)	70–80
Medullary	5–8
Colloid (mucinous)	2–4
Tubular	1–2
Papillary	1–2
Invasive lobular	6–8
Noninvasive	4–6
Intraductal	2–3
Lobular in situ	2–3
Rare cancers	<1
Juvenile (secretory)	...
Adenoid cystic	...
Epidermoid	...
Sudiferous	...

Hormone Receptor Sites

The presence or absence of estrogen receptors in the cytoplasm of tumor cells is of paramount importance in managing patients with recurrent or metastatic disease. Up to 60% of patients with metastatic breast cancer will respond to hormonal manipulation if their tumors contain estrogen receptors. However, fewer than 10% of patients with metastatic, estrogen receptor-negative tumors can be successfully treated with hormonal manipulation.

Progesterone receptors may be an even more sensitive indicator than estrogen receptors of patients who may respond to hormonal manipulation. Up to 80% of patients with metastatic progesterone receptor-positive tumors seem to respond to hormonal manipulation. Receptors probably have no relationship to response to chemotherapy.

Some studies suggest that estrogen receptors are of prognostic significance. Patients whose primary tumors are receptor-positive have a more favorable course after mastectomy than those whose tumors are receptor-negative.

Receptor status is not only valuable for the management of metastatic disease but may help in the selection of patients for adjuvant therapy. Some studies suggest that hormonal therapy (tamoxifen) for patients with receptor-positive tumors treated by mastectomy may improve survival rates.

It is advisable to obtain an estrogen-receptor assay for every breast cancer at the time of initial diagnosis. Receptor status may change after hormonal therapy, radiotherapy, or chemotherapy. The specimen requires special handling, and the laboratory should be prepared to process the specimen correctly.

Curative Treatment

Treatment may be curative or palliative. Curative treatment is advised for clinical stage I and II disease (see Table 12–2). Treatment can only be palliative for patients in stage IV and for previously treated patients who develop distant metastases or unresectable local recurrence.

A. Therapeutic Options: Radical mastectomy involves en bloc removal of the breast, pectoral muscles, and axillary nodes and was the standard curative procedure for breast cancer from the turn of the century until about 10 years ago. Radical mastectomy removes the primary lesion and the axillary nodes with a wide margin of surrounding tissue, including the pectoral muscles. **Extended radical mastectomy** involves, in addition to standard radical mastectomy, removal of the internal mammary nodes. It has been recommended by a few surgeons for medially or centrally placed breast lesions and for tumors associated with positive axillary nodes, because of the known frequency of internal mammary node metastases under these circumstances. **Modified radical mastectomy** (total mastectomy plus axillary dissection) consists of en bloc removal of the breast with the underlying pectoralis major fascia (but not the muscle) and all axillary lymph nodes. Some surgeons remove the pectoralis minor muscle. Others retract or transect the muscle to facilitate removal of the axillary lymph nodes. Except for preservation of the pectoralis major muscle, this procedure is of the same extent as the standard radical mastectomy. Modified radical mastectomy gives superior cosmetic and functional results compared with standard radical mastectomy. **Simple mastectomy** (total mastectomy) consists of removing the entire breast, leaving the axillary nodes intact. Limited procedures such as **segmental mastectomy** (lumpectomy, quadrant excision, partial mastectomy) are becoming more popular as definitive treatment for early breast cancer (eg, stage I). The proved efficacy of **irradiation** in sterilizing the primary lesion and the axillary and internal mammary nodes has made radiation therapy with segmental mastectomy a reasonable option for primary treatment of certain breast cancers.

B. Choice of Primary Therapy: The extent of disease and its biologic aggressiveness are the principal determinants of the outcome of primary therapy. Clinical and pathologic staging help in assessing extent of disease (Table 12–2), but each is to some extent imprecise. Since about two-thirds of patients eventually manifest distant disease regardless of the form of primary therapy, there is a tendency to think of breast carcinoma as being systemic in most patients at the time they first present for treatment.

There is a great deal of controversy regarding the optimal method of primary therapy of stage I, II, and III breast carcinoma, and opinions on this subject have changed considerably in the past decade. Legislation initiated in California and Massachusetts and now adopted in numerous states requires physicians to inform patients of alternative treatment methods in the management of breast cancer.

Radical Mastectomy

For about three-quarters of a century, radical mastectomy was considered standard therapy for this disease. The procedure was designed to remove the primary lesion, the breast in which it arose, the underlying muscle, and, by dissection in continuity, the axillary lymph nodes that were thought to be the first site of spread beyond the breast. When radical mastectomy was introduced by Halsted, the average patient presented for treatment with advanced local disease (stage III), and a relatively extensive procedure was often necessary just to remove all gross cancer. This is no longer the case. Patients present now with much smaller, less locally advanced lesions. Most of the patients in Halsted's original series would now be considered incurable by surgery alone, since they had extensive involvement of the chest wall, skin, and supraclavicular regions.

Although radical mastectomy is extremely effective in controlling local disease, it has the disadvantage of being the most deforming of any of the available treatments for management of primary breast cancer. The surgeon and patient are both eager to find therapy that is less deforming but does not jeopardize the chance for cure.

Less Radical Surgery & Radiation Therapy

A number of clinical trials have been performed in the past decade in which the magnitude of the surgical procedure undertaken for removal of cancer in the breast and adjacent lymph nodes has been varied, with and without the use of local radiotherapy to the chest wall and node-bearing areas.

Radical mastectomy, modified radical mastectomy, and simple mastectomy have been compared in numerous clinical trials. In general, radical mastectomy has a lower local recurrence rate than modified radical or simple mastectomy. Simple mastectomy has the highest regional recurrence rate, since the lymph nodes are not removed, and as many as 30% of patients with clinically negative nodes will have metastatic breast cancer within these nodes. At least half of these patients subsequently develop regional recurrences. Despite these differences in local and regional effect, no significant differences in survival have been consistently demonstrated among these 3 types of treatment. The addition of radiotherapy to mastectomy will also reduce the incidence of local recurrence, but in general, radiotherapy does not improve overall survival rates. Even the removal of occult cancer in axillary lymph nodes generally is not reflected in improvement in overall survival rates, although regional failures will be much lower.

The most significant recent advance in the management of primary breast cancer has been the realization that less than total mastectomy combined with radiotherapy may be as effective as more radical operations alone for certain patients with small primary tumors. Studies are still relatively recent, however, and long-term follow-up is necessary for definitive conclusions. Patients with large or stage III breast cancers may benefit from a combination of surgery, radiotherapy, and systemic chemotherapy.

Radiation therapy alone (without surgery) in the treatment of primary breast cancer fails to achieve local control in about 50% of cases. Small, nonrandomized studies have suggested that removal of the tumor by segmental mastectomy ("lumpectomy") combined with postoperative irradiation is as effective as mastectomy in achieving local control without diminishing long-term survival. A randomized study from Milan compared the results of quadrant resection, axillary dissection, and postoperative radiotherapy with those of a standard Halsted radical mastectomy. The study included only women with lesions less than 2 cm and no palpable axillary lymph nodes. There was no difference in the incidence of local recurrence or survival between the 2 kinds of treatment. Therefore, although the length of follow-up is short, it appears that small, favorable lesions may be controlled by breast-sparing techniques.

A study sponsored by the National Surgical Adjuvant Breast Project in the USA has randomized patients to treatment by segmental resection and axillary dissection, with and without radiation therapy, or to modified radical mastectomy. Patients with lesions up to 4 cm and palpable nodes are being admitted to the study. Consequently, many important questions concerning the advisability of breast-saving operations, the role of radiotherapy, and the biologic significance of multifocal lesions should be answered soon. This study has recently been concluded, and results should be published shortly.

It is important to recognize that axillary dissection is valuable both in planning therapy and in staging of the cancer. Operation is extremely effective in preventing axillary recurrences. In addition, lymph nodes removed during the procedure can be pathologically assessed. This assessment is essential for the planning of adjuvant therapy, which is often recommended for patients with gross or occult involvement of axillary nodes.

Current Recommendations

We believe that total mastectomy plus axillary dissection (modified radical mastectomy) is currently the primary procedure of choice for most patients with potentially curable carcinoma of the breast. Premenopausal patients with involvement of axillary lymph nodes should receive adjuvant chemotherapy. Radical mastectomy may rarely be required for some cases of advanced local disease if the tumor invades the muscle but otherwise is not advisable for the average patient. Extended radical mastectomy would rarely be appropriate and could only be justified for patients with medial lesions and no signs of more distant spread. Treatment of the axillary nodes is not indicated for **noninfiltrating** cancers, because nodal metastases are present in only 1% of such patients.

Preoperatively, full discussion with the patient regarding the rationale for mastectomy and the manner of coping with the cosmetic and psychologic effects of the operation is essential. Patients often have questions about possible alternatives to standard or modified radical mastectomy—eg, local excision, simple mastectomy, and radiotherapy—and wish detailed explanations of the risks and benefits of the various procedures. Women with small tumors (ie, less than 2 cm) and clinically negative axillary nodes should have the option of treatment by segmental mastectomy plus axillary dissection and radiotherapy. However, patients should be cautioned that this treatment is still relatively new and that its long-term results are unknown. Breast reconstruction should be discussed with the patient if this is a realistic possibility. Time spent preoperatively in educating the patient and her family is well spent.

Adjuvant Therapy

Chemotherapy is now being used as adjunctive treatment of patients with curable breast cancer and positive axillary nodes, since there is a great likelihood that these patients harbor occult metastases. Overall, about 75% of such patients eventually succumb within 10 years, even though the initial therapy, either surgery or irradiation, eradicated all neoplasm evident at that time. The objective of adjuvant chemotherapy is to eliminate the occult metastases responsible for late recurrences while they are microscopic and theoretically most vulnerable to anticancer agents.

Numerous clinical trials with various adjuvant chemotherapeutic regimens have been completed. The most extensive clinical experience to date is with the CMF regimen (*c*yclophosphamide, *m*ethotrexate, and *f*luorouracil). The regimen should be repeated every 6–12 months in patients with axillary metastases who were treated with radical or modified radical mastectomy. Follow-up studies at 8 years show that premenopausal women definitely benefit from receiving adjuvant chemotherapy, whereas postmenopausal women probably do not. The recurrence rate in premenopausal patients who received no adjuvant chemotherapy was more than 1½ times that of those who received therapy. No therapeutic effect has been shown in postmenopausal women, perhaps because therapy was modified so often in response to side effects that the total amount of drugs administered was less than planned. Other trials with different agents support the value of adjuvant chemotherapy; in some cases, postmenopausal women appear to benefit. Combinations of drugs are clearly superior to single drugs.

Adjuvant chemotherapy can be offered confidently to premenopausal women with metastases in axillary lymph nodes and no evidence of distant disease, but the use of adjuvant chemotherapy in postmenopausal women is more controversial. It is difficult to determine which regimen is appropriate for which subgroup of women with breast cancer. Some studies show a beneficial effect in premenopausal but not postmenopausal women, while other studies utilizing different combinations of agents show a beneficial effect in postmenopausal but not premenopausal women. In addition, the estrogen receptor status of the tumor must be taken into consideration when chemotherapy is being planned. Some agents were shown to be effective in randomized studies, and others have been shown to be effective when compared to historical controls. In general, comparison with historical controls is less convincing proof of effect than are concurrent randomized prospective trials. For this reason, controversy remains regarding which agents are most beneficial for particular patients with breast cancer.

The addition of hormones may improve the results of adjuvant therapy. For example, tamoxifen has been shown to enhance the beneficial effects of melphalan and fluorouracil in women whose tumors are estrogen receptor-positive. Interestingly, in this study, improvement in disease-free survival rates was seen only in postmenopausal women. Tamoxifen has been used alone with some success as adjuvant treatment for postmenopausal women with estrogen receptor-positive tumors.

The length of time adjuvant therapy must be administered remains uncertain. Several studies suggest that shorter treatment periods may be as effective as longer ones. The Milan group has compared 6 versus 12 cycles of postoperative CMF and found 5-year disease-free survival rates to be comparable. One of the earliest adjuvant trials (Nissen-Meyer) used a 6-day perioperative regimen of intravenous cyclophosphamide alone; follow-up at 15 years shows a 15% improvement in disease-free survival rates for treated patients, suggesting that short-term therapy may be effective.

Patients with estrogen receptor-negative tumors, even without axillary lymph node involvement, may have a recurrence rate as high as 30% within the first 2 years after operation. For this reason, a number of clinical studies are investigating the value of adjuvant chemotherapy in women with estrogen receptor-negative tumors and no evidence of axillary lymph node involvement. Preliminary results suggest that these patients may benefit from adjuvant systemic chemotherapy; however, these studies are not yet conclusive, and we do not routinely employ adjuvant systemic therapy for patients without lymph node involvement.

Important questions remaining to be answered are the timing and duration of adjuvant chemotherapy; which chemotherapeutic agents should be applied for which subgroups of patients; how best to coordinate adjuvant chemotherapy with postoperative radiation therapy; the use of hormonal therapy; the use of combinations of hormonal and chemotherapy; and the value of adjuvant therapy for node-negative patients.

Postoperative Care

A. Immediate Care: Occasional wound complications such as hematoma or serum collection under the skin flaps and necrosis of skin margins are usually easily managed. They are minimized by suction drainage of the wound and avoidance of undue tension on the skin flaps at closure by the use of a skin graft if necessary.

Active motion of the arm and shoulder on the operated side should be encouraged after the first few days, so that by 10–14 days postoperatively there is a full range of motion. Failure of the patient to cooperate or to make progress may necessitate physical therapy. The Service Committee of the American Cancer Society sponsors a rehabilitation program for postmastectomy patients called Reach for Recovery and will provide useful literature upon request. Women who have had a mastectomy may be valuable counselors for the patient before and after operation. The patient's morale is improved by provision of a temporary breast prosthesis held in place by a comfortably fitted brassiere before she leaves the hospital. She should also receive information on where to obtain a more permanent device.

B. Follow-Up Care: After primary therapy, patients with breast cancer should be followed for life for at least 2 reasons: to detect recurrences and to observe the opposite breast for a second carcinoma. Local and distant metastases occur most frequently within the first 3 years. During this period, the patient is examined every 3–4 months. Thereafter, examination is done every 6 months until 5 years postoperatively and then every 6–12 months. Special attention is given to the remaining breast, because of the increased risk of developing a second primary. The patient should examine her own breast monthly, and a mammogram should be obtained annually. In some cases, metastases are dormant for long periods and may appear up to 10–15 years or longer after removal of the primary tumor. Use of estrogen or progestational agents is probably inadvisable in patients free of disease after treatment of primary breast cancer, particularly those patients whose tumor was estrogen receptor-positive.

1. Local recurrence–Recurrence of cancer within the operative field following radical mastectomy is due to incomplete removal of tumor or involved nodes, to cutting across infiltrated lymphatics, to spillage of tumor cells into the wound, or perhaps to blood-borne metastasis implanting in the surgical field. The rate of local recurrence correlates with tumor size, the presence and number of involved axillary nodes, the histologic type of tumor, and the presence of skin edema or skin and fascia fixation with the primary. About 15% of patients develop local recurrence after total mastectomy and axillary dissection. When the axillary nodes are not involved, the local recurrence rate is 5%, but the rate is 25% when they are involved. A similar difference in local recurrence rate was noted between small and large tumors. Local recurrence is even more frequent following operations that do not include an axillary dissection or total mastectomy. Factors that affect the rate of local recurrence in patients who had partial mastectomies are not yet determined. However, early studies show that such things as multifocal cancer, in situ tumors, and positive resection margins are likely to be important.

Chest wall recurrences usually appear within the first 2 years, with a peak incidence in the second year, but may occur as late as 15 or more years after radical mastectomy. Suspect nodules should be biopsied. Local excision or localized radiotherapy may be feasible if an isolated nodule is present. If lesions are multiple or accompanied by evidence of regional involvement in the internal mammary or supraclavicular nodes, the disease is best managed by radiation treatment of the whole chest wall including the parasternal, supraclavicular, and axillary areas.

Local recurrence usually signals the presence of widespread disease and is an indication for bone and liver scans, posteroanterior and lateral chest x-rays, and other examinations as needed to search for evidence of metastases. When there is no evidence of metastases beyond the chest wall and regional nodes, radical irradiation for cure or complete local excision should be attempted. Most patients with locally recurrent tumor will develop distant metastases within 2 years. For this reason, many physicians use systemic therapy for treatment of patients with local recurrence. Although this seems reasonable, it should be pointed out that patients with local recurrence may be cured with local resection or radiation. Systemic chemotherapy or hormonal treatment should be used for patients who develop disseminated disease or those in whom local recurrence occurs following adequate local therapy.

2. Edema of the arm–Significant edema of the arm occurs in 10–30% of patients after radical and in about 5% after modified radical mastectomy.

Late or secondary edema of the arm may develop years after radical mastectomy as a result of axillary recurrence or of infection in the hand or arm, with obliteration of lymphatic channels. There is usually no obvious cause of late arm swelling. After radical mastectomy, the lymphatic drainage of the arm is always compromised, and the extremity becomes more than normally susceptible to infection following minor injuries. The patient should be warned of this, and treatment by antibiotics, heat, rest, and elevation should be instituted promptly if infection occurs. Intravenous infusions and injections for inoculation and immunization should not be given in that extremity. Chronic edema is managed by elevation and by a snugly fitted elastic sleeve that is slipped over the arm from hand to shoulder. A special sleeve designed to provide intermittent compression to the entire arm may be useful in severe cases.

3. Breast reconstruction–Breast reconstruction, with the implantation of a prosthesis, is usually feasible after standard or modified radical mastectomy. Reconstruction should probably be discussed with patients prior to mastectomy, because it offers an important psychologic focal point for recovery. However, most patients who are initially interested in reconstruction decide later that they no longer wish to undergo the procedure. Reconstruction is not an obstacle to the diagnosis of recurrent cancer and should be encouraged if the patient is interested.

4. Risks of pregnancy–Data are insufficient to definitely determine whether interruption of pregnancy improves the prognosis of patients who are discovered during pregnancy to have potentially curable breast cancer and who receive definitive treatment. Theoretically, the increasingly high levels of estrogen produced by the placenta as the pregnancy progresses will be detrimental to the patient with occult metastases of estrogen-sensitive breast cancer. Moreover, occult metastases are present in most patients with positive axillary nodes, and treatment by adjuvant chemotherapy would be potentially harmful to the fetus. Under these circumstances, interruption of early pregnancy seems reasonable, with progressively less rationale for the procedure as term approaches. Obviously, the decision must be highly individualized and will be affected by many factors, including the patient's desire to have the baby and the generally poor prognosis when axillary nodes are involved.

Equally problematic and important is the advice regarding future pregnancy (or abortion in case of pregnancy) to be given to women of child-bearing age who have had a mastectomy or other definitive treatment for breast cancer. Under these circumstances, one must assume that pregnancy will be harmful if occult metastases are present. Experience shows that women with axillary metastases have a relatively poor prognosis for cure and that recurrences continue to appear for up to 10 years or longer after definitive treatment. Hence, pregnancy is generally inadvisable in this group of patients and should probably be interrupted if it occurs, at least until 5 years have passed without recurrence. In principle, the more favorable the stage and pathologic type of disease, the less the possible risk of a stimulating effect by pregnancy on occult metastases. Advice to patients should be individualized accordingly. It should be kept in mind that theoretic considerations—rather than firm clinical evidence from controlled studies—are the basis for the assumption that intercurrent pregnancy will adversely affect prognosis in patients with breast cancer.

In inoperable or metastatic cancer (stage IV disease), induced abortion is usually advisable, because of the possible adverse effects upon the fetus of hormonal treatment, radiotherapy, or chemotherapy.

Prognosis

The stage of breast cancer is the single most reliable indicator of prognosis. Patients with disease localized to the breast and no evidence of regional spread after microscopic examination of the lymph nodes have by far the most favorable prognosis. Estrogen receptors appear to be an important prognostic variable, because patients with estrogen receptor-negative tumors and no evidence of metastases to the axillary lymph nodes have a much higher recurrence rate than do patients with estrogen receptor-positive tumors and no regional metastases. The histologic subtype of breast cancer (eg, medullary, lobular, comedo) seems to have little, if any, significance in prognosis once these tumors are truly invasive.

As mentioned above, several different treatment regimens achieve approximately the same results when given to the appropriate patient. Localized disease can be controlled with local therapy—either surgery alone or limited surgery in combination with radiation therapy. However, the criteria for selection of patients to be treated with conservative resection and radiation therapy require further clarification.

Most patients who develop breast cancer will ultimately die of breast cancer. The mortality rate of breast cancer patients exceeds that of age-matched normal controls for nearly 20 years. Thereafter, the mortality rates are equal, although deaths that occur among the breast cancer patients are often directly the result of tumor. Five-year statistics do not accurately reflect the final outcome of therapy.

When cancer is localized to the breast, with no evidence of regional spread after pathologic examination, the clinical cure rate with most accepted methods of therapy is 75–90%. Exceptions to this may be related to estrogen receptor content of the tumor, tumor size, host resistance, or associated illness. Patients with small estrogen receptor-positive tumors and no evidence of axillary spread probably have a 5-year survival rate of nearly 90%. When the axillary lymph nodes are involved with tumor, the survival rate drops to 40–50% at 5 years and probably less than 25% at 10 years. In general, breast cancer appears to be somewhat more malignant in younger than older women, and this may be related to the fact that fewer younger women have estrogen receptor-positive tumors.

Carcinoma of Female Breast

Baines CJ: Breast self-examination: The doctor's role. *Hosp Pract* (March) 1984;**19**:120.

Bland KI et al: Analysis of breast cancer screening in women younger than 50 years. *JAMA* 1981;**245**:1037.

Bolsen B: Ultrasound breast scanning: (Only) a complement to mammography? *JAMA* 1982;**248**:1025.

Buzdar AU et al: Management of inflammatory carcinoma of breast with combined modality approach: An update. *Cancer* 1981;**47**:2537.

Canellos GP, Hellman S, Veronesi U: The management of early breast cancer. *N Engl J Med* 1982;**306**:1430.

Carter SK: The dilemma of local control of breast cancer. (Editorial.) *West J Med* 1982;**136**:336.

Deffebach RR, Goodman RL, Miller L: Lumpectomy and irradiation in the treatment of early carcinoma of the breast. *West J Med* 1982;**136**:281.

Devitt JE: Clinical benign disorders of the breast and carcinoma of the breast. *Surg Gynecol Obstet* 1981;**152**:437.

Elwood JM, Moorehead WP: Delay in diagnosis and long-term survival in breast cancer. *Br Med J* 1980;**280**:1291.

Ferguson DJ et al: Staging of breast cancer and survival rates: An assessment based on 50 years of experience with radical mastectomy. *JAMA* 1982;**248**:1337.

Fisher B et al: The accuracy of clinical nodal staging and of limited axillary dissection as a determinant of histologic nodal status in carcinoma of the breast. *Surg Gynecol Obstet* 1981;**152**:765.

Goldin BR et al: Estrogen excretion patterns and plasma levels in vegetarian and omnivorous women. *N Engl J Med* 1982;**307**:1542.

Gunby P: Treating breast cancer conservatively: Dissension, contention continues. *JAMA* 1982;**248**:1793.

Hagemeister FB et al: Causes of death in breast cancer: A clinicopathologic study. *Cancer* 1980;**46**:162.

Harris JR, Helman S: Primary radiation therapy for early breast cancer. *Proc Am Soc Clin Oncol* 1983;**2**:104.

Harris JR et al: Clinical-pathologic study of early breast cancer treated by primary radiation therapy. *J Clin Oncol* 1983;**1**:184.

Henderson IC, Canellos GP: Cancer of the breast. (2 parts.) *N Engl J Med* 1980;**302**:17, 78.

Hickey RC et al: Hypercalcemia in patients with breast cancer. *Arch Surg* 1981;**116**:545.

Hornstein E, Skornick Y, Rozin R: The management of breast carcinoma in pregnancy and lactation. *J Surg Oncol* 1982;**21**:179.

Howe GR et al: Estimated benefits and risks of screening for breast cancer. *Can Med Assoc J* 1981;**124**:399.

Huguley CM et al: The value of breast self-examination. *Cancer* 1981;**47**:989.

Kelly PT: Refinements in breast cancer risk analysis. *Arch Surg* 1981;**116**:364.

Kinne DW: Opinion: The case for the one-step biopsy procedure for breast cancer. *CA* 1982;**32**:46.

Lee YTN: Bone scanning in patients with early breast carcinoma: Should it be a routine staging procedure? *Cancer* 1981;**47**:486.

Letton AH et al: Five-year-plus survival of breast screenees. *Cancer* 1981;**48**:404.

Mansour EG et al: Tissue and plasma carcinoembryonic antigen in early breast cancer: A prognostic factor. *Cancer* 1983;**51**:1243.

Martinez A, Clarke D: Irradiation as an alternative to mastectomy for early breast cancer: An important consideration because of changes in laws. *West J Med* 1983;**138**:676.

Minton JP et al: Caffeine and unsaturated fat diet significantly promotes DMBA-induced breast cancer in rats. *Cancer* 1983;**51**:1249.

National Institutes of Health Consensus Development Conference. *JAMA* 1980;**244**:797.

O'Brien RL et al: Breast cancer treatment: Current status. *Postgrad Med* (Sept) 1983;**74**:124.

Paone JF et al: Pathogenesis and treatment of Paget's disease of the breast. *Cancer* 1981;**48**:825.

Pigott J et al: Metastases to the upper levels of the axillary nodes in carcinoma of the breast and its implications for nodal sampling procedures. *Surg Gynecol Obstet* 1984;**158**:255.

Rosen PP et al: Noninvasive breast carcinoma: Frequency of unsuspected invasion and implications for treatment. *Ann Surg* 1979;**189**:377.

Seidman H, Stellman SD, Mushinski MH: A different perspective on breast cancer risk factors: Some implications of the nonattributable risks. *CA* 1982;**32**:301.

Thomas DB, Persing JP, Hutchinson WB: Exogenous estrogens and other risk factors for breast cancer in women with benign breast diseases. *JNCI* 1982;**69**:1017.

Veronesi U et al: Comparing radical mastectomy with quadrantectomy, axillary dissection, and radiotherapy in patients with small cancers of the breast. *N Engl J Med* 1981;**305**:6.

Veronesi U et al: Inefficacy of internal mammary node dissection in breast cancer surgery. *Cancer* 1981;**47**:170.

Webber BL et al: Risk of subsequent contralateral breast carcinoma in a population of patients with in situ breast carcinoma. *Cancer* 1981;**47**:2928.

Westman-Naeser S et al: Multifocal breast carcinoma. *Am J Surg* 1981;**142**:255.

Woods KL, Smith SR, Morrison JM: Parity and breast cancer: Evidence of a dual effect. *Br Med J* 1980;**281**:419.

Mammography

Boyd NF et al: Mammographic signs as risk factors for breast cancer. *Br J Cancer* 1982;**45**:185.

Egan RL: Mammography: Current recommendations and their rationale. *Consultant* 1984;**28**:166.

Gold RH et al: Diagnostic imaging of the breast. *Invest Radiol* 1984;**19**:S43.

Kopans DB, Meyer JE, Sadowsky N: Breast imaging. *N Engl J Med* 1984;**310**:960.

Mammography 1982: A statement of the American Cancer Society. *CA* 1982;**32**:226.

Mann BD et al: Delayed diagnosis of breast cancer as a result of negative mammogram. *Arch Surg* 1983;**118**:23.

Sickles EA et al: Mammography after needle aspiration of palpable breast masses. *Am J Surg* 1983;**145**:395.

Tabar L, Dean PB: Mammographic parenchymal patterns: Risk indicator for breast cancer? *JAMA* 1982;**247**:185.

Hormone Receptors

Gapinski PV, Donegan WL: Estrogen receptors and breast cancer: Prognostic and therapeutic implications. *Surgery* 1980;**88**:386.

Jensen EV: Hormone dependency of breast cancer. *Cancer* 1981;**47**:2319.

Kinne DW et al: Estrogen receptor protein in breast cancer as a predictor of recurrence. *Cancer* 1981;**47**:2364.

Lesser ML et al: Estrogen and progesterone receptors in breast carcinoma: Correlations with epidemiology and pathology. *Cancer* 1981;**48**:299.

McCarty KS Jr et al: Relationship of age and menopausal status to estrogen receptor content in primary carcinoma of the breast. *Ann Surg* 1983;**197**:123.

Steroid receptors in breast cancer. *Cancer* 1980;**46(Suppl)**: 2759. [Entire issue.]

Taylor CR et al: Detection of estrogen receptor in breast and endometrial carcinoma by the immunoperoxidase technique. *Cancer* 1981;**47**:2634.

Adjuvant Chemotherapy

Bonadonna G, Valagussa P: Dose-response effect of adjuvant chemotherapy in breast cancer. *N Engl J Med* 1981;**304**:10.

Bonadonna G et al: Adjuvant chemotherapy in breast cancer. [Letter.] *Lancet* 1983;**21**:1157.

Caprini JA et al: Adjuvant chemotherapy for stage II and III breast carcinoma. *JAMA* 1980;**244**:243.

Fisher B et al: Influence of tumor estrogen and progesterone receptor levels on the response to tamoxifen and chemotherapy in primary breast cancer. *J Clin Oncol* 1983;**1**:227.

Fisher B et al: Treatment of primary breast cancer with chemotherapy and tamoxifen. *N Engl J Med* 1981;**305**:1.

Nissen-Meyer R: The Scandinavian clinical trials. *Experientia* [*Suppl*] 1982;**41**:571.

Rossi A et al: Multimodal treatment in operable breast cancer: Five-year results of the CMF programme. *Br Med J* 1981;**282**:1427.

Tancini G et al: Adjuvant CMF in breast cancer: Comparative 5-year results of 12 versus 6 cycles. *J Clin Oncol* 1983;**1**:2.

Tormey DC et al: A randomized trial of five and three drug chemotherapy and chemoimmunotherapy in women with operable node positive breast cancer. *J Clin Oncol* 1983;**1**:138.

Weiss RB et al: Multimodal treatment of primary breast carcinoma. *Am J Med* 1981;**70**:844.

TREATMENT OF ADVANCED BREAST CANCER

This section covers palliative therapy of disseminated disease incurable by surgery (stage IV).

Radiotherapy

Palliative radiotherapy may be advised for locally advanced cancers with distant metastases in order to control ulceration, pain, and other manifestations in the breast and regional nodes. Radical irradiation of the breast and chest wall and the axillary, internal mammary, and supraclavicular nodes should be undertaken in an attempt to cure locally advanced and inoperable lesions when there is no evidence of distant metastases. A small number of patients in this group are cured in spite of extensive breast and regional node involvement. Adjuvant chemotherapy should be considered for such patients.

Palliative irradiation is also of value in the treatment of certain bone or soft tissue metastases to control pain or avoid fracture. Radiotherapy is especially useful in the treatment of the isolated bony metastasis and chest wall recurrences.

Hormone Therapy

Disseminated disease may respond to prolonged endocrine therapy such as administration of hormones, ablation of the ovaries, adrenals, or pituitary, or administration of drugs that block hormone receptor sites (eg, antiestrogens) or drugs that block the synthesis of hormones (eg, aminoglutethimide). Hormonal manipulation is usually more successful in postmenopausal women. If treatment is based on the presence of estrogen receptor protein in the primary tumor or metastases, however, the rate of response is nearly equal in premenopausal and postmenopausal women. A favorable response to hormonal manipulation occurs in about one-third of patients with metastatic breast cancer. Of those whose tumors contain estrogen receptors, the response is about 60% and perhaps as high as 80% for patients whose tumors contain progesterone receptors as well. Because only 5–10% of women whose tumors do not contain estrogen receptors respond, they should not receive hormonal therapy except in unusual circumstances.

A favorable response to hormonal manipulation may be anticipated also in (1) patients with slowly growing tumors (ie, if there is a long tumor-free interval between diagnosis and the appearance of metastatic disease); (2) patients with metastases to bone and soft tissues or pleura—as opposed to visceral organs such as lung, liver, or brain; (3) very old patients; or (4) patients who have previously shown favorable responses. However, the presence of estrogen receptor protein on the tumor or metastases is the single best predictor of responsiveness. Since the quality of life during a remission induced by endocrine manipulation is usually superior to a remission following cytotoxic chemotherapy, it is usually best to try endocrine manipulation first in cases where the estrogen receptor

status of the tumor is unknown. However, if the estrogen receptor status is unknown but the disease is progressing rapidly or involves visceral organs, endocrine therapy is rarely successful, and introducing it may waste valuable time.

In general, only one type of systemic therapy should be given at a time, unless it is necessary to irradiate a destructive lesion of weight-bearing bone while the patient is on another regimen. The regimen should be changed only if the disease is clearly progressing but not if it appears to be stable. This is especially important for patients with destructive bone metastases, since minor changes in the status of these lesions are difficult to determine radiographically. A plan of therapy that would simultaneously minimize toxicity and maximize benefits is often best achieved by hormonal manipulation.

The choice of endocrine therapy depends on the menopausal status of the patient. Women within 1 year of their last menstrual period are considered to be premenopausal, while women whose menstruation ceased more than a year ago are postmenopausal. The initial choice of therapy is referred to as primary hormonal manipulation; subsequent endocrine treatment is called secondary or tertiary hormonal manipulation.

A. The Premenopausal Patient:

1. Primary hormonal therapy–Bilateral oophorectomy is usually the first choice for primary hormonal manipulation in premenopausal women. It can be achieved rapidly and safely by surgery or, if the patient is a poor operative risk, by irradiation to the ovaries. Ovarian radiation therapy should be avoided in otherwise healthy patients, however, because of the high rate of complications and longer time necessary to achieve results. Oophorectomy presumably works by eliminating estrogens, progestins, and androgens, which stimulate growth of the tumor. The average remission is about 12 months.

The potent antiestrogen tamoxifen has been tried as an alternative to oophorectomy in the premenopausal patient. In limited trials, the response rate to tamoxifen is similar to that of oophorectomy, leading some authorities to recommend tamoxifen as the primary hormonal treatment of metastatic breast cancer in premenopausal women with estrogen receptor–positive tumors. However, only a few premenopausal patients have received tamoxifen without prior oophorectomy, and the optimal dosage remains unclear. In a study in which 40–120 mg/d was given, serum levels of estrone and estradiol were markedly elevated, presumably due to an increased output of pituitary gonadotropins. Although 5 out of 11 women responded to tamoxifen, it appears that either escalating the drug dosage or oophorectomy plus tamoxifen may be necessary in premenopausal patients.

Tamoxifen may eventually become the preferred primary hormonal manipulation in premenopausal women, but experience is presently insufficient to advocate tamoxifen in preference to oophorectomy. The operation is not associated with long-term endocrine dysfunction, as are adrenalectomy and hypophysectomy. Oophorectomy should definitely not be abandoned yet. Randomized trials now being conducted comparing tamoxifen with oophorectomy should clarify this issue.

2. Secondary or tertiary hormonal therapy– Although patients who do not respond to oophorectomy should be treated with cytotoxic drugs, those who respond and then relapse may subsequently respond to another form of endocrine treatment. The initial choice for secondary endocrine manipulation has not been clearly defined. Adrenalectomy or hypophysectomy induces regression in approximately 30–50% of patients who have previously responded to oophorectomy.

Patients who respond initially to oophorectomy but subsequently relapse should receive tamoxifen. If this treatment fails, use of aminoglutethimide (Cytadren) should be considered. Aminoglutethimide is an inhibitor of adrenal hormone synthesis and, when combined with a corticosteroid, provides a therapeutically effective "medical adrenalectomy." Aminoglutethimide causes less morbidity and mortality than surgical adrenalectomy; can be discontinued once the patient improves; and is not associated with the many problems of postsurgical hypoadrenalism, so that patients who require chemotherapy are more easily managed.

B. The Postmenopausal Patient:

1. Primary hormonal therapy–Tamoxifen, 10 mg twice daily, is now the initial therapy of choice for postmenopausal women with metastatic breast cancer amenable to endocrine manipulation. It has fewer side effects than diethylstilbestrol, the former therapy of choice, and is just as effective.

2. Secondary or tertiary endocrine manipulation (postmenopausal)–Postmenopausal patients who do not respond to primary endocrine manipulation should be given cytotoxic drugs. Postmenopausal women who respond initially to tamoxifen but later manifest progressive disease should be given DES. Some authorities use aminoglutethimide, but DES is much easier to administer. Aminoglutethimide should be reserved for patients who respond initially to tamoxifen, progress, respond to DES, and progress for a second time. An alternative, but probably less effective, treatment is use of progestins (eg, megestrol acetate) and androgens. Androgens have many side effects and should rarely be used. In general, hypophysectomy or adrenalectomy is rarely necessary.

Chemotherapy

Cytotoxic drugs should be considered for the treatment of metastatic breast cancer (1) if visceral metastases are present (especially brain or lymphangitic pulmonary); (2) if hormonal treatment is unsuccessful or the disease has progressed after an initial response to hormonal manipulation; or (3) if the tumor is estrogen receptor–negative. The most useful single chemotherapeutic agent to date is doxorubicin (Adriamycin), with a response rate of 40–50%. The remissions tend to be brief, and in general, experience with single-agent chemotherapy in patients with disseminated disease has not been encouraging.

Combination chemotherapy using multiple agents has proved to be more effective, with objectively observed favorable responses achieved in 60–80% of patients with stage IV disease. Various combinations of drugs have been used, and clinical trials are continuing in an effort to improve results and to reduce undesirable side effects. Doxorubicin and cyclophosphamide produced an objective response in 87% of 46 patients who had an adequate trial of therapy. Other chemotherapeutic regimens have consisted of various combinations of drugs, including cyclophosphamide, vincristine, methotrexate, and fluorouracil, with response rates ranging up to 60–70%. Prior adjuvant chemotherapy does not seem to alter response rates in patients who relapse. Few new drugs or combinations of drugs have been sufficiently effective in breast cancer to warrant wide acceptance. However, one new agent, dihydroxyandrostenedione, has been effective enough in heavily pretreated patients to justify phase III trials.

Malignant Pleural Effusion

This condition develops at some time in almost half of patients with breast cancer. When severe and persistent, the effusion is best controlled by closed tube drainage of the chest and intrapleural instillation of a sclerosing agent. An intercostal tube is inserted in a low interspace and placed on suction or water-seal drainage until as much fluid as possible has been removed, and 500 mg of tetracycline dissolved in 30 mL of saline is then injected into the pleural cavity through the tube, which is clamped for 6 hours. The patient's position is changed frequently to distribute the tetracycline within the pleural space. The tube is unclamped and continued on water-seal drainage until drainage has decreased to less than 60 mL in 24 hours. This will usually occur within 5–6 days if the sclerosing action of the tetracycline is effective in causing adherence of visceral to parietal pleura. Transient reaction to the tetracycline such as pleural pain or low-grade fever is treated symptomatically. Fluid reaccumulation is prevented in 50–75% of patients. The procedure may be repeated in a few weeks if fluid recurs. Tetracycline is preferable to various chemotherapeutic agents such as mechlorethamine and thiotepa that may cause nausea, vomiting, or bone marrow depression.

Treatment of Advanced Breast Cancer

Asbury RF et al: Treatment of metastatic breast cancer with aminoglutethimide. *Cancer* 1981;**47**:1954.

Bisel HF: Management of locally advanced and disseminated breast cancer: Chemotherapy. *Cancer* 1980;**46**:1097.

Bitran JD et al: Response to secondary therapy in patients with adenocarcinoma of the breast previously treated with adjuvant chemotherapy. *Cancer* 1983;**51**:381.

Fisher B et al: Disease-free survival at intervals during and following completion of adjuvant chemotherapy. *Cancer* 1981;**48**:1273.

Henderson IC: Less toxic treatment of advanced breast cancer. *N Engl J Med* 1981;**305**:575.

Ingle JN et al: Randomized clinical trial of diethylstilbestrol versus tamoxifen in postmenopausal women with advanced breast cancer. *N Engl J Med* 1981;**304**:16.

Kaufman RJ: Advanced breast cancer: Additive hormonal therapy. *Cancer* 1981;**47**:2398.

Kiang DT et al: Combination therapy of hormone and cytotoxic agents in advanced breast cancer. *Cancer* 1981;**47**:452.

Legha SS et al: Response to hormonal therapy as a prognostic factor for metastatic breast cancer treated with combination chemotherapy. *Cancer* 1980;**46**:438.

Lipton A et al: A randomized trial of aminoglutethimide versus tamoxifen in metastatic breast cancer. *Cancer* 1982; **50**:2265.

Manni A, Pearson OH: Antiestrogen-induced remissions in premenopausal women with stage IV breast cancer: Effects on ovarian function. *Cancer Treat Rep* 1980;**64**:779.

McBride CM et al: Can patients with breast cancer be cured of their disease? *Cancer* 1983;**51**:938.

Minton MJ et al: Corticosteroids for elderly patients with breast cancer. *Cancer* 1981;**48**:883.

Neidhart JA et al: Mitoxantrone versus doxorubicin in advanced breast cancer: A randomized cross-over trial. *Cancer Treat Rev* 1983;**10**(Suppl 3):41.

Powles TJ et al: Failure of chemotherapy to prolong survival in a group of patients with metastatic breast cancer. *Lancet* 1980;**1**:580.

Pritchard KI et al: Tamoxifen therapy in premenopausal patients with breast cancer. *Cancer Treat Rep* 1980;**64**:787.

Santen RJ, Wells SA: The use of aminoglutethimide in the treatment of patients with metastatic carcinoma of the breast. *Cancer* 1980;**46**:1066.

Santen RJ et al: Aminoglutethimide as treatment of postmenopausal women with advanced breast carcinoma. *Ann Intern Med* 1982;**96**:94.

Santen RJ et al: A randomized trial comparing surgical adrenalectomy with aminoglutethimide plus hydrocortisone in women with advanced breast cancer. *N Engl J Med* 1981; **305**:545.

Schweitzer RJ: Oophorectomy/adrenalectomy. *Cancer* 1980; **46**:1061.

Yap HY et al: Dihydroxyandrostenedione: A promising new drug in the treatment of metastatic breast cancer. *Ann Intern Med* 1981;**95**:694.

CARCINOMA OF THE MALE BREAST

Essentials of Diagnosis

- A painless lump beneath the areola in a man, usually over 50 years of age.
- Nipple discharge, retraction, or ulceration may occur.

General Considerations

Breast cancer in men is a rare disease; the incidence is only about 1% of that in women. The average age at occurrence is about 60—somewhat older than the commonest presenting age in women. The prognosis, even in stage I cases, is worse in men than in women. Blood-borne metastases are commonly present when the male patient appears for initial treatment. These metastases may be latent and may not become manifest for many years.

As in women, hormonal influences are probably related to the development of male breast cancer. A high estrogen level, a shift in the androgen-estrogen ratio, or an abnormal susceptibility of breast tissue to normal estrogen concentrations may be of etiologic significance.

There is a high incidence of both breast cancer and gynecomastia in Bantu men, theoretically owing to failure of estrogen inactivation by a damaged liver associated with vitamin B deficiency.

Clinical Findings

A painless lump, occasionally associated with nipple discharge, retraction, erosion, or ulceration, is the chief complaint. Examination usually shows a hard, ill-defined, nontender mass beneath the nipple or areola. Gynecomastia not uncommonly precedes or accompanies breast cancer in men. Nipple discharge is an uncommon presentation for breast cancer in men, as it is in women. However, nipple discharge in a man is an ominous finding associated with carcinoma in nearly 75% of cases.

Breast cancer staging is the same in men as in women. Gynecomastia and metastatic cancer from another site (eg, prostate) must be considered in the differential diagnosis of a breast lesion in a man. Biopsy settles the issue.

Treatment

Treatment consists of modified radical mastectomy in operable patients, who should be chosen by the same criteria as women with the disease. Irradiation is the first step in treating localized metastases in the skin, lymph nodes, or skeleton that are causing symptoms.

Since breast cancer in men is frequently a disseminated disease, endocrine therapy is of considerable importance in its management. Castration in advanced breast cancer is the most successful palliative measure and more beneficial than the same procedure in women. Objective evidence of regression may be seen in 60–70% of men who are castrated—approximately twice the proportion in women. The average duration of tumor growth remission is about 30 months, and life is prolonged. Bone is the most frequent site of metastases from breast cancer in men (as in women), and castration relieves bone pain in most patients so treated. The longer the interval between mastectomy and recurrence, the longer the tumor growth remission following castration. As in women, there is no correlation between the histologic type of the tumor and the likelihood of remission following castration. In view of the marked benefits of castration in advanced disease, prophylactic castration has been suggested in stage II breast cancer in men, but there is no certainty that this approach is warranted, and this should probably not be done.

Bilateral adrenalectomy (or hypophysectomy) has been proposed as the procedure of choice when tumor has reactivated after castration. Aminoglutethimide therapy should replace adrenalectomy in men as it has in women. Corticosteroid therapy is considered by some to be efficacious but probably has no value when compared to major endocrine ablation.

Estrogen therapy—5 mg of diethylstilbestrol 3 times daily orally—may rarely be effective. Androgen therapy may exacerbate bone pain. Castration, bilateral adrenalectomy, and corticosteroids are the main lines of therapy for advanced breast cancer in men at present. Tamoxifen has been reported to be successful in several cases and is becoming increasingly popular and may replace castration as the initial therapy for metastatic disease. Chemotherapy should be administered for the same indications and using the same dose schedules as for women with metastatic disease.

Examination of the cancer for estrogen receptor protein may in future prove to be of value in predicting response to endocrine ablation. Adjuvant chemotherapy for the same indications as in breast cancer in women may be useful, but experience with this form of treatment is lacking at present.

Prognosis

The prognosis of breast cancer is poorer in men than in women. The crude 5- and 10-year survival rates for clinical stage I breast cancer in men are about 58% and 38%, respectively. For clinical stage II disease, the 5- and 10-year survival rates are approximately 38% and 10%. The overall survival rates at 5 and 10 years are 36% and 17%.

Kantarjian H et al: Hormonal therapy for metastatic male breast cancer. *Arch Intern Med* 1983;**143**:237.

Tirelli U et al: Tamoxifen before and after orchiectomy in advanced male breast cancer. *Cancer Treat Rep* 1982;**66**:1883.

Yap HY et al: Chemotherapy for advanced male breast cancer. *JAMA* 1980;**243**:1739.

MAMMARY DYSPLASIA
(Fibrocystic Disease)

Essentials of Diagnosis

- Painful, often multiple, usually bilateral masses in the breast.
- Rapid fluctuation in the size of the masses is common.
- Frequently, pain occurs or increases and size increases during premenstrual phase of cycle.
- Most common age is 30–50. Rare in postmenopausal women.

General Considerations

This disorder, also known as fibrocystic disease or chronic cystic mastitis, is the most frequent lesion of the breast. It is common in women 30–50 years of age but rare in postmenopausal women; this suggests that it is related to ovarian activity. Estrogen hormone is considered a causative factor. The term "mammary dysplasia," or "fibrocystic disease," is imprecise and encompasses a wide variety of pathologic entities. These lesions are always associated with benign changes in the breast epithelium, some of which are found so commonly in normal breasts that they are probably variants of normal breast histology.

The microscopic findings of fibrocystic disease include cysts (gross and microscopic), papillomatosis, adenosis, fibrosis, and ductal epithelial hyperplasia. Although mammary dysplasia has been considered to increase the risk of subsequent breast cancer, it is probable that only the variants in which proliferation of epithelial components is demonstrated represent true risk factors.

Clinical Findings

Mammary dysplasia may produce an asymptomatic lump in the breast that is discovered by accident, but pain or tenderness often calls attention to the mass. There may be discharge from the nipple. In many cases discomfort occurs or is increased during the premenstrual phase of the cycle, at which time the cysts tend to enlarge. Fluctuation in size and rapid appearance or disappearance of a breast tumor are common in cystic disease. Multiple or bilateral masses are not unusual, and many patients will give a past history of transient lump in the breast or cyclic breast pain. Pain, fluctuation in size, and multiplicity of lesions are the features most helpful in differentiation from carcinoma. However, if a dominant mass is present, the diagnosis of cancer should be assumed until disproved by biopsy.

Differential Diagnosis

Pain, fluctuation in size, and multiplicity of lesions help to differentiate these lesions from carcinoma and adenofibroma. Final diagnosis often depends on biopsy. Mammography may be helpful, but the breast tissue in these young women is usually too radiodense to permit a worthwhile study. Sonography is useful in differentiating a cystic from a solid mass.

Treatment

Because mammary dysplasia is frequently indistinguishable from carcinoma on the basis of clinical findings, it is advisable to perform biopsy examination of suspicious lesions, which is usually done under local anesthesia. Surgery should be conservative, since the primary objective is to exclude cancer. Simple mastectomy or extensive removal of breast tissue is rarely, if ever, indicated for mammary dysplasia.

When the diagnosis of mammary dysplasia has been established by previous biopsy or is practically certain, because the history is classic, aspiration of a discrete mass suggestive of a cyst is indicated. The skin and overlying tissues are anesthetized by infiltration with 1% procaine, and a 21-gauge needle is introduced. If a cyst is present, typical watery fluid (straw-colored, gray, greenish, brown, or black) is evacuated and the mass disappears. The patient is reexamined at intervals thereafter. If no fluid is obtained, or if fluid is bloody, if a mass persists after aspiration, or if at any time during follow-up a persistent lump is noted, biopsy should be performed.

Breast pain associated with generalized mammary dysplasia is best treated by avoiding trauma and by wearing (night and day) a brassiere that gives good support and protection. Hormone therapy is not advisable, because it does not cure the condition and has undesirable side effects. Recently, danazol, a synthetic androgen, has been used for patients with severe pain. This treatment suppresses pituitary gonadotropins and should be reserved for the unusual, severe case.

The role of caffeine consumption in the etiology and treatment of fibrocystic disease is controversial. Some studies suggest that eliminating caffeine from the diet is associated with improvement. Many patients are aware of these studies and report relief of symptoms after giving up coffee, tea, and chocolate. However, the observations must be confirmed.

Prognosis

Exacerbations of pain, tenderness, and cyst formation may occur at any time until the menopause, when symptoms subside. The patient should be advised to examine her own breasts each month just after menstruation and to inform her physician if a mass appears. The risk of breast cancer in women with mammary dysplasia is slightly higher than that of women in general. Follow-up examinations at regular intervals should therefore be arranged.

Ernster VL et al: Effects of caffeine-free diet on benign breast disease: A randomized trial. *Surgery* 1982;**91**:263.

Hutchinson WB et al: Risk of breast cancer in women with benign breast disease. *J Natl Cancer Inst* 1980;**65**:13.

Leis HP Jr et al: Fibrocystic breast disease. *The Female Patient* (May) 1983;**8**:56.

Livolsi VA et al: Fibrocystic breast disease in oral-contraceptive users: A histopathological evaluation of epithelial atypia. *N Engl J Med* 1978;**299**:381.

Marshall J, Graham S, Swanson M: Caffeine consumption and benign breast disease: A case control comparison. *Am J Public Health* 1982;**72**:610.

Minton JP et al: Response of fibrocystic disease to caffeine withdrawal and correlation of cyclic nucleotides with breast disease. *Am J Obstet Gynecol* 1979;**135**:157.

Moskowitz M et al: Proliferative disorders of the breast as risk factors for breast cancer in a self-selected screened population: Pathologic markers. *Radiology* 1980;**134**:289.

Oluwole SF, Freeman HP: Analysis of benign breast lesions in blacks. *Am J Surg* 1979;**137**:786.

FIBROADENOMA OF THE BREAST

This common benign neoplasm occurs most frequently in young women, usually within 20 years after puberty. It is somewhat more frequent and tends to occur at an earlier age in black than in white women. Multiple tumors in one or both breasts are found in 10–15% of patients.

The typical fibroadenoma is a round, firm, discrete, relatively movable, nontender mass 1–5 cm in diameter. The tumor is usually discovered accidentally. Clinical diagnosis in young patients is generally not difficult. In women over 30, cystic disease of the breast and carcinoma of the breast must be considered. Cysts can be identified by aspiration. Fibroadenoma does not normally occur after the menopause, but postmenopausal women may occasionally develop fibroadenoma after administration of estrogenic hormone.

Treatment is by excision under local anesthesia as an outpatient procedure, with pathologic examination of the specimen.

Cystosarcoma phyllodes is a type of fibroadenoma with cellular stroma that tends to grow rapidly. This tumor may reach a large size and if inadequately excised will recur locally. The lesion is rarely malignant. Treatment is by local excision of the mass with a margin of surrounding breast tissue. The treatment of malignant cystosarcoma phyllodes is more controversial. In general, complete removal of the tumor and a rim of normal tissue should avoid recurrence. Since these tumors tend to be large, simple mastectomy is often necessary to achieve complete control.

Al-Jurf A, Hawk WA, Crile G Jr: Cystosarcoma phyllodes. *Surg Gynecol Obstet* 1978;**146**:358.

Andersson A, Bergdahl L: Cystosarcoma phyllodes in young women. *Arch Surg* 1978;**113**:742.

Browder W, McQuitty JT, McDonald JC: Malignant cystosarcoma phylloides: Treatment and prognosis. *Am J Surg* 1978;**136**:239.

Pietruszka M, Barnes L: Cystosarcoma phyllodes: A clinicopathologic analysis of 42 cases. *Cancer* 1978;**41**:1974.

Rao BR et al: Most cystosarcoma phyllodes and fibroadenomas have progesterone receptor but lack estrogen receptor. *Cancer* 1981;**47**:2016.

DIFFERENTIAL DIAGNOSIS OF NIPPLE DISCHARGE

In order of increasing frequency, the following are the commonest causes of nipple discharge in the nonlactating breast: carcinoma, intraductal papilloma, mammary dysplasia with ectasia of the ducts. The important characteristics of the discharge and some other factors to be evaluated by history and physical examination are as follows:

(1) Nature of discharge (serous, bloody, or other).

(2) Association with a mass or not.

(3) Unilateral or bilateral.

(4) Single duct or multiple duct discharge.

(5) Discharge is spontaneous (persistent or intermittent) or must be expressed.

(6) Discharge produced by pressure at a single site or by general pressure on the breast.

(7) Relation to menses.

(8) Premenopausal or postmenopausal.

(9) Patient taking contraceptive pills, or estrogen for postmenopausal symptoms.

Unilateral, spontaneous serous or serosanguineous discharge from a single duct is usually caused by an intraductal papilloma or, rarely, by an intraductal cancer. In either case, a mass may not be present. The involved duct may be identified by pressure at different sites around the nipple at the margin of the areola. Bloody discharge is more suggestive of cancer but is usually caused by a benign papilloma in the duct. Cytologic examination of the discharge should be accomplished and may identify malignant cells, but negative findings do not rule out cancer, which is more likely in women over 50. In any case, the involved duct, and a mass if present, should be excised by meticulous technique through a circumareolar incision.

In premenopausal females, spontaneous multiple duct discharge, unilateral or bilateral, most marked just before menstruation, is often due to mammary dysplasia. Discharge may be green or brownish. Papillomatosis and ductal ectasia are also diagnostic possibilities. Biopsy may be necessary to establish the diagnosis of a diffuse nonmalignant process. If a mass is present, it should be removed.

Milky discharge from multiple ducts in the nonlactating breast may occur in certain syndromes (Chiari-Frommel, Argonz–Del Castillo [Forbes-Albright]), presumably as a result of increased secretion of pituitary prolactin. An endocrine workup may be indicated. Drugs of the chlorpromazine type and contraceptive pills may also cause milky discharge that ceases on discontinuance of the medication.

Oral contraceptives may cause clear, serous, or milky discharge from a single duct, but multiple duct discharge is more common. The discharge is more evident just before menstruation and disappears on stopping the medication. If it does not and is from a single duct, exploration should be considered.

Purulent discharge may originate in a subareolar abscess and require excision of the abscess and related lactiferous sinus.

When localization is not possible and no mass is palpable, the patient should be reexamined every week for 1 month. When unilateral discharge persists, even without definite localization or tumor, exploration must be considered. The alternative is careful follow-up at intervals of 1–3 months. Mammography should be done. Cytologic examination of nipple discharge for exfoliated cancer cells may be helpful in diagnosis.

Although none of the benign lesions causing nipple discharge are precancerous, they may coexist with cancer and it is not possible to distinguish them definitely from cancer on clinical grounds. Patients with carcinoma almost always have a palpable mass, but in rare instances a nipple discharge may be the only sign. For these reasons chronic unilateral nipple discharge, especially if bloody, is usually an indication for resection of the involved ducts.

FAT NECROSIS

Fat necrosis is a rare lesion of the breast but is of clinical importance, because it produces a mass, often accompanied by skin or nipple retraction, that is indistinguishable from carcinoma. Trauma is presumed to be the cause, although only about half of patients give a history of injury to the breast. Ecchymosis is occasionally seen near the tumor. Tenderness may or may not be present. If untreated, the mass associated with fat necrosis gradually disappears. As a rule, the safest course is to obtain a biopsy. The entire mass should be excised, primarily to rule out carcinoma. Fat necrosis is common after segmental resection and radiation therapy.

BREAST ABSCESS

During nursing, an area of redness, tenderness, and induration not infrequently develops in the breast. In the early stages, the infection can often be reversed while continuing nursing with that breast and administering an antibiotic. If the lesion progresses to form a localized mass with local and systemic signs of infection, an abscess is present and should be drained, and nursing should be discontinued.

A subareolar abscess may develop (rarely) in young or middle-aged women who are not lactating. These infections tend to recur after incision and drainage unless the area is explored in a quiescent interval with excision of the involved lactiferous duct or ducts at the base of the nipple. Except for the subareolar type of abscess, infection in the breast is very rare unless the patient is lactating. Therefore, findings suggestive of abscess in the nonlactating breast require incision and biopsy of any indurated tissue.

GYNECOMASTIA

Hypertrophy of the male breast may result from a variety of causes. Pubertal hypertrophy is very common during adolescence and is characterized by a tender discoid enlargement 2–3 cm in diameter beneath the areola with hypertrophy of the breast. The changes are usually bilateral and subside spontaneously within a year in the majority of cases.

There is a moderately increased incidence of breast hypertrophy in men past the age of 65, particularly when there is associated weight gain.

Certain organic diseases may be associated with gynecomastia, eg, cirrhosis of the liver, hyperthyroidism, Addison's disease, testicular tumors (especially choriocarcinoma), hypogonadism (eg, Klinefelter's syndrome), feminizing adrenal tumors, testicular tumors, and hepatomas. Gynecomastia may be observed in individuals who recover weight rapidly after prolonged illness or undernutrition.

Many drugs may cause gynecomastia, including estrogens, androgens, human chorionic gonadotropin, antihypertensive agents (reserpine, spironolactone, methyldopa), digitalis, cimetidine, isoniazid, phenothiazines, diazepam, tricyclic antidepressants, amphetamines, and antineoplastic drugs.

If there is uncertainty about the diagnosis of the breast lesion, a biopsy should be done to rule out cancer. Otherwise, the treatment of gynecomastia is nonsurgical unless the patient insists on excision for cosmetic reasons.

Carlson HE: Gynecomastia. *N Engl J Med* 1980;**303**:795.
Teimourian B, Perlman R: Surgery for gynecomastia. *Aesthetic Plast Surg* 1983;**7**:155.
Trump DL, Pavy MD, Staal S: Gynecomastia in men following antineoplastic therapy. *Arch Intern Med* 1982;**142**:511.

PUERPERAL MASTITIS

Postpartum mastitis occurs sporadically in nursing mothers shortly after they return home, or it may occur in epidemic form in the hospital. Hemolytic *Staphylococcus aureus* is usually the causative agent. Inflammation is generally unilateral, and primiparas are more often affected.

In sporadic puerperal mastitis, an acute interlobar inflammation with fever, localized pain, tenderness, and segmental erythema develops via a fissured nipple. The sepsis is in neither the acinar nor the duct system, and the milk is not affected. Hence, the baby should be allowed to nurse (with a nipple shield) to prevent engorgement, which contributes to abscess formation.

Antibiotic therapy against possible penicillinase-resistant organisms (oxacillin, cephalothin, or equivalent) should be given.

In epidemic puerperal mastitis, the infection often can be traced to a carrier. The baby may acquire the pathogen orally from the mother's skin or from someone in the nursery. Epidemic puerperal mastitis is more fulminating than the sporadic type, and infection seems to follow regurgitation of small amounts of milk back into the nipple duct. Thus, the baby harbors the infective organism, which should match bacteria cultured from the milk. Prompt weaning, antibiotic therapy (as above), suppression of lactation, cold packs to the breast, and a snug brassiere to support the breasts are recommended.

If the mother begins antibiotic therapy before suppuration begins, infection can usually be controlled in 24 hours. If delay is permitted, breast abscess often results. Incision and drainage are required for abscess formation. Despite puerperal mastitis of either type, the baby usually thrives without prophylactic antimicrobial therapy.

Prevention consists of proper initial nursing procedure and breast hygiene.

Mahendranath D et al: Study of mastitis with special reference to antibiotic sensitivity. *Indian J Microbiol* 1976;**16**:116.
Niebyl JR, Spence MR, Parmley TH: Sporadic (nonepidemic) puerperal mastitis. *J Reprod Med* 1978;**20**:97.
Thomsen AC, Hansen B, Moller BR: Leukocyte counts and microbiologic cultivation in the diagnosis of puerperal mastitis. *Am J Obstet Gynecol* 1983;**146**:938.

● ● ●

References

Bassett L: *Mammography, Thermography, and Ultrasound in Breast Cancer Detection.* Grune & Stratton, 1982.
Donegan WL, Spratt JS: *Cancer of the Breast,* 2nd ed. Saunders, 1979.
Gallager HS et al (editors): *The Breast.* Mosby, 1978.
Haagensen CD, Bodian C, Haagensen DE Jr: *Breast Carcinoma: Risk and Detection.* Saunders, 1981.
Harris JR, Hellman S, Silen WP (editors): *Conservative Management of Breast Cancer.* Lippincott, 1983.

Gynecology & Obstetrics | 13

Ralph C. Benson, MD, Sadja Greenwood, MD, MPH,
& Alan J. Margolis, MD

GYNECOLOGY

ABNORMAL PREMENOPAUSAL BLEEDING

Abnormal uterine bleeding means either (1) excessive or prolonged bleeding during the normal time of flow (hypermenorrhea, menorrhagia) or (2) any bleeding during the intermenstrual interval (metrorrhagia).

Patterns of Abnormal Uterine Bleeding
Abnormal uterine bleeding usually conforms to one of several distinct patterns.

A. Hypermenorrhea (Menorrhagia): Hypermenorrhea is cyclic menstrual bleeding that is excessive in amount. The cycle may or may not be of normal length.

B. Hypomenorrhea: Hypomenorrhea is an abnormally small amount of menstrual flow. The bleeding may be so slight that it is called "spotting."

C. Polymenorrhea: Polymenorrhea is menstrual-like episodes of bleeding that occur less than 21 days apart. The bleeding may or may not be abnormal in amount.

D. Oligomenorrhea: Oligomenorrhea is menstrual-like episodes of bleeding more than 35 days apart. When the interval is longer than 6 months, the patient is considered to have amenorrhea.

E. Metrorrhagia: Metrorrhagia is uterine bleeding at any time between menstrual periods that are essentially normal in frequency and flow. The bleeding may range from slight spotting to hemorrhagic flow. Metrorrhagia is a common early symptom of uterine cancer, especially endometrial carcinoma, which must be ruled out. Cervical erosions and polyps are characteristically associated with postcoital spotting from the trauma of coitus. "Ovulation bleeding," a single episode of spotting between menses, is quite common.

F. Menometrorrhagia: Menometrorrhagia is uterine bleeding that is totally irregular in frequency and duration of episodes and excessive in amount. Bleeding from any of the conditions that cause metrorrhagia may develop into menometrorrhagia.

Clinical Findings
A. Symptoms and Signs: The diagnosis of the disorders underlying the bleeding usually depends upon (1) a careful description of the duration and amount of flow, related pain, and relationship to the last menstrual period (LMP); (2) a past history of pertinent illnesses; (3) a history of all medications the patient has taken in the past month, so that possible inhibition of ovulation or endometrial stimulation can be assessed; and (4) a careful pelvic examination to look for pregnancy, uterine myomas, adnexal masses, infection, or evidence of endometriosis.

B. Laboratory Studies: Cervical smears should be obtained as needed for cytologic and culture studies. Blood studies should include measurements of hemoglobin or hematocrit, white blood cell count and differential, and sedimentation rate. A test for pregnancy and studies of thyroid function and blood clotting should be considered in the clinical evaluation.

C. Ultrasound Studies: Pelvic ultrasound may be useful to diagnose intrauterine or ectopic pregnancy, uterine myomas, endometriosis, adnexal masses, or other factors related to abnormal uterine bleeding.

D. Cervical Biopsy and Endometrial Curettage: Biopsy, curettage, or aspiration of the endometrium and curettage of the endocervix are often necessary to diagnose the cause of bleeding. Polyps, tumors, and submucous myomas are commonly identified in this way. Obtain cultures for acid-fast bacilli if tuberculosis is suspected. If cancer of the cervix is a possibility, multiple quadrant biopsies (colposcopically directed if possible) and endocervical curettage are indicated as first steps.

Treatment
A. Emergency Measures: For acute blood loss, employ the shock position and give sedation, intravenous fluids, and blood tranfusions when necessary. Hemostasis may require surgical D&C. Definitive treatment of these patients depends on the underlying cause.

B. Management of Dysfunctional Uterine Bleeding: Premenopausal patients with abnormal uterine bleeding include those with early abortion, salpingitis, myomas, or pelvic neoplasms. The history, physical examination, and laboratory findings should identify such patients, who require definitive therapy depending upon the cause of the bleeding. A large group of patients without discernible causes of bleeding remains, most of whom have dysfunctional uterine bleeding.

Dysfunctional uterine bleeding is usually caused by overgrowth of endometrium due to estrogen stimulation without adequate progesterone to stabilize growth; this occurs in anovular cycles. Anovulation associated with high estrogen levels commonly occurs in teenagers, in women aged late 30s to late 40s, and in extremely obese women or those with polycystic ovaries. The use of synthetic estrogen without added progestin is another common cause. Prolonged low levels of unopposed estrogen can cause spotting; high levels can result in profuse or prolonged bleeding.

Such bleeding can usually be treated hormonally; progestins, which limit and stabilize endometrial growth, are generally effective. Routine D&C is usually not necessary. Medroxyprogesterone acetate, 10 mg/d, or norethindrone acetate, 5 mg/d, should be given for 10–14 days starting on day 15 of the ovarian cycle, following which withdrawal bleeding (so-called medical curettage) will occur. The treatment is repeated for several cycles; it can be reinstituted if amenorrhea or dysfunctional bleeding later recurs. Alternatively in young women, oral contraceptives can be given 4 times daily for 5–7 days; after withdrawal bleeding occurs, pills are taken in the usual dosage for 3 cycles.

If the abnormal bleeding is not controlled by hormonal treatment, a D&C is necessary to check for incomplete abortion, polyps, submucous myomas, or endometrial cancer. In women over age 35 with severe or persistent dysfunctional bleeding, a D&C or careful endometrial biopsy is generally indicated to rule out neoplasm before beginning hormonal therapy.

Use of iron supplements, investigation of clotting disorders, and evaluation of the causes of anovulation should be considered as appropriate.

Nonsteroidal anti-inflammatory drugs (ibuprofen, naproxen, mefenamic acid, etc) will often reduce blood loss in menorrhagia, even that associated with an IUD.

Prolonged use of a progestin, as in a minipill, in injectable contraceptives, or in the therapy of endometriosis, can also lead to intermittent bleeding, sometimes severe. In this instance, the endometrium is atrophic and fragile. If bleeding occurs, it should be treated with estrogen as follows: ethinyl estradiol, 20 μg, or conjugated estrogens, 1.25 mg/d for 7 days. In cases of heavy bleeding, intravenous conjugated estrogens, 25 mg every 4 hours for 3–4 doses, can be used, followed by oral estrogen for 1 week or a combination oral contraceptive. This will thicken the endometrium and control the bleeding.

It is useful for the patient and the physician to discuss stressful situations or life-styles that may contribute to anovulation and dysfunctional bleeding, such as prolonged emotional turmoil or excessive use of drugs or alcohol.

C. Use of Thyroid Hormone: Hypermenorrhea or metrorrhagia is often noted in hypothyroidism. Oligomenorrhea or amenorrhea accompanies hyperthyroidism if the periods are altered. Thyroid hormone will improve menstrual function if a deficiency in thyroid hormone production is the only problem. It should not be used for all patients with abnormal menstrual periods.

Prognosis

In the absence of cancer, large tumors, and salpingitis, about 50% of patients with hypermenorrhea will resume normal menstrual periods after curettage alone. The prognosis is even better with the program of hormone therapy described above.

Claessens EA, Cowell CA: Acute adolescent menorrhagia. *Am J Obstet Gynecol* 1981;**139**:277.

Fraser IS et al: Efficacy of mefenamic acid in patients with a complaint of menorrhagia. *Obstet Gynecol* 1981;**58**:543.

POSTMENOPAUSAL VAGINAL BLEEDING

Vaginal bleeding that occurs 6 months or more following cessation of menstrual function may be due to local or systemic causes. Carcinoma of the cervix or endometrium accounts for 35–50% of cases. Administration of estrogens in a noncyclic manner or without added progestin is the second most important cause. Other causes include atrophic vaginitis, trauma, polyps, hypertensive cardiovascular disease, submucous myomas, trophic ulcers of the cervix associated with prolapse of the uterus, blood dyscrasias, and endogenous estrogen production by a feminizing ovarian tumor. Uterine bleeding is usually painless, but pain will be present if the cervix is stenotic, if bleeding is severe and rapid, or if infection or torsion or extrusion of a tumor is present. The patient may report a single episode of spotting or profuse bleeding for days or months.

Diagnosis

The vulva and vagina should be carefully inspected for areas of bleeding, ulcers, or neoplasms. A cytologic smear of the cervix and vaginal pool should be taken; this may disclose exfoliated neoplastic cells. An unstained wet mount of vaginal fluid in saline and potassium hydroxide may reveal white blood cells, infective organisms, or free basal epithelial cells indicative of a low estrogen effect. Endocervical curettage and aspiration curettage of the endometrium should be performed next. These procedures often can be performed in the office with sedation and a paracervical block. A careful search for endometrial polyps should be made. The tissue obtained may reveal polyps, endometrial hyperplasia (with or without an atypical glandular pattern), or cancer.

Treatment

Aspiration curettage (with polypectomy if indicated) will frequently be curative. If simple endometrial hyperplasia is found, give cyclic progestin therapy (medroxyprogesterone acetate, 10 mg/d, or norethindrone acetate, 5 mg/d) for 21 days of each month for 3 months. A repeat D&C can then be performed, and if tissues are normal and estrogen replacement therapy is reinstituted, a progestin should be prescribed (as above) for the last 10–14 days of each estrogen cycle, followed by 5 days with no hormone therapy, so that the uterine lining will be shed. If endometrial hyperplasia with atypical cells or carcinoma of the endometrium is found, hysterectomy is necessary.

Gambrell RD, Bagnell CA, Greenblatt RB: Role of estrogens and progesterone in the etiology and prevention of endometrial cancer: Review. *Am J Obstet Gynecol* 1983;**146:**696.

Grimes DA: Diagnostic dilation and curettage: A reappraisal. *Am J Obstet Gynecol* 1982;**142:**1.

Merrill JA: Management of postmenopausal bleeding. *Clin Obstet Gynecol* 1981;**24:**285.

TOXIC SHOCK SYNDROME

Toxic shock syndrome has occurred in menstruating women using tampons (90% of cases) and occasionally in women with a retained vaginal foreign object (eg, contraceptive diaphragm or sponge), in postpartum or female postsurgical patients, in children, and in men with infected wounds. The disease is most common in women under age 30; it is possible that immunity may develop with older age. The disease may recur during subsequent menses. The probable cause is an exotoxin from certain strains of *Staphylococcus aureus* that enters the bloodstream through vaginal ulcerations produced by tampons or other foreign bodies.

Toxic shock syndrome is a severe multisystem illness with fever, hypotension, diffuse erythroderma, and desquamation of the palms and soles. Intravenous fluids should be given immediately to maintain blood pressure and perfusion of vital organs. Tampons or other vaginal foreign bodies should be removed. Cultures should be made of tissues from focal lesions, tissues of all mucous membranes, and blood samples. A β-lactamase–resistant antibiotic (nafcillin or an appropriate cephalosporin) is specific treatment. Corticosteroids, renal dialysis, mechanical ventilation, and other intensive care treatments may be necessary. (See also Chapter 22.)

Recommendations to women to reduce the risk of toxic shock syndrome might include the following: (1) Avoid using tampons completely, or avoid using them continuously by alternating with menstrual pads. Avoid using tampons overnight. (2) If high fever, vomiting, diarrhea, or other symptoms develop during a menstrual period, stop using tampons. Seek immediate medical care. (3) Women who have had toxic shock syndrome should not use tampons. (4) A contraceptive diaphragm, cap, or sponge should not be left in the vagina for more than 12–18 hours. These devices should not be used during a menstrual period.

Since 1977, many brands of tampons have been made with high-absorbency synthetic compounds (carboxymethylcellulose, polyester, polyacrylates, viscose rayon), which are believed to enhance the risk of toxic shock syndrome by encouraging the growth of *S aureus* and producing vaginal microulcerations. A return to use of cotton or cotton and rayon fibers by tampon manufacturers is being urged by medical and consumer groups.

Wager GP: Toxic shock syndrome: A review. *Am J Obstet Gynecol* 1983;**146:**93.

PREMENSTRUAL SYNDROME
(Premenstrual Tension)

The premenstrual syndrome is a recurrent, variable cluster of troublesome, ill-defined symptoms and signs that develop during the 7–14 days before the onset of menses and subside when menstruation occurs. The syndrome affects about one-third of all premenopausal women, primarily those 25–40 years of age. In about 10% of these, the syndrome may be severe. Although not every woman experiences all the symptoms or signs at one time, many complain of decreased energy; tension; irritability; hostility; depression; behavorial changes; headache; altered libido; mastalgia; backache; and swelling of the abdomen, fingers, and ankles. Patients may also describe increased craving for certain foods. Confusing reports of the spectrum of manifestations have been presented by the media.

The pathogenesis of premenstrual syndrome is still uncertain. Theories include neuroendocrine changes, elevated or lowered levels of estrogen or progesterone, fluid retention, reactive hypoglycemia, and vitamin deficiencies.

It is obvious that further investigation and well-controlled therapeutic studies of this heterogeneous syndrome will be necessary for rational treatment. Current treatment methods are mainly empiric. The physician should provide the best support possible for the patient's emotional and physical distress. This includes the following:

(1) Careful evaluation of the patient, with understanding, explanation, and reassurance, is of first importance.

(2) Advise the patient to keep a daily dairy of all symptoms for 2–3 months, to help in evaluating the timing and characteristics of the syndrome. Psychotherapy may be helpful for some women or couples.

(3) Daily exercise and a diet emphasizing complex carbohydrates (whole grains, vegetables, and fruits) are important. Foods high in sugar content and alcohol should be avoided to minimize reactive hypoglycemia. Salt intake should be restricted to reduce fluid retention. Use of caffeine should be minimized whenever tension and irritability predominate.

(4) Pyridoxine, 100–200 mg/d orally for 2 weeks

before each menstrual period, is said to be helpful by some. Larger doses should be avoided because of possible neurotoxicity.

(5) Natural progesterone, 200–400 mg in rectal or vaginal suppositories daily for 10–14 days before the menstrual period, has been widely heralded to be of therapeutic value. These suppositories must be made up from natural progesterone powder by the pharmacist and are not widely available.

Abplanalp JM: Psychologic components of the premenstrual syndrome: Evaluating the research and choosing the treatment. *J Reprod Med* 1983;**28**:517.

Speroff L: PMS: Looking for new answers to an old problem. *Contemp Obstet Gynecol* (Aug) 1983;**22**:102.

Woods NF, Most A, Dery GK: Prevalence of perimenstrual symptoms. *Am J Public Health* 1982;**72**:1257.

DYSMENORRHEA

1. PRIMARY DYSMENORRHEA
(Spastic Dysmenorrhea)

Primary dysmenorrhea is menstrual pain associated with ovular cycles in the absence of pathologic findings. The pain usually begins within 1–2 years after the menarche and may become more severe with time. The frequency of cases increases up to age 20 and then decreases with age and markedly with parity. Thirty to fifty percent of women are affected at some time, and 5–10% have severe pain.

Primary dysmenorrhea is low, midline, wavelike, cramping pelvic pain often radiating to the back or upper thighs. Cramps may last for 1 or more days and may be associated with nausea, syncope, diarrhea, headache, and flushing. The pain is produced by uterine vasoconstriction, anoxia, and sustained contractions mediated by prostaglandins.

Clinical Findings

The pelvic examination is normal between menses; examination during menses may produce more severe pain, but no pathologic findings are seen.

Treatment

Nonsteroidal anti-inflammatory drugs (ibuprofen, mefenamic acid, naproxen) are generally helpful. Give at the onset of bleeding to avoid inadvertent drug use during early pregnancy. Ovulation can be suppressed and dysmenorrhea usually prevented by oral contraceptives. Women with less severe dysmenorrhea often get relief with aspirin, acetaminophen, or other over-the-counter analgesics. Some patients do not respond to any of these measures and require codeine for pain relief. Acupuncture has been reported to be helpful by some investigators.

Dawood MY: Dysmenorrhoea and prostaglandins: Pharmacological and therapeutic considerations. *Drugs* 1981;**22**:42.

Hanson FW: Naproxen sodium, ibuprofen and a placebo in dysmenorrhea. *J Reprod Med* 1982;**27**:423.

2. SECONDARY DYSMENORRHEA

Secondary dysmenorrhea is menstrual pain for which an organic cause exists. It usually begins well after menarche, sometimes even as late as the third or fourth decade of life.

Clinical Findings

The history and physical examination commonly suggest endometriosis or pelvic inflammatory disease. Other causes may be submucous myoma, IUD use, cervical stenosis with obstruction, or blind uterine horn (rare).

Diagnosis

Laparoscopy is often needed to differentiate endometriosis from pelvic inflammatory disease. Submucous myomas can be detected by passing a sound or curet over the uterine cavity during D&C or by hysterogram or hysteroscopy. Cervical stenosis may result from induced abortion, creating crampy pain at the time of expected menses with no blood flow; this is easily cured by passing a sound into the uterine cavity after administering a paracervical block.

Treatment

A. Specific Measures: Periodic use of analgesics, including the nonsteroidal anti-inflammatory drugs given for primary dysmennorrhea, may be beneficial, and oral contraceptives may give relief, particularly in endometriosis and chronic salpingitis. Danazol is effective in the treatment of endometriosis (see p 461).

B. Surgical Measures: If disability is marked or prolonged, laparoscopy or exploratory laparotomy is usually warranted. Definitive surgery depends upon the degree of disability and the findings at operation.

VAGINITIS

Inflammation and infection of the vagina are common gynecologic problems, resulting from a variety of pathogens, allergic reactions to vaginal contraceptives or other products, or the friction of coitus. The normal vaginal pH is less than 4.5, and *Lactobacillus* is the predominant organism. At the time of the midcycle estrogen surge, clear, elastic, mucoid secretions from the cervical os are often profuse. In the luteal phase and during pregnancy, vaginal secretions are thicker, white, and sometimes adherent to the vaginal walls. These normal secretions can be confused with vaginitis.

Clinical Findings

When the patient complains of vaginal irritation, pain, or unusual discharge, a careful history should be taken, noting the onset of the menstrual period; recent sexual activity; use of contraceptives, tampons, or douches; and the presence of vaginal burning, pain, pruritus, or unusually profuse or malodorous discharge. The physical examination should include careful inspection of the vulva and speculum examination of the vagina and cervix. The cervix should be cultured for gonorrhea or *Chlamydia* if applicable (see pp 878 and 881). The vagina should be cultured for *S aureus* if toxic shock syndrome is suspected (see p 453) or for *Candida* if yeast forms are not demonstrated by wet mount but are strongly suspected. A specimen of vaginal discharge should be examined under the microscope in a drop of saline solution to look for trichomonads, bacteria, white blood cells, and clue cells (stippled or granulated epithelial cells covered with bacteria; see *Gardnerella* below). Discharge from the vaginal walls should be examined in a drop of 10–20% potassium hydroxide to look for *Candida*. The vaginal pH can be tested; it is frequently greater than 4.5 in infections due to trichomonads, *Gardnerella,* or other anaerobes. A bimanual examination to look for evidence of pelvic infection should follow.

A. Candida albicans: Pregnancy, diabetes, and use of antibiotics predispose to *Candida* infections. Heat, moisture, and occlusive clothing also contribute to the risk. Pruritus, vulvovaginal erythema, and a white curdlike discharge that is not malodorous are found. Microscopic examination with 10–20% potassium hydroxide reveals filaments and spores. Cultures with Nickerson's medium may be used if *Candida* is suspected but not demonstrated.

B. Trichomonas vaginalis: This protozoan flagellate infects the vagina, Skene's ducts, and lower urinary tract in women and the lower genitourinary tract in men. It is transmitted through coitus. Pruritus and a malodorous discharge occur, along with diffuse vaginal redness with edematous papillae in severe cases. Motile organisms with flagella are seen by microscopic examination of a wet mount with saline solution. The organism can sometimes be found in a first-morning specimen of urine from an infected male.

C. Gardnerella (Haemophilus) vaginalis: Infection due to these small gram-negative rods and other anaerobes is often associated with increased malodorous discharge without obvious vulvitis or vaginitis. The discharge is grayish and sometimes frothy, with a pH of 5.0–5.5. An aminelike odor is present if a drop of discharge is alkalinized with 10–20% potassium hydroxide. On wet mount in saline, no trichomonads are found; epithelial cells are covered with bacteria and appear stippled or granulated (clue cells).

D. Atrophic Vaginitis: In the absence of estrogen stimulation, the vulvar and vaginal tissues shrink in size, the vaginal walls become thin and dry, and rugal folds disappear. Tenderness and pruritus, with resulting dysuria and dyspareunia, may occur. Fissures and ulcerations of tissue with spotting or bleeding may result from coitus. The wet mount will reveal predominantly parabasal cells.

E. Condylomata Acuminata (Genital Warts): Warty growths on the vulva, perianal area, vaginal walls, or cervix are caused by the human papillomavirus. They are sexually transmitted. Pregnancy and immunosuppression favor growth. Cervical lesions may be visible only by colposcopy and are believed to be related to dysplasia and cervical cancer.

Treatment

A. Candida albicans: Treatment with clotrimazole or miconazole nightly for 1 week is generally effective; nystatin suppositories, gentian violet solution (1–2%), or boric acid capsules (600 mg twice daily) have also been successful. In recurrent cases, prophylaxis may be attempted with use of these fungicides twice weekly or with oral nystatin, 500,000 units 3 times daily for 3 weeks. The sexual partner may be treated with fungicidal creams.

B. Trichomonas vaginalis: Treatment of both partners simultaneously is necessary; metronidazole, 2 g for 1 day (8 tablets at once or 4 tablets in 2 doses) or 250 mg 3 times daily for 7 days, is usually used. Higher doses may be necessary in resistant cases. Metronidazole should be avoided in the first trimester of pregnancy. Patients who refuse metronidazole (see p 897) may obtain relief with daily douches containing 4 tablespoons of vinegar and 2 drops of detergent shampoo in 1 quart of water. The male partner should use a condom during sexual intercourse. Clotrimazole vaginal cream is also said to be useful.

C. Gardnerella (Haemophilus) vaginalis: Treatment of both sexual partners with metronidazole, 500 mg twice daily for 7 days, is effective. However, the wisdom of using a potentially toxic drug for a mild condition that may need repeated treatments is questionable. Either or both of the following treatments may be used alternatively: (1) ampicillin, 500 mg 4 times a day for 7 days, or (2) douching with povidone-iodine solution (1 tablespoon per quart of water), vinegar (3–4 tablespoons per quart of water), or a milky suspension of yogurt to restore *Lactobacillus* levels, plus use of condoms by the sexual partner. The use of vaginal iodine solutions is not recommended in pregnancy.

D. Atrophic Vaginitis: Treatment consists of oral hormone replacement therapy or local applications of estrogen cream. Conjugated estrogen cream, one-eighth applicatorful (0.3 mg of conjugated estrogens), applied daily for 1 week and then every other day, will relieve most symptoms of dyspareunia with minimal systemic effects. Testosterone propionate cream 1% is helpful for individuals unable to use estrogen. For symptomatic relief, this treatment must be maintained indefinitely.

E. Condylomata Acuminata: Both partners should be treated for warts anywhere on their bodies. Treatment for small vulvar warts is with podophyllum resin 20% in tincture of benzoin (do not use during pregnancy or on bleeding lesions) or trichloroacetic acid, carefully applied to avoid the surrounding skin. Podophyllum resin must be washed off after 2–4 hours. Freezing with liquid nitrogen is also effective. Treatment of large warts (> 2 cm) and vaginal warts is with electrodesiccation and curettage of the base, following local or general anesthesia. In all cases, treat any other vaginal infections and sexually transmitted diseases.

Lossick JG: *Gardnerella vaginalis* –associated leukorrhoea: The disease and its treatment. *Rev Infect Dis* 1982;**4**:S793.

Muller M et al: Three metronidazole-resistant strains of *Trichomonas vaginalis* from the US. *Am J Obstet Gynecol* 1980;**138**:808.

Osborne NG, Grubin L, Pratson L: Vaginitis in sexually active women: Relationship to nine sexually transmitted organisms. *Am J Obstet Gynecol* 1982;**142**:962.

Whitehead MI: Dose-related changes in vaginal cytology after topical conjugated equine estrogens. *Br Med J* 1982;**284**:789.

CERVICITIS

Infection of the cervix must be distinguished from physiologic ectopy of columnar epithelium, which is common in young women. True cervicitis is characterized by a red edematous cervix with purulent, often blood-streaked discharge and tenderness on cervical motion. The infection may follow tears during delivery or abortion or may result from a sexually transmitted pathogen such as *Neisseria gonorrhoeae, Chlamydia,* or herpesvirus (which presents with vesicles and ulcers on the cervix during a primary herpetic infection).

The symptoms of cervicitis include leukorrhea, low back pain, dyspareunia, dysmenorrhea, dysuria, urinary frequency and urgency, and spotting or bleeding. Yellow mucopurulent endocervical secretions and the presence of 10 or more polymorphonuclear leukocytes per oil immersion field are suggestive of chlamydial infection.

Cultures should be taken from the cervical os, including cultures for *N gonorrhoeae* and *Chlamydia.* Appropriate antibiotics should be given to the patient (and to her partner in cases of gonorrhea or chlamydial infection). See Chapter 24 for a more detailed discussion.

Brunham RC et al: Mucopurulent cervicitis: The ignored counterpart in women of urethritis in men. *N Engl J Med* 1984;**311**:1.

Holmes KK: The *Chlamydia* epidemic. *JAMA* 1981;**245**:1718.

Rubinstein E: Colposcopic pattern of cervicitis, dysplasia and preinvasive cancer of the uterine cervix. *Acta Obstet Gynecol Scand* 1982;**61**:253.

CYST & ABSCESS OF BARTHOLIN'S DUCT

Gonorrhea and other infections often involve Bartholin's duct, causing obstruction of the gland. Drainage of secretions is prevented, leading to pain, swelling, and abscess formation. The infections usually resolve and pain disappears, but stenosis of the duct outlet with distention often persists. Reinfection causes recurrent tenderness and further enlargement of the duct.

The principal symptoms are periodic painful swelling on either side of the introitus and dys-

pareunia. Fullness in one or both of the labia and soft distortion of the introitus are apparent. A fluctuant swelling 1–4 cm in diameter in the inferior portion of either labium minus is a sign of occlusion of Bartholin's duct. Tenderness is evidence of active infection.

Treat infections with broad-spectrum antibiotics and frequent warm soaks. If an abscess develops, prompt incision and drainage is the simplest form of therapy, but the problem may recur. Marsupialization or incision and drainage with the insertion of an indwelling Word catheter will establish a new duct opening. This can be done at the time of acute enlargement of the gland and abscess formation or as an interval procedure.

Dennefors B, Bergman B: Primary carcinoma of the Bartholin gland. *Acta Obstet Gynecol Scand* 1980;**59**:95.

EFFECTS OF EXPOSURE TO DIETHYLSTILBESTROL IN UTERO

Between 1947 and 1971, diethylstilbestrol (DES) was widely used in the USA for diabetic women during pregnancy and to treat threatened abortion. It is estimated that 2–3 million fetuses were exposed. A relationship between fetal DES exposure and clear cell carcinoma of the vagina was later discovered, and a number of other related anomalies have since been noted. In one-third of all exposed women, there are changes in the vagina (adenosis, septa), cervix (deformities and hypoplasia of the vaginal portion of the cervix), or uterus (T-shaped cavity). In males exposed to DES in utero, testicular and epididymal abnormalities and an increase in oligospermia (although no carcinoma) have been reported.

At present, all exposed women are advised to have an initial colposcopic examination to outline vaginal and cervical areas of abnormal epithelium, followed by cytologic examination of the vagina (all 4 quadrants of the upper half of the vagina) and cervix at 6-month intervals. Lugol's iodine stain of the vagina and cervix will also outline areas of metaplastic squamous epithelium.

Most women are not aware of having been exposed to DES. Examiners should pay attention to structural changes of the vagina and cervix that may signal the possibility of DES exposure and indicate the need for follow-up.

The incidence of clear cell carcinoma is approximately one in 8000 exposed women. Although the frequency of cervical dysplasia is increased, there is no evidence of a larger number of squamous cell carcinomas of the cervix in these patients. These women conceive with regularity but have an increased incidence of early abortion, ectopic pregnancy, and premature births.

Fowler WC et al: Risk of cervical intraepithelial neoplasia among DES-exposed women. *Obstet Gynecol* 1981;**58**:720.

Stillman RJ: In utero exposure to diethylstilbestrol: Adverse effects on the reproductive tract and reproductive performance in male and female offspring. *Am J Obstet Gynecol* 1982; **142**:905.

CERVICAL INTRAEPITHELIAL NEOPLASIA
(CIN; Dysplasia of the Cervix)

The squamocolumnar junction of the uterine cervix represents an area of active squamous cell proliferation. In childhood, this junction is located on the exposed vaginal portion of the cervix. At puberty, because of hormonal influence and possibly because of changes in the vaginal pH, the squamous margin begins to encroach on the single-layered, mucus-secreting epithelium, creating an area of metaplasia (transformation zone). Factors associated with coitus (see Prevention, below) may lead to cellular abnormalities, which over a period of years can result in the development of squamous cell dysplasia or cancer. There are varying degrees of cervical intraepithelial dysplasia (see Table 13–1), defined by the degree of cellular atypia; all types must be observed and treated if they persist or become more severe. At present, the malignant potential of a specific lesion cannot be predicted. Some lesions remain stable for long periods of time; some regress; and others advance.

Clinical Findings

There are no specific signs or symptoms of cervical intraepithelial neoplasia. The diagnosis is made by cytologic screening of an asymptomatic population with no grossly visible cervical changes. All grossly abnormal cervical lesions should be biopsied.

Diagnosis

A. Cytologic Examination (Papanicolaou Smear): All specimens can be spread on one slide and fixed. For optimal screening, specimens should be taken from the vaginal pool, the squamocolumnar junction, and the endocervical canal.

Cytologic reports from the laboratory may describe findings in one of several ways (see Table 13–1). Vaginal infection, cervicitis, and atrophy prevent adequate screening. Repeat smear is indicated after appropriate therapy.

Table 13–1. Classification systems for Papanicolaou smears.

Classification	Dysplasia	Cervical Intraepithelial Neoplasia (CIN)
1	Benign	Benign
2	Benign with inflammation	Benign with inflammation
3	Mild dysplasia	CIN I
3	Moderate dysplasia	CIN II
3	Severe dysplasia	CIN III
4	Carcinoma in situ	CIN III
5	Invasive cancer	Invasive cancer

B. Colposcopy: Viewing the cervix with 10–20 × magnification allows for assessment of the size and margins of an abnormal transformation zone and to see whether it extends into the endocervical canal. The application of 3% acetic acid dissolves mucus, and the acid's desiccating activity sharpens the contrast between normal and actively proliferating thickened squamous epithelium. Abnormal changes include white patches and vascular atypia, which indicate areas of greatest cellular activity. Paint the cervix with Lugol's solution (strong iodine solution [Schiller's test]). Normal squamous epithelium will take the stain; nonstaining squamous epithelum should be biopsied. (The single-layered, mucus-secreting endocervical tissue will not stain either but can readily be distinguished by its darker pink, shinier appearance.)

C. Biopsy: Colposcopically directed punch biopsy and endocervical curettage are office procedures. If colposcopic examination is not performed, the normal-appearing cervix shedding atypical cells can be evaluated by endocervical curettage and multiple punch biopsies of nonstaining squamous epithelium or tissue from each quadrant of the cervix.

Microscopic examination of biopsy specimens is a more exact way of diagnosing the degree of cellular atypia suggested by the cytologic examination. Endocervical curettage will confirm the presence of abnormalities in the endocervical canal. Data from both procedures are important in deciding on treatment.

Prevention

Cervical dysplasia and cancer appear to be initiated by one or more sexually transmitted factors; human papillomavirus and herpes viruses are currently suspected. Cervical cancer almost never occurs in virginal women; it is epidemiologically related to the number of sexual partners a woman has had and the number of other female partners a male partner has had. Use of the contractive diaphragm or condom has been associated with a protective effect. Long-term oral contraceptive users develop more dysplasias and cancers of the cervix than users of other forms of birth control, and smokers are also more at risk. Preventive measures therefore include the following:

(1) Sexually active women should undergo regular cytologic screening to detect abnormalities.

(2) Women should limit the number of sexual partners.

(3) Use of a contraceptive diaphragm by the woman or condom by the man will protect the cervix.

(4) Women should stop smoking.

(5) If a cytologic abnormality is found, the woman should stop using oral contraceptives or other contraceptive methods that leave the cervix exposed and should use a diaphragm or ask her male partner to use a condom.

(6) Prompt treatment of genital warts is advisable for men and women.

Treatment

Treatment varies depending on the degree and

extent of cervical intraepithelial neoplasia. Biopsies should always precede treatment.

A. Cauterization or Cryosurgery: The use of either cauterization or freezing (cryosurgery) is effective for noninvasive small visible lesions without endocervical extension.

B. CO$_2$ Laser: This well-controlled method minimizes tissue destruction. It is colposcopically directed and requires special training. It may be used with large visible lesions.

C. Conization of the Cervix: Conization allows for complete histopathologic assessment and generally results in excision of the lesion. It should be reserved for cases of severe dysplasia or cancer in situ (CIN III), particularly those with endocervical extension.

D. Follow-Up: Because recurrence is possible, especially in the first 2 years after treatment, close follow-up is imperative. Repeat vaginal cytologic examinations at 6-month intervals. After 2 years, yearly examinations suffice.

Skegg DCG et al: Importance of the male factor in cancer of the cervix. *Lancet* 1982;**2**:581.

Trevathan E et al: Cigarette smoking and dysplasia and carcinoma in situ of the uterine cervix. *JAMA* 1983;**250**:499.

CARCINOMA OF THE UTERINE CERVIX

Essentials of Diagnosis

- Abnormal uterine bleeding and vaginal discharge.
- Cervical lesion may be visible on inspection as a tumor or ulceration.
- Vaginal cytology usually positive; must be confirmed by biopsy.

General Considerations

Cancer appears first in the intraepithelial layers (the preinvasive stage, or carcinoma in situ). Preinvasive cancer is a common diagnosis in women 30–40 years of age, but most patients with invasive carcinoma are 40–50 years old. Five to 10 years are usually required for carcinoma to penetrate the basement membrane and invade the tissues. After invasion, death usually occurs in 3–5 years in untreated or unresponsive patients.

Invasion is associated with ulceration and spotting. Sanguineous vaginal discharge or abnormal bleeding does not occur until the cancer has penetrated into the substance of the cervix.

Clinical Findings

A. Symptoms and Signs: The most common signs are metrorrhagia, postcoital spotting, and cervical ulceration. Sanguineous or purulent, odorous, nonpruritic discharge appears after invasion. Bladder and rectal dysfunction or fistulas and pain are late symptoms. Anemia, anorexia, and weight loss are signs of advanced disease.

B. Cervical Biopsy and Endocervical Curettage, or Cold Conization: These procedures are necessary steps after a positive Papanicolaou smear to determine the extent and depth of invasion of the cancer. Even if the smear is positive, treatment is never justified until definitive diagnosis has been established through biopsy studies.

C. "Staging," or Estimate of Gross Spread of Cancer of the Cervix: The depth of penetration of the malignant cells beyond the basement membrane is a reliable clinical guide to the extent of primary cancer within the cervix and the likelihood of secondary or metastatic cancer. It is customary to stage cancers of the cervix under anesthesia as shown in Table 13–2.

D. Other Examinations: Chest x-ray and excretory urography may reveal unexpected metastases. Cystoscopy and sigmoidoscopy should be performed routinely before therapy is started.

Complications

Metastases to regional lymph nodes occur with increasing frequency from stage I to stage IV. Paracervical extension occurs in all directions from the cervix. The ureters are often obstructed lateral to the cervix,

Table 13–2. International classification of cancer of the cervix (1973).*

Preinvasive carcinoma

Stage 0	Carcinoma in situ, intraepithelial carcinoma.

Invasive carcinoma

Stage I	Carcinoma strictly confined to the cervix (extension to the corpus should be disregarded).
Ia	Microinvasive carcinoma (early stromal invasion).
Ib	See other cases of stage I. (Occult cancer should be labeled "occ.")
Stage II	Carcinoma extends beyond the cervix but has not extended onto the pelvic wall. The carcinoma involves the vagina, but not the lower third.
IIa	No obvious parametrial involvement. The vagina has been invaded, but not the lower third.
IIb	Obvious parametrial involvement.
Stage III	Carcinoma has extended onto the pelvic wall. On rectal examination, there is no cancer-free space between the tumor and the pelvic wall. The tumor involves the lower third of the vagina. All cases with hydronephrosis or nonfunctioning kidney.
IIIa	No extension onto the pelvic wall. Vaginal involvement, but not the lower third.
IIIb	Extension onto the pelvic wall and/or hydronephrosis or nonfunctioning kidney.
Stage IV	Carcinoma extended beyond the true pelvis or clinically involving the mucosa of the bladder or rectum. Do not allow a case of bullous edema as such to be allotted to stage IV.
IVa	Spread of growth to adjacent organs (that is, rectum or bladder with positive biopsy from these organs).
IVb	Spread of growth to distant organs.

*Approved by the International Federation of Gynecology and Obstetrics (FIGO). Adopted by American College of Obstetrics and Gynecology (1976).

causing hydroureter and hydronephrosis and consequently impaired kidney function. Almost two-thirds of patients with carcinoma of the cervix die of uremia when ureteral obstruction is bilateral. Pain in the back and in the distribution of the lumbosacral plexus is often indicative of neurologic involvement. Gross edema of the legs may be indicative of vascular and lymphatic stasis due to tumor.

Pelvic infections may complicate cervical carcinoma. Vaginal fistulas to the rectum and urinary tract are severe late complications. Incontinence of urine and feces is a major late complication, particularly in debilitated individuals.

Hemorrhage is the cause of death in 10–20% of patients with extensive invasive carcinoma.

Treatment

A. Emergency Measures: Vaginal hemorrhage originates from gross ulceration and cavitation in stage II–IV cervical carcinoma. Ligation and suturing of the cervix are usually not feasible, but ligation of the uterine or hypogastric arteries may be lifesaving when other measures fail. Styptics such as negatol (Negatan), Monsel's solution, or acetone are effective, although delayed sloughing may result in further bleeding. Wet vaginal packing is helpful. Irradiation usually controls bleeding.

B. Specific Measures:

1. Noninvasive carcinoma (stage 0)–In a woman over 40 with in situ carcinoma of the cervix, total hysterectomy is the surgical treatment of choice; rarely, irradiation may be used alternatively in women who are poor operative risks. In a younger woman who wishes to retain her uterus, conization of the cervix may be acceptable. This is a calculated risk and imposes the absolute necessity of cytologic examinations every 6 months for an indefinite time.

2. Invasive carcinoma–Irradiation is generally the best treatment for invasive squamous cell carcinoma or adenocarcinoma of the cervix. The objectives of irradiation are (1) the destruction of primary and secondary carcinoma within the pelvis and (2) the preservation of tissues not invaded. Gamma emissions derived from x-rays, ^{60}Co, radium, the cyclotron, the linear accelerator, and comparable sources are employed. All stages of cancer may be treated by this method, and there are fewer medical contraindications to irradiation than to radical surgery. Selected stage I cases can be treated satisfactorily with radical surgical procedures by experienced pelvic surgeons.

Prognosis

The overall 5-year arrest rate for squamous cell carcinoma or adenocarcinoma originating in the cervix is about 45% in the major clinics. Percentage arrest rates are inversely proportionate to the stage of cancer: stage 0, 99%; stage I, 77%; stage II, 65%; stage III, 25%; stage IV, about 5%.

Boyce J et al: Prognostic factors in stage I carcinoma of the cervix. *Gynecol Oncol* 1981;**12(2–Part 1)**:154.

Richart RM, Barron BA: Screening strategies for cervical cancer and cervical intraepithelial neoplasia. *Cancer* 1981;**47(5 Suppl)**:1176.

Shingleton HM et al: Adenocarcinoma of the cervix. 1. Clinical evaluation and pathologic features. *Am J Obstet Gynecol* 1981;**139**:799.

CARCINOMA OF THE ENDOMETRIUM
(Corpus or Fundal Cancer)

Adenocarcinoma of the uterine corpus is the second most common cancer of the female genital tract. It occurs most often in women 50–70 years of age. Abnormal uterine bleeding is the presenting sign in 80% of cases. A watery, serous or sanguineous, malodorous vaginal discharge is occasionally present. Pyometra or hematometra may be due to carcinoma of the endometrium. Pain occurs late in the disease, with stasis or infection.

Endocervical curettage and endometrial curettage or aspiration are the only reliable means of diagnosis. Adequate specimens can usually be obtained during an office procedure performed following local anesthesia (paracervical block) and sedation. General anesthesia may sometimes be necessary for a satisfactory examination and safe diagnostic procedure. Simultaneous hysteroscopy can be a valuable addition in order to find localized growth or polyps within the uterine cavity.

Prevention

Routine screening of all women by periodic cervical smears and prompt D&C for patients who report abnormal menstrual bleeding or postmenopausal uterine bleeding will reveal many incipient as well as clinical cases of endometrial cancer. Postmenopausal women taking estrogens or younger women taking estrogens for prolonged anovulation can be given oral progestins for 10 days at the end of each estrogen cycle in order to promote periodic shedding of the uterine lining; this has been associated with a decreased incidence of uterine adenocarcinoma.

Treatment

Treatment usually consists of total hysterectomy and bilateral salpingo-oophorectomy. Preliminary external irradiation or intracavitary radium therapy is indicated if the cancer is poorly differentiated or if the uterus is definitely enlarged in the absence of myomas. If invasion deep into the myometrium has occurred, postoperative irradiation should be considered.

Palliation of advanced or metastatic endometrial adenocarcinoma may be accomplished with large doses of progestins, eg, medroxyprogesterone, 400 mg intramuscularly weekly, or its equivalent.

Prognosis

With early diagnosis and treatment, the 5-year arrest rate is 80–85%.

Barber HPK: Uterine cancer (prevention). *Cancer* 1981;**47(5 Suppl):**1126.

Connelly PJ, Alberhasky RC, Christopherson WM: Carcinoma of the endometrium. 3. Analysis of 865 cases of adenocarcinoma and adenoacanthoma. *Obstet Gynecol* 1982;**59:**569.

CERVICAL POLYPS

Cervical polyps commonly occur after the menarche and are occasionally noted in postmenopausal women. The cause is not known, but inflammation may play an etiologic role. The principal symptoms are discharge and abnormal vaginal bleeding. The polyps are visible in the cervical os on speculum examination.

Cervical polyps must be differentiated from polypoid neoplastic disease of the endometrium, small submucous pedunculated myomas, and endometrial polyps. Cervical polyps rarely contain malignant foci.

Treatment

All cervical polyps should be removed surgically. They can often be removed in the office by avulsion. All tissue recovered should be examined by a pathologist to rule out malignant change. If the cervix is soft, patulous, or definitely dilated and the polyp is large, surgical D&C is required (especially if the pedicle is not readily visible). Exploration of the cervical and uterine cavities with the polyp forceps and curet may reveal multiple polyps.

MYOMA OF THE UTERUS
(Fibroid Tumor, Fibromyoma)

Essentials of Diagnosis

- Irregular enlargement of the uterus (may be asymptomatic).
- Hypermenorrhea, metrorrhagia, dysmenorrhea.
- Acute and recurrent pelvic pain if the tumor becomes twisted on its pedicle or infarcted.
- Symptoms due to pressure on neighboring organs (large tumors).

General Considerations

Myoma is the most common benign neoplasm of the female genital tract. It is a discrete, round, firm uterine tumor composed of smooth muscle and connective tissue. Only 2% are solitary, and several hundred have been found in one uterus. Some myomas become quite large; the largest on record weighed over 45 kg. The most convenient classification is by anatomic location: (1) intramural, (2) submucous, (3) subserous, (4) intraligamentous, (5) parasitic (ie, deriving its blood supply from an organ to which it becomes attached), and (6) cervical. A submucous myoma may become pedunculated and descend through the cervix into the vagina.

Clinical Findings

A. Symptoms and Signs: In nonpregnant women, myomas are frequently asymptomatic. How-

ever, they can cause urinary frequency, dysmenorrhea, menometrorrhagia (often with anemia), or other complications due to the presence of an abdominal mass. Occasionally, degeneration occurs, causing intense pain. Infertility may be due to a myoma that obstructs or distorts the genital tract.

In pregnant women, myomas cause additional hazards: abortion, malpresentation, failure of engagement, premature labor, localized pain (from red degeneration or torsion), dystocia, ineffectual labor, and postpartum hemorrhage.

B. Laboratory Findings: The red blood cell count may be decreased as a result of blood loss, but in occasional cases polycythemia is present, presumably as a result of the production of erythropoietin by the myomas.

C. X-Ray and Ultrasound Findings: A plain film of the pelvis may demonstrate opacities if calcific degeneration has occurred. Hysterography (contraindicated during pregnancy) may reveal a cervical or submucous tumor. Ultrasonography will reveal tumors and can be used sequentially to monitor growth. When multiple subserous or pedunculated myomas are being followed, ultrasonography is important to exclude adnexal disease.

Differential Diagnosis

Irregular myomatous enlargement of the uterus must be differentiated from the similar but regular enlargement that may occur with uterine pregnancy or adenomyosis. Subserous myomas must be distinguished from ovarian tumors. Malignant leiomyosarcoma is a very rare tumor; the average age at onset is 55 years.

Treatment

A. Emergency Measures: Give blood transfusions if necessary. If the patient is markedly anemic as a result of long, heavy menstrual periods, preoperative treatment with depot medroxyprogesterone acetate will slow or stop bleeding, and medical treatment of anemia can be given prior to surgery. Emergency surgery is required for acute torsion of a pedunculated myoma or intestinal obstruction. The only emergency indication for myomectomy during pregnancy is torsion. Abortion is not an inevitable result.

B. Specific Measures:

1. Nonpregnant women–In women who are not pregnant, small asymptomatic myomas should be observed at 6-month intervals. Elective myomectomy can be done to enhance fertility. Elective hysterectomy is justified for pain, abdominal distention, or heavy menses causing anemia. Myomas usually do not require surgery unless they cause significant pressure on the ureters, bladder, or bowel or severe bleeding leading to anemia or are undergoing rapid growth. Cervical myomas larger than 3–4 cm in diameter or pedunculated myomas that protrude through the cervix should be removed.

2. Pregnant patients–If the uterus is no larger than a 6-month pregnancy by the fourth month of gestation, an uncomplicated course may be anticipated. If the mass (especially a cervical tumor) is the size of a 5- or 6-month pregnancy by the second month, abortion will probably occur. If possible, defer surgery until 6 months after delivery, at which time involution of the uterus and regression of the tumor will be complete.

C. Surgical Measures: The measures available for the treatment of myoma are myomectomy and total or subtotal abdominal or vaginal hysterectomy. Myomectomy is the treatment of choice during the childbearing years. The ovaries should be preserved if possible in women under age 50.

Prognosis

Surgical therapy is curative. Future pregnancies are not endangered by myomectomy, although cesarean delivery may be necessary after wide dissection with entry into the uterine cavity. Careful hysterectomy with retention of normal ovaries does not hasten menopause.

Haberstroh WD, Reamer JF, Slate WG: Epithelioid leiomyoma of the uterus. *Obstet Gynecol* 1981;**57(6 Suppl)**:868.

Vardi JR, Tovell HM: Leiomyosarcoma of the uterus: Clinicopathologic study. *Obstet Gynecol* 1980;**56**:428.

CARCINOMA OF THE VULVA

Essentials of Diagnosis

- Occurs most often in the postmenopausal age group.
- History of prolonged vulvar irritation, with pruritus, local discomfort, or slight bloody discharge.
- Early lesions may suggest or include chronic vulvitis.
- Late lesions appear as a mass, an exophytic growth, or a firm, ulcerated area in the vulva.
- Biopsy is necessary to make the diagnosis.

General Considerations

While cancer of the vulva is a disorder of unknown cause, numerous predisposing or contributing factors are recognized, such as chronic granulomatous disorders. The vast majority are squamous carcinomas. More than 50% of patients with this disorder are over age 50 years; the average age is 65 years.

Differential Diagnosis

Biopsy is essential for the diagnosis of vulvar cancer and should be performed with any localized atypical vulvar lesion, including white patches. Multiple skin-punch specimens can be taken in the office under local anesthesia, with care to include tissue from the edges of each lesion sampled.

Benign vulvar disorders that must be excluded in the diagnosis of carcinoma of the vulva include chronic granulomatous lesions (eg, lymphogranuloma venereum, syphilis, vulvar nodulation [due to sebaceous,

inclusion, or Bartholin's cyst], hidradenoma, or neurofibroma). Kraurosis, lichen sclerosis et atrophicus, or other associated leukoplakic changes in the skin should be biopsied but usually are not malignant.

Treatment

A. General Measures: Early diagnosis and treatment of irritative or other predisposing or contributing causes to carcinoma of the vulva should be pursued. Remove prominent or enlarging pigmented moles of the vulva before they become malignant.

B. Surgical Measures:

1. In situ squamous cell carcinoma of the vulva and small, invasive basal cell carcinoma of the vulva should be excised with a wide margin. If the squamous carcinoma in situ is extensive or multicentric, laser therapy or superficial removal of vulvar skin may be required. In this way, the clitoris and uninvolved portions of the vulva may be spared. Skin grafting is possible, and mutilating vulvectomy is avoided.

2. Invasive carcinoma confined to the vulva without evidence of spread to adjacent organs or to the regional lymph nodes will necessitate radical vulvectomy and inguinal lymphadenectomy if the patient is able to withstand surgery. Debilitated patients may be candidates for palliative irradiation only.

Prognosis

Patients with vulvar carcinoma 3 cm in diameter or less without inguinal lymph node metastases who can sustain radical surgery have about a 90% chance of a 5-year arrest of the cancer. If the lesion is greater than 3 cm and has metastasized, the likelihood of 5-year survival is less than 25%.

Morley GW: Cancer of the vulva: A review. *Cancer* 1981;**48(2 Suppl)**:597.

ENDOMETRIOSIS

Aberrant growth of endometrium outside the uterus, particularly in the dependent parts of the pelvis and in the ovaries, is a common cause of abnormal bleeding and secondary dysmenorrhea. This is known as endometriosis. Depending on the location of the endometrial implants, infertility, dyspareunia, or rectal pain with bleeding may result. Aching pain tends to be constant, beginning 2–7 days before the onset of menses to become increasingly severe until flow slackens. Pelvic examination may disclose tender indurated nodules in the cul-de-sac, especially if the examination is done at the onset of menstruation.

Endometriosis must be distinguished from pelvic inflammatory disease, tuberculosis, and myomas and other neoplasms of the reproductive organs. In general, only in salpingitis and endometriosis are the symptoms aggravated by menstruation. Bowel invasion by endometrial tissue may produce clinical findings that must be distinguished from bowel neoplasm;

differentiation in these rare instances depends upon biopsy.

The clinical diagnosis of endometriosis is presumptive and must be confirmed by laparoscopy or laparotomy. Ultrasound examination will often reveal complex fluid-filled masses that cannot be distinguished from neoplasms. Barium enema may delineate colonic involvement of endometriosis.

Treatment

A. Medical Treatment: Young women concerned about fertility with mild but advancing endometriosis should be advised to consider pregnancy without delay to secure a family and perhaps retard the progress of the disease. If the patient does not want a child or cannot become pregnant, exogenous hormone therapy with one of the following regimens is indicated:

1. Danazol (Danocrine), 200–400 mg twice daily for 6–9 months, in the lowest dose necessary to suppress menstruation.

2. Combination estrogen-progestin oral contraceptives, one daily continuously for 6–9 months. Increase the dose only with the onset of breakthrough bleeding.

3. Medroxyprogesterone acetate (Depo-Provera), 100 mg intramuscularly every 2 weeks for 4 doses; then 100 mg every 4 weeks; add oral estrogen or estradiol valerate, 30 mg intramuscularly, for breakthrough bleeding.

4. GnRH analogs are currently being evaluated as treatment for endometriosis because of their ability to suppress ovulation with minimal side effects. Studies are under way to determine the optimal dose to avoid symptoms of hypoestrinism.

5. Analgesics, with or without codeine, may be needed during menses. Nonsteroidal anti-inflammatory drugs may be helpful.

B. Surgical Measures: The surgical treatment of moderately extensive endometriosis depends upon the patient's age and symptoms and her desire to preserve reproductive function. If the patient is under 35, resect the lesions, free adhesions, and suspend the uterus. At least 20% of patients so treated can become pregnant, although some must undergo surgery again if the disease progresses. If the patient is over 35 years old, is disabled by pain, and has involvement of both ovaries, bilateral salpingo-oophorectomy and hysterectomy will probably be necessary.

Extensive endometriosis almost invariably necessitates ablation of both ovaries, both tubes, and the uterus, regardless of the patient's age.

Prognosis

The prognosis for reproductive function in early or moderately advanced endometriosis is good with conservative therapy. Bilateral ovariectomy is curative for patients with severe and extensive endometriosis with pain. Following hysterectomy and oophorectomy, estrogen replacement therapy is indicated.

Buttram VC Jr, Belue JB, Reiter R: Interim report of a study of danazol for the treatment of endometriosis. *Fertil Steril* 1982;**37**:478.

Schenken RS, Malinak LR: Conservative surgery versus expectant management for the infertile patient with mild endometriosis. *Fertil Steril* 1982;**37**:183.

VAGINAL HERNIAS
(Cystocele, Rectocele, Enterocele)

Cystocele, rectocele, and enterocele are vaginal hernias commonly seen in multiparous women. Cystocele is a hernia of the bladder wall into the vagina, causing a soft anterior fullness. Cystocele may be accompanied by urethrocele, which is not a hernia but a sagging of the urethra following its detachment from the symphysis during childbirth. Rectocele is a herniation of the terminal rectum into the posterior vagina, causing a collapsible pouchlike fullness. Enterocele is a vaginal vault hernia containing small intestine, usually in the posterior vagina and resulting from a deepening of the pouch of Douglas. Enterocele may also accompany uterine prolapse or follow hysterectomy, when weakened vault supports or a deep unobliterated cul-de-sac containing intestine protrudes deeply into the vagina. One or more of the 3 types of hernias often occur in combination.

In each type of hernia, laceration or thinning of the endopelvic fascia or its extension down the vagina allows the herniation. This is the result of obstetric injury. Occasionally, vaginal hernias occur in nulliparas who have had lower spinal cord injury or postmenopausal tissue involution or in whom straining or lifting has weakened supporting tissues.

Clinical Findings

A large cystocele may be associated with residual urine, and chronic, recurrent cystitis often follows. Cystocele by itself is not a cause of incontinence.

Patients with cystocele describe (and reveal) anterior vaginal fullness and have a sense of the presence of urine even after voiding. Repeat voiding or manual reduction of the fullness may empty the bladder. Residual urine may become infected.

Rectocele often follows traumatic delivery of a large infant. Constipation or a sense of rectovaginal fullness, often associated with the presence of feces in the rectocele pouch, are typical complaints. Straining at stool increases the size of the rectocele.

Enterocele causes a sense of weight in the pelvis. Constipation may occur. Enterocele is usually seen or felt as a bulge high and above a rectocele, if one is present. The thin enterocele sac usually contains loops of small bowel that are rarely adherent. To distinguish a posterior cul-de-sac hernia, the examiner should place one finger in the rectum and one in the vagina. When the patient strains, the enterocele may be felt in the rectovaginal septum between the fingers. This hernia is more marked when the patient is standing.

Treatment

A. Surgical Measures: The only cure for cystocele, rectocele, or enterocele is corrective surgery.

B. Supportive Measures: Supportive measures include a high-fiber diet for constipation. Weight reduction in obese patients and limitation of straining and lifting are helpful. Pessaries may reduce cystocele, rectocele, or enterocele temporarily.

Prognosis

The prognosis following an uncomplicated surgical procedure for correction of vaginal hernias is good. Hysterectomy without closure of a significant defect in the pelvic floor will be followed by enterocele.

Hendee AE, Berry CM: Abdominal sacropexy for vaginal vault prolapse. *Clin Obstet Gynecol* 1981;**24:**1217.

Kuhn RJ, Hollyock VE: Observations on the anatomy of the rectovaginal pouch and septum. *Obstet Gynecol* 1982;**59:**445.

Zacharin RF: Pulsion enterocele: Review of functional anatomy of the pelvic floor. *Obstet Gynecol* 1980;**55:**135.

UTERINE PROLAPSE

Uterine prolapse most commonly occurs as a delayed result of childbirth injury to the pelvic floor (particularly the transverse cervical and uterosacral ligaments). Unrepaired lacerations of the levator musculature and perineal body augment the weakness. Attenuation of the pelvic structures with aging and congenital weakness can accelerate the development of prolapse.

In slight prolapse, the uterus descends only part way down the vagina; in moderate prolapse, the corpus descends to the introitus and the cervix protrudes slightly beyond; and in marked prolapse (procidentia), the entire cervix and uterus protrude beyond the introitus and the vagina is inverted.

Clinical Findings

A firm mass is palpable in the lower vagina. The patient complains of a sense of heaviness in the pelvis, low backache, and a "dragging" sensation in the inguinal regions.

Pelvic examination with the patient bearing down or straining in either the supine or the standing position will demonstrate downward displacement of a prolapsing cervix and uterus. Herniation of the bladder, rectum, or cul-de-sac is diagnosed in a similar way.

Rectovaginal examination may reveal rectal fullness (rectocele) or hernia of the pouch of Douglas behind and below the cervix.

Intravenous urography may demonstrate bilateral hydronephrosis and hydroureter.

Prevention

Postpartum prolapse may be prevented or minimized by avoiding obstetric trauma (eg, traction on the fetus). Prolonged cyclic hormone therapy for the postmenopausal woman will often conserve the strength of the pelvic floor.

Treatment

The type of surgery depends upon the extent of prolapse and the patient's age and her desire for menstruation, pregnancy, and coitus. The simplest, most effective procedure is vaginal hysterectomy with appropriate repair of the cystocele and rectocele. If the patient desires pregnancy, a partial resection of the cervix with plication of the cardinal ligaments can be attempted. For elderly women who do not desire coitus, partial obliteration of the vagina is surgically simple and effective. Abdominal uterine suspension or ventrofixation will fail in the treatment of prolapse.

Palliative therapy with a well-fitted vaginal pessary (eg, inflatable doughnut type, Gellhorn pessary) may give relief if surgery is refused or contraindicated.

Estrogen supplements improve tissue tone and correct atrophic vaginitis in postmenopausal patients.

Prognosis

Prolapse may remain constant for months or years, but it never regresses and will ultimately become more extreme unless corrected surgically.

PELVIC INFLAMMATORY DISEASE
(PID; Salpingitis, Endoparametritis)

Essentials of Diagnosis

- Abdominal, cervical, and adnexal tenderness.
- One or more of the following:
  Temperature > 38 °C.
  White blood cell count > 10,000/μL.
  Purulent material on culdocentesis.
  Pelvic abscess or inflammatory mass on pelvic examination or ultrasound.
  Gonococci present in endocervix on culture or gram stain.

General Considerations

Pelvic inflammatory disease has increased in incidence in recent years owing to the rise in sexually transmitted disease and in IUD usage. It is most common in young, nulliparous, sexually active women with multiple partners. Use of an IUD is associated with a 2-fold increase in risk; condoms, diaphragms, spermicides, and oral contraceptives provide significant protection. Endoparametritis can result from induced abortion or any other instrumentation of the uterus.

Pelvic inflammatory disease is a polymicrobial infection caused by a variety of aerobic and anaerobic bacteria, including *N gonorrhoeae, Peptostreptococcus, Peptococcus, Bacteroides,* and *Chlamydia.* Organisms present in the endocervix may not be the same ones present in the uterine tubes and peritoneal cavity.

Tuberculous salpingitis is rare in the USA but more common in developing countries; it is characterized by pain and irregular pelvic masses not responsive to antibiotic therapy. Spread of disease is hematogenous from the primary lesion, and the patient may not have been sexually active.

Clinical Findings

A. Symptoms and Signs: Patients with pelvic inflammatory disease often have lower abdominal pain, chills and fever, menstrual disturbances, purulent cervical discharge, and cervical and adnexal tenderness. Right upper quadrant pain may indicate perihepatitis (Fitz-Hugh-Curtis syndrome), which is localized peritonitis involving the anterior surface of the liver and the adjacent peritoneum of the anterior abdominal wall. However, since these findings are not always present and are not specific to pelvic inflammatory disease, the criteria for diagnosis remain as stated above. In chronic pelvic inflammatory disease, dysmenorrhea, dyspareunia, infertility, recurrent low-grade fever, and tender pelvic masses are common.

B. Laboratory Findings: The white blood cell count and sedimentation rate are not consistently elevated. Gram stains and cultures of endocervical material and fluid obtained from culdocentesis are valuable guides to therapy. Gram stains of urethral material and cultures from the sexual partner, if available, are also useful.

C. Ultrasound Findings: Pelvic ultrasound may help to distinguish the masses of pelvic infection from those of endometriosis, uterine myomas, ovarian cysts or tumors, and ectopic pregnancy.

Differential Diagnosis

Appendicitis, ectopic pregnancy, septic abortion, hemorrhagic or ruptured ovarian cysts or tumors, twisted ovarian cyst, degeneration of a myoma, and acute enteritis must be considered. Pelvic inflammatory disease is more likely to occur when there is a history of pelvic inflammatory disease, recent sexual contact, recent onset of menses, or an IUD in place or if the partner has a sexually transmitted disease. Acute pelvic inflammatory disease is highly unlikely when recent intercourse has not taken place or an IUD is not being used. A sensitive serum pregnancy test should be obtained to rule out ectopic pregnancy. Culdocentesis will differentiate between causes of hemoperitoneum (ruptured ectopic pregnancy or hemorrhagic cyst) and pelvic sepsis (salpingitis, ruptured pelvic abscess, or ruptured appendix). Pelvic ultrasound is helpful in the differential diagnosis of ectopic pregnancy of over 6 weeks. Laparoscopy is often utilized to diagnose pelvic inflammatory disease, and it is imperative if the diagnosis is not certain or if the patient has not responded to antibiotic therapy after 48 hours. The appendix should be visualized at laparoscopy to rule out appendicitis. Cultures obtained at the time of laparoscopy are often specific and helpful.

Treatment

A. Hospitalization: Patients with acute pelvic inflammatory disease should be hospitalized if there is fever higher than 38 °C or a possible pelvic abscess, if they are pregnant, if diagnosis is uncertain, or if oral antibiotics are not tolerated.

B. Antibiotics: Early treatment with appropriate antibiotics effective against *N gonorrhoeae, Chla-* *mydia,* and anaerobes is essential to preserve fertility. Treatment of the sexual partner with tetracycline, 500 mg 4 times daily for 7 days, to eradicate *N gonorrhoeae* and *Chlamydia* should be given if possible.

Various treatment regimens for acute pelvic inflammatory disease are effective. Hospitalized patients can be given one of the following regimens: (1) Cefoxitin, 2 g intravenously every 6 hours, plus doxycycline, 100 mg intravenously twice daily. Continue intravenous administration for at least 48 hours after fever has abated. Continue tetracycline, 500 mg 4 times daily, or doxycycline, 100 mg twice daily, orally to complete 10–14 days of therapy. (2) Clindamycin, 600 mg intravenously every 6 hours, plus gentamicin or tobramycin, 2 mg/kg intravenously followed by 1.5 mg/kg intravenously every 8 hours. Continue intravenous administration for at least 48 hours after temperature is normal. Continue clindamycin, 450 mg 4 times daily orally to complete 10–14 days of therapy. (3) Metronidazole, 1 g intravenously every 12 hours, plus doxycycline, 100 mg intravenously every 12 hours. Continue intravenous administration for at least 48 hours after fever has abated. Then continue both drugs orally at the same dosage to complete 10–14 days of therapy.

Outpatients with milder cases of pelvic inflammatory disease should be given cefoxitin, 2 g intramuscularly, or amoxicillin, 3 g orally, or aqueous procaine penicillin G, 4.8 million units intramuscularly—each with probenecid, 1 g orally, followed by doxycycline, 100 mg twice daily orally, for 10–14 days, or tetracycline, 500 mg 4 times daily orally for 10–14 days.

C. General Measures: Fluids, a nutritious diet, and bed rest are advisable. Pain is controlled with simple analgesics. Sexual intercourse should be delayed until recovery is complete, often 2–3 months. Subsequent use of oral contraceptives, condoms, or a diaphragm rather than the IUD will reduce the risk of reinfection. Women who have had pelvic inflammatory disease should ask new or promiscuous partners to use condoms and should avoid coitus during menses, when flare-ups are most common.

D. Surgical Measures: Tubo-ovarian abscesses may require surgical excision. Unless rupture is suspected, institute high-dose antibiotic therapy in the hospital, and monitor therapy with ultrasound. In 70% of cases, antibiotics are effective; in 30%, there is inadequate response in 48–72 hours, and laparotomy is required. Unilateral adnexectomy in the presence of unilateral abscess is acceptable. Hysterectomy and bilateral salpingo-oophorectomy may be necessary for overwhelming infection or in cases of chronic disease with intractable pelvic pain.

Prognosis

One-fourth of women with acute disease develop long-term sequelae, including repeated episodes of infection, chronic pelvic pain, dyspareunia, ectopic pregnancy, or infertility. The risk of infertility increases with repeated episodes of salpingitis: it is estimated at 11% after the first episode, 23% after a second episode, and 54% after a third episode.

Eschenbach DA: Epidemiology and diagnosis of acute pelvic inflammatory disease. *Obstet Gynecol* 1980;**55**(5 **Suppl**): 142S.

Keith LG et al: On the causation of pelvic inflammatory disease. *Am J Obstet Gynecol* 1984;**149**:215.

Kelaghan J et al: Barrier-method contraceptives and pelvic inflammatory disease. *JAMA* 1982;**248**:184.

Shafer MA, Irwin CE, Sweet RL: Acute salpingitis in the adolescent female. *J Pediatr* 1982;**100**:339.

OVARIAN TUMORS

Ovarian tumors are common forms of neoplastic disease in women. Most are benign, but some are malignant. The wide range of types and patterns of ovarian tumors is due to the complexity of ovarian embryology and differences in tissue of origin. Most systems of classification utilize largely the tumor histogenesis, but there may be advantages to employing other criteria such as clinical behavior—functional and nonfunctional, cystic or solid—and always macroscopic or microscopic appearance (see Table 13–3).

The history and physical examination may be supplemented with cervical cytologic studies, ultrasound, and laparoscopy. Upper gastrointestinal series, barium enema, and other studies may help to rule out metastatic origin from other primary sites. An intravenous urogram is important to determine distortion or obstruction of the ureters caused by the tumor.

The treatment of ovarian tumors must be individualized. Small unilocular tumors (as determined by ultrasound) in premenopausal women can be observed for a few months. A 2-month trial of suppression of ovulation with oral contraceptives usually causes functional cysts to disappear. If ultrasound suggests septation or solid components, a neoplasm is more likely, and surgical exploration should be prompt. If a plain film of the abdomen shows calcification, a benign teratoma is likely. Whenever possible in young women, ovarian cystectomy rather than total removal of the ovary is desirable. An enlarged ovary in a postmenopausal woman should be removed promptly.

Malignant ovarian tumors must be removed surgically. Since bilateral involvement is common, the contralateral ovary must be examined at the time of surgery.

The prognosis for benign ovarian tumors after surgical removal is excellent. The outlook for ovarian cancer, unless diagnosed in the earliest stages, is poor.

Requard CK, Mettler FA Jr, Wicks JD: Preoperative sonography of malignant ovarian neoplasms. *AJR* 1981;**137**:79.

PERSISTENT ANOVULATION
(Polycystic Ovary Syndrome, Stein-Leventhal Syndrome)

Essentials of Diagnosis
- Chronic anovulation.
- Infertility.
- Elevated plasma LH values and a reversed FSH/LH ratio.
- Hirsutism (in 70% of patients).

General Considerations
These patients have a relatively steady state of high estrogen, androgen, and LH levels, rather than the fluctuating condition seen in ovulating women. The stromal tissue of the ovary secretes high amounts of androgens, and the peripheral conversion of androstenedione in body fat gives high estrone levels. Sex hormone-binding globulin levels are low, allowing for increased free circulating sex steroids. LH levels are higher than normal; FSH is low or low normal. New follicles in the ovary are continually stimulated but not to the point of ovulation; they may persist for months as follicle cysts. The polycystic ovary has a thickened, pearly white capsule.

Clinical Findings
The patient is anovular, sometimes with amenorrhea and sometimes with irregular heavy bleeding. The ovaries may be enlarged, but this is not a consistent finding. Similarly, she may or may not be obese. Hirsutism occurs in about 70% of patients with this condition. These patients are generally infertile, although they may ovulate occasionally. They have an increased long-term risk of cancer of the breast and endometrium because of unopposed estrogen secretion.

Differential Diagnosis
Anovulation in the reproductive years may also be due to (1) premature menopause (high FSH and LH levels); (2) rapid weight loss or extreme physical exertion (normal FSH and LH levels for age); (3) discontinuation of oral contraceptives (anovulation for 6 months or more occasionally occurs); (4) pituitary adenoma with elevated prolactin (galactorrhea may or may not be present); (5) hyper- or hypothyroidism; (6) Cushing's syndrome or congenital adrenal hyperplasia. Always check FSH, LH, prolactin, and TSH levels when amenorrhea has persisted for 6 months or more without a diagnosis. A 10-day course of progestin (eg, medroxyprogesterone acetate, 10 mg/d) will cause withdrawal bleeding if estrogen levels are adequate; bleeding will not occur if estrogen levels are low. This will aid in the diagnosis and prevent endometrial hyperplasia. In anovular patients over age 35, it is wise to search for an estrogen-stimulated cancer with mammography and endometrial aspiration.

Treatment
If the patient wishes to become pregnant, clomi-

Table 13–3. Ovarian functional and neoplastic tumors.

Tumor	Incidence	Size	Consistency	Menstrual Irregularities	Endocrine Effects	Potential For Malignancy	Special Remarks
Follicle cysts	Rare in childhood; frequent in menstrual years; never in postmenopausal years.	<6 cm, often bilateral.	Moderate	Occasional	Occasional anovulation with persistently proliferative endometrium.	0	Often disappear after a 2-month regimen of oral contraceptives.
Corpus luteum cysts	Occasional.	4–6 cm, unilateral.	Moderate	Occasional delayed period	Prolonged secretory phase.	0	Functional cysts. Intraperitoneal bleeding occasionally.
Theca lutein cysts	Occurs with hydatidiform mole, choriocarcinoma; also with gonadotropin or clomiphene therapy.	To 4–5 cm, multiple, bilateral. (Ovaries may be ≥ 20 cm in diameter.)	Tense	Amenorrhea	hCG elevated.	0	Functional cysts. Hematoperitoneum or torsion of ovary may occur.
Inflammatory (tuboovarian abscess)	Concomitant with acute salpingitis.	To 15–20 cm, often bilateral.	Variable, painful	Menometrorrhagia	Anovulation usual.	0	In acute phase may rupture and cause lethal peritonitis.
Endometriotic cysts	Never in preadolescent or postmenopausal years. Most common in women age 20–40 years.	To 10–12 cm, occasionally bilateral.	Moderate to softened	Rare	0	Very rare	Associated pelvic endometriosis.
Teratoid tumors: Benign teratomas (dermoid cysts)	Childhood to postmenopause.	<15 cm; 15% are bilateral.	Moderate to softened	0	0	Rare	Torsion can occur.
Malignant teratomas	<1% of ovarian tumors. Usually in infants and young adults.	>20 cm, unilateral.	Irregularly firm	0	Occasionally, hCG elevated.	All	Unresponsive to any therapy.
Cystadenoma, cystadenocarcinoma	Common in reproductive years.	Serous: <25 cm, often bilateral. Mucinous; up to 1 meter, occasionally bilateral.	Moderate to softened Moderate to softened	0 0	0 0	>50% for serous. About 5% for mucinous.	Peritoneal implants often occur with serous tumors, rarely occur with mucinous tumors. If mucinous tumor is ruptured, pseudomyxoma peritonei may occur.
Endometrioid carcinoma	15% of ovarian carcinomas.	Moderate.	Firm	0	0	All	Adenocarcinoma of endometrium coexists in 15–30% of cases.
Fibroma	<5% of ovarian tumors.	Usually <15 cm.	Very firm	0	0	Rare	Ascites in 20% (rarely, pleural fluid).
Arrhenoblastoma	Rare. Average age 30 years or more.	Often small (<10 cm), unilateral.	Firm to softened	Amenorrhea	Androgens elevated.	<20%	Recurrences are moderately sensitive to irradiation.
Theca cell tumor (thecoma)	Uncommon.	<10 cm, unilateral.	Firm	Occasionally irregular periods	Estrogens or androgens elevated.	<1%	. . .
Granulosa cell tumor	Uncommon. Usually in prepubertal girls or women older than 50 years.	May be very small.	Firm to softened	Menometrorrhagia	Estrogens elevated.	15–20%	Recurrences are moderately sensitive to irradiation.
Dysgerminoma	About 1–2% of ovarian tumors.	<30 cm, bilateral in one-third of cases.	Moderate to softened	0	. . .	All	Very radiosensitive.
Brenner tumor	About 1% of ovarian tumors.	<30 cm, unilateral.	Firm	0	. . .	Very rare	>50% occur in postmenopausal years.
Secondary ovarian tumors	10% of fatal malignant disease in women.	Varies, often bilateral.	Firm to softened	Occasional	Very rare (thyroid, adrenocortical origin).	All	No therapy is curative.

phene or other drugs can be employed for ovulatory stimulation. Wedge resection of the ovary is often successful in restoring ovulation and fertility, although this procedure is used less commonly now that medical treatments are available.

If the patient does not desire pregnancy, give medroxyprogesterone acetate, 10 mg/d for the first 10 days of each month. This will ensure regular shedding of the endometrium so that hyperplasia will not occur. If contraception is desired, a low-dose combination oral contraceptive can be used; this is also useful in controlling hirsutism, for which treatment must be continued for 6–12 months before results are seen.

Hirsutism may be managed with epilation and electrolysis. If hirsutism is severe, some patients will elect to have a hysterectomy and bilateral oophorectomy followed by estrogen replacement therapy. Spironolactone, an aldosterone antagonist, is also useful for hirsutism. However, since this drug is tumorigenic in rats, its use for a chronic cosmetic condition is questionable.

Goldzieher JW: Polycystic ovarian disease. *Fertil Steril* 1981; **35**:371.

Plymate SR et al: Obesity and its role in polycystic ovary syndrome. *J Clin Endocrinol Metab* 1981;**52**:1246.

URINARY STRESS INCONTINENCE

Involuntary leakage of urine during momentary episodes of increased intra-abdominal pressure is a common gynecologic complaint. Normally, increased pressure is equally distributed to the bladder and urethra, which lie above the urogenital diaphragm. Urine leakage becomes more likely if the urethra is prolapsed and lies below the urogenital diaphragm or if the pelvic muscles of the diaphragm are weakened. In such cases, stress causes a relative decrease in intraurethral pressure, and small amounts of urine escape. Leakage occurs upon coughing, sneezing, laughing, or sudden lifting. Most women with urinary stress incontinence have suffered childbirth injuries or have developed weakness of the pelvic floor structures following menopause. Compression of the bladder by the pregnant uterus, pelvic tumors, or ascites may also impair the patient's ability to retain urine.

A careful history of voiding habits, including amount and timing of urine leakage, is helpful in identifying true stress incontinence. It is important to distinguish loss of urine with stress from overflow incontinence associated with a hypotonic bladder emptying incompletely or urgency loss associated with a hypertonic bladder.

A cystometrogram will identify abnormal detrusor activity, as well as an unusually large or small bladder capacity. Measurement of closing pressure along the length of the urethra will help in determining whether surgical procedures to lengthen and support the urethra will be successful. A voiding cystourethrogram will identify an excessively mobile prolapsing urethra, for which surgical support will be successful.

Treatment

Effective therapy will increase the woman's ability to transmit intravesical pressure to the mid urethra but will not necessarily improve intraurethral pressure per se. A trial of medical treatment is always indicated before surgery is considered. Medical disorders such as diabetes mellitus, extreme obesity, and chronic cough, which aggravate stress incontinence, should be controlled if possible. Postmenopausal women should receive a trial of estrogen replacement (either cyclic oral medication or small doses of vaginal cream). Patients who do not have serious neurologic disorders and have not sustained severe physical injury can be taught to contract the pubococcygeus and sphincter ani muscles repeatedly to reestablish urinary control (Kegel isometric exercises).

Patients who fail to respond to exercises or medical treatment may be candidates for surgery, particularly when cystocele or prolapse of the bladder and uterus is present. A useful surgical prognostic test is to elevate the anterior vaginal wall lateral to the urethra at the urethrovesical junction with the fingers or ring forceps (Bonney test). If loss of urine does not occur with cough, the surgical prognosis is good.

Medical therapy alone is curative in about half of cases. The overall surgical cure rate in patients who require operation is about 85%. The most successful procedure is retropubic suspension of the paravaginal tissues (Burch procedure). Other types of urethral suspension (Pereyra operation) or vaginal urethral plication are occasional alternatives.

Bhatia NN, Ostergard DR: Urodynamic effects of retropubic urethropexy in genuine stress incontinence. *Am J Obstet Gynecol* 1981;**140**:936.

Pereyra AJ et al: Pubourethral supports in perspective: Modified Pereyra procedure for urinary incontinence. *Obstet Gynecol* 1982;**59**:643.

DYSPAREUNIA

Dyspareunia (painful coitus) may be caused by vulvovaginitis; vaginismus; an incompletely stretched hymen; insufficient lubrication of the vagina; or infection, tumors, or other pathologic conditions. Careful history taking and a thorough pelvic examination are essential. During the pelvic examination, the patient should be placed in a half-sitting position and given a hand-held mirror and then asked to point out the site of pain and describe the type of pain. The physician should be able to provide sex counseling and should allow adequate time for a discussion of problems related to sexuality, personal relationships, contraception, and fears of pregnancy.

Etiology

A. Vulvovaginitis: Vulvovaginitis is inflammation or infection of the vagina. For a detailed discussion, see p 454.

B. Vaginismus: Vaginismus is voluntary or involuntary contraction of muscles around the introitus.

It results from fear, sexual trauma, or having learned negative attitudes toward sex during childhood.

C. Remnants of the Hymen: The hymen is usually adequately stretched during initial intercourse, so that pain does not occur subsequently. In some women, the pain of initial intercourse may produce vaginismus. In others, a thin or thickened rim or partial rim of hymen remains after several episodes of intercourse, causing pain.

D. Insufficient Lubrication of the Vagina: Insufficient vaginal lubrication may be due to inadequate time for sexual arousal or to low estrogen effect during lactation or following menopause. When estrogen levels are normal (as evidenced by the occurrence of menstrual periods or the presence of moist, healthy-appearing vaginal mucosa with rugal folds), dyspareunia is probably due to inadequate sexual arousal prior to coitus. Low estrogen levels are evidenced by decreased introital diameter, dry vaginal mucosa, fewer rugal folds, and thinned, reddened epithelium.

E. Infection, Tumors, or Other Pathologic Conditions: Pain occurring with deep thrusting during coitus is usually due to acute or chronic infection of the cervix, uterus, or adnexa; endometriosis; adnexal tumors; or adhesions resulting from prior pelvic disease or operation. Careful history taking and a pelvic examination will generally help in the differential diagnosis.

F. Dyspareunia Due to Unknown Causes: Occasionally, no organic cause of pain can be found. These patients may have psychosexual conflicts or a history of childhood sexual abuse.

Treatment
A. Vulvovaginitis: Infection or inflammation should be treated after careful diagnosis. The sexual partner should also be treated in recurrent cases. Irritation from spermicides may be a factor. The couple may be helped by a discussion of noncoital techniques to achieve orgasm until the infection subsides.

B. Vaginismus: Sexual counseling and education on anatomy and sexual functioning may be appropriate. The patient can be instructed in self-dilation, using a lubricated finger or test tubes of graduated sizes. Before coitus (with adequate lubrication) is attempted, the patient—and then her partner—should be able to easily and painlessly introduce 2 fingers into the vagina. Penetration should never be forced, and the woman should always be the one to control the depth of insertion during dilation or intercourse.

C. Remnants of the Hymen: In rare situations, manual dilation of a remaining hymen under general anesthesia is necessary. Surgery should be avoided.

D. Insufficient Lubrication of the Vagina: If inadequate sexual arousal is the cause, sexual counseling for the woman—and her partner if possible—is helpful. Lubricants may be used during sexual foreplay. For women with low plasma estrogen levels, use of a lubricant during coitus is sometimes sufficient. If not, use conjugated estrogen cream, one-eighth applicatorful daily for 10 days and then every other day. Using the applicator or a finger, the patient can apply the cream directly to the most tender area, usually the hymenal ring. Testosterone cream 1–2% in a water-soluble base is also helpful.

E. Infection, Endometriosis, or Other Pathologic Conditions: Medical treatment of acute cervicitis, endometritis, or salpingitis and temporary abstention from coitus usually relieves pain. Hormonal or surgical treatment of endometriosis may be helpful. Dyspareunia resulting from chronic pelvic inflammatory disease or any condition causing extensive adhesions or fixation of pelvic organs is difficult to treat without extirpative surgery. Couples can be advised to try coital positions that limit deep thrusting and to use manual and oral sexual techniques.

F. Dyspareunia Due to Unknown Cause: Biopsies should be avoided if there is no identifiable lesion. Supportive, understanding discussion may be helpful. Small amounts of topical remedies such as 1% testosterone cream or estrogen cream may relieve pain. Resolution of psychosexual problems or problems relating to traumatic sexual experiences may be necessary.

Fordney DS: Dyspareunia and vaginismus. *Clin Obstet Gynecol* 1978;**21**:205.

Reamy K: The treatment of vaginismus by the gynecologist: An eclectic approach. *Obstet Gynecol* 1982;**59**:58.

INFERTILITY

A couple is said to be infertile if pregnancy does not result after 1 year of normal sexual activity without contraceptives. About 10% of couples are infertile. The male partner contributes to about 40% of cases of infertility. A combination of factors is common.

Diagnostic Survey
A basic infertility study can be performed, usually within a 3-month period, although timing can vary depending on convenience and the desires of the couple. Both partners are evaluated.

During the initial interview, the physician can present an overview of infertility and discuss a plan of study. Separate private consultations are then conducted, allowing appraisal of psychosexual adjustment without embarrassment or criticism. Pertinent details (eg, sexually transmitted disease or prior pregnancies) must be obtained. A complete medical, surgical, occupational, and obstetric history must be taken. The ill effects of cigarettes, alcohol, and other recreational drugs on fertility in both men and women should be discussed. Prescription drugs that impair male potency should be noted. The gynecologic history should include queries regarding the menstrual pattern. The present history includes use and types of contraceptives, douches, libido, sex techniques, frequency and success of coitus, and correlation of intercourse with time of ovulation. Family history includes familial traits, illnesses, repeated abortions, and abnormal children.

General physical and genital examinations are performed on both partners. Basic laboratory studies include complete blood count, urinalysis, serologic test for syphilis, and thyroid function tests.

The woman is instructed to take her basal body temperature orally daily on arising and to record on a graph episodes of coitus and days of menstruation.

The man is instructed to bring a complete ejaculate for analysis. Sexual abstinence for at least 3 days before the semen is obtained is emphasized. A clean, dry, wide-mouthed bottle for collection is preferred. Condoms should not be employed, as the protective powder may be spermicidal. Semen should be examined within 1–2 hours after collection. Semen is considered normal with the following minimum values: volume, 3 mL; concentration, 20 million sperm per milliliter; motility, 50% after 2 hours; and normal forms, 60%.

A. First Testing Cycle: A postcoital test (Sims-Huhner test) is scheduled for just before ovulation (eg, day 12 or 13 in an expected 28-day cycle). The patient is examined within 6 hours after coitus. The cervical mucus should be clear, elastic, and copious owing to the influence of the preovular estrogen surge. (The mucus is scantier and more viscid before and after ovulation.) A good spinnbarkeit (stretching to a fine thread 6 cm or more in length) is desirable. A small drop of cervical mucus should be obtained from within the cervical os and examined under the microscope. The presence of 5 or more active sperm per high-power field constitutes a satisfactory postcoital test. If no spermatozoa are found, the test should be repeated (assuming that active spermatozoa were present in the semen analysis). Sperm agglutination and sperm immobilization tests should be considered if the sperm are immotile or show ineffective tail motility.

The presence of more than 3 white blood cells per high-power field in the postcoital test suggests cervicitis in the woman or prostatitis in the man. When estrogen levels are normal, the cervical mucus dried on the slide will form a fernlike pattern when viewed with a low-power microscope. This type of mucus is necessary for normal sperm transport.

The serum progesterone level should be measured at the midpoint of the secretory phase (21st day); a level of 10–20 ng/mL confirms adequate luteal function.

B. Second Testing Cycle: Hysterosalpingography is performed within 3 days following the menstrual period. This x-ray study will demonstrate uterine abnormalities (septa, polyps, submucous myomas) and tubal obstruction. Ethiodol, an oily radiopaque medium, can be administered through the cervix 24 hours before films are made; dispersion of the dye will help in detection of uterine abnormalities or tubal occlusion. This test has been associated with an increased pregnancy rate by some observers. If the woman has had prior pelvic inflammation, give tetracycline, 2 g/d, beginning immediately before and for 7 days after the x-ray study.

C. Further Testing:

1. Gross deficiencies of sperm (number, motility, or appearance) require repeat analysis.

2. Obvious obstruction of the uterine tubes requires assessment for microsurgery.

3. Absent or infrequent ovulation requires additional laboratory evaluation. Elevated FSH and LH levels indicate ovarian failure causing premature menopause (in women under age 30, karyotyping is indicated to rule out chromosomal abnormalities). Elevated LH levels in the presence of normal FSH levels confirm the presence of polycystic ovaries. Elevation of blood prolactin (PRL) levels suggests pituitary microadenoma.

D. Laparoscopy: Approximately 25% of women whose basic evaluation is normal will have findings on laparoscopy explaining their infertility (eg, peritubal adhesions, endometriotic implants).

Treatment

A. Medical Measures: Fertility may be restored by appropriate treatment in many patients with endocrine imbalance, particularly those with hypo- or hyperthyroidism. Antibiotic treatment of cervicitis is of value. After 6 months of condom protection during intercourse, an antigen-antibody reaction will usually resolve, and sperm agglutination or immobilization should cease to be a problem.

B. Surgical Measures: Excision of ovarian tumors or ovarian foci of endometriosis can restore fertility. Microsurgical relief of tubal obstruction due to salpingitis or tubal ligation will reestablish fertility in a significant number of cases. In special instances of cornual or fimbrial block, the prognosis with newer surgical techniques has become much better. Peritubal adhesions or endometriotic implants often can be treated via laparoscopy or via laparotomy immediately following laparoscopic examination if prior consent has been obtained.

With varicocele in the male, sperm characteristics are often improved following surgical treatment.

C. Induction of Ovulation:

1. Clomiphene citrate (Clomid) –Clomiphene citrate stimulates gonadotropin release, especially LH. Consequently, plasma estrone (E_1) and estradiol (E_2) also rise, reflecting ovarian follicle maturation. If E_2 rises sufficiently, an LH surge occurs to trigger ovulation.

After a normal menstrual period or induction of withdrawal bleeding with progestin, give 50 mg of clomiphene orally daily for 5 days. If ovulation does not occur, increase the dose to 100 mg orally daily for 5 days. If ovulation still does not occur, repeat the course with 150 and then 200 mg daily for 5 days and add chorionic gonadotropin, 10,000 units intramuscularly, 7 days after clomiphene.

The rate of ovulation following this treatment is 90% in the absence of other infertility factors. The pregnancy rate is high. Twinning occurs in 5% of these patients; an increased incidence of congenital anomalies has not been reported. Painful ovarian cyst formation occurs in 8% of patients and may warrant discontinuation of therapy.

In the presence of increased androgen production (DHEA-S > 200 μg/dL), the addition of dexamethasone, 0.5 mg at bedtime, improves the response to clomiphene. Dexamethasone should be discontinued after pregnancy is confirmed.

2. Bromocriptine (Parlodel)–Use only if PRL levels are elevated and there is no withdrawal bleeding following progesterone administration (otherwise use clomiphene). The usual dose is 2.5 mg twice daily. To minimize side effects (nausea, diarrhea, dizziness, headache, fatigue), the dosage can be increased by weekly increments of 1.25–2.5 mg at bedtime. The drug is discontinued once pregnancy has occurred.

3. Human menopausal gonadotropins (hMG) (Pergonal)–hMG is indicated in cases of hypogonadotropism and most other types of anovulation (exclusive of ovarian failure). Because of the complexities, laboratory tests, and expense associated with this treatment, patients who require hMG for the induction of ovulation should be referred to a specialist. Current reports suggest that in the future, hypothalamic amenorrhea unresponsive to clomiphene will be reliably and successfully treated with subcutaneous pulsatile gonadotropin-releasing hormone (GnRH). Use of this substance will avoid the dangerous ovarian complications and the 25% incidence of multiple pregnancy associated with hMG.

4. Ovarian wedge resection–Wedge resection is indicated rarely and only when medical measures are not effective.

D. Treatment of Endometriosis: See p 461.

E. Treatment of Low Midluteal Progesterone Levels: Midluteal progesterone levels of less than 10 ng/mL can be treated with one of the following regimens:

1. Progesterone suppositories, 50 mg twice daily on days 17–31 of the ovarian cycle. If the woman becomes pregnant, continue for 8 weeks.

2. Clomiphene (see above) can also be used for luteal phase insufficiency.

F. Treatment of Inadequate Transport of Sperm:

1. Cervical mucus will provide better transport following administration of 0.325 mg of conjugated equine estrogens from days 5 to 15 of the ovarian cycle (ovulation may be delayed).

2. Intrauterine insemination of concentrated washed sperm has been used to bypass a poor cervical environment. The sperm must be handled by sterile methods, washed in sterile saline or tissue culture solutions, and centrifuged. A small amount of fluid (0.5 mL) containing the sperm is then instilled into the uterus.

3. Artificial insemination can also be used when there is poor sperm penetration of adequate cervical mucus. Intrauterine insemination can be used, or the sperm can be placed in a cervical cap.

G. Azoospermia: If azoospermia is present, artificial insemination by a donor usually results in preg-

nancy, assuming female function is normal. Both partners must consent to this method.

H. In Vitro Fertilization and Implantation of Embryos: This technique is becoming a standard approach to fertility problems involving severe tubal disease and has also been used in cases of premature menopause. A highly organized team of specialists in reproductive function and sophisticated technology are required for successful results.

Prognosis

The prognosis for conception and normal pregnancy is good if minor (even multiple) disorders can be identified and treated; poor if the causes of infertility are severe, untreatable, or of prolonged duration (over 3 years).

It is important to remember that in the absence of severe causes of infertility (azoospermia, prolonged amenorrhea, or bilateral tubal obstruction) 30% of couples will achieve a pregnancy within 3 years. Most of these successes will be unrelated to therapy. Offering appropriately timed information about adoption is considered part of a complete infertility regimen.

Gysler M et al: A decade's experience with an individualized clomiphene treatment regimen including its effect on the postcoital test. *Fertil Steril* 1982;**37**:161.
Hargreave TB: Incidence of serum agglutinating and immobilizing sperm antibodies in infertile couples. *Int J Fertil* 1982;**27**:90.

CONTRACEPTION

Voluntary control of child-bearing benefits women, men, and the children born to them. Contraception should be available to all women and men of reproductive ages. Education about contraception and access to contraceptive pills or devices is especially important for sexually active teenagers and women following childbirth or abortion.

1. ORAL CONTRACEPTIVES

Combined Oral Contraceptives

A. Efficacy and Methods of Use: Oral contraceptives (birth control pills) have a failure rate of less than 0.5% if taken absolutely on schedule. Their primary mode of action is suppression of ovulation. The pills are initially started on the fifth day of the ovarian cycle and taken daily for 21 days, followed by 7 days with no medication, and this schedule is then continued for each cycle. The pills are often started on the first Sunday after the onset of menses, to help patients remember their starting day and to avoid menses on the weekend. If a pill is missed at any time, 2 pills should be taken the next day, and another method of contraception should be used for the rest of the cycle (eg, condoms or foam). A back-up method should also be used during the first cycle if the pills are started later than the fifth day.

B. Benefits of Oral Contraceptives: Besides offering convenient, effective contraception, there are noncontraceptive advantages to oral contraceptives. Menstrual flow is lighter and resultant anemia is less common, and dysmenorrhea is relieved for most women. Functional ovarian cysts generally disappear with oral contraceptive use, and new cysts do not occur. Pain with ovulation and postovulatory aching are relieved. The risk of ovarian and endometrial cancer is decreased. The risk of salpingitis is half the usual rate, and cases that do occur are milder. Acne is usually improved.

C. Selection of an Oral Contraceptive: Most clinicians first prescribe 30–35 μg of estrogen combined with 1 mg or less of progestin. This low dose of estrogen provides highly effective contraception but is also associated with more spotting, breakthrough bleeding, and missed menstrual periods than higher doses, and the patient should be warned of these side effects. Patients taking pills containing more than 50 μg of estrogen should be switched to lower doses whenever possible, since many adverse side effects of the pill are dose-related. The progestins vary in potency and androgenicity. When hirsutism or acne is a problem, it is best to use ethynodiol diacetate (Demulen 1/35 or 1/50) or norethindrone (Norinyl 1/35; Ortho-Novum 1/35, 10/11, 7/7/7, 1/50; Tri-Norinyl). When breakthrough bleeding or dysfunctional bleeding occurs, many clinicians use a compound with norgestrel (Lo/Ovral, Nordette, Ovral).

D. Drug Interactions: Several drugs interact with oral contraceptives to decrease their efficacy by causing induction of microsomal enzymes in the liver, by increasing sex hormone-binding globulin, and by other mechanisms. Some commonly prescribed drugs in this category are the anticonvulsants phenytoin, phenobarbital (and other barbiturates), primidone, and carbamazepine and the antitubercular drug rifampin. Women taking these drugs should use another means of contraception for maximum safety.

E. Contraindications and Adverse Effects: Oral contraceptives have been associated with many adverse effects and are contraindicated in some situations and should be used with caution in others (see Table 13–4).

1. Myocardial infarction–The risk of heart attack is higher with use of oral contraceptives. Age over 35 years; cigarette smoking; obesity; or the presence of hypertension, diabetes, or hypercholesterolemia increases the risk. Young nonsmoking women have minimal increased risk. Smokers over age 30–35 and women with other cardiovascular risk factors should use other methods of birth control.

2. Thromboembolic disease–An increased rate of fatal and nonfatal venous thromboembolism is found in oral contraceptive users. Women who develop thrombophlebitis should stop using this method, as should those at risk of thrombophlebitis because of surgery, fracture, serious injury, or immobilization.

3. Cerebrovascular disease–An increased risk of thrombotic and hemorrhagic stroke and sub-

Table 13–4. Contraindications to use of oral contraceptives.

Absolute contraindications
Pregnancy
Thrombophlebitis or thromboembolic disorders (past or present)
Stroke or coronary artery disease (past or present)
Cancer of the breast (known or suspected)
Undiagnosed abnormal vaginal bleeding
Estrogen-dependent cancer (known or suspected)
Benign or malignant tumor of the liver (past or present)

Relative contraindications
Age over 35 years and heavy cigarette smoking (> 15 cigarettes daily)
Age over 40–45 years
Cervical intraepithelial neoplasia
Migraine or recurrent persistent, severe headache
Hypertension
Cardiac or renal disease
Diabetes
Gallbladder disease
Cholestasis during pregnancy
Active hepatitis or infectious mononucleosis
Sickle cell disease (S/S or S/C type)
Surgery, fracture, or severe injury
Lactation
Uterine myoma
Significant psychologic depression

arachnoid hemorrhage has been found; smoking is associated with increased risk. Women who develop warning symptoms such as severe headache, blurred or lost vision, or other transient neurologic disorders should stop using oral contraceptives. Women with hypertensive disease should not use the pill.

4. Carcinoma–A relationship between long-term (3–4 years) oral contraceptive use and occurrence of cervical dysplasia and cancer has been shown in various studies. No confirmed relationship has been found between use of oral contraceptives and cancer of the breast. Birth control pills appear to protect against endometrial and ovarian cancer. Rarely, oral contraceptives have been associated with the development of benign or malignant hepatic tumors; this may lead to rupture of the liver, hemorrhage, and death. The risk increases with higher dosage, longer duration of use, and older age.

5. Teratogenesis–An increased incidence of defects of arms and legs and cardiovascular defects has been seen in infants born to women who used sex hormones during early pregnancy. The number of twin pregnancies and spontaneous abortions may be increased in women who conceive shortly after stopping use of oral contraceptives.

6. Gallbladder disease–There is an increased risk of gallbladder disease and subsequent cholecystectomy for cholesterol stones in pill users.

7. Metabolic disorders–A decrease in glucose tolerance and an increase in triglyceride levels is seen in pill takers, and women with diabetes should therefore rarely use this method.

8. Hypertension–Oral contraceptives may

cause hypertension in some women; the risk is increased with longer duration of use and older age. Women who have or develop hypertension should use other contraceptive methods.

9. Headache–Migraine or other vascular headaches may occur or worsen with pill use. If severe or frequent, the pill should not be used.

10. Amenorrhea–Postpill amenorrhea lasting a year or longer occurs occasionally, sometimes with galactorrhea. PRL levels should be checked; if elevated, a pituitary prolactinoma may be present.

11. Disorders of lactation–Combined oral contraceptives can impair the quantity and quality of breast milk and should therefore not be given before the infant is weaned. Progestin-only minipills can be used during lactation.

12. Other disorders–Myomas may increase in size with estrogen stimulation. Psychologic depression may occur or be worsened with oral contraceptive use. Fluid retention may lead to worsening of cardiac, renal, or convulsive problems. Asthma may be worsened. Patients who had cholestatic jaundice during pregnancy may develop jaundice while taking birth control pills. Contact lens use may become more difficult.

F. Minor Side Effects: Nausea and dizziness may occur in the first few months of pill use. A weight gain of 2–5 lb commonly occurs. Spotting or breakthrough bleeding between menstrual periods may occur, especially if a pill is skipped or taken late; this may be helped by switching to a pill of slightly greater potency (see ¶ C, above). Missed menstrual periods may occur, especially with low-dose pills. A pregnancy test should be performed if pills have been skipped or if 2 or more menstrual periods are missed. Depression, fatigue, and decreased libido can occur. Chloasma may occur, as in pregnancy, and is increased by exposure to sunlight.

Progestin Minipill

A. Efficacy and Methods of Use: Formulations containing 0.35 mg of norethindrone or 0.075 mg of. norgestrel are available in the USA. Their efficacy is slightly lower than that of combined oral contraceptives, with failure rates of 1–4% being reported. The minipill is believed to prevent conception by causing thickening of the cervical mucus to make it hostile to sperm, alteration of ovum transport (which may account for the higher rate of ectopic pregnancy with these pills), and inhibition of implantation. Ovulation is inhibited inconsistently with this method. The minipill is begun on the first day of a menstrual cycle and then taken continuously for as long as contraception is desired.

B. Advantages: The low dose and absence of estrogen make the minipill safe during lactation; it may increase the flow of milk. It is often tried by women who want minimal doses of hormones and by patients who are over age 35. The minipill can be used by women with uterine myomas or sickle cell disease (S/S or S/C). Like the combined pill, the minipill decreases

the likelihood of pelvic inflammatory disease by its effect on cervical mucus.

C. Complications and Contraindications: Minipill users often have bleeding irregularities (eg, prolonged flow, spotting, or amenorrhea); such patients may need monthly pregnancy tests. Ectopic pregnancies are more frequent, and complaints of abdominal pain should be investigated with this in mind. The absolute contraindications and many of the relative contraindications listed in Table 13–4 apply to the minipill. Exceptions are mentioned in ¶ B, above. Minor side effects of combination oral contraceptives such as weight gain and mild headache may also occur with the minipill.

Rosenfield A: The pill: An evaluation of recent studies (risks and benefits). *Johns Hopkins Med J* 1982;**150**:177.

Sartwell PE, Stolley PD: Oral contraceptives and vascular disease. *Epidemiol Rev* 1982;**4**:95.

2. CONTRACEPTIVE INJECTIONS & IMPLANTS
(Long-Acting Progestins)

Injections of long-acting progestins such as medroxyprogesterone acetate or norethindrone enanthate are widely used in many countries. They are not approved for contraception in the USA because of FDA concerns about animal studies showing an increased incidence of associated breast and genital tract cancer. Injections are given at 3- to 6-month intervals. Pregnancy rates are as low as those of combined oral contraceptives taken conscientiously. Uterine bleeding may be irregular at first, and amenorrhea eventually occurs. Ovulation after the last injection may be delayed. Absolute and relative contraindications are similar to those of the minipill.

Subdermal implants of levonorgestrel or other progestins in polymer-based rods or capsules are undergoing clinical trials in various countries. These implants may be effective for several years.

3. INTRAUTERINE DEVICES
(IUDs)

IUDs in current use in the USA are the Lippes Loop and the Saf-T-Coil (all plastic) and the bioactive devices such as the Copper 7, Copper T, and Progestasert (which secretes progesterone into the uterus). Failure rates are 2–4%; the mechanism of action is thought to be prevention of implantation.

The all-plastic IUDs do not need to be replaced at a specific time, and some women use them for 10 years or more. The copper-bearing IUDs are more suitable for a smaller uterus; they must be replaced every 3 years for maximum efficacy. The progesterone-secreting IUDs must be replaced yearly but have the advantage of causing decreased cramping and menstrual flow.

The IUD is often an excellent contraceptive method for parous women with one sexual partner. It is less desirable for young nulliparas because of the greater threat of pelvic inflammatory disease in young women and the possible impairment of future fertility.

Insertion

Insertion can be performed during or after the menses, at midcycle to prevent implantation, or later in the cycle if the patient has not become pregnant. Immediate postpartum insertion with IUDs designed to minimize expulsion has been successful in some studies; most clinicians wait until 8 weeks postpartum. When insertion is performed during lactation, there is greater risk of uterine perforation or embedding of the IUD. Insertion immediately following abortion is acceptable if there is no sepsis and if follow-up insertion a month later will not be possible; otherwise, it is wise to wait until 4 weeks postabortion.

Contraindications & Complications

Contraindications to use of IUDs are outlined in Table 13–5.

A. Pregnancy: An IUD can be inserted within 5 days following a single episode of unprotected midcycle coitus as a postcoital contraceptive. An IUD should not be inserted into a pregnant uterus. If pregnancy occurs as an IUD failure, there is a greater chance of spontaneous abortion if the IUD is left in situ (50%) than if it is removed (25%). Spontaneous abortion with an IUD in place is associated with a high risk of severe sepsis, and death can occur rapidly. Women using an IUD who become pregnant should have the IUD removed if the string is visible. It can be removed at the time of therapeutic abortion if this is desired. If string is not visible and the patient wants to continue the pregnancy, she should be informed of the serious risk of sepsis and, occasionally, death with such pregnancies. She should be informed that any flulike symptoms such as fever, myalgia, headache, or nausea warrant immediate medical attention for possible septic abortion.

Table 13–5. Contraindications to IUD use.

Absolute contraindications

Pregnancy

Acute or subacute pelvic inflammatory disease or purulent cervicitis

Relative contraindications

Past history of pelvic inflammatory disease or ectopic pregnancy

Multiple sexual partners

Nulliparous woman concerned about future fertility

Lack of available follow-up care

Menorrhagia or severe dysmenorrhea

Cervical or uterine neoplasia

Abnormal size or shape of uterus, including myomas distorting cavity

Valvular heart disease

Diabetes

Since the ratio of ectopic to intrauterine pregnancies is increased among IUD wearers, clinicians should search carefully for adnexal masses in early pregnancy and should always check for remaining placental tissue following abortion.

B. Pelvic Inflammatory Disease: IUD use is associated with double the normal risk of pelvic inflammatory disease, and therefore the IUD should rarely be used by teenagers, women desiring more children, women with multiple sexual partners, and women with a past history of pelvic inflammatory disease or ectopic pregnancy. The IUD should never be inserted in the presence of cervicitis, endometritis, or salpingitis.

If pelvic infection develops, the signs and symptoms may be minimal at first. When infection is strongly suspected, the IUD should be removed and antibiotic treatment begun (see p 464). With pelvic pain in IUD users, it is wise to consider ectopic pregnancy in the differential diagnosis.

IUDs without transcervical tails appear to cause less pelvic inflammatory disease; however, they are more difficult to check at follow-up and require uterine instrumentation at removal.

C. Menorrhagia or Severe Dysmenorrhea: The IUD can cause heavier menstrual periods, bleeding between periods, and more cramping, so it is generally not suitable for women who already suffer from these problems. However, progesterone-secreting IUDs can be tried in these cases, as they often cause decreased bleeding and cramping with menses.

D. Complete or Partial Expulsion: Spontaneous expulsion of the IUD occurs in 10–20% of cases during the first year of use. Remove any IUD if the body of the device can be seen or felt in the cervical os.

E. Missing IUD Strings: If the transcervical tail cannot be seen, this may signify unnoticed expulsion, perforation of the uterus with abdominal migration of the IUD, or simply retraction of the string into the cervical canal or uterus owing to movement of the IUD or uterine growth with pregnancy. Once pregnancy is ruled out, one should probe for the IUD with a sterile sound or forceps designed for IUD removal, after administering a paracervical block. If the IUD cannot be detected, pelvic ultrasound will demonstrate the IUD if it is in the uterus. Alternatively, obtain anteroposterior and lateral x-rays of the pelvis with another IUD or a sound in the uterus as a marker, to confirm an extrauterine IUD. If the IUD is in the abdominal cavity, it should generally be removed by laparoscopy or laparotomy. Open-looped all-plastic IUDs such as the Lippes Loop can be left in the pelvis without danger, but ring-shaped IUDs may strangulate a loop of bowel and copper-bearing IUDs may cause tissue reaction and adhesions.

Perforations of the uterus are less likely if insertion is performed slowly, with meticulous care taken to follow directions applicable to each type of IUD. Once the Lippes Loop has been drawn up into the insertor, it should be used immediately; it should *never* be preloaded and left in the insertor.

Burkman R et al: The relationship of genital tract actinomycetes and the development of pelvic inflammatory disease. *Am J Obstet Gynecol* 1982;**143**:585.

Kaufman DW et al: The effect of different types of intrauterine devices on the risk of pelvic inflammatory disease. *JAMA* 1983;**250**:759.

Tatum HJ: Milestones in intrauterine device development. *Fertil Steril* 1983;**39**:141.

4. DIAPHRAGM & CERVICAL CAP

The diaphragm (with contraceptive jelly) is a safe and effective contraceptive method with features that make it acceptable to some women and not others. Failure rates range from 2 to 20%, depending on the motivation of the woman and the care with which the diaphragm is used. The advantages of this method are that it has no systemic side effects and gives significant protection against pelvic infection and cervical dysplasia as well as pregnancy. The disadvantages are that it must be inserted near the time of coitus and that pressure from the rim predisposes some women to cystitis after intercourse.

The cervical cap (with contraceptive jelly) is similar to the diaphragm but fits snugly over the cervix only (the diaphragm stretches from behind the cervix to behind the pubic symphysis). The cervical cap is more difficult to insert and remove than the diaphragm and is associated with a higher failure rate. The main advantages are that it can be used by women who cannot be fitted for a diaphragm because of a relaxed anterior vaginal wall or by women who have discomfort or develop repeated bladder infections with the diaphragm.

Because of the small risk of toxic shock syndrome, a cervical cap or diaphragm should not be left in the vagina for over 12–18 hours, nor should these devices be used during the menstrual period (see p 453).

Koch JP: The Prentif contraceptive cervical cap: A contemporary study of its clinical safety and effectiveness. *Contraception* 1982;**25**:135.

5. CONTRACEPTIVE SPONGE, FOAM, CREAM, JELLY, & SUPPOSITORY

These products are available without prescription, are easy to use, and are fairly effective, with reported failure rates of 2–29%. All contain the spermicides nonoxynol 9 or octoxynol 9. The contraceptive sponge is inserted before intercourse and can be used for repeated acts of intercourse but should not be left in the vagina for longer than 12–18 hours, because of the risk of toxic shock syndrome (see p 453). Foams, creams, jellies, and suppositories also have the advantages of being simple to use and easily available. Their disadvantage is a slightly higher failure rate than with the diaphragm or condom. Teratogenesis due to spermicides used at the time of conception is under study; no correlation has been proved, but one recent study showed a 25% increase in female births among women using spermicides at the time of conception.

6. CONDOM

The male sheath of rubber or animal membrane affords good protection against pregnancy — equivalent to that of a diaphragm and spermicidal jelly; it also offers protection against sexually transmitted disease and cervical dysplasia. When a spermicide such as vaginal foam is used with the condom, the failure rate approaches that of oral contraceptives. Condoms coated with spermicide are now available in the USA. The disadvantages are dulling of sensation and sperm loss due to tearing, slipping, or leakage with detumescence of the penis.

7. CONTRACEPTION BASED ON AWARENESS OF FERTILE PERIODS

There is renewed interest in methods to identify times of ovulation and avoidance of unprotected intercourse at that time as a means of family planning. These methods are most effective when the couple restricts intercourse to the postovular phase of the cycle or uses a barrier method at other times. Women benefit from learning to identify their fertile periods. Well-instructed, motivated couples may achieve low pregnancy rates with fertility awareness, but in many field trials, the pregnancy rates were as high as 20%.

"Symptothermal" Natural Family Planning
The basis for this approach is patient-observed increase in clear elastic cervical mucus, brief abdominal midcycle discomfort ("mittelschmerz"), and a sustained rise of the basal body temperature about 2 weeks after onset of menstruation. Unprotected intercourse is avoided from shortly after the menstrual period, when fertile mucus is first identified, until 48 hours after ovulation, as identified by a sustained rise in temperature and the disappearance of clear elastic mucus.

Calendar Method
After the length of the menstrual cycle has been observed for at least 8 months (preferably for 1 year), the following calculations are made: (1) The first fertile day is determined by subtracting 18 days from the shortest cycle; (2) the last fertile day is determined by subtracting 11 days from the longest cycle. For example, if the observed cycles run from 24 to 28 days, the fertile period would extend from the sixth day of the cycle (24 minus 18) through the seventeenth day (28 minus 11). It is essential to base the calculations upon a written record of the woman's menstrual periods — not on her memory or testimony alone. Other variations of this method are also used.

Basal Body Temperature Method

Much effort and interest are required by the patient in order to make an accurate basal temperature chart. (The temperature must be taken immediately upon awakening, before any activity.) A slight drop in temperature often occurs 1–1½ days before ovulation, and a rise of about 0.4 °C (0.7 °F) occurs 1–2 days after ovulation. The elevated temperature continues throughout the remainder of the cycle. The second day after the rise marks the end of the fertile period.

Parenteau-Carreau S: The sympto-thermal methods (of family planning). *Int J Fertil* 1981;**26**:170.

Pérez A: Natural family planning: Postpartum period. *Int J Fertil* 1981;**26**:219.

Periodic abstinence: How well do new approaches work? Population Information Program, Johns Hopkins Univ (Sept) 1981; **9**:33.

8. POSTCOITAL CONTRACEPTION

If unprotected intercourse occurs in midcycle and the woman is certain she has not inadvertently become pregnant earlier in the cycle, the following regimens are effective in preventing implantation. The failure rate is less than 1.5%. These methods should be started within 72 hours after coitus. (1) Ethinyl estradiol, 2.5 mg twice daily for 5 days. (2) Diethylstilbestrol, 25 mg twice daily for 5 days. (3) Ovral (50 μg of ethinyl estradiol with 0.5 mg of norgestrel), 2 tablets at once followed by 2 tablets 12 hours later. Antinausea medication may be necessary with these regimens. Bleeding should occur within 3–4 weeks. If pregnancy occurs, abortion is advisable because of fetal exposure to possibly teratogenic doses of sex steroids.

IUD insertion within 5 days after one episode of unprotected midcycle coitus will also prevent pregnancy; copper-bearing IUDs have been tested for this purpose. The disadvantage of this method is possible infection, especially in rape cases; the advantage is ongoing contraceptive protection if this is desired in a patient for whom the IUD is a suitable choice.

Rowlands S, Guilleband J: Postcoital contraception. *Br J Fam Plann* 1981;**7**:3.

Yuzpe AA, Smith RP, Rademaker AW: A multicenter clinical investigation employing ethinyl estradiol combined with dl-norgestrel as a postcoital contraceptive agent. *Fertil Steril* 1982;**37**:508.

9. ABORTION

Since the legalization of abortion in the USA in 1973, the related maternal mortality rate has fallen markedly, because illegal and self-induced abortions have been replaced by safer medical procedures. Abortions in the first trimester of pregnancy are performed by vacuum aspiration under local anesthesia. A similar technique, dilatation and evacuation, is often used in the second trimester, with general or local anesthesia.

Techniques utilizing intra-amniotic instillation of hypertonic saline solution or prostaglandins are also used after 15 weeks from the LMP. Abortions are rarely performed after 20 weeks from the LMP. It is currently believed that fetal viability begins at about 24 weeks. Legal abortion has a mortality rate of 1:100,000. Rates of morbidity and mortality rise with length of gestation. Currently in the USA, 90% of abortions are performed before 12 weeks' gestation and only 3–4% after 17 weeks. Every effort should be made to continue the trend toward earlier abortion.

Complications resulting from abortion include retained products of conception (often associated with infection and heavy bleeding) and unrecognized ectopic pregnancy. Immediate analysis of the removed tissue for placenta can exclude or corroborate the diagnosis of ectopic pregnancy. Women presenting with fever, bleeding, or abdominal pain after abortion should be examined; use of broad-spectrum antibiotics or reaspiration of the uterus (or both) are frequently necessary. Hospitalization is advisable if acute salpingitis requires intravenous administration of antibiotics (see p 464). Complications following illegal abortion often need emergency care for hemorrhage, septic shock, or uterine perforation.

Rh immune globulin should be given to all Rh-negative women following abortion. Contraception should be thoroughly discussed and contraceptive devices or pills supplied at the time of abortion.

Long-term sequelae of repeated induced abortions have been studied, but as yet there is no consensus on whether there are increased rates of fetal loss or premature labor. It is felt that such adverse sequelae can be minimized by performing early abortion with minimal cervical dilatation or by the use of *Laminaria* to induce gradual cervical dilatation.

Cates W: Legal abortion: The public health record. *Science* 1982;**215**:1586.

10. STERILIZATION

In the USA, sterilization is the most popular method of birth control for couples who want no more children. Although sterilization is reversible in some instances, reversal surgery in both men and women is costly, complicated, and not always successful. Therefore, patients should be counseled carefully before sterilization and should view the procedure as final.

Vasectomy is a safe, simple procedure in which the vas deferens is severed and sealed through a scrotal incision under local anesthesia. Long-term follow-up studies on vasectomized men show no excess risk of heart disease, cancer, or immune system problems.

Female sterilization is currently performed via laparoscopic bipolar electrocoagulation or plastic ring application of the uterine tubes or via minilaparotomy with Pomeroy tubal resection. The advantages of laparoscopy are minimal postoperative pain, small incisions, and rapid recovery. The advantages of minilaparotomy are that it can be performed with standard surgical instruments under local or general anesthesia. However, there is more postoperative pain and a longer recovery period. Failure rates after tubal sterilization are less than 0.5%. There is no documented increased incidence of menstrual disturbance after tubal sterilization.

DeStefano F et al: Menstrual changes after tubal sterilization. *Obstet Gynecol* 1983;**62**:673.

Petitti DB et al: Vasectomy and the incidence of hospitalized illness. *J Urol* 1983;**129**:760.

RAPE

Rape, or sexual assault, is legally defined in different ways in various jurisdictions. Physicians and emergency room personnel who deal with rape victims should be familiar with the laws pertaining to sexual assault in their own state. From a medical and psychologic viewpoint, it is essential that persons treating rape victims recognize the nonconsensual and violent nature of the crime. About 95% of reported rape victims are women. Penetration may be vaginal, anal, or oral and may be by the penis, hand, or a foreign object.

"Unlawful sexual intercourse," or statutory rape, is intercourse with a female before the age of majority even with her consent.

Rape represents an expression of anger, power, and sexuality on the part of the rapist. The rapist is usually a hostile man who uses sexual intercourse to terrorize and humiliate a woman. Women neither secretly want to be raped, nor do they expect, encourage, or enjoy rape.

Rape involves severe physical injury in 5–10% of cases and is always a terrifying experience in which most victims fear for their lives. Consequently, all victims suffer some psychologic aftermath. Moreover, some may acquire sexually transmissible disease or become pregnant.

Because rape is a personal crisis, each patient will react differently. The rape-trauma syndrome comprises 2 principal phases:

(1) Immediate or acute–Shaking, sobbing, and restless activity may last from a few days to a few weeks. The patient may experience anger, guilt, shame, and fear of revenge or may repress these emotions. Reactions vary depending on the victim's personality and the circumstances of the attack.

(2) Late or chronic–Problems related to the attack may develop weeks or months later. The life-style and work patterns of the individual may change. Sleep disorders or phobias often develop. Loss of self-esteem can rarely lead to suicide.

Physicians and emergency room personnel who deal with rape victims should work with community rape crisis centers whenever possible to provide ongoing supportive, skilled counseling.

General Office Procedures

The physician who first sees the alleged rape victim should be empathetic. Begin with a statement such as "This is a terrible thing that has happened to you. I want to help."

(1) Secure written consent from the patient, guardian, or next of kin for gynecologic examination; for photographs if they are likely to be useful as evidence; and for notification of police. If police are to be notified, do so, and obtain advice on the transfer of evidence.

(2) Obtain and record the history in the patient's own words. The sequence of events, ie, the time, place, and circumstances, must be included. Note the date of the LMP, whether or not the woman is pregnant, and the time of the most recent coitus prior to the sexual assault. Note the details of the assault such as body cavities penetrated, use of foreign objects, and number of assailants.

Note whether the alleged victim is calm, agitated, or confused (drugs or alcohol may be involved). Record whether the patient came directly to the hospital or whether she bathed or changed her clothing. Record findings but do not issue even a tentative diagnosis lest it be erroneous or incomplete. Do not use the word "rape" in the recorded history.

(3) Have the patient disrobe while standing on a white sheet. Hair, dirt, and leaves; underclothing; and any torn or stained clothing should be kept as evidence. Scrape material from beneath fingernails and comb pubic hair for evidence. Place all evidence in separate clean paper bags or envelopes and label carefully.

(4) Examine the patient, noting any traumatized areas that should be photographed. Examine the body and genitals with a Wood light to identify semen, which fluoresces; positive areas should be swabbed with a premoistened swab and air-dried in order to identify acid phosphatase from prostatic secretions.

(5) Perform a pelvic examination, explaining all procedures and obtaining the patient's consent before proceeding gently with the examination. (In children, general anesthesia may be necessary during the pelvic examination or for repair of vaginal lacerations.) Use a narrow speculum lubricated with water only. Collect material with sterile cotton swabs from the vaginal walls and cervix and make 2 air-dried smears on clean glass slides. Swab the mouth (around molars and cheeks) and anus in the same way, if appropriate. Label all slides carefully. Collect secretions from the vagina, anus, or mouth with a premoistened cotton swab, place at once on a slide with a drop of saline, and cover with a coverslip. Look for motile or nonmotile sperm under high, dry magnification, and record the percentage of motile forms.

(6) Perform appropriate laboratory tests as follows. Culture the vagina, anus, or mouth (as appropriate) for *N gonorrhoeae* and *Chlamydia*. Perform a pregnancy test, Papanicolaou smear of the cervix, and VDRL test. Repeat the pregnancy test if the next menses is missed, and repeat the VDRL test in 6 weeks. Obtain blood (10 mL without anticoagulant)

and urine (100 mL) specimens if there is a history of forced ingestion or injection of drugs or alcohol.

(7) Transfer clearly labeled evidence, eg, laboratory specimens, directly to the clinical pathologist in charge or to the responsible laboratory technician, in the presence of witnesses (never via messenger), so that the rules of evidence will not be breached.

Submit marked clothing, photographs, slides, etc, to the police as evidence, and obtain a written receipt.

Treatment

(1) Give analgesics or tranquilizers if indicated.

(2) Administer tetanus toxoid if deep lacerations contain soil or dirt particles.

(3) Give prophylactic probenecid, 1 g orally, and 30 minutes later aqueous penicillin G, 4.8 million units intramuscularly, to prevent syphilis and gonorrhea. If the victim is allergic to penicillin, give tetracycline, 500 mg 4 times daily for 10 days.

(4) Prevent pregnancy by using one of the methods discussed under Postcoital Contraception, if necessary (see p 475).

(5) Make sure the patient and her family and friends have a source of ongoing psychologic support.

Hicks DJ: Rape: Sexual assault. *Am J Obstet Gynecol* 1980; **137:**931.

MENOPAUSAL SYNDROME

Essentials of Diagnosis

- Cessation of menses due to aging or to bilateral oophorectomy.
- Elevation of FSH and LH levels.
- Hot flushes and night sweats (in 80% of women).
- Decreased vaginal lubrication; thinned vaginal mucosa with or without dyspareunia.

General Considerations

The term "menopause" refers to the final cessation of menstruation, either as a normal part of aging or as the result of surgical removal of both ovaries. In a broader sense, as the term is commonly used, it denotes a 1- to 3-year period during which a woman adjusts to a diminishing and then absent menstrual flow and the physiologic changes that may be associated—hot flushes, night sweats, and vaginal dryness or soreness with coitus.

The average age at menopause in Western societies today is 50–51 years. Premature menopause is defined as ovarian failure and menstrual cessation before age 40; this often has a genetic basis. Surgical menopause due to bilateral oophorectomy is common and can cause more severe symptoms owing to the sudden rapid drop in sex hormone levels.

There is no objective evidence that cessation of ovarian function is associated with increased emotional disturbance or personality changes. However, the time of menopause often coincides with other major life changes, such as departure of children from home, a midlife identity crisis, or divorce. These events, coupled with a sense of the loss of youth, may exacerbate the symptoms of menopause and cause psychologic distress.

Clinical Findings

A. Symptoms and Signs:

1. Cessation of menstruation–Menstrual cycles generally become irregular as menopause approaches. Anovular cycles occur more often, with irregular cycle length and occasional menorrhagia. Menstrual flow usually diminishes in amount owing to decreased estrogen secretion, resulting in less abundant endometrial growth. Finally, cycles become longer, with missed periods or episodes of spotting only. When no bleeding has occurred for one year, the menopausal transition can be said to have occurred. Any bleeding after this time warrants investigation by endometrial curettage or aspiration to rule out endometrial cancer.

2. Hot flushes–Hot flushes (feelings of intense heat over the trunk and face, with flushing of the skin and sweating) occur in 80% of women as a result of the sudden decrease in ovarian hormones. An increase in pulsatile release of gonadotropin-releasing hormone from the hypothalamus is believed to trigger the hot flushes by disturbing the adjacent temperature-regulating area of the brain. Hot flushes are more severe in women who undergo surgical menopause. Flushing is more pronounced late in the day, during hot weather, after ingestion of hot foods or drinks, or during periods of tension. Occurring at night, they often cause sweating and insomnia and result in fatigue on the following day.

3. Dyspareunia–With decreased estrogen secretion, thinning of the vaginal mucosa and decreased vaginal lubrication occur and may lead to dyspareunia. The introitus decreases in diameter. Pelvic examination reveals pale, smooth vaginal mucosa and a small cervix and uterus. The ovaries are not normally palpable after the menopause. Continued sexual activity will help prevent tissue shrinkage; use of lubricants, estrogen or testosterone cream, or oral estrogen therapy can prevent or relieve pain.

4. Osteoporosis–Osteoporosis may occur as a late sequela of menopause, with about 25% of women eventually developing fractures or loss of height and back pain due to vertebral compression. Hip and vertebral fractures with ensuing complications are significant causes of morbidity in elderly women. Risk factors for osteoporosis are listed in Table 13–6. Osteoporosis can be prevented or halted by hormone replacement therapy, calcium therapy, exercise, and other changes in life-style.

B. Laboratory Findings: Vaginal cytologic examination will show a low estrogen effect with predominantly parabasal cells. Serum FSH and LH levels are elevated.

Table 13–6. Risk factors for osteoporosis.

Genetic or Medical Factors	Life-style Factors
All races except blacks	High alcohol use
Previous fractures not due to major trauma	Smoking
	Lack of exercise
Female relatives with osteoporosis	Low dietary intake of calcium
Thin body habitus	
Early menopause (before age 40)	Lack of vitamin D
Inflammatory bowel disease; bowel resection	High-protein or high-salt diet (promotes calciuria)
Prolonged use of cortisone, desiccated thyroid (>2 grains), Dilantin, or aluminum-containing antacids	High caffeine use (more than 5 cups of coffee daily)
Kidney disease necessitating dialysis	

Treatment

A. Natural Menopause: Education and support from health providers, midlife discussion groups, and reading material will help most women having difficulty adjusting to the menopause. Physiologic symptoms can be treated as follows:

1. Vasomotor symptoms–Give conjugated estrogens, 0.625 mg (or ethinyl estradiol, 0.02 mg, or estrone sulfate, 0.625 mg) from days 1 to 25 of each calendar month. If the uterus is intact, add a progestin (medroxyprogesterone acetate, 10 mg, or norethindrone acetate, 2.5–5 mg) on days 16–25, to prevent endometrial hyperplasia or cancer. Withhold hormones from day 26 until the end of the month, when the endometrium will be shed, producing a light, generally painless monthly period. If the patient has had a hysterectomy, a progestin need not be used. Explain to the patient that hot flushes will probably return if the hormone is discontinued. When women wish to stop hormone therapy, the dose should be tapered.

2. Dyspareunia–This problem can be treated with hormone therapy as outlined above. Alternatively, topical use of hormone creams in small doses will often relieve pain with minimal systemic absorption. Use conjugated estrogen vaginal cream, one-eighth applicatorful (0.3 mg of conjugated estrogen) nightly for 7–10 nights. Thereafter, use every other night or twice weekly. Dienestrol cream can also be used. Testosterone propionate 1–2% in a vanishing cream base used in the same manner is also effective if estrogen is contraindicated. A bland lubricant such as unscented cold cream or water-soluble gel can be helpful at the time of coitus.

3. Osteoporosis–Women should ingest at least 800 mg of calcium daily throughout life. In addition, 1 g of elemental calcium (as calcium carbonate) should be taken as a daily supplement at the time of the menopause and thereafter. Vitamin D, 400 IU/d from food, sunlight, or supplements is necessary to enhance calcium absorption. A daily program of energetic walking or other physical exercise helps maintain bone mass. CT scans and photon absorptiometry will detect demineralization of the vertebral bodies and cortical bone, but both tests are expensive. At present, factors indicated in Table 13–6 adequately identify patients most in need of hormone therapy. Dosage is usually the same as for treatment of vasomotor symptoms. Regular follow-up is needed with ongoing treatment.

B. Surgical Menopause: The abrupt hormonal decrease resulting from oophorectomy generally results in severe vasomotor symptoms and rapid onset of dyspareunia and osteoporosis unless treated. Estrogen replacement is generally started immediately after surgery. Conjugated estrogen, 1.25 mg (or ethinyl estradiol 0.05 mg, or estrone sulfate, 1.25 mg), is given for 25 days of each month. After age 45–50 years, this dose can be tapered to 0.625 mg of conjugated estrogen or equivalent.

C. Contraindications to Estrogen Therapy: Women with conditions listed in Table 13–7 should generally not use estrogen. Progestins can be substituted in some cases but are not advisable for patients with diabetes or circulatory disease. At present, there is little evidence that postmenopausal estrogens are associated with breast cancer development. Estrogens must be given with progestins as outlined above in women who have a uterus, to avoid endometrial cancer. Most authorities believe that estrogen in low doses will retard atherosclerosis by raising high-density lipoprotein levels, but progestins have the opposite effect. Estrogen causes growth of uterine myomas, which otherwise shrink after the menopause.

Deutsch S, Ossowski R, Benjamin I: Comparison between degree of systemic absorption of vaginally and orally administered estrogens at different dose levels in postmenopausal women. *Am J Obstet Gynecol* 1981;**139:**967.

Gambrell RD, Gagnell CA, Greenblatt RB: Role of estrogens and progesterone in the etiology and prevention of endometrial cancer: Review. *Am J Obstet Gynecol* 1983;**146:**696.

Judd HL et al: Estrogen replacement therapy: Indications and complications. *Ann Intern Med* 1983;**98:**195.

Table 13–7. Contraindications to estrogen therapy.

Cancer of the breast or uterus
Estrogen-dependent ovarian cancer
History of thromboembolic disease
Hypertension
Diabetes
Hepatic adenoma or other significant liver disease
Gallstones or gallbladder disease
Large uterine myomas

OBSTETRICS

DIAGNOSIS & DIFFERENTIAL DIAGNOSIS OF PREGNANCY

It is advantageous to diagnose pregnancy as promptly as possible when a sexually active woman misses a menstrual period or has symptoms suggestive of pregnancy. In the event of a wanted pregnancy, she can begin prenatal care early and discontinue use of recreational drugs (eg, alcohol, tobacco, marihuana, caffeine) or potentially teratogenic medication in the critical weeks of embryogenesis in the first trimester. In the event of an unwanted pregnancy, she can consider termination of the pregnancy at an early stage.

Pregnancy Tests

Currently available tests permit very early diagnosis of pregnancy, sometimes even before the time of the missed menses. All urine or blood tests rely on the detection of hCG produced by the placenta. hCG levels increase shortly after implantation, reach a peak at 50–90 days, and fall to lower levels in the second and third trimesters. Some pregnancy tests do not distinguish between LH and hCG and may therefore show false-positive results due to the LH surge during ovulation or menopause. A concentrated first morning urine specimen is desirable to prevent false-negative results.

Compared with intrauterine pregnancies, ectopic pregnancies may show lower levels of hCG, which level off or fall in serial determinations. Less sensitive urine tests may not be positive in ectopic pregnancies. Some currently used pregnancy tests and their sensitivities are shown in Table 13–8.

Manifestations of Pregnancy

The following symptoms and signs are usually due to pregnancy, but none are diagnostic. A record or history of time and frequency of coitus may be of considerable value.

A. Symptoms: Amenorrhea, nausea and vomiting, breast tenderness and tingling, urinary frequency and urgency, "quickening" (may be noted at about the 18th week), weight gain.

B. Signs (in Weeks From LMP): Breast changes (enlargement, vascular engorgement, colostrum), abdominal enlargement, cyanosis of vagina and cervical portio (about the seventh week), softening of the cervix (seventh week), softening of the cervico-uterine junction (eighth week), irregular softening and slight enlargement of the fundus (about the sixth week), generalized enlargement and diffuse softening of the corpus (after eighth week).

By 14–15 weeks from the LMP, the uterine fundus is palpable above the pubic symphysis, and by 20–22 weeks, it has reached the umbilicus. By 28 weeks it is usually halfway between the umbilicus and the xiphoid process, and by 38 weeks it has reached the xiphoid process. The fetal heart can be heard at the end of the first trimester with an ultrasonic stethoscope and by 20 weeks with an ordinary fetoscope.

Differential Diagnosis of Pregnancy

The nonpregnant uterus enlarged by myomas can be confused with the gravid uterus, but it is usually very firm and irregular. An ovarian tumor may be found midline, displacing the nonpregnant uterus to the side or posteriorly. Ultrasonography and a pregnancy test will help make an accurate diagnosis in these circumstances.

Khan-Dawood FS, Dawood MY: How early can pregnancy be detected? *Female Patient* (July) 1983;**8:**22.

NUTRITION IN PREGNANCY

Nutrition in pregnancy significantly affects maternal health and infant size and well-being. Pregnant women should have nutrition counseling early in prenatal care and access to supplementary food programs if they lack funds for adequate nutrition. Counseling should stress abstention from alcohol, smoking, and drugs. Caffeine and artificial sweeteners should be used only in small amounts. "Empty calories" should be avoided, and the diet should contain the following foods: protein foods of animal and vegetable origin; milk and milk products; whole-grain cereals and

Table 13–8. Selected diagnostic tests for pregnancy.

Test	Sensitivity (in mIU of hCG/mL)	Comments
Slide test with urine	1000–3000	Hemagglutination (or agglutination) inhibition tests to detect hCG. Convenient for office use. Quick and inexpensive. Accurate 4 weeks after conception. May cross-react with LH.
Tube test with urine	500–1000	As above. May be accurate 2–4 weeks after conception. May cross-react with LH.
Monoclonal antibody test with urine	125–1000	Colorimetric test. Some designed for home use. Accurate 2–4 weeks after conception. Specific for hCG.
Radioreceptor-assay test with serum (RRA)	200	May be accurate 2 weeks after conception. May cross-react with LH.
Radioimmunoassay (RIA)	5–50	Some tests accurate 1 week after conception. Specific for hCG. Also used for quantitative assays in abnormal pregnancies (molar, ectopic, threatened abortion).

breads; and fruits and vegetables, especially green leafy vegetables.

Weight gain in pregnancy should be at least 11 kg, which includes the added weight of the fetus, placenta, and amniotic fluid and of maternal reproductive tissues, fluid, blood, increased fat stores, and increased lean body mass. Maternal fat stores are a caloric reserve for pregnancy and lactation; weight restriction in pregnancy to avoid developing such fat stores may affect the development of other fetal and maternal tissues and is not advisable. Even obese women should gain 9–11 kg. Normally, a pregnant woman gains 1–2 kg in the first trimester and slightly less than 0.5 kg/wk thereafter. She needs approximately an extra 300 kcal/d (depending on energy output) and 30 g/d of additional protein, for a total protein intake of about 75 g/d. Appropriate caloric intake in pregnancy helps prevent infants of low birth weight.

Rigid salt restriction is not necessary. While the consumption of highly salted snack foods and prepared foods is not desirable, 2–3 g/d of sodium is permissible. The increased calcium needs of pregnancy (1200 mg/d) can be met with milk, milk products, green vegetables, soybean products, corn tortillas, and soup stock made with bones and cooked with a small amount of vinegar to release calcium from the bones.

The increased need for iron and folic acid should be met from foods as well as vitamin and mineral supplements. (See section on anemia in pregnancy.) Megavitamins should not be taken in pregnancy, as they may result in fetal malformation or disturbed metabolism. However, a balanced prenatal supplement containing iron, folate, and the recommended daily allowances of various vitamins and minerals is widely used in the USA and is probably beneficial to many women with marginal diets. There is some evidence that prenatal vitamin supplements decrease the risk of neural tube defects in the fetus. Lactovegetarians and ovolactovegetarians do well in pregnancy; vegetarian women who eat neither eggs nor milk products should take oral vitamin B_{12} supplements during pregnancy and lactation.

Smithells RW et al: Possible prevention of neural tube defects by periconceptional vitamin supplementation. *Lancet* 1980; **1**:339.

Susser M: Prenatal nutrition, birth weight, and psychological development: An overview of experiments, quasi experiments and natural experiments in the past decade. *Am J Clin Nutr* 1981;**34**:784.

VOMITING OF PREGNANCY
(Morning Sickness)
& HYPEREMESIS GRAVIDARUM
(Pernicious Vomiting of Pregnancy)

Essentials of Diagnosis

- Morning or evening nausea and vomiting usually begin soon after the first missed period and cease after the fourth to fifth months of gestation.

- Dehydration, acidosis, and nutritional deficiencies may develop with protracted vomiting.

General Considerations

At least half of women, most of them primiparas, complain of nausea and vomiting during early pregnancy. It is common with multiple pregnancy and hydatidiform mole. Persistent severe vomiting during pregnancy—hyperemesis gravidarum—can be disabling and require hospitalization.

The cause of vomiting during pregnancy is believed to be high estrogen levels.

Clinical Findings

A. Symptoms and Signs: Symptoms are most severe in the morning upon arising. Nutritional deficiencies almost never occur in previously well-nourished women. Hyperemesis gravidarum that continues unchecked is characterized by dehydration, acidosis, weight loss, and avitaminosis.

B. Laboratory Findings: Severe vomiting causes hemoconcentration, alkalosis, and electrolyte imbalance. Ketone bodies are present in the concentrated urine specimen.

Differential Diagnosis

Vomiting during pregnancy may be due to any of the diseases with which vomiting is usually associated, eg, infections, poisoning, neoplastic diseases, hyperthyroidism, gastric disorders, gallbladder disease, intestinal obstruction, hiatal hernia, diabetic acidosis, and uremia due to any cause.

Treatment

A. Mild Nausea and Vomiting of Pregnancy: Reassurance and dietary advice are all that is required in many instances. Frequent small meals of nutritious, easily digested low-fat foods should be suggested. Begin prenatal vitamin and mineral supplements as soon as tolerated.

Because of possible teratogenicity, the use of drugs during the first half of pregnancy should be restricted to those of major importance to life and health. Antiemetics, antihistamines, and antispasmodics are generally unnecessary to treat nausea of pregnancy. Vitamin B_6 (pyridoxine), 50–100 mg/d orally, is nontoxic and may be helpful in some patients.

B. Hyperemesis Gravidarum: Hospitalize the patient in a private room at bed rest. Give nothing by mouth for 48 hours, and maintain normal nutrition and electrolyte balance by giving appropriate parenteral fluids and vitamin supplements as indicated. If there is no response after 48 hours, institute nasogastric tube feeding of a well-balanced formula by slow drip. Occasionally, total parenteral nutrition may be necessary. As soon as possible, place the patient on a dry diet consisting of 6 small feedings daily with clear liquids 1 hour after eating. Prochlorperazine rectal suppositories may be useful, and psychosocial consultation is advisable.

If the clinical situation continues to deteriorate, therapeutic abortion may be required.

Prognosis

Vomiting of pregnancy is self-limited, and the prognosis is good. Intractable hyperemesis gravidarum can be a threat to the life of the mother and the fetus.

Hew LR, Deital M: Total parenteral nutrition in gynecology and obstetrics. *Obstet Gynecol* 1980;**55**:464.

Katon WJ et al: Hyperemesis gravidarum: A biopsychosocial perspective. *Int J Psychiatry Med* 1980;**10**:151.

SPONTANEOUS ABORTION

Essentials of Diagnosis

- Vaginal bleeding in a pregnant woman before the 20th week of gestation.
- Uterine cramping.
- Disappearance of symptoms and signs of pregnancy.
- Negative or equivocal pregnancy tests.
- The products of conception may or may not be expelled.

General Considerations

Abortion is defined as termination of gestation before the 20th week of pregnancy. About three-fourths of spontaneous abortions occur before the 16th week of gestation; of these, three-fourths occur before the eighth week. About 15% of all pregnancies terminate in spontaneous abortion.

More than 60% of spontaneous abortions result from ovular defects due to maternal or paternal factors; about 15% are caused by maternal trauma, infections, dietary deficiencies, diabetes mellitus, hypothyroidism, poisoning, or anatomic malformations. There is no reliable evidence that abortion may be induced by psychic stimuli such as severe fright, grief, anger, or anxiety. In about one-fourth of cases, the cause of abortion cannot be determined.

It is important to identify those cases of late abortion (after 16 weeks) that result from cervical incompetence, since this is treatable. Often these women will have a history of late abortions associated with spontaneous rupture of the membranes and minimal labor. Some will have a history of wide cervical dilatation during D&C. In the nonpregnant state, an incompetent cervix will easily admit a dilator 8 mm in diameter.

Clinical Findings

A. Symptoms and Signs:

1. Threatened abortion–Bleeding or cramping occurs, but the pregnancy continues.

2. Inevitable abortion–The passage of some or all of the products of conception is impending. Bleeding and cramping persist, and the cervix is effaced and dilated.

3. Complete abortion–All of the conceptus is expelled. The fetus and the placenta may be expelled separately. When the entire conceptus has been expelled, pain ceases but spotting persists.

4. Incomplete abortion–A significant portion of the pregnancy (usually a placental fragment) remains in the uterus. Only mild cramps are reported, but bleeding is persistent and often excessive.

5. Missed abortion–The pregnancy has ceased to develop for at least 1 month, but the conceptus has not been expelled. Symptoms of pregnancy disappear. There is a brownish vaginal discharge but no free bleeding. Pain does not develop. The cervix is semifirm and slightly patulous; the uterus becomes smaller and irregularly softened; the adnexa are normal.

B. Laboratory Findings:
Pregnancy tests show low or falling levels of hCG. A complete blood count should be obtained if bleeding is heavy. Determine Rh type, and give Rh immune globulin if the type is Rh-negative. All tissue recovered should be assessed by a pathologist.

C. Ultrasonographic Findings:
An expert ultrasonographer can identify a gestational sac at 6 weeks from the LMP and a fetal pole at 7 weeks. Serial observations are often required to evaluate changes in size. A small, irregular sac without a fetal pole is diagnostic of a failing pregnancy.

Differential Diagnosis

The bleeding that occurs in abortion of a uterine pregnancy must be differentiated from the abnormal bleeding of an ectopic pregnancy and anovular bleeding in a nonpregnant woman. The passage of hydropic villi in the bloody discharge is diagnostic of the abortion of a hydatidiform mole.

Complications

Hemorrhage in abortion is a major cause of maternal death. Infection is common after illegally induced abortion or spontaneous abortion associated with an IUD.

Treatment

A. General Measures:

1. Threatened abortion requires 24–48 hours of bed rest followed by gradual resumption of usual activities, with abstinence from coitus and use of douches. Hormonal treatment is contraindicated. Antibiotics should be used only if there are signs of infection.

2. Missed abortion requires counseling regarding the fate of the pregnancy and planning for its elective termination at a time chosen by the patient and physician. Insertion of *Laminaria* stems to dilate the cervix followed by aspiration is the method of choice. Prostaglandin vaginal suppositories are an effective alternative.

B. Emergency Measures:

1. Incomplete abortion requires prompt removal of any products of conception remaining within the uterus. Analgesia and a paracervical block are useful,

followed by uterine exploration with ovum forceps or uterine aspiration.

2. If shock is present, intravenous fluids or blood may be necessary, as well as other intensive care measures.

3. Uterine contraction to expel clots and tissue may be stimulated by oxytocin infusion (40 units in 1000 mL of intravenous fluid). If the uterus is empty, 0.2 mg of methylergonovine maleate (Methergine) may be used to induce uterine spasm.

C. Surgical Measures: In the second trimester of pregnancy, an incompetent cervix can be closed by cerclage using a 5-mm woven Dacron strip (Shirodkar method) or circumsuture with braided silk (McDonald method).

Grimes DA, Cates W Jr, Selik RM: Fatal septic abortion in the United States, 1975–1977. *Obstet Gynecol* 1981;**57**:739.

Ladefoged C: Hydrop degeneration: A histopathological investigation of 260 early abortions. *Acta Obstet Gynecol Scand* 1980;**59**:509.

RECURRENT (HABITUAL) ABORTION

Recurrent, or habitual, abortion has been defined for years as the loss of 3 or more previable (< 500 g) pregnancies in succession. Recurrent or chronic abortion occurs in about 0.4–0.8% of all pregnancies. Abnormalities related to repeated abortion can be identified in approximately half of the couples.

Recurrent abortion is a clinical rather than pathologic diagnosis. The clinical findings are similar to those observed in other types of abortion (see above).

Treatment

The entire program of therapy rather than any single aspect of it will be responsible for success or failure. Most regimens include frequent visits and abundant reassurance.

A. General Measures:

1. Preconception therapy is aimed at detection of maternal or paternal defects that may contribute to abortion. A thorough general and gynecologic examination is essential. Chromosome assessment is indicated when abortion recurs. The competence of the cervical os must be determined. Hysterography (for tumor or congenital anomalies), tests of thyroid function, vaginal smears, and other tests should be performed as indicated. Endometrial tissue should be examined in the postovulation stage of the cycle to determine the adequacy of the response of the endometrium to hormones. Endometrial tissue should be cultured for *Ureaplasma urealyticum* and *Toxoplasma gondii*. Every attempt should be made to restore and maintain good physical and emotional health.

2. Postconception therapy–Provide early prenatal care and schedule frequent office visits. Repeated gentle abdominopelvic examinations are indicated so

that abnormal uterine development can be noted early. Permit unrestricted telephone calls, and offer optimal support by means of weekly visits.

Prescribe a nutritious, well-balanced diet. The patient should strive to achieve and maintain an appropriate pregnancy weight for her height and build. Give thyroid hormone only as indicated.

Coitus should be avoided at the gestational period of prior abortions; some clinicians advise total abstention. Complete bed rest is justified only for bleeding or pain. Empiric steroid sex hormone therapy is contraindicated. Smoking should be curbed, because it interferes with placental circulation.

B. Surgical Measures: Incompetency of the cervix should be corrected surgically. Uterine suspension, myomectomy, and a unification operation (for double uterus) may be justified for treatment of recurrent abortion.

Prognosis

The prognosis is excellent if the cause of abortion can be corrected. If a woman has lost 3 previous pregnancies without identifiable cause, she still has a 70–80% chance of carrying a fetus to viability. If she has aborted 4 or 5 times, the likelihood of a successful pregnancy is 65–70%.

Fitzsimmons J, Wapner RJ, Jackson LG: Repeated pregnancy loss. *Am J Med Genet* 1983;**16**:7.

Stray-Pedersen B, Stray-Pedersen S: Etiologic factors and subsequent reproductive performance in 195 couples with a prior history of habitual abortion. *Am J Obstet Gynecol* 1984;**148**:140.

ECTOPIC PREGNANCY

Essentials of Diagnosis

- Abnormal vaginal bleeding with symptoms suggestive of pregnancy.
- Cramping pains in the lower abdomen.
- A tender mass palpable outside the uterus.
- Pelvic ultrasound finding of empty uterus after seventh week from LMP.
- Failure to recover placental tissue at the time of induced abortion.

General Considerations

Any pregnancy arising from implantation of the ovum outside the cavity of the uterus is ectopic. Ectopic implantation occurs in about one out of 150 live births. About 98% of ectopic pregnancies are tubal. Other sites of ectopic implantation are the peritoneum or abdominal viscera, the ovary, and the cervix. Peritonitis, salpingitis, abdominal surgery, and pelvic tumors may predispose to abnormally situated pregnancy. Combined intra- and extrauterine pregnancy (heterotopic) may occur rarely. Only tubal ectopic pregnancy will be discussed in the following paragraphs.

Clinical Findings

A. Symptoms and Signs: The cardinal symptoms and signs of tubal pregnancy are (1) amenorrhea or irregular bleeding and spotting, followed by (2) pelvic pain, and (3) pelvic (adnexal) mass formation. They may be acute or chronic.

1. Acute (about 40% of tubal ectopic pregnancies)–Severe lower quadrant pain occurs in almost every case. It is sudden in onset, lancinating, intermittent, and does not radiate. Backache is present during attacks. Collapse and shock occur in about 10%, often after pelvic examination. At least two-thirds of patients give a history of abnormal menstruation; many have been infertile.

2. Chronic (about 60% of tubal ectopic pregnancies)–Blood leaks from the tubal ampulla over a period of days, and considerable blood may accumulate in the peritoneum. Slight but persistent vaginal spotting is reported, and a pelvic mass can be palpated. Abdominal distention and mild paralytic ileus are often present.

B. Laboratory Findings: Blood studies show anemia and slight leukocytosis. Quantitative serum pregnancy tests will show levels generally lower than expected for normal pregnancies of the same duration. If pregnancy tests are followed over a few days, there may be a slow rise or a plateau rather than the doubling every 2 days associated with intrauterine pregnancy or the falling levels that occur with early spontaneous abortion.

C. Ultrasonographic Findings: Ultrasonography can reliably demonstrate a gestational sac 6 weeks from the LMP and a fetal pole at 7 weeks if located in the uterus. An empty uterine cavity raises a strong suspicion of extrauterine pregnancy, which can occasionally (but not reliably) be revealed by ultrasound.

D. Special Examinations: Aspiration of the pouch of Douglas (culdocentesis) with an 18-gauge spinal needle will confirm hemoperitoneum. Laparoscopy to confirm an ectopic pregnancy is of great value prior to laparotomy.

Differential Diagnosis

Clinical and laboratory findings suggestive or diagnostic of pregnancy will distinguish ectopic pregnancy from many acute abdominal illnesses such as acute appendicitis, acute pelvic inflammatory disease, ruptured corpus luteum cyst or ovarian follicle, and urinary calculi. Uterine enlargement with clinical findings similar to those found in ectopic pregnancy is also characteristic of an aborting uterine pregnancy or hydatidiform mole.

Treatment

Hospitalize the patient if there is a reasonable likelihood of ectopic pregnancy. Type and cross-match blood. Treat for shock.

Surgical treatment is imperative, since the patient may bleed to death if internal hemorrhage is not promptly brought under control. Generally, salpingec-

tomy will be required if the tube has ruptured. If the condition of the patient permits, assessment of the other tube is important. Patency can be established by the injection of indigo carmine into the uterus, with appropriate compression of the lower uterine segment. Under certain circumstances, a conservative operation may be indicated (removing an unruptured ectopic pregnancy by salpingostomy; simple excision of the ectopic pregnancy, leaving portions of the tube for later microsurgery).

Iron therapy for anemia may be necessary during convalescence. Give Rh_0 (D) immune globulin to Rh-negative patients.

Prognosis

Death due to unrecognized ectopic pregnancy is a leading cause of maternal mortality in the USA.

Tubal pregnancy occurs again in about 12% of cases. This should not be regarded as a contraindication to future pregnancy, but the patient requires careful observation.

Roberts SK: Sonography of ectopic pregnancy: A review. *Med Ultrasound* 1982;**6**:71.

PREECLAMPSIA-ECLAMPSIA
(Pregnancy-Induced Hypertension, Toxemia of Pregnancy)*

Essentials of Diagnosis

- Onset of symptoms in the third trimester of pregnancy.
- Blood pressure > 140/90 mm Hg, or a rise of 30 mm Hg systolic or 15 mm Hg diastolic associated with the following:
  Significant proteinuria (500 mg/dL/24 h).
  Generalized edema, headache, visual disturbances, and epigastric pain.
  Increasing symptoms and signs preceding convulsions.

General Considerations

Preeclampsia-eclampsia usually occurs in the last trimester of pregnancy. It is most often first observed during labor or in the first 24 hours after delivery. The term **preeclampsia** denotes the nonconvulsive form; with the development of convulsions and coma, the disorder is termed **eclampsia**. About 5% of pregnant women in the USA develop preeclampsia. Primigravidas are most commonly affected. The incidence of preeclampsia is increased with multiple pregnancies, essential hypertension, diabetes mellitus, chronic renal disease, collagen disorders, and hydatidiform mole. Uncontrolled eclampsia may cause permanent disability, and it is a significant cause of maternal death. Five percent of cases of preeclampsia progress to eclampsia.

*The term toxemia is a misnomer and is being abandoned in the medical literature.

The cause is not known. Before the syndrome is clinically manifested, there is generalized vasospasm apparently initiated by the presence of chorionic tissue. The longer vasospasm continues, the greater the likelihood of associated pathologic changes in maternal organs, including the placenta; this indirectly affects the fetus.

None of the interventions recommended to reduce the incidence or severity of the process have proved to be of significant value when studied objectively, including diuretics, dietary restriction or enhancement, sodium restriction, and vitamin-mineral supplements. The only cure is termination of the pregnancy at a time as favorable as possible for fetal survival in the light of the medical condition of the mother.

Clinical Findings

A. Preeclampsia:

1. Mild–Symptoms are absent. Diastolic blood pressure is elevated to 90–100 mm Hg. There is minimal proteinuria and no evidence of intrauterine growth retardation.

2. Severe–Headache, visual changes, and upper abdominal pain are present, as is oliguria. Intrauterine growth retardation is present. Blood pressure exceeds 160/110 mm Hg. Ophthalmoscopic examination reveals arteriolar spasm, occasional edema of the optic disks, and cotton-wool exudates. Laboratory findings include proteinuria (> 2000 mg/dL/24 h), evidence of azotemia (increased serum creatinine, uric acid, or urea nitrogen), disseminated intravascular coagulation (thrombocytopenia, decreased fibrinogen, and increased fibrin split products), and hepatocellular damage, including hyperbilirubinemia.

B. Eclampsia: The symptoms of eclampsia usually are engrafted on those of severe preeclampsia and include the following: (1) generalized tonic-clonic convulsions; (2) coma followed by amnesia and confusion; (3) 3–4+ proteinuria; (4) marked hypertension preceding a convulsion, and hypotension thereafter (during coma or vascular collapse); and (5) oliguria or anuria.

Differential Diagnosis

The combination of renal, neurologic, and hypertensive findings in a previously normal pregnant woman distinguishes preeclampsia-eclampsia from primary hypertensive, renal, or neurologic disease.

Treatment

A. Preeclampsia: This condition should be recognized as early as possible by meticulous prenatal care. The objectives of treatment are (1) to prevent eclampsia, abruptio placentae, hepatic rupture, and ocular or vascular accidents; and (2) to deliver a normal baby that will survive. Place the patient at bed rest and give small doses of a benzodiazepine if necessary to make bed rest more acceptable. Delivery should be delayed, if possible, until the disease is under control and the fetus is mature.

1. Home management–Most patients can be managed at home (at bed rest) under alert supervision, including frequent blood pressure readings, daily urine protein determinations, and careful recording of fluid intake and output. Mild sodium restriction (< 3 g of salt per day) is advisable. If improvement does not occur in 48 hours, transfer the patient to a hospital.

2. Hospital care–Determine blood pressure, serum electrolytes, and urine protein at frequent intervals. Examine the ocular fundi every day, noting particularly arteriolar spasm, edema, hemorrhages, and exudates. The diet should be high in calcium, low in fat, high in complex carbohydrate, and moderate in protein content. Sedatives to promote quiet rest are indicated. Intravenous hydralazine is the antihypertensive of choice if diastolic blood pressure goes above 110 mm Hg. When labor ensues, magnesium sulfate is required to prevent seizures.

3. Observation of the fetus–With stabilization of preeclampsia, an optimal time for delivery minimizes perinatal illness and death. Deliver the fetus after 37 weeks by appropriate induction of labor, with cesarian section reserved for obstetric indications. Earlier in the third trimester, the status of the fetus can be followed with nonstress tests and oxytocin challenge tests done at 48-hour intervals. Regular maternal observations of fetal movements (''kick counts'') are also useful. Estriol and human placental lactogen determinations are not mandatory.

B. Eclampsia:

1. Emergency care–If the patient is convulsing, turn her on her side to prevent aspiration of vomitus and mucus and to prevent the caval syndrome. Insert a padded tongue blade or plastic airway between the teeth to prevent biting of the tongue and to maintain respiratory exchange. Aspirate fluid and food from the glottis or trachea. Give oxygen by nasal prongs. Give magnesium sulfate, 4 g (20 mL of a 20% solution) intravenously over a 4-minute period. At the same time, give 10 g of magnesium sulfate (20 mL of a 50% solution), one-half (10 mL) deep in each buttock (1 mL of 2% lidocaine may be added to each syringe to minimize pain). Thereafter, every 4 hours give 5 g of magnesium sulfate (10 mL of a 50% solution) in alternate buttocks as long as (1) knee jerk is present, (2) respirations are regular in rate (not < 16/min), and (3) urine output was at least 100 mL in the previous 4 hours. In cases of overdosage, give calcium gluconate (or equivalent), 20 mL of a 10% aqueous solution intravenously slowly, and repeat every hour until urinary, respiratory, and neurologic depression have cleared.

2. General care–Hospitalize the patient in a darkened, quiet room at absolute bed rest, lying on her side, with side rails for protection during convulsions. Allow no visitors. Do not disturb the patient for unnecessary procedures (eg, baths, enemas), and leave the blood pressure cuff on her arm. Typed and cross-matched blood must be available for immediate use, because patients with eclampsia often develop premature separation of the placenta with hemorrhage and are susceptible to shock.

3. Laboratory evaluation–Insert a retention catheter for accurate measurement of the quantity of urine passed. Determine the protein content of each 24-hour specimen until the fourth or fifth postpartum day. Blood tests to evaluate clotting factors, liver function, and electrolytes should be obtained as often as the severity and progression of the disease indicate. If serum protein is below 5 g/dL, give 250–500 mL of serum albumin. If serum albumin is not available, plasma protein fraction can be used.

4. Physical examination–Check blood pressure frequently during the acute phase and every 2–4 hours thereafter. Monitor the fetal heart constantly, if possible. Perform ophthalmoscopic examination once a day. Examine the face, extremities, and especially the sacrum (which becomes dependent when the patient is in bed) for edema.

5. Diet and fluids–If the patient is convulsing, give nothing by mouth. Record fluid intake and output for each 24-hour period. If she can eat and drink, give a high-carbohydrate, moderate-protein, low-fat diet. If the urine output exceeds 700 mL/d, replace the output plus visible fluid loss with isotonic fluid. If the output is less than 700 mL/d, allow no more than 2000 mL of fluid per day (including parenteral fluid).

6. Diuretics–Because maternal hypovolemia is the rule in patients with preeclampsia-eclampsia, diuretics should be avoided. Hypertonic solutions are also unnecessary. Furosemide may be used in cases of pulmonary edema.

7. Sedatives–Use these agents sparingly if at all.

8. Antihypertensives–Hydralazine given in 5- to 10-mg increments intravenously every 20 minutes is used whenever the diastolic pressure is above 110 mm Hg. A satisfactory response is a decrease to 90–100 mm Hg. Further lowering may impair placental perfusion.

9. Delivery–Because severe hypertensive disease, renal disease, and preeclampsia-eclampsia are usually aggravated by continuing pregnancy, the best method of treatment of any of these disorders is termination of pregnancy, preferably after definite viability. Control eclampsia before attempting induction of labor or delivery. Vaginal delivery is preferred. Induce labor, preferably by amniotomy alone, when the patient's condition permits. Use oxytocin to stimulate labor if necessary. Monitor the fetus carefully. Regional anesthesia is the technique of choice. Nitrous oxide (70%) and oxygen (30%) may be given with contractions, but 100% oxygen should be administered between contractions during the second stage.

Elective cesarean section may be considered if the patient is not at term, if labor is not inducible, if there is bleeding, or if there is evidence of disproportion. Convulsions or coma must be absent for 12 or more hours before cesarean section is performed.

Prognosis

The maternal mortality rate in eclampsia is 10–15%. Most patients improve strikingly in 24–48 hours with appropriate therapy, but early termination of pregnancy is usually required.

Although babies of mothers with preeclampsia-eclampsia are usually small for gestational age (probably because of placental malfunction), they fare better than preterm babies of the same weight born of women who do not develop preeclampsia-eclampsia.

Pritchard JA, Cunningham FG, Pritchard SA: The Portland Memorial Hospital Protocol for Treatment of Eclampsia: Evaluation of 245 cases. *Am J Obstet Gynecol* 1984;**148**:951.

Rolbin SH, Cole AF, Hew EM: Haemodynamic monitoring in the management of severe pre-eclampsia and eclampsia. *Can Anaesth Soc J* 1981;**28**:363.

Wheeler AS, Harris BA: Anesthesia for pregnancy-induced hypertension. *Clin Perinatol* 1982;**9**:95.

GESTATIONAL TROPHOBLASTIC NEOPLASIA
Hydatidiform Mole & Choriocarcinoma

Essentials of Diagnosis

- Uterus often larger than expected for duration of pregnancy.
- Excessively elevated levels of hCG.
- Vesicles passed from vagina.
- Ultrasound findings characteristic of mole.
- Uterine bleeding in pregnancy.

General Considerations

Gestational trophoblastic neoplasia is a spectrum of disease that includes hydatidiform mole, invasive mole, and choriocarcinoma. Cytogenetics has demonstrated that true moles are almost always euploid and sex chromatin-positive, 46,XX with all genetic material of paternal origin. Partial moles are usually triploid but occasionally trisomic, 46,XX or 46,XY.

The highest rates of gestation trophoblastic neoplasia occur in developing countries, with rates of 1:125 pregnancies in certain areas of the Orient. In the USA, the frequency is 1:1500 pregnancies. Risk factors include low socioeconomic status, a prior history of mole, and age below 18 or above 40. Approximately 10% of women require further treatment after evacuation of the mole; 5% develop choriocarcinoma. Choriocarcinoma also presents more subtly after other types of pregnancy (following delivery, abortion, or ectopic pregnancy).

Clinical Findings

A. Symptoms and Signs: Excessive nausea and vomiting occur in over one-third of patients with hydatidiform mole. Uterine bleeding, beginning at 6–8 weeks, is observed in virtually all instances and is indicative of threatened or incomplete abortion. In about one-fifth of cases, the uterus is larger than would be expected in a normal pregnancy of the same duration. Intact or collapsed vesicles may be passed through the vagina. These grapelike clusters of enlarged villi are diagnostic. Bilaterally enlarged cystic ovaries are sometimes palpable. They are the result of ovarian hyperstimulation due to excess hCG.

Preeclampsia-eclampsia, frequently of the fulminating type, may develop during the second trimester of pregnancy, but this is unusual.

Choriocarcinoma may be manifested by continued or recurrent uterine bleeding after evacuation of a mole or following a delivery, abortion, or ectopic pregnancy. The presence of an ulcerative vaginal tumor, pelvic mass, or evidence of distant metastatic tumor may be the presenting observation. The diagnosis is established by pathologic examination of curettings or by biopsy.

B. Laboratory Findings: A serum hCG beta-subunit value above 40,000 mIU/mL or a urinary hCG value in excess of 100,000 IU/24 h increases the likelihood of hydatidiform mole, although such values are occasionally seen with a normal pregnancy (eg, in multiple gestation).

C. Ultrasonography: Ultrasound has virtually replaced all other means of preoperative diagnosis of hydatidiform mole. The multiple echoes indicating edematous villi within the enlarged uterus and the absence of a fetus and placenta are pathognomonic.

D. X-Ray Findings: A preoperative chest film is indicated to rule out pulmonary metastases of trophoblast.

Treatment

A. Specific (Surgical) Measures: Empty the uterus as soon as the diagnosis of hydatidiform mole is established, preferably by suction. Do not resect ovarian cysts or remove the ovaries; spontaneous regression of theca lutein cysts will occur with elimination of the mole.

If malignant tissue is discovered at surgery or during the follow-up examination, chemotherapy is indicated.

Thyrotoxicosis indistinguishable clinically from that of primary thyroid or pituitary origin may occur. Surgical removal of the mole promptly corrects the thyroid overactivity.

B. Follow-up Measures: Weekly quantitative hCG level measurements are required. Moles show a progressive decline in hCG. After 2 negative weekly tests (< 5 mIU/mL), the interval may be increased to monthly for 6 months and then to every 2 months for a year. If levels plateau or begin to rise, the patient should be evaluated by repeat chest film and D&C before the initiation of chemotherapy.

C. Antitumor Chemotherapy: For low-risk patients with a good prognosis, give methotrexate, 0.4 mg/kg intramuscularly over a 5-day period, or dactinomycin, 10–12 μg/kg/d intravenously over a 5-day period (see pp 1062 and 1063). Refer patients with a poor prognosis to a tumor center, where multiple-agent chemotherapy probably will be given. The side effects—anorexia, nausea and vomiting, stomatitis, rash, diarrhea, and bone marrow depression—usually are reversible in about 3 weeks. They can be ameliorated by the administration of folic acid. Death occurs

occasionally from agranulocytosis or toxic hepatitis. Repeated courses of methotrexate 2 weeks apart generally are required to destroy the trophoblast and maintain a zero chorionic gonadotropin titer, as indicated by hCG β-subunit determination.

D. Supportive Measures: Replace blood, give iron, and encourage good nutrition. If infection is suspected, give broad-spectrum antibiotics for 24 hours before and 3–4 days after surgery. Prescribe oral contraceptives (if acceptable) or another reliable birth control method to avoid the hazard and confusion of elevated hCG from a new pregnancy. hCG levels should be negative for a year before pregnancy is again attempted.

Prognosis

A 5-year arrest after courses of chemotherapy, even when metastases have been demonstrated, can be expected in at least 85% of cases of choriocarcinoma. The risk of chronic abortion or fetal anomaly is not greater in women who have had hydatidiform mole.

Fasoli M et al: Management of gestational trophoblastic disease: Results of a cooperative study. *Obstet Gynecol* 1982;**60**:205.

Jones WB: Management of low-risk metastatic gestational trophoblastic disease. *J Reprod Med* 1981;**26**:213.

Lurain JR et al: Gestational trophoblastic disease: Treatment results at the Brewer Trophoblastic Disease Center (Chicago). *Obstet Gynecol* 1982;**60**:354.

THIRD-TRIMESTER BLEEDING

Five to 10% of women have vaginal bleeding in late pregnancy. Multiparas are more commonly affected. Obstetric bleeding is a major cause of maternal mortality and morbidity. The physician must distinguish between placental causes of obstetric bleeding (placenta previa, premature separation of the placenta) and nonplacental causes (systemic disease or disorders of the lower genital tract).

The approach to the problem of bleeding in late pregnancy should be conservative and expectant.

The patient should be hospitalized at once and placed at complete bed rest. Perform a gentle abdominal examination. Significant degrees of premature separation of the placenta (abruptio placentae) cause uterine tetany and tenderness, whereas placenta previa is associated with painless bleeding, abnormal fetal position (breech, transverse lie), and a high presenting part. Inspect the vagina and cervix with a speculum for cancer or infection. Avoid digital rectal or vaginal examination, which may result in excessive bleeding. Typed and cross-matched blood should be ready in case of need during the examination. Ultrasonography is accurate in detecting placental location. Over 90% of patients with third-trimester bleeding will stop bleeding in 24 hours with bed rest alone, although the bleeding may recur at a later time. If bleeding is profuse and persistent, and especially if there are persistent uterine contractions, vaginal examination is indicated after preparation for cesarian section and blood replacement.

If the patient is less than 36 weeks pregnant, it may be necessary to keep her in the hospital or at home at bed rest until the chances of delivering a viable infant improve.

Gillieson MS, Winer-Muram HT, Muram D: Low-lying placenta. *Radiology* 1982;**144**:577.

POSTPARTUM HEMORRHAGE

Postpartum hemorrhage has been defined arbitrarily as the loss of at least 500 mL of blood following delivery. It is a major cause of maternal death in the USA.

The most common causes of postpartum hemorrhage are uterine atony, vaginal or cervical lacerations, uterine rupture, and blood dyscrasias or coagulation defects.

The following types of patients are especially prone to develop postpartum bleeding: women with multiple pregnancies, polyhydramnios, a history of postpartum hemorrhage, primary or secondary uterine inertia, uterine infections, placenta previa, abruptio placentae; women who have had heavy analgesia or anesthesia; and those who are delivered by cesarean section.

Treatment

Reinspect the placenta for missing fragments. Examine for lacerations of the birth canal. Note the quality of contractions of the elevated uterus, determine bleeding and clotting time, and obtain typed and cross-matched blood for transfusion.

Control bleeding promptly by suture of lacerations, manual recovery or expression of the placenta, or intravenous oxytocin (Pitocin) as indicated. Packing the uterus may temporarily control bleeding, eg, during the period of preparation before hysterectomy in cases of rupture of the uterus.

Prognosis

The mortality rate in postpartum hemorrhage depends upon the amount and rapidity of blood loss, the patient's general health, and the speed and adequacy of treatment.

Poole GV et al: Comparison of colloids and crystalloids in resuscitation from hemorrhagic shock. *Surg Gynecol Obstet* 1982;**154**:577.

HIGH-RISK PREGNANCY

Chronic maternal diseases such as congenital heart problems, hypertension, diabetes, and renal disease significantly affect pregnancy and fetal welfare and require special management. In addition, 20% of pregnant women in the USA have other medical, so-

---

High-Risk Obstetric Categories (After Wigglesworth)

History of Any of the Following:

Hereditary abnormality (osteogenesis imperfecta, Down's syndrome, etc).

Premature or small-for-dates neonate (most recent delivery).

Congenital anomaly, anemia, blood dyscrasia, toxemia, etc.

Severe social problem (teen-age pregnancy, drug addiction, alcoholism, etc).

Long-delayed or absent prenatal care.

Age < 18 or > 35 years.

Teratogenic viral illness or dangerous drug administration in the first trimester.

A fifth or subsequent pregnancy, especially when the gravida is > 35 years of age.

Prolonged infertility or essential drug or hormone treatment.

Significant stressful or dangerous events in the present pregnancy (critical accident, excessive exposure to irradiation, etc).

Heavy cigarette smoking.

Pregnancy within 2 months of a previous delivery.

Diagnosis of Any of the Following:

Height under 60 inches or a prepregnant weight of 20% less than or over the standard for height and age.

Minimal or no weight gain.

Obstetric complications (preeclampsia-eclampsia, multiple pregnancy, hydramnios, etc).

Abnormal presentation (breech, presenting part unengaged at term, etc).

A fetus that fails to grow normally or is disparate in size from that expected.

A fetus > 42 weeks' gestation.

---

cial, and obstetric problems that may significantly affect pregnancy (see listing of high-risk categories). All of these women require special care to minimize maternal and fetal morbidity and mortality.

Diagnostic Evaluation

A. Initial Screening: Initial screening of the gravida must include the following:

1. A detailed history including all earlier pregnancies and their outcomes, occupation (plans for work during pregnancy and return postpartum), current physical complaints and drug use, medical history (especially of chronic disease with disability), family history (especially of congenital anomalies, fetal losses, and inheritable diseases), and nutritional habits.

2. A complete general physical examination (including height, weight, development, etc) and diagnosis of systemic disease, dysfunction, or abnormality.

3. Careful abdominopelvic evaluation with special reference to the following:

a. Uterus—Configuration, size, fundal height, fetal size (estimate), fetal presentation, position, engagement, amount of amniotic fluid.

b. Cervix–Position, ulceration, effacement, dilatation.

c. Spine, pelvis, and extremities–Abnormalities, measurement of pelvic diameters.

4. Laboratory tests–Hematocrit, urinalysis, urine culture, serologic test for syphilis, rubella and antibody screening, blood type, Rh determination, cervical culture for gonorrhea and *Chlamydia*, and cervical cytology. Special studies may be required for particular problems (eg, glucose tolerance test, herpes culture, hemoglobin electrophoresis, hepatitis B antigen, tuberculin skin test).

B. Antenatal Visits: Antenatal visits should be more frequent for high-risk than for normal obstetric patients. This allows for more accurate appraisal of the course of the pregnancy and identification and correction of problems (eg, anemia, urinary tract infection). Obstetric disorders that may require special treatment or decision (eg, preeclampsia-eclampsia, uterine bleeding) must be identified early. Visits also provide the opportunity for education about hygiene; nutrition; use of cigarettes, alcohol, and drugs; care of the newborn; and psychologic support.

C. Assessment of Fetal Growth, Maturity, and Well-Being:

1. Indirect (noninvasive) methods–

a. Recalculation of gestational age of the fetus (LMP, basal body temperature, dates of possible conception, date of quickening, first fetal heart tones).

b. Uterine growth (fundal height, estimated fetal weight).

c. Engagement of presenting part.

d. Ultrasonography (fetal biparietal diameter and circumferences of chest and abdomen).

e. Fetal activity pattern as determined by nonstress test and daily kick counts by the mother in the third trimester.

f. Oxytocin challenge test.

2. Direct (invasive) methods–

a. First trimester (eighth week)–Chorionic villus biopsy for cytogenetic evaluation.

b. Second trimester (15th week)–Study of amniotic fluid cells (culture, cytochemistry, chromosome studies, and alpha-fetoprotein concentration).

c. Third trimester–Amniocentesis (amniotic fluid volume, enzyme studies, osmolality, optical den-

Table 13–9. Teratogenic and fetotoxic drugs.

Maternal Medication	Fetal or Neonatal Effect
Established teratogenic agents	
Alcohol	Fetal alcohol syndrome (growth retardation, increase in anomalies)
Anticoagulants (dicumarol, warfarin)	Optic atrophy, mental retardation, hydrocephalus
Anticonvulsants (phenytoin, trimethadione)	Mental and growth retardation, microcephaly
Antineoplastics	Multiple anomalies, abortion
Alkylating agents (cyclophosphamide)	
Folic acid antagonists (methotrexate, aminopterin)	
Hormones	
Estrogens, progestins	Anomalies involving vertebrae, anus, cardiovascular system, trachea, esophagus, renal system, and limbs (VACTERL)
Diethylstilbestrol	Genital anomalies, late development of clear cell carcinoma of the vagina
Androgens	Masculinization of female fetus
Isotretinoin (Accutane)	Multiple anomalies involving central nervous system
Organic mercury	Central nervous system anomalies
Possible teratogens	
Lithium carbonate	Cardiac defects
Sulfonylurea derivatives	Anomalies
Tranquilizers	
Benzodiazepines	Facial cleft deformities
Meprobamate	Multiple anomalies
Fetotoxic drugs	
Analgesics, narcotics	
Heroin, morphine	Neonatal death or convulsions, tremors
Salicylates (excessive)	Neonatal bleeding
Antithyroid drugs	
Radioiodine	Destruction of fetal thyroid
Propylthiouracil, methimazole	Fetal goiter
Sedatives, hypnotics, tranquilizers	
Phenobarbital (excessive)	Neonatal bleeding
Phenothiazines	Hyperbilirubinemia
Tetracyclines	Dental discoloration and abnormalities
Thiazides	Thrombocytopenia
Tobacco smoking	Undersized babies
Vitamin K (excessive)	Hyperbilirubinemia

Table 13–10. Risk of preterm delivery.*

Score†	Socioeconomic Status	Past History	Daily Habits	Current Pregnancy — Mother	Current Pregnancy — Fetus
1	2 children at home. Low socioeconomic status.	One first trimester abortion. Less than 1 year since last birth.	Work outside home.	Unusual fatigue.	...
2	Under 20 years of age. Over 40 years of age. Single parent.	Two first trimester abortions.	More than 10 cigarettes per day. More than 6 cups of coffee per day.	Less than 12 lb weight gain by 32 weeks. Albuminuria. Hypertension. Bacteriuria.	...
3	Low socioeconomic status. Malnourished. Shorter than 150 cm (5 ft). Weighs less than 45 cm (100 lb).	Three first trimester abortions.	Unusual anxiety. Heavy work. Long, tiring travel. Long commute distance.	Weight loss of 2 kg. Febrile illness. Leiomyomas.	Breech position at 32 weeks or unengaged breech at term. Head engaged before 34 weeks.
4	Under 18 years of age.	Pyelonephritis.	...	Uterine bleeding after 12 weeks. Effacement or dilation of cervix before 36 weeks. Uterine irritability.	...
5	...	Uterine anomaly. Second trimester abortion. Cone biopsy.	...	Placenta previa. Hydramnios. Pregnancy beyond 42 weeks.	...
10	...	Premature delivery. DES exposure. Repeated second trimester abortion.	...	Abdominal surgery. Cervical surgery.	Twins. Small-for-dates fetus.

*Modified and reproduced, with permission, from Zuspan FK, Quilligan EJ (editors): *Practical Manual of Obstetric Care.* Mosby, 1982. (Modified from Creasy R: Personal communication.)

†Score is computed by addition of the number of points given any item. 0–5 = minimal risk; 6–9 = moderate risk; 10 or more = high risk.

sity for bilirubinoid pigments, creatinine content, lecithin-sphingomyelin ratio, phosphatidylglycerol determination).

D. Abnormal Uterine Growth: When duration of pregnancy has been validated, a large uterus for dates may indicate multiple pregnancy, hydramnios, uterine myomas, or fetal macrosomia. A small uterus may result from oligohydramnios, fetal disease (eg, rubella, cytomegalic inclusion disease), or anomaly. Maternal causes include hypertension, renal or cardiac disease, hemoglobinopathy, drug or heavy alcohol use, and smoking. In many cases of intrauterine growth retardation, a cause cannot be found. Clinical suspicion should be confirmed by ultrasound examinations repeated at regular intervals.

E. Preterm Delivery: Preterm (premature) delivery is associated with serious perinatal illness and higher death rates. Preventive measures include changing the daily habits shown in Table 13–10, early awareness of contractions, and bed rest for uterine irritability.

Treatment

Maternal disease must be treated cautiously to avoid harm to the fetus. Perinatal mortality and morbidity rates can sometimes be reduced by prolonging gestation—eg, in the case of premature labor, multiple pregnancy, placenta previa, cervical incompetence, slight premature separation of the placenta, or thyroid dysfunction. Judicious early delivery may be necessary to rescue the fetus if the membranes rupture before 34 weeks or in the case of preeclampsia-eclampsia, severe isoimmunization, clinical diabetes mellitus, persistent urinary tract infection, considerable hydramnios, or placental insufficiency.

The reader should consult the references listed below for the diagnosis and treatment of obstetric problems, the course and conduct of labor, and perinatal complications and their therapy.

Prognosis

Although improved obstetric care has reduced the maternal mortality rate in the USA from 660:100,000 births in 1930 to 10:100,000 in 1980, two-thirds to three-fourths of the latter were still probably preventable. Many investigators believe that better nutrition could further reduce the infant mortality rate. Socioeconomic factors undoubtedly play a role. The majority of maternal and perinatal problems can be identified early enough to apply remedial measures.

Bowes WA: Delivery of the very low birth weight infant. *Clin Perinatol* 1981;**8**:183.

Deter RL et al: Longitudinal studies of fetal growth with the use of dynamic image ultrasonography. *Am J Obstet Gynecol* 1982; **143**:545.

Ritchie JW, McClure BG: The "small-for-dates" problem. *Clin Obstet Gynaecol* 1982;**9**:131.

MEDICAL CONDITIONS COMPLICATING PREGNANCY

Hypertensive Disease

Hypertensive disease in women of childbearing age is usually essential hypertension. Other less common but important causes should be looked for: coarctation of the aorta, pheochromocytoma, aldosteronism, and renovascular and renal hypertension.

Preeclampsia is superimposed on 20% of pregnancies in women with hypertensive disease, and in such patients it appears earlier, is more severe, and is more often associated with intrauterine growth retardation. It may be difficult to determine whether or not hypertension in a pregnant woman precedes or derives from the pregnancy if she is not examined until after the 20th week and there is no reliable medical history. When in doubt, treat for preeclampsia. The hypertension of preeclampsia usually recedes 6 weeks after delivery. If it persists for 3 months postpartum, it is probably essential hypertension.

Pregnant women with probable hypertensive disease require antihypertensive drugs only if the diastolic pressure is sustained at or above 110 mm Hg. One should strive to keep the diastolic pressure between 90 and 100 mm Hg. However, if the pressure is over 110 mm Hg, do not attempt to lower it quickly by more than 25%.

If a hypertensive woman is being managed successfully by medical treatment when she registers for antenatal care, one may generally continue the antihypertension medication. Diuretics can be continued in pregnancy; propranolol is best replaced by a more selective β-adrenergic antagonist that is less lipid-soluble (eg, metoprolol). For initiation of treatment, one may begin with hydralazine, 25 mg orally daily, and increase the dosage as indicated. If the response is unsatisfactory or if the patient is not near term, give methyldopa, 250 mg orally twice daily, again building in divided doses as needed to as much as 2 g daily.

The incidence or severity of preeclampsia and the increased perinatal mortality rate associated with hypertensive syndromes are reduced slightly by long-term drug therapy.

Therapeutic abortion may be indicated in cases of severe hypertension during pregnancy. If pregnancy is allowed to continue, the risk to the fetus must be assessed periodically in anticipation of early delivery.

Rubin PC: Beta-blockers in pregnancy. *N Engl J Med* 1981; **305**:1323.

Sibai BM et al: Plasma volume determination in pregnancies complicated by chronic hypertension and intrauterine fetal demise. *Obstet Gynecol* 1982;**60**:174.

Wood SM, Blainey JD: Prescribing in pregnancy: Hypertension and renal disease. *Clin Obstet Gynaecol* 1981;**8**:439.

Anemia

Plasma volume increases approximately 50% during pregnancy, while red cell volume increases 25%, causing hemodilution with lowered hemoglobin and hematocrit values. True anemia in pregnancy is often defined as a hemoglobin measurement below 11 g/dL or hematocrit below 33%. Anemia is very common in pregnancy, causing fatigue, anorexia, dyspnea, and edema. Prevention through optimal nutrition and iron and folic acid supplementation is desirable.

A. Iron Deficiency Anemia: Many women enter pregnancy with low iron stores resulting from heavy menstrual periods, previous pregnancies, or poor nutrition. It is difficult to meet the increased requirement for iron through diet, so that anemia often develops unless iron supplements are given. Red cells may not become hypochromic and microcytic until the hematocrit has fallen far below normal levels. The reticulocyte count is low. A serum iron level below 40 μg/dL and a transferrin saturation less than 16% suggest iron deficiency anemia. Treatment consists of a diet containing iron-rich foods and 60 mg of elemental iron (eg, 300 mg of ferrous sulfate) 3 times a day with meals. Iron is best absorbed if taken with a source of vitamin C (raw fruits and vegetables, lightly cooked greens). For prevention of anemia, all pregnant women should take daily iron supplements containing 60 mg of elemental iron.

B. Folic Acid Deficiency Anemia: Folic acid deficiency anemia is the main cause of macrocytic anemia in pregnancy, since vitamin B_{12} deficiency anemia is rare in the child-bearing years. The daily folate requirement doubles from 400 μg to 800 μg in pregnancy. Twin pregnancies, acute infections, malabsorption syndromes, and use of anticonvulsant drugs such as phenytoin can precipitate folic acid deficiency. The anemia may first be seen in the puerperium owing to the increased need for folate during lactation.

The diagnosis is made by finding macrocytic red cells and hypersegmented neutrophils in a blood smear. However, blood smears in pregnancy may be difficult to interpret, since they frequently show iron deficiency changes as well. Because the deficiency is hard to diagnose and folate intake is inadequate in some socioeconomic groups, 0.8–1 mg of folic acid is routinely given as a supplement in pregnancy. Treat an established deficiency with 1–5 mg/d. Good sources of folate in food are leafy green vegetables, orange juice, peanuts, and beans. Cooking and storage of food destroy folic acid. Strict vegetarians who eat no eggs or milk products should take vitamin B_{12} supplements during pregnancy and lactation.

C. Sickle Cell Anemia: Women with sickle cell anemia are subject to serious complications in pregnancy. The anemia becomes more severe, and crises may occur more frequently. Complications include infections, bone pain, pulmonary infarction, congestive heart failure, and preeclampsia. There is an increased rate of spontaneous abortion and higher maternal and perinatal mortality rates. Newer methods of intensive medical treatment have improved the outcome for mother and fetus. Frequent transfusions of packed cells or leukocyte-poor washed red cells are used to lower the level of hemoglobin S and elevate the level of hemoglobin A; this minimizes the severity of anemia and sickle cell crises. Folic acid supplements should be given, and analgesics and adequate hydration are important.

Parents with sickle cell disease or sickle cell trait may wish to undergo first-trimester chorionic villus biopsy or second-trimester amniocentesis to determine whether sickle cell anemia has been passed on to the fetus. Genetic counseling should be available before pregnancy and postpartum for all patients with hemoglobinopathies and their partners. Elective sterilization and therapeutic abortion should be available if desired. IUDs and oral contraceptives are contraindicated for these patients, but progestin-only contraceptives may be used.

Women with sickle cell trait alone generally have an uncomplicated gestation. Sickle cell–hemoglobin C disease in pregnancy is similar to sickle cell anemia and is treated similarly.

Chang JC, Kan YW: A sensitive new prenatal test for sickle cell anemia. *N Engl J Med* 1982;**307**:30.

Milner PF, Jones BR, Döbler J: Outcome of pregnancy in sickle cell anemia and sickle cell–hemoglobin C disease: An analysis of 181 pregnancies in 98 patients, and a review of the literature. *Am J Obstet Gynecol* 1980;**138**:239.

Palgi A, Levi S, Reshef A: Anemia of pregnancy: Evaluation of the effectiveness of routine dietary supplementation program in an Israeli community. *Am J Public Health* 1981;**71**:736.

Diabetes Mellitus

During pregnancy there is increased tissue resistance to insulin with resultant increased levels of blood insulin as well as glucose and triglycerides. These changes result from secretion of human placental lactogen and increasing levels of estrogen and progesterone. The prevention of common hazards of diabetes, such as hypoglycemia, ketosis, and diabetic coma, requires great effort and attention to detail on the part of both the physician and the patient. Although pregnancy does not appear to alter the ultimate severity of diabetes, retinopathy and nephropathy may appear or become worse during pregnancy. Over the years, the White classification of diabetes during pregnancy (Table 13–11) has allowed for uniform description and comparison of diabetic pregnant women.

Even in carefully managed diabetics, the incidence of obstetric complications such as hydramnios, preeclampsia-eclampsia, infections, and prematurity is increased. The infants are larger than those of nondiabetic women. There is an increase in the number of unexplained fetal deaths in the last few weeks of pregnancy as well as a high rate of neonatal deaths.

The maintenance of euglycemia is improved by

Table 13–11. Classification of diabetes during pregnancy (Priscilla White).*

Class	Characteristics	Implications
Glucose intolerance of pregnancy	Erroneously known as gestational diabetes. Abnormal glucose tolerance during pregnancy; postprandial hyperglycemia during pregnancy.	Diagnosis before 30 weeks' gestation important to prevent macrosomia. Treat with diet adequate in calories to prevent maternal weight loss. Goal is postprandial blood glucose < 130 mg/dL at 1 hour, or < 105 mg/dL at 2 hours. If insulin is necessary, manage as in classes B, C, and D.
A	Chemical diabetes diagnosed before pregnancy; managed by diet alone: any age at onset.	Management as for glucose intolerance of pregnancy.
B	Insulin treatment used before pregnancy; onset at age 20 or older; duration < 10 years.	Some endogenous insulin secretion may persist. Fetal and neonatal risks same as in classes C and D, as is management.
C	Onset at age 10–20, or duration 10–20 years.	Insulin-deficient diabetes of juvenile onset.
D	Onset before age 10, or duration > 20 years, or chronic hypertension (not preeclampsia), or background retinopathy (tiny hemorrhages).	Fetal macrosomia or intrauterine growth retardation possible. Retinal microaneurysms, dot hemorrhages, and exudates may progress during pregnancy, then regress after delivery.
F	Diabetic nephropathy with proteinuria.	Anemia and hypertension common; proteinuria increases in third trimester, declines after delivery. Fetal intrauterine growth retardation common; perinatal survival about 85% under optimal conditions; bed rest necessary.
H	Coronary artery disease.	Serious maternal risk.
R	Proliferative retinopathy.	Neovascularization, with risk of vitreous hemorrhage or retinal detachment; laser photocoagulation useful; abortion usually not necessary. With active process of neovascularization, prevent bearing-down efforts.

*Reproduced, with permission, from Benson RC (editor): *Current Obstetric & Gynecologic Diagnosis & Treatment,* 5th ed. Lange, 1984.

patient-performed blood sugar monitoring at home. Attempts are under way to decrease the number of congenital anomalies associated with diabetic pregnancies. Prepregnancy evaluation and adjustment of insulin control based on glycosylated hemoglobin (A_{1c}) will maintain strict euglycemia in early pregnancy when organogenesis is occurring. The use of a continuous insulin pump is under study for its effect in lowering the frequency of anomalies. Time of delivery is dictated by deterioration of diabetic control, the onset of preeclampsia, decreased fetal reactivity as judged by nonstress or oxytocin challenge tests, or confirmation of lung maturity at or about 38 weeks of pregnancy.

Jovanovic L, Peterson CM: Optimal insulin delivery for pregnant diabetic patient. *Diabetes Care* 1982;**5(Suppl I)**:24.

Tuberculosis

The diagnosis of tuberculosis in pregnancy is made by careful history taking, a physical examination, and skin testing, with special attention to women from ethnic groups with a high prevalence of the disease. Chest films should not be obtained as a routine screening measure in pregnancy but should be used only in patients with a skin test that has converted from negative to positive or with suggestive findings in the history and physical examination. Use abdominal shielding if a chest film is obtained.

If adequately treated, tuberculosis in pregnancy has an excellent prognosis. There is no increase in spontaneous abortion, fetal problems, or congenital anomalies in patients receiving antitubercular chemotherapy. Despite chemotherapy, a patient occasionally becomes ill with meningeal, miliary, or peritoneal involvement. In an untreated mother, congenital tuberculosis can occur in the newborn.

Treatment is with isoniazid and ethambutol or isoniazid and rifampin, in a short course (9–12 months) or standard course (18–24 months). Because isoniazid therapy may result in vitamin B_6 deficiency, a supplement of 50 mg/d of vitamin B_6 should be given simultaneously. Streptomycin, ethionamide, and most other antitubercular drugs should be avoided in pregnancy.

Snider DE Jr et al: Treatment of tuberculosis during pregnancy. *Am Rev Respir Dis* 1980;**122**:65.

Heart Disease

Most cases of heart disease complicating pregnancy in the USA now are of congenital origin. About 5% of maternal deaths are due to heart disease. Pregnancy causes a significant increase in pulse rate, an increase of cardiac output of more than 30%, a rise in plasma and blood volume, and expansion of the red cell mass. Both vital capacity and oxygen consumption rise only slightly.

For practical purposes, the functional capacity of the heart is the best single measurement of cardiopulmonary status.

Class I: Ordinary physical activity causes no discomfort (perinatal mortality rate about 5%).

Class II: Ordinary activity causes discomfort and slight disability (perinatal mortality rate 10–15%).

Class III: Less than ordinary activity causes discomfort or disability; patient is barely compensated (perinatal mortality rate about 35%).

Class IV: Patient decompensated; any physical activity causes acute distress (perinatal mortality rate over 50%).

The physical stress of labor, delivery, and the puerperium imposes moderate to extreme burdens on the maternal heart. These increase to a peak at 32 weeks, when maximal cardiac load must be anticipated.

In general, patients with class I or class II functional disability (80% of pregnant women with heart disease) do well obstetrically. Over 80% of maternal deaths due to heart disease occur in women with class III or IV cardiac disability. Congestive failure is the usual cause of death. Three-fourths of these deaths occur in the early puerperium. Particularly lethal during pregnancy are situations in which there is pulmonary hypertension (eg, large septal shunts and severe mitral stenosis).

Therapeutic abortion and elective sterilization should be offered to patients with class III or IV cardiac disease. Cesarean section should be performed only upon obstetric indications.

McAnulty JH, Metcalfe J, Ueland K: General guidelines in the management of cardiac disease (during pregnancy). *Clin Obstet Gynecol* 1981;**24**:773.

Urinary Tract Infection

The urinary tract is especially vulnerable to infections during pregnancy because the altered secretions of steroid sex hormones and the pressure exerted by the gravid uterus upon the ureters and bladder cause hypotonia and congestion and predispose to urinary stasis. Labor and delivery and urinary retention postpartum also may initiate or aggravate infection. *Escherichia coli* is the offending organism in over two-thirds of cases.

From 2 to 8% of pregnant women have asymptomatic bacteriuria ($\geq$ 100,000 colonies per milliliter of urine), which some believe to be associated with increased risk of prematurity. It is estimated that 20–40% of these women will develop pyelonephritis during pregnancy.

A first-trimester urine culture is indicated in women with a history of recurrent or recent episodes of urinary tract infection. If the culture is positive, treatment should be initiated as a prophylactic measure. Sulfisoxazole, nitrofurantoin, penicillins, and cephalosporins are acceptable medications for 7–10 days. If bacteriuria returns, suppressive medication (one daily dose of an appropriate antibiotic) for the remainder of the pregnancy is indicated. Acute pyelonephritis requires hospitalization for intravenous administration of antibiotics until the patient is afebrile; this is followed by a full course of oral antibiotics.

Gilstrap LC III, Cunningham FG, Whalley PJ: Acute pyelonephritis in pregnancy: An anterospective study. *Obstet Gynecol* 1981;**57**:409.

Syphilis, Gonorrhea, & *Chlamydia trachomatis* Infection (See also Chapters 24 and 25.)

These sexually transmitted diseases have significant consequences for mother and child. Untreated syphilis in pregnancy will cause late abortion or transplacental infection with congenital syphilis. Gonorrhea will produce large-joint arthritis by hematogenous spread as well as newborn eye damage. Maternal chlamydial infections are largely asymptomatic but are manifested in the newborn by inclusion conjunctivitis and, at age 2–4 months, by pneumonia. The diagnosis of each can be reliably made by appropriate laboratory tests, which should be included in all prenatal care. The sexual partners of women with sexually transmitted diseases should be identified and treated also if that can be done.

Herpes Genitalis (See also pp 68 and 829.)

Infection of the lower genital tract by herpesvirus type 2 is a sexually transmissible disease of increasing frequency and seriousness.

Primary infection during pregnancy is responsible for an increased incidence of spontaneous abortion, stillbirth, and neonatal death. Patients with primary infection complain of fever, malaise, anorexia, local genital pain, leukorrhea, dysuria, vaginal bleeding, and variable neurologic symptoms (peripheral nerve pain or paresthesias and difficulty in voiding or defecating). Typical genital lesions are multiple shallow ulcerations, vesicles, and erythematous papules. Painful bilateral inguinal adenopathy is usually present owing to secondary infection of the ulcerations. Clinical diagnosis is generally easy to make and may be confirmed by viral culture or a stained scraping of the base of an ulcer, which will reveal multinucleated giant cells and inclusion bodies.

For topical therapy of the initial attack, give 5% acyclovir (Zovirax) ointment 6 times daily for 1 week. This agent is of no benefit in recurrent herpes. Many topical remedies have been used in an attempt to ease pain, such as cold milk compresses, povidone-iodine, and anesthetic jellies. Topical or systemic corticosteroids are not helpful in vulvovaginal herpes.

Women with a history of recurrent genital herpes attacks should be followed by clinical observation throughout pregnancy and by weekly cervical cultures from the 36th week. If there are active vulvovaginal lesions or if there is a positive culture at the time of rupture of the membranes or labor, cesarean section should be performed to prevent serious neonatal infection. Separation of the newborn from a mother with open lesions is mandatory. For treatment, see p 829 and Chapter 29.

Grossman JH III, Wallen WC, Sever JL: Management of genital herpes simplex virus infection during pregnancy. *Obstet Gynecol* 1981;**58**:1.

Thyrotoxicosis

Thyrotoxicosis during pregnancy may result in fetal anomalies, late abortion, or preterm labor and fetal hyperthyroidism with goiter. Thyroid storm in late pregnancy or labor is a life-threatening emergency.

Radioactive isotope therapy must never be given during pregnancy. The thyroid inhibitor of choice is propylthiouracil, which acts to prevent further thyroxine formation by blocking iodination of tyrosine. There is a 2- to 3-week delay before the pretreatment hormone level begins to fall. The initial dose of propylthiouracil is 100–150 mg 3 times a day; the dose is lowered to 50 mg 4 times a day as the euthyroid state is approached. It is desirable to keep thyroxine (T_4) in the high normal range during pregnancy; it may be necessary to adjust the dose of propylthiouracil to achieve this end. A maintenance dose of 100 mg/d minimizes the chance of fetal hypothyroidism and goiter. Elective thyroidectomy is recommended by some in preference to medical management during and even after pregnancy (see Chapter 19).

Burr WA: Prescribing in pregnancy: Thyroid disease. *Clin Obstet Gynaecol* 1981;**8**:341.

SURGICAL COMPLICATIONS DURING PREGNANCY

Elective major surgery should be avoided during pregnancy. However, normal, uncomplicated pregnancy has no debilitating effect and does not alter operative risk except as it may interfere with the diagnosis of abdominal disorders and increase the technical problems of intra-abdominal surgery. Abortion is not a serious hazard after operation unless peritoneal sepsis or other significant complication occurs.

During the first trimester, congenital anomalies may be induced in the developing fetus by hypoxia. Avoid surgical intervention during this period; if surgery does become necessary, the greatest precautions must be taken to prevent hypotension and hypoxia.

The second trimester is usually the optimal time for elective operative procedures.

McDonald JS, Kryc JJ: Anesthetic considerations in the presence of intrapartum emergencies. *Clin Perinatol* 1981;**8**:145.

Ovarian Tumors

The most common adnexal mass in early pregnancy is the corpus luteum, which may become cystic and enlarge to 6 cm in diameter. Any persistent mass over 5 cm should be evaluated by ultrasound examination; unilocular cysts are likely to be corpus luteum cysts, whereas septated or semisolid tumors are likely to be neoplasms. Ovarian tumors may undergo torsion and cause abdominal pain and nausea and vomiting and must be differentiated from appendicitis, other bowel disease, and ectopic pregnancy. Patients with suspected ovarian cancer should be referred to a gynecologic oncologist to determine whether the pregnancy can progress to fetal viability or whether treatment should be instituted without delay.

Carcinoma of the Breast
(See also p 441 and Chapter 12.)

Cancer of the breast is diagnosed approximately once in 3500 pregnancies. Pregnancy may accelerate the growth of cancer of the breast; however, delay in diagnosis affects the outcome of treatment more significantly. Inflammatory carcinoma is an extremely virulent type of breast cancer that occurs most commonly during lactation.

Breast enlargement obscures parenchymal masses, and breast tissue hyperplasia decreases the accuracy of mammography. Any perceived discrete mass should be promptly evaluated by aspiration to verify cystic structure and then by fine-needle biopsy if it is solid. A definitive diagnosis may require excisional biopsy under local anesthesia. If breast biopsy confirms the diagnosis of cancer, radical or modified radical mastectomy should be done regardless of the stage of the pregnancy. If spread to the regional glands has occurred, irradiation or chemotherapy should be considered. Under these circumstances, termination of an early pregnancy or delay of therapy for fetal maturation is indicated.

The 5-year survival rate in patients with stage I cancer of the breast diagnosed during pregnancy and treated by radical surgery is 60–70%; with stage II breast cancer, the survival rate drops to less than 10% even with radical surgery and x-ray therapy. Long-term survivors of cancer of the breast need not be advised against future pregnancies.

Anderson JM: Mammary cancers and pregnancy. *Br Med J* 1979; **1**:1124.
Sahni K et al: Carcinoma of breast associated with pregnancy and lactation. *J Surg Oncol* 1981;**16**:167.

Choledocholithiasis, Cholecystitis, & Idiopathic Cholestasis of Pregnancy

Severe choledocholithiasis and cholecystitis are not common during pregnancy despite the fact that women tend to form gallstones. When they do occur, it is usually in late pregnancy or in the puerperium. About 90% of patients with cholecystitis have gallstones; 90% of stones will be visualized by ultrasonography.

Symptomatic relief may be all that is required.

Gallbladder surgery in pregnant women should be attempted only in extreme cases (eg, obstruction), because it increases the perinatal mortality rate to about 15%. Cholecystostomy and lithotomy may be all that is feasible during advanced pregnancy, cholecystectomy being deferred until after delivery. On the other hand, withholding surgery when it is definitely needed may result in necrosis and perforation of the gallbladder and peritonitis. Cholangitis due to impacted common duct stone requires surgical removal of gallstones and establishment of biliary drainage.

Idiopathic cholestasis of pregnancy is due to a hereditary metabolic (hepatic) deficiency aggravated by the high estrogen levels of pregnancy. It causes intrahepatic biliary obstruction of varying degrees. The rise in bile acids is sufficient in the third trimester to cause severe, intractable, generalized itching and sometimes clinical jaundice. There may be mild elevations in blood bilirubin and alkaline phosphatase levels. The fetus is generally unaffected, although an increased prematurity rate has been reported. Resins such as cholestyramine (4 g 3 times a day) absorb bile acids in the large bowel and relieve pruritus but are difficult to take and may cause constipation. Their use requires vitamin K supplementation. The disorder is cured once the infant has been delivered, but it recurs in subsequent pregnancies and sometimes with the use of oral contraceptives.

Douwas SG et al: Liver disease and pregnancy. *Obstet Gynecol Surv* 1983;**38**:531.

Hernia

Pregnancy gives protection against symptoms of umbilical, incisional, and inguinal hernia. The enlarging uterus displaces the intestine, so that the bowel will not usually enter a defect in the body wall. Many abdominal hernias are reduced spontaneously during pregnancy. A few irreducible ones may result in obstruction of the involved intestine.

The inguinal rings widen during pregnancy. Rarely, an obvious indirect inguinal hernia will appear. Generally, these are asymptomatic and disappear after delivery, possibly to recur in a subsequent pregnancy.

Incarcerated hernias must be reduced surgically during pregnancy if severe pain or obstruction develops. Elective herniorrhaphy should be deferred until after delivery. The necessity for repair is not an indication for cesarean section.

Appendicitis

Appendicitis occurs in about one of 1200 pregnancies. Management is more difficult than when the disease occurs in nonpregnant persons, since the appendix is carried high and to the right, away from McBurney's point, and localization of pain and infection do not usually occur. The distended uterus displaces the colon and small bowel; uterine contractions prevent abscess formation and walling-off; and the intestinal relationships are disturbed. In at least 20% of obstetric patients, the diagnosis of appendicitis is not made until the appendix has ruptured and peritonitis has become established. Such a delay may lead to premature labor or abortion. With early diagnosis and appendectomy, the prognosis is good for mother and baby.

PREVENTION OF HEMOLYTIC DISEASE OF THE NEWBORN
(Erythroblastosis Fetalis)

The antibody anti-Rh_0 (D) is responsible for most severe instances of hemolytic disease of the newborn (erythroblastosis fetalis). About 15% of whites and much lower proportions of blacks and Asians are Rh_0 (D)-negative. If an Rh_0 (D)-negative woman carries an Rh_0 (D)-positive fetus, she may develop antibodies against Rh_0 (D) when fetal red cells enter her circulation at delivery (or during abortion, ectopic pregnancy, abruptio placentae, or other antepartum bleeding problems). This antibody, once produced, remains in the woman's circulation and poses a serious threat of hemolytic disease for subsequent Rh-positive fetuses.

Passive immunization against hemolytic disease of the newborn now is possible with Rh_0 (D) immune globulin, a purified concentrate of antibodies against Rh_0 (D) antigen. To be maximally effective, the Rh_0 (D) immune globulin should be given within 72 hours after delivery (or spontaneous or induced abortion or ectopic pregnancy). The antibodies in the immune globulin destroy fetal Rh-positive cells so that the mother will not produce anti-Rh_0 (D). During her next Rh-positive gestation, erythroblastosis will be prevented.

The usual dose of Rh_0 (D) immune globulin for prevention of isoimmunization is 1 vial (300 μg) intramuscularly.

It has recently been demonstrated that a rare Rh-negative woman will become sensitized by small feto-maternal bleeding episodes in the early third trimester. An additional safety measure is the administration of the immune globulin at the 28th week of pregnancy. The antibody molecules are too large to pass through the placenta and affect an Rh-positive fetus. The maternal clearance of the globulin is slow enough that protection will continue for 12 weeks.

Bowman JM, Pollack JM: Antenatal prophylaxis of Rh isoimmunization. *Can Med Assoc J* 1978;**118**:627.

Kurtz EM, Pappas AA, Cannon A: Laboratory identification of erythroblastosis fetalis. *Ann Clin Lab Sci* 1982;**12**:388.

Wainscoat JS, Peto TEA, Gunson HH: Maternal anti-D concentrations and outcome in rhesus haemolytic disease of the newborn. *Br Med J* 1982;**285**:327.

PREVENTION OF PRETERM (PREMATURE) LABOR

Preterm (premature) labor is labor that begins before the 37th week of pregnancy; it is responsible for 85% of neonatal illnesses and deaths. Management is critical. The onset of labor is a result of a complex sequence of biologic events involving regulatory factors which are still poorly understood. It is theorized that the delicate balance of hormones and other agents which maintain pregnancy may be upset by maternal changes such as alteration in estrogen-progesterone-prostaglandin production or by fetal factors such as increases in fetal ACTH and cortisol. If these events occur too early, preterm labor may ensue. The most significant risk factors for the onset of preterm labor are a past history of preterm delivery, premature rupture of the membranes, or exposure to diethylstilbestrol. In the current pregnancy, multiple gestation and abdominal or cervical surgery are especially important. To estimate the clinical risk, see Table 13–10.

Low rates of preterm delivery are associated with success in educating patients to identify regular, frequent uterine contractions and in alerting medical and nursing staff to evaluate these patients early and initiate treatment if cervical changes can be identified. Sedation with opiates and hydration with oral or intravenous fluids, if given before uterine contractions have changed the cervix appreciably, will often avert the need for specific drug therapy.

Uterine smooth muscle is largely under sympathetic nervous system control, and stimulation of β_2 receptors relaxes the myometrium. Consequently, inhibition of uterine contractility often can be accomplished by the administration of β-adrenergic drugs such as ritodrine (Yutopar).

Ritodrine may be administered by intravenous infusions of 0.05–0.3 mg/min to decrease the frequency and intensity of uterine contractions. Within several hours after cessation of contractions, ritodrine infusion may be scaled back by 0.05 mg every 15 minutes until a minimum effective dose is established. Oral therapy is started 30 minutes before stopping intravenous ritodrine and is continued in a dose of 10–20 mg every 4–6 hours. A dose-related elevation of heart rate of 20–40 beats/min may occur. An increase of systolic blood pressure up to 10 mm Hg is likely, and the diastolic pressure may fall 10–15 mm Hg during the infusion. Nonetheless, cardiac output increases considerably. Transient elevation of blood glucose, insulin, and fatty acids together with slight reduction of serum potassium have been reported. Fetal tachycardia may be slight or absent. No drug-caused perinatal deaths have been reported. Maternal side effects requiring dose limitation are tachycardia ($\geq$ 140 beats/min), palpitations, and nervousness. Fluids should be limited to 2500 mL/24 h. Serious side effects (pulmonary edema, chest pain with or without electrocardiographic changes) are often idiosyncratic, not dose-related, and warrant termination of therapy.

One must identify cases in which untimely delivery is the sole threat to the life or health of the infant. An effort should be made to eliminate (1) maternal conditions that compromise the intrauterine environment and make premature birth the lesser risk, eg, preeclampsia-eclampsia; (2) fetal conditions that either are helped by early delivery or render attempts to stop premature labor meaningless, eg, severe erythroblastosis fetalis; and (3) clinical situations in which it is likely that an attempt to stop labor will be futile, eg, ruptured membranes, cervix fully effaced and dilated more than 3 cm, strong labor in progress.

In pregnancies of less than 34 weeks' duration, betamethasone (12 mg intramuscularly repeated in 24 hours) is administered to hasten fetal lung maturation and permit delivery 48 hours after initial treatment when prolongation of pregnancy is contraindicated.

Herron M, Katz M, Creasy RK: Evaluation of a preterm birth prevention program. *Obstet Gynecol* 1982;**59**:452.

Katz M, Robertson PA, Creasy RK: Cardiovascular complications associated with terbutaline treatment of preterm labor. *Am J Obstet Gynecol* 1981;**139**:605.

LACTATION

Breast feeding should be encouraged by educative measures throughout pregnancy and the puerperium. Mothers should be told the benefits of breast feeding—it is emotionally satisfying, promotes mother-infant bonding, is economical, and gives significant immunity to the infant. If the mother must return to work, even a brief period of nursing is beneficial.

Transfer of immunoglobulins in breast milk protects the infant against many systemic and enteric infections. Lymphocytes transferred to the infant from breast milk play an immunoprotective role. The intestinal flora of breast-fed infants inhibits the growth of pathogens. Breast-fed infants have fewer bacterial and viral infections, less severe diarrhea, fewer allergy problems, and less subsequent obesity than bottle-fed infants.

Frequent breast feeding on an infant demand schedule enhances milk flow and successful breast feeding. Mothers breast-feeding for the first time need help and encouragement from physicians, nurses, and other nursing mothers or lay groups such as the La Leche League. Milk supply can be increased by increased suckling and increased rest.

Nursing mothers should have a fluid intake of over 2 L/d. WHO suggests 24 g of extra protein (over the 41 g/d baseline for an adult woman) and 550 extra kcal/d in the first 6 months of nursing. Calcium intake should be 1200–1500 mg/d. Continuation of a prenatal vitamin and mineral supplement is wise. Strict vegetarians who eschew both milk and eggs should always take vitamin B_{12} supplements during pregnancy and lactation.

Effects of Drugs in a Nursing Mother

Drugs taken by a nursing mother may accumulate in milk and be transmitted to the infant. The amount of a drug entering the milk depends on the drug's lipid solubility, mechanism of transport, and degree of ionization (see Table 13–12).

Suppression of Lactation

A. Mechanical Suppression: The simplest and safest method of suppressing lactation after it has started is to gradually transfer the baby to a bottle or a cup over a 3-week period. Milk supply will decrease with decreased demand, and minimal discomfort ensues. If nursing must be stopped abruptly, the mother should avoid nipple stimulation, refrain from expressing milk, and use a snug brassiere. Ice packs and analgesics can be helpful. If suppression is desired before nursing has begun, use this same technique. Engorgement will gradually recede over a 2- to 3-day period.

B. Hormonal Suppression: Oral and long-acting injections of hormonal preparations are available to suppress lactation. They are all effective if begun at the time of delivery but have occasional side effects—increased thromboembolic episodes (estrogens) hair growth (androgens, elevated blood pressure and temporary emotional changes (bromocriptine).

1. Suppression with estrogens–Ethinyl estradiol, 0.05 mg, is administered as follows:

a. Four tablets (0.2 mg) twice daily on first postpartum day.

b. Three tablets (0.15 mg) twice daily on second day.

c. Two tablets (0.1 mg) twice daily on third day.

d. One tablet (0.05 mg) twice daily on fourth to seventh days.

2. Suppression with estrogen and androgens–Testosterone enanthate, 180 mg/mL, and estradiol valerate, 8 mg/mL, 2 mL injected intramuscularly immediately after delivery, is very effective.

3. Suppression with bromocriptine–Bromocriptine (Parlodel), 2.5 mg orally twice daily with meals for 10–14 days, will suppress lactation in women who do not wish to nurse their infants or after stillbirth or abortion. The drug should not be started until 4 hours postpartum, when vital signs are stable. Postural hypotension, nausea, headache, dizziness, nasal congestion, and mild constipation have been noted as side effects. These symptoms can be allayed by reducing the dose of the drug temporarily. Hypertension, seizures, and stroke have also been reported in a small number of women.

Committee on Drugs: The transfer of drugs and other chemicals into human breast milk. *Pediatrics* 1983;**72**:375.

Duchesne C, Leke R: Bromocriptine mesylate for prevention of postpartum lactation. *Obstet Gynecol* 1981;**57**:464.

PUERPERAL MASTITIS

Postpartum mastitis occurs sporadically in nursing mothers shortly after they return home, or it may occur in epidemic form in the hospital. Hemolytic *Staphylococcus aureus* is usually the causative agent. Inflammation is generally unilateral, and primiparas are more often affected.

Table 13–12. Drugs or substances to be used cautiously or not at all by nursing mother.*

Drugs or Substances	Effect on Nursing Infant	Drugs or Substances	Effect on Nursing Infant
Alcohol	No harmful effects unless taken in excess, when it can be associated with decreased linear growth and sedation.	Cimetidine†	Concentrated in breast milk; may suppress gastric acidity and cause central nervous system stimulation.
Antibiotics Ampicillin; penicillin; amoxicillin	Very small amounts excreted in milk; safe.	Ergot alkaloids Ergotamine (in doses to treat migraine)†	Causes vomiting, diarrhea, convulsions.
Cephalosporins	Safe.	Bromocriptine†	Suppresses lactation.
Tetracycline	Effects are dose-related; amount infant receives from milk is too small to cause discoloration of teeth. Safe.	Hormones Oral contraceptives†	Contraindicated; may cause reduction of milk supply.
Chloramphenicol†	Neonate may be unable to conjugate the drug; potential harm to bone marrow, leading to anemia, shock, and death.	Laxatives Cascara	Can cause diarrhea in infant.
		Nicotine	Increased respiratory disease in infants exposed to smoke.
Sulfonamides†	May cause jaundice in the neonatal period; may cause hemolytic anemia in infant with glucose-6-phosphate dehydrogenase (G6PD) deficiency.	Radioactive materials for testing Gallium citrate (^{67}G)	Insignificant amount excreted in milk; no nursing for 2 weeks.
Metronidazole	Nursing may be resumed 48 hours after last dose.	^{125}I	Discontinue nursing for 48 hours.
Anticoagulants Heparin; warfarin; dicumarol	Safe.	^{131}I	After a test dose, nursing may be resumed after 24–36 hours; after a treatment dose, nursing may be resumed after 2–3 weeks.
Antihistamines	Not appreciably excreted in milk, but large doses may affect milk supply.	^{99m}Technetium	Discontinue nursing for 72 hours (half-life; 6 hours)
Antineoplastics	Some agents excreted in measurable amounts in milk.	Other drugs Caffeine	Irritability, poor sleep pattern.
Methotrexate	Causes immune suppression.	Cannabis;† cocaine;† polyhalogenated biphenyls† (eg, PCB$_5$, PBB$_5$); D-lysergic acid† (LSD)	Contraindicated; may interfere with mother's caretaking abilities and nutrition.
Cyclophosphamide†	Contraindicated.		
Antithyroids Thiouracil;† methimazole†	Contraindicated; may cause goiter or agranulocytosis.	Sedatives and tranquilizers	Can cause sedation in infant.
Propylthiouracil	Considered safe.	Lithium carbonate†	Contraindicated because of toxicity.
Cardiac drugs Quinidine†	Contraindicated; may cause arrhythmia in infant.		

*Modified and reproduced, with permission, from Sahu S: Drugs and the nursing mother. *Am Fam Physician* (Dec) 1981;24:137.
†Absolutely contraindicated.

In sporadic puerperal mastitis, an acute interlobar inflammation with fever, localized pain, tenderness, and segmental erythema develops via a fissured nipple. The sepsis is in neither the acinar nor the duct system, and the milk is not affected. Hence, the baby should be allowed to nurse (with a nipple shield) to prevent engorgement, which contributes to abscess formation. Antibiotic therapy against possible penicillinase-resistant organisms (dicloxacillin or a cephalosporin) should be given.

If the mother begins antibiotic therapy before suppuration begins, infection can usually be controlled in 24 hours. If delay is permitted, breast abscess can result. Incision and drainage are required for abscess formation. Despite puerperal mastitis, the baby usually thrives without prophylactic antimicrobial therapy.

• • •

References

Beacham DW, Beacham WD: *Synopsis of Gynecology,* 10th ed. Mosby, 1982.

Benson RC (editor): *Current Obstetric & Gynecologic Diagnosis & Treatment,* 5th ed. Lange, 1984.

Benson RC: *Handbook of Obstetrics & Gynecology,* 8th ed. Lange, 1983.

Caplan R: *Principles of Obstetrics.* Williams & Wilkins, 1982.

Cavanagh D et al (editors): *Obstetric Emergencies,* 3rd ed. Harper & Row, 1982.

Danforth DN (editor): *Textbook of Obstetrics and Gynecology,* 4th ed. Harper & Row, 1982.

Dewhurst CJ: *Integrated Obstetrics and Gynaecology for Postgraduates,* 3rd ed. Mosby, 1982.

Ellis J, Beckman C (editors): *Clinical Manual of Obstetrics.* Appleton-Century-Crofts, 1983.

Hatcher RA et al: *Contraceptive Technology 1984–1985.* Irvington, 1984.

Jelliffe DB, Jelliffe EFP: *Human Milk in the Modern World.* Oxford Univ Press, 1981.

Jones HW Jr, Jones GS: *Novak's Textbook of Gynecology,* 10th ed. Williams & Wilkins, 1981.

Kaplan HS: *The New Sex Therapy.* Brunner/Mazel, 1974.

Llewellyn-Jones D: *Fundamentals of Obstetrics and Gynecology,* 3rd ed. Faber & Faber, 1982

Mudaliar AL, Krishna MK: *Clinical Obstetrics.* State Mutual Books, 1982.

Speroff L, Glass R, Kase N: *Clinical Gynecologic Endocrinology and Infertility,* 3rd ed. Williams & Wilkins, 1983.

Worthington-Roberts BS, Vermeersch J, Williams SL: *Nutrition in Pregnancy and Lactation.* Mosby, 1981.

Zuspan FP, Quilligan EJ: *Practical Manual of Obstetric Care.* Mosby, 1981.

Arthritis & Allied Rheumatic Disorders | 14

Martin A. Shearn, MD, & Ephraim P. Engleman, MD

Examination of the Patient

The specific diagnosis of a rheumatic disease can often be made at the bedside or in the office.

The examination depends upon a careful history and physical examination, with special attention to signs of articular inflammation (eg, heat, soft tissue swelling, effusion) and the functional status of the joints (eg, range of motion, deformity). Depending upon the suspected diagnosis, certain laboratory procedures complete the study. These most commonly include a blood count, urinalysis, sedimentation rate, tests for rheumatoid factor and antinuclear antibodies, synovianalysis, and x-rays of affected joints. These studies are important not only for diagnosis but also as a baseline for judging the results of therapy.

Examination of Joint Fluid

Synovial fluid examination (Table 14–1) may provide valuable diagnostic and prognostic information in the management of joint disease. After as much fluid has been removed as possible, the needle is withdrawn and the puncture site is covered with a sterile dressing.

The following studies should then be performed:

(1) Gross examination: Carefully note consistency and appearance. If fluid is green or purulent, examination with Gram's stain is indicated. If grossly bloody, consider a bleeding disorder, trauma, or "traumatic tap." Note if the fluid is xanthochromic.

(2) Microscopic examination:

(a) Cytology: Collect 2–5 mL in a heparinized tube. The red and white cells are counted, using the same equipment and technique as for a standard white count. The diluent, however, should be normal saline solution, since the usual acidified diluent causes the fluid to clot in the pipette (see below). One drop of methylene blue added to the diluent makes the cells distinguishable. Differential counts are performed on thin smears with Wright's stain.

(b) Crystals: Compensated polarized light microscopy identifies the existence and type of crystals. The demonstration of urate or calcium pyrophosphate crystals is most important diagnostically.

(3) Culture: Collect 1 mL of fluid in a sterile culture tube and perform routine cultures as well as special studies for gonococci, tubercle bacilli, or fungi as indicated.

(4) Glucose: Collect 2–3 mL of fluid in a fluoride tube. The patient should be in a fasting state and the blood glucose determined at the time of joint aspiration.

Interpretation. (See Table 14–2.) Synovial fluid studies are not diagnostic unless a specific organism is identified in the culture or unless the urate crystals of gouty synovitis or the calcium pyrophosphate crystals of pseudogout are demonstrated. There is considerable overlap in the cytologic and biochemical values obtained in different diseases. These studies do make possible, however, a differentiation according to severity of inflammation. Thus, joint fluids in inflammatory diseases such as infections and rheumatoid arthritis are often turbid, with an elevated white count (usually well above 3000 cells/μL, with over 50% polynucleated forms) and a synovial fluid sugar con-

Table 14–1. Examination of joint fluid.

Measure	Normal	Group I (Noninflammatory)	Group II (Inflammatory)	Group III (Septic)
Volume (mL) (knee)	< 3.5	Often > 3.5	Often > 3.5	Often > 3.5
Clarity	Transparent	Transparent	Translucent-opaque	Opaque
Color	Clear	Yellow	Yellow to opalescent	Yellow to green
WBC (per μL)	< 200	200–3000	3000–100,000	> 100,000*
Polymorphonuclear leukocytes (%)	< 25%	< 25%	50% or more	75% or more*
Culture	Negative	Negative	Negative	Usually positive
Glucose (mg/dL)	Nearly equal to serum	Nearly equal to serum	> 25, lower than serum	< 25, much lower than serum

*Counts are lower with infections caused by organisms of low virulence or if antibiotic therapy has been started.

Table 14—2. Differential diagnosis by joint fluid groups.*

Group I (Noninflammatory)	Group II (Inflammatory)	Group III (Septic)	Hemorrhagic
Degenerative joint disease	Rheumatoid arthritis	Bacterial infections	Hemophilia or other hemorrhagic diathesis
Trauma†	Acute crystal-induced synovitis		Trauma with or without fracture
Osteochondritis dissecans	(gout and pseudogout)		Neuropathic arthropathy
Osteochondromatosis	Reiter's syndrome		Pigmented villonodular synovitis
Neuropathic arthropathy†	Ankylosing spondylitis		Synovioma
Subsiding or early inflammation	Psoriatic arthritis		Hemangioma and other benign neoplasm
Hypertrophic osteoarthropathy‡	Arthritis accompanying ulcerative		
Pigmented villonodular synovitis†	colitis and regional enteritis		
	Rheumatic fever‡		
	Systemic lupus erythematosus‡		
	Progressive systemic sclerosis (scleroderma)‡		

*Reproduced from Rodnan GP (editor): Primer on the rheumatic diseases, 7th ed. *JAMA* 1973;**224**(Suppl):662.
†May be hemorrhagic.
‡Groups I or II.

tent that is considerably lower than the blood glucose. In diseases characterized by relatively mild articular inflammation, such as degenerative joint disease or traumatic arthritis, the synovial fluid is usually clear, with a low white cell count (usually below $3000/\mu L$), and the synovial fluid and blood glucose levels are within 10 mg/dL of each other.

CONNECTIVE TISSUE (COLLAGEN) DISEASES

The connective tissue disorders are a protean group of acquired diseases in which genetic factors appear to play a role. They have in common widespread immunologic and inflammatory alterations of connective tissue. A variety of other names have been given to the group (eg, collagen diseases, collagenoses, diffuse vascular diseases, collagen vascular diseases, visceral angiitides), but no completely satisfactory term has been found. This group of acquired diseases must be distinguished from rare heritable disorders of connective tissue (see Chapter 21).

The acquired connective tissue diseases generally include the following clinical entities: rheumatoid arthritis, systemic lupus erythematosus, polymyositis, scleroderma, necrotizing vasculitis, rheumatic fever, mixed connective tissue disease, relapsing polychondritis, and Sjögren's syndrome.

These entities have certain features in common, and differentiation among them is often difficult because of overlapping features. Common findings include synovitis, pleuritis, myocarditis, endocarditis, pericarditis, peritonitis, vasculitis, myositis, changes in skin, alterations of connective tissues, and, in some cases, nephritis. Laboratory tests may reveal Coombs-positive hemolytic anemia, thrombocytopenia, leukopenia, B and T cell alterations,

immunoglobulin excesses or deficiencies, impaired or accentuated delayed hypersensitivity, antinuclear antibodies, antibodies to DNA and ENA (extractable nuclear antigen), rheumatoid factors, cryoglobulins, false-positive serologic tests for syphilis, elevated muscle enzymes, antithyroid antibodies, alterations in serum complement, and changes in acute phase reactants.

Although the connective tissue disorders are regarded as acquired diseases, the underlying causes cannot be determined in most instances, and it is unlikely that the established clinical entities have similar causes. Heredity, infection or other environmental antigen, immunoglobulin deficiency or inappropriate control (T cells), drug allergy, antigen-antibody-complement immune complexes, anaphylaxis, cytolysis, or some combination of all of these factors appear to play varying undefined roles. Investigations into the etiologic role of viruses appear promising.

Some of the laboratory alterations that occur in this group of diseases (eg, false-positive serologic tests for syphilis) may also occur in asymptomatic individuals and may suggest the possibility of the presence or future development of one of the connective tissue diseases. It is interesting to note also that these alterations in laboratory values may be demonstrated in certain asymptomatic relatives of patients with connective tissue diseases, in older persons in association with certain drugs and infections, and in patients with abnormalities of the immune system.

RHEUMATOID ARTHRITIS

Essentials of Diagnosis
- A systemic disease.
- Prodromal symptoms: malaise, fever, weight loss, and morning stiffness.
- Onset usually insidious and in small joints; progression is centripetal and symmetric; deformities common.

- X-ray findings: juxta-articular osteoporosis, joint erosions, and narrowing of the joint spaces.
- Rheumatoid factor test usually positive.
- Extra-articular manifestations: vasculitis, atrophy of muscle, subcutaneous and systemic granulomas, pleurisy, pericarditis, pulmonary fibrosis, lymphadenopathy, splenomegaly, and leukopenia.

General Considerations

Rheumatoid arthritis is a chronic systemic inflammatory disease of unknown cause, chiefly affecting synovial membranes of multiple joints. The disease has a wide clinical spectrum with considerable variability in joint and extra-articular manifestations. The prevalence in the general population is 1–3%; female patients outnumber males almost 3:1. The usual age at onset is 20–40 years, although rheumatoid arthritis may begin at any age.

The pathologic findings in the joint include chronic synovitis with pannus formation. The pannus erodes cartilage, bone, ligaments, and tendons. In the acute phase, effusion and other manifestations of inflammation are common. In the late stage, organization may result in fibrous ankylosis; true bony ankylosis is rare. In both acute and chronic phases, inflammation of soft tissues around the joints may be prominent and may be a significant factor in joint damage.

The microscopic findings most characteristic of rheumatoid arthritis are those of the subcutaneous nodule. This is a granuloma with a central zone of necrosis, a surrounding palisade of radially arranged elongated connective tissue cells, and a periphery of chronic granulation tissue. Pathologic alterations indistinguishable from those of the subcutaneous nodule are occasionally seen in the myocardium, pericardium, endocardium, heart valves, visceral pleura, lungs, sclera, dura mater, spleen, and larynx as well as in the synovial membrane, periarticular tissues, and tendons. Nonspecific pericarditis and pleuritis are found in 25–40% of patients at autopsy. Additional nonspecific lesions associated with rheumatoid arthritis include inflammation of small arteries, pulmonary fibrosis, round cell infiltration of skeletal muscle and perineurium, and hyperplasia of lymph nodes. Secondary amyloidosis may also be present.

Clinical Findings

A. Symptoms and Signs: The clinical manifestations of rheumatoid disease are highly variable. The onset of articular signs of inflammation is usually insidious, with prodromal symptoms of malaise, weight loss, vasomotor disturbances (eg, paresthesias, Raynaud's phenomenon), and vague periarticular pain or stiffness. Less often, the onset is acute, apparently triggered by a stressful situation such as infection, surgery, trauma, emotional strain, or the postpartum period. There is characteristically symmetric joint swelling with associated stiffness, warmth, tenderness, and pain. Pain and stiffness are prominent in the morning and subside during the day. Stiffness may recur after daytime inactivity and may be much more severe after strenuous activity. Stiffness is a useful indication of active disease. Although any joint may be affected, the proximal interphalangeal and metacarpophalangeal joints of the fingers as well as the wrists, knees, ankles, and toes are most often involved. Monarticular disease is occasionally seen early. Synovial cysts and rupture of tendons may occur. Entrapment syndromes are not unusual—particularly entrapment of the median nerve at the carpal tunnel of the wrist. Palmar erythema is seen occasionally, as are tiny hemorrhagic infarcts in the nail folds or finger pulps, which are signs of vasculitis. Twenty percent of patients have subcutaneous nodules. These are most commonly situated over bony prominences but are also observed in the bursas and tendon sheaths. A small number of patients have an enlarged spleen and lymph node enlargement. Low-grade fever, anorexia, weight loss, fatigue, and weakness are often present; chills are rare. After months or years, thickening of the periarticular tissue, flexion deformities, subluxation, and ankylosis, usually fibrous, may occur. Atrophy of skin or muscle is common. Dryness of the eyes (also of the mouth and other mucous membranes), with corneal and conjunctival staining characteristic of keratoconjunctivitis sicca, is found especially in advanced disease (see Sjögren's Syndrome). Other ocular manifestations worthy of note include episcleritis, scleromalacia, and scleral nodules. Pericarditis and pleural disease, when present, are frequently unsuspected clinically; these are found commonly at autopsy.

B. Laboratory Findings: Serum protein abnormalities are often present. Various serologic techniques are used to detect certain macroglobulins (antiglobulins) that constitute rheumatoid factor. One of these, the latex fixation test, is positive in 75% of cases. High titers of rheumatoid factor are commonly associated with severe rheumatoid disease. False-positive reactions are not unusual. Titers may be significantly elevated with advanced age, other connective tissue disorders, liver disease, chronic lung disease, syphilis, sarcoidosis, infective endocarditis, leprosy, and parasitic infections. Antinuclear antibodies are often demonstrable, although their titers are usually lower in rheumatoid arthritis than in systemic lupus erythematosus.

During both the acute and chronic phases, the erythrocyte sedimentation rate and the gamma globulins (most commonly IgM and IgG) are usually elevated. A moderate hypochromic normocytic anemia is common. The white cell count is normal or slightly elevated, but leukopenia may occur, especially in the presence of splenomegaly (eg, Felty's syndrome). Joint fluid examination is valuable, reflecting abnormalities that are associated with varying degrees of inflammation. (See Tables 14–1 and 14–2.) Low synovial complement values are found in severe forms of rheumatoid arthritis.

C. X-Ray Findings: Early signs are soft tissue

swelling, osteoporosis around the involved joint, and erosion of the peripheral "bare space" of bone surface that is not covered by cartilage. Later, extensive erosion of cartilage causes joint space narrowing. Bony cysts result from invasion by granulation tissue. Rheumatoid synovium may invade the joint capsule, ligaments, and tendons, and it may add to joint instability induced by destruction of cartilage and bone. After some years, the degenerative changes of secondary osteoarthritis may be superimposed.

Special attention should be directed to the upper cervical spine and especially to C1–2, where subluxation may result in the development of serious neurologic complications.

D. Radionuclide Joint Scanning: Radioisotope joint scintigraphy may help identify or exclude the presence of synovitis in symptomatic patients without objective clinical, laboratory, and x-ray findings. Although a sensitive technique, it lacks specificity.

Differential Diagnosis

The differentiation of rheumatoid arthritis from other diseases of connective tissue can be exceedingly difficult, even impossible. However, certain clinical features are often helpful. Rheumatic fever is characterized by the migratory nature of the arthritis, the dramatic and objective response to salicylates in adequate doses, the more common occurrence of carditis, and the elevated antistreptolysin titer. Butterfly rash, discoid lupus erythematosus, photosensitivity, alopecia, high titer to anti-DNA, and renal disease point to the diagnosis of systemic lupus erythematosus. Degenerative joint disease (osteoarthritis) is not associated with constitutional manifestations, and the joint pain is characteristically relieved by rest, frequently in contrast to the morning stiffness of rheumatoid arthritis. Signs of articular inflammation, prominent in rheumatoid arthritis, are usually minimal in degenerative joint disease. Gouty arthritis may be confused with rheumatoid arthritis, but acute onset in one joint, hyperuricemia, the identification of urate crystals in the joint fluid, the presence of tophi, and the dramatic response to colchicine indicate gout. Pyogenic arthritis can be distinguished by chills as well as fever, the demonstration of the causative organism in the joint fluid, and the frequent presence of a primary focus elsewhere, eg, gonococcal urethritis.

Treatment

A. Basic Program (Conservative Management): Evidence indicates that conservative management offers a long-term prognosis that is often as good as that of more spectacular methods. Since none of the latter measures is curative, and because their administration is often accompanied by undesirable side effects, a conservative approach should be initiated first.

The primary objectives of treatment of rheumatoid arthritis are reduction of inflammation and pain, preservation of function, and prevention of deformity. A simple regimen consisting of rest, physical therapy, and salicylates is the best means of rehabilitating the

patient. These measures constitute the basic program of treatment to which other treatment may be added.

1. Systemic rest–There is a great deal of empiric evidence for the benefits of systemic rest. The amount of rest required depends upon the severity of the disease. Complete bed rest may be desirable and even imperative, particularly in patients with profound systemic and articular involvement. In mild disease, 2 hours of rest each day may suffice. In general, rest should be continued until significant improvement is sustained for at least 2 weeks; thereafter, the program may be liberalized. However, the increase of physical activity must proceed gradually and with appropriate support for any involved weight-bearing joints.

2. Emotional factors–The importance of emotional factors in rheumatoid arthritis and the need for psychologic support cannot be overemphasized. This support depends in part upon rapport between the patient and the doctor and is necessary during all phases of the illness. Patients often need help in dealing with fear, disability, and loss.

3. Articular rest–Decrease of articular inflammation may be expedited by articular rest. Relaxation and stretching of the hip and knee muscles, to prevent flexion contractures, can be accomplished by having the patient lie in the prone position for 15 minutes several times daily in addition to nighttime rest. Sitting in a flexed position for prolonged periods is a poor form of joint rest. Appropriate adjustable supports or splints provide rest for inflamed weight-bearing joints, relieve spasm and thus pain, and prevent or reduce deformities due to muscle spasm, soft tissue contracture, or ligamentous instability. The supports must be removable to permit daily range of motion and exercise of the affected extremities (see below). When ambulation is started, care must be taken to avoid weight bearing, which will aggravate flexion deformities. This is accomplished with the aid of supports such as crutches and braces until the tendency toward contracture has subsided.

4. Exercise–This is the most important measure in the physical therapy of rheumatoid arthritis. The management of rheumatoid arthritis is based on the concomitant administration of rest and therapeutic exercise, always in proper balance. Therapeutic exercises are designed to preserve joint motion and muscular strength and endurance. Most effective are exercises of the active-assistive type. These should be performed, within the limits of pain tolerance, from the outset of management. As tolerance for exercise increases and the activity of the disease subsides, progressive resistance exercises may be introduced. (Specific instructions for exercises are contained in *Home Care Programs in Arthritis,* a booklet published by The Arthritis Foundation, 1314 Spring Street NW, Atlanta 30309.)

5. Heat and cold–These are used primarily for their muscle-relaxing and analgesic effect. Radiant or moist heat is generally most satisfactory. The ambulatory patient will find warm tub baths most convenient. Exercise may be better performed after exposure to heat. Some patients derive more relief of joint pain from local application of cold.

6. Diet–The diet should be well-balanced and adjusted to each individual's requirements. There is no specific food contraindication. If dietary intake is normal, there is usually no need to use supplemental vitamins.

7. Hematinic agents–These are not beneficial in the treatment of the anemia of rheumatoid arthritis. If iron deficiency coexists, however, iron salts are useful—eg, ferrous sulfate, 0.2 g orally 3 times daily. Significant iron deficiency is not unusual following long-term loss of microscopic amounts of blood per rectum associated with the prolonged use of salicylates.

8. Nonsteroidal anti-inflammatory drugs– (See Chapter 1.)

a. Aspirin–Aspirin is generally the first drug employed. Given in adequate and regular dosage, the salicylates exert an anti-inflammatory effect. The proper dose is the amount that provides optimal relief of symptoms without causing toxic reactions. Most adults can tolerate daily doses of 4–6 g, which result in serum levels of 20–30 mg/dL. After 1 week, the salicylate half-life increases to 15 hours; therefore, the patient need not be given aspirin every 4 hours, as is often recommended. Determination of serum salicylate levels is an effective way of monitoring patient compliance. Tinnitus and gastric irritation are early manifestations of toxicity. If tinnitus occurs, the daily dose should be decreased by decrements of 0.6 or 0.9 g until this symptom disappears. Symptoms of gastric irritation may be lessened by the ingestion of salicylates with meals and antacid. The use of enteric-coated tablets may also reduce gastric irritation. Salicylates should not, of course, be used by patients with a history of allergy to aspirin or related products.

b. Other nonsteroidal anti-inflammatory drugs–If aspirin proves ineffective or if intolerable gastrointestinal effects occur, a trial of the newer anti-inflammatory analgesic agents is indicated. Because of a simpler dosage schedule, compliance may be better with these agents. A number of recently introduced nonsteroidal anti-inflammatory analgesic drugs are available: ibuprofen (Motrin), fenoprofen (Nalfon), naproxen (Naprosyn), tolmetin (Tolectin), sulindac (Clinoril), meclofenamate sodium (Meclomen), and piroxicam (Feldene). Many other drugs of this class are available outside the USA, and still others are under investigation. The new drugs themselves are not free of gastroduodenal and other side effects (particularly renal) but tend to cause less gastrointestinal discomfort than does aspirin in full dosage. Renal toxicity may occur, including interstitial nephritis, nephrotic syndrome, and reversible renal failure. Hyperkalemia due to hyporeninemic hypoaldosteronism may also be seen. While more expensive, none of the drugs is superior to salicylates in efficacy. Each of them, however, may be effective in patients who fail to respond to salicylate therapy. Drug toxicity also varies from individual to individual. The relative long-term therapeutic merits of the new nonsteroidal drugs have not been fully established.

Indomethacin is probably no more effective than the salicylates in the treatment of rheumatoid arthritis, and its untoward effects are far greater. Phenylbutazone is not advised for chronic therapy because of its toxicity.

9. Physical therapy–See p 523.

B. Other Anti-inflammatory Drugs:

1. Chloroquines (antimalarials)–Chloroquine phosphate and hydroxychloroquine sulfate have antirheumatic properties in patients with rheumatoid arthritis. A daily dose of only 250 mg (1 tablet) of chloroquine or 200 mg (1 tablet) of hydroxychloroquine minimizes the likelihood of major toxic reactions (eg, retinitis, keratitis). Nevertheless, periodic ophthalmologic examination is required if these drugs are used in the treatment of rheumatoid arthritis.

2. Gold salts (chrysotherapy)–Gold salts in the treatment of rheumatoid arthritis have gained increased popularity in recent years. There is evidence that these agents may retard the bone erosions of rheumatoid arthritis. About 60% of patients may be expected to benefit from gold therapy. The exact mode of action is not known, but the effect of these agents on the functional capacity of macrophages may be significant.

a. Indications–Active disease responding unfavorably to conservative management; erosive disease.

b. Contraindications–Previous gold toxicity; significant renal, hepatic, or hematopoietic dysfunction.

c. Preparations of choice–Gold sodium thiomalate or aurothioglucose.

d. Weekly intramuscular dose–Give 50 mg weekly until toxic reactions appear or there is a clinical response. If there is no response after 800 mg have been given, the drug should be discontinued. If the response is good, a total dose of 1 g should be given, followed by a regimen of 50 mg every 2 weeks and, with continued improvement, every 3 and then every 4 weeks for an indefinite period. Recent studies suggest that smaller doses may be effective.

e. Toxic reactions–About 32% of patients (range in various series: 4–55%) experience toxic reactions to gold therapy; the mortality rate is less than 0.4%. The manifestations of toxicity are similar to those of poisoning by other heavy metals (notably arsenic) and include dermatitis (mild to exfoliative), stomatitis, agranulocytosis and other signs of bone marrow impairment, nephritis, and nitritoid reactions (especially to gold thiomalate and presumably due to its vehicle). In order to prevent or reduce the severity of toxic reactions, do not give gold salts to patients with any of the contraindicating disorders listed above and observe all patients carefully during the course of gold therapy. Before giving injections, ask how the patient has felt since the previous injection; examine the skin and mucous membranes for dermatitis or purpura; examine the urine for protein and microscopic hematuria; determine the hemoglobin and white cell count; and inspect a blood smear for differential white cell count values and for platelets. Platelet counts and liver function tests should be performed periodically. Warn the patient against exposure to strong light.

If signs of toxicity appear, withdraw the drug immediately. Severe toxicity may require corticosteroids for control, but failure to respond to steroids might then be an indication for the cautious use of penicillamine or dimercaprol (BAL) as chelating agents.

3. Corticosteroids–Although corticosteroids usually produce an immediate and dramatic anti-inflammatory effect in rheumatoid arthritis, they do not alter the natural progression of the disease; furthermore, clinical manifestations of active disease commonly reappear when the drug is discontinued. The serious problem of untoward reactions resulting from prolonged corticosteroid therapy greatly limits its long-term use. Another disadvantage that might stem from the use of steroids lies in the tendency of the patient and the physician to neglect the less spectacular but proved benefits derived from general supportive treatment, physical therapy, and orthopedic measures.

The corticosteroids may be used on a short-term basis to tide patients over acute disabling episodes, to facilitate other treatment measures (eg, physical therapy), or to manage serious extra-articular manifestations (eg, pericarditis, perforating eye lesions). Corticosteroids may also be indicated for active and progressive disease that does not respond favorably to conservative management and when there are contraindications to gold salts or therapeutic failure of gold salts and penicillamine.

Give the least amount of steroid that will achieve the desired clinical effect, but not more than 10 mg of prednisone or equivalent per day. Many patients do reasonably well on 5–7.5 mg daily. (The use of 1-mg tablets is to be encouraged.) When the steroids are to be discontinued, they should be phased out gradually on a planned schedule appropriate to the duration of treatment.

Intra-articular corticosteroids may be helpful if one or 2 joints are the chief source of difficulty. Intra-articular hydrocortisone esters, 25–50 mg, may be given for symptomatic relief, but no more often than 4 times a year.

4. Penicillamine–This agent may be used in patients with severe rheumatoid arthritis who have continuing rheumatic activity in spite of therapy with the agents discussed above. Penicillamine may prove effective in a number of such patients, although toxicity is high. The mechanism of action is not understood. Up to one-half of patients experience some side effects, such as oral ulcers, fever, rash, disturbances of taste, thrombocytopenia, leukopenia, and aplastic anemia. Proteinuria and nephrotic syndrome may occur. Immune complex diseases (eg, myasthenia gravis, systemic lupus erythematosus, polymyositis, Goodpasture's syndrome) may be induced by the drug. The drug should not be used during pregnancy.

If penicillamine is employed, one should start

with small doses: 250 mg daily, increasing by 125 mg every 2–3 months up to a maximum of 750 mg–1 g/d. Penicillamine is given between meals to enhance absorption. Careful monitoring for toxicity is essential.

C. Experimental Drugs:

1. Cytotoxic drugs–Cyclophosphamide, methotrexate, azathioprine, and chlorambucil have been used in patients with severe rheumatoid arthritis. Response to treatment is not invariably correlated with laboratory parameters of rheumatoid activity. The toxicity of these drugs and their potential teratogenic and oncogenic capacities are such that they should not be employed except by a physician thoroughly conversant with their use.

2. Other experimental measures–Numerous nonsteroidal anti-inflammatory drugs are currently under study. These include an oral gold preparation and the anthelmintic agent levamisole. The latter drug, like gold salts and penicillamine, appears to have long-acting antirheumatic effects. Its mechanism of action, though not understood, is thought to be in part related to immunoaugmentation. Plasmapheresis, leukapheresis, and nodal irradiation are under investigation.

D. Surgical Measures: See p 524.

Prognosis

The course of rheumatoid arthritis is totally unpredictable, although spontaneous remissions and relapses are common early in the disease. Occasionally, in well-established cases, permanent spontaneous remission occurs, with either return to normal function of the involved joints (if involvement is early and minimal) or some decrease in the degree of disability (if of longer duration). Although the disease is commonly progressive—and although some degree of permanent deformity may result—it must be emphasized that after 10 years half of patients are still capable of self-care and fully employable.

Adams EM, Yocum DE, Bell CL: Hydroxychloroquine in the treatment of rheumatoid arthritis. *Am J Med* 1983;**75**:321.

Chalmers A et al: Systemic lupus erythematosus during penicillamine therapy of rheumatoid arthritis. *Ann Intern Med* 1982;**97**:659.

Fischer M et al: Generalized vasculopathy and finger blood flow abnormalities in rheumatoid arthritis. *J Rheum* 1984;**11**:1.

Million R et al: Long-term study of management of rheumatoid arthritis. *Lancet* 1984;**1**:812.

Mitchell DM, Fries JF: An analysis of the American Rheumatism Association criteria for rheumatoid arthritis. *Arthritis Rheum* 1982;**25**:481.

Olive DM, Stoff JS: Renal syndromes associated with nonsteroidal antiinflammatory drugs. *N Engl J Med* 1984;**310**:563.

Proceedings of the International Symposium on Penicillamine, Miami, Florida, May 8–9, 1980. *J Rheumatol* 1981;**8(Suppl 7)**:1. [Entire issue.]

Scott DEI, Bacon PA, Tribe CR: Systemic rheumatoid vasculitis: A clinical and laboratory study of 50 cases. *Medicine* 1981;**60**:288.

Zimmermann M (editor): Antipyretic analgesic therapy: Current worldwide status. (Symposium.) *Am J Med* 1983;**75**. [Entire issue.]

JUVENILE CHRONIC ARTHRITIS

Rheumatoidlike disease with onset before age 17 is referred to as juvenile chronic arthritis. Synovitis that persists for at least 6 weeks is an essential criterion of diagnosis. Various forms of the disease have been described, including (1) a form with systemic onset; (2) pauciarticular arthritis, often with iritis; (3) polyarticular arthritis, including both seronegative and seropositive types, resembling adult disease; and (4) a form reported chiefly in older boys who later develop ankylosing spondylitis. The various subtypes of juvenile arthritis often manifest different HLA haplotypes. In systemic-onset disease, there is a characteristic evanescent, salmon-colored morbilliform rash, a high spiking fever that may antedate the arthritis by months, and severe systemic disease with hepatosplenomegaly, lymphadenopathy, or pleuropericarditis. Iridocyclitis may be asymptomatic and detected only by slit lamp examination; it occurs commonly in patients with mild arthritis. A clinical presentation with features identical to those of juvenile chronic arthritis may recur in adulthood after an episode before age 17 or may even appear for the first time in adult life.

In many children with chronic arthritis, the apophyseal joints of the cervical spine, especially C2–3, are affected. Abnormalities of bony growth and development are related to active disease and may be transient and reversible or, with chronic disease activity, may be irreversible and result in premature closure of epiphyses or ossification centers.

The differential diagnosis of juvenile chronic arthritis includes idiopathic ankylosing spondylitis, leukemia, and chronic infectious disease. Joint fluid examination, culture, and even synovial biopsy, may be useful in diagnosis. HLA-B27 typing is useful in identifying those patients who may develop spondylarthritis. Antinuclear antibody is often positive in the subgroup that develops iridocyclitis. Rheumatoid factor is positive only in the small subset of patients whose disease resembles adult rheumatoid arthritis.

The treatment of juvenile chronic arthritis must be individualized.

Fink CW: Treatment of juvenile arthritis. *Bull Rheum Dis* 1982;**32**:21.

Gewanter HL, Roghmann KJ, Baum J: The prevalence of juvenile arthritis. *Arthritis Rheum* 1983;**26**:599.

Hanson V: From Still's disease and JRA to JCPA, JCA, and JA: Medical progress or biased ascertainment. *J Rheum* 1982;**9**:819.

Larson EB: Adult Still's disease: Evolution of a clinical syndrome and diagnosis—treatment and follow-up of 17 patients. *Medicine* 1984;**63**:82.

Moore TL, Weiss TD: Immunologic studies in juvenile arthritis. *Bull Rheum Dis* 1982;**32**:25.

SYSTEMIC LUPUS ERYTHEMATOSUS

Essentials of Diagnosis

- Occurs mainly in young women.
- Rash over areas exposed to sunlight.
- Joint symptoms in 90% of patients.
- Multiple system involvement.
- Depression of hemoglobin, white blood cells, platelets.
- Serologic findings: positive antinuclear antibody test and antibodies to DNA.

General Considerations

Systemic lupus erythematosus is an inflammatory autoimmune disorder that may affect multiple organ systems. Its clinical manifestations are thought to be secondary to the trapping of antigen-antibody complexes in capillaries of visceral structures. The clinical course may vary from a mild episodic disorder to a rapidly fulminating fatal illness.

Systemic lupus erythematosus is not uncommon. Figures from a large representative urban community population indicate a prevalence exceeding one in 2000 persons. About 85% of patients are women. Although the disease may occur at any age, most patients are between ages 10 and 50, with greatest clustering between 20 and 40. Blacks are affected more often than members of other races.

Before making a diagnosis of spontaneous systemic lupus erythematosus, it is imperative to ascertain that the condition has not been induced by a drug. Approximately 25 pharmacologic agents have been implicated as causing a lupuslike syndrome, but only a few cause the disorder with appreciable frequency. Procainamide and hydralazine are the most important and best studied of these drugs. While antinuclear antibody tests and other serologic findings become positive in many persons receiving these agents, in only a few do clinical manifestations occur.

Four features distinguish drug-induced lupus from spontaneously occurring disease: (1) in the drug-induced syndrome, the sex ratio is nearly equal; (2) nephritis and central nervous system features are not ordinarily present; (3) depressed serum complement and antibodies to native DNA are absent; and (4) the clinical features and most laboratory abnormalities revert toward normal when the offending drug is withdrawn, although serologic abnormalities may persist for months or years.

The familial occurrence of systemic lupus erythematosus has been repeatedly documented, and the disorder has involved identical twins in a number of instances. Aggregation of serologic features (positive antinuclear antibody test, antibodies to DNA, hypergammaglobulinemia) is seen in asymptomatic family members, and the prevalence of other rheumatic diseases is increased among close relatives of patients. There is increased incidence of HLA-DR2 and -DR3 in patients with this disease. A current hypothesis suggests that there is an underlying genetically determined abnormality in immunologic regulation, related to defective T cell function, resulting in overactivity of B cells. This leads to production of multiple autoantibodies, which causes tissue damage through the mechanism of immune complex deposition.

Viruses are thought to play a role in the induction of this disorder in a genetically disposed host. The New Zealand mouse, in which a clinical syndrome develops that is remarkably similar to idiopathic lupus in humans, harbors the murine leukemia virus. Patients with systemic lupus have increased antibody titers to various viral antigens, including those of measles, rubella, and parainfluenza. In studies of patients with this disorder, electron micrographs of capillary endothelial cells in renal biopsy tissue and of circulating lymphocytes have shown tubular reticular structures thought to be virus-related.

The diagnosis of systemic lupus erythematosus should be suspected in patients having a multisystem disease with serologic positivity (eg, antinuclear antibody, serologic test for syphilis). Differential diagnosis should exclude diseases that may present in a similar manner, such as rheumatoid arthritis, scleroderma, chronic active hepatitis, acute drug reactions, polyarteritis, and drug-induced lupus.

The American Rheumatism Association has proposed that the diagnosis of systemic lupus erythematosus can be made with reasonable probability if 4 of the 11 following criteria are present, serially or simultaneously, during any interval of observation: malar rash; discoid rash; photosensitivity; oral ulcers; nonerosive arthritis; serositis; renal disorder; neurologic disorder; hemolytic anemia, leukopenia, lymphopenia, or thrombocytopenia; positive LE cell preparation, anti-DNA, anti-Sm, or false-positive serologic test for syphilis; positive antinuclear antibody.

Clinical Findings

A. Symptoms and Signs: The systemic features include fever, anorexia, malaise, and weight loss. Most patients have skin lesions at some time; the characteristic "butterfly" rash affects fewer than half of patients. Other cutaneous manifestations include discoid lupus, typical fingertip lesions, periungual erythema, nail fold infarcts, and splinter hemorrhages. Alopecia is commonly seen. Mucous membrane lesions tend to occur during periods of exacerbation. Raynaud's phenomenon, present in about 20% of patients, often antedates other features of the disease.

Joint symptoms, with or without active synovitis, occur in over 90% of patients and are often the earliest manifestation. The arthritis is rarely deforming; erosive changes are almost never noted on x-ray study. Subcutaneous nodules are rare.

Ocular manifestations include conjunctivitis, photophobia, transient blindness, and blurring of vision. Cotton-wool spots on the retina (cytoid bodies) represent degeneration of nerve fibers due to occlusion of retinal blood vessels.

Pleurisy, pleural effusion, bronchopneumonia, and pneumonitis are frequent. Restrictive lung disease is often demonstrated.

The pericardium is affected in the majority of patients. Cardiac failure may result from myocarditis and hypertension. Cardiac arrhythmias are common. Atypical verrucous endocarditis of Libman-Sacks, occasionally seen at autopsy, rarely alters cardiac dynamics during life.

Abdominal pains, ileus, and peritonitis may result from vasculitis. Nonspecific reactive hepatitis or that induced by salicylates may alter liver function.

Neurologic complications of systemic lupus erythematosus are usually observed in patients who have highly active disease. Mental changes, severe depression, and psychosis are sometimes heightened by the administration of large doses of corticosteroids. Convulsive disorders, peripheral neuropathies, transverse myelitis, cerebrovascular accidents, and Guillain-Barré syndrome may be seen.

Several forms of renal disease are observed. Proliferative glomerulonephritis, which may be associated with nephrotic syndrome and renal insufficiency, is the major threat to life in systemic lupus erythematosus. Mesangial nephritis is usually benign but occasionally may progress. A third type, membranous glomerulonephritis, is associated with profuse proteinuria and nephrotic syndrome and tends to be very slowly progressive. With appropriate therapy, the survival rate even for patients with serious renal disease (proliferative glomerulonephritis) is favorable.

Other clinical features include lymphadenopathy, splenomegaly, Hashimoto's thyroiditis, hemolytic anemia, and thrombocytopenic purpura.

B. Laboratory Findings: The LE cell, which is present at some time in over two-thirds of patients, is not specific for systemic lupus erythematosus, since it is present also in rheumatoid arthritis, drug-induced lupus, and other collagen disorders. Antinuclear antibody, which is a less specific indicator, may be detected in about 95% of cases. Serum elevations of antibodies to double-stranded DNA and depressed serum complement—findings suggestive of disease activity—often return toward normal in remission. Hypergammaglobulinemia, a positive Coombs test reaction, and rheumatoid factor may be demonstrable in the serum. Biologically false-positive serologic tests for syphilis occur in about 20% of patients. The fluorescent treponemal antibody absorption test may also be falsely positive; a beaded pattern of immunofluorescence may serve to distinguish it from a true positive reaction. Antibody titers to a wide variety of other cellular tissues and organ tissues may be observed.

There is often mild normocytic, normochromic anemia and occasionally autoimmune hemolytic anemia. The sedimentation rate is almost always elevated when the disease is active. Leukopenia and lymphopenia are common; thrombocytopenia occasionally may be severe, resulting in purpura or bleeding.

Liver function tests are often mildly abnormal. Abnormality of urinary sediment is almost always found in association with renal lesions. Showers of red blood cells and mild proteinuria are frequent during exacerbation of the disease; these usually abate with remission. Profuse proteinuria indicates serious renal involvement.

Treatment

It should be remembered that many patients with systemic lupus erythematosus have a benign form of the disease requiring only supportive care and need little or no medication. Patients with photosensitivity should be cautioned against sun exposure and should apply a protective lotion to the skin while out of doors. Skin lesions often respond to the local administration of corticosteroids. Joint symptoms can usually be alleviated by rest and full salicylate dosage. Every drug that may have precipitated the condition should be withdrawn if possible.

Antimalarials (hydroxychloroquine) may be helpful in treating the joint and skin features. When these are used, the dose should generally not exceed 200 mg/d, and periodic monitoring for retinal changes is necessary. Corticosteroids are required for the control of certain serious complications. These include thrombocytopenic purpura, hemolytic anemia, myocarditis, pericarditis, convulsions, pulmonary manifestations, acute lupus crisis, and nephritis. Forty to 60 mg of prednisone are often needed initially; however, the lowest dose of corticosteroid that controls the condition should be employed. Central nervous system lupus may require higher doses of corticosteroids than are usually given. In lupus nephritis, sequential studies of serum complement and antibodies to DNA often permit early detection of disease exacerbation and thus prompt increase in corticosteroid therapy. Such studies also allow for lowering the dosage of the drugs and withdrawing them when they are no longer needed. Immunosuppressive agents such as cyclophosphamide, chlorambucil, and azathioprine are used in cases resistant to corticosteroids. Patients with proliferative glomerulonephritis may do better when an immunosuppressive agent is added to steroid therapy. Very close follow-up is needed to watch for potential side effects when immunosuppressants are employed. These agents should be given by those experienced in their use. Systemic steroids are not usually given for arthritis, skin rash, leukopenia, or the anemia associated with chronic disease. Positive serologic findings in asymptomatic patients are not an indication for treatment.

Course & Prognosis

The prognosis for patients with systemic lupus appears to be considerably better than older reports implied. From both community settings and university centers, 10-year survival rates exceeding 85% are being reported. In most patients, the illness pursues a mild chronic course, occasionally interrupted by disease activity. With time, the number and intensity of exacerbations decrease and the probability of major insult to visceral structures declines. After 5 years of disease, abnormal laboratory findings such as raised sedimentation rates and anti-DNA titers tend to become normal in many patients. However, there are some in whom the disease pursues a virulent course, leading to serious impairment of vital structures such as lung, heart, brain, or kidneys, and the disease may lead to death. Although such manifestations are more likely to be seen in the early phases of the illness, one must be alert to the possibility of their occurrence at any time. The most frequently observed serious complication is progressive renal disease followed by central nervous system involvement. Another important cause of sickness and death is infection, related in part to the use of corticosteroids. With careful management, however, the outlook for most patients with systemic lupus erythematosus is increasingly favorable.

Coplon NS et al: The long-term clinical course of systemic lupus erythematosus in end-stage renal disease. N Engl J Med 1983;308:186.

Delaney P: Neurologic complications of systemic lupus erythematosus. Am Fam Physician (July) 1983;28:191.

Fine LG et al: Systemic lupus erythematosus in pregnancy. Ann Intern Med 1981;94:667.

Fries JF: Disease criteria for systemic lupus erythematosus. Arch Intern Med 1984;144:252.

Ginzler E et al: A multicenter study of outcome in systemic lupus erythematosus. Arthritis Rheum 1982;25:601.

Gladman DD et al: Haemostatic abnormalities in systemic lupus erythematosus. Q J Med 1983;52:424.

Maddison PJ, Provost TT, Reichler M: Serological findings in patients with "ANA-negative" systemic lupus erythematosus. Medicine 1981;60:87.

Miller MH et al: Systemic lupus erythematosus in males. Medicine 1983;62:327.

Reveille JD et al: Familial systemic lupus erythematosus: Immunogenetic studies in eight families. Medicine 1983;62:21.

Steinberg AD (moderator): Systemic lupus erythematosus: Insights from animal models. Ann Intern Med 1984;100:714.

Whiting-O'Keefe Q et al: The information content from renal biopsy in systemic lupus erythematosus. Ann Intern Med 1982;96:718.

PROGRESSIVE SYSTEMIC SCLEROSIS
(Scleroderma)

Progressive systemic sclerosis is a chronic disorder characterized by diffuse fibrosis of the skin and internal organs. Its cause is unknown, although abnormal serologic features have suggested the possibility of an altered immune status. Symptoms usually appear in the third to fifth decades, and women are affected 2–3 times as frequently as men.

Scleroderma may appear in any of several forms. A localized form of scleroderma (morphea) is benign and unassociated with visceral disease. Eosinophilic fasciitis, which may be a variant of scleroderma, is a rare disorder presenting with skin changes like those of scleroderma. Biopsy of involved tissue shows fasciitis with eosinophilia. Visceral features are generally absent, although aplastic anemia has been an associated feature.

Another group of patients have a relatively benign, slowly progressive disorder characterized by calcinosis, Raynaud's phenomenon, esophageal involvement, sclerodactyly, and telangiectasia (CREST syndrome). In some patients, other organs are involved. Still others have an overlapping syndrome called mixed connective tissue disease that consists of myositis, certain features of systemic lupus erythematosus, and a high titer of extractable nuclear antigen (ENA); this disorder tends to respond to relatively small doses of corticosteroids, usually less than 20 mg of prednisone daily. Systemic sclerosis may take a rapidly progressive course in which the function of major viscera is compromised, leading to death within a few years.

Most frequently, the disease makes its appearance in the skin, although visceral involvement may precede cutaneous alteration. Polyarthralgia and Raynaud's phenomenon (present in 90% of patients) are early manifestations. Subcutaneous edema, fever, and malaise are common. With time the skin becomes thickened and hidebound, with loss of normal folds. Telangiectasia, pigmentation, and depigmentation are characteristic. Ulceration about the fingertips and subcutaneous calcification are seen. Dysphagia due to esophageal dysfunction, which occurs in 90% of patients, results from abnormalities in motility and later from fibrosis. Fibrosis and atrophy of the gastrointestinal tract cause hypomotility and malabsorption. Large-mouthed diverticula occur in the jejunum, ileum, and colon. Diffuse pulmonary fibrosis and pulmonary vascular disease are reflected by low diffusing capacity and decreased lung compliance. Cardiac abnormalities include pericarditis, heart block, myocardial fibrosis, and right heart failure secondary to pulmonary hypertension. Hypertensive-uremic syndrome, resulting from obstruction to smaller renal blood vessels, indicates a grave prognosis.

Mild anemia is often present, and it is occasionally hemolytic because of microangiopathy. Elevation of the sedimentation rate and hypergammaglobulinemia are also common. Proteinuria and cylindruria appear in association with renal involvement. Antinuclear antibody tests are frequently positive, often with a speckled or nucleolar pattern. Rheumatoid factor and a positive LE preparation may be found.

Treatment is symptomatic and supportive. Broad-spectrum antibiotics are useful when intestinal malabsorption occurs. Claims of efficacy of various specific therapeutic modalities are largely unfounded. The prognosis tends to be worse in blacks, in males, and in older patients. In most cases, death results from renal, cardiac, or pulmonary failure or from sepsis.

Catoggio LJ et al: Serological markers in progressive systemic sclerosis: Clinical correlations. *Ann Rheum Dis* 1983;**42**:23.

Follansbee WP et al: Physiologic abnormalities of cardiac function in progressive systemic sclerosis with diffuse scleroderma. *N Engl J Med* 1984;**310**:142.

Hoffman R et al: Diffuse fasciitis and aplastic anemia: A report of 4 cases revealing an unusual association between rheumatologic and hematologic disorders. *Medicine* 1982; **61**:373.

Lee P et al: Nailfold capillary microscopy in the connective tissue diseases: A semiquantitative assessment. *J Rheumatol* 1983;**10**:930.

Medsger TA Jr, Dixon JA, Garwood VF: Palmar fasciitis and polyarthritis associated with ovarian carcinoma. *Ann Intern Med* 1982;**96**:424.

Steen VD, Medsger TA, Rodnan GP: D-Penicillamine therapy in progressive systemic sclerosis (scleroderma): A retrospective analysis. *Ann Intern Med* 1982;**97**:652.

Steen VD et al: Factors predicting development of renal involvement in progressive systemic sclerosis. *Am J Med* 1984; **76**:779.

Thurm RH, Alexander JC: Captopril in the treatment of scleroderma renal crisis. *Arch Intern Med* 1984;**144**:733.

POLYMYOSITIS-DERMATOMYOSITIS

Polymyositis is a systemic disorder of unknown cause whose principal manifestation is muscle weakness. It is the most frequent primary myopathy in adults. When skin manifestations are associated with it, the entity is designated dermatomyositis. The true incidence is not known, since milder cases are frequently not diagnosed. The disease may affect persons of any age group, but the peak incidence is in the fifth and sixth decades of life.

Polymyositis may begin abruptly, although often it is gradual and progressive. A classic rash, occurring in about 40% of patients, is dusky red and may be seen over the butterfly area of the face, neck, shoulders, and upper chest and back. Periorbital edema and a purplish (heliotrope) suffusion over the upper eyelids are classic signs. Subungual erythema, cuticular telangiectases, and scaly patches over the dorsum of the proximal interphalangeal and metacarpophalangeal joints (Gottron's sign) are highly suggestive. Muscle weakness chiefly involves proximal groups, especially of the extremities. Neck flexor weakness occurs in two-thirds of cases. Pain and tenderness of affected muscles are frequent, and Raynaud's phenomenon and joint symptoms may be associated. Atrophy and contractures occur late. Associated myocarditis is not uncommon. Interstitial pulmonary fibrosis is sometimes associated, and calcinosis may be observed, especially in children. Association with malignant neoplasms, particularly in older patients, is well recognized, but the frequency in several large series appears to be less than 10%. Polymyositis may occur in association with Sjögren's syndrome. It may also be a prominent feature of mixed connective tissue disease.

Measurement of serum levels of muscle enzymes, especially creatine phosphokinase and aldolase, is most useful in diagnosis and in assessment of disease activity. Anemia is uncommon. Urinary creatine is elevated, and the urine may contain myoglobin. The sedimentation rate is not usually elevated. Elevated serum gamma globulin concentrations and rheumatoid factor are found in a minority of patients. Electromyographic abnormalities consisting of polyphasic potentials, fibrillations, and high-frequency action potentials are helpful in establishing the diagnosis. Biopsy of carefully selected involved muscle, usually proximal, is a most important procedure; positive findings are necrosis of muscle fibers associated with inflammatory cells, sometimes located near blood vessels. The muscle biopsy may, however, reveal little change in spite of significant muscle weakness.

Most patients respond to corticosteroids. Often a daily dose of 40–60 mg or more of prednisone is required initially. The dose is then adjusted downward according to the response of sequentially observed serum levels. Long-term use of steroids is often needed, and the disease may recur or reemerge when they are withdrawn. Patients with an associated neoplasm have a poor prognosis, although remission may follow treatment of the tumor. In patients resistant or intolerant to corticosteroids, therapy with methotrexate or azathioprine has been advised, but this agent should be used with caution in view of its potential adverse effects.

Gutierrez G, Dagnino R, Mintz G: Polymyositis/dermatomyositis and pregnancy. *Arthritis Rheum* 1984;**27**:291.

Kagen LJ: Approach to the patient with myopathy. *Bull Rheum Dis* 1983;**33**:1.

Strongwater SL, Annesley T, Schnitzer TJ: Myocardial involvement in polymyositis. *J Rheumatol* 1983;**10**:459.

MIXED CONNECTIVE TISSUE DISEASE

Mixed connective tissue disease (MCTD) is a clinical syndrome in which overlapping features of systemic lupus erythematosus, scleroderma, and myositis are present in conjunction with high titers of an extractable nuclear antigen (ENA). The antigen contains ribonucleoprotein and is associated with a speckled pattern on the antinuclear antibody (ANA). Patients with MCTD usually have nondeforming arthritis, swollen hands with taut and thickened skin, Raynaud's phenomenon, and myositis. Abnormal esophageal motility and interstitial pulmonary fibrosis are also common. Renal disease tends to show mesangial or membranous changes. Laboratory findings show exceedingly high titers of ENA of the ribonucleoprotein type, speckled ANA, absent or low anti-DNA titers, and normal complement.

In a multicenter study of MCTD with a mean duration of 6 years, 4% of patients died. Longer-term follow-up has shown that many patients subsequently developed scleroderma. The prognosis of this disorder is generally good if pulmonary involvement and renal involvement are not severe. MCTD treatment is similar to that of systemic lupus erythematosus, although MCTD tends to be milder, with less serious renal and central nervous system disease; patients respond to lower doses of corticosteroids. Mild disease is often controlled with nonsteroidal anti-inflammatory drugs.

Alpert MA et al: Cardiovascular manifestations of mixed connective tissue disease in adults. *Circulation* 1983;**68**:1182.

Nimelstein SH et al: Mixed connective tissue disease: A subsequent evaluation of the original 25 patients. *Medicine* 1980;**59**:239.

Sullivan WD et al: A prospective evaluation emphasizing pulmonary involvement in mixed connective tissue disease. *Medicine* 1984;**63**:92.

SJÖGREN'S SYNDROME

Sjögren's syndrome, an autoimmune disorder, is the result of chronic dysfunction of exocrine glands in many areas of the body. It is characterized by dryness of the eyes, mouth, and other areas covered by mucous membrane and is frequently associated with a rheumatic disease. The disorder is predominantly a disease of women, in a ratio of 9:1, with greatest incidence between age 40 and 60 years.

Keratoconjunctivitis sicca, its ocular feature, results from inadequate tear production caused by lacrimal gland atrophy. Eye symptoms include burning, smarting, and itching. Ropy secretions often occur, and tears are not produced during crying. Parotid enlargement, which may be chronic or relapsing, develops in one-third of patients. Dryness of the mouth (xerostomia) leads to difficulty in speaking, swallowing, and eating and to severe dental caries. There may be loss of taste and smell. Desiccation may involve the nose, throat, larynx, bronchi, vagina, and skin.

Systemic manifestations include dysphagia, pancreatitis, pleuritis, pericarditis, central nervous system involvement, and peripheral neuropathy, vasculitis, and purpura. Renal tubular acidosis (type I, distal) occurs in 20% of patients. A urinary concentrating defect is common. Changes due to chronic interstitial nephritis, which may result in impaired renal function, may be seen. A glomerular lesion is rarely observed but may occur secondary to cryoglobulinemia.

A spectrum of lymphoproliferation ranging from benign to malignant may be found. Malignant lymphomas and Waldenström's macroglobulinemia occur with greater frequency than could be explained by chance in patients with this disorder.

Laboratory findings include mild anemia, leukopenia, and eosinophilia. Rheumatoid factor is found in 70% of patients. Heightened levels of gamma globulin, antinuclear antibodies, and antibodies against RNA, salivary gland, lacrimal duct, and thyroid may be noted. Antibodies against cytoplasmic antigens SS-A and SS-B are found predominantly in Sjögren's syndrome alone (primary SS), whereas antibodies against salivary ducts and the RANA antigen are found in Sjögren's syndrome in association with rheumatoid arthritis (secondary SS).

Disorders with which Sjögren's syndrome is frequently associated include rheumatoid arthritis, systemic lupus erythematosus, chronic hepatobiliary disease, scleroderma, polymyositis, Hashimoto's thyroiditis, panarteritis, and interstitial pulmonary fibrosis. When Sjögren's syndrome occurs without associated connective tissue disease, HLA-DR3 antigen is usually present.

Useful ocular diagnostic tests include the Schirmer test, which measures the quantity of tears secreted, and staining of the conjunctiva with rose bengal solution. An early finding is the low level of lysozyme in tear fluid. The salivary gland may be evaluated by radionuclide scanning, salivary flow measurements, or sialography. Labial biopsy, a simple procedure, is a valuable diagnostic technique with minimal risk; if lymphoid foci are seen, the diagnosis is confirmed. Biopsy of the parotid gland should be reserved for patients with atypical presentations such as unilateral gland enlargement.

The disease is usually benign and may be consistent with a normal life span. The outlook is influenced mainly by the nature of the associated disease.

Treatment is symptomatic and supportive. Artificial tears applied frequently will relieve ocular symptoms and avert further desiccation. The mouth should be kept well lubricated. Drugs such as atropine and decongestants that decrease salivary secretions are best avoided. A program of oral hygiene is essential in order to preserve dentition. If there is an associated rheumatic disease, its treatment is not altered by the presence of Sjögren's syndrome.

Alexander EL, Provost TT, Alexander EE: Neurologic complications of primary Sjögren's syndrome. *Medicine* 1982;**61**:247.

Daniels TE: Labial salivary gland biopsy in Sjögren's syndrome: Assessment as a diagnostic criterion in 362 suspected cases. *Arthritis Rheum* 1984;**27**:147.

Fairfax AJ et al: Pulmonary disorders associated with Sjögren's syndrome. *Q J Med* 1981;**199**:279.

Pavlidis NA, Karsh J, Moutsopoulos HM: The clinical picture of primary Sjögren's syndrome: A retrospective study. *J Rheum* 1982;**9**:685.

VASCULITIC SYNDROMES

The vasculitic syndromes are a heterogenous group of disorders characterized by the pathologic features of inflammation and necrosis of blood vessels. In most disorders characterized as vasculitides, no cause has been found. Hepatitis B is clearly the cause of one form, and other infections have been implicated, as in the vasculitis that occurs in bacterial endocarditis. No common pathogenic link has been identified for these disorders, although the deposition of immune complexes in the vascular system occurs in many.

Although vasculitis is seen in multiple disorders, only the major vasculitides will be discussed here.

POLYARTERITIS
(Periarteritis Nodosa)

Polyarteritis is characterized by focal or segmental lesions of blood vessels, especially arteries of small to medium size, resulting in a variety of clinical presentations depending upon the specific site of the blood vessel involved. The pathologic hallmark of the disease is acute necrotizing inflammation of the arterial media, with fibrinoid necrosis and extensive inflammatory cell infiltration of all coats of the vessel and surrounding tissue. Aneurysmal dilatations occur; hemorrhage, thrombosis, and fibrosis may lead to occlusion of the lumen. Arterial lesions may be seen in all stages—acute, healing, and healed. Such vascular lesions may involve virtually every organ of the body but are especially prominent in the kidney, heart, liver, gastrointestinal tract, muscle, and testes.

The cause of polyarteritis is unknown. The disease occurs in drug abusers and may be induced by the therapeutic use of allopurinol, sulfonamides, and other drugs. A history of allergy is often obtained; hepatitis B surface antigen is seen in over one-third of cases. Immune complex deposition in the walls of involved vessels has been observed.

Polyarteritis affects chiefly young adults but may appear at any age. Men are affected 3 times as frequently as women. The clinical onset is frequently abrupt, often accompanied by fever, chills, and tachycardia. Arthralgia and myositis with muscle tenderness are prominent. Mucous membane lesions and a wide variety of cutaneous abnormalities develop, including livedo reticularis, purpura, petechiae, urticaria, subcutaneous nodules, and skin ulceration. Occlusion of retinal vessels results in cotton-wool spots (cytoid bodies). Hypertension occurs in half of patients; renal involvement in more than 80%. The renal lesion is a segmental necrotizing glomerulonephritis with extracapillary proliferation, often with localized intravascular coagulation. Pulmonary manifestations occur in one-fourth of patients. Abdominal pain and nausea and vomiting are common. Infarction of arteries compromises the function of major viscera and may lead to cholecystitis, appendicitis, and intestinal obstruction. Cardiac involvement is manifested by pericarditis, myocarditis, and arrhythmias; myocardial infarction secondary to coronary arteritis also occurs. Mononeuritis multiplex is a characteristic finding. Almost any site in the nervous system may be affected.

Laboratory findings include proteinuria, hematuria, and cylindruria. Most patients manifest anemia and leukocytosis. Eosinophilia is seen in approximately one-third of patients but is more frequently encountered in association with pulmonary lesions. The sedimentation rate is almost always rapid. Rheumatoid factor, positive antinuclear antibody test, positive serologic test for syphilis, and increased serum concentration of gamma globulin are present inconstantly. Serum complement is often normal or elevated.

Diagnosis may be difficult and should be confirmed, if possible, by histologic evidence of a typical arteritic lesion. Biopsy of a tender muscle is unfortunately positive in only about 30% of cases, and testicular biopsies are positive in a smaller percentage unless the testes are tender. Visceral angiography demonstrating aneurysmal dilatation of renal, mesenteric, and hepatic arteries is useful when positive but has been negative in many proved cases.

The course is variable and unpredictable. Spontaneous remission may occur, but the disease usually runs a fulminant course, with death occurring in months to years.

Corticosteroids in high doses (up to 60 mg of prednisone daily) may control fever and constitutional symptoms and heal vascular lesions. Cyclophosphamide has also proved an effective agent. These drugs may be required for long periods, and relapses are not infrequent when they are withdrawn.

Cupps TR, Moore PM, Fauci AS: Isolated angiitis of the central nervous system: Prospective diagnostic and therapeutic experience. *Am J Med* 1983;**74**:97.

Scott DGI et al: Systemic vasculitis in a district general hospital 1972–1980: Clinical laboratory features, classifications and prognoses of 80 cases. *Q J Med* 1982;**203**:292.

POLYMYALGIA RHEUMATICA & TEMPORAL ARTERITIS

Polymyalgia rheumatica, a disorder affecting middle-aged or elderly persons, is rare before age 50. Women are afflicted more often than men. The disease often develops abruptly, with pain and stiffness of the pelvis and shoulder girdle in association with fever, malaise, and weight loss. Anemia and a markedly accelerated sedimentation rate are almost always present. The course is generally limited to 1–2 years.

Polymyalgia rheumatica bears a close relationship to temporal arteritis. The 2 conditions often coexist, but each may occur independently. The importance of diagnosing temporal arteritis lies in the risk of blindness due to obstruction of the ophthalmic arteries, which may occur unless treatment is given. Symptoms suggestive of temporal arteritis include unilateral throbbing headache, scalp sensitivity, visual symptoms, jaw claudication, and localized thickening or loss of pulsation of the temporal artery, but this disorder may occur without local symptoms. Biopsy of the temporal vessel should be performed whenever the clinical picture is suggestive and will usually reveal inflammation of the vessel, often with giant cells. An adequate biopsy specimen is essential because the disease tends to be segmental. Ten percent of patients have vasculitis of other major arteries.

In the presence of headache and other symptoms suggestive of cranial arteritis, corticosteroids should be administered immediately (eg, prednisone, 60 mg daily) and continued for several months before tapering. Where there is polymyalgia without local cranial symptoms, smaller doses of prednisone (5–15 mg daily) bring almost immediate relief. If such a response does not occur, the diagnosis should be questioned. In adjusting the dosage of steroid, the sedimentation rate is a useful guide to disease activity. One should administer the smallest dose of corticosteroid that normalizes the sedimentation rate. Blindness rarely occurs when this rate has reached the normal range. The drug may be discontinued when disease activity ceases, although the disorder may recur and in some patients remains active for years.

Bengtsson B, Malmvall B: The epidemiology of giant cell arteritis including temporal arteritis and polymyalgia rheumatica. *Arthritis Rheum* 1981;**24**:899.

Chuang T et al: Polymyalgia rheumatica: A 10-year epidemiologic and clinical study. *Ann Intern Med* 1982;**97**:672.

Espinoza LR et al: Polymyalgia rheumatica and giant cell arteritis: Circulating immune complexes. *J Rheumatol* 1982;**9**:556.

Jones JG, Hazleman BL: Prognosis and management of polymyalgia rheumatica. *Ann Rheum Dis* 1981;**40**:1.

Kyle V, Hazleman BL: Polymyalgia rheumatica/giant cell arteritis. *Clin Exp Rheumatol* 1983;**1**:171.

WEGENER'S GRANULOMATOSIS

Wegener's granulomatosis is a rare disorder characterized by vasculitis, necrotizing granulomatous lesions of both upper and lower respiratory tract, and glomerulonephritis. Without treatment it is invariably fatal, most patients surviving less than a year after diagnosis. It occurs most commonly in the fourth and fifth decades of life and affects men and women with equal frequency.

The disorder presents as a febrile illness with weakness, malaise, and weight loss. Symptoms include purulent sinusitis, rhinitis, polyarthralgia, abnormalities of skin and eyes, neuropathies, and ulcerations of the nasal septum. When a granuloma is the presenting sign, differentiation from the entity midline granuloma is difficult. Dyspnea, cough, chest pain, and hemoptysis may dominate the clinical picture. X-ray of the chest often reveals nodular pulmonary lesions, frequently cavitating; histologic examination of the lesions shows necrotizing vasculitis with granuloma formation. Although limited forms of Wegener's granulomatosis have been described in which the kidney is spared, severe progressive renal disease usually ensues and results in rapid deterioration of renal function. In such cases the urinary sediment invariably contains red cells, white cells, and casts. Renal biopsy discloses a segmental necrotizing glomerulonephritis with multiple crescents.

Laboratory studies show anemia (occasionally microangiopathic), leukocytosis, eosinophilia, and a rapid sedimentation rate. Immunologic findings are variable.

It is essential that the diagnosis be made early, since effective treatment is available and may be lifesaving. Remissions lasting as long as 8 years have been induced in a majority of patients treated with cyclophosphamide. Drug therapy should be instituted as soon as the diagnosis is made, before significant damage has been done to vital organs. Corticosteroids are usually of limited value.

Fauci AS et al: Wegener's granulomatosis: Prospective clinical and therapeutic experience with 85 patients for 21 years. *Ann Intern Med* 1983;**98**:76.

Pinching AJ et al: Wegener's granulomatosis: Observations on 18 patients with severe renal disease. *Q J Med* 1983;**52**:435.

HENOCH-SCHÖNLEIN PURPURA

This is a form of anaphylactoid purpura of unknown cause; the underlying pathologic feature is vasculitis, which principally affects small blood vessels. Although the disease is predominantly seen in children, adults are also affected. Hypersensitivity to aspirin and food and drug additives has been reported. The purpuric skin lesions are classically located on the lower extremities and dependent areas but may also be seen on the hands, arms, and trunk. Localized areas of edema, especially common on the dorsal surfaces of the hands, are frequently observed. Joint symptoms are present in the vast majority of patients, the knees and ankles being most commonly involved. Abdominal pain secondary to vasculitis of the intestinal tract is often associated with gastrointestinal bleeding. Hematuria signals the presence of a renal lesion that is usually reversible, although it occasionally may progress to renal insufficiency. Biopsy of the kidney reveals segmental glomerulonephritis with crescents and mesangial deposition of IgA and IgG. Aside from an elevated sedimentation rate, most laboratory findings are noncontributory.

The disease is usually self-limited, lasting 1–6 weeks, and subsides without sequelae if renal involvement is not severe. There is no effective treatment, although immunosuppressive drugs have met with some success in the nephropathy of this disorder.

Casanueva B et al: Increased IgA-producing cells in the blood of patients with active Henoch-Schönlein purpura. *Arthritis Rheum* 1983;**26**:854.

Egido J et al: The role of IgA and IgG immune complexes in IgA nephropathy. *Nephron* 1984;**36**:52.

BEHÇET'S SYNDROME

Named after the Turkish dermatologist who first described it, this disease of unknown cause is characterized by recurrent oral and genital ulcers, uveitis, seronegative arthritis, and central nervous system abnormalities. Other features include ulcerative skin lesions, erythema nodosum, thrombophlebitis, and vasculitis. Arthritis occurs in about two-thirds of patients, most commonly affecting the knees and ankles. Keratitis, uveitis—often with hypopyon—and optic neuritis are observed. The ocular involvement is often fulminant and may result in blindness. Involvement of the central nervous system often results in serious disability or death. Findings include cranial nerve palsies, convulsions, encephalitis, mental disturbances, and spinal cord lesions. Leukocytosis and a rapid sedimentation rate are common.

The clinical course may be chronic but is often characterized by remissions and exacerbations. Corticosteroids and immunomodulating drugs have been used with beneficial results.

Gibson T et al: Synovial histopathology of Behçet's syndrome. *Ann Rheum Dis* 1981;**40**:376.

O'Duffy JD, Robertson DM, Goldstein NP: Chlorambucil in the treatment of uveitis and meningoencephalitis of Behçet's disease. *Am J Med* 1984;**76**:75.

Yurdakul S et al: The arthritis of Behçet's disease: A prospective study. *Ann Rheum Dis* 1983;**42**:505.

RELAPSING POLYCHONDRITIS

This is a rare disease of unknown cause characterized by inflammatory destructive lesions of cartilaginous structures, principally the ears, nose, trachea, and larynx. It may be associated with other rheumatic disorders such as systemic lupus erythematosus, rheumatoid arthritis, or Hashimoto's thyroiditis. The disease, which is usually episodic, affects males and females equally. The cartilage is painful, swollen, and tender during an attack and subsequently becomes atrophic, resulting in permanent deformity. Biopsy of the involved cartilage shows inflammation, loss of basophilia, and chondrolysis. Noncartilaginous manifestations of the disease include fever, episcleritis, uveitis, deafness, and aortic insufficiency. In 85% of patients, an arthropathy is seen that tends to be migratory, asymmetric, and seronegative, affecting both large and small joints and the parasternal articulation.

Corticosteroid therapy is often effective. Involvement of the tracheobronchial tree, leading to its collapse, may cause death if tracheostomy is not done promptly.

Espinoza LR et al: Immune complex–mediated renal involvement in relapsing polychondritis. *Am J Med* 1981;**71**:181.

McCune WF et al: Type II collagen–induced auricular chondritis. *Arthritis Rheum* 1982;**25**:266.

ANKYLOSING SPONDYLITIS

Essentials of Diagnosis

- Chronic low backache in young adults.
- Progressive limitation of back motion and of chest expansion.
- Transient (50%) or permanent (25%) peripheral joint involvement indistinguishable from peripheral rheumatoid arthritis.
- Diagnostic x-ray changes in sacroiliac joints.
- Uveitis in 20–25%.
- Accelerated erythrocyte sedimentation rate and negative serologic tests for rheumatoid factor.
- HLA-B27 usually positive.

General Considerations

Ankylosing spondylitis is a chronic inflammatory disease of the joints of the axial skeleton, manifested clinically by pain and progressive stiffening of the spine. While the synovitis of ankylosing spondylitis is histologically identical with that of peripheral rheumatoid arthritis, certain features tend to distinguish this disease from rheumatoid arthritis: its preponderance among males (approximately 10:1); age at onset (usually in late teens or early 20s); the relatively high incidence of uveitis; a pathologically distinctive lesion of the aorta; and absence of rheumatoid factor. In addition to the synovitis, a second pathologic feature of ankylosing spondylitis is reactive periostitis. The annulus fibrosus may gradually ossify, with fusion of vertebral bodies.

Clinical Findings

A. Symptoms and Signs: The onset is usually gradual, with intermittent bouts of back pain that may radiate down the thighs. As the disease advances, symptoms progress in a cephalad direction and back motion becomes limited, with the normal lumbar curve flattened and the thoracic curvature exaggerated. Atrophy of the trunk muscles is common. Chest expansion is often limited as a consequence of costovertebral joint involvement. Radicular symptoms may occur. Sciatica or the cauda equina syndrome may occur and is frequently progressive. In advanced cases, the entire spine becomes fused, allowing no motion in any direction. Transient acute arthritis of the peripheral joints occurs in about 50% of cases, and permanent changes in the peripheral joints—most commonly the hips, shoulders, and knees—are seen in about 25%.

When it occurs in childhood, ankylosing spondylitis may, at its onset, mimic pauciarticular juvenile rheumatoid arthritis.

Spondylitic heart disease, characterized chiefly by atrioventricular conduction defects and aortic insufficiency occurs in 3–5% of patients with long-standing severe disease. Amyloidosis may also occur in patients with chronic disease. Nongranulomatous anterior uveitis may occur in as many as 25% of cases and may be a presenting feature. Pulmonary fibrosis of the upper lobe, with progression to cavitation and bronchiectasis, may occur. Constitutional symptoms similar to those of rheumatoid arthritis may occasionally be present.

B. Laboratory Findings: The erythrocyte sedimentation rate is accelerated in 85% of cases, but serologic tests for rheumatoid factor are characteristically negative. There may be leukocytosis and anemia.

HLA-B27 is found in 80–90% of patients with ankylosing spondylitis, as opposed to 6–8% among normal individuals. These figures must be modified in different racial groups. Although the cellular membrane antigens determined by the major histocompatibility locus in humans (HLA system) are found with greater than normal frequency in some other diseases, the most striking association is that between HLA-B27 and certain rheumatic diseases—notably ankylosing spondylitis, Reiter's syndrome, and the sacroiliitis and spondylitis associated with psoriasis and inflammatory bowel disease.

Persons with other rheumatic diseases such as rheumatoid arthritis, degenerative joint disease (osteoarthritis), and gout do not show a higher than normal incidence of HLA-B27.

C. X-Ray Findings: Early in the course of ankylosing spondylitis, x-ray shows erosion and sclerosis of the sacroiliac joints; later, involvement of the apophyseal joints of the spine, ossification of the annulus fibrosus, calcification of the anterior and lateral spinal ligaments, and squaring and generalized demineralization of the vertebral bodies may occur. The term "bamboo spine" has been used to describe the late radiographic changes.

Additional x-ray findings include periosteal new bone formation on the iliac crest, ischial tuberosities, and calcanei and alterations of the symphysis pubica and sternomanubrial joint similar to those of the sacroiliacs. Radiologic changes in peripheral joints, when present, may be differentiated from rheumatoid arthritis by their asymmetry, relative lack of demineralization, smaller erosive changes, and marginal periostitis.

Differential Diagnosis

Although rheumatoid arthritis may ultimately involve the spine, it does so characteristically in the cervical region, usually sparing the sacroiliac joints. Other features that differentiate ankylosing spondylitis from rheumatoid arthritis are the rare involvement of the small joints of the hands and feet, the absence of subcutaneous nodules, and the negative serologic tests for rheumatoid factor in spondylitis. The history and physical findings of ankylosing spondylitis serve to distinguish this disorder from other causes of low back pain such as degenerative disk disease, degenerative joint disease, osteoporosis, soft tissue trauma, and tumors. The single most valuable distinguishing radiologic sign of ankylosing spondylitis is the appearance of the sacroiliac joints, although a similar pattern may be seen in Reiter's syndrome and in arthritis associated with inflammatory intestinal diseases and psoriasis. The x-ray appearance of the sacroiliac joints in spondylitis should be distinguished from that in osteitis condensans ilii. In some geographic areas and in persons with appropriate occupations, brucellosis and fluoride poisoning may be important in the differential diagnosis.

Treatment

A. Basic Program: In general, treatment is similar to that of rheumatoid arthritis. The importance of postural and breathing exercises should be stressed.

B. Drug Therapy: Phenylbutazone is a potent anti-inflammatory agent that in small doses is often effective in ankylosing spondylitis and may be used if response to salicylates or other nonsteroidal anti-inflammatory drugs (see p 3) is inadequate. Contraindications include peptic ulcer, cardiac decompensation, or significant renal, hepatic, or hematopoietic dysfunction. Give the least amount that will provide symptomatic improvement. Start with 100 mg daily and increase if necessary to 100 mg every 12 hours or every 8 hours, but do not give more than 300 mg daily except for very short periods during flare-ups. The drug may be continued cautiously as long as required for symptomatic relief unless toxic reactions occur. Special precautions include blood counts twice weekly for 4 weeks, once weekly for the next 4 weeks, and once every 2 or 3 weeks thereafter. Toxic reactions include salt and water retention, rash, agranulocytosis and other hematologic abnormalities, and peptic ulcer. If toxicity occurs, withdraw the drug immediately (see Agranulocytosis, p 337).

Indomethacin is also an effective anti-inflammatory analgesic drug that is less toxic than phenylbutazone. The initial dosage is 25 mg twice daily, increasing weekly to the lowest effective dose (but not to exceed 50 mg 3 times daily). Indomethacin may produce a variety of untoward reactions, including headache, giddiness, nausea and vomiting, peptic ulcer, depression, and psychosis.

Other newer nonsteroidal anti-inflammatory drugs are effective and may be better tolerated.

C. Physical Therapy: See p 523.

Prognosis

Spontaneous remissions and relapses are common and may occur at any stage. Occasionally, the disease progresses to ankylosis of the entire spine. In general, the functional prognosis is good unless the hips are seriously and permanently involved.

Kinsella TD, Fritzler MJ, McNeil DJ: Ankylosing spondylitis: A disease in search of microbes. (Editorial.) *J Rheumatol* 1983;**10:**2.

Lochead JA et al: HLA-B27 haplotypes in family studies of ankylosing spondylitis. *Arthritis Rheum* 1983;**26:**1011.

van der Linden S, Valkenburg HA, Cats A: Evaluation of diagnostic criteria for ankylosing spondylitis: A proposal for modification of the New York criteria. *Arthritis Rheum* 1984;**27:**361.

ARTHRITIS & INFLAMMATORY INTESTINAL DISEASES

Arthritis is a common complication of ulcerative colitis, regional enteritis, and Whipple's disease. Occasionally, such joint disease is indistinguishable from rheumatoid arthritis and may represent a coincidence of the 2 disorders. More commonly, however, intestinal arthritis is asymmetric, affects large joints, parallels the course of the bowel disease, and rarely results in residual deformity. Ankylosing spondylitis, which may accompany inflammatory bowel disease, is indistinguishable from idiopathic ankylosing spondylitis and usually runs a course separate from bowel disease activity.

The synovitis is pathologically nonspecific. Rheumatoid factor is usually absent from the serum. The test for HLA-B27 antigen is often positive in the presence of sacroiliitis or spondylitis. Treatment of the joint disorder that resembles rheumatoid arthritis is the same as for rheumatoid arthritis; that of intestinal arthritis involves control of intestinal inflammation and use of supportive anti-inflammatory drugs; that of ankylosing spondylitis is the same as for idiopathic ankylosing spondylitis.

About 15% of patients who have jejunoileal bypass surgery for morbid obesity develop an inflammatory symmetric polyarticular disorder. The arthritis is usually acute in onset and nonmigratory and may affect the small as well as the large joints. The sedimentation rate is elevated, and antinuclear antibody and rheumatoid factor tests may be positive. Nonsteroidal anti-inflammatory agents are often effective, although some patients require prednisone.

Jorizzi JL: Bowel-associated dermatosis-arthritis syndrome. *Arch Intern Med* 1984;**144:**738.

PSORIATIC ARTHRITIS

In 15–20% of patients with psoriasis, arthritis coexists. The patterns or subsets of arthritis that may accompany psoriasis include the following:

(1) Joint disease that resembles rheumatoid arthritis in which polyarthritis is symmetric. Usually, fewer joints are involved than in rheumatoid arthritis, and rheumatoid factor is absent.

(2) An oligoarticular form that may lead to considerable destruction of the affected joints.

(3) A pattern of disease in which the distal interphalangeal joints are primarily affected. Early, this may be monarticular, and often the joint involvement is asymmetric. Pitting of the nails and onycholysis are frequently associated.

(4) A severe deforming arthritis (arthritis mutilans) in which osteolysis is severe.

(5) A spondylitic form with sacroiliitis and spinal involvement predominating. This form is linked to the presence of HLA-B27, which is seen in 60–85% of cases.

Rheumatoid nodules are not seen in psoriatic arthritis. Although psoriasis usually precedes the onset of arthritis, in 20–25% of patients the arthritis precedes the skin disease. Arthritis is at least 5 times more common in patients with severe skin disease than in those with only mild skin findings. Occasionally, though, patients may have a single patch of psoriasis and be unaware of it. Thus, a careful search for cutaneous lesions is essential. Also, the psoriatic lesions may have cleared when arthritis appears—in such cases, the history is most useful. Nail pitting, a residue of previous psoriasis, is sometimes the only clue. Laboratory studies show an elevation of the sedimentation rate, negative rheumatoid factor, and negative response to other immunologic testing, although gamma globulins may be elevated. Uric acid may be high, reflecting the active turnover of skin affected by psoriasis. There is a correlation between the extent of psoriatic involvement and the level of uric acid.

Radiologic findings are most helpful in distinguishing the disease from other forms of arthritis. There are marginal erosions of bone and irregular destruction of joint and bone, which, in the phalanx, may give the appearance of a sharpened pencil or a pencil-and-cup deformity. Fluffy periosteal new bone may be marked, especially at the insertion of muscles and ligaments into bone. Such productive changes will be seen along the shafts of metacarpals, metatarsals, and phalanges and are seen in other affected areas as well. Paravertebral ossification occurs, which may be distinguished from ankylosing spondylitis by the absence of ossification in the anterior aspect of the spine. Also, the ossification is not closely applied to the vertebral bodies.

Treatment regimens are symptomatic. Nonsteroidal anti-inflammatory drugs are useful. Antimalarials may exacerbate the psoriasis. Gold therapy is often effective. In resistant cases, methotrexate has been used with some success, but it should be used only by those fully conversant with its toxicity.

Bird HA et al: Psoriatic arthritis. *Clin Rheum Dis* 1983;**9**:675.
Green L et al: Arthritis in psoriasis. *Ann Rheum Dis* 1981;**40**:366.
Laurent MR, Panayi GS, Shepherd P: Circulating immune complexes, serum immunoglobulins and acute phase proteins in psoriasis and psoriatic arthritis. *Ann Rheum Dis* 1981;**40**:66.
Willkens RF et al: Randomized, double-blind, placebo controlled trial of low-dose pulse methotrexate in psoriatic arthritis. *Arthritis Rheum* 1984;**27**:376.

REITER'S SYNDROME

Reiter's syndrome is a clinical tetrad of unknown cause consisting of nonspecific urethritis, conjunctivitis (or, less commonly, uveitis), mucocutaneous manifestations, and arthritis. It occurs most commonly in young men. It may follow (within a few days to 4 weeks) chlamydial infection or bacterial diarrhea due to *Shigella* or *Yersinia* and is usually accompanied by a systemic reaction, including fever (without chills). The arthritis is most commonly asymmetric and frequently involves the large weight-bearing joints (chiefly the knee and ankle); sacroiliitis or ankylosing spondylitis is observed in at least 20% of patients, especially after frequent recurrences. The mucocutaneous lesions may include balanitis, stomatitis, and keratoderma blennorrhagica, resembling pustular psoriasis with involvement of the skin and nails. Carditis and aortic regurgitation may occur. While most signs of the disease disappear within days or weeks, the arthritis may persist for several months or even years. The test for HLA-B27 is positive in 80% of white patients and may thus be helpful in diagnosis. These percentages are considerably lower (20–30%) in blacks. (See p 513 for further discussion of HLA-B27.) Characteristically, the initial attack is self-limited and terminates spontaneously.

Recurrences involving any combination of the clinical manifestations are common and are sometimes followed by permanent sequelae, especially in the joints. X-ray signs of permanent or progressive joint disease may be seen in the sacroiliac as well as the peripheral joints.

Reiter's syndrome must be distinguished from gonococcal arthritis, rheumatoid arthritis, idiopathic ankylosing spondylitis, and psoriatic arthritis.

Treatment is symptomatic. As in psoriatic arthritis, the most useful drugs are the nonsteroidal anti-inflammatory agents.

Baldassare AR et al: Immunoprotein deposition in synovial tissue in Reiter's syndrome. *Ann Rheum Dis* 1981;**40**:281.
Ruppert GB, Linday J, Barth WF: Cardiac conduction abnormalities in Reiter's syndrome. *Am J Med* 1982;**73**:335.

• • •

DEGENERATIVE JOINT DISEASE
(Osteoarthritis)

Essentials of Diagnosis

- A degenerative disorder without systemic manifestations.
- Pain relieved by rest.
- Articular inflammation minimal.
- X-ray findings: narrowed joint space, osteophytes, increased density of subchondral bone, bony cysts.
- Commonly secondary to other articular disease.

General Considerations

Degenerative joint disease is a chronic progressive arthropathy characterized by degeneration of cartilage and by hypertrophy of bone at the articular margins. Inflammation is usually minimal, and thus the popular term osteoarthritis is inappropriate. Hereditary and mechanical factors may be variably involved in the pathogenesis.

Degenerative joint disease is traditionally divided into 2 types: (1) primary, which most commonly affects the terminal interphalangeal joints (Heberden's nodes) and less commonly the proximal interphalangeal joints (so-called Bouchard's nodes), the metacarpophalangeal and carpometacarpal joints of the thumb, the hip (malum coxae senilis), the knee, the metatarsophalangeal joint of the big toe, and the cervical and lumbar spine; and (2) secondary, which may occur in any joint as a sequela to articular injury resulting from either intra-articular (including rheumatoid arthritis) or extra-articular causes. The injury may be acute, as in a fracture; or chronic, as that due to overweight, bad posture, occupational overuse of a joint, or metabolic diseases (eg, hyperparathyroidism, hemochromatosis, ochronosis). The articular cartilage is first roughened and finally worn away, and spur formation and lipping occur at the edge of the joint surface. The synovial membrane becomes thickened, with hypertrophy of the villous processes; the joint cavity, however, never becomes totally obliterated, and the synovial membrane does not form adhesions. As indicated above, inflammation is usually minimal except for that observed in acute interphalangeal joint involvement (Heberden's node) and in "primary generalized osteoarthritis," in which many small joints may be affected, especially those of the fingers (exclusive of the metacarpophalangeal joints). There is also a related condition called erosive osteoarthritis in which inflammation is characteristic and the synovial membrane shows changes similar to those seen in rheumatoid disease.

Clinical Findings

A. Symptoms and Signs: The onset is insidious. Initially, there is articular stiffness; this develops later into pain on motion of the affected joint and is made worse by prolonged activity and relieved by rest. Deformity may be absent or minimal; however, bony enlargement is occasionally prominent, and flexion contracture or valgus or varus deformity of the knee is not unusual. There is no ankylosis, but limitation of motion of the affected joint or joints is common. Coarse crepitus may often be felt in the joint. Joint effusion and other articular signs of inflammation are mild. There are no systemic manifestations.

B. Laboratory Findings: Elevated sedimentation rate and other laboratory signs of inflammation or dysproteinemia are not present.

C. X-Ray Findings: X-rays may reveal narrowing of the joint space, sharpened articular margins, osteophyte formation and lipping of marginal bone, and damaged and thickened, dense subchondral bone. Bone cysts may also be present.

Differential Diagnosis

Because articular inflammation is minimal and systemic manifestations are absent, degenerative joint disease should seldom be confused with other arthritides. The appearance of the hands in degenerative joint disease may mimic that in rheumatoid arthritis. Bony rather than soft tissue swelling and lack of involvement of the metacarpophalangeal joints are helpful indications in diagnosis. The neurogenic arthropathy of Charcot is easily distinguished by x-ray and neurologic examination. Degenerative joint disease may coexist with any other type of joint disease. Furthermore, one must be cautious in attributing all skeletal symptoms to degenerative changes in joints, especially in the spine, where metastatic neoplasia, osteoporosis, multiple myeloma, or other bone disease may coexist.

Treatment

A. General Measures:

1. Rest–Physical activity that induces physiologic or traumatic strain should be avoided. Occupational or recreational overuse of an affected joint must be prevented. If weight-bearing joints are involved, such weight-bearing activities as climbing stairs, walking, or prolonged standing should be minimized. Postural strain should be corrected. Supports to pendulous abdomen or breasts should be supplied.

2. Diet should be adjusted to meet the patient's needs. In obese patients, weight reduction helps to diminish stress on the joints.

3. Local heat in any form and other forms of physical therapy are often of symptomatic value.

B. Analgesic and Anti-inflammatory Drugs: Salicylates (as for rheumatoid arthritis) or other nonsteroidal anti-inflammatory drugs (see p 3) are indicated for the relief of pain and inflammation.

C. Intra-articular Corticosteroids (as for rheumatoid arthritis) may give transient relief.

D. Orthopedic Measures: Orthopedic measures to correct developmental anomalies, deformities, disparity in leg length, and severely damaged joint surfaces may be required. (See General Principles in the Physical Management of Arthritic Joints, p 523.)

Prognosis

Although marked disability is less common than in rheumatoid arthritis, symptoms may be quite severe and limit activity considerably. This is especially true of involvement of the hips, knees, and cervical spine. Although there is no cure, proper treatment may greatly relieve symptoms and thereby improve function.

Clinical Pathologic Osteoarthritis Workshop (Queen's University, Kingston, Ontario, Canada). *J Rheumatol* 1983;**10**. [Entire issue.]

Forman MD, Malamet R, Kaplan D: A survey of osteoarthritis of the knee in the elderly. *J Rheumatol* 1983;**10**:282.

Weiss TE: Osteoarthritis: Protective measures that work; other therapies available. *Consultant* (July) 1982;**26**:213.

NEUROGENIC ARTHROPATHY
(Charcot's Joint)

Neurogenic arthropathy is joint destruction resulting from loss or diminution of proprioception, pain, and temperature perception. Although traditionally associated with tabes dorsalis, it is more frequently seen in diabetic neuropathy, syringomyelia, spinal cord injury, subacute combined degeneration of pernicious anemia, leprosy, and peripheral nerve injury. Prolonged administration of hydrocortisone by the intra-articular route may also cause Charcot's joint. As normal muscle tone and protective reflexes are lost, a marked traumatic (secondary) degenerative joint disease ensues; this results in an enlarged, boggy, painless joint with extensive erosion of cartilage, osteophyte formation, and multiple loose joint bodies. X-ray changes, although sometimes "classic," may be degenerative or hypertrophic in the same patient.

Treatment is directed against the primary disease; mechanical devices are used to assist in weight bearing and prevention of further trauma. In some instances, amputation becomes unavoidable.

ACUTE BACTERIAL (SEPTIC) ARTHRITIS

Essentials of Diagnosis

- Sudden onset of acute arthritis, usually monarticular, most often in large weight-bearing joints and wrists, frequently preceded by migratory arthralgia.
- Chills and fever.
- Joint fluid findings often diagnostic.
- Dramatic therapeutic response to appropriate antibiotic.
- Similar infection commonly found elsewhere in body.

General Considerations

The pyogenic cocci (gonococcus, meningococcus, *Staphylococcus, Streptococcus pneumoniae,* and other streptococci), *Haemophilus influenzae,* and gram-negative bacilli are the usual causes of this form of arthritis. The organisms may enter the joints directly, as in local trauma or needling or by extension from adjacent bone, or indirectly, by hematogenous spread. In recent years this type of disease has been seen more commonly as a result of the development of resistant strains of organisms, the increasing therapeutic use of intra-articular injections, intravenous drug abuse, and the increasing survival rate of premature infants, in whom the incidence of septic arthritis is relatively high. Septic arthritis is more apt to localize in previously diseased joints (eg, gouty arthritis, degenerative joint disease). The worldwide increase of gonococcal infections, particularly with antibiotic-resistant gonococci, has posed a special problem. Pathologic changes include varying degrees of acute inflammation, with synovitis, effusion, abscess formation in synovial or subchondral tissues, and, if treatment is not adequate, articular destruction.

Clinical Findings

A. Symptoms and Signs: The onset is usually sudden; the joint becomes acutely painful, hot, and swollen; and chills and fever are often present. In gonococcal infections, disseminated infections may be seen in individuals whose primary infection may be asymptomatic. The large weight-bearing joints and the wrists are most frequently affected. Although only one or 2 joints are affected, there may be a prodromal period of migratory arthralgia that may last for several days; this is especially true during the period of bacteremia.

Special attention is called to the systemic manifestations of gonococcal infection. Disseminated infection is not uncommon in individuals whose anogenital or throat infection may be asymptomatic. Dissemination in women usually occurs during pregnancy or menstruation. The initial bacteremic stage may persist for weeks and may be characterized not only by migratory arthralgia but also by chills and fever or normal temperature and by typical skin lesions. The latter are commonly tiny red papules or petechiae that may disappear or progress through transient vesicular, pustular, and bullous stages. The organism is rarely recovered from these lesions. Tenosynovitis is commonly observed. Less common systemic complications are liver function abnormalities, myocarditis or pericarditis, meningitis, and endocarditis.

B. Laboratory Findings: The leukocyte count of the synovial fluid may be as high as $100,000/\mu L$, with 90% or more polymorphonuclear cells. Synovial fluid sugar is usually low. The organisms are often demonstrated by smear or culture. However, there is increasing evidence that articular infection starts in the periarticular tissues and that organisms do not appear in synovial fluid unless the infective focus ulcerates into the joint cavity. In gonococcal arthritis, for example, the gonococcus is recovered from joint fluid in only half of cases. Throat and anorectal cultures for gonococci as well as blood and genital cultures are required whenever infection with this organism is suspected.

C. X-Ray Findings: X-rays are usually normal early in the disease, but radiologic evidence of demineralization may be present within days of onset. Bony erosions and narrowing of the joint space followed by osteomyelitis and periostitis may be seen within 2 weeks.

Differential Diagnosis

The septic course with chills and fever, the acute systemic reaction, the joint fluid findings, evidence of similar infection elsewhere in the body, and the dramatic response to appropriate antibiotics are diagnostic of bacterial arthritis. Gout and pseudogout are excluded by the failure to find crystals on synovial fluid analysis. Acute rheumatic fever and rheumatoid arthritis commonly involve many joints and are not associated with chills. Pyogenic arthritis may be superimposed on other types of joint disease, notably rheumatoid arthritis, and must be excluded (by joint fluid examination) in any apparent acute relapse of the primary disease, particularly when a joint has been needled or one is more strikingly inflamed than the others.

Treatment

Prompt systemic or oral antibiotic therapy should be based on the best clinical judgment of the causative organism and the results of smear and culture of joint fluid, blood, urine, or other specific sites of potential infection. If the organism cannot be determined clinically, treatment should be started with bactericidal antibiotics effective against staphylococci, pneumococci, gonococci, and gram-negative organisms. Cultures for gonococci require immediate inoculation of Thayer-Martin medium.

Frequent (even daily) local aspiration is sometimes indicated. Incision and drainage are rarely required. Pain can be relieved with local hot compresses and by immobilizing the joint with a splint or traction. Rest, immobilization, and elevation are used at the onset of treatment. Early active motion exercises within the limits of tolerance will hasten recovery.

Prognosis

With prompt antibiotic therapy (within 7–10 days of onset), functional recovery is usually complete. Bony ankylosis and articular destruction commonly occur if treatment is inadequate.

Arthur RE et al: Synovial fluid lactic acid in septic and nonseptic arthritis. *Arthritis Rheum* 1983;**26**:1499.

Ho G Jr, Su EY: Therapy for septic arthritis. *JAMA* 1982; **247**:797.

Rinaldi RZ et al: Penicillin-resistant gonococcal arthritis: A report of four cases. *Ann Intern Med* 1982;**97**:43.

OTHER INFECTIOUS ARTHROPATHIES

Lyme Arthritis

This disease is named after Lyme, Connecticut, the village where the first recognized case occurred. Lyme arthritis is caused by a spirochete transmitted by a tick (*Ixodes dammini* or a related species) that harbors the organism. Clinical manifestations include fever, headache, arthritis, and a characteristic skin lesion at the site of the tick bite (erythema chronicum migrans) as well as involvement of the heart (eg, arrhythmias, myocarditis) and nervous system (eg, neuropathies, meningoencephalitis). The arthritis is often recurrent and may develop into a proliferative erosive synovitis. The condition responds to tetracycline or penicillin.

Tuberculous Arthritis

Tuberculous arthritis is characterized by insidious onset and a slow progression of chronic monoarthritis, usually of a lower extremity. Systemic manifestations may be minimal or absent, and chest x-ray may be normal. Diagnosis is usually confirmed by culture of joint fluid and by culture and biopsy of the synovial membrane. Antituberculosis chemotherapy in the early stage of the disease is usually effective.

Fungal Arthritis

Arthritis due to hematogenous spread of fungi occurs rarely. Diagnosis is established by synovial fluid culture and by synovial biopsy and culture. Successful management often requires amphotericin B, surgical drainage, and other orthopedic procedures.

Viral Arthritis

Arthritis may be a manifestation of many viral infections. It is generally mild and of short duration, and it terminates spontaneously without lasting ill effects. Mumps arthritis may occur in the absence of parotitis. Rubella arthritis, which occurs more commonly in adults than in children, may appear immediately before or during or soon after the disappearance of the rash. Its usual polyarticular and symmetric distribution mimics that of rheumatoid arthritis. However, the seronegative tests for rheumatoid factor and the rising rubella titers in convalescent serum help to confirm the diagnosis. Postrubella vaccination arthritis may have its onset as long as 6 weeks following vaccination and occurs in all age groups.

Polyarthritis may be associated with type B hepatitis and often occurs before the onset of jaundice, or it may occur in the absence of jaundice. Urticaria or other types of skin rash may be present. Serum transaminase levels are elevated, and either hepatitis B surface antigen or its antibody is present. Serum complement levels are usually low during active arthritis and become normal after remission of arthritis. False-positive tests for rheumatoid factor, when present, disappear within several weeks. The arthritis is mild; it rarely lasts more than a few weeks and is self-limiting and without deformity.

Rehm-Graves S et al: Tuberculosis of the greater trochanteric bursa. *Arthritis Rheum* 1983;**26**:77.

Sergent JS: Extrahepatic manifestations of hepatitis B infection. *Bull Rheum Dis* 1983;**33**:1.

Steere AC et al: The spirochetal etiology of Lyme disease. *N Engl J Med* 1983;**308**:733.

Steere AC et al: Treatment of the early manifestations of Lyme disease. *Ann Intern Med* 1983;**99**:22.

INTERMITTENT HYDRARTHROSIS

Intermittent hydrarthrosis is a rare clinical entity of unknown cause that is characterized by episodes of often painless joint effusions, particularly in the knee, usually recurring at regular intervals and lasting several hours to several days. The attacks characteristically begin in adolescent females; the joints appear normal between attacks, and attacks frequently terminate or lessen with pregnancy or advancing age. A significant number of patients will later develop rheumatoid arthritis. Other causes of joint effusion must be carefully excluded before the diagnosis is considered.

Treatment is symptomatic and may include removal of joint fluid.

PALINDROMIC RHEUMATISM

Palindromic rheumatism is a disease of unknown cause characterized by frequent recurring attacks (at irregular intervals) of acutely inflamed joints. Periarticular pain and swelling and transient subcutaneous nodules may also occur. The attacks cease within several hours to several days. The knee and finger joints are most commonly affected, but any peripheral joint may be involved. Systemic manifestations do not occur. Although hundreds of attacks may take place over a period of years, there is no permanent articular damage. Laboratory findings are usually normal. Palindromic rheumatism must be distinguished from acute gouty arthritis and an atypical, acute onset of rheumatoid arthritis.

Symptomatic treatment is usually all that is required during the attacks. Chrysotherapy may be of value in preventing recurrences.

Pines A et al: Familial palindromic rheumatism: A possible association with HLA. *Ann Rheum Dis* 1983;**42**:631.

Schumacher HR: Palindromic onset of rheumatoid arthritis: Clinical, synovial fluid, and biopsy studies. *Arthritis Rheum* 1982;**25**:361.

FIBROMYALGIA

Fibromyalgia is a relatively common form of nonarticular rheumatism. The condition is characterized by diffuse musculoskeletal aching associated with multiple tender points in soft tissues. It affects chiefly women in the sixth decade of life. Associated symptoms include morning stiffness, fatigue, headache, neck pain, and sleep disturbances. Laboratory tests are noncontributory. Although fibromyalgia usually occurs in the absence of any other disease (primary form), it may accompany rheumatoid arthritis, osteoarthritis, or hypothyroidism (secondary form). Attention to the sleep disorder often leads to improvement in the symptom complex.

Campbell SM et al: Clinical characteristics of fibrositis. 1. A "blinded," controlled study of symptoms and tender points. *Arthritis Rheum* 1983;**26**:817.

Yunus MB: Fibromyalgia syndrome: A need for uniform classification. (Editorial.) *J Rheumatol* 1983;**10**:841.

CRYSTAL DEPOSITION ARTHRITIS

1. GOUTY ARTHRITIS

Essentials of Diagnosis

- Acute onset, usually monarticular, involving the metatarsophalangeal joint of the big toe in about 50% of cases.
- Dramatic therapeutic response to colchicine.
- Postinflammatory desquamation and pruritus.
- Hyperuricemia.
- Identification of urate crystals in joint fluid or tophi.
- Asymptomatic periods between acute attacks.
- Urate deposits in subcutaneous tissue, bone, cartilage, joints, and other tissues.
- Familial disease; 90% males.

General Considerations

Gout is a metabolic disease of heterogeneous nature, often familial, associated with abnormal amounts of urates in the body and characterized early by a recurring acute arthritis, usually monarticular, and later by chronic deforming arthritis.

Primary gout is a heritable metabolic disease in which hyperuricemia is usually due to overproduction or underexcretion of uric acid—sometimes both. It is rarely due to a specifically determined genetic aberration (eg, Lesch-Nyhan syndrome). Secondary gout, which may have some latent heritable component, is related to acquired causes of hyperuricemia, eg, myeloproliferative disorders, multiple myeloma, hemoglobinopathies, chronic renal disease, and lead poisoning.

About 90% of patients with gout are men, usually over 30 years of age. In women the onset is usually postmenopausal. The characteristic histologic lesion is the tophus, a nodular deposit of monosodium urate monohydrate crystals, and an associated foreign body reaction. These may be found in cartilage, subcutaneous and periarticular tissues, tendon, bone, the kidneys, and elsewhere. Urates have been demonstrated in the synovial tissues (and fluid) during acute arthritis; indeed, the acute inflammation of gout is believed to be activated by the phagocytosis by polymorphonuclear cells of urate crystals with the ensuing release from the nucleated neutrophils of chemotactic and other substances capable of mediating inflammation. The precise relationship of hyperuricemia to acute gouty arthritis is still obscure, since hyperuricemia may occur in patients who never have gouty arthritis. Recent studies suggest that rapid fluctuations in serum urate levels, either increasing or decreasing, are important factors in precipitating acute gout. The mechanism of the late, chronic stage of gouty arthritis is better understood. This is characterized pathologically by tophaceous invasion of the articular and periarticular tissues, with structural derangement and secondary degeneration (osteoarthritis).

Uric acid kidney stones are present in 10–20% of patients with gouty arthritis. Nephrosclerosis with renal dysfunction is common. The term gouty nephropathy (or "gouty nephritis"), which is much less common, refers to kidney disease due to tophaceous deposition in the renal parenchyma, chiefly the pyramids and the renal vasculature. It is often associated with pyelonephritis.

Hyperuricemia often occurs in patients without arthritis, urinary stones, or tophaceous deposits (Table 14–3). Unless the serum uric acid levels are consistently higher than 11 mg/dL or are associated with rapid breakdown of cellular nucleic acid following aggressive treatment of leukemia or lymphoma, drug treatment need not be instituted until arthritis, renal calculi, or tophi become apparent. Psoriasis, sarcoidosis, and diuretic drugs are commonly overlooked causes of hyperuricemia. An adequate fluid intake and urinary output may suffice as treatment for uncomplicated hyperuricemia. Asymptomatic hyperuricemia need not be treated with drugs.

Clinical Findings

A. Symptoms and Signs: The acute arthritis is characterized by its sudden onset, frequently nocturnal, either without apparent precipitating cause or following rapid fluctuations in serum urate levels from

Table 14–3. Origin of hyperuricemia.*

Primary Hyperuricemia
  A. Increased production of purine:
    1. Idiopathic.
    2. Specific enzyme defects (eg, Lesch-Nyhan syndrome,
       glycogen storage disease).
  B. Decreased renal clearance of uric acid (idiopathic).
Secondary Hyperuricemia
  A. Increased catabolism and turnover of purine:
    1. Myeloproliferative disorders.
    2. Lymphoproliferative disorders.
    3. Carcinoma and sarcoma (disseminated).
    4. Chronic hemolytic anemias.
    5. Cytotoxic drugs.
    6. Psoriasis.
  B. Decreased renal clearance of uric acid:
    1. Intrinsic kidney disease.
    2. Functional impairment of tubular transport:
      a. Drug-induced (eg, thiazides, probenecid).
      b. Hyperlacticemia (eg, lactic acidosis, alcoholism).
      c. Hyperketoacidemia (eg, diabetic ketoacidosis, starva-
        tion).
      d. Diabetes insipidus (vasopressin-resistant).
      c. Bartter's syndrome.

*Modified from Rodnan GP: Gout and other crystalline forms of arthritis. *Postgrad Med* (Oct) 1975;**58**:6.

food and alcohol excess, surgery, infection, diuretics, chemicals (eg, meglumine diatrizoate, Urografin), or uricosuric drugs. The metatarsophalangeal joint of the great toe is the most susceptible joint, although others, especially those of the feet, ankles, and knees, are commonly affected. More than one joint may occasionally be affected during the same attack; in such cases, the distribution of the arthritis is usually asymmetric. As the attack progresses, the pain becomes intense. The involved joints are swollen and exquisitely tender and the overlying skin tense, warm, and dusky red. Fever, headache, malaise, anorexia, and tachycardia are common. Local desquamation and pruritus during recovery from the acute arthritis are almost pathognomonic of gout but are not always present. Tophi may be found in the external ears, hands, feet, olecranon, and prepatellar bursas. They are usually seen only after several attacks of acute arthritis.

Asymptomatic periods of months or years commonly follow the initial acute attack. Later, gouty arthritis may become chronic, with symptoms of progressive functional loss and disability. Gross deformities, due usually to tophaceous invasion, are seen. Signs of inflammation may be absent or superimposed.

Hypertension, renal stones, and renal failure may be associated with gouty arthritis.

B. Laboratory Findings: The serum uric acid is practically always elevated (> 7.5 mg/dL) unless uricopenic drugs are being given (see p 1102). During an acute attack, the erythrocyte sedimentation rate and white cell count are usually elevated. Examination of the material aspirated from a tophus shows the typical crystals of sodium urate and confirms the diagnosis.

Further confirmation is obtained by identification of sodium urate crystals by compensated polariscopic examination of wet smears prepared from joint fluid aspirates. Such crystals are negatively birefringent and needlelike and may be found free or in cells.

C. X-Ray Findings: Early in the disease, x-rays show no changes. Later, punched-out areas in the bone (radiolucent urate tophi) are seen. Although bony punched-out areas may also be seen in rheumatoid arthritis, a punched-out area is diagnostic of gout if it is adjacent to a soft tissue tophus.

Differential Diagnosis

Once the diagnosis of acute gouty arthritis is suspected, it is easily confirmed by the presence of hyperuricemia, dramatic response to full doses of colchicine, local desquamation and pruritus as the edema subsides, positive identification of tophi, a positive family history, and polariscopic examination of joint fluid. Acute gout is often confused with cellulitis. Appropriate bacteriologic studies should exclude acute pyogenic arthritis. Acute chondrocalcinosis (pseudogout) may be distinguished by the identification of calcium pyrophosphate crystals in the joint fluid, usually normal serum uric acid, the x-ray appearance of chondrocalcinosis, and the relative therapeutic ineffectiveness of colchicine.

Chronic tophaceous arthritis may rarely mimic chronic rheumatoid arthritis. In such cases, the diagnosis of gout is established conclusively by the demonstration of urate crystals in the contents of a suspected tophus. Biopsy may be necessary to distinguish tophi from rheumatoid nodules. An x-ray appearance similar to that of gout may be found in rheumatoid arthritis, sarcoid, multiple myeloma, hyperparathyroidism, or Hand-Schüller-Christian disease.

Treatment

A. Acute Attack:

1. Colchicine, which may inhibit the chemotactic property of leukocytosis and thus interfere with the inflammatory response to urate crystals, is the traditional drug; it is used diagnostically as well as therapeutically. It should be given as early as possible in the acute attack or during the prodrome to obtain maximum benefit, since 75% of patients with acute gouty arthritis respond to colchicine, and failure of relief in the remainder may be related to a delay in the initiation of treatment. Trial with colchicine should not replace joint aspiration for diagnosis when an aspirable joint is readily accessible, since 80% of patients receiving colchicine have significant abdominal cramping, diarrhea, nausea, or vomiting. Give 0.5 or 0.6 mg every hour or 1 mg every 2 hours until pain is relieved or until nausea or diarrhea appears, and then stop the drug. The usual total dose required is 4–8 mg. The pain and swelling will subside in 24–72 hours. Once the patient knows how much will produce toxic symptoms, the drug should be given in a dose of about 1 mg less than the toxic dose. Colchicine-induced diarrhea is controlled with diphenoxylate with atropine (Lomotil) or with loperamide (Imodium). The incidence of gastrointestinal side effects of colchicine can be reduced by intravenous administration in an initial dose of 1–3 mg in 10–20 mL of saline solution. This may be repeated in a few hours, but no more than 4 mg should be given intravenously within a period of 24 hours for a single attack. Colchicine may cause local pain and tissue damage from extravasation during injection. This route of administration is rarely necessary and is inadvisable if the oral route can be used. Administration of usual doses of colchicine to patients with significant renal or hepatic disease may result in serious toxicity. Oral colchicine should not be used in patients with inflammatory bowel disease.

2. Phenylbutazone and **oxyphenbutazone** are remarkably effective anti-inflammatory agents in acute gout and are the drugs of choice when the diagnosis is well established. The initial dose is 400 mg, followed by 200 mg every 6 hours until the attack subsides; do not continue for more than 3 days. Toxicity is rarely a problem in such short-term use of phenylbutazone, except in the presence of active ulcer.

3. Indomethacin is as effective as phenylbutazone in acute gout. Give 50 mg every 6 hours for 3–4 doses. When a response occurs, reduce dosage to 25 mg 3–4 times daily for 4–5 days. Active peptic ulcer is a contraindication.

4. Newer nonsteroidal anti-inflammatory agents have been shown to be effective and may be used instead of phenylbutazone and indomethacin.

5. Corticotropin (ACTH) and the corticosteroids often give dramatic symptomatic relief in acute episodes of gout and, if given for a sufficient length of time, will control most acute attacks. However, when corticotropin and corticosteroids are discontinued shortly after termination of attacks, many patients promptly undergo relapse unless colchicine is given. However, since colchicine, phenylbutazone, and indomethacin are as effective as corticotropin and the corticosteroids if not more so, and since they provide a more lasting effect, these agents are preferred.

6. Analgesics–At times the pain of an acute attack may be so severe that analgesia is necessary before a more specific drug becomes effective. In these cases, codeine or meperidine may be given. Cinchophen and neocinchophen should not be used because they cause severe liver damage.

7. Bed rest is very important in the management of the acute attack and should be continued for about 24 hours after the acute attack has subsided. Early ambulation may precipitate a recurrence. **Physical therapy** is of little value during the acute attack, although hot or cold compresses to or elevation of the affected joints makes some patients more comfortable.

B. Management Between Attacks: Treatment during symptom-free periods is intended to minimize urate deposition in tissues, which causes chronic tophaceous arthritis, and to reduce the frequency and severity of recurrences. There is evidence that these objectives are in fact attainable.

1. Diet–From a dietary standpoint, it is most important simply to avoid obesity, fasting, dehydration, and acidosis. Rigid diets fail to influence the hyperuricemia or the course of gouty arthritis. Since dietary sources of purines contribute very little to the causation of the disease, restriction of foods high in purine (eg, kidney, liver, sweetbreads, sardines, anchovies, meat extracts) cannot be expected to contribute significantly to the management of the disease. Specific foods or alcoholic beverages that precipitate attacks should be avoided. However, there is little evidence that alcohol in moderation will precipitate attacks or is otherwise harmful in patients with gout. A high liquid intake and, more importantly, a daily urinary output of 2 L or more will aid urate excretion and minimize urate precipitation in the urinary tract.

2. Colchicine–The daily administration of colchicine in a dose of 0.5 mg 3 times daily should be started simultaneously with uricosuric drugs or allopurinol in order to suppress the acute attack that may be precipitated by these drugs. After several weeks of such treatment, it is usually possible to lower the daily dose of colchicine to 0.5 mg. There is some suggestion that colchicine, even in this small dosage, has preventive value and should be continued indefinitely.

3. Reduction of serum uric acid–Indications include persistent serum uric acid levels greater than 11 mg/dL, frequent acute arthritis not controlled by colchicine prophylaxis, tophaceous deposits, or renal damage. It is emphasized that mild hyperuricemia which is either asymptomatic or associated only with infrequent attacks of arthritis may not require treatment.

Two classes of agents may be used to lower the serum uric acid—the uricosuric drugs and allopurinol (neither is of value in the treatment of acute gout).

a. Uricosuric drugs–These drugs, by blocking tubular reabsorption of filtered urate and reducing the metabolic pool of urates, prevent the formation of new tophi and reduce the size of those already present. Furthermore, when administered concomitantly with colchicine, they may lessen the frequency of recurrences of acute gout. The indication for uricosuric treatment is the increasing frequency or severity of the acute attacks.

The following uricosuric drugs may be employed:

(1) Probenecid (Benemid), starting with 0.5 g daily and gradually increasing to 1–2 g daily.

(2) Sulfinpyrazone (Anturane), starting with 100 mg daily and gradually increasing to 200–400 mg daily. In any case, the maintenance dose is determined by observation of the serum uric acid response and the urinary uric acid response. Ideally, one attempts to maintain a normal serum urate level.

Hypersensitivity to either uricosuric drug in the form of fever and rash occurs in 5% of cases; gastrointestinal complaints occur in 10%.

Precautions with uricosuric drugs. It is important to maintain a daily urinary output of 2000 mL or more in order to minimize the precipitation of uric acid in the urinary tract. This can be further prevented by giving alkalinizing agents to maintain a urine pH of above 6. If a significant uricosuric effect is not obtained in the presence of overt renal dysfunction, do not increase the dose of the drug beyond the limits stated above. Uricosuric drugs are probably contraindicated in patients with a history of uric acid lithiasis. Avoid using salicylates, since they antagonize the action of uricosuric agents.

b. Allopurinol–The xanthine oxidase inhibitor allopurinol (Zyloprim) promptly lowers plasma urate and urinary uric acid concentrations and facilitates tophus mobilization. The drug is of special value in uric acid overproducers (as defined by urinary excretion of uric acid in excess of 800 mg/d while on a purine-free diet); in tophaceous gout; in patients unresponsive to the uricosuric regimen; and in gouty patients with renal insufficiency or uric acid renal stones. It should be used cautiously in patients with renal insufficiency. Hepatotoxicity of a hypersensitivity type has been reported. It is not indicated in asymptomatic hyperuricemia. The most frequent adverse effect is the precipitation of an acute gouty attack. However, the commonest sign of hypersensitivity to allopurinol (occurring in 5% of cases) is a pruritic rash that may progress to toxic epidermal necrolysis. Diffuse angiitis, renal failure, and death may ensue if the drug is not discontinued as soon as signs of sensitivity appear.

The daily dose is determined by the serum uric acid response. A normal serum uric acid level is often obtained with a daily dose of 200–300 mg. Occasionally (and in selected cases) it may be helpful to continue the use of allopurinol with a uricosuric drug. Neither of these drugs is of help in acute gout.

Severe and potentially fatal hypersensitivity reactions associated with allopurinol have been reported.

C. Chronic Tophaceous Arthritis: There is good evidence that in the presence of adequate renal function, tophaceous deposits can be made to shrink in size and occasionally to disappear altogether. The treatment is essentially the same as that outlined for the intervals between acute attacks. Surgical excision of large tophi offers immediate mechanical improvement in selected deformities and may lessen the load on renal function.

Prognosis

Without treatment, the acute attack may last from a few days to several weeks, but proper treatment quickly terminates the attack. The intervals between acute attacks vary up to years, but the asymptomatic periods often become shorter if the disease progresses. Chronic tophaceous arthritis occurs after repeated attacks of acute gout, but only after inadequate treatment. Although the deformities may be marked, only a small percentage of patients become bedridden. The younger the patient at the onset of disease, the greater the tendency to a progressive course. Destructive arthropathy is rarely seen in patients whose first attack is after age 50.

Patients with gout have an increased incidence of hypertension, renal disease (eg, nephrosclerosis,

tophi, pyelonephritis), diabetes mellitus, hypertriglyceridemia, and atherosclerosis, although these relationships are not well understood.

Glynn RJ, Campion EW, Silbert JE: Trends in serum uric acid levels: 1961–1980. *Arthritis Rheum* 1983;**26**:87.
Hande KR, Noone RM, Stone WJ: Severe allopurinol toxicity: Description and guidelines for prevention in patients with renal insufficiency. *Am J Med* 1984;**76**:47.
McCarty DJ: Crystals, joints and consternation. (Heberden oration.) *Ann Rheum Dis* 1983;**42**:243.
McCarty DJ, Lehr JR, Halverson PB: Crystal populations in human synovial fluid: Identification of apatite, octacalcium phosphate, and tricalcium phosphate. *Arthritis Rheum* 1983;**26**:1220.

2. CHONDROCALCINOSIS & PSEUDOGOUT (Calcium Pyrophosphate Dehydrate [CPPD] Deposition Disease)

The term chondrocalcinosis refers to the presence of calcium-containing salts in articular cartilage. It is most often first diagnosed radiologically. It may be familial and is commonly associated with a wide variety of metabolic disorders, eg, hemochromatosis, hyperparathyroidism, ochronosis, diabetes mellitus, hypothyroidism, Wilson's disease, and true gout. Pseudogout, most often seen in persons age 60 or older, is characterized by acute, recurrent and rarely chronic arthritis that usually involves large joints (principally the knees) and is almost always accompanied by chondrocalcinosis of the affected joints. Identification of calcium pyrophosphate crystals in joint aspirates is diagnostic of pseudogout. Like the intra-articular urate crystals of gouty synovitis, calcium pyrophosphate crystals are believed to induce the synovitis of pseudogout. They may be seen with the ordinary light microscope but are best visualized under polarized light, in which they exhibit a weakly positive birefringence; like gouty crystals, they may be intracellular or extracellular. X-ray examination shows not only calcification (usually symmetric) of cartilaginous structures but also signs of advanced degenerative joint disease (osteoarthritis). Unlike gout, pseudogout is usually associated with normal serum urate levels and is not ordinarily benefited by colchicine.

Treatment of chondrocalcinosis is directed at the primary disease, if present. Some of the nonsteroidal anti-inflammatory agents (salicylates, indomethacin, naproxen, and other drugs) are helpful in the treatment of acute episodes of pseudogout. Colchicine may be of benefit. Aspiration of the inflamed joint and intra-articular injection of a hydrocortisone ester is also of benefit in resistant cases.

Lust G et al: Evidence of a generalized metabolic defect in patients with hereditary chondrocalcinosis. *Arthritis Rheum* 1981;**24**:1517.
Rodnan GP: Treatment of the gout and other forms of crystal-induced arthritis. *Bull Rheum Dis* 1982;**32**:43.

3. HYDROXYAPATITE CRYSTAL DEPOSITION

Bicipital tendinitis and rotator cuff tears are often related to the presence of hydroxyapatite deposits. The latter condition tends to affect elderly women and presents with a painful shoulder with decreased mobility and stability.

ARTHRITIS IN SARCOIDOSIS

The frequency of arthritis among patients with sarcoidosis is variously reported between 10% and 37%. It is usually acute in onset, but articular symptoms may appear insidiously and often antedate other manifestations of the disease. Knees and ankles are most commonly involved, but any joint may be affected. Distribution of joint involvement is usually polyarticular and symmetric. The arthritis is commonly self-limiting after several weeks or months; infrequently, the arthritis is recurrent or chronic. Despite its occasional chronicity, the arthritis is rarely associated with joint destruction or significant deformity. Although sarcoid arthritis is often associated with erythema nodosum, the diagnosis is contingent upon the demonstration of other extra-articular manifestations of sarcoidosis and, notably, biopsy evidence of epithelioid tubercles. In chronic arthritis, x-ray shows rather typical changes in the bones of the extremities with intact cortex and cystic changes. Typical sarcoid granulomas may be demonstrated by a biopsy of a chronically involved synovial membrane. Rheumatoid factor is sometimes present in low titers in the serum of patients with sarcoidosis, but the finding is nonspecific and unrelated to the joint disease.

Treatment of arthritis in sarcoidosis is usually symptomatic and supportive. Colchicine may be of value. A short course of corticosteroids may be effective in patients with severe and progressive joint disease.

The occurrence of joint disease is usually a favorable prognostic sign with respect to the course of sarcoidosis.

Scott DGI et al: Chronic sarcoid synovitis in the Caucasian: An arthroscopic and histological study. *Ann Rheum Dis* 1981;**40**:121.

•   •   •

GENERAL PRINCIPLES IN THE PHYSICAL MANAGEMENT OF ARTHRITIC JOINTS

Proper physical management of arthritic joints can improve patient comfort and help preserve joint and muscle function and total well-being. In order to obtain optimal results, as well as to conserve financial resources and time, it is important for the physician to be as specific as possible in instructions to the patient or to the occupational and physical therapists conducting treatment.

Exercise

A. Passive Range of Motion: Since someone other than the patient puts the joints through the range of motion once or twice daily, the patient is not directly involved and maintenance of muscle tone is not assisted. Passive exercises should be ordered infrequently and only for specific purposes.

B. Active Range of Motion: This type of exercise requires the patient to actively contract the muscles in order to put joints through the range of motion. The precribed motions should be repeated 3–10 times once or twice daily. Such active exercise should be encouraged, since it involves the patient, costs no money, protects joint motion, and assists in maintaining muscle tone.

C. Isometric Exercise: With this type of exercise the muscle is contracted but not shortened, while the joint is minimally moved, for 3–10 repetitions several times daily. This maintains or even increases muscle strength and tone; the patient is involved; joint use is minimal; and the cost is nil. Isometric exercise should be used to supplement passive or active range of motion exercises.

D. Isotonic Exercise: In isotonic exercise, the muscle is contracted and shortened and the joint is maximally moved and stressed. This type of exercise should seldom be used (see below).

E. Hydrotherapy: The buoyancy of water permits maximum isotonic and isometric exercise with no more stress on joints than active range-of-motion exercises. Although ideal for arthritic patients, its cost often precludes use and it is generally prescribed only for specific short-term goals.

F. Active-Assistive Exercise: The therapist provides direct supervision, physical support, and exercise guidance. Although this is ideal for arthritic patients, cost again often precludes its use except for specific short-term goals. A member of the family may be taught to assist the patient in exercises on a long-term basis.

Note: Any exercise in the arthritic patient may be associated with some pain, but pain lasting for hours after exercise is an indication for a change in the duration or type of exercise.

Heat, Cold, & Massage

A. Heat: Most patients with chronic arthritis find that some form of heat gives temporary muscle relaxation and relief of pain. Generally, moist heat is more effective than electric pads or heat lamps. Tub baths may require bar supports for ease of entry and exit. Paraffin dips may spare the patient the "dishpan hands" caused by water.

B. Cold: Some patients with particularly acute arthritis or acutely injured arthritic joints find that cold (ice pack or bag) relieves pain more effectively than does heat.

C. Massage: While massage is helpful in relaxing muscles and giving psychologic support, it provides only temporary relief, and its cost is usually high.

Splints

Splints may provide joint rest, reduce pain, and prevent contracture, but certain principles should be adhered to.

(1) Night splints of the hands or wrists (or both) should maintain the extremity in the position of optimum function. The elbow and shoulder lose motion so rapidly that other local measures and corticosteroid injections are usually preferable to splints.

(2) The best "splint" for the hip is prone-lying for several hours a day on a firm bed. For the knee, prone-lying may suffice, but splints in maximum tolerated extension are frequently needed. Ankle splints are of the simple right-angle type.

(3) Splints should be applied for the shortest period needed, should be made of lightweight materials for comfort, and should be easily removable for range-of-motion exercises once or twice daily to prevent loss of motion.

(4) Corrective splints, such as those for overcoming knee flexion contractures, should be used under the guidance of a physician familiar with their proper use.

Note: Avoidance of prolonged sitting or knee pillows may decrease the need for splints.

Braces

Unstable joints—particularly the knee and wrist—can be supported, and the pain of weight bearing may be relieved, by appropriately prescribed braces.

Assistive Devices

Patient-oriented publications, physical therapists, occupational therapists, and home health nurses can help the patient to obtain appropriate gripping bars, raised toilet seats, long-handled reachers, and other devices to help in coping with daily living.

Referral of the Patient for Surgical Opinion by an Orthopedist

A. Synovectomy: This procedure has been used for over 50 years to attempt to retard joint destruction by invasive synovial pannus of rheumatoid arthritis. However, its prophylactic effect has not been documented, and inflammation of regenerated synovial membrane has been demonstrated. Thus, the only indication for synovectomy is intractable pain in an isolated joint, most commonly the knee.

B. Joint Replacement: (See also Total Joint Arthroplasty, p 543.) Total hip replacement by methylmethacrylate has been highly successful. Infection, the major complication, is uncommon. The long-term effects of replacement of the knee—and more recently the ankle, shoulder, and other joints—have not been fully determined.

C. Arthroplasty: Realignment and reconstruction of the knee, wrist, and small joints of the hand are feasible in a small number of selected patients.

D. Tendon Rupture: This is a fairly common complication in rheumatoid arthritis and requires immediate orthopedic referral. The most common sites are the finger flexors and extensors, the patellar tendon, and the Achilles tendon.

E. Arthrodesis: Arthrodesis (fusion) is being used less now than formerly, but a chronically infected, painful joint may be an indication for this surgical procedure.

Joint Protection Program

Physical and occupational therapists can instruct patients in changing their daily habits and their occupational and recreational activities to lessen damage to joints, maintain range of motion, and lessen pain and muscle atrophy.

Delisa JA: Practical use of therapeutic physical modalities. *Am Fam Physician* (May) 1983;**27**:129.

●   ●   ●

References

Blechman WJ et al (editors): The state of the art in arthritis therapy. *Postgrad Med* (May) 1983. [Special report.]

Coles LS et al: From experiment to experience: Side effects of nonsteroidal anti-inflammatory drugs. *Am J Med* 1983; **74**:820.

Moskowitz RW: *Clinical Rheumatology: A Problem-Oriented Approach to Diagnosis and Management,* 2nd ed. Lea & Febiger, 1982.

Rheumatology Committee, American College of Physicians: Rheumatology: An annotated bibliography of recent literature. *Ann Intern Med* 1983;**98**:264.

Shearn MA: Nonsteroidal anti-inflammatory agents; nonopiate analgesics; drugs used in gout. Chapter 34 in: *Basic & Clinical Pharmacology,* 2nd ed. Katzung B (editor). Lange, 1984.

Stites DP et al: *Basic & Clinical Immunology,* 5th ed. Lange, 1984.

Bone & Joint Diseases | 15

Steven S. Fountain, MD, & Floyd H. Jergesen, MD

INFECTIONS OF BONES & JOINTS

Direct microbial contamination of the bones or joints results from open fracture, surgical procedures, gunshot wounds, diagnostic needle aspirations, and therapeutic or self-administered drug injections.

Indirect or secondary infections are first noticed in other areas of the body and extend to the bone or joint by hematogenous routes. The use of immunosuppressive drugs is associated with increasing frequency of hematogenous osteomyelitis.

ACUTE PYOGENIC OSTEOMYELITIS & ARTHRITIS

Essentials of Diagnosis

- Fever, chills, malaise, and sweating.
- Pain, tenderness, or swelling.
- Migratory arthralgia may precede single-joint pyarthrosis, usually of a large weight-bearing type of joint.
- Aspiration of involved bone or joint is usually diagnostic.
- Culture of blood or lesion tissue is essential for precise diagnosis.

General Considerations

Initial bone infections are indirectly seeded by a single strain of pyogenic bacteria about 95% of the time. Direct or primary osteomyelitis may be produced by mixed bacteria. About 75% of hematogenous acute infections of bone are due to staphylococci; group A hemolytic streptococci are the next most common pathogens.

Gonococcal joint infections have increased in frequency, with antibiotic-resistant strains being the most significant. Synovial tissue cultures are often required to recover gonococci. Staphylococci, streptococci, *Haemophilus influenzae,* and some gram-negative bacilli may be found in infected joints.

Salmonellae cause most cases of bacteremia associated with sickle cell disease. Among patients with hemoglobinopathies, osteomyelitis is caused by sal-monellae almost 10 times as often as by other pyogenic bacteria. In otherwise healthy patients with salmonellosis, bone lesions are likely to be solitary. Infections of bones and joints occur as a complication in less than 1% of cases of typhoid fever. See Salmonellosis, p 865.

Bone or joint infection as a complication of brucellosis (see p 869) is uncommon. It may involve the skeletal system or bursae around joints, usually the shoulder or elbow. Bone lesions most commonly occur in the lumbar spine or sacroiliac joints.

Clinical Findings

A. Symptoms and Signs: The onset of acute osteomyelitis in adults is less likely to be striking than the often sudden and alarming presentation seen in children. Generalized toxic symptoms of bacteremia may be absent, and vague or evanescent local pain may be the earliest manifestation. Tenderness may be present or absent, depending upon the extent and duration of bone involvement. Limitations of joint motion may be marked, especially in patients with spinal involvement or lesions occurring near joints. Gonococcal joint infections are often preceded for weeks by migratory arthralgia, with or without chills or fever and red papular skin petechiae. Asymptomatic anogenital and throat infections or menstruation or pregnancy in women may precede systemic dissemination. Other organ systems (eg, liver, heart, nervous system) may be subsequently involved.

Large weight-bearing joints and wrists are the most frequently infected, following migratory arthralgia of several days. The onset is sudden, with associated constitutional symptoms as with acute osteomyelitis. The immunologic response determines the severity of toxic symptoms of bacteremia.

B. Laboratory Findings: Aspiration of bone, synovial tissue, and periosteal or joint fluid to recover organisms for culture is necessary for accurate diagnosis. Blood cultures are frequently positive, and in gonococcal arthritis, synovial and periarticular tissues may be the first tissues to yield the diagnosis. The white count and sedimentation rate are often elevated, and in pyarthrosis, the joint fluid leukocyte count may reach $100,000/\mu L$ (90% polymorphonuclears). Secondary anemia may appear in severe cases of both bone or joint infections.

Infections due to *Salmonella* or *Brucella* can be precisely diagnosed by positive culture of material from the osteoarticular focus. Significant rising serologic agglutination titers support a tentative diagnosis during the acute stage.

C. Radiologic Findings: Early findings may include soft tissue swelling and loss of tissue planes and periarticular demineralization of bone. About 2 weeks after onset of symptoms, bony erosion and alteration of cancellous bone appear, followed by periostitis. If a joint is involved, the surface becomes irregular and narrow.

Xeroradiography and radionuclide imaging may localize occult lesions several days before x-ray studies become diagnostic.

Differential Diagnosis

Acute hematogenous osteomyelitis must be differentiated from suppurative arthritis, rheumatic fever, and cellulitis. Acute form with mixed symptoms and subacute forms must be differentiated from tubercular or mycotic infections of bone and Ewing's sarcoma.

Joint fluid findings will differentiate among septic arthritis; gout; pseudogout; and tuberculous, fungal, and viral arthritis. Care should be taken to avoid contamination of an adjacent joint when passing needles and trocars through tissues involved in pyogenic osteomyelitis and cellulitis. Acute rheumatic fever and rheumatoid arthritis commonly involve more than a single joint and are associated with less severe constitutional symptoms.

Complications

Inadequate treatment of bone or joint infections results in chronicity, and this possibility is increased by delay in diagnosis and treatment. Arthrodesis may be a sequela of destruction and may be extensive. Extension to adjacent bone or joints may complicate acute pyarthrosis or osteomyelitis. Recurrence of bone infections often results in anemia, weight loss, weakness, and amyloidosis. Rarely, pseudoepitheliomatous hyperplasia, squamous cell carcinoma, or fibrosarcoma arises in persistently infected tissues.

Treatment

Appropriate chemotherapeutic agents administered within the first 2 or 3 days may suffice. In gonococcal arthritis, frequent aspiration is sometimes indicated. Surgical decompression (in addition to chemotherapy) is sometimes used in an attempt to minimize progression of the pyogenic process. Cultures and antibiotic sensitivity studies should determine the choice of antibiotic agents; the initial selection of drug is based on clinical assessment of the most probable cause. Serum drug levels should be measured periodically as a guide to dosage, and repeated cultures may be necessary for most effective treatment. Open or closed drainage of the local lesion is important when prompt clinical response to initial treatment does not occur. Antibiotic therapy during the acute stage should be continued for at least 2–3 weeks following repeated

wound cultures while the patient is afebrile. Analgesics, rest, immobilization, and elevation of the part should be used from the beginning of treatment.

Prognosis

If sterility of the joint or lesion is achieved within 2–4 days, a good functional result can be expected in most cases if there is no compromise of the patient's immune defense system.

CHRONIC PYOGENIC OSTEOMYELITIS & ARTHRITIS

Essentials of Diagnosis

- Pain, tenderness, swelling, and redness.
- Sinus tract formation with intermittent drainage.
- X-ray evidence of bone or joint deformity, destruction, and cavitation.
- Mixed pathogens often cultured.

General Considerations

Failure or delay in adequate treatment of the acute pyogenic bone or joint infection results most commonly in chronicity. Symptoms may be sparse, intermittent, and delayed following the acute process by weeks or years, particularly with osteomyelitis.

Clinical Findings

A. Symptoms and Signs: Intermittent drainage from a sinus tract, with or without pain, tenderness, or redness of the bones or joints, may require a wound dressing to avoid soiling clothes. Intermittent treatment often interrupts the course and results in temporary quiescence. A history of surgical operations or implants with postoperative infections is sometimes present.

B. Laboratory Findings: Confirmation of the cause of the infection is often difficult, since the organisms are multiple, most commonly pyogenic cocci and enteric gram-negative rods. Sinus drainage commonly includes skin contaminants, so that areas of synovium and bone not adjacent to the exudate may be confused with the true pathogens.

C. Radiologic Findings: Standard x-rays may demonstrate bone or joint destruction and cavitation. Structural changes and bone or joint deformity are not uncommon. Bone necrosis, sequestra, and focal areas of involvement can be delineated with sinograms and tomography. Occult infections may be found with radionuclide imaging.

Differential Diagnosis

Chronic suppurative arthritis mimics gout and nonpyogenic arthritis (tuberculous, fungal, mycotic, syphilitic). Chronic pyogenic osteomyelitis resembles some types of bone tumor and bone dysplasia radiographically.

Treatment

Dressing changes with or without long-term antibiotic treatment based on identification of the pathogen may be satisfactory for minor recurrences of chronic bone disease.

Patients with progressive osteolysis, bone necrosis, and drainage and joint destruction may require operative treatment. Surgical saucerization, excision of bone, and debridement of healthy tissues is often necessary. Wound closure is often at the surgeon's discretion and experience. Joint arthrodesis and amputation may be required. Combinations of antibiotics based on culture and sensitivity studies are required for successful treatment of chronic infection.

Prognosis

In long-term chronic infection of bone and joints, recurrence is exceedingly likely. Any residual nidus of infected bone, synovium, or soft tissue remains as a source of later infection. With radical excision, if residual tissues are healthy, control of infection and restoration of joint function may be expected.

Armstrong EP, Rush DR: Treatment of osteomyelitis. *Clin Pharm* 1983;**2**:213.

Berg E: The acutely swollen joint: First impressions may mislead. *Postgrad Med* (Jan) 1984;**75**:62.

Blockey NJ: Chronic osteomyelitis. *J Bone Joint Surg* [*Br*] 1983;**65**:120.

Bonakdar-pour A, Gaines VD: The radiology of osteomyelitis. *Orthop Clin North Am* 1983;**14**:21.

Gillespie WJ, Mayo KM: The management of acute hematogenous osteomyelitis in the antibiotic era: A study of the outcome. *J Bone Joint Surg* [*Br*] 1981;**63B**:126.

Glover SC et al: Treatment of pyogenic osteomyelitis. *J Antimicrob Chemother* 1981;**8**:347.

Golimbu C, Firooznia H, Rafii M: CT of osteomyelitis of the spine. *AJR* 1984;**142**:159.

Ho G Jr, Su EY: Therapy for septic arthritis. *JAMA* 1982; **247**:797.

Hughes S: Radionuclides in orthopedic surgery. *J Bone Joint Surg* [*Br*] 1980;**62**:141.

Kern RZ, Houpt JB: Pyogenic vertebral osteomyelitis: Diagnosis and management. *Can Med Assoc J* 1984;**130**:1025.

Lindenbaum S, Alexander H: Infections simulating bone tumors: A review of subacute osteomyelitis. *Clin Orthop* (April) 1984; **184**:193.

Tindall EA et al: Osteomyelitis complicating septic arthritis. *JAMA* 1983;**250**:2671.

Waldvogel FA: Treatment of osteomyelitis and septic arthritis. *Bull NY Acad Med* 1982;**58**:733.

Waldvogel FA, Vasey H: Osteomyelitis: The past decade. *N Engl J Med* 1980;**303**:360.

Zack BG: Acute hematogenous osteomyelitis: A challenge to clinical acumen. *Postgrad Med* (Feb) 1984;**75**:103.

Zbella FA et al: Gonococcal arthritis in pregnancy. *Obstet Gynecol Surv* 1984;**39**:8.

SPECIFIC INFECTIONS OF BONES & JOINTS

MYCOTIC INFECTIONS OF BONES & JOINTS

Fungal infections of the skeletal system are usually secondary to a primary infection in another organ system, frequently the lower pulmonary tract (see Chapter 28). Although skeletal lesions have a predilection for the cancellous extremities of long bones and the bodies of vertebrae, the predominant lesion—a granuloma with varying degrees of necrosis and abscess formation—does not produce a characteristic clinical picture.

Differentiation from other chronic focal infections depends upon culture studies of synovial fluid or tissue obtained from the local lesion. Serologic and skin tests and histologic studies provide presumptive support of the diagnosis.

Coccidioidomycosis

Coccidioidomycosis of bones and joints is usually secondary to primary pulmonary infection (see p 946). During the initial phase of pulmonary infection, arthralgia with periarticular swelling, especially in the regions of the knees and ankles, should be differentiated from organic bone and joint involvement. Osseous lesions commonly occur in cancellous bone of the vertebrae or near the ends of long bones. Local atrophy of bone progresses to focal destruction, which may appear cystic, indicating coalescence of granulomas or abscess formation.

The precise diagnosis depends upon recovery of *Coccidioides immitis* from the lesion or histologic examination of grossly suspicious synovium obtained by open biopsy when the synovial fluid is negative.

Systemic treatment with amphotericin B should be tried for bone and joint infections (see p 947). It may also be of value for instillation into joints during the early stages of infection or after synovectomy. Treatment with miconazole is sometimes effective. Chronic infection of bone may respond to operative excision of dead infected bone and soft tissue. Amputation may be the only solution for stubbornly progressive infections that do not respond to less drastic measures. Immobilization of joints by plaster casts and avoidance of weight bearing provide beneficial rest. Synovectomy, joint debridement, and arthrodesis are reserved for more advanced joint infections. Contaminated dressings and plaster casts should be carefully handled to prevent spread of infection to others.

Hoeprich PD, Lawrence RM, Goldstein E: Treatment of coccidioidomycosis with miconazole. *JAMA* 1980;**243**:1923.

Histoplasmosis

Focal skeletal or joint involvement in histoplasmosis is rare and generally represents dissemination from a primary focus in the lungs (see p 947). Skeletal lesions may be single or multiple and are not characteristic.

SYPHILIS OF BONES & JOINTS

Syphilitic arthritis or osteitis may occur during any stage of the congenital or acquired systemic disease (see Chapter 25). Almost any bone in the body may be involved. Neurotrophic arthropathy (Charcot's joints) can be caused indirectly by syphilitic disease of the spinal cord.

A tertiary manifestation of either congenital or acquired syphilis is granulomatous gumma formation, characterized by localized destruction of bone accompanied by surrounding areas of sclerosis. Gummas are found most frequently in the long bones of the legs, the clavicles, and the skull. Extensive destruction with accompanying rarefaction may cause pathologic fracture because of structural weakening. The x-ray picture of syphilitic osteitis in the adult is not diagnostic, but bone production is generally more pronounced than bone destruction.

Osteoarticular lesions due to other causes that simulate those of *T pallidum* must be differentiated in patients who have received either adequate or inadequate treatment of the systemic disease. When localized clinical symptoms with compatible x-ray studies are supported by a history of congenital or acquired infection, serologic studies will probably provide confirmatory evidence. A favorable response of the bone and joint lesions to specific systemic drug treatment supports the diagnosis.

The only local treatment that is necessary for the skeletal lesion is immobilization to provide comfort or protection from fracture if extensive weakening of bone is judged to be present.

Graudal C et al: Osteitis in early syphilis. *Br J Vener Dis* 1981; **57**:312.

Kelly AP: Syphilis: Update on diagnosis and treatment. *Consultant* (March) 1984;**28**:173.

TUBERCULOSIS OF BONES & JOINTS

Essentials of Diagnosis
- Pain, tenderness, swelling, limitation of joint motion.
- Known primary infection in another organ.

General Considerations
Practically all tuberculous infections in the USA are caused by the human strain of *Mycobacterium tuberculosis* (see Chapter 7). Infection of the musculoskeletal system is commonly caused by hematogenous spread from a primary lesion of the respiratory or gastrointestinal tract. Tuberculosis of the thoracic or lumbar spine may be associated with an active lesion of the genitourinary tract. It is usually a disease of childhood, occurring most commonly before puberty. Adult infection is uncommon except in the debilitated geriatric patient. Tuberculous osteomyelitis secondary to cutaneous inoculation has been reported.

Clinical Findings
A. Symptoms and Signs: The onset of symptoms is generally insidious and not accompanied by alarming general manifestations of fever, sweating, toxicity, or prostration. Pain in an involved joint may be mild at onset, is usually worse at night, and may be accompanied by stiffness. Limping and restriction of joint motion are mechanisms used to protect a weight-bearing joint. As the disease process progresses, limitation of joint motion becomes fixed because of muscle contractures, organic destruction of the joint, and the progressive healing response in soft tissue and bone.

Local findings during the early stages may be limited to tenderness, soft tissue swelling, joint effusion, and increase in skin temperature about the involved area. As the disease progresses without treatment, muscle atrophy and deformity become apparent. Abscess formation with spontaneous drainage externally leads to sinus formation. Progressive destruction of bone in the spine may cause a gibbus, especially in the thoracolumbar region.

B. Laboratory Findings: The precise diagnosis rests upon recovery of the causative acid-fast pathogen from joint fluid, pus, or tissue specimens. Biopsy of the lesion or of a regional lymph node may demonstrate the characteristic histologic picture of caseating necrosis and giant cells but is not specific for tuberculosis.

C. X-Ray Findings: X-ray manifestations are not characteristic. There is a latent period between the onset of symptoms and the initial positive x-ray finding. The earliest changes of tuberculous arthritis are those of soft tissue swelling and distention of the capsule by effusion. Subsequently, bone atrophy causes thinning of the trabecular pattern, narrowing of the cortex, and enlargement of the medullary canal. As joint disease progresses, destruction of cartilage is manifested by narrowing of the joint cleft and focal erosion of the articular surface, especially at the margins. Extensive destruction of joint surfaces causes deformity. As healing takes place, osteosclerosis becomes apparent around areas of necrosis and sequestration. Where the lesion is limited to bone, especially in the cancellous portion of the metaphysis, the x-ray picture may be that of single or multilocular cysts surrounded by sclerotic bone. As intraosseous foci expand toward the limiting cortex and erode it, subperiosteal new bone formation takes place.

Differential Diagnosis
Cutaneous reaction to protein derivatives of various mycobacteria is of presumptive diagnostic value insofar as the local lesion is concerned.

Tuberculosis of the musculoskeletal system must

be differentiated from all subacute and chronic infections, rheumatoid arthritis, gout, and, occasionally, osseous dysplasia.

Complications

Clinical infection probably occurs only in persons with inadequate immunologic defense following massive exposure to this ubiquitous pathogen. In people with inadequate defense mechanisms, children, and elderly people with other systemic disease, tuberculosis is likely to progress rapidly. Destruction of bones or joints may occur in a few weeks or months if adequate treatment is not provided. Deformity due to joint destruction, abscess formation with spread into adjacent soft tissues, and sinus formation are common. Paraplegia is the most serious complication of spinal tuberculosis. As healing of severe joint lesions takes place, spontaneous fibrous or bony ankylosis follows.

Treatment (See also p 147.)

A. General Measures: General care is especially important when prolonged recumbency is necessary and includes skillful nursing care.

B. Surgical Measures: No rigid recommendations can be made for the operative treatment of tuberculosis, because the stage of the infection and the character of the lesion are the determinants. In acute infections where synovitis is the predominant feature, treatment can be conservative, at least initially: Immobilization by splint or plaster, aspiration, and chemotherapy may suffice to control the infection. This treatment is desirable for the management of infections of large joints of the lower extremities in children during the early stage of the infection. Immobilization may also be used in adults either as definitive treatment of early and mild infections or preliminary to operative management. Synovectomy may be valuable for less acute hypertrophic lesions that involve tendon sheaths, bursae, or joints.

Various types of operative treatment are necessary for chronic or advanced tuberculosis of bones and joints depending upon the location of the lesion and the age and general condition of the patient. The availability of effective drugs for systemic use has broadened the indications for synovectomy and debridement. Conversely, the need for more radical surgical procedures such as arthrodesis and amputation has diminished. Even though the infection is active and all involved tissue cannot be removed, supplementary chemotherapy permits healing to proceed. In general, arthrodesis of weight-bearing joints is preferred when useful function cannot be salvaged.

C. Chemotherapy: Combinations of antituberculosis agents are recommended (see p 147).

Babhulkar SS et al: Atypical spinal tuberculosis. *Bone Joint Surg* [Br] 1984;**66:**239.
Glassroth J, Robins AG, Snider DE Jr: Tuberculosis in the 1980s. *N Engl J Med* 1980;**302:**1441.
Halsey JP et al: A decade of skeletal tuberculosis. *Ann Rheum Dis* 1982;**41:**7.
Shea JM: Bilateral tuberculous osteomyelitis of medial humeral condyles: Infection secondary to cutaneous inoculation. *JAMA* 1982;**247:**821.
Versfeld GA, Solomon A: A diagnostic approach to tuberculosis of bones and joints. *J Bone Joint Surg* [Br] 1982;**64:**446.

PAIN SYNDROMES

CERVICOBRACHIAL PAIN SYNDROMES

A large group of articular and extra-articular disorders is characterized by pain that may involve simultaneously the neck, shoulder girdle, and upper extremity. Diagnostic differentiation is often difficult. Some of these entities and clinical syndromes represent primary disorders of the cervicobrachial region; others are local manifestations of systemic diseases. The clinical picture is further complicated when 2 or more of these conditions occur coincidentally.

Clinical Findings

A. Symptoms and Signs: Neck pain may be limited to the posterior neck region or, depending upon the level of the symptomatic joint, may radiate segmentally (sclerotomally) to the occiput, anterior chest, shoulder girdle region, arm, forearm, and hand. It may be intensified by active or passive neck motions. The general distribution of pain and paresthesias, when they are a feature, corresponds roughly to the involved dermatome in the upper extremity. Radiating pain in the upper extremity is often intensified by hyperextension of the neck and deviation of the head to the involved side. Limitation of cervical movements is the most common objective finding. Neurologic signs depend upon the extent of compression of nerve roots or the spinal cord. Severe compression of the spinal cord may cause long-tract involvement resulting in paraparesis or paraplegia.

B. X-Ray Findings: An early x-ray finding is loss of the normal anterior convexity of the cervical curve (loss of cervical lordosis). Comparative reduction in height of the involved disk space is a frequent finding. The most common late x-ray finding is osteophyte formation anteriorly, adjacent to the disk; other late changes occur around the apophyseal joint clefts, chiefly in the lower cervical spine. Myelography is the most valuable x-ray means of demonstrating nerve root or spinal cord compression. Computer-assisted myelography may prove to be a valuable adjunct to diagnosis.

Differential Diagnosis & Treatment

The differential diagnosis of neck pain includes acute and chronic cervical strain or sprains (whiplash injury); herniated nucleus pulposus; inflammatory disorders such as cervical spondylosis (degenerative arthritis, hypertrophic arthritis, osteoarthritis), ankylosing spondylitis, and rheumatoid arthritis; osteomyelitis; neoplasms; spinal stenosis, compression fractures, osteoporosis, and psychoneurotic disorders.

A. Acute or Chronic Cervical Musculotendinous Strain: Cervical strain is generally caused by mechanical postural disorders, overexertion, or minor injury (whiplash injury). Acute episodes are painful and limited in duration, with decreased cervical spine motion and paraspinal muscle spasm, resulting in stiffness of the neck and loss of motion. Muscle trigger points can often be localized. Management includes neck and head immobilization by halter traction or a cervical collar and administration of analgesics and sedation. Gradual return to full activity is permitted.

Patients with chronic symptoms will have few objective findings. Stress due to work or recreational activities is often implicated. Chronic pain, especially that radiating into the upper extremity, usually requires additional treatment such as bracing.

B. Herniated Nucleus Pulposus: Rupture or prolapse of the nucleus pulposus of the cervical disks into the spinal canal may occur in middle-aged patients. Pain radiates to the arms at the level of C6–7. When intra-abdominal pressure is increased owing to coughing, sneezing, or movement, symptoms are aggravated, and cervical muscle spasm may often occur. Neurologic abnormalities may include decreased reflexes of the deep tendons of the biceps and triceps and decreased sensation and muscle atrophy or weakness in the forearm or hand. Cervical halter traction, complete bed rest, and other conservative measures are generally successful. Contrast myelography, CT scans, and electromyography help delineate lesions requiring surgical treatment (laminectomy, fusion). Chemonucleolysis is not a useful treatment alternative in cervical disk disease.

C. Arthritic Disorders: Cervical spondylosis (degenerative arthritis, hypertrophic arthritis) is a collective term describing degenerative changes that occur in the apophyseal joints and intervertebral disk joints, with or without neurologic signs. Osteoarthritis of the articular facets is characterized by progressive thinning of the cartilage, subchondral osteoporosis, and osteophytic proliferation around the joint margins. Degeneration of cervical disks and joints does occur in adolescents but is more common after age 40. Degeneration is progressive and is marked by gradual narrowing of the disk space, as demonstrated by x-ray. Osteocartilaginous proliferation occurs around the margin of the vertebral body and gives rise to osteophytic ridges that may encroach upon the intervertebral foramens and spinal canal, causing compression of the neurovascular contents. A large anterior osteophyte may occasionally cause dysphagia. Musculotendinous strain of varying degrees accounts for most symptoms of cervicobrachial syndrome.

Ankylosing spondylitis is discussed on pp 512 and 532. Rheumatoid arthritis can mimic ankylosing spondylitis, with intervertebral disk and connective tissue involvement. Atlantoaxial subluxation occurs in 25% of patients with rheumatoid arthritis, regardless of the severity of disease. Inflammation of the synovial structures resulting from erosion and laxity of the transverse ligament can lead to neurologic signs of spinal cord disorder.

Management is similar to that of ankylosing spondylitis. Treatment may vary from use of a cervical collar or more rigid bracing to operative treatment, depending on the degree of subluxation and neurologic progression. Surgical treatment may involve stabilization of the cervical spine.

D. Other Disorders: Osteomyelitis is discussed on pp 525 and 532; neoplasms on p 532; spinal stenosis, compression fractures, and osteoporosis on p 533; and psychoneurotic disorders on p 533.

Beetham WP Jr, Hsieh R: Clinical evaluation of neck pain. *Hosp Med* (Sept) 1982;**18**:60.

Hirsh LF: Cervical degenerative arthritis: Possible cause of neck and arm pain. *Postgrad Med* (July) 1983;**74**:123.

Levine AM: Spinal orthoses. *Am Fam Physician* (March) 1984; **29**:277.

LOW BACK PAIN SYNDROME

Low back pain may be associated with a variety of causes, and careful history and physical examination of such a patient may yield important clues regarding the site and cause of the disorders. Such a patient may be subjected to a large number of laboratory, x-ray, and diagnostic procedures with ambiguous or unrevealing results. This may in turn reflect inadequate clinical evaluation and failure to fully utilize information obtained from properly conducted physical examinations.

Clinical Findings

A carefully elicited history of the patient's illness should include age, general health, occupation, possible injuries, onset of symptoms, pattern of pain and relationship to physical activity, aggravating and relieving factors, emotional status, loss of time from work, and possible litigation.

Inspection and palpation of the painful area are important. Since pain from nerve roots or nerves is commonly referred toward the periphery, the physician should explore the entire nerve lengths leading from the painful area and should note the presence of any masses or tenderness and, where possible, the size and consistency of nerves.

Rectal and vaginal examination should be part of the examination to help rule out local lesions and involvement of accessible lumbodorsal plexuses.

Muscle spasm and tenderness to percussion and deep pressure may give evidence suggesting radicular irritation, particularly when associated with local deformity or restriction of spinal motion.

The range of motion of joints and the effect of movement on the pain should be determined, since pain from areas such as the hip may be referred distally, and severe distal peripheral pain may be referred to the entire limb.

The regional blood vessels and those of the extremity should be checked for adequacy of pulsation and aneurysmal dilatation.

Sciatic stretch tests (eg, the straight leg-raising test and Lasègue's sign) should be elicited. With the patient supine, the relaxed, extended lower extremity is gently lifted from the bed or table. The presence and amount of pain and the extent to which the straight leg may be raised are noted. Pain and limitation of motion often accompany radiculopathy, especially that which occurs with herniated lumbar or lumbosacral disks.

Patrick's sign is elicited to differentiate sciatic from hip joint disease. The patient lies supine, and the heel of the lower extremity being tested is passively placed on the opposite knee. The knee on the side being tested is then pressed laterally and downward by the examiner as far as it will go. The test is considered positive if motion is involuntarily restricted, and pain frequently accompanies this limitation of motion. The test is positive in hip joint disease and negative in sciatica. ("F-ab-er-e" is a mnemonic formula: "f" for flexion, "ab" for abduction, "er" for external rotation, and "e" for extension motions of the hip.)

Kernig's sign is elicited with the patient supine. The examiner flexes the hip and then extends the knee as far as possible without producing significant pain. A positive Kernig test consists of involuntary spasm of the hamstring muscles that limits extension of the knee and often causes pain. Its clinical significance is similar to that of a positive straight leg-raising test.

Lumbar paraspinal muscle spasm frequently is noted with local radiculitis, which is due to many causes, including herniated lumbar intervertebral disk.

With the examiner standing behind the patient, the presence of lordosis, scoliosis, or list affecting the lumbar region is noted. The effect of flexion, hyperextension, and lateral flexion of the trunk on the pelvis is observed.

Psoas muscle spasm usually indicates disease of the psoas muscle or of the lumbar vertebrae and soft tissue adjacent to this muscle. It may be tested with the patient prone and the pelvis firmly pressed against the table with one hand by the examiner. With the other hand grasping the ankle, the leg is moved to the vertical position with the knee flexed at a right angle. The hip is passively hyperextended by lifting up on the ankle. Limitation of motion is produced by involuntary psoas muscle spasm.

Limitation of passive lumbar flexion and resulting pain often accompany disease of the lumbar or lumbosacral articulations. With the patient supine, the examiner grasps one lower extremity with both hands, moves the thigh to a position of maximal flexion, and then presses firmly downward toward the table and upward toward the patient's head, passively flexing the lumbar spinal column.

Differential Diagnosis

The cause of back pain may often be established by correlating the findings of a carefully elicited history with a thorough physical examination. When find-ings suggest physical injury or diseases requiring specific treatment, x-rays of the involved area of the spine are often required for diagnostic and legal purposes. X-ray findings may provide a convenient basis for the differentiation of the causes of back pain.

A. Disorders of the Spine Without Essential Radiographic Findings of the Spine:
1. Musculotendinous strain.
2. Herniated nucleus pulposus.
3. Ankylosing spondylitis.
4. Rheumatoid arthritis of the spine.
5. Osteomyelitis.
6. Neoplasm.

B. Disorders of the Spine With Specific Radiographic Findings of the Spine:
1. Spondylosis.
2. Osteoarthritis.
3. Spinal stenosis.
4. Spondylolysis and spondylolisthesis.
5. Facet tropism.
6. Unilateral transitional vertebra.
7. Compression fractures.
8. Untreated scoliosis.
9. Osteoporosis.

C. Other Disorders With Normal Radiographic Findings of the Spine:
1. Abdominal aneurysm.
2. Thrombotic occlusion of the terminal aorta.
3. Gastrointestinal disorders.
4. Genitourinary disorders.
5. Anxiety reactions with back pain.
6. Hysterical reactions with back pain.
7. Malingering with back pain.
8. Compensatory back pain.

Low Back Pain Without Characteristic X-Ray Changes

Disorders of the spine without characteristic x-ray changes causing back pain include musculotendinous strain of the thoracic and lumbar spine, herniated nucleus pulposus, ankylosing spondylitis, osteomyelitis, and primary and metastatic bone tumors.

A. Musculotendinous Strain: Strain is generally related to postural or mechanical causes. Acute episodes of pain are severe and usually limited in duration, with decreased back motion and paraspinal muscle spasm, resulting in a list and loss of lordosis. Muscle trigger points can often be localized. Management includes complete bed rest, local heat, a firm sleeping surface, analgesics, and sedatives. After 24 hours of pain-free recumbency without medication, walking activity is tried, with progression to full activity if symptoms do not recur. Patients with chronic symptoms present few objective findings, and stress of work and play is often implicated. Predisposing factors may include poor posture, obesity, poor muscle tone, pregnancy, and myofasciitis. Management may include daily exercises or sport activities appropriate for age, a firm mattress, and a weight reduction program if needed.

B. Herniated Nucleus Pulposus: This is the most common radicular syndrome manifested in the lumbosacral region and occurs principally in young adult males. Backache, exacerbated by increased intra-abdominal pressure due to coughing, sneezing, and movement, usually antedates the sciatic syndrome. The latter is noted by a positive Lasègue and a negative Patrick sign. Intervertebral disks L4–5 and L5–S1 are most commonly affected, causing weakness or atrophy of the thigh or calf, decreased sensation in a radicular pattern, and hyporeflexia. Except for an occasional narrowed intervertebral space, x-rays are not generally helpful. Pain from a herniated nucleus pulposus is almost always relieved by recumbency at complete bed rest, analgesics, sedation, and a firm sleeping surface. The patient who does not respond to conservative treatment in 14–21 days or who demonstrates progression of neurologic deficits should undergo contrast myelography, electrodiagnostic tests, and CT scan. Based upon these findings, operation may be indicated. The role of extradural corticosteroid injections is controversial. **Chemonucleolysis** is a useful alternative to surgical diskectomy but should not preclude good conservative treatment. Patients who are good candidates for surgical disk excision can benefit from this special technique.

C. Inflammatory Disorders: Ankylosing spondylitis (see p 512) occurs principally in men and rheumatoid arthritis (see p 500) chiefly in women. The former affects mainly the spine and sacroiliac joints and develops acutely, with constitutional symptoms, or insidiously, with stiffness and aching in the lower back. Early findings may consist of decreased lumbar lordosis, decreased back motion, sacroiliac joint tenderness, and decreased chest expansion due to costovertebral joint involvement. No significant x-ray changes are noted during the first 1–2 years following onset of symptoms. These disorders are progressive and may lead to complete calcification of the anterior longitudinal ligament with bony union between vertebral bodies similar to "bamboo spine." Management includes anti-inflammatory agents and postural and breathing exercises that minimize kyphotic deformities. Sleeping in a prone position can also be of benefit if the habit is acquired before complete calcification of the spine occurs. Surgical osteotomies may be of benefit to patients with fixed deformities.

Rheumatoid arthritis can cause severe low back pain in addition to pain in the joints of the hips and hands, resulting in intervertebral disk and connective tissue degeneration. Management is similar to that of ankylosing spondylitis.

D. Osteomyelitis: (See p 525.) Osteomyelitis of the spine produces destructive lesions with localized pain and sensitivity to percussion. In young patients, there is often a history of respiratory tract (staphylococcal or streptococcal) infection; in older patients, there is often a history of manipulation of the genitourinary tract (gram-negative bacilli). X-rays may show localized decalcification of the vertebrae and subperiosteal calcification 10–14 days after an acute pyogenic episode. Postoperative infections following diskectomy may develop in 1–8 weeks. Management by immobilization of the back usually alleviates the pain. If antibiotic therapy does not control the infection, surgical debridement and drainage with or without bone grafting of the defect are required. Chronic pyogenic osteomyelitis resulting from acute septicemia is more common in areas where narcotic addiction is a problem. Brucellosis, coccidioidomycosis, and mycobacterial infection may follow an ill-defined or insidious course with low-grade fever; x-ray changes are evident even later than the symptoms. Back pain, constitutional symptoms, weight loss, and a list develop. Hyperemic osteoporosis of cancellous bone may result in vertebral collapse and granulation tissue, producing neurologic symptoms. Abscesses may form and dissect along fascial planes, especially the psoas muscle, draining into the groin and the gluteal and paravertebral areas. Management is similar to that of acute pyogenic infection. Abscess drainage may be needed. Occasionally, spinal fusion may be necessary for instability or progressive deformity causing neurologic deficit.

E. Neoplasms: Neoplasms may affect the spinal cord or the osseous vertebrae at any level and may be benign or malignant. The patient who complains of constant night pain and progressively worsening sleep difficulties due to pain should be suspected of having a tumor. The most common primary tumor in patients over 40 is multiple myeloma; secondary neoplasms are metastatic carcinoma from the breast, prostate, kidney, or lung. Neck or back pain may be the initial complaint, and x-rays of the spine may be normal until 30% of the bone has been destroyed. Tumors may be bone-producing or bone-destroying, depending upon the origin of the lesion. Measurement of serum acid and alkaline phosphatase, calcium, and phosphorus; determination of the sedimentation rate; and bone scanning may be useful. Neurogenic tumors may not manifest neurologic deficits and may require CT scan and myelography for assessment. Management may include symptomatic treatment, needle or open biopsy, and decompression or stabilization procedures with orthoses, halo casts, or operative means depending on the location of the lesion, the extent of involvement, and the neurologic findings.

Low Back Pain With Characteristic X-Ray Changes

These include osteoarthritis, spondylolisthesis, spinal stenosis, facet tropism, transitional vertebra, untreated scoliosis, and osteoporosis.

A. Degenerative Changes: Degenerative changes of the intervertebral disks (spondylosis) and the posterior articulating facets (osteoarthritis) and spinal stenosis are often interrelated, affecting the entire spine, and occur chiefly in patients of middle age or older. Early morning stiffness and pain aggravated by prolonged sitting and standing that is improved by walking (except for spinal stenosis) are often relieved by recumbency. Sciatic radiation may occur. Fatigue, obesity, and muscle tension or spasm aggravate the problem. A finding of musculotendinous strain may be superimposed. The formation of osteophytes around the periphery of the vertebral body or facet joints may narrow the central and lateral nerve root canals, causing stenosis of the thecal space and entrapment of the peripheral nerves. Herniation of the nucleus pulposus may occur. With osteoarthritic subluxation and enlargement of both facet joints with disk absorption, entrapment of the lateral spinal nerve roots may occur. Early x-ray findings show osteophyte formation lateral and anterior (traction spur) to the vertebral body, with later narrowing of the disk and facet joints and foraminal encroachment. CT scan and myelography confirm the diagnosis. Management includes analgesics, anti-inflammatory agents, weight loss, modification of activities, and decompressive or surgical arthrodesis or both. With a subluxated facet syndrome, manipulation therapy may give some relief.

B. Spondylolysis and Spondylolisthesis: A defect in the pars interarticularis (spondylolysis) and a bilateral defect with vertebral slippage (spondylolisthesis) are believed in most cases to be acquired disorders resulting from stress fractures. Although often asymptomatic, they may cause low back pain with or without sciatic radiation. Involvement of L5 is most common, followed by L4, with a depression above the sacrum on physical examination. X-rays are necessary to confirm the diagnosis, particularly oblique views. Management of acute symptoms remains conservative, with bed rest and analgesics. Recurrent and increasingly severe symptoms with or without neurologic involvement and continuing evidence of slippage radiographically warrant surgical decompression or fusion.

C. Facet Tropism and Transitional Vertebra: Normally, the facets are symmetrically aligned at each vertebral level. Facet tropism occurs with asymmetry and is thought to be of clinical importance, adding rotational stresses to the joint. Asymmetric stress resulting from unilateral transitional vertebra (Bertolotti's syndrome) often causes a herniated nucleus pulposus one level above the sacralized or lumbarized segment. Both are diagnosed by radiography. When conservative measures fail, spinal fusion with or without decompression may be of benefit.

D. Compression Fractures: Compression fractures often result from mild trauma and are diagnosed by x-ray examination. The level and degree of injury determine the degree of neurologic involvement and the necessity for thorough and repeated neurologic examinations. The possibility of cancer or osteoporosis should be considered in patients with a history of fractures resulting from trivial trauma. Stable injuries respond to bed rest and conservative care; unstable ones require prolonged bed rest (approximately 3 months) and orthotic or surgical treatment or both.

E. Untreated Scoliosis: Uncorrected scoliosis in adults can cause back pain. After skeletal maturity has been achieved, spinal curves can progress up to 2 degrees per year and up to 8 degrees per pregnancy or period of exogenous hormone use. Unsound scoliosis may result in an imbalance or list. Degenerative changes develop more rapidly. Symptomatic treatment may be helpful. Adult patients with progressive symptoms of pain in the area of the deformity may get relief from operative treatment.

F. Osteoporosis: Osteoporosis is the most common metabolic disorder causing back pain. If protein synthesis is impaired, bone destroyed by normal metabolism is not replaced, and the result is a decrease in bone density. Osteoporosis affects postmenopausal women more commonly than older men. X-rays reveal a marked decrease in vertebral bone density and decreased height, with thoracic kyphosis or lumbar lordosis. The intervertebral disks often bulge into the vertebral end plate, and compression fractures may be noted. Laboratory values are normal, and cancer must be ruled out. Treatment is directed toward the cause, as noted on p 723. Controlled stress to bone (activity) strengthens bone and favors increased deposition of all bony elements. Orthotic support may be useful. In advanced cases, surgical measures must be considered to minimize neurologic symptoms.

Miscellaneous Causes of Low Back Pain

Other causes of back pain not accompanied by radiographic abnormalities include vascular aneurysms, visceral disorders, and psychoneurotic problems.

A. Vascular Aneurysms: Arteriosclerotic obliteration of the aorta, resulting in abdominal aneurysm or thrombotic occlusion of the terminal aorta, gives rise to intermittent claudication and back pain similar to that of herniated nucleus pulposus or neoplasm. Deep, boring pain in the lumbar or pelvic region with decreased peripheral pulses and skin temperature, a pulsating abdominal mass, and a bruit or a thrill with a history of cold feet and small strokes all suggest such a diagnosis. Surgical resection of the aneurysm is often curative. Thrombotic occlusion of the terminal aorta may produce pain in the buttocks, thighs, or legs, with fatigue, weakness, or muscle atrophy along with male impotence; persistent peripheral pulses may still be present. Vascular surgery by a skilled operator may provide symptomatic relief in some instances.

B. Visceral Disorders: Gastrointestinal and genitourinary disease may be a source of back pain. Pancreatic disease and duodenal ulcer may give rise to left thoracolumbar and midback pain. Flank pain can be caused by renal disease. Lumbosacral pain can be due to prostatitis; gynecologic disorders such as pelvic inflammatory disease, uterine fibroids, and endometriosis; and retrocolic disorders. Gallbladder disease pain is commonly referred to the right infrascapular area. Treatment should be directed primarily at the underlying problem.

C. Psychoneurotic Disorders: Complaints of a tired and weak back and back pain (not necessarily severe), with no objective findings except for moist hands, a tremor, and muscle tension, may suggest anxiety reaction. Hysterical back pain may be severe and dramatically exaggerated. Elicitation of a history of domestic or work-related problems and observation of a flat affect with a bizarre reaction to treatment will further suggest the disorder. Treatment may include reassurance and judicious use of mild analgesics and sedatives. Chronicity of complaints, however, is common, and psychiatric referral may be necessary.

The patient with compensatory back or neck pain is interested in monetary gain only, whereas the malingerer seeks a conscious real or imagined secondary gain but may not be interested in pecuniary gain. Subjective complaints in both types of patients are usually out of proportion to objective findings noted on physical examination. The experienced clinician can usually identify the malingerer or the patient with compensatory back or neck pain. These diagnostic impressions should not be conveyed to the patient. It is best to state simply that no organic disorder can be found that explains the patient's symptoms.

Bradford D, Cooper K, Oegema TR Jr: Chymopapain, chemonucleolysis, and nucleus pulposus regeneration. *J Bone Joint Surg* [*Am*] 1983;**65**:1220.

Cailliet R: *Low Back Pain Syndrome,* 3rd ed. Davis, 1981.

Chafetz N, Genant HK: Computed tomography of the lumbar spine. *Orthop Clin North Am* 1983;**14**:147.

Fredrickson BE et al: The natural history of spondylolysis and spondylolisthesis. *J Bone Joint Surg* [*Am*] 1984;**66**:699.

Javid MJ et al: Safety and efficacy of chymopapain (Chymodiactin) in herniated nucleus pulposus with sciatica: Results of a randomized, double-blind study. *JAMA* 1983;**249**:2489.

Kraus H, Nagler W, Melleby A: Evaluation of an exercise program for back pain. *Am Fam Physician* (Sept) 1983;**28**:153.

Liang M, Komaroff AL: Roentgenograms in primary care patients with acute low back pain: A cost-effectiveness analysis. *Arch Intern Med* 1982;**142**:1108.

McAfee PC et al: The value of computed tomography in thoracolumbar fractures: An analysis of 100 consecutive cases and a new classification. *J Bone Joint Surg* [*Am*] 1983;**65**:461.

Mooney V (editor): Symposium on evaluation and care of lumbar spine problems. *Orthop Clin North Am* 1983;**14**:473.

Simons DG, Travell JG: Myofascial origins of low back pain. 1. Principles of diagnosis and treatment. 2. Torso muscles. 3. Pelvic and lower extremity muscles. *Postgrad Med* (Feb) 1983;**73**:66, 81, 99.

THORACIC OUTLET SYNDROMES

Thoracic outlet syndromes include certain disorders with varied manifestations that are caused by compression of the neurovascular structures supplying the upper extremity: cervical rib syndrome, costoclavicular syndrome, scalenus anticus and scalenus medius syndromes, pectoralis minor syndrome, Wright's syndrome, "effort thrombosis" of the axillary and subclavian veins, and the subclavian steal syndrome. Patients often have a history of trauma to the head and neck areas.

Symptoms and signs may arise from intermittent or continuous pressure on elements of the brachial plexus and the subclavian or axillary vessels by a variety of anatomic structures of the shoulder girdle region. The neurovascular bundle can be compressed between the anterior or middle scalene muscles and a normal first thoracic rib or a cervical rib. Descent of the shoulder girdle may continue during adulthood and cause compression. Faulty posture, chronic illness, occupation, and advancing age are other predisposing factors. The components of the median nerve that encircle the axillary artery may cause compression and vascular symptoms. Sudden or repetitive strenuous physical activity may initiate "effort thrombosis" of the axillary or subclavian vein.

Pain may radiate from the point of compression to the base of the neck, the axilla, the shoulder girdle region, arm, forearm, and hand. Paresthesias are frequently present and are commonly distributed to the volar aspect of the fourth and fifth digits. Sensory symptoms may be aggravated at night or by prolonged use of the extremities for daily tasks. Weakness and muscle atrophy are the principal motor symptoms. Vascular symptoms consist of arterial ischemia characterized by pallor of the fingers on elevation of the extremity, sensitivity to cold, and, rarely, gangrene of the digits or venous obstruction marked by edema, cyanosis, and engorgement.

Deep reflexes are usually not altered. When the site of compression is between the upper rib and clavicle, partial obliteration of subclavian artery pulsation may be demonstrated by abduction of the arm to a right angle with the elbow simultaneously flexed and rotated externally at the shoulder so that the entire extremity lies in the coronal plane. Neck or arm position has no effect on the diminished pulse, which remains constant in the subclavian steal syndrome.

X-ray examination is most helpful in differential diagnosis. The value of clinical plethysmography as an objective method of recording brachial arterial pulsations has been emphasized. When venous or arterial obstruction is thought to be intravascular, venography or arteriography is likely to demonstrate the location of the occlusion. Determinations of the conduction velocities of the ulnar and other peripheral nerves of the upper extremity may help to localize the site of their compression.

Thoracic outlet syndrome must be differentiated from symptomatic osteoarthritis of the cervical spine, tumors of the cervical spinal cord or nerve roots, periarthritis of the shoulder, and other cervicobrachial pain syndromes.

Conservative treatment is directed toward relief of compression of the neurovascular bundle. The patient is instructed to avoid any physical activity that is likely to precipitate or aggravate symptoms. Overhead pulley exercises are useful to improve posture. Shoulder bracing, although uncomfortable to many patients, provides a constant stimulus to improve posture. When the patient is lying down, the shoulder girdle should be bolstered by arranging pillows in an inverted "V" position.

Operative treatment may be necessary when conservative measures are not successful.

Symptoms may disappear spontaneously or may

be relieved by carefully directed conservative treatment. Operative treatment is more likely to relieve the neurologic rather than the vascular component that causes symptoms.

Coccia MR, Satiani B: Thoracic outlet syndrome. *Am Fam Physician* (Feb) 1984;**29**:121.

Crawford FA Jr: Thoracic outlet syndrome. *Surg Clin North Am* 1980;**60**:947.

Young HA, Hardy DG: Thoracic outlet syndrome. *Br J Hosp Med* 1983;**29**:457.

SCAPULOHUMERAL PERIARTHRITIS
(Adhesive Capsulitis, Frozen Shoulder)

Periarthritis of the shoulder joint is an inflammatory disorder involving primarily the soft tissues that may be due to many causes. The condition may be divided into a primary type, in which no obvious cause can be identified, and a secondary type associated with an organic articular lesion (eg, rheumatoid arthritis, osteoarthritis, fracture or dislocation). The primary type is most common in the minor shoulder among women after the fourth decade. It may be manifested as inflammation of the articular synovia, the tendons around the joint, the intrinsic ligamentous capsular bands, the paratendinous bursae (especially the subacromial), and the bicipital tendon sheath. Calcareous tendinitis and attritional disease of the rotator cuff, with or without tears, are incidental lesions.

The onset of pain, which is aggravated by extremes of shoulder joint motion, may be acute or insidious. Pain may be most annoying at night and may be intensified by pressure on the involved extremity when the patient sleeps in the lateral decubitus position. Tenderness upon palpation is often noted near the tendinous insertions into the greater tuberosity or over the bicipital groove. Although a sensation of stiffness may be noted only at onset, restriction of shoulder joint motion soon becomes apparent and is likely to progress unless effective treatment is instituted.

Opinion differs on how best to treat this disorder. Pain can usually be controlled with mild analgesics and nonsteroidal anti-inflammatory agents. Passive exercise of the shoulder by an overhead pulley mechanism should be repeated slowly for about 2 minutes 4 times daily. Forceful manipulation of the shoulder joint during this exercise should be avoided. Injection of tender areas with local anesthetics or corticosteroids gives at best only transitory relief. Some surgeons prefer closed manipulation of the shoulder under anesthesia, but this is likely to aggravate rather than relieve pain and restriction of motion. Operative treatment has been advocated by some but should be reserved for the occasional refractory case.

Neviaser JS: Adhesive capsulitis and the stiff and painful shoulder. *Orthop Clin North Am* 1980;**11**:327.

SCAPULOHUMERAL CALCAREOUS TENDINITIS

Calcareous tendinitis of the shoulder joint is an acute or chronic inflammatory disorder of the capsulotendinous cuff (especially the supraspinatus portion) characterized by deposits of calcium salts among tendon fibers. It is a common cause of acute pain near the lateral aspect of the shoulder joint in men over age 30. The calcium deposit may be restricted to the tendon substance or may rupture into the overlying bursa.

Symptoms consist of pain (at times quite severe), tenderness to pressure over the deposit, and restriction of shoulder joint motion. Chronic symptoms may be intermittent and similar to those of scapulohumeral periarthritis.

X-ray examination confirms the diagnosis and demonstrates the site of the lesion.

Calcareous tendinitis must be differentiated from other cervicobrachial pain syndromes, pyogenic arthritis, osteoarthritis, gout, and tears of the rotator cuff.

The aim of treatment is to relieve pain and restore shoulder joint function. Pain is best treated by multiple needling of the lesion under local anesthesia. In the occasional refractive case, operative evacuation of the calcium deposit is necessary to relieve pain. After either type of treatment, early recovery of shoulder joint function should be fostered by judiciously supervised exercises. Acute symptoms occasionally subside after spontaneous rupture of the calcium deposit into the subacromial bursa. Chronic symptoms may be treated by analgesics, exercises, injection of local anesthetics or corticosteroids with or without needling of the deposit, and x-ray therapy. Large deposits may require surgical evacuation.

When x-ray examination shows that a deposit has disappeared, recurrence of that deposit is rare. Symptoms of periarthritis may persist if shoulder joint motion is not completely regained.

Post M (editor): The painful shoulder. (Symposium.) *Clin Orthop* (March) 1983;**173**:1.

Resnick D: Shoulder pain. *Orthop Clin North Am* 1983;**14**:81.

EPICONDYLITIS
(Tennis Elbow, Epicondylalgia)

Epicondylitis is a pain syndrome affecting the mid portion of the upper extremity; no single causative lesion has been identified. It has been postulated that chronic strain of the forearm muscles due to repetitive grasping or rotatory motions of the forearm causes microscopic tears and subsequent chronic inflammation of the common extensor or common flexor tendon at or near their respective osseous origins from the epicondyles.

Epicondylitis occurs most frequently in the major extremity during middle life. Pain is predominantly on the medial or lateral aspect of the elbow region, may be aggravated by grasping, and may radiate proximally into the arm or distally into the forearm. The point of maximal tenderness to pressure is 1–2 cm distal to the epicondyle but may also be present in the muscle bellies more distally. Resisted dorsiflexion or volar flexion of the wrist may accentuate the pain. X-ray examination generally reveals no significant change.

Epicondylitis must be differentiated from other cervicobrachial pain disorders and entrapment syndromes as well as from arthritic diseases.

Treatment is directed toward relief of pain and tenderness. Most acute or subacute symptoms can be relieved by rest, mild analgesics, and avoidance of repetitive grasping. An elastic bandage applied firmly about the proximal forearm may temporarily ameliorate discomfort when the patient is grasping forcefully. Chronic symptoms may require restrictive immobilization such as that provided by an elbow brace or a volar plaster splint. Infiltration of "trigger points" by local anesthetic solutions with or without corticosteroids may be helpful. Operative treatment is reserved for severe, refractory cases.

Berson BL, McGinniss GH: Common tennis injuries. *Hosp Med* (April) 1983;**19**:122.
Van Rossum J et al: Tennis elbow: A radial tunnel syndrome? *J Bone Joint Surg [Br]* 1978;**60**:197.

CARPAL TUNNEL SYNDROME

Carpal tunnel syndrome is a rather common painful disorder caused by compression of the median nerve between the essentially inelastic carpal ligament and other structures within the carpal tunnel (entrapment neuropathy). The volume of the contents of the tunnel can be increased by organic lesions such as synovitis of the tendon sheaths or carpal joints, recent or malhealed fractures, tumors, and occasionally congenital anomalies. Even though no anatomic lesion is apparent, flattening or even circumferential constriction of the median nerve may be observed during operative section of the ligament. Carpal tunnel syndrome may be due to many causes. The disorder may arise in individuals with a long history of strenuous and repetitive use of the hands, or it may follow injuries of the wrists (fractures, dislocations, and bruises). More frequently there is no history of significant trauma. The syndrome is often idiopathic in postmenopausal women and has been attributed to changes in tissue turgor due to aging. A familial type of carpal tunnel syndrome has been reported in which no single common etiologic factor can be identified. The condition occasionally occurs in advanced pregnancy, when it is felt to be due to fluid retention with local edema.

Carpal tunnel syndrome can be a feature of many systemic diseases: rheumatoid arthritis and other rheumatic disorders (inflammatory tenosynovitis); myxedema, amyloidosis, sarcoidosis, and leukemia (tissue infiltration); acromegaly (connective tissue hypertrophy); and hyperparathyroidism, hypocalcemia, and diabetes mellitus (by unknown mechanisms).

Pain in the distribution of the median nerve, which may be burning and tingling (acroparesthesia), is the initial symptom. Aching pain may radiate proximally into the forearm and even to the shoulder joint, neck, and chest. Pain may be episodic or constant and is exacerbated by manual activity, particularly by extremes of volar flexion or dorsiflexion of the wrist. It may be only nocturnal. Impairment of sensation in the median nerve distribution may not be apparent when symptoms are recent, and subtle disparity between the affected and opposite sides can be demonstrated by requiring the patient to identify different textures of cloth by rubbing them between the tips of the thumb and the index finger. Tinel's sign (tingling or shocklike pain on volar wrist percussion) and Phalen's sign (acute wrist flexion) may be positive. Muscle weakness or atrophy, especially of the abductor pollicis brevis, appears later than sensory disturbances. Useful special examinations include electromyography and determinations of segmental sensory and motor conduction delay. Distal median sensory conduction delay may be evident before motor delay.

This syndrome should be differentiated from other cervicobrachial pain syndromes and from compression syndromes of the median nerve in the forearm or arm.

Treatment is directed toward relief of pressure on the median nerve. Conservative treatment usually relieves mild symptoms of recent onset. When a primary lesion is discovered, specific treatment should be given. When soft tissue swelling is a cause, elevation of the extremity may relieve symptoms. Splinting of the hand and forearm at night may be beneficial. When nonspecific inflammation of the ulnar bursa is thought to be a cause, some authors recommend injection of corticosteroids into the carpal tunnel.

Conservative treatment, especially splinting of the wrist, may be helpful in relieving pain of recent duration but should not be prolonged when median nerve motor or sensory impairment is present.

Operative division of the volar carpal ligament gives lasting relief from pain, which usually subsides within a few days. Muscle strength returns gradually, but complete recovery cannot be expected when atrophy is pronounced.

Bora FW Jr, Osterman AL: Compression neuropathy. *Clin Orthop* (March) 1982;**163**:20.
Gelberman RH et al: The carpal tunnel syndrome: A study of carpal tunnel pressures. *J Bone Joint Surg [Am]* 1981;**63**:380.
Nugent GR: Carpal tunnel syndrome. *Hosp Med* (March) 1983; **19**:31.
Szabo RM, Gelberman RH, Dimick MP: Sensibility testing in patients with carpal tunnel syndrome. *J Bone Joint Surg [Am]* 1984;**66**:60.

DUPUYTREN'S CONTRACTURE

This relatively common disorder is characterized by hyperplasia of the palmar fascia and related structures, with nodule formation and contracture of the palmar fascia. The cause is unknown, but the condition has a genetic predisposition and occurs primarily in white men over 50 years of age. The incidence of Dupuytren's contracture is higher among alcoholics and patients with chronic systemic disorders (eg, cirrhosis, diabetes, epilepsy, tuberculosis). It does not appear to be work-related. The onset may be acute, but slowly progressive chronic disease is more common.

Dupuytren's contracture may manifest itself by nodular or cordlike thickening of one or both hands, with the fourth and fifth fingers most commonly affected. The patient may complain of tightness of the involved digits, with inability to satisfactorily extend the fingers, and on occasion there is tenderness. The resulting functional and cosmetic problems may be extremely disabling. Fasciitis involving other areas of the body may lead to plantar fibromatosis (10% of patients) or Peyronie's disease (1–2%).

Periodic examination of patients in early stages of disease is recommended. If the palmar nodule is growing rapidly, injections of triamcinolone into the nodule may be of benefit. Surgical intervention is indicated in patients with significant flexion contractures, depending on the location. Attention should be given to associated health problems before surgery is undertaken.

In severe cases, recurrence after surgery is not uncommon. Digital amputation is reserved for hopelessly contracted fingers that cannot be corrected surgically.

Hayden JW: Compartment syndromes: Early recognition and management. *Postgrad Med* (July) 1983;**74**:191.
Paletta FX: Dupuytren's contracture. *Am Fam Physician* (May) 1981;**23**:85.

SHOULDER-HAND SYNDROME

Shoulder-hand syndrome (accepted by some as a clinical entity) is a variable complex of symptoms and signs arising from various painful disorders of the shoulder joint and hand of the same extremity. It is considered to be a manifestation of reflex neurovascular (sympathetic) dystrophy. The syndrome is essentially a combination of scapulohumeral periarthritis and Sudeck's atrophy of the hand and wrist.

Shoulder-hand syndrome occurs with increasing frequency during the middle years of life. Pain and restricted motion of the shoulder may precede or follow the ipsilateral painful hand involvement. The incidence of diabetes is reported to be significantly higher in patients with shoulder-hand syndrome related to capsulitis of the shoulder. The elbow joint is usually spared; when the elbow is involved, there is painful restriction of motion.

This syndrome should be differentiated from other cervicobrachial pain syndromes, rheumatoid arthritis, polymyositis, scleroderma, and gout.

In addition to specific treatment of the underlying disorder, treatment is directed toward restoration of function. Therapy described for scapulohumeral periarthritis (see above) and Sudeck's atrophy (see p

290) is given simultaneously. The prognosis depends in part upon the stage in which the lesions of the shoulder joint and hand are encountered and the extent and severity of associated organic disease. Early treatment offers the best prognosis for recovery.

Schutzer SF, Gossling HR: The treatment of reflex sympathetic dystrophy syndrome. *J Bone Joint Surg* [*Am*] 1984;**66**:625.
White RH: Shoulder pain. *West J Med* 1982;**137**:340.

CERVICOBRACHIAL PAIN OF INTRATHORACIC ORIGIN

Pain in the shoulder girdle region and upper extremity due to myocardial ischemia of arteriosclerotic heart disease is discussed in Chapter 9. This is a frequent cause of shoulder-hand syndrome.

Bronchogenic carcinoma (see Chapter 7) in the region of the pulmonary apex is an uncommon cause of cervicobrachial pain. Because of the frequency of bronchogenic carcinoma among older people, it is likely to coexist with other organic lesions that cause pain in the anatomic regions discussed in this chapter. X-ray examination of the upper thorax by lordotic projections or tomography may reveal lesions that are not demonstrated by routine x-ray techniques employed for the diagnosis of lung, shoulder girdle, and cervical spine disorders.

BURSITIS

Inflammation of the synoviumlike cellular membrane overlying bony prominences may be secondary to trauma, infection, or arthritic conditions. The most common locations are the subdeltoid, olecranon, ischial (weaver's bottom), and prepatellar (housemaid's knee) bursae. Clinically and anatomically, this syndrome can be differentiated from adjacent inflammatory disorders of tendons, and the attacks may suggest an arthritic process. On occasion, calcific deposits are noted on x-rays of the involved bursae.

Various methods of treatment have been used, including local heat, immobilization, analgesics, nonsteroidal anti-inflammatory agents, and local steroid injections. Infected bursae usually require surgical drainage or aspiration and antibiotic therapy.

Hoffman GS: Tendinitis and bursitis. *Am Fam Physician* (June) 1981;**23**:103.
Knisely GK, Gibson GR, Reichman RC: *Haemophilus influenzae* bursitis and meningitis in an adult. *Arch Intern Med* 1983;**143**:1465.

Table 15–1. "Primary" bone tumors.

Name and Source	Age and Sex Incidence	Clinical Features*	X-Ray Findings	Treatment	Prognosis
Osteoid osteoma. Osteoblastic connective tissue origin	Older children and adolescents. M 2:1	Small, painful (especially nocturnal), tender tumor of almost any bone, but more often in the femur and tibia.	Dense sclerotic lesion with radiolucent center.	Surgical removal.	Good. Removal is curative.
Osteogenic sarcoma. Osteoblastic connective tissue derivation	Peak incidence 20 years. Rare over 40 years. Slight male preponderance.	Gradually progressive pain with variable swelling, local heat, venous engorgement, and tenderness, commonly at metaphyses of major long bones; about 50% involve the knee region. Other sites include pelvis, slender long bones, and flat bones. Weight loss, anemia, and elevation of serum alkaline phosphatase occur later. Histologic examination of biopsy specimen is the most useful laboratory procedure.	Variable, depending upon the osteolytic or sclerosing nature of the tumor. Penetration of cortical bone usually occurs with periosteal elevation and extension into soft tissues. Bone spicules perpendicular to the normal cortical surface—"sunburst" effect—may appear in sclerosing lesions. Chest x-ray may reveal pulmonary metastases.	Local control by amputation or resection of accessible lesions and adjuvant chemotherapy with multiple drugs. Chemotherapy with or without radiation for palliation if tumor is inoperable.	Poor. Smallest and most distal lesions offer best prognosis. Prognosis less favorable for large tumors and trunk tumors. Five-year overall survival rate is 5–20%. Death due to metastases or toxic effects of drug therapy.
Fibrosarcoma. Nonosteoblastic connective tissue derivation	Adults 30–70 years, but also seen in second decade. M = F	Similar to above. Differentiation from osteogenic sarcoma depends upon histologic findings. May be a history (very rare) of irradiation exposure of bone many years previously.	Similar to above.	Amputation if accessible, with or without preliminary irradiation.	Poor, but perhaps slightly better than for osteogenic sarcoma.
Enchondroma. Cartilaginous derivation	Adults. Rare before 10 years. M = F	Mild pain, tenderness, or swelling or spontaneous fracture of bones of hands or feet or of metaphyses of major long bones or flat bones. Lesions may be multiple. Histologic examination confirms diagnosis.	Discrete foci of radiolucency with mottling and compartmentalization. Cortical expansion occurs without extensive erosion.	Curettement of solitary nodules.	Usually good. Pelvic lesions may become malignant.
Chondromyxoid fibroma. Cartilaginous derivation	Young adults 10–30 years. Rare before 10 years. M = F	Pain, swelling, tenderness at metaphyses of major long bones, bones of hands or feet, and flat bones. Histologic examination confirms the diagnosis.	Not characteristic. Ovoid or elongated focus of rarefaction and cortical expansion with erosion. May be multiple foci of osteolysis.	Thorough curettement or excision.	Good.
Chondrosarcoma. Cartilaginous derivation	Adults 30–60 years, also found in childhood and adolescence. M = F	Slow development of pain and swelling of almost any bone, especially long bones, with delayed tendency to metastasis (compare with osteogenic sarcoma).	Irregularly mottled and calcified interior of long bones with fuzzy localized destruction of cortex. Peripheral lesions present a dense, blotchy peripheral outline.	Radical surgical excision or amputation.	If excision is complete, prognosis is excellent; if incomplete, recurrence and progression.

Giant cell tumor (osteoclastoma) Nonosteoblastic connective tissue derivation	10–50 years. M = F	Pain and swelling at ends of major long bones, especially near knee and lower radius. Also found in other bones of extremities and spine.	Eccentrically located osteolytic focus with expansion and cortical erosion. Roughly spherical foamlike areas in cancellous ends of femur and tibia or in distal radial metaphyses.	Excision preferred to curettement when feasible.	About half are biologically benign and have a favorable outcome regardless of treatment. About a third are aggressive, recur, and require further treatment. The rest are frankly malignant.
Chondroblastoma (epiphyseal giant cell tumor) Cartilaginous derivation	Almost always under 20 years. Predominantly male.	Pain and swelling in epiphyseal areas of major tubular bones and in flat bones.	Ovoid areas of mottled translucency in epiphyses or adjacent metaphyses with demarcating wall of sclerotic bone.	Thorough curettement usually adequate.	Almost always benign. Instances of malignancy reported.
Ewing's sarcoma Mesenchymal connective tissue derivation	Adolescent and young adults, but may occur in children. Slight male preponderance.	Pain, swelling, and tenderness of single or multiple lesions of shafts of major tubular bones, vertebrae, or flat bones of trunk. Later findings include fever, anemia, leukocytosis, and increased sedimentation rate. Biopsy essential for diagnosis. Course may be slow, with remissions and exacerbations to progression with metastases.	Diffuse osteosclerosis of cortex with fusiform configuration, subperiosteal lamination ("onion peel") and, occasionally, "sunburst" periosteal reaction and medullary destruction evidenced by diffuse rarefaction or mottling.	Supervoltage radiation and adjuvant multidrug chemotherapy.	Very poor. Mortality rate about 85% with local radiation alone.
Plasma cell myeloma† (multiple myeloma) Hematopoietic origin	Adults over 40 years. M 2:1	Multifocal skeletal involvement. Local pain, swelling, and tendency to pathologic fractures. Spine involvement can cause kyphosis and decreased stature. Late findings include anemia, hypercalcemia, hypercalciuria, hyperglobulinemia, Bence Jones proteinuria, and hyperuricemia. Marrow aspiration or bone biopsy essential for diagnosis. Course may be slow, with remissions and exacerbations.	Variable. Diffuse osteoporosis. Focal lesions appear as diffuse or circumscribed (punched-out) areas of rarefaction without surrounding sclerosis and sometimes with cortical expansion.	X-ray therapy for relief of pain. Chemotherapy (alkylating agents).	Chemotherapy may relieve symptoms and sometimes prolongs life. Average survival is about 1–2 years but may be much longer.

*Local pain, swelling, and tenderness—and occasionally pathologic fractures—are common features of all bone tumors.
†See p 334.

TUMORS & TUMORLIKE LESIONS OF BONE

Essentials of Diagnosis

- Persistent pain, swelling, or tenderness of a skeletal part.
- Limitation of motion of an affected part.
- Pathologic ("spontaneous") fractures.
- Suspicious areas of bony enlargement, deformity, radiodensity, or radiolucency on x-ray.
- Histologic evidence of bone neoplasm on biopsy specimen.

General Considerations

Primary tumors of bone are relatively uncommon in comparison with secondary or metastatic neoplasms. They are, however, of great clinical significance because of the possibility of cancer and because some of them grow rapidly and metastasize widely.

Although tumors of bone have been categorized classically as primary or secondary, there is some disagreement about which tumors are primary to the skeleton. Tumors of mesenchymal origin that reflect skeletal tissues (eg, bone, cartilage, and connective tissue) and tumors developing in bones that are of hematopoietic, nerve, vascular, fat cell, and notochordal origin should be differentiated from secondary malignant tumors that involve bone by direct extension or hematogenous spread. Because of the great variety of bone tumors, it is difficult to establish a truly satisfactory simple classification of bone neoplasms.

Clinical Findings

Persistent skeletal pain and swelling, with or without limitation of motion of adjacent joints or spontaneous fracture, are indications for prompt clinical, x-ray, laboratory, and possibly biopsy examination. X-rays may reveal the location and extent of the lesion and certain characteristics that may suggest the specific diagnosis. The so-called classic x-ray findings of certain tumors (eg, punched-out areas of the skull in multiple myeloma, "sun ray" appearance of osteogenic sarcoma, and "onion peel" effect of Ewing's sarcoma), although suggestive, are not pathognomonic. Even histologic characteristics of the tumor, when taken alone, cannot provide infallible information about the nature of the process. The age of the patient, the duration of complaints, the site of involvement and the number of bones involved, and the presence or absence of associated systemic disease — as well as the histologic characteristics — must be considered collectively for proper management.

The possibility of benign developmental skeletal abnormalities, metastatic neoplastic disease, or infections (eg, osteomyelitis), collagenoses, posttraumatic bone lesions, or metabolic disease of bone must always be kept in mind. If bone tumors occur in or near the joints, they may be confused with the various types of arthritis, especially monarticular arthritis.

The diagnosis of bone tumors is most precise when it is made in close consultation between the clinician, radiologist, and pathologist.

Treatment

Although prompt action is essential for optimal treatment of certain bone tumors, accurate diagnosis is required because of the great potential for harm that may result either from temporization or from radical or ablative operations or unnecessary irradiation. If conservative treatment is elected, careful clinical and x-ray follow-up and expert consultation are necessary.

The clinical features, treatment, and prognosis of a few primary bone tumors are summarized in Table 15-1.

Freiberger R: Thoughts on the diagnosis of bone tumors. *Radiology* 1984;**150**:276.

Levy RN (editor): Metastatic disease of bone. *Clin Orthop* (Sept) 1982;**169**:1.

Mankin HJ: Advances in diagnosis and treatment of bone tumors. *N Engl J Med* 1979;**300**:543.

Mirra JM: *Bone Tumors: Diagnosis & Treatment.* Lippincott, 1980.

Schocker JD et al: Radiation therapy for bone metastasis. *Clin Orthop* (Sept) 1982;**169**:38.

Simon MA: Causes of increased survival of patients with osteosarcoma: Current controversies. *J Bone Joint Surg [Am]* 1984;**66**:306.

Sweetnam R: Osteosarcoma. (2 parts.) *Br J Hosp Med* (Aug) 1982;**28**:112, 116.

Winzelberg GG: Radionuclide evaluation of nonmalignant bone disorders. *Am Fam Physician* (Feb) 1983;**27**:175.

OTHER DISORDERS OF BONES & JOINTS

PATHOLOGIC FRACTURES

A pathologic fracture is a break in the continuity of bone produced by minimal trauma. Sometimes the fracture may be the result of trivial physical injury. Many local and generalized diseases can predispose to pathologic fracture (see below), and it is essential to determine the cause of all fractures that appear to occur in the absence of trauma.

Classification

A. Generalized or Systemic Disorders:

1. Hereditary developmental abnormalities of bone, eg, osteogenesis imperfecta, marble bone disease.
2. Nutritional and vitamin deficiency disease, eg, rickets, vitamin D-resistant rickets, osteomalacia, scurvy.
3. Endocrine abnormalities, eg, hyperparathyroidism, corticosteroid therapy, Cushing's syndrome, Fröhlich's syndrome.
4. Senile osteoporosis.

5. Osteoporosis of disuse.
6. Hematologic disorders, eg, multiple myeloma, leukemia, histiocytosis (eg, Hand-Schüller-Christian disease), lipidoses (eg, Gaucher's disease).
7. Primary neoplasms of bone (with metastases).
8. Metastatic neoplasms of bone, eg, from breast, prostate, thyroid, kidney.
9. Renal disorders, eg, renal rickets with hyperphosphatemia.
10. Osteitis deformans (Paget's disease).
11. Polyostotic fibrous dysplasia (Albright's disease).

B. Local Disorders of Bone:
1. Bone cysts.
2. Primary benign bone neoplasms.
3. Primary malignant bone neoplasms.
4. Metastatic neoplastic.
5. Osteomyelitis.
6. Radiation injury of bone.
7. Neurotropic dystrophy of bone: diabetes, tabes.

Treatment

Make every attempt to determine the cause of pathologic or spontaneous fractures. Patients with predisposing bony defects or abnormalities should be cautioned against exposure to trauma. Institute treatment of the underlying cause when possible, and correct contributing factors concurrent with appropriate orthopedic management of the fracture. Fractures associated with cancer and advanced disease, particularly when the fracture is unstable, tend not to heal. It is often necessary to utilize internal fixation and methylmethacrylate cement in addition to the usual conservative orthopedic measures.

Bouma WH et al: The surgical treatment of pathologic and impending fractures of the long bones. *J Trauma* 1980;**20**:1043.
Heisterberg L et al: Treatment of pathologic fractures. *Acta Orthop Scand* 1979;**50**:787.

FAT EMBOLIZATION SYNDROME

Fat embolization syndrome is a life-threatening form of acute respiratory failure that may occur following severe trauma, especially long-bone fractures. The pathophysiology is not completely understood, but it is thought that embolic fat released from injured tissues is deposited within the pulmonary capillaries. Release and local accumulation of free fatty acids cause alveolocapillary damage leading to respiratory failure, changes in blood coagulation, and central nervous system dysfunction. Apparently, all degrees of embolization syndrome occur, ranging from minor symptoms to frank respiratory failure. The syndrome may be fatal.

The syndrome may not become clinically apparent until 12 hours to 3 or 4 days after the injury occurs.

Symptoms and signs include tachypnea, tachycardia, fever, skin petechiae, changes in mental status (ranging from restlessness to stupor or coma), and convulsions. Arterial blood gas levels are essential for early detection. Hypoxemia, often clinically inapparent initially, usually occurs early and before the development of other signs and symptoms. Other laboratory findings may include anemia, thrombocytopenia, and lipuria. Chest x-rays are not characteristic but may show diffuse, fluffy infiltrates in both lung fields.

Prompt immobilization of long-bone fractures is considered to be an important factor in prevention of the syndrome. Successful treatment of fat embolization syndrome requires early detection, management of respiratory failure (see Adult Respiratory Distress Syndrome, p 167), restoration of blood volume, and other supportive measures. Current evidence suggests that corticosteroids are useful for prophylaxis of fat embolism, particularly in high-risk patients. The prognosis for fat embolization syndrome is usually good if the disorder can be detected early and proper treatment given promptly.

Gossling HR, Donohue TA: The fat embolism syndrome. *JAMA* 1979;**241**:2740.
Schonfeld SA et al: Fat embolism prophylaxis with corticosteroids: A prospective study in high-risk patients. *Ann Intern Med* 1983;**99**:438.

OSTEOGENESIS IMPERFECTA
(Fragilitas Ossium, Brittle Bones)

Essentials of Diagnosis

- Clinical triad: (1) Fragility of bone manifest by pathologic fracture. (2) Clearness or blue coloration of scleras. (3) Deafness.
- Family history.
- Ligamentous laxity.
- Proneness to bruising.
- Dental defects.

General Considerations

Osteogenesis imperfecta is a heritable disorder of connective tissue usually transmitted as an autosomal dominant, although some cases may be autosomal recessive. Two recognized clinical types may occur: osteogenesis imperfecta congenita (fetal type), in which fractures occur in utero and skeletal deformities are apparent at birth; and osteogenesis imperfecta tarda, in which fractures and deformities occur after birth.

Clinical Findings

A. Symptoms and Signs: Fragility of bones is the single most obvious diagnostic criterion. Repeated long-bone fractures in childhood should suggest the underlying disorder. Clearness or blue coloration of the scleras, conductive deafness, and spinal deformities (scoliosis and kyphosis) are often present.

Defective dentin formation (dentinogenesis imperfecta), joint hypermobility, hernias, and hyperelasticity of the skin suggest a soft tissue dysplasia.

The milder cases of the late form may simulate idiopathic juvenile or menopausal osteoporosis.

B. X-Ray Findings: The cortices of the major long bones in the congenita type are thin, and the marrow cavities are broad. In the late type, the bones may be "slender," with narrow shafts, reduced marrow cavities, and bell-shaped widening of the epiphyses. Callus formation after fracture may be meager or luxuriant. Hyperplastic callus formation may occur with or without apparent fracture.

Treatment

There is no treatment for the inadequate formation of osteoid. Calcitonin may be of some value in the tarda group.

Most fractures require immobilization for the relief of pain and prevention of malhealing. Extensive deformities of the diaphysis of a major long bone require more elaborate surgical treatment (eg, multiple osteotomies and internal fixation). Surgical treatment of kyphoscoliosis may have to be delayed until late adolescence, when skeletal structures are stronger.

Prognosis

Because of the protean manifestations of this disease, the course and prognosis are variable. Transmission of the more severe traits is probably prevented by death before puberty or by prevention of reproduction of invalids. The incidence of fracture and the extent of ligamentous laxity are likely to decrease after puberty, and this favorable turn tends to continue through adolescence into later life.

Moorefield WG, Miller GR: Aftermath of osteogenesis imperfecta: The disease in adulthood. *J Bone Joint Surg [Am]* 1980; **62:**113.
Paterson CR, McAllion S, Miller R: Osteogenesis imperfecta: Dominant inheritance and normal sclera. *J Bone Joint Surg [Br]* 1983;**65:**35.

JOGGING INJURIES

Current enthusiasm for running and jogging for pleasure and physical fitness has resulted in a wide array of musculoskeletal problems in about 75% or more of runners at some time. Jogging may cause overuse stress injuries to the feet, ankles, legs, knees, hips, or back, especially in overweight persons. Some of the injuries may become evident shortly after the individual takes up the sport; others may take weeks or months to develop. There have been many reports of associated medical problems involving other organ systems and even of death.

Exercise is a healthful activity that should be encouraged, but it should be adapted to individual capacities and limitations. Exercise-related physical problems may arise from many factors, including improper conditioning or training, preexisting illness, medications, unfavorable environment (heat or cold,

high altitude), improper running gear (especially footwear), overexertion, carelessness, and unforeseen accidents.

The following is a partial list of disorders that have been reported to result from running or jogging:

(1) Musculoskeletal disorders:

(a) Feet: "Runner's toe" (subungual hematoma), Morton's neuroma (painful enlargement of an interdigital nerve), Morton's foot (callus under the head of the second metatarsal), high rigid arch (cavus) problems, stress fractures (particularly in the region of the second and third metatarsals).

(b) Heels: Plantar fasciitis (heel spur), retrocalcaneal bursitis, Achilles tendinitis.

(c) Legs: Shin splints (pain along the medial and lateral surfaces of the anterior tibias), stress fractures, acute and chronic compartment syndromes (pain and weakness of muscles in the leg compartments), popliteal tendinitis, pes anserinus tendinitis.

(d) Knees: Chondromalacia of the patella, "runner's knee" (patellar tendinitis), medial retinaculitis, degenerative joint disease.

(e) Hips: Anterior-superior iliac apophysitis, trochanteric bursitis, degenerative joint disease.

(f) Back: Low back pain, sciatica, disk disease (often preexisting).

(2) Dermatologic disorders: Urticaria (physical, and essential cold urticaria), dyshidrotic eczematoid dermatitis, calcaneal petechiae ("black heel"), blisters, calluses, frostbite, miliaria, sunburn, skin infections, exacerbations of existing skin problems.

(3) Systemic disorders: Dehydration, heat exhaustion, heat stroke.

(4) Nervous system disorders: Sciatica and other neuropathies.

(5) Cardiorespiratory disorders: (Usually exacerbations of preexisting disease.) Asthma, cardiac arrhythmias, angina, myocardial infarction, sudden death (?).

(6) Genitourinary disorders: Hematuria, menstrual irregularities (oligomenorrhea, amenorrhea).

(7) Altered laboratory values: Physiologic alteration of normal values may cause confusion, eg, microscopic hematuria; low or low-normal hemoglobin; increased serum creatine phosphokinase, glutamic-oxaloacetic transaminase, and lactate dehydrogenase; increased serum uric acid and myoglobin.

Clancy WG Jr (editor): Runners' injuries: A symposium. (2 parts.) *Am J Sports Med* 1980;**8:**137, 287.
Dugan RC, D'Ambrosia R: Fibular stress fractures in runners. *J Fam Pract* 1983;**17:**415.
Hanson PG, Giese MD, Carliss RJ: Clinical guidelines for exercise training. *Postgrad Med* (Jan) 1980;**67:**120.
Norfray JF et al: Early confirmation of stress fractures in joggers. *JAMA* 1980;**243:**1647.
Taunton JE, Clement DB, Webber D: Lower extremity stress fractures in athletes. *Physician Sports Med* 1981;**9:**77.
Thompson PD et al: Incidence of death during jogging in Rhode Island from 1975 through 1980. *JAMA* 1982;**247:**2535.

•   •   •

TOTAL JOINT ARTHROPLASTY

In the last 2 decades, remarkable progress has been made in the replacement of severely damaged joints with prosthetic materials. At present, artificial joint replacement is primarily indicated to relieve pain and only secondarily to restore function. Many patients who have minimal pain, therefore, even with marked destruction of the joint on radiographic examination, are not suitable candidates for joint replacement.

Success of the replacement depends upon the amount of physical stress to which the prosthetic components are subjected. Vigorous impact activity, even with the most advanced biomaterials and design, will result in failure of the prosthesis with time. Revision operations are technically more difficult, and the results may not be as good as with the primary procedure. The patient, therefore, must understand the limitations of joint replacement and the consequences of unrestrained joint usage.

Total Hip Arthroplasty

Hip replacement was originally designed for use in patients over 65 years of age with severe osteoarthritis. In these patients—usually less active physically—the prosthesis not only functioned well but outlasted the patients. Severe arthritis that fails to respond to conservative measures (see p 516) remains the principal indication for hip arthroplasty. Hip arthroplasty may also be indicated in younger patients severely disabled by painful hip disease (eg, rheumatoid arthritis), since in such cases it can be assumed that stress on the prosthetic joint will not be great. Contraindications to the operation include active infec-tion and neurotrophic joint disease. Serious complications may occur in about 1% of patients and include thrombophlebitis, pulmonary embolization, sepsis, and dislocation of the joint. Extensive experience has now been accumulated, and the results are generally successful in properly selected patients.

Total Knee Arthroplasty

The indications and contraindications for total knee arthroplasty are similar to those for hip arthroplasty, but experience with the artificial knee is not as extensive. Results are slightly better in osteoarthritis patients than in those with rheumatoid arthritis. Knee arthroplasty is probably not advisable in younger individuals. Complications are similar to those with hip arthroplasty. The failure rate of knee arthroplasty is slightly higher than that of hip arthroplasty.

Total Arthroplasty

Prostheses are now available for total arthroplasty of every major joint of the extremities, but experience with joints other than the hip and the knee has been limited.

Guyer RD: An update on artificial joint replacement. *Am Fam Physician* (March) 1982;**25**:196.

National Institutes of Health–Consensus Conference: Total hip-joint replacement in Sweden. *JAMA* 1982;**248**:1822.

National Institutes of Health–Consensus Conference: Total hip-joint replacement in the United States. *JAMA* 1982;**248**:1817.

Newton SE: Total ankle arthroplasty: Clinical study of 50 cases. *J Bone Joint Surg* [*Am*] 1982;**64**:104.

Scott WN (editor): Symposium on total knee arthroplasty. *Orthop Clin North Am* 1982;**13**:1.

Weisman BN: The radiology of total joint replacement. *Orthop Clin North Am* 1983;**14**:171.

Wolfgang GL: Total hip arthroplasty: Picking the right candidate helps determine success. *Consultant* (March) 1984;**28**:209.

• • •

References

Dalinka MK (editor): Symposium on orthopedic radiology. *Orthop Clin North Am* 1983;**14**:3.

Drennan JC: *Orthopaedic Management of Neuromuscular Disorders.* Lippincott, 1983.

Edmonson AS, Crenshaw AH (editors): *Campbell's Operative Orthopedics,* 6th ed. 2 vols. Mosby, 1980.

Greenfield GB: *Radiology of Bone Diseases,* 3rd ed. Lippincott, 1980.

Kirchner PT, Simon MA: Radioisotopic evaluation of skeletal disease. *J Bone Joint Surg* [*Am*] 1981;**63**:673.

Korn MW (editor): Symposium on special considerations in sports medicine. *Orthop Clin North Am* 1983;**14**:293.

McCarty DJ (editor): *Arthritis and Allied Conditions,* 10th ed. Lea & Febiger, 1984.

Salter RB: *Textbook of Disorders and Injuries of Musculoskeletal Structure,* 2nd ed. Williams & Wilkins, 1983.

Turek SL: *Orthopaedics,* 4th ed. Lippincott, 1984.

Yachmai I: *Angiography of Bone and Soft Tissue Lesions.* Springer-Verlag, 1979.

16 | Genitourinary Tract

Marcus A. Krupp, MD

NONSPECIFIC MANIFESTATIONS OF DISEASE OR DISORDERS

Pain

The localization, pattern of referral, and type of pain are important clues to the diagnosis of genitourinary tract disease.

(1) Pain caused by **renal disease** is usually felt as a dull ache in the "flanks" or costovertebral angle, often extending along the rib margin toward the umbilicus. Because many renal diseases do not produce sudden distention of the capsules of the kidney, there is often no pain.

(2) **Ureteral pain** is related to obstruction and is usually acute in onset, severe, and colicky and radiates from the costovertebral angle down the course of the ureter into the scrotum or vulva and the inner thigh. The radiation of the pain may be a clue to the site of obstruction. High ureteral pain is usually referred to the testicle or vulva; midureteral pain to the lower quadrants of the abdomen; and low ureteral pain to the bladder.

(3) **Bladder pain** accompanies overdistention of the bladder in acute urinary retention and distention of a bladder wall altered by tuberculosis or interstitial cystitis. Relief comes with emptying the bladder. Pain due to bladder infection is usually referred to the distal urethra and accompanies micturition.

(4) Pain caused by **chronic bladder disease** is uncommon. Acute **prostatic inflammation** may produce perineal or low mid back pain.

(5) Pain caused by **testicular inflammation or trauma** is acute and severe and is occasionally referred to the costovertebral angle. Pain associated with infection of the epididymis is similar to that associated with testicular inflammation.

Urinary Symptoms

Infection, inflammation, and obstruction produce symptoms associated with urination.

(1) **Frequency, urgency, and nocturia** are common when inflammation of the urinary tract is present. Severe infection produces a constant desire to urinate even though the bladder contains only a few milliliters of urine. Frequency and nocturia occur when bladder capacity is diminished by disease or when the bladder cannot be emptied completely, leaving a large volume of residual urine. Nocturia associated with a large urine volume may occur with heart failure, renal insufficiency, mobilization of edema due to any cause, diabetes insipidus, hyperaldosteronism, and ingestion of large amounts of fluid late in the evening.

(2) **Dysuria and burning pain in the urethra on urination** are associated with infection of the bladder and prostate.

(3) **Enuresis** may be due to urinary tract disease but is most often caused by neural or psychogenic disorders.

(4) **Urinary incontinence** may be due to anatomic abnormality, physical stress, the urgency associated with infection or nervous system disease, or the dribbling associated with an overdistended flaccid bladder.

Characteristics of Urine

Urinalysis, an essential part of the examination of all patients, is critical in the study of patients who may have renal disease. Organic and inorganic materials in solution in the urine are diagnostic of metabolic disease (inherited or acquired) and of renal disease.

(1) **Proteinuria (albuminuria)** is an important sign of renal disease. Normally, up to 150 mg/d of protein is excreted in urine. Exercise, febrile illness, or severe dehydration may produce increased proteinuria in persons without renal disease. Rarely, a normal person may have significant proteinuria when in an upright position but none while recumbent (postural or orthostatic proteinuria). Proteinuria in excess of 200–500 mg/d is almost always indicative of renal disease. Increased filtration of protein occurs because of reduction in the density of anionic charges in the glomerular capillary wall, not because of altered epithelial pore size. The "dipstick" test for albumin will usually not detect light-chain globulins (eg, Bence Jones protein) and will be false positive with highly alkaline urine. Tests with sulfosalicylic acid will be false positive with sulfisoxazole metabolites, tolbutamide metabolites, acetazolamide, some penicillins (nafcillin, ampicillin, piperacillin), some cephalosporins, levodopa, and tolmetin and with radiographic contrast media.

(2) **Urinary sediment** provides evidence of renal disease that is not available from other sources, and some elements are characteristic of the type and extent

of renal disease. Whenever possible, the physician should examine the sediment, particularly if renal disease may be present. The significance of elements appearing in the urine will be explained below in the discussion of each disease.

(3) Cloudy urine is most frequently the result of the urates or phosphates that precipitate out as urine collects in the bladder and is usually of no significance.

(4) Hematuria is always of grave significance. It may be due to glomerular disease, neoplasms, vascular accidents, infections, anomalies, stones, coagulation defects, or trauma to the urinary tract. When blood appears only during the initial period of voiding, the most likely source is the anterior urethra or prostate. When blood appears during the terminal period of voiding, the most likely source is the posterior urethra, vesical neck, or trigone. Blood mixed in with the total urine volume is from the kidneys, ureters, or bladder.

The causes of hematuria can be summarized as follows:

A. Localized:

1. Urethra–Trauma, infection.
2. Bladder–Infection, stone, neoplasm, varices (especially of bladder neck with prostatic enlargement), drug reaction (cyclophosphamide), radiation injury, parasite infestation.
3. Ureter–Infection, stone, tumor.
4. Kidney–Glomerular disease, infection, stone, anatomic anomalies (including polycystic disease, arteriovenous malformations), renal vein or artery thrombosis, neoplasms, trauma (including renal biopsy).

B. Systemic:

1. Anticoagulant therapy.
2. Bleeding diathesis–Hemophilia, thrombocytopenia, disseminated intravascular coagulation.
3. Hemolytic disease–Hemoglobinurias, hemolytic-uremic syndrome.
4. Sickle cell crisis.
5. Anaphylactoid purpura with renal involvement.

RENAL FUNCTION TESTS

Diagnosis of renal diseases and evaluation of renal function depend on laboratory determinations. As renal function becomes impaired, laboratory observations provide reliable indices of the capacity of the kidney to meet the demands of excretion, reabsorption, and secretion and to fulfill its role in maintaining homeostasis. Useful tests may be categorized according to the physiologic function measured:

(1) Glomerular filtration rate (GFR): Inulin clearance is the reference method for measuring GFR. After a single intravenous injection of ^{51}Cr edetate, ^{99m}technetium diethylenetriamine penta-acetate, or ^{131}I iothalamate, the slope of decreasing concentration in plasma can be determined to give a precise measure of GFR. For routine clinical use, the less precise endogenous creatinine clearance is adequate. Plasma

creatinine or urea levels reflect GFR, rising as the filtration rate diminishes. GFR may be estimated from the serum creatinine by the following formula:

$$\text{GFR (mL/min)} = \frac{0.014\,(140 - \text{Age}) \times \text{Weight (kg)}}{\text{Serum creatinine (mg/dL)}}$$

The result is for men; for women, decrease by 15%.

Concentrations of serum urea nitrogen and creatinine are used as indicators of adequacy of renal function. Urea nitrogen concentration will vary directly with the quantity of protein in the diet and will increase with increased catabolism following trauma or stressful disease or with decreased renal blood flow (decreased filtration and increased reabsorption). The combination of a high protein load and decreased renal blood flow consequent to bleeding into the upper gastrointestinal tract will result in a transient elevation of serum urea nitrogen. Creatinine is produced at a relatively constant rate independently of diet. It is excreted at a fairly constant rate by glomerular filtration; for clinical purposes, tubular secretion is of little consequence except when renal failure is well advanced and tubular secretion becomes a significant portion of the total creatinine excreted. Creatinine clearance in the presence of chronic renal failure yields higher values than does inulin clearance. The concentration of serum creatinine increases as renal impairment advances; the concentration exceeds the normal level when creatinine clearance reaches about 50% of normal. The ratio of concentration of serum or blood urea nitrogen to creatinine is normally about 10:1. Ratios greater than 15:1 occur with prerenal azotemia, postrenal azotemia due to acute obstructive uropathy, and upper gastrointestinal hemorrhage.

(2) Renal plasma flow (RPF): There is no simple clinical test of RPF. Measurement of clearance of para-aminohippurate or of radioiodine-tagged compounds utilized in urography may be used.

(3) Tubular function: Clinical means of assessing tubular function include the ability to produce urine that is more concentrated or less concentrated than the osmolality of plasma; the ability to acidify the urine; and, of lesser value, the ability to excrete phenolsulfonphthalein (PSP).

RENAL BIOPSY

Renal biopsy is useful to confirm the diagnosis in instances in which choice of therapy depends on tissue diagnosis. Tissue should be prepared for light and electron microscopy and for immunofluorescent stains. Percutaneous renal biopsy is used to distinguish by structural characteristics among the causes of the nephrotic syndrome, the presence of generalized disease (amyloidosis, sarcoidosis, collagen disorder), rapidly progressive glomerulonephritis, and the causes of hematuria and proteinuria. Biopsy occasionally is used to assess rejection response in a transplanted kidney. Confirm the presence of a generalized disease (collagen disorder, amyloidosis, sarcoidosis), and follow rejection response in a transplanted kidney. Absolute contraindications include anatomic presence of only one kidney; severe malfunction of one kidney even though function is adequate in the other; bleeding diathesis; the presence of hemangioma, tumor, or large cysts; perinephric abscess or renal infection; hydronephrosis; and an uncooperative patient. Relative contraindications are the presence of serious hypertension, end-stage chronic renal failure, severe arteriosclerosis, and unusual difficulty in doing a biopsy owing to obesity, anasarca, or inability of the patient to lie flat.

ROENTGENOGRAPHIC EXAMINATION & ULTRASOUND

Renal Radiography

Radiography is an essential resource for the diagnosis and evaluation of renal disease amenable to medical as well as surgical treatment. Kidney size, shape, and position may be critical elements of information. Routine films, tomography, urography, angiography, and computed tomography (CT) scans are sources of anatomic and physiologic data that often are definitive, revealing details of circulation, structure, and calcification available by no other means. Collaboration with the radiologist provides the greatest opportunity for properly performed and interpreted examinations. X-ray contrast agents are hazardous in the presence of severe dehydration, renal disease, diabetic nephropathy, liver failure, and multiple myeloma.

Scanning With Radionuclides

Use of appropriate radioisotope-tagged compounds (iodohippurate sodium I 131, chlormerodrin Hg 203, technetium ^{99m}Tc), sensitive detectors, and scintillation cameras provides ready assessment of renal blood flow and clearance of the compound, as well as visualization of the size and shape of the kidneys, the site of ureteral obstruction, and the presence of dilated ureters and urinary bladder. The 2 kidneys can be compared as a means of identifying unilateral disease.

Ultrasound (Sonography)

Ultrasound is a noninvasive technique that is free of hazard. Radarlike devices utilizing high-frequency sound waves are capable of delineating solid or fluid-filled organs or masses. Kidney size and shape can often be distinguished clearly enough to identify tumors or cysts and anomalies such as horseshoe kidney. Calcification within the kidney and urinary tract can sometimes be demonstrated better in this way than by any other means. It is a useful guide in performing renal biopsy. Dilated renal calices, the renal pelvis, and the ureters can be identified. Bladder and prostatic neoplasms can often be demonstrated.

Abuels JG: Proteinuria: Diagnostic principles and procedures. *Ann Intern Med* 1983;**98**:186.

Fairley KF, Birch DF: Hematuria: A simple method for detecting glomerular bleeding. *Kidney Int* 1982;**21**:105.

Hanglustaine D et al: Detection of glomerular bleeding using a simple staining method for light microscopy. *Lancet* 1982;**2**:761.

Morrin PAF: Urinary sediment in the interpretation of proteinuria. (Editorial.) *Ann Intern Med* 1983;**98**:254.

Stamey T, Kindrachuk RW: *Urinary Sediment and Urinalysis: A Practical Guide for the Health Professional*. Saunders, 1984.

DISORDERS OF THE KIDNEYS

GLOMERULONEPHRITIS

Information obtained from experimentally induced glomerular disease in animals and from correlations with evidence derived by modern methods of examination of tissue obtained by biopsy and at necropsy has provided a new concept of glomerulonephritis.

The clinical manifestations of renal disease are apt to consist only of varying degrees of microscopic hematuria, excretion of characteristic formed elements in the urine, proteinuria, and renal insufficiency and its complications. Alterations in glomerular architecture as observed in tissue examined by light microscopy are also apt to be minimal and difficult to interpret. For these reasons, attempts to correlate clinical syndromes with histologic features of renal tissue have failed to provide a satisfactory basis for precise diagnosis, treatment, and prognosis.

Immunologic techniques for demonstrating a variety of antigens, antibodies, and complement fractions have helped toward understanding the origins and pathogenesis of glomerular disease. Electron microscopy has complemented the immunologic methods.

Briefly, glomerular disease resulting from immunologic reactions may be divided into 2 groups:

(1) Immune complex disease, in which soluble antigen-antibody complexes in the circulation are trapped in the glomeruli. The antigens are not derived from glomerular components; they may be exogenous (bacterial, viral, chemical, including antibiotics and other drugs) or endogenous (circulating native DNA, tumor antigens, thyroglobulin). Factors in the pathogenic potential of the antigen include its origin, quantity, and route of entry and the host's duration of exposure to it. The immune response to the antigen depends partly on the severity of inflammation or infection and partly on the host's capacity to respond (immunocompetency).

In the presence of antigen excess and, in some cases, antibody excess, antigen-antibody complexes form in the circulation and are trapped in the glomeruli as they are filtered through capillaries rendered permeable by the action of vasoactive amines. The antigen-antibody complexes bind components of complement, particularly C3. Activated complement provides chemoactive factors that attract leukocytes whose lysosomal enzymes incite the injury to the glomerulus.

By immunofluorescence methods and by electron microscopy, these complexes appear as lumpy deposits between the epithelial cells and the glomerular basement membrane and in the mesangium. IgG, IgM, occasionally IgA, and C3 have been identified.

(2) Anti-glomerular basement membrane disease, in which antibodies are generated against the glomerular basement membrane of the kidney and often against lung basement membrane, which appears to be antigenically similar to glomerular basement membrane. The autoantibodies may be stimulated by autologous glomerular basement membrane altered in some way or combined with an exogenous agent. The reaction of antibody with glomerular basement membrane is accompanied by activation of complement, the attraction of leukocytes, and the release of lysosomal enzymes. The presence of thrombi in glomerular capillaries is often accompanied by leakage of fibrinogen and precipitation of fibrin in Bowman's space, with subsequent development of epithelial "crescents" in the space.

Immunofluorescence techniques and electron microscopy show the anti-glomerular basement membrane complexes as linear deposits outlining the membrane. IgG and C3 are usually demonstrable.

Classification of Glomerulonephritis

A current classification of glomerulonephritis is based on the immunologic concepts described above. However, the discussions in the following pages are organized according to traditional clinical categories.

I. Immunologic Mechanisms Likely
A. Immune Complex Disease:
Glomerulonephritis clearly poststreptococcal
Glomerulonephritis associated with infectious agents, including staphylococci, pneumococci, infective endocarditis, secondary syphilis, leprosy, malaria, toxoplasmosis, schistosomiasis, viruses of hepatitis (HBAg), measles, and varicella
Lupus erythematosus
Glomerulonephritis associated with other systemic (autoimmune?) disease such as systemic lupus erythematosus, polyarteritis nodosa, scleroderma, anaphylactoid purpura, idiopathic cryoglobulinemia, and tumor antigens (eg, colon, bronchus, kidney, melanoma)
Membranous glomerulonephritis, cause unknown
Membranoproliferative glomerulonephritis, cause unknown
Focal glomerulonephritis
Rapidly progressive glomerulonephritis (some cases)
B. Anti-Glomerular Basement Membrane Disease:
Goodpasture's syndrome
Rapidly progressive glomerulonephritis (some cases)
II. Immunologic Mechanisms Not Clearly Shown
Lipoid nephrosis (minimal lesion)
Focal glomerulonephritis (some cases)
Chronic sclerosing glomerulonephritis
Diabetic glomerulosclerosis
Amyloidosis
Hemolytic-uremic syndrome and thrombotic thrombocytopenic purpura
Wegener's granulomatosis
Alport's syndrome
Sickle cell disease

1. ACUTE GLOMERULONEPHRITIS

Acute nephritis is often related to an antecedent infection with a group A hemolytic streptococcus or, less frequently, to a variety of other infectious agents. The clinical syndrome of acute nephritis occurs with other renal diseases, including systemic lupus erythematosus, idiopathic mesangiocapillary proliferative (membranoproliferative) glomerulonephritis, Henoch-Schönlein purpura, acute interstitial nephritis, and mixed cryoglobulinemia.

The following description of the clinical presentation of poststreptococcal glomerulonephritis applies in whole or in part to the syndrome of acute nephritis due to any other cause.

Essentials of Diagnosis

- History of preceding streptococcal or, rarely, other infection.
- Concurrent systemic vasculitis or hypersensitivity reaction.
- Malaise, headache, anorexia, low-grade fever.
- Mild generalized edema, mild hypertension, retinal hemorrhages.
- Gross hematuria; protein, red cell casts, granular and hyaline casts, white cells, and renal epithelial cells in urine.
- Evidence of impaired renal function, especially nitrogen retention.

General Considerations

Glomerulonephritis is a disease affecting both kidneys. In most cases, recovery from the acute stage is complete; however, progressive involvement may destroy renal tissue, in which case renal insufficiency results. Acute glomerulonephritis is most common in children 3–10 years of age, although 5% or more of initial attacks occur in adults over age 50. By far the most common cause is an antecedent infection of the pharynx and tonsils or of the skin with group A β-hemolytic streptococci, certain strains of which are nephritogenic. In children under age 6, pyoderma (impetigo) is the most common antecedent; in older children and young adults, pharyngitis is a common antecedent and skin infection a rare one. Rarely, nephritis may follow other infections (see above) and exposure to some drugs, including penicillins, sulfonamides, phenytoin, aminosalicylic acid, and aminoglycoside antibiotics. *Rhus* dermatitis and reactions to venom or chemical agents may be associated with renal disease clinically indistinguishable from glomerulonephritis.

The pathogenesis of the glomerular lesion has been further elucidated by the use of new immunologic techniques (immunofluorescence) and electron microscopy. A likely sequela to infection by nephritogenic strains of β-hemolytic streptococci is injury to the mesangial cells in the intercapillary space. The glomerulus may then become more easily damaged by antigen-antibody complexes developing from the immune response to the streptococcal infection. The C3 component of complement is deposited in association with IgG (rarely IgA or IgM) or alone in a granular pattern on the epithelial side of the basement membrane and occasionally in subendothelial sites as well. Similar immune complex deposits in the glomeruli can often be demonstrated when the origin is other than streptococcal.

Gross examination of the involved kidney shows only punctate hemorrhages through the cortex. Microscopically, the primary alteration is in the glomeruli, which show proliferation and swelling of the mesangial and endothelial cells of the capillary tuft. The proliferation of capsular epithelium produces a thickened crescent about the tuft, and in the space between the capsule and the tuft there are collections of leukocytes, red cells, and exudate. Edema of the interstitial tissue and cloudy swelling of the tubule epithelium are common. Immune complexes are demonstrable by means of immunofluorescence techniques. Electron microscopy reveals the dense immune complex deposits as well as altered glomerular structures. As the disease progresses, the kidneys may enlarge. The typical histologic findings in glomerulitis are enlarging crescents that become hyalinized and converted into scar tissue and obstruct the circulation through the glomerulus. Degenerative changes occur in the tubules, with fatty degeneration and necrosis and ultimate scarring of the nephron. Arteriolar thickening and obliteration become prominent.

Clinical Findings

A. Symptoms and Signs: Nephritis begins about 2 weeks after the streptococcal infection or exposure to a drug or other inciting agent. Often the disease is very mild, and there may be no reason to suspect renal involvement unless the urine is examined. In severe cases, the patient develops malaise, headache, mild fever, flank pain, and oliguria. The urine is noted as "bloody," "coffee-colored," or "smoky." Renal salt and water retention result from the diminished GFR and relatively increased tubular reabsorption, accounting for most of the symptoms and signs. Edema appears in the periorbital areas and may include the extremities and pleural and peritoneal spaces. Increased blood volume is accompanied by increased cardiac output and some increase in arterial peripheral

resistance with consequent arterial hypertension. Pulmonary vascular congestion occurs frequently and produces shortness of breath. Frank pulmonary edema may ensue.

B. Laboratory Findings: The diagnosis is confirmed by examination of the urine, which may be grossly bloody or coffee-colored (acid hematin) or may show only microscopic hematuria. Red cell morphology provides a clue as to whether the origin of the red cell is glomerular or nonglomerular. Red cells of glomerular origin are dysmorphic and show a variety of distorted forms and swollen forms. Examine the sediment with phase microscopy or with oil immersion in light microscopy after using one of the commercially available sediment stains. Red cells of nonglomerular origin are not distorted. In addition, the urine contains protein (1–3+) and casts. Hyaline and granular casts are commonly found in large numbers, but the classic sign of glomerulitis, the erythrocyte cast (blood cast), may be rare and require careful search of a centrifuged urinary sediment. The erythrocyte cast resembles a blood clot formed in the lumen of a renal tubule; it is usually of small caliber, intensely orange or red, and under high power with proper lighting may show the mosaic pattern of the packed red cells held together by the clot of fibrin and plasma protein.

With the impairment of renal function (decrease in GFR and blood flow) and with oliguria, plasma or serum urea nitrogen and creatinine become elevated, the levels varying with the severity of the renal lesion. The sedimentation rate is rapid. A mild normochromic anemia may result from fluid retention and dilution. Infection of the throat with nephritogenic streptococci is frequently followed by increasing antistreptolysin O (ASO) titers in the serum, whereas high titers are usually not demonstrable following skin infections. Production of antibody against streptococcal deoxyribonuclease B (anti-DNase B) is more regularly observed following both throat and skin infections. Serum complement levels are usually low.

Confirmation of diagnosis is made by examination of the urine, although the history and clinical findings in typical cases leave little doubt. The finding of erythrocytes that are dysmorphic or contained in a cast is proof of their glomerular origin.

Differential Diagnosis

Although considered to be the hallmark of glomerulonephritis, erythrocyte casts also occur along with other abnormal elements in any disease in which glomerular inflammation and tubule damage are present, ie, polyarteritis nodosa, disseminated lupus erythematosus, dermatomyositis, sarcoidosis, subacute infective endocarditis, "focal" nephritis, Goodpasture's syndrome, Henoch's purpura, or poisoning with chemicals toxic to the kidney.

Complications

In severe cases, signs compatible with cardiac failure appear as a result of salt and water retention rather than of myocardial failure per se: cardiac enlargement, tachycardia, S$_3$ gallop, pulmonary passive congestion, pleural fluid, and peripheral edema.

With severe hypertension, signs of left ventricular failure often develop, and the symptoms and signs of hypertensive encephalopathy may predominate: severe headache, drowsiness, muscle twitchings and convulsions, vomiting, and at times papilledema and retinal hemorrhage.

Any infection in a patient with glomerulonephritis must be seen as a serious complication.

Treatment

A. Specific Measures: There is no specific treatment. Eradication of β-hemolytic streptococci with penicillin or other antibiotic is desirable. Adrenocorticosteroids and corticotropin are of no value and may be contraindicated because they increase protein catabolism, sodium retention, and hypertension. Immunosuppressive and cytotoxic drugs have been ineffective in this form of nephritis. (See Nephrotic Syndrome.)

B. General Measures: In uncomplicated cases, treatment is symptomatic and designed to prevent overhydration and hypertension. Hospitalization is indicated if oliguria, nitrogen retention, and hypertension are present. Bed rest is of great importance and should be continued until clinical signs abate. Excretion of protein and formed elements in the urine will increase with resumption of activity, but such increases should not be great. Erythrocytes may be excreted in large numbers for months, and the rate of excretion is not a good criterion for evaluating convalescence.

In the presence of elevated blood urea nitrogen and oliguria, dietary protein restriction is indicated. If severe oliguria is present, no protein should be given. If no nitrogen retention is apparent, the diet may contain 0.5 g of protein/kg ideal weight. Carbohydrates should be given liberally to provide calories and to reduce the catabolism of protein and prevent starvation ketosis. With severe oliguria, potassium intoxication may occur, requiring dialysis.

The degree of oliguria and fluid retention and the severity of circulatory congestion and edema dictate the degree of restriction of salt and water. Loop diuretics are useful in reduction of fluid overload and of accompanying hypertension. Hemodialysis is performed as indicated by the severity of the acute renal insufficiency.

If anemia becomes severe (hematocrit < 30%), give transfusions of packed red cells.

C. Treatment of Complications:

1. Hypertensive encephalopathy should be treated vigorously as a medical emergency. Drowsiness and confusion accompanied by severe headache, nausea, blurred vision, and twitching progress to stupor and coma. A greatly elevated blood pressure (often > 250/150 mm Hg) and evidence of retinal arteriolar spasm with or without papilledema and hemorrhages are characteristic. The goal of therapy is to reduce blood pressure to near normal levels without

further impairing renal function. The first-line drugs include nitroprusside, diazoxide, hydralazine, and nifedipine.

Treatment for hypertensive crisis requires close monitoring.

a. Sodium nitroprusside intravenously at 2–50 μg/kg/min acts promptly but is of brief duration. Observation in an intensive care unit with intra-arterial blood pressure monitoring is required.

b. Diazoxide, 150–300 mg, may be given rapidly as a bolus and 150 mg repeated as needed every 5–10 minutes. A continuous infusion of 300 mg/min may be substituted. Close monitoring is essential. Diazoxide produces sodium retention, which should be corrected by intravenous furosemide.

c. Hydralazine, 5–10 mg intravenously every 15 minutes or 30–50 mg intravenously every 4–6 hours, is slower to act. Propranolol, 1–5 mg intravenously, may be required to reduce tachycardia.

d. Nifedipine, 10–20 mg sublingually, may be used initially for rapid control under close monitoring.

e. Minoxidil, prazosin, and clonidine may be useful for maintenance therapy.

f. Phenytoin may be of value in controlling seizures.

2. Heart failure should be treated as any case of left ventricular failure, ie, with severe restriction of fluid and sodium intake and the use of agents that reduce peripheral resistance (afterload) and venous return (preload) (see pp 248–250). Oxygen helps relieve respiratory distress. If digitalis is used, its effects must be monitored closely.

3. Infection should be promptly eradicated with appropriate antibiotics.

Prognosis

Most patients with acute disease recover completely within 1–2 years; 5–20% show progressive renal damage. If oliguria, heart failure, or hypertensive encephalopathy is severe, death may occur during the acute attack.

See references under IgA Nephropathy, p 553.

2. CHRONIC GLOMERULONEPHRITIS

If acute glomerulonephritis does not heal within 1–2 years, the vascular and glomerular lesions continue to progress, and tubular changes occur. In the presence of smoldering active nephritis, the patient is usually asymptomatic, and the only evidence of disease is the excretion of abnormal urinary elements.

The urinary excretion of protein, red cells, white cells, epithelial cells, and casts (including erythrocyte casts, granular casts, and hyaline and waxy casts) continues at levels above normal. As renal impairment progresses, signs of renal insufficiency appear (see below).

Treatment

Treat intercurrent infections promptly and vigorously as indicated. Avoid unnecessary vaccinations.

Treat exacerbations as for the acute attack, nephrotic state, or incipient renal insufficiency as indicated. A protein intake of 0.5–1 g/kg is permissible as long as renal function is adequate to maintain a normal blood urea nitrogen. A liberal fluid intake is desirable.

Strenuous exercise may be harmful; otherwise, normal activity is permitted.

Prognosis

Worsening of the urinary findings may occur with infection, trauma, or fatigue. Exacerbations may resemble the acute attack or may be typical of the nephrotic syndrome (see below). Death in uremia is the usual outcome, but the course is variable, and the patient may live a reasonably normal life for 20–30 years.

See references under IgA Nephropathy, p 553.

3. NEPHROTIC SYNDROME

Essentials of Diagnosis

- Massive edema.
- Proteinuria > 3.5 g/d.
- Hypoalbuminemia < 3 g/dL.
- Hyperlipidemia: Cholesterol > 300 mg/dL.
- Lipiduria: Free fat, oval fat bodies, fatty casts.

General Considerations

Because treatment and prognosis vary with the cause of nephrotic syndrome (nephrosis), renal biopsy and appropriate examination of an adequate tissue specimen are important. Light microscopy, electron microscopy, and immunofluorescence identification of immune mechanisms provide critical information for identification of most of the causes of nephrosis.

Glomerular diseases associated with nephrotic syndrome include the following: (See Table 16–1.)

(1) Minimal glomerular lesions: Lipoid nephrosis accounts for about 20% of cases of nephrotic syndrome in adults.

(2) Membranous glomerulonephritis: About 30% of cases.

(3) Diffuse proliferative glomerulonephritis: About 5% of cases.

(4) Focal proliferative glomerulonephritis: About 10% of cases.

(5) Mesangiocapillary (membranoproliferative) glomerulonephritis: About 7% of cases.

(6) Miscellaneous diseases: These include diabetic glomerulopathy, systemic lupus erythematosus, polyarteritis, Wegener's granulomatosis, amyloid disease, multiple myeloma, neoplasms (including lymphomas and carcinomas), hepatitis B, syphilis, reaction to toxins (bee venom, *Rhus* antigen), reaction to drugs (trimethadione, etc), and exposure to heavy metals.

Clinical Findings

A. Symptoms and Signs: Edema may appear insidiously and increase slowly; often it appears suddenly and accumulates rapidly. As fluid collects in the serous cavities, the abdomen becomes protuberant, and the patient may complain of anorexia and become short of breath. Symptoms other than those related to the mechanical effects of edema and serous sac fluid accumulation are not remarkable.

On physical examination, massive edema is apparent. Signs of hydrothorax and ascites are common. Pallor is often accentuated by the edema, and striae commonly appear in the stretched skin of the extremities. Hypertension, changes in the retina and retinal vessels, and cardiac and cerebral manifestations of hypertension may be demonstrated more often when collagen disease, diabetes mellitus, or renal insufficiency is present.

B. Laboratory Findings: The urine contains large amounts of protein, 4–10 g/24 h or more. The sediment contains casts, including the characteristic fatty and waxy varieties; renal tubule cells, some of which contain lipid droplets (oval fat bodies); and variable numbers of erythrocytes. A mild normochromic anemia is common, but anemia may be more severe if renal damage is great. Nitrogen retention varies with the severity of impairment of renal function. The plasma is often lipemic, and cholesterol and triglycerides are usually elevated. Plasma protein is greatly reduced. The albumin fraction is typically decreased to less than 3 g/dL. Some reduction of gamma globulin occurs in pure nephrosis, whereas in systemic lupus erythematosus the protein of the gamma fraction may be greatly elevated. Serum complement is usually low in active disease. The serum electrolyte concentrations are often normal, although the serum sodium may be slightly low; total serum calcium may be low, in keeping with the degree of hypoalbuminemia and decrease in the protein-bound calcium moiety. During edema-forming periods, urinary sodium excretion is very low and urinary aldosterone excretion elevated. If renal insufficiency (see above) is present, the blood and urine findings are usually altered accordingly.

Renal biopsy is essential to confirm the type of lesion and to indicate prognosis.

Differential Diagnosis

Renal vein thrombosis is associated with nephrotic syndrome; it is likely that renal vein thrombosis is secondary to nephrosis rather than a cause of it. Constrictive pericarditis may present with a clinical picture resembling nephrosis.

Treatment

There is no specific treatment except for syphilis or for heavy metal poisoning. Bed rest is indicated for patients with severe edema or those who have infections. Infections should be treated vigorously and promptly with appropriate antibiotics. Hospitalization is desirable when corticosteroid therapy is initiated. The diet should provide a normal protein ration

Table 16–1. Morphologic characteristics of selected glomerulopathies.

	Light Microscopy	Electron Microscopy	Immunofluorescence*				
			IgG	IgA	IgM	C3	FRA
Primary glomerulonephritis							
Diffuse proliferative, including poststreptococcal	Proliferation of mesangial cells, endothelial cells, and/or epithelial cells.	Subepithelial GBM† deposits. Mesangial cells and matrix increased.	Variable and irregular granular deposits along capillary walls and in mesangium.	++	v	v	+	v
Focal proliferative	Focal proliferative changes plus increased mesangial cellularity.	Mesangial deposits.	Segmental granular GBM and mesangial deposits.	++	+	+	++	v
Proliferative with crescent formation	Crescent formation from proliferation of epithelial cells filling Bowman's space.	Subendothelial deposits along GBM with increased mesangial matrix; proliferating epithelial cells.	Diffuse granular or linear deposits involving peripheral capillary loops.	++	+	+	+	+
Mesangiocapillary (membranoproliferative)	Proliferation of mesangial cells, increased mesangial matrix, thickening of capillary walls.	I. Deposits in mesangium; endothelial cells separated from endothelial cells by mesangial matrix. II. Confluent intra-GBM deposit.	I. Granular deposit along GBM. C3 alone in mesangium. II. Intramembranous deposit in GBM and TBM.†	++	v	++	+++	v
Membranous	Thickening of capillary wall. Subepithelial spikes (silver stain).	Dense subepithelial deposits.	Coarse granular deposits along capillary wall.	++	v	v	++	v
Focal sclerosing	Segmental sclerosis with hyaline deposits in subendothelial areas of affected loops, especially of juxtamedullary cortex.	Subendothelial and mesangial dense deposits. Diffuse or segmental alteration of foot processes.	Irregular granular or nodular deposits at site of focal lesions.	+	±	++	++	–
Chronic, end stage	Hyalinization of glomerular tufts, loss of tubules, interstitial fibrosis.	Fibrosis, hyaline deposits, advanced alterations characteristic of primary disease.	Granular deposits in scarred and partially intact glomeruli and in interstitial areas.	±	±	++	+	±
Systemic disease							
Systemic lupus erythematosus	Variable patterns of minimal changes, mesangial proliferative, focal proliferative, membranous lesions. Hematoxylin bodies in capillary loops.	Characteristic massive subendothelial, intramembranous and subepithelial deposits; wire loop lesions. Microtubules in endothelial cells and leukocytes.	Variable. Granular deposits corresponding to type and location of altered glomeruli.	++	+	++	++	+
Disease of uncertain immunologic cause							
Lipoid nephrosis	No alteration, or minimal lesion of proliferative type.	Abnormalities of epithelial cells with smudging of foot processes and obliteration of slit pore membrane.	Minimal irregular clumps in mesangial areas.	±	–	±	±	–
Berger's IgA nephropathy	Segmental to diffuse mesangial proliferation and increase in mesangial matrix.	Deposits in mesangium.	Granular deposits in mesangium.	+	++	–	++	+
Henoch-Schönlein purpura	Focal and diffuse proliferative lesions and mesangial lesions.	Same as focal and proliferative types with increased mesangial deposits.	Diffuse glomerular deposits, largely in mesangium.	+	++	+	++	+
Wegener's granulomatosis	Proliferative and crescent-forming lesions.	Dense GBM deposits.	Variable scattered granular deposits.	+	±	+	+	+

*FRA = Fibrin/fibrinogen-related antigen; v = variable.
†GBM = Glomerular basement membrane; TBM = tubular basement membrane.

(0.75–1 g/kg/d), with adequate calories. Sodium intake should be restricted to 0.5–1 g/d. Potassium need not be restricted. Iron and vitamin supplements may be helpful. If edema, ascites, or pleural effusion becomes disabling, a cautious trial of diuretics is warranted; the physician should watch for reduction of an already diminished plasma volume (postural hypotension, prerenal azotemia, shock).

Adrenocorticosteroids are useful for treatment of the nephrotic syndrome in children and in adults when the underlying disease is the minimal glomerular lesion (lipoid nephrosis), systemic lupus erythematosus, proliferative glomerulonephritis, or idiosyncrasy to toxin or venom. In the adult with minimal glomerular lesion, a trial of corticosteroid therapy is justified, although the advantage over no treatment is uncertain and complications of therapy are more frequent. Prednisone, 1 mg/kg/d orally or 2 mg/kg orally as a single morning dose on alternate days for 4–8 weeks, is an adequate trial. Failure to respond indicates that the cause is probably not minimal lesion disease.

Diuresis and diminishing proteinuria are evidence of response to therapy. The dose of prednisone may then be reduced slowly over a period of a month or more. Failure to respond suggests that the cause may be other than minimal disease.

For treatment of patients with membranous glomerular lesions, the alternate-day prednisone program (120 mg on alternate mornings) may be employed for up to 8 weeks.

Focal glomerulosclerosis, mesangiocapillary (membranoproliferative) glomerulonephritis, and proliferative glomerulonephritis do not respond to steroid alone or to steroid plus immunosuppressive therapy. Treatment is solely symptomatic.

Diuretics are often ineffective. The most useful are the loop diuretics, thiazides, chlorthalidone, and others that may be employed in comparable effective dose levels. Spironolactone may be helpful when employed concurrently with other diuretics. Salt-free albumin, dextran, and other oncotic agents are of little help, and their effects are transient.

Caution: Elevation of serum potassium, development of hypertension, and sudden severe increase in edema contraindicate continuation of corticosteroid therapy. Such complications usually arise during the first 2 weeks of continuous therapy.

Immunosuppressive drugs, including alkylating agents, cyclophosphamide, mercaptopurine, azathioprine, and others, are under trial in the treatment of the nephrotic syndrome. The use of corticosteroids plus immunosuppressive agents is similar to that employed in reversing rejection of homotransplants in humans. Encouraging results have been reported in children and adults with membranous lesions and with systemic lupus erythematosus. Those with minimal lesions refractory to corticosteroid therapy did no better when immunosuppressive agents were added. Improvement was shown in the glomerular changes and renal function in many responding well to treatment. The incidence of improvement has not been established.

Serious side effects related both to corticosteroids and to the cytotoxic agents are common. At present, this form of therapy should be employed only by those experienced in treating the nephrotic syndrome in patients who have proved refractory to well-established treatment regimens.

For renal vein thrombosis, the treatment is directed against progress of thrombus formation with heparin and long-term use of coumarin drugs.

Prognosis

The course and prognosis depend upon the basic disease responsible for the nephrotic syndrome. In about half of cases of childhood nephrosis, the disease appears to run a rather benign course when properly treated and to leave insignificant sequelae. Of the others, most go inexorably into the terminal state, with renal insufficiency. Adults with nephrosis fare less well, particularly when the fundamental disease is glomerulonephritis, systemic lupus erythematosus, amyloidosis, or diabetic nephropathy. In those with minimal lesions, remissions, either spontaneous or following corticosteroid therapy, are common. Treatment is more often unsuccessful or only ameliorative when the other glomerular lesions are present. Hypertension and nitrogen retention are serious signs.

Cogan MG: Nephrotic syndrome. *West J Med* 1982;**136**:411.

Glassock RJ et al: Primary glomerular disease. Page 1407 in: *The Kidney,* 2nd ed. Brenner BM, Rector FC (editors). Saunders, 1981.

Harrington JT: Thrombolytic therapy in renal vein thrombosis. (Editorial.) *Arch Intern Med* 1984;**144**:33.

Kaplan BS et al: Glomerular injury in patients with neoplasia. *Annu Rev Med* 1976;**27**:117.

Llach F, Papper S, Massry SG: The clinical spectrum of renal vein thrombosis: Acute and chronic. *Am J Med* 1980;**69**:819.

Wagoner RD et al: Renal vein thrombosis in idiopathic membranous glomerulopathy and nephrotic syndrome: Incidence and significance. *Kidney Int* 1983;**23**:368.

4. IgA NEPHROPATHY
(Idiopathic Benign Hematuria)

The entity of primary hematuria (idiopathic benign and recurrent hematuria, or Berger's disease) is now included among the immune complex glomerulopathies in which deposition of IgA with C3 and fibrin-related antigens occurs in a granular pattern in the mesangium of the glomerulus.

Recurrent macroscopic and microscopic hematuria and mild proteinuria are characteristically the only manifestations of renal disease. Recent prospective studies have shown progression of renal disease, with destruction of glomeruli and loss of renal function, often with hypertension. Exacerbations have been observed with upper respiratory tract disease. Progression is usually slow, extending over 2–3 decades.

Berger's nephropathy has appeared in siblings and identical twins. It has been shown that HLA-DR4 antigen occurs in 49% of patients, an incidence 2.5 times that of the control population.

Diagnosis is made by renal biopsy and demonstration of the mesangial deposits of IgA often accompanied by C3 and by small amounts of IgG. IgA may be deposited in skin capillaries as well. Similar deposits may be seen in Henoch-Schönlein purpura, disseminated lupus erythematosus, eclampsia, membranous glomerulonephritis, acute postinfectious glomerulonephritis, and other rare causes of glomerulopathy. The urine sediment resembles that of any latent glomerulonephritis, with protein, red cells, and casts, including erythrocyte casts. The paucity of clinical manifestations and slow progress may be determining factors in the diagnosis.

No specific treatment has been advocated for this indolent disease.

Baldwin DS: Chronic glomerulonephritis: Nonimmunologic mechanisms of progressive glomerular damage. *Kidney Int* 1982;**21**:109.

Baldwin DS et al: Poststreptococcal glomerulonephritis: A progressive disease? *Am J Med* 1977;**61**:1.

Couser WG: Mesangial IgA nephropathies: Steady progress. *West J Med* 1984;**140**:89.

Couser WG: What are circulating immune complexes doing in glomerulonephritis? *N Engl J Med* 1981;**304**:1230.

Culpepper RM, Andreoli TE: The pathophysiology of the glomerulopathies. *Adv Intern Med* 1983;**28**:161.

Fairley KF, Birch DF: Hematuria: Simple method for identifying glomerular bleeding. *Kidney Int* 1982;**21**:105.

Hood SA et al: IgA-IgG nephropathy: Predictive indices of progressive disease. *Clin Nephrol* 1981;**16**:55.

5. ANTI–GLOMERULAR BASEMENT MEMBRANE NEPHRITIS
(Goodpasture's Syndrome)

The patient usually gives a history of recent hemoptysis and often of malaise, anorexia, and headache. The clinical syndrome is that of severe acute glomerulonephritis accompanied by diffuse hemorrhagic inflammation of the lungs. The urine shows gross or microscopic hematuria, and laboratory findings of severely suppressed renal function are usually evident. Biopsy shows glomerular crescents, glomerular adhesions, and inflammatory infiltration interstitially. Electron microscopic examination shows an increase in basement membrane material and deposition of fibrin beneath the capillary endothelium. In some cases, circulating antibody against glomerular basement membrane can be identified. IgG and C3 complement can be demonstrated as linear deposits on the basement membranes of the glomeruli and the lung. Anti-glomerular basement membrane antibody also reacts with lung basement membrane.

Only rare cases of survival have been documented. Large doses of corticosteroids in combination with immunosuppressive agents are indicated. In addition, plasmapheresis may be employed to remove circulating antibody. Hemodialysis and nephrectomy with renal transplantation may offer the only hope for rescue. Transplantation should be delayed until circulating antiglomerular antibodies have disappeared.

Occasionally, acute renal disease with a similar clinical and immunologic pattern may occur without associated lung disease. (See next section.)

6. RAPIDLY PROGRESSIVE GLOMERULONEPHRITIS

Rapid deterioration of renal function in the course of a few weeks to a few months is characteristic of fulminant anti-glomerular basement membrane glomerulonephritis. Other glomerular disorders that can follow the same clinical course include poststreptococcal glomerulonephritis, mesangiocapillary (membranoproliferative) glomerulonephritis, Wegener's granulomatosis, systemic lupus erythematosus, polyarteritis, Henoch-Schönlein purpura, mixed cryoglobulinemia, and ventriculovenous shunt nephritis. Scleroderma may produce a similar picture.

Oliguria, hematuria and proteinuria, and mild hypertension may be the only signs. Abdominal pain and nausea and vomiting may be prominent.

Exuberant proliferation of epithelial cells of Bowman's capsule with crescent formation is the main feature of renal biopsy. Immunofluorescent stains show either fine linear deposits of IgG and segmental deposits of C3 related to anti-glomerular basement membrane antibody or granular deposits of IgG and IgM accompanied by C3 related to immune complex disease.

Treatment with corticosteroids and immunosuppressive drugs has not been successful. Plasmapheresis may be helpful. Dialysis and transplantation may be necessary.

Spontaneous recovery is rare. Progression of renal failure is the rule.

Briggs WA et al: Antiglomerular basement membrane antibody-mediated glomerulonephritis and Goodpasture's syndrome. *Medicine* 1979;**58**:348.

Lockwood CM, Peters DK: Plasma exchange in glomerulonephritis and related vasculitides. *Annu Rev Med* 1980;**31**:167.

Myers TJ et al: Thrombotic thrombocytopenic purpura: Combined treatment with plasmapheresis and anti-platelet agents. *Ann Intern Med* 1980;**92**:149.

Oredugba O et al: Pulse methylprednisolone therapy in idiopathic rapidly progressive glomerulonephritis. *Ann Intern Med* 1980;**92**:504.

Ridolfi RL, Bell WR: Thrombotic thrombocytopenic purpura: Report of 25 cases and review of the literature. *Medicine* 1981;**60**:413.

CHRONIC RENAL INSUFFICIENCY

Essentials of Diagnosis

- Weakness and easy fatigability, headaches, anorexia, nausea and vomiting, pruritus, polyuria, nocturia.

- Hypertension with secondary encephalopathy, retinal damage, heart failure.
- Anemia, azotemia, and acidosis, with elevated serum potassium, phosphate, and sulfate and decreased serum calcium and protein.
- Urine specific gravity low and fixed; mild to moderate proteinuria; few red cells, white cells, and broad renal failure casts.

General Considerations

Chronic renal insufficiency may be a consequence of a variety of diseases involving the kidney parenchyma or obstruction of the excretory tract. Causes of chronic renal failure include the following:

1. Primary glomerular disease (immune complex glomerulonephritis)
2. Renal vascular disease
3. Chronic pyelonephritis
4. Metabolic diseases with renal involvement
5. Nephrotoxins
6. Infection
7. Chronic radiation nephritis
8. Tubular disease
9. Chronic obstructive uropathy
10. Congenital anomalies of both kidneys
11. Nephropathy of particular geographic distribution

The pathologic picture varies with the cause of the damage to the kidney. Extensive scarring with decrease in kidney size, hyalinization of glomeruli, and obliteration of some tubules and hypertrophy and dilatation of others produce great distortion of renal architecture. The vascular changes are due to the effects of scar formation and of prolonged hypertension, with thickening of the media, fragmentation of elastic fibers, intimal thickening, and obliteration of the lumens in some areas. In diabetic nephropathy, the typical glomerular lesions of intercapillary sclerosis are often distinct. The vascular lesions of periarteritis or of systemic lupus erythematosus often serve to establish these diagnoses. Obstructive uropathy presents the classic picture of hydronephrosis with compression and destruction of the renal parenchyma. Polycystic disease, multiple myeloma, amyloid disease, persistent hypercalcemia, and other causes of renal failure usually can be identified by characteristic lesions.

Pathophysiology of Uremia

The clinical findings of the uremic syndrome result from loss of nephrons and decreased renal blood flow and glomerular filtration.

With the loss of nephrons, the burden of solute excretion falls on fewer functional units, with subsequent impaired ability of the kidney to maintain body water, osmolality of body fluids, and electrolyte and acid-base balance. The consequences of nephron loss are, briefly, as follows.

A. Water: Increased solute load per nephron produces an osmotic diuresis with associated impaired ability to excrete concentrated or dilute urine. Dehydration is common and hazardous; water intoxication may occur if fluid intake is excessive.

B. Electrolyte:

1. Both excretion and conservation of electrolyte are inadequate. Reduced filtration and excretion of phosphate, sulfate, and organic acid end products of metabolism result in increased concentration of these anions in body fluids, with displacement of bicarbonate. Furthermore, decreased ability to produce H^+ and NH_4^+ for excretion with anion in the urine contributes to acidosis.

2. Sodium loss due to the impaired reabsorption that accompanies osmotic diuresis contributes to a decrease in extracellular fluid volume. With reduction of plasma volume, renal perfusion declines, with exacerbation of renal failure. Since the kidney cannot respond appropriately, a sudden increase in sodium intake cannot be excreted readily, and edema will usually ensue.

3. Potassium regulation is usually not impaired until oliguria is severe or acidosis becomes prominent. Hyperkalemia is a sign of severe insufficiency.

4. Calcium and phosphate metabolism is seriously disturbed as a consequence of reduction of glomerular filtration and tubule function, impairment of 1-hydroxylation of the vitamin D metabolite 25-hydroxy D_3 to 1,25-dihydroxy D_3, and reduced effect of parathyroid hormone on the skeleton. The ensuing hyperphosphatemia and hypocalcemia elicit the development of secondary hyperparathyroidism. The combination of hyperparathyroidism and impaired vitamin D metabolism results in bone disease (renal osteodystrophy) characterized by osteitis fibrosa, osteomalacia, osteoporosis, osteosclerosis, and, in children, impaired growth. Calcification in soft tissue may occur. Rarely, parathyroid secretion cannot be influenced by therapy, a condition termed tertiary hyperparathyroidism. Pertinent laboratory findings include hyperphosphatemia, hypocalcemia (even when corrected for hypoalbuminemia), hypermagnesemia, and elevated parathyroid hormone levels.

C. Nitrogen Retention: High urea, creatinine, and urate levels are manifestations of reduced clearance. Urea load is related to protein metabolism, while creatinine is related to muscle mass and is independent of protein intake.

D. Anemia: Depression of red cell production probably results from reduced secretion of erythropoietin by the kidney. Survival time of red cells is shorter than normal. Size and hemoglobin content of red cells are usually normal.

E. Hypertension: With renal ischemia and increasing destruction of the renal parenchyma, hypertension becomes evident. The consequences of increasing hypertension include cardiovascular damage and further deterioration of the kidney. The coincidence of malignant hypertension and uremia is particularly ominous.

Clinical Findings

A. Symptoms and Signs: Progressive weakness

and lethargy are often prominent. (Easy fatigability and shortness of breath may limit activity.) Thirst, weight loss, anorexia, gastrointestinal irritability, diarrhea, hiccup, and itching are common complaints. Occasionally, a persistent bad or metallic taste annoys the patient. Symptoms of nervous system involvement include paresthesias and burning sensations associated with peripheral neuropathy, myoclonic jerking, and seizures. Headache, visual difficulties, and symptoms of left heart failure result from hypertension. Cerebral hemorrhage, pulmonary edema, and frank heart failure are usually late occurrences. Purpura and bleeding from the nose and gastrointestinal tract may be severe. Bone pain and, in children, retarded growth reflect osteodystrophy.

The history should include a review of familial disease and questions regarding previous renal disease, drug ingestion, and symptoms of lower urinary tract obstruction.

Physical examination of the patient reveals pallor, hyperpnea, uremic breath, dehydration, excoriated skin, and purpura. Hypertension with retinopathy is usually present. Cardiac enlargement, pulmonary edema, and pericarditis may be evident. Evidence of peripheral neuropathy should be sought. Bone deformity and awkwardness of gait are evidence of osteodystrophy.

B. Laboratory Findings: Anemia, azotemia, and acidosis are the principal findings. The anemia is usually normochromic and normocytic, with hemoglobin in the range of 6–9 g/dL. The urine is usually dilute and contains small amounts of protein; few red, white, and epithelial cells; and a few granular and waxy casts, some of which are large (broad renal failure casts). Blood urea nitrogen, serum creatinine, and often serum uric acid concentrations are greatly elevated. Serum sodium may be slightly lower than normal and serum potassium slightly to markedly elevated; serum calcium is decreased; with bone disease, alkaline phosphatase activity in the serum is increased, and circulating parathyroid hormone is often elevated. Serum magnesium may be elevated. With retention of phosphate, sulfate, and, frequently, chloride, plasma bicarbonate concentration is decreased. (Phosphate and sulfate participate in the "anion gap" of uremia.) Both retention of organic acids and impaired tubular secretion of hydrogen ion plus loss of sodium and bicarbonate buffer are accompanied by a decrease in plasma pH. Chest x-ray may show evidence of cardiac enlargement, midzone interstitial edema of the lung, frank pulmonary congestion, or pulmonary edema. The ECG reflects left ventricular strain or hypertrophy and changes due to potassium toxicity. The size of the kidneys should be determined by ultrasonography, plain x-ray films, or tomograms of the abdomen. Intravenous or retrograde urography or selected radionuclide studies may be indicated to rule out obstruction of the lower urinary tract or ureters. Radiologic evidence of bone disease (osteomalacia and osteitis fibrosa) is common long before overt symptoms and clinical signs appear.

Differential Diagnosis

Chronic renal insufficiency presents symptoms and signs related to the functional disability resulting from a reduction in the number of functioning nephrons rather than to the cause of the renal damage. It is often impossible to distinguish between renal insufficiency due to chronic glomerulonephritis, pyelonephritis, malignant hypertension, diabetic nephropathy, and collagen disease. The presence of large kidneys characteristic of polycystic disease should serve to identify this cause of renal failure. The physician must identify remediable causes of renal insufficiency such as obstruction, infection, persistent hypercalcemia, gout, myeloma, and drug toxicity.

Treatment

Hypertension or heart failure should be treated as indicated with agents that sustain renal function and coronary artery blood flow (see below).

A. Diet and Fluids: Limitation of protein of high biologic value to 0.5 g/kg/d helps to reduce azotemia, acidosis, and hyperkalemia. Trials of mixtures of essential amino acids or of amino acid precursors such as α-keto and α-hydroxy acid analogs are promising approaches to protein replacement.

The diet should include adequate calories and a multivitamin product plus folic acid, 1 mg daily, particularly when protein is severely restricted. Sodium need not be restricted. Fluid intake should be sufficient to maintain an adequate urine volume, but no attempt should be made to force diuresis. Obligatory water loss may be quite high because of the large solute load (eg, sodium and urea) that must be excreted by a reduced number of nephrons. Intake of up to 2–3 L may be required when creatinine clearance is reduced to 10–20 mL/min. With decreasing clearance, urine volume decreases. Intake must be sufficient to maintain renal function without causing excessive diuresis or water retention. If edema is present, a cautious trial of furosemide or ethacrynic acid is indicated, with careful monitoring of serum electrolytes. *Caution:* Water restriction for laboratory examination, tests of renal function, or any other reason is hazardous.

B. Electrolyte Replacement:

1. Sodium supplements may be required to restore sodium losses resulting from failure of the kidney to provide NH_4^+ and H^+ for sodium conservation. A mixture of NaCl and $NaHCO_3$ in equal parts, 1–2 g 2–3 times daily with meals, may be required in addition to dietary sources. Weight loss and a decreasing urine volume indicate a need for additional sodium; hypertension and edema are signs that a trial of sodium restriction is in order.

2. Potassium intake may have to be restricted or supplemented. In severe hyperkalemia, active measures to remove potassium may be required (see discussion in Chapter 3). Measurement of the serum potassium concentration will provide indications.

3. Serum phosphate levels may be lowered and secondary hyperparathyroidism ameliorated by reducing absorption of phosphate in the gastrointestinal tract

with administration of aluminum hydroxide gel, 30 mL, or (as tablets) 4–5 g 3–4 times daily.

4. Calcium lactate, 4 g 2–3 times daily, may be given to relieve hypocalcemic tetany. Intravenous administration of calcium gluconate may be required at times.

C. Bone Disease (Renal Osteodystrophy): In the presence of bone disease, phosphate binders and supplemental calcium are employed as above. In addition, vitamin D_3 (cholecalciferol) or, more effectively, its metabolites 25-hydroxy D_3, 1α-hydroxy D_3, and 1,25-dihydroxy D_3 (calcitriol) are useful in correcting osteomalacia and osteitis fibrosa, with some amelioration of myopathy. *Caution:* Close observation is mandatory to prevent hypercalcemia and soft tissue calcification, which may ensue if dosage is too great. Thorough knowledge of indications and hazards must be obtained before using these potent cholecalciferols.

Parathyroidectomy may be required if "tertiary" hyperparathyroidism is present.

D. Anemia: Iron is of little value unless iron deficit exists. Determination of serum ferritin is a reliable test to prove iron deficit. With evidence that transfusion is responsible for improved acceptance of renal allografts, there should be no hesitation in giving blood transfusions to patients whose anemia is symptomatic or if the hematocrit falls to the low 20s. Prolonged bleeding time and difficulty with hemostasis can be corrected transiently with cryoprecipitate. Desmopressin acetate (1-d-amino-8-D-arginine vasopressin; DDAVP), 0.3 μg/kg body weight diluted in 50–100 mL of saline solution, may be infused intravenously over 30 minutes to shorten the bleeding time for about 4 hours. DDAVP is sometimes used to prevent bleeding during minor surgical procedures.

E. General Measures: Nausea and vomiting may be alleviated with chlorpromazine, 15–25 mg orally or 10–20 mg intramuscularly (or equivalent amounts of related compounds). The barbiturate drugs may be used for sedation as required.

Hypertension is a common manifestation of uremia. An expanded extracellular fluid volume is often responsible for hypertension, and the circumstances can be ameliorated by reduction of extracellular fluid volume by hemodialysis. Some cases of hypertension are due to elevated concentrations of renin in peripheral blood. Combinations of hydralazine and propranolol may be effective; methyldopa is useful in patients on hemodialysis; minoxidil, metoprolol, clonidine, and prazosin are useful drugs. Angiotensin-converting enzyme inhibitors may be helpful. Bilateral nephrectomy may be necessary to rescue the patient from persistent hypertension. (See references for details of management of hypertension in the presence of renal failure.)

F. Approach to Drug Therapy: Because the half-life of many drugs is prolonged in patients with renal failure, the physician must monitor the effects of drugs closely. The dosage of drugs must often be reduced and guided by blood levels (see references).

G. Chronic Dialysis and Kidney Transplants: These approaches to the treatment of renal insufficiency due to any cause have been under investigation for many years, and encouraging experience has prompted expansion of facilities for scheduled, repeated extracorporeal dialysis. The growing success of renal transplantation holds promise for extending the lives of patients with chronic renal disease.

Amelioration of complications such as neuropathy, hyperparathyroidism, and anemia can be frequently achieved by dialysis or transplantation.

1. Simplified mechanisms for dialysis with the artificial kidney and ingenious cannulas and arteriovenous fistulas permit periodic dialysis with a minimum of professional supervision in hospital centers and in the patient's home. Patients with creatinine clearances of 0–2 mL/min have been kept alive for 6–10 years in reasonable health and activity by dialysis once or twice a week. The criteria for selection of patients are now clear. Centers have been established for the treatment of chronic renal insufficiency, and home units are generally available, although considerable skill is required to operate the devices. A recent survey indicates a 1-year survival rate on dialysis of 87%, a 2-year survival rate of 73%, and, in the 20- to 45-year age group, a 6-year survival rate of 60%.

Peritoneal dialysis can be used for temporary or long-term therapy. Chronic ambulatory peritoneal dialysis provides less effective clearance of small molecules (urea, creatinine) than does hemodialysis, but clearance is adequate to relieve symptoms of uremia and to accomplish excellent treatment. One to 2 L of dialysate modified to meet the needs of the patient can be exchanged 3–5 times daily. With good technique, the risk of peritonitis is reduced; its occurrence can usually be treated successfully with appropriate antibiotics.

Hemofiltration, a variant of dialysis in which a highly permeable membrane is employed, may prove a useful alternative to conventional dialysis.

2. Transplantation of kidneys from one human to another has been technically feasible for many years. Survival of such grafts has been limited by rejection of the foreign organ by the recipient except when donor and recipient were identical twins. Blood typing and leukocyte typing for histocompatibility antigens have improved the matching of donor and recipient, with an encouraging decrease in the rejection rate. The enhanced survival of cadaver renal grafts in patients who have had 5 or more blood transfusions compared to those who have had none is clear (1-year graft survival > 60% versus 42%). The utility of employing blood transfusion in anticipation of renal transplantation is under study. Further experience with immunosuppressive drugs (azathioprine or cyclophosphamide) and adrenal corticosteroids has improved protection of the homologous transplant from rejection for extended periods. The use of antilymphocytic globulin (ALG) or cyclosporin-A (or both) to suppress immunity has been impressively effective, but evaluation requires more experience. Survival data since January 1970 are much improved over prior experience. When the donor is a

parent or an HLA-matched sibling, recipient survival with the first transplant still functional at 2 years is 80% or greater and at 3 years 70%. When the transplant is a cadaver kidney, recipient survival with the first transplant still functional at 1 year is about 50% and at 3 years 42%. The selection of cadaver kidneys compatible by HLA type and other criteria should improve graft survival.

Adequate dialysis. (Editorial.) *Lancet* 1982;**1**:147.

Anderson RJ, Schrier RW: *Clinical Uses of Drugs in Patients With Kidney and Liver Disease.* Saunders, 1981.

Anemia of chronic renal failure. (Editorial.) *Lancet* 1983;**1**:965.

Bennett WM et al: Drug prescribing in renal failure: Dosing guidelines for adults. *Am J Kidney Dis* 1983;**3**:155.

Brenner BM, Meyer TW, Hostetter TH: Dietary protein intake and the progressive nature of kidney disease. *N Engl J Med* 1982;**307**:652.

Brenner B, Stein J (editors): *Chronic Renal Failure.* Vol 7 of: *Contemporary Issues in Nephrology.* Churchill Livingstone, 1981.

Carpenter CB, Strom TB: Transplantation: Immunogenetic and clinical aspects. (Part 1.) *Hosp Pract* (Dec) 1982;**17**:125.

Carvalho A: Bleeding in uremia: A clinical challenge. (Editorial.) *N Engl J Med* 1983;**308**:38.

Friedman EA: Diabetic nephropathy: Strategies in prevention and management. *Kidney Int* 1982;**21**:780.

Kurtzman NA: Chronic renal failure: Metabolic and clinical consequences. *Hosp Pract* (Aug) 1982;**17**:107.

Lacke C et al: Twelve months' experience with continuous ambulatory and intermittent peritoneal dialysis. *Arch Intern Med* 1981;**141**:187.

Levey AS, Harrington JT: Continuous peritoneal dialysis for chronic renal failure. *Medicine* 1982;**61**:330.

Mannucci PM et al: Deamino-8-D-arginine vasopressin shortens the bleeding time in uremia. *N Engl J Med* 1983;**308**:8.

Mooradian AD, Morley JE: Endocrine dysfunction in chronic renal failure. *Arch Intern Med* 1984;**144**:351.

Opelz G et al: Introduction of high kidney graft survival rate by multiple transfusion. *Lancet* 1981;**1**:1223.

Proceedings of a conference on advances in renal transplantation, Bologna, October 11, 1982. *Kidney Int* 1983;**23(Suppl 14).**

Raskin NH, Fishman RA: Neurologic disorders in renal failure. (2 parts.) *N Engl J Med* 1976;**294**:143, 204.

Rosanski SJ, Sugimoto T: An analysis of the United States renal transplant patient population and organ survival characteristics: 1977 to 1980. *Kidney Int* 1982;**22**:685.

Strom TB: The improving utility of renal transplantation in the management of end-stage renal disease. *Am J Med* 1982; **73**:105.

Strom TB, Carpenter CB: Transplantation: Immunogenetic and clinical aspects. (Part 2.) *Hosp Pract* (Jan) 1983;**18**:135.

Symposium on continuous ambulatory peritoneal dialysis. *Kidney Int* 1983;**23**:2. [Entire issue.]

Walser M: Nutritional support in renal failure: Future directions. *Lancet* 1983;**1**:340.

HEMOLYTIC-UREMIC SYNDROME

This syndrome, though still uncommon, is being recognized with increasing frequency. Many features are similar to thrombotic thrombocytopenic purpura. The essential features include renal microangiopathy (with decreased glomerular filtration, proteinuria, and hematuria), microangiopathic hemolytic anemia, and thrombocytopenia. Endothelial damage involves renal arterioles and glomerular capillaries, with rare extension to other organs. Ischemic necrosis in the renal cortex may occur with obstruction from intravascular coagulation. Acute renal insufficiency is the major threat to life.

Two types of the syndrome have been described. Sporadic cases may be idiopathic or secondary to infections with *Shigella, Salmonella*, or viral agents. This form is more common in children, and the mortality rate is low (under 5%). The syndrome may occur in pregnant women, in women taking oral contraceptives, or as a complication of malignant hypertension or renal transplantation.

A familial, or hereditary, type has been identified in which members of a family may have recurrent episodes over several years. The mortality rate is 30%.

Initial treatment is the conservative management of acute renal failure. Persistent thrombocytopenia and microangiopathic hemolytic anemia and worsening renal disease with serious hypertension are indications for more radical treatment as for thrombotic thrombocytopenic purpura. Heparin, antiplatelet drugs (dipyridamole, aspirin), and corticosteroids (prednisone) have been employed with some success. Plasmapheresis, prednisone, antiplatelet agents, and vincristine have been employed in desperate cases.

The disease in adults has a high mortality rate. Relapses are common. Chronic renal failure is a frequent outcome.

Campos A et al: The hemolytic-uremic syndrome. *The Kidney* 1981;**14**:23.

Ponticelli C et al: Hemolytic uremic syndrome in adults. *Arch Intern Med* 1980;**140**:353.

Shumak KH, Rock GA: Therapeutic plasma exchange. *N Engl J Med* 1984;**310**:762.

ARTERIOLAR NEPHROSCLEROSIS

Intimal thickening of the afferent arteriole of the glomerulus is characteristic. Obliteration of the arteriole or severe narrowing of the lumen deprives the nephron of its blood supply and produces areas of infarction and scar formation. Obliteration of glomeruli is common. If the disease is "malignant" and rapidly progressive, points of hemorrhage are found, and vascular changes, resembling endarteritis with severe intimal thickening associated with malignant hypertension, become marked. Renal insufficiency occurs when the kidney is scarred and contracted.

The symptoms and signs are those of hypertension and renal insufficiency and, occasionally, heart failure and hypertensive encephalopathy.

Treatment is directed against hypertension and chronic renal insufficiency.

The course is progressively downhill. The patient usually succumbs to renal failure, and death is sometimes hastened by intercurrent infection.

DISEASES OF THE RENAL TUBULES & INTERSTITIUM

1. DISORDERS OF PROSTAGLANDIN SYNTHESIS

The roles of prostaglandins PGE_2, $PGF_{2\alpha}$, PGI_2 (prostacyclin), and of TxA_2 (thromboxane), all of which have been isolated from the kidney, are only partially understood. There is evidence that prostaglandin biosynthesis is influenced by bradykinin, angiotensin II, catecholamines, glucocorticoids, and nonsteroidal anti-inflammatory drugs. Prostaglandins modify salt and water excretion by their influence on glomerular filtration rate, proximal tubule fluid reabsorption, gradients in concentration of medullary solute, and reabsorption of water and electrolyte in the distal nephron. Prostaglandins mediate release of renin in response to depletion of intravascular volume. Altered prostaglandin metabolism is seen with hypertension, obstructive uropathy, Bartter's syndrome, and disorders of water reabsorption. Nonsteroidal analgesics can produce acute renal failure, nephrotic syndrome, and interstitial nephritis, all of which may be in part the result of inhibition of prostaglandin synthesis.

Levenson DJ, Simmons CE Jr, Brenner BM: Arachidonic acid metabolism, prostaglandins and the kidney. *Am J Med* 1982;**72:**354.

2. ACUTE RENAL FAILURE

Essentials of Diagnosis

- Sudden onset of oliguria; urine volume 20–200 mL/d. (Oliguria may not occur.)
- Proteinuria and hematuria; isosthenuria with a specific gravity of 1.010–1.016.
- Anorexia, nausea and vomiting, lethargy, elevation of blood pressure. Signs of uremia.
- Progressive increase in serum urea nitrogen, creatinine, potassium, phosphate, sulfate; decrease in sodium, calcium, bicarbonate.
- Spontaneous recovery in a few days to 6 weeks.

General Considerations

Acute renal failure is a term applied to a state of sudden cessation of renal function following a variety of insults to normal kidneys. Emphasis has recently been placed on vasomotor constriction of afferent arterioles as the initial lesion—hence the term vasomotor nephropathy. Among the causes of acute renal failure are the following: (1) Toxic agents, eg, carbon tetrachloride, methoxyflurane, sulfonamides, aminoglycoside antibiotics, amphotericin B, mercury bichloride, arsenic, diethylene glycol, and mushroom poisoning. X-ray contrast materials are hazardous in patients with dehydration, renal disease, diabetic nephropathy, liver failure, or multiple myeloma. (2) Traumatic shock due to severe injury, surgical shock,

or myocardial infarction, and ischemia associated with surgery on the abdominal aorta (vasomotor nephropathy). (3) Tissue destruction due to crushing injury, rhabdomyolysis, burns, intravascular hemolysis (transurethral resection of the prostate, incompatible blood transfusion). (4) Infectious diseases, eg, leptospirosis, hemorrhagic fever, gram-negative bacteremia with shock, toxic shock syndrome, peritonitis. (5) Disseminated intravascular coagulation. (6) Complications of pregnancy, eg, bilateral cortical necrosis. (7) Immunologic mechanisms induced by methicillin, penicillin, phenytoin, and other drugs.

Return of renal function can be expected, but even with the best treatment the mortality rate is high.

Renal tubular necrosis is the characteristic finding. In some instances, after exposure to a specific toxin, the proximal tubule may be primarily damaged; and renal tubule cell disintegration and desquamation with collection of debris in the lumens of the tubules are found uniformly throughout both kidneys. In other cases, tubule cell destruction and basement membrane disruption are scattered throughout both kidneys. In cases due to hemolysis or crushing injury, heme or myoglobin casts may be present, but it is unlikely that such casts produce tubule cell destruction. The spotty distribution of the damage caused by ischemic necrosis is consistent with a great reduction in cortical blood flow in addition to a moderate to marked decrease in total renal blood flow. In bilateral cortical necrosis, ischemic infarcts are distributed throughout both kidneys.

Clinical Findings

The history is critical in identification of the cause. The cardinal sign of acute renal failure is acute reduction of urine output following injury, surgery, a transfusion reaction, or other causes listed above. The daily volume of urine may be reduced to 20–30 mL/d or may be as high as 400–500 mL/d. In some cases, urine volume may always be greater than 600 mL/d. After a few days to 6 weeks of oliguria, the daily urine volume slowly increases. Anorexia, nausea, and lethargy are common symptoms. Other symptoms and signs are related to the causative agent or event.

The course of the disease may be divided into the oliguric and diuretic phases.

A. Oliguric Phase: During the oliguric phase, the urine excretion is greatly reduced. The urine contains protein, red cells, epithelial cells, and characteristic "dirty" brown granular casts; and the specific gravity of the urine is usually 1.010–1.016. The rate of catabolism of protein determines the rate of increase of metabolic end products in body fluids. In the presence of injury, rhabdomyolysis, or fever, the blood urea nitrogen and the serum creatinine, potassium, phosphate, sulfate, and organic acids increase rapidly. Typically, because of dilution and intracellular shifts, the serum sodium concentration drops to 120–130 meq/L. As organic acids and phosphate accumulate, serum bicarbonate concentration decreases. Normochromic anemia is common. With prolonged oliguria, signs of uremia appear, with nausea, vomiting, diarrhea, neuromuscular irritability, convulsions, somnolence, and coma. Hypertension frequently develops and may be associated with retinopathy, left heart failure, and encephalopathy. During this phase of the disease, therapy modifies the clinical picture significantly. Overhydration produces signs of water intoxication, with convulsions, edema, and the serious complication of pulmonary edema. Excess saline administration may produce edema and congestive failure. Failure to restrict potassium intake or to employ agents to remove potassium at the proper time may result in hyperkalemia manifested by neuromuscular depression that progresses to paralysis and interference with the cardiac conduction system, resulting in arrhythmias; death may follow respiratory muscle paralysis or cardiac arrest (see p 36). With proper treatment, potassium intoxication is almost always reversible, and death should seldom occur because of it.

B. Diuretic Phase: After a few days to 6 weeks of oliguria, the diuretic phase begins, signifying that the nephrons have recovered to the point that urine excretion is possible. The urine volume usually increases in increments of a few mL to 100 mL/d until 300–500 mL/d are excreted, after which the rate of increase in flow is usually more rapid. Rarely, the urine volume increases rapidly during the first day or so of diuresis. Diuresis may be the result of impaired nephron function, with loss of water and electrolytes; but this is uncommon, and true deficits of water, sodium, and potassium seldom occur. More often, diuresis represents an unloading of excess extracellular fluid that has accumulated during the oliguric phase as a result of either overhydration during therapy or unusual metabolic production of water. Diuresis usually occurs when the total nephron function is still insufficient to excrete nitrogenous metabolic products, potassium, and phosphate, and the concentration of these constituents in the serum may continue to rise for several days after urine volumes exceed 1 L/d. Renal function returns slowly toward normal, and blood chemical findings usually become normal.

Differential Diagnosis

Because acute glomerulonephritis, collagen disease, acute interstitial nephritis, uric acid nephropathy, myeloma, hepatorenal syndrome, Reye's syndrome, ureteral obstruction due to edema at the ureterovesical junction following ureteral catheterization, ureteral obstruction by neoplasm, bilateral renal artery occlusion due to embolism or dissecting aneurysm, and, rarely, a ruptured bladder may present with symptoms and signs indistinguishable from those of tubular necrosis, appropriate diagnostic procedures (ultrasound examination of kidneys and bladder, x-ray of abdomen, etc) should be employed as suggested by the history and by physical examination. Functional or prerenal azotemia consequent to shock, severe volume depletion, congestive heart failure, pressor agents, or diuretics must be distinguished to assure appropriate immediate therapy.

Table 16–2. Acute renal failure versus prerenal azotemia.

	Acute Renal Failure	Prerenal Azotemia
Urine osmolality (mosm/L)	< 350	> 500
Urine/plasma urea	< 10	> 20
Urine/plasma creatinine	< 20	> 40
Urine Na (meq/L)	> 40	< 20
Renal failure index = $\dfrac{U_{Na}}{U/P_{Cr}}$	> 1	< 1
*$F_{E_{Na}} = \dfrac{U/P_{Na}}{U/P_{Cr}} \times 100$	> 1	< 1

*Excreted fraction of filtered sodium. See Espinel CH: The FENa test: Use in the differential diagnosis of acute renal failure. *JAMA* 1976;**236**:579; and Miller TR et al: Urinary diagnostic indices in acute renal failure: A prospective study. *Ann Intern Med* 1978;**89**:47.

In the differentiation between acute renal failure and prerenal azotemia, the ability to excrete creatinine and urea and to conserve sodium are useful criteria (Table 16–2).

The loss of normal capacity to excrete creatinine and to conserve sodium indicates acute renal failure. The clinical setting must be carefully assessed, for in chronic renal insufficiency the ability to conserve sodium is lost, and after administration of diuretics sodium excretion is elevated.

Treatment

A. Specific Measures: Immediate treatment of the cause of oliguria is essential.

1. Decreased renal perfusion–Diminished circulating blood volume resulting in decreased renal perfusion (prerenal failure) can be ruled out by infusion of 500–1000 mL of 0.9% NaCl solution and use of a loop diuretic. Treatment in the very early period of acute renal shutdown with furosemide, 20–120 mg intravenously, or with rapid intravenous administration of mannitol, 25 g as a 20% solution, may prevent or reduce tubular necrosis.

2. Shock–Vigorous measures to restore normal blood pressure levels are mandatory in order to overcome renal ischemia. *Caution:* When it is apparent that tubular necrosis has occurred, fluid volume must be sharply curtailed; if vasopressor drugs are needed, they must be given in the limited amount of fluid permitted.

3. Transfusion reaction–See Chapter 10.

4. Obstruction of ureters–Cystoscopy and catheterization of ureters may be necessary.

5. Heavy metal poisoning–Dimercaprol (BAL) may be of use in mercury or arsenic poisoning, although by the time the renal lesion is apparent it may be too late.

B. General Measures: Conservative medical management often serves adequately for the uncomplicated case. Indications for dialysis include rapidly increasing blood urea nitrogen, serum creatinine, and potassium, and metabolic acidosis often consequent to severe trauma or infection. Overhydration, usually from too vigorous treatment with intravenous solutions, and oliguria lasting 4–5 days are also indications for dialysis. Hemodialysis is more effective, but peritoneal dialysis may be adequate. Aggressive supportive therapy (combating infection, use of hyperalimentation, etc) should accompany treatment by dialysis.

1. Oliguric phase–The objectives of therapy are to maintain normal body fluid volume and electrolyte concentration, reduce tissue catabolism to a minimum, and prevent infection until healing occurs.

a. Bed rest–"Reverse isolation" to protect the patient from exposure to hospital infections.

b. Fluids–Restrict fluids to a basic ration of 400 mL/d for the average adult. Additional fluid may be given to replace unusual losses due to vomiting, diarrhea, sweating, etc. The metabolism of fat, carbohydrate, and protein provides water of combustion; and catabolism of tissues provides intracellular water. These sources must be included in calculations of water balance, thus leaving only a small ration to be provided as "intake" (see ¶ e, below).

c. Diet–In order to limit sources of nitrogen, potassium, phosphate, and sulfate, no protein should be given. Glucose, 100–200 g/d, should be given to prevent ketosis and to reduce protein catabolism. Although fat may be given as butter or emulsion orally or intravenously, it is usually better if the patient fulfills caloric needs from existing fat deposits.

The fluid and glucose may be given orally or intravenously. When administered intravenously as a 20–50% glucose solution, the 400 mL of fluid should be given continuously throughout the 24-hour period through an intravenous catheter threaded into a large vein to reduce the likelihood of thrombosis. Vitamin B complex and vitamin C should be provided.

For patients on dialysis, parenteral hyperalimentation with a mixture of essential amino acids and nonessential amino acids (particularly those partially synthesized in the kidney) supplemented by glucose and lipid for calories prevents excessive catabolism of tissue and enhances recovery.

d. Electrolyte replacement–Replace preexisting deficits. Otherwise, electrolyte therapy is not necessary unless clear-cut losses are demonstrable, as in vomiting, diarrhea, etc. *Note:* Potassium must not be administered unless proved deficits exist, and then only with caution.

e. Observations–Daily records of fluid intake and output are essential; avoid an indwelling catheter if at all possible. Weight should be recorded daily whenever possible. Because the patient's own tissues are being consumed, weight loss should be about 0.5 kg/d. If weight loss does not occur, too much fluid is being given. Frequent (often daily) measurements of serum electrolytes (especially potassium) and creatinine are essential. The ECG may be helpful in evaluating potassium levels.

f. Infection–Treat vigorously with appropriate antibiotics in doses commensurate with renal failure.

g. Congestive heart failure–See discussion in Chapter 8.

h. Anemia–A hematocrit of less than 30% is an indication for cautious transfusion with a small volume of packed fresh red blood cells.

i. Potassium intoxication–See discussion in Chapter 3.

j. Uremia–Hemodialysis and peritoneal dialysis are effective, but they require expert management in a well-equipped hospital. With appropriate facilities, dialysis has proved to be of great value if employed "prophylactically" before serum creatinine reaches 7–8 mg/dL.

k. Convulsions and encephalopathy–Give paraldehyde rectally. Barbiturates should be restricted to pentobarbital sodium or amobarbital sodium, which are metabolized by the liver. Chlorpromazine and promazine are also effective. Dialysis is useful.

2. Diuretic phase–Unless water and electrolyte deficits clearly exist, no attempt should be made to "keep up" with the diuresis; collections of excess water and electrolyte are usually being excreted. Fluid and diet intake can be liberalized as diuresis progresses until a normal daily intake is reached. Protein restriction should be continued until blood urea nitrogen and serum creatinine levels are declining. Infection is still a hazard. Diuresis is occasionally accompanied by sodium retention, hypernatremia, and hyperchloremia associated with confusion, neuromuscular irritability, and coma. When this happens, water and glucose must be given in sufficient quantities to correct hypernatremia. Serum electrolytes and blood urea nitrogen or serum creatinine should be measured frequently.

Prognosis

If severe complications of trauma and infection are not present, skillful treatment often will tide the patient over the period of oliguria until spontaneous healing occurs. Death may occur as a result of water intoxication, congestive heart failure, acute pulmonary edema, potassium intoxication, and encephalopathy. With recovery, there often is little residual impairment of renal function.

Brenner BM, Lazarus JM (editors): *Acute Renal Failure.* Saunders, 1983.

Miller TR et al: Urinary diagnostic indices in acute renal failure: A prospective study. *Ann Intern Med* 1978;**89**:47.

Oken DE: On the differential diagnosis of acute renal failure. *Am J Med* 1981;**71**:916.

Schrier RW: Acute renal failure: Pathogenesis, diagnosis, and management. *Hosp Pract* (March) 1981;**16**:93.

Smolens P, Stein JH: Pathophysiology of acute renal failure. *Am J Med* 1981;**70**:479.

3. INTERSTITIAL NEPHRITIS

Acute interstitial nephritis may be due to systemic infections from bacteria, viruses, and spirochetes and sensitivity to drugs, including antibiotics (penicillins, cephalosporins, sulfonamides, rifampin, vancomycin), diuretics (thiazides, furosemide), nonsteroidal anti-inflammatory agents, phenindione, allopurinol, cimetidine, and others. Many patients will show other signs of hypersensitivity such as rash, arthralgia, fever, and eosinophilia. In some patients, there is an increase in circulating IgE. Hematuria, proteinuria, and enlargement of the kidneys are commonly demonstrable. Occasionally, acute renal failure may occur. Recovery may be complete.

Chronic interstitial nephritis is characterized by focal or diffuse interstitial fibrosis accompanied by infiltration with inflammatory cells ultimately associated with extensive atrophy of renal tubules. It represents a nonspecific reaction to a variety of causes: analgesic abuse, lead and cadmium toxicity, nephrocalcinosis, urate nephropathy, radiation nephritis, sarcoidosis, Balkan nephritis, and some instances of obstructive uropathy. There are cases in which antitubule basement membrane antibodies have been identified by means of immunofluorescence linear staining of IgG and C3. Most patients with antiglomerular basement membrane disease (Goodpasture's syndrome) and some with rapidly progressive glomerulonephritis will have anti-tubular basement membrane disease as well.

Linton AL, Lindsay RM: Drug-induced acute interstitial nephritis. *The Kidney* 1982;**15**:1.
Nanra RS: Renal effects of antipyretic analgesics: Proceedings of a symposium—antipyretic analgesic therapy. *Am J Med* 1983;**75**:70.

4. ANALGESIC NEPHROPATHY

Renal papillary necrosis has usually been associated with fulminating urinary tract infection in the presence of diabetes mellitus. Since 1953, however, more and more cases have been associated with long-term ingestion of analgesic mixtures. The typical patient habitually consumes large amounts of analgesic mixtures of nonsteroidal anti-inflammatory drugs. The ensuing damage to the kidneys usually is detected late, after renal insufficiency has developed.

The kidney lesion is pathologically nonspecific, consisting of peritubular and perivascular inflammation with degenerative changes of the tubule cells (chronic interstitial nephritis). There are no glomerular changes. Renal papillary necrosis extending into the medulla may involve many papillae.

Hematuria is a common presenting complaint. Renal colic occurs when necrotic renal papillae slough away. Polyuria may be prominent. Signs of acidosis (hyperpnea), dehydration, and pallor of anemia are common. Infection is a frequent complication. The history of excessive use of analgesics may be concealed by the patient.

The urine usually is remarkable only for the presence of blood and small amounts of protein. Hemolytic

anemia is usually evident. Elevated blood urea nitrogen and serum creatinine and the electrolyte changes characteristic of renal failure are typically present.

Urograms show cavities and ring shadows of areas of destruction of papillae.

Treatment consists of withholding analgesic mixtures. Renal failure and infection are treated as outlined elsewhere in this chapter.

Clive DM, Stoff JS: Renal syndromes associated with nonsteroidal antiinflammatory drugs. *N Engl J Med* 1984;**310**:563.
Dunn MJ: Clinical effects of prostaglandins in renal disease. *Hosp Pract* (March) 1984;**19**:99.
Eknoyan G et al: Renal papillary necrosis: An update. *Medicine* 1982;**61**:55.
Hartman GW et al: Analgesia-associated nephropathy. *JAMA* 1984;**251**:1734.
Maker JF: Analgesic nephropathy: Observations, interpretations and perspectives on the low incidence in America. *Am J Med* 1984;**76**:345.

5. URIC ACID NEPHROPATHY

See section on gout, p 519.

Crystals of urate produce an interstitial inflammatory reaction. Urate may precipitate out in acid urine in the calices or distally in the ureters to form uric acid stones. Patients with myeloproliferative disease under treatment may develop hyperuricemia and are subject to occlusion of the upper urinary tract by uric acid crystals. Alkalinization of the urine and a liberal fluid intake will help prevent crystal formation. Allopurinol is a useful drug to prevent hyperuricemia and hyperuricosuria.

6. OBSTRUCTIVE UROPATHY

Interstitial nephritis due to obstruction may not be associated with infection. Tubular conservation of salt and water is impaired. Following relief of obstruction, diuresis may be massive and may require vigorous but judicious replacement of water and electrolyte.

Klahr S: Pathophysiology of obstructive nephropathy. *Kidney Int* 1983;**23**:414.

7. MYELOMATOSIS

Features of myelomatosis that contribute to renal disease include proteinuria (including filtrable Bence Jones protein and κ and λ chains), with precipitation in the tubules leading to accumulation of abnormal proteins in the tubule cells; hypercalcemia; and occasionally increase in viscosity of the blood associated with macroglobulinemia. A Fanconi-like syndrome may develop.

Plugging of tubules, giant cell reaction around tubules, tubular atrophy, and, occasionally, the accumulation of amyloid are evident on examination of renal tissue.

Renal failure may occur acutely or may develop slowly. Hemodialysis may rescue the patient during efforts to control the myeloma with chemical agents.

Cohen DJ et al: Acute renal failure in patients with multiple myeloma. *Am J Med* 1984;**76**:247.

HEREDITARY RENAL DISEASES

The importance of inheritance and the familial incidence of disease warrants inclusion of the classification of hereditary renal diseases suggested by Perkoff. Although relatively uncommon in the population at large, hereditary disease must be recognized to permit early diagnosis and treatment in other family members and to prepare the way for genetic counseling.

Many of the renal diseases that can occur as heritable abnormalities are listed in Chapter 32 (Some Diseases With Known Modes of Inheritance). Selected diseases are discussed briefly below.

1. HEREDITARY CHRONIC NEPHRITIS

Evidence of the disease usually appears in childhood, with episodes of hematuria often following an upper respiratory infection. Renal insufficiency commonly develops in males but only rarely in females. Survival beyond age 40 is rare.

In many families, deafness and abnormalities of the eyes accompany the renal disease. Another form of the disease is accompanied by polyneuropathy. Infection of the urinary tract is a common complication.

The anatomic features in some cases resemble proliferative glomerulonephritis; in others, there is thickening of the glomerular basement membrane or podocyte proliferation and thickening of Bowman's capsule. In a few cases, there are fat-filled cells (foam cells) in the interstitial tissue or in the glomeruli.

Laboratory findings are commensurate with existing renal function.

Treatment is symptomatic.

2. CYSTIC DISEASES OF THE KIDNEY

Congenital structural anomalies of the kidney must always be considered in any patient with hypertension, pyelonephritis, or renal insufficiency. The manifestations of structural renal abnormalities are related to the superimposed disease, but management and prognosis are modified by the structural anomaly.

Polycystic Kidneys

Polycystic kidney disease is familial (autosomal dominant) and often involves not only the kidney but the liver and pancreas as well.

The formation of cysts in the cortex of the kidney is thought to result from failure of union of the collecting tubules and convoluted tubules of some nephrons. New cysts do not form, but those present enlarge and, by pressure, cause destruction of adjacent tissue. Cysts may be found in the liver and pancreas. The incidence of cerebral vessel aneurysms is higher than normal.

Cases of polycystic disease are discovered during the investigation of hypertension, by diagnostic study in patients presenting with pyelonephritis or hematuria, or by investigating the families of patients with polycystic disease. At times, flank pain due to hemorrhage into a cyst will call attention to a kidney disorder. Otherwise, the symptoms and signs are those commonly seen in hypertension or renal insufficiency. On physical examination the enlarged, irregular kidneys are easily palpable.

The urine may contain leukocytes and red cells. With bleeding into the cysts, there may also be bleeding into the urinary tract. The blood chemical findings reflect the degree of renal insufficiency. Examination by echography or x-ray shows the enlarged kidneys, and urography demonstrates the classic elongated calices and renal pelves stretched over the surface of the cysts.

No specific therapy is available, and surgical interference is contraindicated unless ureteral obstruction is produced by an adjacent cyst. Hypertension, infection, and uremia are treated in the conventional manner.

Because persons with polycystic kidneys may live in reasonable comfort with slowly advancing uremia, it is difficult to determine when renal transplantation is in order. Hemodialysis can extend the life of the patient, but recurrent bleeding and continuous pain indicate the need for a transplant.

Although the disease may become symptomatic in childhood or early adult life, it usually is discovered in the fourth or fifth decades. Unless fatal complications of hypertension or urinary tract infection are present, uremia develops very slowly, and patients live longer than with other causes of renal insufficiency.

Cystic Disease of the Renal Medulla

Two syndromes have become more frequent as their diagnostic features have become better known.

Medullary cystic disease is a familial disease (either autosomal dominant or recessive) that may become symptomatic during adolescence. Anemia is usually the initial manifestation, but azotemia, acidosis, and hyperphosphatemia soon become evident. Hypertension may develop. The urine is not remarkable, although there is often an inability to produce a concentrated urine. Many small cysts are scattered through the renal medulla. Renal transplantation is indicated by the usual criteria for the operation.

Sponge kidney is asymptomatic and is discovered by the characteristic appearance of the urogram. Enlargement of the papillae and calices and small cavities within the pyramids are demonstrated by the contrast media in the excretory urogram. Many small calculi often occupy the cysts, and infection may be troublesome. Life expectancy is not affected, and only symptomatic therapy for ureteral impaction of a stone or for infection is required.

Gardner KD Jr (editor): *Cystic Diseases of the Kidney.* Wiley, 1976.

3. ANOMALIES OF FUNCTION OF THE PROXIMAL TUBULE

Defects of Amino Acid Reabsorption
A. Congenital Cystinuria: Increased excretion of cystine results in the formation of cystine calculi in the urinary tract. Ornithine, arginine, and lysine are also excreted in abnormally large quantities. There is also a defect in absorption of these amino acids in the jejunum. Nonopaque stones should be examined chemically to provide a specific diagnosis.

Maintain a high urine volume by giving a large fluid intake. Maintain the urine pH above 7 by giving sodium bicarbonate and sodium citrate plus acetazolamide (Diamox) at bedtime to ensure an alkaline night urine. In refractory cases, a low-methionine (cystine precursor) diet may be necessary. Penicillamine has proved useful in some cases.

B. Aminoaciduria: Hereditary defects of renal tubule function or defects of amino acid metabolism are manifested by loss of a variety of amino acids. Failure to thrive and the presence of other tubular deficits suggest the diagnosis.

There is no treatment.

C. Hepatolenticular Degeneration (Wilson's Disease): In this congenital familial disease, aminoaciduria is associated with cirrhosis of the liver and neurologic manifestations (see p 415).

Multiple Defects of Tubular Function
A. De Toni-Fanconi-Debré Syndrome: Aminoaciduria, phosphaturia, glycosuria, and a variable degree of renal tubular acidosis characterize this syndrome. Osteomalacia is a prominent clinical feature; other clinical and laboratory manifestations are associated with specific tubular defects described above.

The proximal segment of the renal tubule is replaced by a thin tubular structure constituting the swan-neck deformity. The proximal segment also is shortened to less than half the normal length.

Treatment consists of replacing cation deficits (especially potassium), correcting acidosis with bicarbonate or citrate, replacing phosphate loss with isotonic neutral phosphate (mono- and disodium salts) solution, and a liberal calcium intake. Vitamin D is usually helpful, but the dose used must be controlled by monitoring serum calcium and phosphate.

B. Acquired Fanconi Syndrome: Defects in tubular reabsorption resembling those of the Fanconi syndrome can be induced by heavy metal poisoning (cadmium, lead, copper, uranium, mercury), by a degradation product of tetracycline, by cresol poisoning, by galactosemia, by renal tubule damage associated with diseases accompanied by dysproteinemia, and by tubulointerstitial disease, nephrotic syndrome, and amyloidosis.

Treatment is directed at the primary cause and at correction of electrolyte abnormalities.

Defects of Phosphorus & Calcium Absorption
A. Vitamin D-Resistant Rickets: Excessive loss of phosphorus and calcium results in rickets or osteomalacia poorly responsive to vitamin D therapy. Treatment consists of giving large doses of vitamin D calcium supplementation of the diet.

B. Pseudohypoparathyroidism: See p 714.

Defects of Glucose Absorption (Renal Glycosuria)
Relative inability to reabsorb glucose means that glycosuria is present when blood glucose levels are normal. Ketosis is not present. The glucose tolerance test response is usually normal. In some instances, renal glycosuria may precede the onset of true diabetes mellitus.

There is no treatment for renal glycosuria.

Defects of Glucose & Phosphate Absorption (Glycosuric Rickets)
The symptoms and signs are those of rickets or osteomalacia, with weakness, pain, or discomfort of the legs and spine, and tetany. The bones become deformed, with bowing of the weight-bearing long bones, kyphoscoliosis, and, in children, signs of rickets. X-ray shows markedly decreased density of the bone, with pseudofracture lines and other deformities. Nephrocalcinosis may occur with excessive phosphaturia, and renal insufficiency may follow. Urinary calcium and phosphorus are increased, and glycosuria is present. Serum glucose is normal, serum calcium normal or low, serum phosphorus low, and serum alkaline phosphatase elevated.

Treatment consists of giving large doses of vitamin D and dietary calcium supplementation.

4. RENAL TUBULAR ACIDOSIS

Both the proximal tubule and the distal tubule can secrete hydrogen ion (H^+) and reclaim bicarbonate (HCO_3^-) from the luminal fluid. Normally, the preponderance of filtered HCO_3^- is reclaimed in the proximal tubule, leaving a smaller demand on the distal segment of the nephron to provide hydrogen for reabsorption of a small amount of HCO_3^- and excretion of metabolic acids.

Proximal Renal Tubular Acidosis (Type II)
The defect in H^+ secretion in the proximal tubule results in a decrease in absorption of filtered bicarbonate, loss of bicarbonate in the urine, and decreased concentration of bicarbonate in extracellular fluid. Secretion of H^+ in the distal tubule is unimpaired.

As plasma bicarbonate concentration diminishes,

less bicarbonate is filtered, and ultimately an equilibrium is reached. This sets a limit on bicarbonate loss, and the resultant acidosis is only moderate. Accompanying the limitation of hydrogen ion secretion are increased potassium secretion into the urine and retrieval of Cl^- instead of HCO_3^-. The acidosis is therefore associated with hypokalemia and hyperchloremia. Because Cl^- replaces HCO_3^- in the extracellular fluid, there is no anion gap. Hypercalciuria is moderate, and stone formation is uncommon. Transport of glucose, amino acids, phosphate, and urate may be deficient as well and may result in the Fanconi syndrome (see above).

Proximal renal tubular acidosis may be genetic in origin. It is transiently seen with acetazolamide therapy, use of outdated tetracycline, and exposure to some heavy metals (eg, lead). Proximal renal tubular acidosis may occur when the kidney is involved with medullary cystic disease, Sjögren's syndrome, amyloidosis, or multiple myeloma. (See also de Toni-Fanconi-Debré Syndrome, above.)

The pH of the urine is high except if acidosis becomes severe when bicarbonate disappears from the urine and the pH drops to a lower limit of 5.5–5.4.

When treatment is required for the acidosis, it consists of replacement with large amounts of HCO_3^- and replacement of wasted K^+. Bicarbonate in doses of 6–15 mmol/kg/d may be required; some of this should be $KHCO_3$. Shohl's solution, a mixture of sodium citrate and citric acid (1 mL = 1 mmol HCO_3^-), in doses of 20–50 mL 3 times a day, may be substituted for part of the HCO_3^- requirement. Hydrochlorothiazide, to produce slight volume depletion with resultant increased HCO_3^- reabsorption, plus spironolactone, to reduce K^+ excretion, have been employed to ameliorate proximal renal tubular acidosis.

Distal Renal Tubular Acidosis (Type I)

The distal tubule cells, like those of the proximal tubule, generate carbonic acid from CO_2 and H_2O and retrieve the bicarbonate by secreting H^+ to exchange for Na^+ in the tubular fluid. H^+ is excreted with acid anion and buffers in the urine and is also combined with NH_3 to form NH_4^+, an additional cation that accompanies acid anion in the excreted urine.

The defect in distal renal tubular acidosis is either a defect in secretion of H^+ or an inability to transport H^+ against a steep concentration gradient between extracellular fluid and urine in the terminal segments of the nephron (eg, plasma $[H^+]$, 4×10^{-8}, molar versus urine pH 4.5 or 32×10^{-6}, molar $[H^+]$), or both of these. The defect persists no matter how severe the acidosis, and diagnosis depends on the observation that in the presence of acidosis, the urine pH remains greater than 5.5. Potassium excretion is heightened by failure of H^+ secretion and by activation of the secretion of aldosterone; hypokalemia is often apparent clinically. Hypercalciuria with renal stone and nephrocalcinosis and metabolic bone disease are seen in severe and long-standing cases. There is an incomplete

form of distal renal tubular acidosis that is revealed only when it is necessary to excrete a large acid load. To prove that this incomplete form of renal tubular acidosis exists, 0.1 g of NH_4Cl per kilogram is administered orally. Within 6–8 hours, arterial blood pH should be less than 7.35, plasma bicarbonate should be less than 20 mmol/L, and the urine pH should remain greater than 5.5.

Distal renal tubular acidosis may be genetically transmitted. It can occur in association with sickle cell anemia, a variety of autoimmune diseases, chronic pyelonephritis and urolithiasis, cirrhosis of the liver, diseases in which nephrocalcinosis occurs, and therapy with amphotericin B or analgesics.

Treatment of the acute emergency of severe metabolic acidosis includes vigorous bicarbonate replacement supplemented with adequate K^+. The chronic case requires lifelong therapy with enough $NaHCO_3$ or Shohl's solution to neutralize the metabolic acids that must be excreted (50 mmol/d or more) and to correct hypercalciuria. Potassium loss will usually diminish enough so that K^+ replacement is not required, but in some cases, potassium intake may have to be increased.

Appropriate therapy will protect against development of nephrocalcinosis, azotemia, and metabolic bone disease.

Type IV Renal Tubular Acidosis

Recognition of type IV renal tubular acidosis is increasingly common as the clinical manifestations become known. It occurs with hyporeninemic hypoaldosteronism when moderate renal insufficiency is associated with diabetes mellitus; with chronic renal insufficiency from many causes; or as an adverse effect of drugs such as aldactone (especially with cirrhosis) and nonsteroidal anti-inflammatory agents. It also occurs with normal aldosterone activity when there is chronic renal insufficiency (rarely) or urinary obstruction. The characteristics of type IV renal tubular acidosis include impairment of renal acidification accompanied by reduced renal clearance of potassium, which results in hyperkalemia and acidosis. The disorder is related to lack of aldosterone or inability of aldosterone to stimulate H^+ secretion at the cation exchange portion of the distal tubule.

Treatment with fludrocortisone in doses that do not induce hypervolemia and hypertension (0.1–0.3 mg/d) may correct acidosis and hyperkalemia. Alternatively, reducing potassium intake, use of potassium-binding resins, and use of loop diuretics may correct the hyperkalemia. Acidosis may be corrected by small doses of sodium bicarbonate (2 meq/kg/d).

5. ANOMALIES OF THE DISTAL TUBULE

Excess Potassium Secretion (Potassium "Wastage" Syndrome)

Excessive renal secretion or loss of potassium may occur in 4 situations: (1) Chronic renal insufficiency with diminished H^+ secretion. (2) Renal tubular acidosis and de Toni–Fanconi syndrome, with cation loss resulting from diminished H^+ and NH_4^+ secretion. (3) Aldosteronism and hyperadrenocorticism. (4) Excessive tubular secretion of potassium, the cause of which is unknown. Hypokalemia indicates that the deficit is severe. Muscle weakness, metabolic alkalosis, and polyuria with dilute urine are signs of hypokalemia.

Defects of Water Absorption
(Renal Diabetes Insipidus)

Nephrogenic diabetes insipidus occurs more frequently in males. Unresponsiveness to antidiuretic hormone is the key to differentiation from pituitary diabetes insipidus.

In addition to congenital refractoriness to antidiuretic hormone, obstructive uropathy, lithium, methoxyflurane, and demeclocycline may also render the tubule refractory. Impaired water reabsorption may be present with sickle cell anemia, medullary cystic disease, hypokalemia, and hypercalcemia.

Symptoms are related to an inability to reabsorb water, with resultant polyuria and polydipsia. The daily urine volume approaches 12 L, and osmolality and specific gravity are low. Mental retardation, atonic bladder, and hydronephrosis occur frequently.

Treatment consists primarily of an adequate water intake. Chlorothiazide may ameliorate the diabetes; the mechanism of action is unknown, but the drug may act by increasing isosmotic reabsorption in the proximal segment of the tubule secondary to volume contraction.

6. UNSPECIFIED RENAL TUBULAR ABNORMALITIES

In idiopathic hypercalciuria, decreased reabsorption of calcium predisposes to the formation of renal calculi. Serum calcium and phosphorus are normal. Urine calcium excretion is high; urine phosphorus excretion is low.

Treatment is discussed on p 573.

Brenner RJ et al: Incidence of radiographically evident bone disease, nephrocalcinosis, and nephrolithiasis in various types of renal tubular acidosis. *N Engl J Med* 1982;**307**:217.

Hruska KA, Ban D: Renal tubular acidosis. *Arch Intern Med* 1982;**142**:1909.

Mattern WD: Renal tubular acidosis. *The Kidney* 1982;**15**:11.

Morris RC Jr: Renal tubular acidosis. *N Engl J Med* 1981; **304**:418.

Morris RC Jr, Sebastian A: Disorders of renal tubules that cause disorders of fluid, acid-base, and electrolyte metabolism. In: *Clinical Disorders of Fluid and Electrolyte Metabolism*, 3rd ed. Maxwell MH, Kleeman CR (editors). McGraw-Hill, 1980.

Segal S: Disorders of renal amino acid transport. *N Engl J Med* 1976;**294**:1044.

7. CONGENITAL ANOMALIES

Renal Agenesis

Occasionally one kidney, usually the left, is congenitally absent. The remaining kidney is hypertrophied. Before performing a nephrectomy for any reason, it is mandatory to prove the patient has a second kidney.

Horseshoe Kidney

A band of renal tissue or of fibrous tissue may join the 2 kidneys. Associated abnormalities of the ureterocaliceal system, or hydronephrosis resulting from ureteral obstruction by aberrant vessels, predispose to pyelonephritis.

Ectopic Kidney

The kidney may occupy a site in the pelvis, and the ureter may be shorter than normal. Infection is common in ectopic kidneys compromised by ureteral obstruction or urinary reflux.

Nephroptosis

Unusual mobility of the kidney permits it to move from its normal position to a lower one. The incidence of ureteral occlusion due to movement of a kidney is extremely low.

Megaloureter & Hydronephrosis

These anatomic abnormalities may occur congenitally but are more commonly the result of vesicoureteral urinary reflux.

Kissane JM: Congenital malformations. Page 83 in: *Pathology of the Kidney*, 3rd ed. Heptinstall RH (editor). Little, Brown, 1983.

8. RENAL DISEASE INCIDENT TO OTHER DISEASES

Abnormalities of renal function occur with other diseases and may be of therapeutic and prognostic importance. In sickle cell anemia, circulatory changes resulting from sickling and aggregation of red cells contribute to decreased concentrating ability, a defect in acidification of urine, hematuria, renal infarction, glomerulopathy, papillary necrosis, and renal failure. With acute pancreatitis, acute renal failure may occur in the absence of shock. In hepatorenal syndrome, severe renal failure may appear with cirrhosis of the liver and ascites or with severe jaundice of either parenchymatous or obstructive origin. Limited space precludes an adequate discussion. Acute renal failure in pregnancy occurs with toxemia, intrauterine hemorrhage, and complications of abortion and in the immediate postpartum period (hemolytic-uremic syndrome).

Brenner BM, Rector FC Jr: *The Kidney*, 2nd ed. Saunders, 1981.

Wong PY et al: The hepatorenal syndrome. (Clinical Conference.) *Gastroenterology* 1979;**77**:1326.

INFECTIONS OF THE URINARY TRACT*

The term urinary tract infection denotes a wide variety of clinical entities in which the common denominator is the presence of a significantly large number of microorganisms in any portion of the urinary tract. Microorganisms may be evident only in the urine (bacteriuria), or there may be evidence of infection of an organ, eg, urethritis, prostatitis, cystitis, pyelonephritis. At any given time, any one of these organs may be asymptomatic or symptomatic. Infection in any part of the urinary tract may spread to any other part of the tract.

Symptomatic urinary tract infection may be acute or chronic. The term relapse implies recurrence of infection with the same organism; the term reinfection implies infection with another organism.

Pathogenesis

Urine secreted by normal kidneys is sterile until it reaches the distal urethra. Bacteria can reach the urinary tract by the ascending route or by hematogenous spread. The latter occurs during bacteremia (eg, with staphylococci) and results in abscess formation in the cortex or the perirenal fat. Far commoner is ascending infection, where bacteria are introduced into the urethra (from fecal flora on the perineum or the vaginal vestibule, or by instrumentation) and travel up the urinary tract to reach the bladder, ureters, or renal pelvis. The most important factor in aiding or perpetuating ascending infection is anatomic or functional obstruction to free urine flow. Free flow, large urine volume, complete emptying of the bladder, and acid pH are important antibacterial defenses.

Age & Sex Distribution of Urinary Tract Infection

In infants, urinary tract infection occurs more frequently in boys than in girls, in keeping with a higher incidence of obstructive anomalies of the urinary tract. After the first year of life, urinary tract infection is more frequent in girls because of the contamination of the vaginal vestibule with fecal flora, and the short urethra. In surveys of schoolchildren, only 0.05% of boys have bacteriuria, whereas at least 2% of girls have bacteria in their urine specimens. In later life, urinary tract infection is rare among men until the age of prostatic hypertrophy (over 40), but there is a regular increase in incidence among women until age 70, when about 10% of women have urinary tract infection. There is some correlation of the incidence of urinary tract infection with sexual activity in women, as well as with parity.

Infecting Microorganisms

Virtually any microorganism introduced into the urinary tract may cause urinary tract infection. However, the vast majority of cases of urinary tract infection are caused by aerobic members of the fecal flora, especially *Escherichia* (*E coli* O serotypes 1, 2, 6, 7, 8, 11, 15, and 75 are common), *Enterobacter, Klebsiella*, enterococci, *Pseudomonas*, and *Proteus*. Other organisms (eg, *Staphylococcus saprophyticus*) occasionally appear in spontaneous urinary tract infection, but their significance must be assessed as described below. Infections with strict anaerobes are very rare. Viruses may cause immune complex nephritis but—except for adenovirus type 11 in hemorrhagic cystitis of children—do not cause urinary tract infections. Chlamydiae, mycoplasmas, and other organisms causing urethritis, vaginitis, and other genital tract disorders are listed below.

Significant Bacteriuria

The concept of significant bacteriuria is basic to the accurate interpretation of urine cultures. Urine secreted by the normal kidney is sterile and remains so while it travels to the bladder. However, the normal urethra has a microbial flora, and any voided urine in normal persons may therefore contain thousands of bacteria per milliliter derived from this normal flora. To differentiate this smaller number of microorganisms from the larger number commonly found in infections of the urinary tract, it is essential to count the number of bacteria in fresh, properly collected specimens by appropriate methods (quantitative culture). In general, active urinary tract infections are characterized by more than 100,000 bacteria per milliliter. If such numbers are found in 2 consecutive specimens and if the bacteria are of a single type, there is more than a 95% chance that an active infection is present. On the other hand, a significant proportion of acutely dysuric women have pyuria with only $10^3–10^5$/mL bacteria at times but respond promptly to antibacterial treatment. In persons who chronically show low-grade bacteriuria, suprapubic aspiration may help in diagnosis.

Pathology

Acute urinary tract infection shows inflammation of any part of the tract and sometimes intense hyperemia or even bleeding of the mucous membranes. The prominent lesion in the kidney is acute inflammation of the interstitial tissue, which may progress to frank suppuration and patchy necrosis. Chronic urinary tract infection may cause only minimal changes or progessively more severe scarring in any part of the tract. Chronic pyelonephritis may lead to widespread fibrosis and scarring of functional cortical and medullary tissue, resulting in renal insufficiency. Chronic interstitial nephritis may result from bacterial infection or from other causes (eg, hypersensitivity).

Collection of Urine for Culture*

A. Voided Midstream Specimen: This is the

---

*By Ernest Jawetz, MD, PhD.

*See Kunin reference on p 569.

optimal method, involving no risk to the patient. The urethral meatus or vaginal vestibule is cleansed, the labia are spread, and the first part of the stream is discarded. The mid part of the stream is aseptically collected in a sterile container.

B. Specimen Obtained by Catheterization: Each urethral catheter insertion carries a 1–2% risk of introducing microorganisms into the bladder and thus initiating urinary tract infection. Results of quantitative culture from a single catheterized urine specimen yielding more than 100,000 bacteria of a single species per milliliter of urine indicate that active urinary tract infection is present. In persons with indwelling urethral catheters, specimens must be obtained by aseptic needle aspiration of urine through the catheter wall, *not* by disconnecting the closed system.

C. Specimen Obtained by Suprapubic Aspiration: While the bladder is distended, the suprapubic skin is aseptically prepared, and a sterile needle is then thrust into the bladder. This permits aspiration of bladder urine free from urethral contamination. It is especially useful in infants (from whom satisfactory specimens for culture may be difficult to obtain) and in patients with equivocal counts on several occasions.

Examination of Urine

Urine must be cultured or examined microscopically within 1 hour of collection or after no more than 18 hours of refrigeration. Urine is a good culture medium for many microorganisms, and growth can occur at room temperature.

A. Microscopic Examination: A drop of fresh urine or a drop of resuspended sediment from centrifuged fresh urine is placed on a microscope slide, covered with a cover glass, and examined with the high-dry objective under reduced illumination. The prevalence of leukocytes is noted. The presence of more than 10 bacteria (often motile) per field in the unstained specimen suggests a bacteria count of more than 100,000/mL of urine. Smears may also be made from fresh urine, stained with Gram's stain, and examined under the oil immersion objective. Three bacteria or more per field in such stains suggest infection. By immunofluorescence, bacteria in urine are coated with immunoglobulin if they are derived from tissue infection (especially pyelonephritis, prostatitis) but are not so coated if the infection is limited to the outflow system (cystitis, urethritis).

B. Urine Culture: With a calibrated loop, undiluted urine and urine diluted 1:100 are spread on eosinmethylene blue and blood agar plates. After incubation, numbers of colonies are estimated and multiplied by the dilution factor to yield the bacterial count per milliliter. A number of simplified semiquantitative culture methods are available that are readily performed in the physician's office at nominal cost. The dip-slide method and its several variations involve dipping an agar-coated slide or similar device into fresh urine, incubating it, and then comparing the resultant growth with optical density standards.

C. Chemical Tests of Urine: The presence and number of bacteria can also be estimated by various chemical tests that rely on the enzymatic activity of viable bacteria, eg, the reduction of nitrate. These indirect tests are much less reliable than tests employing quantitative estimates of bacterial growth.

D. Identification of Microorganisms: In most cases of acute urinary tract infection, detailed identification of the etiologic organism may not be required. However, in chronic or recurrent urinary tract infection, identification of the organism by standard microbiologic methods is desirable. Antimicrobial drug susceptibility tests are not needed in the first attack of urinary tract infection. Most of these infections are due to coliform organisms and are often treated with sulfonamide, ampicillin, or amoxicillin. In chronic or recurrent urinary tract infection, antimicrobial drug susceptibility tests are needed. It must be kept in mind that many drugs appear in the urine in very high concentration, whereas "standard" disk tests indicate susceptibility only to levels achieved in blood.

ACUTE URINARY TRACT INFECTION

Clinical Findings

A. Lower Tract Involvement:

1. Symptoms and signs–Burning pain on urination, often with turbid, foul-smelling, or dark urine, frequency, and suprapubic or lower abdominal discomfort. There are usually no positive physical findings unless the upper tract is involved also.

2. Laboratory findings–Microscopic examination of a properly collected urine specimen usually shows significant bacteriuria and pyuria and occasionally hematuria. Bacteriuria may be confirmed by "dipslide" or similar test.

B. Upper Tract Involvement:

1. Symptoms and signs–Headache, malaise, vomiting, chills and fever, costovertebral angle pain and tenderness, and abdominal pain. The absence of upper tract signs does not exclude bacterial invasion of the upper tract.

2. Laboratory findings–Significant bacteriuria is often accompanied by proteinuria and pyuria. The bacteria in the urine are often coated with immunoglobulin, as revealed by immunofluorescence. Leukocytosis is common, with a marked shift to the left. Blood culture is only rarely positive.

Differential Diagnosis

Acute urinary tract infection may occasionally present as an "acute abdomen," acute pancreatitis, or basal pneumonia. In all of these circumstances, the presence of significant bacteriuria usually establishes the diagnosis. On the other hand, dysuria, frequency, nocturia, and lower abdominal pain may be the "urethral" or "bladder" syndrome, especially in sexually active women. It may represent vaginitis; urethritis; cervicitis attributable to *Trichomonas, Gardnerella,*

Chlamydia, Neisseria, or *Ureaplasma;* or small numbers of bacteria in bladder urine.

Prevention

Certain women have a high rate of urinary reinfection, sometimes related to sexual activity. In the latter situation, 1 or 2 doses of an effective antimicrobial (eg, trimethoprim-sulfamethoxazole, ampicillin) taken after intercourse tend to prevent establishment of infection. In other women, recurrences can be greatly reduced if the patient takes trimethoprim-sulfamethoxazole, 1 tablet 3 times weekly or one-half tablet daily at bedtime for months.

In patients who must have an indwelling catheter postoperatively and in whom closed sterile drainage is established, the onset of bacteriuria is delayed if antimicrobial drugs (eg, cephalosporins) are given during the first 3 days after insertion. Thereafter, there is no benefit.

Treatment

A. Specific Measures:

1. First attack of urinary tract infection– Acute symptomatic cystitis in women often responds to treatment for just 1–3 days with sulfisoxazole, 4 g/d; ampicillin, 2–4 g/d; amoxicillin, 1–3 g/d; or trimethoprim, 80 mg, plus sulfamethoxazole, 400 mg, 2–4 tablets daily. Oral cephalexin, 2–4 g/d, or cephradine, 2–4 g/d, may be equally effective. Acute infection in men or those suggestive of upper tract involvement should be treated with similar drugs for 7–10 days. Maintain an alkaline urine pH. If symptoms have not improved and the urine has not cleared as shown by microscopy on day 4 of treatment, reexamine the urine for possible resistant microorganisms. Follow-up at 2 and 6 weeks after treatment is stopped should demonstrate absence of bacteriuria; otherwise, re-treat.

2. Recurrence of urinary tract infection– Select an antimicrobial drug on the basis of antimicrobial susceptibility tests of cultured organisms. Give the drug for 10–14 days in doses sufficient to maintain high urine levels. Reexamine the urine 2 and 6 weeks after treatment is stopped.

3. Second recurrence, or failure of bacteriuria to be suppressed– Perform tests of renal function and excretory urograms and consider referral to a urologist for a workup for possible obstruction, reflux, and localization of infection in the upper or lower tract. (For details, see Kunin reference, below.) Men with recurrent urinary tract infection and probable prostatitis as a persistent focus often fail to be cured by 10–14 days of treatment. In these patients, a 12- to 20-week trial of trimethoprim-sulfamethoxazole or ampicillin is indicated if the organism is susceptible to these.

B. General Measures: Forcing fluids may relieve signs and symptoms but should be limited to amounts that will avoid undue dilution of antimicrobials in the urine. Analgesics may be required briefly for pain. Metabolic abnormalities such as diabetes mellitus must be identified and treated.

Prognosis

Initial attacks of acute urinary tract infection, in the absence of obstruction, tend to subside with treatment or spontaneously. The symptoms and bacteriuria often disappear. This is not true in recurrent or chronic urinary tract infection. About 20% of pregnant women with asymptomatic bacteriuria in the first trimester develop symptomatic urinary tract infection—often upper tract infection—later in pregnancy.

CHRONIC URINARY TRACT INFECTION

Essentials of Diagnosis

- Recurrent episodes of lower or upper tract involvement.
- Absence of symptoms or signs referable to the urinary tract, but persistent asymptomatic bacteriuria.
- Possibility of obstruction, focal lesion, or poor drainage in urinary tract.
- Impairment of renal function, with nitrogen retention, anemia, acidosis, uremia, or hypertension.

General Considerations

Chronic or recurrent episodes of urinary tract infection may produce no permanent harm or may lead to dysfunction or scarring of the lower or upper tract. Chronic bacterial pyelonephritis may progress to inflammation of interstitial tissue, scarring, atrophy, and, rarely, progressive renal failure or hypertension. In any patient with hypertension, a search for bacterial pyelonephritis should be made. If unilateral pyelonephritis is present, nephrectomy may be curative. With bilateral pyelonephritis, chronic suppression of infection may permit improved renal function. The end stage of renal failure resulting from chronic bacterial pyelonephritis may be indistinguishable from that resulting from chronic glomerulonephritis or nephrosclerosis. Over a significant extent of its natural history, chronic urinary tract infection is asymptomatic, manifested mainly by bacteriuria or by recurrent episodes of acute urinary tract infection.

Clinical Findings

A. Symptoms and Signs: There are often no positive clinical findings in chronic urinary tract infection except significant bacteriuria. There may be episodes of recurrent acute urinary tract infection with symptoms referable to the lower or to the upper urinary tract. Hypertension, anemia, or uremia may appear in the late stages of chronic pyelonephritis.

Whenever chronic bacteriuria is discovered, it is mandatory to perform a complete urologic study, including excretory urograms, cystograms, and voiding cystourethrograms, followed by procedures to localize the source of bacteriuria to one or both sides and to the lower or upper tract. Surgical correction of any abnormality (reflux, obstruction, etc) found in these studies must be considered while chronic suppression of bacteriuria is undertaken.

B. Laboratory Findings: The white blood count is usually normal, but significant anemia may be present in early renal failure. Blood urea and serum creatinine may be elevated; creatinine clearance may be reduced. Repeated and meticulous urine culture is the crucial laboratory procedure that is a guide to medical treatment. In addition, methods such as "bladder washout" may be used to distinguish infection of the lower from that of the upper tract. If significant bacteriuria is discovered, an attempt may be made to eradicate or suppress it (see below). If no significant bacteriuria is found, infection by tubercle bacilli, anaerobic bacteria, or fungi must be considered.

Immunofluorescence staining usually shows that bacteria derived from tissue infection are coated with immunoglobulin, eg, in pyelonephritis and prostatitis. Bacteria from the ureter or bladder are not stained by this technique.

The concentrating ability of the kidney is one of the earliest functions to be impaired in chronic pyelonephritis. Determination of urine osmolality under controlled fluid intake is a good guide to changes in kidney status under antimicrobial treatment.

Treatment

A. Specific Measures: Specific treatment may consist of surgical correction of functional or anatomic abnormalities by the urologist, or antimicrobial treatment. The latter usually involves attempts to eradicate the infectious agent by short-term treatment and, if bacteriuria recurs, long-term suppression of the bacteria by administration of urinary antiseptics.

1. If the same organism is isolated from at least 2 sequential urine cultures, antimicrobial drug sensitivity tests should be performed. From the group of drugs to which the organism is susceptible in vitro, the least toxic is selected (for choice of drugs, see Chapter 29) and administered daily in full systemic doses orally for 4 weeks. Urine pH must be adjusted to be optimal for the selected drug. The urine must be checked after 3 days of treatment and then at weekly intervals to make certain that bacteriuria is suppressed and that a new infection with another organism has not occurred. At the end of treatment, all drug administration is stopped and, 2 and 6 weeks later, the urine is checked again. If bacteriuria is not found, it may be assumed that the particular organism has been eradicated. Repeated examinations for bacteriuria are necessary to confirm absence of recurrent infection.

2. If the foregoing measures fail to eradicate the infection, chronic suppression of bacteriuria is attempted by daily dosage with a urinary antiseptic, eg, nitrofurantoin, methenamine mandelate or hippurate, nalidixic acid, or acidifying agents (see Chapter 29). Urinary pH must be adjusted to the optimum for the drug selected and usually should be held below pH 6.0. The patient can monitor urine pH with indicator paper once a day. After 1 week of treatment and monthly thereafter, the urine must be examined for bacteria.

Chronic suppression is continued for 6 months or even longer if the patient can tolerate the drug and superinfection does not occur. If the latter should occur, a specific antimicrobial drug may be selected, by laboratory test, for a 14-day course of treatment, and suppression with another urinary antiseptic may then be continued. At the end of 1 year of suppressive treatment, renal function and bacteriuria are reevaluated. During suppressive long-term treatment, instrumentation of the urinary tract should be strenuously avoided.

B. General Measures: Water diuresis may often provide relief from minor discomfort of lower urinary tract symptoms. Water and electrolyte balance must be maintained and renal failure managed as described on pp 559 and 560. For management of hypertension, see Chapter 8. Prevention of infection is all-important, particularly by avoidance of catheterization and instrumentation and by adherence to the principles of good hygiene. In some women, prophylactic administration of ampicillin, a cephalosporin, trimethoprim, or nitrofurantoin, either every day or at the time of sexual intercourse, may prevent recurrences of infection.

Prolonged drug administration should be avoided in patients with neurogenic bladder or long-term indwelling catheter. Removal of the catheter takes priority over drug treatment.

Prognosis

Probably 10% or less of asymptomatic bacteriuria patients develop renal failure attributable to the infection; hypertension is even more rare. Chronic urinary tract infection is eradicated by short-term therapy (2–6 weeks) in about 25–35% of patients. Some of the others have relapses caused by the same organism; some have reinfection caused by other organisms.

Long-term suppression (> 6 months) with urinary antiseptics eradicates bacteriuria in about two-thirds of patients, but some may become reinfected later. Many elderly patients tolerate recurrent urinary tract infection well, and therapy of their asymptomatic bacteriuria is inappropriate. Antimicrobial drugs should be limited to the relief of acute symptoms.

Harding GFK et al: Long-term antimicrobial prophylaxis for recurrent urinary tract infection in women. *Rev Infect Dis* 1982;**4**:438.

Kass EH: Horatio at the orifice: The significance of bacteriuria. *J Infect Dis* 1978;**138**:546.

Kunin CM: *Detection, Prevention and Management of Urinary Tract Infections,* 3rd ed. Lea & Febiger, 1979.

Kunin CM: Duration of treatment of urinary tract infections. *Am J Med* 1981;**71**:849.

Nicolle LE et al: Bacteriuria in elderly institutionalized men. *N Engl J Med* 1983;**309**:1420.

Platt R et al: Mortality associated with nosocomial urinary tract infection. *N Engl J Med* 1982;**307**:637.

Rubin RH et al: Single-dose amoxicillin therapy for urinary tract infection. *JAMA* 1980;**244**:561.

Shapiro ED, Wald ER: Single-dose amoxicillin treatment of urinary tract infections. *J Pediatr* 1981;**99**:989.

Souney P, Polk BF: Single-dose therapy for urinary tract infections in women. *Rev Infect Dis* 1982;**4**:29.

Stamey TA: *The Pathogenesis and Treatment of Urinary Tract Infections.* Williams & Wilkins, 1980.

Stamm WE et al: Diagnosis of coliform infection in acutely dysuric women. *N Engl J Med* 1982;**307**:463.

Stamm WE et al: Treatment of the acute urethral syndrome. *N Engl J Med* 1981;**304**:956.

TUBERCULOSIS OF THE GENITOURINARY TRACT

Essentials of Diagnosis

- Fever, easy fatigability, night sweats, or other signs of systemic infection.
- Symptoms or signs of upper or lower urinary tract infection.
- Urine may contain leukocytes and erythrocytes but no visible bacteria. Routine urine culture is negative.
- Special culture of urine for mycobacteria reveals *Mycobacterium tuberculosis.*
- Excretory urogram may show deformed or "moth-eaten" calices and varying types of kidney tissue destruction.
- Cystoscopy may reveal ulcers or granulomas of bladder wall.

General Considerations

Hematogenous dissemination of tubercle bacilli from foci in the lung or lymph nodes is the usual source of tuberculosis of the kidney; rarely does the infection originate in the genital tract. The genital organs may become infected by hematogenous spread or secondary to kidney infection. The prostate, seminal vesicles, epididymides, and, rarely, the testes may be infected. The oviducts are more frequently involved than the ovaries and uterus.

The kidney and ureter may show little gross change. Caseous nodules in the renal parenchyma and abscess formation with destruction of tissue and fibrosis often produce extensive damage. Calcification in the lesions is common. The ureter and calices are thickened, and stenosis may occur, with total destruction of functioning renal tissue above. The bladder shows mucosal inflammation and submucosal tubercles that become necrotic and form ulcers. Fibrosis of the bladder wall occurs late or upon healing. Tubercles with caseous necrosis and calcification are found in the genital organs. Microscopically, typical tubercles are found, and demonstration of the tubercle bacilli in the lesions is usually easily accomplished.

Note: A complete search must be made for tuberculosis elsewhere in the body whenever urinary tract tuberculosis is found.

Clinical Findings

A. Symptoms and Signs: Symptoms are not characteristic or specific. Manifestations of chronic infection, with malaise, fever, fatigability, and night sweats, may be present. Kidney and ureter infection is usually silent. Bladder infection produces frequency, burning on urination, nocturia, and, occasionally, tenesmus. If bleeding occurs with clot formation, ureteral or vesical colic may occur. Gross hematuria is fairly common. There may be nodular induration of the testes, epididymis, or prostate, and thickened seminal vesicles. Occasionally, pain and tenderness occur in the costovertebral angle. A draining sinus may form from any of these sites.

B. Laboratory Findings: The urine contains "pus without bacteria," red cells, and usually protein. Culture for tubercle bacilli confirms the diagnosis. If renal damage is extensive, signs of renal insufficiency can be demonstrated: elevated blood urea nitrogen and serum electrolyte abnormalities characteristic of uremia. A mild anemia usually is present, and the sedimentation rate is rapid.

C. X-Ray and Cystoscopic Findings: Excretory urograms reveal the moth-eaten appearance of the involved calices or the obliteration of calices, stenosis of calices, abscess cavities, ureteral thickening and stenosis, and the nonfunctioning kidney (autonephrectomy). Calcification of involved tissues is common. Thorough cystoscopic examination is required to determine the extent of bladder wall infection and to provide biopsy material if needed. Culture of urine obtained from ureteral catheters will help establish whether one or both kidneys are affected.

Differential Diagnosis

The "sterile" pyuria of chronic pyelonephritis and chronic nonspecific urethritis and cystitis may mimic tuberculous infection. Culture should serve to distinguish tuberculosis from these.

Treatment

Intensive and prolonged antituberculosis therapy is indicated, employing 2 or 3 drugs simultaneously for 12–18 months (see Chapter 29). In 1984, the drugs of choice (and dosages) appear to be isoniazid, 5–8 mg/kg/d (usually 300 mg daily orally); ethambutol, 15 mg/kg/d as a single oral dose; and rifampin, 10–20 mg/kg/d (usually 600 mg as a single oral dose). Alternative drugs are listed in Chapter 29.

Pyridoxine, 100 mg/d orally, is usually given simultaneously with isoniazid to prevent neurotoxic reactions. Surgical procedures are generally limited to situations where extensive destruction of one kidney makes it unlikely that infection can be eradicated and useful function restored (nephrectomy) or where obstruction in the tract interferes with proper function, or when erosion of a vessel leads to severe bleeding.

Prognosis

The outlook depends largely on the degree of destruction of renal tissue and impairment of renal function. If urinary tract tuberculosis is detected early, prolonged drug treatment can suppress and arrest the infectious process successfully. Structural defects resulting from infection or fibrosis require surgical correction.

Alvarez S, McCabe WR: Extrapulmonary tuberculosis revisited. *Medicine* 1984;**63**:25.

American Thoracic Society: Treatment of tuberculosis and other mycobacterial diseases. *Am Rev Respir Dis* 1983;**127**:790.

Christensen WI: Genitourinary tuberculosis. *Medicine* 1974; **53**:377.

Gow JG: Genitourinary tuberculosis: A 7-year review. *Br J Urol* 1979;**51**:239.

PROSTATITIS

Bacteria may reach the prostate from the bloodstream (eg, tuberculosis) or from the urethra. Prostatitis is thus commonly associated with urethritis (eg, gonococcal, chlamydial, mycoplasmal) or with active bacterial infection of the lower urinary tract. Perineal pain, lumbosacral backache, fever, dysuria, and frequency may be symptoms of prostatic bacterial infection ("prostatosis").

Prostatitis may be acute or chronic. However, acute prostatitis commonly develops into a chronic state, and overmanipulation of chronic prostatitis gives rise to acute stage symptoms.

Clinical Findings

A. Symptoms and Signs: Symptoms of acute prostatitis usually are perineal pain, fever, dysuria, frequency, and urethral discharge. To the palpating finger, the prostate feels enlarged, boggy, and very tender; fluctuation occurs only if an abscess has formed. Even gentle palpation of the prostate results in expression of copious purulent discharge.

Symptoms of chronic prostatitis may include lumbosacral backache, perineal pain, mild dysuria and frequency, and scanty urethral discharge. Palpation reveals an irregularly enlarged, firm, and slightly tender prostate.

B. Laboratory Findings: With acute febrile prostatitis, there is often leukocytosis. The expressed prostatic fluid shows pus cells and bacteria on microscopy and culture. During the acute phase, prostatic palpation may express frank pus. The first glass of urine contains a far larger number of pus cells and bacteria than subsequent urine samples.

Differential Diagnosis

Prostatitis should be differentiated from lower urinary tract infection, although it may form part of it. In the latter case, the infected prostate may serve as a source of recurrent lower urinary tract infections. Other perirectal infections may be considered, as well as epididymitis, gonococcal infection, and tuberculosis.

Complications

Epididymitis and cystitis as well as urethritis commonly accompany acute prostatitis. Chronic prostatitis commonly predisposes to recurrent urinary tract infection and occasionally to urethral obstruction and acute urinary retention.

Treatment

A. Specific Measures: For acute prostatitis, initial treatment may consist of sulfamethoxazole, 400 mg, plus trimethoprim, 80 mg, 6–8 tablets daily; tetracycline, 2 g daily by mouth; or ampicillin, 250 mg 6 times daily, until culture of prostatic fluid and susceptibility tests indicate the drug of choice. Treatment for 2 weeks usually results in subsidence of the acute inflammation, but chronic prostatitis may continue.

Eradication of bacteria in chronically infected prostatic tissue is exceedingly difficult. Antimicrobial drugs diffusing best into prostatic acini must be lipid-soluble and basic (eg, trimethoprim-sulfamethoxazole). Erythromycins are quite active in the prostate but effective mainly against gram-positive organisms, which are rare in urinary tract infections and prostatitis. Conversely, most drugs that are active against gram-negative coliform bacteria (the commonest cause of prostatitis) fail to reach the prostatic acini.

B. General Measures: During the acute phase, the patient must be kept at bed rest, with adequate hydration, and kept comfortable by means of analgesics, stool softeners, and sitz baths. Urethral instrumentation and prostatic massage must be avoided.

Chronic prostatitis should be treated by prolonged antimicrobial therapy accompanied by vigorous prostatic massage once weekly to promote drainage. Total prostatectomy is curative but has a high morbidity and a significant mortality rate. Transurethral prostatectomy offers uncertain benefits. Surgical drainage of an abscess is mandatory.

Prognosis

Although the symptoms of acute prostatitis will usually subside with treatment, the prospects for the eventual elimination of chronic prostatitis are often discouraging.

Meares EM: Prostatitis: Review of pharmacokinetics and therapy. *Rev Infect Dis* 1982;**4**:475.

Paulson DF, White RD: Trimethoprim-sulfamethoxazole and minocycline in the treatment of culture proved bacterial prostatitis. *J Urol* 1978;**120**:184.

URINARY STONES

Urinary stones and calcification in the kidney may be associated with metabolic disease; may be secondary to infection in the urinary tract; may occur in sponge kidney, tuberculosis of the kidney, or papillary necrosis; or may be idiopathic. The incidence of urinary tract calculus is higher in men.

NEPHROCALCINOSIS

Essentials of Diagnosis

- Asymptomatic, or symptoms of primary disease producing hypercalciuria.

- Physical signs of the primary disease.
- Anemia is common.
- Blood chemistry findings of primary disease plus variable degrees of renal insufficiency.

General Considerations

Chronic hypercalciuria and hyperphosphaturia may result in precipitation of calcium salts in the renal parenchyma. The commonest causes are hyperparathyroidism, hypervitaminosis D (particularly with associated high calcium intake), and excess calcium and alkali intake. Chronic pyelonephritis predisposes to nephrocalcinosis. Other causes include acute osteoporosis following immobilization, sarcoidosis, renal tubular acidosis, the de Toni-Fanconi syndrome, and destruction of bone by metastatic carcinoma.

Clinical Findings

The symptoms, signs, and laboratory findings are those of the primary disease. The diagnosis is usually established by x-ray demonstration of calcium deposits in the kidney, which appear as minute calcific densities with linear streaks in the region of the renal papillae. True renal stones may be present as well in these patients.

Differential Diagnosis

Differentiate from renal calculi, renal tuberculosis, and medullary sponge kidney.

Treatment

Specific treatment is directed at the primary disorder. Particular attention is directed to treatment of urinary tract infection and renal insufficiency. When renal tubular acidosis or the de Toni-Fanconi defect is present, it is essential to maintain a high fluid intake, to replace cation deficit, and to alkalinize the urine with sodium bicarbonate. See Renal Tubular Acidosis, p 563.

RENAL STONE

Essentials of Diagnosis

- Often asymptomatic.
- Symptoms of obstruction of calix or ureteropelvic junction, with flank pain and colic.
- Nausea, vomiting, abdominal distention.
- Hematuria.
- Chills and fever and bladder irritability if infection is present.

Etiology

A. Excessive Excretion of Relatively Insoluble Urinary Constituents:

1. **Calcium –**
   a. Hypercalciuria with normocalcemia.
      (1) Idiopathic hypercalciuria (30–40% of stone formers).

   (2) Renal tubular acidosis, type I; distal tubule deficit (see p 564).
   b. Hypercalciuria with hypercalcemia or normocalcemia.
      (1) Primary hyperparathyroidism (see p 717). (Five to 7% of stone formers.)
      (2) High vitamin D intake.
      (3) Renal tubular acidosis, type I.
      (4) Excessive intake of milk and alkali.
      (5) Destructive bone disease due to neoplasm or of metabolic origin (corticosteroid excess, thyrotoxicosis).
      (6) Sarcoidosis.
      (7) Prolonged immobilization.

2. **Oxalate –** Over half of urinary stones are composed of calcium oxalate or calcium oxalate mixed with phosphate.
   a. Congenital or familial oxaluria (rare).
   b. Ileal disease; ileal resection or bypass.
   c. High oxalate intake (tea, cocoa, spinach, beets, rhubarb, parsley, nuts). Vitamin C is an oxalate precursor.
   d. Methoxyflurane anesthesia.

3. **Uric acid –**
   a. Gout – Stones may form spontaneously or as a result of treatment with uricosuric agents.
   b. Hyperuricosuria with or without hyperuricemia. Idiopathic or secondary to high purine intake (see C, below).
   c. Anticancer therapy with agents that cause rapid destruction of cells, resulting in increased excretion of uric acid.
   d. Myeloproliferative disease (leukemia, lymphoma, myeloid metaplasia, etc).

4. **Cystine –** Hereditary cystinuria (see p 574).

B. Physical Changes in the Urine:

1. Increased concentration of urine solute as a consequence of low intake of fluid and low urine volume.
2. Urinary pH –
   a. Low pH – Organic substances less soluble (uric acid, cystine).
   b. High pH – Inorganic salts usually less soluble (calcium phosphate and mixed calcium phosphate–calcium oxalate stones).
   c. High pH associated with urinary tract infection with organisms containing urease (especially *Proteus*). Hydrolysis of urea yields ammonia, which produces an increase in pH. $Mg + NH_4 + PO_4^{3-}$ precipitates as magnesium ammonium phosphate (struvite) to form stones.

C. Nucleus (Nidus) for Stone Formation:

1. Uricosuria – Crystals of uric acid or sodium hydrogen urate may initiate precipitation of calcium oxalate from solution.
2. Bits of necrotic tissue, blood clots, and clumps of bacteria, particularly in the presence of stasis or infection, may serve as a nucleus for stone formation.

D. Congenital or Acquired Deformities of the Kidneys:

1. Sponge kidney.
2. Horseshoe kidney.
3. Local caliceal obstruction or defect.

General Considerations

The location and size of the stone and the presence or absence of obstruction determine the changes that occur in the kidney and caliceal system. The pathologic changes may be modified by ischemia due to pressure or by infection.

Clinical Findings

A. Symptoms and Signs: Often a stone trapped in a calix or in the renal pelvis is asymptomatic. If a stone produces obstruction in a calix or at the ureteropelvic junction, dull flank pain or even colic may occur. Hematuria and symptoms of accompanying infection may be present. Nausea and vomiting may suggest enteric disease. Flank tenderness and abdominal distention may be the only findings.

B. Laboratory Findings: Urinalysis is the most important laboratory test. In addition to gross or microscopic hematuria, the presence of pyuria suggests associated urinary tract infection. Crystals may provide a lead to the composition of the stone and the underlying metabolic disorder (hypercalciuria, gout, cystinuria, renal tubular acidosis, oxaluria). Chemical analysis of serum with a broad biochemical profile will assist in confirming the metabolic disorder. Always obtain a stone for analysis.

C. Imaging Procedures: A plain abdominal x-ray film (kidney, ureter, and bladder) will assist in discovering symptomatic and asymptomatic radiopaque stones and related bone lesions (eg, hyperparathyroidism). If the stone has not passed within a day or 2 after the acute onset of symptoms, radionuclide renography may reveal the presence of persistent obstruction. Ultrasonography will usually define renal size and caliceal and ureteral dilatation above the site of obstruction. Excretory and retrograde urograms help to delineate the site and degree of obstruction and to confirm the presence of nonopaque stones (uric acid).

Differential Diagnosis

Differentiate from acute pyelonephritis, renal tumor, renal tuberculosis, and infarction of the kidney.

Complications

Infection and hydronephrosis may destroy renal tissue.

Prevention of Further Stone Formation

(1) Obtain a stone for analysis whenever possible. Useful for diagnosis and therapy.

(2) Review the family history to identify metabolic causes (cystinuria, gout, hypercalcemia, renal tubular acidosis, hyperoxaluria).

(3) Treat predisposing diseases such as hyperparathyroidism, gout, cystinuria, renal tubular acidosis, infection, sarcoidosis, hypercortisolism, and hyperoxaluria and anatomic defects of the urinary tract.

(4) Instruct the patient to maintain a high fluid intake to produce a dilute urine, ie, urine volume of more than 2000 mL/d with a specific gravity less than 1.015.

(5) Maintain urine pH at a suitable level: (a) Above pH 6.5 for uric acid stones; above 7.5 for cystine stones: Use Shohl's solution (see p 564), 10–30 mL 5 times a day, ie, after each meal, at bedtime, and during the night. (b) Below pH 6.5 for struvite stones: There is no practical long-term therapy that will not produce metabolic acidosis. For a brief trial, one may use ascorbic acid, 3 g/d or more, or methionine, 8–12 g/d.

(6) If hyperuricosuria is present in those who form calcium stones, allopurinol, 100 mg twice a day, plus restriction of intake of purine-containing foods will often reduce stone formation.

(7) If idiopathic hypercalciuria is present, the patient should reduce calcium intake by avoiding milk and milk products, calcium-containing medications, and vitamin D-fortified foods. A high fluid intake is essential. Chronic use of thiazide diuretics in modest doses (hydrochlorothiazides, 50 mg twice daily, or equivalent) plus modest restriction of salt intake will reduce calcium excretion and may enhance excretion of magnesium, which has an inhibitory effect on stone formation. Inorganic orthophosphate has proved beneficial when used alone or with thiazides. Combinations of dibasic and monobasic phosphate salts of sodium and potassium provide a mix of neutral pH. Most formulations provide 250 mg phosphorus per capsule or tablet. Give in divided doses 3 or 4 times a day to provide a total of 1250–1500 mg of phosphorus per day. Cellulose phosphate chelates cations and may be used to reduce intestinal absorption of calcium. When used, it should be accompanied by a low-calcium diet and magnesium supplementation.

(8) Magnesium oxide inhibits calcium salt precipitation. If stones consist of calcium oxalate, a reduction of oxalate intake is in order. Cocoa, tea, rhubarb, spinach, Swiss chard, beets, parsley, nuts, and excess vitamin C should be avoided.

(9) Treat patients who are "idiopathic calcium stone formers" according to paragraphs 7 and 8 above.

(10) In the presence of urinary tract infection with urease-containing organisms, suppression of struvite stone formation is difficult. Infection must be eradicated or reduced with appropriate antibiotics (see pp 568 ff).

(11) Prevention of uric acid stones by inhibiting the formation of uric acid is now possible by blocking the conversion of xanthine to uric acid with the xanthine oxidase inhibitor allopurinol. The usual adult dose of allopurinol is 600 mg/d (300 mg every 12 hours). This will reduce elevated serum uric acid to normal levels and markedly reduce the excretion of uric acid. It is effective even in the presence of renal failure associated with gouty nephropathy. The drug is

well tolerated and apparently produces no alteration of renal function. Treatment should be continued indefinitely in patients with gout (see Chapter 14) or myeloproliferative disorders. Allopurinol may be used in association with antileukemia and anticancer agents. While the allopurinol effect is developing, treatment should include a high fluid intake and alkalinization of the urine with sodium bicarbonate, 10–12 g/d in divided doses, or Shohl's solution, 50–150 mL/d.

(12) Cystine stone formation can be reduced by forcing fluids to produce a urine output of 3–4 L daily and alkalinizing the urine with sodium bicarbonate or sodium citrate and acetazolamide at bedtime. Urine pH should be maintained at 7.5 or higher, at which levels cystine solubility is greatly increased. A low-methionine diet may help, but protein deprivation must be avoided. Patients with severe cystinuria may require penicillamine, which complexes cystine and reduces the total excretion of cystine. There are many side effects of penicillamine that appear to be dose-related.

Treatment

Small stones may be passed. They do no harm if infection is not present. Larger stones may be removed by percutaneous nephrostomy plus mechanical, ultrasonic, or electrohydraulic disintegration of the stone to permit easy removal of the debris. Surgical removal may be required. Nephrectomy may be necessary.

Combat infection with appropriate antibiotics. Drainage of an abscess may be required.

Prognosis

If obstruction can be prevented and infection eradicated, the prognosis is good.

URETERAL STONE

Essentials of Diagnosis

- Obstruction of ureter produces severe colic with radiation of pain to regions determined by the position of the stone in the ureter.
- Gastrointestinal symptoms common.
- Urine usually contains fresh red cells.
- May be asymptomatic.
- Exacerbations of infection when obstruction occurs.

General Considerations

Ureteral stones are formed in the kidney but produce symptoms as they pass down the ureter.

Clinical Findings

A. Symptoms and Signs: The pain of ureteral colic is intense. The patient may be in mild shock, with cold, moist skin. There is marked tenderness in the costovertebral angle. Abdominal and back muscle spasm may be present. Referred areas of hyperesthesia may be demonstrated.

B. Laboratory Findings: As for renal stone.

C. X-Ray and Instrumental Examination: X-rays may show the stone lodged in the ureter or at the ureterovesical junction. Nonopaque stones can be demonstrated by radionuclide renography, ultrasonography, or excretory urograms, which reveal the site of obstruction and the dilated ureteropelvic system above it. Because of the danger of infection, cystoscopy and ureteral catheterization should be avoided unless retrograde urography is essential.

Differential Diagnosis

Differentiate from clots due to hemorrhage, and from tumor, acute pyelonephritis, and acute cholecystitis.

Prevention

Proceed as for renal stone. Every effort should be made to obtain a stone for analysis.

Treatment

A. Specific Measures: Most stones will pass spontaneously if spasm of the ureter is relieved and fluids are forced. By a cystoscopic or percutaneous approach, removal of stones may be accomplished with baskets or by ultrasound lithotripsy. Surgical ureterolithotomy may be necessary.

B. General Measures: Morphine or other opiates should be given in doses adequate to control pain. Morphine sulfate, 8 mg (or equivalent dosage of other drugs), may be given intravenously and repeated in 5–10 minutes if necessary. Thereafter, subcutaneous administration is usually adequate. Atropine sulfate, 0.8 mg subcutaneously, or methantheline bromide, 0.1 g intravenously, may be used as an antispasmodic.

Prognosis

If obstruction and infection can be treated successfully, the outlook is excellent.

VESICAL STONE

Essentials of Diagnosis

- Bladder irritability, with dysuria, urgency, and frequency.
- Interruption of urinary stream as stone occludes urethra.
- Hematuria.
- Pyuria.

General Considerations

Vesical stones occur most commonly when there is residual urine infected with urea-splitting organisms (eg, *Proteus,* staphylococci). Thus, bladder stones are associated with urinary stasis due to bladder neck or urethral obstruction, diverticula, neurogenic bladder, and cystocele. Foreign bodies in the bladder act as foci for stone formation. Ulceration and bladder inflammation predispose to stone formation.

Most vesical stones are composed of calcium phosphate, calcium oxalate, or magnesium ammonium phosphate. Uric acid stones are common in the presence of an enlarged prostate and uninfected urine.

Clinical Findings

A. Symptoms and Signs: Symptoms of chronic urinary obstruction or stasis and infection are usually present. Dysuria, frequency and urgency, and interruption of the urinary stream (causing pain in the penis) when the stone occludes the urethra are common complaints. Physical findings include prostatic enlargement, evidence of distended (neurogenic) bladder, and cystocele. The stone may be palpable.

B. Laboratory Findings: The urine usually shows signs of infection and contains red cells.

C. X-Ray and Cystoscopic Examination: X-ray examination shows the calcified stone, and urograms show the bladder abnormalities and upper urinary tract dilatation due to long-standing back pressure. Direct cystoscopic examination may be necessary.

Treatment & Prognosis

Stones can be removed by fragmentation using ultrasound, mechanical, or electrohydraulic lithotripsy. Surgical lithotomy may be necessary.

Urethral obstruction, cystocele, and other contributing anatomic factors must be eliminated by appropriate surgery.

Give analgesics as required, and treat infection with appropriate antibiotics.

The prognosis is excellent.

Brenner RJ et al: Incidence of radiographically evident bone disease, nephrocalcinosis and nephrolithiasis in various types of renal tubular acidosis. *N Engl J Med* 1982;**307**:217.

Broadus AE, Thier SO: Metabolic basis of renal-stone disease. *N Engl J Med* 1979;**300**:839.

Coe FL: Prevention of kidney stones. *Am J Med* 1981;**71**:514.

Smith DR: *General Urology,* 11th ed. Lange, 1984.

Smith LH: Medical treatment of idiopathic calcium urolithiasis. *The Kidney* 1983;**16**:9.

Symposium on surgery of stone disease. *Urol Clin North Am* 1983;**10**:583. [Entire issue.]

• • •

URETERAL OBSTRUCTION

Obstruction of one or both ureters may be due to a variety of acquired diseases, including injury to ureters during pelvic surgery; postirradiation fibrosis; compression by extrinsic neoplastic disease; occlusion of the ureterovesical junction by cancer of the bladder, prostate, uterine cervix, or rectum; endometriosis; chronic infections of the urinary tract; retroperitoneal fasciitis; and chronic vesical outlet obstruction from prostatic hyperplasia or cancer, urethral stricture, or vesical stone.

Although rare, retroperitoneal fasciitis (fibroplasia) warrants further discussion. Chronic inflammatory disease of retroperitoneal tissues over the lower lumbar vertebrae may compress one or both ureters, with consequent dilatation of the ureter and renal pelvis proximal to the site of obstruction. The vena cava and, occasionally, the aorta or other major arteries in the area may be occluded. Rarely, extension upward may extend to the mediastinum, with occlusion of retroperitoneal viscera.

The reaction occurs in some patients taking methysergide for migraine or beta-blocker drugs (propranolol, atenolol, oxyprenolol) for the usual indications. Retroperitoneal fibrosis may accompany sclerosing Hodgkin's disease. Lymphomas and spread of metastatic tumor retroperitoneally may simulate the disease by occluding the ureters and great vessels.

Symptoms and signs include low back pain, abdominal pain, anorexia, weight loss, fever, urinary frequency, and, depending on the degree of renal insufficiency, polyuria or anuria. Occlusion of arteries trapped in the fibrotic reaction can produce claudication and weakness of the legs and impotence. A mass is often palpable over the promontory of the sacrum.

Laboratory findings are those of impaired renal function secondary to chronic obstruction, with elevated blood urea nitrogen and serum creatinine, metabolic acidosis, and anemia (see Chronic Renal Insufficiency). Excretory urograms show medial deviation of the ureters and dilatation of the excretory tract proximal to the obstruction.

Therapy includes abstaining from the offending drug and a trial of corticosteroid. Give prednisone, 30–60 mg/d orally, until evidence of improvement permits reduction to a maintenance dose of 5–15 mg/d. Operation may be required to relieve ureteral obstruction.

URINARY INCONTINENCE

Urinary incontinence can be an embarrassing and distressing condition. The causes of incontinence include congenital defects of bladder and urethra; injury to urethral sphincters during childbirth or after surgery on or adjacent to the bladder exit; urinary tract infection; diminished bladder capacity resulting from intrinsic disease; chronic dilatation of the bladder resulting from bladder neck obstruction (overflow incontinence); upper motor neuron lesions (spinal cord injury, stroke, etc); and stress incontinence. The history, a complete urologic examination, and vesical function tests will delineate the diagnosis and proper therapy.

Finkbeiner AE, Bissada NK: Drug therapy for lower urinary tract dysfunction. *Urol Clin North Am* 1980;**7**:3.

Smith DR: *General Urology,* 11th ed. Lange, 1984.

TUMORS OF THE GENITOURINARY TRACT

ADENOCARCINOMA OF KIDNEY
(Hypernephroma)

Essentials of Diagnosis
- Painless gross hematuria.
- Fever.
- Enlarged kidney may be palpable.
- Evidence of metastases.

General Considerations
The commonest malignant tumor of the kidney is adenocarcinoma, which occurs more frequently in men. It rarely occurs before age 35 and more commonly after age 50. This tumor metastasizes early to the lungs, liver, and long bones.

Adenocarcinoma of the kidney apparently arises from renal tubule cells or adenomas. It invades blood vessels early. On microscopic examination, the cells resemble renal tubule cells arranged in cords and varying patterns.

Clinical Findings
A. Symptoms and Signs: Gross hematuria is the most frequent sign. Fever is often the only symptom. A flank mass may be palpable. Pain of renal or ureteral origin may occur with bleeding into the tumor or renal pelvis. Vena caval occlusion may produce characteristic patterns of collateral circulation and edema of the legs.

A hypernephroma may not produce classic symptoms of renal tumor. It may produce symptoms and signs suggesting a wide variety of diseases: fever of obscure origin, leukemoid reaction, refractory anemia, erythrocytosis, hypercalcemia, hypoglycemia, peripheral neuropathy, and increased production of gonadotropins and prostaglandins.

B. Laboratory Findings: Polycythemia occasionally develops as a result of increased secretion of erythropoietin by the tumor. Anemia is more commonly found. Hematuria is almost always present. The erythrocyte sedimentation rate is rapid.

C. X-Ray Findings: X-ray examination may show an enlarged kidney. Metastatic lesions of bone and lung may be revealed. Excretory or retrograde urography (sometimes both) are necessary to establish the presence of a renal tumor. CT scans with contrast medium often can differentiate renal cyst or anomaly from tumor, define tumor size and consistency, and document any extension of tumor into the renal vein and vena cava. Radionuclide renography is also useful.

D. Ultrasonic Scan: Renal size and contour can be determined by ultrasound records. Cysts can often be differentiated from solid tumors. With visualization by real time ultrasound scan, an experienced operator may perform "thin needle" biopsy of the renal mass.

Presence of tumor in the renal vein and vena cava can often be demonstrated.

Differential Diagnosis
Differentiate from focal nephritis, hydronephrosis, polycystic kidneys, renal cyst, and renal tuberculosis.

Treatment
Nephrectomy is indicated if no metastases are present. Even when metastases are present, nephrectomy may be indicated for intractable bleeding or pain.

X-ray irradiation of metastases may be of value, although the lesions are usually fairly radioresistant. Isolated single pulmonary metastases can occasionally be removed surgically. At present, chemotherapy is ineffective. Palliation may be achieved with medroxyprogesterone.

Prognosis
The course is variable. Some patients may not develop metastases for 10–15 years after removal of the primary tumor. About 35% of patients live more than 5 years.

Cherukuri SV et al: Systemic effects of hypernephroma. *Urology* 1977;**10**:93.

McDonald MW: Current therapy for renal cell carcinoma. *J Urol* 1982;**127**:211.

EMBRYOMA OF THE KIDNEY
(Wilms' Tumor)

Embryoma is a highly malignant mixed tumor that occurs almost exclusively in children under 6 years of age. It metastasizes early to the lungs, liver, and brain.

Weight loss and anorexia are the most common signs. Pain occurs rarely. The enlarged kidney is usually easily palpable. Metastases produce an enlarged liver. Hypertension is common. Anemia may be present. The urine is not remarkable. X-ray examination demonstrates the tumor and metastases in the lung. Excretory urograms and gastrointestinal examination help to determine the size of the tumor.

Wilms' tumor must be differentiated from hydronephrosis, polycystic kidney disease, and neuroblastoma of the adrenal medulla.

Treatment consists of nephrectomy followed by local irradiation and irradiation of metastases. Antitumor chemotherapy with dactinomycin increases the cure rate and is usually effective in controlling local recurrences and metastases. Vincristine and doxorubicin have also been effective. (See Chapter 33.)

Cure can be achieved if metastases have not occurred before nephrectomy.

D'Angio GJ et al: Wilms' tumor: An update. *Cancer* 1980; **45(Suppl)**:1791.

TUMORS OF THE RENAL PELVIS & URETER

Epithelial tumors of the renal pelvis and ureter are relatively rare. They are usually papillary and tend to metastasize along the urinary tract. Epidermoid tumors are highly malignant and metastasize early. Transitional cell tumors have occurred in cases of interstitial nephritis and papillary necrosis due to phenacetin abuse.

Painless hematuria is the most common complaint. Colic occurs with obstruction due to blood clot or tumor. Tenderness in the flank may be found. Anemia due to blood loss occurs. The urine contains red cells and clots; white cells and bacteria are present when infection is superimposed. Urography should reveal the filling defect in the pelvis or show obstruction and dilatation of the ureter. At cystoscopy, the bleeding from the involved ureter may be seen and satellite tumors identified. Exfoliative cytologic studies should be done.

Radical removal of the kidney, the involved ureter, and the periureteral portion of the bladder should be done unless metastases are extensive.

Irradiation of metastases is usually of little value.

The prognosis depends upon the type of tumor. With anaplastic neoplasms, death usually occurs within 2 years.

TUMORS OF THE BLADDER

Essentials of Diagnosis

- Hematuria.
- Suprapubic pain and bladder symptoms associated with infection.
- Visualization of tumor at cystoscopy.

General Considerations

Bladder tumors are second to prostatic tumors in frequency. At least 75% of bladder tumors occur in men over age 50. Tumors usually arise at the base of the bladder and involve ureteral orifices and the bladder neck. The common tumor is papillomatous of low-grade malignancy; epidermoid tumors, adenocarcinomas, and sarcomas are rare. Metastases involve regional lymph nodes, bone, liver, and lungs.

Clinical Findings

A. Symptoms and Signs: Hematuria is the commonest symptom. Cystitis with frequency, urgency, and dysuria is a frequent complication. With encroachment of the tumor on the bladder neck, the urinary stream is diminished. Suprapubic pain occurs as the tumor extends beyond the bladder. Obstruction of the ureters produces hydronephrosis, frequently accompanied by renal infection, in which case the signs of urinary tract infection may be present. Physical examination is not remarkable. The bladder tumor may be palpable on bimanual (abdominorectal or abdominovaginal) examination.

B. Laboratory Findings: Anemia is common. The urine contains red cells, white cells, and bacteria. Exfoliative cytology is usually confirmatory.

C. X-Ray and Instrumental Examination: Excretory urography may reveal ureteral obstruction. Cystograms usually show the tumor. Cystoscopy and biopsy confirm the diagnosis.

Differential Diagnosis

Hematuria and pain can be produced by other tumors of the urinary tract, urinary calculi, renal tuberculosis, acute cystitis, or acute nephritis.

Treatment

A. Specific Measures: Tumor staging is required to serve as a guide to selection of treatment. Transurethral resection may be adequate to remove local and superficial tumors. Cystectomy with ureterosigmoidostomy or another urinary diversion procedure is required for invasive tumors. Radiation therapy may be useful for more anaplastic tumors. Thiotepa instillations may be effective in eradicating superficial and papillary bladder epithelial tumors. For metastatic disease, fluorouracil, cisplatin, and doxorubicin may be effective.

B. General Measures: Urinary tract infection should be controlled with appropriate antibiotics. Anastomosis of ureters to an isolated loop of ileum or sigmoid colon, one end of which is brought to the skin to act as a conduit, is relatively free of renal complications and of alteration of body fluid electrolytes. An isolated loop of ileum or sigmoid colon can be used as a urinary conduit when anastomosed to the ureters.

Prognosis

There is a tendency toward recurrence and increasing malignancy. With infiltrating carcinomas the outlook is poor even with radical resection.

Grossman HB: Current therapy of bladder carcinoma. *J Urol* 1979;**121**:1.

Soloway MS: Rationale for intensive intravesical chemotherapy for superficial bladder cancer. *J Urol* 1980;**123**:461.

BENIGN PROSTATIC HYPERPLASIA

Essentials of Diagnosis

- Prostatism: hesitancy and straining to initiate micturition, reduced force and caliber of the urinary stream, nocturia.
- Acute urinary retention.
- Enlarged prostate.
- Uremia follows prolonged obstruction.

General Considerations

Hyperplasia of the prostatic lateral and subcervical lobes that are invaded by periurethral glands results in enlargement of the prostate and urethral obstruction.

Clinical Findings

A. Symptoms and Signs: The symptoms of prostatism increase in severity as the degree of urethral obstruction increases. Symptoms may be overlooked or not reported when the progression of obstruction is slow. On rectal examination, the prostate is usually found to be enlarged. The bladder may be seen and palpated as retention of urine increases. Infection commonly occurs with stasis and retention of "residual urine." Hematuria may occur. Uremia may result from prolonged back pressure and severe bilateral hydronephrosis. Determination of blood urea nitrogen may provide the only clue to slowly advancing and relatively asymptomatic obstructive disease. Residual urine can be measured by postvoiding catheterization. In the presence of prostatism, ganglionic blocking agents and parasympatholytic drugs used in the treatment of hypertension, as well as tranquilizers, weaken the power of detrusor contraction, thus causing symptoms simulating vesical neck obstruction and in some cases urinary retention.

B. X-Ray and Cystoscopic Examination: Excretory urograms reveal the complications of back pressure: ureteral dilatation, hydronephrosis, and postvoiding urinary retention. Cystoscopy will reveal enlargement of the prostate and secondary bladder wall changes such as trabeculation, diverticula, inflammation due to infection, and vesical stone.

Differential Diagnosis

Other causes of urethral obstruction include urethral stricture, vesical stone, bladder tumor, neurogenic bladder, or carcinoma of the prostate.

Treatment

A. Specific Measures: Conservative (nonsurgical) management should be undertaken only in collaboration with a urologist. Relieve acute urinary retention by catheterization. Maintain catheter drainage if the degree of obstruction is severe. Surgery is usually necessary. There are various indications for each of the 4 approaches: transurethral resection, or prostatectomy by suprapubic, retropubic, and perineal procedures.

B. General Measures: Treat infection of the urinary tract with appropriate antibiotics. The patient who develops postobstructive diuresis must be sustained with appropriate water and electrolyte replacement.

Prognosis

Surgical resection will relieve symptoms. The surgical mortality rate is low.

CARCINOMA OF THE PROSTATE

Essentials of Diagnosis

- Prostatism.
- Hard consistency of the prostate.
- Metastases to bone produce pain, particularly in the low back.

- Anemia. Elevated serum acid phosphatase with extension of the cancer beyond the prostatic capsule.

General Considerations

Cancer of the prostate is rare before age 60. It metastasizes early to the bones of the pelvis and locally may produce urethral obstruction with subsequent renal damage. The growth of the tumor is increased by androgens and inhibited by estrogens. The prostatic tissue is rich in acid phosphatase, and when cancer has extended beyond the prostate to the periprostatic tissue or to bone, the serum acid phosphatase is increased. The serum acid phosphatase concentration thus provides a good index of extension and growth of the tumor.

Clinical Findings

A. Symptoms and Signs: Obstructive symptoms similar to those of benign prostatic hyperplasia are common. Rectal examination reveals a stone-hard prostate that is often nodular and fixed. Low back pain occurs with metastases to the bones of the pelvis and spine. Pathologic fractures may occur at the sites of metastases. Obstruction may produce renal damage and the symptoms and signs of renal insufficiency. An enlarged nodular liver and an enlarged supraclavicular sentinel lymph node are late signs of metastatic disease.

B. Laboratory Findings: Anemia may be extreme if bone marrow is replaced by tumor. The urine may show evidence of infection. Serum prostatic acid phosphatase is increased when metastases have occurred, and serum alkaline phosphatase may be elevated as new bone is formed at the site of metastases. Biopsy by transurethral resection or by needle aspiration through the perineum establishes the diagnosis.

C. X-Ray Findings: Very early experience with nuclear magnetic resonance (NMR) imaging shows it to be a sensitive indicator of the presence of cancer within the prostate. X-ray examination of the bones of the pelvis, spine, ribs, and skull will reveal the typical osteoblastic metastases. Excretory urograms delineate changes secondary to urethral obstruction and the back pressure of urine retention. Lymphangiography may demonstrate metastases to pelvic nodes. Radionuclide bone scan with technetium Tc 99m polyphosphate delineates bone metastases.

Differential Diagnosis

Differentiate from benign prostatic hyperplasia, urethral stricture, vesical stone, bladder tumor, and neurogenic bladder.

Treatment

Every effort must be made to ascertain the stage of disease by anatomic extent and histologic characteristics in order to apply appropriate therapy. Before metastasis has occurred, cure may be obtained by radical resection of the prostate, including the seminal vesicles and a portion of the bladder neck, with or without lymph node dissection. Palliative therapy includes transurethral resection to relieve obstruction. Interstitial implantation of radioactive iodine (^{125}I) has proved useful in selected cases of localized cancer. Radiotherapy with the linear accelerator or radioactive cobalt has provided good remission. Irradiation of bone metastases may afford relief. In late stages (stage D), antiandrogen therapy slows the rate of growth and extension of the cancer. Orchiectomy or estrogen therapy alone is often effective in reducing symptoms and extending survival. Chemotherapy is of little use.

The effectiveness of therapy can be judged by clinical response and by periodic measurements of the serum acid and alkaline phosphatase.

Prognosis

Palliative therapy is often not effective for long. Most patients die within 3 years; a few survive for 5–10 years.

Klein LA: Prostatic carcinoma. *N Engl J Med* 1979;**300**:824.
Murphy GP: Prostate cancer: Continuing progress. *CA* 1981; **31**:96.

TUMORS OF THE TESTIS
(See also Chapter 19.)

Essentials of Diagnosis

- Painless enlargement of the testis.
- Mass does not transilluminate.
- Evidence of metastases.

General Considerations

The incidence of testicular tumors is about 0.5% of all types of cancer in males. Tumors occur most frequently between ages 18 and 35 and are often malignant. Classification of tumors of the testes is based upon their origin from germinal components or from nongerminal cells. The most common are the germinal tumors: seminomas; embryonal tumors, including embryoma, choriocarcinoma, embryonal carcinoma, teratocarcinoma, and adult teratoma; and the gonadoblastomas of intersexes. Nongerminal tumors include those of interstitial cell, Sertoli cell, and stromal origin. Rarely, lymphomas, leukemias, plasmacytomas, and metastatic carcinoma may involve the testis.

Seminomas, the most common testicular tumors, tend to spread slowly via the lymphatics to the iliac and periaortic nodes and disseminate late. Embryonal tumors invade the spermatic cord and metastasize early, particularly to the lungs. Seminomas are usually radiosensitive; embryonal tumors are usually radioresistant. Chemotherapy may be helpful in choriocarcinoma.

Secretion of gonadotropic hormones occurs with only about 10% of tumors. The literature on tumor-hormonal relationships is limited and confusing, but gonadotropin secretion is usually indicative of a carcinomatous tumor.

Gynecomastia may be associated with testicular tumors. Interstitial cell tumors, which occur at any age and are rarely malignant, are occasionally associated with gynecomastia and with sexual precocity and virilization.

Clinical Findings

A. Symptoms and Signs: Painless enlargement of the testes is typical. The enlarged testis may produce a dragging inguinal pain. The tumor is usually symmetric and firm, and pressure does not produce the typical testicular pain. The tumors do not transilluminate. Attachment to the scrotal skin is rare. Gynecomastia may be present. Virilization may occur in preadolescent boys with Leydig cell tumors. Hydrocele may develop.

Metastases commonly go to regional lymph nodes and then to those of the mediastinum and supraclavicular region. The lungs and the liver are often sites of metastases.

B. Laboratory Findings: Gonadotropins may be present in high concentrations in urine and plasma in cases of choriocarcinoma, and pregnancy tests are positive. Radioimmunoassay for the beta unit of human chorionic gonadotropin is the test of choice for diagnosis and follow-up assessment. Urinary 17-ketosteroids are normal or low in Leydig cell tumors. Estrogens may be elaborated in both Sertoli cell and Leydig cell tumors. Alpha-fetoprotein is a useful tumor marker for diagnosis and assessment of the tumor burden of teratocarcinoma and embryonal carcinoma (derivatives of the extraembryonic primitive yolk sac).

C. X-Ray Findings: Pulmonary metastases are demonstrated by chest films. Lymphangiography will reveal enlarged iliac and periaortic nodes. Displacement of ureters by enlarged lymph nodes can be demonstrated by use of urography or venacavograms.

Differential Diagnosis

Tuberculosis, syphilitic orchitis (gumma of the testicle), hydrocele, spermatocele, and tumors or granulomas of the epididymis may produce similar local manifestations.

Treatment

The testicle should be removed and the lumbar and inguinal nodes examined. Radical resection of iliac and lumbar nodes is usually indicated except for seminoma, which is radiosensitive. Radiation is the treatment of choice following removal of the testis bearing a seminoma. Radiation is employed following radical surgery for other malignant tumors. Chemotherapy (Table 33–2) is effective against chorionic tumors (choriocarcinoma). Metastatic disease may be curable with combination chemotherapy, including cisplatin, vinblastine, and bleomycin. Other drugs that may be effective in various combinations include vincristine, dactinomycin, doxorubicin, and cyclophosphamide.

Prognosis

The presence of metastases or high gonadotropin secretion indicates a poor prognosis. Seminomas are least malignant, with 90% 5-year cures. Almost all patients with choriocarcinoma are dead within 2 years. Less than half of those with other tumors will live 5 years.

Braunstein GD et al: Germ cell tumors of the testes. *West J Med* 1977;**126**:362.

Drasga RE, Einhorn LE, Williams SD: The chemotherapy of testicular cancer. *CA* 1982;**32**:66.

Fraley EE, Lange PH, Kennedy BJ: Germ-cell testicular cancer in adults. (2 parts.) *N Engl J Med* 1979;**301**:1370, 1420.

•   •   •

References

Black DAK (editor): *Renal Disease*, 4th ed. Lippincott, 1978.

Brenner BM, Rector FC Jr: *The Kidney*, 2nd ed. Saunders, 1981.

Coe FL (editor): Symposium on renal therapeutics. *Med Clin North Am* 1978;**62**:1145. [Entire issue.]

Heptinstall RH: *Pathology of the Kidney*, 3rd ed. Little, Brown, 1983.

Klahr S: Pathophysiology of obstructive nephropathy. *Kidney Int* 1983;**23**:414.

Kunin CM: *Detection, Prevention, and Management of Urinary Tract Infections*, 3rd ed. Lea & Febiger, 1979.

Leaf A, Cotran RS: *Renal Pathophysiology*, 2nd ed. Oxford Univ Press, 1980.

Massry SG, Glassock RJ (editors): *Textbook of Nephrology*. Williams & Wilkins, 1983.

Maxwell MH, Kleeman CR (editors): *Clinical Disorders of Fluid and Electrolyte Metabolism*, 3rd ed. McGraw-Hill, 1980.

Schrier RW (editor): *Renal and Electrolyte Disorders*, 2nd ed. Little, Brown, 1980.

Smith DR: *General Urology*, 11th ed. Lange, 1984.

Stanbury JB et al (editors): *The Metabolic Basis of Inherited Disease*, 5th ed. McGraw-Hill, 1983.

Nervous System | 17

Michael J. Aminoff, MD, FRCP

HEADACHE

Headache is such a common complaint and can occur for so many different reasons that its proper evaluation may be difficult. Although underlying structural lesions are not present in most patients presenting with headache, it is nevertheless important to bear this possibility in mind. About one-third of patients with brain tumors, for example, present with a primary complaint of headache.

The intensity, quality, and site of pain—and especially the duration of the headache and the presence of associated neurologic symptoms—may provide clues to the underlying cause. The onset of severe headache in a previously well patient is more likely than chronic headache to relate to an intracranial disorder such as subarachnoid hemorrhage or meningitis. Headaches that disturb sleep, exertional headaches, and late-onset paroxysmal headaches are also more suggestive of an underlying structural lesion, as are headaches accompanied by neurologic symptoms such as drowsiness, visual or limb problems, seizures, or altered mental status. Chronic headaches are commonly due to migraine, tension, or depression, but they may be related to intracranial lesions, head injury, cervical spondylosis, dental or ocular disease, temporomandibular joint dysfunction, sinusitis, hypertension, and a wide variety of general medical disorders. All patients should be examined fully for these and other neurologic and medical problems. Depending on the initial clinical impression, the need for such investigations as CT scan of the head, electroencephalography, and lumbar puncture must be assessed on an individual basis. The diagnosis and treatment of primary neurologic disorders associated with headache are considered separately under these disorders.

Tension Headache

Patients frequently complain of poor concentration and other vague nonspecific symptoms, in addition to constant daily headaches that are often viselike or tight in quality and may be exacerbated by emotional stress, fatigue, noise, or glare. The headaches are usually generalized, may be most intense about the neck or back of the head, and are not associated with focal neurologic symptoms.

When treatment with simple analgesics does not suffice, diazepam or chlordiazepoxide may be helpful. If these are not effective, a trial of antimigrainous agents (see Migraine, below) is worthwhile. Techniques to induce relaxation are also useful and include massage, hot baths, and biofeedback. Psychologic counseling to explore underlying causes of chronic anxiety is often rewarding.

Depression Headache

Depression headaches are frequently worse on arising in the morning and may be accompanied by other symptoms of depression. Headaches are occasionally the focus of a somatic delusional system (eg, fear that the brain is "rotting"). Tricyclic antidepressant drugs are often helpful in conjunction with psychiatric consultation.

Migraine

Classic migrainous headache is a lateralized throbbing headache that occurs episodically following its onset in adolescence or early adult life. In many cases, however, the headaches do not conform to this pattern, although their associated features and response to antimigrainous preparations nevertheless suggest that they have a similar basis. In this broader sense, migrainous headaches may be lateralized or generalized, may be dull or throbbing, and are sometimes associated with anorexia, nausea, vomiting, photophobia, and blurring of vision (so-called sick headaches). They usually build up gradually and may last for several hours or longer. They have been related to dilatation and excessive pulsation of branches of the external carotid artery. Photopsia or other focal disturbances of neurologic function may precede or accompany the headaches and have been attributed to constriction of branches of the internal carotid artery.

Patients often give a family history of migraine. Attacks may be triggered by emotional or physical stress, lack or excess of sleep, missed meals, specific foods (eg, chocolate), alcoholic beverages, menstruation, or use of oral contraceptives.

An uncommon variant is so-called basilar artery migraine, in which blindness or visual disturbances throughout both visual fields are initially accompanied or followed by dysarthria, dysequilibrium, tinnitus, and paresthesias periorally and distally and are sometimes followed by transient loss or impairment of consciousness or by a confusional state. This, in turn, is followed by a throbbing (usually occipital) headache, often with nausea and vomiting.

In ophthalmoplegic migraine, lateralized pain—often about the eye—is accompanied by nausea, vomiting, and diplopia due to transient external ophthalmoplegia. The ophthalmoplegia is due to third nerve palsy, sometimes with accompanying sixth nerve involvement, and may outlast the orbital pain by several days or even weeks. The ophthalmic division of the fifth nerve has also been affected in some patients. Ophthalmoplegic migraine is rare; more common causes of a painful ophthalmoplegia are internal carotid artery aneurysms and diabetes.

In rare instances, the neurologic or somatic disturbance accompanying typical migrainous headaches becomes the sole manifestation of an attack ("migraine equivalent"). On other occasions, the patient may be left with a permanent neurologic deficit following a migrainous attack, presumably because of irreversible cerebral ischemic damage.

Management of migraine consists of avoidance of any precipitating factors, together with prophylactic or symptomatic pharmacologic treatment if necessary.

During acute attacks, many patients find it helpful to rest in a quiet, darkened room until symptoms subside. A simple analgesic (eg, aspirin or propoxyphene) taken right away often provides relief, but treatment with extracranial vasoconstrictors or other drugs is sometimes necessary. Cafergot, a combination of ergotamine tartrate and caffeine, is often particularly helpful; 1–4 tablets are taken at the onset of headache or warning symptoms and more are taken after about 20 minutes if symptoms have not begun to subside. Ergonovine maleate, up to 5 tablets (1 mg) taken at the onset of symptoms, may also provide relief. Because of impaired absorption or vomiting during acute attacks, oral medication sometimes fails to help. Cafergot given rectally as suppositories, ergotamine tartrate given intramuscularly (0.25–0.5 mg), or dihydroergotamine mesylate given either intramuscularly or intravenously (0.5–1 mg) may be useful in such cases. Ergotamine-containing preparations may affect the gravid uterus and thus should be avoided during pregnancy.

Prophylactic treatment may be necessary if migrainous headaches occur frequently. Some of the more common drugs used for this purpose are listed in Table 17–1. Drugs that are least likely to produce severe or disabling side effects should be tried first. Several drugs may have to be tried in turn, however, before the headaches are brought under control. Once a drug has been found to help, it should be continued for several months. If the patient remains headache-free, the dose can then be tapered and the drug eventually withdrawn. Many patients have spontaneous remission, so that medication can be discontinued, at least for a while.

Cluster Headache (Migrainous Neuralgia)

Cluster headache affects predominantly middle-aged men. There is often no family history of headache or migraine. Episodes of severe unilateral periorbital pain occur daily for several weeks and are often accompanied by one or more of the following: ipsilateral nasal congestion, rhinorrhea, lacrimation, redness of the eye, and Horner's syndrome. Episodes usually occur at night, awaken the patient from sleep, and last for less than 2 hours. Spontaneous remission then occurs, and the patient remains well for weeks or months before another bout of closely spaced attacks occurs. During a bout, many patients report that alcohol triggers an attack; others report that stress, glare, or ingestion of specific foods occasionally precipitates attacks. In experimental studies, sublingual nitroglycerin or subcutaneous histamine was found to provoke attacks in some patients.

In occasional patients, typical attacks of pain and associated symptoms recur at intervals without remission. This variant has been referred to as chronic cluster headache.

Clinical examination reveals no abnormality apart from Horner's syndrome that either occurs transiently during an attack or, in long-standing cases, remains as a residual deficit between attacks.

Treatment of an individual attack with oral drugs

Table 17–1. Prophylactic treatment of migraine.*

Drug	Usual Adult Daily Dose (mg)	Common Side Effects
Propranolol	80–240	Fatigue, lassitude, depression, insomnia, nausea, vomiting, constipation.
Amitriptyline	10–150	Sedation, dry mouth, constipation, weight gain, blurred vision, edema, hypotension, urinary retention.
Ergonovine maleate	0.6–2	Nausea, abdominal pain, diarrhea.
Cyproheptadine	12–20	Sedation, dry mouth, epigastric discomfort, gastrointestinal disturbances.
Clonidine	0.2–0.6	Dry mouth, drowsiness, sedation, headache, constipation.
Methysergide	4–8	Nausea, vomiting, diarrhea, abdominal pain, cramps, weight gain, insomnia, edema, peripheral vasoconstriction. Retroperitoneal and pleuropulmonary fibrosis and fibrous thickening of cardiac valves may occur; patients must be closely supervised.

*Reproduced, with permission, from Aminoff MJ: Neurologic disorders. In: *Handbook of Medical Treatment*, 17th ed. Watts HD (editor). Jones, 1983.

is generally unsatisfactory, but use of ergotamine tartrate aerosol or inhalation of 100% oxygen (7 L/min for 15 minutes) is often effective. Drugs should be given to prevent further attacks until the ongoing bout is over. Ergotamine tartrate is an effective prophylactic and can be given as rectal suppositories (0.5–1 mg at night or twice daily), by mouth (2 mg daily), or by subcutaneous injection (0.25 mg 3 times daily for 5 days per week). Various prophylactic agents that have been found to be effective in individual patients are propranolol, amitriptyline, cyproheptadine, lithium carbonate (monitored by plasma lithium determination), prednisone (20–40 mg daily or on alternate days for 2 weeks, followed by gradual withdrawal), and methysergide (4–6 mg daily).

Giant Cell (Temporal or Cranial) Arteritis

The superficial temporal, vertebral, ophthalmic, and posterior ciliary arteries are often the most severely affected pathologically. The major symptom is headache, sometimes associated with myalgia, malaise, anorexia, masticatory claudication, weight loss, and other nonspecific complaints. Clinical examination commonly reveals tenderness of the scalp and over the temporal arteries, which may become thrombosed. Further details, including approaches to treatment, are given in Chapter 14.

Posttraumatic Headache

A variety of nonspecific symptoms may follow a closed head injury, regardless of whether or not consciousness is lost. Headache is often a conspicuous feature. Some authorities believe that psychologic factors bear on the development of the syndrome, because its development does not correlate with the severity of the injury and neurologic signs are lacking. Support for this view has been sought in reports that early settlement of litigation contributes to ultimate recovery. However, litigation is often not an issue, and most patients show no evidence of underlying psychopathologic disorder.

The headache itself usually appears within a day or so following injury, may worsen over the ensuing weeks, and then gradually subsides. It is usually a constant dull ache, with superimposed throbbing that may be localized, lateralized, or generalized. It is sometimes accompanied by nausea, vomiting, or scintillating scotomas.

Dysequilibrium, sometimes with a rotatory component, may also occur in the posttraumatic syndrome and is often enhanced by postural change or head movement. Impaired memory, poor concentration, emotional instability, and increased irritability are other common complaints and occasionally are the sole manifestations of the syndrome. The duration of symptoms relates in part to the severity of the original injury, but even trivial injuries are sometimes followed by symptoms that persist for months.

Special investigations are usually not helpful. The electroencephalogram may show minor nonspecific changes, while the electronystagmogram sometimes suggests either peripheral or central vestibulopathy. CT scans of the head usually show no abnormal findings.

Treatment is difficult, but optimistic encouragement and graduated rehabilitation, depending upon the occupational circumstances, are advised. Headaches often respond to simple analgesics, but severe headaches may necessitate treatment with amitriptyline, propranolol, or ergot derivatives.

Cough Headache

Severe head pain may be produced by coughing (and by straining, sneezing, and laughing) but, fortunately, usually lasts for only a few minutes or less. The pathophysiologic basis of the complaint is not known, and often there is no underlying structural lesion. However, intracranial lesions, usually in the posterior fossa (eg, Arnold-Chiari malformation, basilar impression), are present in about 10% of cases, and brain tumors or other space-occupying lesions may certainly present in this way. Accordingly, CT scanning should be undertaken in all patients and repeated annually, since a small structural lesion may not show up initially.

The disorder is usually self-limited, although it may persist for several years. For unknown reasons, symptoms sometimes clear completely after lumbar puncture. Indomethacin may provide relief.

Headache Due to Other Neurologic Causes

Intracranial mass lesions of all types may cause headache owing to displacement of vascular structures. Posterior fossa tumors often cause occipital pain, and supratentorial lesions lead to bifrontal headache, but such findings are too inconsistent to be of value in attempts at localizing a pathologic process. The headaches are nonspecific in character and may vary in severity from mild to severe. They may be worsened by exertion or postural change and may be associated with nausea and vomiting, but this is true of migraine also. Headaches are also a feature of pseudotumor cerebri (see p 603). Signs of focal or diffuse cerebral dysfunction or of increased intracranial pressure will indicate the need for further investigation. Similarly, a progressive headache disorder or the new onset of headaches in middle or later life merits investigation if no cause is apparent.

Cerebrovascular disease may be associated with headache, but the mechanism is unclear. Headache may occur with internal carotid artery occlusion or carotid dissection and after carotid endarterectomy. Diagnosis is facilitated by the clinical accompaniments and the circumstances in which the headache developed.

Acute severe headache accompanies subarachnoid hemorrhage and meningeal infections, but the accompanying signs of meningeal irritation and the frequent impairment of consciousness then indicate the need for further investigations. A dramatically severe headache may also occur in association with paroxysmal hypertension in patients with pheochromocytoma.

Dull or throbbing headache is a frequent sequela of lumbar puncture and may last for several days. It is aggravated by the erect posture and alleviated by recumbency. The exact mechanism is unclear, but it is commonly attributed to leakage of cerebrospinal fluid through the dural puncture site.

Caviness VS, O'Brien P: Headache. *N Engl J Med* 1980; **302**:446.

Couch JR, Hassanein RS: Amitriptyline in migraine prophylaxis. *Arch Neurol* 1979;**36**:695.

Diamond S, Dalessio DJ: *The Practicing Physician's Approach to Headache,* 3rd ed. Williams & Wilkins, 1982.

Diamond S, Medina JL: Benign exertional headache: Successful treatment with indomethacin. *Headache* 1979;**19**:249.

Kelly R: The post-traumatic syndrome. *J R Soc Med* 1981; **74**:242.

Kudrow L: *Cluster Headache: Mechanisms and Management.* Oxford Univ Press, 1980.

Kudrow L: Response of cluster headache attacks to oxygen inhalation. *Headache* 1981;**21**:1.

Lance JW: Headache. *Ann Neurol* 1981;**10**:1.

Lance JW: *Mechanism and Management of Headache,* 3rd ed. Butterworth, 1978.

Martin MJ: Psychogenic factors in headache. *Med Clin North Am* 1978;**62**:559.

Pearce JMS: Chronic migrainous neuralgia: A variant of cluster headache. *Brain* 1980;**103**:149.

Raskin NH, Appenzeller O: *Headache.* Vol 19 of: *Major Problems in Internal Medicine.* Saunders, 1980.

Saper JR: Migraine. (2 parts.) *JAMA* 1978;**239**:2380, 2480.

Ziegler DK: Tension headache. *Med Clin North Am* 1978; **62**:495.

FACIAL PAIN

Trigeminal Neuralgia

Trigeminal neuralgia may begin at any age but is most common in middle and later life. It affects women more frequently than men. The disorder is characterized by momentary episodes of sudden lancinating facial pain that commonly arises near one side of the mouth and then shoots toward the ear, eye, or nostril on that side. The pain may be triggered or precipitated by such factors as touch, movement, drafts, and eating. Indeed, in order to lessen the likelihood of triggering further attacks, many patients try to hold the face still while talking. Spontaneous remissions for several months or longer may occur. As the disorder progresses, however, the episodes of pain become more frequent, remissions become shorter and less common, and a dull ache may persist between the episodes of stabbing pain. Symptoms remain confined to the distribution of the trigeminal nerve (usually the second or third division) on one side only.

The characteristic features of the pain in trigeminal neuralgia usually distinguish it without difficulty from other causes of facial pain. In general, neurologic examination shows no abnormality except in a few patients in whom trigeminal neuralgia is symptomatic of some underlying lesion, such as multiple sclerosis or a brain stem neoplasm, in which case the finding

will depend on the nature and site of the lesion. Similarly, CT scans and radiologic contrast studies are normal in patients with classic trigeminal neuralgia.

In a young patient presenting with trigeminal neuralgia, multiple sclerosis must be suspected even if there are no other neurologic signs. In such circumstances, findings on evoked potential testing and examination of cerebrospinal fluid may be corroborative (see p 612). When the facial pain is due to a posterior fossa tumor, CT scanning and arteriography generally reveal the lesion, which should then be surgically removed if possible.

The drug most helpful for treatment of trigeminal neuralgia is carbamazepine, given in a dose of up to 1200 mg/d and monitored by serial blood counts and liver function tests. If carbamazepine is ineffective or cannot be tolerated by the patient, phenytoin should be tried.

In the past, various surgical and other means of providing symptomatic relief (eg, alcohol injection of the affected nerve, rhizotomy, or tractotomy) were recommended if pharmacologic treatment was unsuccessful. More recently, however, posterior fossa exploration has frequently revealed some structural cause for the neuralgia (despite normal findings on CT scans or arteriograms), such as an anomalous artery or vein impinging on the trigeminal nerve root. In such cases, simple decompression and separation of the anomalous vessel from the nerve root produce lasting relief of symptoms. In elderly patients with a limited life expectancy, radio-frequency rhizotomy is sometimes preferred because it is easy to perform, has few complications, and provides symptomatic relief for a period of time. Surgical exploration generally reveals no abnormality and is inappropriate in patients with trigeminal neuralgia due to multiple sclerosis.

Atypical Facial Pain

Facial pain without the typical features of trigeminal neuralgia is generally a constant, often burning pain that may have a restricted distribution at its onset but soon spreads to the rest of the face on the affected side and sometimes involves the other side, the neck, or the back of the head as well. The disorder is especially common in middle-aged women, many of them emotionally depressed, but it is not clear whether depression is the cause of or a reaction to the pain. Most forms of treatment are either unhelpful or provide benefit for only a limited period. Simple analgesics should be given a trial, as should tricyclic antidepressants, carbamazepine, and phenytoin. Opiate analgesics should be avoided, since addiction is a very real danger in patients with this disorder. Attempts at surgical treatment should be avoided.

Glossopharyngeal Neuralgia

Glossopharyngeal neuralgia is an uncommon disorder in which pain similar in quality to that in trigeminal neuralgia occurs in the throat, about the tonsillar fossa, and sometimes deep in the ear and at the back of the tongue. The pain may be precipitated by swallowing, chewing, talking, or yawning and is sometimes accompanied by syncope. In most instances, no underlying structural abnormality is present. Carbamazepine is the treatment of choice and should be tried before any surgical procedures are considered.

Postherpetic Neuralgia

About 10% of patients who develop shingles suffer from postherpetic neuralgia. This complication seems especially likely to occur in the elderly and when the first division of the trigeminal nerve is affected. A history of shingles and the presence of cutaneous scarring resulting from shingles aid in the diagnosis.

The incidence of postherpetic neuralgia is reduced by the treatment of shingles with steroids. Management of the established complication is essentially medical. If simple analgesics fail to help, a trial of a tricyclic drug (eg, amitriptyline, up to 100–150 mg/d) in conjunction with a phenothiazine (eg, perphenazine, 2–8 mg/d) is often effective. Many patients derive benefit from using a vibrator on the affected area and gradually increasing the frequency of application and the intensity of vibration with time, as tolerance increases.

Facial Pain Due to Other Causes

Facial pain may be caused by temporomandibular joint dysfunction in patients with malocclusion, abnormal bite, or faulty dentures. There may be tenderness of the masticatory muscles, and an association between pain onset and jaw movement is sometimes noted. Treatment consists of correction of the underlying problem.

A relationship of facial pain to chewing or temperature changes may suggest a dental disturbance. Facial swelling and trismus, when present, help to establish the diagnosis. Nevertheless, the cause is sometimes not obvious, and diagnosis requires careful dental examination and x-rays.

Sinusitis and ear infections causing facial pain are usually recognized by the history of respiratory tract infection and fever and, in some instances, aural discharge. There may be localized tenderness. Radiologic evidence of sinus infection or mastoiditis is confirmatory.

Glaucoma is an important ocular cause of facial pain, usually localized to the periorbital region. The underlying cause should be treated.

Facial pain may also be due to cluster headache (see above).

Jannetta PJ, Sweet WH: Trigeminal neuralgia. In: *Current Surgical Management of Neurological Disease*. Wilson CB, Hoff JT (editors). Churchill Livingstone, 1980.

Tomsen T et al: Carbamazepine therapy in trigeminal neuralgia. *Arch Neurol* 1980;**37**:699.

Wilson CB, Yorke C, Prioleau G: Microsurgical vascular decompression for trigeminal neuralgia and hemifacial spasm. *West J Med* 1980;**132**:481.

EPILEPSY

The term epilepsy denotes any disorder characterized by recurrent seizures. A seizure is a transient disturbance of cerebral function due to an abnormal paroxysmal neuronal discharge in the brain. Epilepsy is common, affecting approximately 0.5% of the population in the USA.

Etiology

Epilepsy has several causes. Its most likely cause in individual patients relates to the age of onset.

A. Idiopathic or Constitutional Epilepsy: Seizures usually begin between 5 and 20 years of age but may start later in life. No specific cause can be identified, and there is no other neurologic abnormality.

B. Symptomatic Epilepsy: There are many causes for recurrent seizures.

1. Congenital abnormalities and perinatal injuries may result in seizures presenting in infancy or childhood.

2. Metabolic disorders such as hypocalcemia, hypoglycemia, pyridoxine deficiency, and phenylketonuria are major treatable causes of seizures in neonates or infants. In adults, alcoholism and drug dependence are common causes of recurrent seizures, and other metabolic disorders such as renal failure and diabetes may also be responsible.

3. Trauma is an important cause of seizures at any age, but especially in young adults. Posttraumatic epilepsy is more likely to develop if the dura mater was penetrated and generally becomes manifest within 2 years following the injury. However, seizures developing in the first week after head injury do not necessarily imply that future attacks will occur. There is suggestive evidence that prophylactic anticonvulsant drug treatment reduces the incidence of posttraumatic epilepsy.

4. Tumors and other space-occupying lesions may lead to seizures at any age, but they are an especially important cause of seizures in middle and later life, when the incidence of neoplastic disease increases. The seizures are commonly the initial symptoms of the tumor and often are partial (focal) in character. They are most likely to occur with structural lesions involving the frontal, parietal, or temporal regions. Tumors must be excluded by appropriate laboratory studies in all patients with onset of seizures after 30 years of age, focal seizures or signs, or a progressive seizure disorder.

5. Vascular diseases become increasingly frequent causes of seizures with advancing age and are the most common cause of seizures with onset at age 60 years or older.

6. Degenerative disorders are a cause of seizures in later life.

7. Infectious diseases must be considered in all age groups as potentially reversible causes of seizures. Seizures may occur in the context of an acute infective or inflammatory illness, such as herpes encephalitis, or in patients with more long-standing or chronic disorders such as neurosyphilis or cerebral cysticercosis. Seizures are a common sequela of supratentorial brain abscess, developing most frequently in the first year after treatment.

Classification of Seizures

Seizures can be categorized in various ways, but the descriptive classification proposed by the International League Against Epilepsy is clinically the most useful. Seizures are divided into those that are generalized and those affecting only part of the brain (partial seizures).

A. Partial Seizures: The initial clinical and electroencephalographic manifestations of partial seizures indicate that only a restricted part of one cerebral hemisphere has been activated. The ictal manifestations depend upon the area of the brain involved. Partial seizures are subdivided into simple seizures, in which consciousness is preserved, and complex seizures, in which it is impaired. Partial seizures of either type sometimes become secondarily generalized, leading to a tonic, clonic, or tonic-clonic attack.

1. Simple partial seizures – Simple seizures may be manifested by focal motor symptoms (convulsive jerking) or somatosensory symptoms (eg, paresthesias or tingling) that spread (or "march") to different parts of the limb or body depending upon their cortical representation. In other instances, special sensory symptoms (eg, light flashes or buzzing) indicate involvement of visual, auditory, olfactory, or gustatory regions of the brain, or there may be autonomic symptoms or signs (eg, abnormal epigastric sensations, sweating, flushing, pupillary dilatation). When psychic symptoms occur, they are usually accompanied by impairment of consciousness, but the sole manifestations of some seizures are phenomena such as dysphasia, dysmnesic symptoms (eg, *déjà vu, jamais vu*), affective disturbances, illusions, or structured hallucinations.

2. Complex partial seizures – Impaired consciousness may be preceded, accompanied, or followed by the psychic symptoms mentioned above, and automatisms may occur. Such seizures may also begin with some of the other simple symptoms mentioned above.

B. Generalized Seizures: There are several different varieties of generalized seizures, as outlined below. In some circumstances, seizures cannot be classified because of incomplete information or because they do not fit into any category.

1. Absence (petit mal) seizures – These are characterized by impairment of consciousness, sometimes with mild clonic, tonic, or atonic components (ie, reduction or loss of postural tone), autonomic components (eg, enuresis), or accompanying automatisms. Onset and termination of attacks are abrupt. If attacks occur during conversation, the patient may miss a few words or may break off in mid sentence for a few seconds. The impairment of external awareness is so brief that the patient is unaware of it. Absence seizures almost always begin in childhood and frequently cease by the age of 20 years, although occasionally they are then replaced by other forms of generalized seizure. If very frequent, they may interfere with learning at school. Electroencephalographically, such attacks are associated with bursts of bilaterally synchronous and symmetric 3-Hz spike-and-wave activity. A normal background in the electroencephalogram and normal or above-normal intelligence imply a good prognosis for the ultimate cessation of these seizures.

2. Atypical absences – There may be more marked changes in tone, or attacks may have a more gradual onset and termination than in typical absences.

3. Myoclonic seizures – Myoclonic seizures consist of single or multiple myoclonic jerks.

4. Tonic-clonic (grand mal) seizures – In these seizures, which are characterized by sudden loss of consciousness, the patient becomes rigid and falls to the ground. Respiration is arrested, and the patient becomes cyanotic. This tonic phase, which usually lasts for less than a minute, is followed by a clonic phase in which there is jerking of the body musculature that may last for 2 or 3 minutes and is then followed by a stage of flaccid coma. During the seizure, the tongue or lips may be bitten, urinary or fecal incontinence may occur, and the patient may be injured. Immediately after the seizure, the patient may either recover consciousness, drift into sleep, have a further convulsion without recovery of consciousness between the attacks (**status epilepticus**), or after recovering consciousness have a further convulsion (**serial seizures**). In other cases, patients will behave in an abnormal fashion in the immediate postictal period, without subsequent awareness or memory of events (**postepileptic automatism**). Headache, disorientation, confusion, drowsiness, nausea, soreness of the muscles, or some combination of these symptoms commonly occurs postictally.

5. Tonic, clonic, or atonic seizures – Loss of consciousness may occur with either the tonic or clonic accompaniments described above, especially in children. Atonic seizures (**epileptic drop attacks**) have also been described.

Clinical Findings

A. Symptoms and Signs: Nonspecific changes such as headache, mood alterations, lethargy, and myoclonic jerking alert some patients to an impending seizure hours before it occurs. These prodromal symptoms are distinct from the aura which may precede a generalized seizure by a few seconds or minutes and which is itself a part of the attack, arising locally from a restricted region of the brain.

In most patients, seizures occur unpredictably at any time and without any relationship to posture or ongoing activities. Occasionally, however, they occur at a particular time (eg, during sleep) or in relation to external precipitants such as lack of sleep, missed meals, emotional stress, menstruation, alcohol ingestion (or alcohol withdrawal; see below), or use of certain drugs. Fever and nonspecific infections may also precipitate seizures in known epileptics; in infants and young children, it may be hard to distinguish such attacks from febrile seizures. In a few patients, seizures are provoked by specific stimuli such as flashing lights or a flickering television set (**photosensitive epilepsy**), music, or reading.

Clinical examination between seizures shows no abnormality in patients with idiopathic epilepsy, but in the immediate postictal period, extensor plantar responses may be seen. The presence of lateralized or focal signs postictally suggests that seizures may have a focal origin. In patients with symptomatic epilepsy, the findings on examination will reflect the underlying cause.

B. Laboratory, X-Ray, and Other Studies: In patients older than 10 years, initial investigations should always include a full blood count, blood glucose determination, liver and renal function tests, and serologic tests for syphilis. The hematologic and biochemical screening tests are important both in excluding various causes of seizures and in providing a baseline for subsequent monitoring of long-term effects of treatment.

Electroencephalography should be performed. The findings may support the clinical diagnosis of epilepsy (by demonstrating paroxysmal abnormalities containing spikes or sharp waves), may provide a guide to prognosis, and may help classify the seizure disorder. Classification of the disorder is important for determining the most appropriate anticonvulsant drug with which to start treatment. For example, absence (petit mal) and complex partial seizures may be difficult to distinguish clinically, but the electroencephalographic findings and treatment of choice differ in these 2 conditions. Finally, the electroencephalographic findings are important in evaluating candidates for surgical treatment.

A CT scan should be performed in all patients with focal neurologic symptoms or signs, focal seizures, or electroencephalographic findings of a focal disturbance. It should also be performed in patients with clinical evidence of a progressive disorder and in those presenting with seizures after the age of 30 years, because of the possibility of an underlying neoplasm. A chest x-ray should also be performed in such patients, since the lungs are a common site for primary or secondary neoplasms.

Differential Diagnosis

The distinction between the various disorders likely to be confused with generalized seizures is usually made on the basis of the history. The importance of obtaining an eyewitness account of the attacks cannot be overemphasized.

A. Differential Diagnosis of Partial Seizures:

1. Transient ischemic attacks–These attacks are distinguished from seizures by their longer duration, lack of spread, and symptomatology. There is a loss of motor or sensory function (eg, weakness or numbness) with transient ischemic attacks, whereas positive symptomatology (eg, convulsive jerking or

paresthesias) characterizes seizures.

2. Rage attacks–Rage attacks are usually situational and lead to goal-directed aggressive behavior.

3. Panic attacks–These may be hard to distinguish from simple or complex partial seizures unless there is evidence of psychopathologic disturbances between attacks and the attacks have a clear relationship to external circumstances.

B. Differential Diagnosis of Generalized Seizures:

1. Syncope–Episodes of syncope usually occur while the patient is standing or after a sudden change in posture to the erect position, especially in patients with autonomic insufficiency. Syncope may occur in healthy individuals in hot weather, after pain or blood loss, during intense emotional stimulation, and following prolonged coughing or straining (which impedes venous return to the heart). Premonitory symptoms such as nausea, sweating, unsteadiness, yawning, and graying of vision are followed by loss of consciousness during which the patient is pale, sweaty, and flaccid and may experience one or 2 convulsive jerks. Injury is rare. Incontinence may occur and does not reliably distinguish seizures from syncope. Recovery is rapid once the patient is recumbent, but residual headache, nausea, sweatiness, and unsteadiness are common. If the patient is unable to fall into the recumbent position but is maintained upright (for example, by room fixtures and fittings), more conspicuous convulsive movements will occur.

2. Cardiac dysrhythmias–Cerebral hypoperfusion due to a disturbance of cardiac rhythm should be suspected in patients with known cardiac or vascular disease or in elderly patients who present with episodic loss of consciousness. Preceding palpitations or marked pallor followed by flushing during attacks will support the clinical diagnosis. A relationship of attacks to physical activity is also suggestive of cardiac dysrhythmia or outflow obstruction. Holter monitoring may be necessary to establish the diagnosis with confidence and may need to be continued for several days, because normal findings do not exclude the diagnosis unless the recording encompasses at least one episode in which consciousness is lost.

3. Brain stem ischemia–Loss of consciousness is preceded or accompanied by other brain stem signs. Basilar migraine is discussed on p 581 and vertebrobasilar vascular disease on p 593.

4. Pseudoseizures–The term pseudoseizures is used to denote both hysterical conversion reactions and attacks due to malingering when these simulate epileptic seizures. Many patients with pseudoseizures also have true seizures or a family history of epilepsy. Although pseudoseizures tend to occur at times of emotional stress, this may also be the case with true seizures.

Clinically, the attacks superficially resemble tonic-clonic seizures, but there may be obvious preparation before pseudoseizures occur. Moreover, there is usually no tonic phase; instead, there is a wild and asynchronous thrashing about of the limbs, which increases if restraints are imposed and which rarely leads to injury or incontinence. Consciousness may be normal or "lost," but in the latter context the occurrence of goal-directed behavior or of shouting, swearing, etc, indicates that loss of consciousness is feigned. Postictally, there are no changes in behavior or neurologic findings, and the patient may vaguely recall some incident that occurred while consciousness was supposedly lost.

Encephalography and laboratory studies may help in the recognition of pseudoseizures. In patients with epileptic seizures accompanied by loss of consciousness, electroencephalographic changes during the ictal event are to be expected. In contrast, there are no electrocerebral changes during pseudoseizures. More recently, the level of serum prolactin has been found to increase dramatically between 15 and 30 minutes after a tonic-clonic convulsion in most patients, whereas it is unchanged after a pseudoseizure.

Pseudoseizures are best managed by indicating to patients that the attacks are not epileptic in nature but have some other basis. Psychiatric evaluation, individual or group therapy, and rehabilitation may be helpful.

Treatment

A. General Measures: For patients with recurrent seizures, drug treatment is prescribed with the goal of preventing further attacks and is usually continued until there have been no seizures for at least 4 years. Epileptic patients should be advised to avoid activities or situations that provoke attacks (eg, alcohol ingestion or prolonged periods of food or sleep deprivation) and situations that could be dangerous or life-threatening if further seizures should occur. State legislation may require physicians to report to the authorities any patients with seizures or other episodic disturbances of consciousness.

1. Choice of medication–The drug with which treatment is best initiated depends upon the type of seizures to be treated (Table 17–2). The dose of the selected drug is gradually increased until seizures are controlled, blood levels reach the upper limit of the optimal therapeutic range, or side effects prevent further increases. If seizures continue despite treatment at the maximal tolerated dose, a second drug is added and the dose increased until its blood levels are in the therapeutic range; the first drug is then gradually withdrawn. In most patients with seizures of a single type, satisfactory control can be obtained with a single anticonvulsant drug. Treatment with more than 2 drugs is almost always unhelpful unless the patient is having seizures of different types. If the drugs shown in Table 17–2 are ineffective, a number of second-line anticonvulsant drugs can be tried, but these have more frequent and troublesome side effects, which limit their use.

2. Monitoring–Monitoring plasma drug levels has led to major advances in the management of seizure disorders. The same daily dose of a particular drug leads to markedly different blood concentrations

in different patients, and this will affect the therapeutic response. Steady-state drug levels in the blood should therefore be measured when treatment is initiated, dosage is changed, or another drug is added to the therapeutic regimen and when seizures are poorly controlled. Dose adjustments are then guided by the laboratory findings. The most common cause of a lower concentration of drug than expected for the prescribed dose is poor patient compliance. Compliance can be improved by encouragement and explanation and by limiting to a minimum the number of daily doses. Recurrent seizures or status epilepticus may result if drugs are taken erratically, and in some circumstances noncompliant patients may be better off without any medication.

All anticonvulsant drugs have side effects, and some of these are shown in Table 17–2. A complete blood count should be performed at least annually in all patients because of the risk of anemia or blood dyscrasia. Treatment with certain drugs may require more frequent monitoring or use of additional screening tests. For example, periodic tests of hepatic function are necessary if valproic acid or carbamazepine is used, and serial blood counts are important with carbamazepine or ethosuximide.

3. Discontinuation of medication–Only when patients have been seizure-free for several (at least 4) years should withdrawal of medication be considered. Unfortunately, there is no way of predicting which patients can be managed successfully without treatment, although seizure recurrence is more likely in patients who initially failed to respond to therapy, those with seizures having focal features or of multiple types, and those with continuing electroencephalographic abnormalities. Mental subnormality is also associated with increased risk of recurrence. Dose reduction should be gradual over a period of weeks or months, and drugs should be withdrawn one at a time. If seizures recur, treatment is reinstituted with the same drugs used previously. Seizures are no more difficult to control after a recurrence than before.

B. Special Circumstances:

1. Solitary seizures–In patients who have had only one seizure, investigation should exclude an underlying cause requiring specific treatment. Prophylactic anticonvulsant drug treatment is generally not required unless further attacks occur. The risk of seizure recurrence varies in different series, but in one recent survey it was only 27% over 3 years, with none occurring thereafter. Epilepsy should not be diagnosed on the basis of a solitary seizure, since the diagnosis of epilepsy is based on a history of repeated attacks in a patient expected to have further attacks. Similarly, if seizures occur only in the context of a transient, nonrecurrent systemic disorder, such as acute cerebral anoxia, the diagnosis of epilepsy should be avoided, and long-term prophylactic anticonvulsant drug treatment is unnecessary.

2. Alcohol withdrawal seizures–One or a few generalized tonic-clonic seizures may occur within 48 hours or so of withdrawal from alcohol after a period of

Table 17-2. Drug treatment for seizures.[*]

	Usual Adult Daily Dose (mg/kg)	Usual Adult Daily Dose (mg)	Minimum Number of Daily Doses	Time to Steady-State Drug Levels (days)	Optimal Blood Level (per mL)	Selected Side Effects and Idiosyncratic Reactions
Generalized tonic-clonic (grand mal) or partial (focal) seizures						
Phenytoin	4-8	200-400	1	5-10	10-20 μg	Nystagmus, ataxia, dysarthria, sedation, confusion, gingival hyperplasia, hirsutism, megaloblastic anemia, blood dyscrasias, skin rashes, fever, systemic lupus erythematosus, lymphadenopathy, peripheral neuropathy, dyskinesias.
Carbamazepine	5-25	600-1200	2	3-4	4-8 μg	Nystagmus, dysarthria, diplopia, ataxia, drowsiness, nausea, blood dyscrasias, hepatotoxicity.
Phenobarbital	2-5	100-200	1	14-21	10-40 μg	Drowsiness, nystagmus, ataxia, skin rashes, learning difficulties, hyperactivity.
Primidone	5-20	750-1500	3	4-7	5-15 μg	Sedation, nystagmus, ataxia, vertigo, nausea, skin rashes, megaloblastic anemia, irritability.
Valproic acid	10-60		3	2-4	50-100 μg	Nausea, vomiting, diarrhea, drowsiness, alopecia, weight gain, hepatotoxicity, thrombocytopenia.
Absence (petit mal) seizures						
Ethosuximide	20-35	100-1500	2	5-10	40-100 μg	Nausea, vomiting, anorexia, headache, lethargy, unsteadiness, blood dyscrasias, systemic lupus erythematosus, urticaria, pruritus.
Valproic acid	10-60		3	2-4	50-100 μg	See above.
Clonazepam	0.05-0.2		2	?	20-80 ng	Drowsiness, ataxia, irritability, behavioral changes, exacerbation of tonic-clonic seizures.
Myoclonic seizures						
Valproic acid	10-60		3	2-4	50-100 μg	See above.
Clonazepam	0.05-0.2		2	?	20-80 ng	See above.

[*]Reproduced, with permission, from Aminoff MJ: Neurologic disorders. In: *Handbook of Medical Treatment,* 17th ed. Watts HD (editor). Jones, 1983.

high or chronic intake. If the seizures have consistently focal features, the possibility of an associated structural abnormality, often traumatic in origin, must be considered. Treatment with anticonvulsant drugs is generally not required for alcohol withdrawal seizures, since they are self-limited. Status epilepticus may rarely follow alcohol withdrawal and is managed along conventional lines (see below). Long-term prophylactic anticonvulsant drug treatment is unnecessary and may even be hazardous if the patient is poorly compliant. Further attacks will not occur if the patient abstains from alcohol.

3. Tonic-clonic status epilepticus–Poor compliance with the anticonvulsant drug regimen is the most common cause of tonic-clonic status epilepticus. Other causes include alcohol withdrawal, intracranial infection or neoplasms, metabolic disorders, and drug overdose. The mortality rate may be as high as 20%, and among survivors the incidence of neurologic and mental sequelae may be high. The prognosis relates to the length of time between onset of status epilepticus and the start of effective treatment.

Status epilepticus is a medical emergency. Management includes maintenance of the airway to ensure adequate pulmonary ventilation. In adults, unless the cause of the seizures is obvious, 50% dextrose (25-50 mL) is routinely given intravenously in case hypoglycemia is responsible. If seizures continue, 10 mg of diazepam is given intravenously over the course of 2 minutes, and the dose is repeated after 10 minutes if necessary. This is usually effective in halting seizures for a brief period, but a long-acting anticonvulsant must also be given to provide continuing control. Regardless of the response to diazepam, therefore, phenytoin (15 mg/kg) is given intravenously at a rate of 50 mg/min, which permits therapeutic levels to be reached in the brain within a few minutes. The drug is best injected directly but can also be given in saline; it precipitates, however, if injected into glucose-containing solutions. Because cardiac arrhythmias may develop during rapid administration of large doses of phenytoin, electrocardiographic monitoring during administration is indicated.

If seizures continue, phenobarbital is then given in a loading dose of 10-15 mg/kg intravenously by slow or intermittent injection. Equipment for assisted respiration should be available for immediate use if required, since respiratory depression and hypotension are common complications. In refractory cases, one or more of the following may be necessary: lidocaine,

50–100 mg intravenously; paraldehyde, 5–10 mL intravenously (as a 4% solution in normal saline), by deep intramuscular injection, or rectally (in mineral oil); and amobarbital, 200–1000 mg by infusion. Since paraldehyde will dissolve plastic syringes and nasogastric tubes, they should not be used for its administration.

If these measures fail, general anesthesia with ventilatory assistance and neuromuscular junction blockade may be required.

Intravenous diazepam sometimes leads to respiratory depression and hypotension, and these complications become more probable as additional drugs are given. It is therefore important to monitor vital signs frequently during the course of treatment. Because diazepam has a short half-life, other benzodiazepines have also been used in the immediate management of status epilepticus. Lorazepam given intravenously has been effective in several studies and has more prolonged clinical effects than diazepam. It is unclear whether lorazepam is as safe and as rapidly effective as diazepam, but ongoing comparative studies may clarify the issue.

After status epilepticus is controlled, an oral drug program for the long-term management of seizures is started, and investigations into the cause of the disorder are pursued.

4. Nonconvulsive status epilepticus–Absence (petit mal) and complex partial status epilepticus are characterized by fluctuating abnormal mental status, confusion, impaired responsiveness, and automatism. Electroencephalography is helpful both in establishing the diagnosis and in distinguishing the 2 varieties. Initial treatment with intravenous diazepam is usually helpful regardless of the type of status epilepticus, but phenytoin, phenobarbital, carbamazepine, and other drugs may also be needed to obtain and maintain control in complex partial status epilepticus.

Aminoff MJ, Simon RP: Status epilepticus: Causes, clinical features and consequences in 98 patients. *Am J Med* 1980;**69**:657.

Bleck TP: Therapy for status epilepticus. *Clin Neuropharmacol* 1983;**6**:255.

Bruni J, Albright PS: The clinical pharmacology of antiepileptic drugs. *Clin Neuropharmacol* 1984;**7**:1.

Delgado-Escueta AV, Treiman DM, Walsh GO: The treatable epilepsies. (2 parts.) *N Engl J Med* 1983;**308**:1508, 1576.

Delgado-Escueta AV et al: Current concepts in neurology: Management of status epilepticus. *N Engl J Med* 1982;**306**:1337.

Desai BT, Porter RJ, Penry JK: Psychogenic seizures: A study of 42 attacks in six patients, with intensive monitoring. *Arch Neurol* 1982;**39**:202.

Engel J Jr et al: Recent developments in the diagnosis and therapy of epilepsy. *Ann Intern Med* 1982;**97**:584.

Hauser WA et al: Seizure recurrence after a first unprovoked seizure. *N Engl J Med* 1982;**307**:522.

King DW et al: Pseudoseizures: Diagnostic evaluation. *Neurology* 1982;**32**:18.

Reynolds EH, Elwes RDC, Shorvon SD: Why does epilepsy become intractable? Prevention of chronic epilepsy. *Lancet* 1983;**2**:952.

Weiss GH et al: Prognostic factors for the occurrence of post-traumatic epilepsy. *Arch Neurol* 1983;**40**:7.

TRANSIENT ISCHEMIC ATTACKS

Transient ischemic attacks are characterized by focal ischemic cerebral neurologic deficits that last for less than 24 hours (usually less than 1–2 hours). Patients with recent onset of attacks are at high risk for cerebral infarction, myocardial infarction, or death. About 30% of patients with stroke have a past history of transient ischemic attacks, and proper treatment of the attacks is an important means of preventing strokes. The incidence of stroke does not relate either to the number or duration of individual attacks but is increased in patients with hypertension, diabetes, or pathologic changes (atherosclerotic plaques or ulcers) in the carotid artery.

Etiology

An important cause of transient cerebral ischemia is embolization. In many patients with these attacks, a source of embolization is readily apparent in the heart or a major extracranial artery to the head, and emboli sometimes are visible in the retinal arteries. Moreover, an embolic phenomenon explains why separate attacks may affect different parts of the territory supplied by the same major vessel. Cardiac causes of embolic ischemic attacks include rheumatic heart disease, mitral valve disease, cardiac dysrhythmia, infective endocarditis, atrial myxoma, and mural thrombi complicating myocardial infarction. In patients with stenosis or ulceration of a major artery to the brain, a mural thrombus may form and serve as a source of emboli. In the anterior circulation, atherosclerotic changes occur most commonly in the region of the carotid bifurcation extracranially, and these changes may cause a bruit. In some patients with transient ischemic attacks or strokes, an acute or recent hemorrhage is found to have occurred into this atherosclerotic plaque, and this finding may have pathologic significance.

Other (less common) abnormalities of blood vessels that may cause transient ischemic attacks include fibromuscular dysplasia, which affects particularly the cervical internal carotid artery; inflammatory arterial disorders such as giant cell arteritis, systemic lupus erythematosus, polyarteritis, and granulomatous angiitis; and meningovascular syphilis. Transient severe hypotension (eg, due to blood loss, cardiac dysrhythmia, or postural change) may cause a reduction of cerebral blood flow if a major extracranial artery to the brain is markedly stenosed, but this is a rare cause of transient ischemic attack.

Hematologic causes of ischemic attacks include polycythemia, sickle cell disease, hyperviscosity syndromes, leukocytosis, and thrombocytosis. Severe anemia may also lead to transient focal neurologic deficits in patients with preexisting cerebral arterial disease.

The **subclavian steal syndrome** may lead to transient vertebrobasilar ischemia. Symptoms develop when there is localized stenosis or occlusion of one subclavian artery proximal to the source of the vertebral artery, so that blood is "stolen" from this artery. A bruit in the supraclavicular fossa, unequal radial pulses, and a difference of 20 mm Hg or more between the systolic blood pressures in the arms should suggest the diagnosis in patients with vertebrobasilar transient ischemic attacks.

Clinical Findings

A. Symptoms and Signs: The symptoms of transient ischemic attacks vary markedly among patients; however, the symptoms in a given individual tend to be constant in type. Onset is abrupt and without warning, and recovery usually occurs rapidly, often within a few minutes.

If the ischemia is in the carotid territory, common symptoms are weakness and heaviness of the contralateral arm, leg, or face, singly or in any combination. Numbness or paresthesias may also occur either as the sole manifestation of the attack or in combination with the motor deficit. There may be slowness of movement, dysphasia, or monocular visual loss in the eye contralateral to affected limbs. During an attack, examination may reveal flaccid weakness with pyramidal distribution, sensory changes, hyperreflexia or an extensor plantar response on the affected side, dysphasia, or any combination of these findings. Subsequently, examination reveals no neurologic abnormality, but the presence of a carotid bruit or cardiac abnormality may provide a clue to the cause of symptoms.

Vertebrobasilar ischemic attacks may be characterized by vertigo, ataxia, diplopia, dysarthria, dimness or blurring of vision, perioral numbness and paresthesias, and weakness or sensory complaints on one, both, or alternating sides of the body. These symptoms may occur singly or in any combination. Drop attacks due to bilateral leg weakness, without headache or loss of consciousness, may occur, sometimes in relation to head movements.

The natural history of attacks is variable. Some patients will have a major stroke after only a few attacks, whereas others may have frequent attacks for weeks or months without having a stroke. Attacks may occur intermittently over a long period of time, or they may stop spontaneously. In general, carotid ischemic attacks are more liable than vertebrobasilar ischemic attacks to be followed by stroke.

B. Laboratory, X-Ray, and Other Studies: Clinical and laboratory evaluation must include assessment for hypertension, heart disease, and diffuse vascular disease.

Investigations are directed at identifying the cause of attacks and should include complete blood count, blood glucose determination, serologic tests for syphilis, and an electrocardiogram and chest x-ray. Echocardiography is performed in patients with heart murmurs, and blood cultures are undertaken if endocarditis is suspected. Holter monitoring is indicated if a transient, paroxysmal disturbance of cardiac rhythm is suspected. CT scan of the head will exclude the possibility of a small cerebral hemorrhage or a cerebral tumor masquerading as a transient ischemic attack. A number of noninvasive techniques, such as ultrasonography, have been developed for studying the cerebral circulation and imaging the major vessels to the head, but they have not replaced arteriography as a means of demonstrating the status of the cerebrovascular system. Accordingly, if findings on CT scan are normal, if there is no cardiac source of embolization, and if age and general condition indicate that the patient is a good operative risk, bilateral carotid arteriography should be undertaken in the further evaluation of carotid ischemic attacks.

Differential Diagnosis

Focal seizures must be distinguished. They usually cause abnormal motor or sensory phenomena such as clonic limb movements, paresthesias, or tingling, rather than weakness or loss of feeling. Symptoms generally spread ("march") up the limb and may lead to a generalized tonic-clonic seizure. The electroencephalogram may help in detecting the epileptogenic source.

Classic migraine is easily recognized by the visual premonitory symptoms, followed by nausea, headache, and photophobia, but less typical cases may be hard to distinguish. The patient's age and medical history (including family history) may be helpful in this regard. Patients with migraine commonly have a history of episodes since adolescence and report that other family members have a similar disorder.

Focal neurologic deficits may occur during periods of hypoglycemia in diabetic patients receiving treatment, and the lack of general hypoglycemic symptoms does not exclude this possibility.

Treatment

When arteriography reveals a surgically accessible lesion on the side appropriate to carotid ischemic attacks and there is relatively little atherosclerosis elsewhere in the cerebrovascular system, operative treatment (carotid thromboendarterectomy) need not be delayed. When more extensive atherosclerotic disease is angiographically evident in the cerebral circulation, the benefits of surgery are less clear and the operative risks greater.

In patients with carotid ischemic attacks who are poor operative candidates (and thus have not undergone arteriography) or who are found to have extensive vascular disease, medical treatment should be instituted. Similarly, patients with vertebrobasilar ischemic attacks are treated medically and are not subjected to arteriography unless there is clinical evidence of stenosis or occlusion in the carotid or subclavian arteries.

Medical treatment is aimed at preventing further attacks and stroke. Cigarette smoking should be stopped, and cardiac sources of embolization, hypertension, diabetes, arteritis, or hematologic disorders should be treated appropriately. If anticoagulants are indicated for the treatment of embolism from the heart, they should be started immediately, provided there is no contraindication to their use. There is no advantage in delay, and the common fear of causing hemorrhage into a previously infarcted area is misplaced, since there is a far greater risk of further embolism to the cerebral circulation if treatment is withheld. Treatment is initiated with intravenous heparin while warfarin sodium is introduced.

In patients with presumed or angiographically verified atherosclerotic changes in the extracranial or intracranial cerebrovascular circulation, antithrombotic medication is prescribed. The treatment selected will depend upon the patient's age, the likelihood of compliance in taking the drug, and the ready availability of medical and laboratory services. Some physicians prefer to use anticoagulant drugs (eg, warfarin, with temporary heparinization until the dose of warfarin is adequate) unless they are medically contraindicated, continuing them for 3–6 months before they are tapered and ultimately replaced with aspirin (300 mg/d) or, in women, dipyridamole, which is continued for another year. Other physicians prefer aspirin or dipyridamole from the onset.

The evidence supporting a therapeutic role for aspirin and other agents suppressing platelet aggregation is incomplete. Platelets adhere to and aggregate around an atherosclerotic plaque and release various substances including thromboxane A_2. In a double-blind prospective study performed in Canada, it was found that treatment with aspirin significantly reduced the frequency of transient ischemic attacks and the incidence of stroke or death in men. A number of other studies in which different doses of aspirin were used similarly suggest a beneficial effect and suggest also that men and women respond differently to treatment. The optimal daily dose remains to be established. Dipyridamole may act by enhancing the production of prostacyclin (which has antithrombotic activities) in the vessel wall.

In recent years, many patients with transient ischemic attacks associated with stenotic lesions of the distal internal carotid or the proximal middle cerebral arteries have undergone surgical extracranial-intracranial arterial anastomosis. Most commonly, a connection is made between the superficial temporal and middle cerebral arteries, and the operative mortality rate is generally low. The indications for and results of such surgery are difficult to determine at present.

Canadian Cooperative Study Group: A randomized trial of aspirin and sulfinpyrazone in threatened stroke. *N Engl J Med* 1978;**299**:53.

Dyken ML: Anticoagulant and platelet-antiaggregating therapy in stroke and threatened stroke. *Neurol Clin* 1983;**1**:223.

Ross Russell RW: Pathogenesis of transient attacks. *Neurol Clin* 1983;**1**:279.

Sandok BA et al: Guidelines for the management of transient ischemic attacks. *Mayo Clin Proc* 1978;**53**:665.

Whisnant JP, Cartlidge NEF, Elveback LR: Carotid and vertebral-basilar transient ischemic attacks: Effect of anticoagulants, hypertension, and cardiac disorders on survival and stroke occurrence—a population study. *Ann Neurol* 1978; **3**:107.

Yatsu FM, Mohr JP: Anticoagulation therapy for cardiogenic emboli to brain. *Neurology* 1982;**32**:274.

STROKE

In the USA, stroke remains the third leading cause of death, despite a general decline in the incidence of stroke in the last 30 years. The precise reasons for this decline are uncertain, but increased awareness of risk factors (hypertension, diabetes, hyperlipidemia, cigarette smoking, cardiac abnormalities, family history of stroke) and improved prophylactic measures and surveillance of those at increased risk have been contributory. A previous stroke makes individual patients more susceptible to further strokes.

For years, strokes have been subdivided pathologically into infarcts (thrombotic or embolic) and hemorrhages, and clinical criteria for distinguishing between these possibilities have been emphasized. However, in one autopsy study of 1000 cases of stroke, a clinical diagnosis of cerebral hemorrhage was confirmed in only 65% of cases and that of cerebral infarction in only 58%. Similar findings have been reported in other studies. These findings indicate the difficulty in determining on clinical grounds the pathologic basis of stroke.

1. LACUNAR INFARCTION

Lacunar infarcts are among the most common cerebral vascular lesions. They are small infarcts (usually < 5 mm in diameter) that occur in the distribution of short penetrating arterioles in the basal ganglia, pons, cerebellum, anterior limb of the internal capsule, and, less commonly, the deep cerebral white matter. Lacunar infarcts may be associated with hypertension or diabetes and have been found in conjunction with several clinical syndromes, including contralateral pure motor or pure sensory deficit, ipsilateral ataxia with crural paresis, and dysarthria with clumsiness of the hand. The neurologic deficit may progress over 24–36 hours before stabilizing.

Lacunar infarcts are sometimes visible on CT scans as small, punched-out, hypodense areas, but in other patients no abnormality is seen. In some instances, patients with a clinical syndrome suggestive of lacunar infarction are found on CT scanning to have a severe hemispheric infarct.

The prognosis for recovery from the deficit produced by a lacunar infarct is usually good, with partial or complete resolution occurring over the following 4–6 weeks in many instances. Hypertension or diabetes should be treated, if present. The role of anticoagulant treatment in the prevention of further lacunar infarction has not been systematically studied.

Fisher CM: Lacunar stroke and infarcts: A review. *Neurology* 1982;**32**:871.

Miller VT: Lacunar stroke: A reassessment. *Arch Neurol* 1983;**40**:129.

Mohr MP: Lacunes. *Neurol Clin* 1983;**1**:201.

2. CEREBRAL INFARCTION

Thrombotic or embolic occlusion of a major vessel leads to cerebral infarction. Causes include the disorders predisposing to transient ischemic attacks (see above) and atherosclerotic degeneration of cerebral arteries. The resulting deficit depends upon the particular vessel involved and the extent of any collateral circulation.

Clinical Findings

A. Symptoms and Signs: Onset is usually abrupt, and there may then be very little progression except that due to brain swelling. Clinical evaluation always includes examination of the heart and auscultation over the subclavian and carotid vessels to determine whether there are any bruits.

1. Obstruction of carotid circulation–Occlusion of the ophthalmic artery is probably symptomless in most cases because of the rich orbital anastomoses, but its transient embolic obstruction leads to amaurosis fugax—sudden and brief loss of vision in one eye.

Occlusion of the anterior cerebral artery distal to its junction with the anterior communicating artery causes weakness and cortical sensory loss in the contralateral leg and sometimes mild weakness of the arm, especially proximally. There may be a contralateral grasp reflex, paratonic rigidity, and abulia or frank confusion. Urinary incontinence is not uncommon, particularly if behavioral disturbances are conspicuous. Bilateral anterior cerebral infarction is especially likely to cause marked behavioral changes and memory disturbances. Unilateral anterior cerebral artery occlusion proximal to the junction with the anterior communicating artery is generally well tolerated because of the collateral supply from the other side.

Middle cerebral artery occlusion leads to dense contralateral hemiplegia, hemisensory loss, and homonymous hemianopia, and the eyes are deviated to the side of the lesion. If the dominant hemisphere is involved, global aphasia is also present. It may be impossible to distinguish this clinically from occlusion of the internal carotid artery. With occlusion of either of these arteries, there may also be considerable swelling of the hemisphere, leading to drowsiness, stupor, and coma in extreme cases. Occlusions of different branches of the middle cerebral artery cause more limited findings. For example, involvement of the anterior main division leads to a predominantly expressive dysphasia and to contralateral paralysis and loss of sensations in the arm, the face, and to a lesser extent, the leg. Posterior branch occlusion produces a receptive (Wernicke's) aphasia and a homonymous visual field defect. With involvement of the nondominant hemisphere, speech and comprehension are preserved, but there may be a confusional state, dressing apraxia, and constructional and spatial deficits.

Capsular hemiplegia results from obstruction of a lenticulostriate vessel. Infarction occurs in the posterior limb of the internal capsule and the adjacent corona radiata and leads primarily to a motor deficit; disturbances of speech, vision, or sensation are uncommon accompaniments. This is the clinical picture of lacunar stroke, which is described above.

2. Obstruction of vertebrobasilar circulation–Occlusion of the posterior cerebral artery may lead to a thalamic syndrome in which contralateral hemisensory disturbance occurs, followed by the development of spontaneous pain and hyperpathia. There is often a macular-sparing homonymous hemianopia and sometimes a mild, usually temporary, hemiparesis. Depending on the site of the lesion and the collateral circulation, the severity of these deficits varies and other deficits may also occur, including involuntary movements and alexia. Occlusion of the main artery beyond the origin of its penetrating branches may lead solely to a macular-sparing hemianopia.

Vertebral artery occlusion distally, below the origin of the anterior spinal and posterior inferior cerebellar arteries, may be clinically silent because the circulation is maintained by the other vertebral artery. If the remaining vertebral artery is congenitally small or severely atherosclerotic, however, a deficit similar to that of basilar artery occlusion is seen unless there is good collateral circulation from the anterior circulation through the circle of Willis. When the small paramedian arteries arising from the vertebral artery are occluded, contralateral hemiplegia and sensory deficit occur in association with an ipsilateral cranial nerve palsy at the level of the lesion. An obstruction of the posterior inferior cerebellar artery or an obstruction of the vertebral artery just before it branches to this vessel leads ipsilaterally to spinothalamic sensory loss involving the face, ninth and tenth cranial nerve lesions, limb ataxia and numbness, and Horner's syndrome, combined with contralateral spinothalamic sensory loss involving the limbs.

Occlusion of both vertebral arteries or the basilar artery leads to coma with pinpoint pupils, flaccid quadriplegia and sensory loss, and variable cranial nerve abnormalities. With partial basilar artery occlusion, there may be diplopia, visual loss, vertigo, dysarthria, ataxia, weakness or sensory disturbances in some or all of the limbs, and discrete cranial nerve palsies. In patients with hemiplegia of pontine origin, the eyes are often deviated to the paralyzed side, whereas in patients with a hemispheric lesion, the eyes commonly deviate from the hemiplegic side.

Occlusion of any of the major cerebellar arteries produces vertigo, nausea, vomiting, nystagmus, ipsilateral limb ataxia, and contralateral spinothalamic sensory loss in the limbs. If the superior cerebellar artery is involved, the contralateral spinothalamic loss also involves the face; with occlusion of the anterior inferior cerebellar artery, there is ipsilateral spinothalamic sensory loss involving the face, usually in conjunction with ipsilateral facial weakness and deafness. Massive cerebellar infarction may lead to coma, tonsillar herniation, and death.

3. Coma–Infarction in either the carotid or vertebrobasilar territory may lead to loss of consciousness. For example, an infarct involving one cerebral hemisphere may lead to such swelling that the function of the other hemisphere or the rostral brain stem is disturbed and coma results. Similarly, coma occurs with bilateral brain stem infarction when this involves the reticular formation, and it occurs with brain stem compression after cerebellar infarction.

B. Laboratory, X-Ray, and Other Studies: Investigations should include a complete blood count (including platelets), sedimentation rate, blood glucose determination, and serologic tests for syphilis. Electrocardiography will help exclude a cardiac dysrhythmia or recent myocardial infarction that might be serving as a source of embolization. Plain x-ray of the chest may reveal cardiomegaly or valvular calcification; the presence of a neoplasm would suggest that the neurologic deficit is due to metastasis rather than stroke. Blood cultures should be performed if endocarditis is suspected, echocardiography if heart murmur is present, and Holter monitoring if paroxysmal cardiac dysrhythmia requires exclusion. A CT scan of the head is important in excluding cerebral hemorrhage, but it may not permit distinction between a cerebral infarct and tumor. Examination of the cerebrospinal fluid is not always necessary but may be helpful if there is diagnostic uncertainty; it should be delayed until after CT scanning.

Treatment

The patient must be examined in detail, and if the neurologic deficit progresses over the following minutes or hours, heparinization may be of value in limiting or arresting further deterioration. Since the signs of progressing stroke may be simulated by an intracerebral hematoma, the latter must be excluded by immediate CT scanning or angiography before the patient is heparinized.

Early management of a completed stroke consists of general supportive measures, with maintenance of adequate ventilation, nutrition, fluid and electrolyte balance, and care of the bladder and bowels. During the acute stage, there may be marked brain swelling and edema, with symptoms and signs of increasing intracranial pressure, an increasing neurologic deficit, or herniation syndrome. Corticosteroids have been prescribed in an attempt to reduce vasogenic cerebral edema. Prednisone (up to 100 mg/d) or dexamethasone (16 mg/d) has been used, but the evidence that corticosteroids are of any benefit is conflicting. Dehydrating hyperosmolar agents have also been prescribed in efforts to reduce brain swelling, but there is little evidence of any major benefit.

There is no convincing evidence of clinical benefit from treatment with vasodilators such as papaverine, which have been given in order to enhance blood flow to ischemic brain. Similarly, neither hypercapnia nor hypocapnia, which influences cerebral perfusion, has been shown to have any benefit. Barbiturates are known to decrease neuronal metabolism and energy requirements and have been reported to improve functional recovery in experimental stroke models; their use in humans, however, is experimental and premature at present. Attempts to lower the blood pressure of hypertensive patients during the acute phase of a stroke should be avoided, since there is loss of cerebral autoregulation and since lowering the blood pressure may further compromise ischemic areas.

Anticoagulant drugs have no role in the management of patients with a completed stroke, except when there is a cardiac source of embolization. Treatment is then started with intravenous heparin while warfarin is introduced. If the CT scan shows no evidence of hemorrhage and the cerebrospinal fluid is clear, anticoagulant treatment may be started without delay. Many physicians, however, prefer to wait for about 5–7 days (to reduce any risk of cerebral hemorrhage) before initiating anticoagulant treatment. There are insufficient data to indicate which of these alternatives is preferable.

Physical therapy has an important role in the management of patients with impaired motor function. Passive movements at an early stage will help prevent contractures. As cooperation increases and some recovery begins, active movements will improve strength and coordination. In all cases, early mobilization and active rehabilitation are important. Occupational therapy may improve morale and motor skills, while speech therapy may be beneficial in patients with expressive dysphasia or dysarthria. When there is a severe and persisting motor deficit, a device such as a leg brace, toe spring, frame, or cane may help the patient move about, and the provision of other aids to daily living may improve the quality of life.

Prognosis

The prognosis for survival after cerebral infarction is better than after cerebral or subarachnoid hemorrhage. Loss of consciousness after a cerebral infarct implies a poorer prognosis than otherwise. The extent of the infarct governs the potential for rehabilitation. Patients who have had a cerebral infarct are at risk for further strokes and for myocardial infarcts.

Barnett HJM: Heart in ischemic stroke: A changing emphasis. *Neurol Clin* 1983;**1**:291.

Buonanno F, Toole JF: Management of patients with established ("completed") cerebral infarction. *Stroke* 1981;**12**:7.

Ross Russell RW (editor): *Vascular Disease of the Central Nervous System,* 2nd ed. Churchill Livingstone, 1983.

Whisnant JP: Indications for medical and surgical therapy for ischemic stroke. Vol 16 of: *Stroke: Advances in Neurology.* Thompson RA, Green JR (editors). Raven Press, 1977.

Wolf PA, Kannel WB, Verter J: Current status of risk factors for stroke. *Neurol Clin* 1983;**1**:317.

3. INTRACEREBRAL HEMORRHAGE

Spontaneous intracerebral hemorrhage in patients with no angiographic evidence of an associated vascular anomaly (eg, aneurysm or angioma) is usually due to hypertension. The pathologic basis for hemorrhage is probably the presence of microaneurysms that are now known to develop on perforating vessels of 100–300 μm in diameter in hypertensive patients. Hypertensive intracerebral hemorrhage occurs most frequently in the basal ganglia and less commonly in the pons, thalamus, cerebellum, and cerebral white matter. Hemorrhage may extend into the ventricular system or subarachnoid space, and signs of meningeal irritation are then found. Hemorrhages usually occur suddenly and without warning, often during activity.

In addition to its association with hypertension, nontraumatic intracerebral hemorrhage may occur with hematologic and bleeding disorders (eg, leukemia, thrombocytopenia, hemophilia, or disseminated intravascular coagulation), anticoagulant therapy, liver disease, cerebral amyloid angiopathy, and primary or secondary brain tumors. Bleeding is primarily into the subarachnoid space when it occurs from an intracranial aneurysm or arteriovenous malformation (see below), but it may be partly intracerebral as well. In some cases, no specific cause for cerebral hemorrhage can be identified.

Clinical Findings

A. Symptoms and Signs: With hemorrhage into the cerebral hemisphere, consciousness is initially lost or impaired in about one-half of patients. Vomiting occurs very frequently at the onset of bleeding, and headache is sometimes present. Focal symptoms and signs then develop, depending on the site of the hemorrhage. With hypertensive hemorrhage, there is generally a rapidly evolving neurologic deficit with hemiplegia or hemiparesis. A hemisensory disturbance is also present with more deeply placed lesions. With lesions of the putamen, loss of conjugate lateral gaze may be conspicuous. With thalamic hemorrhage, there may be a loss of upward gaze, downward or skew deviation of the eyes, lateral gaze palsies, and pupillary inequalities.

Cerebellar hemorrhage may present with sudden onset of nausea, vomiting, dysequilibrium, headache, and loss of consciousness that may terminate fatally within 48 hours. Less commonly, the onset is gradual and the course episodic or slowly progressive—clinical features suggesting an expanding cerebellar lesion. In yet other cases, however, the onset and course are intermediate, and examination shows lateral conjugate gaze palsies to the side of the lesion; small reactive pupils; contralateral hemiplegia; peripheral facial weakness; ataxia of gait, limbs, or trunk; periodic respiration; or some combination of these findings.

B. Laboratory, X-Ray, and Other Studies: A complete blood count, platelet count, bleeding time, prothrombin and partial thromboplastin times, and liver function tests may reveal some predisposing cause for the hemorrhage. Peripheral leukocytosis is a common nonspecific finding.

The cerebrospinal fluid may be bloodstained and under increased pressure. Clear fluid does not exclude an intracerebral hemorrhage, since the hematoma may not have extended into the ventricular system or subarachnoid space. Moreover, lumbar puncture is not without risk of precipitating a herniation syndrome in patients with a large hematoma and is unnecessary if facilities for CT scanning are available.

CT scanning is important not only in confirming that hemorrhage has occurred but also in determining the size and site of the hematoma. Unless the cause of hemorrhage is obvious or the patient is comatose, cerebral angiography is undertaken to determine if an aneurysm or arteriovenous malformation is present.

Treatment

Neurologic management is generally conservative and supportive, regardless of whether the patient has a profound deficit with associated brain stem compression, in which case the prognosis is grim, or a more localized deficit not causing increased intracranial pressure or brain stem involvement. Attention is directed to maintaining fluid and electrolyte balance and ensuring adequate ventilation. In patients with cerebellar hemorrhage, however, prompt surgical evacuation of the hematoma is appropriate because spontaneous unpredictable deterioration may otherwise lead to a fatal outcome and because operative treatment may lead to complete resolution of the clinical deficit.

In patients with a bleeding tendency, the cause must be recognized and replacement therapy given as appropriate. The treatment of underlying structural lesions depends upon their nature.

Drury I, Whisnant JP, Garraway WM: Primary intracerebral hemorrhage: Impact of CT on incidence. *Neurology* 1984; **34:**653.

Ojemann RG, Heros RC: Spontaneous brain hemorrhage. *Stroke* 1983;**14:**467.

Richardson A: Spontaneous intracerebral hemorrhage. In: *Vascular Disease of the Central Nervous System.* Ross Russell RW (editor). Churchill Livingstone, 1983.

4. SUBARACHNOID HEMORRHAGE

Between 5 and 10% of strokes are due to subarachnoid hemorrhage. Although hemorrhage is usually from rupture of an aneurysm or arteriovenous malformation, no specific cause can be found in 20% of cases.

Clinical Findings

A. Symptoms and Signs: Subarachnoid hemorrhage has a characteristic clinical picture. Its onset is with sudden headache of a severity never experienced previously by the patient. This may be followed by nausea and vomiting and by a loss or impairment of consciousness that can either be transient or progress inexorably to deepening coma and death. If consciousness is regained, the patient is often confused and irritable and may show other symptoms of an altered mental status. Neurologic examination generally reveals nuchal rigidity and other signs of meningeal irritation, except in deeply comatose patients. A focal neurologic deficit is occasionally present and may suggest the site of the underlying lesion.

B. Laboratory, X-Ray, and Other Studies: A CT scan should be performed immediately to confirm that hemorrhage has occurred and to search for clues regarding its source. Findings sometimes are normal in patients with suspected hemorrhage, and the cerebrospinal fluid must then be examined before the possibility of subarachnoid hemorrhage is discounted.

In patients with verified subarachnoid hemorrhage, cerebral arteriography is undertaken to determine the source of bleeding. Since arteriography is a prerequisite of surgery, it is not performed unless or until the patient's condition has stabilized and is good enough so that operative treatment is feasible. In deeply comatose patients, for example, arteriography should usually not be performed. In general, bilateral carotid and vertebral arteriography are necessary because aneurysms are often multiple, while arteriovenous malformations may be supplied from several sources.

Treatment

The medical management of patients is important. The measures outlined on p 614 must be applied to comatose patients. Conscious patients are confined to bed, advised against any exertion or straining, treated symptomatically for headache and anxiety, and given laxatives or stool softeners to prevent straining. If there is severe hypertension, the blood pressure can be lowered gradually, but not below a diastolic level of 100 mm Hg. Phenytoin or phenobarbital is generally prescribed routinely to prevent seizures. Further comment concerning the specific operative management of arteriovenous malformations and aneurysms follows.

5. INTRACRANIAL ANEURYSM

Saccular aneurysms ("berry" aneurysms) tend to occur at arterial bifurcations, are considerably more common in adults than in children, are frequently multiple (20% of cases), and are usually asymptomatic. They may be associated with polycystic kidney disease and coarctation of the aorta. Most aneurysms are located on the anterior part of the circle of Willis—particularly on the anterior or posterior communicating arteries, at the bifurcation of the middle cerebral artery, and at the bifurcation of the internal carotid artery.

Clinical Findings

A. Symptoms and Signs: Aneurysms may cause a focal neurologic deficit by compressing adjacent structures. However, most are asymptomatic or produce only nonspecific symptoms until they rupture, at which time subarachnoid hemorrhage results. There is often a paucity of focal neurologic signs in patients with subarachnoid hemorrhage, but when present such signs may relate either to a focal hematoma or to ischemia in the territory of the vessel with the ruptured aneurysm. Hemiplegia or other focal deficit sometimes occurs after a delay of 4–14 days and is due to focal arterial spasm in the vicinity of the ruptured aneurysm. This spasm is of uncertain, probably multifactorial, cause, but it sometimes leads to significant cerebral ischemia or infarction, and it may further aggravate any existing increase in intracranial pressure. Subacute hydrocephalus due to interference with the flow of cerebrospinal fluid may occur after 2 or more weeks, and this leads to a delayed clinical deterioration that is relieved by shunting.

In some patients, "warning leaks" of a small amount of blood from the aneurysm precede the major hemorrhage by a few hours or days. They lead to headaches, sometimes accompanied by nausea and neck stiffness, but the true nature of these symptoms is often not appreciated until massive hemorrhage occurs.

B. Laboratory, X-Ray, and Other Studies: The CT scan generally confirms that subarachnoid hemorrhage has occurred, but occasionally the findings are normal despite rupture of the aneurysm. Examination of cerebrospinal fluid in such cases shows it to be grossly bloodstained. The electroencephalogram sometimes indicates the side or site of hemorrhage but frequently shows only a diffuse abnormality. Electrocardiographic changes suggesting myocardial ischemia are well described and have been attributed to release of catecholamines by the stress of the hemorrhage. Peripheral leukocytosis and transient glycosuria are also common findings.

Angiography (bilateral carotid and vertebral studies) generally indicates the size and site of the lesion, sometimes reveals multiple aneurysms, and may show arterial spasm. If arteriograms show no abnormality, the examination should be repeated after 2 weeks because vasospasm may have prevented detection of an aneurysm during the initial study.

Treatment

The major aim of treatment is to prevent further hemorrhages. Definitive treatment requires a surgical approach to the aneurysm and ideally consists of clipping of the aneurysmal base. If surgery is not feasible, medical management as outlined above for subarachnoid hemorrhage is continued for about 6 weeks and is followed by gradual mobilization.

The optimal time for surgery depends upon the clinical status of the patient. Although some surgeons now favor early operation, others have shown that the operative morbidity and mortality rates are decreased by delaying surgery for at least 10 days after the hemorrhage. (The optimal timing of surgery is currently being investigated in a multicenter study that is nearing completion.) Unfortunately, the risk of further hemorrhage is greatest within a few days of the first hemorrhage; approximately 20% of patients will have further bleeding within 2 weeks and 40% within 6 months. Accordingly, attempts have been made to reduce this risk pharmacologically. Since antifibrinolytic drugs prevent lysis of any blood clot that has formed near the site of rupture, aminocaproic acid (Amicar) is often given for the first 2 weeks or so, or until surgery, to reduce the incidence of early recurrence of bleeding. The daily dose is 24–36 g (5 g initially, followed by 1–1.25 g hourly) given intravenously for the first week and then orally, while the streptokinase clot lysis time is monitored. Outside of the USA, use of tranexamic acid is preferred. Potential complications include venous thrombosis, pulmonary embolism, and enhanced cerebral vasospasm, but data from published studies indicate that these have not caused major problems. Whether these substances really do lower the incidence of further hemorrhage remains controversial, and a random controlled trial to settle the issue is in progress.

There is currently no specific treatment for cerebral vasospasm, but calcium channel blocking agents have helped to reduce or reverse experimental vasospasm, and results of a clinical study in which nimodipine was given orally to neurologically normal patients after subarachnoid hemorrhage indicate that it significantly reduced the incidence of ischemic deficits from arterial spasm without producing any side effects. The initial dose of nimodipine was 0.7 mg/kg, followed by 0.35 mg/kg every 4 hours for 21 days.

With regard to unruptured aneurysms, those that are symptomatic merit prompt surgical treatment, whereas small asymptomatic ones discovered incidentally are often followed arteriographically and corrected surgically only if they increase in size to over 5 mm. The natural history of unruptured aneurysms is not clearly defined, however, and the age and condition of the patient and experience of the surgeon will clearly bear on any therapeutic decisions.

Adams HP et al: Antifibrinolytic therapy in patients with aneurysmal subarachnoid hemorrhage: A report of the Cooperative Aneurysm Study. *Arch Neurol* 1981;**38**:25.

Allen GS et al: Cerebral arterial spasm: A controlled trial of nimodipine in patients with subarachnoid hemorrhage. *N Engl J Med* 1983;**308**:619.

Kassell NF, Drake CG: Review of the management of saccular aneurysms. *Neurol Clin* 1983;**1**:73.

Sundt TM, Whisnant JP: Subarachnoid hemorrhage from intracranial aneurysms: Surgical management and natural history of disease. *N Engl J Med* 1978;**299**:116.

Weibers DO, Whisnant JP, O'Fallon WM: The natural history of unruptured intracranial aneurysms. *N Engl J Med* 1981;**304**:696.

6. ARTERIOVENOUS MALFORMATIONS

Arteriovenous malformations are congenital vascular malformations that result from a localized maldevelopment of part of the primitive vascular plexus and consist of abnormal arteriovenous communications without intervening capillaries. They vary in size ranging from massive lesions that are fed by multiple vessels and involve a large part of the brain to lesions so small that they are hard to identify at arteriography, surgery, or autopsy. In approximately 10% of cases, there is an associated arterial aneurysm, while 1–2% of patients presenting with aneurysms have associated arteriovenous malformations. Clinical presentation may relate to hemorrhage from the malformation or an associated aneurysm or may relate to cerebral ischemia due to diversion of blood by the anomalous arteriovenous shunt or due to venous stagnation. Regional maldevelopment of the brain, compression or distortion of adjacent cerebral tissue by enlarged anomalous vessels, and progressive gliosis due to mechanical and ischemic factors may also be contributory. In addition, communicating or obstructive hydrocephalus may occur and lead to symptoms.

Clinical Findings
A. Symptoms and Signs:
1. Supratentorial lesions–Most cerebral arteriovenous malformations are supratentorial, usually lying in the territory of the middle cerebral artery. Initial symptoms consist of hemorrhage in 30–60% of cases, epilepsy in 20–40%, headache in 5–25%, and miscellaneous complaints (including focal deficits) in 10–15%. Up to 70% of arteriovenous malformations bleed at some point in their natural history, most commonly before the patient reaches the age of 40 years. This tendency to bleed is unrelated to the lesion site or to the patient's sex, but small arteriovenous malformations are more likely to bleed than large ones. Arteriovenous malformations that have bled once are more likely to bleed again. Hemorrhage is commonly intracerebral as well as into the subarachnoid space, and it has a fatal outcome in about 10% of cases. Focal or generalized seizures may accompany or follow hemorrhage, or they may be the initial presentation, especially with frontal or parietal arteriovenous malformations. Headaches are especially likely when the external carotid arteries are involved in the malformation. These sometimes simulate migraine but more commonly are nonspecific in character, with nothing about them to suggest an underlying structural lesion.

In patients presenting with subarachnoid hemorrhage, examination may reveal an abnormal mental status and signs of meningeal irritation. Additional findings may help to localize the lesion and sometimes indicate that intracranial pressure is increased. A cranial bruit always suggests the possibility of a cerebral arteriovenous malformation, but bruits may also be found with aneurysms, meningiomas, acquired arteriovenous fistulas, and arteriovenous malformations involving the scalp, calvarium, or orbit. Bruits are best heard over the ipsilateral eye or mastoid region and are of some help in lateralization but not in localization. Absence of a bruit in no way excludes the possibility of arteriovenous malformation.

2. Infratentorial lesions–Brain stem arteriovenous malformations are often clinically silent, but they may hemorrhage, cause obstructive hydrocephalus, or lead to progressive or relapsing brain stem deficits. Cerebellar arteriovenous malformations may also be clinically inconspicuous but sometimes lead to cerebellar hemorrhage (see p 595).

B. Laboratory, X-Ray, and Other Studies: In patients presenting with suspected hemorrhage, CT scanning indicates whether subarachnoid or intracerebral bleeding has recently occurred, helps to localize its source, and may reveal the arteriovenous malformation. If the CT scan shows no evidence of bleeding but subarachnoid hemorrhage is diagnosed clinically, the cerebrospinal fluid should be examined.

When intracranial hemorrhage is confirmed but the source of hemorrhage is not evident on the CT scan, arteriography is necessary to exclude aneurysm or arteriovenous malformation. Even if the findings on CT scan suggest arteriovenous malformation, arteriography is required to establish the nature of the lesion with certainty and to determine its anatomic features, so that treatment can be planned. The examination must generally include bilateral opacification of the internal and external carotid arteries and the vertebral arteries. Arteriovenous malformations typically appear as a tangled vascular mass with distended tortuous afferent and efferent vessels, a rapid circulation time, and arteriovenous shunting.

Electroencephalography is usually indicated in patients presenting with seizures and may show consistently focal or lateralized abnormalities resulting from the underlying cerebral arteriovenous malformation. This should be followed by CT scanning. Findings on plain x-rays of the skull are often normal unless an intracerebral hematoma is present.

Treatment

Surgical treatment to prevent further hemorrhage is justified in patients with arteriovenous malformations that have bled, provided that the lesion is accessible and the patient has a reasonable life expectancy. Surgical treatment is also appropriate if intracranial pressure is increased or if there is cardiac decompensation, as occurs in children, and to prevent further progression of a focal neurologic deficit. In patients presenting solely with seizures, anticonvulsant drug treatment is usually sufficient and operative treatment unnecessary unless there are further developments.

Definitive operative treatment consists of excision of the arteriovenous malformation if it is surgically accessible and is not in a critical location. Arteriovenous malformations that are inoperable because of their location are sometimes treated solely by embolization; although the risk of hemorrhage is not reduced, neurologic deficits may be stabilized or even reversed by this procedure. Two other new techniques

for the treatment of intracerebral arteriovenous malformations are injection of a vascular occlusive polymer through a flow-guided microcatheter and permanent occlusion of feeding vessels by positioning detachable balloon catheters in the desired sites and then inflating them with quickly solidifying contrast material. A recent study suggests that proton beam therapy may be useful in the management of inoperable cerebral arteriovenous malformations.

Aminoff MJ: Angiomas and fistulae involving the nervous system. In: *Vascular Disease of the Central Nervous System.* Ross Russell RW (editor). Churchill Livingstone, 1983.

Drake CG: Arteriovenous malformations of the brain: The options for management. *N Engl J Med* 1983;**309**:308.

Graf CJ, Perret GE, Torner JC: Bleeding from cerebral arteriovenous malformations as part of their natural history. *J Neurosurg* 1983;**58**:331.

Stein BM, Wolpert SM: Arteriovenous malformations of the brain. (2 parts). *Arch Neurol* 1980;**37**:1, 69.

7. SPINAL CORD VASCULAR DISEASES

Infarction of the Spinal Cord

Infarction of the spinal cord is rare. It occurs only in the territory of the anterior spinal artery because this vessel, which supplies the anterior two-thirds of the cord, is itself supplied by only a limited number of feeders. Infarction usually results from interrupted flow in one or more of these feeders, eg, by dissecting aortic aneurysm, aortography, polyarteritis, and hypotensive crisis. The paired posterior spinal arteries, by contrast, are supplied by numerous arteries at different levels of the cord.

Since the anterior spinal artery receives numerous feeders cervically, infarcts almost always occur more caudally. Clinical presentation is characterized by acute onset of flaccid, areflexive paraplegia that evolves after a few days or weeks into a spastic paraplegia with extensor plantar responses. There is an accompanying dissociated sensory loss, with impairment of appreciation of pain and temperature but preservation of sensations of vibration and position. Treatment is symptomatic.

Hematomyelia

Hematomyelia, a rare disorder, is usually related to trauma, vascular malformation, bleeding disorder, or anticoagulant therapy. A severe cord syndrome develops rapidly and is associated with blood in the cerebrospinal fluid.

Epidural or Subdural Hemorrhage

Epidural or subdural hemorrhage may lead to sudden severe back pain and an acute compressive myelopathy necessitating urgent myelography and surgical evacuation. It may occur in patients with bleeding disorders or those who are taking anticoagulant drugs, sometimes following trauma or lumbar puncture. Epidural hemorrhage may also be related to vascular malformation or tumor deposit.

Arteriovenous Malformation of the Spinal Cord

Arteriovenous malformations of the cord are congenital lesions that present with spinal subarachnoid hemorrhage or myeloradiculopathy. Since most of these malformations are located in the thoracolumbar region, they lead to motor and sensory disturbances in the legs and to sphincter disorders. Pain in the legs or back is often severe. Examination reveals an upper, lower, or mixed motor deficit in the legs; sensory deficits are also present and are usually extensive, although occasionally they are confined to radicular distribution. The signs thus indicate an extensive lesion in the longitudinal axis of the cord. Cervical arteriovenous malformations lead also to symptoms and signs in the arms. A spinal bruit is sometimes audible, and cutaneous angioma may be related to the spinal malformation. In general, the diagnosis is suggested at myelography (performed with the patient prone and supine) when serpiginous filling defects due to enlarged vessels are found. Selective spinal arteriography confirms the diagnosis. Most lesions are extramedullary, are posterior to the cord (lying either intra- or extradurally), and can easily be treated by ligation of feeding vessels and excision of the fistulous anomaly. If treatment is not given, the patient is likely to become increasingly disabled or to die from recurrent subarachnoid hemorrhage.

Aminoff MJ: *Spinal Angiomas.* Blackwell, 1976.

Henson RA, Parson M: Ischaemic lesions of the spinal cord: An illustrated review. *Q J Med* 1967;**36**:205.

INTRACRANIAL & SPINAL TUMORS

1. PRIMARY INTRACRANIAL TUMORS

Approximately half of all primary intracranial neoplasms (Table 17–3) are gliomas, and the remainder are meningiomas, pituitary adenomas, neurofibromas, and other tumors. Certain tumors, especially neurofibromas, hemangioblastomas, and retinoblastomas, may have a familial basis, and congenital factors bear on the development of craniopharyngiomas. Tumors may occur at any age, but certain gliomas show particular age predilections (Table 17–3).

Clinical Findings

A. Symptoms and Signs: Intracranial tumors may lead to a generalized disturbance of cerebral function and to symptoms and signs of increased intracranial pressure. In consequence, there may be personality changes, intellectual decline, emotional lability, seizures, headaches, nausea, and malaise. If the pressure is increased in a particular cranial compartment, brain tissue may herniate into a compartment with lower pressure. The most familiar syndrome is herniation of the temporal lobe uncus through the tentorial hiatus, which causes compression of the third cranial nerve, midbrain, and posterior cerebral artery. The earliest sign of this is ipsilateral pupillary dilatation, followed by stupor, coma, decerebrate posturing, and respiratory arrest. Another important herniation syndrome consists of displacement of the cerebellar tonsils through the foramen magnum, which causes medullary compression leading to apnea, circulatory collapse, and death. Other herniation syndromes are less common and of less clear clinical importance.

Intracranial tumors also lead to focal deficits depending on their location.

1. Frontal lobe lesions--Tumors of the frontal lobe often lead to progressive intellectual decline, slowing of mental activity, personality changes, and contralateral grasp reflexes. They may lead to expressive aphasia if the posterior part of the left inferior frontal gyrus is involved. Anosmia may also occur as a consequence of pressure on the olfactory nerve. Precentral lesions may cause focal motor seizures or contralateral pyramidal deficits.

2. Temporal lobe lesions–These lesions may produce a variety of disturbances. Tumors of the uncinate region may be manifest by seizures with olfactory or gustatory hallucinations, motor phenomena such as licking or smacking of the lips, and some impairment of external awareness without actual loss of consciousness. Temporal lobe lesions also lead to depersonalization, emotional changes, behavioral disturbances, sensations of *déjà vu* or *jamais vu,* micropsia or macropsia, visual field defects (crossed upper quadrantanopia), and auditory illusions or hallucinations. Left-sided lesions may lead to dysnomia and receptive aphasia, while right-sided involvement sometimes disturbs the perception of musical notes and melodies.

3. Parietal lobe lesions–Tumors in this location characteristically cause contralateral disturbances of sensation and may cause sensory seizures, sensory loss or inattention, or some combination of these symptoms. The sensory loss is cortical in type and involves postural sensibility and tactile discrimination, so that the appreciation of shape, size, weight, and texture is impaired. Objects placed in the hand may not be recognized (astereognosis). Extensive parietal lobe lesions may produce contralateral hyperpathia and spontaneous pain (thalamic syndrome). Involvement of the optic radiation leads to a contralateral homonymous field defect that sometimes consists solely of lower quadrantanopia. Lesions of the left angular gyrus cause Gerstmann's syndrome (a combination of alexia, agraphia, acalculia, right-left confusion, and finger agnosia), whereas involvement of the left submarginal gyrus causes ideational apraxia. Anosognosia (the denial, neglect, or rejection of a paralyzed limb) is seen in patients with lesions of the nondominant (right) hemisphere. Constructional apraxia and dressing apraxia may also occur with right-sided lesions.

4. Occipital lobe lesions–Tumors of the occipi-

Table 17–3. Primary tumors of the brain.

Tumor	Clinical Features	Treatment and Prognosis
Glioblastoma multiforme	Presents commonly with nonspecific complaints and increased intracranial pressure. As it grows, focal deficits develop.	Course is rapidly progressive, with poor prognosis. Total surgical removal is usually not possible, and response to radiation therapy is poor.
Astrocytoma	Presentation similar to glioblastoma multiforme but course more protracted, often over several years. Cerebellar astrocytoma, especially in children, may have a more benign course.	Prognosis is variable. By the time of diagnosis, total excision is usually impossible; tumor often is not radiosensitive. In cerebellar astrocytoma, total surgical removal is often possible.
Medulloblastoma	Seen most frequently in children. Generally arises from roof of fourth ventricle and leads to increased intracranial pressure accompanied by brain stem and cerebellar signs. May seed in subarachnoid space.	Treatment consists of surgery combined with radiation therapy and chemotherapy.
Ependymoma	Glioma arising from the ependyma of a ventricle, especially the fourth ventricle; leads early to signs of increased intracranial pressure. Arises also from central canal of cord.	Tumor is not radiosensitive and is best treated surgically if possible.
Oligodendroglioma	Slow-growing. Usually arises in cerebral hemisphere in adults. Calcification may be visible on skull x-ray.	Treatment is surgical, which is usually successful.
Brain stem glioma	Presents during childhood with cranial nerve palsies and then with long-tract signs in the limbs. Signs of increased intracranial pressure occur late.	Tumor is inoperable; treatment is by irradiation and shunt for increased intracranial pressure.
Cerebellar hemangioblastoma	Presents with dysequilibrium, ataxia of trunk or limbs, and signs of increased intracranial pressure. Sometimes familial. May be associated with retinal and spinal vascular lesions, polycythemia, and hypernephromas.	Treatment is surgical.
Pineal tumor	Presents with increased intracranial pressure, sometimes associated with impaired upward gaze (Parinaud's syndrome) and other deficits indicative of midbrain lesion.	Ventricular decompression by shunting is followed by surgical approach to tumor; irradiation is indicated if tumor is malignant. Prognosis depends on histopathologic findings and extent of tumor.
Craniopharyngioma	Originates from remnants of Rathke's pouch above the sella, depressing the optic chiasm. May present at any age but usually in childhood, with endocrine dysfunction and bitemporal field defects.	Treatment is surgical, but total removal may not be possible.
Acoustic neurinoma	Ipsilateral hearing loss is most common initial symptom. Subsequent symptoms may include tinnitus, headache, vertigo, facial weakness or numbness, and long-tract signs. (May be familial and bilateral when related to neurofibromatosis.) Most sensitive screening test is brain stem auditory evoked potential.	Treatment is excision by translabyrinthine surgery, craniectomy, or a combined approach. Outcome is usually good.
Meningioma	Originates from the dura mater or arachnoid; compresses rather than invades adjacent neural structures. Increasingly common with advancing age. Tumor size varies greatly. Symptoms vary with tumor site—eg, unilateral exophthalmos (sphenoidal ridge); anosmia and optic nerve compression (olfactory groove). Tumor is usually benign and readily detected by CT scanning; may lead to calcification and bone erosion visible on plain x-rays of skull.	Treatment is surgical. Tumor may recur if removal is incomplete.

tal lobe characteristically produce crossed homonymous hemianopia or a partial field defect. With left-sided or bilateral lesions, there may be visual agnosia both for objects and for colors, while irritative lesions on either side can cause unformed visual hallucinations. Bilateral occipital lobe involvement causes cortical blindness in which there is preservation of pupillary responses to light. There may also be loss of color perception, prosopagnosia (inability to identify a familiar face), simultagnosia (inability to integrate and interpret a composite scene as opposed to its individual elements), and Balint's syndrome (failure to turn the eyes to a particular point in space, despite preservation of spontaneous and reflex eye movements). The denial of blindness or a field defect constitutes Anton's syndrome.

5. Brain stem and cerebellar lesions–Brain stem lesions lead to cranial nerve palsies, ataxia, incoordination, nystagmus, and pyramidal and sensory deficits in the limbs on one or both sides. Intrinsic brain stem tumors, such as gliomas, tend to produce an increase in intracranial pressure only late in their course. Cerebellar tumors produce marked ataxia of the trunk if the vermis cerebelli is involved and produce ipsilateral appendicular deficits (ataxia, incoordination, and hypotonia of the limbs) if the cerebellar hemispheres are affected.

6. False localizing signs–Tumors may lead to neurologic signs other than by direct compression or infiltration, thereby leading to errors of clinical localization. These false localizing signs include third or sixth nerve palsy produced by herniation syndromes, bilateral extensor plantar responses, and an extensor plantar response occurring ipsilateral to a hemispheric tumor as a result of compression of the opposite cerebral peduncle against the tentorium.

B. Laboratory, X-Ray, and Other Studies: Diagnosis of intracranial neoplasms has been facilitated by CT scanning, which may not only detect the lesion but may also define its location, shape, and size; the extent to which normal anatomy is distorted; and the degree of any associated cerebral edema or mass effect. Although CT scanning is not so helpful in the evaluation of tumors in the posterior fossa, magnetic resonance imaging (MRI) promises to be of particular value in this regard. The characteristic appearance of meningiomas on CT scanning is virtually diagnostic; ie, a lesion in a typical site (parasagittal and sylvian regions, olfactory groove, sphenoidal ridge, tuberculum sellae) that appears as a homogeneous area of increased density in non-contrast CT scans and enhances uniformly with contrast.

Arteriography may show stretching or displacement of normal cerebral vessels by the tumor and the presence of tumor vascularity. The presence of an avascular mass is a nonspecific finding that could be due to tumor, hematoma, abscess, or any space-occupying lesion. In patients with normal hormone levels and an intrasellar mass, angiography is necessary to distinguish with confidence between a pituitary adenoma and an arterial aneurysm.

Isotopic brain scans may occasionally be diagnostic when a clinically suspected tumor is not detected by CT scanning. The electroencephalogram, formerly an important noninvasive screening procedure, has had a lesser role since the advent of CT scanning but can be used to provide complementary information concerning cerebral function rather than structure. It may show either a focal disturbance due to the neoplasm or a more diffuse change reflecting altered mental status.

Cerebrospinal fluid is frequently abnormal in patients with intracranial tumors, but the findings are rarely diagnostic. Because of the risk of herniation, lumbar puncture should generally be delayed until after CT scanning has been performed in patients with suspected intracranial mass lesions. The findings on CT scan often remove the need for lumbar puncture.

Hormonal studies, outlined in Chapter 19, will help document endocrine disturbances that occur with pituitary tumors and craniopharyngiomas.

Treatment

Treatment depends on the type and site of the tumor (Table 17–3) and the condition of the patient. Complete surgical removal may be possible if the tumor is extra-axial (eg, meningioma, acoustic neuroma) or is not in a critical or inaccessible region of the brain (eg, cerebellar hemangioblastoma). Surgery also permits the diagnosis to be verified and may be beneficial in reducing intracranial pressure and relieving symptoms even if the neoplasm cannot be completely removed. Clinical deficits are sometimes due in part to obstructive hydrocephalus, in which case simple surgical shunting procedures often produce dramatic benefit. In patients with malignant gliomas, radiation therapy increases median survival rates regardless of any preceding surgery, and its combination with chemotherapy provides additional benefit. Indications for irradiation in the treatment of patients with other primary intracranial neoplasms depend upon tumor type and accessibility, the feasibility of complete surgical removal, and local custom. Corticosteroids help reduce cerebral edema and are usually started before surgery. Herniation is treated with intravenous dexamethasone and intravenous mannitol (20%). Symptomatic treatment with analgesic and anticonvulsant drugs is given as necessary.

Baker HL, Houser OW, Campbell JK: National Cancer Institute Study: Evaluation of computed tomography in the diagnosis of intracranial neoplasms. *Radiology* 1980;**136**:91.

Lieberman A, Ransohoff J: Treatment of primary brain tumors. *Med Clin North Am* 1979;**63**:835.

Wilson CB: Current concepts in cancer: Brain tumors. *N Engl J Med* 1979;**300**:1469.

Wilson CB, Fulton DS, Seager ML: Supportive management of the patient with malignant brain tumor. *JAMA* 1980;**244**:1249.

2. METASTATIC INTRACRANIAL TUMORS

Cerebral Metastases

Metastatic brain tumors present in the same way as other cerebral neoplasms, ie, with increased intracranial pressure, with focal or diffuse disturbance of cerebral function, or with both of these manifestations. Indeed, in patients with a single cerebral lesion, the metastatic nature of the lesion may only become evident on histopathologic examination. In other patients, there is evidence of widespread metastatic disease, or an isolated cerebral metastasis develops during treatment of the primary neoplasm.

The most common source of intracranial metastasis is carcinoma of the lung; other common sources are neoplasms of the breast, kidney, and gastrointestinal tract. Most cerebral metastases are located supratentorially. The laboratory and radiologic studies used to evaluate patients with metastases are similar to those described in the preceding section on primary neoplasms. CT scanning should be performed both with and without contrast material. On rare occasions, the results of radionuclide scanning are positive when results of CT scanning are negative. Lumbar puncture is not undertaken routinely and may lead to cerebral herniation, but it will be necessary in patients with suspected carcinomatous meningitis (see below). There is some controversy concerning the extent to which patients with verified cerebral metastasis from an unknown primary should be investigated to determine its source.

In patients with only a single cerebral metastasis who are otherwise well, it may be possible to remove the lesion, depending upon its site, and then treat with irradiation. Alternatively, irradiation may be selected as the sole means of treatment. In patients with multiple metastases or widespread systemic disease, the long-term outlook is gloomy, and treatment by radiation therapy or chemotherapy must be considered on an individualized basis.

Leptomeningeal Metastases (Carcinomatous Meningitis)

The neoplasms metastasizing most commonly to the leptomeninges are carcinoma of the breast, lymphomas, and leukemia. Leptomeningeal metastases lead to multifocal neurologic deficits, which may be associated with infiltration of cranial and spinal nerve roots, direct invasion of the brain or spinal cord, obstructive hydrocephalus, or some combination of these factors.

The diagnosis is confirmed by examination of the cerebrospinal fluid. Findings may include elevated cerebrospinal fluid pressure, pleocytosis, increased protein concentration, and decreased glucose concentration. Cytologic studies may indicate that malignant cells are present; if not, spinal tap should be repeated at least twice to obtain further samples for analysis.

CT scans showing contrast enhancement in the basal cisterns or showing hydrocephalus without any evidence of a mass lesion support the diagnosis. Myelography may show deposits on multiple nerve roots.

Treatment is by irradiation to symptomatic areas, combined with intrathecal methotrexate. The long-term prognosis is poor—only about 10% of patients survive for a year.

Cairncross JG, Kim J-H, Posner JB: Radiation therapy for brain metastases. *Ann Neurol* 1980;7:529.

Henson RA, Urich H: *Cancer and the Nervous System.* Blackwell, 1982.

3. PRIMARY & METASTATIC SPINAL TUMORS

Approximately 10% of spinal tumors are intramedullary. Ependymoma is the most common type of intramedullary tumor; the remainder are other types of glioma. Extramedullary tumors may be extradural or intradural in location. Among the primary extramedullary tumors, neurofibromas and meningiomas are relatively common, are benign, and may be intra- or extradural. Carcinomatous metastases, lymphomatous or leukemic deposits, and myeloma are usually extradural.

Tumors may lead to spinal cord dysfunction by direct compression, by ischemia secondary to arterial or venous obstruction, and, in the case of intramedullary lesions, by invasive infiltration.

Clinical Findings

A. Symptoms and Signs: Symptoms usually develop insidiously. Pain is often conspicuous with extradural lesions; is characteristically aggravated by coughing or straining; may be radicular, localized to the back, or felt diffusely in an extremity; and may be accompanied by motor deficits, paresthesias, or numbness, especially in the legs. When sphincter disturbances occur, they are usually particularly disabling.

Examination may reveal localized spinal tenderness. A segmental lower motor neuron deficit or dermatomal sensory changes (or both) are sometimes found at the level of the lesion, while an upper motor neuron deficit and sensory disturbance are found below it. The combination of signs may constitute Brown-Séquard syndrome or central cord syndrome, in some instances.

B. Laboratory, X-Ray, and Other Studies: The cerebrospinal fluid is often xanthochromic and contains a greatly increased protein concentration with normal cell content and glucose concentration; Queckenstedt's test at lumbar puncture may reveal a partial or complete block. Findings on plain x-ray of the spine may be normal but are commonly abnormal when there are metastatic deposits. Myelography, CT scanning with metrizamide, or both procedures may be necessary to identify and localize the site of cord compression. If a complete block is present at lumbar myelography, a cisternal myelogram is performed to determine the upper level of the block.

Treatment

Intramedullary tumors are treated by decompression and surgical excision (when feasible), and irradiation. The prognosis depends upon the cause and severity of cord compression before it is relieved.

In the past, treatment of epidural spinal metastases consisted of surgical decompression of the spinal cord followed by irradiation, but a recent study has shown that irradiation alone is equally effective. Dexamethasone is also given in a high dosage (eg, 25 mg 4 times daily for 3 days, followed by rapid tapering of the dosage, depending on response) to reduce cord swelling and relieve pain. Surgical decompression is best reserved for patients with tumors that are unresponsive to irradiation or have previously been irradiated and for cases in which there is some uncertainty about the diagnosis. The long-term outlook is poor, but radiation treatment may at least delay the onset of major disability. Analgesics are given as necessary for pain.

Posner JB, Gilbert RW: Epidural spinal cord compression from metastatic tumor. *Ann Neurol* 1978;3:40.

4. NONMETASTATIC NEUROLOGIC COMPLICATIONS OF MALIGNANT DISEASE

A variety of nonmetastatic neurologic complications of malignant disease can be recognized:

(1) Metabolic encephalopathy due to electrolyte abnormalities, infections, drug overdose, or the failure of some vital organ may be reflected by drowsiness, lethargy, restlessness, insomnia, agitation, confusion, stupor, or coma. The mental changes are usually associated with tremor, asterixis, and multifocal myoclonus. The electroencephalogram is generally diffusely slowed. Laboratory studies are necessary to detect the cause of the encephalopathy, which must then be treated appropriately.

(2) Immune suppression resulting from either the malignant disease or its treatment (eg, by chemotherapy) predisposes patients to brain abscess, progressive multifocal leukoencephalopathy, meningitis, herpes zoster infection, and other infectious diseases. Moreover, an overt or occult cerebrospinal fluid fistula, as occurs with some tumors, may also increase the risk of infection. CT scanning aids in the early recognition of a brain abscess, but metastatic brain tumors may have a similar appearance. Examination of the cerebrospinal fluid is essential in the evaluation of patients with meningitis but is of no help in the diagnosis of brain abscess. Treatment is of the infective organism.

(3) Cerebrovascular disorders that cause neurologic complications in patients with systemic cancer include nonbacterial thrombotic endocarditis and septic embolization. Cerebral, subarachnoid, or subdural hemorrhages may occur in patients with myelogenous leukemia and may be found in association with metastatic tumors, especially malignant melanoma. Spinal subdural hemorrhage sometimes occurs after lumbar puncture in patients with marked thrombocytopenia.

Diffuse intravascular coagulation occurs most commonly in patients with leukemia or lymphoma and is characterized by a fluctuating encephalopathy, often with associated seizures, that frequently progresses to coma or death. There may be few accompanying neurologic signs.

Venous sinus thrombosis, which usually presents with convulsions and headaches, may also occur in patients with leukemia or lymphoma. Examination commonly reveals papilledema and focal or diffuse neurologic signs. Treatment is with anticonvulsants and drugs to lower the intracranial pressure. The role of anticoagulants is controversial.

(4) Encephalopathy characterized by impaired recent memory, disturbed affect, hallucinations, and seizures occurs in some patients with carcinomas. The cerebrospinal fluid is often abnormal. Electroencephalograms may show diffuse slow-wave activity, especially over the temporal regions. Pathologic changes are most marked in the inferomedian portions of the temporal lobes. There is no specific treatment.

(5) Subacute cerebellar degeneration occurs most commonly in association with carcinoma of the lung. Symptoms may precede those due to the neoplasm itself, which may be undetected for several months or even longer. Typically, there is a pancerebellar syndrome causing dysarthria, nystagmus, and ataxia of the trunk and limbs. Mild pleocytosis and increased protein concentration may be found in the cerebrospinal fluid. Treatment is of the underlying malignant disease.

(6) Malignant disease is more commonly associated with sensorimotor polyneuropathy than with pure sensory neuropathy (ie, dorsal root ganglionitis) or autonomic neuropathy (see p 622).

(7) Dermatomyositis or myasthenic syndrome may be seen in patients with underlying carcinoma (see Chapter 14 and p 628).

(8) A syndrome similar to amyotrophic lateral sclerosis or progressive spinal muscular atrophy is encountered occasionally in patients with neoplastic disease. Whether this is more than fortuitous is unclear.

5. BRAIN ABSCESS

Infectious disorders are considered elsewhere in this book, but brief comment will be made here concerning cerebral abscess, which presents as an intracranial space-occupying lesion. Brain abscess may arise as a sequela of disease of the ear or nose, may be a metastatic complication of infection elsewhere in the body, or may result from infection introduced intracranially by trauma or surgical procedures. The most common infective organisms are streptococci and staphylococci. Headache, drowsiness, inattention, confusion, and seizures are early symptoms, followed by signs of increasing intracranial pressure and then a focal neurologic deficit. There may be little or no evidence of systemic infection.

A CT scan of the head characteristically shows an area of increased contrast surrounding a low-density core. Similar abnormalities may, however, be found in patients with metastatic neoplasms. Arteriography indicates the presence of a space-occupying lesion, which appears as an avascular mass with displacement of normal cerebral vessels, but this procedure provides no clue to the nature of the lesion.

Treatment consists of intravenous antibiotics, combined with surgical drainage (aspiration or excision) if necessary to reduce the mass effect.

Rosenblum ML et al: Nonoperative treatment of brain abscesses in selected high-risk patients. *J Neurosurg* 1980;**52:**217.

6. PSEUDOTUMOR CEREBRI (Benign Intracranial Hypertension)

Symptoms of pseudotumor cerebri consist of headache, diplopia, and other visual disturbances due to papilledema and abducens nerve dysfunction. Examination reveals the papilledema and some enlargement of the blind spots, but patients otherwise look well. Investigations reveal no evidence of a space-occupying lesion, and the CT scan shows small or normal ventricles. Lumbar puncture confirms the presence of intracranial hypertension, but the cerebrospinal fluid is normal.

There are many causes of pseudotumor cerebri. Thrombosis of the transverse venous sinus as a noninfectious complication of otitis media or chronic mastoiditis is an important cause, and sagittal sinus thrombosis may lead to a clinically similar picture. Other causes include chronic pulmonary disease, endocrine disturbances such as hypoparathyroidism or Addison's disease, vitamin A toxicity, and the use of nalidixic acid, tetracycline, or oral contraceptives. Cases have also followed withdrawal of corticosteroids after long-term use. In many instances, however, no specific cause can be found, and the disorder remits spontaneously after several months. This idiopathic variety is said to be especially common in overweight young women.

Untreated pseudotumor cerebri leads to secondary optic atrophy and permanent visual loss. Repeated lumbar punctures to lower the intracranial pressure by removal of cerebrospinal fluid is effective, but pharmacologic approaches to treatment are now more satisfactory. Acetazolamide reduces formation of cerebrospinal fluid and can be used to start treatment; furosemide serves the same function and can be added to the treatment regimen if necessary. Oral corticosteroids have also been used. Obese patients should be advised to lose weight. Treatment is monitored by checking visual acuity, funduscopic appearance, and pressure of the cerebrospinal fluid.

If medical treatment fails to control the intracranial pressure, surgical placement of a lumboperitoneal or other shunt should be undertaken to preserve vision.

In addition to the above measures, any specific cause of pseudotumor cerebri requires appropriate treatment. Thus, hormone therapy should be initiated if there is an underlying endocrine disturbance. Discontinuing the use of nalidixic acid, tetracycline, oral contraceptives, or vitamin A will allow for resolution of pseudotumor cerebri due to these agents. If corticosteroid withdrawal is responsible, the medication should be reintroduced and then tapered more gradually.

Rush JA: Pseudotumor cerebri. *Br J Hosp Med* 1983;**29**:320.

SELECTED NEUROCUTANEOUS DISEASES

Tuberous Sclerosis

Tuberous sclerosis may occur sporadically or on a familial basis with autosomal dominant inheritance. Its pathogenesis is unknown. Neurologic presentation is with seizures and progressive psychomotor retardation beginning in early childhood. The cutaneous abnormality, adenoma sebaceum, becomes manifest usually between 5 and 10 years of age and typically consists of reddened nodules on the face (cheeks, nasolabial folds, sides of the nose, and chin) and sometimes on the forehead and neck. Other typical cutaneous lesions include subungual fibromas, shagreen patches, and leaf-shaped hypopigmented spots. Associated abnormalities include retinal lesions and tumors, benign rhabdomyomas of the heart, lung cysts, benign tumors in the viscera, and bone cysts.

The disease is slowly progressive and leads to increasing mental deterioration. There is no specific treatment, but anticonvulsant drugs may help in controlling seizures.

Neurofibromatosis (Recklinghausen's Disease)

Neurofibromatosis may occur either sporadically or on a familial basis with autosomal dominant inheritance. Neurologic presentation is usually with symptoms and signs of tumor. Multiple neurofibromas characteristically are present and may involve spinal or cranial nerves, especially the eighth cranial nerve. Examination of the superficial cutaneous nerves usually reveals palpable mobile nodules. In some cases, there is an associated marked overgrowth of subcutaneous tissues (plexiform neuromas), sometimes with an underlying bony abnormality. Associated cutaneous lesions include axillary freckling and patches of cutaneous pigmentation (café au lait spots). Malignant degeneration of neurofibromas occasionally occurs and may lead to peripheral sarcomas. Meningiomas, gliomas (especially optic nerve gliomas), bone cysts, pheochromocytomas, scoliosis, and obstructive hydrocephalus may also occur.

It may be possible to correct disfigurement by plastic surgery. Intraspinal or intracranial tumors and tumors of peripheral nerves should be treated surgically if they are producing symptoms.

Sturge-Weber Syndrome

Sturge-Weber syndrome consists of a congenital, usually unilateral, cutaneous capillary angioma involving the upper face, leptomeningeal angiomatosis, and, in many patients, choroidal angioma. It has no sex predilection and usually occurs sporadically. The cutaneous angioma sometimes has a more extensive distribution over the head and neck and is often quite disfiguring, especially if there is associated overgrowth of connective tissue. Focal or generalized seizures are the usual neurologic presentation and may commence at any age. There may be contralateral homonymous hemianopia, hemiparesis and hemisensory disturbance, ipsilateral glaucoma or buphthalmos, and mental subnormality. Skull x-rays taken after the first 2 years of life usually reveal gyriform ("tramline") intracranial calcification, especially in the parieto-occipital region, due to mineral deposition in the cortex beneath the intracranial angioma.

Treatment is aimed at controlling seizures pharmacologically. Ophthalmologic advice should be sought concerning the management of choroidal angioma and of increased intraocular pressure.

Hereditary Hemorrhagic Telangiectasia (Rendu-Osler-Weber Syndrome)

Rendu-Osler-Weber syndrome is inherited in an autosomal dominant manner. Recurrent hemorrhage results from multiple cutaneous, mucosal, and visceral telangiectasias that occur in this disorder. Neurologic presentation is commonly associated with some complication of the pulmonary arteriovenous fistulas that also occur as part of the syndrome; these complications include cerebral abscess, hypoxia, and embolic phenomena. Various types of vascular anomalies (eg, telangiectasias, cavernous angiomas, arteriovenous malformations, and aneurysms) may also occur in the brain or spinal cord.

Riccardi VM: Von Recklinghausen neurofibromatosis. *N Engl J Med* 1981;**305**:1617.

Roman G et al: Neurological manifestations of hereditary hemorrhagic telangiectasia (Rendu-Osler-Weber disease): Report of 2 cases and review of the literature. *Ann Neurol* 1978;**4**:130.

MOVEMENT DISORDERS

1. BENIGN ESSENTIAL (FAMILIAL) TREMOR

The cause of benign essential tremor is uncertain, but it is sometimes inherited in an autosomal dominant manner. Tremor may begin at any age and is enhanced by emotional stress. The tremor usually involves one or both hands, the head, or the hands and head, while the legs tend to be spared. Examination reveals no other abnormalities. A small quantity of alcohol commonly provides remarkable but short-lived relief by an unknown mechanism.

Although the tremor may become more conspicuous with time, it generally leads to little disability other than cosmetic and social embarrassment, and treatment is often therefore unnecessary. Occasionally, however, it interferes with manual skills and leads to impairment of handwriting. Speech may also be affected if the laryngeal muscles are involved. In such circumstances, treatment with propranolol, unless contraindicated, may be helpful but will need to be continued indefinitely in daily doses of 60–240 mg. It is not clear whether the response to propranolol depends on central or peripheral mechanisms. Primidone may be helpful when propranolol is ineffective.

Jankovic J, Fahn S: Physiologic and pathologic tremors: Diagnosis, mechanism, and management. *Ann Intern Med* 1980;**93**:460.

Larsen TA, Calne DB: Essential tremor. *Clin Neuropharmacol* 1983;**6**:185.

2. PARKINSONISM

Parkinsonism is a relatively common disorder that occurs in all ethnic groups, with an approximately equal sex distribution. The most common variety, idiopathic Parkinson's disease (paralysis agitans), begins most often between 45 and 65 years of age.

Etiology

Parkinsonism occasionally has a familial basis, but this is uncommon. In the past, the disorder often developed within 10 years of encephalitis lethargica, but since this type of infection is not now encountered, postencephalitic parkinsonism is becoming increasingly rare. Exposure to certain toxins (eg, manganese dust, carbon disulfide) and severe carbon monoxide poisoning may lead to parkinsonism. Recently, typical parkinsonism was reported in a group of individuals who had attempted to make a narcotic drug related to meperidine but actually synthesized and then took 1-methyl-4-phenyl-1,2,5,6-tetrahydropyridine (MPTP). This compound selectively destroys dopaminergic neurons in the substantia nigra. Reversible parkinsonism may develop in patients receiving neuroleptic drugs (see Chapter 18). Only rarely is hemiparkinsonism the presenting feature of a brain tumor or some other progressive space-occupying lesion.

In idiopathic parkinsonism, there is cell loss in the substantia nigra, globus pallidus, putamen, and certain other brain stem centers, and Lewy bodies are present in the basal ganglia, brain stem, spinal cord, and sympathetic ganglia. Dopamine depletion due to degeneration of the dopaminergic nigrostriatal system leads to an imbalance of dopamine and acetylcholine, which are neurotransmitters normally present in the corpus striatum. Treatment is directed at redressing this imbalance by blocking the effect of acetylcholine with anticholinergic drugs or by the administration of levodopa, the precursor of dopamine.

Clinical Findings

Tremor, rigidity, bradykinesia, and postural instability are the cardinal features of parkinsonism and may be present in any combination. The tremor of about 4–6 cycles per second is most conspicuous at rest, is enhanced by emotional stress, and is often less severe during voluntary activity. Although it may ultimately be present in all limbs, the tremor is commonly confined to one limb or to the limbs on one side for months or years before it becomes more generalized.

Rigidity (an increase in resistance to passive movement) is responsible for the characteristically flexed posture seen in many patients, but the most disabling symptoms of parkinsonism are due to bradykinesia, manifested as a slowness of voluntary movement and a reduction in automatic movements such as swinging of the arms while walking. Curiously, however, effective voluntary activity may briefly be regained during an emergency (eg, the patient is able to leap aside to avoid an oncoming motor vehicle).

Clinical diagnosis of the well-developed syndrome is usually simple. The patient has a relatively immobile face with widened palpebral fissures, infrequent blinking, and a certain fixity of facial expression. There is often mild blepharoclonus, and a tremor may be present about the mouth and lips. Repetitive tapping (about twice per second) over the bridge of the nose produces a sustained blink response (Myerson's sign). Other findings may include saliva drooling from the mouth, perhaps due to impairment of swallowing; soft and poorly modulated voice; a variable rest tremor and rigidity in some or all of the limbs; slowness of voluntary movements; impairment of fine or rapidly alternating movements; and micrographia. There is typically no muscle weakness (provided that sufficient time is allowed for power to be developed) and no alteration in the tendon reflexes or plantar responses. It is difficult for the patient to arise from a sitting position and begin walking. The gait itself is characterized by small shuffling steps and a loss of the normal automatic arm swing; there may be unsteadiness on turning and difficulty in stopping.

Differential Diagnosis

Diagnostic problems may occur in mild cases. For example, mild hypokinesia or slight tremor is commonly attributed to old age. Depression, with its associated expressionless face, poorly modulated voice, and reduction in voluntary activity, can be difficult to distinguish from mild parkinsonism, especially since the 2 disorders may coexist; in some cases, a trial of antidepressant drug therapy may be necessary. The family history, the character of the tremor, and lack of other neurologic signs should distinguish essential tremor from parkinsonism. Wilson's disease can be distinguished by its early age at onset, the presence of other abnormal movements and Kayser-Fleischer rings, and abnormal levels of serum and urinary copper and serum ceruloplasmin. Huntington's disease presenting with rigidity and bradykinesia may be mistaken for parkinsonism unless the family history and accompanying dementia are recognized. In Shy-Drager syndrome, the clinical features of parkinsonism are accompanied by autonomic insufficiency (leading to postural hypotension, anhidrosis, disturbances of sphincter control, impotence, etc) and more widespread neurologic deficits (pyramidal, lower motor neuron, or cerebellar signs). In progressive supranuclear palsy, bradykinesia and rigidity are accompanied by a supranuclear disorder of eye movements, pseudobulbar palsy, and axial dystonia. Creutzfeldt-Jakob disease may be accompanied by features of parkinsonism, but dementia is usual, myoclonic jerking is common, ataxia and pyramidal signs may be conspicuous, and the electroencephalographic findings are usually characteristic.

Treatment

A. Medical Measures: Drug treatment is not required early in the course of parkinsonism, but the nature of the disorder and the availability of medical treatment for use when necessary should be discussed with the patient.

1. Amantadine–Patients with mild symptoms but no disability may be helped by treatment with amantadine. This drug improves all of the clinical features of parkinsonism, but its mode of action is unclear. Side effects include restlessness, confusion, depression, skin rashes, edema, nausea, constipation, anorexia, postural hypotension, and disturbances of cardiac rhythm. However, these are relatively uncommon with the usual dose (100 mg 2 times daily).

2. Anticholinergic drugs–Anticholinergic drugs are more helpful in alleviating tremor and rigidity than bradykinesia. Treatment is started with a small dose of one preparation (Table 17–4), and the dose is gradually increased until benefit occurs or side effects limit further increments. If treatment is ineffective, the drug is gradually withdrawn and another preparation then tried. Ethopropazine is probably the most helpful drug in this group for the relief of tremor.

Common side effects include dryness of the mouth, nausea, constipation, palpitations, cardiac arrhythmias, urinary retention, confusion, agitation, restlessness, drowsiness, mydriasis, increased intraocular pressure, and defective accommodation.

Anticholinergic drugs are contraindicated in patients with prostatic hypertrophy, closed-angle glaucoma, or obstructive gastrointestinal disease.

3. Levodopa–Levodopa, which is converted in the body to dopamine, improves all of the major features of parkinsonism, including bradykinesia. Long-term levodopa therapy does not stop progression of the disorder; moreover, its effectiveness may decline after 2 or 3 years, and certain complications or adverse reactions to it may develop with time. Levodopa is therefore best reserved for patients with definite disability. The commonest early side effects of levodopa are nausea, vomiting, and hypotension, but cardiac irregularities may also occur. Dyskinesias, restlessness, confusion, and other behavioral changes tend to occur somewhat later and become more common with time. Levodopa-induced dyskinesias may take any conceivable form, including chorea, athetosis, dystonia, tremor, tics, and myoclonus. An even later complication is the "on-off phenomenon," in which

Table 17–4. Anticholinergic drugs for treatment of parkinsonism.*

Drug	Usual Daily Dose (mg)
Benztropine mesylate (Cogentin)	1–6
Biperiden (Akineton)	2–12
Chlorphenoxamine (Phenoxene)	150–400
Cycrimine (Pagitane)	5–20
Ethopropazine (Parsidol)	150–300
Orphenadrine (Disipal, Norflex)	150–400
Procyclidine (Kemadrin)	7.5–30
Trihexyphenidyl (Aphen, Artane, Tremin; others)	6–20

*Reproduced, with permission, from Katzung BG (editor): *Basic & Clinical Pharmacology*, 2nd ed. Lange, 1984.

abrupt but transient fluctuations in the severity of parkinsonism occur unpredictably but frequently during the day. The "off" period of marked bradykinesia has been shown to relate in some instances to falling plasma levels of levodopa. During the "on" phase, dyskinesias are often conspicuous but mobility is increased.

Carbidopa, which inhibits the enzyme responsible for the breakdown of levodopa to dopamine, does not cross the blood-brain barrier. When levodopa is given in combination with carbidopa, the extracerebral breakdown of levodopa is largely prevented. This reduces the amount of levodopa required daily for beneficial effects, and it lowers the incidence of nausea, vomiting, hypotension, and cardiac irregularities. Such a combination does not prevent the development of the "on-off phenomenon," and the incidence of other side effects (dyskinesias or psychiatric complications) may actually be increased.

Sinemet, a commercially available preparation that contains carbidopa and levodopa in a fixed ratio (1:10 or 1:4), is generally used. Treatment is started with a small dose—eg, one tablet of Sinemet 10/100 (containing 10 mg of carbidopa and 100 mg of levodopa) 3 times daily—and gradually increased depending on the response. Most patients require Sinemet 25/250, taken 3 or 4 times daily.

The dyskinesias and behavioral side effects of levodopa are dose-related, but reduction in dose may eliminate any therapeutic benefit. In such circumstances, a drug holiday may be helpful. Levodopa medication is gradually withdrawn over several days and not reinstated for 1–2 weeks. When it is reintroduced, up to two-thirds of patients show improved responsiveness and so derive benefit at a lower daily dose than previously required. The "on-off phenomenon" may also be improved by a drug holiday, but any benefit in this regard is usually short-lived. Unfortunately, there is no way of predicting which patients will benefit from a drug holiday, and it is a distressing and difficult experience that generally necessitates hospitalization.

Levodopa therapy is contraindicated in patients with psychotic illness or closed-angle glaucoma. It should not be given to patients taking monoamine oxidase A inhibitors or within 2 weeks of their withdrawal, because hypertensive crises may result. Levodopa should be avoided in patients with suspected malignant melanomas, which may be activated, and in patients with active peptic ulcers, which may bleed.

4. Bromocriptine–This ergot derivative acts directly on dopamine receptors and has been used as adjunctive therapy in parkinsonism. It is best reserved for patients who have either become refractory to levodopa or who have developed the "on-off phenomenon." Patients who have never responded to levodopa generally fail to respond to bromocriptine as well. The initial dosage of bromocriptine is 1.25 mg twice daily; this is increased by 2.5 mg every 2 weeks until benefit occurs or side effects limit further increments. The usual daily maintenance dose in patients with parkinsonism is between 10 and 30 mg.

Side effects include anorexia, nausea, vomiting, constipation, postural hypotension, digital vasospasm, cardiac arrhythmias, various dyskinesias and mental disturbances, headache, nasal congestion, erythromelalgia, and pulmonary infiltrates.

Bromocriptine is contraindicated in patients with a history of mental illness or recent myocardial infarction and is probably best avoided in those with peripheral vascular disease or peptic ulcers (bleeding from peptic ulcers has been reported).

5. Other drugs–A number of other dopamine agonists, including lisuride and pergolide, have been used to treat parkinsonism, but these are still under study.

B. General Measures: Physical therapy or speech therapy helps many patients. The quality of life can often be improved by the provision of simple aids to daily living, eg, rails or banisters placed strategically about the home, special table cutlery with large handles, nonslip rubber table mats, and devices to amplify the voice.

C. Surgical Measures: Surgical treatment (thalamotomy) is generally reserved for the patient who is relatively young, has predominantly unilateral tremor and rigidity that have failed to respond to medication, and has no evidence of diffuse vascular disease.

Calne DB et al: Advances in the neuropharmacology of parkinsonism. *Ann Intern Med* 1979;**90**:219.

Current concepts and controversies in Parkinson's disease. *Can J Neurol Sci* 1984;**11(Suppl)**. [Entire issue.]

Langston JW et al: Chronic parkinsonism in humans due to a product of meperidine-analog synthesis. *Science* 1983; **219**:979.

Lesser RP et al: Analysis of the clinical problems in parkinsonism and the complications of long-term levodopa therapy. *Neurology* 1979;**29**:1253.

Lieberman AN et al: Long-term efficacy of bromocriptine in Parkinson disease. *Neurology* 1980;**30**:518.

Markham CH, Diamond SG: Evidence to support early levodopa therapy in Parkinson disease. *Neurology* 1981;**31**:125.

Parkes JD: Adverse effects of antiparkinsonian drugs. *Drugs* 1981;**21**:341.

3. HUNTINGTON'S DISEASE

Huntington's disease is characterized by chorea and dementia. It is inherited in an autosomal dominant manner and occurs throughout the world, in all ethnic groups, with a prevalence rate of about 5 per 100,000. Symptoms do not usually develop until after 30 years of age. Thus, by the time of diagnosis the patient has usually had children, and so the disease continues from one generation to the next. The cause of Huntington's disease is unknown.

Clinical onset is usually between 30 and 50 years of age. The disease is progressive and usually leads to a fatal outcome within 15–20 years. The initial symptoms may consist of either abnormal movements or intellectual changes, but ultimately both occur. The earliest mental changes are often behavioral, with irritability, moodiness, antisocial behavior, or a psychiatric disturbance, but a more obvious dementia subsequently develops. The dyskinesia may initially be no more than an apparent fidgetiness or restlessness, but eventually choreiform movements and some dystonic posturing occur. Progressive rigidity and akinesia (rather than chorea) sometimes occur in association with dementia, especially in cases with childhood onset. CT scanning or pneumoencephalography usually demonstrates cerebral atrophy and atrophy of the caudate nucleus in established cases.

Chorea developing with no family history of choreoathetosis should not be attributed to Huntington's disease, at least until other causes of chorea have been excluded clinically and by appropriate laboratory studies. If a patient presents solely with progressive intellectual failure, it may not be possible to distinguish Huntington's disease from other causes of dementia unless there is a characteristic family history or a dyskinesia develops.

There is no cure for Huntington's disease, progression cannot be halted, and treatment is purely symptomatic. The reported biochemical changes suggest a relative underactivity of neurons containing gamma-aminobutyric acid (GABA) and acetylcholine or a relative overactivity of dopaminergic neurons. Treatment with drugs blocking dopamine receptors, such as phenothiazines or haloperidol, may control the dyskinesia and any behavioral disturbances. Haloperidol treatment is usually begun with a dose of 1 mg once or twice daily, which is then increased every 3 or 4 days depending on the response. Tetrabenazine, a drug that depletes central monoamines, is widely used in Europe to treat dyskinesia but is not yet available in the USA. Reserpine is similar in its actions to tetrabenazine and may be helpful; the daily dose is built up gradually to between 2 and 5 mg, depending on the response. Attempts to compensate for the relative GABA deficiency by enhancing central GABA activity or to compensate for the relative cholinergic underactivity by giving choline chloride have not been therapeutically helpful.

Patients should be advised about the risk of passing on the disorder, and any existing offspring should be offered genetic counseling. There is no certain way of determining whether asymptomatic offspring have inherited the disease.

Bird ED: Chemical pathology of Huntington's disease. *Ann Rev Pharmacol Toxicol* 1980;**20**:533.

Martindale B, Yale R: Huntington's chorea: Neglected opportunities for preventive medicine. *Lancet* 1983;**1**:634.

Shoulson I, Fahn S: Huntington disease: Clinical care and evaluation. *Neurology* 1979;**29**:1.

4. SYDENHAM'S CHOREA

Sydenham's chorea, a complication of infection with group A hemolytic streptococci, occurs primarily in children and young adults. It is probably caused by an arteritis. Symptoms develop 2–3 months after rheumatic fever or polyarthritis in about one-third of cases. They may have an acute or insidious onset and usually clear over the following 4–6 months. Symptoms may recur during pregnancy (chorea gravidarum) or in those taking oral contraceptive drugs.

Symptoms consist of unilateral or bilateral choreiform movements. When mild, these may be mistaken for restlessness or fidgetiness. There may be accompanying behavioral changes. Evidence of cardiac involvement is present in about 30% of cases, but there is usually no history of sore throat, no fever, and a normal sedimentation rate and ASO titer.

Treatment consists of bed rest, sedation, and prophylactic antibiotic therapy even if there are no other signs of acute rheumatic fever. A course of intramuscular penicillin is followed by continuous prophylactic oral penicillin daily until about the age of 20 years to prevent further streptococcal infections. The dyskinesia is usually so mild that its pharmacologic management is unnecessary.

Nausieda PA et al: Chorea induced by oral contraceptives. *Neurology* 1979;**29**:1605.

Nausieda PA et al: Sydenham chorea: An update. *Neurology* 1980;**30**:331.

5. IDIOPATHIC TORSION DYSTONIA

Idiopathic torsion dystonia may occur sporadically or on a hereditary basis, with autosomal dominant, autosomal recessive, and X-linked recessive modes of transmission. It may begin in childhood or later and persists throughout life.

The disorder is characterized by the onset of abnormal movements and postures in a patient with a normal birth and developmental history, no relevant past medical illness, and no other neurologic signs. Investigations (including CT scan) reveal no cause for the abnormal movements. Dystonic movements of the head and neck may take the form of torticollis, blepharospasm, facial grimacing, or forced opening or closing of the mouth. The limbs may also adopt abnormal but characteristic postures. The age at onset influences both the clinical findings and the prognosis. With onset in childhood, there is usually a family history of the disorder, symptoms commonly commence in the legs, and progression is likely until there is severe disability from generalized dystonia. In contrast, when onset is later, a positive family history is unlikely, initial symptoms are often in the arms or axial structures, and severe disability does not usually occur, although generalized dystonia may ultimately develop in some patients. If all cases are considered together, about one-third of patients eventually become so severely disabled that they are confined to chair or bed, while another one-third are affected only mildly.

Before a diagnosis of idiopathic torsion dystonia is made, it is imperative to exclude other causes of dystonia. For example, perinatal anoxia, birth trauma, and kernicterus are common causes of dystonia, but abnormal movements usually then develop before the age of 5, the early development of the patient is usually abnormal, and a history of seizures is not unusual. Moreover, examination may reveal signs of mental retardation or pyramidal deficit in addition to the movement disorder. Dystonic posturing may also occur in Wilson's disease, Huntington's disease, or parkinsonism; as a sequela of encephalitis lethargica or previous neuroleptic drug therapy; and in certain other disorders. In these cases, diagnosis is based on the history and accompanying clinical manifestations.

Idiopathic torsion dystonia usually responds poorly to drugs. Diazepam, baclofen, carbamazepine, amantadine, or anticholinergic medication (in high dosage) is occasionally helpful; if not, a trial of treatment with phenothiazines, haloperidol, or tetrabenazine (not available in USA) may be worthwhile. However, the doses of these latter drugs that are required for benefit lead usually to mild parkinsonism. Stereotactic thalamotomy is sometimes helpful in patients with predominantly unilateral dystonia, especially when this involves the limbs.

Eldridge R, Fahn S (editors): *Dystonia: Advances in Neurology.* Vol 14. Raven Press, 1976.
Fahn S: High dosage anticholinergic therapy in dystonia. *Neurology* 1983;**33:**1255.

6. FOCAL TORSION DYSTONIA

A number of the dystonic manifestations that occur in idiopathic torsion dystonia may also occur as isolated phenomena. They are best regarded as focal dystonias that either occur as formes frustes of idiopathic torsion dystonia in patients with a positive family history or represent a focal manifestation of the adult-onset form of that disorder when there is no family history. Medical treatment is generally unsatisfactory. A trial of the drugs used in idiopathic torsion dystonia is worthwhile, however, since a few patients do show some response.

Both **blepharospasm** and **oromandibular dystonia** may occur as an isolated focal dystonia. The former is characterized by spontaneous involuntary forced closure of the eyelids for a variable interval. Oromandibular dystonia is manifested by involuntary contraction of the muscles about the mouth causing, for example, involuntary opening or closing of the mouth, roving or protruding tongue movements, and retraction of the platysma.

Spasmodic torticollis, usually with onset between 25 and 50 years of age, is characterized by a tendency for the neck to twist to one side. This initially occurs episodically, but eventually the neck is held to the side. Spontaneous resolution may occur in the first year or so. The disorder is otherwise usually lifelong. Selective section of the spinal accessory nerve and the upper cervical nerve roots is sometimes helpful if medical treatment is unsuccessful.

Writer's cramp is characterized by dystonic posturing of the hand and forearm when the hand is used for writing and sometimes when it is used for other tasks, eg, playing the piano, using a screwdriver or eating utensils. Drug treatment is usually unrewarding, and patients are often best advised to learn to use the other hand for activities requiring manual dexterity.

Eldridge R, Fahn S (editors): *Dystonia.* Vol 14 of *Advances in Neurology.* Raven Press, 1976.
Jankovic J, Havins WE, Wilkins RB: Blinking and blepharospasm: Mechanism, diagnosis, and management. *JAMA* 1982;**248:**3160.
Lal S: Pathophysiology and pharmacotherapy of spasmodic torticollis: A review. *Can J Neurol Sci* 1979;**6:**427.

7. MYOCLONUS

Occasional myoclonic jerks may occur in anyone, especially when drifting into sleep. General or multifocal myoclonus is common in patients with idiopathic epilepsy and is especially prominent in certain hereditary disorders characterized by seizures and progressive intellectual decline, such as the lipid storage diseases and Lafora's disease. It is also a feature of various rare degenerative disorders, notably Ramsay Hunt syndrome, and is common in subacute sclerosing panencephalitis and Creutzfeldt-Jakob disease. Generalized myoclonic jerking may accompany the metabolic encephalopathies, result from levodopa therapy, occur in alcohol or drug withdrawal states, or follow anoxic brain damage. It also occurs on a hereditary or sporadic basis as an isolated phenomenon in otherwise healthy subjects.

Segmental myoclonus is a rare manifestation of a focal spinal cord lesion. It may also be the clinical expression of **epilepsia partialis continua,** a disorder in which a repetitive focal epileptic discharge arises in the contralateral sensorimotor cortex, sometimes from an underlying structural lesion. An electroencephalogram is often helpful in clarifying the epileptic nature of the disorder, and CT scan may reveal the causal lesion.

Myoclonus may respond to certain anticonvulsant drugs, especially valproic acid, or to one of the benzodiazepines, particularly clonazepam. Myoclonus following anoxic brain damage is often responsive to 5-hydroxytryptophan, the precursor of 5-hydroxytryptamine, and sometimes to clonazepam. In patients with segmental myoclonus, a localized lesion should be searched for and treated appropriately.

Goldberg MA, Dorman JD: Intention myoclonus: Successful treatment with clonazepam. *Neurology* 1976;**26:**24.
Kelly JJ, Sharbrough FW, Daube JR: A clinical and electrophysiological evaluation of myoclonus. *Neurology* 1981;**31:**581.

Thal LJ et al: Treatment of myoclonus with L-5-hydroxytrypto-
phan and carbidopa: Clinical, electrophysiological, and biochemical observations. *Ann Neurol* 1980;7:570.

8. WILSON'S DISEASE

In this metabolic disorder, abnormal movements
and postures of all sorts may occur with or without
coexisting signs of liver involvement. It is discussed in
detail in Chapter 11.

9. DRUG-INDUCED ABNORMAL MOVEMENTS

Phenothiazines and butyrophenones may produce
a wide variety of abnormal movements, including parkinsonism, akathisia, acute dystonia, chorea, and tardive dyskinesia. These complications are discussed in
Chapter 18. Chorea may also develop in patients receiving levodopa, anticholinergic drugs, phenytoin,
lithium, amphetamines, or oral contraceptives, and it
resolves with withdrawal of the offending substance.
Parkinsonism that is reversible may be produced by
reserpine.

10. GILLES DE LA TOURETTE'S SYNDROME

Symptoms begin in childhood, between 2 and 15
years of age. Motor tics are the initial manifestation in
80% of cases and most commonly involve the face,
whereas in the remaining 20%, the initial symptoms
are phonic tics; all patients ultimately develop a combination of different motor and phonic tics. The former
occur especially about the face, head, and shoulders
(eg, sniffing, blinking, frowning, shoulder shrugging,
head thrusting, etc). Phonic tics commonly consist of
grunts, barks, hisses, throat-clearing, coughs, etc, but
sometimes also of verbal utterances including cop-
rolalia. There may also be echolalia, echopraxia, and
palilalia. Some tics may be self-mutilating in nature,
such as severe nail-biting, hair-pulling, or biting of the
lips or tongue. The disorder is chronic, but the course
may be punctuated by relapses and remissions.

Examination usually reveals no abnormalities
other than the multiple tics. Psychiatric disturbances
may occur, however, because of the cosmetic and
social embarrassment produced. Investigations are unrevealing except that the electroencephalogram may
show minor nonspecific abnormalities of no diagnostic
relevance.

The diagnosis of the disorder is often delayed for
years, the tics being interpreted as psychiatric illness or
some other form of abnormal movement. Patients are
thus often subjected to unnecessary and expensive
treatments before the true nature of the disorder is
recognized. The ticlike character of the abnormal
movements and the absence of other neurologic signs

should differentiate this disorder from other movement
disorders presenting in childhood. Wilson's disease,
however, can simulate the condition and should be
excluded.

Treatment is symptomatic and may need to be
continued indefinitely. Haloperidol is generally regarded as the drug of choice. It is started in a low daily
dose (0.25 mg) that is gradually increased (by 0.25 mg
every 4 or 5 days) until there is maximum benefit with
a minimum of side effects, or until side effects limit
further increments. A total daily dose of between 2 and
8 mg is usually optimal, but higher doses are sometimes necessary. More recently, treatment with clonazepam or clonidine has been found to be helpful, and it
seems sensible to begin treatment with one of these
drugs in order to avoid some of the long-term extrapyramidal side effects of haloperidol. Phenothiazines,
such as fluphenazine, have also been used, but patients
unresponsive to haloperidol are usually unresponsive
to these as well.

Cohen DJ et al: Clonidine ameliorates Gilles de la Tourette
syndrome. *Arch Gen Psychiatry* 1980;**37**:1350.
Lees AJ et al: A clinical study of Gilles de la Tourette syndrome in
the United Kingdom. *J Neurol Neurosurg Psychiatry* 1984;
47:1.
Shapiro AK et al: Gilles de la Tourette's syndrome: Summary of
clinical experience with 250 patients and suggested nomenclature for tic syndromes. In: *Dystonia: Advances in Neurology.*
Vol 14. Eldridge R, Fahn S (editors). Raven Press, 1976.

DEMENTIA

Dementia, the symptom complex of progressive
global impairment of intellectual function, is a major
medical, social, and economic problem that is worsening as the number of elderly people in the general
population increases. In the USA, more than 20 million people were more than 65 years old in 1970; 10%
of these were mildly demented and another 5% so
severely demented that they could not cope with the
tasks of independent daily life. By the turn of the
century, a 50% increase in the number of demented
elderly persons has been projected. Nevertheless, the
clinical features of dementia are often not recognized
at an early stage, so that investigations are delayed and
treatment is withheld.

It is clinically important to distinguish dementia
from other disturbances of cognitive function.

(1) It is sometimes difficult to distinguish between dementia and a confusional state. In general,
however, a **confusional state,** which represents the
mildest level of a disturbance in consciousness, has an
acute or subacute onset and fluctuating course, is frequently reversible, and is characterized by short attention span and variable degrees of disorientation; if
there is excessive agitation, the term **delirium** is often
used. In dementia, by contrast, there is no alteration in
the level of consciousness, and the course is usually
chronic and progressive, although it may be possible to
arrest or reverse it in some cases.

(2) The global cognitive impairment in dementia clearly distinguishes it from disorders characterized by focal, circumscribed deficits of higher cortical function. Nevertheless, **aphasia,** and especially the fluent, articulate, but meaningless speech (jargon aphasia) that occurs with lesions in Wernicke's area, is often mistaken for dementia. Similarly, patients with memory disturbances may be held to be demented until it is recognized that their difficulties result from a selective **amnestic syndrome.**

(3) Psychiatric disorders may masquerade as dementia. **Depression** is especially likely to cause a so-called pseudodementia, because it leads to retardation, withdrawal, lack of spontaneity, and paucity of ideas. However, such a pseudodementia generally has a more abrupt onset and rapid progression and is accompanied by a variety of somatic complaints (eg, anorexia, insomnia, headaches, constipation, weight loss) in addition to a depressed affect; moreover, patients make little attempt to respond to tests of intellectual function, and there may be a past history of depressive illness. **Schizophrenic disturbances** generally begin before the age of 40 years and are considered in detail in Chapter 18.

(4) **Mental retardation** is distinguished by the age and history, since it represents a failure of development rather than a deterioration from a previous level of intellectual functioning.

Reversible or treatable causes of dementia include normal pressure hydrocephalus, intracranial mass lesions, vascular disease (multi-infarct dementia), hypothyroidism, vitamin B_{12} deficiency, Wilson's disease, drug toxicity, hepatic or renal failure, and any of the chronic meningitides, including neurosyphilis. Investigations in all patients should be undertaken with this in mind.

The clinical findings, laboratory investigations, and management of Alzheimer's disease and other disorders presenting with dementia are discussed in Chapters 2 and 18.

VERTIGO

Dysfunction of the vestibular system leads to vertigo, a feeling of rotatory dysequilibrium. The vertigo that results from peripheral vestibulopathy is usually of sudden onset, may be so severe that the patient is unable to walk or stand, and is frequently accompanied by nausea and vomiting. Tinnitus and deafness may be associated and provide strong support for a peripheral origin. Nystagmus is found on examination and is usually horizontal with a rotatory component, the fast phase being toward the intact side. Visual fixation tends to inhibit both the nystagmus and the complaint of vertigo.

With central nervous system lesions, vertigo may develop gradually and then become progressively more severe. Nystagmus is not always present, can occur in any direction, and may be dissociated in the 2 eyes; vertical nystagmus always indicates a central lesion.

Episodic vertigo can occur in patients with diplopia from external ophthalmoplegia and is maximal when the patient looks in the direction where the separation of images is greatest. Cerebral lesions involving the temporal cortex may also produce vertigo, which is sometimes the initial symptom of a seizure. Finally, vertigo may be a feature of a number of systemic disorders and can occur as a side effect of certain anticonvulsant, antibiotic, hypnotic, analgesic, and tranquilizing drugs and alcohol.

Common Syndromes With Conspicuous Vertigo
A. Vertigo Due to Peripheral Lesions:
1. Benign positional vertigo–This form of vertigo is usually peripheral in origin, although it occasionally occurs with central lesions. Vertigo and nystagmus occur as posture-dependent phenomena and are especially likely to occur when the patient is lying down or the head is tilted backward. Typically with peripheral lesions, there is a latency period of up to about 45 seconds before they develop, and after another 10–60 seconds they subside and then cease; they habituate with constant repetition of the positional change that induces them. In central lesions, there is no latent period, fatigability, or habituation of the symptoms and signs.

2. Meniere's disease–Meniere's disease is characterized by vertiginous episodes lasting up to several hours and occurring on a background of increasing hearing loss, tinnitus, and vertigo. Caloric testing commonly reveals loss or impairment of thermally induced nystagmus on the involved side. The disorder and its treatment are discussed in detail in Chapter 6.

3. Vestibular Neuronitis–In vestibular neuronitis, a paroxysmal, usually single attack of vertigo occurs without accompanying impairment of auditory function, and may persist for several weeks before clearing. Examination reveals nystagmus and absent responses to caloric stimulation on one or both sides. The cause of the disorder is unclear. Treatment is symptomatic.

4. Labyrinthitis–Acute or chronic labyrinthitis is accompanied by severe vertigo, as discussed in Chapter 6.

5. Acoustic neuromas–These tumors may produce vertigo but usually not as an initial manifestation of the lesion. They are considered further in Table 17–3.

B. Vertigo Due to Central Nervous System Lesions:
Central nervous system causes of vertigo include brain stem vascular disease, arteriovenous malformations or tumors, multiple sclerosis, and vertebrobasilar migraine. There are usually other signs of brain stem dysfunction (eg, cranial nerve palsies; motor, sensory, or cerebellar deficits in the limbs) or of increased intracranial pressure. Auditory function is generally spared. The underlying cause should be treated.

Treatment

Investigations such as audiologic evaluation, caloric stimulation, electronystagmography, CT scan, and brain stem auditory evoked potential studies will help to distinguish between central and peripheral lesions and to identify causes requiring specific therapy. Medical treatment is otherwise symptomatic. Bed rest may reduce the severity of vertigo, and treatment with antihistamines such as meclizine, cyclizine, or dimenhydrinate (25–50 mg 4 times daily) is sometimes helpful. If these fail, scopolamine, ephedrine, or diazepam is worthy of trial. A combination of drugs sometimes helps when the response to one drug is disappointing.

Brandt T, Daroff RB: The multisensory physiological and pathological vertigo syndromes. *Ann Neurol* 1980;**7**:195.
Price NM et al: Transdermal scopolamine in the prevention of motion sickness at sea. *Clin Pharmacol Ther* 1981;**29**:414.
Slater R: Benign recurrent vertigo. *J Neurol Neurosurg Psychiatry* 1979;**42**:363.

MULTIPLE SCLEROSIS

This common neurologic disorder of unknown cause has its greatest incidence in young adults. Epidemiologic studies indicate that multiple sclerosis is much more common in certain parts of the world than in others. No population with a high risk for multiple sclerosis exists between latitudes 40 °N and 40 °S. Genetic, dietary, and climatic factors cannot account for these differences. There may be a familial incidence of the disease. The strong association between multiple sclerosis and specific HLA antigens provides support for a theory of genetic predisposition. Many believe that the disease has an immunologic basis, but verification of this is awaited. Pathologically, focal—often perivenular—areas of demyelination with reactive gliosis are found scattered in the white matter of brain and spinal cord and in the optic nerves.

Clinical Findings

A. Symptoms and Signs: The common initial presentation is weakness, numbness, tingling, or unsteadiness in a limb; spastic paraparesis; retrobulbar neuritis; diplopia; dysequilibrium; or a sphincter disturbance such as urinary urgency or hesitancy. Symptoms may disappear after a few days or weeks, although examination often reveals a residual deficit.

In most patients, there is an interval of months or years after the initial episode before new symptoms develop or the original ones recur. Eventually, however, relapses and usually incomplete remissions lead to increasing disability, with weakness, spasticity, and ataxia of the limbs, impaired vision, and urinary incontinence. The findings on examination at this stage commonly include optic atrophy, nystagmus, dysarthria, and pyramidal, sensory, or cerebellar deficits in some or all of the limbs.

Less commonly, symptoms are steadily progressive from their onset, and disability develops at a relatively early stage. The diagnosis cannot be made with confidence unless the total clinical picture indicates involvement of different parts of the central nervous system at different times.

A number of factors (eg, infection, trauma) may precipitate or trigger exacerbations. Relapses are also more likely during the 2 or 3 months following pregnancy, possibly because of the increased demands and stresses that occur in the postpartum period.

B. Laboratory, X-Ray, and Other Studies: Investigations may help to support the clinical diagnosis and exclude other disorders, but a definitive diagnosis can never be based solely on the laboratory findings. If there is clinical evidence of only a single lesion in the central nervous system, multiple sclerosis cannot properly be diagnosed unless it can be shown that other regions are affected subclinically. The electrocerebral responses evoked in the clinical neurophysiology laboratory by monocular visual stimulation with a checkerboard pattern stimulus, by monaural click stimulation, and by electrical stimulation of a sensory or mixed peripheral nerve have been used to detect subclinical involvement of the visual, brain stem auditory, and somatosensory pathways, respectively.

There may be mild lymphocytosis or a slightly increased protein concentration in the cerebrospinal fluid, especially soon after an acute relapse. Of more help in diagnosis is the fact that the IgG level in cerebrospinal fluid may be increased, and protein electrophoresis characteristically shows the presence of discrete bands of IgG, called oligoclonal bands, in many patients. The presence of such bands is not specific, however, since they have been found in a variety of inflammatory neurologic disorders and occasionally in patients with vascular or neoplastic disorders of the nervous system.

CT scanning, especially with high doses of contrast medium and delayed scanning techniques, is sometimes helpful in demonstrating the presence of a multiplicity of lesions. Magnetic resonance imaging can detect a multiplicity of lesions even when CT scans are normal.

In patients presenting with myelopathy alone and in whom there is no clinical or laboratory evidence of more widespread disease, myelography may be necessary to exclude a congenital or acquired surgically treatable lesion. The foramen magnum region must be visualized to exclude the possibility of Arnold-Chiari malformation, in which part of the cerebellum and the lower brain stem are displaced into the cervical canal and produce mixed pyramidal and cerebellar deficits in the limbs.

Treatment

At least partial recovery from acute exacerbations can reasonably be expected, but further relapses may occur without warning, and there is no means of preventing progression of the disorder. Some disability is likely to result eventually, but about half of all patients are without significant disability even 10 years after onset of symptoms.

Recovery from acute relapses may be hastened by treatment with corticosteroids, but the extent of recovery is unchanged. A high dose (eg, prednisone, 60 or 80 mg) is given daily for a week, after which medication is tapered over the following 2 or 3 weeks. Long-term treatment with steroids provides no benefit and does not prevent further relapses.

Several recent studies have suggested that intensive immunosuppressive therapy with cyclophosphamide given intravenously in high doses may help to arrest the course of chronic progressive active multiple sclerosis. Results of further clinical trials are now awaited. Hyperbaric oxygen treatment, recently shown in a preliminary study to have a beneficial but transient effect in patients with advanced chronic multiple sclerosis, cannot be recommended without confirmatory studies and longer periods of follow-up. The use of interferon in the prevention of relapses has recently been studied, and a detailed report of the findings is awaited.

Treatment for spasticity (see below) and for neurogenic bladder may be needed in advanced cases. In all cases, care of the general health is important. Excessive fatigue must be avoided, and patients should rest during periods of acute relapse.

Ebers GC: Genetic factors in multiple sclerosis. *Neurol Clin* 1983;**1**:645.

Fischer BM et al: Hyperbaric-oxygen treatment of multiple sclerosis: A randomized, placebo-controlled, double-blind study. *N Engl J Med* 1983;**308**:181.

Hauser SL et al: Intensive immunosuppression in progressive multiple sclerosis: A randomized, three-arm study of high-dose intravenous cyclophosphamide, plasma exchange, and ACTH. *N Engl J Med* 1983;**308**:173.

Lukes SA et al: Nuclear magnetic resonance imaging in multiple sclerosis. *Ann Neurol* 1983;**13**:592.

McFarlin DE: Treatment of multiple sclerosis. (Editorial.) *N Engl J Med* 1983;**308**:215.

McFarlin DE, McFarland HF: Multiple sclerosis. (2 parts.) *N Engl J Med* 1982;**307**:1183, 1246.

Oger J, Roos R, Antel JP: Immunology of multiple sclerosis. *Neurol Clin* 1983;**1**:655.

Reder AT, Antel JP: Clinical spectrum of multiple sclerosis. *Neurol Clin* 1983;**1**:573.

ACUTE DISSEMINATED ENCEPHALOMYELITIS

Acute disseminated encephalomyelitis is characterized by perivascular areas of demyelination scattered throughout the brain and spinal cord, with an associated inflammatory reaction. Clinically, there is a monophasic illness, with neurologic deficits developing over a few days and then resolving, at least in part, over the following weeks. Onset of the disorder is often related to a viral infection, especially measles or chickenpox. Headache, fever, and confusion are early symptoms, and seizures may also occur; signs of meningeal irritation are found on examination. Common signs of cord involvement are flaccid weakness and sensory disturbances of the legs, extensor plantar responses, and urinary retention. There may also be signs of involvement of the optic nerves, cerebral hemispheres, brain stem, or cerebellum. The cerebrospinal fluid may contain an increased number of mononuclear cells, with normal protein and sugar concentrations. Treatment with corticosteroids is often prescribed, but there is little evidence of benefit. A mortality rate between 5 and 30% is reported in different series. Many survivors are left with severe residual deficits.

Lukes SA, Norman D: Computed tomography in acute disseminated encephalomyelitis. *Ann Neurol* 1983;**13**:567.

SPASTICITY

The term "spasticity" is commonly used for an upper motor neuron deficit, but it properly refers to a velocity-dependent increase in resistance to passive movement that affects different muscles to a different extent, is not uniform in degree throughout the range of a particular movement, and is commonly associated with other features of pyramidal deficit. It is often a major complication of stroke, cerebral or spinal injury, and multiple sclerosis.

Spasticity should be treated when it interferes with daily activities or causes distress or disability. Asymptomatic spasticity requires no treatment. Treatment may increase functional disability when increased extensor tone is providing additional support for patients with weak legs.

Physical therapy with appropriate stretching programs is important during rehabilitation after the development of an upper motor neuron lesion and in subsequent management of the patient. The aim is to prevent joint and muscle contractures and, perhaps, to modulate spasticity.

Drug management is important in reducing spasticity that interferes with function or causes distress. Dantrolene weakens muscle contraction by interfering with the role of calcium. It may be helpful in the treatment of spasticity but is best avoided in patients with poor respiratory function or severe myocardial disease. Treatment is begun with 25 mg once daily, and the daily dose is built up by 25-mg increments every 3 days, depending on tolerance, to a maximum of 100 mg 4 times daily. The drug should be withdrawn if no benefit has occurred after treatment with the maximum tolerated dose for about 2 weeks. Side effects include diarrhea, nausea, weakness, hepatic dysfunction (that may rarely be fatal, especially in women older than 35), drowsiness, lightheadedness, and hallucinations.

Diazepam may modify spasticity by its action on spinal interneurons and perhaps also by influencing supraspinal centers. Its efficacy in the treatment of spasticity due to complete cord lesions has been questioned. Treatment is started in low dose and increased depending upon the response; doses on the order of 10 mg 3 or 4 times daily are not uncommon. Side effects include drowsiness, lightheadedness, increased weakness, fatigue, unsteadiness, hallucinations, and hypotension. Withdrawal symptoms including seizures may follow abrupt discontinuation of treatment after prolonged administration of high doses.

Baclofen seems to be the most effective drug for treating spasticity of spinal origin. It is particularly helpful in relieving painful flexor (or extensor) spasms. The maximum recommended daily dose is 80 mg; treatment is started with a dose of 5 or 10 mg twice daily and then built up gradually. Side effects include gastrointestinal disturbances, lassitude, fatigue, sedation, unsteadiness, confusion, and hallucinations.

Motor-point blocks by intramuscular phenol have been used to reduce spasticity selectively in one or a few important muscles and may permit return of function in patients with incomplete myelopathies. Intrathecal injection of phenol or absolute alcohol may be helpful in more severe cases, but greater selectivity can be achieved by nerve root or peripheral nerve neurolysis. These procedures should not be undertaken until the spasticity syndrome is fully evolved, ie, only after about 1 year or so, and only if long-term drug treatment either has been unhelpful or carries a significant risk to the patient.

A number of surgical procedures, eg, adductor or heel cord tenotomy, may help in the management of spasticity. Neurectomy may also facilitate patient management. For example, obturator neurectomy is helpful in patients with marked adductor spasms that interfere with personal hygiene or cause gait disturbances. Posterior rhizotomy reduces spasticity, but its effect may be short-lived, whereas anterior rhizotomy produces permanent wasting and weakness in the muscles that are denervated.

Spasticity may be exacerbated by decubitus ulcers, urinary or other infections, and nociceptive stimuli, which must therefore be prevented.

SUBACUTE COMBINED DEGENERATION OF THE SPINAL CORD

Subacute combined degeneration of the spinal cord is due to vitamin B_{12} deficiency, such as occurs in pernicious anemia. It is characterized by myelopathy with predominant pyramidal and posterior column deficits, sometimes in association with polyneuropathy, mental changes, or optic neuropathy. Megaloblastic anemia may also occur, but this does not parallel the neurologic disorder, and the former may be obscured if folic acid supplements have been taken. Treatment is with vitamin B_{12}.

WERNICKE'S ENCEPHALOPATHY

Wernicke's encephalopathy is characterized by confusion, ataxia, and ophthalmoplegia (nystagmus, lateral rectus muscle weakness, and conjugate gaze palsies); peripheral neuropathy may also be present. It is due to thiamine deficiency and in the USA occurs most commonly in alcoholics. It may have a fatal outcome if treatment is delayed. In suspected cases, thiamine (50 mg) is given intravenously immediately and then intramuscularly on a daily basis until a satisfactory diet can be assured. The diagnosis is confirmed by the response to treatment, which must not be postponed while laboratory confirmation is obtained (by the finding of reduced blood transketolase activity and a marked thiamine pyrophosphate effect).

STUPOR & COMA

The patient who is stuporous is unresponsive except when subjected to repeated vigorous stimuli, while the comatose patient is unrousable and unable to respond to external events or inner needs, although reflex movements and posturing may be present.

Coma is a major complication of serious central nervous system disorders. It can result from seizures, metabolic disturbances, or structural lesions causing bilateral cerebral hemispheric dysfunction or a disturbance of the brain stem reticular activating system. A mass lesion involving one cerebral hemisphere may cause coma by compression of the brain stem.

Assessment & Emergency Measures

The diagnostic workup of the comatose patient must proceed concomitantly with immediate management. In particular, immediate steps must be taken to evaluate and maintain vital functions, with supportive therapy for respiration or blood pressure being initiated if necessary. The patient can be positioned on one side with the neck partly extended, dentures removed, and secretions cleared by suction; if necessary, the patency of the airways is maintained with an oropharyngeal airway. In order to determine the cause of the coma, blood is then drawn for determination of serum glucose, electrolyte, and calcium levels; arterial blood gases; liver and renal function tests; and toxicologic studies if necessary. Dextrose 50% (25 g), naloxone (0.4–1.2 mg), and thiamine (50 mg) to counteract possible hypoglycemia, opiate overdosage, or thiamine deficiency should be given intravenously without delay. The intravenous line is left in place to facilitate further access to the circulation.

After these initial measures, further details are obtained from attendants of the patient's medical history, the circumstances surrounding the onset of coma, and the time course of subsequent events. Abrupt onset of coma suggests subarachnoid hemorrhage, brain stem stroke, or intracerebral hemorrhage, whereas a slower onset and progression occur with other structural or mass lesions. A metabolic cause is suggested by a preceding intoxicated state or agitated delirium. A detailed general and neurologic examination is undertaken, with particular attention to the behavioral response to painful stimuli, the pupils and their response to light, the position of the eyes and their movement in response to passive movement of the head and ice-water caloric stimulation, and the respiratory pattern.

A. Response to Painful Stimuli: Purposive limb withdrawal from painful stimuli implies that sensory pathways from and motor pathways to the stimulated limb are functionally intact, at least in part. Unilateral absence of responses despite application of stimuli to both sides of the body in turn implies a corticospinal lesion; bilateral absence of responsiveness suggests brain stem involvement, bilateral pyramidal tract lesions, or psychogenic unresponsiveness. Inappropriate responses may also occur. Decorticate posturing may occur with lesions of the internal capsule and rostral cerebral peduncle, decerebrate posturing with dysfunction or destruction of the midbrain and rostral pons, and decerebrate posturing in the arms accompanied by flaccidity or slight flexor responses in the legs in patients with extensive brain stem damage extending down to the pons at the trigeminal level.

B. Ocular Findings:

1. Pupils–Hypothalamic disease processes may lead to unilateral Horner's syndrome, while bilateral diencephalic involvement or destructive pontine lesions may lead to small but reactive pupils. Ipsilateral pupillary dilatation with no direct or consensual response to light occurs with compression of the third cranial nerve, eg, with uncal herniation. The pupils are slightly smaller than normal but responsive to light in many metabolic encephalopathies; however, they may be fixed and dilated following overdosage with atropine, scopolamine, or glutethimide, and pinpoint (but responsive) with opiates. Pupillary dilatation for several hours following cardiopulmonary arrest implies a poor prognosis.

2. Eye movements–Conjugate deviation of the eyes to the side suggests the presence of an ipsilateral hemispheric lesion or a contralateral pontine lesion. A mesencephalic lesion is suggested by downward conjugate deviation. Dysconjugate ocular deviation in coma suggests a structural brain stem lesion unless there was preexisting strabismus.

The oculomotor responses to passive head turning and to caloric stimulation relate to each other and provide complementary information. In response to brisk rotation of the head from side to side and to flexion and extension of the head, normally conscious patients with open eyes do not exhibit contraversive conjugate eye deviation (doll's-head eye response) unless there is voluntary visual fixation or bilateral frontal pathology. With cortical depression in lightly comatose patients, a brisk doll's-head eye response is seen. With brain stem lesions, this oculocephalic reflex becomes impaired or lost, depending on the site of the lesion.

The oculovestibular reflex is tested by caloric stimulation using irrigation with ice water. In normal

subjects, jerk nystagmus is elicited for about 2 minutes, with the slow component toward the irrigated ear. In unconscious patients with an intact brain stem, the fast component of the nystagmus disappears so that the eyes tonically deviate toward the irrigated side for 2–3 minutes before returning to their original position. With impairment of brain stem function, the response becomes perverted and finally disappears. In metabolic coma, oculocephalic and oculovestibular reflex responses are preserved, at least initially.

C. Respiratory Patterns: Diseases causing coma may lead to respiratory abnormalities. Cheyne-Stokes respiration may occur with bihemispheric or diencephalic disease or in metabolic disorders. Central neurogenic hyperventilation occurs with lesions of the brain stem tegmentum; apneustic breathing suggests damage at the pontine level (eg, due to basilar artery occlusion); and atactic breathing (a completely irregular pattern of breathing with deep and shallow breaths occurring randomly) is associated with lesions of the lower pontine tegmentum and medulla.

Continuing Care

The continuing care of patients with impaired consciousness includes maintenance of a clear airway and removal of secretions by suction as necessary. Patients are kept on their side and turned regularly, and pressure is avoided on bony prominences such as the heels. Bladder function is controlled by catheterization and bowel function by nursing care. Fluid and nutrients can be given intravenously or by nasogastric tube depending on the duration of the disorder, and metabolic parameters are monitored. The prognosis depends on the underlying disorder.

Bates D et al: A prospective study of nontraumatic coma: Methods and results in 310 patients. *Ann Neurol* 1977;**2**:211.

Plum F, Posner JB: *The Diagnosis of Stupor and Coma*, 3rd ed. Davis, 1980.

Sigsbee B, Plum F: The unresponsive patient. *Med Clin North Am* 1979;**63**:813.

1. STUPOR & COMA DUE TO STRUCTURAL LESIONS

Supratentorial mass lesions tend to affect brain function in an orderly way. There may initially be signs of hemispheric dysfunction, such as hemiparesis. As coma develops and deepens, cerebral function becomes progressively disturbed, producing a predictable progression of neurologic signs that suggest rostrocaudal deterioration.

Thus, as a supratentorial mass lesion begins to impair the diencephalon, the patient becomes drowsy, then stuporous, and finally comatose. There may be Cheyne-Stokes respiration; small but reactive pupils; doll's-head eye responses with side-to-side head movements, but sometimes an impairment of reflex upward gaze with brisk flexion of the head; tonic ipsilateral deviation of the eyes in response to vestibular stimulation with cold water; and initially a positive response to pain but subsequently only decorticate posturing. With further progression, midbrain failure occurs. Motor dysfunction progresses from decorticate to bilateral decerebrate posturing in response to painful stimuli, Cheyne-Stokes respiration is gradually replaced by sustained central hyperventilation; the pupils become mid-sized and fixed; and the oculocephalic and oculovestibular reflex responses become impaired, perverted, or lost. As the pons and then the medulla fail, the pupils remain unresponsive; oculovestibular responses are unobtainable; respiration is rapid and shallow; and painful stimuli may lead only to flexor responses in the legs. Finally, respiration becomes irregular and stops, the pupils often then dilating widely.

In contrast, a subtentorial (ie, brain stem) lesion may lead to an early, sometimes abrupt disturbance of consciousness without any orderly rostrocaudal progression of neurologic signs.

A structural lesion should always be suspected if the findings suggest dysfunction at a particular level of the nervous system. In such circumstances, a CT scan or cerebral angiogram should be performed before, or instead of, a lumbar puncture in order to avoid any risk of cerebral herniation. Further management is of the causal lesion and is considered separately under the individual disorders.

2. STUPOR & COMA DUE TO METABOLIC DISTURBANCES

Patients with a metabolic cause of coma generally have signs of patchy, diffuse, and symmetric neurologic involvement that cannot be explained by loss of function at any single level or in a sequential manner, although focal or lateralized deficits may occur in hypoglycemia. Moreover, pupillary reactivity is usually preserved, while other brain stem functions are often grossly impaired. Comatose patients with meningitis, encephalitis, or subarachnoid hemorrhage may also have little in the way of focal neurologic signs, however, and clinical evidence of meningeal irritation is sometimes very subtle in comatose patients. Examination of the cerebrospinal fluid in such patients is essential to establish the correct diagnosis.

Treatment of metabolic encephalopathy is of the underlying disturbance and is considered in other chapters. Any concomitant chest infection should be treated and cerebral oxygenation and blood flow ensured. Disturbances of blood glucose, acid-base balance, and electrolytes must be corrected, infection vigorously treated, and body temperature controlled. If the cause of the encephalopathy is obscure, all drugs except essential ones may have to be withdrawn in case they are responsible for the altered mental status.

3. BRAIN DEATH

The definition of brain death is controversial, and diagnostic criteria have been published by many dif-

ferent professional organizations. In order to establish brain death, the irreversibly comatose patient must be shown to have lost all brain stem reflex responses, including the pupillary, corneal, oculovestibular, oculocephalic, oropharyngeal, and respiratory reflexes, and should have been in this condition for at least 6 hours. Spinal reflex movements do not exclude the diagnosis, but ongoing seizure activity or decerebrate or decorticate posturing is not consistent with brain death. The apnea test (presence or absence of spontaneous respiratory activity at a P_{aCO_2} of at least 60 mm Hg) serves to determine whether or not the patient is capable of respiratory activity.

Reversible coma simulating brain death may be seen with hypothermia (temperature < 32 °C), overdosage with central nervous system depressant drugs, or shock, and these conditions must be excluded. Certain ancillary tests may assist the determination of brain death but are not essential. An isoelectric electroencephalogram, when the recording is made according to the recommendations of the American Electroencephalographic Society, is especially helpful in confirming the diagnosis. Alternatively, the demonstration of an absent cerebral circulation by angiography of the 4 major vessels to the brain can be confirmatory.

Black PM: Brain death. (2 parts.) *N Engl J Med* 1978;**299**:338, 393.

Chatrian GE: Electrophysiologic evaluation of brain death: A critical appraisal. In: *Electrodiagnosis in Clinical Neurology.* Aminoff MJ (editor). Churchill Livingstone, 1980.

Korein J (editor): Brain death: Interrelated medical and social issues. *Ann NY Acad Sci* 1978;**315**. [Entire issue.]

Schafer JA, Caronna JJ: Duration of apnea needed to confirm brain death. *Neurology* 1978;**28**:661.

4. PERSISTENT VEGETATIVE STATE

Patients with severe bilateral hemispheric disease may show some improvement from an initially comatose state, so that, after a variable interval, they appear to be awake but lie motionless and without evidence of awareness or higher mental activity. This persistent vegetative state has been variously referred to as akinetic mutism, apallic state, or coma vigil. Most patients in this persistent vegetative state will die in months or years, but partial recovery has occasionally occurred and in rare instances has been sufficient to permit communication or even independent living.

Levy DE, Knill-Jones RP, Plum F: The vegetative state and its prognosis following nontraumatic coma. *Ann NY Acad Sci* 1978;**315**:293.

5. LOCKED-IN SYNDROME
(De-efferented State)

Acute destructive lesions (eg, infarction, hemorrhage, demyelination, encephalitis) involving the ventral pons and sparing the tegmentum may lead to a mute, quadriparetic but conscious state in which the patient is capable of blinking and of voluntary eye movement in the vertical plane, with preserved pupillary responses to light. Such a patient can mistakenly be regarded as comatose. Prognosis is variable, but recovery has occasionally been reported, in some cases including resumption of independent daily life, though this may take up to 2 or 3 years.

HEAD INJURY

Trauma is the most common cause of death in young people, and head injury accounts for almost half of these trauma-related deaths. The prognosis following head injury depends upon the site and severity of brain damage. Some guide to prognosis is provided by the mental status, since loss of consciousness for more than 1 or 2 minutes implies a worse prognosis than otherwise. Similarly, the degree of retrograde and posttraumatic amnesia provides an indication of the severity of injury and thus of the prognosis. Absence of skull fracture does not exclude the possibility of severe head injury. After the history has been obtained, the patient must be examined in detail, with particular attention directed at the level of consciousness and extent of any brain stem dysfunction (p 614).

Note: In general, patients who have lost consciousness for 2 minutes or more following head injury should be admitted to the hospital for observation, as should patients with focal neurologic deficits, lethargy, or skull fractures. If patients are not to be detained, responsible family members should be given clear instructions about the need for, and manner of, checking on them at regular (hourly) intervals and for obtaining additional medical help if necessary. Progressive deterioration is an important indication for further investigation.

Laboratory Studies

Skull x-rays may provide evidence of fractures. An air-fluid level in the frontal or sphenoidal sinuses suggests the possibility of basilar fractures. Because injury to the spine may have accompanied head trauma, cervical spine x-rays (especially in the lateral projection) should always be obtained in comatose patients and in patients with severe neck pain or a deficit possibly related to cord compression. CT scanning has an important role in demonstrating focal intracranial hemorrhage and may also provide evidence of cerebral edema or contusion and displacement of midline structures. If a CT scanner is not available, arteriography may be necessary to exclude the possibility of a subdural or epidural hemorrhage or an intracerebral lesion.

Cerebral Injuries

These are summarized in Table 17–5, where treatment is also indicated.

Scalp Injuries & Skull Fractures

Scalp lacerations and depressed or compound depressed skull fractures should be treated surgically as appropriate. Simple skull fractures require no specific treatment.

The clinical signs of basilar skull fracture include bruising about the orbit, blood in the external auditory meatus, and leakage of cerebrospinal fluid (which can be identified by its glucose content) from the ear or nose. Cranial nerve palsies (involving especially the first, second, third, fourth, fifth, seventh, and eighth nerves in any combination) may also occur. Prophylactic antibiotics should be given if there is any leakage of cerebrospinal fluid. Conservative treatment, with elevation of the head, restriction of fluids, and administration of acetazolamide (250 mg 4 times daily) is often helpful, but if the leak continues for more than a few days lumbar subarachnoid drainage may be necessary. Only very occasional patients require intracranial repair of the dural defect because of persistence of the leak or recurrent meningitis.

Late Complications of Head Injury

The relationship of **chronic subdural hemor-**

Table 17–5. Acute cerebral sequelae of head injury.

Sequelae	Clinical Features	Pathology
Concussion	Transient loss of consciousness with bradycardia, hypotension, and respiratory arrest for a few seconds followed by retrograde and posttraumatic amnesia. Occasionally followed by transient neurologic deficit.	Bruising on side of impact (coup injury) or contralaterally (contrecoup injury).
Cerebral contusion/laceration	Loss of consciousness longer than with concussion. May lead to death or severe residual neurologic deficit.	Cerebral contusion, edema, hemorrhage, and necrosis. May have subarachnoid bleeding.
Acute epidural hemorrhage	Headache, confusion, somnolence, seizures, and focal deficits occur several hours after injury and lead to coma, respiratory depression, and death unless treated by surgical evacuation.	Tear in meningeal artery, vein, or dural sinus, leading to hematoma visible on CT scan.
Acute subdural hemorrhage	Similar to epidural hemorrhage, but interval before onset of symptoms is longer. Treatment is by surgical evacuation.	Hematoma from tear in veins from cortex to superior sagittal sinus or from cerebral laceration, visible on CT scan.
Cerebral hemorrhage	Generally develops immediately after injury. Clinically resembles hypertensive hemorrhage. Surgical evacuation is sometimes helpful.	Hematoma, visible on CT scan.

rhage to head injury is not always clear. In many elderly persons there is no history of trauma, but in other cases a head injury, often trivial, precedes the onset of symptoms by several weeks. The clinical presentation is usually with mental changes such as slowness, drowsiness, headache, confusion, memory disturbances, personality change, or even dementia. Focal neurologic deficits such as hemiparesis or hemisensory disturbance may also occur but are less common. CT scan is an important means of detecting the hematoma, which is sometimes bilateral. Treatment is by surgical evacuation to prevent cerebral compression and tentorial herniation.

Normal-pressure hydrocephalus may follow head injury, subarachnoid hemorrhage, or meningoencephalitis, but in many instances there are no specific antecedents. Hydrocephalus occurs because flow and absorption of cerebrospinal fluid is interrupted. The resulting clinical syndrome is characterized by intellectual deterioration, urinary incontinence, and an apraxic gait. CT scan reveals enlarged ventricles without evidence of cortical atrophy. Radionuclide cisternography helps to confirm the diagnosis by demonstrating the obstruction to flow of cerebrospinal fluid. Surgical shunting procedures may be of clinical benefit, especially in the presence of the full clinical triad and typical appearance on CT scan.

Other late complications of head injury include posttraumatic seizure disorder (see p 585) and posttraumatic headache (see p 583).

Cameron MM: Chronic subdural haematoma: A review of 114 cases. *J Neurol Neurosurg Psychiatry* 1978;**41**:834.

Rose J, Valtonen S, Jennett B: Avoidable factors contributing to death after head injury. *Br Med J* 1977;**2**:615.

Seelig JM et al: Traumatic acute subdural hematoma: Major mortality reduction in comatose patients treated within four hours. *N Engl J Med* 1981;**304**:1511.

SPINAL TRAUMA

While spinal cord damage may result from whiplash injury, severe injury usually relates to fracture-dislocation causing compression or angular deformity of the cord either cervically or in the lower thoracic and upper lumbar region. Extreme hypotension following injury may also lead to cord infarction (see p 598).

Total cord transection results in immediate flaccid paralysis and loss of sensation below the level of the lesion. Reflex activity is lost for a variable period, and there is urinary and fecal retention. As reflex function returns over the following days and weeks, spastic paraplegia or quadriplegia develops, with hyperreflexia and extensor plantar responses, but a flaccid atrophic (lower motor neuron) paralysis may be found depending on the segments of the cord that are affected. The bladder and bowels also regain some reflex function, permitting urine and feces to be expelled at intervals. As spasticity increases, flexor or

extensor spasms (or both) of the legs become troublesome, especially if the patient develops bed sores or a urinary tract infection. Paraplegia with the legs in flexion or extension may eventually result.

With lesser degrees of injury, patients may be left with mild limb weakness, distal sensory disturbance, or both. Sphincter function may also be impaired, urinary urgency and urgency incontinence being especially common. More particularly, a unilateral cord lesion leads to an ipsilateral motor disturbance with accompanying impairment of proprioception and contralateral loss of pain and temperature appreciation below the lesion (Brown-Séquard syndrome). A central cord syndrome may lead to a lower motor neuron deficit and loss of pain and temperature appreciation, with sparing of posterior column functions. A radicular deficit may occur at the level of the injury—or, if the cauda equina is involved, there may be evidence of disturbed function in several lumbosacral roots.

Treatment of the injury consists of immobilization and—if there is cord compression—decompressive laminectomy and fusion. Anatomic realignment of the spinal cord by traction and other orthopedic procedures is also important. Subsequent care of the residual neurologic deficit—paraplegia or quadriplegia—may involve treatment of spasticity and care of the skin, bladder, and bowels.

Sussman BJ: Fracture dislocation of the cervical spine: A critique of current management in the United States. *Paraplegia* 1978;**16**:15.

Yashon D: *Spinal Injury.* Appleton-Century-Crofts, 1978.

SYRINGOMYELIA

Destruction or degeneration of gray and white matter adjacent to the central canal of the spinal cord leads to cavitation and accumulation of fluid within the spinal cord. The precise pathogenesis is unclear, but many cases are associated with Arnold-Chiari malformation, in which there is displacement of the cerebellar tonsils, medulla, and fourth ventricle into the spinal canal, sometimes with accompanying meningomyelocele. In such circumstances, the cord cavity connects with and may merely represent a dilated central canal. In other cases, the cause of cavitation is less clear. There is a characteristic clinical picture, with segmental atrophy and areflexia and loss of pain and temperature appreciation in a "cape" distribution owing to the destruction of fibers crossing in front of the central canal. Thoracic kyphoscoliosis is usually present. With progression, involvement of the long motor and sensory tracts occurs as well, so that a pyramidal and sensory deficit develops in the legs. Upward extension of the cavitation (syringobulbia) leads to dysfunction of the lower brain stem and thus to bulbar palsy, nystagmus, and sensory impairment over one or both sides of the face.

Syringomyelia, ie, cord cavitation, may also occur in association with an intramedullary tumor or following severe cord injury, and the cavity then does not communicate with the central canal.

In patients with Arnold-Chiari malformation, there are commonly abnormalities on plain x-rays of the skull and cervical spine. CT scans show caudal displacement of the fourth ventricle. Positive contrast myelography may demonstrate Arnold-Chiari malformation, whereas with gas myelography the cord cavity may vary in size depending on the position of the patient. Focal cord enlargement is found at myelography in patients with cavitation related to past injury or intramedullary neoplasms.

Treatment of Arnold-Chiari malformation with associated syringomyelia is by suboccipital craniectomy and upper cervical laminectomy, with the aim of decompressing the malformation at the foramen magnum. The cord cavity should be drained, and if necessary an outlet for the fourth ventricle can be made. In cavitation associated with intramedullary tumor, treatment is surgical, but radiation therapy may be necessary if complete removal is not possible. Post-traumatic syringomyelia is also treated surgically if it leads to increasing neurologic deficits or to intolerable pain.

MOTOR NEURON DISEASES

This group of disorders is characterized clinically by weakness and variable wasting of affected muscles, without accompanying sensory changes. Certain of these disorders, such as Werdnig-Hoffman disease and Kugelberg-Welander syndrome, occur in infants or children and are not considered further here.

Motor neuron disease in adults generally commences between 30 and 60 years of age. There is degeneration of the anterior horn cells in the spinal cord, the motor nuclei of the lower cranial nerves, and the corticospinal and corticobulbar pathways. The disorder is usually sporadic, but familial cases may occur.

Classification

Five varieties have been distinguished on clinical grounds.

A. Progressive Bulbar Palsy: Bulbar involvement predominates owing to disease processes affecting primarily the motor nuclei of the cranial nerves.

B. Pseudobulbar Palsy: Bulbar involvement predominates in this variety also, but it is due to bilateral corticobulbar disease and thus reflects upper motor neuron dysfunction.

C. Progressive Spinal Muscular Atrophy: This is characterized primarily by a lower motor neuron deficit in the limbs due to degeneration of the anterior horn cells in the spinal cord.

D. Primary Lateral Sclerosis: There is a purely upper motor neuron deficit in the limbs.

E. Amyotrophic Lateral Sclerosis: A mixed upper and lower motor neuron deficit is found in the limbs. This disorder is sometimes associated with dementia, parkinsonism, and other neurologic diseases.

Clinical Findings

A. Symptoms and Signs: Difficulty in swallowing, chewing, coughing, breathing, and talking (dysarthria) occur with bulbar involvement. In progressive bulbar palsy, there is drooping of the palate, a depressed gag reflex, pooling of saliva in the pharynx, a weak cough, and a wasted, fasciculating tongue. In pseudobulbar palsy, the tongue is contracted and spastic and cannot be moved rapidly from side to side. Limb involvement is characterized by motor disturbances (weakness, stiffness, wasting, fasciculations) reflecting lower or upper motor neuron dysfunction; there are no objective changes on sensory examination, though there may be vague sensory complaints. The sphincters are generally spared.

The disorder is progressive and usually fatal within 3–5 years; death usually results from pulmonary infections. Patients with bulbar involvement generally have the poorest prognosis.

B. Laboratory, X-Ray, and Other Studies: Electromyography may show changes of chronic partial denervation, with abnormal spontaneous activity in the resting muscle and a reduction in the number of motor units under voluntary control. Motor conduction velocity is usually normal but may be slightly reduced, and sensory conduction studies are also normal. Biopsy of a wasted muscle shows the histologic changes of denervation. The serum creatine phosphokinase may be slightly elevated but never reaches the extremely high values seen in some of the muscular dystrophies. The cerebrospinal fluid is normal.

There have been recent reports of juvenile spinal muscular atrophy due to hexosaminidase deficiency, with abnormal findings on rectal biopsy and reduced hexosaminidase A in serum and leukocytes.

Treatment

There is no specific treatment. Symptomatic and supportive measures may include prescription of anticholinergic drugs (such as trihexyphenidyl, amitriptyline, or atropine) if drooling is troublesome, braces or a walker to improve mobility, and physical therapy to prevent contractures. Spasticity may be helped by baclofen or diazepam. A semiliquid diet or nasogastric tube feeding may be needed if dysphagia is severe. Gastrostomy or cricopharyngomyotomy is sometimes resorted to in extreme cases of predominant bulbar involvement, and tracheostomy may be necessary if respiratory muscles are severely affected; but in the terminal stages of these disorders, the aim of treatment should be to keep patients as comfortable as possible.

Hudson AJ: Amyotrophic lateral sclerosis and its association with dementia, parkinsonism and other neurological disorders: A review. *Brain* 1981;**104**:217.

Johnson WG et al: Juvenile spinal muscular atrophy: A new hexosaminidase deficiency phenotype. *Ann Neurol* 1982; **11**:11.

Rowland LP (editor): *Human Motor Neuron Diseases.* Vol 36 of *Advances in Neurology.* Raven Press, 1982.

Sinaki M, Mulder DW: Rehabilitation techniques for patients with amyotrophic lateral sclerosis. *Mayo Clin Proc* 1978; 53:173.

PERIPHERAL NEUROPATHIES

Peripheral neuropathies can be categorized on the basis of the structure primarily affected. The predominant pathologic feature may be axonal degeneration (axonal or neuronal neuropathies) or paranodal or segmental demyelination. The distinction may be possible on the basis of neurophysiologic findings. Motor and sensory conduction velocity can be measured in accessible segments of peripheral nerves. In axonal neuropathies, conduction velocity is normal or reduced only mildly and needle electromyography provides evidence of denervation in affected muscles. In demyelinating neuropathies, conduction may be slowed considerably in affected fibers, and in more severe cases, conduction is blocked completely, without accompanying electromyographic signs of denervation.

Peripheral neuropathies may also occur as a result of disorders affecting the connective tissues of the nerves or the blood vessels supplying the nerves, but these are much less common than the preceding varieties.

Nerves may be injured or compressed by neighboring anatomic structures at any point along their course. Common mononeuropathies of this sort are considered on p 624. A similar clinical disturbance is produced by peripheral nerve tumors, but these are rare except in patients with Recklinghausen's disease. Multiple mononeuropathies suggest a patchy multifocal disease process such as vasculopathy (eg, diabetes, arteritis), an infiltrative process (eg, leprosy, sarcoidosis), radiation damage, or an immunologic disorder (eg, brachial plexopathy). Diffuse polyneuropathies lead to a symmetric deficit, often most marked distally. They include the hereditary, metabolic, and toxic disorders, idiopathic inflammatory polyneuropathy (Guillain-Barré syndrome), and the peripheral neuropathies that may occur as a nonmetastatic complication of malignant diseases.

1. POLYNEUROPATHIES & MONONEURITIS MULTIPLEX

The cause of polyneuropathy or mononeuritis multiplex may be suggested by the mode of onset and predominant clinical manifestations. A full laboratory workup includes a complete blood count and sedimentation rate; liver and thyroid function tests; determination of plasma urea and electrolytes and serum proteins and electrophoresis; a serologic test for syphilis; tests for antinuclear antibody and rheumatoid factor; fasting blood glucose level; screening of blood and urine for heavy metal poisoning; cerebrospinal fluid examina-

tion; and chest x-ray. Measurement of nerve conduction velocity is important in confirming the peripheral nerve origin of symptoms and providing a means of following clinical changes, as well as indicating the likely disease process (ie, axonal or demyelinating neuropathy). Cutaneous nerve biopsy may help establish a precise clinical diagnosis. In about half of cases, however, no specific cause can be established.

Treatment is of the underlying cause, when feasible, and is discussed below under the individual disorders. Symptomatic and general measures are also important, especially in advanced cases. Physical therapy helps prevent contractures, and splints can maintain a weak extremity in a position of useful function. Anesthetic extremities must be protected from injury. To guard against burns, patients should check the temperature of water and hot surfaces with a portion of skin having normal sensation, measure water temperature with a thermometer, and use cold water for washing or lower the temperature setting of their hot-water heaters. Shoes should be examined frequently during the day for grit or foreign objects in order to prevent pressure lesions.

Patients with polyneuropathies or mononeuritis multiplex are subject to additional nerve injury at pressure points and should therefore avoid such behavior as leaning on elbows or sitting with crossed legs for lengthy periods.

Neuropathic pain is sometimes troublesome and may respond to simple analgesics such as aspirin. Narcotics or narcotic substitutes may be necessary for severe hyperpathia or pain induced by minimal stimuli, but their use should be avoided as far as possible. The use of a frame or cradle to reduce contact with bedclothes may be helpful. Many patients experience episodic stabbing pains, which sometimes respond to phenytoin, carbamazepine, or tricyclic antidepressant drugs.

Symptoms of autonomic dysfunction are occasionally troublesome. Postural hypotension is often helped by wearing waist-high elastic stockings and sleeping in a semierect position at night. Fludrocortisone reduces postural hypotension, but doses as high as 1 mg/d are sometimes necessary in diabetics and may lead to recumbent hypertension. Indomethacin has been found helpful by some but has been disappointing in the author's experience. Impotence, diarrhea, and bladder dysfunction are difficult to treat, but a flaccid neuropathic bladder may respond to parasympathomimetic drugs such as bethanechol chloride, 10–50 mg 3 or 4 times daily.

Inherited Neuropathies

A. Charcot-Marie-Tooth Disease: Several distinct varieties of Charcot-Marie-Tooth disease can be recognized. There is usually an autosomal dominant mode of inheritance, but occasional cases occur on a sporadic, recessive, or X-linked basis. Clinical presentation may be with foot deformities or gait disturbances in childhood or early adult life. Slow progression leads to the typical features of polyneuropathy, with distal weakness and wasting that begin in the legs, a variable amount of distal sensory loss, and depressed or absent tendon reflexes. Tremor is a conspicuous feature in some instances. Pathologic examination reveals segmental demyelination and remyelination of peripheral nerves, an increase in their transverse fascicular area, and hyperplasia of Schwann cells. Electrodiagnostic studies show a marked reduction in motor and sensory conduction velocity (hereditary motor and sensory neuropathy [HMSN] type I).

In other instances (HMSN type II), motor conduction velocity is normal or only slightly reduced, sensory nerve action potentials may be absent, and signs of chronic partial denervation are found in affected muscles electromyographically. The predominant pathologic change is axonal loss rather than segmental demyelination.

A clinically similar disorder may occur in patients with progressive spinal muscular atrophy, but there is no sensory loss; electrophysiologic investigation reveals that motor conduction velocity is normal or only slightly reduced, and nerve action potentials are normal.

B. Dejerine-Sottas Disease (HMSN Type III): Both recessive and dominantly inherited forms of this disorder have been described. The recessive form has its onset in infancy or childhood and leads to a progressive motor and sensory polyneuropathy with weakness, ataxia, sensory loss, and depressed or absent tendon reflexes. The peripheral nerves may be palpably enlarged and are characterized pathologically by segmental demyelination, Schwann cell hyperplasia, and thin myelin sheaths. Electrophysiologically, there is slowing of conduction, and sensory action potentials may be unrecordable. Cases with a dominant mode of inheritance are best classified with neuropathies of the Charcot-Marie-Tooth type.

C. Friedreich's Ataxia: Patients generally present in childhood or early adult life with this autosomal recessive disorder. The gait becomes atactic, the hands become clumsy, and other signs of cerebellar dysfunction develop accompanied by weakness of the legs and extensor plantar responses. Involvement of peripheral sensory fibers leads to sensory disturbances in the limbs and depressed tendon reflexes. There is bilateral pes cavus. Pathologically, there is a marked loss of cells in the posterior root ganglia and degeneration of peripheral sensory fibers. In the central nervous system, changes are conspicuous in the posterior and lateral columns of the cord. Electrophysiologically, conduction velocity in motor fibers is normal or only mildly reduced, but sensory action potentials are small or absent.

D. Refsum's Disease (HMSN Type IV): This autosomal recessive disorder is due to a disturbance in phytanic acid metabolism. Clinically, pigmentary retinal degeneration is accompanied by progressive sensorimotor polyneuropathy and cerebellar signs. Auditory dysfunction, cardiomyopathy, and cutaneous manifestations may also occur. The cerebrospinal fluid contains an increased protein but normal cell content.

Motor and sensory conduction velocity is reduced, often markedly, and there may be electromyographic evidence of denervation in affected muscles. Dietary restriction of phytanic acid and its precursors may be helpful therapeutically.

E. Porphyria: Peripheral nerve involvement may occur during acute attacks in both variegate porphyria and acute intermittent porphyria. The general clinical features of these disorders are discussed in Chapter 32. Motor symptoms usually occur first, and weakness is often most marked proximally and in the upper limbs rather than the lower. Sensory symptoms and signs may be proximal or distal in distribution. Autonomic involvement is sometimes pronounced. The electrophysiologic findings are in keeping with the results of neuropathologic studies suggesting that the neuropathy is axonal in type.

Neuropathies Associated With Systemic & Metabolic Disorders

A. Diabetes Mellitus: In this disorder, involvement of the peripheral nervous system may lead to symmetric sensory polyneuropathy, asymmetric motor neuropathy (diabetic amyotrophy), thoracoabdominal neuropathy, autonomic neuropathy, or isolated lesions of individual nerves. These may occur singly or in any combination.

Sensory polyneuropathy, the most common manifestation, may lead to no more than depressed tendon reflexes and impaired appreciation of vibration in the legs. When symptomatic, there may be pain, paresthesias, or numbness in the legs, but in severe cases distal sensory loss occurs in all limbs. Diabetic amyotrophy is characterized by asymmetric weakness and wasting involving predominantly the proximal muscles of the legs, accompanied by local pain. Thoracoabdominal neuropathy leads to pain over the trunk. In patients with autonomic neuropathy, postural hypotension, impaired thermoregulatory sweating, constipation, flatulence, diarrhea, impotence, urinary retention, and incontinence may occur, and there may be abnormal pupillary responses. Isolated lesions of individual peripheral nerves are common and in the limbs tend to occur at sites of compression or entrapment.

B. Uremia: Uremia may lead to a symmetric sensorimotor polyneuropathy that tends to affect the lower limbs more than the upper limbs and is more marked distally than proximally. The diagnosis can be confirmed electrophysiologically, for motor and sensory conduction velocity is moderately reduced. The neuropathy improves both clinically and electrophysiologically with prolonged dialysis or renal transplantation.

C. Alcoholism and Nutritional Deficiency: Many alcoholics have an axonal distal sensorimotor polyneuropathy that is frequently accompanied by painful cramps, muscle tenderness, and painful paresthesias and is often more marked in the legs than in the arms. Symptoms of autonomic dysfunction may also be conspicuous. Motor and sensory conduction velocity may be slightly reduced, even in subclinical cases, but gross slowing of conduction is uncommon. A similar distal sensorimotor polyneuropathy is a well-recognized feature of beriberi. In vitamin B_{12} deficiency, distal sensory polyneuropathy may develop but is usually overshadowed by central nervous system manifestations (eg, myelopathy, optic neuropathy, or intellectual changes). Treatment is by vitamin B_{12} supplementation.

D. Paraproteinemias: A symmetric sensorimotor polyneuropathy that is gradual in onset, progressive in course, and often accompanied by pain and dysesthesias in the limbs may occur in patients (especially men) with multiple or solitary myeloma. The neuropathy is of the axonal type in classic lytic myeloma, but segmental demyelination (primary or secondary) and axonal loss occur in sclerotic myeloma and lead to predominantly motor clinical manifestations. The neuropathy of classic multiple myeloma is unresponsive to any treatment, but in sclerotic and solitary myeloma radiation of bone lesions leads to improvement in the polyneuropathy. Focal peripheral nerve lesions may also be found in multiple myeloma.

Polyneuropathy may also occur in association with macroglobulinemia and cryoglobulinemia. Entrapment neuropathy, such as carpal tunnel syndrome, is more common than polyneuropathy in patients with primary (nonhereditary) generalized amyloidosis. When polyneuropathy does occur, sensory and autonomic symptoms are especially conspicuous, whereas distal wasting and weakness occur later. The manner in which the hereditary amyloid neuropathies present depends upon the type of amyloidosis.

Neuropathies Associated With Infectious & Inflammatory Diseases

A. Leprosy: Leprosy is an important cause of peripheral neuropathy in certain parts of the world. Sensory disturbances are mainly due to involvement of intracutaneous nerves. In tuberculoid leprosy, they develop at the same time and in the same distribution as the skin lesion but may be more extensive if nerve trunks lying beneath the lesion are also involved. In lepromatous leprosy, there is more extensive sensory loss, and this develops earlier and to a greater extent in the coolest regions of the body, such as the dorsal surfaces of the hands and feet, where the bacilli proliferate most actively. Motor deficits result from involvement of nerves in sites where they run superficially and where their temperature therefore is lowest, eg, the ulnar nerve in the region proximal to the olecranon groove, the median nerve as it emerges from beneath the forearm flexor muscle to run toward the carpal tunnel, the peroneal nerve at the head of the fibula, and the posterior tibial nerve in the lower part of the leg; patchy facial muscular weakness may also occur owing to involvement of the superficial branches of the seventh cranial nerve.

Motor disturbances in leprosy are suggestive of multiple mononeuropathy, whereas sensory changes resemble those of distal polyneuropathy. Careful examination, however, relates the distribution of sensory deficits to the temperature of the tissues; in the legs, for example, sparing frequently occurs between the toes and in the popliteal fossae, where the temperature is higher. Treatment is with antileprotic agents.

B. Sarcoidosis: Sarcoidosis may affect the central nervous system. In addition, cranial nerve palsies (especially facial palsy), multiple mononeuropathy, and, less commonly, symmetric polyneuropathy may all occur, the latter sometimes preferentially affecting either motor or sensory fibers. Improvement may occur with use of corticosteroids.

C. Rheumatoid Arthritis: Compressive or entrapment neuropathies, mild distal sensory polyneuropathy, and severe progressive sensorimotor polyneuropathy can occur in rheumatoid arthritis. The polyneuropathies are predominantly axonal in type and probably ischemic in origin.

Toxic Neuropathies

Axonal polyneuropathy may follow exposure to industrial agents or pesticides such as acrylamide, organophosphorus compounds, hexacarbon solvents, methyl bromide, and carbon disulfide; metals such as arsenic, thallium, mercury, and lead; and drugs such as phenytoin, perhexiline, isoniazid, nitrofurantoin, and vincristine and massive doses of pyridoxine. Detailed occupational, environmental, and medical histories and recognition of clusters of cases are important in suggesting the diagnosis. Treatment is by preventing further exposure to the causal agent. Isoniazid neuropathy is prevented by pyridoxine supplementation.

Diphtheritic neuropathy results from a neurotoxin released by the causative organism and is common in many areas. Palatal weakness may develop 2–4 weeks after infection of the throat, and infection of the skin may similarly be followed by focal weakness of neighboring muscles. Disturbances of accommodation may occur about 4–5 weeks after infection and distal sensorimotor demyelinating polyneuropathy after 1–3 months.

Neuropathies Associated With Malignant Diseases

Both a sensorimotor and a purely sensory polyneuropathy may occur as a nonmetastatic complication of malignant diseases. The sensorimotor polyneuropathy may be mild and occur in the course of known malignant disease; or it may have an acute or subacute onset, lead to severe disability, and occur before there is any clinical evidence of the cancer, occasionally following a remitting course, with relapses occurring in some instances.

Acute Idiopathic Polyneuropathy (Guillain-Barré Syndrome)

This acute or subacute polyradiculoneuropathy sometimes follows infective illness, inoculations, or surgical procedures but often occurs in a previously well person. It probably has an immunologic basis, but the precise mechanism is unclear. The main complaint is of weakness that varies widely in severity in different patients and often has a proximal emphasis and symmetric distribution. It usually begins in the legs, spreading to a variable extent but frequently involving the arms and often one or both sides of the face. The muscles of respiration or deglutition may also be affected. Sensory symptoms are usually less conspicuous than motor ones, but distal paresthesias and dysesthesias are common, and neuropathic or radicular pain is present in many patients. Autonomic disturbances are also common, may be severe, and are sometimes life-threatening; they include tachycardia, cardiac irregularities, hypotension or hypertension, facial flushing, abnormalities of sweating, pulmonary dysfunction, and impaired sphincter control.

The cerebrospinal fluid characteristically contains a high protein concentration with a normal cell content, but these changes may take 2 or 3 weeks to develop. Electrophysiologic studies may reveal marked abnormalities, which do not necessarily parallel the clinical disorder in their temporal course. Pathologic examination has shown that primary demyelination occurs in regions infiltrated with inflammatory cells, and it seems probable that myelin disruption has an autoimmune basis.

When the diagnosis is made, the history and appropriate laboratory studies should exclude the possibility of porphyric, diphtheritic, or toxic (heavy metal, hexacarbon, organophosphate) neuropathies. Poliomyelitis, botulism, and tick paralysis must also be considered. The presence of pyramidal signs, a markedly asymmetric motor deficit, a sharp sensory level, or early sphincter involvement should suggest a focal cord lesion.

Most patients eventually make a good recovery, but this may take many months, and 10–20% patients are left with persisting disability. Treatment is controversial. Corticosteroids were often prescribed in the past, but a prospective randomized trial has now shown that early treatment with prednisone is ineffective and may actually affect the outcome adversely by prolonging recovery time. Anecdotal reports of the value of plasmapheresis have prompted a collaborative multi-institutional controlled study that is nearing completion. For the present, the recommended treatment is supportive care with the aim of preventing or treating complications such as respiratory failure, vascular collapse, pulmonary emboli, hypertension, and cardiac arrhythmias. Severely affected patients are best managed in intensive care units where respiratory and circulatory function can be monitored and respiration assisted if necessary. Patients should be admitted to such units if they are continuing to deteriorate and their forced vital capacity is declining, and intubation should be considered if the forced vital capacity reaches 15 mL/kg, dyspnea becomes evident, or the blood oxygen saturation declines. Careful respiratory toilet and chest physical therapy help prevent bronchial obstruction and atelectasis. Preparations must also be made to maintain the blood pressure if necessary. Marked hypotension may respond to volume replacement or pressor agents. Frequent turning of the patient helps prevent decubitus ulcers, and physical therapy helps prevent contractures.

Approximately 3% of patients with acute idiopathic polyneuropathy have one or more relapses, sometimes several years after the initial illness. Relapses are clinically similar to the original illness. Plasma exchange therapy may produce improvement in chronic and relapsing inflammatory polyneuropathy.

Chronic Inflammatory Polyneuropathy

Chronic inflammatory polyneuropathy, an acquired immunologically mediated disorder, is clinically similar to Guillain-Barré syndrome except that it has a relapsing or steadily progressive course over months or years. In the relapsing form, partial recovery may occur after some relapses, but in other instances there is no recovery between exacerbations. Although remission may occur spontaneously with time, the disorder frequently follows a progressive downhill course leading to severe functional disability.

Electrodiagnostic studies show marked slowing of motor and sensory conduction, and focal conduction block. Signs of partial denervation may also be present owing to secondary axonal degeneration. Nerve biopsy may show chronic perivascular inflammatory infiltrates in the endoneurium and epineurium, without accompanying evidence of vasculitis. However, a normal nerve biopsy result or the presence of nonspecific abnormalities does not exclude the diagnosis.

Corticosteroids may be effective in arresting or reversing the downhill course. Treatment is usually begun with prednisone, 60 mg daily, continued for 2–3 months or until a definite response has occurred. If no response has occurred despite 3 months of treatment, a higher dose may be tried. In responsive cases, the dose is gradually tapered, but most patients become corticosteroid-dependent, often requiring prednisone, 20 mg daily on alternate days, on a long-term basis. Patients unresponsive to corticosteroids may benefit instead from treatment with a cytotoxic drug such as azathioprine. Anecdotal reports of benefit with plasmapheresis have been published.

Asbury AK: Diagnostic considerations in Guillain-Barré syndrome. *Ann Neurol* 1981;**9(Suppl):**1.

Asbury AK: Proximal diabetic neuropathy. *Ann Neurol* 1977; **2:**179.

Chad D et al: The pathogenesis of cryoglobulinemic neuropathy. *Neurology* 1982;**32:**725.

Davis CJF, Bradley WG, Madrid R: The peroneal muscular atrophy syndrome: Clinical, genetic, electrophysiological and nerve biopsy studies. *J Genet Hum* 1978;**26:**311.

Delaney P: Neurologic manifestations in sarcoidosis. *Ann Intern Med* 1977;**87:**336.

Dowling PC, Cook SD, Prineas JW (editors): Guillain-Barré syndrome: Proceedings of a conference sponsored by the Kroc Foundation. *Ann Neurol* 1981;**9(Suppl).** [Entire issue.]

Dyck PJ et al: Chronic inflammatory polyradiculoneuropathy. *Mayo Clin Proc* 1975;**50:**621.

Ewing DJ, Campbell IW, Clarke BF: The natural history of

diabetic autonomic neuropathy. *Q J Med* 1980;**49**:95.

Harding AE, Thomas PK: The clinical features of hereditary motor and sensory neuropathy types I and II. *Brain* 1980; **103**:259.

Hughes RAC et al: Controlled trial of prednisolone in acute polyneuropathy. *Lancet* 1978;**2**:750.

Kelly JJ et al: The natural history of peripheral neuropathy in primary systemic amyloidosis. *Ann Neurol* 1979;**6**:1.

Kelly JJ et al: The spectrum of peripheral neuropathy in myeloma. *Neurology* 1981;**31**:24.

Loffel NB et al: The Landry-Guillain-Barré syndrome: Complications, prognosis, and natural history in 123 cases. *J Neurol Sci* 1977;**33**:71.

Lotti M et al: Occupational peripheral neuropathies. *West J Med* 1982;**137**:493.

Oh SJ et al: Rapid improvement in nerve conduction velocity following renal transplantation. *Ann Neurol* 1978;**4**:369.

Prineas JW: Pathology of the Guillain-Barré syndrome. *Ann Neurol* 1981;**9(Suppl)**:6.

Prineas JW, McLeod JG: Chronic relapsing polyneuritis. *J Neurol Sci* 1976;**27**:427.

Sabin TD, Swift TR: Leprosy. In: *Peripheral Neuropathy.* Dyck PJ et al (editors). Saunders, 1984.

Stanbury JB et al (editors): *The Metabolic Basis of Inherited Disease,* 5th ed. McGraw-Hill, 1983.

Sun SF, Streib EW: Diabetic thoracoabdominal neuropathy: Clinical and electrodiagnostic features. *Ann Neurol* 1981;**9**:75.

2. MONONEUROPATHIES

An individual nerve may be injured along its course, or compressed, angulated, or stretched by neighboring anatomic structures, especially at a point where it passes through a narrow space (entrapment neuropathy). The relative contributions of mechanical factors and ischemia to the local damage are not clear. With involvement of a sensory or mixed nerve, pain is commonly felt distal to the lesion. Symptoms never develop with some entrapment neuropathies, resolve rapidly and spontaneously in others, and become progressively more disabling and distressing in yet other cases. The precise neurologic deficit depends on the nerve involved. Percussion of the nerve at the site of the lesion may lead to paresthesias in its distal distribution.

Entrapment neuropathy may be the sole manifestation of subclinical polyneuropathy, and this must be borne in mind and excluded by nerve conduction studies. Such studies are also indispensable for the accurate localization of the focal lesion.

In patients with acute compression neuropathy such as Saturday night palsy, no treatment is necessary. Complete recovery generally occurs, usually within 2 months, presumably because the underlying pathology is demyelination. However, axonal degeneration can occur in severe cases, and recovery then takes longer and may never be complete.

In chronic compressive or entrapment neuropathies, treatment consists of the avoidance of any aggravating factors, the correction of any underlying contributory systemic condition, and in some instances, local infiltration of the region about the nerve with corticosteroids. Surgical decompression may help some patients, especially if there is a progressively increasing neurologic deficit or if electrodiagnostic studies show evidence of partial denervation in weak muscles.

Peripheral nerve tumors are uncommon, except in Recklinghausen's disease, but also give rise to mononeuropathy. This may be distinguishable from entrapment neuropathy only by noting the presence of a mass along the course of the nerve and by demonstrating the precise site of the lesion with appropriate electrophysiologic studies. Treatment of symptomatic lesions is by surgical removal if possible.

Carpal Tunnel Syndrome
See p 536.

Pronator Teres or Anterior Interosseous Syndrome

The median nerve gives off its motor branch, the anterior interosseous nerve, below the elbow as it descends between the 2 heads of the pronator teres muscle. A lesion of either nerve may occur in this region, sometimes after trauma or owing to compression from, for example, a fibrous band. With anterior interosseous nerve involvement, there is no sensory loss, and weakness is confined to the pronator quadratus, flexor pollicis longus, and the flexor digitorum profundus to the second and third digits. Weakness is more widespread and sensory changes occur in an appropriate distribution when the median nerve itself is affected. The prognosis is variable. If improvement does not occur spontaneously, decompressive surgery may be helpful.

Ulnar Nerve Lesions

Ulnar nerve lesions are likely to occur in the elbow region as the nerve runs behind the medial epicondyle and descends into the cubital tunnel. In the condylar groove, the ulnar nerve is exposed to pressure or trauma. Moreover, any increase in the carrying angle of the elbow, whether congenital, degenerative, or traumatic, may cause excessive stretching of the nerve when the elbow is flexed. Ulnar nerve lesions may also result from thickening or distortion of the anatomic structures forming the cubital tunnel, and the resulting symptoms may also be aggravated by flexion of the elbow, because the tunnel is then narrowed by tightening of its roof or inward bulging of its floor. A severe lesion at either site causes sensory changes in the medial 1½ digits and along the medial border of the hand. There is weakness in the ulnar-innervated muscles in the forearm and hand. With a cubital tunnel lesion, however, there may be relative sparing of the flexor carpi ulnaris muscle. Electrophysiologic evaluation using nerve stimulation techniques allows more precise localization of the lesion.

If conservative measures (eg, avoidance of factors liable to cause compression or stretch of the nerve) are unsuccessful in relieving symptoms and preventing further progression, surgical treatment may be necessary. This consists of nerve transposition if the lesion is in the condylar groove, or a release procedure if it is in the cubital tunnel.

Ulnar nerve lesions may also develop at the wrist or in the palm of the hand, usually owing to repetitive trauma or to compression from ganglia or benign tumors. They can be subdivided depending upon their presumed site. Compressive lesions are treated surgically. If repetitive mechanical trauma is responsible, this is avoided by occupational adjustment or job retraining.

Radial Nerve Lesions

The radial nerve is particularly liable to compression or injury in the axilla (eg, by crutches or by pressure when the arm hangs over the back of a chair). This leads to weakness or paralysis of all the muscles supplied by the nerve, including the triceps. Sensory changes may also occur but are often surprisingly inconspicuous, being marked only in a small area on the back of the hand between the thumb and index finger. Injuries to the radial nerve in the spiral groove occur characteristically during deep sleep, as in intoxicated individuals (Saturday night palsy), and there is then sparing of the triceps muscle, which is supplied more proximally. The nerve may also be injured at or above the elbow; its purely motor posterior interosseous branch, supplying the extensors of the wrist and fingers, may be involved immediately below the elbow, but then there is sparing of the extensor carpi radialis longus, so that the wrist can still be extended. The superficial radial nerve may be compressed by handcuffs or a tight watch strap.

Femoral Neuropathy

The clinical features of femoral nerve palsy consist of weakness and wasting of the quadriceps muscle, with sensory impairment over the anteromedian aspect of the thigh and sometimes also of the leg to the medial malleolus, and a depressed or absent knee jerk. Isolated femoral neuropathy may occur in diabetics or from compression by hematomas or retroperitoneal neoplasms. In the latter circumstances, decompressive surgery may be helpful. Femoral neuropathy may also result from pressure from the inguinal ligament when the thighs are markedly flexed and abducted, as in the lithotomy position.

Meralgia Paresthetica

The lateral femoral cutaneous nerve, a sensory nerve arising from the L2 and L3 roots, may be compressed or stretched in obese or diabetic patients and during pregnancy. The nerve usually runs under the outer portion of the inguinal ligament to reach the thigh, but the ligament sometimes splits to enclose it. Hyperextension of the hip or increased lumbar lordosis—such as occurs during pregnancy—leads to nerve compression by the posterior fascicle of the ligament. However, entrapment of the nerve at any point along its course may cause similar symptoms, and several other anatomic variations predispose the nerve to damage when it is stretched. Pain, paresthesia, or numbness occurs about the outer aspect of the thigh, usually unilaterally, and is sometimes relieved by sitting. Examination shows no abnormalities except in severe cases when cutaneous sensation is impaired in the affected area. Symptoms are usually mild and commonly settle spontaneously, so patients can be reassured about the benign nature of the disorder. Hydrocortisone injections about the nerve where it lies medial to the anterosuperior iliac spine often relieve symptoms temporarily, while nerve decompression by transposition may provide more lasting relief.

Sciatic & Common Peroneal Nerve Palsies

Misplaced deep intramuscular injections are probably still the most common cause of sciatic nerve palsy. Trauma to the buttock, hip, or thigh may also be responsible. The resulting clinical deficit depends on whether the whole nerve has been affected or only certain fibers. In general, the peroneal fibers of the sciatic nerve are more susceptible to damage than those destined for the tibial nerve. A sciatic nerve lesion may therefore be difficult to distinguish from peroneal neuropathy, unless there is electromyographic evidence of involvement of the short head of the biceps femoris muscle. The common peroneal nerve itself may be compressed or injured in the region of the head and neck of the fibula. There is weakness of dorsiflexion and eversion of the foot, accompanied by numbness or blunted sensation of the anterolateral aspect of the calf and dorsum of the foot.

Tarsal Tunnel Syndrome

The tibial nerve, the other branch of the sciatic, supplies several muscles in the lower extremity, gives origin to the sural nerve, and then continues as the posterior tibial nerve to supply the plantar flexors of the foot and toes. It passes through the tarsal tunnel behind and below the medial malleolus, giving off calcaneal branches and the medial and lateral plantar nerves that supply small muscles of the foot and the skin on the plantar aspect of the foot and toes. Compression of the posterior tibial nerve or its branches between the bony floor and ligamentous roof of the tarsal tunnel leads to pain, paresthesias, and numbness over the bottom of the foot, especially at night, with sparing of the heel. Muscle weakness may be hard to recognize clinically. Compressive lesions of the individual plantar nerves may also occur more distally, with similar clinical features to those of the tarsal tunnel syndrome. Treatment is surgical decompression.

Dawson DM, Hallett M, Millender LH: *Entrapment Neuropathies.* Little, Brown, 1983.
Nakano KK: The entrapment neuropathies. *Muscle Nerve* 1978; **1:**264.

3. BELL'S PALSY

Bell's palsy is an idiopathic facial paresis of lower motor neuron type that has been attributed to an inflammatory reaction involving the facial nerve near the stylomastoid foramen or in the bony facial canal. A relationship of Bell's palsy to reactivation of herpes simplex virus has recently been suggested, but there is little evidence to support this.

The clinical features of Bell's palsy are characteristic. The facial paresis generally comes on abruptly, but it may worsen over the following day or so. Pain about the ear precedes or accompanies the weakness in many cases but usually lasts for only a few days. The face itself feels stiff and pulled to one side. There may be ipsilateral epiphora, restricted eye closure, and difficulty with eating and fine facial movements. A disturbance of taste is common, owing to involvement of chorda tympani fibers, and hyperacusis due to involvement of fibers to the stapedius occurs occasionally.

The management of Bell's palsy is controversial. Approximately 60% of cases recover completely without treatment, presumably because the lesion is so mild that it leads merely to conduction block. Considerable improvement occurs in most other cases, and only about 10% of all patients are seriously dissatisfied with the final outcome because of permanent disfigurement or other long-term sequelae. Treatment is unnecessary in most cases but is indicated for patients in whom an unsatisfactory outcome can be predicted.

It is generally accepted that treatment must be commenced within 5 or 6 days if it is to be effective. The best clinical guide to prognosis within this time frame is the severity of the palsy. Patients with clinically complete palsy when first seen are less likely to make a full recovery than those with an incomplete one. A poor prognosis for recovery is also associated with advancing age, hyperacusis, and severe initial pain. Electromyography and nerve excitability or conduction studies provide a guide to prognosis but not early enough to aid in the selection of patients for treatment.

Whether there is any effective treatment is questionable. The only medical treatment that may influence the outcome is administration of corticosteroids, but studies supporting this concept have been criticized on methodologic grounds, and recent rigorously controlled trials have shown no convincing benefit. Many physicians nevertheless routinely prescribe corticosteroids for patients with Bell's palsy seen within 5 days of onset. Others prescribe them only when the palsy is clinically complete or there is severe pain. Treatment with prednisone, 60 or 80 mg daily in divided doses for 4 or 5 days, followed by tapering of dose over the next 7–10 days, is a satisfactory regimen. It is helpful to protect the eye with a patch if eye closure is not possible. There is no evidence that surgical procedures to decompress the facial nerve are of benefit.

Adour KK: Current concepts in neurology: Diagnosis and management of facial paralysis. N Engl J Med 1982;**307**:348.
May M et al: The use of steroids in Bell's palsy: A prospective controlled study. Laryngoscope 1976;**86**:1111.
Wolf SM et al: Treatment of Bell palsy with prednisone: A prospective, randomized study. Neurology 1978;**28**:158.

ACUTE INTERVERTEBRAL DISK PROLAPSE
(See p 532.)

CERVICAL SPONDYLOSIS
(See p 530.)

BRACHIAL PLEXUS LESIONS

Brachial Plexus Neuropathy

Brachial plexus neuropathy may be idiopathic, sometimes occurring in relationship to a number of different nonspecific illnesses or factors. In other instances, brachial plexus lesions follow trauma or result from congenital anomalies, neoplastic involvement, or injury by various physical agents. In rare instances, the disorder occurs on a familial basis.

Idiopathic brachial plexus neuropathy (neuralgic amyotrophy) characteristically begins with severe pain about the shoulder, followed within a few days by weakness, reflex changes, and sensory disturbances involving especially the C5 and C6 segments. Symptoms and signs are usually unilateral but may be bilateral. Wasting of affected muscles is sometimes profound. The disorder relates to disturbed function of cervical roots or part of the brachial plexus, but its precise cause is unknown. Recovery occurs over the ensuing months but may be incomplete. Treatment is purely symptomatic.

Cervical Rib Syndrome

Compression of the C8 and T1 roots or the lower trunk of the brachial plexus by a cervical rib or band arising from the seventh cervical vertebra leads to weakness and wasting of intrinsic hand muscles, especially those in the thenar eminence, accompanied by pain and numbness in the medial 2 fingers and the ulnar border of the hand and forearm. The subclavian artery may also be compressed, and this forms the basis of Adson's test for diagnosing the disorder; the radial pulse is diminished or obliterated on the affected side when the seated patient inhales deeply and turns the head to one side or the other. Electromyography, nerve conduction studies, and somatosensory evoked potential studies may help confirm the diagnosis. X-rays sometimes show the cervical rib or a large transverse process of the seventh cervical vertebra, but normal findings do not exclude the possibility of a cervical band. Treatment of the disorder is by surgical excision of the rib or band.

Gilliatt RW et al: Peripheral nerve conduction in patients with cervical rib and band. *Ann Neurol* 1978;**4**:124.

Kori SH, Foley KM, Posner JB: Brachial plexus lesions in patients with cancer: 100 cases. *Neurology* 1981;**31**:45.

Lascelles RG et al: The thoracic outlet syndrome. *Brain* 1977; **100**:601.

DISORDERS OF NEUROMUSCULAR TRANSMISSION

1. MYASTHENIA GRAVIS

General Considerations

Myasthenia gravis occurs at all ages, sometimes in association with a thymic tumor or thyrotoxicosis. It is more common in females than males. Onset is usually insidious, but the disorder is sometimes unmasked by a coincidental infection that leads to exacerbation of symptoms. Exacerbations may also occur before the menstrual period or during or shortly after pregnancy. Symptoms are due to a variable degree of block of neuromuscular transmission. This probably has an immunologic basis, and autoantibodies binding to acetylcholine receptors are found in most patients with the disease. These antibodies have a primary role in reducing the number of functioning acetylcholine receptors. Clinically, this leads to weakness; initially powerful movements fatigue readily. The external ocular muscles and certain other cranial muscles, including the masticatory, facial, and pharyngeal muscles, are especially likely to be affected, and the respiratory and limb muscles may also be involved.

Clinical Findings

A. Symptoms and Signs: Patients present with ptosis, diplopia, difficulty in chewing or swallowing, respiratory difficulties, limb weakness, or some combination of these problems. Weakness may remain localized to a few muscle groups or may become generalized. Symptoms often fluctuate in intensity during the day, and this diurnal variation is superimposed on a tendency to longer-term spontaneous relapses and remissions that may last for weeks. Nevertheless, the disorder follows a slowly progressive course and may have a fatal outcome owing to respiratory complications such as aspiration pneumonia.

Clinical examination confirms the weakness and fatigability of affected muscles. In most cases, the extraocular muscles are involved, and this leads to ocular palsies and ptosis, which are commonly asymmetric. Pupillary responses are normal. The bulbar and limb muscles are often weak, but the pattern of involvement is variable. Sustained activity of affected muscles increases the weakness, which improves after a brief rest. Sensation is normal, and there are usually no reflex changes.

The diagnosis can generally be confirmed by the response to a short-acting anticholinesterase. Edrophonium (Tensilon) can be given intravenously in a dose of 10 mg (1 mL), 2 mg being given initially and the remaining 8 mg about 30 seconds later if the test dose is well tolerated; in myasthenic patients, there is an obvious improvement in strength of weak muscles lasting for about 5 minutes. Alternatively, 1.5 mg of neostigmine can be given intramuscularly, and the response then lasts for about 2 hours; atropine sulfate (0.6 mg) should be available to reverse muscarinic side effects.

B. Laboratory, X-Ray, and Other Studies: Lateral and anteroposterior x-rays of the chest and CT scans should be obtained to demonstrate a coexisting thymoma, but normal studies do not exclude this possibility.

Electrophysiologic demonstration of a decrementing muscle response to repetitive 2- or 3-Hz stimulation of motor nerves indicates a disturbance of neuromuscular transmission. Such an abnormality may even be detected in clinically strong muscles with certain provocative procedures. Needle electromyography of affected muscles shows a marked variation in configuration and size of individual motor unit potentials, and single-fiber electromyography reveals an increased jitter, or variability in the time interval between 2 muscle fiber action potentials from the same motor unit.

Assay of serum for elevated levels of circulating acetylcholine receptor antibodies is another approach to the laboratory diagnosis of myasthenia gravis, but laboratory facilities for performing the test are not widely available.

Treatment

Anticholinesterase drugs provide symptomatic benefit without influencing the course of the disease. Neostigmine, pyridostigmine, or both can be used, the dose being determined on an individual basis. Overmedication may temporarily increase weakness, which is then unaffected or enhanced by intravenous edrophonium.

Thymectomy usually leads to symptomatic benefit or remission and should be undertaken in patients younger than age 60, unless weakness is restricted to the extraocular muscles. If the disease is of recent onset and only slowly progressive, operation is sometimes delayed for a year or so, in the hope that spontaneous remission will occur.

Treatment with corticosteroids is indicated for patients who have responded poorly to anticholinesterase drugs and have already undergone thymectomy. It is introduced with the patient in the hospital, since weakness may initially be aggravated. Once weakness has stabilized after 2–3 weeks or any improvement is sustained, further management can be on an outpatient basis. Alternate-day treatment is usually well tolerated, but if weakness is enhanced on the nontreatment day it may be necessary for medication to be taken daily. The dose of corticosteroids is determined on an individual basis, but an initial high daily dose can gradually be tapered to a relatively low maintenance level as improvement occurs. Treatment with azathioprine may also be effective, and the relative merit of this approach is currently under investigation.

In patients with major disability in whom conventional treatment is either unhelpful or contraindicated, plasmapheresis may be beneficial.

Lennon VA: Myasthenia gravis: Diagnosis by assay of serum antibodies. *Mayo Clin Proc* 1982;**57**:723.

Lisak RP, Barchi RL: *Myasthenia Gravis: Major Problems in Neurology.* Vol 11. Saunders, 1982.

Seybold ME: Myasthenia gravis: A clinical and basic science review. *JAMA* 1983;**250**:2516.

2. NEONATAL MYASTHENIA

Infants born to myasthenic women should be carefully watched during the first postnatal week for signs of neonatal myasthenia, which occurs in about 10–15% cases. Such signs include a poor cry, respiratory difficulties, weakness in sucking, a weak Moro reflex, and feeble limb movements. They are usually not evident immediately after birth but become apparent within the first 72 hours of postnatal life. Neonatal myasthenia is a transient disorder that presumably relates to placental transfer of maternal antibody against acetylcholine receptors. It is unrelated to the duration or severity of the maternal illness, except that the latter is usually generalized rather than localized. The neonatal disorder can be treated with anticholinesterase drugs and usually resolves within 6 weeks following delivery. It may, however, have a fatal outcome owing to aspiration or respiratory failure, and facilities should be available for the immediate resuscitation of affected infants or those at risk of being affected.

3. MYASTHENIC SYNDROME (Eaton-Lambert Syndrome)

Myasthenic syndrome is often associated with an underlying carcinoma, sometimes developing before the tumor is diagnosed, and occasionally occurs with certain autoimmune diseases. There is defective release of acetylcholine in response to a nerve impulse, and this leads to weakness especially of the proximal muscles of the limbs. Unlike myasthenia gravis, however, power steadily increases with sustained contraction. The diagnosis can be confirmed electrophysiologically, because the muscle response to stimulation of its motor nerve increases remarkably if the nerve is stimulated repetitively at high rates, even in muscles that are not clinically weak.

Treatment with plasmapheresis and immunosuppressive drug therapy (prednisone and azathioprine) may lead to clinical and electrophysiologic improvement. Guanidine hydrochloride (25–50 mg/kg/d in divided doses) is occasionally helpful in seriously disabled patients, but adverse effects of the drug include marrow suppression. The response to treatment with anticholinesterase drugs such as pyridostigmine or neostigmine, either alone or in combination with guanidine, is variable.

Dau PC, Denys EH: Plasmapheresis and immunosuppressive drug therapy in the Eaton-Lambert syndrome. *Ann Neurol* 1982;**11**:570.

Newsom-Davis J et al: Lambert-Eaton myasthenic syndrome: Electrophysiological evidence for a humoral factor. *Muscle Nerve* 1982;**5**:S17.

4. BOTULISM

The toxin of *Clostridium botulinum* prevents the release of acetylcholine at neuromuscular junctions and autonomic synapses. Botulism occurs most commonly following the ingestion of contaminated home-canned food and should be suggested by the development of sudden, fluctuating, severe weakness in a previously healthy person. Symptoms begin within 72 hours following ingestion of the toxin and may progress for several days. Typically, there is diplopia, ptosis, facial weakness, dysphagia, and nasal speech, followed by respiratory difficulty and finally by weakness that appears last in the limbs. Blurring of vision (with unreactive dilated pupils) is characteristic, and there may be dryness of the mouth, constipation (paralytic ileus), and postural hypotension. Sensation is preserved, and the tendon reflexes are not affected unless the involved muscles are very weak. If the diagnosis is suspected, the local health authority should be notified and a sample of serum and contaminated food (if available) sent to be assayed for toxin. Support for the diagnosis may be obtained by electrophysiologic studies; with repetitive stimulation of motor nerves at fast rates, the muscle response increases in size progressively.

Patients should be hospitalized in case respiratory assistance becomes necessary. Treatment is with trivalent antitoxin, once it is established that the patient is not allergic to horse serum. Guanidine hydrochloride (25–50 mg/kg/d in divided doses) to facilitate release of acetylcholine from nerve endings sometimes helps to increase muscle strength. Anticholinesterase drugs are of no value. Respiratory assistance and other supportive measures should be provided as necessary.

5. DISORDERS ASSOCIATED WITH USE OF AMINOGLYCOSIDES

Large doses of certain antibiotics, eg, kanamycin and gentamicin, may produce a clinical disturbance similar to botulism by preventing the release of acetylcholine from nerve endings, but symptoms subside rapidly as the responsible drug is eliminated from the body. These antibiotics are particularly dangerous in patients with preexisting disturbances of neuromuscular transmission and are therefore best avoided in patients with myasthenia gravis.

MYOPATHIC DISORDERS

Muscular Dystrophies

These inherited myopathic disorders are characterized by progressive muscle weakness and wasting. They are subdivided by mode of inheritance, age at onset, and clinical features, as shown in Table 17–6. In the Duchenne type, pseudohypertrophy of muscles frequently occurs at some stage; intellectual retardation is common; and there may be skeletal deformities, muscle contractures, and cardiac involvement. The serum creatine phosphokinase level is increased, especially in the Duchenne and Becker varieties, and mildly increased also in limb-girdle dystrophy. Electromyography may help to confirm that weakness is myopathic rather than neurogenic. Similarly, histopathologic examination of a muscle biopsy specimen may help to confirm that weakness is due to a primary disorder of muscle and to distinguish between various muscle diseases.

There is no specific treatment, but it is important to encourage patients to lead as normal lives as possible. Prolonged bed rest must be avoided, as inactivity often leads to worsening of the underlying muscle disease. Physical therapy and orthopedic procedures may help to counteract deformities or contractures.

Congenital Myopathies

These are a group of myopathic disorders that present in infancy with hypotonia and weakness. They are usually nonprogressive. Distinct entities have been defined by the ultrastructural appearance of the muscles. There is no specific treatment.

Myotonic Dystrophy

Myotonic dystrophy, a slowly progressive, dominantly inherited disorder, usually manifests itself in the third or fourth decade but occasionally appears early in childhood. Myotonia leads to complaints of muscle stiffness and is evidenced by the marked delay that occurs before affected muscles can relax after a contraction. This can often be demonstrated clinically by delayed relaxation of the hand after sustained grip or by percussion of the belly of a muscle. In addition, there is weakness and wasting of the facial, sternocleidomastoid, and distal limb muscles. Associated clinical features include cataracts, frontal baldness, testicular atrophy, diabetes mellitus, cardiac abnormalities, and intellectual changes. Electromyographic sampling of affected muscles reveals myotonic discharges in addition to changes suggestive of myopathy.

Myotonia can be treated with quinine sulfate (300–400 mg 3 times daily), procainamide (0.5–1 g 4 times daily), or phenytoin (100 mg 3 times daily). In myotonic dystrophy, phenytoin is preferred, since the other drugs may have undesirable effects on cardiac conduction. Neither the weakness nor the course of the disorder is influenced by treatment.

Myotonia Congenita

Myotonia congenita is commonly inherited as a dominant trait. Generalized myotonia without weakness is usually present from birth, but symptoms may not appear until early childhood. Patients complain of muscle stiffness that is enhanced by cold and inactivity and relieved by exercise. Muscle hypertrophy, at times pronounced, is also a feature. A recessive form with later onset is associated with slight weakness and atrophy of distal muscles. Treatment with quinine sulfate, procainamide, or phenytoin may help the myotonia, as in myotonic dystrophy.

Polymyositis, Dermatomyositis, & Polymyalgia Rheumatica

See Chapter 14.

Myopathies Associated With Other Disorders

Myopathy may occur in association with chronic hypokalemia, osteomalacia, hyper- or hypothyroidism, hyper- or hypoparathyroidism, hyper- or hypoadrenalism, hypopituitarism, and acromegaly and in patients taking corticosteroids, chloroquine, colchicine, bretylium tosylate, or drugs causing potassium

Table 17–6. The muscular dystrophies.

Disorder	Inheritance	Age at Onset (years)	Distribution	Prognosis
Duchenne type	X-linked recessive	1–5	Pelvic, then shoulder girdle; later, limb and respiratory muscles.	Rapid progression. Death within about 15 years after onset.
Becker's	X-linked recessive	5–25	Pelvic, then shoulder girdle.	Slow progression. May have normal life span.
Limb-girdle (Erb's)	Autosomal recessive (may be sporadic or dominant)	10–30	Pelvic or shoulder girdle initially, with later spread to the other.	Variable severity and rate of progression. Possible severe disability in middle life.
Facioscapulo-humeral	Autosomal dominant	Any age	Face and shoulder girdle initially; later, pelvic girdle and legs.	Slow progression. Minor disability. Usually normal life span.
Distal	Autosomal dominant	40–60	Onset distally in extremities; proximal involvement later.	Slow progression.
Ocular	Autosomal dominant	Any age	External ocular muscles. May also be mild weakness of face, neck, and arms.	
Oculopharyngeal	Autosomal dominant	Any age	As the ocular form, but with dysphagia.	

depletion. Treatment is of the underlying cause. My-opathy also occurs with chronic alcoholism, whereas acute reversible muscle necrosis may occur shortly after acute alcohol intoxication.

PERIODIC PARALYSIS SYNDROME

Periodic paralysis may have a familial (dominant inheritance) basis. Episodes of flaccid weakness or paralysis occur, sometimes in association with abnor-malities of the plasma potassium level. Strength is normal between attacks. The **hypokalemic** variety is characterized by attacks that tend to occur on awaken-ing, after exercise, or after a heavy meal and may last for several days. Patients should avoid excessive exer-tion. A low-carbohydrate and low-salt diet may help

prevent attacks, as may acetazolamide, 250–750 mg/d. An ongoing attack may be aborted by potassium chloride given orally or intravenously, provided the ECG can be monitored and renal function is satisfac-tory. It is sometimes associated with hyperthyroidism, and treatment of the endocrine disorder may then pre-vent recurrences. In **hyperkalemic** periodic paralysis, attacks also tend to occur after exercise but usually last for less than an hour. Severe attacks may be terminated by intravenous calcium gluconate (1–2 g) or by intra-venous diuretics (chlorothiazide, 50 mg), glucose, or glucose and insulin; daily acetazolamide or chlorothiazide may prevent recurrences. In **nor-mokalemic** periodic paralysis, the patient may be un-able to move his or her limbs in severe attacks; fortu-nately, respiration and swallowing are rarely affected, because treatment with acetazolamide is not always helpful.

• • •

References

Adams RD, Victor M: *Principles of Neurology,* 2nd ed. McGraw-Hill, 1981.

Aminoff MJ (editor): *Electrodiagnosis in Clinical Neurology.* Churchill Livingstone, 1980.

Baraitser M: *The Genetics of Neurological Disorders.* Oxford, 1982.

Blackwood W, Corsellis JAN (editors): *Greenfield's Neuropathology,* 3rd ed. Arnold, 1976.

Dyck PJ et al (editors): *Peripheral Neuropathy,* 2nd ed. Saunders, 1984.

Fishman RA: *Cerebrospinal Fluid in Diseases of the Nervous System.* Saunders, 1980.

Rowland LP (editor): *Merritt's Textbook of Neurology,* 7th ed. Lea & Febiger, 1984.

Ross Russell RW (editor): *Vascular Disease of the Central Nervous System,* 2nd ed. Churchill Livingstone, 1983.

Walton JN (editor): *Brain's Diseases of the Nervous System,* 8th ed. Oxford, 1977.

Walton JN (editor): *Disorders of Voluntary Muscle,* 4th ed. Churchill Livingstone, 1981.

Psychiatric Disorders | 18

James J. Brophy, MD

Psychiatric disorders may result from disturbance of one or more of the following interrelated factors: (1) biologic function, (2) psychodynamic adaptation, (3) learned behavior, and (4) social and environmental conditions. Although the clinical situation at a given time determines which area of dysfunction will be emphasized, proper patient care requires an approach that simultaneously encompasses all factors. With such an integrated approach, a psychiatric diagnostic label will not obscure possible correctable physical illness.

(1) Biologic function. Psychiatric disorders of biologic origin may be secondary to identifiable physical illness or caused by as yet unexplained biochemical disturbances of the brain. A wide variety of psychiatric disorders (eg, psychosis, depression, delirium, anxiety), as well as nonspecific symptoms frequently considered to be of psychogenic origin, may be caused by organic brain disease or by derangement of cerebral metabolism caused by illness, nutritional deficiencies, or toxic agents (see p 676). Psychopharmacologic research is progressively elucidating the roles of certain amino acids (eg, phenylalanine, tryptophan), acetylcholine, and the monoamines (eg, dopamine, norepinephrine, serotonin, peptides) in neurotransmission and neuroendocrine function. This information has expanded knowledge of neurochemical changes in psychiatric conditions and has made it possible to more selectively tailor drugs for specific disorders. Neuroendocrine studies have shown that the hypothalamic-pituitary-adrenal (HPA) system is altered in a significant number of patients with depression and other psychiatric problems. This has led to some newer investigational techniques (eg, dexamethasone suppression test, thyrotropin-releasing hormone test). There is some evidence that changes in the immune system occur following psychic trauma, with effects on morbidity and mortality.

Newer neuroradiologic techniques (eg, CT scan, nuclear magnetic resonance [NMR] imaging) are revealing unexpected structural brain abnormalities in certain cases of such conditions as schizophrenia and bipolar affective disorders.

(2) Psychodynamic maladaptation involves intrapsychic aberrations (see p 646) and is usually treated by a psychotherapeutic approach. There are over 100 alleged forms of psychotherapy, excluding behavioral approaches. Depending on the therapist's approach, psychotherapy can be classified as supportive, interpretive, persuasive, educative, or some combination of these. Depth, duration, intensity, and frequency of sessions may vary. Various theoretic frameworks may be employed—freudian, jungian, adlerian, sullivanian, kleinian, etc. The "dynamic" approaches have their roots in classic freudian psychoanalysis, whereas "experiential" psychotherapy is of more recent origin, including many tenuous offshoots currently popular but of dubious long-term significance.

(3) Learned behavior is part of the pathogenetic mechanism in all psychiatric disorders. Although a biochemical abnormality may be the matrix of a schizophrenic process, the content of the psychotic material is to a great degree learned and socially relevant. Paranoid delusions reflect current concerns (eg, radar, electronic eavesdropping). In the case of anxiety disorders, many behavioral scientists feel that learned behavior alone is the major consideration. Appropriate parenting consists in great part of utilizing proper behavioral practices, rewarding correct behavior, and punishing delinquent behavior. Personality disorders are examples of failure to learn and incorporate patterns of behavior acceptable in societal surroundings. Just as the use of pharmacologic agents spurred the research necessary for understanding brain chemistry, the use of behavioral techniques adapted from animal studies has stimulated research in conditioning and its effect on human behavior.

(4) Social and environmental conditions have always been considered vital factors in the mental balance of the individual. Without the encounter with the environment, there can be no socially recognized illness: the exigencies of everyday life contribute both to the development of a stable personality and to the deviations from the norm. There is a constantly changing cultural influence that determines which types of behavior will be tolerated or considered deviant. In recent years, the cultural norms of acceptance have broadened. The principal vehicle for modeling and learning in our social structure is the family unit, which has shifted from an extended group with numerous relatives to a smaller nuclear group consisting of one or both parents and their children. Changes in the family unit have coincided with changes in work patterns of parents and in schooling and work patterns of young adults. The changes are complex and generally have lengthened the period of dependency and increased stresses in the family unit; this, in turn, affects the underlying social fabric. Although such issues as poverty, crime, equality, freedom of action, and political priorities may not be immediate medical considerations, indirectly they have a major impact on the psychobiologic organism that we call the human being.

Mollica RF: From asylum to community: The threatened disintegration of public psychiatry. *N Engl J Med* 1983;**308**:367.
Snyder SH: Drug and neurotransmitter receptors in the brain. *Science* 1984;**224**:22.
Wurtman RJ: Nutrients that modify brain function. *Sci Am* (April) 1982;**246**:50.

PSYCHIATRIC ASSESSMENT

Psychiatric diagnosis rests upon the established principles of a thorough history and examination. All of the forces contributing to the individual's life situation must be identified, and this can only be done if the examination includes the history; mental status; medical conditions; and pertinent social, cultural, and environmental factors impinging on the individual.

Interview

The manner in which the history is taken is important not only because it affects success in eliciting pertinent data but also because it may be of therapeutic value in itself. The setting should be quiet, and patients should initially be allowed to tell about their problems in an unstructured way without interruption. At some point an instruction such as "Tell me about yourself" will be productive. The interviewer should minimize writing, unnecessary direct questioning, and interpretive comments. Long, rambling discussions may be controlled by subtly interjecting questions relevant to the topic, although the patient's digressions sometimes provide important clues to his or her mental status. The first few minutes are often the most important part of the interview.

The interviewer should be alert for key words or phrases that can be used to help the patient develop the theme of the main difficulty. For example, if the patient says, "Doctor, I hurt, and when we have marital problems, things just get worse"—the words "hurt" and "marital problems" are important clues that need amplification when the physician makes another comment. Nonverbal clues may be as important as words, and one should notice gestures, tones of voice, and facial expressions. Obvious omissions, shying away from painful subjects, and sudden shifts of subject matter give important clues to unconscious as well as conscious sources of difficulty.

Every psychiatric history should cover the following points: (1) complaint, from the patient's viewpoint; (2) the present illness, or the evolution of the complaints; (3) previous disorders and the nature and extent of treatment; (4) the family history—important for genetic aspects and family influences; (5) personal history—childhood development, adolescent adjustment, and adult coping patterns; (6) sexual history; and (7) current life functioning, with attention to vocational, social, educational, and avocational areas.

It is often essential to obtain additional information from the family. Observing interactions of significant other people with the patient in the context of a family interview may give significant diagnostic information and may even underscore the nature of the problem and suggest a therapeutic approach.

The Mental Status Examination

Observation of the patient and the content of the remarks made during the interview constitute the informal part of the mental status examination, ie, that which is obtained indirectly. The remainder of the information comes from direct questioning, which really is intended only to fill in the gaps.

The mental status examination includes the following: (1) Appearance: Note unusual modes of dress, makeup, etc. (2) Activity and behavior: Gait, gestures, coordination of bodily movements, etc. (3) Affect: Outward manifestation of emotions such as depression, anger, elation, fear, resentment, or lack of emotional response. (4) Mood: Inward feelings, sum of statements, and observable emotional manifestations. (5) Speech: Coherence, spontaneity, articulation, hesitancy in answering, and duration of response. (6) Content of thought: Associations, preoccupations, obsessions, depersonalization, delusions, hallucinations, paranoid ideation, anger, fear, or unusual experiences. (7) Sensorium: (a) orientation to person, place, time, and circumstances; (b) remote and recent memory and recall; (c) calculations, digit retention (forward and backward), serial 7s and 3s; (d) general fund of knowledge (presidents, states, distances, events); (e) abstracting ability, often tested with common proverbs or with analogies and differences (eg, how are a lie and a mistake the same, and how are they different?). (8) Judgment regarding commonsense problems such as what to do when one runs out of medicine. (9) Insight into the nature and extent of the current difficulty and its ramifications in the patient's daily life.

The mental status examination is important in establishing a diagnosis and must be recorded clearly and completely in the chart. A change can provide valuable clues to diagnosis and treatment.

Medical Examination

The examination of a psychiatric patient must include a complete medical history and physical examination as well as all necessary laboratory and other special studies. Physical illness may frequently present as psychiatric disease, and vice versa. It is hazardous to assign a "functional" cause to symptoms simply because they arose during an emotional crisis.

Special Diagnostic Aids

Many tests and evaluation procedures are available that can be used to support and clarify initial diagnostic impressions.

A. Psychologic Testing: Psychologic testing by a trained psychologist may measure intelligence; provide information about personality, feelings, psychodynamics, and psychopathology; and differentiate psychic problems from organic ones. The place of such tests is similar to that of other tests in medicine—helpful in diagnostic problems but a useless expense when not needed.

1. Objective tests—These tests provide quantitative evaluation compared to standard norms.

a. Intelligence tests—The test most frequently used is the Wechsler Adult Intelligence Scale-Revised Form (WAIS-R). Intelligence tests often reveal more than IQ. The results, given expert interpretation, can lend objective support to the ultimate psychiatric diagnosis. Mood disturbances, thought disorders, and organic brain disease can be differentially reflected in the results from a combination of the verbal and nonverbal sections of the test.

b. Minnesota Multiphasic Personality Inventory (MMPI)—This test measures the individual's answers against the response patterns of the general population in the following categories: hypochondriacal, depressive, hysterical, psychopathic, paranoid, psychasthenic, schizophrenic, and hypomanic.

c. Bender Gestalt Test—This test is used to elicit evidence of psychomotor dysfunction in persons with organic disorders.

d. Vocational aptitude and interest tests—Several are available and may be used as a source of advice regarding vocational plans.

2. Projective tests—These tests are unstructured, so that the subject is forced to respond in ways that reflect fantasies and individual modes of adaptation. Conscious and unconscious attitudes may be deduced from the subject's responses. Projective tests are of very limited usefulness even when done by an expert.

a. Rorschach Psychodiagnostics—This test utilizes 10 inkblots. It requires expert interpretation and is not fully standardized.

b. Thematic Apperception Test (TAT)—This test uses 20 pictures of people in different situations. Interpretation is based on psychoanalytic theory concerning defenses against feelings of anxiety and reflects areas of interpersonal conflicts.

c. Sentence completion tests, Draw-a-Person tests, etc—The dubious value of these tests varies according to the skill of the evaluator.

B. Neurologic Evaluation: Consultation is often necessary and may include specialized tests such as electroencephalography, echoencephalography, brain scan, cerebral angiography, pneumoencephalography, CT scan, positron emission transaxial tomography (PETT), and nuclear magnetic resonance (NMR) imaging.

C. Amobarbital Interviews: The success of any of the sedative agents in eliciting clinically useful information is quite limited. The suggestive force of giving substances by injection is helpful, as judged from a comparison of amobarbital and saline interviews. The procedure can be helpful in differentiating psychosis from delirium; the former improves with amobarbital, whereas the latter worsens. Some cases of conversion disorders or dissociative disorders respond to this approach. Hypnosis can provide similar relief in selected subjects.

D. Biologic Markers: The dexamethasone suppression test (DST) and the thyrotropin-releasing hormone (TRH) test have been used as aids in the diagnosis, treatment, and follow-up of patients with depressive illness. Clinical usefulness of the tests is limited, but they represent progress in the search for reliable biologic markers.

Formulation of the Diagnosis

A psychiatric diagnosis must be based upon positive evidence accumulated by the above techniques. It must not be based simply on the exclusion of organic findings.

A thorough psychiatric evaluation has therapeutic as well as diagnostic value and should be expressed in ways best understood by the patient, family, and other physicians. The problem-oriented medical record is applicable to psychiatric disorders.

Hoeper EW: The usefulness of screening for mental illness. *Lancet* 1984;**1**:33.

Martin AR: Exploring patient beliefs: Steps to enhancing physician-patient interaction. *Arch Intern Med* 1983;**143**:1773.

Perry JC, Jacobs D: Overview: Clinical applications of the Amytal interview in psychiatric emergency settings. *Am J Psychiatry* 1982;**139**:552.

Watts FN: Strategies of clinical listening. *Br J Med Psychol* 1983;**56**:113.

TREATMENT APPROACHES

The approaches to treatment of psychiatric patients are, in a broad sense, similar to those in other branches of medicine. For example, the internist treating a patient with heart disease uses not only **medical measures** such as digitalis and pacemakers but also **psychologic** techniques (in an attempt to promote insight and self-realization in the patient), **social** and environmental manipulation, and **behavioral** techniques (to change behavior patterns).

The psychiatrist may utilize the same general therapeutic categories (conceptual models), but there is a shift of emphasis in treatment methods and the methods are less explicit. The **medical** approaches used by the psychiatrist include, for example, medications (the taking of which may be a psychosocial event) and convulsive therapy. The **psychologic** techniques include individual, group, and family therapies. **Social** interventions relate to the patient's environment by means of milieu therapy, partial hospitalization, day care, halfway house placement, or alteration in job or living situation. **Behavioral** therapy is directed toward identifying specific behavior patterns, factors determining such behavior, and ways of modifying it.

Regardless of the methods employed, treatment must be directed toward an objective, ie, **goal-oriented.** This usually involves (1) obtaining active cooperation on the part of the patient; (2) establishing reasonable goals and modifying the goal downward if failure occurs; (3) emphasizing positive behavior (goals) instead of symptom behavior (problems); (4) delineating the method; and (5) setting a time frame (which can be modified later).

The physician must resist pressures for prescribed treatment and instantaneous results, on the part of either the patient or relatives or close friends. The physician's own rigid resistance must not be substituted for that of the patient. The physician should be flexible and find ways to modify and work around patient resistance. Beware of unrealistic demands by the patient or the patient's family for a speedy resolution to a complex psychiatric problem. In almost all cases, psychiatric treatment involves the *active participation* of the significant people in the patient's life. It takes time to unravel the complex interrelationships between the psyche, the soma, and the sociocultural milieu of the patient. Time must be spent with the patient, but the frequency and duration of appointments are highly variable and should be adjusted to meet both the patient's psychologic needs and financial restrictions. The physician can unwittingly promote chronic illness by prescribing inappropriate medication, particularly the simultaneous use of multiple drugs. The patient comes to believe that problems respond only to medication, and the more drugs prescribed, the stronger the misconception becomes.

Psychiatric Referrals

All physicians have always treated psychiatric problems and are in an excellent position to meet their patients' emotional needs in an organized and competent way, referring to psychiatrists for consultation *or* treatment those patients who represent particularly complex problems. The most difficult problems involve evaluation of suicidal or assaultive potential and diagnostic differentiation in affective disorders and psychoses. A particularly vexing problem that has treatment ramifications is the differentiation between atypical bipolar affective disorder and schizophrenia. The psychiatric problems associated with unusual psychopharmacologic therapy and with medications used in other branches of medicine may require expert pharmacologic consultation. When a psychiatric referral is made, it should be conducted like any other referral: in an open manner, with full explanation of the problem to the patient and the referral appointment made while the patient is still in the office.

Barsky AJ: Nonpharmacologic aspects of medication. *Arch Intern Med* 1983;**143**:1544.

Nicholi AN Jr: The nontherapeutic use of psychoactive drugs: A modern epidemic. *N Engl J Med* 1983;**308**:925.

Perl M, Shelp EE: Sounding board: Psychiatric consultation masking moral dilemmas in medicine. *N Engl J Med* 1982;**307**:618.

MEDICAL APPROACHES

1. ANTIPSYCHOTIC DRUGS
(Neuroleptics, "Major Tranquilizers")

This group of drugs includes the **phenothiazines, thioxanthenes** (both similar in structure), **butyrophenones, dihydroindolones,** and **dibenzoxazepines.** Table 18–1 lists the drugs in order of increasing milligram potency and decreasing side effects (with the exception of extrapyramidal symptoms). Thus, chlorpromazine has lower milligram potency and causes more severe side effects and fewer extrapyramidal complications than fluphenazine.

Table 18–1. Commonly used antipsychotics.

	Chlor-promazine Ratio	Usual Daily Oral Dose	Usual Daily Maximum Dose*
Phenothiazines			
Chlorpromazine (Thorazine and other trade names)	1:1	100–200 mg	1 g
Thioridazine (Mellaril)	1:1	100–200 mg	600 mg
Mesoridazine (Serentil)	1:2	50–100 mg	400 mg
Piperacetazine (Quide)	1:8	20 mg	160 mg
Butaperazine (Repoise)†	1:8	20–50 mg	150 mg
Perphenazine (Trilafon)†	1:10	8–16 mg	64 mg
Trifluoperazine (Stelazine)†	1:20	5–15 mg	60 mg
Fluphenazine (Permitil, Prolixin)†	1:50	2–10 mg	60 mg
Thioxanthenes			
Chlorprothixene (Taractan)	1:1	100–200 mg	600 mg
Thiothixene† (Navane)	1:20	5–10 mg	80 mg
Butyrophenone			
Haloperidol (Haldol)	1:50	2–5 mg	80 mg
Dihydroindolone			
Molindone (Lidone, Moban)	1:15	50–100 mg	225 mg
Dibenzoxazepine			
Loxapine (Daxolin, Loxitane)	1:10	50–75 mg	200 mg

*Can be higher in some cases.
†Indicates piperazine structure.

The only butyrophenone commonly used in the USA is haloperidol, which is totally different in structure but very similar in action and extrapyramidal side effects to the piperazine phenothiazines such as fluphenazine, perphenazine, and trifluoperazine. Haloperidol has a paucity of autonomic side effects, markedly lowers hyperactivity and psychotic ideation, and is particularly effective in movement disorders such as those seen in Gilles de la Tourette's syndrome. Molindone and loxapine are similar in action, side effects, and safety to the piperazine phenothiazines.

None of the antipsychotics produce true physical dependency, and they have a wide safety margin between therapeutic and toxic effects.

Clinical Indications

The antipsychotics are used to treat the **schizophrenias, organic brain psychoses, psychotic depression, mania,** and **other psychoses.** They may be effective in psychedelic abuse, amphetamine psychosis, and selected cases of delirium. They quickly lower the arousal (activity) level and, perhaps indirectly, gradually improve socialization and thinking.

Symptoms that are ameliorated by these drugs include hyperactivity, hostility, delusions, hallucinations, negativism, and poor sleep. Individuals with acute psychosis and good premorbid function respond quite well. The most common cause of failure in the treatment of acute psychosis is inadequate dosage, and the most common cause of relapse is noncompliance. A simple regimen, preferably one dose given at bedtime, is usually the most effective plan. Patients with long-standing symptoms and unusual variations often respond poorly.

Dosage Forms & Patterns

The dosage range is quite broad. For example, chlorpromazine, 25 mg orally at bedtime, may be sufficient for the elderly person with a mild organic brain syndrome, whereas 1000 mg/d may be used in a young schizophrenic patient. For this reason, it is misleading to depend on static dosage levels. Haloperidol, 10 mg intramuscularly, is quite effective in the very active patient, particularly in mania, acute delirium, or acute schizophrenic disorder. Psychomotor agitation, racing thoughts, and auditory hallucinations are the symptoms most responsive to this initial treatment. Intramuscular medication is absorbed rapidly and uniformly. It achieves an initial 10-fold plasma level advantage over equal oral doses. This advantage levels off after 24 hours of haloperidol administration, and oral doses are then usually quite effective. Observe the response over the first hour, and repeat the dose every 1–2 hours until the patient is under control. Most patients will not require more than 80 mg in a 24-hour period. The potency of intramuscular administration is 1.5 times that of the oral form. The onset of action occurs in 30 minutes. Dystonia occurs in about 30% of patients, mostly in the 20- to 40-mg dosage range, but the incidence of autonomic and cardiovascular complications is quite low. Intra-

Table 18–2. Antipsychotic drug interactions with other drugs.

Drug	Effects
Barbiturates	Central nervous system depression and decreased antipsychotic drug levels.
Antacids	Decreased absorption of antipsychotic drugs.
All anticholinergics	Increased anticholinergic effects.
Cyclic antidepressants	Increased antidepressant blood levels.
Phenytoin	Increased phenytoin levels.
Trihexyphenidyl	Decreased antipsychotic levels.
Levodopa	Decreased antiparkinson effect.
Thiazide diuretics	Increased hypotensive effect.
Methyldopa	Decreased hypotensive effect.
Guanethidine	Decreased hypotensive effect.

venous use of haloperidol (the only neuroleptic used in this manner) is reserved for special situations (eg, severely burned patients, postsurgical agitation).

The philosophy of administration of these drugs is similar to that which governs the use of insulin in acute diabetic coma. Insulin is given until the glucose level approaches normal. In the acute psychotic patient, the antipsychotic drug is given until behavior becomes as near normal as possible. After the acute diabetic situation is resolved, insulin is titrated to maintain a reasonable glucose level, and patients vary widely in their required dosage. After the acute psychiatric situation is resolved, the psychiatric patient will require *only enough medication* to help maintain reasonable behavior. In the case of the chronic schizophrenic patient— like the brittle diabetic patient—the drugs may be required indefinitely and on a varying dosage schedule related to the patient's needs.

Psychiatric patients—particularly paranoid individuals—often neglect to take their medication. In these cases, the enanthate and decanoate (the latter is slightly longer lasting and has fewer extrapyramidal side effects) forms of fluphenazine may be given subcutaneously or intramuscularly to achieve an effect that will usually last 10–21 days. A patient who cannot be depended on to take oral medication will generally agree to come to the physician's office for a "shot." The usual dose of these long-acting preparations is 25 mg (1 mL) every 2 weeks. Dosage and frequency of administration vary from about 100 mg weekly to 12.5 mg monthly. Use the smallest amount as infrequently as possible. A relatively crude conversion estimate is that 17 mg of fluphenazine decanoate every 2 weeks is equivalent to 200 mg of chlorpromazine daily. A biweekly injection of 35 mg of fluphenazine decanoate is equivalent to 5 mg of oral fluphenazine daily. The principal side effects are extrapyramidal reactions. Antiparkinsonism drugs usually need not be used prophylactically, particularly with the low-potency antipsychotic drugs. Most patients taking *depot* neuroleptic drugs will require ongoing treatment with antiparkinsonism agents.

In most cases, oral medications are adequate. The concentrate is best absorbed, the tablet next best. Various factors play a role in the absorption of oral medications. Of particular importance are previous gastrointestinal surgery and concomitant administration of other drugs, eg, antacids. Cigarette smoking tends to increase catabolism of the drugs, thus requiring higher dosages.

Divided daily doses are not necessary after a maintenance dose has been established, and most patients can then be maintained on a single daily dose, usually taken at bedtime. This is particularly appropriate in a case where the sedative effect of the drug is desired for nighttime sleep, and undesirable sedative effects can be avoided during the day. Costs of medication, nursing time, and patient unreliability are reduced when either a single daily dose or a large bedtime/smaller morning dose schedule is utilized.

Side Effects

The side effects *decrease* as one goes from the sedating, lower milligram potency drugs such as chlorpromazine to those of higher milligram potency such as fluphenazine and haloperidol (see Table 18–1). However, the extrapyramidal effects *increase* as one goes down the list (consider chlorprothixene as similar to chlorpromazine).

The most common side effects are autonomic. Anticholinergic effects include dry mouth, blurred vision, urinary retention (particularly in elderly men with enlarged prostates), delayed gastric emptying, ileus, and precipitation of acute glaucoma in patients with narrow anterior chamber angles. Other autonomic effects include orthostatic hypotension, impotence, and inhibition of ejaculation. Cardiac arrhythmias may occur frequently as electrocardiographic findings and less frequently as clinical conditions, usually in the elderly. Thioridazine, which has the fewest extrapyramidal side effects, has the most cardiac effects. One should avoid the concomitant use of thioridazine and sympathomimetic drugs. The most frequently seen electrocardiographic changes include diminution of the T wave amplitude, appearance of prominent U waves, depression of the ST segment, and prolongation of the QT interval. These electrocardiographic findings do not alter treatment.

Metabolic and endocrine effects include weight gain, hyperglycemia, infrequent temperature irregularities (particularly in hot weather), and water intoxication that may be due to inappropriate antidiuretic hormone function. An increased incidence of antinuclear antibodies has been reported in patients taking more than 400 mg of chlorpromazine a day. Lactation and menstrual irregularities are common, as are problems in achieving erection, ejaculation (including retrograde ejaculation), and orgasm in males (approximately 50% of cases) and orgasm in females (approximately 30%). Delay in achieving orgasm is sometimes a factor in noncompliance with drug taking. Both antipsychotic and antidepressant drugs inhibit sperm motility. Bone marrow depression and cholestatic jaundice occur infrequently; these are sensitivity reactions, and they usually appear in the first 2 months of treatment. They subside on discontinuance of the drug.

There is cross-sensitivity among all of the phenothiazines, and a drug from a different group must be used when allergic reactions occur.

Photosensitivity is commonly related to chlorpromazine use. Retinopathy and hyperpigmentation are associated with use of fairly high dosages of chlorpromazine and thioridazine. The appearance of particulate melanin deposits in the lens of the eye is related to the total dose given, and patients on long-term medication should have eye examinations every year. Teratogenicity has not been causally related to these drugs, but prudence is indicated in the first trimester of pregnancy. The seizure threshold is lowered, particularly in older patients taking higher dosages. It is safe to use these medications in epileptics controlled by anticonvulsants.

The **neuroleptic malignant syndrome** of extrapyramidal signs, blood pressure changes, altered consciousness, and hyperpyrexia is an uncommon but serious complication of neuroleptic treatment. Rigidity, involuntary movements, dysarthria, and dysphagia are accompanied by pallor, cardiovascular instability, pulmonary congestion, and diaphoresis and may result in stupor, coma, and death. The cause may be related to a number of factors, including poor dosage control of neuroleptic medication and increased sensitivity of dopamine receptor sites. Dantrolene, 50 mg every 12 hours, has been of some value in the treatment of this condition. Bromocriptine mesylate, 5 mg 3 times a day, has been reported to be effective.

Extrapyramidal symptoms. Akathisia is the most common so-called extrapyramidal symptom. It occurs early in treatment (but may persist after neuroleptics are discontinued) and is characterized by a subjective desire to be in constant motion followed by an inability to sit or stand still and consequent pacing. It may include feelings of fright, rage, terror, or sexual torment. Antiparkinsonism drugs such as trihexyphenidyl, 2–5 mg orally 3 times daily, or benztropine mesylate, 1–2 mg twice daily, are usually effective. There are increasing reports of the abuse of the antiparkinsonism agents (see Substance Use Disorders, p 670). In resistant cases, diazepam, 5 mg 3 times daily, or amantadine, 100 mg orally 3 times daily, may alleviate the symptoms where the antiparkinsonism agents have failed. Infrequently, an adverse response occurs, characterized by dramatic exacerbations of the psychosis, restlessness, aggressiveness, feelings of terror, and subtle extrapyramidal symptoms. Biperiden, 5 mg intramuscularly every 2–3 hours for several doses, usually relieves the symptoms promptly. Reevaluate the dosage level of the neuroleptic drug.

Acute dystonias are often of sudden onset early in treatment and most commonly produce bizarre muscle spasms of the head, neck, and tongue. Frequently present are torticollis, oculogyric crises, swallowing difficulties, and masseter spasms. Occasionally the back, arm, or leg muscles may be affected. Diphenhydramine, 50 mg intramuscularly, is effective for the acute crisis; then give benztropine mesylate, 2 mg twice daily, or biperiden, 2 mg 3 times daily, for several weeks; then discontinue gradually, since few of the extrapyramidal symptoms require long-term use of the antiparkinsonism drugs (all of which are about equally efficacious), although trihexyphenidyl tends to be mildly stimulating and benztropine mildly sedating. Neuroleptic-induced catatonia is similar to catatonic stupor with rigidity, drooling, urinary incontinence, and cogwheeling. It usually responds slowly to withdrawal of the offending medication and use of antiparkinsonism agents.

Drug-induced parkinsonism is indistinguishable from idiopathic parkinsonism, but it occurs later in treatment than the preceding extrapyramidal symptoms. The condition includes the typical signs of apathy and reduction of facial and arm movements (akinesia, which can mimic depression), festinating gait, rigidity, loss of postural reflexes, and the pill-rolling tremor. This extrapyramidal symptom also responds to the aforementioned antiparkinsonism drugs in the same dosages. After 4–6 weeks, the drugs can often be discontinued with no recurrent symptoms. In any of the extrapyramidal symptoms, amantadine, 100–400 mg daily, may be used instead of the antiparkinsonism drugs if anticholinergic effects are a problem. Anticholinergic toxicity is characterized by impaired attention and short-term memory, disorientation, anxiety, visual and auditory hallucinations, and other psychotic ideation. Physostigmine, 2–4 mg intramuscularly, can reverse this central anticholinergic organic mental state.

Tardive dyskinesia is a syndrome of abnormal involuntary stereotyped movements of the face, mouth, tongue, and limbs that may occur after months or (usually) years of treatment with neuroleptic agents. The reported prevalence varies widely, different reports indicating from 3 to 50% of patients who have undergone long-term neuroleptic therapy. There are indications that the incidence is increasing, although this may represent increased awareness of the problem. *The physician must weigh the risk factors of any drugs versus the benefits.*

Early manifestations include fine wormlike movements of the tongue at rest, difficulty in sticking out the tongue, facial tics, increased blink frequency, or jaw movements of recent onset. Later manifestations include bucco-linguo-masticatory movements, lip smacking, chewing motions, mouth opening and closing, puffing of the cheeks, eye blinking, and choreoathetoid movements of the extremities (the last being more prevalent in younger patients).

The incidence of tardive dyskinesia increases with age (3 times more common in patients over 40) and is higher in women. Brain damage is said to be predisposing, although conclusive studies are lacking. The psychiatric diagnosis is not a major consideration in itself. Exposure to neuroleptic drugs certainly plays a role, although tardive dyskinesia does not develop in about 80% of the patients at risk. The symptoms have been reported in patients undergoing long-term anticonvulsant drug therapy. It is estimated that approximately 25% of neuroleptic-treated patients with an abnormal movement disorder develop the disorder due to reasons other than drug therapy. There may be other predisposing factors not evident at this time. Such factors may explain why some patients develop the dyskinesia after only a few months of medication while others never do. There may also be subgroups of dyskinesias that are not yet well defined.

The dyskinesias do not occur during sleep and can be voluntarily suppressed for short periods. Stress and movements in other parts of the body will often aggravate the condition. Tardive dyskinesia is not alleviated by antiparkinsonism agents and may be worsened by them. There is concern that the chronic use of antiparkinsonism drugs may contribute to the development of the dyskinesia, either by masking early signs or by altering neurochemical balance, but this has not been proved. There is no known difference among any of the antipsychotic drugs in the development of this syndrome. There is a correlation between the incidence of tardive dyskinesia and interruption of drug therapy; thus, the concept of drug holidays as a beneficial treatment plan is in doubt.

Early signs of dyskinesia must be differentiated from those reversible signs produced by ill-fitting dentures or nonneuroleptic drugs such as levodopa, tricyclic antidepressants, antiparkinsonism agents, anticonvulsants, and antihistamines. Other neurologic conditions such as Huntington's chorea can be differentiated by history and examination.

At present, the emphasis is on prevention. When the tardive dyskinesic syndrome is first noted, gradually discontinue all neuroleptic drugs if possible. In about one-third of cases, symptoms will gradually disappear over several months. In cases that do not improve with discontinuation of the antipsychotic drugs and those in which psychotic symptoms necessitate the use of neuroleptics, a rauwolfia derivative such as reserpine can be given instead. This is an effective antipsychotic agent, although the depressive and gastrointestinal side effects limit usage. There is evidence that the benzodiazepines may alleviate the syndrome through their action on the GABA neurotransmitter system. Pure lecithin, lithium, and sodium valproate have been helpful only in a limited number of cases. In some cases, one must weigh the advantages against the side effects, and, with the consent of the patient, continue the antipsychotic drug therapy at the lowest therapeutic dosage.

Appleton WS: Fourth psychoactive drug usage guide. *J Clin Psychiatry* 1982;**43**:12.

Kane JM, Smith JM: Tardive dyskinesia: Prevalence and risk factors 1959–1979. *Arch Gen Psychiatry* 1982;**39**:473.

Kessler KA, Waletzky JP: Clinical use of the antipsychotics. *Am J Psychiatry* 1981;**138**:202.

Mueller PS, Vester JW, Fermaglich J: Neuroleptic malignant syndrome: Successful treatment with bromocriptine. *JAMA* 1983;**249**:386.

2. LITHIUM

The use of lithium over the last 35 years has dramatically affected both diagnosis and treatment in psychiatry. Large areas of neurochemical research have been affected by use of this drug, which is one of the 3 major advances in psychopharmacology, along with use of antipsychotic and antidepressant drugs. The discovery of lithium's effectiveness in affective disorders has shown that many of these patients were erroneously diagnosed as having a schizophrenic disorder. It has also become evident that some alcohol-dependent individuals have affective disorders and can be successfully treated with lithium. This has led to further research on a number of poorly defined and treated conditions, including aggressive states, movement disorders, and organic brain syndromes.

The precise manner in which lithium exerts its therapeutic effects has yet to be defined, although it probably involves ionic processes at the cell membrane that in turn affect the flow of neurotransmitters mediated by adenylate cyclase or cAMP. It differs from the other psychopharmacologic drugs in that it is a salt and is used only in one form, and its dosage is guided by blood serum level.

Clinical Indications

As a prophylactic drug for bipolar affective disorder, lithium significantly decreases the frequency and severity of both manic and depressive attacks in about 80% of patients. A positive response is more predictable if the patient has a low frequency of episodes (no more than 2 per year with intervals free of psychopathology). A positive response occurs more frequently in individuals who have blood relatives with a diagnosis of manic or hypomanic attacks. Patients who swing rapidly back and forth between manic and depressive attacks (at least 4 cycles per year) usually respond poorly to lithium prophylaxis initially, but some improve with continued long-term treatment.

Acute manic or hypomanic symptoms will respond to lithium therapy. It is common to use neuroleptic drugs or electroconvulsive therapy to treat the excited or psychotic manic stage and then make a decision with the patient and family about the feasibility of long-term prophylactic lithium therapy. The decision is usually based on the severity of the condition. Schizoaffective disorders and some types of schizophrenia are probably psychotic symptoms of bipolar affective disorder, for which lithium treatment may be effective.

Lithium alone and combined with cyclic antidepressants in the acute phases is useful in the prophylaxis of some recurrent unipolar depressions. Its use in the treatment of acute depression is not warranted except in depressions occurring in a bipolar patient who has previously responded to the drug. Lithium is compatible with other commonly used psychotherapeutic drugs, although the concomitant use of an antipsychotic drug may worsen lithium toxicity. Lithium is not effective in primary alcoholism, seda-

tive abuse, hyperkinesis, or obsessive compulsive neurosis unless there is an underlying primary affective disorder. Because of the lag period of 4–10 days until therapeutic serum levels of 0.8–1.2 meq/L are attained, it is desirable to give an antipsychotic drug initially in order to achieve prompt control of the manic symptoms. Haloperidol, 5–30 mg orally daily, can be used and then gradually discontinued over the first week as therapeutic lithium levels are established. Most patients with bipolar disease can be managed with lithium alone, though some will require continued or intermittent use of a neuroleptic or antidepressant medication.

Dosage Forms & Patterns

Lithium carbonate (Eskalith, Lithane, Lithonate, Lithotabs, Lithobid) is available in the USA in 300-mg capsules. Capsules are usually preferred because they are associated with less nausea and less metallic taste. Tablets (Lithotabs), which can be broken, are used in patients requiring a more exact dosage than a multiple of 300 mg. Side effects can be mitigated by taking the drug with food or by use of Lithobid (slow release). Lithium citrate is available as a syrup for patients in whom compliance is a problem. The dosage is that required to maintain blood levels in the therapeutic range. For acute attacks this ranges from 1 to 1.6 meq/L, whereas the prophylactic dose is 0.4–1 meq/L. Maintenance levels should be kept as low as clinically feasible. The dose required to meet this need will vary in individuals and should be determined by giving a test dose of 600 mg of lithium carbonate after the clinical workup, which should include a medical history and physical examination; complete blood count; T_4, blood urea nitrogen, creatinine, and electrolyte determinations; urinalysis; and ECG. Twenty-four hours after the administration of the test dose, a blood sample is drawn for lithium determination. (See Table 18–3 for dosage requirements based on a test dose.) The usual practice is to administer lithium twice a day.

Further lithium determinations should be made weekly until the lithium level remains stable in the desired therapeutic range. Serum levels are then checked every several weeks, then monthly. After the patient has been stable for several months to a year, blood for lithium level determinations can then be drawn according to the clinician's judgment (usually at 3–4 month intervals). Lithium is readily absorbed,

Table 18–3. Predicted lithium daily dosage necessary to produce therapeutic levels.

24-h Lithium Level (meq/L)	Total Daily Dose (mg)
< 0.05	3600
0.05–0.09	2700
0.10–0.14	1800
0.15–0.19	1200
0.20–0.23	900
0.24–0.30	600
> 0.30	300

with peak serum levels occurring within 1–3 hours and complete absorption in 8 hours. Half of the total body lithium is excreted in 18–24 hours. *The blood for the lithium levels should be drawn 12 hours after the last dose.* Serum levels should be determined when clinically indicated, particularly when there is any condition that may lower sodium levels (eg, diarrhea; dehydration; use of diuretics). Adequate hydration is important. Patients receiving lithium should use diuretics with caution and only under close medical supervision. Lithium is 95% excreted in urine. The thiazide diuretics cause increased lithium reabsorption from the proximal renal tubules, resulting in increased serum lithium levels, and adjustment of lithium intake must be made to compensate for this. Reduce lithium dosage by 25–40% when the patient is receiving 50 mg/d of hydrochlorothiazide. Potassium-sparing diuretics (spironolactone, amiloride, triamterene) may also cause increased serum lithium levels and require careful monitoring of lithium intake. Loop diuretics (furosemide, ethacrynic acid, bumetanide) appear not to alter serum lithium levels.

Side Effects

A. Early: Mild gastrointestinal symptoms (take lithium with food), fine tremors (treat with propranolol, 20–60 mg/d orally, only if persistent), slight muscle weakness, and some degree of somnolence are early side effects that are usually transient. Moderate polyuria (reduced renal responsiveness to antidiuretic hormone) and polydipsia (associated with increased plasma renin concentration) are occasionally present. Weight gain (often a result of calories in fluids taken for polydipsia) and leukocytosis are fairly common.

B. Lithium Toxicity: Frank toxicity usually occurs at blood levels above 2 meq/L. This is often a result of sodium loss, since sodium and lithium are reabsorbed at the same loci in the proximal renal tubules. Any sodium loss such as that which occurs with diarrhea, use of diuretics, or excessive perspiration results in increased lithium levels. Symptoms and signs include vomiting and diarrhea, the latter exacerbating the problem since more sodium is lost. Other signs and symptoms include tremors, marked muscle weakness, confusion, dysarthria, vertigo, ataxia, hyperreflexia, rigidity, seizures, opisthotonos, and coma. Toxicity is higher in the elderly, who should be maintained on slightly lower serum levels. Lithium overdosage may be accidental or intentional or may occur as a result of poor monitoring. Compliance with lithium therapy is adversely affected by the loss of some hypomanic experiences valued by the patient. These include social extroversion and a sense of heightened enjoyment in many activities such as sex and business dealings, often with increased productivity in the latter. There is no evidence that creativity is suppressed with the use of lithium therapy. Kidney disease is a major factor in toxic alterations of sodium/lithium balance.

C. Other Side Effects: These include weight gain, goiter (3%; often euthyroid), occasionally hypothyroidism (5%; concomitant administration of lithium and iodide enhances the hypothyroid and goitrogenic effect of either drug), changes in the glucose tolerance test toward a diabeticlike curve, edema, and leukocytosis. Thyroid and kidney function should be checked at 3- to 6-month intervals. Most of these side effects subside when lithium is discontinued; when residual side effects exist, they are usually not serious. Most clinicians treat lithium-induced hypothyroidism with thyroid hormone while continuing lithium therapy. Hypercalcemia and elevated parathyroid hormone levels occur in some patients. Electrocardiographic abnormalities (principally T wave flattening or inversion) may occur during lithium administration but are not of clinical significance. Sinoatrial block may occur, particularly in the elderly. It is important that other drugs which prolong intraventricular conduction, such as tricyclic antidepressants, be used with caution in conjunction with lithium. Lithium may precipitate or exacerbate psoriasis in some patients. Lithium-induced delirium with therapeutic lithium levels is an infrequent complication and often persists for several days after serum levels have become negligible. Encephalopathy has occurred in patients on combined lithium/neuroleptic therapy. Patients receiving long-term lithium therapy may have cogwheel rigidity and, occasionally, other extrapyramidal signs. A wide variety of neurologic sequelae have been reported; most remit quickly when lithium therapy is discontinued.

The long-term use of lithium has adverse effects on renal function (with interstitial fibrosis, tubular atrophy, and glomerulosclerosis) in some patients (sometimes connected with a history of lithium toxicity and concomitant neuroleptic use) that are not always completely reversible. Lithium-induced nephrogenic diabetes insipidus occasionally occurs. A rise in serum creatinine levels is an indication for in-depth evaluation of renal function. Lithium increases parathyroid hormone levels, with increased serum calcium and decreased serum phosphate. Long-term lithium therapy has also been associated with a relative lowering of the level of memory and perceptual processing. Some impairment of attention and emotional reactivity has also been noted.

Lithium exposure in early pregnancy increases the frequency of congenital anomalies, with a marked shift toward major cardiovascular anomalies. *It is advisable for women using lithium either to avoid pregnancy or to not use lithium at all during a planned pregnancy, particularly during the first trimester.* If there has been exposure in the first trimester, especially between the eighth and twelfth weeks, the possibility of teratogenic defect is highest. Bottle-feeding should be considered in mothers using lithium, since concentration in breast milk is one-third to one-half that in serum.

Patients with massive ingestions of lithium or levels above 3 meq/L should be treated with induced emesis and gastric lavage. In normal renal function, osmotic and saline diuresis increases renal lithium clearance. Urinary alkalinization is also helpful, since

Table 18–4. Lithium interactions with other drugs.

Drug	Effects
Thiazide diuretics	Increased lithium levels.
Potassium-sparing diuretics (spironolactone, amiloride, triamterene)	Increased lithium levels.
Osmotic diuretics (urea, mannitol)	Increased lithium excretion.
Theophylline, aminophylline	Increased lithium excretion.
Sodium bicarbonate	Increased lithium excretion.
Succinylcholine	Increased succinylcholine duration of action.
Iodine	Enhanced goitrogenic effect.
Methyldopa	Rigidity, mutism, fascicular twitching.
Indomethacin	Increased lithium levels.
Phenylbutazone	Increased lithium levels.

sodium bicarbonate decreases lithium reabsorption in the proximal tubule, as does acetazolamide also. Aminophylline potentiates the diuretic effect by increasing the glomerular filtration rate of lithium. Drugs affecting the distal loop have no effect on lithium reabsorption. In exceptional cases, hemodialysis and peritoneal dialysis decrease plasma concentration; this gradually shortens recovery time.

Donaldson IM, Cuningham J: Persisting neurologic sequelae of lithium carbonate therapy. *Arch Neurol* 1983;**40**:747.

Jefferson JW, Greist JH: Some hazards of lithium use. *Am J Psychiatry* 1981;**138**:93.

Mitchell JE, Mackenzie TB: Cardiac effects of lithium therapy in man: A review. *J Clin Psychiatry* 1982;**43**:47.

Ramsey TA, Cox M: Lithium and the kidney: A review. *Am J Psychiatry* 1982;**139**:443.

3. ANTIDEPRESSANT DRUGS

Antidepressant drugs are classified in 3 groups: (1) monoamine oxidase inhibitors (MAOI); (2) tricyclic antidepressants; and (3) the new cyclic, or so-called new generation, antidepressant drugs, which include maprotiline and trazodone (already in clinical use in the USA) and bupropion, mianserin, and nomifensine (expected to be released soon). The monoamine oxidase inhibitors were first used for the treatment of depression in the early 1950s. The tricyclic antidepressants were discovered as the result of molecular manipulation of the phenothiazine molecule in the search for more effective antipsychotic drugs. The emergence of diet-related complications of monoamine oxidase inhibitors coincided with the development of the tricyclic antidepressants and was one of the factors favoring the use of the latter drugs. The first 2 groups of drugs support the catecholamine concept of major mental disorders, which postulates that depression is associated with relative availability of catecholamines (dopamine, norepinephrine, epinephrine) and indoleamines (serotonin, histamine).

Clinical Indications

Tricyclic antidepressants are the drugs of choice for the treatment of severe depressions of any sort, but particularly those classified as major depressive disorders (see Affective Disorders, p 663). Tricyclic antidepressants are also effective in depressions associated with bipolar affective disorders, although they may occasionally precipitate a manic episode. It is also fairly common to use a tricyclic antidepressant to treat a developing depression in a bipolar patient who is receiving lithium prophylaxis. The depressions associated with reactive and adjustment disorders generally do not require medication and can be treated with psychotherapy and the passage of time, although some of these depressions become rather severe. In these cases, *particularly when vegetative signs are present,* a tricyclic antidepressant will often prevent further deepening of the depression and provide some relief. The major depressive disorders and the reactive depressions respond differently to tricyclic antidepressants: patients with major depressive disorders may experience a marked and, at times, astonishing improvement, whereas patients with reactive depressions improve, but not dramatically. Tricyclic antidepressants have also been used in the treatment of enuresis, catalepsy, chronic pain, hyperkinetic disorders, and peptic ulcer disease. The monoamine oxidase inhibitors have been relegated to a secondary role in the USA, although they are used to a much greater extent in Great Britain. They clearly have an important role in the treatment of major depressions, alone or in combination with other drugs. Newer antidepressants soon to be released in the USA (eg, bupropion, nomifensine) tend to be more stimulating than the older drugs and have no anticholinergic effects and no known relationship to serotonin or norepinephrine.

In the patient with severe depression, it is customary to start a tricyclic drug appropriate to the symptoms. For example, a sedative drug such as amitriptyline is indicated in patients with disrupted sleep or some degree of anxiety or mild agitation, but a non-sedative drug such as desipramine is indicated for patients showing withdrawal but having minimal sleep problems and little anxiety. If the patient fails to respond, consider prescribing a tricyclic with the opposite neurotransmitter effect (see Table 18–5). If, after a full trial, this also is ineffective, consider using a monoamine oxidase inhibitor antidepressant. It is common practice to stop the tricyclic antidepressant and allow a "washout time" of 1–2 weeks before starting the monoamine oxidase inhibitor. Combined tricyclic–monoamine oxidase inhibitor therapy should be given very carefully under close medical supervision by a physician experienced with combined drug therapy. There is a small subgroup of severe depressions that do not respond to any antidepressant drugs. Although these disorders are not classified as bipolar affective disorders, some cases respond to lithium therapy. There is evidence that a subgroup of depressions with somatic complaints and obsessive-compulsive-phobic components responds best to the

Table 18–5. Commonly used antidepressants.

	Usual Daily Oral Dose (mg)	Usual Daily Maximum Dose (mg)	Sedative Effects*	Anticholinergic Effects*	Serotonin Uptake*	Norepinephrine Uptake*
Tricyclic compounds						
Amoxapine	150–200	400	2	2	1	4
Amitriptyline	150–200	300	3	4	4	0
Desipramine	150–200	300	1	1	0	4
Doxepin	150–200	300	4	3	1	1
Imipramine	150–200	300	2	2	3	2
Nortriptyline	100–150	200	2	1	2	2
Protriptyline	15–40	60	1	2	–	–
Trimipramine	75–150	200	4	4		
Monoamine oxidase inhibitors						
Isocarboxazid	10–20	30	–	–	–	–
Phenelzine	45–60	90	–	–	–	–
Tranylcypromine	20	30	–	–	–	–
New cyclic compounds						
Maprotiline	150–200	300	4	1	0	4
Trazodone	200–400	600	4	0	–	–

*4 = strong effect; 1 = weak effect; 0 = no effect.

monoamine oxidase inhibitors. Depressions with atypical vegetative signs such as increased appetite, weight gain, and increased sleep; agorophobia with secondary depression; and pain syndromes with depression are considered responsive to the monoamine oxidase inhibitors. Panic reactions with agoraphobias have responded to both monoamine and tricyclic antidepressants.

Electroconvulsive therapy has consistently been more effective than either of the antidepressant groups of drugs (see Other Organic Therapies, p 645). Convenience, expense, and public opinion have been major factors in the use of electroconvulsive therapy. It should be considered in those who are at risk of suicide and in those who fail to respond to adequate trials of medication. Stimulants have little, if any, place in the treatment of depression. Their uses are in the treatment of childhood hyperkinesis and narcolepsy.

Dosage Forms & Patterns

The tricyclic antidepressants are characterized more by their similarities than by their differences. Side effects and neurotransmitter activity of these drugs are outlined in Table 18–5. The dosages tend to be quite similar, except for protriptyline. The newer cyclic antidepressants are generally about as effective as the tricyclic drugs; side effects and time of onset of action may differ. Side effects also dictate the choice of drugs; for example, trazodone is the drug of choice in older men with some degree of prostatic hypertrophy, because it has significantly less anticholinergic effect.

The lag in clinical response (less with amoxapine and maprotiline) may be as much as several weeks; however, the side effects of these drugs limit the clinician's ability to increase the dosage rapidly. The lag time is apparently related to delays in achieving therapeutic blood levels and the interval required to

affect neurotransmitter systems. Even though they receive similar dosages, individuals vary considerably (up to 30-fold) in concentration of the drug in plasma. There is evidence that a plasma steady state of approximately 100 ng/mL is the optimum level for most of the tricyclic antidepressants. Absorption plays a role in the blood level of these drugs, and patients who have had gastrointestinal surgery often have lower levels. Early responses include relief of both anxiety and insomnia. Even though the patient may state that the depression has not lifted, there is usually increased energy and less preoccupation with somatic concerns in the first several weeks of therapy. Mood depression and sexual dysfunction are often the last problems to be relieved.

The 2 most common reasons for clinical failure in the treatment of depression are (1) poor selection of treatable depressions and (2) inadequate trial of medication (including noncompliance, which is frequently related to poor instruction about side effects). An adequate trial includes adequate dosages over an appropriate period of time. Usually, treatment starts with a moderate dose (eg, amitriptyline, 100 mg at bedtime) that is increased by 25–50 mg every several days depending on side effects and clinical response to maximum dosage. (See Table 18–5.) The drug should be tried for several weeks at maximum dosages before it is considered a failure. Most patients respond when the dosage is in the range of 150–200 mg. Once clinical relief of symptoms is achieved, the dosage is maintained for several months, and thereafter the drug is given in the lowest effective dose for as long as the depression continues. This involves a gradual downward adjustment of the dosage until the patient requires no medication—a process that usually takes several months from the start of the depression. Some patients will require medication for considerably longer periods. Patients with bipolar affective disorders respond best to lithium, whereas the recurrent major depressive disorders respond better to antidepressants. Patients with bipolar disorders are at high risk for precipitation of the manic phase when taking a tricyclic antidepressant; the manic phase usually occurs within 12 weeks of the onset of therapy. Bipolar patients also tend to cycle more rapidly when treated with tricyclic antidepressants. Either of these occurrences should alert the physician to possible bipolar illness, and the patient should be evaluated for lithium treatment. Relapses in bipolar patients maintained on lithium may be related to gradual onset of hypothyroidism (a side effect of lithium). If this is not the case, they may be treated concomitantly with antidepressants; dosage requirements tend to be lower than in uncomplicated acute depression. Maintenance dosages of tricyclic antidepressants are one-half to one-third the amount needed by the individual for treatment of an acute episode.

Except for some early adjustments, it is not necessary to use divided doses of tricyclic antidepressants: a single dose at bedtime is adequate (particularly when the clinician takes advantage of the sedative side effects to help treat associated insomnia). Doxepin, amitriptyline, and trazodone are the most sedating of the antidepressants. The bedtime dose helps achieve compliance, since people tend to take drugs at bedtime and not during the day. Frightening dreams can be alleviated by using divided doses. Alcohol and smoking increase dosage requirements because of increased catabolism of the drug.

Essentially the same procedures apply to the use of the monoamine oxidase inhibitors. There is less lag time and a narrower range of dosages, so that therapeutic levels are more quickly achieved. With these drugs it is vital to instruct patients about dietary restrictions (see Side Effects, below). Combined antipsychotic-antidepressant drug therapy is needed only in unusual cases, and in those instances, the fixed dosage of the commercial combinations is a disadvantage. Triiodothyronine, 25–50 μg/d orally, is sometimes empirically useful in patients who are nonresponsive to tricyclic antidepressants.

Severe depression involves a high risk of suicide, and these groups of drugs have a narrow margin of safety in overdoses. Since most people who commit suicide with drugs take what is at hand, it is important that the amount of medication dispensed be less than the lethal dose, ie, less than a week's supply. Since the clinician will see the severely depressed patient frequently, the medication can be given at each visit, and the reasons for this can be discussed with the patient. Rather than being annoyed at this supposed lack of trust, most suicidal patients are relieved that the physician cares.

Side Effects

Most of the tricyclic and newer cyclic antidepressants, with the exception of trazodone, have strong **anticholinergic effects,** commonly including dry mouth (the most persistent side effect), blurred vision, constipation, and urinary retention to varying degrees, the worst occurring in men with prostatic hypertrophy. The anticholinergic effects predispose to other medical problems such as heat stroke or dental problems. Orthostatic hypotension occasionally occurs and does not remit with continued use of a drug. Cardiac effects include altered rate, rhythm, and contractility. The cardiac abnormality is a function of the anticholinergic effect, direct myocardial depression, and interference with adrenergic neurons. Electrocardiographic changes range from benign ST segment and T wave changes and sinus tachycardia to a variety of complex and serious arrhythmias, the latter requiring a change in medication. The seizure threshold is lowered, and a patient will occasionally become psychotic. Loss of libido and decreased orgasm occur. Erectile and ejaculatory disturbances are fairly common. Photosensitivity is infrequent. Delirium and severe agitation are infrequent complications, as are extrapyramidal reactions similar to those caused by the phenothiazines. Amitriptyline has the most side effects and maprotiline and trazodone the fewest.

Long-term monoamine oxidase inhibitor therapy can cause a craving for sweets (with resultant weight gain), insomnia, and anorgasmia. **Sympathomimetic symptoms** of tachycardia, sweating, and tremor are frequently noted. In patients past age 50, less of the drug is protein-bound, and dosage requirements are lower. The monoamine oxidase inhibitors frequently cause orthostatic hypotension. One advantage is the lack of anticholinergic effects, but nausea, insomnia, or drowsiness is common. **Central nervous system** side effects include agitation and toxic psychoses. Great care must be taken to avoid the ingestion of sympathomimetic amines, since the reduction of effective monoamine oxidase leaves the individual vulnerable to the effects of exogenous amines, including those foods containing tyramine, eg, liver of all types, sausage and bologna, aged cheeses, pickled herring, concentrated yeast extract, Chinese pea pods, and English bean pods. Beer, ale, wines (particularly red wine and sherry), sardines, and anchovies contain varying amounts of tyramine. Avocados and overripe fruits are to be avoided. All stimulants should be avoided, including both prescribed and over-the-counter decongestants, most of which contain phenylpropanolamine. (See Table 18–6.) Treatment of a hypertensive crisis is the same as that for pheochromocytoma (see p 739); give phentolamine, 1.2 mg intravenously every 5 minutes as needed to lower blood pressure.

Overdoses of tricyclic antidepressants are dangerous and must be considered a medical emergency. Major complications include coma with shock, respiratory depression, seizures, hyperpyrexia, smooth muscle paralysis, delirium, and severe cardiac arrhythmias. The drug should be removed from the gastrointestinal tract as soon as possible after insertion of a cuffed endotracheal tube if the patient is comatose. Ventilatory support should be provided. Shock is treated with fluids and hyperpyrexia by cooling tech-

Table 18-6. Antidepressant drug interactions with other drugs.

Drug	Effects
Tricyclic and cyclic antidepressants	
Antacids	Decreased absorption of antidepressants.
Clonidine	Decreased antihypertensive effect.
Cimetidine	Increased antidepressant blood levels.
Methyldopa	Decreased antihypertensive effect.
Guanethidine	Decreased antihypertensive effect.
Sympathomimetic drugs	Increased pressor effect.
Quinidine	Decreased ventricular conduction.
Procainamide	Decreased ventricular conduction.
Digitalis	Increased incidence of heart block.
Propranolol	Increased hypotension.
Insulin	Decreased blood sugar.
Rauwolfia derivatives	Increased stimulation.
Anticoagulants	Increased hypoprothrombinemic effect.
Sedatives	Increased sedation.
Other anticholinergic drugs	Marked anticholinergic responses.
Monoamine oxidase inhibitors	
Levodopa	Increased blood pressure.
Sympathomimetic drugs	Increased blood pressure.
Belladonnalike drugs	Increased blood pressure.
Antihistamines	Increased sedation.
Meperidine	Increased mood lability.
Succinylcholine	Increased neuromuscular blockade.
Sulfonylureas	Decreased blood sugar.
Insulin	Decreased blood sugar.
Guanethidine	Decreased blood pressure.
Methyldopa	Decreased blood pressure.

niques. Arterial blood gases and pH must be monitored for early correction of any abnormalities, particularly since these contribute to cardiac complications. Seizures should be treated with intravenous anticonvulsants. Cardiac complications are treated on the basis of electrocardiographic findings. Physostigmine in repeated doses of 0.5 mg *given slowly* intravenously may be used to reverse the central anticholinergic effect.

Feighner JP: The new generation of antidepressants. *J Clin Psychiatry* 1983;**44(5-Part 2)**:49.

Goodwin FK et al: Potentiation of antidepressant effects by L-triiodothyronine in tricyclic nonresponders. *Am J Psychiatry* 1982;**139**:34.

Richardson JW III, Richelson E: Antidepressants: A clinical update for medical practitioners. *Mayo Clin Proc* 1984;**59**:330.

Tollefson GD: Monoamine oxidase inhibitors: A review. *J Clin Psychiatry* 1983;**44**:280.

Veith RC et al: Cardiovascular effects of tricyclic antidepressants in depressed patients with chronic heart disease. *N Engl J Med* 1982;**306**:954.

See also general references under Antipsychotic Drugs.

4. SEDATIVE-HYPNOTIC DRUGS
(Anxiolytic Agents, "Minor Tranquilizers")

The sedatives are a heterogeneous group of drugs that differ in chemical structure but have quite similar pharmacologic and behavioral effects. They are often marketed as "minor tranquilizers" or "antianxiety agents," and all have hypnotic properties when given in adequate dosage. Ethanol is the most commonly used antianxiety drug. The various sedatives differ mainly in milligram potency, dose-response curves, and onset and duration of action. All are general depressants of brain function and decrease anxiety, producing disinhibition and a lowering of passive avoidance in sufficient dosage. To varying degrees, all have the potential for dependency with tolerance and severe withdrawal symptoms. Short-acting drugs may present a greater risk of withdrawal reactions than longer-acting agents. They are additive and have cross-tolerance and cross-dependence. Some have anticonvulsant and muscle relaxant properties, although muscle relaxation usually occurs in the ataxic dosage range.

The highly addicting drugs with a narrow margin of safety such as glutethimide, methaqualone, ethchlorvynol, methyprylon, meprobamate, and the barbiturates (with the exception of phenobarbital) should be avoided. Phenobarbital, in addition to its anticonvulsant properties, is a reasonably safe and very cheap sedative but has the aforementioned disadvantage of enzyme stimulation, which markedly reduces its usefulness if any other medications are being used by that patient. Although its effect on dicumarol is the most widely known, it increases the catabolism of practically all other drugs, including antipsychotics and antidepressants.

The benzodiazepines are the latest in a long line of sedatives that were initially regarded as safe, effective, and not likely to cause dependency. However, like its predecessors, the benzodiazepine group has potential for abuse and complex metabolic actions. When ingested by themselves, these agents are safer than other drugs used in suicide attempts. Despite the fact that the "safer" benzodiazepines are replacing barbiturates for purposes of sedation, there has been no significant reduction in suicides caused by drugs. Furthermore, many attempted suicides involve not only multiple drug use but also alcohol. It is clear that carelessly dispensing drugs for obscure complaints and persistent patient demands is a part of the problem.

All of the benzodiazepines are similar in chemical structure and clinical properties. Benzodiazepine receptors in the brain occur in great numbers in the limbic system, hippocampus, and olfactory bulb. The receptors act in concert with gamma-aminobutyric acid (GABA) inhibitory neurotransmitters. They vary in milligram potency and duration of action, the latter being a function of lipid solubility and activity of metabolites.

The benzodiazepines are not believed to increase hepatic microsomal activity, and they therefore do not increase the catabolism of other drugs in this way as do the barbiturates and other sedatives. Onset of action does not differ significantly among the benzodiazepines, although the relatively quick absorption and high lipid solubility of diazepam have enhanced its popularity. The length of action of the benzodiazepines varies as a function of the active metabolites they produce. Short-acting benzodiazepines, which do not produce active metabolites, have half-lives of 5–20 hours. The other benzodiazepines produce active metabolites and have half-lives of 1–8 days. The long-acting sedatives are poorly absorbed when given intramuscularly, while the short-acting benzodiazepines are rapidly absorbed by this route. The antihistamines hydroxyzine and diphenhydramine are often prescribed for their sedative properties even though the effect is limited.

Clinical Indications

The sedatives are used clinically for the treatment of anxiety, which may be the result of many factors, eg, transient situational problems, acute and chronic stresses of life, chronic medical problems, intractable pain exacerbated by apprehension and depression, and problems that people cannot or will not resolve (unhappy marriages, unsatisfactory jobs, etc). In higher doses these drugs act as hypnotics. Whether the indications are anxiety or insomnia, the drugs should be used judiciously. There are no indications for sedatives that cannot be met by one of the benzodiazepines.

The first nonsedative anxiolytic drug scheduled to be marketed soon in the USA is buspirone (Buspar). It is structurally different from the sedatives, lacks anticonvulsant activity, and does not impair motor performance. It may provide anxiolytic action with low abuse potential and little or no synergism with alcohol.

Dosage Forms & Patterns
(See Table 18–7.)

All of the sedatives may be given orally, and several are available in parenteral form. There is evidence that the benzodiazepines are slowly and erratically absorbed when given intramuscularly. The intravenous use of such benzodiazepines as diazepam and chlordiazepoxide produces rapid clinical results but occasional complications of pain and phlebitis. Antacids significantly alter the absorption of benzodiazepines, an important consideration, since many anxious individuals suffer from gastrointestinal disturbances and use both types of drugs concomitantly. Food also modifies the absorption of diazepam (and possibly the other benzodiazepines), initially slowing absorption but resulting in higher levels over many hours. In the average case of anxiety, diazepam, 5–10 mg orally every 4–6 hours as needed, is a reasonable starting regimen. Since people vary widely in their response and since the drugs are long-lasting, one must individualize the dosage. Once this is established, an *adequate* dose early in the course of symptom development will obviate the need for "pill-popping," which contributes to dependency problems.

Table 18–7. Commonly used sedatives.

	Usual Oral Sedative Dose (mg)	Usual Oral Hypnotic Dose (mg)	Usual Maximum Daily Oral Dose (mg)
Benzodiazepines			
Alprazolam* (Xanax)	0.5		4
Chlordiazepoxide (Librium)	5–30	50–100	75–100
Clorazepate (Tranxene)	3.25–15	30	60
Diazepam (Valium)	2–10	20–30	40
Flurazepam (Dalmane)		15	60
Halazepam (Paxipam)	20	40–60	160
Lorazepam* (Ativan)	2		
Oxazepam* (Serax)	10–30	30–60	90
Prazepam (Centrax)	10		60
Temazepam* (Restoril)		15	30
Triazolam* (Halcion)		0.25–0.5	
Miscellaneous			
Chloral hydrate (Noctec)*	250	500–1000	2000
Hydroxyzine pamoate (Vistaril)	25–50	100	300
Phenobarbital	15–30	90	300

*Shorter-acting sedatives.

Side Effects

The side effects are mainly behavioral and depend on patient reaction and dosage. As the dosage exceeds the levels necessary for sedation, the side effects include disinhibition, ataxia, dysarthria, nystagmus, errors of commission (machinery should not be operated until the patient is well stabilized), and excessive sedation, with sleep followed by coma and death if large doses are taken. Elderly or debilitated patients usually require much smaller doses for sedation. Use the shorter-acting drugs, eg, lorazepam or temazepam, in the elderly. Clorazepate and prazepam require gastric acid for conversion to active compounds. Thus, they should not be used in patients with anacidity or those who use antacids regularly. Bradycardia, hypotension, and respiratory arrest have occurred after the intravenous use of diazepam, but this has usually happened in patients with preexisting cardiopulmonary diseases and is also thought to be related to the propylene glycol solvent.

A serious side effect of chronic excessive dosage is drug dependency, which may involve tolerance, and physiologic dependency with withdrawal symptoms similar in morbidity and mortality to alcohol withdrawal. Abrupt withdrawal of sedative drugs may cause serious and even fatal convulsive seizures. Duration of usage is also a factor as is length of action. Withdrawal symptoms are more gradual in the longer-acting benzodiazepines. These include perceptual distortions, anxiety, faintness, and hyperreactivity to external stimuli, with seizures as late as the twelfth day of withdrawal. In the case of the benzodiazepines, several months of overusage have usually preceded the development of dependency; in the case of the less safe

Table 18–8. Benzodiazepine interactions with other drugs.

Drug	Effects
Antacids	Decreased absorption of benzodiazepines.
Disulfiram	Increased duration of action of sedatives.
Cimetidine	Increased half-life of benzodiazepines.
Levodopa	Inhibition of antiparkinson effect.
Contraceptives	Increased half-life of diazepam.
Rifampin	Decreased plasma diazepam.
Isoniazid	Increased plasma diazepam.

drugs, such as the barbiturates, overusage for a period of weeks may result in a dependent state requiring planned withdrawal.

The sedatives produce cumulative clinical effects with repeated dosage (especially if the patient has not had time to metabolize the previous dose); additive effects when given with other classes of sedatives or alcohol (many "accidental" deaths are the result of concomitant use of sedatives and alcohol); and residual effects after termination of treatment (particularly in the case of drugs that undergo slow biotransformation).

Consensus Conference: Drugs and insomnia: The use of medications to promote sleep. *JAMA* 1984;**251**:2410.

Greenblatt DJ, Shader RI, Abernethy BR: Drug therapy: Current status of benzodiazepines. (2 parts.) *N Engl J Med* 1983;**309**:354, 410.

Lader M: Dependence on benzodiazepines. *J Clin Psychiatry* 1983;**44**:121.

Mellinger GD, Balter MB, Uhlenhuth EH: Prevalence and correlates of the long-term use of anxiolytics. *JAMA* 1984;**251**:375.

5. OTHER ORGANIC THERAPIES

Electroconvulsive therapy (ECT) causes a central nervous system seizure (peripheral convulsion is not necessary) by means of electric current. The key objective is to exceed the seizure threshold, which can be accomplished by a variety of means. Electrical stimulation is more reliable and simpler than the use of chemical convulsants such as pentylenetetrazol (Metrazol) or hexafluorodiethyl ether (Indoklon). The mechanism of action is not known, but it is thought to involve major neurotransmitter responses at the cell membrane. Current insufficient to cause a seizure produces no therapeutic benefit and causes more postictal confusion.

Electroconvulsive therapy is the most effective (about 70%) treatment of severe depression, particularly depression with psychotic ideation and agitation commonly seen in the involutional period. Comparative controlled studies of electroconvulsive therapy in severe depression show that it is slightly more effective than chemotherapy. It is also very effective in the manic disorders. It has not been shown to be helpful in chronic schizophrenic disorders, and it is generally not used in acute schizophrenic episodes unless drugs are not effective and it is urgent that the psychosis be controlled (eg, a catatonic stupor complicating an acute medical condition).

Before electroconvulsive therapy is administered, a history and physical examination are performed, along with indicated laboratory tests. Lateral spine films and an electroencephalogram (EEG) are frequently done, particularly in elderly patients. Occasionally, the EEG will reveal a clinically silent intracranial lesion that may be a factor in the depression and is a contraindication to electroconvulsive therapy. The patient should not eat or drink for at least 8 hours before treatment. Dentures are removed prior to electroconvulsive therapy. An empty bladder is desirable because of incontinence resulting from the seizure. Atropine sulfate, 0.6–1 mg intramuscularly, is given for its vagolytic effect. A short-acting barbiturate such as methohexital, 40–70 mg, is given carefully intravenously (extravasation is very irritating to tissues) to cause unconsciousness. Succinylcholine, 30–60 mg intravenously, will produce a flaccid paralysis, and the anesthesiologist can then ventilate the patient with 100% oxygen from the onset of unconsciousness until spontaneous respiration resumes. Succinylcholine is contraindicated if the patient is using echothiophate iodide for glaucoma, since the latter is absorbed in amounts sufficient to interfere with the hydrolysis of succinylcholine and can thus precipitate prolonged apnea. Chronic renal dialysis, excessive supported ventilation, and congenital pseudocholinesterase deficiency may also result in prolonged apnea.

Placement of electrodes may be bitemporal or unilateral on the nondominant side. The latter is considered to produce less impairment of memory, although it may be slightly less effective and require more than the usual 9–12 treatments. Electroconvulsive therapy may be performed every few days (3 per week is usual), or all of the treatments may be given in 1–3 sessions under electrocardiographic monitoring of seizure activity (multiple-monitored electroconvulsive therapy).

A seizure usually lasts 5–20 seconds, with a brief postictal state. The patient can resume activity in about an hour. The most common side effects are memory disturbance and headache. Memory loss or confusion is usually related to number and frequency of electroconvulsive therapy treatments. Some memory loss is occasionally permanent, but most memory faculties return to full capacity within several weeks. There have been reports that lithium administration concurrent with electroconvulsive therapy resulted in greater memory loss. Before anesthesia was used, spinal compression fractures and severe anticipatory anxiety were common.

An intracranial lesion is a positive contraindication. Other problems such as cardiac disorders are not major contraindications and must be evaluated in light of the severity of the medical problem versus the need for electroconvulsive therapy. Serious complications arising from electroconvulsive therapy occur in less than one in a thousand cases. Most of these problems are cardiovascular or respiratory in nature (eg, aspiration of gastric contents). Patient education and acceptance of the technique and public opinion are the biggest obstacles to the use of electroconvulsive therapy.

Psychosurgery has a limited place in selected cases of severe, unremitting anxiety and depression, obsessional neuroses, and, to a lesser degree, some of the schizophrenias. The stereotactic techniques now being used, including modified bifrontal tractotomy, are great improvements over the crude methods of the past. In the controversial area of **megavitamin treatment** for the schizophrenic patient, the overall therapeutic efficacy of nicotinic acid or nicotinamide as the sole or adjuvant medication is no better than that of an inactive placebo. **Acupuncture** and **electrosleep,** while currently of interest, are of unproved usefulness for any psychiatric conditions.

Abrams R et al: Bilateral versus unilateral electroconvulsive therapy: Efficacy in melancholia. *Am J Psychiatry* 1983;**140**:463.

Frith CD et al: Effects of ECT and depression on various aspects of memory. *Br J Psychiatry* 1983;**142**:610.

Hansen H et al: Stereotactic psychosurgery: A psychiatric and psychological investigation of the effects and side effects of the interventions. *Acta Psychiatr Scand [Suppl]* 1982;**301**:1.

Kerr RA et al: ECT: Misconceptions and attitudes. *Aust NZ J Psychiatry* 1982;**16**:43.

Mills MJ et al: Electroconvulsive therapy in Massachusetts. *Am J Psychiatry* 1984;**141**:534.

6. HOSPITALIZATION

The need for hospital care may range from admission to a medical bed in a general hospital for an acute situational stress reaction to admission to a psychiatric ward when the patient is in the throes of an acute psychosis. The trend over recent years has been to admit patients to general hospitals in the community, treat patients aggressively, and discharge them promptly to the next appropriate level of treatment— day hospital, halfway house, outpatient therapy, etc. Involuntary hospitalization should be objectively determined on the basis of patient and society welfare. Sixty percent of admissions are readmissions. The total "in residence" population (hospital plus residential) is the same as the hospital total of 20 years ago.

Hospital care may be indicated when patients are too sick to care for themselves or when they present serious threats to themselves or others; when observation and diagnostic procedures are necessary; or when specific kinds of treatment such as electroconvulsive therapy, complex medication trials, or hospital environment (milieu) are required.

The disadvantages of psychiatric hospitalization include decreased self-confidence as a result of needing hospitalization; the stigma of being a "psychiatric patient"; possible increased dependency and regression; and the expense. Generally, there is no advantage to prolonged hospital stays for most psychiatric disorders.

Chodoff P: Involuntary hospitalization of the mentally ill as a moral issue. *Am J Psychiatry* 1984;**141**:384.

Goldman HH et al: The multiple functions of the state mental hospital. *Am J Psychiatry* 1983;**140**:296.

Gudeman JE, Shore MF, Dickey B: Day hospitalization and an inn instead of inpatient care for psychiatric patients. *N Engl J Med* 1983;**308**:749.

Kiesler CA, Sibulkin AE: Episodic rate of mental hospitalization: Stable or increasing? *Am J Psychiatry* 1984;**141**:44.

PSYCHOLOGIC APPROACHES

Psychotherapy is a process whereby a socially sanctioned healer seeks to help persons overcome or alleviate psychologically caused distress and disability by a systematic procedure linked to a theory of the source and the nature of the sufferer's difficulties. Although there are over 100 alleged forms of psychotherapy, all of them (excluding behavioral approaches) fall into one of 2 broad categories: dynamic or experiential. Negative as well as positive effects can occur in any psychotherapeutic endeavor. Negative effects are usually a result of inexperience, poor judgment, and inflexibility of therapists.

Dynamic psychotherapy. The basic concepts of dynamic psychotherapy rest in the role of the unconscious with drives and conflicts that remain out of awareness and in the importance of determinism, which emphasizes that each psychic event is determined by the ones that preceded it.

Although some of the postulates have not stood the test of time, other basic tenets such as the defense mechanisms (which are ways of dealing with anxiety) are of major importance in explaining many facets of behavior and are helpful in the practice of psychotherapy. The common ones include the following: **(1) Sublimation,** wherein the drive is turned into a new but useful and more acceptable channel. *Example:* A childish desire to exhibit oneself may be sublimated into a theatrical career. **(2) Repression** is the unconscious purposeful forgetting of urgings or events that would be painful if allowed to become conscious. *Example:* Forgetting well-known dates, etc. **(3) Projection** is the mechanism whereby painful feelings or ideas are projected outward upon persons or things in the environment and are felt to be external to the individual. *Example:* A person with unconscious homosexual impulses feels he must defend himself by assuming that others are making homosexual accusations. **(4) Denial** is used by the individual to treat obvious reality factors as if they did not exist. *Example:* The plumbing is not working properly, but the person does not accept the fact and goes on as if nothing is wrong. **(5) Introjection** (the opposite of projection) is the incorporation by a person of traits that are characteristic of another. *Example:* A depressed person may incorporate another person's affects and attitudes and so, if he is disliked by that other person, comes to dislike himself. **(6) Regression** is the return to a more infantile level of function. *Example:*

Children commonly retreat to a more childish level when siblings are born and demonstrate more immature behavior such as thumb-sucking and bed-wetting. **(7) Undoing** is the mechanism by which a person performs some activity which "undoes" or neutralizes something objectionable that occurred previously. *Example:* A person with a sick mother replaces every thought of her with the thought that she is as healthy as any other woman. **(8) Reaction formation** serves to prevent a painful thought from emerging by immediately substituting a pleasant thought. *Example:* A person who cannot acknowledge disliking someone never shows any hostility and always presents a pleasant demeanor. **(9) Isolation** is a separation of the original memory and its affect. *Example:* A beloved wife is killed in a serious accident, yet the husband discusses the details with a complete lack of emotion. **(10) Displacement** is a condition in which not only is the affect connected with a particular person or incident separated from it but the affect is then attached to another. *Example:* The factory worker having problems with his supervisor that cannot be expressed goes home and becomes angry with his wife. **(11) Rationalization** is substitution of an acceptable reason for an unacceptable one. *Example:* A student cannot face studying for an examination and decides that one should be relaxed for examinations, which thus justifies going to a movie instead of studying.

The focus is rooted in the subjective past, and the mode of change is to make the unconscious conscious, ie, to achieve insight with an understanding of the early past and its connection with conflicts. To achieve reduction of the conflicts, the therapist in a dyadic relationship uses free associations, interpretations, and analysis of both resistance and transference of feelings (a repetition of the past that is inappropriate to the present) onto the therapist. The process is long-term (in classic analysis, daily sessions; in later modifications, weekly or twice-weekly meetings) and is set in a doctor-patient relationship with the expectation of a major reorganization of the psyche.

Experiential psychotherapy. This includes gestalt therapy, client-centered psychotherapy, existential analysis, and structural analysis. Experiential therapy evolved from the concepts of fragmentation of the self, existential despair, and the lack of unity with one's own experiences. The focus of therapy is on the present. The mode of change is in the immediate experiencing of one's emotions. The past is not significant in the therapeutic process. The therapist uses intense interactions in a comfortable setting that stimulates self-expression. The sharing is an important element in the encounter to ameliorate the feelings of isolation and alienation and emphasize the possibility of unlimited psychic growth. The goals in this short-term process (weekly meetings for weeks or months) are self-determination; creativity; and self-affirmation within a setting of adult, humanistic, peer-oriented relationships. Any of the ideologic themes can be modified to change the technical aspects of therapy.

Supportive psychotherapy usually denotes a friendly relationship with the patient, strengthening of existing defenses, and an emphasis on the here and now, with little effort to make substantial changes in personality or in coping techniques. It frequently entails good role modeling and practical guidance.

Group therapy. The decision for group versus individual therapy is usually based on the patient's need to improve interpersonal relationships, and the group setting may provide the "laboratory" for improvisation and practice of new behaviors that can then be generalized to everyday activities. Therapy groups are usually composed of individuals who have no outside connection with one another, but groups may be made up of couples or families.

The various schools of therapy often purport to be unique, or more effective, or of more lasting value than others. In reality, they have many similarities and common derivations, with about the same results. The attitude of the patient and the skill of the therapist rather than the ideology are usually the major factors in producing change.

Bennet MJ: Focal psychotherapy: Terminable and interminable. *Am J Psychother* 1983;**37**:365.

Chevron ES, Rounsaville BJ: Evaluating the clinical skills of psychotherapists: A comparison of techniques. *Arch Gen Psychiatry* 1983;**40**:1129.

Crown S: Contraindications and dangers of psychotherapy. *Br J Psychiatry* 1983;**143**:436.

DeWitt KN et al: Judging change in psychotherapy. *Arch Gen Psychiatry* 1983;**40**:1121.

Pilkonis PA et al: A comparative outcome study of individual, group, and conjoint psychotherapy. *Arch Gen Psychiatry* 1984;**41**:431.

SOCIAL APPROACHES

In contrast to psychologic techniques, which deal principally with intrapsychic phenomena and interpersonal problems, the social approaches to psychiatric treatment attempt to modify attitudes and behavior by altering the **environmental** factors contributing to the patient's maladaptation. The scope of the attempt may range from provision of a therapeutic milieu—eg, in a day hospital or residential community—to minor alterations in school procedures or daily family activities. Various psychologic and behavioral techniques are used within social approaches.

Part-Time Hospitalization

The patient either participates in the hospital milieu during the day (day hospitals—going home at night), or stays the night (night hospitals—going to work or school during the day), or spends several hours a day in the hospital for up to 5 or 6 days a week.

Self-Help Communities

These are usually sponsored by nongovernmental agencies for the purpose of helping people with a particular type of difficulty. The individual lives-in full time for varying periods and usually continues to be affiliated with the group after leaving. Examples of self-help communities include halfway houses, residences for alcoholics, Salvation Army, and church-sponsored agencies.

Substitute Homes

Substitute homes provide shelter and treatment-related programs for longer periods of time. Examples of "substitute" homes are foster homes, usually for children; board and care homes, primarily for people who are disabled and unlikely to return to productive function; mental hygiene homes, providing special services for the mentally disabled who are unable to live in board and care homes; family care homes, similar to foster homes but taking adults—usually several at one time; residential treatment centers, taking a number of children and offering fairly intensive treatment programs; and shelters for young people—who are often in the process of withdrawing from drugs.

Nonresidential Self-Help Organizations

The following are examples of organizations usually administered by people who have survived similar problems and have banded together to help others cope with the same problem: Alcoholics Anonymous (and Al-Anon, to help families of alcoholics); Recovery Inc., organized and run by people who have had an emotional problem that required hospitalization; Schizophrenics Anonymous; Gamblers Anonymous; Overeaters Anonymous; colostomy clubs; mastectomy clubs; the Epilepsy Society; the American Heart Association's Stroke Clubs of America; burn recovery groups; other groups organized to help people deal with practical and psychologic problems of a particular illness; and friendship centers that assist people in their efforts to find specific kinds of help. At times, the best support for a patient is contact with another patient who has conquered a similar problem.

Special Professional & Paraprofessional Organizations

Examples of special organizations of this type are Homemaker Service, made up of individuals who come into the home to help the partially disabled maintain the household; Visiting Nurse Associations, which usually provide more than medical assistance; adult protective services for the elderly; genetic counseling services; family service agencies, for marriage counseling and family problems; Travelers Aid, for rendering assistance to new residents and transients; legal aid societies; Big Brothers Inc., to provide a masculine figure when one is lacking in the family (or Big Sisters for girls); consumer credit organizations, to help the financially naive organize their financial problems; crisis centers, eg, "free clinics" and county-sponsored satellite clinics; and church-sponsored agencies. Medication groups exist, in which physicians, nurses, and pharmacists provide education regarding drugs and help patients to accept the need for long-term medication.

Stress Reduction Techniques

Social and environmental factors are major aids in lowering stress and should be part of the activities of daily living. Both active recreation (sports, physical exercise, participant hobbies) and passive recreation (reading, music, painting) are necessary for a balanced life and alleviation of stress. Although they are major factors in causing stress, job pressures and uncertainty about vocational goals are frequently ignored. Family structure and dynamics must be evaluated, and there will be occasions (eg, adult children living at home, presence of in-laws) when a social restructuring is in order.

Brady JP: Social skills training for psychiatric patients. 1. Concepts, methods and clinical results. *Am J Psychiatry* 1984;**141**:333.

Greenblatt M, Becerra RM, Serafetinides EA: Social networks and mental health: An overview. *Am J Psychiatry* 1982;**139**:977.

Johnson HA: Stroke clubs: Undervalued and underused. *JAMA* 1984;**251**:1881.

BEHAVIORAL APPROACHES

Behavior therapy has its foundations in theories of the learning process. The role of the behavior therapist is that of a teacher who attempts to bring about change in the patient's maladaptation. The specific problem and the factors that play a role in precipitating or perpetuating the problem must first be identified. An attempt can then be made to alter those factors that perpetuate unwanted behavior.

The emphasis of behavior therapy is on "here and now" and **direct** change. The goal is to "unlearn" those destructive or unproductive types of behavior that result from faulty learning and to enhance the individual's repertoire of useful social and adaptive skills. Great emphasis is placed on identifying and then obliterating whatever is maintaining the maladaptive behavior.

Whereas **conditioning** is understood by some to be synonymous with a specific type of learning (eg, Pavlov's dogs), behavior therapy is much broader. It includes the relationship with the therapist, utilizes verbal techniques to a lesser degree than other therapies, and interprets "behavior" in a broad sense that includes thoughts and feelings.

Many of the techniques of behavior therapy require a cooperative effort on the part of a number of people who must all understand and be consistent in their responses to specified behaviors. Thus, a cooperative social setting such as a milieu ward or the patient's own home and family is important in implementing many of the following techniques.

Techniques of Behavior Therapy

A. Modeling: Much learning occurs by imitation. From the earliest years of childhood, the individual's behavior is modeled after parents, teachers, peers, employers, public personalities, historical figures, etc ("significant others"). The therapist makes a conscious effort to serve as a model of particular kinds of behavior that are significant to and attainable by the patient. This device is particularly useful in treating patients with low self-esteem.

B. Operant Conditioning: Operant conditioning is the deliberate implementation of a system of rewards to encourage repetition of specific desired behaviors. A voluntary behavior is singled out for a specific reward every time the behavior is used. The objective is to develop a habit in the use of that behavior. Like modeling, operant conditioning is a common procedure in families, and the child soon learns that "good" behavior is rewarded. "Token economies" (tokens are given for acceptable behavior, and these tokens can be redeemed for foods, outings, etc) in centers for retarded or autistic patients and those with behavioral problems are effective, particularly where verbal techniques have little meaning.

C. Aversive Conditioning: Aversive conditioning is the opposite of operant conditioning but is a less potent shaper of behavior. Undesirable behavior results in an unpleasant consequence (eg, vomiting induced by apomorphine, mild electric or sound shock), whereas satisfactory alternative responses are operantly encouraged. The most common conditions treated by this technique have been enuresis, smoking, alcoholism, and homosexuality. The results have been varied, but some successes have been reported, particularly in enuresis.

D. Extinction: Extinction is the process of refusing to reinforce behavior on the theory that behavior cannot be sustained without some sort of reinforcement. Temper tantrums and noxious behavior, usually contrived to gain attention of any sort, are "extinguished" in this way.

E. Desensitization: Familiarity lessens anxiety and reduces the tendency to avoid exposure to the feared object, person, or situation. The subject is repeatedly exposed to the feared stimulus (eg, looking at a picture of an elevator when the fear has been riding in elevators) at such a low level of intensity that the fear response is minimal. Exposures are then gradually increased (eg, walking past a real elevator) until the subject is able to tolerate the real experience with markedly reduced fear. This technique has been most effective in the treatment of phobias and a variety of situations (such as frigidity or impotence) that engender fears of failure, disapproval, and embarrassment.

F. Emotive Imagery: Deliberate evocation of mental images that arouse certain feelings can be used as a way of warding off painful emotions resulting from stress-inducing circumstances. Noxious imagery can be used in aversive conditioning and "pleasant thoughts" in operant training. In "mental imagery" desensitization, the phobic or sensitive situation is reproduced in graded quantities and the patient learns to handle minor upsetting imagined situations without anxiety before proceeding to the more difficult ones.

G. Flooding: Flooding (implosion) consists of overwhelming the individual, in a safe setting, with anxiety-producing stimuli. The anxiety responses gradually lessen (law of diminishing returns) until extinction occurs. In some ways, flooding is a desensitization technique without the graded approach. It has been used in treatment of obsessive compulsive patients and those with such behavior problems as compulsive hoarding.

H. Role Playing: In the role-playing technique, patients can practice various types of behaviors in anxiety-producing but "safe" situations. For example, the therapist may assume the role of an angry friend and the patient uses different ways of handling the situation. Role reversal—where the therapist and the patient change roles—then gives the patient a chance to experience the other's feelings and attitudes. Assertiveness training for inhibited individuals is a variant to help people learn to be more spontaneous.

Klein DF et al: Treatment of phobias. 2. Behavior therapy and supportive psychotherapy: Are there any specific ingredients? *Arch Gen Psychiatry* 1983;**40**:139.

Messer SB: Integrating psychoanalytic and behavior therapy: Limitations, possibilities and trade offs. *Br J Clin Psychol* 1983;**22**(Part 2):131.

Rapp MS, Thomas MR, Reyes EC: Mega-doses of behavior therapy for treatment-resistant agoraphobics. *Can J Psychiatry* 1983;**28**:105.

Schmidt MM et al: Amount of therapist contact and outcome in a multidimensional depression treatment program. *Acta Psychiatr Scand* 1983;**67**:319.

COMMON PSYCHIATRIC DISORDERS

STRESS & ADJUSTMENT DISORDERS
(Situational Disorders)

Stress exists when the adaptive capacity of the individual is overwhelmed by events. The event may be an insignificant one objectively considered, and even favorable changes (eg, promotion and transfer) requiring adaptive behavior can produce stress. For each individual, stress is subjectively defined, and the response to stress is a function of each person's personality and physiologic endowment.

Classification & Clinical Findings

Opinion differs about what events are most apt to produce stress reactions. The Holmes/Rahe studies of psychosocial factors provide some insights into the stress-inducing potential of marriage, family relationships, work and social relationships, financial problems, illness and injury, etc. The causes of stress are different at different ages—eg, in young adulthood, the sources of stress are found in the marriage or parent-child relationship, the employment relationship, and the struggle to achieve financial stability; in the middle years, the focus shifts to changing spousal relationships, problems with aging parents, and problems associated with having young adult offspring who themselves are encountering stressful situations; in old age, the principal concerns are apt to be retirement, loss of physical capacity, thoughts of death, and major personal losses.

An individual may react to stress by becoming anxious or depressed, by developing a physical symptom, by running away, by having a drink or starting an affair, or in limitless other ways. Common subjective responses are fear (of repetition of the stress-inducing event), rage (at frustration), guilt (over aggressive impulses), and shame (over helplessness). Acute stress may be manifested by restlessness, irritability, fatigue, the startle reaction, and a feeling of tension. Inability to concentrate, sleep disturbances (insomnia, bad dreams), and somatic preoccupations often lead to self-medication, most commonly with alcohol or other central nervous system depressants. Maladaptive behavior to stress is called adjustment disorder, with the major symptom specified (eg, "adjustment disorder with depressed mood").

Posttraumatic stress disorder (eg, the so-called post-Vietnam syndrome) is a syndrome with symptoms of reexperiencing the traumatic event (eg, rape, military combat), along with decreased responsiveness to current events and autonomic manifestations of sleep problems, nightmares, difficulties in concentration, and hyperalertness. The symptoms may be precipitated or exacerbated by distant events that are a reminder of the original stress. Symptoms frequently arise after a long latency period. The sooner the symptoms arise after the initial trauma and the sooner therapy is initiated, the better the prognosis.

Differential Diagnosis

Adjustment disorders must be distinguished from anxiety disorders, affective disorders, and personality disorders exacerbated by stress and from primarily somatic disorders with psychic overlay.

Treatment

A. Behavioral: Stress reduction techniques include immediate symptom reduction (eg, rebreathing in a bag for hyperventilation) or early recognition and removal from a stress source before full-blown symptoms appear. It is often helpful for the patient to keep a daily log of stress precipitators, responses, and alleviators. Techniques for general tension reduction are also helpful in reducing the reaction to stressful events. Some of the more common and successful procedures include regularly performed physical exercise, meditation, yoga, and ritualistic relaxation techniques. Some stress-related somatic problems, such as hypertension, respond to exercise programs. A balance of therapeutic approaches is usually best.

Specific behavioral techniques such as desensitization are indirectly helpful in anxiety reduction of stress reactions. For example, alleviation of a phobia can lead to a general reduction of tension and thus raise the response threshold to stress stimuli.

B. Medical: Judicious use of sedatives (eg, lorazepam, 1–2 mg orally daily) for a limited time and as a part of an overall treatment plan can provide relief from acute anxiety symptoms. Problems arise when the situation becomes chronic through inappropriate treatment or when the treatment approach supports the development of chronicity (see Sedatives, p 643).

C. Psychologic: Formal psychotherapy is seldom necessary in the isolated stress response or adjustment disorder. Supportive psychotherapy, with an emphasis on the here and now and strengthening of existing defenses, is a helpful approach while time and the patient's own resiliency allow a restoration to the previous level of function. A more formal psychotherapeutic approach is helpful in patients with poor coping patterns, repetitive symptom patterns, and marked susceptibility to life's vicissitudes. Posttraumatic stress syndromes respond to catharsis and dynamic psychotherapy oriented toward acceptance of the event. Marital problems are a major area of concern, and it is important that the physician have available a dependable referral source when marriage counseling is indicated.

D. Social: The stress reactions of life crisis problems are, more than any other category, a function of psychosocial upheaval, and it is patients responding to these problems who so frequently present with somatic symptoms. While it is not easy for the patient to make necessary changes (or they would have been made long ago), it is important for the physician to establish the framework of the problem, since the patient's denial system may obscure the issues. Clarifying the problem allows the patient to begin viewing it within the proper context and facilitates the sometimes very difficult decisions the patient eventually must make (eg, change of job or eviction of mother-in-law). It is important that the physician *not dictate what changes must be made.*

Prognosis

Return to satisfactory function after a short period is part of the clinical picture of this syndrome. Resolution may be delayed if others' responses to the patient's difficulties are thoughtlessly harmful or if the secondary gains appear to the patient to outweigh the advantages of recovery.

Andreasen NC, Hoenk PR: The predictive value of adjustment disorders: A follow-up study. *Am J Psychiatry* 1982;**139:**584.
Van Putten T, Yager J: Posttraumatic stress disorder: Emerging from the rhetoric. *Arch Gen Psychiatry* 1984;**41:**411.

ANXIETY DISORDERS & DISSOCIATIVE DISORDERS
(Neuroses)

Essentials of Diagnosis

- Overt anxiety or an overt manifestation of a defense mechanism (such as a phobia) or both.
- No apparent situational basis for the symptoms.

- Somatic symptoms referable to the autonomic nervous system or to a specific organ system (eg, dyspnea, palpitations, paresthesias).
- Not a result of physical disorders, psychiatric conditions (eg, schizophrenia), or drugs.

General Considerations

Anxiety includes psychologic and somatic symptoms with or without an ascertainable cause. It is ubiquitous and can be a transient symptom or a chronic debilitated state. Anxiety may reflect the result of a maladaptive attempt to resolve internal conflicts. These conflicts usually include unresolved childhood problems such as dependency, insecurity, hostility, excessive need for affection, concerns about intimacy, and overly strong drives for power and control.

Principal components of anxiety are **psychologic** (tension, fears, difficulty in concentration, apprehension) and **somatic** (tachycardia, palpitations, tremor, sweating). Sympathomimetic symptoms of anxiety are both a response to a central nervous system state and a reinforcement of further anxiety. Anxiety can become self-generating, since the symptoms reinforce the reaction, causing it to spiral.

The resultant anxiety is handled in different ways. Anxiety may be free-floating, resulting in acute anxiety attacks, occasionally becoming chronic. When one or several defense mechanisms (see p 646) are functioning, the consequences are well-known problems such as phobias, conversion reactions, dissociative states, obsessions, and compulsions. Lack of structure is frequently a contributing factor, as noted in those people who have "Sunday neuroses." They do well during the week with a planned work schedule but cannot tolerate the unstructured weekend. Planned-time activities tend to bind anxiety, and many people have increased difficulties when this is lost, as in retirement.

Some believe that various manifestations of anxiety are not a result of unconscious conflicts but are "habits"—persistent patterns of nonadaptive behavior acquired by learning. The "habits," being non-adaptive, are unsatisfactory ways of dealing with life problems—hence the resultant anxiety, which is often handled by the individual. Help is sought only when the anxiety becomes too painful. Exogenous factors such as stimulants (eg, caffeine) must be considered as causative or contributing factors. Mitral valve prolapse has been found to be a cause in some people with prominent anxiety and cardiac manifestations.

The treatment approach adopted in the management of the neuroses tends to reflect the philosophic bias of the therapist. Results do not differ significantly among various treatment methods.

Clinical Findings

A. Anxiety and Panic Disorders: Acute anxiety attacks are characterized by a sudden onset of tension, restlessness, and breathlessness; a sense of impending doom; hyperventilation; and variable somatic symptoms. There is marked fatigue after the acute attack.

Chronic anxiety takes the form of repeated attacks and long-lasting autonomic reactivity (eg, increased blood pressure, perspiration, frequent palpitations). Chronic irritability and fatigue are common.

B. Phobic Disorders: Phobic ideation can be considered a mechanism of "displacement" in which the patient transfers feelings of anxiety from their true object to one that can be avoided so as not to feel anxiety. However, since phobias are ineffective defense mechanisms, there tends to be an increase in the scope, intensity, and number of phobias. Some believe that phobias are thought disorders with as yet undiscovered biochemical or neurophysiologic aberrations. Agoraphobia (fear of open places and public areas) is frequently associated with severe panic attacks. Patients often develop the syndrome in early adult life, making a normal life-style difficult.

C. Obsessive Compulsive Disorders: In the obsessive compulsive reaction, the irrational idea or the impulse persistently intrudes into awareness. Obsessions (constantly recurring thoughts such as fears of hitting somebody) and compulsions (repetitive actions such as washing hands many times prior to peeling a potato) are recognized by the individual as absurd and are resisted, but anxiety is alleviated only by ritualistic performance or mechanical impulse or entertainment of the idea. The primary underlying concern of the patient is to not lose control. These patients are usually predictable, orderly, conscientious, and intelligent, traits that are seen in many compulsive behaviors such as anorexia and compulsive running.

D. Dissociative Disorders: Fugue, amnesia, somnambulism, and multiple personality are the usual dissociative states. The reaction is precipitated by emotional crisis, and although the primary gain is anxiety reduction, the secondary gain is a temporary solution of the crisis. Mechanisms include repression and isolation as well as particularly limited concentration such as seen in hypnotic states. This condition, which is similar in many ways to temporal lobe dysfunction and may be related, may last for hours or days.

Treatment

A. Psychologic: Traditional psychotherapy is still the customary way of treating these disorders. Irrespective of the therapist's philosophic orientation, the relationship with the therapist in individual therapy is anxiety-reducing and effective when the therapy deals with the conflict producing the anxiety. The therapist who can help the patient delineate specific problems and goals is helping the patient find specific alternatives to unproductive or harmful ways of dealing with problems. When economically feasible, psychoanalysis can be helpful, particularly when the patient is motivated to deal with the past events that have laid the groundwork for the present problem. Other individual approaches such as reality therapy or transactional analysis are particularly helpful when interpersonal relationships are a major factor. Group therapy is the treatment of choice when the anxiety is clearly a function of the patient's difficulties in dealing with others, and if these other people are part of the family it is appropriate to include them and initiate family or couples therapy.

B. Behavioral: Behavioral approaches are widely used in various anxiety disorders. Relaxation techniques, including meditation, can sometimes be helpful in reducing anxiety. Desensitization, by exposing the patient to graded doses of a phobic object or situation, is an effective technique and one that the patient can practice outside of the therapy session. Emotive imagery, wherein the patient imagines the anxiety-provoking situation while at the same time learning to relax, helps to decrease the anxiety when the patient faces the real life situation. Some compulsions are treated by "flooding," ie, saturating the person with the anxiety-producing situation or phobic object. This changes the relationship of the compulsion to the anxiety, and the compulsion is given up, since it no longer serves to ward off anxiety. "Modeling" techniques are used when anxiety is related to lack of confidence and the patient looks to the therapist as a model of how to handle anxiety-provoking situations. Any of the behavioral techniques (see above) can be used beneficially in altering the contingencies (precipitating factors or rewards) supporting any anxiety-provoking behavior.

C. Medical: Sedatives are effective in reducing anxiety. Benzodiazepines are the sedatives of choice in most cases (eg, chlordiazepoxide, 5–30 mg/d orally). Other classes of drugs, such as antipsychotic agents, and the older sedatives, such as the barbiturates, have no advantages over the benzodiazepines but have numerous disadvantages (diverse side effects and more dependency problems, respectively). Beta-blockers such as propranolol have been helpful in reduction of peripheral somatic symptoms. Ethanol is the most frequently self-administered drug, but it has no proper role in the treatment of anxiety.

Tricyclic and new cyclic antidepressants as well as monoamine oxidase inhibitors have been quite effective in the treatment of panic attacks (eg, imipramine, 75–150 mg/d orally) but less so in blocking phobic-avoidant behavior. Studies comparing tricyclics and monoamine oxidase inhibitors have shown no advantage for either group, although the monoamine oxidase inhibitors require strict dietary regulations. High-dose alprazolam therapy (about 10 mg daily) has been effective in some patients with panic disorders.

D. Social: Social modification may require measures such as family counseling to aid acceptance of the patient's symptoms. Any help in maintaining the social structure is anxiety-alleviating, and work, school, and social activities should be maintained. School and vocational counseling may be provided by professionals, who often need help from the physician in defining the patient's limitations.

Prognosis

Anxiety disorders are usually of long standing and may be quite difficult to treat. Some, such as

obsessions and compulsions, tend to be most resistant. All can be relieved to varying degrees with psychotherapy and behavioral techniques.

Anderson DJ, Noyes R, Crowe RR: A comparison of panic disorders and generalized anxiety disorder. *Am J Psychiatry* 1984;**141:**572.

Brown JT, Mulrow CD, Stoudemire GA: The anxiety disorders: Review. *Ann Intern Med* 1984;**100:**558.

Matuzas W, Glass RM: Treatment of agoraphobia and panic attacks. *Arch Gen Psychiatry* 1983;**40:**220.

Noyes R Jr: Beta-blocking drugs and anxiety. *Psychosomatics* 1982;**23:**155.

SOMATOFORM DISORDERS
(Psychophysiologic Disorders, Psychosomatic Disorders)

Essentials of Diagnosis

- Symptoms may involve one or more organ systems.
- Subjective complaints exceed objective findings.
- Correlations of symptom development and psychosocial stresses.
- Matrix of biogenetic and developmental patterns.

General Considerations

A major source of diagnostic confusion in medicine has been to assume cause-and-effect relationships when parallel events have been observed. This post hoc ergo propter hoc reasoning has been particularly vexing in many situations where the individual exhibits psychosocial distress that could well be secondary to a chronic illness but has been assumed to be primary and causative. An example is the person with a chronic bowel disease who becomes querulous and demanding. Is this a result of problems of coping with a chronic disease, or is it a personality pattern that causes the gastrointestinal problem?

People react differently to illness. Emotional stress often exacerbates or precipitates an acute illness. Vulnerability in one or more organ systems plays a major role in the development of particular symptoms, and the "functional" versus "organic" dichotomy is a hindrance to good treatment.

In any patient presenting with a condition judged to be somatoform, depression must be considered in the diagnosis.

Clinical Findings

A. Conversion Disorder: "Conversion" of psychic conflict into physical symptoms in parts of the body innervated by the sensorimotor system (eg, paralysis, aphonia) is a disorder that is more common in unsophisticated individuals and certain cultures. The term "hysterical conversion" was previously used to describe this condition. The defense mechanisms utilized in this condition are repression (a barring from consciousness) and isolation (a splitting of the affect from the idea). The somatic manifestation that takes the place of anxiety is typically paralysis, and in some instances the organ dysfunction may have symbolic meaning (eg, arm paralysis in marked anger). Hysterical seizures (''pseudoseizures'') are usually difficult to differentiate from intoxication states or panic attacks. Retention of consciousness, random flailing with asynchronous movements of the right and left sides, and resistance to having the nose and mouth pinched closed during the attack all point toward a hysterical event. Electroencephalography *during the attack* is the most helpful diagnostic aid in excluding seizure states. Serum prolactin levels rise abruptly in the postictal state but not in pseudoseizures. There is usually a past history of other conversion situations. The conversion may temporarily ''solve the problem.'' La belle indifférence is not a significant characteristic (as commonly believed). Important criteria in diagnosis include a history of conversion or somatization disorder, modeling, a serious precipitating emotional event, associated psychopathology (eg, schizophrenia, personality disorders), a temporal correlation between the precipitating event and the symptom, and a temporary ''solving of the problem'' by the conversion.

B. Somatization Disorder (Briquet's Syndrome, Hysteria): This disorder denotes individuals who have multiple physical complaints referrable to several organ systems (particularly genital, gastrointestinal, spinal, cardiopulmonary, and neurologic). It usually occurs before age 30 and is more frequent in women. Polysurgery is common. Preoccupation with medical and surgical modalities constitutes a life-style that excludes most other activities. The symptoms are a reflection of adaptive patterns, coping techniques, and reactivity of the particular organ system. There is often evidence of long-standing somatic reactivity, often with a history of similar organ system involvement in other family members. Multiple symptoms that constantly change and inability of more than 3 doctors to make a diagnosis are strong clues to the problem.

C. Psychogenic Pain Disorder: This involves a long history of complaints of severe pain not consonant with anatomic and clinical signs. This diagnosis should be made only after extended evaluation has established a clear correlation of psychogenic factors with exacerbations and remissions of complaints. Furthermore, there should be evidence that the pain confers some secondary gain. This diagnosis must not be made by exclusion but must be supported by positive psychologic factors.

D. Hypochondriasis: This is a fear of disease and preoccupation with the body, with perceptual amplification and heightened responsiveness. A process of social learning is usually involved, frequently with a role model who was a member of the family and may be a part of the underlying psychodynamic etiology.

E. Factitious Disorders: These are characterized by self-induced symptoms or false physical and laboratory findings for the purpose of deceiving physicians or other hospital personnel. The deceptions may involve self-mutilation, fever, hemorrhage, hypoglycemia, seizures, and an almost endless variety of manifestations—often presented in an exaggerated and dramatic fashion (Munchausen's syndrome). The duplicity may be either simple or extremely complex and difficult to recognize. The patients are frequently connected in some way with the health professions, they are often migratory, and their motivation in complex cases is usually unclear.

Complications

The main reason a patient sees the doctor is for diagnosis, but closely allied to this is a need for reassurance, acceptance, attention, and affection. What can be done specifically to alleviate the complaint is often secondary to the reassurance and support of the physician. Misunderstanding of these priorities adversely affects the doctor-patient relationship. Many patients feel relieved when told after careful examination that there is nothing wrong. Others react quite differently, believing that being told there is nothing wrong means they will receive no care. This is often true; the doctor prescribes one medicine after another, usually different brands of the same class of ''tranquilizer,'' and various tests and procedures are ordered, reinforcing the patient's belief that the problem is purely organic. There is no acknowledgment of the influence of emotional conflicts. ''Doctor shopping'' engenders more procedures and increased risk. Secondary gains such as disability payments cloud the picture. In many cases, simple psychotherapeutic approaches by the physician would help the patient. Referral to a psychiatrist is often interpreted by the patient to mean that the physician has ''given up.'' The patient often regards the psychiatrist as someone who is there not for the ultimate purpose of cure but chiefly to provide comfort or even to offer help with the process of dying. In any event, the reactions of the patient are anger at abandonment, fear of the referral, and a continued search for succor.

Treatment

A. Medical: Medical support with careful attention to building a therapeutic doctor-patient relationship is the mainstay of treatment. *It must be accepted that the patient's distress is real.* Diligent attempts should be made to relate symptoms to adverse developments in the patient's life. It may be useful to have the patient keep a meticulous diary, paying particular attention to various pertinent factors evident in the history. Regular, frequent, short appointments may be helpful. Drugs should not be prescribed to replace appointments. One doctor should be the primary physician, and consultants should be used only for evaluation. An emphatic, realistic, optimistic approach must be maintained in the face of the expected ups and downs.

B. Psychologic: Psychologic approaches can be used by the primary physician when it is clear that the patient is ready to make some changes in life-style in order to achieve symptomatic relief. This is often best approached on a here and now basis and oriented toward pragmatic changes rather than an exploration of early experiences that the patient frequently fails to relate to current distress. Individual group therapy with others who have similar problems is sometimes of value to improve coping, allow ventilation, and focus on interpersonal adjustment. Hypnosis and amobarbital interviews used early are helpful in resolving conversion disorders. If the primary physician has been working with the patient on psychologic problems related to the physical illness, the groundwork is often laid for successful psychiatric referral.

C. Behavioral: Behavioral therapy is probably best exemplified by the current efforts in biofeedback techniques that have a behavioral basis. In biofeedback, the particular abnormality (eg, increased peristalsis) must be recognized and monitored by the patient and therapist (eg, by an electronic stethoscope to amplify the sounds). This is immediate feedback, and after learning to recognize it the patient can then learn to identify any change thus produced (eg, a decrease in bowel sounds) and so become a conscious originator of the feedback instead of a passive recipient. Relief of the symptom operantly conditions the patient to utilize the maneuver that relieves symptoms (eg, relaxation causing a decrease in bowel sounds). With emphasis on this type of learning, the patient is able to identify symptoms early and initiate the countermaneuvers, thus decreasing the symptomatic problem. Migraine and tension headaches have been particularly responsive to biofeedback methods.

D. Social: Social endeavors include family, work, and other interpersonal activity. Family members should come for some appointments with the patient so that they can learn how best to live with the patient. This is particularly important in treatment of the somatization and psychogenic pain disorders. Ileostomy clubs and similar groups provide a climate for encouraging the patient to accept and live with the problem. Ongoing communication with the employer may be necessary to encourage long-term continued interest in the employee. Employers can become just as discouraged as physicians in dealing with employees who have chronic problems.

Prognosis

The prognosis is much better if the primary physician is able to intervene early before the situation has deteriorated. After the problem has crystallized into chronicity, it is very difficult to effect change.

Barsky AJ, Klerman GL: Overview: Hypochondriasis, bodily complaints and somatic styles. *Am J Psychiatry* 1983; **140:**273.

DeSouza C, Othmer E: Somatization disorders and Briquet's syndrome. *Arch Gen Psychiatry* 1984;**41:**334.

Folks DG, Ford CV, Regan WM: Conversion symptoms in a general hospital. *Psychosomatics* 1984;**25:**285.

Henker FO: Psychosomatic illness: Biochemical and physiologic foundations. *Psychosomatics* 1984;**25:**19.

Scoggin CH: Factitious illness: Dramatic deceit versus reality. *Postgrad Med* (Nov) 1983;**74:**259.

CHRONIC PAIN DISORDERS

Essentials of Diagnosis
- Chronic complaints of pain.
- Symptoms frequently exceed signs.
- Minimal relief with standard treatment.
- History of many physicians.
- Frequent use of many nonspecific medications.

General Considerations

A problem in the management of pain is the lack of distinction between acute and chronic pain syndromes. Most physicians are adept at dealing with acute pain problems but have difficulty handling the patient with chronic pain. This type of patient frequently takes too many medications, stays in bed a great deal, has had many physicians, has lost skills, and experiences little joy in either work or play. All relationships suffer (including those with physicians), and life becomes a constant search for succor. The search results in complex physician-patient relationships that usually include many drug trials, particularly sedatives. Treatment failures provoke angry responses and depression from both the physician and the patient, and the pain syndrome is exacerbated. When frustration becomes too great, a new physician is found, and the cycle is repeated. The longer the existence of the pain, the more important the psychologic factors of anxiety and depression, which are often a consequence rather than a cause of chronic pain. As with all other conditions, it is counterproductive to speculate about whether the pain is "real." It is real to the patient, and acceptance of the problem underlines a mutual endeavor to alleviate the disturbance.

Clinical Findings

Components of the chronic pain syndrome include **anatomic changes, chronic anxiety and depression,** and **changed life-style.** Usually, the anatomic problem is irreversible, since it has already been subjected to many interventions with increasingly unsatisfactory results.

Chronic anxiety and depression produce heightened irritability and overreaction to stimuli. A marked decrease in pain threshold is apparent. This pattern develops into a hypochondriacal preoccupation with the body and a constant need for reassurance. The pressure on the doctor becomes wearing and often leads to covert rejection devices, such as not being available or making referrals to other physicians. This is perceived by the patient, who then intensifies the effort to get help, and the typical cycle is under way. Anxiety and depression are seldom discussed, almost as if there is a tacit agreement not to deal with these issues.

Changes in life-style involve some of the so-called "pain games." These usually take the form of a family script in which the patient accepts the role of being sick, and this role then becomes the focus of most family interactions and may become important in maintaining the family, so that neither the patient nor the family wants the patient's role to change. Demands for attention and efforts to control the behavior of others revolve around the central issue of control of other people (including physicians). Cultural factors frequently play a role in the behavior of the patient and how the significant people around the patient cope with the problem. Some cultures encourage demonstrative behavior, while others value the stoic role. The physician's recognition of this fact is important, since overt dramatization of the discomfort is sometimes helpful in alleviating the problem.

Another secondary gain that frequently maintains the patient in the sick role is financial compensation ("green poultice") or other benefits. Frequently, such systems are structured so that they reinforce the maintenance of sickness and discourage any attempts to give up the role. Physicians unwittingly reinforce this role because of the very nature of the practice of medicine, which is to respond to complaints of illness. Helpful suggestions are often met with responses like "Yes, but. . . ." Medications then become the principal approach, and drug dependency problems may develop.

Treatment

A. Behavioral: The cornerstone of a unified approach to chronic pain syndromes is a comprehensive behavioral program. This is necessary to identify and eliminate pain reinforcers, to decrease drug use, and to use effectively those positive reinforcers that shift the focus from the pain. It is critical that the patient be made a partner in the effort to alleviate pain. (Avoid the concept of cure.) The patient should agree to discuss the pain only with the physician and not with family members; this tends to stabilize the patient's personal life, since the family is usually tired of the subject. At the beginning of treatment, the patient should be assigned self-help tasks graded up to maximal activity, as a means of positive reinforcement. The tasks should not exceed capability. The patient can also be asked to keep a self-rating chart to log accomplishments, so that progress can be measured and remembered. Instruct the patient to record degrees of pain on a self-rating scale in relation to various situations and mental attitudes so that similar circumstances can be avoided or modified.

Avoid negative reinforcers such as sympathy and attention to pain. Emphasize a positive response to productive activities, which remove the focus of attention from the pain. Activity is also desensitizing, since the patient learns to tolerate increasing activity levels.

Biofeedback techniques (see Somatoform Disorders, p 652) and hypnosis have been successful in ameliorating some pain syndromes. Hypnosis tends to be most effective in those patients with a high level of denial, who are more responsive to suggestion. Hypnosis can be used to lessen anxiety, alter perception of the length of time that pain is experienced, and encourage relaxation.

B. Medical: A *single physician* in charge of the multiple treatment approach is the highest priority. Consultations as indicated and technical procedures done by others are appropriate, but the care of the patient should remain in the hands of the primary physician. Referrals should not be allowed to raise the patient's hopes unrealistically or to become a way for the physician to reject the case. The attitude of the doctor should be one of honesty, interest, and hopefulness—not for a cure but for alleviation of symptoms and continuing improvement.

Medications, nerve stimulation, and surgery should be used appropriately, not out of desperation (see Chapter 1). Sedatives can be a useful adjunct in the treatment plan, with due regard taken for the dependency problem associated with all sedatives. Physical means of relief (heat, cold) should be part of the daily routine; this tends to encourage compliance. Neither analgesics nor sedatives should be given on an "as needed" schedule. A fixed schedule lessens the conditioning effects of these drugs. Tricyclic antidepressants in doses smaller than those used in depression may be helpful by blocking central nervous system pain interpretation. They are used in full doses when depression is significant. Major factors in a positive drug response include expectations and positive attitudes of both patient and physician.

C. Social: Involvement of family members and other significant persons in the patient's life should be an early priority. The best efforts of both patient and therapists can be unwittingly sabotaged by other persons who may feel that they are "helping" the patient. They frequently tend to reinforce the negative aspects of the pain syndrome. The patient becomes more dependent and less active, and the pain syndrome becomes an immutable way of life. The more destructive "pain games" described by many experts in chronic pain syndromes are results of well-meaning but misguided efforts of family members. Ongoing therapy with the family can be most helpful in the early identification and elimination of these behavior patterns.

Alteration of behavior in others (including employers and friends) requires repetition of instructions and fairly frequent contact. The tendency is to slip back into behavior patterns that impede progress. Group instruction by a nurse or physician's assistant is valuable and is enhanced by interchanges of people in the group. Repetition and group interaction tend to fix the instructions.

D. Psychologic: In addition to group therapy with family members and others, groups of patients can be helpful if properly led. The major goal, whether of individual or group therapy, is to gain patient *involvement*. A group can be a powerful instrument for achieving this goal, with the development of group loyalties and cooperation. People will frequently make efforts with group encouragement that they would never make alone. Individual therapy should be directed toward strengthening existing defenses and improving self-esteem. The rapport between patient and physician, as in all psychotherapeutic efforts, is the major factor in therapeutic success.

Bakris GL et al: Chronic pain: A pharmacologic review and behavior modification approach. *Postgrad Med* (May) 1983;**73**:119.

Hendler N: Depression caused by chronic pain. *J Clin Psychiatry* 1984;**45**(Section 2):30.

Swanson DW: Chronic pain as a third pathologic emotion. *Am J Psychiatry* 1984;**141**:211.

Webb WL Jr: Chronic pain: Psychosomatic illness review. *Psychosomatics* 1983;**24**:1053.

PSYCHOSEXUAL DISORDERS

General Considerations

The stages of sexual activity include **excitement** (arousal), **plateau, orgasm,** and **resolution.** The precipitating excitement or arousal is psychologically determined. Arousal response leading to plateau is a physiologic and psychologic phenomenon of vasocongestion, a parasympathetic reaction causing erection in the male and labial/clitoral congestion in the female. The orgasmic response includes emission in the male and clonic contractions of the analogous striated perineal muscles of both male and female. Resolution is a gradual return to normal physiologic status.

While the arousal stimuli—vasocongestive and orgasmic reponses—constitute a single response in a well-adjusted person, they can be considered as separate stages that can produce different syndromes responding to different treatment procedures.

Clinical Findings

There are 3 major groups of sexual disorders.

A. Paraphilias (Sexual Arousal Disorders): In these conditions, formerly called "deviations" or "variations," the excitement stage of sexual activity is associated with sexual objects or orientations different from those usually associated with adult heterosexual stimulation. The stimulus may be a woman's shoe, a child, the genitalia of persons of the same sex, animals, instruments of torture, or incidents of aggression. The pattern of sexual stimulation is usually one that has early psychologic roots. Poor experiences with heterosexual activity frequently reinforce this pattern over time.

Exhibitionism is the impulsive behavior of exposing the genitalia in order to achieve sexual excitation. It is a childhood sexual behavior carried into adult life, and it is limited as a clinical condition to males.

Transvestism is the wearing of clothes and the enactment of a role of the opposite sex for the purpose of sexual excitation. Such fetishistic cross-dressing can be part of masturbation foreplay in heterosexual men who in all other respects behave in a masculine way. Transvestism in homosexuality and transsexualism is not done to cause sexual excitement but is a function of the gender disorder.

Voyeurism achievment of sexual arousal by secretly watching the activities of women, usually in various stages of undress or sexual activity. In both exhibitionism and voyeurism, excitation leads to masturbation as a **replacement** for heterosexual activity.

Pedophilia is the use of a child of either sex to achieve sexual arousal and, in many cases, gratification. Contact is frequently oral, with either participant being dominant, but pedophilia includes intercourse of any type. Adults of both sexes engage in this behavior, but because of social and cultural factors it is more commonly identified with males. The pedophile has difficulty in adult sexual relationships, and males who perform this act are frequently impotent.

Incest involves a sexual relationship with a person in the immediate family, most frequently a child. In many ways it is similar to pedophilia (intrafamilial pedophilia). Incestuous feelings are fairly common, but cultural mores are usually sufficiently strong to act as a barrier to the expression of sexual feelings.

Bestiality is the attainment of sexual gratification by intercourse with an animal. The intercourse may involve penetration or simply contact with the human genitalia by the tongue of the animal. The practice is more common in rural or isolated areas and is frequently a substitute for human sexual contact rather than an expression of preference.

Sadism is the attainment of sexual arousal by inflicting pain upon the sexual object, and **masochism** is the attainment of sexual excitation by enduring pain. Much sexual activity has aggressive components (eg, biting, scratching). Forced sexual acquiescence (eg, rape) is considered to be primarily an act of aggression.

Bondage is the achievement of erotic pleasure by being humiliated, enslaved, physically bound, and restrained. It is life-threatening, since neck binding or partial asphyxiation usually forms part of the ritual.

Necrophilia is sexual intercourse with a dead body or the use of parts of a dead body for sexual excitation, often with masturbation.

B. Gender Identity Variations: *Core gender identity* reflects a biologic self-image—the conviction that "I am a male" or "I am a female." While this is a fixed self-image, *gender role identity* is a dynamic, changing self-representation. Variances of core gender identity are rare, while those of gender role identity are common. The 3 major conditions in which the gender variation is overt include transvestism, homosexuality, and transsexualism.

Homosexuality is romantic love or overt sexual activity between members of the same sex and is often considered a gender role problem. In the clinical condition there is further implication that it is the *preferred* sexual outlet. A large percentage of individuals of both sexes have had transient homosexual contacts but prefer heterosexual activity and are thus not categorized as homosexuals. The particular mode of homosexual intercourse is incidental. There are 2 major groupings of homosexuals. One consists of apparently well-adjusted individuals whose life-style revolves around "gay" activities and friends, and the other of those whose life-style is predominantly "straight," with furtive homosexual activity. The latter group includes many so-called bisexuals who have suppressed their homosexual behavior and have not revealed their sexual preference. The physician must be aware of any special medical or psychosocial problems the homosexual patient may have and must take pains to be nonjudgmental.

Transsexualism (a core gender identity problem) is an attempt to deny and reverse biologic sex by maintaining sexual identity with the opposite gender. Transsexuals do not alternate between gender roles; rather, they assume a fixed role of attitudes, feelings, fantasies, and choices consonant with those of the opposite sex, all of which clearly date back to early development. For example, male transsexuals in early childhood behave, talk, and fantasize as if they were girls. They do not grow out of feminine patterns, they do not work in professions traditionally considered to be masculine, and they have no interest in their own penises either as evidence of maleness or as organs for erotic behavior. The desire for sex change starts early and may culminate in assumption of a feminine lifestyle, hormonal treatment, and use of surgical procedures, including castration and vaginoplasty.

C. Psychosexual Dysfunction: This category includes a large group of vasocongestive and orgasmic disorders. Often, they involve problems of sexual adaptation, education, and technique that are often initially discussed with, diagnosed by, and treated by the family physician.

There are 2 conditions common in the male: impotence and ejaculation disturbances.

Impotence (erectile dysfunction) is the inability to attain or maintain an erection firm enough for satisfactory intercourse. Causes for this vasocongestive disorder can be psychologic, physiologic, or both. After the onset of the problem, a history of repeated erections (particularly nocturnal penile tumescence, which may be evaluated in a sleep laboratory) is evidence that the dysfunction is psychologic in origin. Psychologic impotence is caused by either interpersonal or intrapsychic factors (eg, marital disharmony, depression). Organic factors include diabetes mellitus, drug abuse (alcohol, narcotics, stimulants), pharmacologic agents (anticholinergic drugs, antihypertensive medication, all psychotherapeutic drugs, narcotics, estrogens), organ system failure (circulatory, cardiorespiratory, renal), surgical complications (prostatectomy, vascular and back surgery), trauma (disk and spinal cord injuries), endocrine disturbances (pituitary, thyroid, adrenal), neurologic disorders (multiple sclerosis, tumors, peripheral neuropathies, pernicious anemia, syphilis), urologic problems (phimosis, Peyronie's disease, priapism), and congenital abnormalities (Klinefelter's syndrome).

Ejaculation disturbances include premature ejaculation, inability to ejaculate, and retrograde ejaculation. (One may ejaculate even though impotent.) Ejaculation is usually connected with orgasm, and ejaculatory control is an acquired behavior that is minimal in adolescence and increases with experience. Pathogenic factors are those that interfere with learning control, most frequently sexual ignorance. Intrapsychic factors (anxiety, guilt, depression) and interpersonal maladaptation (marital problems, unrespon-

siveness of mate, power struggles) are also common. Organic causes include interference with sympathetic nerve distribution, often due to surgery or trauma, or the effects of pharmacologic agents on sympathetic tone. Postcoital cephalalgia is common and may be a variant of migraine.

In females, the 2 most common forms of sexual dysfunction are vaginismus and frigidity.

Vaginismus is a conditioned response in which a spasm of the perineal muscles occurs if there is any stimulation of the area. The desire is to avoid penetration. Sexual responsiveness and vasocongestion may be present, and orgasm from clitoral stimulation is common.

Frigidity is a complex condition in which there is a general lack of sexual responsiveness. The woman has difficulty in experiencing erotic sensation and does not have the vasocongestive response. Sexual activity varies from active avoidance of sex to an occasional orgasm. Orgasmic dysfunction—in which a woman has a vasocongestive response but varying degrees of difficulty in reaching orgasm—is sometimes differentiated from frigidity. Causes for the dysfunctions include poor sexual techniques, early traumatic sexual experiences, interpersonal disharmony (marital struggles, use of sex as a means of control), and intrapsychic problems (anxiety, fear, guilt). Organic causes include any conditions that might cause pain in intercourse, pelvic pathology, mechanical obstruction, or neurologic deficits.

Disorders of sexual desire refer to reduction or absence of sexual desire in either sex and may be a function of organic or psychologic difficulties. Any chronic illness can sap desire, but cerebral problems such as partial complex seizures, panhypopituitarism, Cushing's syndrome, and parkinsonism frequently cause a decrease in sexual drive. Hormonal variations, including use of antiandrogen compounds such as cyproterone acetate, and chronic renal failure contribute to deterioration in sexual activity. Alcohol, sedatives, narcotics, marihuana, and psychotherapeutic agents may affect sexual drive.

Treatment

A. Paraphilias and Gender Identity Disorders:

1. Psychologic–Sexual arousal disorders involving variant sexual activity (paraphilia), particularly those of a more superficial nature (eg, voyeurism) and those of recent onset, are responsive to psychotherapy in a moderate percentage of cases. The prognosis is much better if the motivation comes from the individual rather than the legal system; unfortunately, however, court intervention is frequently the only stimulus to treatment because the condition persists and is reinforced until conflict with the law occurs. The new therapies frequently focus on barriers to normal arousal response; the expectation is that the variant behavior will decrease as normal behavior increases.

2. Behavioral–Aversive and operant conditioning techniques have been tried frequently in gender role disorders but have been only occasionally successful. In some cases, the sexual arousal disorders improve with modeling, role-playing, and conditioning procedures. Emotive imagery is occasionally helpful in lessening anxiety in fetish problems.

3. Social–Although they do not produce a change in sexual arousal patterns or gender role, self-help groups such as "gay" clubs and churches have facilitated adjustment to an often hostile society. Attention to the family is particularly important in helping persons in such groups to accept their situation and alleviate their guilt about the role they think they had in creating the problem.

4. Medical–After careful evaluation, some transsexuals are treated with hormones and genital surgery. The surgical procedures include penectomy in the male, with preservation of the invaginated penile skin for vaginoplasty. The meatus is occasionally partially preserved as a cervix substitute, and the scrotal skin is used in the construction of labia. Surgical procedures—particularly the construction of a penis—are more complicated in female-to-male conversion.

B. Psychosexual Dysfunction:

1. Medical–Identification of a contributory reversible cause is most important. Even if the condition is not reversible, identification of the specific cause helps the patient to accept the condition. Marital disharmony, with its exacerbating effects, may thus be avoided. Of all the sexual dysfunctions, impotence is the condition most likely to have an organic basis. When the condition is irreversible, penile implants may be considered. One type is an inserted pump device that offers the patient a choice of flaccidity or erection, but this is costly, complex, and subject to mechanical problems. Another type of implant results in permanent erection but is simple and relatively trouble-free. Revascularization, using the inferior epigastric artery, has been done in patients with impotence due to circulatory problems.

2. Behavioral–Syndromes resulting from conditioned responses have been treated by conditioning techniques with excellent results. Vaginismus responds well to desensitization with graduated Hegar dilators along with relaxation techniques. Masters and Johnson have used behavioral approaches in all of the sexual dysfunctions, with concomitant supportive psychotherapy and with improvement of the communication patterns of the couple.

3. Psychologic–The use of psychotherapy by itself is best suited for those cases in which interpersonal difficulties or intrapsychic problems predominate. Anxiety and guilt about parental injunctions against sex constitute the most frequent psychopathology contributing to sexual dysfunction. Even in these cases, however, a combined behavioral-psychologic approach usually produces results most quickly.

4. Social–The proximity of other people (eg, a mother-in-law) in a household is frequently an inhibiting factor in sexual relationships. In such cases, some social engineering may alleviate the problem.

Kaplan JH et al: Impotence: A four-article symposium. *Postgrad Med* (Oct) 1983;**74**:181.

Pardridge WM et al: UCLA Conference: Androgens and sexual behavior. *Ann Intern Med* 1982;**96**:488.

Segraves RT: Male sexual dysfunction and psychoactive drug use: Review of a common relationship. *Postgrad Med* (Jan) 1982;**71**:227.

Spark RF: Neuroendocrinology and impotence. (Editorial.) *Ann Intern Med* 1983;**98**:103.

Wise TN: Sexual dysfunction in the medically ill. *Psychosomatics* 1983;**24**:787.

PERSONALITY DISORDERS

Essentials of Diagnosis

- Long history dating back to childhood.
- Recurrent maladaptive behavior.
- Low self-esteem and lack of confidence.
- Minimal introspective ability.
- Major difficulties with interpersonal relationships or society.
- Depression with anxiety when maladaptive behavior fails.

General Considerations

Personality—a hypothetical construct—is the result of the prolonged interaction of an individual with personal drives and with outside influences, the sum being the enduring and unique patterns of behavior which are adopted in order to cope with the environment and which characterize one as an individual. Obviously, the more satisfactory the early development of a person, the stronger the personality development. The personality structure, or character, is an integral part of self-image and is important to one's sense of identity. People who fail to integrate satisfactory early experiences tend to have personality structures that manifest more primitive responses.

Lack of a self-identity is characteristic and is manifested by marked dependence on others and a tendency to imitate someone who may be important at a given time. There are repeated attempts to move toward another person, often in this dependent fashion, followed by the inevitable rejections that elicit the overreactive response.

The ambiguity of the term is one of the principal characteristics that perpetuates its use. It implies a developmental maladaption from an early age, with subsequent problems of behavior that are repetitive, personally handicapping, and annoying to others. The individual does not learn from bad experiences and feels little anxiety unless the pathologic coping pattern fails.

The classification of subtypes depends upon the predominant symptoms and their severity. The most severe disorders—those that bring the patient into greatest conflict with society—tend to be classified as antisocial (psychopathic).

Classification & Clinical Findings

Paranoid: Defensive, oversensitive, secretive,

suspicious, hyperalert, with limited emotional response.—**Schizoid:** Shy, introverted, withdrawn, avoids close relationships.—**Compulsive:** Perfectionist, egocentric, indecisive, with rigid thought patterns and need for control.—**Histrionic (hysterical):** Dependent, immature, seductive, histrionic, egocentric, vain, emotionally labile (a mnemonic device describing these traits is *dishevel*).—**Schizotypal:** Superstitious, socially isolated, suspicious, with limited interpersonal ability and odd speech.—**Narcissistic:** Exhibitionist, grandiose, preoccupied with power, lacks interest in others, with excessive demands for attention.—**Avoidant:** Fears rejection, hyperreacts to rejection and failure, with poor social endeavors and low self-esteem.—**Dependent:** Passive, overaccepting, unable to make decisions, lacks confidence, with poor self-esteem.—**Passive-aggressive:** Stubborn, procrastinating, argumentative, sulking, helpless, clinging, negative to authority figures.—**Antisocial:** Selfish, callous, promiscuous, impulsive, unable to learn from experience, has legal problems.—**Borderline:** Impulsive, lacks self-control and self-fullfillment, with identity problems, affective instability, suicidal and aggressive behaviors, feelings of emptiness, and occasional psychotic decompensation.

Differential Diagnosis

Patients with the less severe types of personality disorders tend to show anxiety and depression when pathologic techniques fail, and their symptoms can be similar to those occurring with neurotic problems. Occasionally, the more severe cases may decompensate into psychosis under stress.

Treatment

A. Social: Social and therapeutic environments such as day hospitals, halfway houses, and self-help communities utilize peer pressures to modify the self-destructive behavior. The patient with a personality disorder often has failed to profit from experience, and difficulties with authority impair the learning experience. The use of peer relationships and the repetition possible in a structured setting of a helpful community enhances the educational opportunities and increases learning. When one's companions note every flaw in one's character and insist that it be corrected immediately, a powerful learning environment is being created. When problems are detected early, both the school and the home can serve as foci of intensified social pressure to change the behavior, particularly with the use of behavioral techniques.

B. Behavioral: The behavioral techniques used are principally operant and aversive conditioning. The former simply emphasizes the recognition of acceptable behavior and reinforcement of this with praise or other tangible rewards. Aversive responses usually mean punishment, although this can range from ignoring the person to some specific punitive responses such as verbal abuse. Extinction plays a role in that an attempt is made not to respond to inappropriate behavior, and the lack of response eventually causes the person to abandon that type of behavior. Pouting and tantrums, for example, diminish quickly when such behavior elicits no reaction.

C. Psychologic: Psychologic intervention is most usefully accomplished in group settings. Group therapy is helpful when specific interpersonal behavior needs to be improved (eg, schizoid and inadequate types, where involvement with people is markedly impaired). This mode of treatment also has a place with so-called acting-out patients, ie, those who frequently act in an impulsive and inappropriate way. Do not display anger with this type of patient. Act within known limits, limit the time spent on the case, and be flexible in approach. The peer pressure in the group tends to impose restraints on rash behavior. The group also quickly identifies the patient's types of behavior and helps to improve the validity of the patient's self-assessment, so that the antecedents of the unacceptable behavior can be effectively handled, thus decreasing its frequency. Individual therapy is of limited usefulness even in motivated patients.

D. Medical: Hospitalization in a milieu setting is occasionally indicated, but in most cases treatment can be accomplished in the day treatment center or self-help community. Antipsychotics may be required for short periods in conditions that have temporarily decompensated into transient psychoses (eg, haloperidol, 2–5 mg orally every 3–4 hours until the patient has quieted down and is regaining contact with reality). In most cases, these drugs are required only for several days and can be discontinued after the patient has regained a previously established level of adjustment. Sedatives (eg, diazepam, 5–10 mg orally several times a day) can be used when a decrease of passive avoidance is desired to allow the patient to learn and practice new kinds of behavior in a therapeutic setting (eg, in the very fearful schizoid patient who passively avoids people and is attempting to learn to interact in a group therapy setting).

Prognosis

Antisocial and borderline categories generally have a poor prognosis, whereas persons with mild schizoid or passive-aggressive tendencies have a good prognosis if appropriate treatment is given.

Barrash J et al: Discriminating borderline disorders from other personality disorders. *Arch Gen Psychiatry* 1983;**40**:1297.

Chodoff P: Hysteria and women. *Am J Psychiatry* 1982;**139**:545.

Koenigsberg HW et al: Diagnosing borderline conditions in an outpatient setting. *Arch Gen Psychiatry* 1983;**40**:49.

Stoudemire A, Thompson TL: The borderline personality in the medical setting. *Ann Intern Med* 1982;**96**:76.

SCHIZOPHRENIC & OTHER PSYCHOTIC DISORDERS

Essentials of Diagnosis (Schizophrenia)

- Social withdrawal, usually slowly progressive, often with deterioration in personal care.

- Loss of ego boundaries, with inability to perceive oneself as a separate entity.
- Loose thought associations, often with slowed thinking or rapid shifting from topic to topic.
- Autism with absorption in inner thoughts and frequent sexual or religious preoccupations.
- Auditory hallucinations, often of a derogatory nature.
- Delusions, frequently of a grandiose or persecutory nature.
- Symptoms of at least 6 months' duration.

Frequent additional signs:

- Flat affect and rapidly alternating mood shifts irrespective of circumstances.
- Hypersensitivity to environmental stimuli, with a feeling of enhanced sensory awareness.
- Variability or changeable behavior incongruent with the external environment.
- Concrete thinking with inability to abstract; inappropriate symbolism.
- Impaired concentration worsened by hallucinations and delusions.
- Depersonalization, wherein one behaves like a detached observer of one's own actions.

General Considerations

The schizophrenic disorders are a group of syndromes manifested by massive disruption of thinking, mood, and overall behavior. According to *DSM-III* criteria, the onset of illness occurs before age 45; signs must be continuous for at least 6 months; the illness is not preceded by a full depressive or manic syndrome; and symptoms are not due to mental retardation or organic mental disorder. The characterization and nomenclature of the disorders are quite arbitrary and are influenced by sociocultural factors and schools of psychiatric thought.

Other psychotic disorders are conditions that are similar to schizophrenic illness in their acute symptoms but have a less pervasive influence over the long term. The individual usually attains higher levels of functioning. The acute psychotic episodes tend to be less disruptive of the person's life-style, with a fairly quick return to previous levels of functioning.

It is currently believed that the schizophrenic disorders are of multifactorial etiology with genetic, environmental, neuroendocrine, and pathophysiologic components. At present, there is no laboratory method to confirm the diagnosis of schizophrenia. There may or may not be a history of a major disruption in the individual's life (failures, losses, physical illness) before gross psychotic deterioration is evident. History obtained from others may indicate a long-standing "strange" premorbid personality.

Classifications

A. Schizophrenic Disorders: Schizophrenic disorders are subdivided on the basis of certain prominent phenomena that are frequently present. **Disorganized (hebephrenic) schizophrenia** is characterized by marked incoherence and an incongruous or silly affect. **Catatonic schizophrenia** is distinguished by a marked psychomotor disturbance of either excitement (purposeless and stereotyped) or rigidity with mutism. Infrequently, there may be rapid alternation between excitement and stupor (see under catatonic syndrome, p 661). **Paranoid schizophrenia** includes marked persecutory or grandiose delusions often consonant with hallucinations of similar content. **Undifferentiated schizophrenia** denotes a category in which symptoms are not specific enough to warrant inclusion of the illness in the other subtypes. **Residual schizophrenia** is a classification that includes persons who have clearly had an episode warranting a diagnosis of schizophrenia but who at present have no overt psychotic symptoms, although they show milder signs such as social withdrawal, flat affect, and eccentric behaviors.

B. Paranoid Disorders: Paranoid disorders are psychoses in which the predominant symptoms are persistent persecutory delusions, with minimal impairment in daily function (the schizophrenic disorders show significant impairment). Intellectual and occupational activities are little affected, whereas social and marital functioning tend to be markedly involved. Hallucinations are not usually present. The category includes such states as paranoia, shared paranoid disorder (folie à deux), and paranoid state, the last being characterized by its transitory nature, whereas the others are more chronic.

C. Schizoaffective Disorders: Schizoaffective disorders are those cases that fail to fit comfortably either in the schizophrenic or in the affective categories. They are usually cases with affective symptoms that precede or develop concurrently with psychotic manifestations. They were formerly included under the heading of schizoaffective schizophrenia and more recently have been labeled by some as atypical bipolar affective disorders.

D. Schizophreniform Disorders: Schizophreniform disorders are similar in their symptoms to the schizophrenic disorders except that the duration of the illness is less than 6 months but more than 1 week.

E. Brief Reactive Psychotic Disorders: These disorders last less than 1 week. They are the result of psychologic stress. The shorter duration is significant and correlates with a more acute onset and resolution as well as a much better prognosis.

Clinical Findings

The signs and symptoms vary markedly among individuals as well as in the same person at different times. **Appearance** may be bizarre, although the usual finding is a mild to moderate unkempt blandness. **Motor activity** is generally reduced, although extremes ranging from catatonic stupor to frenzied excitement occur. **Social behavior** is characterized by marked withdrawal, coupled with disturbed interpersonal relationships and a reduced ability to experience pleasure. Dependency and a poor self-image are common. **Verbal utterances** are variable, the language being concrete yet symbolic, with unassociated rambling statements (at times interspersed with mutism) during an acute episode. Neologisms (made-up word or phrases), echolalia (repetition of words spoken by others), and verbigeration (repetition of senseless words or phrases) are occasionally present. **Affect** is usually flattened and shallow, with occasional inappropriateness. **Depression** is ubiquitous but may be less apparent during the acute psychotic episode and become more obvious during recovery. It is sometimes confused with akinetic side effects of antipsychotic drugs.

Cognitive dysfunction is the rule, and thought content may vary from a paucity of ideas to a rich complex of delusional fantasy with archaic thinking. One frequently notes after a period of conversation that little if any information has actually been conveyed. Incoming stimuli produce varied responses. In some cases a simple question may trigger explosive outbursts, whereas at other times there may be no overt response whatsoever (catatonia). When paranoid ideation is present, the patient is often irritable and less cooperative. Delusions (false beliefs) are characteristic of paranoid thinking, and they usually take the form of a preoccupation with the supposedly threatening behavior exhibited by other individuals. This ideation may cause the patient to adopt active countermeasures such as locking doors and windows, taking up weapons, covering the ceiling with aluminum foil to counteract radar waves, and other bizarre efforts. Somatic delusions revolve around issues of bodily decay or infestation. **Perceptual distortions** usually include auditory hallucinations—visual hallucinations are more commonly associated with organic mental states—and may include illusions (distortions of reality) such as figures changing in size or lights varying in intensity. Lack of humor, feelings of dread, depersonalization (a feeling of being apart from the self), and fears of annihilation may be present. Any of the above symptoms generates higher anxiety levels, with heightened arousal and occasional panic, as the individual fails to cope.

Ventricular enlargement, as seen on CT scan, has been correlated with a chronic course, severe cognitive impairment, and nonresponsiveness to neuroleptic medications.

The development of the acute episode in schizophrenia frequently is the end product of a gradual decompensation. Frustration and anxiety appear early, followed by depression and alienation, along with decreased effectiveness in day-to-day coping. This often leads to feelings of panic and increasing disorganization, with loss of the ability to test and evaluate the reality of perceptions. The stage of so-called "psychotic resolution" includes delusions, autistic preoccupations, and psychotic insight, with acceptance of the decompensated state.

Differential Diagnosis

First and foremost should be a reconsideration of the diagnosis of schizophrenia in any person who has been so diagnosed in the past, particularly when the clinical course has been atypical. A number of these patients have been found to actually have atypical episodic affective disorders that have responded well to lithium. Manic episodes often mimic schizophrenia. Also, many individuals have been diagnosed as schizophrenic because of inadequacies in psychiatric nomenclature. Thus, persons with brief reactive psychoses and schizophreniform disorders were often inappropriately diagnosed as having schizophrenia. Toxic reactions to drugs have also been incorrectly diagnosed as schizophrenia in many instances.

Psychotic depressions, psychotic organic mental states, and any illness with psychotic ideation tend to be confused with schizophrenia, partly because of the regrettable tendency to use the terms interchangeably. Adolescent phases of growth and counterculture behaviors constitute another area of diagnostic confusion. It is particularly important to avoid a misdiagnosis in these groups because of the long-term implications arising from having such a serious diagnosis made in a formative stage of life.

Medical disorders such as thyroid dysfunction, adrenal and pituitary disorders, and practically all of the organic mental states in the early stages must be ruled out. Complex partial seizures, especially when psychosensory phenomena are present, are an important differential consideration. Toxic drug states arising from prescription, over-the-counter, and street drugs may mimic all of the psychotic disorders. The chronic use of amphetamines and other stimulants frequently produces a psychosis that is almost identical to the acute paranoid schizophrenic episode. Stimulants may precipitate acute psychiatric symptoms in the compensated schizophrenic. The presence of formication and stereotypy suggests the possibility of stimulant abuse. Phencyclidine (see p 674) has become a very common street drug, and in many cases an adverse reaction to it is difficult to distinguish from other psychotic disorders. Cerebellar signs, excessive salivation, dilated pupils, and increased deep tendon reflexes should alert the physician to the possibility of a toxic psychosis. Industrial chemicals, both organic and metallic; degenerative disorders; and metabolic deficiencies must be considered in the differential diagnosis.

Catatonic syndrome, frequently assumed to exist solely as a component of schizophrenic disorders, is actually the end product of a number of illnesses, including various organic conditions. Neoplasms, viral encephalopathies, central nervous system hemorrhage, metabolic derangements such as diabetic ketoacidosis, sedative withdrawal, and hepatic and renal malfunction have all been implicated. It is particularly important to realize that drug toxicity (eg, overdoses of antipsychotic medications such as fluphenazine enanthate or fluphenazine decanoate) can cause catatonic syndrome, which may be misdiagnosed as a catatonic schizophrenic disorder and inappropriately treated with more antipsychotic medication.

Treatment

A. Medical: Hospitalization is often necessary, particularly when the patient's behavior shows gross disorganization. The presence of competent family members lessens the need for hospitalization, and each case should be judged individually. The major considerations are to prevent self-inflicted harm or harm to others and to provide the patient's basic needs. Antipsychotic medications are the treatment of choice. Evidence to date suggests that all of the antipsychotic drugs are similarly effective in treating psychoses, with the differences being in milligram potency and side effects. The latter are the principal reason for choosing one drug over another (see Antipsychotic Drugs, p 634). The long-acting injectable (depot) neuroleptics are used in the noncompliant patient. About 30–60% of schizophrenics eventually receives this form of medication therapy.

A high-potency drug such as haloperidol, thiothixene, or fluphenazine may be selected for treatment of the acute case. The major aim of treatment is rapid alleviation of the psychotic state. Haloperidol, 10–15 mg orally or 5–10 mg intramuscularly, may be given every hour until agitation and psychotic symptoms subside and the patient is noticeably calmer. The total amount administered the first day gives a clue about the daily amount that will be required for the first several days, after which the patient will usually require less medication. After the condition of the patient has been stabilized and symptoms are adequately controlled, it is necessary to give medication only once a day, preferably at bedtime to take advantage of any sedative effects. If the patient remains stable, very gradually lower the dosage. The amount of medication should be the least amount necessary to control psychotic symptoms. The length of time a patient will require medication varies widely. Chronically ill patients with a history of recurrent illness may need drugs indefinitely, whereas others will need medication for only a few months after the acute episode. Relapse rates are markedly lowered (to about 50%) when medications are used appropriately over the longer term in the schizophrenic patient.

Undertreatment is the usual cause of treatment failure in the early part of the acute period. Side effects, particularly drug-induced parkinsonism, are often secondary to inadequate downward adjustment of medication as the patient improves. It is not usually necessary to use prophylactic antiparkinsonism drugs, particularly when the patient is hospitalized. In outpatients it is sometimes desirable to do so when the probability of an extrapyramidal reaction is greater (eg, with fluphenazine enanthate or haloperidol) and when a reaction may adversely influence compliance. Antiparkinsonism agents need not be continued indefinitely. In many cases, a decrease in the antiparkinsonism drug is well tolerated, and it can be gradually discontinued. The majority of patients on depot neuroleptics will need long-term antiparkinsonism medication. Hemodialysis has no proved benefit in schizophrenia.

B. Social: Environmental considerations are most important in the individual with a chronic illness, who usually has a history of repeated hospitalizations, a continued low level of functioning, and symptoms that never completely remit. This type of patient has usually never lived up to basic potential and frequently has been rejected by family members. When the patient lives with the family, conjoint psychotherapy with the family reduces exacerbations of the psychosis. The work record has frequently been poor, with a disability pension being the usual means of financial support. In these cases, board and care homes experienced in caring for psychiatric patients are most important. There is frequently an inverse relationship between stability of the living situation and the amounts of required antipsychotic drugs.

Psychosocial and psychopharmacologic measures tend to be positively interactive. In those cases in which there is potential for improved performance or the need for specific adjunctive therapies (eg, occupational therapy, basic training skills), a day treatment center or part-time hospitalization may be helpful. Flexibility in the use of part-time hospitalization, day treatment, and other ongoing social care methods is desirable, since the amount of medication necessary is often inversely proportional to the stability of the work and living situation. Nonresidential self-help groups such as Recovery, Inc. should be utilized whenever possible. They provide a setting for sharing, learning, and mutual support and are frequently the only social involvement with which this type of patient is comfortable. Work agencies (eg, Goodwill Industries, Inc.) and vocational rehabilitation departments provide assessment, training, and job opportunities at a level commensurate with the person's clinical condition.

C. Psychologic: The need for psychotherapy varies markedly depending on the patient's current status and past history. Patients with a long history of chronic disability do not benefit appreciably from the usual verbal, insight-oriented therapies. A person with a single psychotic episode and a previously good level of adjustment may do very well with psychologic therapy after the acute phase has been resolved with medication and the passage of time. This is particularly true in those cases in which the psychosis was a result of psychologic stress. The complexity of the treatment must be appropriate to the status of the patient; obviously, a person just recovering from a severe psychotic episode is usually not ready to deal with anxiety-laden material about oedipal conflicts. On the other hand, psychotherapy dealing with the here and now of everyday problems and the daily concerns of living is quite appropriate. With improvement, the patient may be ready for more insight-oriented therapy (either individual or group) and may be receptive to experiential therapeutic approaches. Generally, psychotherapy is helpful in assisting the patient to reintegrate the experience, gain some insight into antecedent problems, and become a more self-observant individual who can recognize early signs of stress. Family therapy should be given concomitantly to help alleviate the patient's stress and to assist relatives in coping with the patient.

D. Behavioral: Behavioral techniques are most frequently used in therapeutic settings such as day treatment centers, but there is no reason why they cannot be incorporated into family situations or any therapeutic setting. Many behavioral techniques are used unwittingly (eg, positive reinforcement— whether it be a word of praise or an approving nod— after some positive behavior), and with some careful thought, this approach can be a most powerful instrument for helping a person learn behaviors that will facilitate social acceptance. The family or board and care situation is the most important place for practice of such techniques, since so much of the patient's time is spent in such settings. Operant conditioning has been used successfully in formal ways (eg, token economies) as well as informally, as occurs in daily living situations. Extinction occurs as inappropriate behaviors are not reinforced and the person can gradually abandon the behavior (eg, outbursts, temper tantrums). A chronic psychotic process usually includes many odd and primitive techniques used mainly to gain attention. Giving these up is a combination of learning new behavior and not being rewarded for the old.

Abrams R, Taylor MA: The genetics of schizophrenia: A reassessment using modern criteria. *Am J Psychiatry* 1983; **140:**171.

Guze SB et al: A follow-up and family study of schizophrenia. *Arch Gen Psychiatry* 1983;**40:**1273.

Manschreck TC: Current concepts in psychiatry: Schizophrenic disorders. *N Engl J Med* 1981;**305:**1628.

Manschreck TC: Drug treatment of schizophrenia: Principles and limitations. *Drug Ther* (Sept) 1983;**13:**185.

Stoudemire A, Nelson A, Houpt JL: Interictal schizophrenia-like psychoses in temporal lobe epilepsy. *Psychosomatics* 1983;**24:**331.

Taylor MA, Abrams R: Cognitive impairment in schizophrenia. *Am J Psychiatry* 1984;**141:**197.

AFFECTIVE DISORDERS
(Depression & Mania)

Essentials of Diagnosis

Present in most depressions:

- Lowered mood, varying from mild sadness to intense feelings of guilt and hopelessness.
- Difficulty in thinking, including inability to concentrate and lack of decisiveness.
- Loss of interest, with diminished involvement in work and recreation.
- Somatic complaints such as headache; disrupted, lessened, or excessive sleep; change in appetite; decreased sexual drive.
- Anxiety.

Present in some severe depressions:

- Psychomotor retardation or agitation.
- Delusions of a hypochondriacal or persecutory nature.
- Withdrawal from activities.

- Physical symptoms of major severity, eg, anorexia, insomnia, reduced sexual drive, weight loss, and various somatic complaints.
- Suicidal ideation.

General Considerations

Depression, like anxiety, is ubiquitous and is a reality of everyday life. It frequently presents in the form of somatic complaints with negative findings. It can be a normal reaction to a wide variety of events and must be evaluated as such. When the depression is appropriate to a life event and is not of major magnitude, specific treatment is not necessary. In many cases the patient comes to the physician to find out if the depression is abnormal, and in a significant number of cases all that is needed is reassurance. Not every depression requires treatment, and the inappropriate use of antidepressant medications is a direct result of the physician's failure to appreciate this.

The whole issue of depression is further confused by the fact that the word is used as an expression of a mood, a symptom, a syndrome, or a disease. Furthermore, the classifications are totally different and do not necessarily relate to each other. So-called neurotic versus psychotic classifications are not well differentiated, and treatment is not predicated on the distinction.

There are 4 basic theoretic models of depression:

(1) The "aggression-turned-inward" construct, which is apparent in many clinical cases of depression but has no substantial proof.

(2) The "loss" model, which postulates that depression is a reaction to loss of a person, thing, status, self-esteem, or even a habit pattern.

(3) The "interpersonal relationship" approach, which utilizes behavioral concepts. The person who is depressed may use depression as a means of controlling other people (including doctors). It can be an extension and outgrowth of such simple behavior as pouting, silence, or ignoring something or someone. It fails to serve the need and the problem worsens.

(4) The "biogenic amine" hypothesis, which stresses biochemical derangements characterized by a depletion of biogenic amines. Indirect clinical evidence for this model includes low spinal fluid concentrations of the major metabolite of brain norepinephrine and somatostatin, increased cortisol, and increased REM sleep, along with abnormalities on the dexamethasone suppression test and thyrotropin-releasing hormone test. Biologic markers are as yet of limited usefulness (see p 633). To date, it has not been possible to correlate depression subtype with serotonin, norepinephrine, or dopamine abnormalities.

Clinical Findings

In general, there are 3 major groups of depressions, with similar symptoms in each group.

A. Reactive: Depression may occur in reaction to some outside (exogenous) adverse life situation, usually loss of a person by death, divorce, etc; financial reversal; or loss of an established role, such as being needed. Anger and its repression are frequently associated with the loss, and this in turn often produces a feeling of guilt. The loss, anger, and guilt are readily apparent as the patient discusses the depression with the physician, who should be particularly alert to these components. Adjectives such as reactive and neurotic (implying anxiety, which is often present in these depressions) are often used in this group of depressions. The symptoms range from mild sadness, anxiety, irritability, worry, lack of concentration, discouragement, and somatic complaints to the more severe symptoms of the next group.

B. Major Affective Disorders: The subclassifications include major depressive episodes, manic episodes, and bipolar (manic-depressive) disorders.

1. A major depressive episode (endogenous unipolar disorder, involutional melancholia) is a period of mood depression that occurs relatively independently of the patient's life situations or events. Complaints vary widely but most frequently include a loss of interest and pleasure in living (anhedonia), withdrawal from activities, and feelings of guilt. Also included are inability to concentrate, anxiety, chronic fatigue, feelings of worthlessness, somatic complaints (unidentifiable somatic complaints frequently indicate depression), and loss of sexual drive. Diurnal variation with improvement as the day progresses is common. Vegetative signs that frequently occur are insomnia (particularly early morning awakening), anorexia with weight loss, and constipation. Occasionally, severe agitation and psychotic ideation (paranoid thinking, somatic delusions) are present. Paranoid symptoms may range from general suspiciousness to ideas of reference with delusions. The somatic delusions frequently revolve around feelings of impending annihilation or hypochondriacal beliefs that the body is rotting away with cancer. Hallucinations are uncommon. Major depressive disorders may occur at any time from childhood through adult life. The incidence is somewhat higher in women, and there is a greater chance of occurrence during the involutional period. Acuteness of onset is correlated with earlier recovery. Puerperal psychosis may be linked to the major affective disorders.

2. A manic episode is a mood change characterized by elation with hyperactivity, overinvolvement in life activities, low irritability threshold, flight of ideas, easy distractibility, and little need for sleep. The overenthusiastic quality of the mood and the expansive behavior initially attract others, but the irritability, mood lability, aggressive behavior, and grandiosity usually lead to marked interpersonal difficulties. Activities may occur that are later regretted, eg, excessive spending, resignation from a job, a hasty marriage, sexual acting out, and exhibitionistic behavior, with alienation of friends and acquaintances. Atypical manic episodes can include gross delusions, paranoid ideation of severe proportions, and auditory hallucinations usually related to some grandiose perception. Most hospitalized manic patients show bizarre idiosyncratic thought processes. The episodes begin

abruptly (sometimes precipitated by life stresses) and may last from several days to months. Generally, the manic episodes are of shorter duration than the depressive episodes. In almost all cases, the manic episode is part of a broader bipolar (manic-depressive) disorder.

3. Bipolar disorders (manic *and* depressive episodes) and individual manic episodes usually occur earlier (late teens or early adult life) than major depressive episodes. Cyclothymic disorders are milder forms of bipolar disorders. The rapidity of cycling varies markedly and tends to be related to 48-hour sleep-wake cycles. There is an intimate relationship between affective disorders and sleep patterns. Atypical episodes must be differentiated from schizophrenic and other psychotic disorders that also have an onset about this time. Manic patients differ from schizophrenics in that the former use more effective interpersonal maneuvers, are more sensitive to the social maneuvers of others, and are more able to utilize weakness and vulnerability in others to their own advantage. Schizophrenics are more withdrawn, less sensitive to nuances, and less flexible, and unlike the manic, seldom if ever function on an efficient interpersonal level.

4. Dysthymic disorders differ from the major affective disorders in the magnitude of symptomatology. Severity and duration vary, and there are no psychotic features. These conditions in the past were frequently called depressive neuroses.

C. Secondary to Illness and Drugs: Any illness, severe or mild, can cause significant depression. Conditions such as rheumatoid arthritis, multiple sclerosis, and chronic heart disease are particularly likely to be associated with depression, as are all other chronic illnesses. Estrogens clearly play a role in some depressions. Varying degrees of depression occur at various times in schizophrenic disorders and organic mental states. **Alcohol dependency** frequently coexists with serious depression. Any patient overusing alcohol should be evaluated for an affective disorder before any other diagnosis is considered. Conversely, any patient with symptoms of depression should be questioned carefully for problems of alcohol abuse.

The classic model of drug-induced depression occurs with the use of reserpine, both in a clinical and a neurochemical sense. Corticosteroids and oral contraceptives are commonly associated with affective changes. Antihypertensive medications such as alpha methyldopa, guanethidine, clonidine, and propranolol have been associated with the development of depressive syndromes. Infrequently, disulfiram and anticholinesterase drugs may be associated with symptoms of depression. The appetite-suppressing drugs, while initially stimulating, often result in a depressive syndrome when the drug is withdrawn. Alcohol, sedatives, opiates, and most of the psychedelic drugs are depressants and, paradoxically, are often used in self-treatment of depression. They inevitably worsen the problem; the suicide rate is highest with the use of these drugs.

Differential Diagnosis

Since depression may be a part of any illness—either reactively or as a secondary symptom—careful attention must be given to personal life adjustment problems, the role of medications (eg, reserpine), schizophrenia, and brain syndromes.

Complications

The longer the depression continues, the more crystallized it becomes, particularly when there is an element of secondary reinforcement. The most important complication is *suicide,* which always includes some elements of aggression. There are 4 major groups of people who make suicide attempts:

(1) Those who are overwhelmed by problems in living. By far the greatest number fall into this category. There is often great ambivalence; they don't really want to die, but they don't want to go on as before either.

(2) Those who are clearly attempting to control others. This is the blatant attempt in the presence of a significant other person in order to hurt or control that person.

(3) Those with severe depressions. This group includes both exogenous and endogenous conditions. A patient may seem to make a dramatic improvement, but the lifting of depression may be due to the patient's decision to commit suicide. Hopelessness and guilt tend to be the 2 major symptom determinants.

(4) Those with psychotic illness. These individuals tend not to verbalize their concerns, are unpredictable, and are often successful but comprise a small percentage of the total.

The immediate goal of psychiatric evaluation is to assess the current suicidal risk and the need for hospitalization versus outpatient management. The intent is less likely to be truly suicidal, for example, if small amounts of poison were ingested or scratching of wrists was superficial; if the act was performed in the presence of others or with early notification of others; or if the attempt was arranged so that early detection would be anticipated. There is a significant correlation between suicide and delusional thoughts. Other risk factors are previous suicide attempts, male sex, older age, contemplation of violent methods, drug and alcohol use, severe depression, and psychosis.

The patient's current mood status is best evaluated by direct evaluation of plans and concerns about the future, personal reactions to the attempt, and thoughts about the reactions of others. The patient's immediate resources should be assessed—people who can be significantly involved (most important), family support, job situation, financial resources, etc.

If hospitalization is not indicated, the physician must formulate and institute a treatment plan or make an adequate referral. Medication should be dispensed in small amounts to at-risk patients. The problem is often worsened by the long-term complications of the suicidal attempt, eg, brain damage due to hypoxia; peripheral neuropathies caused by staying for long periods in one position, causing nerve compressions;

and uncorrectable medical or surgical problems such as esophageal strictures and tendon dysfunctions.

The reasons for self mutilation, most commonly wrist-cutting but also autocastration, autoamputation, and autoenucleation, may be very different from the reasons for a suicide attempt. The initial treatment plan, however, should presume suicidal ideation, and conservative treatment should be initiated as for attempted suicide.

Sleep disturbances in the depressions are discussed on p 666.

Treatment

A. Medical: Hospitalization with suicidal precautions is required when the patient is suicidal or seriously incapacitated. It is important to rule out underlying disease and drug usage. **Thyroid function** should be carefully evaluated. If the suicide risk is high, electroconvulsive therapy should be considered as a treatment of choice (see Other Organic Therapies, p 645). Cyclic antidepressants (see Antidepressant Drugs, p 640) are effective in most severe depressions and should be used in adequate dosage and given a sufficient period of trial. An example would be imipramine, 100 mg daily to start, increased by 25 mg daily every several days until remission occurs or until 300 mg daily are being given. When psychotic ideation (usually paranoia or somatic delusions) is present, the response to antidepressants is variable. In these cases, antipsychotic drugs, eg, trifluoperazine, 5–10 mg daily initially with dosage increasing by 5 mg each day, may be used until psychotic symptoms are ameliorated. It may be necessary later to add an antidepressant if the psychosis is controlled but the depression persists. Loxapine (which is metabolized to amoxapine) may be useful in the treatment of psychotic depression. In resistant depressions, a trial of monoamine oxidase inhibitors can be cautiously attempted. Lithium is sometimes effective in acute depressions and decreases the recurrence rate of depressions in bipolar disorders and some unipolar cases. Stimulants can be useful in geriatric patients with apathy who are not significantly depressed.

Manic episodes are treated with haloperidol, 10 mg orally or intramuscularly every 1–2 hours, until the symptoms subside. At the same time, appropriate laboratory tests are done prior to *considering* treatment with lithium carbonate (see Lithium, p 638). Over a period of about 1 week, haloperidol can be gradually discontinued and lithium blood levels stabilized.

Carbamazepine, 800–1600 mg daily, has sometimes, but not always, been effective in patients for whom lithium is contraindicated. Hematologic monitoring is required. Conjoint use of these 2 drugs has been reported to cause neurologic symptoms in some patients.

The question of how long one should continue medications has not been satisfactorily answered. In general, the patient should be continued on the smallest amount of drug necessary to prevent relapse. This warrants a very gradual reduction in dosage over a period of months until the drug can be stopped. It will be necessary to maintain some patients indefinitely on medication.

B. Psychologic: It is seldom possible to engage an individual in penetrating psychotherapeutic endeavors during the acute stage of a severe depression. While medications may be taking effect, a supportive approach to strengthen existing defenses and appropriate consideration of the patient's continuing need to function at work, to engage in recreational activities, etc, are necessary as the severity of the depression lessens. If the patient is not seriously depressed, it is often quite appropriate to initiate intensive psychotherapeutic efforts, since flux periods are a good time to effect change. A catharsis of repressed anger and guilt may be beneficial. Therapy during or just after the acute stage may focus on coping techniques, with some practice of alternative choices. When lack of self-confidence and identity problems are factors in the depression, individual psychotherapy can be oriented to ways of improving self-esteem, increasing assertiveness, and lessening dependency. Group therapy techniques are particularly valuable not only with interpersonal dysfunction but also with problems rooted in family dynamics. It is usually helpful to involve the spouse or other significant family members early in treatment. Timing is important—the particular therapeutic approach should be initiated when the patient is ready. Inflexible dedication to any particular treatment modality can be counterproductive. Good clinical judgment may dictate early psychotherapy in a patient with mild to moderate depression, whereas in another patient the initial approach might be medical. The sensitivity of the clinician to the patient's needs is, in itself, of great psychotherapeutic importance.

C. Social: Flexible use of appropriate social services can be of major importance in the treatment of depression. Since alcohol is often associated with depression, early involvement in alcohol treatment programs such as Alcoholics Anonymous can be important to future success (see Alcohol Dependency, p 670). The structuring of daily activities during severe depression is often quite difficult for the patient. The help of family, employer, or friends is often necessary to mobilize the patient who experiences no joy in daily activities and tends to remain uninvolved and to deteriorate. Insistence on sharing activities will help involve the patient in simple but important daily functions. In some severe cases, the use of day treatment centers or support groups of a specific type (eg, mastectomy groups) is indicated. It is not unusual for a patient to have multiple legal, financial, and vocational problems. As the depression lifts, support agencies that provide legal aid and vocational rehabilitation can be of great assistance.

D. Behavioral: When depression is a function of self-defeating coping techniques such as passivity, the role-playing approach can be useful. Behavioral techniques including desensitization may be used in problems such as phobias where depression is a by-product. When depression is a regularly used interpersonal style, behavioral counseling to family members or others can help in extinguishing the behavior in the patient.

Prognosis

Reactive depressions are usually time-limited, and the prognosis with treatment is good if suicide or a pathologic pattern of adjustment does not intervene. Major affective disorders frequently respond well to effective drug treatment given early and in adequate amounts for a reasonable period of time.

Bolwig TG: Treatment approaches in depression. *Acta Psychiatr Scand* 1983;**302**:52.

Keller MB et al: Predictors of relapse in major depressive disorder. *JAMA* 1983;**250**:3299.

Lehmann HE: Clinical evaluation and natural course of depression. *J Clin Psychiatry* 1983;**44**(5–Part 2):5.

Lieberman PB, Strauss JS: The recurrence of mania: Environmental factors and medical treatment. *Am J Psychiatry* 1984;**141**:77.

Pokorny AD: Prediction of suicide in psychiatric patients. *Arch Gen Psychiatry* 1983;**40**:249.

Watts CAH: Depressive disorders in the community: The scene in Great Britain, 1965. *J Clin Psychiatry* 1984;**45**:70.

SLEEP DISORDERS

Sleep disturbances occur commonly in psychiatric disorders, particularly in depression. The complaints are difficult to evaluate, since approximately 30% of a normal population sample will complain of "insomnia": trouble falling asleep, waking up during the night (the most common), or early final awakening. There are 2 distinct states of sleep as shown on electroencephalographic studies: REM (rapid eye movement) sleep, also called dream sleep, D state sleep, and paradoxic sleep; and NREM (nonREM) sleep, which is also known as slow (delta) wave sleep or S state sleep and is divided into stages 1, 2, 3, and 4. Dreaming occurs in both REM and NREM sleep. There is no clear evidence that REM sleep deprivation is harmful or productive of mental disorder. The stages of NREM sleep have been less well studied because of technical problems in selectively evaluating a particular stage, but stage 4 disturbances are related to clinical syndromes and are differentiated by electroencephalographic delta wave patterns.

In the general population, complaints of sleep disturbance tend to increase with age, with a decrease in stage 3 and 4 sleep (including a decline of delta wave amplitude) and an increase in stage 1 electroencephalographic patterns. REM sleep falls to less than 20% of total sleep time in the person above 70 years of age. Disordered sleep is frequently related to daytime naps or changes in sleep habits. In such cases, the obvious answer is to rearrange sleep schedules and avoid sedatives. Barbiturates and nonbarbiturate sedative-hypnotics such as glutethimide are *not* desirable sedatives; they are initially effective, but they reduce REM sleep and are quickly tolerated. About a week is required for return to baseline levels. Chronic use of multiple doses of these drugs produces a more marked decrease of both REM sleep and slow wave sleep, with rebound increase of both types when the drug is withdrawn. The benzodiazepines do not significantly alter REM sleep but do suppress stage 4 sleep.

Insomnia is usually considered to be sleep deprivation or a marked change in the perceived sleep pattern.

Factors contributing to insomnia include (1) situational problems such as transient stress, job pressures, and marital discord; (2) aging; (3) medical disorders that inevitably include pain and physical discomfort; (4) drug-related episodes, including withdrawal from alcohol or sedatives; and (5) psychologic conditions, particularly the major mental illnesses such as schizophrenia and affective disorders (see pp 659 and 663).

Caffeine is a cortical stimulant that prolongs sleep onset, lightens sleep, and increases morning drowsiness. Over-the-counter decongestants also tend to delay the onset and disrupt the continuity of sleep.

Schizophrenics vary markedly in the degree of sleep disturbance they endure. In acute episodes the disruption is severe, even to the point of total insomnia. The chronic schizophrenic or the patient in remission often does not have any complaints, and an electroencephalographic pattern is not remarkably abnormal. Antipsychotic drugs decrease sleep latency (interval between going to bed and going to sleep), increase overall sleep time, and increase REM sleep. Most (except chlorpromazine) reduce delta sleep and increase spindle sleep. Sedating antipsychotic drugs such as chlorpromazine given at bedtime obviate the need for sedatives in the schizophrenic with sleep problems.

Sleep disturbance is one of the most common symptoms of **affective disorders.** Some bipolar patients sleep more when they are depressed and less when they are manic, but there is much variation. Primary depressions usually show sleep continuity disturbances with decreased auditory arousal threshold, shortened REM stage latency, more REM sleep at the beginning of the night than in early morning hours, and a marked reduction in stages 3 and 4 sleep. In the manic phase, REM sleep is decreased, but there are varying reports on slow wave sleep. Both unipolar and bipolar patients in the depressed phase usually have a decreased total sleep time. The incidence of excess sleep in depression is low—about 8%. Unfortunately, there is no specific correlation of particular types of depression to clinical type of sleep problem. Antidepressants decrease REM sleep (with marked rebound on drug withdrawal) and have varying effects on slow wave sleep. The effect on REM sleep correlates positively with reports that reductions in REM sleep tend to parallel improvement of the depression. Use of the more sedating tricyclic antidepressants such as amitriptyline, given at bedtime in full dosage, frequently eliminates the need to use a sedative. Lithium significantly reduces REM sleep and increases delta and spindle sleep.

Hypersomnias are clinical syndromes such as narcolepsy, the Kleine-Levin syndrome, and sleep apnea.

Narcolepsy is a sleep disturbance that usually occurs before age 40 and includes one or more of the following 4 conditions: (1) Sleep attacks are sudden, reversible, short-lasting (about 15 minutes) episodes occurring during any type of activity. Electroencephalographic recordings usually show a direct progression to REM sleep. The patient awakens refreshed, and there is a refractory period of 1–5 hours before another attack can occur. Amphetamines are the treatment of choice in sleep attacks. Give amphetamine sulfate (or an equivalent drug), 10 mg each morning, and increase the dosage as required. The average dose is 10–20 mg 3 times daily. (2) Cataplexy is a sudden loss of muscle tone ranging from specific small muscle groups to general muscle weakness that causes the person to slump to the floor, unable to move. Cataplexy is often initiated by an emotional outburst (laughing, crying, anger) and lasts from several seconds to 30 minutes. Tricyclic antidepressants such as imipramine, 75–100 mg daily, are effective in cataplexy but not in sleep attacks. (3) Sleep paralysis involves acquisition of flaccid muscle tone with full consciousness, either during awakening or while falling asleep. There is usually intense fear and occasional auditory hallucinations. The attack is terminated by touching or calling the patient. (4) Hypnagogic hallucinations, either visual or auditory, may precede sleep or occur during the sleep attack. If the hallucinations occur during awakening, they are called hypnopompic hallucinations. The occurrence of the symptoms of the narcoleptic tetrad are as follows: sleep attacks, almost 100%; sleep attacks and cataplexy, about 70%; sleep paralysis alone, about 5%.

The **Kleine-Levin syndrome** involves hypersomnic attacks lasting up to 2 days and occurring infrequently (3–4 times per year). There is confusion upon awakening. It is a separate entity from narcolepsy, and there is no specific treatment.

Sleep apnea constitutes apneic episodes in both REM and NREM sleep. Noisy, stertorous snoring and hypersomnolence the next day are common. Intellectual and personality changes include decreased attention span, decreased memory, and hyperirritability. There are 2 types of sleep apnea: central apnea, in which there is a cessation of respiratory movement with loss of air flow, and obstructive apnea, in which there is persistent respiratory effort but an upper airway blockage. Diaphragmatic pacing and clomipramine can be helpful in the central nervous system condition, while tracheostomy, pharyngoplasty, or a tongue-restraining device is the current treatment of choice for the obstructive type. Studies with protriptyline indicate that it decreases daytime somnolence and increases nocturnal oxygenation, but apnea duration and frequency are not significantly decreased. Hypertension is seen in most of these patients. Any patient evaluated for hypertension should be questioned about sleep apnea. Consultation with sleep specialists is recommended in the treatment of this complex disorder.

Stage 4 sleep disorders are conditions that occur during that stage of sleep. **Enuresis** is the most common, usually in children and with variable nightly occurrence. While it often seems that the wetting occurred during dream sleep, it is actually seen most frequently in stage 4 sleep, with some preponderance in the first third of the night. Imipramine, 50–100 mg daily, is the preferred treatment. Behavioral techniques of aversive conditioning (eg, a wet sheet causing a bell to ring) are sometimes effective. **Somnambulism** also occurs mostly in children during stage 3 and 4 sleep. Protecting the environment (latches on windows and doors) has been the most common approach. Any of the benzodiazepines suppress stage 4 sleep and can help in preventing sleepwalking. **Pavor nocturnus** (night terrors) usually occurs in young children, predominantly in stage 4 sleep. As in somnambulism, amnesia for the episode occurs, and stage 4 suppressants such as benzodiazepines may be used for the condition.

The benzodiazepine and barbiturate sedatives increase total sleep time, decrease sleep latency, decrease the number of nocturnal awakenings, initially reduce REM sleep, and increase spindle sleep. There are variable effects on delta sleep. Symptoms of abstinence from the sedatives (withdrawal symptoms) include insomnia, frequent awakenings, and REM sleep rebound. Chloral hydrate and its derivatives have little known effect on sleep patterns or stages. Alcohol in a single dose shortens sleep latency and decreases nocturnal awakenings, but increased dosage increases nocturnal awakenings. Alcohol use tends to decrease REM sleep and increase delta sleep, while in withdrawal both REM and delta sleep are increased.

Amphetamines increase sleep latency, increase nocturnal awakenings, decrease REM and delta sleep, and increase spindle sleep. High caffeine intake increases REM and spindle sleep but decreases delta sleep. Cigarette smoking disrupts the regular sleep patterns. Cocaine effects are quite variable. Chronic marihuana usage increases sleep latency, increases most REM sleep factors, and decreases delta sleep.

Coleman RM et al: Sleep-wake disorders based on a polysomnographic diagnosis: A national cooperative study. *JAMA* 1982; **247**:997.

Crick F, Mitchison G: The function of dream sleep. *Nature* 1983;**304**:111.

Gillin JC: Sleep studies in affective illness: Diagnostic, therapeutic, and pathophysiological implications. *Psychiatr Ann* 1983;**13**:369.

McNamara E et al: EEG sleep evaluation of depression in borderline patients. *Am J Psychiatry* 1984;**141**:182.

DISORDERS OF AGGRESSION

Acts performed with the deliberate intent of causing physical harm to persons or property have a wide variety of causative factors. Aggression and violence are symptoms rather than diseases, and most frequently they are *not* associated with an underlying medical condition. In terms of demographic characteristics, the perpetrator of an act of aggression is often a male under age 25, a member of a minority group, a person in socially and economically deprived circumstances, and a resident of an inner city area.

Those who commit acts of aggression fall into 2 general personality types. The more common is a person with a pattern of physically aggressive behavior from an early age, with a poor capacity for peer relationships; truancy; and a family member (usually the father) who has a history of brutality or antisocial behavior. The less common type is the overcontrolled, chronically frustrated person who seethes inside until some event precipitates a violent overreaction. Some clues to the dangerous patient include statements that they feel powerless, feel humiliated, have headaches, or feel that they are "going to explode" or have "something terribly wrong with my body." In both types, disinhibiting drugs (most commonly alcohol) play a role in the aggressive outburst.

Drugs play a significant role in aggressive behavior. Although any mind-altering drug may be associated with aggression, the sedatives, especially alcohol, are the most prevalent. In the USA, 50% of all violent deaths are alcohol-related. The ingestion of even small amounts of alcohol can result in pathologic intoxication that resembles an acute organic mental condition. Amphetamines or other stimulants are frequently associated with aggressive behavior. Barbiturates and, increasingly, the benzodiazepines (both of which are often combined with alcohol) are frequent factors in the outburst. Phencyclidine, which has seen a phenomenal upsurge in usage, is becoming a drug commonly associated with violent behavior that is occasionally of a bizarre nature. Treatment of the acute situation is the same as for any instance of substance abuse (see Substance Use Disorders, p 670). Psychotherapy is not successful in modifying the underlying personality problems. It has long been known that this type of individual does better with strong external controls to replace the lack of inner controls. Close probationary supervision and court-mandated restrictions can be most helpful. There should be a major effort to help the individual avoid drug usage (eg, Alcoholics Anonymous).

Episodic dyscontrol syndrome is a descriptive term for a cluster of behaviors that may or may not warrant the use of the term "syndrome." The disorder is characterized by physical abuse, usually of wife or children, pathologic intoxication, impulsive sexual activities, and automobile misuse.

Wife-beating and rape (see p 476) are much more widespread than heretofore recognized. Awareness of the problem is to some degree due to increasing recognition of the rights of women and the understanding by women that they do not have to accept abuse. Women frequently have remained in violent home situations because of financial, legal, and cultural restraints. Acceptance of this kind of aggression inevitably leads to more, with the ultimate aggression being murder—20–50% of murders in the USA occur within the family. Police are involved in more domestic disputes than *all other criminal incidents combined*. The woman is by far the most frequent victim of intrafamily strife—3:1 in the case of family homicide. Such violent behavior is clearly more prevalent in succeeding generations of families who have indulged in it. Paternal violence (often associated with alcohol abuse) toward a daughter who marries during the teens to escape the home (often accompanied by premarital pregnancy) and acceptance of violence from the new husband set the stage for replication of violent behavior by the next generation. Extreme jealousy in men, often exacerbated by alcohol, is frequently used as an excuse for aggression. This jealousy may lead to attempts to limit the wife's activities outside the home, thus furthering her financial dependency. Interspersed periods of "sobriety" encourage the wife's hope for change and delay any efforts she might make to break the cycle. Children who are a part of such relationships inevitably become victims. The majority of abused children come from this type of household.

Presenting symptoms of victims frequently are depression, anxiety, and somatic complaints, and it is often only after overcoming the patient's great reluctance by means of gentle questioning that one is able to elicit the truth. The physician should be suspicious about the origin of any injuries not fully explained, particularly if such incidents recur. Any history of alcohol excess warrants further careful questioning. If depression seems related to suppressed aggression, it is important to discuss the reasons for such feelings. Feelings of powerlessness often contribute to depression and acceptance of further violence.

Attempts to correlate brain dysrhythmias with episodic discontrol syndrome have not been successful. Clinicians are unable to predict dangerous behavior beyond the level of chance.

Major mental disorders such as affective disorders, schizophrenic disorders, and organic mental states are seldom a factor in violent behavior. However, young paranoid schizophrenics are the most dangerous of mentally disordered persons. Although it has been reported that manic-depressive conditions are underdiagnosed in the criminal population in the USA, there is no clear evidence linking mania or other psychotic disorders to a pattern of aggressive behavior. When violence does occur in this group, it is frequently associated with attempts to control a person who is in the throes of an acute psychotic state.

Treatment

Management of any violent individual includes appropriate *psychologic* maneuvers. Move slowly, talk slowly with clarity and reassurance, and evaluate the situation. Strive to create a setting that is minimally disturbing and eliminate people or things threatening to the violent individual. Do not threaten or abuse and do not touch or crowd the person. For purposes of negotiation, use an individual whom the violent person can relate to most comfortably. Honesty is important. Make no false promises, and continue to engage the subject verbally until the situation is under control.

Pharmacologic means are often necessary whether or not psychologic approaches have been successful. This is particularly true in the agitated or psychotic patient. The drug of choice in psychotic aggressive states is haloperidol, 10 mg intramuscularly every hour until symptoms are alleviated. Droperidol is another butyrophenone that acts very rapidly and can be given intramuscularly or intravenously (eg, 5–10 mg hourly to a maximum of 45 mg in 24 hours). Benzodiazepine sedatives (eg, diazepam, 5 mg orally or intravenously every several hours) can be used for agitation, but an antipsychotic drug is preferred for management of the seriously violent and psychotic patient.

Physical management is necessary if psychologic and pharmacologic means are not sufficient. It requires the active and visible presence of an adequate number of personnel to reinforce the idea that the situation is under control despite the patient's lack of inner controls. Such an approach often precludes the need for actual physical restraint. If it becomes necessary, however, 2 people shielded by a single bed size mattress can usually corner and subdue the patient without injury to anyone. Seclusion rooms and restraints should be used only when necessary, and the patient must then be observed at *frequent* intervals. Design of corridors and seclusion rooms is important. Narrow corridors, small spaces, and crowded areas exacerbate the potential for violence in an anxious patient.

The treatment of beaten wives is a frustrating experience, chiefly because of the woman's reluctance to leave the situation. Reasons for staying vary, but common themes include the fear of more violence because of leaving; the hope that the situation may ameliorate (in spite of steady worsening); and the financial aspects of the situation, which are seldom to the woman's advantage. An early step is to get the woman into a therapeutic situation that provides the support of others in similar straits. Al-Anon is frequently a valuable asset and quite appropriate when alcohol is one of the factors in the abuse of the woman. The group can support the victim while she gathers strength to consider alternatives without being paralyzed by fear. Many cities now offer temporary emergency centers and counseling. "Rescue" attempts by physicians and other well-meaning individuals are often unsuccessful and discourage the would-be assistor from ever again dealing with such problems. *Use the available resources*, attend to any medical or psychiatric problems, and maintain a compassionate interest.

Devinsky O, Bear D: Varieties of aggressive behavior in temporal lobe epilepsy. *Am J Psychiatry* 1984;**141**:651.

Monahan J: The prediction of violent behavior: Toward a second generation of theory and policy. *Am J Psychiatry* 1984;**141**:10.

Phillips P, Nasr SJ: Seclusion and restraint and prediction of violence. *Am J Psychiatry* 1983;**140**:229.

Viken RM: Family violence: Aids to recognition. *Postgrad Med* (May) 1982;**71**:115.

SUBSTANCE USE DISORDERS
(Drug Dependency, Drug Abuse)

The term "drug dependency" is used in a broad sense here to include both addictions and habituations. It involves the triad of compulsive drug use referred to as drug addiction, which includes (1) a **psychologic craving** or dependence, and the behavior included in the procurement of the drug ("the life"); (2) **physiologic dependence,** with withdrawal symptoms on discontinuance of the drug; and (3) **tolerance,** ie, the need to increase the dose to obtain the desired effects. Drug dependency is a function of the amount of drug used and the duration of usage. The amount needed to produce dependency varies with the nature of the drug and the idiosyncratic nature of the user. The frequency of use is usually daily, and the duration is inevitably greater than 2–3 weeks. Dependency increases with increased amount and duration of drug usage. Transgenerational continuity of drug abuse is common.

The physician faces 2 problems with substance abuse: (1) the prescribing of substances such as sedatives, stimulants, or narcotics that might produce dependency, and (2) the treatment of individuals who have already abused drugs, most commonly alcohol. It is critical that the physician be aware of the abuse potential of drugs and prescribe them accordingly. Furthermore, patient education must be given a high priority. Finally, members of the medical profession must educate fellow physicians and exercise restraint in prescribing substances that are subject to abuse when other measures might be preferable.

It is first necessary to identify the drugs and treat the specific condition. With the exception of narcotic antagonists and physostigmine in anticholinergic poisoning, the treatments are symptomatic. Detoxification is required in patients for whom drug dependency is marked and in whom abrupt withdrawal might precipitate dangerous withdrawal symptoms. The most serious problems are with alcohol and sedatives, particularly barbiturates and the very dangerous glutethimide, ethchlorvynol, methyprylon, and methaqualone. The drug used in detoxification should be a member of the same group as the offending drug and should be fairly long-acting. Gradual withdrawal minimizes symptoms and provides an opportunity to change the attitude of the user toward drug abuse.

Fawzy FI, Coombs RH, Gerber B: Generational continuity in the use of substances: The impact of parental substance use on adolescent substance use. *Addict Behav* 1983;**8**:109.

Tsuang MT, Simpson JC, Kronfol Z: Subtypes of drug abuse with psychosis: Demographic characteristics, clinical features, and family history. *Arch Gen Psychiatry* 1982;**39**:141.

ALCOHOL DEPENDENCY & ABUSE
(Alcoholism)

Essentials of Diagnosis
Major criteria:
- Physiologic dependence as manifested by evidence of withdrawal when intake is interrupted.
- Tolerance to the effects of alcohol.
- Evidence of alcohol-associated illnesses, such as alcoholic liver disease, cerebellar degeneration.
- Continued drinking despite strong medical and social contraindications and life disruptions.
- Impairment in social and occupational functioning.
- Depression.
- Blackouts.

Other signs:
- Alcohol stigmas: Alcohol odor on breath, alcoholic facies, flushed face, tremor, ecchymoses, peripheral neuropathy.
- Surreptitious drinking.
- Unexplained work absences.
- Frequent accidents, falls, or injuries of vague origin; in smokers, cigarette burns on hands or chest.

General Considerations
Alcoholism is a syndrome consisting of 2 phases: problem drinking and alcohol addiction. Problem drinking is the repetitive use of alcohol, often to alleviate tension or solve other emotional problems. Alcohol addiction is a true addiction similar to that which occurs following the repeated use of barbiturates or similar drugs. Concurrent dependence on sedative-hypnotics is very common. It may occur in an attempt to control the anxiety generated by heavy alcohol abuse or in the mistaken belief that control by other pharmacologic agents will stop the alcohol abuse. Adoption and twin studies indicate some genetic influence, particularly in male alcoholics. Depression is often present and should be evaluated carefully. The majority of suicides involve alcohol usage.

Clinical Findings
A. Acute Intoxication: The signs of alcoholic intoxication are the same as those of overdosage with any other central nervous system depressant: drowsiness, errors of commission, disinhibition, dysarthria, ataxia, and nystagmus. For a 70-kg person, an ounce of whiskey, a glass of wine, or a 12-oz bottle of beer raises the level of alcohol in the blood by 25 mg/dL. Blood levels below 50 mg/dL rarely cause significant motor dysfunction. Intoxication as manifested by ataxia, dysarthria, and nausea and vomiting indicates a blood level above 150 mg/dL, and lethal blood levels range from 350 to 900 mg/dL. In severe cases, overdosage is marked by respiratory depression, stupor, shock syndrome, coma, and death. Serious overdoses are frequently due to a combination of alcohol with other sedatives.

B. Withdrawal: There is a wide spectrum of manifestations of alcoholic withdrawal, ranging from anxiety and tremulousness through increasing irritability and hyperreactivity to full-blown **delirium tremens** (see p 644). The latter is an acute organic psychosis that is usually manifest within 24–72 hours after the last drink (but may occur up to 7–10 days later). It is characterized by mental confusion, tremor, sensory hyperacuity, visual hallucinations (often of snakes, bugs, etc), autonomic hyperactivity, diaphoresis, dehydration, electrolyte disturbances (hypokalemia, hypomagnesemia), seizures, and cardiovascular abnormalities. The acute withdrawal syndrome is often completely unexpected and occurs when the patient has been hospitalized for some unrelated problem and presents as a diagnostic problem. *Suspect alcohol withdrawal in every unexplained delirium.* Seizures occur early (the first 24 hours) and are more prevalent in persons who have a history of withdrawal syndromes. The mortality rate from delirium tremens may be as high as 25%.

C. Alcoholic Hallucinosis: This syndrome occurs either during heavy drinking or on withdrawal and is characterized by a paranoid psychosis without the tremulousness, confusion, and clouded sensorium seen in withdrawal syndromes. The patient appears normal except for the auditory hallucinations, which are frequently persecutory and may cause the patient to behave aggressively.

D. Chronic Alcoholic Brain Syndromes: These encephalopathies are characterized by increasing erratic behavior, memory and recall problems, and emotional instability—the usual signs of organic brain syndrome due to any cause (see p 676). Early recognition and treatment of Wernicke's encephalopathy with intravenous thiamine and parenteral B complex vitamins can prevent irreversible damage.

Differential Diagnosis

The differential diagnosis of problem drinking is essentially between primary alcoholism (when no other major psychiatric diagnosis exists) and secondary alcoholism, when alcohol is used as self-medication for major underlying psychiatric problems such as schizophrenia or depression. The differentiation is important, since the latter group requires treatment for the specific psychiatric problem.

The differential diagnosis of alcoholic withdrawal consists of the possible use of other sedatives. Acute alcoholic hallucinosis must be differentiated from other acute paranoid states such as amphetamine psychosis or acute paranoid schizophrenia. An accurate history is the most important differentiating factor. The history is also the most important feature in differentiating chronic organic brain syndromes due to alcohol from those due to other causes. The form of the brain syndrome is of little help, eg, chronic brain syndromes from lupus erythematosus may be associated with confabulation similar to that resulting from long-standing alcoholism.

Complications

The medical and psychosocial problems of alcoholism are staggering. The central and peripheral nervous system complications include chronic brain syndromes, cerebellar degeneration, and peripheral neuropathies. The effects on the liver result not only in cirrhosis with its direct complications such as liver failure and esophageal varicosities but also in the systemic effects of altered metabolism, protein abnormalities, and coagulation defects.

Fetal alcohol syndrome includes one or more of the following developmental defects in the offspring of alcoholic women: (1) low birth weight and small size with failure to catch up in size or weight; (2) mental retardation, with an average IQ in the 60s; and (3) a variety of birth defects, with a large percentage of cardiac abnormalities. The fetuses are very quiet in utero, and there is an increased frequency of breech presentations. There is a higher incidence of delayed postnatal growth and behavior development. The risk factors are appreciably higher when more than 6 drinks are ingested each day. With lesser amounts, the risk is not precisely established.

Treatment of Problem Drinking

A. Psychologic Treatment: The most important consideration for the physician is to suspect the problem early and take a nonjudgmental attitude, though this does not mean a passive one. The physician who only sits and listens is actually reinforcing the patient's feelings of being rejected. There must be an active, nonauthoritarian interest in the problem, with emphasis on the things that can be done. This approach emphasizes the fact that the physician cares and strikes a positive and hopeful note early in treatment.

Valuable time should not be wasted trying to find out why the patient drinks; come to grips early with the immediate problem of *how to stop the drinking.* Total abstinence (not "controlled drinking") should be the primary goal. This often means early involvement of the spouse and elucidation of specific ways in which he or she can be helpful in stopping the drinking. In fact, if there is a spouse or family, the prognosis is much better, and working with both of the marriage partners—alone or together—should be started immediately.

B. Social Methods of Treatment: Get the patient into Alcoholics Anonymous (AA), the spouse into Al-Anon, and any children age 12–20 into Al-Ateen. Success is usually proportionate to the utilization of AA, other social agencies, religious counseling, and other resources. The patient should be seen frequently for short periods and charged an appropriate fee.

Do not underestimate the importance of religion, particularly since the alcoholic is often a dependent person who needs a great deal of support. Early enlistment of the help of a concerned religious adviser can often provide the turning point for a personal conversion to sobriety.

One of the most important considerations is the

job; it is usually lost or in jeopardy. In the latter case, some specific recommendations to employers can be offered: (1) Avoid placement in jobs where the alcoholic must be alone, eg, traveling buyer or sales executive. (2) Use supervision but not surveillance. (3) Keep competition with others to a minimum. (4) Avoid positions that require quick decision making on important matters.

C. Medical Treatment: Hospitalization is not usually necessary or even desirable at this stage, which is not an acute one. It is sometimes used to dramatize a situation and force the patient to face the problem of alcoholism, but generally it should be used only on medical indications.

Because of the many medical complications of alcoholism, a complete physical examination with appropriate laboratory tests is mandatory, with special attention to the liver and nervous system. Use of sedatives as a replacement for alcohol is not desirable. Usually the result is a concomitant use of sedatives *and* alcohol and a worsening of the problem.

The medical deterrent drug disulfiram can be of critical importance in helping the alcoholic to make the essential decision to *stop drinking*. There should be nothing surreptitious about the use of disulfiram (no slipping the drug into the coffee by the spouse, etc). It should be discussed with the patient, with full disclosure of its side effects, mode of action, and dangers (organic brain syndrome is an infrequent complication). The initial dosage schedule of disulfiram (after a minimum of 12 hours' abstention from alcohol) is 500 mg/d in a single dose in the morning. This can be decreased to a maintenance dose of 250 mg/d, continued indefinitely. Reports of liver damage due to disulfiram warrant baseline hepatic studies and monitoring. Any sedative or narcotic should be used cautiously when there is concomitant disulfiram administration. Disulfiram impairs elimination of caffeine. A disulfiram regimen need not interfere with other treatment approaches such as AA.

D. Behavioral Treatment: Conditioning approaches have been used in many settings in the treatment of alcoholism, most commonly as a type of aversion therapy. For example, the patient is given a drink of whisky and then a shot of apomorphine, and proceeds to vomit. In this way a strong association is built up between the vomiting and the drinking. Although this kind of treatment has been successful in some cases, many people do not retain the learned aversive response.

Treatment of Withdrawal & Hallucinosis
A. Medical Treatment:
1. Alcoholic hallucinosis–Alcoholic hallucinosis, which can occur either during or on cessation of a prolonged drinking period, is not a typical withdrawal syndrome and is handled differently. Since the symptoms are primarily those of a psychosis in the presence of a clear sensorium, they are handled like any other psychosis: hospitalization (in most cases) and adequate amounts of antipsychotic drugs.

Haloperidol, 5 mg orally twice a day for the first day or so, usually ameliorates symptoms quickly, and the drug can be decreased and discontinued over several days as the patient improves. It then becomes necessary to deal with the chronic alcohol abuse, which has been discussed.

2. Withdrawal symptoms–Withdrawal symptoms, ranging from a mild syndrome to the severe state usually called **delirium tremens,** are a medical problem with a significant morbidity and mortality rate. They usually occur when an intake of at least 7–8 pints of beer or 1 pint of spirits daily for several months has been stopped. The patient should be hospitalized and given adequate central nervous system depressants to counteract the excitability resulting from the sudden cessation of alcohol. Monitoring of vital signs and fluids and electrolyte levels is essential for the severely ill patient. Antipsychotic drugs such as chlorpromazine should *not* be used. The choice of the specific sedative is less important than using adequate amounts to bring the patient to a level of moderate sedation, and this will vary from person to person. A common regimen is to use diazepam, 10 mg intravenously initially and then 5 mg intravenously every 5 minutes until the patient is calm. Then give the drug orally in a dosage of 5–10 mg every 1–4 hours depending on the clinical need. After stabilization, the amount of diazepam required to maintain a sedated state may be given orally every 8–12 hours. If restlessness, tremulousness, and other signs of withdrawal persist, the dosage is increased until moderate sedation occurs. The dosage is then gradually reduced until withdrawal is complete. This usually requires a week or so of treatment. Clonidine, 5 μg/kg orally every 2 hours, suppresses cardiovascular signs of withdrawal and also has some anxiolytic effect.

Meticulous examination for other medical problems is necessary. Alcoholics commonly have liver disease and associated clotting problems and are also prone to injury—and the combination all too frequently leads to undiagnosed subdural hematoma.

Anticonvulsant drugs are not needed unless there is a history of seizures. In these situations, phenytoin can be given in a loading dose—500 mg orally and, several hours later, another 500 mg orally (ie, 1 g over 4–6 hours). This drug is then continued in a dosage of 300 mg daily, which is checked by serum drug level.

A general diet should be given, and vitamins in high doses: thiamine, 100 mg 3 times a day; pyridoxine, 100 mg/d; folic acid, 5 mg 3 times a day; and ascorbic acid, 100 mg twice a day. Intravenous glucose solutions should not be given prior to the vitamins. Concurrent administration is satisfactory, and hydration should be meticulously assessed on an ongoing basis. Magnesium levels often decline, and replacement by magnesium sulfate solution intravenously several times a day for several days is desirable.

Chronic brain syndromes secondary to a long history of alcohol intake are not responsive to any specific measures. Attention to the social and environmental care of this type of patient is paramount.

B. Psychologic and Behavioral Techniques:
The comments in the section on problem drinking apply here also; these methods of treatment become the primary consideration after the successful treatment of withdrawal or alcoholic hallucinosis. Psychologic and social measures should be initiated in the hospital shortly before discharge. This increases the possibility of continued posthospitalization treatment.

Crowley TJ: Alcoholism: Identification, evaluation and early treatment. *West J Med* 1984;**140**:461.

Gordis E, Dole VP, Ashley MJ: Regulation of alcohol consumption: Individual appetite and social policy. *Am J Med* 1983;**74**:322.

Hoffman NG, Harrison PA, Belille CA: Alcoholics Anonymous after treatment: Attendance and abstinence. *Int J Addict* 1983;**18**:311.

Keiter RH: Principles of disulfiram use. *Psychosomatics* 1983;**24**:483.

Schuckit MA: An evaluation of primary alcoholics with histories of violence. *J Clin Psychiatry* 1984;**45**:3.

Sherlock S: Alcohol and disease. *Br Med Bull* 1982;**8**:1. [Entire issue.]

West LJ et al: Alcoholism. *Ann Intern Med* 1984;**100**:405.

OTHER DRUG & SUBSTANCE DEPENDENCIES

Narcotics

The terms "opiates" and "narcotics" are used interchangeably and include a group of drugs with actions that mimic those of morphine. The group includes natural derivatives of opium, synthetic surrogates, and a number of polypeptides, some of which have been discovered to be natural neurotransmitters. The principal narcotic of abuse is heroin (metabolized to morphine), which is not used as a legitimate medication. The other common narcotics are prescription drugs and differ in milligram potency, duration of action, and agonist and antagonist capabilities (see Chapter 1). All of the narcotic analgesics can be reversed by the narcotic antagonist naloxone.

The clinical signs of mild narcotic intoxication include needle tracks; changes in mood, with feelings of euphoria; drowsiness; nausea with occasional emesis; and miosis. Overdosage causes respiratory depression, peripheral vasodilatation, pinpoint pupils, pulmonary edema, coma, and death.

Dependency is a major concern when continued use of narcotics occurs, although withdrawal causes only moderate morbidity (about the severity of a bout with the "flu"). Addicts sometimes consider themselves more addicted than they really are and may not require a withdrawal program. Grades of withdrawal are categorized from 0–4: grade 0 includes craving and anxiety; grade 1, yawning, lacrimation, rhinorrhea, and perspiration; grade 2, previous symptoms plus mydriasis, piloerection, anorexia, tremors, and hot and cold flashes with generalized aching; grades 3 and 4, increased intensity of previous symptoms and signs,

with increased temperature, blood pressure, pulse, and respiratory rate and depth. In withdrawal from the most severe addiction, vomiting, diarrhea, weight loss, hemoconcentration, and spontaneous ejaculation or orgasm commonly occur.

Treatment for overdosage (or suspected overdosage) is naloxone (Narcan), 0.4 mg intravenously. If an overdose has been taken, the results are dramatic and occur within 2 minutes. Effects of naloxone are quickly dissipated, and administration of the drug can be repeated at 5- to 10-minute intervals. Since the length of action of naloxone is much shorter than that of the narcotics, the patient must be under close observation. Hospitalization, supportive care, naloxone administration, and observation for withdrawal from other drugs should be maintained for as long as necessary. Complications include infections (eg, pneumonia, septic emboli, hepatitis), traumatic insults (eg, arterial spasm due to drug injection, gangrene), and pulmonary edema (50% of patients).

Treatment for withdrawal begins if grade 2 signs develop. If a withdrawal program is necessary, use methadone, 10 mg orally (use parenteral administration if the patient is vomiting), and observe. If signs (piloerection, mydriasis, cardiovascular changes) persist for more than 4–6 hours, give another 10 mg; continue to administer methadone at 4- to 6-hour intervals until signs are not present (rarely more than 40 mg of methadone in 24 hours). Divide the total amount of drug required over the first 24-hour period by 2 and give this dose every 12 hours. Each day, reduce the total 24-hour dose by 5–10 mg. Thus, a moderately addicted patient initially requiring 30–40 mg of methadone could be withdrawn over a 4-day period. Clonidine, 0.1 mg in several divided doses over a 10- to 14-day period, is an alternative to methadone detoxification; it is not necessary to taper the dose. Clonidine is helpful in alleviating cardiovascular symptoms but does not significantly relieve anxiety, insomnia, or generalized aching.

Methadone maintenance programs are of some value in chronic recidivism. Under carefully controlled supervision, the narcotic addict is maintained on fairly high doses of methadone (40–120 mg/d) that satisfy craving and block the effects of heroin to a great degree. Methadyl acetate is longer lasting and is replacing methadone in some programs. Abrupt withdrawal from methadyl acetate does not result in more severe withdrawal problems than gradual withdrawal. Narcotic antagonists (eg, naltrexone) can be used successfully if the drug can be given on a sufficiently frequent schedule. Treatment for both overdosage and withdrawal is medically straightforward but frustrating because of the many associated social problems.

Sedatives (Anxiolytics)

This group includes all of the so-called minor tranquilizers, antianxiety drugs, and sleeping medications (see Sedatives, p 643). The benzodiazepines, barbiturates, and assorted hypnotic agents (eg, Doriden, Quaalude) are the most commonly used sedatives. They can all produce dependency and resemble alcohol in their behavioral manifestations. They are all additive (mixed usage along with alcohol is common), with cross dependency. Thus, selective sedatives may be used to withdraw a patient from other sedative addiction.

Acute intoxication states are manifested by drowsiness, errors of commission (which may result in accidents), slowed speech and thinking, impaired memory, disinhibition, nystagmus, ataxia, dysarthria, and sleep.

Overdosage is characterized by respiratory depression, severe hypotension, decreased gastrointestinal activity, stupor, shock syndrome, coma, and death.

Manifestations of withdrawal vary, depending on the nature of the sedative and the degree of dependency (the latter a function of dosage and length of dependency). Usually, withdrawal is more severe in the short-acting barbiturates and milder in the long-acting benzodiazepines. The signs and symptoms range from mild restlessness to death. In a patient strongly dependent (> 1000 mg/d) on short-acting barbiturates, manifestations include restlessness, anxiety (12–16 hours), intolerance to loud noise and bright lights, seizures, muscular weakness, and orthostatic hypotension (16–36 hours). Delirium is occasionally present, accompanied by visual hallucinations, disorientation, and paranoid ideation; this may last up to 1 week. The longer-acting sedatives have a longer withdrawal pattern, and the symptoms tend to be milder.

Complications of sedative abuse include pneumonia, septicemia with injected drugs, bullous cutaneous lesions with barbiturates, renal failure secondary to muscle necrosis in overdoses, peripheral neuropathies related to extended time in pressure positions during coma, and the results of associated trauma.

Treatment of overdoses (see p 1007) and withdrawal states are medical emergencies. Unlike withdrawal from narcotics, which is relatively benign, sedative withdrawal is as dangerous as alcohol withdrawal and is treated in the same manner. Treatment of sedative dependency is also handled in much the same way as treatment of alcohol dependency. Recognition of the problem and use of supporting treatment organizations are most important.

Psychedelics

About 6000 species of plants have psychoactive properties. All of the common psychedelics (LSD, mescaline, psilocybin, dimethyltryptamine, and other derivatives of phenylalanine and tryptophan) produce similar behavioral and physiologic effects. An initial feeling of tension is followed by emotional release such as crying or laughing (1–2 hours). Later, perceptual distortions occur, with visual illusions and hallucinations, and occasionally there is fear of ego disintegration (2–3 hours). Major changes in time sense and mood lability then occur (3–4 hours). A feeling of detachment and a sense of destiny and control occur (4–6 hours). Of course, reactions vary among individ-

uals, and some of the current street drugs such as phencyclidine ("angel dust," PCP, Sernyl) produce markedly different time frames. Occasionally, the acute episode is terrifying (a "bad trip") and may not remit for long periods of time. The attitude of the user and the setting where the drug is used affect the experience. Most of the street drugs peddled as mescaline, LSD, and THC are really phencyclidine, the use of which has reached epidemic proportions (see below). Psychedelic usage in women during the first trimester of pregnancy is connected with an increased incidence of spontaneous abortion and congenital defects.

Treatment of the acute episode primarily involves protection of the individual from erratic behavior that may lead to injury or death. A structured environment is usually sufficient until the drug is metabolized. In severe cases, antipsychotic drugs with minimal side effects (eg, haloperidol, 5 mg intramuscularly) may be given every several hours until the individual has regained control. In cases where "flashbacks" occur (mental imagery from a "bad trip" that is later triggered by mild stimuli such as marihuana, alcohol, or psychic trauma), a short course of an antipsychotic drug (eg, trifluoperazine, 5 mg orally) for several days is sufficient.

Phencyclidine

Phencyclidine (PCP, angel dust, peace pill, hog, Sernyl), developed as an anesthetic agent in veterinary practice, first appeared as a street drug deceptively sold as tetrahydrocannabinol (THC). Because it is simple to produce and mimics to some degree the traditional psychedelic drugs, it has become a common deceptive substitute for LSD and mescaline. It is available in crystals, capsules, and tablets to be inhaled, injected, swallowed, or smoked (it is commonly sprinkled on marihuana).

Absorption after smoking is rapid, with onset of symptoms in several minutes and peak symptoms in 15–30 minutes. Mild intoxication produces a euphoria accompanied by a feeling of numbness. Moderate intoxication (5–10 mg) results in disorientation, detachment from surroundings, distortion of body image, combativeness, unusual feats of strength, and loss of ability to integrate sensory input, especially touch and proprioception. Physical symptoms include dizziness, ataxia, dysarthria, nystagmus, hyperreflexia, and tachycardia. There are increases in blood pressure, respiration, muscle tone, and urine production. Severe intoxication (20 mg or more) produces an increase in degree of moderate symptoms, with the addition of seizures, deepening coma, hypertensive crisis, and severe psychotic ideation. The drug is particularly long lasting (several days to several weeks) owing to high lipid solubility, gastroenteric recycling, and the production of active metabolites. Overdosage may be directly fatal, with the major causes of death being hypertensive crisis, respiratory arrest, and convulsions. Acute rhabdomyolysis has been reported and can result in myoglobinuric renal failure.

Differential diagnosis involves the whole spectrum of street drugs, since in some ways phencyclidine mimics sedatives, psychedelics, and marihuana in its effects.

Treatment is discussed on p 1014.

Marihuana

Cannabis sativa, a hemp plant, is the source of marihuana. The parts of the plant vary in potency. The resinous exudate of the flowering tops of the female plant (hashish, charas) is the most potent, followed by the dried leaves and flowering shoots of the female plant (bhang) and the resinous mass from small leaves of inflorescence (ganja). The least potent parts are the lower branches and the leaves of the female plant and all parts of the male plant. The drug is usually inhaled by smoking. Effects occur in 10–20 minutes and last 2–3 hours. "Joints" of good quality contain about 500 mg of marihuana (which contains approximately 5–10 mg of tetrahydrocannabinol with a half-life of 7 days). Some new hybrids and varieties contain up to 13% tetrahydrocannabinol. The user and the setting, as in psychedelic use, are important factors in the effect of the drug.

With moderate dosage, marihuana produces 2 phases: mild euphoria followed by sleepiness. In the acute state, the user has an altered time perception, less inhibited emotions, impaired immediate memory, and conjunctival infection. High doses produce transient psychotomimetic effects. No specific treatment is necessary except in the case of the occasional "bad trip," in which case the person is treated in the same way as for psychedelic usage. Marihuana frequently aggravates existing mental illness and slows the learning process in children.

Studies of long-term effects have conclusively shown abnormalities in the pulmonary tree. Laryngitis and rhinitis are related to prolonged use, along with chronic obstructive pulmonary disease. Electrocardiographic abnormalities are common, but no long-term cardiac disease has been linked to marihuana use. Chronic usage has resulted in depression of plasma testosterone levels and reduced sperm counts. Abnormal menstruation and failure to ovulate have occurred in some female users. Psychologic effects of chronic marihuana usage are still unclear.

Stimulants

The abuse of stimulants has increased markedly since World War II, partly because of the proliferation of drugs marketed for weight reduction. The **amphetamines,** including methedrine ("speed"), methylphenidate, and phenmetrazine, are gradually being placed under control, but street availability remains high. Moderate usage of any of the stimulants produces hyperactivity, a sense of enhanced physical and mental capacity, and sympathomimetic effects. Tolerance develops quickly and, as the dosage is increased, paranoid ideation (with delusions of parasitosis), stereotypy, bruxism, and full-blown psychoses occur.

People who have used stimulants chronically (eg, anorexigenics) occasionally become sensitized to future use of stimulants. In these individuals, even small amounts of mild stimulants such as caffeine can cause symptoms of paranoia and auditory hallucinations. The clinical picture of acute stimulant intoxication includes sweating, tachycardia, elevated blood pressure, mydriasis, hyperactivity, and an acute brain syndrome with confusion and disorientation.

Cocaine is a stimulant, not a narcotic. Its use has been steadily increasing in recent years. Cocaine has generally been used by snorting (complications include septal ulceration) or by injecting intravenously. The latter produces marked euphoria but is more toxic and has the problems associated with parenteral use of any street drug. Recently, coca (the first extraction product in the preparation of cocaine) has been increasingly used, mostly because it is much cheaper than cocaine. Usage of the free base form of cocaine, which is prepared by the consumer by alkalinization and solvent extraction, has increased. The free base form produces a powerful high lasting several minutes and many associated problems, including wide mood swings, a marked craving for more cocaine, paranoia, and, possibly, lung damage caused by the vasoconstrictive action of the drug. The rare person with plasma pseudocholinesterase deficiency is particularly susceptible to small doses of cocaine. Overdoses may cause cardiac arrest, fatal hyperpyrexia, or exacerbation of angina symptoms.

The stimulants may be discontinued abruptly (unlike sedatives), and the withdrawal usually results in sleep disturbances, lassitude, hyperphagia, and depression (sometimes with suicidal ideation) lasting several days to several weeks. Occasionally, an abstinence syndrome develops consisting of delirium, sleeplessness, and increased motor activity. It may arise 3–10 days after cessation of amphetamines. A short course of moderate doses of antipsychotics constitutes effective treatment in psychoses due to stimulants.

Caffeine

The most popular mind-affecting drugs are caffeine, nicotine, and alcohol. Some 10 billion pounds of coffee (the richest source of caffeine) are consumed yearly throughout the world. Tea, cocoa, and cola drinks also contribute to an intake of caffeine that is often astoundingly high in a large number of people. The content of caffeine in a (180-mL) cup of beverage is as follows: brewed coffee, 80–140 mg; instant coffee, 60–100 mg; decaffeinated coffee, 1–6 mg; leaf tea, 30–80 mg; tea bags, 25–75 mg; instant tea, 30–60 mg; cocoa, 10–50 mg; and 12-oz cola drinks, 30–65 mg. Sunkist orange drink is the only noncola drink to contain significant amounts of caffeine. A 1-oz chocolate candy bar has about 20 mg. Caffeine-containing analgesics usually contain approximately 30 mg per unit, exceptions being Excedrin, with 60 mg, and Cafergot, with 100 mg. Symptoms of caffeinism include anxiety, agitation, restlessness, insomnia, a feeling of being "wired," and somatic symptoms referable to the heart and gastrointestinal tract. It is common for a case of caffeinism to present as an anxiety disorder. It is also common for caffeine and other stimulants to precipitate severe symptoms in compensated schizophrenic and manic-depressive patients. Chronically depressed patients often use caffeine drinks as self-medication. This diagnostic clue may help distinguish some major affective disorders. A number of patients with these disorders respond well to monoamine oxidase inhibitors. Withdrawal from caffeine (more than 500 mg/d) can produce headaches, irritability, and occasional nausea.

Miscellaneous Drugs & Solvents

The principal over-the-counter drugs of concern are phenylpropanolamine and an assortment of antihistaminic agents. Frequently, these drugs are sold in combination as cold remedies (eg, Contac, Dristan, Triaminic). Not infrequently, a mild analgesic is added to the preparation. Most appetite suppressant drugs are combinations of phenylpropanolamine and caffeine; these drugs are also heavily marketed as "stay-awake" drugs. Practically all of the so-called sleep aids are now antihistamines. Scopolamine and bromides have generally been removed from the over-the-counter market.

The major problem in the use of all these drugs relates to phenylpropanolamine, which has all the side effects of any stimulant, including precipitation of anxiety states, auditory and visual hallucinations, paranoid ideation, and, occasionally, delirium. Aggressiveness and some loss of impulse control have been reported. Sleep disturbances are common even with reasonably small doses.

Antihistamines usually produce some central nervous system depression—thus their use as over-the-counter sedatives. Drowsiness is usually a problem only with the operation of machinery. Antihistamine intoxication can produce excitement. The mixture of antihistamines with alcohol usually exacerbates the central nervous system effects.

The abuse of laxatives sometimes can lead to electrolyte disturbances that may contribute to the manifestations of an organic brain syndrome. The greatest use of laxatives tends to be in the elderly, who are most vulnerable to physiologic changes.

Many of the so-called street drugs are strong anticholinergics. For this reason, sedating phenothiazines should generally not be used, and physostigmine may be considered when the clinical signs of atropinism are present.

Amyl nitrite, a drug useful in angina pectoris, has been used in recent years as an "orgasm expander." The changes in time perception caused by the drug prompted its nonmedical use, and popular lore concerning the effects of inhalation just prior to orgasm has led to increased use. Tolerance develops readily, but there are no known withdrawal symptoms. Abstinence for several days reestablishes the previous level of responsiveness. Long-term effects are unknown.

Sniffing of solvents and inhaling of gases (including aerosols) produce a form of inebriation similar to that of the volatile anesthetics. Agents include gasoline, toluene, petroleum ether, lighter fluids, cleaning fluids, paint thinners, and nail polish. Typical intoxication states include euphoria, slurred speech, and confusion, and with high doses, acute manifestations are unconsciousness and cardiorespiratory depression or failure; chronic exposure produces a variety of symptoms related to the liver, kidney, or bone marrow. Lead encephalopathy can be associated with sniffing leaded gasoline. In addition, studies of workers chronically exposed to jet fuel showed significant increases in neurasthenic symptoms, including fatigue, anxiety, mood changes, memory difficulties, and somatic complaints. These same problems have been noted in long-term solvent abuse.

AMA Council on Scientific Affairs: Marijuana: Its health hazards and therapeutic potentials. *JAMA* 1981;**246**:1823.

Cornelius JR, Soloff PH, Reynolds CF: Paranoia, homicidal behavior, and seizures associated with phenylpropanolamine. *Am J Psychiatry* 1984;**141**:120.

Curatolo PW, Robertson D: The health consequences of caffeine. *Ann Intern Med* 1983;**98**:641.

Dole VP: Performance-based rating of methadone maintenance programs. *N Engl J Med* 1982;**306**:169.

Gardner ER, Hall RCN: Psychiatric symptoms produced by over-the-counter drugs. *Psychosomatics* 1982;**23**:186.

Halikas JA et al: Regular marijuana use and its effect on psychosocial variables. *Compr Psychiatry* 1983;**24**:229.

Hollister L: Drugs of abuse. Chap 30, pp 353–364, in Katzung BG (editor): *Basic & Clinical Pharmacology*, 2nd ed. Lange, 1984.

Judson BA, Goldstein A, Inturrisi CE: Methadyl acetate (LAAM) in the treatment of heroin addicts. 2. Double-blind comparison of gradual and abrupt detoxification. *Arch Gen Psychiatry* 1983;**40**:834.

McCarron MM et al: Short-acting barbiturate overdosage. *JAMA* 1982;**248**:55.

McLellan AT et al: Is treatment for substance abuse effective? *JAMA* 1982;**247**:1423.

Nichols AM: The inhalants: An overview. *Psychosomatics* 1983;**24**:914.

Sato M et al: Exacerbation of paranoid psychotic state after long-term abstinence in patients with previous methamphetamine psychosis. *Biol Psychiatry* 1983;**18**:429.

Stern TA, Mulley AG, Thibault GE: Life-threatening drug overdose: Precipitants and prognosis. *JAMA* 1984;**251**:1983.

Van Dyke C, Byck R: Cocaine. *Sci Am* (March) 1982;**246**:128.

ORGANIC MENTAL DISORDERS
(Organic Brain Syndrome [OBS])

Essentials of Diagnosis

- Cognitive impairment: disorientation, defective sensation and perception, impairment of capacity for recall and recent memory, impaired thinking and logical reasoning.
- Emotional disturbances: depression, shame, anxiety, irritability.
- Behavioral disturbances: decreased impulse control, exhibitionism, sexual acting-out, aggression.

- History or findings to indicate one or more of the etiologic factors listed below.

General Considerations

The organic problem may be a primary brain disease or a secondary manifestation of some general disorder, including central nervous system syphilis.

All of the brain syndromes show some degree of cognitive impairment depending on the site of involvement, the rate of onset and progression, and the duration of the underlying brain lesion. Emotional disturbances are often inversely proportionate to the severity of the cognitive disorder. The behavioral disturbances tend to be more common with chronicity, more directly related to the underlying personality, and not necessarily correlated with cognitive dysfunction.

Etiology

A. Intoxications: Alcohol, sedatives, bromides, anticholinergic drugs, antidepressants, analgesics (eg, pentazocine), pollutants, chronic salicylate use, solvents, a wide variety of over-the-counter and prescribed drugs (see Psychiatric Complications of Nonpsychiatric Drugs, p 684), and household, agricultural, and industrial chemicals.

B. Drug Withdrawal: Alcohol, sedative-hypnotics, and corticosteroids.

C. Long-Term Effects of Alcohol: Wernicke-Korsakoff syndrome.

D. Infections: Septicemia; meningitis and encephalitis due to bacterial, viral, fungal and tuberculosis organisms; and central nervous system syphilis. Acute and chronic infections due to the entire range of microbiologic pathogens, including syphilis.

E. Endocrine: Thyrotoxicosis, hypothyroidism, adrenocortical dysfunction (including Addison's disease and Cushing's syndrome), pheochromocytoma, insulinoma, insulin overdose, hyperparathyroidism, hypoparathyroidism, and panhypopituitarism.

F. Respiratory: Hypoxia, hypocapnia, any imbalance in respiratory exchange.

G. Metabolic Disturbances: Fluid and electrolyte, acid-base, hepatic disease (hepatic encephalopathy, Wilson's disease), renal failure, porphyria.

H. Nutritional Deficiencies: Vitamin B_1 (beriberi), vitamin B_{12} (pernicious anemia), nicotinic acid (pellagra), protein-calorie malnutrition.

I. Trauma: Subdural hematoma, subarachnoid hemorrhage, intracerebral bleeding, concussion syndrome.

J. Cardiovascular Disorders: Cardiac infarctions, arrhythmias, cerebrovascular spasms, hemorrhage, embolism, and occlusions.

K. Neoplasms: Primary or metastatic lesions of the central nervous system, cancer-induced hypercalcemia.

L. Idiopathic Epilepsy: Grand mal and postictal, temporal lobe dysfunction.

M. Collagen and Immunologic Disorders: Systemic lupus erythematosus.

N. Degenerative Diseases: Alzheimer's disease, Pick's disease, multiple sclerosis, parkinsonism, Huntington's chorea, and normal pressure hydrocephalus.

O. Miscellaneous: Tourette's syndrome.

Clinical Findings

The manifestations are many and varied and include problems with orientation, short or fluctuating attention span, loss of recent memory and recall, impaired judgment, emotional lability, lack of initiative, impaired impulse control, inability to reason through problems, depression (worse in mild to moderate types), confabulation (not limited to alcohol organic brain syndrome), constriction of intellectual functions, visual hallucinations, and delusions. Physical findings will naturally vary according to the cause. The electroencephalogram is often abnormal. The so-called catastrophic reaction occurs when the patient realizes the deficit and reacts with anger and denial.

A. Delirium: Delirium is a disorder of attention. Onset is usually rapid. The mental status fluctuates (impairment is usually least in the morning), with varying inability to concentrate, maintain attention, and sustain purposeful behavior. There is a marked deficit of short-term memory and recall. Amnesia is retrograde (impaired recall of past memories) and anterograde (inability to recall events after the onset of the delirium). Orientation problems follow the inability to retain information. Perceptual disturbances (often visual hallucinations) and psychomotor restlessness with insomnia are common. Autonomic changes include tachycardia, dilated pupils, and sweating. The average duration is about 1 week, with full recovery in most cases.

B. Dementia: Dementia is characterized by chronicity and deterioration in all mental functions. It is usually progressive, more common in the elderly (although not an inevitable sign of aging), and rarely reversible even if underlying disease can be corrected. Memory failure is severe, with retrograde and anterograde amnesia (more remote events tend to be best preserved). Loss of intellectual abilities and impairment of abstract thinking, along with personality disintegration, tend to markedly impair social and occupational function. Loss of impulse control (sexual and language) is common. The tenuous level of function makes the individual most susceptible to minor physical and psychologic stresses. The course depends on the underlying cause, and the general trend is steady deterioration.

There are 3 types of dementia: (1) primary degenerative dementia, accounting for about 50% of cases; (2) atherosclerotic dementia, 15–20% of cases; and (3) mixtures of the first 2 types, 15–20% of cases (see also Chapter 2). Examples of primary degenerative dementia are Alzheimer's dementia (most common) and Pick, Parkinson, Creutzfeldt-Jacob, and Huntington dementias (less common). Alzheimer's dementia has a slow onset and tends to occur after 40 years of age. It is associated with a relative cholinergic deficiency, principally of choline acetyltransferase. The diagnosis can be established clinically only by exclusion of other known organic causes of dementia. At present, the definitive diagnosis can be established only on the basis of characteristic pathologic findings on postmortem examination. The symptoms of all types of early dementia include recent memory defects, multiple somatic and psychologic complaints, a muddled history, and easily precipitated delirium.

Pseudodementia is a term applied to depressed patients who appear to be demented. It is occasionally used to include other reversible conditions that mimic dementia (eg, mass lesions, effects of medication). Depression should be considered in every apparent case of dementia. (See Table 18–9.)

C. Amnestic Syndrome: This is a short-term memory disturbance without delirium or dementia. It is usually associated with thiamine deficiency and chronic alcohol use. It impairs selective areas of cognitive functioning. The onset is usually sudden, but the course is usually chronic.

D. Organic Hallucinosis: This condition is characterized by persistent or recurrent hallucinations (usually auditory) without the other symptoms usually found in delirium or dementia. Alcohol or hallucinogens are often the cause, and some people seem to be particularly susceptible to stimulants. There does not have to be any other mental disorder, and there may be complete spontaneous resolution.

E. Organic Personality Syndrome: This syndrome is characterized by emotional lability and loss of impulse control along with a general change in personality. Social inappropriateness is common. Loss of interest and lack of concern with the consequences of one's actions are often present. The individual does not have symptoms referable to other conditions such as delirium or dementia. The course depends on the underlying cause (eg, frontal lobe contusion may resolve completely).

Differential Diagnosis

Patients with nonorganic ("functional") psy-

choses often remain oriented; the onset is usually gradual; hallucinations are usually auditory rather than visual; and intellectual functions are relatively intact, with good memory and a normal electroencephalogram and no demonstrable organic disease. The differentiation of pseudodementia and dementia are categorized in Table 18–9.

Complications

Chronicity is sometimes a function of early nonreversal, eg, subdural hematoma, low-pressure hydrocephalus. Prompt correction of reversible causes improves recovery of mental function. Accidents secondary to impulsive behavior and poor judgment are a major consideration. Secondary depression and impulsive behavior not infrequently lead to suicide attempts. Drugs, particularly sedatives, may worsen thinking abilities and contribute to the overall problems.

Treatment

A. Medical: Provide a pleasant, comfortable, nonthreatening, and physically safe environment with adequate nursing or attendant services. *Correct underlying medical problems.* Do not overlook any possibility of reversible organic disease. The CT scan, with its noninvasive diagnostic capabilities, has helped immeasurably. Give antipsychotics in small doses at first (eg, thioridazine, 25 mg orally at bedtime) and increase according to the need to reduce psychotic ideation or excessive irritability. Aggressiveness and rage states in central nervous system lesions can be reduced with propranolol, 320–520 mg/d. Bedtime administration obviates the need for sedatives, which often worsen organic brain syndrome.

Cerebral vasodilators were originally used on the assumption that cerebral arteriosclerosis and ischemia were the principal causes of the dementias. Although there is a slight reduction of blood flow in primary degenerative dementia (probably as a result of the basic disorder), there is no evidence that this is a major factor in this group of disorders or that vasodilators are of value. Ergotoxine alkaloids (Hydergine) have been studied, with mixed results; improvement in ambulatory self-care and depressed mood has been noted, but there has been no improvement of cognitive functioning on any standardized tests. Hyperbaric oxygen treatment has not produced significant improvement. Drugs having a stimulatory effect, such as methylphenidate, may cause affective improvement without a change in cognitive function. Physostigmine has shown some promise in improving memory function in Alzheimer's disease. The affective improvement can benefit the patient and family by providing some improvement in the quality of life. Numerous investigational drugs have been used, but there is no clear-cut evidence of benefit.

Failing sensory functions should be supported as necessary, with hearing aids, cataract surgery, etc.

B. Social: Substitute home care, board care, or convalescent home care may be most useful when the family is unable to care for the patient. The setting

Table 18–9. Differentiation of pseudodementia and dementia.

Pseudodementia	Dementia
Rapid onset	Slow onset
Rapid progress	Usually slow course
Early loss of social skills	Social skills retained for a long time
Patient emphasizes disability	Patient conceals disability
Complaints of memory loss	Few complaints
Recent and remote memory equally affected	Loss of recent memory
More often previous psychiatric history	No previous psychiatric history
Vegetative symptoms common	Fewer vegetative symptoms
Inconsistency on examination	Consistent manifest deficiencies
Same problems night and day	Worse at night

should include familiar people and objects, lights at night, and a simple schedule. Family counseling may help the family to cope with problems that may occur and may help keep the patient at home as long as possible. Volunteer services, including homemakers, visiting nurse, and adult protective services may be required if the patient is left at home.

C. Behavioral: Behavioral techniques include operant responses that can be used to induce positive behaviors, eg, paying attention to the patient who is trying to communicate appropriately, and extinction by ignoring inappropriate responses.

D. Psychologic: Formal psychologic therapies are not usually helpful and may make things worse by taxing the patient's limited cognitive resources.

Prognosis

The prognosis is good in acute (reversible) cases, fair in moderate cases, and poor in deteriorated states.

Blass JP, Weksler ME: Toward an effective treatment of Alzheimer's disease. *Ann Intern Med* 1983;**98**:251.

Coyle JT, Price DL, DeLong MR: Alzheimer's disease: A disorder of cortical cholinergic innervation. *Science* 1983;**219**:1184.

Dubin WR et al: Organic brain syndrome: The psychiatric imposter. *JAMA* 1983;**249**:60.

Hollister LE, Yesavage J: Ergoloid mesylates for senile dementias: Unanswered questions. *Ann Intern Med* 1984;**100**:894.

McAllister TW: Overview: Pseudodementia. *Am J Psychiatry* 1983;**140**:528.

Seltzer B, Sherwin I: A comparison of clinical features in early- and late-onset primary degenerative dementia. *Arch Neurol* 1983;**40**:143.

GERIATRIC PSYCHIATRIC DISORDERS
(See also Chapter 2.)

Essentials of Diagnosis

- Some degree of organic brain syndrome often present.
- Depression, paranoid ideation, and easy irritability are common.
- High frequency of medical problems.
- Patient is frequently worsened by a wide variety of medications.
- Fear of death is often a major factor.

General Considerations

There are 3 basic factors in the process of aging: biologic, sociologic, and psychologic.

The complex **biologic** changes depend on inherited characteristics (the best guarantee of long life is to have long-lived parents), nutrition, declining sensory functions such as hearing or vision, disease, trauma, and life-style. As a person ages, the central nervous system becomes less hardy, and relatively minor disorders or combinations of disorders may cause deficits in cognition and affective response. Hypochondriasis is frequently a mechanism of compensating for de-

creased function. A definite correlation between hearing loss and paranoid ideation exists in the elderly. (See Organic Brain Syndrome, p 676).

The **sociologic** factors derive from stresses connected with occupation, family, and community. Any or all of these areas may be disrupted in a general phenomenon of "disengagement" that older people experience as friends die, the children move away, and the surroundings become less familiar. Retirement commonly precipitates a major disruption in a well-established life structure. This is particularly stressful in the person whose compulsive devotion to a job has precluded other interests, so that sudden loss of this outlet leaves a void that is not easily filled.

The **psychologic** withdrawal of the elderly person is independent of the cultural rejection (the USA tends to be a youth-oriented society). It is frequently related to a loss of self-esteem, which is based on the economic insecurity of older age with its congruent loss of independence, the realization of decreasing physical and mental ability, and the fear of approaching death. The process of aging is often poorly accepted, and the real or imagined loss of physical attractiveness may have a traumatic impact that the plastic surgeon can only soften for a time. In a culture that stresses physical and sexual attractiveness, it is difficult for most people to accept the change. Sexual problems tend to be overlooked, since the elderly person is frequently embarrassed to raise questions about them.

Clinical Findings & Complications

The most common psychiatric syndrome in the elderly is organic brain syndrome of varying degree (see Chapter 2). Psychotic ideation (usually paranoid) may coexist with the organic brain syndrome. Frequently, in the milder cases, the individual is aware of the deficiency in sensorium and becomes depressed about actual or threatened loss of function. Depression becomes the most obvious symptom. Unless the examination is done with great care, the organic brain syndrome is missed and the patient is treated for the secondary symptom of depression without evaluation of the organic problem. Anxiety is often associated with organic illness. In organic brain syndrome, anxiety heightens preexisting confusion.

Depression in the absence of a brain syndrome is frequently manifested in the elderly as a somatic complaint without the overt signs of depression (see Affective Disorders, p 663). Night awakenings are common in depression in the elderly person. This is often diagnosed as hypochondriasis, which is also more frequent in older people (eg, preoccupation with bowel function). This leads to a high usage of over-the-counter drugs. The increased and varied complaints are often an attempt to compensate and divert attention from decreased mental function. Overt depression is often related to life exigencies (80% of people over age 65 have some kind of medical problem). Alcoholism is present in approximately 15% of older patients presenting with psychiatric symptoms. The incidence of suicide is higher in elderly people—loneliness, age, and medical problems being directly related to the higher number of successful suicides. Because of somatic complaints hiding a "masked depression," it is necessary to be alert to suicidal ideation in this group. Direct questioning about suicidal intent is always warranted when any suspicion exists.

Treatment

A. Social: Socialization, a structured schedule of activities, familiar surroundings, continued achievement, and avoidance of loneliness (probably the most important factor) are some of the major considerations in prevention and amelioration of the psychiatric problems of older age. Whenever possible, the patient should remain in a familiar setting or return to one for as long as possible. An inexorable downhill trend frequently follows dislocation, with the accompanying disengagement from adaptable activities. The patient can be supported in the primary environment by various agencies that can help avoid a premature change of habits. For patients with disabilities that make it difficult to cope with the problems of living alone, homemaker services can assist in continuing the day-to-day activities of the household; visiting nurses can administer medications and monitor the physical condition of the patient; and geriatric social groups can help maintain socialization and human contacts. In the hospital, attention to the kinds of people placed in the same room is most important. All too often, the 4-bed ward is peopled by 4 withdrawn, nonfunctioning people who provide no stimulation for each other, and the resultant isolation increases the degree of depression; occasionally, a florid psychosis develops. Attention to the proper mixture of active and inactive people can help relieve the loneliness that so often pervades such wards.

B. Medical: Treatment of any reversible components of an organic brain syndrome is obviously the major medical consideration. One commonly overlooked factor is self-medication, frequently with over-the-counter drugs that further impair the patient's already precarious functioning. Frequent culprits are antihistamines and anticholinergic drugs.

Any signs of psychosis, such as paranoid ideation and delusions, respond very well to *small amounts* of antipsychotics. Trifluoperazine, 2–5 mg orally once a day, or fluphenazine, 1–2 mg orally daily, will usually decrease psychotic ideation markedly. Associated agitation is usually ameliorated. The use of long-acting fluphenazine for acute paranoid ideation or agitation is appropriate if it is used initially in low dosage (2.5–5 mg) every week to 10 days with close attention to the possibility of extrapyramidal side effects, which are more frequent in the geriatric population.

The astute use of the antipsychotics can often maintain the older person in the home environment and delay the traumatic dislocation that usually worsens the patient's condition. Because of sensitivity to anticholinergic effects, avoid nonpiperazine phenothiazines and unnecessary antiparkinsonism drugs. Seda-

tives frequently have a worsening effect and should generally be avoided. All psychoactive drugs have a higher incidence of side effects and are metabolized and excreted more slowly in the elderly. Antidepressants are used when indicated in depression. Trazodone is particularly useful, since anticholinergic side effects tend to be fewer than with other antidepressants. When sedatives are to be used, consider oxazepam or lorazepam, since they have no active metabolites and thus have a shorter half-life. Infrequently, a stimulant in small doses (eg, methylphenidate, 5–10 mg orally daily) can be used to treat apathy. The stimulant may help increase the patient's energy for social involvement and help the patient to maintain life activities. Lithium is helpful in the treatment of severe mood swings but has a narrow margin of neurotoxicity in the elderly. The appropriate use of wine and beer for mild sedative effects is quite rewarding in the hospital and other care facilities as well as at home. Attention must be given to possible abuses.

C. Behavioral: The impaired cognitive abilities of the geriatric patient necessitate simple behavioral techniques. Positive responses to appropriate behavior encourage the patient to repeat desirable kinds of behavior, and frequent repetition offsets to some degree the defects in recent memory and recall. It also results in participation—a most important element, since there is a tendency in the older population to withdraw, thus increasing isolation and functional decline.

One must be careful not to reinforce and encourage obstreperous behavior by responding to it; in this way, extinction or at least gradual reduction of inappropriate behavior will occur. At the same time, the obstreperous behavior often represents a nondirective response to frustration and inability to function, and a structured program of activity is necessary.

D. Psychologic: Patients may require help in adjusting to changing roles and commitments and in finding new goals and viewpoints. The older person steadily loses an important commodity—the future—and may attempt to compensate for this by preoccupation with the past. Involvement with the present and psychotherapy on a here and now basis can help make the adjustment easier.

Ban T: Chronic disease and depression in the geriatric population. *J Clin Psychiatry* 1984;**45(Section 2)**:18.

Beck JC et al: Dementia in the elderly: The silent epidemic. *Ann Intern Med* 1982;**97**:231.

Blazer DG: Impact of late-life depression on the social network. *Am J Psychiatry* 1983;**140**:162.

Cutler NR et al: Brain imaging: Aging and dementia. *Ann Intern Med* 1984;**101**:355.

O'Malley TA et al: Identifying and preventing family-mediated abuse and neglect of elderly persons. *Ann Intern Med* 1983;**98**:998.

Salzman C et al: Long vs short half-life benzodiazepines in the elderly. *Arch Gen Psychiatry* 1983;**40**:293.

Thompson TL, Moran MG, Nies AS: Psychotropic drug use in the elderly. (2 parts.) *N Engl J Med* 1983;**308**:134, 194.

DEATH & DYING

As Thomas Browne said, "The long habit of living indisposeth us for dying." It is only when death comes close to us that we really begin to respond to the possibility of our own death.

Death means different things to different people. For some it may represent an escape from unbearable suffering or other difficulties; for others, entrance into a new transcendental life. Death may come as a narcissistic attempt to find lasting fame or importance in martyrdom or heroic adventure, or it may be an atonement for real or imagined guilt or a means of extorting from others posthumously the affection that was not forthcoming during life.

Often the process is more shattering to those whose charge it is to maintain life, and there is a good deal of question about the so-called agony of death. Some observers, including Sir William Osler, take the view that there is no such thing, and the experiences of people who have been resuscitated from cardiac standstill seem to substantiate his view. They describe a sensation of detachment, a final peaceful "letting go"; and one is at times impressed with the fact that the dying patient resents any interference with the process by physicians and nurses.

How each individual responds to imminent death is a function not only of what death means to that person but also of the mechanisms used to deal with problems—and these are usually the same as those used throughout life. Patients frequently worry more about *how* they will die than about death itself. Responses frequently seen in the dying patient include denial, anger, bargaining, depression, and acceptance—stages that are seen in many people as they go through any significant flux or loss. Seldom are these stages seen in isolation, and the complexity of the process contributes to the juxtaposition of the stages and the noted lability of mood and attitude in the dying patient.

An ill person may at first deny any concern with dying and then later admit to a fear of going to sleep because of the possibility of not waking up. This is often demonstrated by a need to keep the light on and to call frequently during the night with minor complaints. Some find it necessary to deny impending death to the end. Their families and doctors will often join in the conspiracy of denial, either out of sympathy or for their own reasons. It is important not to force the patient to realize the truth but to allow the opportunity, *when the patient is ready,* to discuss and deal with the problem of impending death. Frank discussion can mitigate the terror some patients feel. For many it is a comfort to be actively involved in the process of dying, sharing in the anticipation of death, and making whatever plans may be important. Alleviation of pain is a primary concern of many patients. The physician should not be concerned about addiction to narcotics when treating a dying patient.

The reactions of the family are often a combination of pain, anger, sadness, and depression. They react to each other and to the personnel caring for the patient. The problem to be resolved with the survivors is the guilt feelings they may have—that they continue to exist while the other person has died. Also to be reconciled are the vague sense of being responsible for the death and the subconscious refusal to believe that the person is really dead. The staff must be careful not to alienate the family, because this can result in less than optimum care. Some emotional investment in the patient by the staff is proper and inevitable, but it must be handled with insight and professional restraint. An insecure staff member may respond to a patient's death as if it were a professional failure. If the emotional investment is too little, the staff member may seem to be aloof and insensitive, while overconcern may lead to depression and despair, further impairing the person's capacity to serve as a source of support for the patient and the family in a time of distress.

The physician and staff must be aware of their own anxieties; maintain an appropriate level of involvement (a change of physicians may be necessary when this is impossible); allow for free and ongoing communication between patient, physician, and family; and share as a group—staff and family—the impending and unavoidable loss.

Bayer R et al: The care of the terminally ill: Mortality and economics. *N Engl J Med* 1983;**309**:1490.

Friel PB: Death and dying. *Ann Intern Med* 1982;**97**:767.

Hilfiker D: Allowing the debilitated to die: Facing our ethical choices. *N Engl J Med* 1983;**308**:716.

Lewis JM: Dying with friends: Implications for the psychotherapist. *Am J Psychiatry* 1982;**139**:261.

PSYCHIATRIC PROBLEMS ASSOCIATED WITH MEDICAL & SURGICAL DISORDERS

Essentials of Diagnosis

Acute problems:

- Psychotic organic brain syndrome secondary to the medical or surgical problem, or the effect of the environment (eg, intensive care unit).
- Acute anxiety, often related to ignorance and fear of the immediate problem as well as uncertainty about the future.
- Anxiety as an intrinsic aspect of the medical problem (eg, hyperthyroidism).

Intermediate problems:

- Depression as a function of the illness or acceptance of the illness, often associated with realistic or fantasied hopelessness about the future.
- Behavioral problems, often related to denial of illness and, in extreme cases, causing the patient to leave the hospital against medical advice.

Recuperative problems:

- Decreasing cooperation as the patient sees improvement and is not compelled to follow orders closely.

- Readjustment problems with family, job, and society.

General Considerations
A. Acute Problems:

1. "Intensive care unit psychosis" is a type of delirium that is frequently accompanied by psychotic ideation. It is an expression of organic (frequently including a preexisting organic brain syndrome), psychologic, and environmental factors. Some factors include sleep deprivation, sedative and analgesic medications, alcohol withdrawal, metabolic fluctuations (particularly hypoxemia and hyponatremia), fear, and overstimulation. It is important to consider and recognize the problem early when it is more easily corrected. (See Organic Mental Disorders, p 676.)

2. Pre- and postsurgical anxiety states are common—and commonly ignored. Presurgical anxiety is ubiquitous and is principally a fear of death (note the high number of surgical patients who make out their wills). Patients may be fearful of anesthesia (improved by the preoperative anesthesia interview), the mysterious operating room, and the disease processes that might be uncovered by the surgeon. Such fears frequently cause people to delay examinations that might result in earlier surgery and a greater incidence of cure.

The opposite of this is **surgery proneness,** the quest for surgery to escape from overwhelming life stresses. Polysurgery patients are not easily categorized. Dynamic motivations include unconscious guilt, a masochistic need to suffer, an attempt to deal with another family member's illness, and psychogenic pain. More apparent reasons may include an attempt to get relief from pain and a life-style that has become almost exclusively medically oriented, with all of the risks entailed in such an endeavor.

Postsurgical anxiety states are usually related to pain, procedures, and loss of body image. Acute pain problems are quite different from chronic pain disorders (see Chronic Pain Disorders, p 654); the former are readily handled with *adequate* analgesic medication. Problems usually are due to inadequate dosage and overly long time intervals between administration, eg, meperidine is commonly administered every 4 hours even though the duration of action is closer to 3 hours. Anxiety about procedures can be eased by actually introducing the patient to the procedures *before* surgery, in effect desensitizing the patient to the forthcoming trauma. The alteration in body image is particularly difficult for mastectomy patients. Any procedure that results in a stoma has the attendant ramification of odor, excretion bag, and concern about intimate relationships with others.

3. Iatrogenic problems usually pertain to medications, complications of diagnostic and treatment procedures, and impersonal and unsympathetic staff behavior. Polypharmacy is often a factor. Patients with unsolved diagnostic problems are at higher risk. They are desirous of relief, and the quest engenders more diagnostic procedures with a higher incidence of complications. The upset patient and family may be very demanding. Negative responses or a lack of attention by the staff to excessive demands may result in complications that escape the attention of the staff. Experience teaches medical personnel to appreciate that excessive demands or obstreperous behavior usually result from anxiety. Such behavior is best handled with calm and measured responses.

B. Intermediate Problems:

1. Prolonged hospitalization presents unique problems in certain hospital services, eg, burn units, orthopedic services, and tuberculosis wards. The acute problems of the severely burned patient have been discussed and frequently are medical complications. The intermediate problems often are behavioral difficulties related to length of hospitalization and necessary procedures. Pain is a major problem in addition to anxiety about procedures. Debridement and grafting seem never-ending to the patient, who is angry about and becoming resistant to immobilization, boredom, and apparent lack of progress. This is especially true for people who have led an unencumbered lifestyle. Disputes with staff are common and often concern pain medication or ward privileges. Some patients regress to infantile behavior and dependency. Staff members must agree about their approach to the patient in order to ensure the smooth functioning of the unit.

2. Depression frequently intervenes during this period. It can contribute to irritability and overt anger. Severe depression can lead to anorexia, which further complicates healing and metabolic balance. It is during this period that the issue of disfigurement arises. Relief at survival gives way to concern about future function and appearance.

C. Recuperative Problems:

1. Anxiety about return to the outside world can cause regression to a dependent position. Complications increase, and staff forbearance again is tested. Anxiety at this stage usually is handled more easily than previous behavior problems.

2. Posthospital adjustment is related to the severity of the deficits and the use of outpatient facilities (eg, physical therapy, rehabilitation programs, psychiatric outpatient treatment). Lack of appropriate follow-up can contribute to depression in the patient, who may feel that he or she is making poor progress and may have thoughts of "giving up." Reintegration into work, educational, and social endeavors may be painfully slow. Life is simply much more difficult when one is disfigured or disabled.

Clinical Findings

The symptoms that occur in these patients are similar to those discussed in previous sections of this chapter, eg, organic brain syndrome, anxiety, and depression. Behavior problems may include lack of cooperation, increased complaints, demands for medication, sexual approaches to nurses, threats to leave the hospital, and actual signing out against medical recommendations.

Differential Diagnosis

Organic brain syndrome must always be ruled out, since it often presents with symptoms resembling anxiety, depression, or psychosis. The schizophrenias may present with any of the above complaints. Personality disorders existing prior to hospitalization often underlie the various behavior problems, but particularly the management problems.

Complications

Prolongation of hospitalization causes increased expense, deterioration of patient-staff relationships, and increased probabilities of iatrogenic and legal problems. The possibility of increasing posthospital treatment problems is enhanced.

Treatment

A. Medical: The most important consideration by far is to have *one* physician in charge, a physician whom the patient trusts and who is able to oversee multiple treatment approaches. In the acute problems, attention must be paid to metabolic imbalance, alcohol withdrawal, and previous drug use—prescribed, recreational, or over-the-counter. Adequate sleep and analgesia are important in the prevention of delirium.

Most physicians are attuned to the early detection of the surgery-prone patient. Plastic and orthopedic surgeons are at particular risk. Appropriate consultations may help detect some problems and mitigate future ones.

Postsurgical anxiety states can be alleviated by personal attention from the surgeon. Anxiety is not so effectively lessened by ancillary medical personnel, whom the patient perceives as lesser authorities, until after the physician has reassured the patient. Inappropriate use of "as needed" analgesia places an unfair burden on the nurse.

Depression should be recognized early. If severe, it may be treated by antidepressant medications (see Antidepressant Drugs, p 640). In the majority of cases, early consideration leads to early diagnosis and treatment by psychotherapeutic measures without the need for medication.

B. Psychologic: Prepare the patient for what is to come. This includes the types of units where the patient will be quartered, the procedures that will be performed, and any disfigurements that will result from surgery. Often because of anxiety, a great number of patients do not really listen to these explanations and are greatly surprised after surgery. Explanations with other family members present *on several occasions* may be necessary. The nursing staff can be helpful, since patients frequently confide a lack of understanding to a nurse but are reluctant to do so to the physician.

Time taken to elicit and discuss the patient's fears goes far in reducing the normal anxiety experienced by most patients. Repetition gives the patient time to digest information and ask further questions. Valid concerns and distorted understandings often relate to the death of a relative.

Denial of illness is frequently a block to acceptance of treatment. This, too, should be handled with family members present (to help the patient face the reality of the situation) in a series of short interviews (for reinforcement). Dependency problems resulting from long hospitalization are best handled by focusing on the changes to come as the patient makes the transition to the outside world. Key figures are teachers, vocational counselors, and physical therapists. Challenges should be realistic and practical and handled in small steps.

Depression is usually related to the loss of familiar hospital supports, and the outpatient therapists and counselors help to lessen the impact of the loss. The effect of depression on the family can delay resolution. Some of the impact can be alleviated by anticipating, with the patient and family, the signal features of the common depression to help prevent the patient from assuming a permanent sick role (invalidism).

Communication with the patient must be done with tact and under the best possible conditions. Suicide is always a concern when a patient is faced with despair. Be honest and compassionate, and make it clear by your actions that you are on the patient's side. Do not give unrealistic reassurances. Try to see the situation from the patient's position. Help the patient maintain hope, and nurture your relationship.

C. Behavioral: Prior desensitization can significantly allay anxiety about medical procedures. A "dry run" can be done to reinforce the oral description. Cooperation during acute problem periods can be enhanced by the use of appropriate reinforcers such as a favorite nurse or *helpful* family member. People who are positive reinforcers are even more helpful during the intermediate phases when the patient becomes resistant to the seemingly endless procedures (eg, debridement of burned areas). Other small pleasures such as wine or beer with hospital meals or after procedures can improve cooperation. Analgesic medications should be used effectively (see Chronic Pain Disorders, p 654).

Specific situations (eg, psychologic dependency on the respirator) can be corrected by weaning with appropriate reinforcers (eg, a loved one allowed in the room whenever the patient is disconnected from the respirator). Behavioral approaches should be done in a positive and optimistic way for maximal reinforcement.

D. Social: A change in environment requires adaptation. Because of the illness, admission and hospitalization may be more easily handled than discharge. Reintegration into society can be difficult. In some cases, the family is a negative influence. A predischarge evaluation must be made to determine whether the family will be able to cope with the physical or mental changes in the patient. Working with the family while the patient is in the acute stage may presage a successful transition later on.

A positive work situation is critical to the restoration of self-esteem. In many cases, the previous form of employment is no longer available. Vocational counseling can provide new career directions. It should be started in the hospital as early as possible and may include the occupational therapists.

Development of a new social life can be facilitated by various self-help organizations (eg, the stoma club). Sharing problems with others in similar circumstances eases the return to a social life which may be quite different from that prior to the illness.

Prognosis

The prognosis is good in all patients who have reversible medical and surgical conditions. It is guarded when there is serious functional loss that impairs vocational, educational, or societal possibilities—especially in the case of progressive and ultimately life-threatening illness.

Brodsky L, Brodsky V: Reconciling silent psychosis accompanying medical or surgical problems. *Psychosomatics* 1984;**25**:191.

Carpenter WT, Gruen PH: Cortisol's effects on human mental functioning. *J Clin Psychopharmacol* 1982;**2**:91.

Corradi RB: Psychological regression with illness. *Psychosomatics* 1983;**24**:353.

Dalos NP et al: Disease activity and emotional state in multiple sclerosis. *Ann Neurol* 1983;**13**:573.

Derogatis LR et al: The prevalence of psychiatric disorders among cancer patients. *JAMA* 1983;**249**:751.

DeVaul RA, Faillace LA: Surgery-proneness: A review and clinical assessment. *Psychosomatics* 1980;**21**:295.

Engels WD: Psychosomatic illness review. 4. Dermatologic disorders. *Psychosomatics* 1982;**23**:1209.

Hall RCW: Psychosomatic illness review. 5. Psychiatric effects of thyroid hormone disturbance. *Psychosomatics* 1983;**24**:7.

Jacobson AM, Leibovich JB: Psychological issues in diabetes mellitus: Psychosomatic illness review. *Psychosomatics* 1984;**25**:7.

Latimer PR: Psychosomatic illness review. 7. Irritable bowel syndrome. *Psychosomatics* 1983;**24**:205.

Lennard-Jones JE: Current concepts: Functional gastrointestinal disorders. *N Engl J Med* 1983;**308**:431.

Lloyd GG, Cawley RH: Distress or illness? A study of psychological symptoms after myocardial infarction. *Br J Psychiatry* 1983;**142**:120.

Margolis GJ et al: Psychological aspects of primary radiation therapy for breast carcinoma. *Am J Clin Oncol* 1983;**6**:533.

Martin MJ: Psychosomatic illness review. 8. Muscle-contraction (tension) headache. *Psychosomatics* 1983;**24**:319.

Nadelson C, Wotman MT, Ellis EA: Psychosomatic aspects of obstetrics and gynecology. *Psychosomatics* 1983;**24**:871.

Raskin NH: Psychosomatic illness review. 1. Migraine. *Psychosomatics* 1982;**23**:897.

Reich P et al: Acute psychological disturbances preceding life-threatening ventricular arrhythmias. *JAMA* 1981;**246**:233.

Rivinus TM: Psychiatric effects of the anticonvulsant regimens. *J Clin Psychopharmacol* 1982;**2**:165.

Rogers MP, Liang MH, Partridge AJ: Psychological care of adults with rheumatoid arthritis. *Ann Intern Med* 1982;**96**:344.

Sharfstein SS et al: Relationship between alternate-day corticosteroid therapy and behavioral abnormalities. *JAMA* 1982;**248**:2987.

Sneddon J: Myasthenia gravis: A study of social, medical, and emotional problems. *Lancet* 1980;**1**:526.

Taylor CB, Fortmann SP: Essential hypertension. *Psychosomatics* 1983;**24**:433.

Walker WJ: Changing US life style and declining vascular mortality: A retrospective. (Editorial). *N Engl J Med* 1983;**308**:649.

PSYCHIATRIC COMPLICATIONS OF NONPSYCHIATRIC DRUGS

Psychiatric manifestations can occur as adverse effects or side effects of practically every known therapeutic drug. It is not always easy, however, to determine if psychiatric symptoms arising during drug therapy of patients with physical disorders are due to the drug, based simply upon its known propensity to produce such symptoms. There is always the possibility of predisposing individual psychologic factors, as well as the psychologic and physical effects of the illness itself.

Although even the least noxious of drugs may produce unexpected psychiatric symptoms, there are some commonly used drugs and classes of drugs that, by virtue of the frequency or severity of the reactions associated with their use, deserve special mention:

(1) Anticholinergic drugs: Scopolamine, benztropine, trihexyphenidyl—restlessness, confusion, delirium, paranoid ideation.

(2) Cardiovascular drugs: Reserpine, methyldopa—depression, agitation; digitalis compounds—drowsiness, confusion, toxic psychosis; propranolol—lethargy, nightmares, confusion; lidocaine—restlessness, agitation; disopyramide—aggressive behavior; clonidine—depression; tocainide—confusion, psychosis.

(3) Antihistamine drugs: Diphenhydramine—sedation; cimetidine—confusion, toxic psychosis.

(4) Antidiabetic drugs: Insulin—hypoglycemia with restlessness, confusion, delirium.

(5) Hormones: Prednisone, other corticosteroids—mood swings, depression, mania; estrogens—depression, irritability; bromocriptine—paranoia.

(6) Antituberculosis drugs: Isoniazid, cycloserine—insomnia, restlessness, toxic psychosis.

(7) Antimalarial drugs: Chloroquine, quinacrine (also anthelmintic)—toxic psychosis; niridazole—hyperactivity, delirium.

(8) Muscle relaxants: Baclofen, cyclobenzaprine—confusion, depression, hallucinations.

(9) Analgesics: Pentazocine—hallucinations, confusion; indomethacin—depression.

(10) Miscellaneous: Levodopa—euphoria, anxiety, toxic psychosis; disulfiram—depression, delirium, psychotic ideation.

• • •

References

Dubovsky SL, Weissberg MP: *Clinical Psychiatry in Primary Care,* 2nd ed. Williams & Wilkins, 1982.

Goldman HH (editor): *Review of General Psychiatry.* Lange, 1984.

Goodwin DW, Guze SB: *Psychiatric Diagnosis,* 3rd ed. Oxford Univ Press, 1984.

Hall RCW (editor): *Psychiatric Presentations of Medical Illness.* SP Medical & Scientific Books, 1980.

Hollister LE: *Clinical Pharmacology of Psychotherapeutic Drugs,* 2nd ed. Churchill Livingstone, 1983.

Kalinowsky LB, Hippius H, Klein HE: *Biological Treatments in Psychiatry.* Grune & Stratton, 1982.

Kolb LC, Brodie HKH: *Modern Clinical Psychiatry,* 10th ed. Saunders, 1982.

Lerman F, Weibert RT: *Drug Interactions Index.* Medical Economics Books, 1982.

Rowe JW, Besdine RW: *Health and Disease in Old Age.* Little, Brown, 1982.

Tavris C: *Anger: The Misunderstood Emotion.* Simon & Shuster, 1983.

Weller M (editor): *The Scientific Basis of Psychiatry.* Baillière Tindall, 1983.

19 | Endocrine Disorders

Carlos A. Camargo, MD, & Felix O. Kolb, MD

Our concepts of the endocrine system, the mechanisms of action of hormones, the complex interrelationships among hormones in maintaining our internal milieu, and the diagnosis and therapy of disorders of the endocrine glands have all undergone radical changes during the last decade. The line separating a hormone from other information-carrying molecules is becoming a tenuous one. This chapter, however, deals with the classically accepted hormonal systems.

It is now clear that all hormones regulate intracellular mechanisms responsible for the production of cellular proteins and that the induction or activation of these proteins is responsible for the effects of the hormones. The process whereby these new proteins are formed is quite complex. We have learned that many hormones have predecessors without biologic activity and that these "prohormones" must be transformed into active moieties. These changes may take place inside the endocrine gland itself (eg, many pituitary hormones), in other tissues peripheral in location such as liver or kidney (eg, vitamin D transformations), or inside the target organ cell (eg, testosterone-dihydrotestosterone transformation in prostatic cells). It is also possible for a hormone to exert all of its actions via a mediator formed in another organ (growth hormone–somatomedin).

Hormones attach to cells via specific receptors found either in the surface of the cells (most peptide hormones) or inside the cellular cytoplasm (steroid hormones). The importance of these receptors in modern concepts of endocrine function cannot be overemphasized. Our understanding of disease processes in endocrinology is currently being greatly enhanced by knowledge of the dynamic aspects of hormone receptors, their modulation and control, and endocrine abnormalities.

The Challenges of Diagnosis of Endocrine Diseases

The diagnosis of endocrine disorders is complicated by the following factors:

A. Interrelationships of the Endocrine Glands: Because the endocrine glands are so closely interrelated, the presenting symptoms and signs of any endocrine disorder may represent a secondary disturbance in another gland or even in more than one gland. The diagnostic clue may therefore be in an organ that is secondarily affected by hypofunction or hyperfunction of the gland in question. For example, amenorrhea may be due to an abnormality of the pituitary or adrenal gland rather than to a primary ovarian lesion.

B. Homeostatic (Compensatory) Mechanisms: A well-balanced system of homeostasis often disguises the existence of a functional change in an endocrine gland, eg, partial pituitary suppression by cortisol administration. Special stress tests may be required to clarify the diagnosis.

C. Size of Lesion Versus Magnitude of Effect: The metabolic effect of an endocrine disturbance is not necessarily proportionate to the size of the lesion. A small tumor may cause extensive disturbance, whereas a striking enlargement may have only modest pathologic significance.

D. Physiologic Versus Pathologic States: The line between a physiologic aberration and a pathologic state may be quite tenuous. For example, when does the delay in appearance of signs of puberty become pathologic? Family background, judicious use of statistical data, and evaluation of nonendocrine problems such as state of nutrition and general health often help suggest when a search for an endocrine abnormality should be started.

E. Neurologic Integration: Many of the endocrine glands are regulated by neuroendocrine factors elaborated in the hypothalamus that control the secretion of the pituitary hormones. The synthesis of TSH- and LH-releasing factors and somatostatin has proved to be of diagnostic value and has opened new vistas for treatment in the future.

F. Multiple and Nonendocrine Involvement: The increasing number of recognized syndromes of multiple endocrine tumors and autoimmune deficiencies (often familial) and the endocrinopathies associated with nonendocrine gland cancers has complicated the problems of diagnosis. A patient may present with renal stone as the main complaint and be found to have not only hypercalcemia due to hyperparathyroidism but also an enlarged sella turcica due to a prolactin-secreting tumor (multiple endocrine neoplasia type I). Conversely, failure of multiple endocrine glands may be due to poorly understood autoimmune mechanisms (eg, simultaneous primary thyroid and adrenal insufficiencies [Schmidt's syndrome]).

A tumor of a nonendocrine organ may also produce, at the same time, several "ectopic" hormones (eg, oat cell carcinoma of the lung secreting ACTH and vasopressin simultaneously).

G. Difficulties of Laboratory Diagnosis: Direct chemical and radioimmunoassays of many hormones in blood, urine, saliva, and other biologic fluids have been developed. The concentration of hormones in these fluids, however, often varies from subject to subject and from hour to hour, making interpretation of data difficult on occasion. Bedside observation and sensitive indirect procedures are still required to establish the diagnosis of many endocrine disorders.

Baxter JD, Funder JW: Hormone receptors. *N Engl J Med* 1979; **301**:1149.

Clayton RN (editor): Receptors in health and disease. *Clin Endocrinol Metab* 1983;**12**:1. [Entire issue.]

Eisenbarth GS et al: The polyglandular failure syndrome: Disease inheritance, HLA type, and immune function. *Ann Intern Med* 1979;**91**:528.

Pollet RJ, Levey GS: Principles of membrane receptor physiology and their application to clinical medicine. *Ann Intern Med* 1980;**92**:663.

Schimke RN: Multiple endocrine adenomatosis syndromes. *Adv Intern Med* 1976;**21**:249.

COMMON PRESENTING COMPLAINTS

Delayed Growth

Growth delays due to endocrine and metabolic disorders are at times difficult to distinguish from familial or genetic dwarfism. Often there is an association with delayed genital development. Rule out bone diseases and nutritional, metabolic, emotional, and chronic cardiorespiratory or renal disorders that may delay growth. Look for associated stigmas such as polydactyly and webbing. Plotting of the growth rate will demonstrate whether growth has been delayed since birth or only during a specific period in childhood. Hypothyroidism must be excluded, as it is at times subtle and can be diagnosed only by sensitive tests of thyroid function. Epiphyseal dysgenesis (stippling) may be the telltale sign of juvenile hypothyroidism. The differentiation of hypopituitarism from delayed adolescence will usually become apparent in adult life. Dwarfism due to isolated lack of pituitary growth hormone is not uncommon. Dwarfism is seen also with gonadal dysgenesis in Turner's syndrome and with pseudohypoparathyroidism. A rapid growth spurt with eventual short stature is typical of sexual precocity and of the adrenogenital syndromes. Glucocorticoid excess (endogenous source or iatrogenic) can result in prompt cessation of growth; a fall in growth rate with simultaneous increase in rate of weight gain is suggestive of Cushing's syndrome.

Excessive Growth

Excessive growth may be a familial or racial characteristic or a physiologic event (eg, the growth spurt of puberty) as well as a sign of endocrine disease. If precocious genital development occurs, consider true precocity due to pituitary or hypothalamic disorders, or pseudoprecocious puberty due to excess of adrenal, ovarian, or testicular hormones (often due to tumors). These patients, if not treated rapidly, will eventually be of short stature as a result of premature closure of their epiphyses. Pituitary tumors secreting excess growth hormone cause gigantism if present before puberty and acromegaly if growth hormone excess takes place after closure of the epiphyseal plates of long bones. A few cases of nonpituitary "cerebral gigantism" have been described. Purely hypogonadal individuals tend to grow taller, with eunuchoid proportions (span exceeds height; excessive length of floor-to-pubis segment of body).

Obesity

Although obesity is a common presenting "endocrine" complaint, most cases are due to physical inactivity and excessive food intake. A rapid onset of massive obesity associated with lethargy or polyuria suggests a hypothalamic lesion (rare). Many cases of extreme obesity are associated with delayed puberty. Hypothyroidism is usually not associated with marked obesity. In Cushing's disease or syndrome, there is roundness of the face with a characteristic "buffalo hump" and trunk obesity with thin extremities. Striae are common with any type of obesity. They are wider (over 10 mm) and more violaceous in Cushing's syndrome. Amenorrhea, hypertension, and glycosuria or a diabetic glucose tolerance curve are commonly associated with obesity and often improve after adequate weight loss. Insulin-secreting adenomas are often associated with weight gain, but these are quite rare. In most instances, the obese patient requires increased activity and reduction in caloric intake, and all such patients require sympathetic understanding and reinforcement of motivation.

Wasting & Weakness

Contrary to old beliefs, hypopituitarism is only rarely associated with cachexia. Always rule out nonendocrine causes and consider anorexia nervosa and dietary fanaticism before looking for endocrine disturbances. Consider diabetes mellitus, thyrotoxicosis, pheochromocytoma, and Addison's disease if weight loss is progressive. Occult cancer and depressive reactions should also be ruled out.

Abnormal Skin Pigmentation or Color

First consider normal individual, familial, and racial variations. Hyperpigmentation may coexist with depigmentation (vitiligo) in Addison's disease, which must be ruled out by standard tests. Search carefully for pigmentary spots on mucous membranes, gums, and nipples. Differentiate Addison's disease from sprue, hemochromatosis, and argyria. Severe malnutrition is often associated with hyperpigmentation. It may be confined to skin areas exposed to sunlight, as in pellagra. Pregnancy and thyrotoxicosis are at times associated with spotty brown pigmentation, especially over the face (chloasma). A similar type of pigmentation has been seen occasionally with oral contraceptive administration. Other drugs (eg, diethylstilbestrol) will cause localized brown-black pigmentation over the nipples. Brown pigment spots with a ragged border are typical of Albright's syndrome (associated with fibrous dysplasia and precocious sexual development in the female); smooth pigmented nevi are seen in neurofibromatosis. Acanthosis nigricans may be associated with acromegaly and other endocrine tumors but is also often seen in patients with severe obesity. Patients with Cushing's disease usually have a ruddy complexion. Hyperpigmentation, especially after adrenalectomy, suggests a pituitary tumor or, more rarely, an extra-adrenal cancer. Carotenemia with yellowish skin is characteristic of primary myxedema. Sudden flushing and skin discoloration suggest the carcinoid syndrome. Vitiligo is often associated with autoimmune endocrinopathies.

Hirsutism

Marked normal variations in the amount of body hair occur on a racial, familial, or genetic nonendocrine basis. Hirsutism is one of the common presenting complaints of women, but occasionally it may be the first sign of a serious neoplastic disease. It is rarely completely reversible even if a tumor is removed. Hirsutism is of greater significance if it occurs other than at puberty, with pregnancy, or at the menopause; if it is associated with other features of virilization, such as voice changes, balding, or enlargement of the clitoris; and if the onset is sudden. Always investigate the patient's adrenal status and rule out tumor and hyperplasia. Ovarian causes include polycystic ovaries (Stein-Leventhal syndrome), hilar cell tumors, arrhenoblastoma, and theca cell luteinization. As a minimum screening procedure, a urinary 17-ketosteroid determination and plasma testosterone level should be obtained. The patient with an adrenal disorder will often have elevated 17-ketosteroids, whereas the patient with a testosterone-producing tumor such as an arrhenoblastoma will have abnormally high plasma testosterone level but usually normal 17-ketosteroids. The presence of obesity, amenorrhea, and hirsutism with elevated plasma testosterone and high tonic levels of LH is highly suggestive of polycystic ovary syndrome. It is important to make certain that the patient has not received androgenic medication. Certain drugs (eg, phenytoin, diazoxide) and an occasional malignant tumor will cause a generalized increase in body hair.

Change in Appetite

Polyphagia (associated with polydipsia and polyuria) is classically found in uncontrolled diabetes mellitus. However, excessive eating is usually not an endocrine problem but a compulsive personality trait. Only rarely is it due to a hypothalamic lesion, in which case it is associated with somnolence and other signs of the hypothalamic disease, eg, hypogonadism and also congenital abnormalities. Excessive appetite with weight loss is observed in thyrotoxicosis; polyphagia with weight gain may rarely indicate acromegaly or hypoglycemia due to an insulin-secreting islet cell adenoma.

Anorexia and nausea associated with weight loss and diarrhea may occur at the onset of addisonian crisis or uncontrolled diabetic acidosis. Weight loss due to anorexia plus increased metabolic rate is often seen in patients with pheochromocytoma. Anorexia and nausea with constipation are found with any state of hypercalcemia, eg, hyperparathyroidism, and may be indistinguishable from the same symptoms occurring in peptic ulcer (which may coexist with hyperparathyroidism). Recurrent peptic ulceration with high gastrin levels is diagnostic of pancreatic gastrinoma (Zollinger-Ellison syndrome).

Polyuria & Polydipsia

Polyuria, commonly associated with polydipsia, is usually of nonendocrine etiology, due to a habit of drinking excessive water (psychogenic). However, if it is severe and of sudden onset, it suggests diabetes mellitus or diabetes insipidus. Diabetes insipidus may develop insidiously or may appear suddenly after head trauma or brain surgery. Always attempt to rule out an organic lesion in or about the posterior pituitary-supraoptic tract. In children, the physician must consider nephrogenic diabetes insipidus and eosinophilic granuloma. Lithium and demeclocycline may induce polyuria by interfering with the renal action of ADH.

Polyuria and polydipsia are frequently seen in any state of hypercalcemia, such as hyperparathyroidism, and are also part of the syndrome of primary hyperaldosteronism, in which they are typically nocturnal. Polyuria may occur in renal tubular disorders, such as renal tubular acidosis and Fanconi's syndrome, as well as in a multitude of renal diseases associated with damage to the medullary interstitium that is responsible for establishing the osmotic gradient required for concentration of urine.

Gynecomastia

Enlargement of one or both breasts, usually painless and of rapid onset, is a common finding in adolescent boys. It may also be seen in old men. It is often transient and of little significance. One must differentiate between true glandular enlargement and simple fat pads or ballooning of the areolar tissue. Any painless hard lump, especially if unilateral, may be carcinoma.

True gynecomastia is found in many endocrine and nonendocrine disorders, eg, thyrotoxicosis, liver disease, paraplegia, and adrenal tumors. If associated with small testicles and lack of sperm, it may be part of Klinefelter's syndrome. A buccal smear may indicate a positive chromatin nuclear pattern.

Breast enlargement and tenderness may be due to estrogen therapy but occur also after the administration of androgens (especially to eunuchoid patients), and in some patients taking spironolactone, cimetidine, digitalis, reserpine, or chlorpromazine. They have been described in heavy marihuana and heroin users.

Gynecomastia may be the presenting sign of serious testicular tumors, such as choriocarcinoma, which may be too small to be palpable yet may metastasize widely. It may occur in bronchogenic carcinomas that produce gonadotropic hormones. It has been observed after hemodialysis.

Starvation states may also be associated with gynecomastia during the "refeeding" phase. The mechanisms of breast enlargement are not totally understood, but a common pathway is an increase in the estrogen/androgen ratio.

Breast enlargements may be transitory or may persist even after the cause (eg, exogenous estrogen) is removed; plastic surgical removal is often necessary for cosmetic reasons.

Abnormal Lactation

Lactation is a physiologic phenomenon when seen in the newborn ("witch's milk"); it may occur before menstruation or may persist for prolonged periods after recent delivery, and is part of the syndrome of pseudocyesis. It is frequently present in acromegaly and, more rarely, in thyrotoxicosis and myxedema. A common cause of the galactorrhea-amenorrhea syndrome is a prolactin-secreting tumor of the pituitary gland. The level of serum prolactin is usually above 100 ng/mL in these patients. Current techniques of computerized tomography (CT scan) allow visualization of small pituitary adenomas. Galactorrhea may also occur after pituitary stalk section. It can occur after thoracotomy or other injuries to the chest wall as well as after breast surgery. Abnormal lactation occurs rarely with estrogen-secreting adrenal tumors and quite rarely with corpus luteum cysts and choriocarcinoma. Many drugs (phenothiazines, antihypertensive agents such as reserpine and methyldopa, estrogen-containing medications such as oral contraceptives, etc) may produce lactation. Serum prolactin levels are high in most patients with galactorrhea, and they can be used to evaluate the response to therapy.

Precocious Puberty (in Both Sexes)

Precocious puberty is often a normal variant or a familial trait, but it may indicate serious organic disease. One must differentiate true precocity (caused by release of pituitary gonadotropins) from pseudoprecocity. At times there is only premature breast development ("thelarche") or only premature appearance of pubic and axillary hair ("adrenarche") with normal subsequent menarche. Hypothalamic lesions, encephalitis, and certain tumors (eg, hamartoma of the tuber cinereum, pineal tumors) may cause true sexual precocity. Precocious puberty also occurs in girls who have associated fibrous dysplasia of bone and pigment spots (Albright's syndrome). Adrenal hyperplasia or tumor and gonadal tumors usually cause pseudoprecocious puberty with virilization or feminization.

Hepatomas may rarely cause isosexual precocity. Reversible precocity with lactation and pituitary enlargement may be seen in juvenile hypothyroidism. The cause must be detected early, since all children with precocious puberty will eventually be short or even dwarfed as a result of premature closure of the epiphyses, and because many of the tumors responsible for precocious puberty are potentially malignant.

Sexual Infantilism & Delayed Puberty

It is often difficult to differentiate between simple functional delay of puberty (often a familial trait) and organic causes for such delays. Any type of gonadal or genetic defect may manifest itself primarily by failure of normal sexual development. Many patients grow to eunuchoid proportions, with span exceeding height. Consider hypothalamic lesions, especially if familial and associated with loss of sense of smell (Kallmann's syndrome), craniopharyngioma, pituitary tumors, and defective testes or ovaries, and look for associated stigmas (webbed neck of Turner's syndrome, gynecomastia of Klinefelter's syndrome). The serum gonadotropins are very helpful in determining the site of disease. If high, they point to the gonad as the defective organ. Chromosomal disorders should be ruled out by chromosomal analysis. Buccal smear for chromatin sex pattern is less expensive but does not exclude mosaicism.

Lack of Potency & Libido in Males

Many cases are psychogenic in origin and are not helped by hormone therapy. Occasionally, however, lessening of sexual desire or impairment of function may be the presenting sign of pituitary adenoma, Addison's disease, or testicular damage. The earlier in life the deficiency makes its appearance, the more pronounced is loss of libido associated with genital hypoplasia. Diabetes mellitus (especially with neuropathy) and thyrotoxicosis may first become manifest with this complaint. Chronic alcoholism, use of sedative and hypnotic drugs, some antihypertensive agents, and, occasionally, central nervous system lesions may be responsible. Measurement of plasma testosterone, LH, and prolactin may be helpful in differentiating organic and functional states. Plasma testosterone is low in hypogonadal states. An exception is thyrotoxicosis, where the level of plasma testosterone is high because of increased circulating levels of testosterone-binding globulin; however, the "free," non-protein-bound fraction is low. Hyperprolactinemia (of whatever origin) is often associated with impotence and decreased libido. Be sure to rule out estrogenic or feminizing tumors of the testis or adrenal and search for other signs of feminization, such as gynecomastia. Psychologic problems are difficult to rule out in the evaluation of impotence, since even the most "organic" impotence may be accompanied by secondary psychologic alterations. Fear of performance failure is a common phenomenon that may be helped by psychotherapy. Determinations of nocturnal penile tumescence are often useful in separating primary psychologic from organic causes.

Cryptorchism

Failure of descent of the testes is a common but poorly understood phenomenon. Not infrequently, spontaneous descent takes place at the time of puberty.

There is no agreement about when hormonal therapy should be instituted. If the testes are present, gonadotropic hormone will bring them down unless a hernia or blockage of the passageway prevents their descent. If there is doubt about whether the testes are present or not, determine testosterone and gonadotropin levels and obtain a buccal smear to determine the sex chromatin pattern.

Early surgical repair is advisable because intra-abdominal testes may later fail to produce sperm normally and because the incidence of malignancy in intra-abdominal testes is high. Cryptorchism may be associated with hypogonadism or may be part of pseudohermaphroditism.

A new approach to cryptorchism is therapy with gonadorelin (gonadotropin-releasing hormone). The use of synthetic gonadorelin in a nasal spray for 4 weeks has resulted in successful descent of the testes in a significant proportion of cases. This preparation is not commercially available at present in the USA.

Bone & Joint Pains & Pathologic Fractures

If the onset is at an early age and if there is a family history of similar disorders, consider osteogenesis imperfecta (look for blue scleras). Bowing of the bone and pseudofractures suggest rickets or osteomalacia, due either to intestinal or, more commonly, renal tubular disorders. Always consider hyperparathyroidism, specifically if bone pain, bone cysts, and fractures are associated with renal stones. Back pain with involvement of the spine suggests osteoporosis, especially when it occurs after the menopause. In cases of osteopenia of unknown cause, hyperthyroidism and Cushing's syndrome should always be considered and ruled out by appropriate tests. Aches and pains in the extremities are suggestive of rickets or osteomalacia. Rule out metastatic tumors, multiple myeloma, and Paget's disease in elderly patients by scintiscan and other tests. In doubtful cases, bone biopsy is indicated. Bone densitometry measurements are often more accurate than x-ray in determining minor mineral losses from the skeleton.

Renal Colic; Gravel & Stone Formation

A metabolic cause must be sought for recurrent stone formation and for kidney stones in children. If there is a family history, cystinuria and uric acid stones must be considered, or renal tubular acidosis with nephrocalcinosis. About 5% of stones are due to hyperparathyroidism, which must be ruled out in every instance of calcium stones. Look for bone disease, especially subperiosteal resorption of the bones of the fingers, and obtain a parathormone assay. Look also for signs of osteomalacia associated with excessive renal loss of calcium. Vitamin D intoxication, sarcoidosis, and excessive intake of milk and alkali must be considered. Any rapid bone breakdown may give rise to renal calcium stones, eg, in Cushing's syndrome. Uric acid stones may occur in patients with gouty arthritis, but often they occur simply because the urinary pH is very acid; they occur also after any type of intensive therapy for leukemia or polycythemia. Idiopathic hypercalciuria is the most common metabolic cause of recurrent calcium stones in males. Primary hyperoxaluria is a rare cause of severe renal calcification and may be associated with deposition of oxalate in soft tissues (oxalosis). Oxalate stones are seen frequently in patients with intestinal disorders (eg, ileitis, shunt procedures for obesity). At times, stones form in a structurally abnormal kidney (eg, medullary sponge kidney). Metabolic causes of renal stones must be corrected early before renal damage due to infection and obstruction occurs, since this may not be reversed upon removal of the initiating factor. The keys to proper diagnosis are careful stone analysis and chemical tests in blood and urine for calcium, phosphate, and uric acid.

Tetany & Muscle Cramps

Mild tetany with paresthesias and muscle cramps is usually due to hyperventilation with alkalosis resulting from an anxiety state. If tetany occurs in children, rule out idiopathic hypoparathyroidism or pseudohypoparathyroidism. Look for calcification in the lens, poor teeth, and x-ray evidence of basal ganglia calcification. Consider latent hypoparathyroidism in the post-thyroidectomy patient. Tetany may be the presenting complaint of osteomalacia or rickets or of acute pancreatitis. Neonatal tetany is probably due to the high phosphate content of milk and relative hypoparathyroidism. A similar mechanism has been considered responsible for leg cramps during pregnancy. Neonatal tetany may rarely indicate maternal hyperparathyroidism. Severe hypocalcemic tetany will occasionally produce convulsions and must be differentiated from "idiopathic" epilepsy. Classic signs of tetany are Chvostek's sign and Trousseau's phenomenon. If tetany is associated with hypertension, hypokalemia, and polyuria, consider primary hyperaldosteronism. Leg cramps may occur in some diabetic patients. Magnesium deficiency must be considered in tetany unresponsive to calcium.

Mental Changes

Disturbances of mentation are often subtle and may be difficult to recognize, but they may be important indications of underlying endocrine disorders. Nervousness, flushing, and excitability are characteristic of the menopause, hyperthyroidism, and anxiety states. Convulsions with abnormal electroencephalographic findings may occur in hypocalcemic tetany or in hypoglycemia, either spontaneously or induced by insulin. Islet cell tumors may cause sudden loss of consciousness, somnolence and prolonged lethargy, or coma. Diabetic acidosis may progress gradually into coma. Hypercalcemia leads to somnolence and lethargy, with marked weakness. Mental confusion may occur in hypopituitarism or Addison's disease or in long-standing myxedema. Confusion, lethargy, and nausea may be the presenting symptoms of water intoxication due to inappropriate or excessive secretion of antidiuretic hormone. Mental deterioration is the rule in long-standing and untreated hypoparathyroidism and hypothyroidism (cretinism). Insomnia and psychosis are part of Cushing's syndrome, either spontaneous or induced. A rapid change in glucocorticoid status (either a sudden increase or a sudden decrease) may be associated with acute psychosis. Mental deficiency may be associated with abnormal excretion of amino acids in the urine (eg, phenylketonuria) and with chromosomal abnormalities.

DISEASES OF THE HYPOTHALAMUS & OF THE PITUITARY GLAND

The function of the pituitary gland is controlled by regulating hormones (factors) produced by the hypothalamus. These releasing and release-inhibiting hormones are relatively simple polypeptides, several of which have been identified and synthesized (Table 19–1). Corticotropin-releasing factor has been recently isolated and characterized as a 41-amino acid peptide. A clinical disorder may be due to lack or excess of a pituitary hormone or, more commonly, to lack of releasing or inhibiting factor of the hypothalamus. Isolated or multiple defects may occur. Accurate radioimmunoassays and stimulation tests have made it possible to classify accurately the location of the defect. The exciting work of Guillemin and Schally in isolating and synthesizing these hypothalamic factors is proving of great value in the control of pituitary functional disorders. Clinical use of synthetic hypothalamic factors and their agonist or antagonist analogs is a new and promising development (eg, use of GnRH and analogs in cryptorchism, delayed puberty, induction of ovulation, management of precocious puberty). It is not true that chromophobe tumors of the pituitary are hormonally inactive. Some have been found to secrete excessive ACTH, growth hormone, prolactin, thyrotropin, LH, and FSH. A certain degree of overlap in function has been noted, eg, pituitary enlargement and lactation in juvenile myxedema reversed by the administration of thyroid hormone. Prolactin assays may be most important for the early diagnosis of pituitary lesions.

McCann SM (editor): Hypophysiotropic hormones. *Annu Rev Physiol* 1979;**41**:553.

Sandow J: Clinical applications of LHRH and its analogues. *Clin Endocrinol (Oxf)* 1983;**18**:571.

Scanlon MF: Neuroendocrinology. *Clin Endocrinol Metab* 1983;**12**:3. [Entire issue.]

Schally AV: Aspects of hypothalamic regulation of the pituitary gland. *Science* 1978;**202**:18.

Schlechte J et al: Prolactin-secreting pituitary tumors in amenorrheic women: A comprehensive study. *Endocr Rev* 1980; **1**:295.

Vale W et al: Characterization of a 41-residue ovine hypothalamic peptide that stimulates secretion of corticotropin and β-endorphin. *Science* 1981;**213**:1394.

Yen SSC: Clinical applications of gonadotropin-releasing hormone and gonadotropin-releasing hormone analogs. *Fertil Steril* 1983;**39**:257.

Table 19–1. The pituitary hormones and their hypothalamic regulatory factors (hormones).*

Hormones	Regulatory Factors (Hormones)
Growth hormone (somatotropin, STH)	Somatotropin-releasing factor (SRF, GH-RH, GH-RF); somatotropin release–inhibiting hormone (SIF, somatostatin)†
Corticotropin (ACTH)	Corticotropin-releasing factor (CRF or CRH)†
Thyrotropin (TSH)	Thyrotropin-releasing hormone (TRF, TRH)†
Follicle-stimulating hormone (FSH)	FSH and LH share a common hypothalamic peptide, gonadotropin-releasing hormone or gonadorelin (FSH-RH, LH-RH, LH-RF, LRH, GnRH)†
Luteinizing hormone (LH)	
Prolactin (LTH, mammotropin)	Prolactin-releasing factor (PRF, PRH); prolactin release–inhibiting hormone (PRIH or PIF)
Melanocyte-stimulating hormone	MSH-releasing factor (MRH, MRF); MSH release–inhibiting factor (MRIH, MIF)

*Modified from Schally AV et al: Hypothalamic regulatory hormones. *Science* 1973;**179**:341.

†Presently fully identified and synthesized.

PANHYPOPITUITARISM & HYPOPITUITARY CACHEXIA
(Simmonds' Disease)

Essentials of Diagnosis

- Sexual dysfunction; weakness; easy fatigability; lack of resistance to stress, cold, and fasting; axillary and pubic hair loss.
- Low blood pressure; may have visual field defects.
- All low: T_4, ^{123}I uptake, FSH, LH, TSH, urinary 17-ketosteroids and hydroxycorticosteroids, growth hormone. Prolactin level may be elevated.
- X-ray may reveal sellar lesion.

General Considerations

Hypopituitarism is a relatively rare disorder in which inactivity of the pituitary gland leads to insufficiency in the target organs. All or several of the tropic hormones may be involved. Isolated defects, eg, of the gonadotropins, are not rare. There is also great variation in the severity of the lesions, from those merely involving pathways (hypothalamic lesions) to almost complete destruction of the gland itself. The etiology of this disorder includes circulatory collapse due to hemorrhage following delivery and subsequent pituitary necrosis (Sheehan's syndrome), granulomas, hemochromatosis, cysts and tumors (chromophobe adenomas and craniopharyngiomas are most common), surgical hypophysectomy, external irradiation to the skull, trauma, metastatic disease, and aneurysms involving the sella turcica. True pituitary cachexia (Simmonds' disease) is quite rare.

The pituitary tumor may be part of the syndrome of multiple endocrine adenomatosis (type I), with concomitant involvement of the parathyroid glands and pancreatic islets. Isolated or partial deficiencies of anterior pituitary hormones (eg, FSH, LH, TSH) or their releasing factors may occur and may be detected by refined techniques.

Clinical Findings

These vary with the degree of pituitary destruction, and are related to the lack of hormones from the "target" endocrine glands.

A. Symptoms and Signs: Weakness; lack of resistance to cold, to infections, and to fasting; and sexual dysfunction (lack of development of primary and secondary sex characteristics, or regression of function) are the most common symptoms. In expanding lesions of the sella, interference with the visual tracts may produce loss of temporal vision, whereas a craniopharyngioma may cause blindness. Short stature is the rule if the onset is during the growth period. Amenorrhea and galactorrhea may be the first indications of a pituitary tumor. In men, impotence is usually an early complaint.

In both sexes there is sparseness or loss of axillary and pubic hair, and there may be thinning of the eyebrows and of the head hair, which is often silky.

The skin is often dry, with lack of sweating, and the patient appears pale. Pigmentation is lacking even after exposure to sunlight. Fine wrinkles are seen, and the facies presents a "sleepy" appearance.

The heart is small and the blood pressure low. Orthostatic hypotension is often present. Cerebrovascular symptoms or abnormal lactation may occur.

B. Laboratory Findings: The fasting blood glucose may be low. Dilutional hyponatremia is often present. Hyperkalemia does not occur, since aldosterone production, which is mainly controlled by the renin-angiotensin system, is not affected. The insulin tolerance test (use only 0.05 unit/kg intravenously) shows marked insulin sensitivity and is dangerous in these patients, since severe hypoglycemic reactions may occur. The T_4 level is low, and the TSH is not elevated (as in primary myxedema). Urinary 17-ketosteroids and 17-hydroxycorticosteroids and plasma cortisol are low but rise slowly after corticotropin administration (this does not occur in primary Addison's disease). Both TSH and corticotropin may

have to be given for several days. The metyrapone (Metopirone) test has been used to demonstrate limited pituitary ACTH reserve. Plasma levels of sex steroids (testosterone and estradiol) are low, and so are the urinary and serum gonadotropins. Anemia is common. Direct assay of growth hormone levels in blood by immunochemical methods shows low levels with little response to insulin hypoglycemia, to arginine infusion, or to levodopa. ACTH, TSH, LH, and FSH levels are low. TSH response to repeated intravenous infusions of thyrotropin-releasing hormone (TRH) may be of help in differentiating hypothalamic from pituitary lesions. Elevated prolactin levels may be an early finding in chromophobe adenomas.

The demonstration of a low level of a hormone secreted by a target gland in the presence of a low level of a trophic hormone is strongly suggestive of hypothalamic or pituitary disease (low plasma cortisol *and* ACTH, T_4 *and* TSH, estradiol or testosterone *and* LH).

C. X-Ray Findings: X-rays of skull may show a lesion in or above the sella. Craniopharyngiomas are often calcified and may be seen in a plain film. CT scan is helpful in ascertaining the degree of suprasellar extension of a tumor, the presence of cysts, "empty sella," etc. In growing children, one may find delay in bone age.

D. Eye Examination: Visual field defects (bitemporal hemianopia) may be present.

Differential Diagnosis

Anorexia nervosa may simulate hypopituitarism. In fact, severe malnutrition may give rise to functional hypopituitarism. By and large, cachexia is far more common in anorexia nervosa, and loss of axillary and pubic hair is rare; at times mild facial and body hirsutism is seen in anorexia nervosa. The 17-ketosteroids are low normal or not as low as in hypopituitarism; plasma and urinary cortisol may be high and may respond rapidly to corticotropin stimulation; and the gonadotropins are usually present at low levels. Thyroid function tests are not abnormal in anorexia nervosa except for low T_3. Pituitary growth hormone assays may show high levels in anorexia nervosa and very low levels in hypopituitarism.

Primary Addison's disease and primary myxedema are at times difficult to differentiate from pituitary insufficiency, but the response to corticotropin and TSH often helps. Direct radioimmunoassays of ACTH and TSH are more accurate diagnostic methods, since they are invariably elevated in primary insufficiency of the adrenal or thyroid glands.

Enlargement of the sella may require CT scans to rule out "empty sella syndrome," where minimal endocrine abnormalities are present and radiation or surgery is not indicated.

The severe hypoglycemia after fasting may cause confusion with hyperinsulinism.

The mental changes of hypopituitarism may be mistaken for a primary psychosis.

Complications

In addition to those of the primary lesion (eg, tumor), complications may develop at any time as a result of the patient's inability to cope with minor stressful situations. This may lead to high fever, shock, coma, and death. Sensitivity to thyroid may precipitate an adrenal crisis when thyroid is administered. Rarely, acute hemorrhage may occur in large pituitary tumors with rapid loss of vision, headache, and evidence of acute pituitary failure requiring emergency decompression of the sella.

Treatment

The pituitary lesion, if a tumor, is treated by surgical removal (either through craniotomy or, more recently, through a transsphenoidal approach using microsurgery), x-ray irradiation, or both. Endocrine substitution therapy must be used before, during, and often permanently after such procedures.

Recently, new therapeutic vistas have been provided by the development of purified pituitary hormones and of hypothalamic releasing factor or their analogs. Some of these materials, however, are not extensively available yet. The mainstay of substitution therapy for pituitary insufficiency remains the replacement of the end-organ deficiencies (adrenal, thyroid, and gonadal). This must be continued throughout life. Almost complete replacement therapy can be carried out with corticosteroids, thyroid hormone, and sex steroids.

A. Corticosteroids: Give hydrocortisone tablets, 15–25 mg/d orally in divided doses. Most patients do well with 15 mg in the morning and 5–10 mg in the late afternoon. A mineralocorticoid is rarely needed, since the adrenal conserves the capacity to secrete aldosterone. Additional amounts of rapid-acting corticosteroids must be given during states of stress, eg, during infection, trauma, or surgical procedures.

B. Thyroid: Thyroid (and insulin) should rarely, if ever, be used in panhypopituitarism unless the patient is receiving corticosteroids. Because of lack of adrenal function, patients may be exceedingly sensitive to these drugs. For this reason one should exercise special care in differentiating primary myxedema from hypopituitarism—sometimes a difficult problem.

Begin with small doses of desiccated thyroid, eg, 15–30 mg daily, and gradually increase to tolerance: 60–120 mg is usually adequate. Levothyroxine, 0.1–0.175 mg daily, is preferred.

C. Sex Hormones:

1. If gonadal failure is present, appropriate sex steroid replacement should be instituted. For males, testosterone enanthate, cypionate, or any other long-acting ester is given parenterally every 3–4 weeks (200–400 mg/dose). Because of hepatic complications, the long-term use of oral androgens is not recommended.

2. Estrogens are useful in the female for their mild anabolic effect and their effect on secondary sex characteristics. Give diethylstilbestrol, 0.5–1 mg daily orally; ethinyl estradiol, 0.02–0.05 mg daily orally; or conjugated estrogenic substances (eg, Premarin), 0.625–1.25 mg daily orally. Three weeks of estrogen therapy are usually followed by 5 days of a progestational agent such as medroxyprogesterone acetate, 10 mg daily.

3. Chorionic gonadotropic hormone (hCG) in combination with human pituitary FSH or postmenopausal urinary gonadotropin may be used in an attempt to produce fertility.

4. Clomiphene citrate and LH-releasing factor are sometimes useful with hypothalamic hypogonadism.

Note: Sex hormones, especially estrogens, should be employed cautiously in young patients with panhypopituitarism, or else the epiphyses will close before maximum growth is achieved. Most androgens also share this property—especially when given in large doses.

D. Human Growth Hormone: This hormone is by far the most effective agent for increasing height, but it is available for only a few patients. New methods of production of hGH (human growth hormone) using recombinant DNA techniques promise increased availability of this hormone. It has been used to increase the stature of some children who do *not* have clear-cut growth hormone deficiency. (See Rudman reference, below). A better understanding of growth hormone-releasing factors may offer alternative forms of treatment in the future.

E. Other Drugs: Bromocriptine has been used successfully in the treatment of pituitary lesions producing lactation and amenorrhea.

Prognosis

This depends on the primary cause. If it is due to postpartum necrosis (Sheehan's syndrome), partial or even complete recovery may occur. Functional hypopituitarism due to starvation and similar causes may also be corrected. The recent observation that some patients with hypopituitarism may suffer from failure of hypothalamic releasing factor offers hope for simpler therapy in the near future.

If the gland has become permanently destroyed, the problem is to replace target hormones, since chronic replacement with pituitary tropic hormones is not yet feasible. With appropriate therapy, a patient with hypopituitarism can expect a normal life span. Major improvements in pituitary surgical techniques in the last decade have resulted in safe and satisfactory removal of many pituitary tumors.

Berke JP et al: The "empty" sella. *Neurology* 1975;**25**:1137.

Frasier SD: Human pituitary growth hormone (hGH) therapy in growth hormone deficiency. *Endocr Rev* 1983;**4**:155.

Nabarro JDN: Pituitary surgery for endocrine disorders. *Clin Endocrinol* 1980;**13**:285.

Preece MA: Diagnosis and treatment of children with growth hormone deficiency. *Clin Endocrinol Metab* 1982;**11**:1.

Rudman D et al: Children with normal variant short stature: Treatment with human growth hormone for six months. *N Engl J Med* 1981;**305**:123.

Veldhuis JD, Hammond JM: Endocrine function after spontaneous infarct of the anterior pituitary: Report, review and reappraisal. *Endocr Rev* 1980;**1**:100.

Wass JAH, Besser GM: The medical management of hormone-secreting tumors of the pituitary. *Annu Rev Med* 1983;**34:** 283.

Zervas NT, Martin JB: Management of hormone-secreting pituitary adenomas. *N Engl J Med* 1980;**302**:210.

ACROMEGALY & GIGANTISM

Essentials of Diagnosis

- Excessive growth of hands (increased glove size), feet (increased shoe size), jaw (protrusion of lower jaw), and internal organs; or gigantism before closure of epiphyses.
- Amenorrhea, headaches, visual field loss, sweating, weakness.
- Elevated serum inorganic phosphorus and BMR; T_4 normal; glycosuria.
- Elevated serum growth hormone with failure to suppress after glucose.
- X-ray: Sellar enlargement and terminal phalangeal "tufting." Increased heel pad.

General Considerations

Growth hormone seems to exert its peripheral effects through the release of several somatomedins produced in the liver.

An excessive amount of growth hormone is most often produced by a benign pituitary adenoma. The disease may be associated with adenomas elsewhere, such as in the parathyroids or pancreas (multiple endocrine neoplasia type I). Acromegaly may also rarely occur as a result of secretion of ectopic growth hormone releasing factor (GHRF) by tumors such as bronchial and intestinal carcinoids, pancreatic islet cell adenomas, and lung carcinomas. If the onset is before closure of the epiphyses, gigantism will result. If the epiphyses have already closed at onset, only overgrowth of soft tissues and terminal skeletal structures (acromegaly) results. At times the disease is transient ("fugitive acromegaly") and followed by pituitary insufficiency.

Clinical Findings

A. Symptoms and Signs: Crowding of other hormone-producing cells, especially those concerned with gonadotropic hormones, causes amenorrhea and loss of libido. Production of excessive growth hormone causes doughy enlargement of the hands with spadelike fingers, large feet, jaw, face, tongue, and internal organs, wide spacing of the teeth, and an oily, tough, "furrowed" skin and scalp with multiple fleshy tumors (mollusca). Hoarse voice is common. Sleep apnea may occur. At times, acanthosis nigricans is present. Pressure of the pituitary tumor causes headache, bitemporal hemianopia, lethargy, and diplopia. In long-standing cases secondary hormonal changes take place, including diabetes mellitus, goiter, and abnormal lactation. Less commonly, these may be the presenting picture in acromegaly. Excessive sweating may be the most reliable clinical sign of activity of the disease.

B. Laboratory Findings: Serum inorganic phosphorus may be elevated (over 4.5 mg/dL) during the active phase of acromegaly. Serum gonadotropins are normal or low. Glycosuria and hyperglycemia may be present, and there is resistance to the administration of insulin. Hypercalciuria is common. The basal metabolic rate may be elevated. The T_4 is normal or low. 17-Ketosteroids and hydroxycorticosteroids may be high or low, depending upon the stage of the disease. In the active phase of the disease, serum levels of growth hormone are elevated above 7 ng/mL. Administration of glucose fails to suppress the serum level (as it does in normal individuals). Intravenous infusion of TRH or LRH often results in stimulation of growth hormone secretion, whereas in normal individuals there is no such effect. The plasma levels of immunoreactive somatomedin C have been reported to correlate closely with disease activity. (See Clemmons reference, below.)

C. X-Ray Findings: X-ray of the skull may show a large sella with destroyed clinoids, but a sella of usual size does not rule out the diagnosis. The frontal sinuses may be large. One may also demonstrate thickening of the skull and long bones, with typical overgrowth of vertebral bodies and severe spur formation. Dorsal kyphosis is common. Typical "tufting" of the terminal phalanges of the fingers and toes may be demonstrated, with increase in size of the sesamoid bone. A lateral view of the feet demonstrates increased thickness of the heel pad. Modern techniques of CT scanning can demonstrate even small pituitary tumors.

D. Eye Examination: Visual field examination may show bitemporal hemianopia.

Differential Diagnosis

Growth hormone excess is to be considered if there is rapid growth or resumption of growth once stopped (eg, change in shoe size or ring size). Consider the diagnosis also in unexplained amenorrhea, insulin-resistant diabetes mellitus, or goiter with elevated basal metabolic rate that does not respond to antithyroid drugs. Physiologic spurts of growth and increase in tissue size from exercise, weight gain, or certain occupations enter into the differential diagnosis. The syndrome of cerebral gigantism with mental retardation and ventricular dilatation but normal growth hormone levels resembles acromegalic gigantism. Myxedema and, rarely, pachydermoperiostosis may resemble acromegaly. Serial photographs are of help in differentiating familial nonendocrine gigantism and facial enlargement. Other conditions causing visceromegaly must be considered.

Complications

Complications include pressure of the tumor on surrounding structures, rupture of the tumor into the brain or sinuses, the complications of diabetes, cardiac enlargement, and cardiac failure. The carpal tunnel syndrome, due to compression of the median nerve at the wrist, may cause disability of the hand. Cord compression due to large intervertebral disks may be seen. Weakness due to myopathy often affects the limbs.

Treatment

The treatment of choice of active tumors without visual field loss used to be pituitary irradiation. Today, surgery is the treatment of choice. Transsphenoidal microsurgery has removed the hyperfunctioning tissue while preserving anterior pituitary function in most patients. Pituitary irradiation is useful if surgical therapy fails to return the elevated growth hormone levels to normal. Periodic reassessment of pituitary function after these procedures is advisable. In the "burnt out" case, hormonal replacement as for hypopituitarism may be required. Medical treatment of active acromegaly with progesterone and chlorpromazine has been disappointing. Reports of medical treatment with bromocriptine offer a novel approach, but long-term results must be awaited.

Prognosis

Prognosis depends upon the age at onset and, more particularly, the age at which therapy is begun. Menstrual function may be restored. Severe headaches may persist even after treatment. Secondary tissue and skeletal changes do not respond completely to removal of the tumor. The diabetes may be permanent in spite of adequate pituitary ablation. The patient may succumb to the cardiovascular complications. The tumor may "burn out," causing symptoms of hypopituitarism, or it may appear as an "empty" sella.

Christy NP: Choosing the best treatment for acromegaly. (Editorial.) *JAMA* 1982;**247**:320.

Clemmons DR et al: Evaluation of acromegaly by radioimmunoassay of somatomedin-C. *N Engl J Med* 1979;**301**:1138.

Melmed S et al: Pathophysiology of acromegaly. *Endocr Rev* 1983;**4**:271.

Moses AC et al: Bromocriptine therapy in acromegaly: Use in patients resistant to conventional therapy and effect on serum levels of somatomedin C. *J Clin Endocrinol Metab* 1981; **53**:752.

Pickett JBE III et al: Neuromuscular complications of acromegaly. *Neurology* 1975;**25**:638.

Schuster LD et al: Acromegaly: Reassessment of the long-term therapeutic effectiveness of transsphenoidal pituitary surgery. *Ann Intern Med* 1981;**95**:172.

Wilson C et al: Transsphenoidal microsurgical removal of 250 pituitary adenomas. *J Neurosurg* 1978;**48**:13.

CLINICAL DISORDERS OF PROLACTIN SECRETION

Normal Physiology

Although the existence of prolactin has been known for over 40 years, it was only in the 1970s that a significant amount of knowledge accumulated concerning clinical disorders associated with this hormone. Prolactin is a peptide hormone with a molecular weight of 21,000 which is secreted by the pituitary and in the mammalian species has as its main role that of inducing lactation. The hormone is hypersecreted during pregnancy, and the levels in plasma increasingly rise until the time of delivery. Under the combined effect of prolactin, increased estrogen, and progesterone, further breast development takes place, with eventual formation of milk in the acini. After parturition, the sudden withdrawal of estrogen caused by the expulsion of the placenta results in the onset of lactation. Estrogens play a synergistic role along with prolactin to promote the differentiation and development of the breast, but they antagonize prolactin in inhibiting the actual secretion of milk. The presence of prolactin is absolutely essential for lactation. During the puerperal period, the act of suckling constitutes a powerful stimulus for the continued production of prolactin. Lactation will cease if prolactin secretion is interrupted by prolactin-lowering drugs or by pituitary destruction. Prolactin is an unusual hormone in terms of control of secretion in that it is under a predominantly inhibitory control. Thus, section of the pituitary stalk will result in marked increases in prolactin secretion. Also, a pituitary transplanted to another anatomic site will abundantly secrete prolactin. There is mounting evidence that the prolactin inhibitory factor (PIF) is dopamine and that the control of prolactin secretion is primarily modulated by secretion of PIF. A prolactin-stimulating factor also exists, but its physiologic role is less clear. Prolactin, like other peptide hormones, is secreted episodically, and its concentration in blood is not stable (0–20 ng/mL).

Elevated serum prolactin is found in association with multiple physiologic and pathologic causes (see Table 19–2). Estrogens increase serum prolactin levels slowly by increasing the number of prolactin-secreting cells in the anterior pituitary gland. Many drugs inhibit prolactin inhibitory factor, thereby raising the production of prolactin.

Clinical Consequences of Prolactin Excess

In women, prolactin excess produces (1) disturbances of pituitary ovarian function with anovulatory

Table 19–2. Causes of hyperprolactinemia.

Physiologic Causes	Pharmacologic Causes	Pathologic Causes
Sleep (REM phase)	Phenothiazines	Pituitary stalk section
Exercise	Tricyclic antidepressants	Hypothalamic disease
Stress (trauma, surgery)	Reserpine	Prolactin-secreting tumors
Pregnancy	Methyldopa	Nelson's syndrome
Puerperium	Amphetamines	Acromegaly
Suckling	Anesthetic agents	Hypothyroidism
	Estrogens	Renal failure
	Metoclopramide	Chronic chest wall stimulation (postthoractomy; postmastectomy; herpes zoster, etc)

cycles, oligomenorrhea, or (frequently) amenorrhea; (2) galactorrhea (less common); and (3) hirsutism (rare). (See p 744.)

In men, excess prolactin is associated with (1) impotence and decreased libido (very common), (2) hypogonadism (less common), and (3) galactorrhea (very rare). (See p 689.)

Of all patients with secondary amenorrhea, as many as 28% may have elevated prolactin levels. In men, increased prolactin concentrations are usually not associated with galactorrhea, because the male breast tissue has not been primed by estrogens and progesterone.

Most women with hyperprolactinemia have amenorrhea or manifestations of a short luteal phase. Several syndromes are characterized in part by clinical associations of galactorrhea-amenorrhea: Argonz-del Castillo syndrome (galactorrhea-amenorrhea in nulliparous women), Chiari-Frommel syndrome (galactorrhea-amenorrhea following normal parturition), and Forbes-Albright syndrome (galactorrhea-amenorrhea accompanied by pituitary enlargement). It is now clear that these syndromes are not different clinical entities and may represent transitional phases of the same basic problem. Recent studies indicate that amenorrhea is much more common than galactorrhea.

The most important cause of high serum prolactin is a pituitary tumor. As many as 65% of all pituitary tumors may be associated with hyperprolactinemia. The tumors may be small (microadenomas) or produce clear-cut enlargement of the sella (macroadenomas). A great number of tests have been devised in the last few years to separate a prolactin-secreting tumor from other causes of hyperprolactinemia. Most of them are unreliable. A possible exception may be the response of serum prolactin to the administration of thyrotropin-releasing hormone (TRH). In normal individuals, there is a significant increase in serum prolactin following the intravenous administration of 400 μg of TRH. In most patients with prolactin-secreting tumors, this increase in prolactin levels does not occur. More useful, however, is the actual level of circulating prolactin. In patients with proved pituitary tumors, plasma levels of prolactin are usually over 100 ng/mL. Tomograms of the sella have been helpful in diagnosing small prolactin-secreting tumors that may produce subtle bony deformities. CT scan of the pituitary may also demonstrate small prolactinomas. Differentiation from normal variants, however, is not always possible.

Treatment

The treatment of a hyperprolactinemic state obviously depends upon the cause. If the problem is due to administration of exogenous estrogens, discontinuation of these drugs will produce improvement after a period of several months. Discontinuation of psychotropic agents usually results in a much faster recovery and resumption of menses. Most prolactin-secreting tumors are not responsive to radiation therapy, and surgical removal via the transsphenoidal route is the treatment of choice. In expert hands, surgical removal

results in complete disappearance of the symptoms (amenorrhea-galactorrhea and hypogonadism, or impotence and decreased libido in the male). A follow-up period of several years, however, is necessary to determine if a "cure" has been achieved, since some patients show a tendency toward relapse of increased prolactin secretion. If hyperprolactinemia is due to hypothyroidism, administration of thyroid hormone will rapidly correct the situation. Bromocriptine, a drug that binds to the pituitary dopamine receptor, thus inhibiting both spontaneous as well as TRH-provoked secretion from the gland, is useful in the medical therapy of hyperprolactinemic syndromes. In doses of 2.5–10 mg/d, it promptly reduces the levels of circulating prolactin, with rapid resumption of menses and cessation of galactorrhea. The role of bromocriptine in the treatment of prolactin-secreting pituitary tumors is debatable at present, but the drug is certainly helpful where surgery fails to correct the problem. Bromocriptine has been shown to inhibit the growth of prolactin-secreting tumors both in vivo and in vitro. Dramatic reductions in size of prolactinomas can occur during bromocriptine administration. Unfortunately, discontinuation of therapy usually results in reappearance of hyperprolactinemia and galactorrhea-amenorrhea. Since the patient's fertility is usually promptly restored with bromocriptine therapy, many pregnancies have resulted, with no clear evidence that the drug is teratogenic. Pregnancy, however, with its concomitant hypersecretion of estrogens, may result in marked increase in pituitary tumor size with danger of sudden development of visual disturbances. Close supervision of these patients is imperative.

Frantz AG: Prolactin. N Engl J Med 1978;298:201.

Hardy J: The transsphenoidal surgical approach to the pituitary. Hosp Pract (June) 1979;14:81.

Jewelewicz R, Van de Wiele RL: Clinical course and outcome of pregnancy in 25 patients with pituitary microadenomas. Am J Obstet Gynecol 1980;136:339.

Kleinberg DL, Noel GL, Frantz AG: Galactorrhea, a study of 235 cases, including 48 with pituitary tumors. N Engl J Med 1977; 296:589.

Koppelman MCS et al: Hyperprolactinemia, amenorrhea and galactorrhea. Ann Intern Med 1984;100:115.

March CM et al: Longitudinal evaluation of patients with untreated prolactin-secreting pituitary adenomas. Am J Obstet Gynecol 1981;139:835.

Prescott RW et al: Hyperprolactinaemia in men: Response to bromocriptine therapy. Lancet 1982;1:245.

Schlechte J et al: Prolactin-secreting pituitary tumors in amenorrheic women: A comprehensive study. Endocrine Rev 1980; 1:295.

Spark RF, Dickstein G: New drugs: Bromocriptine and endocrine disorders. Ann Intern Med 1979;90:949.

Spark RF et al: Hyperprolactinaemia in males with and without pituitary macroadenomas. Lancet 1982;2:129.

Thorner MO et al: Rapid regression of pituitary prolactinomas during bromocriptine treatment. J Clin Endocrinol Metab 1980;51:438.

Tucker H St G et al: Galactorrhea-amenorrhea syndrome: Follow-up of forty-five patients after pituitary tumor removal. Ann Intern Med 1981;94:302.

Wass JAH, Besser JM: The medical management of hormone-secreting tumors of the pituitary. *Annu Rev Med* 1983;**34**:283.

DIABETES INSIPIDUS

Essentials of Diagnosis

- Polydipsia (4–20 L/d); excessive polyuria.
- Urine specific gravity < 1.006.
- Inability to concentrate urine on fluid restriction.
- Hyperosmolality of plasma.
- Vasopressin reduces urine output (except in nephrogenic diabetes insipidus).

General Considerations

Diabetes insipidus is an uncommon disease characterized by an increase in thirst and the passage of large quantities of urine of a low specific gravity. The urine is otherwise normal. The disease may occur acutely, eg, after head trauma or surgical procedures near the pituitary region, or may be chronic and insidious in onset. It is due to insufficiency of the posterior pituitary or impaired function of the supraoptic pathways that regulate water metabolism. Partial forms of the disease exist. More rarely, it is due to unresponsiveness of the kidney to vasopressin (nephrogenic diabetes insipidus).

The causes may be classified as follows:

A. Due to Deficiency of Vasopressin:

1. Primary diabetes insipidus, due to a defect inherent in the gland itself (no organic lesion), may be familial, occurring as a dominant trait; or, more commonly, sporadic or "idiopathic."

2. Secondary diabetes insipidus is due to destruction of the functional unit by trauma, infection (eg, encephalitis, tuberculosis, syphilis), primary tumor or metastatic tumors from the breast or lung (common), vascular accidents (rare), and xanthomatosis (eosinophilic granuloma or Hand-Schüller-Christian disease).

Postpartum diabetes insipidus with amenorrhea and galactorrhea has been reported.

B. "Nephrogenic" Diabetes Insipidus: This disorder is due to a defect in the kidney tubules that interferes with water reabsorption and occurs as an X-linked recessive trait. Patients with this type of the disease are the so-called "water babies." In adults it may be associated with hyperuricemia. At times this type is acquired, eg, after pyelonephritis, potassium depletion, or amyloidosis. Certain drugs (eg, demeclocycline, lithium) may induce nephrogenic diabetes insipidus. The disease is unresponsive to vasopressin.

Clinical Findings

A. Symptoms and Signs: The outstanding signs and symptoms of the disease are intense thirst, especially with a craving for ice water, and polyuria, the volume of ingested fluid varying from 4 to 20 L daily, with correspondingly large urine volumes. Restriction of fluids causes marked weight loss, dehydration, headache, irritability, fatigue, muscular pains, hypothermia, tachycardia, and shock.

B. Laboratory Findings: Polyuria of over 6 L daily with a specific gravity below 1.006 is highly suggestive of diabetes insipidus. Simple water deprivation with measurement of urine osmolality may be diagnostic. Special tests have been devised to distinguish true diabetes insipidus from psychogenic polydipsia. The latter will often respond (with reduction in urine flow and increase in urinary specific gravity) to administration of hypertonic (3%) saline solution; true diabetes insipidus does not. Hypertonic saline infusions may be dangerous to patients with abnormal cardiovascular status. Although a positive response tends to rule out true diabetes insipidus, a negative result must be followed by careful prolonged dehydration and measurement of both urine and plasma osmolality and body weight under hospital conditions. Plasma osmolality is normally maintained in the range of 285–290 mosm/kg associated with ADH concentrations of 1–3 μU/mL in plasma and 11–30 μU/h in urine. Impaired ability to either synthesize or release ADH results in diminished ability of the kidney to conserve water. Patients with severe diabetes insipidus minimally concentrate urine following dehydration. After administration of 5 units of vasopressin, urine osmolality promptly rises. Patients with milder degrees may fail to release ADH in response to hypertonicity but retain the ability to release hormone following nonosmotic stimuli. Some patients respond to an osmotic stimulus only when the plasma osmolality exceeds normal levels ("high set osmoreceptor"). The presence of intact thirst perception results in polydipsia and polyuria. Failure to respond to vasopressin (Pitressin) indicates "nephrogenic" diabetes insipidus if the serum calcium and potassium levels are normal. A recently developed radioimmunoassay for arginine vasopressin will facilitate the differential diagnosis of diabetes insipidus and psychogenic polydipsia. The high levels of plasma vasopressin in nephrogenic diabetes insipidus are diagnostic.

If true primary diabetes insipidus seems likely on the basis of these tests, search for a possible brain lesion with x-rays of the skull, visual field tests, and CT scan of the pituitary hypothalamic area. Search also for associated bone lesions of xanthomatosis and obtain biopsy for confirmation. Look for a primary tumor in the lung or breast. In nephrogenic diabetes insipidus, rule out pyelonephritis or hydronephrosis and demeclocycline and lithium administration.

Differential Diagnosis

The most important differentiation is from the "psychogenic" water-drinking habit (see above). This may be difficult, since patients with long-standing polydipsia develop a true defect in renal concentrating ability. The baseline serum osmolality is helpful, since subjects with psychogenic polydipsia have low values, whereas the serum osmolality is normal or high in patients with diabetes insipidus. Polydipsia and polyuria may also be seen in diabetes mellitus, chronic nephritis, hypokalemia (eg, in primary hyperaldosteronism), and in hypercalcemic states such as hyperparathyroidism. The low fixed specific gravity of the urine in chronic nephritis does not rise after administration of vasopressin. On the other hand, in spite of the inability of patients with diabetes insipidus to concentrate urine, other tests of renal function yield essentially normal results.

Complications

If water is not readily available, the excessive output of urine will lead to severe dehydration, which rarely proceeds to a state of shock. Insomnia and dysphagia may occur. All the complications of the primary disease may eventually become evident. In patients who also have a disturbed thirst mechanism and who are receiving effective antidiuretic therapy, there is a danger of induced water intoxication. In untreated subjects, the passage of large volumes of urine for many years may be associated with dilatation of the ureters and urinary bladder.

Treatment

A. Specific Measures: Vasopressin tannate (Pitressin Tannate) suspension in oil, 0.5–1 mL intramuscularly, has been the standard treatment for many years. It is effective for 24–72 hours. It is usually best to administer the drug in the evening so that maximal results can be obtained during sleep. Patients learn to administer the drug themselves, and the dosage is adjusted as necessary. Warn the patient to shake the vial well before filling the syringe. Aqueous vasopressin injection is rarely used in continuous treatment because of its short duration of action (1–4 hours). A synthetic substitute, lysine-8 vasopressin, is available as a nasal spray (lypressin). This form of treatment may be preferred by patients with mild disease. It is free of local side effects, and water intoxication, which is not unusual with vasopressin tannate in oil, does not occur. A recently synthesized analog of arginine vasopressin (desmopressin acetate [DDAVP]) is longer-acting and has become the treatment of choice, although it is quite expensive at present.

B. Other Measures: Mild cases require no treatment other than adequate fluid intake. Hydrochlorothiazide (Hydrodiuril), 50–100 mg/d (with potassium chloride), is of some help in reducing the urine volume of true or nephrogenic diabetes insipidus. Chlorpropamide (Diabinese) has been found to be an effective antidiuretic and may be tried in mild cases. It has no effect in the nephrogenic type. After an initial dose of 250 mg twice daily, many patients can be maintained on 125–250 mg daily. Side effects include nausea, skin allergy, hypoglycemia, and a disulfiramlike reaction to alcohol. Other drugs under investigation are clofibrate, halofenate, and carbamazepine (Tegretol). Solute restriction (low-sodium, no-excess protein diet) may be of additional help. Psychotherapy is required for most patients with compulsive water drinking.

C. X-Ray Therapy: This may be used in the treatment of some cases due to tumor (eg, eosinophilic granuloma).

Prognosis

Diabetes insipidus may be latent, especially if there is associated lack of anterior pituitary function; and may be transient, eg, following head trauma. The ultimate prognosis is essentially that of the underlying disorder. Since many cases are associated with organic brain disease, the prognosis is often poor. Surgical correction of the primary brain lesion rarely alters the diabetes insipidus.

If the disease is due to an eosinophilic granuloma of the skull, temporary amelioration or even complete cure may be effected with x-ray therapy.

The prognosis of the "nephrogenic" type is only fair, since intercurrent infections are common, especially in infants affected with the disease. The acquired forms of this type may be reversible—eg, if urinary tract infection or obstruction is alleviated.

Cobb WE, Spare S, Reichlin S: Neurogenic diabetes insipidus: Management with dDAVP (1-desamino-8-D arginine vasopressin). *Ann Intern Med* 1978;**88**:183.

Hays RM: Antidiuretic hormone. *N Engl J Med* 1976;**295**:659.

Miller M et al: Recognition of partial defects in antidiuretic hormone secretion. *Ann Intern Med* 1970;**73**:721.

Moses AM, Notman DD: Diabetes insipidus and syndrome of inappropriate antidiuretic hormone secretion (SIADH). *Adv Intern Med* 1982;**27**:73.

INAPPROPRIATE SECRETION OF ANTIDIURETIC HORMONE

This syndrome, which is essentially water intoxication, may be mild and may only be manifested as asymptomatic hyponatremia, or it may be accompanied by irritability, lethargy, confusion, and seizures. It may lead to coma and death if not recognized. Laboratory findings include hyponatremia (which usually suggests the diagnosis) and hypo-osmolarity of the serum, continued renal excretion of sodium, formation of hyperosmolar urine, and expanded fluid volume. Adrenal and renal function are normal. Plasma arginine vasopressin levels are elevated or high normal but are inappropriate for plasma osmolality.

The disorder is most commonly caused by oat cell bronchogenic carcinoma, but it may also be present in pulmonary tuberculosis, porphyria, acute leukemia, acute myocardial infarction, myxedema, and central nervous system disorders. In children, it may be a complication of pneumoencephalography. It may be induced by chlorpropamide, vincristine, cyclophosphamide, and potassium-depleting diuretics.

Treatment is best accomplished by water restriction, which succeeds if the syndrome is recognized early. In severe cases of hyponatremia, when rapid correction is required, the use of furosemide diuresis with electrolyte replacement may be tried. Lithium carbonate has been found to be effective in this syndrome, but lithium intoxication may occur. Demeclocycline may be a safer drug to correct antidiuresis. Urea may be a safe and effective drug. A search for the primary cause of the disorder must also be undertaken.

The prognosis is often poor because of the advanced stage of the syndrome at the time of recognition and the serious primary disorder causing it (see Chapter 3).

Cooke CR et al: The syndrome of inappropriate antidiuretic hormone secretion (SIADH): Pathophysiologic mechanisms in solute and volume regulation. *Medicine* 1979;**58**:240.

Forrest JN et al: Superiority of demeclocycline over lithium in treatment of chronic syndrome of inappropriate secretion of antidiuretic hormone. *N Engl J Med* 1978;**298**:173.

Newsome HH: Vasopressin: Deficiency, excess and the syndrome of antidiuretic hormone secretion. *Nephron* 1979;**23**: 125.

DISEASES OF THE THYROID GLAND

Thyroid hormone affects cellular oxidative processes throughout the body. It is normally elaborated within the follicles of the gland by a combination of inorganic iodine, which is trapped by the gland under the influence of pituitary TSH, and tyrosine, forming monoiodotyrosine and diiodotyrosine, which further combine to form thyroxine (T_4) and triiodothyronine (T_3), the principal hormones of the gland. The "storage" form of the hormone is thyroglobulin, a combination of thyroxine and thyroid globulin, and it is in this colloidal form that the hormone is found within the follicles.

Under the influence of TSH, the active hormones are released from the gland as the need arises. Most of the circulating T_3, however, results from extra thyroidal metabolism of T_4. Circulating thyroxine is bound to plasma proteins, primarily thyroxine-binding globulins, and prealbumin. High levels of estrogen (eg, in pregnancy or in women taking oral contraceptives) increase the thyroxine-binding globulin levels and thus also the total level of T_4. The binding can be inhibited by certain compounds, eg, phenytoin and high doses of aspirin, which lower the T_4. The free (unbound) levels of circulating hormones regulate TSH release. The physiologic importance of triiodothyronine in clinical disorders is now well established. The availability of synthetic TSH-releasing hormone has been helpful in the evaluation of pituitary reserve and in the diagnosis of both hyper- and hypothyroidism.

The requirements for iodine are minimal (about 20–200 μg/d), but if a true deficiency arises or if the demand for iodine is increased (eg, during puberty), hormone production will be insufficient and circulating levels will be low. This leads to increase in pituitary TSH output, and thyroid hyperplasia follows.

The peripheral metabolism of the thyroid hormones, especially by the liver, and its alteration in disease states are significant. Most circulating T_3 derives from peripheral conversion of T_4, which is also metabolized to a biologically inactive compound, reverse T_3. In many chronic illnesses, starvation, etc, the proportion of T_3 formed decreases and that of reverse T_3 increases. The importance of this peripheral conversion, as well as the hypothalamic-pituitary regulation altered by the adrenergic nervous system, is becoming apparent. In addition, an autoregulatory mechanism within the thyroid gland itself seems to maintain the constancy of thyroid hormone stores.

Thyroid disorders may occur with or without diffuse or nodular enlargement of the gland (goiter). Symptoms may be due to pressure alone or to hyperfunction or hypofunction. A strong genetic predisposition to thyroid disease is being recognized.

Since thyroid hormone affects all vital processes of the body, the time of onset of a deficiency state is most important in mental and physical development. Prolonged insufficiency that is present since infancy (cretinism) causes irreversible changes. Milder degrees of hypofunction, especially in adults, may go unrecognized or may masquerade as symptoms of disease of another system, eg, menorrhagia. Diagnosis will then depend to a large extent upon laboratory aids, especially the finding of an elevated TSH level.

In any age group, whenever an isolated thyroid nodule is felt that is not associated with hyperfunction—and especially if there is any change in size of the nodule—the possibility of neoplasm must be considered.

Chopra IJ et al: Thyroid function in nonthyroidal illnesses. *Ann Intern Med* 1983;**98**:946.

Doniach D: Humoral and genetic aspects of thyroid autoimmunity. *Clin Endocrinol Metabol* 1975;**4**:267.

Sterling K: Thyroid hormone action at the cell level. (2 parts.) *N Engl J Med* 1979;**300**:117, 173.

Van Herle AJ, Vassart G, Dumont JE: Control of thyroglobulin synthesis and secretion. (2 parts.) *N Engl J Med* 1979;**301**: 239, 307.

TESTS OF THYROID FUNCTION

The more specific tests of thyroid function, now widely available, have gradually replaced most of the older ones such as the BMR, PBI, BEI, and T_4 by column. The tests most widely used in clinical practice are T_4 and "free" T_4 radioimmunoassays. When the latter is not available, the resin uptake of T_3 and determination of free thyroxine index (FTI) are useful. The TSH (RIA) assay has been of great help in diagnosis.

1. THYROID HORMONES IN SERUM

T_4 (RIA)

Normal: 5–13 μg/dL.

This test measures thyroxine by radioimmunoassay. It is affected by states of altered thyroxine binding.

"Free" Thyroxine Determination (FT$_4$)

Normal: 0.8–2.3 ng/dL.

This test measures the metabolically effective

fraction of circulating T_4. If properly performed, it is the best measurement of thyroid hormones, since it is not affected by binding problems, chronic illness, etc. It is not yet generally available.

Radioactive T_3 Uptake of Resin
  Normal (varies with methods): 25–35%.
  This test is not dependent upon exogenous organic or inorganic iodides. It is an indirect measure of thyroxine-binding protein and is of value in certain patients, eg, in pregnancy when the T_4 is high due to increased thyroxine-binding while T_3 uptake is low. In general, T_3 uptake parallels the T_4 except in the rare euthyroid patient with deficient thyroxine-binding protein, where the T_4 is low but the T_3 uptake normal or high. A test for T_4 should be done at the same time.

Free Thyroxine Index (FTI)
  The normal range varies in different laboratories.
  The product of T_4 and resin T_3 uptake ($T_4 \times T_3$ uptake) usually (not always) corrects for abnormalities of thyroxine binding. If a free T_4 determination is available, this calculation is unnecessary.

Thyroxine-Binding Globulin (TBG-RIA)
  Normal: 2–4.8 mg/dL.
  This is a direct and specific test for abnormal

thyroxine binding and is not affected by alterations in other serum proteins.

T_3 by Radioimmunoassay
  Normal: 80–200 ng/mL.
  This test is of value in the diagnosis of thyrotoxicosis with normal T_4 values (T_3 thyrotoxicosis) and in some cases of toxic nodular goiter. It decreases rapidly in states of malnutrition, chronic illnesses, weight reduction diets, etc.

2. IN VIVO UPTAKE OF THYROID GLAND

Radioiodine (^{123}I) Uptake of Thyroid Gland
  Normal: 5–35% in 24 hours. The normal range has been lowered in the USA because of increase of dietary intake of iodine.
  A. Elevated: Thyrotoxicosis, hypofunctioning large goiter, iodine lack; at times, chronic thyroiditis.
  B. Low: Administration of iodides, T_4, antithyroid drugs, thyroiditis, hypothyroidism.
  A scintiscan over the gland outlines areas of increased and decreased activity. If the uptake of ^{123}I is blocked, technetium Tc 99m may be used to obtain a scintiscan. Suppression of uptake after administration

Table 19–3. Typical results of some blood thyroid function tests in various conditions.*
(N = Normal range. ↑ = Elevated. ↓ = Decreased. V = Variable.)

Note: The more direct tests are subject to technical variables. They should be used when the more standard tests do not give decisive information, since many drugs cause interference with these thyroid tests.

	T_4(RIA)	T_3 Resin	Free T_4 Index	T_3 Serum	RAI (^{123}I) Uptake	Other Useful Tests and Comments
Hyperthyroidism	↑	↑	↑	↑	↑	TSH ↓
Hypothyroidism	↓	↓	↓	↓	↓	TSH ↑ in primary myxedema, ↓ in pituitary myxedema
Euthyroid, or hypothyroid therapy with: T_4	N	N	N	V	↓	TSH ↓ with 0.1–0.2 mg T_4
T_3 (1)	↓	↓	↓		↓	TSH ↓ with 50 µg T_3
Desiccated thyroid (2)	N	N	N		↓	TSH ↓ with 120–200 mg
Euthyroid following (3) Radiographic contrast dyes	N	N	N or ↑	N	↓	Effects may persist for 2 weeks to years
Pregnancy Hyperthyroid	↑	N or ↑	↑	↑	↑	Effects persist for 6–10 weeks after termination
Euthyroid	↑	↓	N	↑	↑	
Hypothyroid	N or ↓	↓	↓	↓	↓	
Birth control pills	↑	↓	N	↑	N	TSH normal
Nephrotic syndrome (4)	↓	↑	N	N	N	Low TP and TBG
Phenytoin, high doses of salicylates, testosterone	↓	↑	N	↓	N	TSH normal
Iodine deficiency	N	N	N	N	↑	^{123}I ↓ by T_4 or T_3
Iodide ingestion	N	N	N	N	↓	^{123}I ↑ with TSH

*Modified and reproduced, with permission, from Leeper RD: *Current Concepts* 1972;1:1. Courtesy of the Upjohn Co., Kalamazoo, Mich.

(1) T_3 causes decreased measurements of serum thyroxine because T_4 secretion is depressed or absent. T_3 resin uptake is decreased because of decreased saturation of TBG with T_4.

(2) Assuming normal T_3:T_4 ratio. Different batches of thyroid extract may vary.

(3) Free T_4 index may be increased if measurement for serum T_4 is elevated by contamination.

(4) TBG is lost in this disease, which accounts for decreased serum thyroxine.

of 100 μg of T_3 daily for several days will determine if the area in the gland is autonomous or TSH-dependent. Administration of TSH for 2 or more days, with increase in ^{123}I uptake over low control levels, indicates the presence of thyroid tissue and hence shows that low uptake was due to lack of TSH; the availability of plasma TSH measurements has made this test largely obsolete.

3. MISCELLANEOUS TESTS OF THYROID FUNCTION

Serum Cholesterol

Normal: 150–250 mg/dL. This test is nonspecific, as many factors may influence cholesterol level. The absolute level is less significant than the change after institution of therapy.

A. Relatively Elevated: Hypothyroidism.

B. Relatively Low: Thyrotoxicosis (occasionally).

Achilles Tendon Reflex

The relaxation time is often prolonged in hypothyroidism, but also in pregnancy, diabetes, old age, etc. It is rapid in hyperthyroidism. Although it lacks specificity for diagnosis, this test may be of value in following response to therapy.

Thyrotropin Immunoassay & Response to TRF

Normal: TSH-RIA less than 10 μU/mL; TRF response: doubling of TSH within 40 minutes after administration of 400 μg intravenously.

Radioimmunoassay of serum TSH is the most sensitive test for the early detection of primary hypothyroidism. TSH elevations may occur in subclinical hypothyroidism (eg, after destructive thyroid treatment), in iodine deficiency goiter, and in some dyshormonogenic goiters. It may also be elevated in rare cases of thyroid hormone resistance (Refetoff syndrome). T_4 treatment is rational in patients with goiter and elevated TSH. After adequate T_4 replacement, patients with myxedema should have undetectable or low TSH levels. A normal TSH response to TRF rules out pituitary hypothyroidism. A prolonged and exaggerated rise in TSH after administration of thyrotropin-releasing factor (TRF) in patients with borderline elevations of TSH may provide further evidence of primary thyroid failure. Patients with hyperthyroidism fail to respond to TRF, and a normal response virtually excludes hyperthyroidism.

Serologic Tests

Antibodies against several thyroid constituents (antithyroglobulin and antimicrosomal) are most commonly found in Hashimoto's thyroiditis but are also found in most patients with Graves' disease, a few patients with goiters or thyroid carcinomas, and in an occasional normal patient. Thyroid-specific stimulating autoantibodies such as LATS (long-acting thyroid stimulator) and LATS protector (which is probably

Table 19–4. Appropriate use of thyroid tests.

Purpose	Test	Comment
For screening	Free T_4	Best test if available.
	T_4 (RIA)	Varies with TBG.
	T_3 resin uptake	Varies with TBG.
	Free thyroxine index	Useful combination.
For hypo-thyroidism	Serum TSH	Primary vs secondary hypothyroidism. "Feedback" with T_4 and T_3.
	TRH stimulation	Differentiates pituitary and hypothalamic disorders.
	Antithyroglobulin and antimicrosomal antibodies	Elevated in Hashimoto's thyroiditis.
For hyper-thyroidism	Serum TSH	Usually suppressed.
	T_3 (RIA)	Elevated.
	^{123}I uptake and scan	Increased diffuse vs "hot" areas.
	Suppression test (100 μg T_3 for 7 days)	Autonomy. For atypical Graves' disease with normal uptake.
	TRH stimulation	No response; safer than suppression test.
	Antithyroglobulin and antimicrosomal antibodies	Elevated in Graves' disease.
	TSH displacing immunoglobulin (TDI)	Positive in Graves' disease (not always).
For nodules	^{123}I uptake and scan	"Warm" vs "cold."
	^{99m}Tc scan	Vascular vs avascular.
	Echo scan	Solid vs cystic. Pure cysts are not malignant.
	Thyroglobulin (TG)	High in metastatic, papillary, or follicular carcinomas.
	Calcitonin	High in medullary carcinoma.

identical with human-specific thyroid stimulator [HSTS]) are found in Graves' disease. A generic test for these and other thyroid-stimulating immunoglobulins (TSI) measures their displacement of TSH in thyroid cell membranes. A serum thyroglobulin radioimmunoassay has been recently introduced. The serum thyroglobulin level is high in thyroid cancer and may help in the differential diagnosis of benign and malignant lesions. Most of these factors can be measured as yet only in research laboratories.

Echo Scan (Ultrasound)

This simple technique has been used to determine if thyroid lesions are solid or cystic. Cysts are less likely to be malignant, since thyroid carcinomas rarely undergo cystic degeneration. One should remember, however, that most solid lesions are benign.

Fine-Needle Aspiration

Aspiration of thyroid tissue with a fine-gauge (21–26) needle has been shown to be helpful in the diagnosis of thyroid disorders, especially nodular lesions. Reading by an experienced cytopathologist is mandatory.

Calcitonin Assay
Elevated in medullary carcinoma.

Borst GC et al: Euthyroid hyperthyroxinemia. *Ann Intern Med* 1983;**98**:366.

Brown J et al: Autoimmune thyroid diseases: Graves' and Hashimoto's. *Ann Intern Med* 1978;**88**:379.

Colacchio TA, LoGerfo P, Feind CR: Fine-needle cytologic diagnosis of thyroid nodules: Review and report of 300 cases. *Am J Surg* 1980;**140**:568.

Frable WJ: *Fine Needle Aspiration Biopsy.* Saunders, 1983.

Melmed S et al: A comparison of methods for assessing thyroid function in nonthyroidal illness. *J Clin Endocrinol Metab* 1982;**54**:300.

Refetoff S: Syndromes of thyroid hormone resistance. *Am J Physiol* 1982;**243**:E88.

Schimmel M, Utiger RD: Thyroidal and peripheral production of thyroid hormones: Review of recent findings and their clinical implications. *Ann Intern Med* 1977;**87**:760.

SIMPLE & NODULAR GOITER

Essentials of Diagnosis
- Enlarged thyroid gland in a patient living in an endemic area.
- No symptoms except those associated with compression by large gland.
- T_4 and serum cholesterol normal; radioactive iodine uptake normal or elevated.
- TSH may be elevated.

General Considerations
Simple goiter in many parts of the world is due to iodine lack, and occurs in endemic areas away from the seacoast. Relative insufficiency of the iodine leads to functional overactivity and hyperplasia of the gland, which becomes filled with colloid poor in iodine. If the deficiency is corrected, the enlargement may subside. In long-standing cases, the goiter persists and is often nodular. In the USA, the ingestion of iodine is now so high (due to iodates in bread and other iodine sources in the diet) that iodine deficiency due to lack of ingestion is extremely rare. Unknown factors other than iodine lack play a role in the genesis of goiter. Simple goiter may occur transiently when there is greater demand for thyroid hormone, eg, with the onset of puberty or during pregnancy. Rarely, goiter may occur in spite of adequate iodine intake when there is interference with formation of thyroid hormones, eg, due to excess intake of certain goitrogenic vegetables (rutabagas, turnips), exposure to thiocyanate, or congenital lack of certain enzyme systems. Goitrogens occurring in contaminated water supplies have been described. Goiter is more easily prevented than cured; it is rarer since the introduction of iodized salt. Simple goiters may show chronic thyroiditis on biopsy.

Clinical Findings
A. Symptoms and Signs: The gland is visibly enlarged and palpable. There may be no symptoms, or symptoms may occur as a result of compression of the structures in the neck or chest: wheezing, dysphagia, respiratory embarrassment. (*Note:* Recurrent laryngeal compression is rare.) There may be associated congenital deafness (Pendred's syndrome) and disorders of taste.

B. Laboratory Findings: The T_4 and serum cholesterol are usually normal. The radioiodine uptake of the gland may be normal or high. Radioactive uptakes over nodules show them to be low in activity (in contrast to toxic nodular goiters).

With special techniques it is possible to demonstrate enzymatic defects in thyroid hormone production or abnormal circulating compounds in a considerable number of patients with goiters, especially the familial types. The TSH levels may be elevated. Antimicrosomal and antithyroglobulin antibody titers are not elevated.

C. Ultrasound Examination: The technique of thyroid echography has enabled the physician to evaluate thyroid nodules. Echograms are safe and rapidly obtained, and they can show whether a thyroid mass of 1–4 cm is a cystic or a solid lesion. A cystic nodule is much less likely to contain a malignant lesion than is a solid nodule. An echogram can also be used to follow the development of thyroid nodules while the patient is being maintained on thyroid hormone.

Differential Diagnosis
It may be difficult, by examination alone, to differentiate simple goiter from toxic diffuse or nodular goiter, especially in a patient with a great many nervous symptoms. A history of residence in an endemic area, a family history of goiter, or onset during stressful periods of life (eg, puberty or pregnancy) will often help. Thyroid function tests are usually normal in simple goiter. High titers of antithyroid antibodies point to the presence of autoimmune thyroid disease (Hashimoto's thyroiditis or Graves' disease). If the lesion is nodular, and especially if only a single nodule is present, neoplasm must be considered. Echography is often helpful in differentiating benign from malignant nodules.

Prevention
With a dietary intake of 100–200 μg of iodine daily, simple goiter due to iodine deficiency should not occur. During times of stress (puberty, pregnancy, and lactation), the upper limits of this dose may be necessary. This amount is provided in 1–2 g of iodized salt daily. Iodinated oil has been introduced in certain areas of the world as a prophylactic agent for goiter.

Treatment
A. Specific Measures:

1. Thyroid–Levothyroxine, 0.1 mg or more, or thyroid, 120–180 mg or more—especially if the goiter is multinodular—appears to be of value in most cases. The goiter will stop growing and often will decrease in size. As a guide to therapy, T_4 should be maintained in the high normal range. TSH levels should be suppressed by adequate replacement therapy.

2. Iodine therapy–If the enlargement is discovered early and is due to iodine deficiency, it may disappear completely with adequate iodine administration. Five drops daily of saturated solution of potassium iodide or strong iodine solution (Lugol's solution) in one-half glass of water is sufficient. Continue therapy until the gland returns to normal size, and then place the patient on a maintenance dosage or use iodized table salt.

B. Indications for Surgery:

1. Signs of pressure–If signs of local pressure are present that are not helped by medical treatment, the gland should be removed surgically.

2. Potential cancer–Surgery should be considered for any thyroid gland with a single "cold" (low ^{123}I or ^{99m}Tc uptake) noncystic nodule, for the chances of a single nodule being malignant are high. This is particularly true in younger people and in any case when there is no decrease in size or abnormal growth in spite of thyroid therapy after a period of 3–6 months. Nodules can be aspirated for cytopathologic study.

Prognosis

Simple goiter may disappear spontaneously or may become large, causing compression of vital structures. Multinodular goiters of long standing, especially in people over 50 years of age, may become toxic. This often happens after ingestion of large amounts of iodine (jodbasedow phenomenon). Whether they ever become malignant is not established.

Hamburger JI: Evolution of toxicity in solitary nontoxic autonomously functioning thyroid nodules. *J Clin Endocrinol Metab* 1980;**50**:1089.
Lever EG et al: Inherited disorders of thyroid metabolism. *Endocr Rev* 1983;**4**:213.
Stanbury JB, Hetzel BS (editors): *Endemic Goiter and Endemic Cretinism.* Wiley, 1980.
Studer H, Ramelli F: Simple goiter and its variants: Euthyroid and hyperthyroid multinodular goiters. *Endocr Rev* 1982;**3**:40.

HYPOTHYROIDISM

In view of the profound influence exerted on all tissues of the body by thyroid hormone, lack of the hormone may affect virtually all body functions. The degree of severity ranges from mild and unrecognized hypothyroid states to striking myxedema.

A state of hypothyroidism may be due to primary disease of the thyroid gland itself, or lack of pituitary TSH or hypothalamic TRF. A true end-organ insensitivity to normal amounts of circulating hormone has been postulated but is rarely observed. Although gross forms of hypothyroidism, ie, myxedema and cretinism, are readily recognized on clinical grounds alone, the far more common mild forms often escape detection without adequate laboratory facilities.

1. CRETINISM & JUVENILE HYPOTHYROIDISM

Essentials of Diagnosis
- Dwarfism; mental retardation; dry, yellow, cold skin; "pot belly" with umbilical hernia.
- T_4 low; serum cholesterol elevated.
- Delayed bone age; "stippling" of epiphyses.
- TSH elevated.

General Considerations

The causes of cretinism and juvenile hypothyroidism are as follows (after Wilkins):

A. Congenital (Cretinism):

1. Thyroid gland absent or rudimentary (embryonic defect; most cases of sporadic cretinism).

2. Thyroid gland present but defective in hormone secretion, goitrous, or secondarily atrophied. Due to extrinsic factor (deficient iodine, goitrogenic substances, in most cases of endemic cretinism); or due to maternal factors (some cases of congenital goiter). Many cases are familial, and enzymatic defects in thyroid hormone synthesis may be demonstrated.

B. Acquired (Juvenile Hypothyroidism): Atrophy of the gland or defective function may be due to unknown causes, thyroiditis, or operative removal (lingual thyroid or toxic goiter), or secondary to pituitary deficiency.

Clinical Findings

A. Symptoms and Signs: All degrees of dwarfism may be seen, with delayed skeletal maturation; apathy; physical and mental torpor; dry skin with coarse, dry, brittle hair; constipation; slow teething; poor appetite; large tongue; "pot belly" with umbilical hernia; deep voice; cold extremities and cold sensitivity; and true myxedema of subcutaneous and other tissues. A yellow, carotenemic skin is not infrequent. The thyroid gland is usually not palpable, but a large goiter may be present that may be diffuse or nodular. Sexual development is retarded but maturation eventually occurs. Menometrorrhagia or amenorrhea may be seen in older girls. Rarely, sexual precocity and galactorrhea with pituitary enlargement may occur. Deafness is occasionally associated with goiters. Nephrocalcinosis is a rare finding in cretinism.

B. Laboratory Findings: The basal metabolic rate is probably the least reliable (especially in infants and children) and the T_4 (see above) the most reliable index of thyroid activity; the latter is usually under 3 μg/dL. Serum cholesterol is frequently elevated. Radioactive iodine uptake is very low in athyroid individuals, but it may be high in some goitrous cretins where the iodine is not bound in the gland and is released. By special techniques, abnormal circulating iodine compounds and enzymatic defects in thyroid hormone production and release are demonstrable in some patients. Others show circulating autoantibodies to thyroid constituents. TSH by radioimmunoassay is invariably elevated; this may be the best screening test if readily available, especially in newborns.

C. X-Ray Findings: Delayed skeletal maturation is a constant finding, often with "stippling" of the epiphyses (especially of the femoral head), with flattening; widening of the cortices of the long bones, absence of the cranial sinuses, and delayed dentition may also be noted.

Differential Diagnosis

It is of practical interest to differentiate primary hypothyroidism from pituitary failure because in the latter instance a search for a pituitary lesion must be undertaken. Treatment with thyroid hormone must be instituted cautiously when hypothyroidism is secondary to pituitary failure, since it may occasionally precipitate adrenal crisis. Radioiodine uptake studies before and after exogenous TSH administration will often show whether a gland is present or not. TSH assay will help greatly in the differentiation of primary hypothyroidism from pituitary hypothyroidism. Cretinism is most often confused with Down's syndrome, although retarded skeletal development is rare in mongoloid infants. Macroglossia may be due to tumor, eg, lymphangioma. The dry skin of ichthyosis may be misleading. All causes of stunted growth and skeletal development (see above) must be considered as well. Rather than risk the development of full-blown cretinism in the questionable case, a trial of thyroid therapy is reasonable. Recent screening programs have led to earlier diagnosis. (See Fisher reference, below.)

Treatment

See Myxedema, below.

Prognosis

The progress and outcome of the disease depend largely upon the duration of thyroid deficiency and the adequacy and persistence of treatment. Since mental development is at stake, it is of utmost importance to start treatment early.

The prognosis for full mental and physical maturation is much better if the onset of disease occurs later in life. Congenital cretins almost never attain full mental development. Skeletal and sexual maturation, though often retarded, do take place normally under continued thyroid therapy.

By and large, the response to thyroid therapy is gratifying, but therapy usually must be maintained throughout life.

Fisher DA et al: Recommendations for screening programs for congenital hypothyroidism. *Am J Med* 1976;**61**:932.

Postellon DC: Diagnosis and treatment of congenital hypothyroidism. *Compr Ther* 1983;**9**:41.

Stanbury JB, Dumont JE: Familial goiter and related disorders. Chapter 11 in: *The Metabolic Basis of Inherited Disease*, 5th ed. Stanbury JB et al (editors). McGraw-Hill, 1983.

2. ADULT HYPOTHYROIDISM & MYXEDEMA

Essentials of Diagnosis

- Weakness, fatigue, cold intolerance, constipation, menorrhagia, hoarseness.
- Dry, cold, yellow, puffy skin; scant eyebrows; thick tongue; bradycardia; delayed return of deep tendon reflexes.
- Anemia (often macrocytic).
- T_4 and radioiodine uptake low.
- TSH elevated in primary myxedema.

General Considerations

Primary thyroid deficiency is much more common than secondary hypofunction due to pituitary insufficiency. Primary myxedema occurs after thyroidectomy, eradication of thyroid by radioactive iodine, ingestion of goitrogens (eg, thiocyanates, rutabagas, lithium carbonate), or chronic thyroiditis. It can also happen after external x-ray irradiation of the neck (as in patients with lymphoma). Most cases, however, are due to atrophy of the gland from unknown causes, probably due to an autoimmune mechanism. This may also involve other endocrine glands, eg, adrenals, in the same patient (Schmidt's syndrome).

Secondary hypothyroidism may follow destructive lesions of the pituitary gland, eg, chromophobe adenoma or postpartum necrosis (Sheehan's syndrome). It is usually manifested by associated disorders of the adrenals and gonads. Since thyroid hormone is necessary for all glandular functions, primary myxedema may lead to secondary hypofunction of the pituitary, adrenals, and other glands, making diagnosis difficult.

Clinical Findings

These may vary from the rather rare full-blown myxedema to mild states of hypothyroidism, which are far more common and may escape detection unless a high index of suspicion is maintained.

A. Symptoms and Signs:

1. Early–The principal symptoms are weakness, fatigue, cold intolerance, lethargy, dryness of skin, headache, and menorrhagia. Nervousness is a common finding. Physical findings may be few or absent. Outstanding are thin, brittle nails; thinning of hair, which may be coarse; and pallor, with poor turgor of the mucosa. Delayed return of deep tendon reflexes is often found.

2. Late–The principal symptoms are slow speech, absence of sweating, modest weight gain, constipation, peripheral edema, pallor, hoarseness, decreased sense of taste and smell, muscle cramps, aches and pains, dyspnea, anginal pain, and deafness. Some women have amenorrhea; others have menorrhagia. Galactorrhea may also be present. Physical findings include puffiness of the face and eyelids, typical carotenemic skin color and occasional purpura, thinning of the outer halves of the eyebrows, thickening of the tongue, hard pitting edema, and effusions into the pleural, peritoneal, and pericardial cavities, as well as into joints. Cardiac enlargement ("myxedema heart") is often due to pericardial effusion. The heart rate is slow; the blood pressure is more often normal than low, and even hypertension that reverses with treatment may be found. Pituitary enlargement due to hyperplasia of TSH-secreting cells, which may be reversible following thyroid therapy, may be seen in long-standing hypothyroidism. (*Note:* Obesity is not common in hypothyroidism.)

B. Laboratory Findings: The T_4 is under 3.5 μg/dL. Radioiodine uptake is decreased (below 10% in 24 hours), but this test is not always reliable. The radioactive T_3 resin uptake is usually low. Plasma cholesterol is elevated in primary and, less commonly, in secondary hypothyroidism (decrease on thyroid therapy is a sensitive index). Anemia is often present; it may be macrocytic, owing to associated pernicious anemia, or hypochromic microcytic, owing to iron deficiency in women with menorrhagia. Serum creatine phosphokinase (CPK) is often elevated. Increase in ^{123}I uptake and T_4 after administration of 10–20 units of thyrotropic hormone (given for several days) suggests secondary hypothyroidism rather than primary myxedema. 17-Hydroxysteroids and 17-ketosteroids in urine are low but plasma cortisol is normal unless the patient has associated autoimmune Addison's disease or the hypothyroidism is secondary to pituitary disease with associated adrenal insufficiency. Serum prolactin is elevated in some patients with primary hypothyroidism, presumably due to hypersecretion of hypothalamic thyrotropin-releasing hormone (TRH). The radioimmunoassay of TSH is a most useful test, since it is consistently elevated in primary hypothyroidism and low in pituitary hypothyroidism. Antithyroid antibody titers (antimicrosomal and antithyroglobulin) are high in patients with Hashimoto's thyroiditis and idiopathic primary myxedema.

Differential Diagnosis

Mild hypothyroidism must be considered in all states of neurasthenia, menstrual disorders without grossly demonstrable pelvic disease, unexplained weight gain, and anemia. Myxedema enters into the differential diagnosis of unexplained heart failure that does not respond to digitalis or diuretics, "idiopathic" hyperlipemia, and unexplained ascites. The protein content of myxedematous effusions is high. The thick tongue may be confused with that seen in primary amyloidosis. Pernicious anemia may be suggested by the pallor and the macrocytic type of anemia seen in myxedema. It enters into the differential diagnosis of myasthenic and rheumatic syndromes. Some cases of primary psychosis and cerebral arteriosclerosis or even brain tumors must be differentiated from profound myxedema. (*Note:* The cerebrospinal fluid proteins may be elevated in myxedema.)

Complications

Complications are mostly cardiac in nature, oc-

curring as a result of advanced coronary artery disease and congestive failure, which may be precipitated by too vigorous thyroid therapy. There is an increased susceptibility to infection. Megacolon has been described in long-standing hypothyroidism. Organic psychoses with paranoid delusions may occur ("myxedema madness"). Rarely, adrenal crisis may be precipitated by thyroid therapy of pituitary myxedema. Hypothyroidism is a rare cause of infertility, which may respond to thyroid medication. Sellar enlargement and even well-defined TSH-secreting tumors may develop in untreated cases. These tumors decrease in size after replacement therapy is instituted.

A rare complication of severe hypothyroidism is deep stupor, at times progressing to **myxedema coma,** with severe hypothermia, hypoventilation, hypoxia, hypercapnia, and hypotension. Water intoxication and severe hyponatremia are common. Convulsions and abnormal central nervous system signs may occur. Myxedema coma is often induced by an underlying infection; cardiac, respiratory, or central nervous system illness; cold exposure; or drug use. The mortality rate is high.

Caution: Myxedematous patients are unusually sensitive to opiates and may die from average doses.

Refractory hyponatremia is often seen in severe myxedema, possibly due to inappropriate secretion of antidiuretic hormone; however, a defect in distal tubular reabsorption of sodium and water has been demonstrated in this disorder.

Treatment

A. Specific Therapy: Thyroid or a synthetic preparation is used. The initial dosage varies with the severity of the hypothyroidism.

1. *Caution*–When treating patients with severe myxedema or myxedema heart disease, or elderly patients with hypothyroidism with other associated heart disease, begin with small doses of levothyroxine, 25–50 μg daily for 1 week, and increase the dose every week by 25 μg daily up to a total of 100–150 μg daily. This dosage should be continued until signs of hypothyroidism have vanished or mild toxic symptoms appear, and the dosage then stabilized to maintain the T_4 at normal levels.

2. Patients with early hypothyroidism may be started with larger doses, 50–100 μg daily, increasing by 25 μg every week to the limit of tolerance.

3. Maintenance–Each patient's dose must be adjusted to obtain the optimal effect. Most patients require 100–150 μg daily for maintenance. Optimal dosage can be estimated by following the T_4 and TSH levels, but clinical judgment is often the best guide.

4. Desiccated thyroid may be used for replacement therapy, although it is not as well standardized or as predictable as crystalline levothyroxine. One grain (65 mg) of desiccated thyroid is equivalent to 100 μg of levothyroxine or 25 μg of triiodothyronine.

5. When a rapid response is necessary, sodium liothyronine (T_3 [Cytomel]) may be employed. Begin with very low doses because of its speed of action.

Begin with 5 μg and increase slowly (see p 753). *Note:* Serum T_4 cannot be used as a guide to T_3 therapy.

6. Mixtures of T_4 and T_3 in a ratio of 4:1 —liotrix (Euthroid, Thyrolar)—have been introduced as "complete" replacement therapy. Since T_4 is normally converted to T_3 in extrathyroidal tissues, there is no need for this preparation.

7. **Myxedema coma** is a medical emergency with a high mortality rate. Triiodothyronine, 10–25 μg or more given by stomach tube every 8 hours, or, preferably, levothyroxine sodium, 200–400 μg intravenously as a single injection and repeated once in a dose of 100–200 μg in 12 hours, with the addition of hydrocortisone, 100 mg every 8 hours, may be lifesaving. The patient must not be warmed, adequate pulmonary ventilation must be provided, and fluid and electrolyte replacement must be carefully monitored. Infection is often present and must be vigorously treated.

8. Suppression of serum TSH has become a useful test of adequate maintenance or replacement therapy in hypothyroidism.

B. Needless Use of Thyroid: The use of thyroid medication as nonspecific stimulating therapy is mentioned only to be condemned. It has been shown that the doses usually employed merely suppress the activity of the patient's own gland.

"Metabolic insufficiency" is a questionable entity. The use of thyroid in cases of amenorrhea or infertility warrants consideration only if the patient is likely to be hypothyroid.

Prognosis

The patient may succumb to the complications of the disease if treatment is withheld too long, eg, myxedema coma. With early treatment, striking transformations take place both in appearance and mental function. Return to a normal state is possible, but relapses will occur if treatment is interrupted. On the whole, response to thyroid treatment is most satisfactory in true hypothyroidism, and complete rehabilitation of the patient is possible if treatment is adequate and maintained indefinitely. Chronic maintenance therapy with unduly large doses of thyroid hormone may lead to subtle but important side effects (eg, bone demineralization).

Christianson HB: Cutaneous manifestations of hypothyroidism including purpura and ecchymoses. *Cutis* 1976;**17**:45.

Khaleeli AA: Myxedema coma: Report on five successfully treated cases. *Postgrad Med J* 1978;**54**:825.

Klein I, Levey GS: Unusual manifestations of hypothyroidism. *Arch Intern Med* 1984;**144**:123.

Levine HD: Compromise therapy in the patient with angina pectoris and hypothyroidism: A clinical assessment. *Am J Med* 1980;**69**:411.

HYPERTHYROIDISM
(Thyrotoxicosis)

Essentials of Diagnosis

- Weakness, sweating, weight loss, nervousness, loose stools, heat intolerance.
- Tachycardia; warm, thin, soft, moist skin; exophthalmos; stare; tremor.
- Goiter, bruit.
- T_4, radio-T_3 resin uptake, and radioiodine uptake elevated. Failure of suppression by T_3 administration.

General Considerations

Thyrotoxicosis is one of the most common endocrine disorders. Its highest incidence is in women between the ages of 20 and 40. When associated with ocular signs or ocular disturbances and a diffuse goiter, it is called **Graves' disease** (known as Basedow's disease in Europe). Instead of a diffuse goiter, there may be a nodular toxic goiter, or all the metabolic features of thyrotoxicosis may occasionally be present without visible or palpable thyroid enlargement. The latter form is quite common in the elderly patient, who may even lack some of the hypermetabolic signs ("apathetic Graves' disease") but may present with a refractory cardiac illness. Lastly, a poorly understood syndrome of marked eye signs, often without hypermetabolism, may precede, accompany, or follow treatment of thyrotoxicosis, and has been termed exophthalmic Graves' disease, exophthalmic ophthalmoplegia, and malignant (progressive) exophthalmos (infiltrative ophthalmopathy). Current thinking on the pathogenesis of Graves' disease involves the formation of autoantibodies that bind to the TSH receptor in thyroid cell membranes and stimulate the gland to hyperfunction. These thyroid-stimulating immunoglobulins (TSI) are demonstrable by special techniques in the plasma of most (but not all) patients with Graves' disease.

Other causes of hyperthyroidism include the following: **(1) Plummer's disease,** or autonomous toxic adenoma of the thyroid, which may be single or multiple. This is not an autoimmune disease and is not accompanied by infiltrative ophthalmopathy or dermopathy. Antithyroid antibodies are not present in the plasma, and tests for TSI are negative. **(2) Jodbasedow disease,** or iodine-induced hyperthyroidism, which may occur in patients with multinodular goiters after ingestion of large amounts of iodine. **(3) Thyrotoxicosis factitia,** due to ingestion of excessive amounts of exogenous thyroid hormone. **(4) Struma ovarii** or **hydatidiform mole** causes rare cases of clinical hyperthyroidism, although asymptomatic elevation of T_4 may be seen in chorionic tumors, presumably due to ectopic production of a TSH-like material. **(5) TSH-secreting tumor** of the pituitary is an extremely rare cause of hyperthyroidism. Much more commonly, these tumors are the consequence of long-standing **hypothyroidism. (6) Thyroiditis** may be associated with transient hyperthyroidism during the initial phase.

Clinical Findings

A. Symptoms and Signs: Restlessness, nervousness, irritability; easy fatigability, especially toward the latter part of the day; and unexplained weight loss in spite of ravenous appetite are often the early features. There is usually excessive sweating and heat intolerance, and quick movements with incoordination varying from fine tremulousness to gross tremor. Less commonly, patients' primary complaints are difficulty in focusing their eyes, pressure from the goiter, diarrhea, or rapid, irregular heart action.

The patient is quick in all motions, including speech. The skin is warm and moist and the hands tremble. A diffuse or nodular goiter may be seen or felt with a thrill or bruit over it. The eyes appear bright, there may be a stare, at times periorbital edema, and commonly lid lag, lack of accommodation, exophthalmos, and even diplopia. The hair and skin are thin and of silky texture. At times there is increased pigmentation of the skin, but vitiligo may also occur. Spider angiomas and gynecomastia are common. Cardiovascular manifestations vary from tachycardia, especially during sleep, to paroxysmal atrial fibrillation and congestive failure of the "high-output" type. At times a harsh pulmonary systolic murmur is heard (Means' murmur). Lymphadenopathy and splenomegaly may be present. Wasting of muscle and bone (osteoporosis) are common features, especially in long-standing thyrotoxicosis. Rarely, one finds nausea, vomiting, and even fever and jaundice (in which case the prognosis is poor). Mental changes are common, varying from mild exhilaration to delirium and exhaustion progressing to severe depression.

Associated with severe or malignant exophthalmos is at times a localized, bilateral, hard, nonpitting, symmetric swelling ("pretibial myxedema") over the tibia and dorsum of the feet (infiltrative dermopathy). At times there is clubbing and swelling of the fingers (acropachy). It often subsides spontaneously.

Thyroid "storm," rarely seen today, is an extreme form of thyrotoxicosis that may occur after stress, thyroid surgery, or radioactive iodine administration and is manifested by marked delirium, severe tachycardia, vomiting, diarrhea, dehydration, and in many cases, very high fever. The mortality rate is high.

B. Laboratory Findings: The T_4 level and radioiodine and T_3 resin uptakes are increased. On rare occasions, the T_4 level may be normal but the serum T_3 elevated ("T_3 thyrotoxicosis"). The radioiodine uptake cannot be suppressed by T_3 administration (see p 700). In toxic nodular goiter, a high radioiodine uptake in the nodule may be diagnostic if combined with elevated T_4 or T_3 and low TSH levels. Serum cholesterol levels are low (variable). Postprandial glycosuria is occasionally found. Urinary creatine is increased. Lymphocytosis is common. Urinary and, at times, serum calcium and phosphate are elevated. Serum alkaline phosphatase is often elevated. In patients with Graves' disease, thyroid-stimulating immunoglobulins (TSI) are often present in serum and tests for antithyroid antibodies (antimicrosomal and antithyroglobulin) are also positive. TSH is low and fails to rise after TRF administration.

C. X-Ray Findings: Skeletal changes include diffuse demineralization or, at times, resorptive changes (osteitis). Hypertrophic osteoarthropathy with proliferation of periosteal bone may be present, especially in the hands (acropachy).

D. Electrocardiographic Findings: Electrocardiography may show tachycardia, atrial fibrillation, and P and T wave changes.

Differential Diagnosis

A difficult differentiation is between hyperthyroidism and anxiety neurosis, especially in the menopause. Subacute thyroiditis may present with toxic symptoms, and the gland is usually quite tender. The thyroid antibody tests may be positive; T_4 may be elevated, but radioiodine uptake is very low. Exogenous thyroid administration will present the same laboratory features as thyroiditis. A rare pituitary tumor may produce the picture of thyrotoxicosis with high levels of TSH.

A hypermetabolic state due mainly to overproduction of T_3 has been described ("T_3 thyrotoxicosis"). The T_4 is normal or low and the radioiodine uptake is normal or moderately elevated but fails to be suppressed by T_3 administration. Serum T_3 is elevated.

Some states of hypermetabolism without thyrotoxicosis, notably severe anemia, leukemia, polycythemia, and cancer, rarely cause confusion. Pheochromocytoma and acromegaly, however, may be associated with hypermetabolism, enlargement of the thyroid, and profuse sweating. Appropriate laboratory tests will easily distinguish these entities.

Cardiac disease (eg, atrial fibrillation, failure) refractory to treatment with digitalis, quinidine, or diuretics suggests the possibility of underlying hyperthyroidism. Other causes of ophthalmoplegia (eg, myasthenia gravis) and exophthalmos (eg, orbital tumor) must be considered. Thyrotoxicosis must also be considered in the differential diagnosis of muscle wasting diseases and diffuse bone atrophy. Hypercalciuria and bone demineralization may resemble hyperparathyroidism. The 2 diseases may be present in the same patient. Diabetes mellitus and Addison's disease may coexist with thyrotoxicosis.

Complications

The ocular and cardiac complications of long-standing thyrotoxicosis are most serious. Severe malnutrition and wasting with cachexia may become irreversible. If jaundice is present, the mortality rate increases. Episodes of periodic paralysis induced by exercise or heavy carbohydrate ingestion and accompanied by hypokalemia may complicate thyrotoxicosis in Orientals. Thyroid "storm" (see p 710) is rarely seen but may be fatal. Malignancy rarely accompanies toxic goiter. Complications of treatment for goiter include drug reactions following iodine and thiouracil treatment, hypoparathyroidism and laryngeal palsy after surgical treatment, and progressive exophthalmos. The exophthalmos may progress despite adequate therapy to the point of corneal ulceration and destruction of the globe unless orbital decompression is done. Hypercalcemia and nephrocalcinosis may occur. Decreased libido, impotence, decreased sperm count, and gynecomastia are often found in men with Graves' disease. (See Kidd reference, below.)

Treatment

Treatment is aimed at halting excessive secretion of the thyroid hormone. Several methods are available; the method of choice is still being debated and varies with different patients. The most widely accepted method in the past has been subtotal removal after adequate preparation. There is a greater tendency toward trying long-term medical treatment with antithyroid drugs to achieve remission of the disease and to use radioactive iodine therapy rather than surgical thyroidectomy for thyroid ablation except for large multinodular glands. The age of the patient and reproductive history and wishes are important considerations. Children and young adults who have not yet had children are better treated with antithyroid drugs rather than with radioactive iodine. If medical therapy fails or the gland is very large, subtotal thyroidectomy should be strongly considered, subject to the availability of a skilled and experienced thyroid surgeon. It should be pointed out that even among experts, there is wide divergence of opinion as to the "definitive" treatment of Graves' disease, especially in the young (see Dunn reference, below).

A. Subtotal Thyroidectomy: Adequate preparation is of the utmost importance. One or 2 drugs are generally necessary for adequate preparation: one of the thiouracil group of drugs alone, or, preferably, a thiouracil plus iodine. The sympatholytic agent propranolol has been used successfully as the sole agent before surgery. This drug, however, does not return the patient to a normal metabolic rate, and most experts prefer to render the patient euthyroid prior to surgery.

1. Preoperative use of thiouracil and similar drugs–Several thiouracil drugs are available: propylthiouracil, methimazole, and carbimazole. The modes of action are probably identical. These agents block the intrathyroidal synthesis of hormone. Propylthiouracil has also been shown to impede the peripheral conversion of T_4 to T_3, and carbimazole has been recently described as decreasing autoimmune response in Graves' disease. (See McGregor reference, below.)

Propylthiouracil has been most widely used and appears to be the least toxic. It is the thiouracil preparation of choice. The T_4 invariably falls, the rate of fall depending upon the total quantity of previously manufactured hormone available from the gland or in the circulating blood. (More hormone is present if iodine has been given previously.) The average time required for the T_4 to return to normal is about 4–6 weeks. If the drug is continued, the T_4 will continue to fall until the patient becomes myxedematous.

Preparation is usually continued and surgery deferred until the T_4 and T_3 uptake are normal. There is no need to rush surgery and no danger of "escape" as with iodine. In severe cases, 100–200 mg 4 times daily (spaced as close to every 6 hours as possible) is generally adequate. Larger doses (eg, for patients with very large glands) are occasionally necessary. In milder cases, 100 mg 3 times daily is sufficient.

Propylthiouracil appears to be an ideal drug except for 2 disadvantages: the danger of toxic reactions (especially agranulocytosis) and interference with surgery. Toxic reactions to propylthiouracil are rare, however. In practice, patients are instructed to watch for fever, sore throat, or rash and to notify their physicians immediately if any of these occurs, so that blood count and examination can be performed. If the white count falls below 3000/μL or if less than 45% granulocytes are present, therapy should be discontinued. Other rare reactions are drug fever, rash, and jaundice. The second objection is of a technical nature; since the gland may remain hyperplastic and vascular, surgical removal is more difficult. For this reason, combined therapy, using propylthiouracil and iodine, is the method of choice in preparing patients for thyroidectomy (see below).

Methimazole (Tapazole) has a mode of action similar to that of the thiouracils. The average dose is 10–15 mg every 8 hours. The smaller dosage is no guarantee against toxic reactions, especially skin rash, which are more common with this drug than with the thiouracils.

Carbimazole (not available in the USA but commonly used in Europe) is rapidly converted to methimazole and is similar in action. The average dose is 10–15 mg every 8 hours. Toxic side effects are slightly more common with this drug.

2. Preoperative use of iodine–Iodine is given in daily dosages of 5–10 drops of strong iodine solution (Lugol's solution) or saturated solution of potassium iodide with nonspecific therapy (see below) until the T_4 has dropped toward normal, the signs and symptoms have become less marked, and the patient has begun to gain weight. The disadvantages of preparation with iodine are that (1) a few patients may not respond, especially those who have received iodine recently; (2) sensitivity to iodides may be present; (3) if there is too long a wait before surgery, the gland may "escape" and the patient may develop a more severe hyperthyroidism than before; and (4) it is generally impossible to reduce the T_4 to normal with iodine alone.

3. Combined propylthiouracil-iodine therapy–The advantage of this method is that one obtains the complete inhibition of thyroid secretion with the involuting effect of iodine. This can be done in one of 2 ways:

Propylthiouracil followed by iodine appears at present to be the preoperative method of choice. Begin therapy with propylthiouracil; about 10–21 days before surgery is contemplated (when all thyroid tests have returned to normal or low normal range), begin the iodine and *continue* for 1 week after surgery.

Concomitant administration of the 2 drugs from the start in dosages as for the individual drugs, ie, 100–200 mg propylthiouracil 4 times daily and strong iodine solution, 10–15 drops daily. This method is less commonly used and less desirable than sequential administration (outlined above).

Patients who fail to be euthyroid after subtotal thyroidectomy can be re-treated with propylthiouracil or with radioiodine.

4. Propranolol–This drug may be used alone for the preoperative preparation of the patient in doses of 80–240 mg daily. It is the most rapid way of reversing some of the seemingly catecholamine-mediated toxic manifestations of the disease, and less time is necessary to prepare the patient for thyroidectomy. It has been suggested as the treatment of choice for thyrotoxicosis in pregnancy. Since it does not reverse the hypermetabolic state itself, escape and even thyroid storm may occur in patients so prepared. It should not be used in patients with bronchial asthma, and it should be employed with extreme caution if congestive heart failure seems likely to develop.

B. Continuous Propylthiouracil Therapy (Medical Treatment): Control of hyperthyroidism with propylthiouracil alone is often the treatment of choice, especially in young people, who are not good candidates for ^{131}I therapy. The advantage is that it avoids the risks and postoperative complications of surgery, eg, myxedema, hypoparathyroidism. The disadvantage is the remote possibility of toxic reactions plus the necessity of watching the patient carefully for signs of hypothyroidism. Since the advent of propylthiouracil, it appears that the incidence of toxic reactions is slight.

Begin with 100–200 mg every 6–8 hours and continue until the T_4 and T_3 uptake are normal and all signs and symptoms of the disease have subsided; then place the patient on a maintenance dose of 50–150 mg daily, observing the thyroid function tests periodically to avoid hypothyroidism.

An alternative method is to continue with doses of 50–200 mg every 6–8 hours until the patient becomes hypothyroid and then maintain the T_4 at normal levels with thyroid hormone. (This may be the preferred treatment of exophthalmic goiter.)

The duration of therapy and the recurrence rate with nonsurgical therapy have not been completely worked out. At present it would seem that of the patients kept on propylthiouracil between 18 and 24 months (the dosage slowly decreased), about 50–70% will have no recurrence. Patients with large thyroid glands that fail to decrease in size with medical therapy have a greater chance of recurrence of thyrotoxicosis after cessation of therapy. In some laboratories, the levels of thyroid-stimulating immunoglobulins (TSI) have been helpful in predicting outcome of medical therapy. Those having recurrences after cessation of treatment may be treated again with propylthiouracil, with radioiodine, or with surgery.

C. Radioactive Iodine (^{131}I): The administration of radioiodine has proved to be an excellent method for destruction of over-functioning thyroid tissue (either diffuse or toxic nodular goiter). The rationale of treatment is that the radioiodine, being concentrated in the thyroid, will destroy the cells that concentrate it. The only objections to date to radioiodine therapy are the possibility of carcinogenesis and the possibility of damage to the genetic pool of the individual treated. Studies to date have failed to show evidence of these effects. Nevertheless, the use of radioiodine is generally limited to older age groups (30 or above); however, the age level is not absolute, and some children may be best treated with radioiodine. *Do not use this drug in pregnant women.* A high incidence of hypothyroidism several years after this form of treatment has recently been recognized, but this has also been found in patients treated in other ways and may be the natural course of the disease. Prolonged follow-up, preferably with T_4 and TSH measurements, is therefore mandatory. There is a greater tendency toward higher-dosage radioiodine ablation of the toxic gland, with subsequent permanent replacement therapy with thyroid hormone, rather than using smaller doses initially, which may require re-treatment and may still fail to prevent appearance of myxedema several years later.

D. General Measures:

1. The patient with hyperthyroidism should not engage in strenuous activities. In severe cases, bed rest may be necessary. Mild cases may be treated with propylthiouracil or radioiodine on an ambulatory basis.

2. Diet should be high in calories, proteins, and vitamins. Hyperthyroid patients consume great quantities of food, are generally in negative nitrogen and calcium balance, and need the excess foods and vitamins because of their increased metabolic needs. Supplemental vitamin B complex should be given.

3. Sedation–When first seen, these patients are often very nervous. Sedation is sometimes necessary, eg, phenobarbital, 30 mg 3–6 times daily.

4. Since many signs resemble the effects of catecholamines, sympathetic blocking agents (reserpine, guanethidine, propranolol) have been recommended. Propranolol is especially useful in rapidly controlling tachycardia and cardiac irregularities, but it must be used cautiously in incipient or frank failure. It is especially effective in patients with neuromuscular signs, eg, periodic paralysis or upper motor neuron signs.

E. Treatment of Complications:

1. **Exophthalmos**–The exact cause of exophthalmos in hyperthyroidism is still not known. It has been shown that exophthalmos is due to edema and cellular infiltration of the orbital muscles, probably because of an autoimmune reaction that may be facilitated by lymphatic channel communication between the thyroid gland and the ocular orbits. Removing the thyroid secretion (extirpation or administration of propylthiouracil) does not necessarily help this condition and may possibly even aggravate it, leading to malignant exophthalmos. It has been suggested that

this is because the thyroid secretion exerts an inhibitory effect on the anterior pituitary, and removal of the gland allows the anterior pituitary to secrete more hormones and aggravate the condition. However, since the pituitary TSH levels are *always* low in thyrotoxicosis due to Graves' disease, it is questionable whether thyroid therapy is of use unless the patient is becoming hypothyroid.

a. Dark glasses, protection from dust, eye shields, tarsorrhaphy, and other measures may be necessary to protect the eyes. Elevation of the head of the bed at night, diuretics, and local use of methylcellulose solution (1%) to prevent drying of the protruding eyes are helpful. Ophthalmologic consultation should be requested.

b. Corticotropin (ACTH) or corticosteroids in large doses have proved helpful in some cases. They act by reducing the inflammatory reaction in the periorbital tissues. They may also reduce the level of autoimmune activity.

c. Surgery for malignant exophthalmos–Every patient with exophthalmos should be measured periodically with an exophthalmometer; do not rely upon clinical judgment to determine whether or not exophthalmos is present or progressing. In severe progressive cases, where corneal edema or ulceration, limitation of extraocular muscle movements, and failing vision occur, orbital decompression may be necessary to save the eyesight.

d. Orbital irradiation is often helpful and should be considered in severe cases (see Kriss reference, below). Immunosuppressive therapy has also been suggested.

2. Cardiac complications–A number of cardiac complications are at times associated with hyperthyroidism.

a. Some degree of tachycardia is almost always found if normal rhythm is present in thyrotoxicosis. This requires only the treatment of the thyrotoxicosis. Severe tachycardia responds promptly to propranolol therapy.

b. Congestive failure tends to occur in longstanding thyrotoxicosis, especially in the older age groups. Treatment is the same as for congestive failure due to any cause.

c. Atrial fibrillation may occur in association with thyrotoxicosis. Treat as any other atrial fibrillation, but do not try to convert the atrial fibrillation in a toxic patient. Most cases will revert to normal rhythm soon after toxicity is removed. However, if fibrillation remains for 2 weeks after surgery or for 2–4 weeks after T$_4$ or other thyroid function tests have returned to normal with propylthiouracil therapy, and if no contraindications are present, one should consider conversion to a normal rhythm.

3. "Crisis" or "storm"–Fortunately, this condition is rare with modern therapy. It occurs now mainly in patients inadequately prepared with propylthiouracil and iodine, those with complicating infection, immediately after subtotal thyroidectomy, or, rarely, after ^{131}I therapy. It can occur spontaneously or after any sudden stress in an untreated patient with thyrotoxicosis. It is characterized by high fever, tachycardia, central nervous system irritability, and delirium. The cause is uncertain, but relative adrenocortical insufficiency may be a contributing factor. Large doses of the rapidly acting corticosteroids may be lifesaving. Give additional large doses of propylthiouracil by nasogastric tube. Sodium iodide, 1–2 g intravenously and repeated every 12–24 hours, has also been advocated. Large doses of propranolol intravenously have been the most effective means of rapidly controlling thyroid storm. Plasmapheresis has been used in cases not responsive to the above measures. Cholestyramine, which binds thyroid hormone in the gut, is an alternative drug. General measures consist of oxygen, cold packs, sedation, glucose infusions, multivitamins, and careful monitoring of the state of hydration, electrolyte balance, etc. Therapy is best carried out in an intensive care unit.

4. Dermopathy–Severe pretibial myxedema, an uncommon complication of Graves' disease, responds well to local glucocorticoid therapy.

Prognosis

Graves' disease is a cyclic entity and may subside spontaneously. More commonly, however, it progresses, especially with recurrent psychic trauma, and other types of stress. The ocular, cardiac, and psychic complications often are more serious than the chronic wasting of tissues and may become irreversible even after treatment. Progressive exophthalmos is perhaps more common after surgical than after medical treatment. Permanent hypoparathyroidism and vocal cord palsy are risks of surgical thyroidectomy. With any form of therapy, unless radical thyroidectomy or large dosage ^{131}I therapy is used, recurrences are common. With adequate treatment and long-term follow-up, the results are good. It is perhaps wiser to speak of induced remission rather than cure. Posttreatment hypothyroidism is common. It may occur several years after radioactive iodine therapy or subtotal thyroidectomy. Although benign and even malignant thyroid neoplasms may occur following radioiodine treatment, a recent survey shows that the incidence is no greater than after subtotal thyroidectomy.

Patients with jaundice and fever have a less favorable prognosis. Thyrotoxic periodic paralysis with hypokalemia—to which males of Oriental background are predisposed—may alter the prognosis. Periorbital swelling and chemosis often precede serious and progressive malignant exophthalmos leading to blindness, and they must be watched for carefully.

Although it is rare, thyroid storm has the worst prognosis. It is best avoided by careful preoperative preparation of the patient rather than treated once it appears.

Burrow GN: Hyperthyroidism during pregnancy. *N Engl J Med* 1978;**298**:150.

Dobyns BM: Prevention and management of thyroid storm. *World J Surg* 1978;**2**:293.

Dunn JT: Choice of therapy in young adults with hyperthyroidism of Graves' disease. *Ann Intern Med* 1984;**100**:891.

Fradkin JE, Wolff J: Iodide-induced thyrotoxicosis. *Medicine* 1983;**62**:1.

Jacobson DH, Gorman CA: Endocrine ophthalmopathy: Current ideas concerning etiology, pathogenesis and treatment. *Endocr Rev* 1984;**5**:200.

Kidd GS et al: The hypothalamic-pituitary-testicular axis in thyrotoxicosis. *J Clin Endocrinol Metab* 1979;**48**:798.

Kriss JP, McDougall IR, Donaldson SS: Graves' ophthalmopathy. In: *Current Therapy in Endocrinology 1983–1984.* Krieger DT, Bardin CW (editors). Mosby, 1983.

McClung MR, Greer MA: Treatment of hyperthyroidism. *Annu Rev Med* 1980;**31**:385.

McDevitt DG: Propranolol in treatment of thyrotoxicosis: Review. *Postgrad Med J* 1976;**52 (Suppl 4)**:157.

McGregor AM et al: Carbimazole and the autoimmune response in Graves' disease. *N Engl J Med* 1980;**303**:302.

Smallridge RC et al: Hyperthyroidism due to TSH-secreting pituitary tumors. *Arch Intern Med* 1983;**143**:503.

Sugrue D et al: Hyperthyroidism in the land of Graves: Results of treatment by surgery, radio-iodine and carbimazole in 837 cases. *Q J Med* 1980;**49**:51.

Weetman AP, McGregor AM: Autoimmune thyroid disease: Developments in our understanding. *Endocr Rev* 1984;**5**:309.

THYROID NODULES & THYROID CANCER

Essentials of Diagnosis

- Painless swelling in region of thyroid, or thyroid nodule not responding to suppression. Normal thyroid function tests.
- Past history of irradiation to neck, goiter, or thyroiditis.

General Considerations (Table 19–5.)

Although carcinoma of the thyroid is rarely associated with functional abnormalities, it enters into the differential diagnosis of all types of thyroid lesions. It is common in all age groups, but especially in patients who have received radiation therapy to the neck structures (eg, thymus gland). The cell type determines to a large extent the type of therapy required and the prognosis for survival. The most common varieties are papillary and follicular carcinomas, which are usually associated with prolonged survival. The anaplastic tumor is rare and carries a very bad prognosis. Finally, the medullary carcinoma of the thyroid originates in the parafollicular cells derived from the last branchial pouch, contains amyloid deposits, and secretes calcitonin. It is familial and often associated with pheochromocytomas (multiple endocrine neoplasia type II) and with the syndrome of multiple mucosal neuromas (multiple endocrine neoplasia type III).

Clinical Findings

A. Symptoms and Signs: The principal signs of thyroid cancer are a painless nodule, a hard nodule in an enlarged thyroid gland, so-called lateral aberrant thyroid tissue, or palpable lymph nodes with thyroid enlargement. Signs of pressure or invasion of the neck structures are present in anaplastic or long-standing tumors.

B. Laboratory Findings: With very few exceptions, all thyroid function tests are normal unless the disease is associated with thyroiditis. The scintiscan usually shows a "cold" nodule. Serum thyroid autoantibodies are sometimes found. Thyroglobulin levels are high in metastatic papillary and follicular tumors. In medullary carcinoma the calcitonin levels are elevated, especially after a calcium infusion. Calcitonin assay is a reliable clue to silent medullary carcinoma, especially in the familial syndrome, although an occasional extrathyroidal tumor (eg, lung) may also produce calcitonin.

C. X-Ray Findings: Extensive bone and soft tissue metastases (some of which may take up radioiodine) may be demonstrable.

Differential Diagnosis (Table 19–6.)

Since nonmalignant enlargements of the thyroid gland are far more common than carcinoma, it is at times most difficult to establish the diagnosis except by biopsy (which may be an open biopsy or a needle biopsy). Echography may be helpful in differentiating cystic and solid nodules. Purely cystic lesions are

Table 19–5. Some characteristics of thyroid cancer.

	Papillary	Follicular	Amyloidic Solid	Anaplastic
Incidence*(%)	61	18	6	15
Average age*	42	50	50	57
Females*(%)	70	72	56	56
Deaths due to thyroid cancer*†(%)	6	24	33	98
Invasion: Juxtanodal	+++++	+	++++++	+++
Blood vessels	+	+++	+++	+++++
Distant sites	+	+++	++	++++
Resemblance to normal thyroid	+	+++	+	±
^{123}I uptake	+	++++	0	0
Degree of malignancy	+	++ to +++	+++	++++++++

*Data based upon 885 cases analyzed by Woolner et al; figures have been rounded to the nearest digit. (After Woolner.)

†Some patients have been followed up to 32 years after diagnosis.

Table 19–6. Differential diagnosis of thyroid nodules.*

Clinical Evidence	Low Index of Suspicion	High Index of Suspicion
History	Familial history of goiter Residence in area of endemic goiter	Previous therapeutic irradiation of head, neck, or chest Hoarseness
Physical characteristics	Older women Soft nodule Multinodular goiter	Children, young adults; men Solitary, firm, dominant nodule Vocal cord paralysis Enlarged lymph nodes Distant metastatic lesions
Serum factors	High titer of antithyroid antibody	Elevated serum calcitonin
Scanning techniques Uptake of ^{123}I Echo scan Thermography Roentgenogram	"Hot" nodule Cystic lesion Cold Shell-like calcification	"Cold" nodule Solid lesion Warm Punctate calcification
Technetium flow	Avascular	Vascular
Thyroxine therapy	Regression after 0.2 mg/d for 3 months or more	No regression

*Reproduced, with permission, from Greenspan FS: Thyroid nodules and thyroid cancer. *West J Med* 1974;**121**:359.

almost always benign. The incidence of malignancy is much greater in single than in multinodular lesions, and far greater in nonfunctioning than in functioning nodules. The differentiation from chronic thyroiditis is at times most difficult, and the 2 lesions may occur together. Any nonfunctioning lesion in the region of the thyroid that does not decrease in size on thyroid therapy or increases rapidly must be considered carcinoma until proved otherwise. Percutaneous needle aspiration biopsy has been very useful when an experienced cytopathologist is available.

Complications

The complications vary with the type of carcinoma. Papillary tumors invade local structures, such as lymph nodes; follicular tumors metastasize through the bloodstream; anaplastic carcinomas invade local structures, causing constriction and nerve palsies, as well as leading to widespread metastases. The complications of radical neck surgery often include permanent hypoparathyroidism, vocal cord palsy, and myxedema.

Treatment

Surgical removal, if possible, is the treatment of choice for most thyroid carcinomas. The appropriate extent of surgical removal is debatable. In recent years, conservative surgery has been shown to be as effective as radical neck dissection, with a much lower

incidence of complications. Papillary tumors respond to thyroid suppressive treatment, which may also be of value in other types (especially after most of the functioning gland has been removed). Some follicular tumors have been treated with radioiodine; metastases may take up radioactive iodine after thyroidectomy or iodide depletion. External irradiation may be useful for local as well as distant metastases. Postoperative myxedema and hypoparathyroidism must be treated in the usual manner.

Reports of chemotherapy of inoperable tumors with doxorubicin are encouraging, but the drug is fairly toxic.

Prognosis

The prognosis is directly related to the cell type. The anaplastic carcinomas advance rapidly in spite of early diagnosis and treatment, while papillary tumors—in spite of frequent bouts of recurrence—are almost never fatal. Early detection and removal of medullary carcinomas by finding elevated calcitonin levels may lead to a better prognosis. In general, the prognosis is less favorable in elderly patients.

Beaugie JM et al: Primary malignant tumours of the thyroid: The relationship between histological classification and clinical behaviour. *Br J Surg* 1976;**63**:173.

Blum M: The diagnosis of the thyroid nodule using aspiration biopsy and cytology. (Editorial.) *Arch Intern Med* 1984;**144**:1140.

Favus MJ et al: Thyroid cancer occurring as a late consequence of head and neck irradiation. *N Engl J Med* 1976;**294**:1019.

Frable WJ: *Fine Needle Aspiration Biopsy.* Saunders, 1983.

Goltzman D et al: Calcitonin as a tumor marker in patients with medullary thyroid carcinoma. *N Engl J Med* 1974;**290**:1035.

Mazzaferri EI, Young RL: Papillary thyroid carcinoma: A 10-year follow-up report of the impact of therapy in 576 patients. *Am J Med* 1981;**70**:511.

Molitch ME et al: The cold thyroid nodule: An analysis of diagnostic and therapeutic options. *Endocr Rev* 1984;**5**:185.

Van Herle AJ et al: The thyroid nodule. *Ann Intern Med* 1982; **96**:221.

THYROIDITIS

Essentials of Diagnosis

- Swelling of thyroid gland, causing pressure symptoms in acute and subacute forms; painless enlargement in chronic form.
- Thyroid function tests variable; discrepancy in T_4 and radioiodine uptake common.
- Serologic autoantibody tests often positive.

General Considerations

Thyroiditis has been more frequently diagnosed in recent years, since special serologic tests for thyroid autoantibodies became available. This heterogeneous group can be divided into 2 groups: (1) due to a specific cause (usually infection), and (2) due to unknown, often autoimmune factors. The second is the more common form.

Clinical Findings

A. Symptoms and Signs:

1. Thyroiditis due to specific causes (pyogenic infections, tuberculosis, syphilis)–A rare disorder causing severe pain, tenderness, redness, and fluctuation in the region of the thyroid gland.

2. Nonspecific (?autoimmune) thyroiditis–

a. Acute or subacute nonsuppurative thyroiditis (de Quervain's thyroiditis, granulomatous thyroiditis, giant cell thyroiditis, giant follicular thyroiditis)–An acute, usually painful enlargement of the thyroid gland, with dysphagia. The pain radiates into the ears. The manifestations may persist for several weeks and may be associated with signs of thyrotoxicosis and malaise. Middle-aged women are most commonly affected. Viral infection has been suggested as the cause. Transient irradiation thyroiditis may be seen after radioactive iodine therapy.

b. Lymphocytic subacute thyroiditis (lymphocytic thyroiditis with hyperthyroidism, atypical subacute thyroiditis)–This form of thyroiditis, characterized by a silent (painless) swelling of the thyroid and associated with symptoms and signs of hyperthyroidism, is being increasingly recognized in the USA. The clinical manifestations are similar to those of moderate Graves' disease, and the differential diagnosis is not simple. Both may present with symmetric, painless, modest enlargement of the thyroid, tremor, weight loss, stare, lid lag, etc, as well as elevated levels of serum T_4. Antibody titers (antithyroglobulin and antithyroid microsomal) are higher in Graves' disease. The ^{123}I uptake is *low* in this form of thyroiditis and *high* in Graves' disease. The hyperthyroid symptoms abate spontaneously, and normalcy is restored within a few months. The transient hyperthyroid state is due to leakage of preformed thyroid hormone from the inflamed gland and not to hyperactivity of the thyroid cells. These patients, therefore, should *not* receive propylthiouracil. Propranolol is useful for symptomatic control of the hyperthyroid phase. The etiology of this entity is unknown.

c. Hashimoto's thyroiditis (struma lymphomatosa, lymphadenoid goiter, chronic lymphocytic thyroiditis)–The most common form of thyroiditis and probably the most common thyroid disorder. Evidence for an autoimmune cause is uniformly present. Onset of enlargement of the thyroid gland is insidious, with few pressure symptoms. The gland is firm, symmetrically enlarged, lobulated, and nontender to palpation. Signs of thyroid dysfunction seldom appear, but rarely the disease may progress to myxedema or even present as thyrotoxicosis ("hashitoxicosis"), which may be transient.

d. Riedel's thyroiditis (chronic fibrous thyroiditis, Riedel's struma, woody thyroiditis, ligneous thyroiditis, invasive thyroiditis)–This is the rarest form of thyroiditis and is found only in middle-aged women. Enlargement is often asymmetric; the gland is stony hard and adherent to the neck structures, causing signs of compression and invasion, including dysphagia, dyspnea, and hoarseness.

B. Laboratory Findings: The PBI, T_4, and T_3 resin uptake are usually markedly elevated in acute and subacute thyroiditis and normal or low in the chronic forms. Radioiodine uptake is characteristically very low in subacute thyroiditis; it may be high with an uneven scan in chronic thyroiditis with enlargement of the gland, and low in Riedel's struma. The TSH stimulation test shows lack of response in most forms of thyroiditis. Leukocytosis, elevation of the sedimentation rate, and increase in serum globulins are common in acute and subacute forms. Thyroid autoantibodies are most commonly demonstrable in Hashimoto's thyroiditis but are also found in the other types. The serum TSH level is elevated if inadequate amounts of biologically active thyroid hormones are elaborated by the thyroid gland.

Complications

In the suppurative forms of thyroiditis any of the complications of infection may occur; the subacute and chronic forms of the disease are complicated by the effects of pressure on the neck structures: dyspnea and, in Riedel's struma, vocal cord palsy. Hashimoto's thyroiditis often leads to hypothyroidism. Carcinoma or lymphoma may be associated with chronic thyroiditis and must be considered in the diagnosis of uneven painless enlargements that continue in spite of treatment. Hashimoto's thyroiditis may be associated with Addison's disease (Schmidt's syndrome), hypoparathyroidism, diabetes, pernicious anemia, various collagen diseases, biliary cirrhosis, vitiligo, and other autoimmune conditions.

Differential Diagnosis

Thyroiditis must be considered in the differential diagnosis of all types of goiters, especially if enlargement is rapid. In the acute or subacute stages it may simulate thyrotoxicosis, and only a careful evaluation of several of the laboratory findings will point to the correct diagnosis. The very low radioiodine uptake in subacute thyroiditis with elevated T_4 and T_3 uptake and a rapid sedimentation rate is of the greatest help. Chronic thyroiditis, especially if the enlargement is uneven and if there is pressure on surrounding structures, may resemble carcinoma, and both disorders may be present in the same gland. The subacute and suppurative forms of thyroiditis may resemble any infectious process in or near the neck structures; and the presence of malaise, leukocytosis, and a high sedimentation rate is confusing. The thyroid autoantibody tests have been of help in the diagnosis of chronic thyroiditis, but the tests are not specific and may also be positive in patients with goiters, carcinoma, and thyrotoxicosis. Biopsy may be required for diagnosis.

Treatment

A. Suppurative Thyroiditis: Antibiotics, and surgical drainage when fluctuation is marked.

B. Subacute Thyroiditis:

1. DeQuervain's thyroiditis–All treatment is empiric and must be maintained for several weeks, since the recurrence rate is high. The drug of choice is aspirin, which relieves pain and inflammation. Severe cases may require a brief course of prednisone therapy: 10 mg 3 times a day for 1 or 2 weeks is effective, but symptoms and signs may recur after the drug is tapered off. Levothyroxine, propylthiouracil, and external x-ray neck irradiation have been used in the past, but there are no convincing data to justify their use.

2. Lymphocytic thyroiditis with hyperthyroidism does not require the use of anti-inflammatory agents. The symptoms of hyperthyroidism may be treated with propranolol. If hypothyroidism develops later, thyroid replacement therapy is indicated.

C. Hashimoto's Thyroiditis: Thyroid, thyroxine, or triiodothyronine in full doses may reduce the size of the gland markedly; since the disease will often progress to myxedema, this treatment probably should be continued indefinitely.

D. Riedel's Struma: Partial thyroidectomy is often required to relieve pressure; adhesions to surrounding structures make this a difficult operation.

Prognosis

The course of this group of diseases is quite variable. Spontaneous remissions and exacerbations are common in the subacute form, and therapy is nonspecific. The disease process may smolder for months. Thyrotoxicosis may occur. The chronic form may be part of a systemic collagen disease (eg, lupus erythematosus, Sjögren's syndrome) with all of the complications of that disease. Recurrent subacute and, more often, chronic thyroiditis lead to permanent destruction of the thyroid gland in a large number of patients and to myxedema. Continuous thyroid replacement therapy, by suppressing TSH, may shrink the gland. It may also lessen the tendency of malignant transformation in chronic thyroiditis, although this belief is controversial at present.

Fisher DA et al: The diagnosis of Hashimoto's thyroiditis. *J Clin Endocrinol Metab* 1975;**40**:795.

Gordin A, Lamberg BA: Natural course of symptomless autoimmune thyroiditis. *Lancet* 1975;**2**:1234.

Kidd A et al: Immunologic aspects of Graves' and Hashimoto's diseases. *Metabolism* 1980;**29**:80.

Klein I et al: Silent thyrotoxic thyroiditis. *Ann Intern Med* 1982;**96**:242.

Nikolai TF et al: Lymphocytic thyroiditis with spontaneously resolving hyperthyroidism (silent thyroiditis). *Arch Intern Med* 1980;**140**:478.

Woolf PD: Transient painless thyroiditis with hyperthyroidism: A variant of lymphocytic thyroiditis? *Endocr Rev* 1980;**1**:411.

THE PARATHYROIDS

HYPOPARATHYROIDISM & PSEUDOHYPOPARATHYROIDISM

Essentials of Diagnosis

- Tetany, carpopedal spasms, stridor and wheezing, muscle and abdominal cramps, urinary frequency, personality changes, mental torpor.
- Positive Chvostek's sign and Trousseau's phenomenon; defective nails and teeth; cataracts.
- Serum calcium low; serum phosphate high; alkaline phosphatase normal; urine calcium (Sulkowitch) negative.
- Basal ganglia calcification on x-ray of skull.

General Considerations

Hypoparathyroidism is most commonly seen following thyroidectomy or, more rarely, following surgery for parathyroid tumor. Very rarely it follows x-ray irradiation to the neck or massive radioactive iodine administration for cancer of the thyroid. Partial hypoparathyroidism occurs in a significant number of patients after thyroidectomy. It is rarely associated with hemochromatosis or metastatic cancer.

Transient hypoparathyroidism may be seen in the neonatal period, presumably due to a relative underactivity of the parathyroids, to magnesium deficiency, or to extraordinary demands on the parathyroids by the intake of cow's milk containing a great deal of phosphate. A similar mechanism may operate in the tetany of pregnancy. Hypomagnesemia may cause failure of release of parathyroid hormone and also resistance to hormonal action on bone, resulting in hypocalcemia reversible by magnesium repletion.

Neonatal tetany may be a manifestation of maternal hyperparathyroidism.

Idiopathic hypoparathyroidism, often associated with candidiasis, may be familial and may be associated with Addison's disease and thyroiditis due to an autoimmune disorder (multiple endocrine deficiency, autoimmune, candidiasis [MEDAC] syndrome).

Pseudohypoparathyroidism is a genetic defect associated with short stature, round face, obesity, short metacarpals, hypertension, and ectopic bone formation. The parathyroids are present and often hyperplastic, but the renal tubules do not respond to the hormone. This resistance, probably due to a receptor defect, may be incomplete and may disappear spontaneously or after restoration of serum calcium to normal. Recent evidence suggests a selective lack of 1,25-dihydroxyvitamin D in pseudohypoparathyroidism. Various unusual syndromes have been described that have some features of Albright's original report (Albright's osteodystrophy) but lack others (pseudopseudohypoparathyroidism, pseudohypoparathyroidism type II, pseudoidiopathic hypoparathyroidism). In some patients, high levels of parathormone lead to osteitis fibrosa, which is reversible with treatment with vitamin D. (See Nusynowitz reference, below.) Resistance to other hormones (TSH, gonadotropins, glucagon) may be present in pseudohypoparathyroid patients.

Clinical Findings (See Table 19–7.)

A. Symptoms and Signs: Acute hypoparathyroidism causes tetany, with muscle cramps, irritability, carpopedal spasm, and convulsions; stridor, wheezing, dyspnea; photophobia and diplopia; abdominal cramps; and urinary frequency. Symptoms of the chronic disease are lethargy, personality changes, anxiety state, blurring of vision due to cataracts, and mental retardation.

Chvostek's sign (facial contraction on tapping the facial nerve near the angle of the jaw) is positive, and Trousseau's phenomenon (carpal spasm after application of a cuff) is present. Cataracts may occur; the nails may be thin and brittle; the skin dry and scaly, at times with fungus infection (candidiasis) and loss of hair (eyebrows); and deep reflexes may be hyperactive. Choreoathetosis may be found in an occasional patient but is reversible with adequate therapy. Choking of the optic disks is rarely found. Teeth may be defective if the onset of the disease occurs in childhood. Branchial anomalies (eg, cleft palate) may be found. In pseudohypoparathyroidism the fingers and toes are short, with absence of the knuckles of the fourth and fifth fingers on making a fist; ectopic soft tissue calcification may be seen and felt.

B. Laboratory Findings: Serum calcium is low, serum phosphate high, urinary phosphate low (tubular reabsorption of phosphate [TRP] above 95%), urinary calcium low to absent, and alkaline phosphatase normal. Alkaline phosphatase may be elevated in pseudohypoparathyroidism. Creatinine clearance is normal. Parathormone level is low or absent in idiopathic or postsurgical hypoparathyroidism but normal or even markedly elevated in pseudohypoparathyroidism.

C. X-Ray Findings: X-rays of the skull may show basal ganglia calcifications; the bones may be denser than normal (in pseudohypoparathyroidism short metacarpals and ectopic bone may be seen, and bones may be demineralized).

D. Other Examinations: Slit lamp examination may show early cataract formation. The ECG shows generalized dysrhythmia (partially reversible) and may show prolonged QT intervals.

Complications

Acute tetany with stridor, especially if associated with vocal cord palsy, may lead to respiratory obstruction requiring tracheostomy. Severe hypocalcemia may lead to cardiac dilatation and failure and cardiac irregularities resistant to digitalis. The complications of chronic hypoparathyroidism depend largely upon the duration of the disease and the age at onset. If it starts early in childhood, there may be stunting of growth, malformation of the teeth, and retardation of mental development. There may be associated sprue syndrome, pernicious anemia, and Addison's disease, probably on the basis of an autoimmune mechanism. In pseudohypoparathyroidism, hypothyroidism is often found. In long-standing cases, cataract formation and calcification of the basal ganglia are seen. Permanent brain damage with convulsions or psychosis may lead to admission to mental institutions. There may be complications of overtreatment with calcium and vitamin D, with renal impairment and calcinosis.

Differential Diagnosis

The symptoms of hypocalcemic tetany are most commonly confused with or mistaken for tetany due to metabolic or respiratory alkalosis, in which the serum calcium is normal. Symptoms of anxiety are common in both instances, and fainting is not uncommon in the hyperventilation syndrome. The typical blood and urine findings should differentiate the 2 disorders. This holds true also for less common causes of hypocalcemic tetany, such as rickets and osteomalacia in the

Table 19–7. Principal findings in the various parathyroid syndromes.*

Syndrome	Low Serum Ca With High Serum P	Serum Alkaline Phosphatase	Cataracts; Calcification of Basal Ganglia	Microdactylia; Ectopic Bone	Subperiosteal Resorption (Osteitis)	Parathyroid Hyperplasia	Ellsworth-Howard Test†	PTH Assay
Hypoparathyroidism	+	Normal	+	0	0	0	+	0
Pseudohypoparathyroidism	+	Normal	+	+	0	+	0	Normal or ↑
Pseudopseudohypoparathyroidism	0	Normal	0	+	0	0	+	Normal
Secondary (renal) hyperparathyroidism	+ (NPN↑)	↑	0	0	+	+	±	↑
Pseudohypoparathyroidism with secondary hyperparathyroidism	+ (NPN normal)	↑	±	+	+	+	0	↑

*Modified and reproduced, with permission, from Kolb FO, Steinbach HL: Pseudohypoparathyroidism with secondary hyperparathyroidism and osteitis fibrosa. *J Clin Endocrinol Metab* 1962;**22**:68.

†Responsiveness to parathyroid hormone.

early stages and acute pancreatitis. In these conditions the serum phosphorus is usually low or low normal; rarely high. Confusion might arise with the tetany due to magnesium deficiency or in chronic renal failure, in which retention of phosphorus will produce a high serum phosphorus with low serum calcium, but the differentiation should be obvious on clinical grounds (eg, uremia, azotemia).

In primary hyperaldosteronism with tetany (due to alkalosis) there is associated hypertension and hypokalemia with inability to concentrate the urine. Hypomagnesemia must be considered if tetany fails to respond to calcium.

The physical signs of pseudohypoparathyroidism without the abnormal blood chemical findings are seen in certain dysplasias ("pseudopseudohypoparathyroidism").

In order to differentiate true hypoparathyroidism, which responds to parathyroid extract, from pseudohypoparathyroidism, which does not respond, the Ellsworth-Howard test (phosphaturia after administration of parathyroid hormone intravenously) may be performed. The parathyroid hormone resistance has been demonstrated to be due to failure of activation of renal adenylate cyclase with defective excretion of cAMP after administration of parathyroid hormone. Medullary carcinoma of the thyroid is rarely associated with hypocalcemia in spite of excess calcitonin.

At times hypoparathyroidism is misdiagnosed as idiopathic epilepsy, choreoathetosis, or brain tumor (on the basis of brain calcifications, convulsions, choked disks) or, more rarely, as "asthma" (on the basis of stridor and dyspnea). Other causes of cataracts and basal ganglia calcification also enter into the differential diagnosis.

Treatment

A. Emergency Treatment for Acute Attack (Hypoparathyroid Tetany): This usually occurs after surgery and requires immediate treatment.

1. Be sure an adequate airway is present.

2. Calcium chloride, 5–10 mL of 10% solution intravenously slowly until tetany ceases, or calcium gluconate, 10–20 mL of 10% solution intravenously, may be given. Ten to 50 mL of either solution may be added to 1 L of 5% glucose in water or saline and administered by slow intravenous drip. The rate should be so adjusted that the serum calcium is raised above 7 mg/dL and maintained between 8 and 9 mg/dL. *Note:* Do not treat tetany too vigorously, or irreversible tissue calcification will occur.

3. Calcium salts should be given orally as soon as possible to supply 1–2 g of calcium daily: calcium gluconate, 8 g 3 times daily; calcium lactate powder, 4–8 g 3 times daily (some patients prefer tablet form); or calcium chloride, 2–4 g 3 times daily (as 30% solution). Calcium carbonate is effective in smaller doses than either calcium gluconate or lactate and is better tolerated than calcium chloride. It is the calcium salt of choice at present. OsCal, a preparation of cal-

cium carbonate containing 250 mg of calcium, is well tolerated. Dosage is 4–8 tablets per day.

4. Dihydrotachysterol (Hytakerol, AT 10) and calciferol–Give either compound as soon as oral calcium is begun. Pure crystalline preparations of dihydrotachysterol in tablets of 0.125, 0.2, and 0.4 mg are available. The initial dose is 0.8–2.4 mg daily for several days. Calciferol, 80–160 thousand units (2–4 mg) daily, is almost as effective (though slower to act) and probably should be used in most patients. 1,25-Dihydroxycholecalciferol (calcitriol, Rocaltrol) is highly effective in hypoparathyroid tetany in doses of 1–3 μg/d. (See Table 19–9.)

5. Phenytoin and phenobarbital have been shown to control overt and latent tetany without alteration in calcium levels. These agents may be used as adjuncts in the management of refractory patients.

B. Maintenance Treatment:

1. High-calcium, low-phosphate diet (omit milk and cheese).

2. Calcium salts (as above except chloride) are continued.

3. Dihydrotachysterol, 0.2–1 mg daily, to maintain blood calcium at normal level.

4. Calciferol, 40–200 thousand units (1–5 mg) daily, is the drug of choice at present for the majority of patients. In some cases, up to 7 or 8 mg of calciferol daily may be needed. Its action is probably similar to that of dihydrotachysterol, and it can certainly be substituted adequately clinically. The initial action of vitamin D appears to be slower. However, the cost to the patient is less than with dihydrotachysterol. It accumulates in the body over prolonged periods, and serum calcium levels should be checked periodically. *Note:* Corticosteroids are effective antidotes in vitamin D intoxication. The active metabolites of vitamin D (see above) may be used if there is unusual resistance to calciferol and in pseudohypoparathyroidism.

5. Aluminum hydroxide gels may be employed to help lower the serum phosphate level in the initial stages of treatment. They are rarely required for chronic therapy.

6. Chlorthalidone, 50 mg/d, combined with a low-sodium diet, may control mild hypoparathyroidism without the use of vitamin D, which would cause more complications. (See Porter reference, below).

Caution: Phenothiazine drugs should be administered with caution in hypoparathyroid patients, since they may precipitate dystonic reactions. Furosemide should be avoided, since it may enhance hypocalcemia.

Prognosis

The outlook is fair if prompt diagnosis is made and treatment instituted. Some changes (eg, in the electroencephalogram) are reversible, but the dental changes, cataracts, and brain calcifications are permanent. They may be in part genetically determined and not related to hypocalcemia per se. Although treatment of the immediate acute attack is simple and effective, long-term therapy is tedious and expensive, since a good preparation of parathormone is not available. Adequate control by a fairly intelligent patient is required to avoid undertreatment or overtreatment. Periodic blood chemical evaluation is required, since sudden changes in calcium levels may call for modification of the treatment schedule. Sudden appearance of hypercalcemia, especially in children, may be due to Addison's disease.

Unrecognized or late cases may find their way into mental institutions.

Breslau NA, Pak CYC: Hypoparathyroidism. *Metabolism* 1979; **28:**1261.

Burckhardt P: Idiopathic hypoparathyroidism and autoimmunity. *Horm Res* 1982;**16:**304.

Hall FM et al: Pseudohypoparathyroidism presenting as renal osteodystrophy. *Skeletal Radiol* 1981;**6:**43.

Haussler MR, Cordy PE: Metabolites and analogues of vitamin D: Which for what? *JAMA* 1982;**247:**841.

Juan D: Hypocalcemia: Differential diagnosis and mechanisms. *Arch Intern Med* 1979;**139:**1166.

Levine MA et al: Resistance to multiple hormone in patients with pseudohypoparathyroidism: Association with deficient activity of guanine nucleotide regulatory protein. *Am J Med* 1983; **74:**545.

Nusynowitz ML, Frame B, Kolb FO: The spectrum of the hypoparathyroid states: A classification based on physiologic principles. *Medicine* 1976;**55:**105.

Okano K et al: Comparative efficacy of various vitamin D metabolites in the treatment of various types of hypoparathyroidism. *J Clin Endocrinol Metab* 1982;**55:**238.

Porter RH et al: Treatment of hypoparathyroid patients with chlorthalidone. *N Engl J Med* 1978;**298:**577.

Rude RK, Oldham SB, Singer FR: Functional hypoparathyroidism and parathyroid hormone end-organ resistance in human magnesium deficiency. *Clin Endocrinol (Oxf)* 1976; **5:**209.

Spiegel AM et al: Pseudohypoparathyroidism: The molecular basis for hormone resistance—A retrospective. (Editorial.) *N Engl J Med* 1982;**307:**679.

Van Dop C, Bourne HR: Pseudohypoparathyroidism. *Annu Rev Med* 1983;**34:**259.

HYPERPARATHYROIDISM

Essentials of Diagnosis

- Renal stones, nephrocalcinosis, polyuria, polydipsia, hypertension, uremia, intractable peptic ulcer, constipation.
- Bone pain, cystic lesions, and, rarely, pathologic fractures.
- Serum and urine calcium elevated; urine phosphate high with low to normal serum phosphate; alkaline phosphatase normal to elevated.
- "Band keratopathy" on slit lamp examination of cornea.
- X-ray: subperiosteal resorption, loss of lamina dura of teeth, renal parenchymal calcification or stones, bone cysts, chondrocalcinosis.
- Elevated levels of parathyroid hormone.

General Considerations

Primary hyperparathyroidism is a relatively rare disease, but its incidence appears to be increasing; it is potentially curable if detected early. Recent surveys suggest that hyperfunction of the parathyroids, often as asymptomatic hypercalcemia, may be present in 0.1% of patients examined. (*Note:* It should always be suspected in obscure bone and renal disease, especially if nephrocalcinosis or calculi are present.) At least 5% of renal stones are associated with this disease. A past history of neck radiotherapy may be of etiologic importance in some cases.

About 80% of cases of primary hyperparathyroidism are caused by a single adenoma (or, in rare cases, 2 adenomas); 15–20% are caused by primary hypertrophy and hyperplasia of all 4 glands; and 2% are caused by carcinoma of one gland. Recent findings suggest that chief cell hyperplasia may be more common than previously reported. Multiple neoplasms, often familial, of the pancreas, pituitary, thyroid, and adrenal glands may be associated with primary hyperparathyroidism due to tumor or, more commonly, due to hyperplasia of the parathyroids (multiple endocrine adenomatosis types I and IIa and IIb; see Table 19–14).

Secondary hyperparathyroidism is almost always associated with hyperplasia of all 4 glands, but on rare occasions an autonomous tumor may arise in hyperplastic glands ("tertiary hyperparathyroidism"). It is most commonly seen in chronic renal disease, but is also found in rickets, osteomalacia, and acromegaly.

Hyperparathyroidism causes excessive excretion of calcium and phosphate by the kidneys; this eventually produces either calculus formation within the urinary tract or, less commonly, diffuse parenchymal calcification (nephrocalcinosis). (The 2 types rarely coexist.) If the excessive demands for calcium are met by dietary intake, the bones may not become drained. If calcium intake is not adequate, bone disease may occur. This may show either diffuse demineralization, pathologic fractures, or cystic bone lesions throughout the skeleton ("osteitis fibrosa cystica"). Factors other than the calcium intake, eg, the level of circulating 1,25-dihydroxyvitamin D, may determine whether bone or stone disease will be present in hyperparathyroidism.

Clinical Findings

A. Symptoms and Signs: The manifestations of hyperparathyroidism may be divided into those referable to (1) skeletal involvement, (2) renal and urinary tract damage, and (3) hypercalcemia per se. Since the adenomas are small and deeply located, only about 5% are palpable. Hyperparathyroidism may be associated with a thyroid adenoma or carcinoma. Some patients have surprisingly few symptoms, and the disease is discovered fortuitously by blood chemical findings.

1. Skeletal manifestations–These may vary from simple back pain, joint pains, painful shins, and similar complaints, to actual pathologic fractures of the spine, ribs, or long bones, with loss of height and progressive kyphosis. At times an epulis of the jaw (actually a "brown tumor") may be the telltale sign of osteitis fibrosa. "Clubbing" of the fingers due to fracture and telescoping of the tips occur more rarely.

2. Urinary tract manifestations–Polyuria and polydipsia occur early in the disease. Sand, gravel, or stones containing calcium oxalate or phosphate may be passed in the urine. Secondary infection and obstruction may cause nephrocalcinosis and renal damage, leading eventually to renal failure.

3. Manifestations of hypercalcemia–Thirst, anorexia, and nausea and vomiting are outstanding symptoms. Often one finds a past history of peptic ulcer, with obstruction or even hemorrhage. There may be stubborn constipation, asthenia, anemia, and weight loss. Hypertension is commonly found. Some patients present primarily with neuromuscular disorders such as muscle weakness, easy fatigability, or paresthesias. Depression and psychosis may occur. Of unusual interest is hypermotility of joints. The fingernails and toenails may be unusually strong and thick. Calcium may precipitate in the corneas ("band keratopathy"). In secondary (renal) hyperparathyroidism, calcium also precipitates in the soft tissues, especially around the joints. Recurrent pancreatitis occurs in some patients.

B. Laboratory Findings: Serum calcium is usually high (adjust for serum protein); the serum phosphate is low or normal; the urinary calcium is often high, but at times is normal or low. There is an excessive loss of phosphate in the urine in the presence of low to low normal serum phosphate (low tubular reabsorption of phosphate; TRP below 89–90%); the alkaline phosphatase is elevated only if clinical bone disease is present (in about 25% of cases). The plasma chloride and uric acid levels may be elevated. (In secondary hyperparathyroidism the serum phosphate is high as a result of renal retention, and the calcium is usually low or normal.) Radioimmunoassays for parathormone are available to confirm the diagnosis in most cases and to establish the diagnosis of "normocalcemic hyperparathyroidism"; however, since the circulating hormone is heterogeneous, there are still technical problems with any assay procedure. (See Habener reference, below.)

A great number of special tests have been devised to demonstrate abnormal phosphate dynamics in primary hyperparathyroidism. None of these are as consistently reliable as several accurately performed serum calcium determinations combined with a good parathyroid hormone assay, which demonstrate hypercalcemia for which no other cause can be detected. Control of the dietary phosphate is important, since high phosphate intake may normalize borderline high serum calcium levels. Measurement of nephrogenous cyclic adenosine monophosphate can be used as a biologic test of parathyroid hormone function.

C. X-Ray Findings: X-ray rarely demonstrates the tumor on barium swallow; at times, special angiography may demonstrate it. If bone disease is present, one may see diffuse demineralization, subperiosteal resorption of bone (especially in the radial aspects of the fingers), and often loss of the lamina dura of the teeth. There may be cysts throughout the skeleton, mottling of the skull ("salt and pepper appearance"), or pathologic fractures. Articular cartilage calcification (chondrocalcinosis) is sometimes found. One may find calculi in the urinary tract or diffuse stippled calcifications in the region of the kidneys (nephrocalcinosis). Soft tissue calcifications around the joints and in the blood vessels may be seen in renal osteitis.

D. Other Examinations: Electrocardiography may show a shortened QT interval. Slit lamp examination of the eye may show corneal calcification ("band keratopathy").

The localization of parathyroid tumors by selenomethionine scanning or in vivo parathyroid staining is of little value; selective radioimmunoassay via venous catheter to localize hyperfunctioning glands is usually done only after an unsuccessful prior neck exploration. Angiography may locate ectopic and intrathoracic tumors. Bone densitometry may show loss of trabecular bone not seen on routine x-ray.

Thermography and ultrasonography may help locate fair-sized adenomas; CT scan may locate aberrant tumors. Recently enlarged parathyroid glands have been located with the technetium-thallium subtraction scan (see Ferlin et al reference, below).

Complications

Although the striking complications are those associated with skeletal damage (eg, pathologic fractures), the serious ones are those referable to renal damage. Urinary tract infection due to stone and obstruction may lead to renal failure and uremia. If the serum calcium level rises rapidly (eg, due to dehydration or salt restriction), "parathyroid poisoning" may occur, with acute cardiac and renal failure and rapid precipitation of calcium throughout the soft tissues. Peptic ulcer and pancreatitis may be intractable before surgery. Pancreatic islet cell adenoma with hypoglycemia may be associated, or ulcerogenic pancreatic tumor may coexist. Hypertension is frequently found. Reversible changes in glucose tolerance and insulin secretion have been reported. There may be associated hyperthyroidism, thyroiditis, or thyroid carcinoma. There is also an increased incidence of hyperuricemia and gouty arthritis. Pseudogout may complicate hyperparathyroidism both before and after surgical removal of tumors. Subcutaneous, soft tissue, and extensive vascular calcification—as well as dermal necrosis—may occur in secondary hyperparathyroidism due to renal insufficiency.

Differential Diagnosis (See Table 19–10.)

The combination of high calcium and low phosphate in the serum, high urinary phosphate and calcium, and normal or high serum alkaline phosphatase is almost pathognomonic of hyperparathyroidism. Only rarely has this combination been seen in multiple myeloma, metastatic cancer (kidney, bladder, thyroid), and hyperthyroidism. The most common problem is the differentiation of idiopathic hypercalciuria with renal stones from primary hyperparathyroidism with borderline serum calcium levels. If renal damage is present, the typical picture may be obscured, ie, the serum phosphate may not be low. Other causes of hypercalcemia (eg, sarcoidosis, vitamin D intoxication) usually respond to the administration of corticosteroids, which usually does not affect the hypercalcemia of primary hyperparathyroidism. Chlorothiazides may raise the serum calcium level. Hypercalcemia due to hypervitaminosis A must be considered as a possibility. If bone disease is present, the typical subperiosteal resorption may differentiate osteitis fibrosa from nonmetabolic bone disease (eg, neoplasm) and from osteoporosis. Bone biopsy may at times settle the diagnosis.

Nonmetastasizing carcinomas (eg, of the lung, kidney, or ovary) have been described with blood chemical changes identical with those seen in hyperparathyroidism; these changes are often reversible upon removal or chemotherapy of these tumors, which appear to produce a parathyroidlike humoral agent or a prostaglandin. If significant hypercalcemia is produced by a disorder other than hyperparathyroidism, the PTH level should be low or undetectable, since the parathyroid glands are suppressed. In actual practice, this is not always the case because of difficulties with the assay and the fact that disorders producing hypercalcemia may coexist with hyperparathyroidism (eg, sarcoidosis, hyperthyroidism, breast carcinoma). Familial hyperplasia of the parathyroids and of other endocrine glands requiring surgical treatment has been seen. Another syndrome, **familial hypocalciuric hypercalcemia,** runs a relatively benign course, is not reversed by subtotal resection of the parathyroid glands, and is best treated conservatively.

Treatment

A. Surgical Measures: A parathyroid tumor, the usual cause, should be removed surgically. The surgeon must be aware that multiple tumors may be present; the tumor may be in the thyroid gland or in an ectopic site, eg, the mediastinum. Hyperplasia of all glands requires removal of 3 glands and subtotal resection of the fourth before cure is assured. Success is related to the expertness of the surgery and follow-up care. Total parathyroidectomy with transplantation of a normal amount of functioning parathyroid tissue into the forearm is a new experimental approach. It is useful when total thyroidectomy is required and in instances of severe primary or secondary parathyroid hyperplasia. It simplifies the management of recurrent hypercalcemia and permits avoidance of permanent hypocalcemia, which is common in such situations. After surgery the patient may in the course of several hours or days develop tetany (usually transient) as a result of rapid fall of blood calcium even though the calcium level may fall only to the normal or low normal range. *Caution:* Be certain that an adequate airway is present. Therapy is as for hypoparathyroid tetany (see p 716). Prolonged hypocalcemia due to recalcification of the "hungry" skeleton may require large amounts of calcium and vitamin D. Additional magnesium salts may have to be given postoperatively.

B. Fluids: A large fluid intake is necessary so that a diluted urine will be excreted to minimize the formation of calcium phosphate renal stones.

C. Treatment of Hypercalcemia: Force fluids both orally and parenterally (sodium chloride given intravenously is most helpful); mobilize the patient; reduce calcium intake; and add extra phosphate orally. Cortisone therapy is usually not effective in this type of hypercalcemia. Sodium sulfate and sodium and potassium phosphate as slow intravenous infusions have been used successfully in patients with hypercalcemia but are hazardous. Furosemide is especially effective; ethacrynic acid may be helpful. Chlorothiazides should not be given. If renal function is impaired, hemodialysis may be lifesaving if only for a short time. Mithramycin effectively reduces the hypercalcemia due to hyperparathyroidism or malignancy, but this drug is quite toxic. Calcitonin combined with glucocorticoids has been used in the treatment of hypercalcemia, but its value is uncertain. The patient with hypercalcemia is very sensitive to the toxic effects of digitalis. Propranolol may be useful in preventing the adverse cardiac effects of hypercalcemia.

D. Medical Treatment of Mild Hyperparathyroidism: Since this disorder is more frequently recognized by routine chemical screening procedures, a number of patients with relatively mild hypercalcemia and few symptoms are encountered. They are best managed by forcing fluids; avoiding immobilization and chlorothiazides; adding phosphate preparations if renal function is good; and giving estrogenic hormones if postmenopausal. Recent reports suggest that cimetidine may lower the markedly elevated parathormone levels in uremic patients without altering the serum calcium level, while long-term administration of propranolol may lower both elevated serum calcium and parathormone levels in primary hyperparathyroidism. If the patient cannot be followed periodically or becomes symptomatic—eg, passes a stone—neck exploration must be considered.

Prognosis

The disease is usually a chronic progressive one unless treated successfully by surgical removal of the abnormal parathyroid glands. There are at times unexplained exacerbations and partial remissions. Completely asymptomatic patients with mild hypercalcemia may be followed by means of serial calcium determinations and treated medically as outlined above. (See Scholz reference, below.)

Spontaneous cure due to necrosis of the tumor has been reported but is exceedingly rare. The prognosis is directly related to the degree of renal impairment. The bones, in spite of severe cyst formation, deformity, and fracture, will heal completely if a tumor is successfully removed, but this may take several years. Significant renal damage, however, progresses even after removal of an adenoma, and life expectancy is materially reduced. Secondary hyperparathyroidism not infrequently results due to irreversible renal impairment. In carcinoma of the parathyroid (rare), the prognosis is not necessarily hopeless. The presence of pancreatitis increases the mortality. If hypercalcemia is severe, the patient may suddenly die in cardiac arrest or may develop irreversible acute renal failure. However, early diagnosis and cure of this disease in an increasing number of patients have led to dramatic recovery. In some patients, reversal of bizarre neuromuscular disorders (neuropathy, asthenia) occurs. Improvement in mentation is often but not always seen after successful surgery. Prolonged postoperative follow-up must be stressed to ensure that the state of hyperparathyroidism has been reversed.

The distressing bone disease of secondary hyperparathyroidism due to renal failure (renal osteodystrophy) can be partially prevented and treated by careful monitoring of the phosphate and parathormone levels. Resistance to vitamin D can now be overcome by the newer biologically active derivatives, eg, 1,25-dihydroxycholecalciferol and 1α-hydroxycholecalciferol. "Tertiary hyperparathyroidism," ie, hypercalcemia following correction of renal failure, is rarely seen in patients so managed, and parathyroidectomy is rarely required nowadays for this disorder.

Bilezikian JP: The medical management of primary hyperparathyroidism. Ann Intern Med 1982;96:198.

Binstock ML, Mundy GR: Effect of calcitonin and glucocorticoids in combination on the hypercalcemia of malignancy. Ann Intern Med 1980;93:269.

Broadus AE et al: A detailed evaluation of oral phosphate therapy in selected patients with primary hyperparathyroidism. J Clin Endocrinol Metab 1983;56:953.

Ferlin G et al: New perspectives in localizing enlarged parathyroids by technetium-thallium subtraction scan. J Nucl Med 1983;24:438.

Gaz RD, Wang CA: Management of asymptomatic hyperparathyroidism. Am J Surg 1984;147:498.

Habener JF, Segre GV: Parathyroid hormone radioimmunoassay. (Editorial.) Ann Intern Med 1979;91:782.

Hanley DA, Sherwood LM: Secondary hyperparathyroidism in chronic renal failure: Pathophysiology and treatment. Med Clin North Am 1978;62:1319.

Hodgson SF, Heath H III: Asymptomatic primary hyperparathyroidism: Treat or follow? (Editorial.) Mayo Clin Proc 1981;56:521.

Jacob AI et al: Reduction by cimetidine of serum parathyroid hormone levels in uremic patients. N Engl J Med 1980;302:671.

Kinder BK et al: Diagnostic and therapeutic approaches to primary hyperparathyroidism. Surg Clin North Am 1980;60:1285.

Lafferty FW: Primary hyperparathyroidism: Changing clinical spectrum, prevalence of hypertension, and discriminant analysis of laboratory tests. Arch Intern Med 1981;141:1761.

Lee DBN, Kleeman CR, Zawada ET: The pathophysiology and clinical aspects of hypercalcemic disorders. West J Med 1978;129:278.

Marcus R et al: Conjugated estrogens in the treatment of postmenopausal women with hyperparathyroidism. Ann Intern Med 1984;100:633.

Marx SJ et al: Familial hypocalciuric hypercalcemia: The relation to primary parathyroid hyperplasia. N Engl J Med 1982;307:416.

Mundy GR, Martin TJ: The hypercalcemia of malignancy: Pathogenesis and treatment. Metabolism 1982;73:1247.

Netelenbos C, Lips P, van der Meer C: Hyperparathyroidism following irradiation of benign diseases of the head and neck. Cancer 1983;52:458.

Saxe AW, Brennan MF: Reoperative parathyroid surgery for primary hyperparathyroidism caused by multiple-gland disease: Total parathyroidectomy and autotransplantation with cryopreserved tissue. Surgery 1982;91:616.

Scholz DA, Purnell DC: Asymptomatic primary hyperparathyroidism: 10-year prospective study. Mayo Clin Proc 1981;56:473.

Shane E, Bilezikian JP: Parathyroid carcinoma: A review of 62 patients. Endocr Rev 1982;3:218.

Stark DD et al: Parathyroid imaging: Comparison of high-resolution CT and high-resolution sonography. AJR 1983;141:633.

METABOLIC BONE DISEASE

(See Table 19–10.)

OSTEOMALACIA & RICKETS

Essentials of Diagnosis

- Muscular weakness, listlessness.
- Aching and "bowing" of bones.
- Serum calcium low to normal; serum phosphate low; alkaline phosphatase elevated.
- "Pseudofractures" and "washed out" bone on x-ray.

General Considerations (See Table 19–8.)

Osteomalacia is the adult form of rickets. It is a condition resulting from a calcium or phosphorus deficiency (or both) in the bone. It may be caused by insufficient absorption from the intestine, due either to a lack of calcium alone, or a lack of or resistance to the action of vitamin D. In adults, this form of osteomalacia is almost always found in association with disorders of fat absorption (diarrhea, sprue, pancreatitis, gastrectomy). The other more common variety of osteomalacia is found in association with renal phosphorus losses ("vitamin D-resistant rickets"), which is often a familial disorder. In this disorder, osteomalacia is the result of renal tubular losses of phosphate or calcium often associated with renal tubular acidosis. There may be associated glycosuria and aminoaciduria (Fanconi's syndrome). Cases of osteomalacia have been described that are due to chronic phosphate depletion from prolonged use of aluminum hydroxide gels or to long-term anticonvulsant therapy. A rare case of vitamin D-resistant rickets may be due to a mesenchymal tumor or fibrous dysplasia of bone. Almost all forms of osteomalacia are associated

Table 19–8. Disorders of vitamin D metabolism associated with bone disease: Etiology and pathogenesis.*

Osteomalacia/rickets

1. Inadequate amounts of vitamin D in the diet and/or failure of formation from precursors in the skin.
2. Malabsorption of vitamin D from the intestine.
3. Defects in the metabolism of vitamin D.
   a. Failure of formation of 25-hydroxyvitamin D as in hepatic disorders.
   b. Failure of formation of 1,25-dihydroxyvitamin D as in renal disease.
   c. Enhanced metabolism of vitamin D or its metabolites to other nonactive compounds as in long-term anticonvulsant therapy.
   d. Type I vitamin D–dependent hypophosphatemic rickets (autosomal recessive), responsive to minute amounts of 1,25-dihydroxyvitamin D_3.
   e. Type II vitamin D–dependent rickets—end-organ unresponsiveness to 1,25-dihydroxyvitamin D_3.
4. Renal tubular disorders resulting in hypophosphatemia, hypophosphatemic rickets (X-linked), nonresponsive to physiologic amounts of 1,25-dihydroxyvitamin D_3.
5. Hypophosphatemia associated with neoplasia; therapy with phosphate binders.
6. Acidosis—possibly as a result of decreased 1,25-dihydroxyvitamin D_3 synthesis or increased 1,25-dihydroxyvitamin D_3 metabolism.

Other disorders associated with defects in vitamin D metabolism and bone disease

1. Hypoparathyroidism.
2. Hyperparathyroidism.
3. Pseudohypoparathyroidism.
4. Nephrotic syndrome.
5. Osteoporosis.

*Reproduced, with permission, from Kumar R, Riggs BL: Vitamin D in the therapy of disorders of calcium and phosphorus metabolism. *Mayo Clin Proc* 1981;**56:**327.

with compensatory, secondary hyperparathyroidism initiated by the low calcium level. It is for this reason that most patients will show only slightly low serum calcium levels (compensated osteomalacia). In chronic uremic states, a mixed picture of osteomalacia and secondary hyperparathyroidism is seen ("renal osteodystrophy"). Aluminum intoxication incident to chronic dialysis therapy may be an important factor. (See Walker reference, below.) Resistance to the action of vitamin D due to failure of its conversion to the biologically active forms, 25-hydroxycholecalciferol and 1,25-dihydroxycholecalciferol, by the liver and kidney, respectively, has been demonstrated in many clinical states as outlined in Table 19–8.

A special form of osteomalacia is the so-called **Milkman's syndrome,** an x-ray diagnosis of multiple bilaterally symmetric pseudofractures that may represent the shadows of calluses near arterial blood vessels traversing and eroding the soft skeleton. Rickets, which is the counterpart of osteomalacia in the growing child, shows additional features, especially around the epiphyses, which are widened and "moth-

eaten" on x-ray. Beading of the ribs, Harrison's groove, bowlegs, and disturbances in growth also occur.

In contrast to osteoporosis, where fractures are more common, osteomalacia is more often associated with bowing of bones.

Clinical Findings

A. Symptoms and Signs: Manifestations are variable, ranging from almost none in mild cases to marked muscular weakness and listlessness in advanced cases. There is usually mild aching of the bones, especially of long bones and ribs, and a tendency to bowing. In the very early and acute osteomalacias, a rapidly falling calcium level may be associated with clinical tetany, although this is rare. As compensation takes place, tetanic features are absent. Malabsorption syndromes may include osteomalacia. A low-potassium syndrome with muscular weakness and paralysis may be present with renal tubular disorders.

B. Laboratory Findings: Serum calcium is low or normal but never high. Serum phosphate is low (may be normal in early stages). The alkaline phosphatase is elevated except in the early phase. Urinary calcium and phosphate are usually low in absorptive disorders and high in renal lesions. The intravenous calcium infusion test demonstrates avidity of bone for calcium (80–90% retained) in osteomalacia due to malabsorption. The blood level of 25-hydroxycholecalciferol may be low. There is decrease in bone mass as measured by more sophisticated techniques. Laboratory findings of the primary steatorrhea or renal disease may be present. Characteristics of renal tubular acidosis are described on p 563. Hypomagnesemia is common in disorders of malabsorption.

C. X-Ray Findings: Involvement of the pelvis and long bones, with demineralization and bowing, is seen; less often, the spine and skull are involved as well. Fractures are rare except for "pseudofractures." Nephrocalcinosis may be seen in patients with renal tubular acidosis.

D. Bone Scintiscan: Bone scans may show increased uptake of tracer material and may locate lesions not visualized on conventional radiograms, eg, pseudofractures.

E. Bone Biopsy: This may be the only way to make a diagnosis. Undecalcified sections must be used with special staining methods to show undecalcified osteoid and osteoblastic overactivity.

Differential Diagnosis (See Table 19–8.)

It is most important to recognize osteomalacia and consider it in the differential diagnosis of bone disease, since it is a potentially curable disease. The childhood forms may be mistaken for osteogenesis imperfecta or other nonmetabolic bone disorders.

The acute forms must be differentiated from other forms of tetany. The long-standing disease enters into the differential diagnosis of any metabolic or generalized nonmetabolic bone disease. The pseudofracture is often the only outstanding sign of latent osteomalacia. Osteoporosis may exist as well and may obscure the osteomalacia. At times the diagnosis is confirmed by a rise and subsequent fall of the serum alkaline phosphatase after treatment with vitamin D and calcium. Renal tubular acidosis is a cause of nephrocalcinosis and must be considered in the differential diagnosis of kidney calcifications with bone disease such as hyperparathyroidism. Other causes of hypophosphatemia, eg, chronic alcoholism, enter into the differential diagnosis. The joint aches and pains may be mistaken for some form of arthritis. The cachexia suggests malignancy. Bone biopsy (eg, of the rib or iliac crest) with tetracycline labeling may establish the diagnosis of latent osteomalacia.

Treatment

A. Specific Measures:

1. Rickets–Vitamin D, even in small doses, is specific; 2000–5000 units daily are adequate unless resistance to vitamin D is present.

2. Adult osteomalacia and renal rickets–Vitamin D is specific, but very large doses are necessary to overcome the resistance to its calcium absorptive action and to prevent renal loss of phosphate. Give until an effect is noted on the blood calcium. The usual dose is 25–100 thousand units daily. Doses up to 300,000 units or more daily may be necessary, but if the doses are over 100,000 daily, they must be used cautiously with periodic determination of serum and urine calcium; the serum phosphate may remain low. Crystalline dihydrotachysterol in doses of 0.4–1 mg daily may be an alternative medication in states associated with fat malabsorption.

3. Pancreatic insufficiency–See Chapter 11.

4. Sprue syndrome–See Chapter 11.

5. Some rare forms of renal disease–See Chapter 16.

B. General Measures:
High-calcium diet and calcium gluconate or calcium lactate, 4–20 g daily, or preferably, calcium carbonate, 4–8 g daily. A high-phosphate diet or phosphate salts may be of value in

certain types of renal rickets. Magnesium salts may have to be added.

C. Vitamin D Metabolites: The increasing availability of the biologically active metabolites of calciferol, 25-hydroxycholecalciferol and 1,25-dihydroxycholecalciferol, will help in the treatment of osteomalacia resistant to vitamin D (eg, chronic liver disease and renal failure). (See Table 19–9.)

Prognosis

The prognosis is usually excellent in the absorptive disorders if diagnosed early. This does not hold for certain of the vitamin D–resistant forms of osteomalacia or rickets or for Fanconi's syndrome, which respond slowly or not at all unless huge amounts of vitamin D are given. Calcitriol may heal the bone disease. Hypercalcemia may occur as a complication of therapy. It can be prevented by carefully monitoring the serum and urine calcium periodically; treat with corticosteroids once the disorder has become established. In the renal forms, the ultimate prognosis is that of the basic kidney disease. Respiratory paralysis due to hypokalemia may prove fatal. The greater availability of the metabolically active metabolites of vitamin D will greatly improve the ultimate outlook in this disorder.

Alfrey AC: Aluminum intoxication. (Editorial.) *N Engl J Med* 1984;**17**:1113.

Avioli LV (editor): Vitamin D metabolites: Their clinical importance. *Arch Intern Med* 1978;**138**:835. [Special issue.]

Brenner RJ et al: Incidence of radiographically evident bone disease, nephrocalcinosis, and nephrolithiasis in various types of renal tubular acidosis. *N Engl J Med* 1982;**307**:217.

DeLuca HF: New developments in the vitamin D endocrine system. *J Am Diet Assoc* 1982;**80**:231.

Frame B, Parfitt AM: Osteomalacia: Current concepts. *Ann Intern Med* 1978;**89**:966.

Frame B, Potts JT Jr (editors): *Clinical Disorders of Bone and Mineral Metabolism.* Excerpta Medica, 1983.

Glorieux FH et al: Bone response to phosphate salts, ergocalciferol, and calcitriol in hypophosphatemic vitamin D–resistant rickets. *N Engl J Med* 1980;**303**:1023.

Table 19–9. Comparison of various vitamin D preparations.*

	How Supplied	Physiologic Dose	Pharmacologic Dose†	Onset of Maximal Effect
Ergocalciferol (calciferol, vitamin D_2, Drisdol)	Capsules, 1200 μg	10 μg/d.	1200 μg/d	30 days
Dihydrotachysterol	Tablets, 125 μg, 200 μg, and 400 μg	20 μg/d	400 μg/d	15 days
Calcifediol (25-hydroxycholecalciferol; Calderol)	Capsules, 20 μg and 50 μg	5 μg/d	50 μg/d	15 days
Calcitriol (1,25-dihydroxycholecalciferol; Rocaltrol)	Capsules, 0.25 μg and 0.5 μg	0.5 μg/d	1 μg/d	3 days

*Modified and reproduced, with permission, from Kumar R, Riggs BL: Vitamin D in the therapy of disorders of calcium and phosphorus metabolism. *Mayo Clin Proc* 1981;**56**:327.

†Usual dose for treating hypoparathyroidism, osteomalacia due to malabsorption or vitamin D resistance, and renal osteodystrophy. One microgram of vitamin D_2 has an activity of 40 IU; 1200 μg is approximately 50,000 IU.

Insogna KL et al: Osteomalacia and weakness from excessive antacid ingestion. *JAMA* 1980;**244**:2544.

Meredith SC, Rosenberg IH: Gastrointestinal-hepatic disorders and osteomalacia. *Clin Endocrinol Metab* 1980;**9**:131.

Norman AW, Roth J, Orci L: The vitamin D endocrine system: Steroid metabolism, hormone receptors, and biological response (calcium binding proteins). *Endocr Rev* 1982;**3**:331.

Parfitt AM, Oliver I, Villanueva AR: Bone histology in metabolic bone disease: The diagnostic value of bone biopsy. *Orthop Clin North Am* 1979;**10**:329.

Spencer H, Kramer L: Antacid-induced calcium loss. (Editorial.) *Arch Intern Med* 1983;**143**:657.

Streck WF, Waterhouse C, Haddad JG: Glucocorticoid effects in vitamin D intoxication. *Arch Intern Med* 1979;**139**:974.

Walker GS et al: Dialysate aluminium concentration and renal bone disease. *Kidney Int* 1982;**21**:411.

OSTEOPOROSIS

Essentials of Diagnosis

- Asymptomatic to severe backache.
- Spontaneous fractures and collapse of vertebrae without spinal cord compression, often discovered "accidentally" on x-ray; loss of height.
- Calcium, phosphorus, and alkaline phosphatase normal.
- Demineralization of spine and pelvis.

General Considerations

Osteoporosis is the most commonly seen metabolic bone disease in the USA. It is characterized by an absolute decrease in the amount of bone present to a level below which it is capable of maintaining the structural integrity of the skeleton. There is a greater loss of trabecular bone than compact bone, accounting for the primary features of the disease, ie, crush fractures of vertebrae, fractures of the neck of the femur, and fractures of the distal end of the radius. Whatever bone is present is normally mineralized. Osteoporosis may be produced secondarily by a number of disorders (see below), but more commonly it is primary and of unknown cause. Since the usual form of the disease is clinically evident in middle life and beyond—and since women are more frequently affected than men—it is often termed "postmenopausal" and "senile" osteoporosis. The serum calcium, phosphate, and alkaline phosphatase are normal, and the bone formation rate is usually normal whereas the bone resorption rate is increased. The inheritance of low skeletal mass in young adult life (especially in white females), loss of sex hormones at the time of the menopause, the effects of aging, lack of activity, inadequate dietary calcium intake, impaired intestinal calcium absorption, a high phosphate intake, acid ash diet, inappropriate secretion of parathyroid hormone or calcitonin, or some combination of these factors have been considered as possible contributing causes. Excessive cigarette smoking may be important.

Etiology

A. Principal Causes:

1. Lack of activity, eg, immobilization as in paraplegia or rheumatoid arthritis. (Osteoblasts depend upon strains and stresses for proper function.)

2. Lack of estrogens ("postmenopausal osteoporosis"). (Females are deprived of estrogens relatively early in life. About 30% of women over 60 years of age have clinical osteoporosis. Some degree of osteoporosis is almost always present in senility.)

3. A chronic low intake of calcium has been suggested as of etiologic importance.

4. Malabsorption, at times with intestinal lactase deficiency, may be an important factor in elderly patients with osteoporosis.

5. Deficient production of 1,25-dihydroxyvitamin D may be a cause of some types.

B. Less Common Causes:

1. Developmental disturbances (eg, osteogenesis imperfecta).

2. Nutritional disturbances (eg, protein starvation or excess, ascorbic acid deficiency, alcohol or caffeine excess).

3. Chronic calcium depletion is claimed by some investigators to cause osteoporosis.

4. Endocrine diseases—Lack of androgens (eunuchoidism, senility in men), hypopituitarism (causes secondary gonadal failure), acromegaly (cause unknown; possibly due to hypogonadism), thyrotoxicosis (not constant; causes excessive catabolism of skeletal tissue), excessive exogenous or endogenous ACTH or corticosteroids causing catabolism of bone (eg, Cushing's disease), and long-standing uncontrolled diabetes mellitus (rare).

5. Bone marrow disorders—The presence of abnormal cells in the bone marrow, such as in myeloma or leukemia, may stimulate osteoclastic activity and cause osteoporosis. This is in addition to the active replacement of the marrow with tumor cells. A bone marrow factor may also play an etiologic role in senile osteoporosis.

6. Prolonged use of heparin may lead to osteoporosis. Tobacco may be an important factor (see Seeman reference, below).

7. Idiopathic osteoporosis occurs most commonly in young men and women and occasionally in older people. It does not respond well to therapy.

8. Idiopathic juvenile osteoporosis is rare and usually shows spontaneous remission after puberty.

Clinical Findings

A. Symptoms and Signs: Osteoporosis may first be discovered accidentally on x-ray examination. It may present as backache of varying degrees of severity or as a spontaneous fracture or collapse of a vertebra.

B. Laboratory Findings: Serum calcium, phosphate, and alkaline phosphatase are normal. The alkaline phosphatase may be slightly elevated in osteogenesis imperfecta and also in other forms of osteoporosis if there has been a recent fracture. Urinary calcium is high early, normal in chronic forms. Urinary hydroxyproline may be elevated in active osteoporosis and in adult osteogenesis imperfecta.

C. X-Ray Findings: The principal areas of demineralization are the spine and pelvis, especially in the femoral neck and head; demineralization is less marked in the skull and extremities. Compression of vertebrae is common. The lamina dura is preserved. Kidney stones may occasionally be seen in acute osteoporosis.

D. Bone Densitometry Measurements: These are helpful in the early detection of bone mineral loss and in following the progression of the disease.

Differential Diagnosis

It is important not to confuse this condition with other metabolic bone diseases, especially osteomalacia and hyperparathyroidism; or with myeloma and metastatic bone disease, especially of the breast and uterus, which may be aggravated by estrogens. (See Table 19–10.) Bone scintiscans and biopsy may be required, since these conditions may coexist in the postmenopausal patient.

A rare case of hypophosphatasia may appear as "osteoporosis."

Treatment

A. Specific Measures: Specific treatment varies with the cause; combined hormone therapy is usually used, although its effectiveness may be in preventing bone loss rather than increasing bone mass.

1. Postclimacteric (mostly in females)–Estrogens appear to decrease bone resorption. Before beginning estrogen therapy in a postmenopausal woman, perform a careful pelvic examination to rule out neoplasm or other abnormality and warn the patient or a relative that vaginal bleeding may occur. Administer estrogen daily except for the first 5–7 calendar days of each month, and then repeat the cycle. Any of the following may be used: (1) Estradiol (Estrace), 1–2 mg orally. (2) Ethinyl estradiol, 0.02–0.05 mg orally daily as tolerated. (3) Estrone sulfate and conjugated estrogenic substances (Amnestrogen, Premarin, etc) are well tolerated and widely used. The dosage is 0.625–1.25 mg orally daily. The long-acting injectable estrogen preparations may be useful. The addition of a progestin, eg, medroxyprogesterone acetate (Provera), 10 mg daily for the last week to 10 days of each estrogen cycle, may reduce some of the side effects. See discussion of menopause (p 477) regarding dangers of estrogen therapy (increased incidence of endometrial carcinoma, phlebitis, etc).

Anabolic steroids, eg, methandrostenolone (Dianabol), commonly used in the past, are of questionable benefit except in the debilitated patient. The dose must be kept low in order to avoid undesirable side effects (eg, hirsutism, hoarseness, clitoral enlargement, and liver impairment). A recent study has shown beneficial effects of stanozolol (Winstrol) in increasing bone mass. (See Chestnut reference, below.) Estradiol valerate and testosterone enanthate (Deladumone) may be the preferable preparation.

2. Old age and idiopathic–As for postclimacteric; both testosterone and estrogens may be used in both males and females. Use with caution in very old people.

3. Patients with malnutrition–Adequate diet is of great importance. However, hormones may be used as above if response to diet alone is poor.

4. Cushing's syndrome–See p 732.

5. Sodium fluoride has recently been tried in refractory osteoporotic patients, but it must be considered still an experimental procedure. Combined with calcium and vitamin D, it appears to enhance bone formation. Recurrent fracture rates have been reduced. (See Bikle reference, below.)

6. Phosphate supplements may be of value in certain types of osteoporosis (eg, after fracture, myeloma), especially if combined with calcium.

7. The efficacy of calcitonin, growth hormone, or diphosphonates is still under study.

B. General Measures: The diet should be high in protein and adequate in calcium (milk and milk products are desirable except in lactose intolerance) and vitamin D. Increased calcium intake by use of supplementary calcium salts (eg, calcium carbonate), up to 1–2 g calcium per day, may be warranted. Additional vitamin D (2000–5000 units/d) may be needed if there is associated malabsorption or osteomalacia. A rare patient may require 1,25-dihydroxycholecalciferol. Thiazides may be useful if hypercalciuria is present. Patients should be kept active; bedridden patients should be given active or passive exercises. The spine must be adequately supported (eg, with a Taylor brace or corset), but rigid or excessive immobilization must be avoided.

Prognosis

The prognosis is good for postclimacteric osteoporosis if therapy is started early and maintained for years. Spinal involvement is not reversible on x-ray, but progression of the disease is often halted. In general, osteoporosis is a crippling rather than a killing disease, and the prognosis is essentially that of the underlying disorder (eg, Cushing's syndrome). The idiopathic variety does not respond appreciably to any form of therapy except possibly fluoride. Careful periodic records of the patient's height will indicate if the disease has become stabilized. In the future, periodic measurements of bone mass in a given individual, using modern techniques (eg, bone densitometry), may alert the physician to a progressive bone loss before clinical or x-ray evidence of osteoporosis occurs. Measures to prevent progressive resorption of bone may be more effective than treatment of clinical disease.

Avioli LV (editor): *The Osteoporotic Syndrome: Detection, Prevention, and Treatment*. Grune & Stratton, 1983.

Baylinck DJ: Glucocorticoid-induced osteoporosis. (Editorial.) *N Engl J Med* 1983;**309**:306.

Bikle DD: Fluoride treatment of osteoporosis: A new look at an old drug. (Editorial.) *Ann Intern Med* 1983;**98**:1013.

Chestnut CH III: Treatment of postmenopausal osteoporosis: Some current concepts. *Scott Med J* 1981;**26**:72.

DeLuca HF et al (editors): *Osteoporosis: Recent Advances in*

Table 19–10. Differential diagnosis of disorders of mineral metabolism.* (TRP = tubular reabsorption of phosphate.)

Disease	Serum					Urine			Comment
	Calcium	Phosphorus	Alkaline Ptase	Urea or Creatinine	Parathyroid Hormone	Calcium	TRP	Hydroxy-proline	
Hyperparathyroidism									
Primary	↑	↓	↑ or N	N or ↑	↑	↑ or N	↓	↑	Phalangeal subperiosteal resorption.
Secondary	↓ or N	↑	↑ or N	↑	↑	N or ↓	↓	↑	
"Tertiary"	↑	N or ↓	↑ or N	↑ or N	↑	↑ or N	↓	↑	Tends to appear after renal transplantation.
Cancer	↑	↑ or N or ↓	↑ or N	↑ or N	↑ or N or ↓	↑	N or ↓	↑	May be abnormal PTH in serum, or prostaglandin.
Sarcoid	↑ or N	N or ↓	↑ or N	↑ or N	↓	↑	N or ↑	↑	Good response to corticosteroids.
Vitamin D intoxication	↑	↑ or N	N	↑ or N	↓	↑	N or ↑	↑	Good response to corticosteroids.
Hyperthyroidism	↑ or N	N or ↑	N or ↑	N	N or ↓	↑	N	↑	Serum thyroxine increased.
Acute bone atrophy (immobilization)	↑ or N	↑ or N	N	N	N or ↓	N	N or ↓	N or ↑	Alkalosis despite renal insufficiency.
Milk-alkali syndrome	↑	↑ or N	↑	↑	N or ↓	↑	N or ↓	↑	"Elfin" facies.
Idiopathic hypercalcemia of infancy	↑	↑	↑	↑	?	↑ or N			
Rickets and osteomalacia									
Vitamin D deficiency	↓	↓	↑↑	N	↑	↓	↓	N	Irritability, muscular hypotonia.
Vitamin D "refractory"	N	↓	↑↑	↑ or N	↑ or N	↓	↓	N	Pseudofractures, short stature.
Hypophosphatasia	↑ or N	N	↓	N	?	↑ or N	N	N	Urinary phosphorylethanolamine increased; rickets.
Hypoparathyroidism	↓	↑	N	N	↓	↓	↑	N or ↑	Short ulnar metacarpals.
Pseudohypoparathyroidism	↓	↑	↑ or N	N	↑ or N	↓	↑	N	Short ulnar metacarpals.
Pseudopseudohypoparathyroidism	N	N	N	N	N	N	N	N	Short ulnar metacarpals, short stature.
Osteoporosis, idiopathic or senile	N	N	N or ↑	N	N	N	N	↑ or N	
Osteogenesis imperfecta	N	N	N or ↑	N	N	N or ↓	N	N or ↓	Blue scleras; deafness.
Osteopetrosis	N	N	N	N	N	N	N	N or ↓	Acid phosphatase increased.
Paget's disease	N	N	↑↑	N	N	N	N	↑↑↑	Cardiac output increased.
Fibrous dysplasia	N	N or ↓	↑ or N	N	N	N	N	↑ or N	Brown spots.

*Modified and reproduced, with permission, from Goldsmith RS: Laboratory aids in the diagnosis of metabolic bone disease. Orthop Clin North Am 1972;3:546.

Pathogenesis and Treatment. Proceedings of 10th Steenbock Symposium, University of Wisconsin, June 1980. University Park Press, 1981.

Gallagher JC, Riggs BL, DeLuca HF: Effect of estrogen on calcium absorption and serum vitamin D metabolites in postmenopausal osteoporosis. *J Clin Endocrinol Metab* 1980; **51**:1359.

Gambrell RD: The menopause: Benefits and risks of estrogen-progestogen replacement therapy. *Fertil Steril* 1982;**37**:457.

Genant HK, Gordan GS, Hoffman PG Jr: Osteoporosis. 2. Prevention of bone loss and fractures in women and risks of menopausal estrogen therapy. *West J Med* 1983;**139**:204.

Genant HK et al: Osteoporosis. 1. Advanced radiologic assessment using quantitative computed tomography. *West J Med* 1983;**139**:75.

Health and Public Policy Committee, American College of Physicians: Radiologic methods to evaluate bone mineral content. *Ann Intern Med* 1984;**100**:908.

Heath H III: Progress against osteoporosis. (Editorial.) *Ann Intern Med* 1983;**98**:1011.

Horsman A et al: The effect of estrogen dose on postmenopausal bone loss. *N Engl J Med* 1983;**309**:1405.

Hutchinson TA et al: Postmenopausal estrogens protect against fractures of hip and distal radius. *Lancet* 1979;**2**:705.

Perry HM III et al: Osteoporosis in young men: A syndrome of hypercalciuria and accelerated bone turnover. *Arch Intern Med* 1982;**142**:1295.

Raisz LG: What marrow does to bone. (Editorial.) *N Engl J Med* 1981;**304**:1485.

Riggs BL, Melton LJ: Evidence for two distinct syndromes of involutional osteoporosis. (Editorial.) *Am J Med* 1983; **75**:899.

Riggs BL et al: Effect of the fluoride/calcium regimen on vertebral fracture occurrence in postmenopausal osteoporosis: Comparison with conventional therapy. *N Engl J Med* 1982; **306**:446.

Seeman E et al: Risk factors for spinal osteoporosis in men. *Am J Med* 1983;**75**:977.

Slovik DM et al: Deficient production of 1,25-dihydroxyvitamin D in elderly osteoporotic patients. *N Engl J Med* 1981; **305**:372.

Smith R: Idiopathic osteoporosis in the young. *J Bone Joint Surg* [*Br*] 1980;**62**:417.

Wasnich RD et al: Thiazide effect on the mineral content of bone. *N Engl J Med* 1983;**309**:344.

NONMETABOLIC BONE DISEASE

POLYOSTOTIC FIBROUS DYSPLASIA
(Osteitis Fibrosa Disseminata)

Essentials of Diagnosis
- Painless swelling of involved bone or fracture with minimal trauma.
- Bone cysts or hyperostotic lesions; usually multiple, but occasionally single, in segmental distribution.

General Considerations
Polyostotic fibrous dysplasia is a rare disease that is frequently mistaken for osteitis fibrosa generalisata due to hyperparathyroidism, since both are manifested by bone cysts and fractures. Polyostotic fibrous dysplasia is not a metabolic disorder of bone but a congenital dysplasia in which bone and cartilage do not form but remain as fibrous tissue.

Polyostotic fibrous dysplasia with "brown spots" with ragged margins and true precocious puberty in the female is called **Albright's syndrome.** Hyperthyroidism and acromegaly may be present also.

Clinical Findings
A. Symptoms and Signs: The manifestations are painless swelling of the involved bone (usually the skull, upper end of femur, tibia, metatarsals, metacarpals, phalanges, ribs, and pelvis), either singly or in multiple distribution, with cysts or hyperostotic lesions and at times with brown pigmentation of the overlying skin. Involvement is segmental and may be unilateral. True sexual precocity may occur in females, with early development of secondary sex characteristics and rapid skeletal growth.

B. Laboratory Findings: Calcium and phosphorus are normal; the alkaline phosphatase and urinary hydroxyproline may be elevated.

C. X-Ray Findings: X-rays reveal rarefaction and expansion of the affected bones or hyperostosis (especially of base of the skull). Fractures and deformities may also be visible.

Differential Diagnosis
The bone cysts and fractures should, by their distribution and skin pigmentation, be distinguished from those of hyperparathyroidism and neurofibromatosis. All other types of bone cyst and tumor must be considered also. The hyperostotic lesions of the skull must be distinguished from those of Paget's disease. Biopsy of bone may be required to settle the diagnosis.

Complications
Shortening of the extremity or deformity (eg, shepherd's crook deformity of femur) may follow extensive involvement of bone. The involvement of the orbit may cause proptosis or even blindness. Thyrotoxicosis, hyperparathyroidism, Cushing's syndrome, acromegaly, and gynecomastia may be associated features. Osteomalacia may be present also, as a result of renal phosphaturia. It may be reversed by removal of dysplastic bone.

Treatment
There is no treatment except for surgical correction of deformities, eg, fractures, expanding cyst in the orbit. Calcitonin has been used in active disease, but the results are not conclusive.

Prognosis
Most lesions heal and the progression is slow. Since precocity is of the isosexual type, girls are sus-

ceptible to early pregnancy. They will ultimately be of short stature. On rare occasions, sarcomatous transformation of bone occurs.

Bell NH et al: Effect of calcitonin in Paget's disease and polyostotic fibrous dysplasia. *J Clin Endocrinol Metab* 1970;**31**:283.

Benedict PH et al: Melanotic macules in Albright's syndrome and in neurofibromatosis. *JAMA* 1968;**205**:618.

McArthur RG, Hayles AB, Lambert PW: Albright's syndrome with rickets. *Mayo Clin Proc* 1979;**54**:313.

PAGET'S DISEASE
(Osteitis Deformans)

Essentials of Diagnosis

- Often asymptomatic. Bone pain may be the first symptom.
- Kyphosis, bowed tibias, large head, waddling gait, and frequent fractures that vary with location of process.
- Serum calcium and phosphate normal; alkaline phosphatase elevated; urinary hydroxyproline elevated.
- Dense, expanded bones on x-ray.

General Considerations

Paget's disease is a nonmetabolic bone disease of unknown etiology, although it is believed that it may represent a benign neoplasm of bone-forming cells. A possible viral etiology has recently been suggested. It causes excessive bone destruction and repair—with associated deformities, since the repair takes place in an unorganized fashion. Up to 3% of persons over age 50 will show isolated lesions, but clinically important disease is much less common. There is a strong familial incidence of Paget's disease.

Clinical Findings

A. Symptoms and Signs: Often mild or asymptomatic. Deep "bone pain" is usually the first symptom. The bones become soft, leading to bowed tibias, kyphosis, and frequent fractures with slight trauma. The head becomes larger, and headaches are a prominent symptom. Increased vascularity over the involved bones causes increased warmth.

B. Laboratory Findings: The blood calcium and phosphorus are normal, but the alkaline phosphatase is usually markedly elevated. Urinary hydroxyproline and calcium are elevated in active disease.

C. X-Ray Findings: On x-ray the involved bones are expanded and denser than normal. Multiple fissure fractures may be seen in the long bones. The initial lesion may be destructive and radiolucent, especially in the skull ("osteoporosis circumscripta").

D. Bone Scans: Fluoride or technetium pyrophosphate bone scans are helpful in delineating activity of bone lesions.

Differential Diagnosis

Differentiate from primary bone lesions such as osteogenic sarcoma, multiple myeloma, and fibrous dysplasia and from secondary bone lesions such as metastatic carcinoma and osteitis fibrosa cystica. If serum calcium is elevated, hyperparathyroidism may be present in some patients as well.

Complications

Fractures are frequent and occur with minimal trauma. If immobilization takes place and there is an excessive calcium intake, hypercalcemia and kidney stones may develop. Associated hyperparathyroidism may also be present. Bony overgrowth may impinge on vital structures, especially nerves, causing deafness and blindness. Vertebral collapse may lead to spinal cord compression. Osteosarcoma may develop in long-standing lesions. The increased vascularity, acting like multiple arteriovenous fistulas, may give rise to high-output cardiac failure. Rheumatic manifestations and hyperuricemia with acute and chronic joint pain often complicate this disease, especially in joints near involved bone.

Treatment

Mild cases require no treatment.

Supply a high-protein diet with adequate vitamin C intake. A high-calcium intake is desirable also unless the patient is immobilized, in which case calcium must be restricted. Vitamin D, 50,000 units 3 times a week, is helpful in some patients with marked osteoblastic overactivity (high serum alkaline phosphatase but low urinary calcium). Anabolic hormones, eg, estradiol valerate and testosterone enanthate (Deladumone), 1–3 mL/mo, may be given as for osteoporosis.

Three new therapeutic agents have been introduced to reduce excessive bone resorption, with consequent fall of serum alkaline phosphatase and urinary hydroxyproline. They should be reserved for active and progressive disease. The calcitonins (porcine, human, and salmon) act by reducing osteoclastic activity. **Synthetic salmon calcitonin (Calcimar)** must be used parenterally in doses of 50–100 IU daily or 3 times weekly for several months to years. Aside from local sensitivity reactions, systemic side effects—eg, flushing—are rare. It is expensive, and antibody formation is common. Escape from treatment (return of abnormal laboratory features or symptoms even though treatment is maintained) commonly occurs. The diphosphonate EHDP (ethane-1-hydroxy-1-1-diphosphonic acid) is available as **etidronate disodium (Didronel)** in 200-mg tablets. The safest dose is 5 mg/kg daily for 90–180 days. In severe disease, 10 mg/kg/d may be used for 90 days, with rest periods before another course is given. The diphosphonates coat the bone crystal, making it less subject to excessive resorption. Etidronate disodium is effective orally with minor side effects, but it must only be used for short periods of time and in low dosage in order to avoid adverse effects on normal bone, eg, spontaneous fractures due to a mineralizing defect. The newer diphosphonates (eg, 3-amino-1-hydroxypropylidene-1,1-bisphosphonate [A.D.P.]) are equally effective agents but are not generally available. **Mithramycin,** an antitumor agent, works most rapidly in reducing activity of the bone disease, with rapid fall of the serum alkaline phosphatase level. It must be used as a slow intravenous infusion and is fairly toxic. Blood counts and liver function tests must be obtained throughout treatment. Response is at times so rapid that hypocalcemia occurs. Patients may respond to one agent after they have escaped from the beneficial effects of another. Combined or sequential therapy using several agents is under investigation. The choice of the best agent and the duration of treatment must be individualized.

Prognosis

The prognosis of the mild form is good, but sarcomatous changes (in 1–3%) or renal complications secondary to hypercalciuria (in 10%) alter the prognosis unfavorably. In general, the prognosis is worse the earlier in life the disease starts. Fractures usually heal well. In the severe forms, marked deformity, intractable pain, and cardiac failure are found. The recently introduced therapeutic agents may improve the prognosis significantly.

Alexandre CM et al: Treatment of Paget's disease of bone with ethane-1,hydroxy-1,1 diphosphonate (EHDP) at a low dosage (5 mg/kg/d). Clin Orthop 1983;174:193.

Altman RD, Singer F (editors): Proceedings of the Kroc Foundation Conference on Paget's Disease of Bone. Arthritis Rheum 1980;10(Suppl):23.

Cawley MI: Complications of Paget's disease of bone. Gerontology 1983;29:276.

Deftos LJ, First BP: Calcitonin as a drug. Ann Intern Med 1981;95:192.

Kanis JA, Russell RGG: Diphosphonates and Paget's disease of bone. Metab Bone Dis Relat Res 1981;3:217.

Krane SM: Etidronate disodium in the treatment of Paget's disease. Ann Intern Med 1982;96:619.

Perry HM 3rd, Droke DM, Avioli LV: Alternate calcitonin and etidronate disodium therapy for Paget's bone disease. Arch Intern Med 1984;144:929.

Schajowicz F, Santini AE, Berenstein M: Sarcoma complicating Paget's disease of bone: A clinicopathological study of 62 cases. J Bone Joint Surg [Br] 1983;65:299.

Singer FR, Mills BG: Evidence for a viral etiology of Paget's disease of bone. Clin Orthop 1983;178:245.

Siris ES, Canfield RE: Paget's disease of bone: Current concepts as to its nature and management. Orthop Rev 1982;11:43.

Siris ES, Jacobs TP, Canfield RE: Paget's disease of bone. Bull NY Acad Med 1980;56:285.

Strewler GJ: Paget's disease of bone. West J Med 1984;140:763.

Wallach S: Treatment of Paget's disease. Adv Intern Med 1982;27:1.

DISEASES OF THE ADRENAL CORTEX

Total destruction of both adrenal cortices is not compatible with human life. The cortex regulates a variety of metabolic processes by means of secretion of some 30 steroid hormones, of which 2, cortisol and aldosterone, are of paramount importance.

The main stimulus for release of steroid hormones from the adrenal cortex appears to be adrenocorticotropic hormone (ACTH) from the anterior pituitary, which, in turn, is under the control of the hypothalamic corticotropin-releasing factor. The plasma free cortisol level, in turn, is one of the factors that regulates ACTH secretion. Aldosterone secretion, in contrast, is principally controlled by volume receptors, by angiotensin II, and also by the plasma potassium concentration. Clinical syndromes of adrenal insufficiency or excess may thus be due to primary lesions of the adrenal glands themselves or may be secondary to pituitary disorders. Although the differentiation is often important from the diagnostic standpoint, treatment is usually directed toward the cortical disorder itself, whether primary or secondary. Many of the steroids isolated from the adrenal cortex are not active, and some have more than one action. Transcortin, a plasma globulin, avidly binds cortisol and thus inactivates it. Estrogens increase transcortin levels. An active equilibrium exists between bound and free unbound cortisol. In general, the adrenocortical hormones have 3 types of activity:

(1) Catabolic (glucocorticoids): Cortisol and related steroids, the "stress hormones" of the adrenal cortex, are vital for survival. These steroids have a general "catabolic" action, increasing protein breakdown, inducing hyperaminoacidemia, and causing a negative nitrogen balance. They also increase gluconeogenesis and have an "anti-insulin" effect. They possess significant anti-inflammatory properties and alter the body's immune response.

(2) Electrolyte-regulating (mineralocorticoids): The principal hormone in this group is aldosterone. Its primary role is in retaining sodium and excreting potassium and thus "regulating" the extracellular fluid compartment and the blood pressure. It has minor effects on carbohydrate metabolism.

Most of the clinical features of both adrenal insufficiency and excess can be explained on the basis of the above types of activity. Since mixed pictures occur, however, and since excess of one type of activity may coexist with deficiency of another (eg, congenital adrenal virilism), exact physiologic correlation is difficult. Some phenomena, eg, the pigmentation of adrenal insufficiency, are not yet fully explained, and may be due to a pituitary intermedin or ACTH excess.

(3) Anabolic (sex steroids): Androstenedione and related C_{19} steroids are protein builders and are also virilizing and androgenic, and represent the principal source of androgens in the female.

Improved chemical and radioimmunoassays of various hormones, stimulation and suppression tests, and refined radiologic procedures have facilitated accurate diagnosis of adrenal disorders. An unusual problem being seen with increased frequency is that of the patient who has no obvious symptoms of adrenal dysfunction but who is found to have an adrenal mass in a CT scan of the abdomen performed for an unrelated reason. Careful history taking, physical examination, and judicious use of the laboratory often allow the physician to determine the best course of therapy.

Besser GM, Jeffcoate WJ: Endocrine and metabolic diseases: Adrenal diseases. *Br Med J* 1976;**1**:448.

Copeland PM: The incidentally discovered adrenal mass. *Ann Intern Med* 1983;**98**:40.

Munck A et al: Physiological actions of glucocorticoids in stress and their relation to pharmacological actions. *Endocr Rev* 1984;**5**:25.

ADRENOCORTICAL HYPOFUNCTION
(Adrenocortical Insufficiency)

1. ACUTE ADRENAL INSUFFICIENCY (Adrenal Crisis)

Essentials of Diagnosis

- Onset of weakness, abdominal pain, high fever, confusion, nausea, vomiting, and diarrhea, with infection, or adrenal destruction, or cortisone withdrawal.
- Low blood pressure, dehydration, and increased skin pigmentation.
- Serum sodium low, serum potassium high, blood and urine corticosteroids low.
- Eosinophilia, elevated blood urea nitrogen.

General Considerations

Acute adrenal insufficiency is a true medical emergency caused by sudden marked deprivation or insufficient supply of adrenocortical hormones. Crisis may occur in the course of chronic insufficiency in a known addisonian patient out of control, or it may be the presenting manifestation of adrenal insufficiency. It may be a temporary exhaustion or may go on to permanent insufficiency. Acute crisis is more commonly seen in diseases of the cortex itself than in disorders of the pituitary gland causing secondary adrenocortical hypofunction.

Adrenal crisis may occur in the following situations: (1) Following stress, eg, trauma, surgery, infection, or prolonged fasting in a patient with latent insufficiency. (2) Following sudden withdrawal of adrenocortical hormone after replacement in a patient with chronic insufficiency or in a patient with normal adrenals but with temporary insufficiency due to suppression by exogenous glucocorticoids. (3) Following bilateral adrenalectomy or removal of a functioning adrenal tumor that had suppressed the other adrenal. (4) Following sudden destruction of the pituitary gland (pituitary necrosis), or when thyroid or insulin is given to a patient with panhypopituitarism. (5) Following injury to both adrenals by trauma, hemorrhage, anticoagulant therapy, thrombosis, infection, or, rarely, metastatic carcinoma. In overwhelming sepsis (principally meningococcemia), massive bilateral adrenal hemorrhage may occur (Waterhouse-Friderichsen syndrome).

Clinical Findings

A. Symptoms and Signs: The patient complains of headache, lassitude, nausea and vomiting, abdominal pain, and often diarrhea. Confusion or coma may be present. Fever may be 40.6 °C (105 °F) or more. The blood pressure is low. Other signs include cyanosis, petechiae (especially with meningococcemia), dehydration, abnormal skin pigmentation with sparse axillary hair, and lymphadenopathy.

B. Laboratory Findings: A high eosinophil count is often found in adrenal failure, but it is not specific. The blood glucose and serum sodium levels are low. Serum potassium and blood urea nitrogen are high. Hypercalcemia may be present. Blood culture may be positive (usually meningococci). Urinary and blood cortisol levels are very low. Plasma ACTH is markedly elevated if the patient has primary adrenal disease (generally higher than 200 pg/mL).

C. Electrocardiographic Findings: The ECG may show decreased voltage.

Differential Diagnosis

This condition must be differentiated from other causes of coma and confusion, such as diabetic coma, cerebrovascular accident, and acute poisoning, and from other causes of high fever. Eosinophilia, which is usually absent in other emergencies, and low plasma cortisol help in the differentiation. (*Note:* If the diagnosis is suspected, draw blood sample for cortisol and treat with hydrocortisone, 100–300 mg intravenously, and saline *immediately* without waiting for the results of laboratory tests.)

Complications

Any of the progressive complications of the initiating disease may occur. The complications of treatment or those occurring during the course of treatment are discussed below.

When treatment is instituted, certain complications may be observed. Hyperpyrexia, loss of consciousness, generalized edema with hypertension, and flaccid paralysis due to low potassium have followed excessive use of intravenous fluids and corticosteroids. Psychotic reactions may occur with cortisone therapy.

Treatment

The patient must be treated vigorously and observed constantly until well out of danger. (*Note:* It is better to overtreat than to undertreat.)

A. Severe Crisis:

1. Emergency treatment–Institute appropriate antishock measures (see Chapter 1), especially intravenous fluids and plasma, vasopressor drugs, and oxygen. Do not give narcotics or sedatives.

Give hydrocortisone phosphate or hydrocortisone sodium succinate, 100 mg intravenously immediately and continue intravenous infusions of 50–100 mg every 6 hours for the first day. Give the same amount every 8 hours on the second day and then gradually reduce the dosage every 8 hours.

If hydrocortisone sodium succinate or hydrocortisone phosphate is not available, give cortisone acetate, 10–25 mg intramuscularly in 4 different sites (to a total of 40–100 mg), following with single injections of cortisone, 25–50 mg intramuscularly every 6 hours, and gradually lengthen the intervals of administration to 25 mg every 8 hours.

Give anti-infective agents as needed, eg, as for meningococcal meningitis.

2. Convalescent treatment–When the patient is able to take food by mouth, give oral hydrocortisone, 10–20 mg every 6 hours, and reduce dosage to maintenance levels as needed.

B. Moderate Crisis: If the patient's physical condition does not appear to be critical and is not associated with a significant degree of shock, the treatment outlined above may be modified by appropriate reduction in dosage. However, it is generally best to overtreat the patient in moderate crisis during the first 24 hours rather than risk undertreatment.

C. Complications During Treatment: Excessive use of intravenous fluids and corticosteroids may cause generalized edema with hypertension; flaccid paralysis due to potassium depletion and psychotic reactions may occur. Monitor blood pressure and ECGs throughout treatment.

1. Overhydration, usually due to sodium retention, may result in cerebral edema (with unconsciousness or convulsions) or pulmonary edema. Withhold sodium and fluids temporarily and treat for these conditions.

2. Hypokalemia–Flaccid paralysis, with low serum potassium, usually occurring on the second to fourth days of treatment, must be treated with potassium salts.

3. Hyperpyrexia is rare with present treatment methods.

4. For other complications of adrenal steroid therapy (eg, psychotic reactions), see p 755.

Prognosis

Before replacement therapy and antibiotics became available, acute adrenal crisis was often rapidly fatal. Even today, if treatment is not early and vigorous, death occurs in several hours. Once the crisis has passed, the patient must be observed carefully to assess the degree of permanent adrenal insufficiency.

2. CHRONIC ADRENOCORTICAL INSUFFICIENCY
(Addison's Disease)

Essentials of Diagnosis

- Weakness, easy fatigability, anorexia; frequent episodes of nausea and vomiting and diarrhea.
- Sparse axillary hair; increased skin pigmentation of creases, pressure areas, and nipples.
- Hypotension, small heart.
- Serum sodium and chloride and urinary 17-ketosteroids and 17-hydroxycorticosteroids are

low. Serum potassium and nonprotein nitrogen are elevated. Eosinophilia and lymphocytosis are present.
- Plasma cortisol levels are low to absent and fail to rise after administration of corticotropin.
- Plasma ACTH level elevated.

General Considerations

Addison's disease is a rare disorder due to progressive destruction of the adrenal cortices. It is characterized by chronic deficiency of hormones concerned with gluconeogenesis and with mineral metabolism, and causes unexplained and often striking skin pigmentation. Electrolyte deficiencies may be the dominant manifestation. If chronic adrenal insufficiency is secondary to pituitary failure (atrophy, necrosis, tumor), lack of glycostasis is more commonly seen than electrolyte deficiencies, and skin pigmentary changes are not encountered. A rare syndrome of isolated aldosterone lack has been described with persistent hyperkalemia, periodic paralysis, salt wasting, and acidosis. The majority of these patients have hypoaldosteronism on the basis of reduced renin production or release.

The term Addison's disease should be reserved for adrenal insufficiency due to adrenocortical disease. Tuberculosis of the adrenals is no longer the most common cause, accounting today for less than one-third of cases. Idiopathic atrophy accounts for most of the other cases. There may be associated thyroiditis, hypoparathyroidism, hypogonadism, diabetes mellitus, pernicious anemia, and candidiasis. An autoimmune mechanism has been postulated for these and other causes of idiopathic atrophy.

Rare causes include metastatic carcinoma (especially of the breast or lung), coccidioidomycosis of the adrenal gland, syphilitic gummas, scleroderma, amyloid disease, and hemochromatosis. Bilateral adrenal hemorrhage may occur in patients taking anticoagulants, in patients in shock, or during open heart surgery, resulting in Addison's disease.

Clinical Findings

A. Symptoms and Signs: The symptoms are weakness and fatigability, anorexia, nausea and vomiting, diarrhea, nervous and mental irritability, and faintness, especially after missing meals. Pigmentary changes consist of diffuse tanning over nonexposed as well as exposed parts or multiple freckles; or accentuation of pigment over pressure points and over the nipples, buttocks, perineum and recent scars. Black freckles may appear on the mucous membranes of the mouth. Seven to 15% of patients have associated vitiligo.

Other findings include hypotension with small heart, hyperplasia of lymphoid tissues, stiffness and calcification of the cartilages of the ear, scant to absent axillary and pubic hair (especially in women), absence of sweating, and at times costovertebral angle tenderness.

B. Laboratory Findings: The white count

shows moderate neutropenia (about 5000/μL), lymphocytosis (35–50%), and a total eosinophil count over 300/μL. Hemoconcentration is present. Serum potassium and urea nitrogen are elevated; serum sodium is low. The serum sodium:potassium ratio is less than 30. Urinary 17-ketosteroid and 17-hydroxycorticosteroid excretion is low. Fasting blood glucose is low. Hypercalcemia may be present.

Low plasma cortisol (less than 5 μg/dL) at 8 AM is diagnostic, especially if accompanied by simultaneous elevation of the plasma ACTH level.

Adrenal calcification on x-ray may be found in about 10% of cases, most frequently in granulomatous diseases such as tuberculosis and coccidioidomycosis.

C. Special Tests:

1. The **8-hour intravenous corticotropin** test is the most specific and reliable diagnostic test. It consists of giving, every day for 3–4 consecutive days, 25 units of corticotropin or 0.25 mg of the synthetic cosyntropin (Cortrosyn) in 1000 mL of physiologic saline by intravenous infusion; in primary Addison's disease, the 24-hour urine 17-hydroxycorticosteroid values fail to rise; in adrenal insufficiency secondary to pituitary insufficiency or in patients who have had suppressive corticosteroid therapy, there is a slow, stepwise rise of 17-hydroxycorticosteroid levels after several days of stimulation. (*Note:* The patient suspected of having Addison's disease should be protected from untoward reactions during the test by the administration of 0.5 mg of dexamethasone without materially altering the urinary steroid levels.)

2. A more rapid test is the **plasma cortisol response to ACTH.** Plasma cortisol samples are obtained in the basal state and 30 minutes after intramuscular injection of 25 units of corticotropin or 0.25 mg of cosyntropin (Cortrosyn). If the plasma cortisol does not rise by at least 10 μg/dL, the diagnosis of primary or secondary adrenal insufficiency is likely.

3. Autoimmune antibodies to adrenal tissue may be found in idiopathic adrenal atrophy.

4. Plasma ACTH levels are high in primary adrenal insufficiency ($>$ 200 pg/mL).

Differential Diagnosis

Differentiate from anorexia nervosa, sprue syndrome, and malignant tumors. Weakness must be differentiated from that due to hyperparathyroidism, hyperthyroid myopathy, and myasthenia gravis; skin pigmentation from that of primary skin diseases, argyria, and hemochromatosis.

Complications

Any of the complications of the underlying disease (eg, tuberculosis) are more likely to occur, and the patient is susceptible to intercurrent infections that may precipitate crisis. Diabetes mellitus and, rarely, thyrotoxicosis may be associated. Thyroiditis, hypoparathyroidism, pernicious anemia, and ovarian failure, probably caused by an autoimmune disorder, may be associated with idiopathic adrenal failure. Hypercalcemia is most apt to occur in children, especially when the adrenocortical level is suddenly reduced.

The dangers of overzealous treatment as well as inadequate replacement must be guarded against. Psychoses, gastric irritation, and low-potassium syndrome may occur with corticosteroid treatment. Corticosteroid treatment may impair the patient's resistance to tuberculosis, which may spread. Excessive desoxycorticosterone administration is rare today but formerly led to hypertension, edema, anasarca, muscular weakness, and tendon contractures.

Treatment

A. Specific Therapy: Ideal replacement therapy should include a combination of glucocorticoids, mineralocorticoids, and anabolic steroids. In mild cases, hydrocortisone alone—or a combination of hydrocortisone and a mineralocorticoid—is adequate.

1. Hydrocortisone is the drug of choice. Most addisonian patients are well maintained on 15–25 mg of hydrocortisone orally daily in 2–3 divided doses. On this dosage, most of the metabolic abnormalities are corrected. Many patients, however, do not obtain sufficient salt-retaining effect and require desoxycorticosterone or fludrocortisone supplementation or extra dietary salt.

2. Fludrocortisone acetate has a potent sodium-retaining effect. The dosage is 0.05–0.1 mg orally daily or every other day, added to cortisone or hydrocortisone. If postural hypotension, hyperkalemia, or weight loss occurs, raise the dose. If weight gain, edema, hypokalemia, or hypertension ensues, lower the dose.

3. Desoxycorticosterone acetate controls electrolyte balance, and, since it has no other significant metabolic effect, it must be used in combination with cortisone or hydrocortisone. It is given intramuscularly initially. The usual dose is 1–4 mg intramuscularly daily. Desoxycorticosterone acetate is now rarely used for chronic therapy.

Caution: When using desoxycorticosterone acetate or fludrocortisone, avoid overdosage. Patients receiving these drugs should not be on low-potassium diets because potassium deficiency may develop.

4. Sodium chloride in large doses (5–20 g daily) may be used to supplement hydrocortisone therapy instead of desoxycorticosterone acetate or if desoxycorticosterone acetate or fludrocortisone is not available.

B. General Measures: Give a high-carbohydrate, high-protein diet. Frequent small feedings tend to be better tolerated than 3 large ones. If replacement therapy is adequate, most patients need no special diets or precautions. Prevent exposure to infection and treat all infections immediately and vigorously and raise the dose of cortisone appropriately. The dose of glucocorticoid should also be raised in case of trauma, surgery, complicated diagnostic procedures, or other forms of stress. Patients are well advised to carry at all times a card or bracelet giving information about their disease and their need for hydrocortisone. This can be lifesaving.

C. Treatment of Complications: Treat spread of tuberculosis (especially renal tuberculosis) and intercurrent infections. The treatment of complications due to inadequate dosage or overdosage of corticosteroids consists of adjusting the dosage or changing the type or mixture of replacement steroids.

Criteria of Adequate Therapy & Overdosage
A. Adequate Therapy:
1. Return of blood pressure to normal.
2. Maintenance of normal fasting blood glucose level.
3. Return of serum electrolytes to normal levels.
4. Weight gain (usually due to fluid).
5. Improvement of appetite and strength.
6. Increase in size of heart to normal.

B. Overdosage: Excessive administration of cortisone or desoxycorticosterone acetate must be avoided, especially in patients with cardiac or renal complications.

1. Signs and symptoms of cortisone overdosage are discussed on p 755.
2. Development of dependent edema, or excessive weight gain.
3. Development of hypertension.
4. Increase of diameter of heart above normal.
5. Development of signs of potassium deficiency (weakness followed by loss of muscle power and finally paralysis), especially if the patient is on a low-potassium diet.

Prognosis
With adequate replacement therapy the life expectancy of patients with Addison's disease is markedly prolonged. Active tuberculosis responds to specific chemotherapy. Withdrawal of treatment or increased demands due to infection, trauma, surgery, or other types of stress may precipitate crisis with a sudden fatal outcome unless large doses of parenteral corticosteroids are employed. Pregnancy may be followed by exacerbation of the disease. Psychotic reactions may interfere with management. Hyperkalemic paralysis is a rare but serious complication if potassium intake is not monitored.

The ultimate prognosis depends largely upon the intelligence of the patient and the availability of medical supervision. A fully active life is now possible for the majority of patients.

Irvine WJ: Autoimmunity in endocrine disease. *Recent Prog Horm Res* 1980;**36**:509.
Schambelan M, Sebastian A: Hyporeninemic hypoaldosteronism. *Adv Intern Med* 1979;**24**:385.

ADRENOCORTICAL OVERACTIVITY

Overactivity of the adrenal secretions is caused either by bilateral hyperplasia or by adenoma or, more rarely, carcinoma of one adrenal. The clinical picture will vary with the type of secretion produced, but in general 3 clinical disorders can be differentiated: (1) Cushing's syndrome, in which the glucocorticoids predominate; (2) the adrenogenital syndrome, in which the adrenal androgens predominate (feminizing tumors are rare); and (3) hyperaldosteronism, with mineralocorticoid excess. The clinical picture is most apt to be mixed in cases of malignant tumor and in bilateral hyperplasia. All syndromes of adrenal overactivity are far more common in females than in males.

1. CUSHING'S SYNDROME
(Adrenocortical Hyperfunction)

Essentials of Diagnosis
- Centripetal obesity, easy bruisability, psychosis, hirsutism, purple striae.
- Osteoporosis, hypertension, glycosuria.
- Elevated 17-hydroxycorticosteroids, low serum potassium and chloride, low total eosinophils, and lymphocytopenia.
- Failure of suppression of cortisol secretion by exogenous dexamethasone.
- Special x-ray studies may reveal a tumor or hyperplasia of the adrenals.

General Considerations
The term Cushing's syndrome refers to hypercortisolism due to any cause. The primary lesion may be in the pituitary or the hypothalamus, with resultant hypersecretion of ACTH and anatomic or functional bilateral adrenal hyperplasia. This is the most common form of the disorder (about 70%) and is usually referred to as Cushing's disease. Hypercortisolism may also be due to an autonomous adrenal tumor (adenoma or carcinoma) or to ectopic secretion of an ACTH-like material by a nonpituitary neoplasm.

Hypercortisolism due to a tumor of one adrenal is usually associated with atrophy of the contralateral gland. Carcinoma of the adrenal (5%) is always unilateral and often metastasizes late. A mixed picture with virilization is often present.

Adrenal rest tumors in the ovary rarely cause Cushing's syndrome; they are more commonly associated with virilizing syndromes. Carcinoma of the anterior pituitary is a rare cause of Cushing's disease.

Administration of corticotropin causes adrenal hyperplasia; administration of glucocorticoid causes adrenal atrophy associated with most features of Cushing's syndrome. These effects are partially reversible when medication is withdrawn.

Certain extra-adrenal malignant tumors (eg, bronchogenic oat cell carcinoma) may secrete ACTH or, more rarely, corticotropin-releasing factor and produce severe Cushing's syndrome with bilateral adrenal hyperplasia. Severe hypokalemia and hyperpigmentation are commonly found in this group.

Clinical Findings
A. Symptoms and Signs: Cushing's syndrome

causes "moon face" and "buffalo hump," obesity with protuberant abdomen, and thin extremities; a plethoric appearance; oligomenorrhea or amenorrhea (or impotence in the male); weakness, backache, headache; hypertension; mild acne and superficial skin infections; chloasmalike pigmentation (especially on the face), hirsutism (mostly of the lanugo hair over the face and upper trunk, arms, and legs), purple striae (especially around the thighs, breasts, and abdomen), and easy bruisability (eg, hematoma formation following venipuncture). Mental symptoms may range from increased lability of mood to frank psychosis.

B. Laboratory Findings: Glucose tolerance is low, often with glycosuria. The patient is resistant to the action of insulin. Urinary 17-hydroxycorticosteroids and plasma cortisol are high (the latter over 20 μg/dL). (*Note:* In patients receiving estrogens—eg, contraceptive pills—the plasma cortisol levels are elevated due to increase in cortisol-binding globulin.) The usual diurnal variation in plasma cortisol levels is absent in Cushing's syndrome. Urinary free cortisol is always elevated. Urinary 17-ketosteroids are often low or normal in Cushing's syndrome due to adenoma; normal or high if the disorder is due to hyperplasia; and very high if due to carcinoma. Total eosinophils are low (under 50/μL), lymphocytes are under 20% and red and white blood cell counts are elevated. Serum CO_2 is high and serum Cl^- and K^+ are low in some cases, especially those associated with malignant tumors.

C. X-Ray Findings: Osteoporosis of the skull, spine, and ribs is common. Nephrolithiasis may be seen. Intravenous urograms or retroperitoneal pneumograms may show a tumor of the adrenal or bilateral enlargement. X-rays are usually not helpful, since basophilic adenomas are very small, but polytomography may show a pituitary microadenoma.

Recent improvements in CT scanning instrumentation have made this technique the most revealing in the evaluation of possible adrenal masses. Adrenal angiography or [131]I-19-iodocholesterol scanning may demonstrate small adrenal tumors or hyperplastic glands.

D. Electrocardiographic Findings: The ECG may show signs of hypertension and hypokalemia and a short PR interval.

E. Special Tests: (*Note:* Exceptions to the following rules are occasionally seen.)

1. Dexamethasone suppression tests–These tests, originally described by Grant Liddle, are still very useful. Administering dexamethasone in low doses (0.5 mg every 6 hours for 2 days) separates patients with all forms of Cushing's syndrome from those who do not have the disorder. (A common problem is to decide whether an obese, hypertensive, slightly hirsute woman does or does not have hypercortisolism.) In patients with Cushing's syndrome, the 24-hour urinary 17-hydroxycorticosteroids are not reduced to less than 3.5 mg in the second day of dexamethasone administration.

Once it is clear that the patient has hypercorti-

solism, one proceeds to the high-dose dexamethasone suppression test (2 mg every 6 hours for 2 days). In patients with Cushing's *disease,* the urinary 17-hydroxycorticosteroids are lowered to less than 50% of the baseline value. This does not occur in those with adrenal tumors or ectopic ACTH production.

A faster, less accurate screening test for Cushing's syndrome is administration of 1 mg of dexamethasone at midnight. In most normal subjects, plasma cortisol levels are suppressed the following morning to less than 5 μg/dL.

2. ACTH stimulation test–The administration of ACTH causes marked hypersecretion of plasma cortisol and urinary 17-hydroxycorticosteroids and 17-ketosteroids in Cushing's disease and often also in cases due to adenoma but does not stimulate secretion in cases due to carcinoma.

3. Metyrapone (Metopirone) stimulation test–Failure of corticosteroids to rise after a 4-hour infusion or after an oral dose of 500 mg every hour for 6 doses favors neoplasm rather than hyperplasia.

4. Direct assay of plasma ACTH–ACTH is detectable in the plasma in bilateral adrenal hyperplasia but not in adrenal tumors. It is markedly elevated in ACTH-secreting ectopic tumors producing Cushing's syndrome, and in Nelson's syndrome (see below).

5. The urinary free cortisol test–This test is very useful for the diagnosis of Cushing's syndrome, since, unlike the 17-hydroxycorticosteroids, free cortisol is not affected by drugs, obesity, hyperthyroidism, etc.

Differential Diagnosis

A frequent problem is differentiating true Cushing's syndrome from obesity associated with diabetes mellitus, especially if there are hirsutism and amenorrhea. The distribution of fat, the presence or absence of muscle atrophy in the extremities, and the color and width of the striae often help but are not infallible signs. Dexamethasone suppression tests often clarify the diagnosis. Cushing's syndrome must be differentiated from the adrenogenital syndrome (see below), since the latter may be amenable to medical treatment unless it is caused by tumor. The 2 diseases may coexist. An elderly woman with osteoporosis, diabetes, and mild hirsutism may present a difficult problem in differentiation. Exogenous administration of corticosteroids must be kept in mind. Recently, hypercortisolism secondary to alcoholism has been reported (pseudo-Cushing's syndrome).

In rare cases the outstanding manifestation of Cushing's disease or syndrome may be only diabetes, osteoporosis, hypertension, or psychosis. Adrenal disease must be ruled out in patients with these disorders, especially in insulin-resistant diabetes mellitus, since early treatment may be curative. The dexamethasone suppression tests (see above) are most helpful in differentiation.

Complications

The patient may suffer from any of the complications of hypertension, including congestive failure, cerebrovascular accidents, and coronary attacks, or of diabetes. Susceptibility to infections, especially of the skin and urinary tract, is increased. Compression fractures of the osteoporotic spine may cause marked disability. Renal colic may occur. Intractable gastric ulcer may be present. Most serious, perhaps, are the psychotic complications not infrequently observed in this disease. After adrenalectomy, hypercalcemia and pancreatitis may complicate the recovery. Pituitary enlargement (due to chromophobe adenomas) and deepening skin pigmentation have been observed following adrenalectomy for hyperplasia (Nelson's syndrome), causing, at times, visual field abnormalities.

Treatment
A. Specific Measures:
1. Adrenal tumors are removed surgically. Total resection of both adrenals in patients with diffuse bilateral hyperplasia was the treatment of choice for rapidly advancing Cushing's disease. At present, the preferred initial therapy is transsphenoidal surgical removal of the ACTH-secreting pituitary adenoma. In selected cases pituitary irradiation may be used, and there are a few patients who may respond well to pharmacologic inhibition of ACTH secretion. If these measures fail to produce a remission of the disease, total adrenalectomy is performed. Adequate preoperative medication and care are of utmost importance. The patient should receive all general measures listed below, plus adequate hormonal supplementation.

If bilateral adrenalectomy is contemplated, give high doses of cortisone, eg, cortisone acetate, 100–300 mg intramuscularly, or, preferably, 100–300 mg of Solu-Cortef in divided doses intramuscularly or intravenously, on the day of surgery; continue the intramuscular dosage for 1–2 days after surgery, then gradually decrease the dose and maintain on oral hydrocortisone as for Addison's disease. Because of the danger of precipitating heart failure, care must be taken to avoid excessive fluids and sodium.

In cases of unilateral tumor, the patient is prepared as for total adrenalectomy. After surgery, cortisol must be provided. Treatment with cortisol may have to be continued for weeks or months, since the contralateral gland may be slow to recover function.

2. X-ray therapy to the pituitary is the treatment of choice in children with Cushing's disease. It may be tried initially; if not successful, total adrenalectomy must be performed. Partial destruction of the pituitary by other means (proton beam, yttrium implant, cryotherapy) has been attempted. Hypophysectomy may be required for large chromophobe adenomas.

Recent reports of a successful "cure" of Cushing's disease by removal of ACTH-secreting pituitary microadenomas via a transsphenoidal approach are very encouraging. An experienced neurosurgeon is required. Long-term follow-up of these cases is lacking, but reports of recurrences are disturbing.

3. Removal of a malignant tumor producing Cushing's syndrome by ectopic secretion of ACTH should be attempted if feasible.

4. Chemical treatment by means of adrenocortical inhibitors has been largely unsuccessful. The least toxic of these, mitotane (Lysodren; *o,p'*-DDD), has limited use in inoperable carcinomas. Metyrapone and aminoglutethimide have been used to reduce adrenocortical overactivity, but the results are erratic. The antiserotonin drug cyproheptadine has been reported to induce remission of the disease, but this has not been universally confirmed.

B. General Measures:
A high-protein diet should be given, although dietary attempts to correct the negative nitrogen balance are never successful. Testosterone or one of the newer anabolic agents may be of value in reversing the negative nitrogen balance. Potassium chloride administration may replace losses before and after surgery.

Insulin is usually unnecessary as the diabetes is mild; however, if the hyperglycemia is severe, it should be given in spite of the insulin resistance usually present.

Prognosis
This is a chronic disease that is subject to cyclic exacerbations (especially with pregnancy) and rare spontaneous remissions; it is a serious and often fatal disease unless discovered and treated early. A rather rapid course suggests a malignant tumor, but these may be dormant for years.

The best prognosis for eventual recovery is for patients in whom a benign adrenal adenoma has been removed and who have survived the postadrenalectomy state of adrenal insufficiency. About 25–50% of patients with bilateral hyperplasia may respond to pituitary irradiation alone. Microsurgery of the pituitary, involving removal of small adenomas, may favorably alter the prognosis in the future. The pituitary tumors that occur in about 10–20% of patients after bilateral adrenalectomy (Nelson's syndrome) are among the most aggressive, involving rapid growth, visual failure, and sometimes malignant transformation. If extensive hypophysectomy is necessary to remove the ACTH-secreting tumor, panhypopituitarism supervenes. Diabetes insipidus, transient or permanent, may also ensue. The more extensive the surgical procedure, the more frequent will be the rate of postoperative complications.

Complete adrenalectomy necessitates chronic replacement therapy with glucocorticoid and mineralocorticoid hormones. A small number of patients with Cushing's disease treated with bilateral adrenalectomy have a subsequent recurrence of hypercortisolism. It is postulated that a small piece of adrenal tissue, either ectopic tissue or tissue left inadvertently by the surgeon, undergoes hyperplasia in response to the very high ACTH levels that are found after adrenalectomy.

Malignant extra-adrenal tumors are usually rapidly fatal, even after such drastic attempts at treatment as total adrenalectomy.

Aron DC et al: Cushing's syndrome: Problems in management. *Endocr Rev* 1982;**3**:229.

Bigos ST et al: Cushing's disease: Management by transsphenoidal pituitary microsurgery. *J Clin Endocrinol Metab* 1980; **50**:348.

Daughaday WH: Cushing's disease and basophilic microadenomas. (Editorial.) *N Engl J Med* 1984;**310**:919.

Krieger DT: Physiopathology of Cushing's disease. *Endocr Rev* 1983;**4**:22.

Orth DN: The old and the new in Cushing's syndrome. *N Engl J Med* 1984;**310**:649.

Tyrrell JB et al: Cushing's disease: Selective transsphenoidal resection of pituitary microadenomas. *N Engl J Med* 1978; **298**:753.

2. THE ADRENOGENITAL SYNDROME: PREPUBERTAL

Adrenal virilizing syndromes in infancy or childhood are of great interest to the pediatrician and may be due to excessive production of androgens by a tumor (benign or malignant) or, more commonly, to congenital adrenal hyperplasia.

Congenital Adrenal Hyperplasia

The term congenital adrenal hyperplasia refers to a complex series of rare but well-studied enzymatic errors of metabolism, with deficient levels of different enzymes involved in the synthesis of cortisol. By far the most common forms are 21- and 11β-hydroxylase deficiencies, both characterized by excessive formation of adrenal androgens under the ACTH drive induced by hypocortisolism. This excess of androgens results in masculinization in the female (ranging from mild hirsutism and clitoral hypertrophy to frank pseudohermaphroditism) and in premature virilization in the male. In both entities, there is a variable degree of clinical hypocortisolism. In untreated 11β-hydroxylase deficiency, there is hypertension due to excessive formation of desoxycorticosterone, a metabolic precursor with potent mineralocorticoid activity. Hypertension never occurs in untreated 21-hydroxylase deficiency; on the contrary, a salt-losing form with clear-cut mineralocorticoid deficiency is present in approximately 50% of cases. In both enzymatic deficiencies, one finds high ACTH levels, plasma androgens, urinary pregnanetriol, and 17-ketosteroids. Specific diagnosis is made by demonstrating elevated plasma levels of the metabolic precursor immediately before the enzymatic block: 11-deoxycortisol in 11β-hydroxylase deficiency and 17-hydroxyprogesterone in 21-hydroxylase deficiency.

The fundamental step in the treatment of congenital adrenal hyperplasia is the administration of enough glucocorticoid to suppress ACTH and reverse the metabolic abnormalities. A mineralocorticoid is required in the salt-losing form. Plastic surgery may be necessary in females with ambiguous genitalia. It should be performed early in life.

New M, Levine LS: Congenital adrenal hyperplasia and related conditions. Chapter 47 in: *The Metabolic Basis of Inherited*

Disease, 5th ed. Stanbury JB et al (editors). McGraw-Hill, 1983.

3. ADRENOGENITAL SYNDROME & VIRILIZING DISEASES OF WOMEN

Essentials of Diagnosis

- Menstrual disorders and hirsutism.
- Regression or reversal of primary and secondary sex characteristics with balding, hoarse voice, acne, and enlargement of the clitoris.
- Occasionally a palpable pelvic tumor.
- 17-Ketosteroids elevated in adrenal disorders, variable in others.
- Urinary and plasma testosterone elevated.

General Considerations

The diagnosis of virilizing disorders in adult females is more difficult than in young girls, since sources of abnormal androgens other than the adrenal exist, principally the ovaries. There is no interference with formation of the female genital tract or secondary sex characteristics, but rather a regression or sex reversal of varying degree. Although the diagnosis is readily apparent in a complete state of the virilizing syndrome (eg, the adult form of the congenital adrenogenital syndrome), the milder forms, presenting primarily with defeminization or merely excessive hirsutism, may be caused by equally serious adrenal and ovarian disorders such as tumors. A sudden change in amount of hair (other than at puberty, pregnancy, or menopause) is of greater importance than hirsutism that has been present throughout life.

Besides adrenal hyperplasia and tumors, syndromes of androgen excess may be caused by the following disorders:

(1) Ovarian disorders: Stein-Leventhal syndrome (large, polycystic ovaries, most common), theca luteinization (thecosis ovarii), arrhenoblastoma, hilar cell tumor or hyperplasia, adrenal cell rests, dysgerminoma (rare).

(2) Hypothalamic-pituitary disorders: Acromegaly (eosinophilic adenoma), hyperostosis frontalis (Stewart-Morgagni-Morel syndrome).

(3) Placental causes: Pregnancy, choriocarcinoma.

(4) Miscellaneous causes: True hermaphroditism, thymic tumors, drugs (eg, testosterone).

Clinical Findings

A. Symptoms and Signs: Symptoms include scant menstrual periods or amenorrhea, acne and roughening of the skin, odorous perspiration, and hoarseness or deepening of voice. Hirsutism is present over the face, body, and extremities, with thinning or balding of head hair. Musculature is increased and feminine contours are lost. The breasts and genitalia are atrophied, the clitoris and larynx enlarged. A tumor may rarely be palpable on pelvic examination (arrhenoblastoma, polycystic ovaries).

B. Laboratory Findings: Urinary 17-ketosteroid determination is the most important single test in the diagnosis of adrenogenital syndrome. It helps differentiate constitutional hirsutism from adrenal disorders, in which the 17-ketosteroids are significantly elevated. Very high levels favor a diagnosis of adrenal tumor. In arrhenoblastoma or Stein-Leventhal syndrome, 17-ketosteroids may be normal or moderately elevated. The dexamethasone suppression test may help distinguish between adrenal tumors, adrenal hyperplasia, and ovarian lesions. Elevated pregnanetriol levels suggest an adrenal lesion. LH levels are often elevated in the Stein-Leventhal syndrome. Plasma 11-deoxycortisol (compound S) and 17-hydroxyprogesterone assays, when more generally available, will be more accurate in determining enzymatic adrenal defects than the urinary 17-ketosteroid and pregnanetriol determinations.

The assay of the most potent androgen (testosterone) in the blood is the screening procedure of choice for virilized women.

C. X-Ray Findings: Ultrasonography is an accurate and noninvasive procedure to demonstrate ovarian enlargement. CT scan, intravenous urograms with adrenal tomography, or adrenal angiograms may reveal an adrenal tumor. Pelvic pneumography has been a valuable tool to demonstrate ovarian enlargement.

D. Laparoscopy is often helpful.

Differential Diagnosis

Since hirsutism may be the only sign of adrenal tumor, all of the disorders characterized by excessive hair have to be considered in the differential diagnosis. From the practical standpoint, however, the diagnosis commonly depends upon whether one is dealing simply with racial, familial, or idiopathic hirsutism, where an unusual end organ sensitivity to endogenous androgen exists; or whether excessive amounts of male hormone are being produced. Recent evidence suggests that most cases of idiopathic hirsutism may be due to an ovarian abnormality in testosterone and androstenedione production and that the dexamethasone test is not reliable in differentiating between adrenal and ovarian sources of excess androgen. In general, if hirsutism is associated with enlargement of the clitoris, deepening of the voice, frontal baldness, development of heavy musculature, or breast atrophy and amenorrhea and if the onset is rapid, one can assume that a tumor of the adrenal or ovary is present. In these circumstances, exploratory operation may be necessary in spite of equivocal laboratory findings. Although virilization is not the rule with Cushing's syndrome, a mixed picture is at times seen in malignant adrenal tumors and, more rarely, in hyperplasia.

Complications

Aside from the known high incidence of malignancy in tumors causing virilization, the interference with femininity and consequent sterility may be irreversible. Diabetes and obesity may be complicating

features. At times, mental disorders accompany states of defeminization.

Treatment

Treatment varies with the cause of the androgen excess.

When ovarian or adrenal tumors are present, surgical removal is the treatment of choice. In some cases of adrenal hyperplasia, especially starting in infancy, there may be associated manifestations of hypoadrenocorticism (eg, excessive salt and water loss and failure to maintain a fasting blood sugar). This condition is due to a congenital absence of hydroxylating enzymes of the adrenals. The "androgenic" compounds formed have no cortisol activity and are unable to suppress endogenous ACTH; hence the continued adrenal stimulation and large glands. Treatment with corticosteroids has proved valuable in reducing the activity of the glands (by suppressing endogenous ACTH) and in supplying exogenously needed corticosteroids. In adults the drugs of choice appear to be prednisone or prednisolone, 5–15 mg daily orally, or dexamethasone, 0.5–1.5 mg daily orally, in divided doses; use the smallest dose that keeps the 17-ketosteroid, pregnanetriol, and testosterone levels within the normal range.

The response of congenital adrenal hyperplasia to long-term corticosteroid therapy is gratifying, with lessening of virilization and hirsutism and eventually normal cyclic menstruation. Plastic repair (removal of the clitoris and repair of a urogenital sinus) is required. Corticosteroid therapy of milder forms of androgen excess (eg, simple hirsutism) is less successful. Estrogen therapy may be of some value but must be used in large dosage. A combination of estrogen-progestogen may be used for long-term suppression of ovarian androgens.

Measurement of the free, non-protein-bound fraction of serum testosterone is helpful in determining the optimal regimen in many cases of hirsutism of unclear origin.

New and still unproved forms of therapy include spironolactone and cimetidine. Androgen antagonists such as cyproterone acetate have been used successfully in experimental clinical trials but are not available in the USA for use in virilizing disorders.

Prognosis

The outlook is favorable if a malignant tumor is removed early, since metastasis often occurs late. Glucocorticoid therapy may be of help in adrenal hyperplastic lesions. Fertility is often restored.

The ultimate fate of the virilized woman depends not only upon the underlying cause (ie, tumor or hyperplasia), but more particularly upon the age at onset of the virilizing influence and its duration. If virilization is of long standing, restoration of normal femininity or loss of hirsutism is unlikely even though the causative lesion is successfully removed.

Note: Many cases of simple hirsutism in females are not due to a readily demonstrable endocrine disease but to hereditary or racial factors and cannot be treated effectively with systemic medications or surgery. Epilation, preferably by electrolysis, is the treatment of choice.

Braithwaite SS et al: Hirsutism. *Arch Dermatol* 1983;**119**:279.

Givens JR: Hirsutism and hyperandrogenism. *Adv Intern Med* 1976;**21**:221.

Shapiro G, Evron S: A novel use of spironolactone: Treatment of hirsutism. *J Clin Endocrinol Metab* 1980;**51**:429.

Strickler RC, Warren JC: Hirsutism: Diagnosis and management. Page 311 in: *Year Book of Obstetrics & Gynecology.* Pitkin M (editor). Year Book, 1979.

PRIMARY HYPERALDOSTERONISM

Essentials of Diagnosis

- Hypertension, polyuria, polydipsia, muscular weakness.
- Hypokalemia, hypernatremia, alkalosis.
- Elevated urinary aldosterone level and low plasma renin level.

General Considerations

Primary hyperaldosteronism is a relatively rare disorder caused by aldosterone excess. It accounts for less than 2% of cases of hypertension. It is more common in females. The two main types of primary hyperaldosteronism are those due to adrenocortical adenoma and those due to macro- or micronodular cortical hyperplasia. Edema is rarely seen in primary hyperaldosteronism, but secondary hyperaldosteronism is often found in edematous states such as cardiac failure and hepatic cirrhosis.

Clinical Findings

A. Symptoms and Signs: Hypertension (usually benign), muscular weakness (at times with paralysis simulating periodic paralysis), paresthesias with frank tetanic manifestations, headache, polyuria (especially nocturnal), and polydipsia are the outstanding complaints. Edema is rarely present. On the other hand, some patients have only diastolic hypertension, without other signs or symptoms.

B. Laboratory Findings: Low serum potassium, hypernatremia, and alkalosis are characteristic, but at times the potassium level is normal. Various degrees of renal damage are manifested by proteinuria, alkaline urine, nephrocalcinosis, and low urine specific gravity unresponsive to vasopressin. If spironolactone, 50–75 mg 4 times daily for 5–8 days, restores serum potassium to normal, suspect hyperaldosteronism. Urinary and plasma aldosterone levels are markedly elevated and plasma renin levels are low.

The best screening test in a patient with hypertension in whom primary aldosteronism is suspected is the determination of plasma renin after sodium depletion (diet or diuretic) and after several hours of being in the upright position. These stimuli normally increase renin production. In primary aldosteronism, the renin level characteristically remains *low.*

A high-sodium diet, saline infusion, or desoxycorticosterone acetate administration fails to suppress the elevated aldosterone levels.

C. Electrocardiographic Findings: Electrocardiographic changes are due to prolonged hypertension and hypokalemia.

D. X-Ray Findings: Cardiac hypertrophy due to hypertension is present. The tumors are usually too small to be visualized, except by adrenal angiography or ^{131}I-19-iodocholesterol scanning. These sophisticated procedures—as well as adrenal vein aldosterone measurements via a venous catheter—for localization of the lesion may become generally available in the future. New techniques of CT scanning, with sharper resolution images, may prove to be best for localization of these small tumors.

E. Other Findings: The plasma volume is increased 30–50% above normal.

Differential Diagnosis

This important reversible cause of hypertension must be considered in the differential diagnosis in any patient who shows muscular weakness and tetanic manifestations; and in the differential diagnosis of periodic paralysis, potassium- and sodium-losing nephritis, nephrogenic diabetes insipidus, and hypokalemia (be certain the patient has not been receiving diuretic agents). Excessive ingestion of licorice or laxatives may simulate hyperaldosteronism. The oral contraceptives may raise aldosterone secretion in some patients. Unilateral renal vascular disease producing secondary hyperaldosteronism with severe hypertension must be ruled out. Plasma renin activity is low in primary hyperaldosteronism and elevated in renal vascular disease. Excessive secretion of desoxycorticosterone and corticosterone may produce a similar clinical picture. Low renin levels are found in about 25% of cases of essential hypertension. Their response to diuretics and their prognosis are better than those of patients with hypertension associated with high renin levels. Excess of an as yet unidentified mineralocorticoid is thought by some to be responsible. Aldosteronism due to a malignant ovarian tumor has been reported. A rare cause of secondary hyperaldosteronism is juxtaglomerular cell hyperplasia (Bartter's syndrome) or a renin-secreting kidney tumor.

It is important to differentiate primary aldosteronism due to an adenoma and that due to bilateral nodular hyperplasia, since the hypertension can be cured or greatly ameliorated by removal of the adenoma, whereas it usually does not respond after bilateral adrenalectomy in patients with hyperplasia. Subjects with adenoma tend to have lower serum potassiums, higher aldosterone levels, and lower renal vein renins. Catheterization of adrenal veins for aldosterone levels is often helpful.

Complications

All of the complications of chronic hypertension

are encountered in primary hyperaldosteronism. Progressive renal damage is less reversible than hypertension.

Treatment

The specific treatment for primary hyperaldosteronism is surgical removal of adenomas. Nodular bilateral hyperplasia is better treated with spironolactone and antihypertensive agents.

An occasional patient responds to dexamethasone suppression.

Prognosis

The hypertension is reversible in about two-thirds of cases but persists or returns in spite of surgery in the remainder.

The prognosis is much improved by early diagnosis with chemical tests and scanning procedures.

Ferriss JB et al: Primary aldosteronism. *Clin Endocrinol Metab* 1981;**10**:419.

Gill JR: Bartter's syndrome. *Annu Rev Med* 1980;**31**:405.

Herf SM et al: Identification and differentiation of surgically corrected hypertension due to primary aldosteronism. *Am J Med* 1979;**67**: 397.

Loriaux DL et al: Spironolactone and endocrine dysfunction. *Ann Intern Med* 1976;**85**:630.

White EA et al: Use of computed tomography in diagnosing the cause of primary aldosteronism. *N Engl J Med* 1980;**303**: 1503.

DISEASES OF THE ADRENAL MEDULLA

PHEOCHROMOCYTOMA

Essentials of Diagnosis

- "Spells" or "attacks" of headache, visual blurring, severe sweats, vasomotor changes in a young adult, weight loss.
- Hypertension, often paroxysmal ("spells") but frequently sustained.
- Postural tachycardia and hypotension; cardiac enlargement.
- Hypermetabolism with normal T_4.
- Elevation of plasma and urinary catecholamines or their metabolites.

General Considerations

Pheochromocytoma is a rare disease characterized by paroxysmal or sustained hypertension due to a tumor of pheochrome tissue, most commonly located in either or both adrenals (90%) or anywhere along the sympathetic nervous chain, and rarely in such aberrant locations as the thorax, bladder, or brain. Most cases occur in sporadic distribution, but about 10–15% are familial. Most tumors are single; multiple tumors are present in only 10% of patients, more commonly in familial cases than sporadic ones.

The following familial syndromes have been identified:

(1) Familial pheochromocytoma without other abnormalities.

(2) Pheochromocytoma associated with calcitonin-secreting medullary carcinoma of the thyroid and hyperparathyroidism (multiple endocrine neoplasia type II).

(3) In association with medullary carcinoma of the thyroid and the syndrome of multiple mucosal neuromas, without hyperparathyroidism (multiple endocrine neoplasia type III).

(4) With neurofibromatosis (Recklinghausen's disease).

(5) With Hippel-Lindau disease (hemangioblastomas of retina, cerebellum, and other parts of the nervous system).

Clinical Findings

A. Symptoms and Signs: Pheochromocytoma is manifested by attacks of severe headache, palpitation or tachycardia, profuse sweating, vasomotor changes (including pallor or flushing of the face or extremities), precordial or abdominal pain, nausea and vomiting, visual disturbances (including blurring or blindness), aphasia and loss of consciousness (rarely), increasing nervousness and irritability, increased appetite, dyspnea, angina, and loss of weight. Physical findings include hypertension, either in attacks or sustained, with cardiac enlargement; postural tachycardia (change of more than 20 beats/min) and postural hypotension; mild elevation of basal body temperature. Retinal hemorrhage or papilledema occurs occasionally.

B. Laboratory Findings: The cold pressor response is negative (blood pressure fall, or a rise of less than 20/15); hypermetabolism exists; T_4 is normal; and glycosuria or hyperglycemia (or both) may be present. Blood volume is usually contracted.

C. Special Tests: Pharmacologic provocative and suppressive tests have become obsolete and are not recommended.

1. Assay of urinary catecholamines on a 24-hour urine specimen—and the simpler tests for 3-methoxy-4-hydroxymandelic acid (vanillylmandelic acid, VMA), or total metanephrines—are now generally available. Urinary catecholamines are usually elevated. One should remember that stress, catecholamine-containing topical nasal medications, many bronchodilators, and methyldopa will also produce abnormally high values. Since VMA determinations can also be affected by a number of drugs, avoidance of drug-taking during the urine collection is desirable. Antihypertensive agents such as thiazides, clonidine, and ganglionic blockers do *not* elevate VMA, metanephrines, or catecholamines.

Most patients with pheochromocytoma have clear-cut elevations of urinary catecholamines (normal range up to 130 μg/24 h) and VMA (normal range, 2–7 mg/24 h). Occasionally there are patients with large tumors that have normal excretion of catecholamines but high VMA, presumably due to intratumoral metabolism of the catecholamines. Conversely, a very small, actively catecholamine-releasing tumor may be associated with normal VMA and very high urinary catecholamines. In any patient with pheochromocytoma, the secretion of catecholamines may be sporadic and intermittent.

2. The most reliable test for pheochromocytoma associated with paroxysmal hypertension is direct **assay of epinephrine and norepinephrine** in the blood and urine during or following an attack. High epinephrine levels favor tumor localization within the adrenal gland. Proper collection of specimens is essential. Determination of blood catecholamines via a venous catheter—a research procedure—will help localize ectopic lesions and paragangliomas.

3. X-ray visualization of the tumor after preparation with blocking agents (see Treatment, below), or intravenous urogram or angiography is often successful. CT scan is safer and has been shown to be very accurate in the diagnosis of these tumors. Ultrasonography is useful in demonstrating adrenal or paraadrenal masses.

A radioactive scanning procedure has recently been described. Results seem encouraging, but experience is limited. (See Sisson reference, below.)

Differential Diagnosis

Pheochromocytoma should always be suspected in any patient with labile hypertension, especially if some of the other features such as hypermetabolism or glycosuria are present in a young person. Because of such symptoms as tachycardia, tremor, palpitation, and hypermetabolism, pheochromocytoma may be confused with thyrotoxicosis. It should be considered in patients with unexplained acute anginal attacks. About 10% are mistakenly treated for diabetes mellitus because of the glycosuria. Pheochromocytoma may also be misdiagnosed as essential hypertension, myocarditis, glomerulonephritis or other renal lesions, toxemia of pregnancy, eclampsia, and psychoneurosis. It rarely masquerades as gastrointestinal hemorrhage and abdominal disorders of an emergency nature. Although false-positive tests are not uncommon with pharmacologic agents and may lead to unnecessary explorations, the occasional false-negative test may permit a potentially curable fatal disease to go unrecognized. Catecholamine determination has made the diagnosis much more accurate.

Complications

All of the complications of severe hypertension may be encountered. Hypertensive crises with sudden blindness or cerebrovascular accidents are not uncommon. These may be precipitated by sudden movement, by manipulation during or after pregnancy, by emotional stress or trauma, or during surgical removal of the tumor. Cardiomyopathy may develop.

After removal of the tumor, a state of severe hypotension and shock (resistant to epinephrine and norepinephrine) may ensue with precipitation of renal failure or myocardial infarction. These complications can be avoided by judicious preoperative and operative use of catecholamine blocking agents such as phentolamine and phenoxybenzamine and by the use of blood or plasma to restore blood volume. Hypotension and shock may occur from spontaneous infarction or hemorrhage of the tumor; emergency surgical removal of the tumor is necessary in these cases.

On rare occasions, a patient dies as a result of the complications of diagnostic tests or during surgery. No patient with suspected pheochromocytoma should be subjected either to an invasive diagnostic procedure or to surgery unless there has been adequate blockade with phenoxybenzamine and, if necessary, with propranolol.

Cholelithiasis is often associated.

Treatment

Surgical removal of the tumor or tumors is the treatment of choice. This may require exploration of the entire sympathetic chain as well as both adrenals. Administration of phenoxybenzamine and blood or plasma before and during surgery has made this type of surgery a great deal safer in recent years. *After* appropriate alpha-adrenergic receptor blockade with phenoxybenzamine, the beta-blocker propranolol can be employed to control tachycardia and other arrhythmias.

Since there may be multiple tumors, it is essential to recheck urinary catecholamine levels postoperatively.

Long-term treatment with phentolamine is not successful. Oral phenoxybenzamine (Dibenzyline) has been successfully used as chronic treatment in inoperable carcinoma and preoperatively in all patients. It should be used in every patient before any invasive diagnostic procedure (such as arteriography) to prevent sudden dangerous increases in blood pressure. Its routine use for 10 days or longer prior to surgery allows the blood pressure to stabilize and blood volume to return to normal, thus reducing surgical and postoperative mortality rates. If the patient has electrocardiographic evidence of myocarditis, phenoxybenzamine therapy should be continued until maximal improvement has occurred. (*Note:* Monitor blood pressure carefully to avoid severe hypotension.)

Alpha-methyl-L-tyrosine (metyrosine, Demser), recently marketed in the USA, is a competitive blocker in the synthesis of catecholamines. It is useful in the medical management of malignant or inoperable tumors.

Prognosis

The prognosis depends entirely upon how early the diagnosis is made. If the tumor is successfully removed before irreparable damage to the cardiovascular system has occurred, a complete cure is usually achieved. Complete cure (or improvement) may follow removal of a tumor that has been present for many years. Rarely, hypertension persists or returns in spite of successful surgery. Only a small percentage of tumors are malignant.

Before the advent of blocking agents, the surgical mortality rate was as high as 30%, but this is rapidly being reduced.

If after removal of a tumor a satisfactory fall of blood pressure does not occur, always consider the presence of another tumor.

It has been estimated that in the USA alone about 800 deaths a year may be due to unrecognized pheochromocytoma.

Bravo EL et al: Circulating and urinary catecholamines in pheochromocytoma: Diagnostic and pathophysiologic implications. N Engl J Med 1979;**301**:682.

Carney JA, Sizemore GW, Tyce GM: Bilateral adrenal medullary hyperplasia in multiple endocrine neoplasia, type 2: The precursor of bilateral pheochromocytoma. Mayo Clin Proc 1975; **50**:3.

Cryer PE: Physiology and pathophysiology of the human sympathoadrenal neuroendocrine system. N Engl J Med 1980; **303**:436.

Engelman K: Phaeochromocytoma. Clin Endocrinol Metab 1977;**6**:769.

Pullerits J et al: Pheochromocytoma: A clinical review with emphasis on pharmacologic aspects. Clin Invest Med 1982; **5**:259.

Schimke RN: Multiple endocrine adenomatosis syndromes. Adv Intern Med 1976;**21**:249.

Sisson JC et al: Scintigraphic localization of pheochromocytoma. N Engl J Med 1981;**305**:12.

DISEASES OF THE PANCREATIC ISLET CELLS*

ISLET CELL FUNCTIONING PANCREATIC TUMORS

The pancreatic islet is composed of several types of cells, each with distinct chemical and microscopic features: the A cell, B cell, and D cell.† The A cells (20%) secrete glucagon, the B cells (75%) secrete insulin, and the D cells (5%) secrete somatostatin. A fourth type, secreting "human pancreatic polypeptide," has been described recently. Each cell may give rise to benign or malignant neoplasms that are often multiple and usually present with a clinical syndrome related to hypersecretion of a native or ectopic hormonal product. Diagnosis of the tumor depends principally on specific assay of the hormone produced. In malignant insulinoma, an increase in plasma proinsulin—and, in the Zollinger-Ellison syndrome, "big" gastrin—may be the most specific finding. The exact

---

*Diabetes mellitus and the hypoglycemic states are discussed in Chapter 20.

†Formerly called α, β, and δ cells.

hormone responsible for the "pancreatic cholera" syndrome remains unknown, but a biologically active substance called vasoactive intestinal peptide (VIP) is often found both in the plasma and in the tumors of patients with this condition. Glucagon-secreting A cell tumors are the rarest of the functional tumors and present with mild diabetes, migratory necrolytic erythema, and stomatitis.

In addition to the native hormones, aberrant or ectopic hormones may be secreted by islet cell tumors, including ACTH, melanocyte-stimulating hormone, serotonin, and chorionic gonadotropin, with a variety of clinical syndromes. Islet cell tumors may be part of the syndrome of multiple endocrine adenomatosis type I (with pituitary and parathyroid adenomas).

Direct resection of the tumor (or tumors), which often spreads locally, is the primary form of therapy for all types of islet cell neoplasm except Zollinger-Ellison syndrome, where treatment choices include blockade of acid secretion by the gastric mucosa with cimetidine or removal of the end organ (total gastrectomy). Palliation of functioning malignancies often requires both antihormonal and anticancer chemotherapy. The use of streptozocin, doxorubicin, and asparaginase, especially for malignant insulinoma, has produced some encouraging results, although these drugs are quite toxic.

Prognosis in these neoplasms is variable. Long-term survival in spite of widespread metastases has been reported. Earlier diagnosis by hormonal assay may lead to earlier detection and a higher cure rate.

Friesen SR: Tumors of the endocrine pancreas. N Engl J Med 1982;**306**:580.

Graham DY et al: Islet cell carcinoma, pancreatic cholera and vasoactive intestinal peptide. Ann Intern Med 1975;**83**:782.

Jaspan JB et al: Clinical features and diagnosis of islet cell tumor. Page 469 in: Tumors of the Pancreas. Moossa AR (editor). Williams & Wilkins, 1980.

Jensen RT et al: Zollinger-Ellison syndrome: Current concepts and management. Ann Intern Med 1983;**98**:59.

Kahn CR et al: Pancreatic cholera: Beneficial effects of treatment with streptozotocin. N Engl J Med 1975;**292**:941.

Stacpoole PW et al: A familial glucagonoma syndrome: Genetic, clinical and biochemical manifestations. Am J Med 1981;**70**:1017.

Stadil F, Stage JG: The Zollinger-Ellison syndrome. Clin Endocrinol Metab 1979;**8**:433.

DISEASES OF THE TESTES

MALE HYPOGONADISM

Male hypogonadism may be classified according to time of onset, ie, prepubertal or postpubertal. It may also be classified as primary or secondary, depending on whether the lesion is in the testes (hypergonadotropic) or in the hypothalamic-pituitary area (hypogonadotropic).

Table 19–11. Causes of hypogonadism.

Primary hypogonadism (hyper-gonadotropic)	Secondary hypogonadism (hypogonadotropic)
Klinefelter's syndrome	Kallmann's syndrome
Anorchia	Pituitary tumors
Surgical or accidental castration	Craniopharyngiomas
	Hypothalamic lesions
Viral infections (mumps)	Hemochromatosis
Tuberculosis	Prader-Willi syndrome
Leprosy	
Myotonic dystrophy	
Ionizing radiation injury	
Chemotherapeutic agents	

The etiologic diagnosis of hypogonadism (eg, primary or secondary) is based on a careful history and physical examination and is confirmed by laboratory tests (Table 19–11).

1. PREPUBERTAL HYPOGONADISM

The diagnosis of hypogonadism cannot usually be made in boys under age 16 or 17, since it is difficult to differentiate from "physiologic" delay of puberty.

Prepubertal hypogonadism is most commonly due to a specific gonadotropic deficiency of the pituitary. It may be familial and associated with anosmia (Kallmann's syndrome) or hyposmia. It may also occur as a result of destructive lesions near the pituitary region (eg, suprasellar cyst) or, more rarely, as a result of destruction or malformation of the testes (prepubertal castration). Rare causes include Prader-Willi syndrome (obesity, hypogonadism, mental retardation, and hypotonia), Laurence-Moon-Biedl syndrome (obesity, hypogonadism, polydactyly, retinitis pigmentosa), and Alström's syndrome (hypogonadism, nerve deafness, obesity, and retinitis pigmentosa).

In cases associated with a complete pituitary defect, the patient is of short stature or fails to grow and mature. Otherwise the patient is strikingly tall due to overgrowth of the long bones due to delay in closure of epiphyseal plates. The external genitalia are underdeveloped, the voice is high-pitched, the beard does not grow, and the patient lacks libido and potency. In adult life he presents a youthful appearance, with obesity (often in girdle distribution), disproportionately long extremities (span exceeds height), lack of temporal recession of the hairline, and a small Adam's apple. Gynecomastia is occasionally seen (but apparent gynecomastia may be merely fat). The skin is fine-grained, wrinkled, and sallow, especially on the face. There is no acne or sebum production. The penis is small and the prostate undeveloped. Pubic and axillary hair are scant. The testes may be absent from the scrotum (cryptorchism) or may be in the scrotum but very small. Rarely, and for unknown reasons, they may be entirely absent (anorchia).

Bone age is retarded. Skull x-rays may show a lesion of the sella or above the sella (eg, craniopharyngioma). Anemia may be present. Urinary 17-ketosteroids are low or normal in testicular failure; very low or absent in primary pituitary failure. Urinary FSH is absent in primary pituitary failure, elevated in castration or testicular failure. Plasma testosterone and serum FSH and luteinizing hormone (LH) measurements are more specific than urinary 17-ketosteroids and urinary gonadotropins.

The response to chorionic gonadotropin injections in cases due to pituitary failure will be maturation, elevation of plasma testosterone, and occasionally descent of cryptorchid testes. (In primary testicular failure, no such response occurs.) Testicular biopsy shows immature tubules and Leydig cells in hypopituitary patients.

Adequate testosterone therapy can make these individuals into apparently normal males except that they usually cannot produce sperm. To produce spermatogenesis, a combination of an FSH preparation, eg, human menopausal gonadotropin (hMG [Pergonal]), with human chorionic gonadotropin (hCG) is usually required. This treatment is expensive. Spermatogenesis can occasionally be achieved with the use of hCG alone. Patients with prepubertal hypogonadism must be placed on testosterone and maintained for life on adequate doses. Long-acting testosterone preparations, 200–300 mg intramuscularly every 2–4 weeks, may be employed. The use of oral synthetic androgenic preparations is less desirable, since they have a significant hepatotoxicity, especially when used for long periods of time. In cases of delayed puberty, clomiphene citrate has been effective in accelerating sexual maturation (see Dickerman reference, below). Recent reports demonstrating a dramatic response of FSH and LH to LH-releasing factor (GnRH, LHRH) seem to locate the defect in isolated hypogonadotropic hypogonadism to the hypothalamus and offer renewed hope for future treatment. Experimental use of pulsatile LHRH infusion to induce both puberty and spermatogenesis has been described.

Bray GA et al: The Prader-Willi syndrome: A study of 40 patients and review of the literature. *Medicine* 1983;**62**:59.

Dickerman Z et al: Acceleration of puberty in boys with delayed puberty by clomiphene citrate. *Acta Endocrinol* 1980;**94**:117.

Lieblich JM et al: Syndrome of anosmia with hypogonadotropic hypogonadism (Kallmann's syndrome): Clinical and laboratory studies in 23 cases. *Am J Med* 1982;**73**:506.

Rayner PHW: Puberty: Precocious and delayed. *Br Med J* 1976; **1**:1385.

Snyder PF, Lawrence DA: Treatment of male hypogonadism with testosterone enanthate. *J Clin Endocrinol Metab* 1980;**51**: 1335.

2. KLINEFELTER'S SYNDROME

The most common primary developmental abnormality causing hypogonadism is Klinefelter's syndrome (seminiferous tubule dysgenesis). It afflicts one out of every 400–500 males. It is caused by the presence of one or more supernumerary X chromosomes and is usually recognized at or shortly after puberty. It is at times familial. Most commonly, there is only failure of the tubules with permanent sterility. The secretory function of the Leydig cells ranges from normal to definite failure. An abnormality in the LH feedback control as well as a disorder in steroidogenesis has recently been demonstrated in Klinefelter's syndrome.

The clinical findings are swelling of the breasts (gynecomastia), sterility, lack of libido and potency (rare), and at times lack of development of body hair, and female escutcheon. Excessive growth of long bones is present. There may be associated mental retardation. The testes are usually small and firm. The penis and prostate are usually normal. The ejaculate usually contains no spermatozoa, although an occasional case with spermatogenesis in a mosaic variant has been described. Urinary 17-ketosteroids are low normal or normal. Serum testosterone is usually low to normal. LH and FSH levels are invariably elevated. Serum estradiol is higher than normal. Testicular biopsy shows sclerosis of the tubules, nests of Leydig cells, and no spermatozoa. The cell karyotype is most commonly 47,XXY, with a chromatin-positive buccal smear. Mosaicism may have clinical features ranging from normal to the classic picture just described here. Chromosomal analysis is necessary to diagnose the condition. In mosaics with a normal 46,XY cell line, spermatogenesis may be present.

All causes of gynecomastia must be differentiated from Klinefelter's syndrome. The plasma FSH and the buccal smear will settle the diagnosis.

Testosterone replacement should be given if secondary sexual characteristics have failed to appear or if impotence and low blood testosterone develop later in life. There is no treatment for the infertility. If gynecomastia is disfiguring, plastic surgical removal is indicated.

Hsueh WA et al: Endocrine features of Klinefelter's syndrome. *Medicine* 1978;**57**:447.

3. POSTPUBERTAL HYPOGONADISM

Any pituitary lesion (eg, tumor, infection, necrosis) may lead to lack of gonadotropin; often hypogonadism is an early sign. The testes may be damaged by trauma, x-ray irradiation, infection, or in other ways. Viral (mumps) and bacterial (gonorrhea, leprosy) orchitis usually affects only the seminiferous tubules and spermatogenesis, leaving Leydig cell function intact. Occasionally, low plasma testosterone and high LH are seen. Many drugs can affect testicular function. Cyclophosphamide rapidly causes azoospermia, and hepatic and renal failure are often associated with low testosterone levels. Myotonic dystrophy (Steinert's disease) should be considered if myotonia, frontal baldness, and diabetes are present. States of malnutrition, anemia, and similar disorders

may lead to functional gonadal underactivity. The male climacteric, although a disputed syndrome, probably does exist; it makes its appearance about 20 years later than the female menopause.

The symptoms of acquired adult hypogonadism are varying degrees of loss of libido and potency; retardation of hair growth, especially of the face; vasomotor symptoms (flushing, dizziness, chills); lack of aggressiveness and interest; sterility; and muscular aches and back pain. Atrophy or hypoplasia of external genitalia and prostate is rare. The skin of the face is thin and finely wrinkled, and the beard is scant. Girdle type obesity and kyphosis of the spine are present.

Urinary and plasma testosterone levels are low. Urinary and serum FSH or LH are low in cases due to pituitary lesions and elevated in primary testicular failure. Serum prolactin is often elevated in hypothalamic or pituitary lesions, especially in pituitary tumors. In fact, the first manifestation of a prolactin-secreting pituitary tumor in a male may be impotence. The sperm count is low, or spermatozoa may be absent.

True adult hypogonadism must be differentiated from the far more commonly seen psychogenic lack of libido and potency. Measurement of plasma testosterone is useful in this regard. Confusion may also arise in men who are obese and have a sparse beard and small genitalia but normal sperm counts and urinary FSH ("fertile eunuchs"). These patients may represent examples of end-organ unresponsiveness or isolated lack of LH. The usual form of male infertility is "spermatogenic arrest." The disorder can only be diagnosed by testicular biopsy. Most of these patients have normal gonadotropin levels and are not benefited by therapy.

Oral methyltestosterone or fluoxymesterone is effective. Because of lack of hepatic toxicity and more effective androgenic activity, the long-acting injectable preparations of testosterone (cypionate, enanthate) are preferred. The dose used is 200–400 mg every 3 weeks. Treatment of long-standing hypogonadism with androgens may precipitate anxiety and acute emotional problems that often require concomitant psychotherapy. Watch for acute urinary retention in older patients. In cases of hypogonadism due to hyperprolactinemia, excellent results may be achieved by administration of bromocriptine or, more permanently, with removal of a pituitary prolactin-secreting tumor.

•   •   •

Prognosis of Hypogonadism

If hypogonadism is due to a pituitary lesion, the prognosis is that of the primary disease (eg, tumor, necrosis). The prognosis for restoration of virility is good if testosterone is given. The sooner administration is started, the fewer stigmas of eunuchoidism remain (unless therapy is discontinued).

The prognosis for fertility is usually not good. It is only feasible in instances where the testicular elements are present but are unstimulated due to lack of pituitary tropic hormones. This therapy may become practical with the greater availability of gonadotropin from postmenopausal urine (human menopausal gonadotropins [hMG]). Synthetic LHRH and LHRH analogs have been successfully used in the treatment of hypogonadotropic hypogonadism. They are not available at present in the USA.

Cryptorchism should be corrected early, since the incidence of malignant testicular tumors is higher in ectopic testicles and the chance of ultimate fertility is lessened in long-standing cases, even after orchiopexy.

Carter JN et al: Prolactin-secreting tumors and hypogonadism in 22 men. *N Engl J Med* 1978;**299**:847.

Davidson J et al: Effects of androgen on sexual behavior in hypogonadal men. *J Clin Endocrinol Metab* 1979;**48**:955.

Lipsett MB: Physiology and pathology of the Leydig cell. *N Engl J Med* 1980;**303**:682.

Skarin G et al: Chronic pulsatile low dose GnRH therapy for induction of testosterone production and spermatogenesis in a man with secondary hypogonadotropic hypogonadism. *J Clin Endocrinol Metab* 1982;**51**:1335.

Snyder PJ: Clinical use of androgens. *Annu Rev Med* 1984;**35**:207.

Spark RF et al: Impotence is not always psychogenic: Newer insights into hypothalamic-pituitary-gonadal dysfunction. *JAMA* 1980;**243**:750.

MALE HYPERGONADISM & TESTICULAR TUMORS*

In adults, almost all lesions causing male hypergonadism are functioning testicular tumors, which quite frequently are malignant. In children, male hypergonadism may take the form of true precocious puberty, due to pituitary or hypothalamic lesions; or pseudoprecocious puberty, due to lesions of the testes or adrenal glands.

1. PREPUBERTAL HYPERGONADISM
(See Table 19–12.)

The symptoms and signs are premature growth of pubic and axillary hair, beard, and external genitalia and excessive muscular development. In true precocity due to pituitary or hypothalamic lesions, pituitary gonadotropins (FSH and LH) are secreted, the testicles enlarge, testosterone is secreted, and spermatogenesis occurs. In adrenal virilization or testicular tumor there is testicular atrophy, with or without palpable nodules; spermatogenesis does not take place. In childhood, interstitial cell tumors are the principal testicular tumors to be considered. Bilateral interstitial cell nodules are also rarely seen with adrenal hyperplasia. Deficiency of 11- or 21-hydroxylase causes isosexual precocity in the male only. Cases of hepatoma with true isosexual precocity due to gonadotropin secretion

*See also Tumors of the Testis in Chapter 16.

Table 19–12. Sexual precocity along isosexual pattern.

Types and Causes	Characteristics
Neurogenic Brain tumor Encephalitis Congenital defect with hypothalamic involvement **Pituitary** Idiopathic activation; "constitutional" type	Testes mature normally; spermatogenesis occurs; secondary characteristics normal; sex hormones excreted in normal adult amounts.
Gonadal Interstitial cell tumor of testis	Tumor in one gonad, the other gonad immature or atrophic; spermatogenesis does not occur; sex hormones excreted in excessive amounts.
Adrenal Embryonic hyperplasia or tumor	Testes usually small and immature, occasionally containing aberrant adrenal tissue; no spermatogenesis; often results in adrenocortical insufficiency in males.

by the tumor have been reported. Rarely, severe hypothyroidism may be associated with precocious puberty.

If the cause of precocity is "constitutional" (ie, cause unknown), it is usually a harmless disorder, although the sexual activities of these children must be controlled to prevent socially undesirable conceptions. If precocity is due to hypothalamic or pituitary lesions, the prognosis is poor, since most of these tumors are not removable. Adrenal tumors and testicular tumors are often malignant.

Most patients with this syndrome who survive into adulthood will be short as a result of premature maturation and closure of their epiphyses.

Treatment

In cases where the tumor is accessible, surgical removal is the treatment of choice. Bilateral adrenal hyperplasia that causes pseudoprecocious puberty can be successfully treated with cortisone, and normal development and spermatogenesis will occur following treatment. Thyroxine replacement therapy stops precocious development in the rare patient with hypothyroidism having this complication. Medroxyprogesterone (Depo-Provera) is the most frequently used drug in true isosexual precocity. This treatment may lead to permanent damage to testicular tissue. The antiandrogen cyproterone acetate has also been used, with similar results. LHRH (GnRH) analogs have been synthesized and successfully used as antagonists to prevent release of gonadotropins, thus halting the process of precocious puberty. This is still experimental.

Ducharme JR, Collu R: Pubertal development: Normal, precocious and delayed. *Clin Endocrinol Metab* 1982;**11**:57.

Luder AS et al: Intranasal and subcutaneous treatment of central precocious puberty in both sexes with a long-acting analog of luteinising hormone–releasing hormone. *J Clin Endocrinol Metab* 1984;**58**:966.

Styne DM, Grunbach MM: Puberty in the male and female: Its physiology and disorders. Pages 189–240 in: *Reproductive Endocrinology.* Yen SSC, Jaffe RB (editors). Saunders, 1978.

2. NEOPLASMS OF THE TESTES IN ADULTS
(See also Chapter 16.)

Many or most testicular neoplasms are functioning (ie, productive of androgenic, estrogenic hormones, or of chorionic gonadotropin), and the majority are highly malignant. They are at times quite small and are clinically recognized because of their hormonal effects or because of the presence of metastases. The sudden appearance of gynecomastia in an otherwise healthy male should raise the possibility of testicular tumor. In general, once hormonal manifestations have become pronounced, cure by surgical removal is very unlikely. Some tumors are bilateral, eg, interstitial cell tumors. Often a mixed picture is present. Gonadotropin-secreting bronchogenic carcinomas have been recently described.

The incidence of cancer in cryptorchism is high.

Treatment

If the diagnosis is made early, surgical removal may be curative; radiotherapy is feasible as a palliative measure in radiosensitive types. Chemotherapy may control the growth of choriocarcinomas.

The serum concentration of the beta subunit of human chorionic gonadotropin (hCG) is elevated in choriocarcinomas and, less commonly, in other testicular tumors. The response to therapy can be monitored in such cases by following the level of this glycoprotein.

Fraley EE, Lange PH, Kennedy BJ: Germ-cell testicular cancer in adults. (2 parts.) *N Engl J Med* 1979;**301**:1370, 1420.

DISEASES OF THE OVARIES*

FEMALE HYPOGONADISM

The outstanding symptom of female hypogonadism is amenorrhea (see below). Partial deficiencies, principally corpus luteum failure, may occur; these do not always cause amenorrhea but more often produce anovulatory periods or metrorrhagia.

Estrogenic failure has far-reaching effects, especially if it begins early in life (eg, Turner's syndrome).

Primary pituitary disorders are much less common causes of hypogonadism in the female than primary ovarian disorders and are often associated with other signs of pituitary failure.

Ovarian failure starting in early life will lead to delayed closure of the epiphyses and retarded bone age, often resulting in tall stature with long extremities. On the other hand, in ovarian agenesis, dwarfism is the rule (see below). In adult ovarian failure, changes are more subtle, with some regression of secondary sex characteristics. In estrogenic deficiency of long standing in any age group, osteoporosis, especially of the spine, is almost always found, since estrogen protects bone against excessive resorption.

A relatively rare form of ovarian failure is seen in states of androgen excess originating in the adrenal cortex or ovary, when estrogens, though present in the body, are suppressed by the presence of large amounts of androgens (see p 747).

1. AMENORRHEA

Since regular menstruation depends upon normal function of the entire physiologic axis extending from the hypothalamus and pituitary to the ovary and the uterine lining, it is not surprising that menstrual disorders are among the most common presenting complaints of endocrine disease in women. Correct diagnosis depends upon proper evaluation of each component of the axis, and nonendocrine factors must also be considered.

If menstruation is defined as shedding of endometrium which has been stimulated by estrogen or by estrogen and progesterone which are subsequently withdrawn, it is obvious that amenorrhea can occur either when hormones are deficient or lacking (the hypohormonal or ahormonal type) or when these hormones, though present in adequate amounts, are never withdrawn (the continuous hormonal type).

Primary amenorrhea implies that menses have never been established. This diagnosis is not usually made before the age of about 16. Secondary amenorrhea means that menses once established have ceased (temporarily or permanently).

The most common type of hypohormonal amenorrhea is the menopause, or physiologic failure of ovarian function. The most common example of continuous hormonal amenorrhea is that due to pregnancy, when cyclic withdrawal is prevented by the placental secretions. These 2 conditions should always be considered before extensive diagnostic studies are undertaken.

The principal diagnostic aids that are used in the study of amenorrhea are as follows: (1) vaginal smear for estrogen effect; (2) endometrial biopsy; (3) "medical D&C" (see below); (4) basal body temperature determination; (5) urine determinations of 17-ketosteroids, FSH, pregnanediol, and pregnanetriol; (6) culdoscopy and gynecography; (7) chromosomal studies; (8) pelvic exploratory operation or laparos-

*See also Chapter 13.

copy and gonadal biopsy; (9) radioimmunoassays of FSH, LH, and prolactin, which are now available for specific diagnosis of certain types of amenorrhea; (10) plasma testosterone assay; (11) x-ray studies of the hypothalamic and pituitary areas; and (12) in young females, bone age.

Baird DT (editor): Abnormalities of gonadotropin secretion in women. *Clin Obstet Gynecol* 1976;**3**:465.

Davajan V et al: Symposium on adolescent gynecology and endocrinology. 2. Secondary amenorrhea, hirsutism in adolescents and the clinical consequences of stilbestrol exposure in utero. *West J Med* 1979;**131**:516.

Odell WD, Federman DD: Symposium on adolescent gynecology and endocrinology. 1. Physiology of sexual maturation and primary amenorrhea. *West J Med* 1979;**131**:401.

Speroff L: The ovary. Chapter 17 in: *Endocrinology and Metabolism.* Felig F et al (editors). McGraw-Hill, 1981.

Yen SSC: Chronic anovulation. In: *Reproductive Endocrinology.* Yen SSC, Jaffe RB (editors). Saunders, 1978.

Primary Amenorrhea

Because of the frequency with which "delayed puberty" is found in otherwise normal females, the diagnosis of primary amenorrhea usually is not made until the patient is clearly beyond the age at which normal menarche occurs. In the USA, the mean age at menarche is 12½ years. If menses have not started by age 16, primary amenorrhea is definitely present, and the cause should be investigated.

Most cases of primary amenorrhea are of the hypohormonal or ahormonal type. Exact diagnosis is essential to rule out organic lesion along the hypothalamic-pituitary-gonadal axis. The chromosomal sex pattern must be determined in many cases. Laparoscopy or pelvic exploration may be required to establish the diagnosis. In large series, the most common cause has always been Turner's syndrome.

The causes are as follows:

(1) Hypothalamic causes: Constitutional delay in onset, debility, serious organic illness, lack of LHRH (GnRH).

(2) Pituitary causes (with low or absent FSH): Suprasellar cyst, pituitary tumors (eosinophilic adenomas, chromophobe adenomas, basophilic adenomas), isolated lack of pituitary gonadotropins.

(3) Ovarian causes (with high FSH): Ovarian agenesis (Turner's syndrome), destruction of ovaries (eg, due to infection or, possibly, autoimmunity).

(4) Uterine causes: Malformations, congenital müllerian dysgenesis, imperforate hymen, hermaphroditism, unresponsive or atrophic endometrium.

(5) Miscellaneous causes: All forms of male pseudohermaphroditism (enzymatic defects in testosterone synthesis, androgen resistance syndromes), androgen excess syndromes (adrenal or ovarian tumors, polycystic ovaries).

Since primary amenorrhea is only a manifestation of multiple and often complex underlying defects, treatment must be individualized according to the specific cause.

Secondary Amenorrhea

Temporary cessation of menses is extremely common and usually does not require extensive endocrine investigation. In the childbearing age, pregnancy must be ruled out. In women beyond the childbearing age, menopause should be considered first. States of emotional stress, malnutrition, anemia, and similar disorders may be associated with temporary amenorrhea and correction of the primary disorder will usually also reestablish menses. Some women fail to menstruate regularly for prolonged intervals after stopping oral contraceptive pills. Lactation may be associated with amenorrhea, either physiologically or for abnormally prolonged periods after delivery. An increasing number of small prolactin-secreting pituitary tumors causing secondary amenorrhea and often lactation have been discovered by means of prolactin assays and pituitary tomography (see prolactin, p 695).

By the use of the "medical D&C" (see p 759), ie, the administration of progesterone with subsequent withdrawal, these amenorrheas can be arbitrarily divided into amenorrhea with negative D&C and amenorrhea with positive D&C. The former (with the exception of pregnancy) show an atrophic or hypoestrin type of endometrium; the latter show an endometrium of the proliferative type but lacking progesterone.

(1) Secondary amenorrhea with negative medical D&C may be due to the following causes: premature ovarian failure, pituitary tumor, pituitary infarction (Sheehan's syndrome). The measurement of serum FSH and LH is extremely helpful in separating ovarian causes (high gonadotropins) from hypothalamic-pituitary origin (low gonadotropins). Serum prolactin levels must be measured. Less common causes include virilizing syndromes such as arrhenoblastoma, Cushing's disease, Addison's disease, and miscellaneous causes such as anorexia nervosa, profound myxedema, and irradiation of the uterine lining.

(2) Secondary amenorrhea with positive medical D&C may be due to metropathia hemorrhagica, Stein-Leventhal syndrome, estrogen medication, estrogenic tumors, ie, granulosa cell tumors (rare), hyperthyroidism, and perhaps liver disease. A common cause is "psychogenic amenorrhea" related to emotional trauma (divorce, going to college, stressful new job, etc). Menses usually return in a few months without any specific therapy. Tonic elevation of serum LH with normal FSH is helpful in the diagnosis of polycystic ovary syndrome. Amenorrhea or oligomenorrhea is also often found in athletes (long-distance runners, dedicated ballet dancers, etc). Depletion of body fat due to exercise may play a role in the pathogenesis of this problem.

Some degree of overlap in these 2 groups is sometimes found.

The aim of therapy is not only to reestablish menses (although this is valuable for psychologic reasons) but also to attempt to establish the cause (eg, pituitary tumor) of the amenorrhea and to restore reproductive function.

Treatment depends upon the underlying disease. It is not necessary to treat all cases, especially temporary amenorrhea or irregular menses in unmarried girls or women. These cases usually are corrected spontaneously after marriage or the first pregnancy.

In patients whose response to progesterone is normal, the administration of this hormone during the last 5–10 days of each month, orally or parenterally (see p 759), will correct the amenorrhea.

In patients who are unresponsive to progesterone and whose urinary gonadotropin levels are low, treatment of a pituitary lesion may restore menstruation; gonadotropins would appear to be of value, and human pituitary FSH has been used with some success experimentally. This, or gonadotropins from postmenopausal urine (menotropins, hMG), has given good results in secondary amenorrhea. Clomiphene citrate (Clomid) has been extensively and often successfully tried for the treatment of these patients. However, in current clinical practice, if attainment of pregnancy is not desirable, estrogen alone or in combination with progesterone is more commonly used. If gonadotropin levels are high, gonadotropins are of no value; treat with estrogens alone or with estrogens and progesterone. A commonly used schedule is the oral administration of 1.2 mg of conjugated estrogens from days 1 to 20 of each month and 10 mg of medroxyprogesterone daily during days 21 to 25. Corticosteroids may restore menstruation in virilizing disorders that are due to enzymatic abnormalities in cortisol biosynthesis. Wedge resection of the ovaries often restores regular menstruation in the polycystic ovary syndrome. The use of LHRH (GnRH) is under investigation at present and appears promising. In patients with the galactorrhea-amenorrhea syndromes associated with elevated prolactin levels, restoration of ovulatory menses has been achieved with the ergot derivative bromocriptine (bromoergocryptine). Transsphenoidal resection of small prolactin-producing pituitary adenomas likewise has resulted in restoration of fertility.

General measures include dietary management as required to correct overweight or underweight; psychotherapy in cases due to emotional disturbance; and correction of anemia and any other metabolic abnormality that may be present (eg, mild hypothyroidism).

Hypothalamic Amenorrhea

Secondary hypothalamic amenorrhea, due to emotional or psychogenic causes, is far more common in young women than amenorrhea due to organic causes (except for pregnancy). It is probably mediated by a hypothalamic block of the release of pituitary gonadotropic hormones, especially LH. Pituitary FSH is still produced and is found in normal or low levels in the urine. Since some LH is necessary in the production of estrogen as well as FSH, a state of hypoestrinism with an atrophic endometrium will eventually result.

A history of psychic trauma just preceding the onset of amenorrhea can usually be obtained. The urinary FSH level is normal or low normal, and the 17-ketosteroid level is low normal. Plasma LH is low. Vaginal smear and endometrial biopsy show mild hypoestrin effects. The response to progesterone (medical D&C) is variable. The endometrium responds to cyclic administration of estrogens.

Menses often return spontaneously, after weight gain, or after several induced "cycles." Psychotherapy may be of value. Clomiphene citrate (Clomid) may be tried to reestablish menses. If amenorrhea persists for many years, signs of severe estrogen deficiency will appear and must be treated.

It is most important to recognize this syndrome and not to mistake it for an organic type of amenorrhea with a very different prognosis.

Jewelewicz R: The diagnosis and treatment of amenorrheas. *Fertil Steril* 1976;**27**:1347.
Kletzy OA et al: Classification of secondary amenorrhea based on distinct hormonal patterns. *J Clin Endocrinol Metab* 1975; **41**:660.
Mason P et al: Induction of ovulation with pulsatile luteinising hormone–releasing hormone. *Br Med J* 1984;**288**:181.
Spark RF et al: Galactorrhea-amenorrhea syndromes: Etiology and treatment. *Ann Intern Med* 1976;**84**:532.

2. TURNER'S SYNDROME
(Primary Ovarian Agenesis, Gonadal Dysgenesis)

Turner's syndrome is a chromosomal disorder associated with congenital absence of the ovaries and with dwarfism and other anomalies. Patients with this syndrome lack one of the two X chromosomes.

The principal features include bilateral streak gonads, genital hypoplasia with infantile uterus, vagina, and breasts and primary amenorrhea; scant axillary and pubic hair; short stature, usually between 122 and 142 cm (48 and 56 inches); increased carrying angle of arms; webbing of neck (quite common); stocky "shield" chest with widely spaced nipples; cardiovascular disorders, especially coarctation of the aorta, congenital valve defects; osteoporosis and other skeletal anomalies (short fourth metacarpals, exostosis of tibia, etc) with increasing age; and prematurely senile appearance. Nevi are common. Lymphedema of hands and feet is seen in infants. There is an increased incidence of autoimmune thyroiditis and diabetes.

Serum FSH and LH are high. Bone age is retarded. The chromatin sex pattern most often shows a "negative" buccal smear and 45,X chromosomal pattern. Mosaicism is common; most frequent is the 45,X, 46,XX chromosomal pattern.

Exploratory operation shows a "streak ovary" and, at times, islands of interstitial cells. The genital apparatus is entirely female but infantile in development.

The principal disorder to be differentiated is pituitary dwarfism. In this disorder, urinary and serum FSH is low or absent, and other signs of pituitary failure are present. Other forms of constitutional dwarfism, such as Laurence-Moon-Biedl syndrome, are ruled out by the FSH levels and lack of stigmas such as polydactyly, retinitis pigmentosa, and other signs of the disease. The short stature and occasional metacarpal deformities may resemble pseudohypoparathyroidism, but these patients menstruate normally. In Noonan's syndrome, a rare inherited disorder, the female patient has many similar phenotypic characteristics (short stature, shield chest, short neck), but cardiac lesions are in the right side of the heart (pulmonary stenosis is common), the ovaries are normal, the chromosomal pattern is 46,XX, and the serum FSH and LH are not elevated.

With administration of estrogens, some increase in height can be achieved, but this is almost never enough to increase stature significantly; androgens may also promote growth, especially fluoxymesterone in low doses. Some cases respond to administration of growth hormone.

Without treatment, growth will eventually cease, since the epiphyses will close spontaneously (though late). The administration of estrogen will develop the breasts and uterus and lead to anovulatory menses upon cyclic withdrawal. *Note:* Endometrial carcinoma has been reported after diethylstilbestrol therapy. Fertility can never be achieved.

The associated congenital cardiovascular anomalies may cause early death or may require surgical correction (eg, coarctation). Webbing of the neck can be corrected by plastic surgery.

Similar syndromes with different chromosomal patterns have been described. "Pure gonadal dysgenesis" has only "streak" gonads and sexual infantilism, with normal stature and normal 46,XX chromosomal pattern. "Mixed" or "atypical" gonadal dysgenesis, a form of hermaphroditism, has a "streak" gonad on one side and an abnormal gonad, prone to neoplasm, on the other side, making prophylactic removal a reasonable procedure. It is very often associated with XY mosaicism.

Hall JG et al: Turner's syndrome. *West J Med* 1982;**137:**62.
Zah W et al: Mixed gonadal dysgenesis. *Acta Endocrinol [Suppl]* 1975;**79:**3.

3. MENOPAUSAL SYNDROME
(See p 477.)

FEMALE HYPERGONADISM

Excesses of ovarian hormones are often encountered during the normal reproductive life of women, and most frequently give rise to irregular or excessive menstrual bleeding and, more rarely, to amenorrhea. Excesses before the age of puberty or after the menopause, however, should be thoroughly investigated, since the possibility of malignant lesions is great. Estrogen excess is more common than progesterone excess, which is seen in pregnancy and in chorioepithelioma. Other extra-ovarian sources of estrogens are malignant tumors of the adrenals, which secrete abnormal amounts of estrogens. Since these tumors usually produce excesses of androgens as well, their hyperestrogenic effects are rarely detectable clinically in the female. Another cause of hyperestrogenism is the ingestion or other use of hormones (eg, in face or vaginal creams).

1. PREPUBERTAL FEMALE HYPERGONADISM

It is important to differentiate organic lesions of the pituitary-hypothalamic region, which cause true precocious puberty in females, from pseudoprecocity due to granulosa cell tumors and choriocarcinoma. Constitutional true sexual precocity may be partial, consisting only of precocious breast development and early growth of pubic hair, or it may be associated with premature menarche as well. It is often familial. Albright's syndrome causes true precocity with fibrous dysplasia of bone (osteitis fibrosa disseminata) and pigmentary changes of the skin (see Chapter 4).

Granulosa cell tumors of the ovary cause uterine bleeding by virtue of their estrogenic secretions, but they do not cause ovulation and these girls are not fertile. The same is usually true of choriocarcinoma. Both of these tumors are highly malignant.

Simple follicle cysts of the ovary, at times easily palpable, may cause precocity.

Pseudoprecocious puberty may also be caused by ingestion of estrogens. Androgenic agents cause early growth of pubic hair.

The significance of the differentiation between true and pseudoprecocious puberty is that in true precocity ovulatory cycles may occur and the patient must be protected from pregnancy. The most useful guide to the differentiation is the urinary and serum FSH determination. FSH is not present in significant levels in girls before puberty and is absent in pseudoprecocious puberty, whereas girls with true precocious puberty may secrete significant levels of FSH and LH.

The diagnosis of either true or pseudoprecocious puberty is important because many cases are due to tumors that must be found and removed if possible (Table 19–13). Unfortunately, most estrogen-secreting tumors are highly malignant, and tumors of the third ventricle and other lesions near the hypothalamus are quite difficult to remove.

Precocious development of breasts and early onset of menses may cause psychic disturbances. Short stature in adult life is the rule, since bone age is advanced and the epiphyses close prematurely. As adults these patients may suffer from excessive menstrual bleeding, which may cause anemia unless it is checked. Cystic mastitis is a chronic problem, and

Table 19–13. Hormones elaborated by actively secreting ovarian tumors.

Type	Secretion
Feminizing	
Granulosa	Estrogen +++
Theca cell	Estrogen ++
Luteoma?	Estrogen + and/or progesterone
Virilizing*	
Arrhenoblastoma	Androgen +++
Adrenal rest (lipoid cell)	Androgen ++ and corticosteroids
Hilar cell	Androgen +++
Miscellaneous	
Choriocarcinoma	Gonadotropins ++++ and estrogens; TSH
Dysgerminoma*	Gonadotropins + and androgens?
Gynandroblastoma	Androgens ++ and estrogens +++
Struma ovarii	Thyroxine +

*Most women have complete amenorrhea with negative medical D&C, since the endometrium is atrophic.

the incidence of uterine adenofibromas is high. It is not definitely known whether long-standing hyperestrinism causes a higher incidence of breast and genital tract cancer, but it may be an aggravating factor.

The only treatment is surgical removal of tumors, but most are malignant and metastasize early. The prognosis for simple constitutional precocity is not so unfavorable, although these girls must be watched to prevent pregnancy. Recent reports on the use of progesterone (Depo-Provera) are encouraging but the response is variable and the possible adverse long-term effects of such treatment are uncertain. Long-acting analogs of LHRH (GnRH) have been used successfully to halt true precocious puberty in both girls and boys. These agents are not yet available in the USA.

Luder AS et al: Intranasal and subcutaneous treatment of central precocious puberty in both sexes with a long-acting analog of luteinising hormone–releasing hormone. J Clin Endocrinol Metab 1984;58:966.
Orr PS et al: Ovarian tumours in childhood: A 27-year review. Br J Surg 1976;63:367.
Styne DM, Grumbach M: Puberty in the male and female: Its physiology and disorders. In: Reproductive Endocrinology. Yen SSC, Jaffe RB (editors). Saunders, 1978.

2. ADULT FEMALE HYPERGONADISM

Adult female hypergonadism may be due to estrogen excess alone or to combined excess of estrogen and progesterone. Estrogen excess is characterized by menorrhagia or, rarely, amenorrhea. The vaginal smear shows estrogen excess. Lack of ovulation is demonstrated by the absence of mid-cycle temperature rise and LH rise. Sterility is the rule. The medical D&C is positive, ie, bleeding starts after a short course of progesterone. Endometrial biopsy shows a proliferative endometrium. The urinary and serum FSH levels are low.

Adult female hyperestrogenism may be caused by (1) states in which ovulation does not occur, leading to "metropathia hemorrhagica" or dysfunctional uterine bleeding; (2) liver disease, which interferes with the catabolism of estrogens; (3) drug administration (eg, estrogen creams or tablets); (4) granulosa cell and theca cell tumors (both types are usually present); and (5) polycystic ovary syndrome (see below).

Estrogen and progesterone excess often causes amenorrhea without other evidence of hypogonadism. Excess of both hormones may be due to the following: (1) Pregnancy. (2) Choriocarcinoma or teratoma. (3) Luteoma. (4) Malignant adrenal tumors (possibly). D&C is negative. Pregnanediol is found in the urine. Secretory endometrium is demonstrated on biopsy. The LH and FSH levels (actually chorionic gonadotropin) may be high and pregnancy tests positive. (5) Hyperhormonal effects with stromal luteinization may occur in postmenopausal women because of metastatic tumors in the ovaries (Krukenberg tumor) or as a result of ectopic production of chorionic gonadotropin by neoplasms.

Treatment depends upon the cause. Cyclic administration of progesterone, wedge resection of the ovary, or surgical removal of functioning tumors at times restores normal cyclic ovarian function. Recent reports of treatment of functional anovulation with human pituitary or urinary FSH, clomiphene, and LHRH (GnRH) are encouraging.

The prognosis is that of the underlying disease. Treatment with progesterone alone or with estrogen in cyclic fashion is usually quite effective in temporary disorders of ovulation. Stubborn anovulation may persist, however, after cessation of therapy.

Braunstein GD et al: Ectopic production of human chorionic gonadotropin by neoplasms. Ann Intern Med 1973;78:309.
Shane JM, Naftolin F: Aberrant hormone activity in tumors of gynecologic importance. Am J Obstet Gynecol 1975;121:131.

VIRILIZING DISORDERS OF THE OVARY
(See also under Adrenogenital Syndrome, p 735, and in Chapter 13.)

Polycystic Ovary Syndrome
This term is used to denote a heterogeneous group of disorders all characterized by bilateral polycystic ovaries but with variable incidence and degree of hirsutism, amenorrhea, and obesity. Patients may have only mild hirsutism or may present with signs and symptoms of virilization. Some women have normal menses; in others, anovulatory cycles and infertility are present. An occasional patient presents with primary amenorrhea. Conditions found to be associated with this syndrome include adrenal defects in the synthesis of cortisol, central nervous system lesions, thyroid diseases, and adrenal and ovarian tumors. In

most cases, however, no associated disorder is found, and the exact mechanism of the syndrome remains unclear.

The eponym **Stein-Leventhal syndrome** is usually reserved for patients who have amenorrhea, hirsutism, and obesity associated with polycystic ovaries without other associated endocrine disease.

Patients with polycystic ovary syndrome usually have normal or elevated estrogen levels; frequently show a tonic elevation of serum LH; and often have elevated levels of plasma testosterone. Gonadal steroid-binding globulin levels in plasma are decreased, so that the free (active) fraction of testosterone is elevated even if the level of total testosterone is normal.

Urinary 17-ketosteroids are usually normal or modestly elevated. FSH is normal or low. Administration of progesterone results in withdrawal bleeding. The hirsutism has been shown to be related to abnormal production of testosterone and related compounds by the ovaries and possibly also by the adrenals. Hereditary factors may be involved. Pelvic sonography is helpful in demonstrating bilateral enlargement of the ovaries. At operation, the enlarged ovaries are found to have many follicles on the surface and are surrounded by a thick capsule ("oyster ovaries").

Therapy must be individualized depending on the severity of the disorder, the presenting complaint, and any associated endocrine disease. Excess hair usually responds to oral contraceptive steroids. Glucocorticoid suppression (with small doses of dexamethasone at bedtime) is sometimes helpful. Combined adrenal and ovarian suppression has been reported to have additional beneficial effect. If children are desired, several procedures are available. Wedge resection often restores ovulatory periods and fertility, but hirsutism is not helped by this procedure unless large doses of estrogens are also used. Recently, ovulation followed by pregnancy has been produced by human pituitary or urinary FSH and also by clomiphene. There is danger of rapid enlargement of the ovaries due to cyst formation and rupture if the dosage is not carefully controlled. Multiple pregnancies may occur.

Diffuse Theca Luteinization

This disorder is similar to the Stein-Leventhal syndrome, but many follicles are not found in the ovaries. Hirsutism and often more marked virilization are associated with amenorrhea.

Excessive testosterone and androstenedione production has been demonstrated recently in ovarian slices removed surgically and also in blood and urine in these patients, which may explain the virilization.

There is a greater incidence of endometrial carcinoma in these patients, possibly related to continued estrogen stimulation.

Ovarian Tumors

Several ovarian tumors can produce significant hirsutism and virilization: hilar cell tumors, teratomas, luteomas, and (most frequently) **arrhenoblastoma.**

Arrhenoblastoma is associated with very high levels of serum testosterone. The 17-ketosteroids in urine are usually normal. Regional venous catheterization may be of great value in localization of the tumor before surgery.

Forbes AP: Endocrine function in hirsute women. (Editorial.) *N Engl J Med* 1976;**294**:665.

Goldzieher JW: Polycystic ovarian disease. *Fertil Steril* 1981; **35**:371.

Strickler RC, Warren JC: Hirsutism: Diagnosis and management. Page 311 in: *Year Book of Obstetrics & Gynecology.* Pitkin M (editor). Year Book, 1979.

Yen SCC: The polycystic ovary syndrome. *Clin Endocrinol* 1980;**12**:177.

DISORDERS OF PLURIGLANDULAR INVOLVEMENT

Involvement of multiple endocrine glands in the same patient is becoming recognized with increasing frequency. Many of these disorders are familial, although sporadic cases are also seen. The syndromes may consist of excessive hormone formation, usually due to the presence of hormone-secreting tumors, or they may consist of failure of multiple endocrine glands.

1. DISORDERS OF HORMONE EXCESS

Several familial syndromes with multiple gland involvement have been described in the last 3 decades. The most common one is multiple endocrine neoplasia (or adenomatosis) type I (MEN I or MEA I). In this condition, tumors of the pituitary gland, the parathyroid gland, and the pancreatic islets occur in the same patient, although not necessarily at the same time. The disorder is inherited as an autosomal dominant, but there is considerable phenotypic variability. Some individuals in the same family express the abnormality as children, whereas in others the clinical manifestations may not appear until late in adult life. The clinical manifestations of this syndrome are extremely variable, since the glandular tumors may secrete a variety of different hormones. The most common finding is hypercalcemia due to primary hyperparathyroidism. Either hyperplasia or adenoma of the parathyroid glands may be found. The clinical manifestations and laboratory findings are identical to those found in spontaneously occurring primary hyperparathyroidism. The pituitary gland tumors may secrete **prolactin** (galactorrhea-amenorrhea syndrome) or **growth hormone** (producing gigantism or acromegaly). The tumors of the pancreatic islets may produce **insulin,** giving all of the clinical manifestations found in a spontaneously occurring insulinoma, or **gastrin,** giving rise to gastric acid hypersecretion (Zollinger-Ellison syndrome). Elevation of serum gastrin (measured by radioimmunoassay) is characteristic of Zollinger-Ellison syndrome and is associated with in-

Table 19–14. Multiple endocrine gland hyperplasia or adenomatosis (MEA).*

	Tissue Affected	Clinical Presentation
Type I (MEA I)	Parathyroid	Adenoma or hyperplasia
	Pancreas	Adenoma (often multiple) of islet cells, gastrinoma
	Pituitary	Adenoma (acromegaly, prolactinoma)
	Adrenal	Adenoma (cortical)
	Miscellaneous	Lipomas, thyroid tumors (other than medullary carcinoma)
Type II or IIa (MEA II)	Thyroid	Medullary carcinoma or C cell hyperplasia
	Adrenal	Pheochromocytomas
	Parathyroid	Hyperplasia or adenoma
Type III or IIb (MEA III)	Thyroid	Medullary carcinoma or C cell hyperplasia
	Adrenal	Pheochromocytomas (adenoma or hyperplasia)
	Neural tissue	Ganglioneuromas
	Somatic manifestations	Marfanoid habitus, thick lips, "blubbery tongue," megacolon

*Modified after Deftos LJ: Calcitonin in clinical medicine. *Adv Intern Med* 1978;**23**:159.

creased hydrochloric acid secretion. Tumors of the pancreatic islets have also been described as secreting additional peptide hormones such as substance P, secretin, vasoactive intestinal peptide (VIP), glucagon, and others. The glucagon-producing tumors are associated with a typical skin rash (migratory necrolytic erythema) with diabetes mellitus, and with very low levels of amino acids in plasma.

A separate disorder of familial hypersecretion of hormones is the so-called multiple endocrine neoplasia type II (MEN II or MEA II) or Sipple's syndrome. In this syndrome, one finds pheochromocytomas (often bilateral) associated with medullary carcinoma of the thyroid, a tumor that originates in the C cells of the thyroid. These cells are the remnants of the ultimobranchial body found in lower species, and they secrete calcitonin. The baseline levels of calcitonin in blood are often markedly elevated and are helpful in the diagnosis of these tumors as well as in monitoring the response to therapy. In members of affected families, one can demonstrate the presence of small calcitonin-producing tumors by stimulatory tests such as calcium infusion or pentagastrin administration that result in markedly elevated levels of calcitonin. In patients with MEA II, one may also find hypercalcemia, which is often due to parathyroid hyperplasia.

A few families have been described with the so-called MEA type III syndrome, which consists of pheochromocytomas and medullary carcinomas of the thyroid associated with multiple mucosal neuromas and a peculiar phenotypic appearance: bumpy lips, enlarged tongue, visible corneal nerves, marfanlike habitus, muscular hypotonia, etc.

Although many theories have been proposed to explain the existence of these syndromes, none are consistent with the facts known at present (see references at end of next section).

2. DISORDERS OF MULTIPLE ENDOCRINE DEFICIENCIES

It has long been known that primary adrenal insufficiency and primary thyroid failure could occur simultaneously in the same patient for unclear reasons (Schmidt's syndrome). It has recently been demonstrated that many of these patients have an autoimmune disorder, with formation of antibodies against cellular fractions of many endocrine glands. In addition to adrenal and thyroid failure, patients with these syndromes may have failure of the gonads, of the parathyroids, of the pituitary gland, of the insulin-secreting cells of the pancreatic islets, etc. There is often an association with pernicious anemia and with vitiligo and nontropical sprue as well as other autoimmune disorders.

The basic mechanisms for the formation of autoantibodies are not clear at present. Although a familial tendency is often seen, many patients present with a sporadic disorder. An increased association of certain HLA antigens has been described in some of the afflicted individuals. No treatment other than hormone replacement is known at present.

Eisenbarth G et al: HLA type and occurrence of disease in familial polyglandular failure. *N Engl J Med* 1978;**298**:92.

Holst JJ: Gut endocrine tumour syndromes. *Clin Endocrinol Metab* 1979;**8**:413.

Leichter SB: Clinical and metabolic aspects of glucagonoma. *Medicine* 1980;**59**:100.

Pont A: Multiple endocrine neoplasia syndromes. *West J Med* 1980;**132**:301.

Schimke RN: Genetic aspects of multiple endocrine neoplasia. *Annu Rev Med* 1984;**35**:25.

HORMONES & HORMONELIKE AGENTS

ANTERIOR PITUITARY & HYPOTHALAMIC HORMONES

All of the anterior pituitary hormones are protein substances and must therefore be administered parenterally to be effective; if taken by mouth, they are digested by the digestive enzymes. In general, with the exception of growth hormone and prolactin, the anterior pituitary hormones have a regulatory function on other glands of internal secretion. The anterior pituitary in turn is regulated to a great extent by hypothalamic-pituitary humoral "releasing factors" as well as "release-inhibiting factors."

Several of these hormones have been prepared in pure or almost pure form: adrenocorticotropin (ACTH, corticotropin); growth hormone; prolactin; and follicle-stimulating (FSH), luteinizing (LH, interstitial cell-stimulating), and thyroid-stimulating (TSH) hormones. Other factors in the anterior pituitary have not yet been fully identified. Of the pure preparations, only corticotropin and thyrotropin are commercially available. The hypothalamic TSH-releasing factor, LHRH, and somatostatin (GH release-inhibiting factor) have been isolated and synthesized, but they are not generally available. Their use has been limited, for the most part, to diagnostic testing. Synthetic analogs, both agonists and antagonists, have been developed and tested clinically, but they are not available at present in the USA.

Corticotropin (ACTH)

Corticotropin is alleged to have remarkable effects in arresting many disease processes that are not satisfactorily influenced by other therapeutic agents. These claims are controversial. The effect of corticotropin is principally mediated by the stimulation of the adrenal cortex. Corticotropin is a protein of small molecular size, and certain peptides derived from it have been found to have similar and as marked physiologic effects as the hormone itself (cosyntropin, Synacthen).

A. Metabolic Effects in Humans: ACTH in adequate doses in normal human beings produces the following metabolic effects through stimulation of cortisol and other adrenal hormones: increased excretion of nitrogen, potassium, and phosphorus; retention of sodium and secondary retention of water; elevation of fasting blood glucose and diabetic glucose tolerance curve; increased urinary excretion of uric acid, calcium, 17-ketosteroids, and corticosteroids; fall of circulating eosinophils and lymphocytes; and elevation of polymorphonuclear neutrophils.

B. Clinical Effects, Uses, and Dosages: See p 754.

Growth Hormone (GH, STH, Somatotropin)

"Purified" GH has been employed in normal humans, pituitary dwarfs, and panhypopituitary individuals. Only the material prepared from human and possibly monkey pituitary glands has a growth-promoting effect in hypopituitary humans. Because the amount of these materials produced is very small, they are available for limited purposes only. The advent of recombinant DNA technology promises unlimited supplies of this and other peptide hormones. This synthetic material has now been used in clinical trials, but it is not yet generally available.

Prolactin

This hormone has not been employed extensively in human research. Its presence is necessary for the initiation and apparently for the continuation of lactation in breasts that have been prepared for lactation by estrogen and progesterone during pregnancy. There have been reports of a "growth hormone-like activity" in humans with the use of ovine prolactin.

Follicle-Stimulating Hormone (FSH)

FSH has different actions in male and female. In the female, FSH stimulates the development of ovarian follicles. Human pituitary FSH and FSH from the urine of menopausal women (Pergonal, hMG, menotropins), followed by chorionic gonadotropin, have been used in patients with amenorrhea to induce ovulation. Clomiphene citrate (Clomid), a synthetic analog of the nonsteroidal estrogen chlorotrianisene (TACE), has been less effective in inducing ovulation. FSH in the male stimulates the germinal epithelium of the testis to produce spermatozoa. It apparently has no effect on the Leydig cells and thus does not influence testosterone secretion.

Luteinizing Hormone
(LH; Interstitial Cell-Stimulating Hormone)

In the female, LH apparently has a dual action, ie, it stimulates the growth of theca lutein cells and transforms the mature follicles into corpora lutea. In the male, it stimulates the Leydig cells of the testis to secrete testosterone, and possibly also estrogen.

There is no good commercially available pituitary LH. hCG, which has a similar action, is used clinically.

Thyroid-Stimulating Hormone
(TSH, Thyrotropin, Thytropar)

TSH is exceedingly efficient in stimulating the thyroid gland. It has limited clinical usefulness at present; its principal uses have been to differentiate pituitary hypothyroidism from primary hypothyroidism or from low radioiodine uptake due to exogenous thyroid hormone or iodine. Availability of TSH measurements has rendered these tests obsolete. It has also been used in an attempt to "stimulate" metastatic thyroid cancer to take up radioiodine for therapeutic purposes.

Note: Allergic and, more rarely, anaphylactic reactions may occur and should be anticipated and promptly treated.

POSTERIOR PITUITARY HORMONES
(See Table 19–15.)

The posterior pituitary hormones, vasopressin and oxytocin, are polypeptides composed of 9 amino acids. Their exact chemical structures have been determined and they have been synthesized. Like the anterior pituitary hormones, they are effective only when administered parenterally, but they can also be absorbed through the nasal mucous membranes. They exert 3 actions: They (1) raise blood pressure (pressor action); (2) cause fluid retention without osmotically equivalent sodium retention (antidiuretic action); and (3) cause uterine contractions (oxytocic action).

Vasopressin has both antidiuretic and pressor actions. Oxytocin may likewise have some pressor effect.

Table 19–15. Posterior pituitary hormones: Preparations available.

Name	Action	Average Dose
Vasopressin tannate (Pitressin Tannate)	Antidiuretic; pressor	0.3–1 mL IM every 12–72 hours
Vasopressin injection (Pitressin)		0.25–0.5 mL IM every 3–4 hours
Posterior pituitary powder (snuff)		5–20 mg 3–4 times daily
Lypressin (Diapid, lysine-8 vasopressin nasal spray)	Antidiuretic (weak pressor)	1–2 sprays in each nostril 3–5 times daily
Desmopressin acetate (DDAVP)		0.1–0.4 mL daily as single dose or in 2–3 doses
Oxytocin injection (Pitocin), synthetic oxytocin (Syntocinon)	Oxytocic	1 mL dissolved in 1 L saline; give by *slow* continuous IV drip
Nasal spray (Pitocin)		1–2 sprays in each nostril every 4–6 hours

Clinical Indications

A. Vasopressin: Vasopressin is used primarily for the treatment of diabetes insipidus. Chlorpropamide potentiates the action of vasopressin and can be used in mild cases of diabetes insipidus.

B. Obstetric Use: Oxytocin is employed in obstetrics for induction of uterine contractions, and after delivery to facilitate expulsion of the placenta and control postpartum bleeding.

PITUITARYLIKE HORMONES ELABORATED BY THE PLACENTA

The most important of the pituitarylike hormones elaborated by the placenta is referred to as "chorionic gonadotropin" (hCG). Its physiologic action is almost identical with that of LH (see above). It is of little value by itself in inducing spermatogenesis or ovulation or maintaining a functional corpus luteum, but it may be effective for these purposes if preceded by pituitary or urinary FSH. Many of its alleged effects have been due to the presence of FSH, whose action may be potentiated by chorionic gonadotropin.

Clinical Indications

In the male, chorionic gonadotropin may induce descent of cryptorchid testes in some cases and is useful in some types of hypogonadism (although testosterone is generally preferred). In the female, chorionic gonadotropin may aid in inducing ovulation and maintaining corpus luteum in a few cases of sterility (if adequate FSH is present). Low daily doses of chorionic gonadotropin in the treatment of obesity have no rational basis except for a placebo effect.

Preparations Available

A. Chorionic gonadotropin, derived from the urine of pregnant women, is available commercially under a variety of trade names (eg, APL, Follutein).

B. Equine gonadotropins (eCG) are derived from the serum of pregnant mares. This preparation is a mixture of FSH and LH. It is not generally recommended, because of its marked sensitizing effect and because antihormones are produced by protracted use. Equine gonadotropins are no longer used to treat the clinical indications given above. eCG has been replaced by **menotropins** (see p 741).

Average Doses

The usual doses of hCG are 200–2000 units intramuscularly every day or every other day; 5000–10,000 units intramuscularly for several days may be needed to induce ovulation.

THYROID HORMONES

The active principles of the thyroid gland appear to be the iodine-containing amino acids, thyroxine (T4) and triiodothyronine (T3). Thyroid hormones act as a general cellular metabolic stimulant with resultant increased oxygen consumption (ie, increased metabolic rate). Their exact mode of action is not known.

Method of Administration

Thyroid hormone, either in the form of thyroglobulin (desiccated thyroid), T4, or T3, is effective when taken orally. There is a marked difference in rates of metabolic responses between T3 and thyroid or T4. In the case of T4, little effect is noted after a single dose for about 24 hours, and the maximal effect is not reached for several days. After the medication is stopped there is a slow loss of the effect, depending upon the initial T4 level and the level reached during thyroid medication. In general, at least 3–6 weeks must elapse after thyroid medication has been discontinued before one can be reasonably certain that the effects have been dissipated. In the case of T3, the peak effect is reached in 12–24 hours and the effect is over in about 6–14 days or less.

Clinical Indications

Thyroid hormone is indicated only in thyroid deficiency states. It is not indicated as a general metabolic stimulant. Patients with thyroid deficiencies rarely require over 0.2 g of desiccated thyroid daily. In patients with heart disease, coronary insufficiency or failure may be precipitated by even small amounts of thyroid.

Preparations & Dosages

A. Levothyroxine (T4, Synthroid, Levothroid,

Etc): The principal advantage of this compound over desiccated thyroid is its assured constant potency. Because it is about 600 times as potent as thyroid, small changes in dose may lead to toxic levels. Dosage must be appraised by clinical response and by periodic T_3 or T_4 determinations. Levothyroxine is metabolically transformed to T_3, and normal values of both hormones can be achieved during replacement therapy. The average dose is 0.1–0.2 mg daily. About 50% of ingested T_4 is absorbed. With a daily dose of 0.15 mg, the absorbed amount matches well the known daily production rate of T_4 by the thyroid gland (about 80 μg). One-tenth milligram is equivalent to 60 mg of desiccated thyroid. This compound is gradually replacing most other preparations for maintenance therapy.

Levothyroxine is also available for injection. Use a 10-mL vial containing 500 μg of lyophilized active substance with 10 mg of mannitol. Dilute with 5 mL of sodium chloride just prior to use. Synthroid is used intravenously in myxedema coma. The dosage is 200–400 μg intravenously on the first day and 100–200 μg intravenously on the second day.

B. Desiccated Thyroid USP: This is a good compound for thyroid replacement. The chief difficulty is that the official assay is for iodine content, which may or may not represent active thyroid hormone so that there may be variations in metabolic effect. Pure beef thyroid (Thyrar) is available. Thyroglobulin (Proloid) is more stable in hormonal content. Replacement therapy may be periodically appraised with T_4 and resin T_3 uptake determinations, but this may not be reliable because of variable iodine content, and adequacy of replacement must be assessed clinically. The dose is 90–150 mg daily.

C. Liothyronine Sodium (T_3, Cytomel): This preparation has a more rapid action and disappearance of effect than thyroid or thyroxine, and is 3–4 times as calorigenic as T_4. Its disadvantage is that the usual thyroid function tests (T_4, T_3 uptake) cannot be used to determine dosage when this drug is used in replacement therapy. The average maintenance dose of sodium liothyronine is 0.05–0.075 mg daily in divided doses.

D. Liotrix (Euthroid, Thyrolar): Liotrix, a 4:1 mixture of T_4 and T_3, is now available as replacement therapy in 4 potencies (Table 19–16). T_4 and T_3 uptake can be used to follow therapy. These preparations are not superior to levothyroxine.

PARATHYROID HORMONES

Parathyroid hormone is a protein substance derived from parathyroid glands. It is only effective when given parenterally.

Parathyroid hormone has a major effect on calcium and phosphorus and hence bone metabolism. Its effect is to cause increased renal excretion of phosphorus and direct decalcification of bone through stimulation of the osteoclasts, leading to mobilization of calcium and phosphorus from bone.

Because of the high cost and general unavailability of parathyroid hormone, 2 other preparations—dihydrotachysterol and vitamin D—are employed in its place. Both of these are sterols and are effective by mouth. Vitamin D, which is less expensive, is almost as effective as dihydrotachysterol, but its action is slower in onset and persists for prolonged periods of time.

Clinical Indications

Parathyroid hormone is rarely used in acute postsurgical hypoparathyroid tetany (after accidental removal of the parathyroid glands) and for special tests (see Ellsworth-Howard test, p 716).

Preparations Available for Treatment of Hypoparathyroidism (See also Table 19–9.)

A. Parathyroid Injection: The average dose is 50–100 units (0.5–1 mL) in aqueous solution 3–5 times daily intramuscularly as indicated.

A single injection of 200 units intravenously is used for the Ellsworth-Howard test.

B. Dihydrotachysterol (AT 10, Hytakerol, Dygratyl): For dosage, see p 716.

C. Calciferol (Vitamin D₂): This preparation has a potency of 40,000 units/mg. The dosage is 1–5 mg daily.

D. Calcitriol (Rocaltrol): 1,25-Dihydroxycholecalciferol is the most potent and rapidly acting vitamin D metabolite. It is available as 0.25- and 0.5-μg capsules for the treatment of hypocalcemia. The dosage is 0.25–1 μg daily.

E. Calcifediol (Calderol): 25-hydroxycholecalciferol is available as 20 μg and 50 μg capsules. The dosage is 50–100 μg daily.

Table 19–16. Equivalency of thyroid preparations.

Desiccated Thyroid	Approximate Equivalent In		
	Levothyroxine, Sodium (Levothroid, Synthroid, Etc)	Liothyronine Sodium (T_3, Cytomel)	Liotrix (Euthroid, Thyrolar)
30 mg	0.05 mg	12.5 μg	Code: ½
65 mg	0.1 mg	25 μg	1
130 mg	0.2 mg	50 μg	2
200 mg	0.3 mg	75 μg	3

CALCITONIN
(Thyrocalcitonin)

Calcitonin, a calcium-lowering hormone derived from special "C" cells of thyroid and parathyroid glands that decreases bone resorption, has been recently isolated and synthesized from several species. It is highly effective in active Paget's disease.

Synthetic salmon calcitonin is now available as Calcimar in 2-mL vials containing 400 Medical Research Council (MRC) units. The recommended dosage is 50–100 MRC units (0.25–0.5 mL) daily intramuscularly or subcutaneously. After treatment for 6–12 months, the dose may be reduced to 50 MRC units 3 times a week. (Prior skin sensitivity testing with a dilute solution is required.)

Synthetic human calcitonin is not yet available in the USA.

ADRENOCORTICAL HORMONES & THEIR ANTAGONISTS

The hormones of the adrenal cortex are all steroids. To date over 30 different steroids have been isolated and identified from animal adrenal glands or adrenal venous blood. Only a few of these have demonstrable metabolic effects. They can be grouped into (1) glucocorticoids, which are the most important pharmacologic agents; (2) mineralocorticoids; and (3) androgenic and estrogenic steroids.

Isolation of hormones from blood obtained by catheterization of adrenal veins shows that about 90% of the glucocorticoids of the adrenal cortex are cortisol and about 10% corticosterone. In general, the best demonstration of the effects of adrenocortical hormone or hormones is seen following corticotropin (ACTH) administration (see below).

Aldosterone, the principal mineralocorticoid has been isolated from adrenals. This hormone has primarily sodium- and water-retaining and potassium-losing effects. It is about 20 times as potent as desoxycorticosterone.

Clinical Effects & Indications

A. Desoxycorticosterone Acetate: The only significant metabolic effects of this hormone are sodium and water retention and increased urinary potassium excretion. In this respect it is about 20 times as potent as cortisone. It has little effect on carbohydrate or protein metabolism.

B. Cortisone Acetate: Cortisone is not an active glucocorticoid, but it is rapidly transformed by the liver to hydrocortisone (cortisol), the most active glucocorticoid produced by the human adrenal. The principal metabolic effects include retention of some sodium and water; increased excretion of nitrogen, potassium, and phosphorus; increased blood glucose and ability to maintain blood glucose levels during fasting in addisonian patients; and return of the electroencephalographic pattern to normal in addisonian

patients. One of the most important effects is the adrenocortical atrophy that results with prolonged use; this is due to endogenous ACTH inhibition and may interfere with the "normal" response of the pituitary-adrenal axis to stress. For clinical effects and use, see below.

C. Hydrocortisone: This compound is available for oral, intravenous, and local (eg, intra-articular) use. Its actions are similar to those of cortisone and its metabolic effects appear to be identical. It is somewhat more potent than cortisone on a weight basis. Hydrocortisone phosphate and hydrocortisone sodium succinate are also available for intravenous or intramuscular use.

D. Cortisone and Hydrocortisone Analogs: Many modifications have been made in the cortisone-hydrocortisone molecule to decrease side reactions in relationship to therapeutic effect. The only beneficial effects of these modifications have been to decrease the sodium-retaining and potassium-losing effects of the compounds. All of these preparations are more potent on a weight basis than are their parent compounds.

E. Fludrocortisone Acetate and Fluprednisolone: These potent anti-inflammatory drugs have been found useful in Addison's disease and also in dermatologic disorders. They have powerful sodium-retaining as well as glucocorticoid effects. Except in Addison's disease, they must be used locally only; and even with local use their absorption may cause excessive sodium retention.

CLINICAL USE OF CORTICOTROPIN (ACTH) & THE CORTICOSTEROIDS

Both pituitary adrenocorticotropin (ACTH), acting by adrenal stimulation, and the C-11-oxygenated adrenal steroids (corticosteroids) have been shown to have profound modifying effects on many pathologic processes, especially those associated with immunologic problems and inflammation. These effects cannot be entirely explained at present on the basis of the known metabolic and immunologic activities of these compounds.

These agents do not appear to "cure." Their action is primarily anti-inflammatory and appears to be related to multiple effects upon blood vessels, leukocytes, macrophages, fibroblasts, cell membrane permeability, etc, rather than to one discrete, all-encompassing effect. They suppress the inflammatory process but do not deal with the underlying cause of the disease process. When they are discontinued, the disease often recurs.

In general, these agents are interchangeable, and there is no support for the claim that a patient or a disease process may be responsive to one and not to another. Their duration of action varies. Both cause varying degrees of pituitary suppression, while the corticosteroids lead to adrenal atrophy after prolonged use as well. They should not be stopped suddenly, and during periods of stress (eg, surgery, trauma) additional amounts of rapidly acting steroids must be provided. Some patients become dependent on corticosteroids, and withdrawal is difficult.

Toxicity & Side Reactions

These agents are potentially dangerous, but with proper precautions most of these dangers can be avoided. (See below.) Corticosteroids are generally contraindicated during early pregnancy, except in the adrenogenital syndromes.

A. Hyperglycemia and glycosuria (diabetogenic effect) is of major significance in the early or potential diabetic.

B. Marked retention of sodium and water, with subsequent edema, increased blood volume, and hypertension, is minimized by the use of the newer agents.

C. Negative nitrogen and calcium balance may occur, with loss of body protein and consequent osteoporosis.

D. Potassium loss may lead to hypokalemic alkalosis.

E. Hirsutism and acne are cosmetic problems that may be of greater concern to females. Amenorrhea may occur.

F. Cushing's features or facies may develop with prolonged administration.

G. Peptic ulcer may be produced or aggravated.

H. Resistance to infectious agents is lowered.

Techniques Employed to Correct or Minimize Dangers

(1) Always reduce the dosage as soon as consistent with the clinical response. Intermittent alternate-day use may be a preferable and safer method of treatment. This method works well with prednisone or prednisolone but not with longer-acting drugs such as dexamethasone.

(2) During the first 2 weeks of therapy, blood pressure and weight should be carefully observed. Take an initial complete blood count and sedimentation rate and repeat as indicated. Determine the urine glucose; if reducing substances are found in the urine, determine fasting blood glucose. Serum potassium, CO_2, and chloride should be checked occasionally if large doses of these hormones are to be given over a period of more than several days. Measurement of plasma or urinary steroid levels is indicated if any question of lack of adrenal response to corticotropin arises.

(3) All patients should be on high-protein diets (100 g or more of protein daily) with adequate calcium intake.

(4) If edema develops, place the patient on a low-sodium diet (200–400 mg of sodium daily). Diuretics may be employed when strict sodium restriction is impossible.

(5) Potassium chloride, as 10% or 20% solution,

Table 19–17. Systemic versus topical activity of corticosteroids.
(Hydrocortisone = 1 in potency.)

	Systemic Activity	Topical Activity
Prednisolone	4–5	1–2
Fluprednisolone	8–10	10
Triamcinolone	5	1
Triamcinolone acetonide	5	40
Dexamethasone	30	10
Betamethasone	30	5–10
Betamethasone valerate		50–150
Methylprednisolone	5	5
Fluocinolone acetonide		40–100
Flurandrenolone acetonide		20–50
Fluorometholone	1–2	40

effervescent tablets, or powder, 3–15 g daily in divided doses, should be administered if prolonged use or high dosage is employed.

(6) In cases of long-continued administration, anabolic preparations may be used to counteract the negative protein, calcium, and potassium balance. Unfortunately, the distressing osteoporosis cannot be prevented.

(7) Do not stop either ACTH or corticosteroids abruptly, since sudden withdrawal may cause a severe "rebound" of the disease process or a malignant necrotizing vasculitis. Also remember that glucocorticoids cause atrophy of the adrenal cortex through endogenous ACTH inhibition; sudden withdrawal may lead to symptoms of adrenal insufficiency.

(8) When treating mild disorders, giving corticosteroids during the daytime only or on alternate days causes less suppression of endogenous ACTH. When discontinuing therapy, withdraw evening dose first.

Contraindications & Special Precautions

A. Stress in Patients Receiving Maintenance Corticosteroids: Patients receiving corticosteroids, especially the oral preparation (or even ACTH), must be carefully watched because suppression of endogenous ACTH interferes with the normal response to stressful situations (eg, surgery or infections). Patients should be warned of this danger, and should carry identification cards showing what drug they are taking, the dosage, and the reason for taking it. Whenever such a situation occurs or is about to occur, the dosage of cortisone or hydrocortisone should be increased or parenteral corticosteroids given (or both). If oral cortisone or hydrocortisone can be administered, it must be administered in larger doses at least every 6 hours.

B. Heart Disease: These agents should be used with caution in patients with cardiac disease or hypertension. Blood pressure may be increased by sodium retention or by increases in plasma renin substrate. The increase in extracellular fluid may lead to cardiac decompensation. Always begin with small doses and place the patient on a low-sodium diet.

C. Predisposition to Psychosis: These drugs cause a sense of well-being and euphoria in most persons, but in predisposed patients an acute psychotic reaction may occur. (Insomnia may be the presenting symptom.) In these cases the drug should be stopped or the dosage reduced, and the patient should be carefully observed and protected. Persons have committed suicide under the influence of these drugs.

D. Effect on Peptic Ulcer: Active peptic ulcer is a contraindication to the use of these drugs because of the danger of perforation or hemorrhage. These agents also tend to activate ulcers, and should be used only in emergency situations or with optimal antiulcer therapy in patients who have a history of peptic ulcer. Acute pancreatitis has been reported as well.

E. Tuberculosis: Active or recently healed tuberculosis is a contraindication to the use of these drugs unless intensive antituberculosis therapy is also carried out. A chest x-ray should be taken before and periodically during prolonged treatment with corticosteroids.

F. Infectious Diseases: Because these drugs tend to lower resistance and therefore to promote dissemination of infections, they must be used with caution, even when appropriate antibiotics are being given, in any acute or chronic infection.

G. Myopathy: A peculiar steroid myopathy has been reported, especially with the substituted steroids.

H. Fatty Liver: Fatty liver and fat embolism may occur.

I. Diagnostic Errors: Administration of these drugs may interfere with certain immune mechanisms that are of diagnostic value, eg, in skin tests and agglutination tests; they produce leukocytosis and lymphopenia, which may be confusing. The potent substituted corticosteroids (eg, dexamethasone) will suppress the urinary ketosteroids and hydroxycorticosteroid values. The signs and symptoms of infection may be masked by corticosteroid therapy. These drugs may also interfere with normal pain perception (eg, joint pain), which may lead to Charcot-like disintegration of the weight-bearing joints after local or systemic corticosteroid therapy.

J. Withdrawal of Corticosteroids: Prolonged use of these agents leads to combined pituitary-adrenal gland suppression that may last for as long as 1 year after stopping the drug. In the presence of infection, trauma, surgery, or other forms of stress, the patient may have signs of adrenal insufficiency unless given supplemental hydrocortisone.

Always withdraw corticosteroids *slowly* to minimize both flare-ups of the original disease and to prevent "steroid withdrawal reactions" (arthralgias, aches and pains, fatigue, nausea, fine desquamation of skin with a "chalky" appearance, etc).

ADRENAL MEDULLARY HORMONES & ANTAGONISTS OR BLOCKING AGENTS

The adrenal medulla contains 2 closely related hormones, epinephrine (about 80%) and norepinephrine (about 20%). They have different actions, as outlined below.

Since epinephrine may be synthetic or derived from natural sources (usually the latter) and thus contaminated with norepinephrine, the reason for some of the apparently paradoxic physiologic effects of the present preparation becomes clearer.

Epinephrine causes an immediate elevation of blood glucose by inducing glycogenolysis in liver and muscle.

Epinephrine
A. Clinical Uses: Epinephrine is used in a great many clinical disorders, including allergic conditions (eg, bronchial asthma, urticaria, angioneurotic edema); for control of superficial bleeding, especially from mucous membranes; with local anesthetics to slow down absorption; rarely, in cardiovascular disorders (eg, Stokes-Adams syndrome, cardiac arrest); and in tests of hepatic glycogen storage.

B. Preparations Available:
1. Epinephrine injection is usually administered subcutaneously but may be given intramuscularly and even intravenously if diluted in 1 L of solution. The dosage is 0.2–1 mL of 1:1000 solution as indicated.
2. Epinephrine inhalation, 1:100, for inhalation only.
3. Epinephrine in oil injection, 1:500, administered only intramuscularly. Usual dose: 0.2–1 mL.

Norepinephrine (Levarterenol)
A. Clinical Indications: Norepinephrine is used almost exclusively for its vasopressor effect in acute hypotensive states (surgical and nonsurgical shock, central vasomotor depression, and hemorrhage; see Chapter 1), and in the postoperative management of pheochromocytoma.

B. Preparations Available: Norepinephrine bitartrate (Levophed), 0.2% solution containing 1 mg free base/mL (1:1000) in ampules containing 4 mL.

C. Mode of Administration: Add 4–16 mL of norepinephrine (or occasionally more) to 1 L of any isotonic solution and give intravenously. Determine response and then maintain flow at a rate calculated to maintain blood pressure (usual rate, 0.5–1 mL/min). (*Note:* Norepinephrine is a very potent drug, and great care must be employed in its use. Do not allow the solution to infiltrate the tissues, since slough may result.)

Angiotensin Amide (Hypertensin)
This octapeptide apparently plays a role in normal blood pressure regulation. It is a potent vasopressor. It

may be of use in some cases that are refractory to norepinephrine.

Blocking Agents
   A. Alpha-Adrenergic Blocking Agents: These drugs reverse the vasoconstricting effects of epinephrine and norepinephrine.
   1. Phentolamine (Regitine)–Available in 5-mg ampules. Formerly used for diagnostic test for pheochromocytoma. Still useful in operative management of pheochromocytoma.
   2. Phenoxybenzamine (Dibenzyline)–Available in 10-mg capsules. A very useful drug for preoperative management of pheochromocytoma. Also used in the chronic treatment of inoperable or malignant pheochromocytoma. Usual dose is 20–100 mg daily.
   B. Beta-Adrenergic Blocking Agents: These drugs reverse the catecholamine-induced vasodilatation and cardiac acceleration. They have been used together with alpha-adrenergic blocking agents in the management of patients with pheochromocytoma and in thyrotoxicosis for the control of cardiac irregularities and thyroid storm.
   Propranolol, metoprolol, timolol, atenolol, nadolol, and pindolol are drugs of this class now marketed in the USA.
   C. Metabolic Blockers: A recently marketed drug, metyrosine (Demser), blocks the first step in catecholamine biosynthesis and is thus useful in decreasing the levels of circulating catecholamines. The dosage is 250 mg 4 times daily, with daily increments of 250–500 mg to a maximum of 4 g/d. Patients should continue to receive the optimal effective dose for at least 5–7 days before surgery.

GONADAL HORMONES

TESTOSTERONE
(Male Sex Hormone)

Of the many steroid hormones isolated from the testis, the most potent androgen is testosterone. It is believed, therefore, that testosterone is "the male sex hormone." Testosterone is responsible for the development of secondary sex characteristics in the male (ie, facial hair, deep voice, development of penis, prostate, and seminal vesicles). Administration of testosterone to the female causes development of male secondary sex characteristics. In the female, the adverse androgenic effects can only be partially overcome by the simultaneous administration of estrogens.

Also important is the protein anabolic (tissue building) effect of testosterone. Testosterone also has mild sodium-, chloride-, and water-retaining effects. It should be used with caution in children to prevent premature closure of the epiphyses.

Free testosterone and testosterone propionate are not effective when swallowed. The only way to administer these agents effectively is parenterally, by intramuscular injection or as implanted pellets. Testosterone preparations that do not occur naturally, eg, methyltestosterone, are effective orally.

Clinical Indications
   Testosterone may be indicated in debilitating disease, in osteoporosis, or in states of delayed growth and development (in both sexes) for its protein anabolic function. It may be of value in large doses in certain refractory anemias. In addition, there are certain uses specific to each sex.
   A. Males: Testosterone is used as replacement therapy in failure of endogenous testosterone secretion (eg, primary or secondary hypogonadism).
   B. Females: Testosterone has been used in women for functional uterine bleeding, endometriosis, dysmenorrhea, premenstrual tension, advanced breast carcinoma, chronic cystic mastitis, and suppression of lactation. There is disagreement about its use in many of these conditions. The virilizing effects limit the total amount that can be used. Even small doses may virilize a susceptible patient or her fetus, if she is pregnant.

Preparations & Dosages
   Many androgenic preparations are now available. Long-acting esters of testosterone (cypionate, enanthate) are preferred; they are injected intramuscularly. The usual dose for androgen replacement in adults is 300 mg every 3 weeks. The oral synthetic preparations (methyltestosterone, fluoxymesterone, etc) are less effective as virilizing agents and have the capacity for producing hepatic injury. Their toxicity ranges from asymptomatic elevation of liver enzymes to carcinoma of the liver in rare but well-documented cases. For these reasons, oral synthetic preparations are less desirable than the parenteral agents.
   Caution: Men receiving testosterone should be observed carefully for prostatic and breast cancer. The virilizing effect of testosterone in women and children may become permanent even after withdrawal of testosterone. Androgenic steroids are contraindicated in pregnant women or women who may become pregnant during the course of therapy, since this may virilize the fetus. These hormones alter serum lipids and could conceivably increase susceptibility to atherosclerotic disease.

Wilson JD, Griffin JE: The use and misuse of androgens. *Metabolism* 1980;**29:**1278.

ESTROGENS

Estrogens control proliferation of endometrium and growth of uterine muscle, changes in vaginal cells (cornification and lowering of vaginal pH below 4), and ductal proliferation of breasts. They decrease the rate of bone resorption and have a slight protein anabolic effect and a moderate calcium-, sodium-, and water-retaining effect. They may also have a choles-terol-lowering effect.

Clinical Indications

Estrogens are used in the treatment of osteoporosis. In women, estrogen is used as replacement therapy in cases of ovarian failure. In men, it is used as an adjunct in the treatment of carcinoma of the prostate.

Preparations & Dosages

Many substances have estrogenic activity, including some nonsteroids (eg, diethylstilbestrol, dienestrol, hexestrol). However, only some of the steroids are useful clinically. There is no evidence that any of the estrogens are less "toxic" than others. Toxicity (eg, nausea and vomiting) is usually due to overdosage. Most of the estrogens exert profound physiologic effects in very small doses, and their therapeutic and toxic dosages are quite similar. The physician should be familiar with the use of one or 2 preparations and resist the tendency to try out new ones.

There is little need at present to administer estrogens by any but the oral route; absorption in the gastrointestinal tract seems to be complete, and there is no evidence that nausea and vomiting can be minimized by parenteral administration. There is likewise no evidence that the "naturally occurring" estrogens are any more effective than the synthetic ones, although they may be better tolerated. *Caution:* Recent reports show the occurrence of adenocarcinoma of the vagina in young women whose mothers were treated with large doses of diethylstilbestrol early in pregnancy. Therefore, the administration of this drug should be avoided in pregnant women.

Estrogens play a role in mammary tumors of animals, and there is increasing evidence that they may cause breast or uterine cancer in humans; therefore, they must be used with care. It is advisable to perform periodic breast examinations and Papanicolaou smears in patients receiving prolonged estrogen therapy. *Cyclic* administration of the *lowest effective dose* is always preferable when estrogens must be given over long periods. Estrogens should be avoided in patients with known carcinoma of the uterus or breast and in patients with liver disease, hypertension, migraine, hyperlipidemia, or a history of thromboembolic disorder. Any unusual genital bleeding during estrogen administration must be reported and must be checked by means of a D&C.

A. Nonsteroidal Estrogens:

1. Diethylstilbestrol–A synthetic nonsteroid estrogen; an effective, inexpensive preparation, but no longer generally available. Give 0.5–1 mg daily orally.

2. Hexestrol, dienestrol, benzestrol, chlorotrianisene (TACE), methallenestril–These preparations have no advantage over diethylstilbestrol and are more expensive.

3. Diethylstilbestrol diphosphate–For treatment of prostatic carcinoma; well tolerated in large doses. Dosage is 1 tablet (50 mg) 3 times daily to 4 or more tablets 3 times daily, depending on tolerance.

B. Steroidal Estrogens for Oral Use:

1. Ethinyl estradiol–An excellent synthetic estrogen. The dosage is 0.02–0.05 mg daily orally.

2. Conjugated estrogenic substances (mostly estrone sulfate)–A "natural" estrogen that is well tolerated. The dosage is 0.3–2.5 mg daily orally.

3. Piperazine estrone sulfate–The dose is 1.5–5 mg/d.

4. 17β-Estradiol–This agent has recently been used more frequently in view of the adverse long-term side effects reported with the use of estrone preparations and diethylstilbestrol (see above). The dose is 0.5–2 mg/d.

C. Estrogens for Injection:

1. Estrone–Little used at present; the conjugated estrogens listed above are preferred. The dosage is 1 mg 2–3 times weekly or 1000 units daily intramuscularly.

2. Estradiol benzoate injection in oil–The dosage is 0.5–1 mg every other day intramuscularly.

3. Estradiol dipropionate injection–This preparation has a slightly longer duration of effect than estradiol benzoate. The dosage is 2–5 mg intramuscularly 1–2 times weekly.

4. Estradiol valerate in sesame oil–A long-acting estrogen. The dosage is 10–20 mg intramuscularly every 2–3 weeks.

5. Estradiol cypionate–1 and 5 mg/mL in oil. Long-acting. The dosage is 2–5 mg intramuscularly every 3–4 weeks.

6. Conjugated estrogenic substances (estrone sulfate)–2.5 mg daily intramuscularly. Premarin Intravenous (20 mg) is a rapid-acting preparation that is given to stop bleeding in menorrhagia.

7. Diethylstilbestrol diphosphate–A 5-mL ampule, containing 0.25 g, is used intravenously in prostatic carcinoma.

D. Estrogens for Topical Use:

1. Diethylstilbestrol vaginal suppositories, 0.1, 0.25, and 0.5 mg.

2. Dienestrol vaginal cream, 0.01%.

3. Premarin lotion, 1 mg/mL, and cream, 0.625 mg/g.

PROGESTINS
(Gestagens)

Up to the present time, progesterone has had a limited use in clinical medicine. Recently, a number of new compounds with progestational activity have been introduced. However, these new compounds also have other actions, which are summarized below.

Progesterone leads to the secretory phase of endometrium. In the absence of estrogens it does not have any significant effect on the uterus, ie, the uterus must be stimulated (proliferated) by estrogens before progesterone can act. Progesterone also causes acinar proliferation of breasts.

Clinical Indications

A. Menstrual Irregularities: Progesterone may be used with estrogens to maintain cyclic menstrual function in women who otherwise do not menstruate. In women with functional disorders who have adequate estrogen production but anovulatory cycles and irregular bleeding, regular menstrual cycles can be induced by the monthly administration of progestins (ie, medroxyprogesterone acetate, 10 mg daily for 5 days every month).

B. "Medical D&C": Progesterone is used to produce the so-called "medical dilatation and curettage," which is actually a test of adequacy of endogenous estrogen production, and it is a useful test in the workup of patients with secondary amenorrhea. If withdrawal bleeding does not occur, it may also indicate that the patient is pregnant. The test may be performed in one of 3 ways.

1. Give 100 mg of progesterone in oil intramuscularly. If menstrual bleeding occurs within 2–10 days, endogenous estrogen production is adequate.

2. Give 20 mg of norethindrone or 10 mg of medroxyprogesterone orally daily for 4–5 days. If menstrual bleeding occurs within 2–3 days, endogenous estrogen production is adequate.

3. Give 250–275 mg of hydroxyprogesterone caproate intramuscularly once. If menstrual bleeding occurs within 10–16 days, endogenous estrogen production is adequate.

C. Use as Contraceptive: Some of the newer agents are being used effectively as contraceptives; they act primarily by preventing ovulation. These drugs consist of progestational agents combined with various estrogens. They are usually given daily beginning on the fifth day after onset of menses and continued for 20 days; then resumed on the fifth day of the cycle, etc. If breakthrough bleeding occurs, the dose may have to be increased. A small dose of a synthetic progesterone (norethindrone) used continuously ("the mini-pill") has been recently introduced as a contraceptive pill. These agents are contraindicated in women with a history of thromboembolism, preexisting genital or breast cancer, liver disease, or cerebrovascular accident.

D. Endometriosis: In endometriosis, the progestins, at times combined with estrogens, are used in large doses. A derivative of ethisterone, danazol, which inhibits synthesis of sex steroids and also blocks their peripheral effects, has recently become the drug of choice for therapy of endometriosis.

E. Precocious Puberty: The progestins have been used recently in children with precocious puberty, but they must be used with caution.

Preparations & Dosages

A. Progesterone, 5–10 mg daily intramuscularly, or 100–200 mg daily orally or intramuscularly (for threatened or habitual abortion).

B. Hydroxyprogesterone caproate, 125–250 mg intramuscularly every 2 weeks.

C. Ethisterone, 60-100 mg daily orally.

D. Medroxyprogesterone, 10–30 mg/d orally, or 100 mg intramuscularly every 2 weeks (for endometriosis only).

E. Dydrogesterone is a synthetic progesterone that does not inhibit ovulation and is nonthermogenic. Give 10–20 mg daily in divided doses.

F. Norethindrone, 5–20 mg daily.

G. Norethindrone acetate, 2.5–10 mg daily.

H. dl-Norgestrel, 0.075 mg daily as antifertility drug.

I. Megestrol acetate, 20- and 40-mg tablets for the treatment of advanced endometrial and breast cancer. Dose: 160–320 mg/d in divided doses.

Side Effects of Progesterone & Progesterone Plus Estrogen Treatment

Prolonged progesterone plus estrogen therapy may cause abdominal distention, weight gain, nausea, acne, skin pigmentation, masculinization of a female fetus, and decidual casts ("pseudomalignant changes") of the endometrium. Some of these side effects may be prevented by lower dosage or sequential therapy (see above). There may be a significant increase in gallbladder disease. Prolonged amenorrhea may occur after stopping these drugs.

The following adverse reactions have been observed in varying incidence in patients receiving oral contraceptives:

Nausea
Vomiting
Gastrointestinal symptoms
Breakthrough bleeding
Spotting
Change in menstrual flow
Amenorrhea
Edema
Chloasma
Breast changes: tenderness, enlargement, secretion
Loss of scalp hair, hirsutism, and acne
Change in weight (increase or decrease)
Changes in cervical erosion and cervical secretions
Suppression of lactation when given immediately postpartum
Cholestatic jaundice
Gallbladder disease
Erythema multiforme
Erythema nodosum
Hemorrhagic eruption
Migraine
Rash (allergic)
Itching
Rise in blood pressure in susceptible individuals
Cerebral thrombosis and hemorrhage
Mental depression

Serious occurrences have been observed in users of oral contraceptives (a cause-and-effect relationship has not been established uniformly). Examination for early signs of these disorders is prudent:

Thrombophlebitis
Pulmonary embolism
Myocardial infarction and coronary thrombosis
Ischemic colitis
Neuro-ocular lesions
Carcinogenic potential, especially liver tumors
    with or without intra-abdominal bleeding

The following laboratory results may be altered
by the use of oral contraceptives:
    Bromsulphalein (BSP) retention and results of
        other hepatic function tests: increased
    Coagulation tests: increase in prothrombin, fac-
        tors VII, VIII, IX, and X
    Thyroid function: increase in PBI, BEI, and T_4,
        and decrease in T_3 resin uptake values
        (radioiodine uptake not affected)
    Metyrapone test
    Pregnanediol determinations

Glucose tolerance test
Blood lipids
Plasma cortisol (increase in cortisol-binding
    globulin)

At the present time it is best to advise the use of an
agent containing the lowest dose of estrogen that will
avoid breakthrough bleeding, to advise the patient to
have periodic health examinations, and to avoid continuous administration beyond 5 years and in the elderly patient.

Note: Janerich et al and Heinonen et al reported a
possible association of the use of synthetic sex steroids
with birth defects, which makes the safety of the use of
oral contraceptives as withdrawal-type pregnancy tests
doubtful, since adequate alternative methods are available. It is prudent to be certain of the absence of
pregnancy before starting a woman on oral contraceptives.

• • •

References

Bondy PK, Rosenberg LE (editors): *Metabolic Control and Dis-
    ease,* 8th ed. Saunders, 1980.

DeGroot LJ et al: *Endocrinology.* 3 vols. Grune & Stratton,
    1979.

Dillon RS: *Handbook of Endocrinology: Diagnosis and Man-
    agement of Endocrine and Metabolic Disorders,* 2nd ed. Lea
    & Febiger, 1980.

Felig P et al (editors): *Endocrinology and Metabolism.*
    McGraw-Hill, 1981.

Greenspan FS, Forsham PH (editors): *Basic & Clinical Endocri-
    nology.* Lange, 1983.

Heinonen OP et al: Cardiovascular birth defects and antenatal
    exposure to female sex hormones. *N Engl J Med* 1977;**296:**67.

Hershman JM: *Endocrine Pathophysiology: A Patient Oriented
    Approach,* 2nd ed. Lea & Febiger, 1982.

Mazzaferri EL: *Endocrinology: A Review of Clinical Endocri-
    nology,* 2nd ed. Medical Examination Publishing Co., 1980.

Ryan WG: *Endocrine Disorders,* 2nd ed. Year Book, 1980.

Smith R: *Biochemical Disorders of the Skeleton.* Butterworth,
    1979.

Speroff L et al: *Clinical Gynecologic Endocrinology and Infertil-
    ity,* 3rd ed. Williams & Wilkins, 1983.

Stanbury JB et al (editors): *The Metabolic Basis of Inherited
    Disease,* 5th ed. McGraw-Hill, 1983.

Tepperman J: *Metabolic & Endocrine Physiology,* 4th ed. Year
    Book, 1980.

Troen P, Nankin HR (editors): *The Testis in Normal and Infertile
    Men.* Raven Press, 1977.

Williams RH (editor): *Textbook of Endocrinology,* 6th ed. Saun-
    ders, 1981.

Yen SSC, Jaffe RB (editors): *Reproductive Endocrinology,*
    Saunders, 1978.

Diabetes Mellitus, Hypoglycemia, & Lipoprotein Disorders | 20

John H. Karam, MD

DIABETES MELLITUS

Classification & Pathogenesis

Clinical diabetes mellitus represents a syndrome with disordered metabolism and inappropriate hyperglycemia due to either an absolute deficiency of insulin secretion or a reduction in its biologic effectiveness or both. Because the etiologic mechanisms are poorly understood, a workshop of the National Institutes of Health convened in 1979 and decided to defer the formulation of a pathophysiologic classification of diabetes (based upon insulin secretion characteristics or insulin sensitivity). Instead, they suggested a "therapeutic" classification, which has been endorsed by the American Diabetes Association. It recommends classifying diabetes mellitus into 2 major types in which age of onset is no longer a criterion (Table 20–1).

A. Type I: Insulin-Dependent Diabetes Mellitus (IDDM): This severe form is associated with ketosis in the untreated state. It occurs most commonly in juveniles but occasionally in adults, especially the nonobese and those who are elderly when hyperglycemia first appears. It is a catabolic disorder in which circulating insulin is virtually absent, plasma glucagon is elevated, and the pancreatic B cells fail to respond to all insulinogenic stimuli. Exogenous insulin is therefore required to reverse the catabolic state, prevent ketosis, reduce the hyperglucagonemia, and bring the elevated blood glucose level down.

Certain HLA antigens—B8, B15, DR3, and DR4—are strongly associated with the development of type I diabetes, particularly in northern Europeans. A DR2 antigen is associated with a reduced incidence of disease. The genetic determinants of all of these antigens located on the sixth human chromosome adjacent to immune response genes show increased linkage to the genetic determinants of type I diabetes. Recently, a polymorphic region of DNA flanking the 5′ end of the insulin gene on chromosome 11 was shown to have an association with type I diabetes in a white population. In addition, circulating islet cell antibodies have been detected in as many as 85% of patients tested in the first few weeks of their diabetes.

Because of these immune characteristics, type I diabetes is felt to result from an infectious or toxic environmental insult to pancreatic B cells of genetically predisposed persons. Extrinsic factors that affect B cell function include damage caused by viruses such as mumps or coxsackie B4 virus, by toxic chemical agents, or by destructive cytotoxins and antibodies released from sensitized immunocytes. An underlying genetic defect on chromosome 6 relating to B cell replication or function may predispose to development of B cell failure after viral infection; alternatively, specific HLA genes may increase susceptibility to a diabetogenic virus or be linked to certain immune response genes that predispose patients to a destructive autoimmune response against their own islet cells (auto-aggression).

The rodenticide Vacor has been implicated in the development of type I diabetes associated with acute neurotoxicity in over 30 cases of attempted suicide. Its selective destruction of pancreatic B cells (sparing the

Table 20–1. Clinical classification of idiopathic diabetes mellitus syndromes.

Type	Ketosis	Islet Cell Antibodies	HLA Association	Treatment
(I) Insulin-dependent (IDDM)	Present	Present at onset	Positive	Insulin (mixtures of rapid- and intermediate-acting, at least twice daily) and diet
(II) Non–insulin-dependent (NIDDM) (a) Nonobese	Absent	Absent	Negative	(1) Eucaloric diet alone (2) Diet plus insulin or sulfonylureas
(b) Obese				(1) Weight reduction (2) Hypocaloric diet, plus sulfonylureas or insulin for symptomatic control only

A cells) results in severe insulinopenic diabetes associated with ketoacidosis and the development of islet cell antibodies in some but not all cases. These patients represent a unique human model of acquired type I diabetes whose study has important implications concerning the pathogenesis and long-term sequelae of diabetes mellitus.

B. Type II: Non-Insulin-Dependent Diabetes Mellitus (NIDDM): This represents a heterogeneous group comprising milder forms of diabetes that occur predominantly in adults but occasionally in juveniles. Circulating endogenous insulin is sufficient to prevent ketoacidosis but is often either subnormal or relatively inadequate in the face of increased needs due to tissue insensitivity. Type II diabetes is defined in essentially negative terms: It is a *non*ketotic form of diabetes that is *not* linked to HLA markers on the sixth chromosome; it has *no* islet cell antibodies; and it is *not* dependent on exogenous insulin therapy to sustain life, thereby being termed ''*non*-insulin-dependent diabetes mellitus'' (*N*IDDM). An element of tissue insensitivity to insulin has been noted in most NIDDM patients irrespective of weight. In this ''non-type I'' group of diabetes is a wide assortment of heterogeneous disorders that include several rare instances in which a defective insulin gene produces a biologically inadequate insulin; however, in most patients with this type of diabetes, the cause is presently undefined. Recent demonstration that the human insulin gene is present on chromosome 11 focuses attention on that chromosome as containing factors which determine proper insulin synthesis and might affect its storage and release.

Two subgroups of patients with type II diabetes are currently distinguished by the absence or presence of obesity:

1. Nonobese NIDDM patients–These patients generally show an absent or blunted early phase of insulin release in response to glucose; however, it may often be elicited in response to other insulinogenic stimuli such as acute intravenous administration of sulfonylureas, glucagon, or secretin. Among this heterogeneous subgroup may be certain unrecognized patients with a milder expression of type I diabetes who retain enough B cell function to avoid ketosis. Also included within this subgroup are those with diabetes characterized as ''maturity-onset diabetes of the young,'' or ''Mason type,'' whose strongly positive family history of a mild form of diabetes suggests an autosomal dominant transmission.

The hyperglycemia in this subgroup of patients often responds to oral hypoglycemic agents or, at times, to dietary therapy alone. Occasionally, insulin therapy is required to achieve satisfactory glycemic control even though it is not needed to prevent ketoacidosis.

An element of tissue insensitivity to insulin can be detected by sensitive investigative techniques in most NIDDM patients regardless of weight. However, this does not seem to be clinically relevant to the treatment of nonobese NIDDM patients, who generally respond

Table 20–2. Factors reducing response to insulin.

Prereceptor inhibitors: Anti-insulin antibodies

Receptor inhibitors:

Insulin receptor antibodies

''Down regulation'' of receptors by hyperinsulinism:

Primary hyperinsulinism (B cell adenoma)

Hyperinsulinism secondary to a postreceptor defect (obesity, Cushing's syndrome, acromegaly, pregnancy) or prolonged glycemia (diabetes mellitus, post-glucose tolerance test)

Postreceptor influences:

Poor responsiveness of principal target organs; obesity; hepatic disease; muscle inactivity

Hormonal excess: glucocorticoids, growth hormone, oral contraceptive agents, progesterone, human chorionic somatomammotropin, catecholamines, thyroxine

---

to appropriate therapeutic supplements of insulin in the absence of rare associated conditions such as lipoatrophy or acanthosis nigricans.

2. Obese NIDDM patients–This form of diabetes is secondary to extrapancreatic factors that produce insensitivity to endogenous insulin. It is characterized by nonketotic mild diabetes, mainly in adults but occasionally also in children. The primary problem is a ''target organ'' disorder resulting in ineffective insulin action (Table 20–2) that can secondarily influence pancreatic B cell function. Hyperplasia of pancreatic B cells is often present and probably accounts for the fasting hyperinsulinism and exaggerated insulin responses to glucose and other stimuli seen in the milder forms of this disorder. In more severe cases, secondary (but potentially reversible) failure of B cell secretion may result after exposure to prolonged fasting hyperglycemia. Obesity is common in this type of diabetes as a result of excessive caloric intake, perhaps facilitated by hunger resulting from mild postprandial hypoglycemia after excess insulin release. In obese patients, insulin insensitivity is positively correlated with the presence of distended adipocytes, but liver and muscle cells also resist the deposition of additional glycogen and triglycerides in their storage depots.

Two major mechanisms have been proposed to account for the observed tissue insensitivity to insulin in obesity: Chronic overfeeding may lead to either (1) sustained B cell stimulation and hyperinsulinism, which in itself induces receptor insensitivity to insulin; or (2) a postreceptor defect associated with overdistended storage depots and a reduced ability to clear nutrients from the circulation. Consequent hyperinsulinism induces receptor insensitivity to insulin.

Regardless of the mechanism, a reduction in overfeeding can interrupt the cycle. In the first case, restricted diet would reduce islet stimulation of insulin release, thereby restoring insulin receptor sites and improving tissue sensitivity to insulin, whereas in the second situation normal tissue sensitivity returns as storage depots become less saturated.

Not enough data exist at present to determine whether obese diabetics have a primary genetic defect of B cell secretion in addition to their peripheral tissue insensitivity to insulin. Careful characterization of insulin release in obese diabetics who have achieved normal weight, will be essential for resolution of this question. Genetic studies of obese diabetics from various racial groups (Nauru Islanders, Pima Indians, American blacks, and whites) have failed to demonstrate the linkage equilibrium to the polymorphic locus flanking the insulin gene on chromosome 11 that is associated with type I diabetes.

In addition to obesity, chronic muscle inactivity or disease and liver disease have been associated with carbohydrate intolerance and hyperinsulinism in response to glucose.

Other secondary causes of carbohydrate intolerance include endocrine disorders—often specific endocrine tumors—associated with excess production of growth hormone, glucocorticoids, catecholamines, or glucagon. In all 4 situations, peripheral responsiveness to insulin is impaired. With excess of glucocorticoids, catecholamines, or glucagon, increased hepatic output of glucose is a contributory factor; in the case of catecholamines, decreased insulin release is an additional factor in producing carbohydrate intolerance.

A rare syndrome of extreme insulin resistance associated with acanthosis nigricans is divided into 2 groups on the basis of clinical and laboratory manifestations: Group A consists of younger women with androgenic features (hirsutism, amenorrhea, polycystic ovaries) in whom insulin receptors are deficient in number. Group B consists of older people, mostly women, in whom immunologic disease is suspected (high erythrocyte sedimentation rate, anti-DNA antibodies, and a circulating immunoglobulin that binds to insulin receptors, reducing their affinity to insulin).

Epidemiologic Considerations

The above comments emphasize the heterogeneity of the disorder termed diabetes mellitus, especially in the "adult-onset" diabetic. Attempts to define diabetes on the basis of abnormal carbohydrate tolerance alone contributed to much of the confusion and controversy regarding its prevalence, genetic transmission, relationship of complications to control, and recommended therapeutic approaches.

An estimated 5.5 million people in the USA are known to have diabetes, of which 440,000 have the insulin-dependent type.

Use of the current "therapeutic" classification has been widely accepted throughout the world, but its deficiencies are apparent in many individual cases. For example, a 22-year-old nonobese woman whose mild diabetes is presently responding adequately to diet alone and who shows a low normal C-peptide response to stimuli had presented with severe diabetes with ketosis and required insulin for several weeks following diagnosis. In addition, she has an associated autoimmune disorder, myasthenia gravis. From an etiologic standpoint, she has type I diabetes, but her present clinical status is "non-insulin dependent." The National Diabetes Data Group is reviewing the

Table 20–3. Clinical features of diabetes.

	Diabetes Type I (IDDM)	Diabetes Type II (NIDDM)
Polyuria and thirst	++	+
Weakness or fatigue	++	+
Polyphagia with weight loss	++	–
Recurrent blurred vision	+	++
Vulvovaginitis or pruritus	+	++
Peripheral neuropathy	+	++
Nocturnal enuresis	++	--
Often asymptomatic	–	++

present classification system so that such cases may be incorporated. Information about the epidemiology of mild adult-onset diabetes was a major contribution of the University Group Diabetes Program (UGDP). This study revealed that the vast majority of persons with mild adult-onset diabetes were obese and thus may well have represented a type of diabetes in which tissue insensitivity to insulin was a fundamental pathologic feature.

Clinical Findings

Regardless of whether the primary defect is an absolute or relative lack of insulin, features of insulin deficiency may arise. In type I, increased catabolism and ketosis occur.

A. Symptoms: (See Table 20–3.) The classic symptoms of polyuria, thirst, recurrent blurred vision, paresthesias, and fatigue are manifestations of hyperglycemia and thus are common to both major types of diabetes. Nocturnal enuresis may signal the onset of diabetes in children; likewise, pruritus vulvae and vaginitis are frequent initial complaints of adult females with hyperglycemia and glycosuria due to either absolute or relative deficiencies of insulin. Weight loss despite normal or increased appetite is a feature of IDDM, whereas weight loss is unusual in obese patients with NIDDM who have normal or increased levels of circulating insulin. These latter patients with the insulin-insensitive type of diabetes may be relatively asymptomatic and may be detected only after glycosuria or hyperglycemia is noted during a routine examination. Diabetes should be suspected in obese patients, in those with a positive family history of diabetes, in patients presenting with peripheral neuropathy, and in women who have delivered large babies or had polyhydramnios, preeclampsia, or unexplained fetal losses.

B. Physical Signs:

1. Acute diabetes syndrome–The IDDM patient presenting with advanced insulin deficiency shows apparent weight loss from a combination of dehydration, loss of subcutaneous fat, and muscle wasting.

The patient with NIDDM is most often obese and, except for vaginitis in females, may have no characteristic physical abnormalities related to diabetes.

However, evidence of neuropathy, which is not an uncommon late complication of diabetes, may be apparent early in the disease.

2. Chronic diabetes syndrome–

a. Ocular signs–Premature cataracts and refractive changes occur in the lens. Retinopathy may be of the "background" variety, consisting of microaneurysms, intraretinal hemorrhages, and hard exudates; or of the "proliferative" type, which includes also the formation of new capillaries and duplication of small veins. Complications of proliferative retinopathy include preretinal or vitreous hemorrhage and fibrosis, which can result in retinal detachment and blindness.

b. Cardiovascular signs–Occlusive vascular disease of the lower extremities is a combination of microangiopathy and atherosclerosis of large and medium-sized arteries. It occurs more commonly after age 40, and diabetics have 20 times the incidence of gangrene of the feet as nondiabetics. If both feet feel cool, a good blood supply might still be present; but if one is cooler than the other, occlusive arterial disease is usually present in the cooler one.

Hypertension develops with progressive renal involvement, and the process of coronary and cerebral atherosclerosis with all of the sequelae of those disorders seems to be accelerated in diabetics.

c. Neurologic signs–The general features of peripheral neuropathy are present, usually predominantly sensory in type, with dulled perception of vibration, pain, and temperature, particularly in the lower extremities. However, bilateral atrophy of the first interosseous muscles of the hand is characteristic of diabetic neuropathy. The ankle jerk is often absent, but the knee jerk may be retained. Both motor and sensory nerve conduction are delayed in peripheral nerves. Autonomic neuropathy includes evidence of postural hypotension, resting tachycardia, decreased cardiovascular responses to Valsalva's maneuver, alternating bouts of diarrhea (particularly nocturnal) and constipation, inability to empty the bladder, and impotence. Impotence due to neuropathy differs from the psychogenic variety in that the latter may be intermittent (erections occur under special circumstances), whereas diabetic impotence is usually persistent.

d. Skin and mucous membrane signs–Chronic pyogenic infections of the skin may occur, especially in poorly controlled diabetic patients. Likewise, eruptive xanthomas can develop in long-standing uncontrolled cases. An unusual lesion termed "necrobiosis lipoidica diabeticorum" occurs more commonly in females and is usually located over the anterior surfaces of the legs or the dorsal surfaces of the ankles.

"Shin spots" are not uncommon in adult diabetics. They are brownish, rounded, painless atrophic lesions of skin in the pretibial area, found in males more commonly than in females. Candidal infection can produce erythema and edema of intertriginous areas below the breasts, in the axillas, and between the fingers. It causes vulvovaginitis in most chronically uncontrolled diabetic females and is a frequent cause of pruritus.

C. Laboratory Findings: These involve tests of glucose and ketone bodies in the urine as well as glucose levels in plasma under basal conditions and after glucose administration. In certain circumstances, measurement of circulating levels of insulin as well as other hormones involved in carbohydrate homeostasis, such as glucagon or growth hormone, may be useful. In view of the serious consequences of atherosclerosis in diabetics, estimates of serum cholesterol and triglycerides are helpful both in evaluating and in controlling the disease.

1. Urinalysis–

a. Glycosuria–The Clinitest tablet placed in 5 drops of urine with 10 drops of water provides a rapid, easy, and semiquantitative estimate of the degree of glycosuria. A glucose level of 0.25% in the urine is required to show a trace reaction (green), and colors progress from yellow through orange until a brick-red color indicates a glucose concentration of 2% or more.

A more specific and convenient method is the paper strip impregnated with glucose oxidase and a chromogen system (Clinistix, Diastix, TesTape), which is sensitive to as little as 0.1% glucose in urine. Diastix can be directly applied to the urinary stream, and differing color responses of the indicator strip reflect glucose concentration. This is sufficiently accurate in most patients to eliminate the need for the more cumbersome Clinitest tablets.

Certain common therapeutic agents interfere with both of these methods. When taken in large doses, ascorbic acid, salicylates, methyldopa (Aldomet), and levodopa (Dopar, etc) can give false-positive Clinitest measurements, as can the presence of alkaptonuria; they give false-negative results when glucose oxidase paper strips are used, since these powerful reducing agents interfere with the color reaction and thus prevent accurate estimation of glucose in the urine of diabetics. Both of these methods are dependent upon a normal renal threshold for glucose as well as reliable bladder emptying for proper interpretation.

b. Ketonuria–Qualitative detection of ketone bodies can be accomplished by nitroprusside tests (Acetest or Ketostix). Although these do not detect the β-hydroxybutyric acid, which lacks a ketone group, the semiquantitative estimation of ketonuria thus obtained is usually adequate for clinical purposes.

2. Blood testing procedures–

a. Glucose tolerance test–

(1) Methodology and normal fasting glucose–Plasma or serum from venous blood samples may be used and has the advantage over whole blood of providing values for glucose which are independent of hematocrit and which reflect the glucose concentration to which body tissues are exposed. For these reasons, and because plasma and serum are more readily measured on automated equipment, they are rapidly replacing the whole blood glucose determinations used heretofore. Fluoride anticoagulant in the collecting tube prevents enzymatic glycolysis by blood corpuscles. If serum is used, samples should be refrigerated and separated from corpuscles within an hour after collection. Glucose oxidase and *o*-tolidine methods are most reliable, with normal plasma values ranging from 70 to 105 mg/dL; serum or plasma methods dependent on reduction of copper or iron give slightly higher values (up to 110 mg/dL).

(2) Criteria for laboratory confirmation of diabetes mellitus–If the fasting plasma glucose is over 140 mg/dL on more than one occasion, further evaluation of the patient with a glucose challenge is unnecessary. However, when fasting plasma glucose is less than 140 mg/dL in suspected cases, a standardized oral glucose tolerance test may be done. The National Diabetes Data Group recommends giving a 75-g glucose dose dissolved in 300 mL of water for adults (1.75 g per kg ideal body weight for children) after an overnight fast in subjects who have been receiving at least 150–200 g of carbohydrate daily for 3 days before the test.

Normal glucose tolerance is considered to be present when the 2-hour plasma glucose is less than 140 mg/dL, with no value between zero time and 2 hours exceeding 200 mg/dL. However, a diagnosis of diabetes mellitus requires plasma glucose levels to be above 200 mg/dL both at 2 hours and at least one other time between zero time and 2 hours. Values above the normal standard that do not meet the criteria for diabetes are considered nondiagnostic. For proper evaluation of the test, the subjects should be normally active and free from acute illness. Medications that may impair glucose tolerance include diuretics, contraceptive drugs, glucocorticoids, nicotinic acid, and phenytoin.

Because of difficulties in interpreting oral glucose tolerance tests and the lack of standards related to aging, they are generally being replaced by documentation of fasting hyperglycemia as a means of diagnosing diabetes mellitus.

(3) Insulin levels during glucose tolerance test–Serum or plasma is separated within 30 minutes after collection and frozen. Normal immunoreactive insulin levels range from less than 10 to 25 μU/mL in the fasting state and 50–130 μU/mL at 1 hour and usually return to levels below 100 μU/mL by 2 hours. Insulin levels during glucose tolerance testing are seldom useful clinically in distinguishing subclasses of NIDDM. When fasting plasma glucose exceeds 120 mg/dL, pancreatic B cells generally do not respond well to added glucose in the face of chronic hyperglycemia regardless of whether the glycemia results from insulin resistance predominantly or from sluggish early insulin release in cases of primary pancreatic B cell dysfunction. Also, when fasting hyperglycemia is milder (110–120 mg/dL), a *late* hyperinsulinism may be present as a consequence of persistent hyperglycemic stimulation of pancreatic B cells regardless of whether the late hyperglycemia results from primary insulin resistance (eg, obesity) or from sluggish early insulin release to a glucose load (eg, nonobese subjects with B cell dysfunction).

b. Glycosylated hemoglobin (hemoglobin A₁) measurements–Glycosylated hemoglobin has re-

cently been discovered to be abnormally high in diabetics with chronic hyperglycemia and to reflect their metabolic control. The major form of glycohemoglobin is termed hemoglobin A_{1c}, which normally comprises only 4–6% of the total hemoglobin. It is produced by a reaction between glucose and the N-terminal amino acid of both β chains of the hemoglobin molecule. The remaining glycohemoglobins (2–4% of the total) consist of phosphorylated glucose or fructose and are termed hemoglobin A_{1a} and hemoglobin A_{1b}. Because separate measurement of hemoglobin A_{1c} is at present technically difficult and appears to offer no special advantage in clinical practice, most laboratories measure the sum of these 3 glycohemoglobins and report it as hemoglobin A_1.

Since glycohemoglobins have a long half-life, they generally reflect the state of glycemia over the preceding 8 weeks, thereby providing an improved method of assessing diabetic control.

Occasionally, fluctuations in hemoglobin A_1 are due to an acutely generated, reversible, intermediary (aldamine-linked) product that can falsely elevate glycohemoglobins when measured with "short-cut" chromatographic methods. This can be eliminated by using more intricate methods or by dialysis of the hemolysate before chromatography. When hemoglobin variants are present, such as negatively charged hemoglobin F, acetylated hemoglobin from high-dose aspirin therapy, or carbamylated hemoglobin produced by the complexing of urea with hemoglobin in uremia, falsely *high* "hemoglobin A_1" values are obtained with commonly used chromatographic methods. In the presence of positively charged hemoglobin variants such as hemoglobin S or C, or when the life span of red blood cells is reduced by increased hemolysis or hemorrhage, falsely *low* values for "hemoglobin A_1" result.

c. Self glucose monitoring–Capillary blood glucose measurements performed by patients themselves, as outpatients, are extremely useful, particularly in IDDM patients in whom "tight" metabolic control is attempted. A portable battery-operated Glucometer (Ames Co.) or Glucoscan (Lifescan, Inc.) provides a digital readout of the intensity of color developed when glucose oxidase paper strips (Dextrostix) are exposed to a drop of capillary blood for 60 seconds. Similar diagnostic strips made by Ames Co. (Visidex) or by Biodynamics Corp. (Chemstrip-bG) have 2 chromogen indicators that permit *visual* estimation of the glucose concentration when compared to a series of color standards. The Chemstrip-bG can be read by a reflectance meter (Accu-chek). In self-monitoring of blood glucose, patients must prick their finger with a small lancet (Monolet, Ames Co.), which can be facilitated by a small plastic trigger device such as an Autolet (Ames Co.), Autoclix (Bio-Dynamics), or Penlet (Lifescan, Inc.).

3. Capillary morphometry (biopsy of the quadriceps muscle)–The basement membrane of capillaries from skeletal muscle tissue of the quadriceps area is abnormally thickened in cases of overt spontaneous diabetes in adults with fasting hyperglycemia of 140 mg/dL or more. Capillary morphometry appears to be less useful in diabetic children, being normal in as many as 60% of those below age 18. Controversy persists about whether basement membrane thickening in diabetics is a consequence of hyperglycemia or is genetically determined, either directly or as an inherited susceptibility to glucotoxicity.

Differential Diagnosis

A. Melituria: Although melituria reflects hyperglycemia in over 90% of patients, 2 major classes of nondiabetic melituria must be considered.

1. Nondiabetic glycosuria (renal glycosuria)–This is a benign, asymptomatic condition wherein glucose appears in the urine despite a normal amount of glucose in the blood, either basally or during a glucose tolerance test. Its cause may vary from an autosomally transmitted genetic disorder to one associated with dysfunction of the proximal renal tubule (Fanconi's syndrome, chronic renal failure), or it may merely be a consequence of the increased load of glucose presented to the tubules by the elevated glomerular filtration rate during pregnancy. As many as 50% of pregnant women normally have demonstrable sugar in the urine, especially during the third and fourth months. This sugar is practically always glucose except during the late weeks of pregnancy, when lactose may be present.

2. Melituria other than glycosuria–Occasionally, a sugar other than glucose is excreted in the urine. The most common of these meliturias is the lactosuria of the late stages of pregnancy and during postpartal lactation; much rarer are other conditions due to inborn errors of metabolism wherein fructose, galactose, or a pentose (L-xylulose) may be excreted in the urine. Testing the urine with paper strips impregnated with glucose oxidase will help differentiate true glycosuria from other meliturias.

B. Hyperglycemia: When hyperglycemia is demonstrated, the diabetic syndrome is present. Causes of hyperglycemia associated with end organ insensitivity to insulin include obesity, acromegaly, Cushing's syndrome, liver disease, muscle disorders (myotonic dystrophy), glucagonoma, lipoatrophy, hemochromatosis, and thyrotoxicosis. Pheochromocytoma can induce hyperglycemia by a variety of mechanisms, including end organ resistance, inhibition of insulin release, and hypersecretion of glucagon. Chronic pancreatitis reduces the number of functioning B cells and can result in a metabolic derangement very similar to that of genetic diabetes mellitus except that a concomitant reduction in pancreatic A cells may reduce glucagon secretion despite insulin deficiency, which often raises glucagon levels. Insulin-dependent diabetes is occasionally associated with Addison's disease and chronic thyroiditis (Schmidt's syndrome). This occurs particularly in females and probably represents an autoimmune disorder in which there are circulating antibodies to adrenocortical and thyroid tissue, thyroglobulin, and gastric parietal cells.

Treatment

A. Principles of Treatment of Diabetes: Rational therapy of diabetes requires the application of principles derived from current knowledge concerning (1) the nature of the disease and (2) the mechanism of action and the efficacy and safety of available treatment regimens (diet, oral hypoglycemic drugs, and insulin). Unfortunately, current knowledge about these matters is not always accurate or complete, and controversy exists about what constitutes the best therapeutic regimen. Fundamental to this controversy is the conflicting evidence about whether microangiopathy is related to the existence and duration of hyperglycemia or whether it reflects a separate, coexisting genetic disorder. Unfortunately, present methods of administering available insulin preparations are generally inadequate to effectively achieve control of blood glucose concentrations within normal limits in order to settle this question. In an attempt to ascertain whether microangiopathy relates to the degree of metabolic derangement in IDDM, the NIH has initiated a multicenter trial incorporating insulin infusion devices and home glucose monitoring. This study will determine whether acceptable control of hyperglycemia in diabetics can be safely and effectively maintained for 7–10 years and whether this prevents vascular complications in these patients. Until this conflict is resolved, the therapeutic objective recently endorsed by the Executive Committee of the American Diabetes Association is to attempt to restore known metabolic derangements to normal in the hope that this approach will impede if not prevent the progression of microvascular disease.

The general principles of therapy emphasized in this chapter will be based on the classification of diabetes outlined in Table 20–1.

Diet will be prescribed individually to meet the needs of each type: caloric restriction for obese patients and regular spaced feedings with a bedtime snack for patients receiving hypoglycemic agents, especially insulin.

Exercise will also be encouraged as an adjunct to diet and insulin replacement in reducing hyperglycemia in the insulinopenic diabetic and to help achieve weight reduction in the insulin-insensitive obese diabetic.

Treatment of the insulinopenic diabetic will be directed toward normalization of the endocrine and metabolic abnormalities. In more severe cases, exogenous insulin replacement will be required, whereas in milder degrees of insulinopenia an attempt to restore endogenous insulin release with sulfonylureas will have the advantage of causing insulin to be released intraportally and will not introduce the immunogenic foreign protein of animal insulin. Potential disadvantages of sulfonylurea therapy will be discussed in the section on safety of oral hypoglycemic agents.

Treatment of insulin-insensitive diabetes will be directed at the cause of tissue resistance, eg, weight reduction in cases of obesity and reduction of endocrine hypersecretion in cases of acromegaly or Cushing's syndrome.

B. Treatment Regimens:

1. Diet–A well-balanced, nutritious diet remains a fundamental element of therapy. However, in more than half of cases, diabetic patients fail to follow their diet. The reasons for this are varied and include unnecessary complexity of the prescription as well as lack of understanding of the goals by both the patient and the physician. In prescribing a diet, it is important to relate dietary objectives to the type of diabetes. In obese patients with mild hyperglycemia, the major goal of diet therapy is weight reduction by caloric restriction. Thus, there is less need for exchange lists, emphasis on timing of meals, or periodic snacks, all of which are so essential in the treatment of insulin-requiring nonobese diabetics.

Because of the prevalence of obese patients with mild diabetes among the population of diabetics receiving therapy, this type of patient represents the most frequent and thus one of the most important challenges for the physician. Treatment requires an energetic, vigorous program directed by persons who are aware of the mechanisms by which weight reduction is known to effectively lower hyperglycemia and who are convinced of the profoundly beneficial effects of weight control on blood lipid levels as well as on hyperglycemia in obese diabetics. Weight reduction is an elusive goal that can only be achieved by close supervision of the obese patient.

a. ADA diet–Exchange lists for meal planning can be obtained from the American Diabetes Association and its affiliate associations or from the American Dietetic Association, 430 North Michigan Avenue, Chicago 60611. The ADA diet stresses the major goal of caloric restriction as a means of achieving or maintaining ideal weight. A prudent diet is recommended, which includes restriction of fat intake to 35% or less of the total calories and suggests that saturated fat be reduced to only one-third of this by substituting poultry, veal, and fish for red meats as a major protein source. At the same time, cholesterol is restricted to less than 300 mg daily. Carbohydrates may be consumed liberally (as much as 50–60% of total calories) as long as refined and simple sugars are avoided as snacks. A recent study (Bantle et al) contends that dietary sucrose need not aggravate postprandial hyperglycemia in diabetic patients if consumed as part of a mixed meal and in exchange for other carbohydrate components of the meal. Unrefined carbohydrates with a fiber content sufficient to provide 15–20 g of fiber daily are recommended for both type I and type II diabetic patients.

b. Dietary fiber–Plant components such as cellulose, gum, and pectin are indigestible by humans and are termed dietary "fiber." It has been clearly demonstrated that when fiber accompanies ingested carbohydrates, glucose absorption is slower and hyperglycemia is diminished. Although the ADA diet does not include fiber supplements such as added bran, it recommends foods such as grain cereals and beans with relatively high fiber content as staple components of the diet in diabetics.

c. Artificial sweeteners–The nonnutritive sweetener saccharin continues to be available in certain foods and beverages despite recent warnings by the FDA about its potential long-term carcinogenicity to the bladder. In March 1979, after an appraisal of all relevant scientific data, a committee of the National Academy of Sciences recommended a restriction on the use of saccharin in children and pregnant women; however, in patients with diabetes or obesity, the panel felt that physicians might best be suited to determine on an individual basis its comparative benefit versus risk.

Nutritive sweeteners such as sorbitol and fructose have recently increased in popularity. Except for acute diarrhea induced by ingestion of large amounts of sorbitol-containing foods, their relative risk has yet to be established. Fructose represents a "natural" sugar substance that is a highly effective sweetener which induces only slight increases in plasma glucose levels.

Aspartame, which has recently been approved for use, may prove to be the optimal sweetener for diabetic patients. It consists of 2 amino acids (aspartic acid and phenylalanine) that combine to produce a nutritive sweetener 180 times as sweet as sucrose.

2. Oral hypoglycemic drugs–These are of 2 major types: sulfonylureas and biguanides. Their modes of action are quite different, and considerable controversy exists over their mechanisms of action, therapeutic indications, and especially their safety in long-term use. In 1977, the US Department of Health, Education, and Welfare recommended discontinuing general use of phenformin (DBI, Meltrol), the only biguanide available in the USA. It was considered to be an imminent hazard to health because of its reported association with lactic acidosis. In many countries, however, phenformin and another biguanide, metformin, continue to be used, although in some of these the indications for biguanide therapy in diabetes are being reevaluated. Only the sulfonylureas remain in use as oral hypoglycemic drugs in the USA.

a. Sulfonylureas–This group of drugs contains a sulfonic acid–urea nucleus which can be modified by chemical substitutions to produce agents that have similar qualitative actions but differ widely in potency. The mechanism of action of the sulfonylureas when they are acutely administered is due to their insulinotropic effect on pancreatic B cells. However, it remains unclear whether this well-documented *acute* action requires additional extrapancreatic effects such as an increase in insulin binding to receptors to explain more adequately the hypoglycemic effect of sulfonylureas during chronic administration.

Sulfonylureas are presently not indicated in the juvenile type ketosis-prone insulin-dependent diabetic, since these drugs seem to depend on functioning pancreatic B cells to produce their effect on blood glucose. In a recent prospective trial comparing sulfonylureas with placebo in insulin-treated type I diabetics, Goldman and coworkers found no apparent potentiation of insulin effectiveness on long-term glycemic control when sulfonylureas were added.

The sulfonylureas seem most appropriate for use in the nonobese insulinopenic mild maturity-onset diabetic in whom acute administration restores the early phase of insulin release that is refractory to acute glucose stimulation. In obese mild diabetics and others with peripheral insensitivity to levels of circulating insulin, primary emphasis should be on weight reduction. When hyperglycemia in obese diabetics has been more severe, with consequent impairment of pancreatic B cell function, sulfonylureas may improve glycemic control until concurrent measures such as diet, exercise, and weight reduction can sustain the improvement without the need for oral-drugs.

(1) Tolbutamide (Orinase) is supplied in tablets of 500 mg. It is rapidly oxidized in the liver to an inactive form, and its approximate duration of effect is relatively short (6–10 hours). Tolbutamide is probably best administered in divided doses (eg, 500 mg before each meal and at bedtime); however, some patients require only 1 or 2 tablets daily. Acute toxic reactions are rare, with skin rashes occurring infrequently. Because of its short duration of action, which is independent of renal function, tolbutamide is probably the safest agent to use in elderly patients, in whom hypoglycemia would be a particularly serious risk. Prolonged hypoglycemia has been reported rarely, mostly in patients receiving certain drugs (eg, dicumarol, phenylbutazone, or some of the sulfonamides). The latter compounds apparently compete with sulfonylureas for oxidative enzyme systems in the liver, resulting in maintenance of high levels of unmetabolized, active sulfonylureas in the circulation.

(2) Chlorpropamide (Diabinese) is supplied in tablets of 100 and 250 mg. This drug, with a half-life of 32 hours, is slowly metabolized, with approximately 20–30% excreted unchanged in the urine. It can also interact with the drugs cited above that depend on hepatic oxidative catabolism and is contraindicated in patients with hepatic or renal insufficiency. The average maintenance dose is 250 mg daily, given as a single dose in the morning. Chlorpropamide is a potent agent that is occasionally effective in controlling hyperglycemia in NIDDM despite the failure of maximum therapeutic doses of other less potent sulfonylureas such as tolbutamide, tolazamide, and acetohexamide. Prolonged hypoglycemic reactions are more common than with tolbutamide, particularly in elderly patients, in whom chlorpropamide therapy should be monitored with special care. Doses in excess of 500 mg daily increase the risk of jaundice, which does not occur with the usual dose of 250 mg/d or less. A hyperemic flush may occur when alcohol is ingested by patients taking chlorpropamide. This alcohol flush appears within 8 minutes of ingesting the alcohol and lasts for 10–12 minutes and is believed to relate to the plasma level of chlorpropamide. Patients taking this drug chronically have a higher frequency of flushing after alcohol than persons given a single-dose challenge with chlorpropamide.

Dilutional hyponatremia is a complication of chlorpropamide therapy in some patients, apparently because chlorpropamide both stimulates vasopressin secretion and potentiates its action at the renal tubule. The antidiuretic effect of chlorpropamide is relatively unique, since 3 other sulfonylureas (acetohexamide, tolazamide, and glyburide) facilitate water excretion in humans. Hematologic toxicity (transient leukopenia, thrombocytopenia) occurs in less than 1% of patients.

(3) Acetohexamide (Dymelor) is supplied in tablets of 250 and 500 mg. Its duration of action is about 10–16 hours, being intermediate in action between tolbutamide and chlorpropamide. Give 0.25–1.5 g daily in one or 2 doses. Liver metabolism is rapid, but the metabolite produced remains active. Side effects are similar to those of the other sulfonylurea drugs.

(4) Tolazamide (Tolinase) is supplied in tablets of 100, 250, and 500 mg. It is comparable to chlorpropamide in potency but has a shorter duration of action and does not cause water retention. Tolazamide is more slowly absorbed than the other sulfonylureas, with effects on blood glucose not appearing for several hours. Its duration of action may last up to 20 hours, with maximal hypoglycemic effect occurring between the fourth and 14th hours. Tolazamide is metabolized to several compounds that retain hypoglycemic effects. If more than 500 mg/d is required, the dose should be divided and given twice daily. Doses larger than 1000 mg daily do not improve the degree of glycemic control.

(5) Second-generation sulfonylureas–In April 1984, the FDA approved 2 potent sulfonylurea compounds, glyburide and glipizide. These agents have similar chemical structures, with cyclic carbon rings at each end of the sulfonylurea nucleus; this causes them to be highly potent (100-fold more so than tolbutamide). Initial use of these drugs in other countries (glyburide in 1969, glipizide in 1971) was associated with a high rate of severe hypoglycemic reactions and even some deaths. This was probably due to lack of familiarity with their potent effects. These drugs should be used with caution in patients with cardiovascular disease or in elderly patients, in whom hypoglycemia would be especially dangerous.

Occasionally, diabetic patients who have not responded to the more potent first-generation sulfonylureas such as chlorpropamide have responded to second-generation sulfonylureas. Unfortunately, substantial benefit has not always resulted when a maximum therapeutic dose of chlorpropamide or tolazamide has been replaced with that of a second-generation drug.

(a) Glyburide (Glibencamide; Diaβeta, Micronase)–Glyburide is available in 1.25-, 2.5-, and 5-mg tablets. The usual starting dose is 2.5 mg/d, and the average maintenance dose is 5–10 mg/d given as a single morning dose; maintenance doses higher than 20 mg/d are not recommended. Glyburide is metabolized in the liver into products with such low hypoglycemic activity that they are considered clinically unimportant. Although assays specific for the unmetabolized compound suggest a plasma half-life of only 1–2 hours, the biologic effects of glyburide are clearly persistent 24 hours after a single morning dose in diabetic patients.

Glyburide has few adverse effects other than its potential for causing hypoglycemia. Flushing has rarely been reported after ethanol ingestion. It does not cause water retention, as chlorpropamide does, but rather slightly enhances free water clearance.

(b) Glipizide (Glucotrol)–Glipizide is available in 5- and 10-mg tablets. For maximum effect in reducing postprandial hyperglycemia, this agent should be ingested 30 minutes before breakfast, since rapid absorption is delayed when the drug is taken with food. The recommended starting dose is 5 mg/d with up to 15 mg/d given as a single daily dose. When higher daily doses are required, they should be divided and given before meals. The maximum recommended dose is 40 mg/d.

At least 90% of glipizide is metabolized in the liver to inactive products, and 10% is excreted unchanged in the urine. Glipizide therapy is therefore contraindicated in patients with hepatic or renal impairment, who would therefore be at high risk for hypoglycemia.

b. Efficacy and safety of the oral hypoglycemic agents–The University Group Diabetes Program (UGDP) reported that the number of deaths due to cardiovascular disease in diabetic patients treated with tolbutamide or phenformin was excessive compared to either insulin-treated patients or those receiving placebos. Controversy persists about the validity of the conclusions reached by the UGDP because of the heterogeneity of the population studied, with its preponderance of obese subjects, and certain features of the experimental design such as the use of a fixed dose of oral drug.

In 1979, the ADA withdrew its 1970 endorsement of the UGDP findings and suggested that choice of therapy should be left to the judgment of the physician after discussion with the patient. The US Supreme Court has rejected attempts to prevent the FDA from inserting a special package warning stating that oral hypoglycemic agents may be associated with increased cardiovascular mortality rates as compared to treatment with diet alone or diet plus insulin. This warning label has been included in all packages of second-generation sulfonylureas since their introduction in April 1984.

3. Insulin–Insulin is indicated for type I (IDDM) diabetics as well as for nonobese type II diabetics with insulinopenia whose hyperglycemia does not respond to diet therapy either alone or combined with oral hypoglycemic drugs.

With the development of highly purified porcine insulin preparations, immunogenicity has been markedly reduced, and it might well be eliminated once adequate supplies of human insulin become available from recombinant DNA biosynthesis or from enzymatic conversion of pork insulin to that of human

insulin structure. However, the problem of achieving optimal insulin delivery systems remains unsolved with the present state of technology. It has not been possible to reproduce the physiologic patterns of intraportal insulin secretion with subcutaneous injections of soluble or longer-acting insulin suspensions. Even so, with the help of appropriate modifications of diet and exercise and careful monitoring of capillary blood glucose levels at home, it has often been possible to achieve acceptable control of blood glucose by using portable insulin infusion pumps or variable mixtures of short- and longer-acting insulins injected at least twice daily.

a. Characteristics of available insulin preparations–Commercial insulin preparations differ with respect to the animal species from which they are obtained, their purity and solubility, and the time of onset and duration of their biologic action. In the fall of 1984, more than 40 different formulations of insulin were available in the USA (Table 20–4).

(1) Species of insulin–Because the supply of pork insulin has been too limited to satisfy the insulin requirements of all diabetic patients, most commercial insulins contain the slightly more antigenic beef insulin, which differs by 3 amino acids from human insulin (in contrast to the single amino acid distinguishing pork and human insulins). Standard preparations of Iletin I (Eli Lilly) are mixtures containing 70% beef and 30% pork insulin. However, a limited supply of monospecies pork or beef insulin (Iletin II) has been available for use in certain patients with insulin allergy or immune insulin resistance. The production of highly purified insulins by Danish manufacturers has resulted in a substantial increase in the availability of porcine insulin. Human insulin can now be produced by recombinant DNA techniques (biosynthetic human insulin) or by enzymatic conversion of pork insulin to human insulin structure (semisynthetic human insulin), in which alanine, the terminal amino acid on the beta chain of pork insulin, is replaced by threonine. Human insulin prepared by the recombinant DNA method has recently been introduced for clinical use as Humulin (Eli Lilly) and dispensed as either Regular or NPH Humulin. Human insulin prepared by enzymatic conversion of pork insulin is marketed by Squibb-Novo as Actrapid Human Insulin or Monotard Human Insulin. Lilly's Humulin and Squibb-Novo human insulin have been approved for general use by the FDA.

(2) Purity of insulin–Recent improvements in purification techniques with Sephadex gel columns have reduced or eliminated contaminating insulin precursors which had molecular weights greater than that of insulin and which were biologically inactive yet capable of inducing anti-insulin antibodies. The degree of purification in which proinsulin contamination is greater than 10 but less than 50 ppm merits the present label of **new improved "single peak" insulin,** and this is currently the main form of insulin produced commercially in the USA by Eli Lilly as Iletin I. When proinsulin content is reduced to less than 10 ppm, manufacturers are entitled by FDA regu-

Table 20—4. Insulin preparations available in the USA.

Preparation	Species Source	Concentration
Rapid-acting		
Standard*		
Regular Iletin I (Lilly)	Beef and pork	U40, U100
Regular (Squibb-Novo)	Beef and pork	U40, U100
Semilente Iletin I (Lilly)	Beef and pork	U40, U100
Semilente (Squibb-Novo)	Beef	U40, U100
"Purified"†		
Regular Humulin (Lilly)	Human	U100
Regular Iletin II (Lilly)	Pork or beef	U100, U500‡
Actrapid (Squibb-Novo)	Pork or human	U100
Velosulin (Nordisk)	Pork	U100
Semitard (Squibb-Novo)	Pork	U100
Intermediate-acting		
Standard		
NPH Iletin I (Lilly)	Beef and pork	U40, U100
Lente Iletin I (Lilly)	Beef and pork	U40, U100
Isophane NPH (Squibb-Novo)	Beef and pork	U40, U100
Lente (Squibb-Novo)	Beef	U40, U100
"Purified"		
NPH Humulin (Lilly)	Human	U100
NPH Iletin II (Lilly)	Pork or beef	U100
Lente Iletin II (Lilly)	Pork or beef	U100
Protaphane NPH (Squibb-Novo)	Pork	U100
Lentard (Squibb-Novo)	Beef and pork	U100
Monotard (Squibb-Novo)	Pork or human	U100
Insulatard NPH (Nordisk)	Pork	U100
Mixtard (Nordisk)	Pork	U100
Long-acting		
Standard		
Ultralente Iletin I (Lilly)	Beef and pork	U40, U100
PZI Iletin I (Lilly)	Beef and pork	U40, U100
Ultralente (Squibb-Novo)	Beef	U100
PZI (Squibb-Novo)	Beef and pork	U40, U100
"Purified"		
PZI Iletin II (Lilly)	Pork or beef	U100
Ultratard (Squibb-Novo)	Beef	U100

*Greater than 10 but less than 25 ppm proinsulin.
†Less than 10 ppm proinsulin.
‡U500 available only as pork insulin.

lations to label the insulin as "purified." Such highly purified insulins are presently marketed in the USA by Eli Lilly, Squibb-Novo, and Nordisk. Because they are relatively free of impurities including even those whose molecular weight is comparable to that of insulin, they have been termed **single component** or **monocomponent insulin.** The Eli Lilly product is called Iletin II to identify this highly purified insulin, and it presently is available only as a monospecies pork or beef insulin. All human insulins are also highly purified.

The more purified insulins that have recently become available seem to preserve their potency quite well, so that refrigeration is recommended but not crucial. During travel, reserve supplies of insulin can thus be readily transported for weeks without losing potency if protected from extremes of heat or cold.

(3) Concentration of insulin–At present, most insulins are available in a concentration of 100 units/mL (U100), and all are dispensed in 10-mL vials. To accommodate children and occasional adults who may require small quantities, a U40 insulin continues to be available. However, with the popularity of "low-dose" (0.5-mL) disposable insulin syringes, there is less need for U40 insulin, since U100 can now be measured with acceptable accuracy in doses as low as 1–2 units. For use in rare cases of severe insulin resistance in which large quantities of insulin are required, a limited supply of U500 regular porcine insulin (Iletin II) is available from Eli Lilly.

b. Insulin preparations–Three principal types of insulins are available: (1) short-acting, with rapid onset of action; (2) intermediate-acting; and (3) long-acting, with slow onset of action (Fig 20–1). Short-acting insulin (unmodified insulin) is a crystalline zinc insulin provided in soluble form and thus is dispensed as a clear solution. All other commercial insulins have been specially modified to retain more prolonged action and are dispensed as turbid suspensions at neutral pH with either protamine in phosphate buffer (protamine zinc insulin and NPH) or varying concentrations of zinc in acetate buffer (ultralente and semilente). The use of protamine zinc insulin and semilente preparations is currently decreasing, and almost no indications for their use exist. Conventional insulin therapy can presently be accomplished with regular insulin dispensed in an infusion device or administered as multiple injections in association with any of 3 insulin suspensions (NPH, lente, or ultralente) whose duration of action is prolonged.

(1) Regular insulin (Regular Iletin I or II or Humulin [Eli Lilly], Insulin Injection and Actrapid [Squibb-Novo], Velosulin [Nordisk]) is a short-acting soluble crystalline zinc insulin whose effect appears within 15 minutes after subcutaneous injection and lasts 5–7 hours. It is the only type of insulin that can be administered intravenously or by infusion pumps. It is particularly useful in the treatment of diabetic ketoacidosis and when the insulin requirement is changing rapidly, such as after surgery or during acute infections.

(2) Lente insulin is a mixture of 30% semilente (an amorphous precipitate of insulin with zinc ions) with 70% ultralente insulin (an insoluble crystal of zinc and insulin)—Lente Iletin I or II (Eli Lilly), Lente Insulin and Monotard (Squibb-Novo). Its onset of action is delayed (Fig 20–1), and because its duration of action often is less than 24 hours (with a range of 18–24 hours), most patients require at least 2 injections daily to maintain a sustained insulin effect. Lente insulin has its peak effect in most patients between 8 and 12 hours, but individual variations in peak response time must be considered when interpreting unusual or unexpected patterns of glycemic responses in individual patients. While lente insulin is the most widely used of the lente series, particularly in combination with regular insulin, there has recently been a resurgence of the use of ultralente in combination with

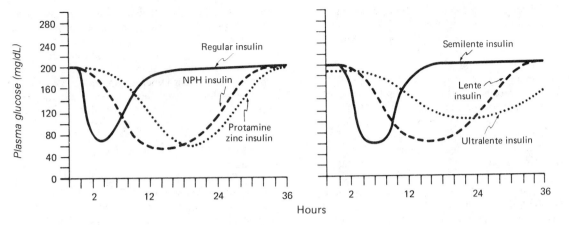

Figure 20-1. Extent and duration of action of various types of insulin (in a fasting diabetic).

multiple injections of regular insulin as a means of attempting optimal control in IDDM patients. Ultralente has a very slow onset of action with a prolonged duration (Fig 20–1), and its administration once or twice daily has been advocated to provide a basal level of insulin comparable to that achieved by basal endogenous secretion or the overnight infusion rate programmed into insulin pumps.

(3) NPH (neutral protamine Hagedorn or isophane) insulin (NPH Iletin I and II or Humulin [Eli Lilly], NPH Insulin and Protaphane [Squibb-Novo], Insulatard NPH [Nordisk]) is an intermediate-acting insulin whose onset of action is delayed by combining 2 parts soluble crystalline zinc with 1 part protamine zinc insulin. This produces equivalent amounts of insulin and protamine, so that neither is present in an uncomplexed form ("isophane").

The onset and duration of action of NPH insulin are comparable to those of lente insulin (Fig 20–1); it is usually mixed with regular insulin and given at least twice daily for insulin replacement in IDDM patients.

(4) Mixtures of insulin – Since intermediate insulins require several hours to reach adequate therapeutic levels, their use in IDDM patients requires supplements of regular insulin preprandially. For convenience, these may be mixed together in the same syringe and injected subcutaneously in split dosage before breakfast and supper. When mixing insulin, it is necessary to inject into both bottles a quantity of air equivalent to the volume of insulin to be subsequently withdrawn. It is recommended that the regular insulin be withdrawn first, then the intermediate insulin. No attempt should be made to mix the insulins in the syringe, and the injection is preferably given immediately after loading the syringe.

Recent reports caution that insulin mixtures containing increased proportions of lente or NPH to regular insulins may retard the rapid action of admixed regular insulin, particularly if not injected immediately after mixing. They suggest that the excess zinc in lente insulin or excess protamine in NPH insulin binds the soluble insulin and partially blunts its action, particu-

larly when a relatively small proportion of regular insulin is mixed with lente or NPH (eg, 1 part regular to 2 or more parts lente or NPH).

c. Methods of insulin administration –

(1) Insulin syringes and needles – Plastic disposable syringes with needles attached are available in 1-mL and 0.5-mL sizes. In cases where very low insulin doses are prescribed, as in young children, the specially calibrated 0.5-mL disposable syringe facilitates accurate measurement of U100 insulin in doses up to 50 units. The "low-dose" syringes have become increasingly popular, because diabetics generally should not take more than 50 units of insulin in a single injection, except in rare instances of extreme insulin resistance. Several recent reports have indicated that "disposable" syringes may be reused until blunting of the needle occurs (usually after 3–5 injections). Sterility adequate to avoid infection with reuse appears to be maintained by refrigerating syringes between uses.

(2) Site of injection – Any part of the body covered by loose skin can be used, such as the abdomen, thighs, upper arms, flanks, and upper buttocks. Rotation of sites continues to be recommended to avoid delayed absorption when fibrosis or lipohypertrophy occurs from repeated use of a single site. However, as more highly purified insulins have become available, fibrosis is less of a problem. Moreover, considerable variability of absorption rates from different sites, particularly with exercise, may contribute to the instability of glycemic control in certain IDDM patients if injection sites are rotated too frequently in different areas of the body.

(3) Insulin delivery systems – Efforts to administer soluble insulin by "closed-loop" systems (glucose-controlled insulin infusion system) have been successful for acute situations such as diabetic ketoacidosis or for administering insulin to diabetics during surgery. However, chronic use is precluded by the need for continually aspirating blood to reach an external glucose sensor and the large size of the computerized pump system.

Current research into smaller "open-loop"

means of insulin delivery (insulin reservoir and pump programmed to deliver regular insulin at a calculated rate without a glucose sensor) has developed several relatively small pumps for subcutaneous, intravenous, or intraperitoneal infusion. With improving methods for patients' self-monitoring of blood glucose, these pump systems have become more useful for managing diabetics. However, at present, conventional methods of insulin administration with multiple subcutaneous injections of soluble, rapid-acting insulin and a single injection of long-acting insulin usually can provide as effective glycemic control as the more expensive open-loop systems.

Although pancreatic islet cells have been successfully transplanted in genetically similar strains of rodents with experimental diabetes, this approach has not yet been successful in humans because of immunologic rejection. Likewise, whole pancreas transplants have generally been unsatisfactory in treating the insulin-dependent diabetic patient.

C. General Considerations in Treatment of Diabetes: Patients with diabetes can have a full and satisfying life. However, "free" diets and unrestricted activity are still not advised for insulin-requiring diabetics. Until new methods of insulin replacement are developed that provide more normal patterns of insulin delivery in response to metabolic demands, multiple feedings will continue to be recommended, and certain occupations potentially hazardous to the patient or others will continue to be prohibited.

Exercise increases the effectiveness of insulin, and moderate exercise is an excellent means of improving utilization of fat and carbohydrate in diabetic patients. A judicious balance of the size and frequency of meals with moderate regular exercise can often stabilize the insulin dosage in diabetics who tend to slip out of control easily. Strenuous exercise could precipitate hypoglycemia in an unprepared patient, and diabetics must therefore be taught to reduce their insulin dosage in anticipation of strenuous activity or to take supplemental carbohydrate. Injection of insulin into a site farthest away from the muscles most involved in exercise may help ameliorate exercise-induced hypoglycemia, since insulin injected proximal to exercising muscle is much more rapidly mobilized. With more knowledge regarding the relationships between caloric intake and expenditure and insulin requirements, the patient can become more liberated from the regimentation imposed by the disorder.

All diabetic patients must receive adequate instruction on personal hygiene, especially with regard to care of the feet (see p 773), skin, and teeth. All infections—but especially pyogenic infections with fever and toxemia—provoke the release of high levels of insulin antagonists such as catecholamines or glucagon and thus bring about a marked increase in insulin requirements. This is a common precipitating cause of ketosis and acidosis and should be treated promptly and vigorously. Supplemental regular insulin is often required to correct hyperglycemia during infection.

Psychologic factors are of great importance in the control of diabetes, particularly when the disease is difficult to stabilize. One reason the diabetic may be particularly sensitive to emotional upset is that A cells of diabetics are hyperresponsive to physiologic levels of epinephrine, producing excessive levels of glucagon with consequent hyperglycemia.

Counseling should be directed at avoiding extremes of compulsive rigidity or self-destructive neglect.

Steps in the Management of the Diabetic Patient

A. Diagnostic Examination: A complete history and physical examination is performed for diagnostic purposes and to rule out the presence of coexisting or complicating disease. Nutritional assessment should determine whether catabolic features dominate despite a history of normal or increased food intake. Any features of the clinical picture that suggest end organ insensitivity to insulin, such as obesity, must be identified. The family history should document not only the incidence of diabetes in other members of the family but also the age at onset, whether it was associated with obesity, and whether insulin was required. Other factors that increase cardiac risk, such as smoking history, presence of hypertension or hyperlipidemia, or oral contraceptive pill use, should be documented.

Laboratory diagnosis should document fasting plasma glucose levels above 140 mg/dL or postprandial values consistently above 200 mg/dL and whether ketonuria accompanies the glycosuria. A glycohemoglobin measurement is useful for assessing the effectiveness of future therapy.

Baseline values of any observation that may help in the evaluation of future complications should be recorded. These include plasma triglycerides and cholesterol, electrocardiography, chest x-ray, renal function studies, peripheral pulses, and neurologic and ophthalmologic examinations.

B. Patient Education: Since diabetes is a lifelong disorder, education of the patient is probably the most important obligation of the physician who provides initial care. The best persons to manage a disease that is affected so markedly by daily fluctuations in environmental stress, exercise, diet, and infections are the patients themselves and their families. Patients must be helped to accept the fact that they have diabetes; until this difficult adjustment has been made, efforts to cope with the disorder are usually futile. The "teaching curriculum" should include explanations by the physician of the nature of diabetes and its potential acute and chronic hazards and how they can be recognized early and prevented or treated. The importance of regular recording of tests for glucose on either capillary blood or double-voided urine specimens should be stressed and instructions on proper testing provided. Advice on personal hygiene, including detailed instructions on foot care (see p 773), as well as individual instruction on diet and specific hypoglycemic therapy, should be provided. Patients

Instructions in the Care of the Feet
for Persons With Diabetes Mellitus or Vascular Disturbances

Hygiene of the Feet

(1) Wash feet daily with mild soap and lukewarm water. Dry thoroughly between the toes by pressure. Do not rub vigorously, as this is apt to break the delicate skin.

(2) When feet are thoroughly dry, rub well with vegetable oil to keep them soft, prevent excess friction, remove scales, and prevent dryness. Care must be taken to prevent foot tenderness.

(3) If the feet become too soft and tender, rub them with alcohol about once a week.

(4) When rubbing the feet, always rub upward from the tips of the toes. If varicose veins are present, massage the feet very gently; never massage the legs.

(5) If the toenails are brittle and dry, soften them by soaking for one-half hour each night in lukewarm water containing 1 tbsp of powdered sodium borate (borax) per quart. Follow this by rubbing around the nails with vegetable oil. Clean around the nails with an orangewood stick. If the nails become too long, file them with an emery board. File them straight across and no shorter than the underlying soft tissues of the toe. Never cut the corners of the nails. (The podiatrist should be informed if a patient has diabetes.)

(6) Wear low-heeled shoes of soft leather that fit the shape of the feet correctly. The shoes should have wide toes that will cause no pressure, fit close in the arch, and grip the heels snugly. Wear new shoes one-half hour only on the first day and increase by 1 hour each day following. Wear thick, warm, loose stockings.

Treatment of Corns & Calluses

(1) Corns and calluses are due to friction and pressure, most often from improperly fitted shoes and stockings. Wear shoes that fit properly and cause no friction or pressure.

(2) To remove excess calluses or corns, soak the feet in lukewarm (not hot) water, using a mild soap, for about 10 minutes and then rub off the excess tissue with a towel or file. Do not tear it off. Under no circumstances must the skin become irritated.

(3) Do not cut corns or calluses. If they need attention it is safer to see a podiatrist.

(4) Prevent callus formation under the ball of the foot (a) by exercises, such as curling and stretching the toes several times a day; (b) by finishing each step on the toes and not on the ball of the foot; and (c)

by wearing shoes that are not too short and that do not have high heels.

Aids in Treatment of Impaired Circulation (Cold Feet)

(1) Never use tobacco in any form. Tobacco contracts blood vessels and so reduces circulation.

(2) Keep warm. Wear warm stockings and other clothing. Cold contracts blood vessels and reduces circulation.

(3) Do not wear circular garters, which compress blood vessels and reduce blood flow.

(4) Do not sit with the legs crossed. This may compress the leg arteries and shut off the blood supply to the feet.

(5) If the weight of the bedclothes is uncomfortable, place a pillow under the covers at the foot of the bed.

(6) Do not apply any medication to the feet without directions from a physician. Some medicines are too strong for feet with poor circulation.

(7) Do not apply heat in the form of hot water, hot water bottles, or heating pads without a physician's consent. Even moderate heat can injure the skin if circulation is poor.

(8) If the feet are moist or the patient has a tendency to develop athlete's foot, a prophylactic dusting powder should be used on the feet and in shoes and stockings daily. Change shoes and stockings at least daily or oftener.

Treatment of Abrasions of the Skin

(1) Proper first-aid treatment is of the utmost importance even in apparently minor injuries. Consult a physician immediately for any redness, blistering, pain, or swelling. Any break in the skin may become ulcerous or gangrenous unless properly treated by a physician.

(2) Dermatophytosis (athlete's foot), which begins with peeling and itching between the toes or discoloration or thickening of the toenails, should be treated immediately by a physician or podiatrist.

(3) Avoid strong irritating antiseptics such as tincture of iodine.

(4) As soon as possible after any injury, cover the area with sterile gauze, which may be purchased at drugstores. Only fine paper tape or cellulose tape (Scotch Tape) should be used on the skin if adhesive retention of the gauze is required.

(5) Elevate and, as much as possible until recovery, avoid using the foot.

should be told about community agencies, such as Diabetes Association chapters, that can serve as a continuing source of instruction.

C. Self-Monitoring of Blood Glucose: Monitoring of blood glucose by patients has allowed greater flexibility in management while achieving improved glycemic control. It involves educating the patient to perform 3 essential steps.

1. The obtaining of a drop of capillary blood from the fingertip by means of a specially designed lancet. Automatic spring-loaded devices (see p 765) facilitate finger-pricking and ensure an adequate blood sample.

2. Application of the sample to the test strip and removal at the proper time.

3. Accurate quantitation of the color developed (either visually or with a portable colorimeter [see p 765]).

Self-monitoring of blood glucose is particularly indicated in brittle diabetics, those attempting ''ideal'' glycemic control such as during pregnancy, patients who have little or no early warning of hypoglycemic attacks, and those with dysfunctional bladders from diabetic neuropathy or altered renal thresholds for glucose. It is useful in educating patients on the glycemic effects of specific foods in their diet and reduces the likelihood of unexpected episodes of severe hypoglycemia in insulin-treated diabetics. It has proved to be an effective and safe clinical tool that in compliant patients can be a valuable component of their therapeutic options.

D. Initial Therapy: Treatment must be individualized on the basis of the type of diabetes and specific needs of each patient. However, certain general principles of management can be outlined for hyperglycemic states of different types.

1. The obese patient–The most common type of diabetic patient is obese and has hyperglycemia because of insensitivity to normal or elevated circulating levels of insulin (insulinoplethoric diabetes).

a. Weight reduction–Treatment is directed toward achieving weight reduction, and prescribing a diet is only one means to this end. Cure can be achieved by reducing adipose stores, with consequent restoration of tissue sensitivity to insulin. The presence of diabetes with its added risk factors may motivate the obese diabetic to greater efforts to lose weight.

b. Hypoglycemic agents–All hypoglycemic agents, including insulin as well as oral hypoglycemic drugs, are not indicated for long-term use in the obese patient with mild diabetes. The weight reduction program can be upset by real or imagined hypoglycemic reactions when insulin therapy is used; it is also possible that administration of insulin to an obese patient who already has excessive circulating levels may have the ill effects of maintaining insulin insensitivity of receptor sites as well as interfering with catabolic mechanisms during caloric deprivation. The obese diabetic who has been previously treated with insulin—often in interrupted fashion—and who requires high doses both to offset excess caloric intake

and to overcome tissue insensitivity may develop immune insulin resistance. This not only increases the requirements for exogenous insulin but also impairs the effectiveness of endogenous insulin and may even precipitate ketosis.

Oral sulfonylureas have a role in the management of obese patients with hyperglycemia that does not respond to dietary measures and, particularly, of those with severe diabetes causing nocturia, blurred vision, or (in women) candidal vulvovaginitis. Insulin injections may be required if a trial of sulfonylurea therapy is ineffective. In such cases, short-term therapy (weeks or months) with either sulfonylureas or insulin may be indicated to ameliorate symptoms until simultaneous caloric restriction leading to weight reduction can occur.

2. The nonobese patient–In the nonobese diabetic, mild to severe hyperglycemia is usually due to refractoriness of B cells to glucose stimulation (insulinopenic diabetes). Treatment depends on whether insulinopenia produces ketoacidosis.

a. Diet therapy–If hyperglycemia is mild, normal metabolic control can occasionally be restored by means of multiple feedings of a diet limited in simple sugars and with a caloric content sufficient to maintain ideal weight. Restriction of saturated fats and cholesterol is also strongly advised.

b. Oral hypoglycemic agents–When diet therapy is not sufficient to correct hyperglycemia, a trial of sulfonylureas to improve insulin release is often successful in nonobese patients with mild nonketotic diabetes. Once the dosage of sulfonylurea reaches the upper recommended limit in a compliant patient without maintaining blood glucose below 200 mg/dL during the day, insulin therapy is indicated.

c. Insulin treatment–The patient requiring insulin therapy should be initially regulated under conditions of optimal diet and normal daily activities. In patients with IDDM, information and counseling should be provided about the advantages of taking multiple injections of insulin in conjunction with self blood glucose monitoring. If tight control is attempted, urine glucose measurements are not sufficient, and at least 3 measurements of capillary blood glucose are required daily to avoid frequent hypoglycemic reactions. A typical initial dose schedule in a 70-kg patient taking 2200 kcal divided into 6 or 7 feedings might be 10 units of regular and 20 units of NPH insulin in the morning and 5 units of regular and 5 units of NPH insulin in the evening. The morning urine or capillary blood glucose (or both) gives a measure of the effectiveness of NPH insulin administered the previous evening; the noon urine or blood glucose reflects the effects of the morning regular insulin; and the 5:00 PM and 9:00 PM sugars represent the effects of the morning NPH and evening regular insulins, respectively. A properly educated patient might be taught to adjust insulin dosage by observing the pattern of glycemia and glycosuria and correlating it with the approximate duration of action and the time of peak effect after injection of the various insulin preparations

(Fig 20–1). Adjustments should be made gradually and preferably not more often than every 3 days if possible. Limited data are available concerning the level of glucose control needed to avoid diabetic complications. Postprandial blood glucose levels below 200 mg/dL have been advocated by retrospective analysis of 2 populations of NIDDM-patients. A reasonable aim of therapy is to approach normal glycemic excursions without provoking severe or frequent hypoglycemia. What has been considered "acceptable" control includes blood glucose levels of 60–130 mg/dL before meals and after an overnight fast and levels no higher than 180 mg/dL 1 hour after meals and 140 mg/dL 2 hours after meals. In NIDDM patients with milder forms of insulinopenia who require insulin therapy, a single morning injection of a small dose of intermediate insulin may suffice to supplement their own endogenous insulin secretion.

Indications for Purified Insulins

Purified insulins or human insulin are indicated when insulin of conventional purity has been associated with allergy, immune resistance, or lipoatrophy. Also, they would seem to be preferable in any patient undergoing insulin therapy for the first time, since the absence of anti-insulin antibodies would facilitate the measurement of therapeutic levels of circulating insulin as a guide for optimal management. In patients with NIDDM whose therapy with insulin is to be for a limited time (eg, in gestational diabetes or during acute infections or surgery), human insulin or purified insulin would reduce the risks of immunologic sensitization to future exposures to insulin.

Complications of Insulin Therapy

A. Hypoglycemia: Hypoglycemic reactions, the most common complication of insulin therapy, may result from delay in taking a meal or unusual physical exertion. With more patients attempting "tight" control without frequent capillary glucose home monitoring, this complication is likely to become even more frequent. In older diabetics, in those taking only longer-acting insulins, and often in those maintaining euglycemia on infusion pumps, autonomic responses are less frequent, and the manifestations are mainly from impaired function of the central nervous system, ie, mental confusion, bizarre behavior, and ultimately coma. More rapid development of hypoglycemia from the effects of regular insulin causes signs of autonomic hyperactivity, both adrenergic (tachycardia, palpitations, sweating, tremulousness) and parasympathetic (nausea, hunger), that may progress to coma and convulsions.

Because of the potential danger of insulin reactions, the diabetic patient should carry packets of table sugar or a candy roll at all times for use at the onset of hypoglycemic symptoms. An ampule of glucagon (1 mg) should be provided to every diabetic receiving insulin therapy, and family or friends should be instructed as to how to inject it in the event that the patient is unconscious or refuses food. An identifica-

tion bracelet, necklace, or card in the wallet or purse should be carried by every diabetic receiving hypoglycemic drug therapy (see box below).

All of the manifestations of hypoglycemia are rapidly relieved by glucose administration. In a case of mild hypoglycemia in a patient who is conscious and able to swallow, orange juice, glucose, or any sugar-containing beverage or food may be given. If more severe hypoglycemia has produced unconsciousness or stupor, the treatment of choice is to give 20–50 mL of 50% glucose solution by intravenous infusion over a period of 2–3 minutes. If intravenous therapy is not available, 1 mg of glucagon injected intramuscularly will usually restore the patient to consciousness within 15 minutes to permit ingestion of sugar. If the patient is stuporous and glucagon is not available, small amounts of honey or syrup can be inserted within the buccal pouch, but, in general, oral feeding is contraindicated in unconscious patients. Rectal administration of syrup or honey (30 mL per 500 mL of warm water) has been effective.

B. Immunopathology of Insulin Therapy: At least 5 molecular classes of insulin antibodies are produced during the course of insulin therapy in diabetes, including IgA, IgD, IgE, IgG, and IgM.

1. Insulin allergy–Insulin allergy, or immediate type hypersensitivity, is a rare condition in which local or systemic urticaria is due to histamine release from tissue mast cells sensitized by adherence of anti-insulin IgE antibodies. In severe cases, anaphylaxis results. A subcutaneous nodule appearing several hours later at the site of insulin injection and lasting for up to 24 hours has been attributed to an IgG-mediated complement-binding Arthus reaction. Because sensitivity is often to noninsulin protein contaminants, the new highly purified insulins have reduced markedly the incidence of insulin allergy, especially of the local

---

I Am a Diabetic and Take Insulin

If I am behaving peculiarly but am conscious and able to swallow, give me sugar or hard candy or orange juice slowly. If I am unconscious, call an ambulance immediately, take me to a physician or a hospital, and notify my physician. *I am not intoxicated.*

My name _____

Address _____

Telephone _____

Physician's name _____

Physician's address _____

Telephone _____

variety. When allergy to beef or, more rarely, pork insulin is present, a species change (eg, to pure pork or human insulin) may correct the problem. Antihistamines, corticosteroids, and even desensitization may be required, especially for systemic hypersensitivity. A kit containing various dilutions of pure beef or pork insulin is distributed by the Eli Lilly Co. for allergy testing and insulin desensitization (not commercially available).

2. Immune insulin resistance–All insulin-treated patients develop a low titer of circulating IgG anti-insulin antibodies that neutralize to a small extent the action of insulin. In some diabetic patients, principally those with some degree of tissue insensitivity to insulin (such as in the obese) and with a history of interrupted exposure to insulin therapy, a high titer of circulating IgG anti-insulin antibodies develops. This results in extremely high insulin requirements—often more than 200 units daily. This is often a self-limited condition and may clear spontaneously after several months. However, in cases where the circulating antibody is specifically more reactive with beef insulin—a more potent immunogen in humans than pork insulin—changing the patient to a less antigenic insulin (pork or human) may make possible a dramatic reduction in insulin dosage or at least may shorten the duration of immune resistance. Other forms of therapy include sulfated beef insulin (a chemically modified form of beef insulin containing an average of 6 sulfate groups per molecule) and immunosuppression with corticosteroids. In some adults, the foreign insulin can be completely discontinued and the patient maintained on diet along with oral sulfonylureas. This is possible only when the circulating antibodies do not effectively neutralize endogenous (human) insulin.

C. Lipodystrophy at Injection Sites: Atrophy of subcutaneous fatty tissue leading to disfigurement and scarring may rarely occur at the site of injection. This complication may represent an immune reaction, since it has become rarer with the development of highly concentrated, pure insulin preparations of neutral pH. Injection of these preparations directly into the atrophic area often results in restoration of normal contours. Hypertrophy of fat tissue at the local injection site continues to occur with the same frequency despite use of highly purified insulins and may be caused by anabolic build-up from high local concentrations of insulin.

Chronic Complications of Diabetes

A. Diabetic Retinopathy: Two main categories exist: background, or "simple," retinopathy, consisting of microaneurysms, hemorrhages, exudates, and retinal edema; and proliferative, or "malignant," retinopathy, consisting of newly formed vessels. Proliferative retinopathy is a leading cause of blindness in the USA. Its current treatment of choice, photocoagulation, was recently evaluated by a report from a large-scale clinical trial conducted on a random basis and known as the Diabetic Retinopathy Study. This involved more than 1700 patients from 15 medical centers on whom 10 years of follow-up are presently available. Findings suggest that extensive "scatter" xenon or argon photocoagulation and focal treatment of new vessels reduce severe visual loss in those cases in which proliferative retinopathy is associated with *recent* vitreous hemorrhages or in which extensive new vessels are located on or near the optic disk.

B. Diabetic Nephropathy: Capillary basement membrane thickening of renal glomeruli produces varying degrees of glomerulosclerosis and renal insufficiency. The clinical syndrome of progressive diabetic nephropathy consists of proteinuria of varying severity occasionally leading to the full-blown nephrotic syndrome with hypoalbuminemia, edema, and an increase in circulating betalipoproteins. In contrast to all other renal disorders, the proteinuria associated with diabetic nephropathy does not diminish with progressive renal failure (patients continue to excrete 10–11 g daily as creatinine clearance diminishes). As renal failure progresses, there is an elevation in the renal threshold at which glycosuria appears.

Dialysis has been of limited value in the treatment of renal failure due to diabetic nephropathy. At present, experience in renal transplantation—especially from related donors—is more promising and is the treatment of choice in cases where there are no contraindications such as severe cardiovascular disease.

C. Gangrene of the Feet in Diabetes: The incidence of gangrene of the feet in diabetics is 20 times the incidence in matched controls. The factors responsible for its development are ischemia, peripheral neuropathy, and secondary infection. Ischemia involves small arteries in all cases; however, in as many as one-third of cases of diabetic gangrene, pedal pulses are palpable, indicating sparing of medium-sized and larger arteries. Cigarette smoking should be avoided, and prevention of foot disease (see p 773) should be emphasized, since treatment is difficult once ulceration and gangrene have developed. Amputation of the lower extremities is sometimes required.

Propranolol is contraindicated in patients with ischemic foot ulcers, because the drug reduces peripheral blood flow.

D. Diabetic Neuropathy: Peripheral and autonomic neuropathy, the 2 most common chronic complications of diabetes, are poorly understood. There is no consistently effective treatment other than optimal control of the diabetes. Ophthalmoplegias inevitably resolve within 6–9 weeks. Diarrhea associated with autonomic neuropathy has occasionally responded to broad-spectrum antibiotic therapy, although it often undergoes spontaneous remission. Gastric atony may be so severe as to require gastrojejunal anastomosis. Metoclopramide may be used orally or intravenously to improve gastric motility when cholinergic activity is diminished but not when it is absent. The physician should be familiar with side effects of metoclopramide; somnolence is a common adverse effect. Impotence is usually permanent. Bethanechol (Urecholine) has occasionally improved emptying of the atonic urinary bladder. Mineralocorticoid therapy and pressure suits have reportedly been of some help in patients with orthostatic hypotension occurring as a result of loss of postural reflexes. Fluphenazine, up to 1 mg 3 times daily, and amitriptyline, 50–75 mg at bedtime, have been recommended for nocturnal pains in the lower extremity. Dramatic relief has often resulted within 48–72 hours. Mild to moderate drowsiness is a side effect that generally improves with time. These drugs should not be continued if improvement has not occurred after 5 days of therapy.

Prognosis of Diabetes

The effect of diabetic control on the development of complications remains an unresolved controversy. The observation that supposedly well-controlled diabetics often have elevated levels of hemoglobin A_{1c}, a result of sustained hyperglycemia, indicates the ineffectiveness of present conventional therapeutic methods for controlling hyperglycemia. Until pancreatic islet transplants or improved insulin delivery systems are available, this important question of control affecting complications may not be resolved. The patient with juvenile-onset insulin-dependent diabetes is at greater risk of developing microangiopathy of the kidneys and retina than the obese diabetic, whose major complications are more apt to be related to disease of the medium-sized and large arteries. Recent intervention trials in small groups of IDDM patients with background or proliferative retinopathy have shown that despite 1 year of "tight" glycemic control with insulin pumps, worsening of the retinopathy continued. A large-scale prevention trial involving 20 centers in the USA is under way to determine if "tight" glycemic control in IDDM can delay or prevent the *onset* of retinopathy.

Until these questions are resolved, the prognosis remains uncertain. A few guidelines, however, are available. In one series of 164 juvenile-onset diabetics with a median age at onset of 9 years, the following outcome was noted after follow-up for 25 years: Out of every 5 diabetics on standard dietary and insulin control, one had died and one was incapacitated with severe proliferative retinopathy and renal failure. However, 2 others were active, contributing members of society despite mild background retinopathy, mild nephropathy, neuropathy, and some degree of ischemia of the feet, and one was completely free of complications (Knowles, 1971). Time will tell whether these statistics will improve with the proper use of insulin mixtures given twice daily and, especially, with improved monitoring by use of portable colorimeters to measure "finger-stick" blood glucose in the home.

The period between 10 and 20 years after onset of diabetes seems to be a critical one. If the patient survives this period without fulminating complications, there is a strong likelihood that reasonably good health will continue. It is clear that the diabetic patient's intelligence, motivation, and awareness of the potential complications of the disease contribute significantly to the ultimate outcome.

Bantle JP et al: Postprandial glucose and insulin responses to meals containing different carbohydrates in normal and diabetic subjects. *N Engl J Med* 1983;**309**:7.

Bell GI, Horita S, Karam JH: A polymorphic locus near the human insulin gene is associated with insulin-dependent diabetes mellitus. *Diabetes* 1984;**33**:176.

Bennett PH: The diagnosis of diabetes: New international classification and diagnostic criteria. *Annu Rev Med* 1983;**34**:295.

Berger M et al: Absorption kinetics and biologic effects of subcutaneously injected insulin preparations. *Diabetes Care* 1982;**5**:77.

Binder C et al: Insulin pharmacokinetics. *Diabetes Care* 1984;**7**:188.

Christlieb AR: The hypertensions of diabetes. *Diabetes Care* 1982;**5**:50.

Cogan DG et al: Aldose reductose and complications of diabetes. *Ann Intern Med* 1984;**101**:82.

Fineberg SE et al: Effects of species of origin, purification levels, and formulation on insulin immunogenicity. *Diabetes* 1983;**32**:592.

Flier JS: Insulin receptors and insulin resistance. *Annu Rev Med* 1983;**34**:145.

Gerich JE: Assessment of insulin resistance and its role in non-insulin-dependent diabetes mellitus. *J Lab Clin Med* 1984;**103**:497.

Goldman J et al: Effect of glyburide on metabolic control and insulin binding in insulin-dependent diabetes mellitus. *Diabetes Care* 1984;**7(Suppl 1)**:106.

Goldstein DE et al: Clinical application of glycosylated hemoglobin measurements. *Diabetes* 1982;**31(Suppl 3)**:70.

Herman WH et al: An approach to the prevention of blindness in diabetes. *Diabetes Care* 1983;**6**:608.

Kadowaki T et al: Chlorpropamide-induced hyponatremia: Incidence and risk factors. *Diabetes Care* 1983;**6**:468.

Kereiakes DJ et al: The heart in diabetes. *West J Med* 1984;**140**:583.

Knowles HC Jr: Long-term juvenile diabetes treated with unmeasured diet. *Trans Assoc Am Physicians* 1971;**84**:95.

Kolterman OG et al: The acute and chronic effects of sulfonylurea therapy in type II diabetic subjects. *Diabetes* 1984;**33**:346.

Lauritzen T et al: Effect of 1 year of near-normal blood glucose levels on retinopathy in insulin-dependent diabetics. *Lancet* 1983;**1**:200.

Mirouze J: Insulin treatment: A non-stop revolution. *Diabetologia* 1983;**25**:209.

Murphy J et al: Conservative management of pregnancy in diabetic women. *Br Med J* 1984;**288**:1203.

Nolte MS et al: Reduced solubility of short-acting soluble insulins when mixed with longer-acting insulins. *Diabetes* 1983;**32**:1177.

Nuttal FQ: Diet and the diabetic patient. *Diabetes Care* 1983;**6**:197.

Peden N, Newton RW, Feely J: Oral hypoglycemic agents. *Br Med J* 1983;**286**:1564.

Pfeifer MA et al: Acute and chronic effects of sulfonylurea drugs on pancreatic islet function in man. *Diabetes Care* 1984;**7(Suppl 1)**:25.

Polonsky KS, Rubenstein AH: C-peptide as a measure of the secretion and hepatic extraction of insulin: Pitfalls and limitations. *Diabetes* 1984;**33**:486.

Reeves ML et al: Comparison of methods for blood glucose monitoring. *Diabetes Care* 1981;**4**:404.

Revers RR et al: Lack of in vivo insulin resistance in controlled insulin-dependent type I diabetic patients. *J Clin Endocrinol Metab* 1984;**58**:353.

Richter EA, Ruderman NB, Schneider SH: Diabetes and exercise. *Am J Med* 1981;**70**:201.

Rosenbloom AL et al: Limited joint mobility in childhood diabetes: Family studies. *Diabetes Care* 1983;**6**:370.

Sidenius P: The axonopathy of diabetic neuropathy. *Diabetes* 1982;**31**:356.

Sutherland DER et al: Improved patient and primary renal allograft survival in uremic diabetic recipients. *Transplantation* 1982;**34**:319.

Tager HS: Abnormal products of the human insulin gene. *Diabetes* 1984;**33**:693.

Unger RH: Special comment: Meticulous control of diabetes: Benefits, risks, and precautions. *Diabetes* 1982;**31**:479.

Viberti G, Keen H: The patterns of proteinuria in diabetes mellitus: Relevance to pathogenesis and prevention of diabetic nephropathy. *Diabetes* 1984;**33**:686.

Ward JD: The diabetic leg. *Diabetologia* 1982;**22**:141.

DIABETIC COMA

Coma may be due to a variety of causes not directly related to diabetes, eg, cerebrovascular accidents, alcohol or other drug toxicity, and head trauma. However, certain major causes of coma directly related to diabetes require differentiation: (1) Hypoglycemic coma resulting from excessive doses of insulin or oral hypoglycemic agents. (2) Hyperglycemic coma associated with either severe insulin deficiency (diabetic ketoacidosis) or mild to moderate insulin deficiency (hyperglycemic nonketotic hyperosmolar coma). (3) Lactic acidosis associated with diabetes, particularly when phenformin is administered to patients with renal insufficiency or taken during suicide attempts, and in diabetics stricken with severe infections or cardiovascular collapse.

A careful physical examination is essential to resolve the differential diagnosis. Patients in deep coma due to hypoglycemia are generally flaccid and hypothermic and have quiet breathing—in contrast to patients with acidosis, who appear dehydrated and whose respirations are rapid and deep if the pH of

arterial blood has dropped to 7.1 or less. The laboratory remains the final arbiter in confirming the diagnosis, but a rapid estimation can be made of blood glucose concentration with paper strips (Chemstrips bG, Visidex, or Dextrostix) and of plasma ketones with either crushed Acetest tablets or Ketostix paper strips.

Adrogué HJ et al: Plasma acid-base patterns in diabetic ketoacidosis. *N Engl J Med* 1982;**307**:1603.

Cohen RD, Woods HF: Lactic acidosis revisited. *Diabetes* 1983;**32**:181.

Fisher JN, Kitabchi AE: A randomized study of phosphate therapy in the treatment of diabetic ketoacidosis. *J Clin Endocrinol Metab* 1983;**57**:177.

Flexner CW et al: Repeated hospitalization for diabetic ketoacidosis: The game of "Sartoris." *Am J Med* 1984;**76**:691.

Foster DW, McGarry JD: The metabolic derangements and treatment of diabetic ketoacidosis. *N Engl J Med* 1983;**309**:159.

Fulop M: The treatment of severely uncontrolled diabetes mellitus. *Adv Intern Med* 1984;**29**:327.

Kreisberg RA: Pathogenesis and management of lactic acidosis. *Annu Rev Med* 1984;**35**:181.

Lever E, Jaspan JB: Sodium bicarbonate therapy in severe diabetic ketoacidosis. *Am J Med* 1983;**75**:263.

Park R, Arieff AI: Lactic acidosis: Current concepts. *Clin Endocrinol Metab* 1983;**12**:339.

Peden NR, Braaten JT, McKendry JBR: Diabetic ketoacidosis during long-term treatment with continuous subcutaneous insulin infusion. *Diabetes Care* 1984;**7**:1.

Schade DS, Eaton RP: Diabetic ketoacidosis: Pathogenesis, prevention and therapy. *Clin Endocrinol Metab* 1983;**12**:321.

1. DIABETIC KETOACIDOSIS

Diabetic ketoacidosis may be the initial manifestation of type I diabetes or may result from increased insulin requirements in type I diabetes patients during the course of infection, trauma, or surgery. Recently, diabetic ketoacidosis has been found to be one of the

Table 20-5. Laboratory diagnosis of coma in diabetic patients.

	Urine		Plasma		
	Sugar	Acetone	Glucose	Bicarbonate	Acetone
Related to diabetes					
Hypoglycemia	0*	0 or +	Low	Normal	0
Diabetic ketoacidosis	++++	++++	High	Low	++++
Hyperglycemic nonketotic	++++	0	High	Normal or slightly low	0
Lactic acidosis	0 or +	0 or +	Normal or low or high	Low	0 or +
Unrelated to diabetes					
Alcohol or other toxic drugs	0 or +	0 or +	May be low	Normal or low†	0 or +
Cerebrovascular accident or head trauma	+ or 0	0	Often high	Normal	0
Uremia	0 or +	0	High or normal	Low	0 or +

*Leftover urine in bladder might still contain sugar from earlier hyperglycemia.
†Alcohol can elevate plasma lactate as well as ketoacids to reduce pH.

more common serious complications of insulin pump therapy, occurring in approximately one per 80 patient months of treatment. Many patients who monitor capillary blood glucose regularly ignore urine ketone measurements, which would signal the possibility of insulin leakage or pump failure before serious illness develops. Poor compliance, either for psychologic reasons or because of inadequate patient education, is one of the most common causes of diabetic ketoacidosis, particularly when episodes are recurrent.

Clinical Findings

A. Symptoms and Signs: As opposed to the acute onset of hypoglycemic coma, the appearance of diabetic ketoacidotic coma is usually preceded by a day or more of polyuria and polydipsia associated with marked fatigue, nausea and vomiting, and, finally, mental stupor that can progress to frank neurologic coma. On physical examination, evidence of dehydration in a stuporous patient with rapid deep breathing and a "fruity" breath odor of acetone would strongly suggest the diagnosis. Hypotension with tachycardia indicates profound dehydration and salt depletion.

B. Laboratory Findings: Glycosuria of 4+ and strong ketonuria with hyperglycemia, ketonemia, low arterial blood pH, and low plasma bicarbonate are typical of diabetic ketoacidosis. Serum potassium is usually slightly elevated despite total body potassium depletion resulting from protracted polyuria or vomiting. Lipidemia may be present only if the rate of development of ketoacidosis was relatively slow (over several weeks or more of poor control). Elevation of serum amylase is common but often represents salivary as well as pancreatic amylase, thereby correlating poorly as an indicator of acute pancreatitis. Multichannel chemical analysis of serum creatinine (SMA-6) is falsely elevated by nonspecific chromogenicity of ketoacids and glucose. Most laboratories can correct for these interfering substances on request.

Pathophysiology

The 2 major metabolic aberrations of diabetic ketoacidosis are hyperglycemia and ketoacidemia, both due to insulin lack associated with hyperglucagonemia.

A. Hyperglycemia: Hyperglycemia results from increased hepatic production of glucose as well as diminished glucose uptake by peripheral tissues. Hepatic glucose output is a consequence of increased gluconeogenesis resulting from insulinopenia as well as from an associated hyperglucagonemia. Hyperglycemia produces an osmotic overload in the kidney, causing diuresis, with a critical loss of electrolytes and a disproportionate loss of free water in the urine with intracellular dehydration.

B. Ketoacidemia: Ketoacidemia represents the effect of insulin lack at multiple enzyme loci. Insulin lack associated with elevated levels of growth hormone and glucagon contributes to an increase in lipolysis from adipose tissue and in hepatic ketogenesis. In addition, there is evidence that reduced

ketolysis by insulin-deficient peripheral tissues contributes to the ketoacidemia. The only true "keto" acid present is acetoacetic acid, which, along with its by-product acetone, is measured by nitroprusside reagents (Acetest and Ketostix). The sensitivity for acetone, however, is poor, requiring over 10 mmol, which is seldom reached in the plasma of ketoacidotic subjects—although this detectable concentration is readily achieved in urine. Thus, in the plasma of ketotic patients, only acetoacetate is measured by these reagents. The more prevalent β-hydroxybutyric acid has no ketone group and is therefore not detected by conventional nitroprusside tests. This takes on special importance with associated circulatory collapse, wherein an increase in lactic acid can shift the redox state to increase β-hydroxybutyric acid at the expense of the readily detectable acetoacetic acid. Bedside diagnostic reagents would then be unreliable, suggesting no ketonemia in cases where β-hydroxybutyric acid is a major factor in producing the acidosis.

Treatment

A. Prevention: Education of diabetic patients to recognize the early symptoms and signs of ketoacidosis has done a great deal to prevent severe acidosis. Urine ketones should be measured in patients with signs of infection or in insulin pump-treated patients when capillary blood glucose is unexpectedly and persistently high. When heavy ketonuria and glycosuria persist on several successive examinations, supplemental regular insulin should be administered and liquid foods such as lightly salted tomato juice and broth should be ingested to replenish fluids and electrolytes. The patient should be instructed to contact the physician if ketonuria persists, and especially if vomiting develops or if appropriate adjustment of the infusion rate on an insulin pump does not correct the hyperglycemia and ketonuria. In juvenile-onset diabetics, particularly in the teen years, recurrent episodes of severe ketoacidosis often indicate poor compliance with the insulin regimen, and these patients will require intensive family counseling.

B. Emergency Measures: If ketosis is severe, the patient should be placed in the hospital for correction of the hyperosmolarity as well as the ketoacidemia. Severe hyperosmolarity correlates closely with central nervous system depression and coma, whereas prolonged acidosis can compromise cardiac output and reduce vascular tone; this contributes to circulatory collapse in the dehydrated patient.

1. Therapeutic flow sheet–One of the most important steps in initiating therapy is to start a flow sheet listing vital signs and the time sequence of diagnostic laboratory values in relation to therapeutic maneuvers. Indices of the metabolic defects include urine glucose and ketones as well as arterial pH, plasma glucose, acetone, bicarbonate, and electrolytes. One physician should be responsible for maintaining this therapeutic flow sheet and prescribing therapy. An indwelling catheter is required in all comatose patients but should be avoided if possible in a fully cooperative diabetic because of the risk of introducing bladder infection. Fluid intake and output should be carefully recorded, and details of the quantity and composition of all fluids and medications should be listed carefully. Gastric intubation and lavage with sodium bicarbonate solution are recommended in the comatose patient with acidosis to correct any gastric retention that may lead to vomiting and aspiration. The patient should not receive sedatives or narcotics. Each case must be managed individually depending on the specific deficits present and subsequent responses to initial therapy.

2. Insulin replacement–Only regular insulin should be used initially in all cases of severe ketoacidosis, and it should be given immediately after the diagnosis is established. Replacement of insulin deficiency helps correct the acidosis by reducing the flux of fatty acids to the liver, reducing ketone production by the liver, and also improving removal of ketones from the blood. Insulin treatment reduces the hyperosmolarity by reducing the hyperglycemia. It accomplishes this by increasing removal of glucose through peripheral utilization as well as by decreasing production of glucose by the liver. This latter effect is accomplished by direct inhibition of gluconeogenesis and glycogenolysis, as well as by lowered amino acid flux from muscle to liver and reduced hyperglucagonemia.

Recent reports suggest that doses of insulin as low as 5–10 units/h, given either by slow intravenous drip or intramuscularly, are as effective in most cases as the much higher doses previously recommended and have even been claimed by some to be superior. For optimal effects, continuous low-dose insulin infusions should always be preceded by a rapid intravenous loading dose of 15–20 units of regular insulin to prime the tissue insulin receptors. During low-dose insulin infusion, at least 3.5 g of human albumin can be added to each liter of intravenous solution to avoid adsorption loss of insulin onto the container or tubing. However, without albumin, loss of insulin can be minimized if the first 50 mL of a 500-mL intravenous bottle containing 25 or more units of insulin are discarded prior to starting the infusion. A loading dose of 0.3 unit/kg body weight of regular insulin as an intravenous bolus followed by 0.1 unit/kg/h, either continuously infused or injected intramuscularly, is sufficient in most patients to replace the insulin deficit. If the plasma glucose level fails to fall at least 10% in the first hour, a repeat loading dose is recommended. Insulin therapy is greatly facilitated when plasma glucose can be measured within a few minutes of sampling. The availability of instruments for rapid and accurate glucose analysis (Beckman or Yellow Springs glucose analyzer) has contributed much to achieving optimal insulin replacement. Rarely, a patient with insulin resistance is encountered, and this requires doubling the insulin dose every 2–4 hours if hyperglycemia does not improve after the first 2 doses of insulin. One must be alert to the danger of anaphylactic shock in resistant patients requiring very high doses of insulin if it is given intravenously. Somatostatin's effective inhibition of growth hormone and glucagon secretion may be a valuable adjunct to insulin therapy in treatment of diabetic ketoacidosis, but it is seldom needed in patients without severe insulin resistance.

3. Fluid and electrolyte replacement–In most patients, the fluid deficit is 4–5 L. Initially, normal saline solution is the solution of choice to help reexpand the contracted vascular volume in the dehydrated patient, thereby improving renal capability to excrete hydrogen ions. The use of sodium bicarbonate has been questioned by some because of the following potential consequences: (1) Hypokalemia from rapid potassium shifts into cells. (2) Tissue anoxia from reduced dissociation of oxygen from hemoglobin when acidosis is rapidly reversed. (3) Cerebral acidosis resulting from a reduction of cerebrospinal fluid pH. However, these considerations are relatively less important in certain clinical settings, and 1–2 ampules of sodium bicarbonate (44 meq per 50-mL ampule) added to a bottle of *hypotonic* saline solution should probably be administered whenever the blood pH is 7 or less or blood bicarbonate is below 9 meq/L. Once the pH reaches 7.2, no further bicarbonate should be given, since it aggravates rebound metabolic alkalosis as ketones are metabolized. Alkalosis causes potassium shifts that increase the risk of cardiac arrhythmias. In the first hour, at least 1 L of normal saline should be infused, and fluid should be given thereafter at a rate of 300–500 mL/h with careful monitoring of serum potassium. If the blood glucose is above 500 mg/dL, 0.45% saline solution may be used after the first hour, since the water deficit exceeds the sodium loss in uncontrolled diabetes with osmotic diuresis. When blood glucose falls to 250 mg/dL or less, 5% glucose solutions should be used to maintain blood glucose between 200 and 300 mg/dL and insulin therapy continued every 2–4 hours until ketonemia has cleared. Glucose administration has the dual advantage of preventing hypoglycemia and also of reducing the likelihood of cerebral edema, which could result from too rapid a decline in hyperglycemia.

4. Potassium and phosphate replacement– Total body potassium loss from polyuria as well as from vomiting may be as high as 200 meq. However, because of shifts from cells due to the acidosis, serum potassium is usually normal or high until after the first few hours of treatment, when acidosis improves and serum potassium returns into cells. Potassium in doses of 20–30 meq/h should be infused within 3–4 hours after beginning therapy, or sooner if initial serum potassium is inappropriately low. An ECG can be of help in monitoring the patient and reflecting the state of potassium balance at the time, but it should not replace accurate laboratory measurements.

Because severe hypophosphatemia also develops during insulin therapy of diabetic ketoacidosis, some potassium can be replaced as the phosphate salt. These 2 ions must be replaced separately rather than as potassium phosphate alone, since the potassium need is several times that of phosphate. Replacing phosphorus ions too rapidly while meeting potassium requirements can precipitate serum calcium and induce tetany.

A significant therapeutic benefit of phosphate replacement has not been documented in at least 2 clinical trials. However, certain potential advantages have been demonstrated. Treatment of hypophosphatemia helps to restore the buffering capacity of the plasma, thereby facilitating renal excretion of hydrogen; and it corrects the impaired oxygen dissociation from hemoglobin by regenerating 2,3-diphosphoglycerate. To minimize the risk of inducing tetany from an overload of phosphate replacement, an average deficit of 40–50 mmol phosphate in adults with diabetic ketoacidosis should be replaced with intravenous infusion *at no greater rate than 3 mmol/h*. A stock solution available from Abbott Laboratories provides a mixture of 1.12 g KH_2PO_4 and 1.18 g K_2HPO_4 in a 5-mL single-dose vial representing 22 meq potassium and 15 mmol phosphate (27 meq).

Five milliliters of this stock solution in 2 L of either 0.45% saline or 5% dextrose in water, infused at 400 mL/h, will replace the phosphate at the optimal rate of 3 mmol/h and will provide 4.4 meq of potassium per hour. Additional potassium should be administered as potassium chloride to provide a total of 10–30 meq of potassium per hour, depending on the serum potassium levels. If serum phosphate remains below 2.5 mg/dL, a repeat 5-hour infusion of potassium phosphate at a rate of 3 mmol/h would be reasonable. Although it remains controversial whether phosphate replacement is beneficial, the total body deficit can be safely replaced in the above manner without risk of tetany.

Foods high in potassium content can be prescribed when the patient has recovered sufficiently to take food orally. (Tomato juice and grapefruit juice contain 14 meq of potassium per 240 mL, and a medium-sized banana 10 meq.)

5. Treatment of associated infection – Appropriate antibiotics should be given if acute bacterial infection, often a precipitating cause, is present.

Prognosis

The frequency of deaths due to diabetic ketoacidosis has been dramatically reduced by improved therapy of young diabetics, but this complication remains a significant risk in the aged and in patients in profound coma in whom treatment has been delayed. Acute myocardial infarction or infarction of the bowel following prolonged hypotension has a high mortality rate. A serious prognostic sign is renal shutdown, and prior kidney dysfunction worsens the prognosis considerably because the kidney plays a key role in compensating for massive shifts of pH and electrolytes. Cerebral edema has been reported to occur rarely as metabolic deficits return to normal. This is best prevented by avoiding sudden reversal of marked hyperglycemia to hypoglycemia, since massive fluid shifts into cerebral tissue can occur as a consequence of osmotically active particles accumulating within neurons during hyperglycemia.

See references on p 778.

2. NONKETOTIC HYPERGLYCEMIC COMA

This second most common form of hyperglycemic coma is characterized by severe hyperglycemia in the absence of significant ketosis, with hyperosmolarity and severe dehydration. It occurs in patients with mild or occult diabetes, and most patients are at least middle-aged to elderly. Underlying renal insufficiency or congestive heart failure is common, and the presence of either worsens the prognosis. A precipitating event such as pneumonia, burns, cerebrovascular accident, or recent operation is often present. Certain drugs such as phenytoin, diazoxide, glucocorticoids, and diuretics have been implicated in its pathogenesis, as have procedures such as peritoneal dialysis.

Pathogenesis

A partial or relative insulin deficiency may initiate the syndrome by reducing glucose utilization of muscle, fat, and liver while inducing hyperglucagonemia and increasing hepatic glucose output. With massive glycosuria, obligatory water loss ensues. If a patient is unable to maintain adequate fluid intake because of an associated acute or chronic illness or has suffered excessive fluid loss (eg, from burns or therapy with diuretics), marked dehydration results. As plasma volume contracts, renal insufficiency develops, and the resultant limitation of glucose loss leads to increasingly high blood glucose concentrations. A severe hyperosmolarity develops that causes mental confusion and finally coma. It is not clear why ketosis is virtually absent under these conditions of insulin insufficiency, although reduced levels of growth hormone may be associated along with portal vein insulin concentrations sufficient to restrain ketogenesis.

Clinical Findings

A. Symptoms and Signs: Onset may be insidious over a period of days or weeks, with weakness, polyuria, and polydipsia. The lack of toxic features of ketoacidosis may retard recognition of the syndrome and delay therapy until dehydration becomes more profound than in ketoacidosis. Reduced intake of fluid is not an uncommon historical feature, due to either inappropriate lack of thirst, gastrointestinal upset, or inaccessibility of fluids to elderly, bedridden patients. Lethargy and confusion develop, progressing to convulsions and deep coma. Physical examination confirms the presence of profound dehydration in a lethargic or comatose patient without Kussmaul respirations.

B. Laboratory Findings: Severe hyperglycemia is present, with blood glucose values ranging from 800 to 2400 mg/dL. In mild cases, where dehydration is less severe, dilutional hyponatremia as well as urinary sodium losses may reduce serum sodium to 120–125 meq/L, which protects to some extent against extreme hyperosmolarity. However, once dehydration progresses further, serum sodium can exceed 140 meq/L, producing serum osmolarity readings of 330–440 mosm/kg. Ketosis and acidosis are usually absent or mild. Prerenal azotemia is the rule, with blood urea nitrogen elevations to 90 mg/dL being typical.

A convenient method of estimating serum osmolality is as follows (normal values in humans are 280–300 mosm/L):

$$mosm/L = 2[Na^+] + \frac{Glucose\ (mg/dL)}{18} + \frac{BUN\ (mg/dL)}{2.8}$$

These calculated estimates are usually 10–20 meq/L lower than values recorded by standard cryoscopic techniques in patients with diabetic coma.

Treatment

Fluid replacement is of paramount importance in treating nonketotic hyperglycemic coma. If circulatory collapse is present, fluid therapy should be initiated with isotonic saline. In all other cases, hypotonic (0.45%) saline appears to be preferable as the initial replacement solution because the body fluids of these patients are markedly hyperosmolar. As much as 4–6 L of fluid may be required in the first 8–10 hours. As long as blood pressure and urine output are maintained, hypotonic saline can be continued; however, as insulin therapy further lowers plasma glucose concentration, a reduced solute content of the vascular compartment may necessitate isotonic saline to avoid hypotension. Careful monitoring of the patient is required for proper sodium and water replacement. Once blood glucose reaches 250 mg/dL, fluid replacement should include 5% dextrose in either water, 0.45% saline solution, or 0.9% saline solution. An important end point of fluid therapy is to restore urine output to 50 mL/h or more.

With the absence of acidosis, there is no initial hyperkalemia; thus, much less potassium is lost in the urine during the initial stages of glycosuria. This results in less severe total potassium depletion than in diabetic ketoacidosis, and less potassium replacement is therefore needed. However, because initial serum potassium is usually not elevated and because it declines rapidly as a result of the sensitivity of the nonketotic patient to insulin, it has been recommended that potassium replacement be initiated earlier than in ketotic patients. Potassium chloride (10 meq/L) can be added to the initial bottle of fluids administered if the patient's serum potassium is not elevated.

When hypophosphatemia develops during insulin therapy, phosphate replacement can be given as described for ketoacidotic patients (at 3 mmol/h).

Less insulin may be required to reduce the hyperglycemia in nonketotic patients as compared to those with diabetic ketoacidotic coma. In fact, fluid replacement alone can reduce hyperglycemia considerably. An initial dose of only 15 units intravenously and 15 units subcutaneously of regular insulin is usually quite effective, and in most cases subsequent doses need not be greater than 10–25 units subcutaneously every 4 hours.

Prognosis

The overall mortality rate of hyperglycemic, hyperosmolar, nonketotic coma is more than 10 times that of diabetic ketoacidosis, chiefly because of its higher incidence in older patients, who may have compromised cardiovascular systems or associated major illnesses. (When patients are matched for age, the prognoses of these 2 hyperglycemic emergencies are reasonably comparable. When prompt therapy is instituted, the mortality rate can be reduced from nearly 50% to that related to the severity of coexistent disorders. A blood urea nitrogen in excess of 90 mg/dL has a worse prognosis for recovery than a blood urea nitrogen below 50 mg/dL, perhaps reflecting the degree of hydration.

See references on p 778.

LACTIC ACIDOSIS

Lactic acidosis is characterized by accumulation of excess lactic acid in the blood. Normally, the principal sources of this acid are the erythrocytes (which lack enzymes for aerobic oxidation), skeletal muscle, skin, and brain. Conversion to glucose and oxidation principally by the liver but also by the kidneys represent the chief pathways for its removal. Overproduction of lactic acid (tissue hypoxia), deficient removal (hepatic failure), or both (circulatory collapse) can cause accumulation of excess lactic acid. Lactic acidosis is not uncommon in any severely ill patient suffering from cardiac decompensation; respiratory or hepatic failure; acute septicemia; acute infarction of lung, bowel, or extremities; leukemia; or terminal metastatic cancer. Hyperlactanemia has been produced by toxic overdoses of phenformin or alcohol. It has been reported with therapeutic doses of phenformin in patients with predisposing factors affecting lactate metabolism or phenformin disposal, eg, renal dysfunction, liver disease, alcoholism, or cardiopulmonary decompensation. With the discontinuation of phenformin therapy in the USA, lactic acidosis in patients with diabetes mellitus has become extremely rare.

Clinical Findings

A. Symptoms and Signs: The main clinical features of lactic acidosis are marked hyperventilation and mental confusion leading to stupor and coma. When lactic acidosis is secondary to tissue hypoxia or vascular collapse, the clinical presentation is variable, being that of the prevailing catastrophic illness. However, in the idiopathic, or spontaneous, variety, the onset is rapid (usually over a few hours), blood pressure is normal, peripheral circulation is good, and there is no cyanosis.

B. Laboratory Findings: Plasma bicarbonate and blood pH are quite low, indicating the presence of severe metabolic acidosis. Ketones are usually absent from plasma and urine or at least not prominent. The first clue may be a high anion gap (serum sodium minus the sum of chloride and bicarbonate anions [in meq/L] should be no greater than 15). A higher value indicates the existence of an abnormal compartment of anions. If this cannot be clinically explained by an excess of keto acids (diabetes), inorganic acids (uremia), or anions from drug overdosage (salicylates, methyl alcohol, ethylene glycol), then lactic acidosis is probably the correct diagnosis. In the absence of azotemia, hyperphosphatemia may be a clue to the presence of lactic acidosis. The diagnosis is confirmed by demonstrating, in a sample of blood that is promptly chilled and separated, a plasma lactic acid concentration of 7 mmol/L or higher (values as high as 30 mmol/L have been reported). Normal plasma values average 1 mmol/L, with a normal lactate/pyruvate ratio of 10:1. This ratio is greatly exceeded in lactic acidosis.*

Treatment

Aggressive treatment of the precipitating cause of lactic acidosis is the main component of therapy. An adequate airway and good oxygenation should be assured. If hypotension is present, fluids and, if appropriate, pressor agents must be given to restore tissue perfusion. Empiric antibiotic coverage should be given after culture samples are obtained in any patient in whom the cause of the lactic acidosis is not apparent.

Alkalinization with intravenous sodium bicarbonate to keep the pH above 7.2 is generally needed in the emergency treatment of severe lactic acidosis. Massive doses may be required (as much as 2000 meq in 24 hours has been used). Hemodialysis may be useful in cases where large sodium loads are poorly tolerated and is particularly useful when phenformin is the precipitating agent, since phenformin as well as lactate is dialyzable. Dichloroacetate, an anion that facilitates pyruvate removal by activating pyruvate dehydrogenase, reverses certain types of lactic acidosis in animals and may prove useful in treating some types of lactic acidosis in humans. Methylene blue, a redox dye, has not been as useful as early reports suggested. If hypoxemia is the precipitating factor, vigorous treatment is indicated.

Prognosis

The mortality rate of spontaneous lactic acidosis approaches 80%. It is slightly lower when lactic acidosis is due to potentially reversible causes such as phenformin, when alkalinization need be maintained only until the drug effect is dissipated. The prognosis

*In collecting samples, it is essential to rapidly chill and separate the blood to remove red cells, whose continued glycolysis at room temperature is a common source of error in reports of high plasma lactate. Frozen plasma remains stable for subsequent assay.

in cases induced by hypoxemia is that of the primary disorder that produced the tissue hypoxia.

See references on p 778.

THE HYPOGLYCEMIC STATES

Spontaneous hypoglycemia in adults is of 2 principal types: fasting and postprandial. Fasting hypoglycemia is often subacute or chronic and usually presents with neuroglycopenia as its principal manifestation; postprandial hypoglycemia is relatively acute and is often heralded by symptoms of adrenergic discharge (sweating, palpitations, anxiety, tremulousness).

Differential Diagnosis (See Table 20–6.)

Fasting hypoglycemia may occur in certain endocrine disorders, such as hypopituitarism, Addison's disease, or myxedema, and in disorders related to liver disease, such as acute alcoholism or liver failure. These conditions are usually obvious, with hypoglycemia being only a secondary feature. When hypoglycemia is a primary manifestation developing in adults without apparent endocrine disorders or inborn metabolic diseases from childhood, the principal diagnostic possibilities include (1) hyperinsulinism, due to either pancreatic B cell tumors or surreptitious administration of insulin (or sulfonylureas); and (2) hypoglycemia due to non-insulin-producing extrapancreatic tumors.

Postprandial (reactive) hypoglycemia may be classified as early (within 2–3 hours after a meal) or late (3–5 hours after eating). Early, or alimentary, hypoglycemia occurs when there is a rapid discharge of ingested carbohydrate into the small bowel followed by rapid glucose absorption and hyperinsulinism. It may be seen after gastrointestinal surgery and is par-

Table 20–6. Common causes of hypoglycemia in the absence of clinically obvious endocrine or hepatic disorders.

Fasting hypoglycemia
  Hyperinsulinism
    Pancreatic B cell tumor
    Surreptitious administration of insulin or sulfonylureas
  Extrapancreatic tumors
Postprandial (reactive) hypoglycemia
  Early hypoglycemia (alimentary)
    Postgastrectomy
    Functional (increased vagal tone)
  Late hypoglycemia (occult diabetes)
    Delayed insulin release due to B cell dysfunction
  Counterregulatory deficiency
  Idiopathic
Alcohol hypoglycemia
Immunopathologic hypoglycemia
  Idiopathic anti-insulin antibodies (which release their bound insulin)
  Antibodies to insulin receptors (which act as agonists)

ticularly associated with the dumping syndrome after gastrectomy. In some cases, it is functional and may represent overactivity of the parasympathetic nervous system mediated via the vagus nerve. Rarely, it results from defective counterregulatory responses such as deficiencies of growth hormone, glucagon, cortisol, or autonomic responses.

Alcohol hypoglycemia may occur after a period of fasting or within several hours after drinking ethanol in combination with sugar-containing mixers. In either case, blood ethanol may be below levels usually associated with legal standards relating to being "under the influence."

Immunopathologic hypoglycemia is an extremely rare condition in which anti-insulin antibodies or antibodies to insulin receptors develop spontaneously. In the former case, the mechanism is unclear, but it may relate to increasing dissociation of insulin from circulating pools of bound insulin. When antibodies to insulin receptors are found, most patients do not have hypoglycemia but rather severe insulin-resistant diabetes and acanthosis nigricans. However, during the course of the disease in these patients, certain anti-insulin receptor antibodies with agonist activity mimicking insulin action predominate, producing severe hypoglycemia.

1. HYPOGLYCEMIA DUE TO PANCREATIC B CELL TUMORS

Fasting hypoglycemia in an otherwise healthy adult is most commonly due to an adenoma of the islets of Langerhans. Ninety percent of such tumors are single and benign, but multiple adenomas can occur as well as malignant tumors with functional metastases. B cell hyperplasia as a cause of fasting hypoglycemia is not well documented in adults. Adenomas may be familial and have been found in conjunction with tumors of the parathyroids and pituitary (Wermer's syndrome; multiple endocrine adenomatosis type I).

Clinical Findings
A. Symptoms and Signs: The signs and symptoms are those of subacute or chronic hypoglycemia, which may progress to permanent and irreversible brain damage. Delayed diagnosis has often resulted in prolonged psychiatric care or treatment for psychomotor epilepsy before the true diagnosis was established. In long-standing cases, obesity can result as a consequence of overeating to relieve symptoms.

Whipple's triad is characteristic of hypoglycemia regardless of the cause. It consists of (1) a history of hypoglycemic symptoms, (2) an associated fasting blood glucose of 40 mg/dL or less, and (3) immediate recovery upon administration of glucose. The hypoglycemic symptoms in insulinoma often develop in the early morning or after missing a meal. Occasionally, they occur after exercise. They typically begin with evidence of central nervous system glucose lack and can include blurred vision or diplopia, headache, feel-

ings of detachment, slurred speech, and weakness. Personality and mental changes vary from anxiety to psychotic behavior, and neurologic deterioration can result in convulsions or coma. Sweating and palpitations may not occur with subacute hypoglycemia until a profound degree of hypoglycemia develops.

B. Laboratory Findings: B cell adenomas do not reduce secretion in the presence of hypoglycemia, and the critical diagnostic test is to demonstrate inappropriately elevated serum insulin levels at a time when hypoglycemia is present. A reliable serum insulin level of 11 μU/mL or more in the presence of blood glucose values below 40 mg/dL is diagnostic of inappropriate hyperinsulinism. Quantitation of insulin receptors is of no diagnostic use. However, the observation of reduced receptor concentration in these patients, as well as elevated levels of proinsulin, provides further insight into the variable hypoglycemic effects of hyperinsulinism among individual patients with insulinoma. Other causes of hyperinsulinemic hypoglycemia must be considered, including factitious administration of insulin or sulfonylureas. An elevated circulating proinsulin level is characteristic of most B cell adenomas and does not occur in factitious hyperinsulinism.

C. Diagnostic Tests:
1. Prolonged fasting under hospital supervision until hypoglycemia is documented is probably the most dependable means of establishing the diagnosis, especially in males. In patients with insulinoma, the blood glucose levels often drop below 40 mg/dL after an overnight fast. In normal male subjects, the blood glucose does not fall below 55–60 mg/dL during a 3-day fast. In contrast, in premenopausal women who have fasted for only 24 hours, the plasma glucose falls normally to such an extent that it must drop to values lower than 35 mg/dL (and to less than 30 mg/dL by 36 hours) to be significant. After 36 hours of fasting, premenopausal females normally achieve such low levels of glucose that clinical evaluation of this test for insulinoma becomes quite difficult. In these cases, however, the women are not symptomatic, presumably owing to the development of sufficient ketonemia to supply energy needs to the brain. Insulinoma patients, on the other hand, become symptomatic when plasma glucose drops to subnormal levels, since inappropriate insulin secretion restricts ketone formation. Moreover, the demonstration of a nonsuppressed insulin level ($\geq$ 11 U/mL) in the presence of hypoglycemia and of an *increasing* ratio of insulin to glucose (ie, glucose falls more rapidly than does insulin) suggests the diagnosis of insulinoma, since normal females show a falling insulin-to-glucose ratio during a fast. If hypoglycemia does not develop in a male patient after 72 hours of fasting terminated with moderate exercise, insulinoma must be considered an unlikely diagnosis.

2. Suppression of C peptide during insulin-induced hypoglycemia is the basis of a recently developed diagnostic test for insulinoma. This small peptide connecting A and B chains of insulin is released in

equimolar quantities with endogenous insulin and thus reflects endogenous insulin secretion, which cannot be directly monitored during insulin infusion. Whereas normal persons suppress their C peptide levels to 50% or more during hypoglycemia induced by 0.1 unit of insulin per kilogram body weight per hour, absence of suppression suggests the presence of an autonomous insulin-secreting tumor.

3. Stimulation tests with pancreatic B cell secretagogues such as tolbutamide, glucagon, or leucine are generally not needed in most cases if basal insulin is found to be nonsuppressible and therefore inappropriately elevated during fasting hypoglycemia. However, in occasional patients with a relatively fixed level of circulating insulin that is only barely inappropriate, stimulation may be helpful, bearing in mind that false-negative results can occur if the tumor is poorly differentiated and agranular.

Tolbutamide testing (1 g of sodium tolbutamide in 20 mL of water rapidly infused over 1–2 minutes) is hazardous and should be reserved for difficult diagnostic problems. Severe hypoglycemia may be avoided by performing the test only when plasma glucose is above 50 mg/dL and terminating it with glucose administration after 20 minutes. A rise in plasma insulin of 200 μU/mL or higher at 5, 10, or 20 minutes after intravenous tolbutamide in patients without obvious causes for hyperinsulinism (such as obesity or acromegaly) would strongly support the diagnosis of insulinoma. However, the greatest value of this test is in ruling out insulinoma in cases where the diagnosis seems unlikely from the clinical presentation. In these circumstances the test may be extended to 90 minutes under supervision; if plasma glucose rebounds from a hypoglycemic nadir at 30 minutes to the basal level by 60–90 minutes, and if peak insulin levels at 5, 10, and 20 minutes do not show a rise above 120 μU/mL, the diagnosis of insulinoma is unlikely and the patient may be spared prolonged fasting in a hospital setting.

Intravenous glucagon (1 mg over 1 minute) can be useful in ruling out insulinoma in patients with "borderline" fasting inappropriate hyperinsulinemia. A rise above baseline of 200 μU/mL or more at 5 and 10 minutes strongly suggests insulinoma, although, as with tolbutamide, poorly differentiated tumors may not respond. Glucagon has the advantage over tolbutamide of correcting rather than provoking hypoglycemia during the test period.

4. Glucose tolerance tests have not been of help in the diagnosis of insulinomas because the variable responsiveness of the adenoma to glucose gives a confusing variety of results. Most adenomas respond poorly to glucose, and a diabetic type of oral glucose tolerance test results. In the rarer tumors that release insulin in response to glucose, difficulty in maintaining blood glucose can be anticipated at surgery.

5. Pancreatic arteriography can occasionally locate tumors preoperatively, but because of the small size of B cell adenomas (1 cm or less in most cases), arteriography has an accuracy rate of only 20% and a false-positive rate of about 5%. CT scan has not proved helpful in the diagnosis of insulinoma because of its inability to distinguish small tumors within the pancreas. Percutaneous transhepatic pancreatic vein catheterization with insulin assay is currently proving useful as a means of localizing small insulinomas.

6. Factitious hypoglycemia may be difficult to document. A suspicion of self-induced hypoglycemia is supported when the patient is associated with the health professions or has access to insulin or sulfonylurea drugs taken by a diabetic member of the family. The triad of hypoglycemia, high immunoreactive insulin, and suppressed plasma C peptide immunoreactivity is pathognomonic of exogenous insulin administration. Demonstration of circulating antibodies supports this diagnosis in suspected cases. When sulfonylureas are suspected as a cause of factitious hypoglycemia, a chemical test of the plasma to detect the presence of these drugs may be required to distinguish laboratory findings from those of insulinoma.

Treatment

A. Surgical Measures: Operation is the treatment of choice, preferably by a surgeon who is experienced at mobilizing the pancreas and exploring adequately the posterior surface of the head and body as well as the tail. Blood glucose should be monitored throughout surgery, and 10% dextrose in water should be infused at a rate of 100 mL/h or faster. In cases where the diagnosis has been established but no adenoma is located, subtotal pancreatectomy is usually indicated, including the entire body and tail of the pancreas. Total pancreatectomy is seldom required now in view of the efficacy of long-term therapy with diazoxide in most patients with insulinomas. Recent development of the "closed loop" artificial pancreas permits monitoring of plasma glucose and infusion of dextrose. This not only protects against hypoglycemia but also may aid in determining whether all insulin-secreting tumors have been removed, at which time the dextrose infusion stops and blood glucose rises.

B. Diet and Chemotherapy: In patients with inoperable functioning islet cell carcinoma or in patients in whom subtotal removal of the pancreas has failed to produce cure, reliance on frequent feedings is necessary. Since most tumors are not responsive to glucose, carbohydrate feedings every 2–3 hours are usually effective in preventing hypoglycemia, although obesity may become a problem. Glucagon should be available for emergency use as indicated in the discussion of treatment of diabetes. Diazoxide, 300–600 mg daily orally, has been useful with concomitant thiazide diuretic therapy to control sodium retention characteristic of diazoxide. Streptozocin is useful in decreasing insulin secretion in islet cell carcinomas, and effective doses have been achieved without the undue renal toxicity that characterized early experience.

Prognosis

When insulinoma is diagnosed early and cured

surgically, complete recovery is likely, although brain damage following severe hypoglycemia is not reversible. A significant increase in survival rate has been shown in streptozocin-treated patients with islet cell carcinoma, with reduction in tumor mass as well as decreased hyperinsulinism.

2. HYPOGLYCEMIA DUE TO EXTRAPANCREATIC TUMORS

These rare causes of hypoglycemia include mesenchymal tumors such as retroperitoneal sarcomas, hepatomas, adrenocortical carcinomas, and miscellaneous epithelial type tumors. The tumors are frequently large and readily palpated or visualized on urograms.

Laboratory diagnosis depends upon fasting hypoglycemia associated with serum insulin levels that are generally below 10 μU/mL. The mechanism of these tumors' hypoglycemic effect remains obscure. Although they do not release immunoreactive insulin, it has been suggested that they may produce certain insulinlike substances similar to the somatomedins or growth factors.

The prognosis for these tumors is generally poor, and surgical removal should be attempted when feasible. Dietary management of the hypoglycemia is the mainstay of medical treatment, since diazoxide is usually ineffective.

3. POSTPRANDIAL HYPOGLYCEMIA (Reactive Hypoglycemia)

Postgastrectomy Alimentary Hypoglycemia

Reactive hypoglycemia following gastrectomy is a consequence of hyperinsulinism resulting from rapid gastric emptying of ingested food that produces overstimulation of vagal reflexes and overproduction of beta-cytotropic gastrointestinal hormones. Symptoms result from adrenergic hyperactivity in response to the hypoglycemia. Treatment is properly directed at avoiding this sequence of events by more frequent feedings with smaller portions of less rapidly assimilated carbohydrate and more slowly absorbed fat and protein. In addition, anticholinergic drugs such as propantheline, 15 mg orally 4 times daily, may be useful in reducing vagal overactivity.

Functional Alimentary Hypoglycemia

This syndrome is classified as functional when no postsurgical explanation exists for the presence of early alimentary type reactive hypoglycemia. It is most often associated with chronic fatigue, anxiety, irritability, weakness, poor concentration, decreased libido, headaches, hunger after meals, and tremulousness. However, most patients with these symptoms do not have hypoglycemia; furthermore, even in those who have documented early hypoglycemia, it is likely to be only a secondary manifestation of their nervous imbalance, with consequent vagal overactivity causing increased gastric emptying and early hyperinsulinism.

Indiscriminate use and overinterpretation of glucose tolerance tests have led to an unfortunate tendency to overdiagnose functional hypoglycemia. As many as a third or more of *normal* subjects have hypoglycemia with or without symptoms during a 4-hour glucose tolerance test. Thus, the nonspecificity of glucose tolerance testing makes it a highly unreliable tool for evaluating patients with suspected episodes of postprandial hypoglycemia. Accordingly, to increase diagnostic reliability, hypoglycemia should preferably be documented during a spontaneous symptomatic episode accompanying routine daily activity, with clinical improvement following feeding. Personality evaluation suggesting hyperkinetic compulsive behavior in thin, anxious patients, particularly females, supports this diagnosis in patients with a compatible history.

In patients with documented postprandial hypoglycemia on a functional basis, there is no harm and occasional benefit in reducing the proportion of carbohydrate in the diet while increasing the frequency and reducing the size of meals; however, it should not be expected that these maneuvers will cure the neurasthenia, since the reflex response to hypoglycemia may be only one component of a generalized primary nervous hyperactivity. Counseling and support and mild sedation should be the mainstays of therapy, with dietary manipulation only an adjunct. Oral anticholinergics have helped in certain advanced cases.

Late Hypoglycemia (Occult Diabetes)

This condition is characterized by a delay in early insulin release from pancreatic B cells, resulting in initial exaggeration of hyperglycemia during a glucose tolerance test. In response to this hyperglycemia, an exaggerated insulin release produces a late hypoglycemia 4–5 hours after ingestion of glucose. These patients are usually quite different from those with early hypoglycemia, being more phlegmatic, often obese, and frequently having a family history of diabetes mellitus.

In obese patients, treatment is directed at weight reduction to achieve ideal weight. Like all patients with postprandial hypoglycemia, regardless of cause, these patients often respond to reduced carbohydrate intake with multiple, spaced, small feedings high in protein. They should be considered early diabetics and advised to have periodic medical evaluations.

4. ALCOHOL HYPOGLYCEMIA

Fasting Hypoglycemia After Ethanol

During the postabsorptive state, normal plasma glucose is maintained by hepatic glucose output derived from both glycogenolysis and gluconeogenesis. With prolonged starvation, glycogen reserves become depleted within 18–24 hours and hepatic glucose output becomes totally dependent on gluconeogenesis.

Under these circumstances, a blood concentration of ethanol as low as 45 mg/dL (considerably below the California legal "under the influence" level of 100 mg/dL) can induce profound hypoglycemia by blocking gluconeogenesis. Neuroglycopenia in a patient whose breath smells of alcohol may be mistaken for alcoholic stupor. Prevention consists of adequate food intake during ethanol ingestion and avoidance of excess ethanol, which could lead to vomiting or anorexia. Therapy consists of glucose administration to replenish glycogen stores until gluconeogenesis resumes.

Postethanol Reactive Hypoglycemia

When sugar-containing soft drinks are used as mixers to dilute alcohol in beverages (gin and tonic, rum and cola), there seems to be a greater insulin release than when the soft drink alone is ingested and a tendency for more of a late hypoglycemic overswing to occur 3–4 hours later. Prevention would consist of avoiding sugar mixers while ingesting alcohol or ensuring supplementary food intake to provide sustained absorption.

5. IMMUNOPATHOLOGIC HYPOGLYCEMIA

This rare cause of hypoglycemia, documented in isolated case reports, may occur as 2 distinct disorders: one associated with spontaneous development of circulating anti-insulin antibodies and another associated with antibodies to insulin receptors, in which the antibodies apparently have agonist capabilities.

Hypoglycemia due to anti-insulin antibodies was first described in Japanese patients and since then has been reported in whites. The diagnosis is difficult to confirm, since most patients found to have "spontaneous" hypoglycemia due to anti-insulin antibodies are also found to have factitious hypoglycemia due to surreptitious administration of insulin. There are rare cases in which administration of exogenous insulin cannot be documented and antibodies to bovine or porcine proinsulin cannot be demonstrated (such antibodies would confirm factitious hypoglycemia). Both fasting hypoglycemia and postprandial hypoglycemia can result from mechanisms that may include the periodic release of pools of endogenous insulin bound to circulating antibody. Frequent small, spaced feedings have been helpful in management, but no specific therapy has been found for this poorly defined syndrome.

Hypoglycemia due to anti-insulin receptor antibodies is an extremely rare syndrome reported in only 6 patients with acanthosis nigricans and who also have had episodes of insulin-resistant diabetes. The hypoglycemia may improve spontaneously though it contributed to the deaths of at least 3 patients. Hypoglycemia was found to respond to prednisone but not to plasmapheresis or immunosuppression. The mechanism of hypoglycemia is attributed to an agonist action of the antibody on the insulin receptor. The balance between the antagonistic and agonistic effects of the antibody determines whether insulin-resistant diabetes or hypoglycemia occurs.

Berger M et al: Functional and morphologic characterization of human insulinomas. *Diabetes* 1983;**32**:921.

Daggett PR et al: Is preoperative localization of insulinomas necessary? *Lancet* 1981;**1**:483.

Hogan MJ et al: Oral glucose tolerance test compared with a mixed meal in the diagnosis of reactive hypoglycemia: A caveat on stimulation. *Mayo Clin Proc* 1983;**58**:491.

Johnson DD et al: Reactive hypoglycemia. *JAMA* 1980;**243**:1151.

Kahn CR: The riddle of tumour hypoglycaemia revisited. *Clin Endocrinol Metab* 1980;**9**:335.

Marks V, Rose FC (editors): *Hypoglycemia.* Blackwell, 1981.

Roche A, Raisonnier A, Gillon-Savouret MC: Pancreatic venous sampling and arteriography in localizing insulinomas and gastrinomas. *Radiology* 1982;**145**:621.

Service FJ (editor): *Hypoglycemia Disorders: Pathogenesis, Diagnosis and Treatment.* Hall, 1983.

Smith LH, Feingold KR: Hypoglycemia: A pitfall of insulin therapy. *West J Med* 1983;**139**:688.

Taylor SI et al: Hypoglycemia associated with antibodies to the insulin receptor. *N Engl J Med* 1982;**307**:1422.

Unger RH: Insulin-glucagon relationships in the defense against hypoglycemia. *Diabetes* 1983;**32**:575.

Williams HE: Alcoholic hypoglycemia and ketoacidosis. *Med Clin North Am* 1984;**68**:33.

DISTURBANCES OF LIPID METABOLISM

The principal circulating lipids in humans are of 4 types: (1) triglycerides, (2) free cholesterol, (3) cholesteryl esters, and (4) phospholipids. These are transported as spherical macromolecular complexes termed **lipoproteins,** wherein an inner core of hydrophobic lipids (triglycerides and cholesteryl esters) is encased by a membrane of unimolecular thickness consisting of various proteins (apolipoproteins, or simply apoproteins) in association with hydrophilic lipids (free cholesterol and phospholipids).

Classification of Lipoproteins

Specific differences among the various lipoprotein classes depend on the amount each class contains of each of the 4 lipids (this affects their size and density), and on the nature of the apoprotein in their membrane. These differences allow for classification of lipoproteins on the basis of ultracentrifugal density, with those containing mostly triglyceride being termed **very low density lipoproteins (VLDL)** and those containing mostly cholesterol called **low-density lipoproteins (LDL);** when the total lipid content is slightly less than the weight of protein in the membrane, the density is **high (HDL).**

When classified on the basis of their mobility on paper electrophoresis, LDL are termed betalipoproteins; VLDL, prebetalipoproteins; and HDL, alphalipoproteins. These 3 classes of lipoproteins are normally present in fasting sera. Chylomicrons constitute a fourth class, normally present only after ingestion of fat. These are of such low density that they float even without centrifugation, and because of their large size and proportionately low protein content, they fail to migrate on paper electrophoresis.

Metabolism of Lipoproteins

Chylomicrons, which carry ingested fat, and VLDL, which contain triglyceride converted from endogenous fatty acids and ingested carbohydrate, are transported in plasma to fat depots, where they are cleared by an enzyme, lipoprotein lipase, attached to capillary endothelium. The normal end products of both chylomicrons and VLDL are "remnant" particles of very low density that contain different B apoproteins in their membranes. The B apoprotein of chylomicron remnants (B-48) is smaller than that of VLDL remnants (B-100), and studies of apoprotein metabolism indicate that chylomicron remnants are completely metabolized by the liver, while VLDL remnants are further hydrolyzed by hepatic lipase, converted to LDL, and then returned to the circulation. Low-density lipoproteins are responsible for transporting cholesteryl esters to peripheral tissues where the transported cholesterol can be used for membrane synthesis, thus sparing these tissues in their endogenous production of cholesterol. High-density lipoproteins

contribute to lipid transport by assisting in activating the lipoprotein lipase as well as in facilitating the removal of cholesterol either from aging cell membranes or from tissue deposits by activating a circulating enzyme, lecithin-cholesterol acyltransferase (LCAT). This produces cholesteryl esters that are subsequently removed by the HDL and either recycled via remnant lipoproteins and LDL for resynthesis of cell membrane or taken to the liver for excretion as biliary cholesterol or bile salts.

Lipoprotein Disorders

An excess or deficiency of certain lipoproteins can result from primary genetic disorders or may be secondary to acquired metabolic dysfunction. Until more information becomes available to permit classification on the basis of cause, the use of electrophoresis to define various phenotypes has been accepted by WHO (Table 20–7). These phenotypes, together with their acquired (secondary) counterparts, probably include the main types of hyperlipidemia seen clinically. These "types" should not be considered disease entities but may be useful for determining the most rational therapy.

A. Primary Genetic Hyperlipoproteinemias:

1. Type I hyperlipoproteinemia (hyperchylomicronemia; Bürger-Grütz disease)–This autosomal recessive condition is the rarest form of familial

Table 20–7. Major categories of primary hyperlipidemia.*

Type	Lipoprotein Abnormalities and Defect	Appearance of Serum†	Cholesterol Elevation‡	Triglyceride Elevation‡	Clinical Presentation	Rule Out
I	Fasting chylomicronemia (due to lipoprotein lipase or apoprotein C-II deficiency). Rare.	Creamy layer over clear infranate	Elevated (to about 10% of triglyceride level)	Often 1000–10,000 or more	Creamy blood, lipemic retina, eruptive xanthomas, hepatosplenomegaly, recurrent abdominal pain; onset in childhood.	Pancreatitis, diabetes.
IIA	Hyperbetalipoproteinemia (lack of a cell surface receptor involved in degrading LDL). Common.	Clear	Usually 300–600 but may be higher	None	Xanthelasma, tendon xanthomas, accelerated atherosclerosis; detectable in childhood.	Hypothyroidism, nephrotic syndrome, hepatic obstruction.
IIB	Familial combined lipidemia (both LDL and VLDL elevation). Quite common.	Turbid	Usually 250–600	Usually 200–600	Relatively common. Severe forms are like IIA; milder forms associated with obesity or diabetes.	Same as IIA.
III	Dysbetalipoproteinemia (lipidemia due to excess of remnants; apoprotein E abnormality). Rare.	Turbid	Highly variable (from near normal to over 1000)	High variable (175–1500 in same patient)	Planar xanthomas, tuberous xanthomas appear in adult. Relatively uncommon. Hyperglycemia, hyperuricemia.	Hepatic disease, diabetes.
IV	Hyperprebetalipoproteinemia (delay in clearance or overproduction of VLDL). Common.	Turbid	300–800	200–5000	Most common, usually in adults. Eruptive xanthomas; accelerated vascular disease, mild glucose intolerance, hyperuricemia.	Nephrotic syndrome, hypothyroidism, glycogen storage disease; oral contraceptives.
V	Mixed lipemia (both chylomicronemia and VLDL); defects similar to I and IV. Rare.	Creamy layer over turbid infranate	300–1000	Usually 500–10,000 or more	Adulthood mainly; recurrent abdominal pain, eruptive xanthomas, hepatosplenomegaly.	Insulin-deficient diabetes, pancreatitis, alcoholism.

*Modified from Levy RI, Morganroth J, Rifkind BM: Treatment of hyperlipidemia. *N Engl J Med* 1974;**290**:1295.
†Refrigerated serum overnight at 4 °C.
‡mg/dL. Normal cholesterol, 150–250 mg/dL; triglycerides, < 150 mg/dL.

hyperlipoproteinemia and is characterized by massive chylomicronemia when a patient is on a normal diet and complete disappearance of the chylomicronemia a few days after fat is eliminated from the diet. Postheparin lipolytic activity is absent in the serum, indicating that the defect is a deficiency of lipoprotein lipase. Lipemia retinalis is seen when serum triglycerides exceed 2500 mg/dL. Serum cholesterol is often quite high, since it accounts for as much as 10% of the weight of chylomicron particles; however, LDL cholesterol is subnormal. Spurious hyponatremia may result from displacement of plasma water by high fat content during routine blood sampling. Pancreatitis is the major hazard, and patients with this disorder may not have accelerated atherosclerosis despite hypercholesterolemia. The diagnosis is suspected in children with recurrent abdominal pain, especially when hepatosplenomegaly is present. Eruptive xanthomas and creamy serum that separates into a creamy supernate and a clear infranate confirm the diagnosis.

Treatment consists of a fat-restricted diet (10–20 g daily), and the response is usually good.

2. Type IIA (hyperbetalipoproteinemia) – This disorder results from the presence of defective cell receptors in homozygotes and a lesser number of such receptors in heterozygotes; this interferes with clearance of betalipoproteins. This receptor defect also prevents normal feedback inhibition of cholesterol synthesis by cholesterol released after internalization of betalipoproteins. It is one of the commonest of familial hyperlipoproteinemias and is transmitted as an autosomal dominant, at least in the severe variety. Milder forms may be caused by dietary indiscretion. The major clinical manifestations of this disorder include an accelerated atherosclerosis, early myocardial infarction, and the presence of tendon xanthomas and xanthelasma. The diagnosis is based on hypercholesterolemia in the presence of clear serum after overnight incubation at 4 °C. Dietary restriction of saturated fat and cholesterol is seldom of help in severe cases; vigorous measures, including oral administration of combinations of bile acid–binding resins with either nicotinic acid or with inhibitors of hydroxymethyl glutaryl-coenzyme A reductase (Compactin) have recently been shown to restore serum cholesterol to normal in highly compliant patients. Jejunoileal bypass surgery has been reported to reduce serum cholesterol by 50% or more but in general, this procedure has produced discouraging results. Chronic plasma-exchange therapy is expensive and inconvenient but can lower cholesterol and reduce the size of xanthomas. In mild cases, dietary management alone may be satisfactory.

3. Type IIB (mixed hyperbeta- and hyperprebetalipoproteinemia) – This familial combined hyperlipidemia is quite common and often alternates with the IIA pattern in affected relatives. In some cases, hyperlipidemia is particularly sensitive to caloric intake and the composition of the diet and may represent several different disorders. When the combined pattern is present in affected members, both the

triglyceride/cholesterol ratio and the electrophoretic pattern are indistinguishable from those of type III disease, as is the character of serum turbidity after overnight incubation at 4 °C. Ultracentrifugal analysis confirms the diagnosis by showing both an LDL and a VLDL elevation, whereas in type III, a "floating beta" particle is obtained. Patients with this disorder are at high risk for coronary artery disease.

4. Type III (hyper-"remnant"-lipoproteinemia; dysbetalipoproteinemia) – This rare disorder results from absence of the apoprotein E_3, which normally activates hepatic lipase to clear chylomicron remnants and transforms VLDL remnants to LDL. In its place is an abnormal isoform (E_2) that binds poorly to hepatic lipase. This results in accumulation of lipoprotein remnants of intermediate density (IDL), which have flotation characteristics on ultracentrifugation in the lower range of VLDL but have the electrophoretic mobility of betalipoproteins (B-VLDL, or floating betas). A reduction in LDL concentration is a consequence of the impairment of VLDL-remnant catabolism and is characteristic of this disorder.

The genetic mode of transmission of dysbetalipoproteinemia suggests a mendelian-recessive trait; however, its expression as hyperlipidemia seems to require precipitating factors such as obesity or hypothyroidism. It occurs predominantly in adults and is rare in premenopausal women, since estrogens seem to reduce accumulation of the "remnant" particles. Patients are often obese and may have tuberous xanthomas, xanthelasma, and accelerated atherosclerosis. Planar xanthomas on the palms have been considered diagnostic. Treatment is especially gratifying in type III disease. Reduction to ideal weight in the obese patient and maintenance on a low-cholesterol diet may produce dramatic improvement, and total correction of hyperlipoproteinemia may result, especially in response to the addition of clofibrate, 1 g twice daily, to the dietary regimen. Estrogen therapy can also produce a dramatic increase in removal of these remnant particles, even though it does not affect the abnormal apoprotein E distribution.

5. Type IV (hyperprebetalipoproteinemia) – This type of lipemia is endogenous as compared to type I hyperlipoproteinemia and represents a failure in removal of prebetalipoproteins produced by the liver, either in normal amounts or excessively.

Since carbohydrate intake induces production of this lipoprotein from esterification of endogenous fatty acids, it has been termed carbohydrate-induced hyperlipemia. It is a common disorder, usually in adults, and often associated with caloric excess, obesity, and hyperuricemia. Chylomicronemia can occasionally develop, especially if alcohol or fat intake is excessive, and eruptive xanthomas may occur. Treatment is directed at weight reduction in the obese, avoiding high carbohydrate or alcohol intake and caloric excess. Although clofibrate, 1 g twice daily, is occasionally beneficial, recent concern about its long-term toxicity precludes its use in this disorder, where slight benefits do not justify the overall risk.

6. Type V (mixed lipemia)–This is a rare disorder wherein excessive prebetalipoproteins and chylomicrons are present. Onset is usually in early adult life and is characterized by recurrent abdominal pain, pancreatitis, hepatosplenomegaly, eruptive xanthomas, and glucose intolerance. The disorder is markedly aggravated by alcohol excess.

Therapy is similar to that for type IV except that fat restriction is necessary as in type I.

B. Secondary Hyperlipoproteinemias: In uncontrolled diabetes mellitus, circulating levels of lipoprotein are often elevated along with glucose. Since lipoprotein lipase is an insulin-dependent enzyme, elevated levels of both chylomicrons and VLDL result from diabetes in which insulin levels are low (insulinopenic diabetes) or ineffective (insulin-insensitive diabetes). Replacement of deficient insulin or restriction of caloric intake to restore effectiveness of endogenous insulin in obese diabetics facilitates clearance of these lipoproteins. In addition, when lipemia is resolving after insulin replacement in insulin-deficient diabetics, an increase of betalipoproteins inevitably follows clearance of the larger triglyceride-carrying particles because of the much longer half-life of the betalipoproteins. Hyperbetalipoproteinemia is commonly a consequence of hypothyroidism or mild forms of nephrotic syndrome.

Hyperprebetalipoproteinemia and mixed lipemia can result from hypopituitarism, lipodystrophy, renal failure with azotemia, severe hypothyroidism, hypergammaglobulin disorders, or advanced nephrotic syndrome (with serum albumin below 2 g/dL). These lipemic manifestations are seen in genetically predisposed persons with mild diabetes mellitus or hyperestrogenemia (as in pregnancy or with oral contraceptive therapy) or in those who use alcohol excessively.

Dysbetalipoproteinemia can become apparent during hypothyroidism and revert to a latent state with thyroid replacement.

In all cases of hyperlipoproteinemia, secondary forms should be ruled out before a diagnosis of primary genetic hyperlipoproteinemia is made.

Relationship of Lipoproteins to Atheroma
(See Fig 20–2.)

Studies suggest that the arterial wall intima is permeable to small molecular complexes in inverse proportion to their size. Elastin, a component of arterial wall, has a demonstrable affinity for apoprotein B, which is present on all lipoproteins except HDL. Accordingly, small lipoproteins such as HDL, LDL, and certain of the smaller VLDL and remnants may enter through defects and tears in the intimal walls of arteries, where all except HDL adhere to elastin, which retards their exit and allows their accumulation. This concept would explain why chylomicrons, owing to their large size, are not considered atherogenic in type I disorders despite severe hypercholesterolemia and why hypertension, aging, and hyperlipidemia, either individually or (especially) in combination, could exaggerate normal atherogenic processes.

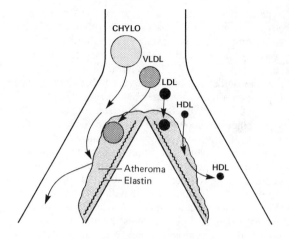

Figure 20–2. Lipoproteins and atheromas.

A number of recent studies have documented a consistent negative correlation between plasma concentration of HDL cholesterol and clinically evident atherosclerosis. In its transit through the wall of the artery, HDL may incorporate cholesteryl esters into its central core for recycling onto cell membranes or for transport to excretory systems in the liver. The presumed role of HDL in clearing cholesterol from tissues may account for the observed increase in risk of atherosclerosis when HDL levels are relatively low, as in obesity, diabetes, and hyperlipidemic disorders and in males, especially when physically inactive. Conversely, in persons with a lower than normal risk of atherosclerosis, such as chronic alcoholics, women of childbearing age, and marathon runners, there is a high level of HDL. The ''scavenger'' role of HDL in clearing cholesterol from tissues could slow down atherogenesis and thereby contribute to the apparent protective effect of high plasma HDL in relation to atherosclerosis.

Treatment

Treatment of the secondary hyperlipoproteinemias consists, where possible, of treatment of the primary disorder, eg, hypothyroidism, nephrotic syndrome, obstructive jaundice, or estrogen excess due to use of oral contraceptives. In primary hyperlipoproteinemia, no one diet is effective in all the lipid transport disorders. Similarly, none of the pharmacologic agents are universally effective. An understanding of lipid transport mechanisms and drug actions has improved the therapeutic approach to the hyperlipidemic patient.

A. Diet Therapy: When chylomicrons are elevated, total fat intake should be reduced (including polyunsaturated fats). In all other hyperlipidemias, certain general principles apply: Restrict calories to achieve or maintain ideal body weight, avoid alcohol, and limit daily cholesterol intake to 300 mg. Reduction of saturated fatty acids in the diet to no more than 10% of the total caloric intake is recommended, with a shift of the ratio of polyunsaturated to saturated fatty acid from the usual 1:5 to 2:1. Polyunsaturated fats improve palatability when saturated fats have to be restricted and may have a beneficial role in reducing platelet factors that promote an increased coagulability of blood.

Application of the above principles of diet to the general population as a means of reducing the risk of atherosclerosis remains a controversial subject, supported by most lipidologists and many cardiologists but rejected by others as an unproved hypothesis. In May 1980, the Food and Nutrition Board of the National Academy of Sciences reported that it found no reason for average healthy people to restrict cholesterol consumption or fat intake except to achieve or maintain normal weight.

B. Hypolipidemic Drugs: Three major classes of drugs are currently in use:

1. Nicotinic acid –Nicotinic acid reduces lipolysis and diminishes production of VLDL and is equally effective at lowering LDL. The dosage is 100 mg 3 times daily initially, gradually building up to a level of 3–7 g daily taken with meals. Cutaneous flushing and pruritus, as well as gastrointestinal upsets, are major side effects. It is particularly useful in primary hyperbetalipoproteinemia when combined with resins that bind bile acids, but it may be effective in all types of primary hyperlipoproteinemia except type I.

2. Clofibrate (chlorphenoxyisobutyrate) –Clofibrate has many known effects in the body and both decreases the synthesis of VLDL and increases its catabolism. It is most effective in type III remnant excess but is of occasional value also in disorders with increased VLDL (IIB, IV, V). In cases of hyperbetalipoproteinemia, its effects have been less impressive. The dosage is 1.5–2 g daily. Side effects are few, but myositis has been reported, especially if hypoalbuminemia is present, as in lipidemia associated with nephrotic syndrome. Pharmacokinetic interactions with anticoagulants may occur. A major risk is increased frequency of cholelithiasis and a possible association with gastrointestinal cancer. The National Collaborative Coronary Drug Project in the USA showed no beneficial effects of clofibrate on mortality rates in men recovering from myocardial infarction; in fact, more arrhythmias occurred in those receiving this drug. Although an international WHO study of 5000 men documented its slight efficacy in reducing the incidence of nonfatal myocardial infarctions, use of clofibrate was associated with a 36% greater mortality rate due to noncardiovascular causes. For these reasons, West Germany has banned the drug, and in the USA the FDA has recommended label revision to include a special warning on clofibrate's risk.

3. Resins to absorb bile acids (cholestyramine, colestipol) –Cholestyramine is an insoluble resin that absorbs bile acids and is thus able to increase cholesterol catabolism and enhance LDL removal. It is not very palatable, and 16–32 g/d is required in 2–4 divided doses, preferably in orange juice or applesauce. Gastrointestinal side effects, especially constipation,

are common. Similar doses of colestipol, a recently introduced resin, are as effective as cholestyramine while being more palatable. VLDL excess is not helped and may be aggravated by these agents. They are the drugs of choice in treating types IIA and IIB, particularly when combined with nicotinic acid. In a recent prospective cross-over trial of patients with type IIA hypercholesterolemia, combined therapy with colestipol and nicotinic acid resulted in complete and sustained normalization of LDL levels.

Hypolipoprotein Disorders

A. Tangier Disease (Deficiency of HDL): This autosomal recessive disorder is characterized by low plasma cholesterol, normal or elevated triglyceride levels, and enlargement of the tonsils, with distinctive orange-yellow deposits of cholesteryl esters. Other features include peripheral neuropathy, hepatosplenomegaly, and corneal deposits of lipid. HDL is deficient or absent.

VLDL and chylomicrons may be increased, since in the absence of HDL, the activation of lipoprotein lipase is reduced (one of the minor HDL apoproteins, apo-Lp-glutamic, is the activator of lipoprotein lipase). Because of its rarity, the prognosis of Tangier disease is poorly characterized.

B. Abetalipoproteinemia (Bassen-Kornzweig Syndrome): This rare disorder is characterized by inability to synthesize VLDL or chylomicrons. Accordingly, it presents a malabsorption of fat and is associated with thinness. Acanthocytosis has been found in all cases, and retinitis pigmentosa and ataxia are associated. Growth is often retarded. The diagnosis is confirmed by finding a plasma cholesterol below 80 mg/dL and triglycerides that are lower than in any other disorder and often undetectable. LDL is absent, as are VLDL and chylomicrons. The prognosis is poor, and progressive severe disability with muscular and skeletal deformities results. Fat-restricted diets are necessary, with medium-chain triglycerides recommended.

Hypobetalipoproteinemia, either on a genetic basis or acquired secondary to severe malabsorption, has also been described.

A recently discovered variant has been reported in which the B-100 apoprotein is not produced by the liver, so that only the gut-derived B-48 apoprotein is present. These patients are not cachectic, and they have normal plasma triglycerides but essentially absent LDL.

C. Familial Lecithin-Cholesterol Acyltransferase (LCAT) Deficiency: LCAT is a plasma enzyme responsible for transferring a fatty acid from lecithin to cholesterol to form a cholesteryl ester. HDL acts as the normal substrate for LCAT and provides a major source of lecithin. In LCAT deficiency, cholesteryl ester formation is impaired and unesterified cholesterol and phospholipids accumulate in the kidney, spleen, liver, arterial walls, and cornea. The prognosis is poor in this rare disorder because of severe renal failure and vascular degeneration.

Carlson LA, Böttiger LE: Serum triglycerides, to be or not to be a risk factor for ischemic heart disease? *Atherosclerosis* 1981; **39**:287.

Connor WE, Connor SL: The dietary treatment of hyperlipidemia. *Med Clin North Am* 1982;**66**:485.

Dobiasova M: Lecithin:cholesterol acyltransferase and the regulation of endogenous cholesterol transport. *Adv Lipid Res* 1983;**20**:107.

Eder HA, Gidez LJ: The clinical significance of the plasma high density lipoproteins. *Med Clin North Am* 1982;**66**:431.

Goldstein JL, Brown MS: LDL receptor defect in familial hypercholesterolemia. *Med Clin North Am* 1982;**66**:335.

Goldstein JL, Kita T, Brown MS: Defective lipoprotein receptors and atherosclerosis: Lessons from an animal counterpart of familial hypercholesterolemia. *N Engl J Med* 1983;**309**:288.

Havel RJ: Treatment of hyperlipidemias: Where do we stand? *Am J Med* 1982;**73**:301.

Kane JP, Malloy MJ: Treatment of hypercholesterolemia. *Med Clin North Am* 1982;**66**:537.

Kostner GM: Apolipoproteins and lipoproteins of human plasma: Significance in health and disease. *Adv Lipid Res* 1983;**20**:1.

Kreisberg RA: Lipids, lipoproteins, apolipoproteins, and atherosclerosis. *Ann Intern Med* 1983;**99**:713.

Mabuchi H et al: Reduction of serum cholesterol in heterozygous patients with familial hypercholesterolemia. *N Engl J Med* 1983;**308**:609.

Mahley RW, Angelin B: Type III hyperlipoproteinemia: Recent insights into the genetic defect of familial dysbetalipoproteinemia. *Adv Intern Med* 1984;**29**:385.

Malloy MJ, Kane JP: Hypolipidemia. *Med Clin North Am* 1982;**66**:469.

Norum KR et al: Transport of cholesterol. *Physiol Rev* 1983; **63**:1343.

Samuel P, McNamara DJ, Shapiro J: The role of diet in the etiology and treatment of atherosclerosis. *Annu Rev Med* 1983;**34**:179.

Schonfeld G: Disorders of lipid transport: Update 1983. *Prog Cardiovasc Dis* 1983;**26**:89.

Steinbrecher UP, Witztum JL: Glucosylation of low-density lipoproteins to an extent comparable to that seen in diabetes slows their catabolism. *Diabetes* 1984;**33**:130.

Zimmerman BR, Palumbo PJ: Lipid disorders and diabetes. *Diabetes Care* 1983;**6**:417.

• • •

References

Brownlee M (editor): *Handbook of Diabetes Mellitus.* (Vol 1: Etiology/Hormone Physiology; Vol 2: Islet-cell Function/Insulin Action; Vol 3: Intermediary Metabolism and Its Regulation; Vol 4: Biochemical Pathology; Vol 5: Current and Future Therapies.) Garland STPM Press, 1980.

Ellenberg M, Rifkin H (editors): *Diabetes Mellitus: Theory and Practice,* 3rd ed. Excerpta Medica, 1983.

Felig P et al (editors): *Endocrinology and Metabolism.* McGraw-Hill, 1981.

Hansen B (editor): *Controversies in Obesity.* Vol 5. *Endocrinology and Metabolism Series.* Praeger, 1983.

Havel RJ (editor): Symposium on lipid disorders. *Med Clin North Am* 1982;**66**:317. [Entire issue.]

Kaplan SA et al: Diabetes mellitus. *Ann Intern Med* 1982; **96**:635.

Keen H, Jarrett J (editors): *Complications of Diabetes,* 2nd ed. Arnold, 1982.

Kobberling J, Tattersal R (editors): *Genetics of Diabetes Mellitus.* Academic Press, 1982.

Lockwood DH, Gerich JE, Goldfine I (editors): Symposium on effects of oral hypoglycemic agents on receptor and postreceptor actions of insulin. *Diabetes Care* 1984;**7(Suppl 1)**:1. [Entire issue.]

Nattrass M, Santiago JV (editors): *Recent Advances in Diabetes:* Vol 1. Churchill Livingstone, 1984.

Peterson CM (editor): *Diabetes Management in the 80's.* Praeger, 1982.

Raskin P (editor): Symposium on diabetes mellitus. *Med Clin North Am* 1982;**66**. [Entire issue.]

Rifkin H (editor): *The Physician's Guide to Type II Diabetes (NIDDM): Diagnosis and Treatment.* American Diabetes Association, 1984.

Rifkin H, Raskin P (editors): *Diabetes Mellitus,* 5th ed. American Diabetes Association, 1981.

Schade DS et al: *Diabetic Coma: Ketoacidotic and Hyperosmolar.* Univ of New Mexico Press, 1981.

Schilfgaarde RV, Persijn GG, Sutherland DER: *Organ Transplantation in Diabetics.* Grune & Stratton, 1984.

Nutrition; Nutritional & Metabolic Disorders | 21

Milton J. Chatton, MD, & Phyllis M. Ullman, MA, RD

Nutrition is a science concerned with foods and their digestion, absorption, assimilation, and excretion. Foods provide for the production of heat and energy, the building and maintenance of tissues, and the regulation of body functions. In order for nutrition to be adequate, the qualitative and quantitative metabolic needs of the body must be met under varying conditions of growth, development, physical activity, environmental stress, and illness and during periods of pregnancy and lactation.

Diet signifies a group of foods essential for the maintenance of health. In **dietary therapy,** this group may be modified to eliminate nutrients perceived as detrimental to health. Prevention of disease by modification of diet is currently receiving considerable attention.

Malnutrition can result from dietary deficiency, imbalance, or excess. It may reflect biochemical alterations at every level of nutrition, ranging from variations in the composition of foods through the entire process of digestion, absorption, and ultimate utilization by the body at the molecular level (see p 816). Inadequate food supplies result in nutritional deficiency leading to marked physical and mental impairment in many persons throughout the world. Even where the food supply is adequate, nutritional deficiencies may occur among persons undergoing unusual stress (eg, persons working at heavy labor or in a hot, dry climate; athletes undergoing rigorous training; or persons who are elderly or ill) or when proper nutritional practices are not followed.

Nutritional Requirements

A well-balanced diet (USA) consists of 7 basic categories of foods: (1) breads, cereals, and starches; (2) fruits and vegetables; (3) meats and alternative proteins; (4) dairy products or alternatives; (5) fats and oils; (6) sugars; and (7) beverages (see Table 21–1). Selection of a wide variety of foods in each of these categories has been recommended. This diet may be altered by choice or circumstance yet remain nutritionally adequate if the correct combinations and quantity of natural foodstuffs are ingested. Individual requirements may vary considerably, particularly for certain groups such as young children, pregnant and lactating women, joggers, athletes, the elderly, and persons with medical illnesses. Unfortunately, as a result of poverty, ignorance in matters of food selection and preparation, dietary faddism, and confusion regarding the nutritive value of processed foods, total nutritional needs are often unmet. The presumed benefit of many of the so-called health foods, organic foods, and "natural" vitamins is unsupported by credible scientific evidence.

A rational look at the modern Western diet suggests that it would be advantageous to return to diets that have (1) more vegetable protein and less animal protein; (2) more complex carbohydrates (eg, whole grain breads, cereals, fiber), more naturally occurring sugars (eg, fruits and vegetables), and less refined sugars; (3) less total fat and cholesterol; (4) less salt; (5) and less alcohol. The diet should contain only sufficient calories to maintain desirable weight and should be supplemented with regular physical exercise.

The criteria for determining the nutritional adequacy of foods, therefore, are subject to continuous reappraisal. The quantity and quality of proteins, fats, carbohydrates, minerals, and vitamins may vary not only with the class of foodstuff but also with the specific type and source of food (see Tables 21–2, 21–5, and 21–6). Furthermore, the roles of food combinations, processed foods, chemical additives, new or unknown micronutrients, and food-drug combinations are receiving deserved attention.

Proteins

Proteins, sufficient in both quantity and quality, are indispensable in the daily diet to provide for growth and maintenance of active body tissues that are undergoing constant destruction and synthesis.

The quality ("biologic value") of the protein depends upon its content of essential (indispensable) amino acids. For example, dairy products and eggs contain all of the essential amino acids and are of high "biologic value"; meat, poultry, fish, and potatoes may be relatively deficient in certain essential amino acids and therefore have somewhat less "biologic value"; and cereals, breads, and most root vegetables taken individually have only fair "biologic value." Proper combination of foods that have only fair protein value, however, may result in adequate protein nutrition if all of the essential amino acids are provided.

Table 21–1. Basic food groups: The daily food guide.

Food	Nutrients Provided	Recommended Daily Amounts
Breads, cereals, and starches	Carbohydrate Protein Vitamin B complex Fiber	Four or more servings. One serving equals: 1/2 cup cooked potato 1 slice bread 1 oz (1 cup) ready-to-eat flake or puffed cereal 1/2–3/4 cup cooked cereal or rice 1/2–3/4 cup cooked pastes (macaroni, spaghetti, noodles) 5 saltines 2 graham crackers
Fruits and vegetables	Carbohydrate Protein Vitamins A, B complex, C Minerals (iron, calcium, phos- phorus, potassium, sodium, and trace elements) Fiber	Four or more servings, at least one to be a citrus fruit or to- mato daily and one to be a dark green or deep yellow vegetable. One serving equals: 1/2 cup vegetable or fruit 1 medium orange or apple 1/2 cup (4 oz) juice
Meats (beef, lamb, pork, veal, poul- try, game), fish, eggs, and legumes (dried peas, beans, lentils, nuts, and seeds)	Protein Fat Vitamin B complex Iron Trace elements Fiber (in vegetables, nuts, and seeds only)	Two or more servings. One serving equals: 3 oz cooked lean, boneless meat or fish (1/4 lb raw) 1/4 chicken or 1/2 cup cooked meat 2 eggs 1 cup cooked dry beans, peas, or lentils 4 tbsp peanut butter 1/2 cup cottage cheese
Milk and dairy products: Yogurt, cheese, ice cream, and any product made with milk (whole, low-fat, nonfat)	Protein Fat Carbohydrate Riboflavin Vitamin A Calcium	Adults: 1–2 cups (8–16 oz) Teenagers: 4 or more cups Children, 9–12: 3 or more cups Under 9: 2–3 cups Pregnant women: 3 or more cups Lactating women: 4 or more cups One serving equals: 1 oz cheese 1/2 cup cottage cheese 1/2 cup ice cream
Fats and oils: Butter, margarine, cream, oils, salad dressings, nuts, avocado	Fat Vitamins A, D, E	6–12 tsp or more per day depending upon caloric needs. At least 1 tbsp oil or margarine daily. One serving equals: 2 tbsp cream 1/8 avocado 6 small nuts
Sugars, syrups, honey, jellies, etc	Carbohydrate	As needed for caloric requirements
Beverages: Coffee, tea, carbonated sweet- ened or diet drinks, juices, alco- holic beverages (beer, whiskey, wine), water	Carbohydrate in juices and sweetened soft drinks only. Calories only in alcoholic bev- erages.	4–8 cups liquid per day. Limit beverages containing caffeine (coffee, tea, soft drinks) to 5 or fewer cups per day. See appendix for caffeine content.

Fats

Aside from the calories and the flavor they add to the diet, fats also provide essential fatty acids, energy storage, and transportation for fat-soluble vitamins. In the USA, fat provides about 40% of the total calories in the average diet, an amount many nutritionists consider to be excessive. It is now recommended that dietary fat be decreased to 30% of total calories. In large population groups throughout the world, fat consumption appears to be adequate at about 20%.

Qualitative differences in the type of fat in foods may be of importance in nutrition. Comparison of the relatively high content of saturated fats in coconut and palm oils and hydrogenated or solid vegetable short-enings with the high content of polyunsaturated fats in safflower oil and certain other unsaturated vegetable oils provides an example of qualitative differences in fats that may have a significant application to the dietary prevention and treatment of certain types of hyperlipidemia (see Chapter 20). Essential fatty acid (linoleic acid) deficiency, although uncommon in individuals who are able to take food by mouth, has been well documented in both infants and adults maintained on conventional fat-free solutions for parenteral hyperalimentation.

Carbohydrates

Carbohydrates are the principal dietary energy source for people throughout the world. They provide an efficient and inexpensive source of energy. They also serve a "protein-sparing" function (ie, they spare protein for vital functions other than energy produc-

Table 21–2. Nutrient content of foods.

Food Group	Average Serving Volume	Weight (g)	Carbohydrate (g)	Protein (g)	Fat (g)	Calories
Milk and dairy products						
Whole milk (3.4–4%)	1 cup	240	12	8	10	170
Low-fat (2%)	1 cup	240	12	8	5	125
Nonfat (less than 1%)	1 cup	240	12	8	–	80
Powdered, skim (dry)	¼ cup	20	12	8	–	80
Yogurt, buttermilk	1 cup	240	13	8	4	125
Ice cream	½ cup	75	14	3	7	130
Protein foods						
Lean meats, cooked	3⅓ ounces	100	–	31	17	277
Fish	3⅓ ounces	100	–	30	8	202
Poultry	3⅓ ounces	100	–	31	3–4	166
Cheese, cheddar type	1 ounce	28	1	7	9	113
Cottage cheese	½ cup	100	3	14	4	106
Egg	1	50	–	6	6	78
Vegetables						
Group A*	½ cup	100	3	1		16
Group B†	½ cup	100	7	2	–	36
Fruits (unsugared)						
All kinds	½ cup	100	10	0–1	–	40
Breads, cereals						
Bread, all kinds	1 slice	20	15	2	–	68
Cereal, prepared						
Dry, flake	¾ cup	28	13	2	–	60
Cooked	½ cup	120	13	2	–	60
Starches (cooked)						
Potatoes, rice, pastes	½ cup	100	16–20	3	–	76–92
Corn, dried peas, beans	½ cup	100	15	3	0.4–1	72
Fats and oils						
Butter, margarine	1 tsp	5	–	–	4	36
Cooking fats (shortening)	1 tsp	5	–	–	4	36
Oils (salad or cooking)	1 tsp	5	–	–	5	45

*Includes all leafy, watery type vegetables or those not listed in group B or as starches.

†Includes beets, carrots, onions, green peas, turnips, yellow squash, artichokes.

tion). It is usually recommended that a minimum of 40% of the total calories in the diet come from carbohydrates—cereals, starches, whole-grain breads, fruits and vegetables. Carbohydrates provide about 50% of the total daily calories in the USA, a percentage much less than that for many other countries and disproportionately high in refined sugars.

Calories

Caloric requirements vary considerably from person to person, in health and in disease. Even under basal conditions, different individuals may have unexplained differences in caloric need. The rate of energy consumption by healthy adults engaged in various levels of physical activity is shown in Table 21–3.

Table 21–3. Average energy calories expended per hour by adults at selected weights engaged in various activities.*

Activity	54 kg (120 lbs)	64 kg (140 lbs)	73 kg (160 lbs)	82 kg (180 lbs)	91 kg (200 lbs)	100 kg (220 lbs)
Sleeping: Reclining	50	58	69	78	86	99
Very light: Sitting	73	83	103	115	127	150
Light: Walking on level, shopping, light housekeeping	143	166	200	225	250	290
Moderate: Cycling, dancing, skiing, tennis	226	262	307	345	382	430
Heavy: Walking uphill, shoveling, swimming, playing basketball or football	440	512	598	670	746	840

Note: Range of rate of expenditure of calories per minute of activity (for a 70-kg man or a 58-kg woman): Sleeping—0.9–1.2; very light—1.5–2.5; light—2–4.9; moderate—5–7.4; heavy—6–12.

*Data from: *Recommended Dietary Allowances,* 9th ed. National Academy of Sciences–National Research Council, 1980. Adapted from McArdle WD, Katch FI, Katch VL: *Exercise Physiology: Energy, Nutrition and Human Performance.* Lea & Febiger, 1981.

Caloric requirements may also be significantly increased in hypermetabolic states (eg, fever, hyperthyroidism, burns); periodic monitoring of weight is essential when these disorders are severe.

Vitamins (See Table 21–4.)

There are wide individual variations in the requirements for vitamins. Markedly decreased as well as increased physiologic requirements have been described. Proposals to prevent or treat clinical disorders with massive doses of vitamins must be evaluated by the same rigorous clinical testing procedures required in the evaluation of new drugs. It should be recognized that large doses of some vitamins (eg, vitamins A, D, K, and niacin) are decidedly toxic to humans.

Trace Elements (See Table 21–5.)

Although the roles of iron, cobalt, iodine, zinc, and selenium are well recognized, the roles of copper, chromium, and manganese are not so clearly understood. Even more obscure are the roles of cadmium,

strontium, nickel, silicon, and molybdenum, which have been studied in lower animals.

Zinc is essential to nucleic acid metabolism and protein synthesis and plays a role in collagen formation, glycolysis, and oxidative phosphorylation. Manifestations of zinc deficiency include growth retardation, hypogonadism, altered sense of taste and smell, and poor wound healing. Zinc deficiency has been reported recently in patients with sickle cell disease. Both hereditary and acquired forms of acrodermatitis enteropathica, a serious skin disorder, have been found to be associated with a zinc deficiency that responds successfully to zinc supplements.

Copper deficiency may cause leukopenia, anemia, bone demineralization, and failure of erythropoiesis in malnourished infants; the deficiency is correctable by copper supplements. Manganese and chromium have been shown to be essential micronutrients in experimental animals, but deficiencies of these and certain other trace elements in humans are largely inferential at present.

Table 21–4. Food sources of vitamins.*

Vitamin	Recommended Allowances	Food Sources
Vitamin A activity	Men: 1000 RE†/d Women: 800 RE†/d Pregnant and lactating women: 1000–1200 RE†/d	Milk; butter; fortified margarines; liver; carotene precursors: carrots, sweet potatoes, apricots, cantaloupe, and yellow vegetables
Vitamin B$_1$ (thiamine)	Men: 1.2–1.4 mg/d Women: 1–1.1 mg/d Pregnant and lactating women: 1.4–1.5 mg/d	Enriched white and whole-grain breads and cereals, liver, meats, egg yolks, yeast, legumes, nuts
Vitamin B$_2$ (riboflavin)	Men: 1.4–1.7 mg/d Women: 1.2–1.3 mg/d Pregnant and lactating women: 1.5–1.7 mg/d	Milk, meat, liver, eggs, enriched white and whole-grain breads and cereals, yeast
Niacin equivalents‡	Men: 16–19 mg/d Women: 13–15 mg/d Pregnant and lactating women: 15–18 mg/d	Enriched white and whole-grain breads and cereals, liver, meat, bran, yeast
Vitamin B$_6$ (pyridoxine)	Men: 1.8–2.2 mg/d Women: 1.8–2 mg/d Pregnant and lactating women: 2.3–2.4 mg/d	Bananas, whole-grain cereals, chicken, legumes, egg yolk, most dark green leafy vegetables, most fish and shellfish, meats, organ meats, nuts, peanut butter, potatoes, sweet potatoes, prunes, raisins, yeast
Vitamin B$_{12}$ (cyanocobalamin)	Men and women: 3 μg/d Pregnant and lactating women: 4 μg/d	Present in foods of animal origin only: liver, kidney, meats, milk, most cheeses, most fish, shellfish, eggs
Folacin (pteroylglutamic acid, PGA)	Men and women: 400 μg/d Pregnant and lactating women: 500–800 μg/d	Green leafy vegetables, liver and organ meats, milk, eggs, dry beans, peas, peanuts, wheat germ
Pantothenic acid	Men and women: 4–7 mg/d	Liver, organ meats, eggs, peanuts, legumes, mushrooms, salmon, whole grains, citrus fruits
Vitamin C (ascorbic acid)	Men and women: 50–60 mg/d Pregnant and lactating women: 70–90 mg/d	Citrus fruits, tomatoes, parsley, green peppers, radishes, green leafy raw vegetables, melons, strawberries, cabbage, potatoes, kale, turnip greens
Vitamin D	Men and women: 5–10 μg cholecalciferol§/d Pregnant and lactating women: 10–15 μg cholecalciferol§/d	Butter, fortified margarines, milk, fish liver oils, saltwater fish, liver, egg yolk
Vitamin E activity	Men and women: 8–10 mg d-α-tocopherol**/d Pregnant and lactating women: 10–11 mg d-α-tocopherol**/d	Vegetable oils, margarines, salad dressings, whole-grain cereals, peanuts, wheat germ
Vitamin K	Men and women: 70–140 μg/d	Cabbage, cauliflower, spinach, other leafy vegetables, pork liver, vegetable oils

*Data from: *Recommended Dietary Allowances*, 9th ed. National Academy of Sciences–National Research Council, 1980.
†One retinol equivalent (RE) equals 1 μg retinol or 6 μg β-carotene.
‡One niacin equivalent equals 1 mg niacin or 60 mg dietary tryptophan.
§One μg cholecalciferol equals 40 IU.
**One mg d-α-tocopherol equals 1.5 IU.

As information accumulates about the possible effects of deficiencies of trace elements in the human diet, and with continued improvement in microchemical quantitation of trace elements, it seems likely that the nutritional importance of the trace elements will be more clearly established in the future. Data obtained from work with patients who receive prolonged therapeutic nutrition by intravenous hyperalimentation or amino acid formula diets will be especially helpful.

Influence of Drugs (See Table 21–6.)

The interaction of drugs and dietary factors was perhaps first recognized in the case of chronic alcoholism and vitamin B complex deficiency. It is now known that long-term therapy with many drugs may induce malnutrition through varied mechanisms, including appetite suppression, intestinal malabsorption, altered vitamin synthesis, increased nutritional requirements, and vitamin depletion. Folate deficiency may be caused by chronic alcoholism and by chronic use of oral contraceptives and anticonvulsants. The corticosteroids are known to deplete muscle protein, lower glucose tolerance, and induce osteoporosis. Vitamin K deficiency can be caused by oral antibiotics, especially if the diet is inadequate. It should also be mentioned that certain nutrients can either decrease the effectiveness of drugs (eg, pyridoxine reverses the antiparkinsonism effect of levodopa) or they can markedly enhance the toxicity of drugs (eg, tyramine-containing substances such as cheese, beer, and red wine can induce hypertensive crises in patients receiving monoamine oxidase inhibitors).

Causes of Malnutrition

Given an abundant available supply of nutritionally adequate food, many factors remain that can result in malnutrition. Examples are given below.

(1) **Failure to take the proper quantity and quality of foods to meet individual requirements:**
   (a) Economic.
   (b) Psychologic (anorexia nervosa, psychiatric disorders).
   (c) Psychosocial (dietary fads, "crash diets," reliance on snack foods).
   (d) Cultural (regional or national food habits).
   (e) Educational (ignorance of essentials).
   (f) Inability to obtain, prepare, and serve foods to self (elderly or physically handicapped persons).
   (g) Chronic alcoholism and drug addiction.
   (h) Iatrogenic (protracted use of unbalanced or restrictive therapeutic diets).
   (i) Anorexigenic drugs (amphetamines).

(2) **Inadequate intake of food because of gastrointestinal disorders:**
   (a) Anorexia following major surgery, especially gastrointestinal surgery.
   (b) Loss of sense of taste or smell.
   (c) Difficulty or inability to swallow food (neurologic or obstructive lesions).
   (d) Pain on ingestion of food (oral, esophageal, or gastric lesions).
   (e) Chronic nausea and vomiting.
   (f) Postgastrectomy dumping syndrome.
   (g) Afferent loop (postgastrectomy) pain.

Table 21–5. Food sources of minerals.*

Mineral	Recommended Allowances	Food Sources
Calcium	Adults: 0.8 g/d. Ages 11–18 and pregnant or lactating women: 1.2 g/d.	Milk (1 g calcium/quart), milk products, cheeses, leafy green vegetables
Phosphorus	Adults: 0.8 g/d. Ages 11–18 and pregnant or lactating women: 1.2 g/d.	Milk, whole-grain cereals, cheeses, legumes, eggs, meat, peanut butter, nuts, liver
Iron	Women: 18 mg/d.† Men: 10 mg/d.	Liver, meat, legumes, whole or enriched grains, potatoes, egg yolk, green vegetables, dried fruits
Sodium	100–300 meq/d or 2.5–7 g/d.	Table salt, seafoods, milk, vegetables, prepared foods
Potassium	50–150 meq/d or 2–6 g/d.	Meats, cereals, vegetables, legumes, fruits (particularly dried), cream of tartar
Copper	1–2 mg/d.	Liver, egg yolk, almonds, legumes, whole grains, oatmeal
Magnesium	300–450 mg/d.	Bananas, whole-grain cereals, legumes, milk, nuts, most dark green leafy vegetables, peanuts
Iodine	150 µg/d.	Iodized salt, seafoods, vegetables grown in iodine-rich soil
Chloride	0.5 g/d.	Table salt, seafoods, animal products
Sulfur	Adequate if protein intake is adequate.	Protein foods: Meats, fish, poultry, eggs, cheeses, milk
Zinc	15 mg/d.	Widespread in foodstuffs
Trace minerals (chromium, cobalt, manganese, molybdenum, selenium, fluoride)	Minute traces.	Leafy green vegetables, whole grains, fruits, legumes, meats, seafoods, organ meats

*Data from: *Recommended Dietary Allowances*, 9th ed. National Academy of Sciences–National Research Council, 1980; and *Nutritive Value of Foods*. Home & Garden Bulletin No. 72 (revised). US Department of Agriculture, 1977.

†Supplemental iron recommended during pregnancy.

(3) Defective absorption or utilization of food because of gastrointestinal disorders:
  (a) Chronic diarrhea due to any cause.
  (b) Malabsorption syndromes (postsurgical short bowel, with loss of mucosal surface and bile salt depletion; hepatic insufficiency, pancreatic insufficiency, tropical and nontropical sprue, lactase deficiency).
  (c) Protein-losing enteropathy.
  (d) Intestinal parasitism.
  (e) Interference by drugs (eg, antacids).
(4) Increased need for food:
  (a) Increased physical activity (heavy labor or exercise).
  (b) Chronic febrile states.
  (c) Increased metabolism (hyperthyroidism).
  (d) Abnormal excretion (impairment of renal function).
(5) Impaired metabolism of nutrients:
  (a) Hereditary biochemical disorders.

  (b) Acquired biochemical disorders (liver damage, drugs).
(6) Interaction of drugs and nutrients.

The human diet, therefore, must meet the caloric needs and the quantitative and qualitative nutrient requirements of the individual based upon age, weight, physical activity, pregnancy, lactation, state of health, intake of alcohol, and medications. Special therapeutic diets may be necessary to correct acquired or hereditary nutritional and metabolic abnormalities. In certain instances when patients are unable to take food by mouth, enteral or parenteral alimentation may be necessary.

Nutrition of Cancer Patients
Patients with cancer may develop malnutrition as a result of almost any of the effects (frequently multiple) mentioned in the above outline. The nutritional status of cancer patients can be adversely affected not only by the local and systemic effects of the neoplasm

Table 21-6. Effect of drugs on nutrient absorption and metabolism.*

Drug	Effect
Antacids	
Aluminum antacids	Decrease absorption of phosphate.
Others	Alkaline destruction of thiamine; some decrease absorption of vitamin A, iron; steatorrhea.
Anticonvulsants	
Phenobarbital	Decreases serum folate, vitamins B_6, B_{12}; increases catabolism of vitamin D and metabolites.
Phenytoin	Decreases serum folate, vitamins B_6, B_{12}, calcium; increases catabolism of vitamin D and metabolites.
Primidone	Decreases serum folate, vitamins B_6, B_{12}; decreases calcium absorption; increases catabolism of vitamin D and metabolites.
Antimicrobials	
Neomycin	Binds bile acids; decreases absorption of fat, carotene, vitamins A, D, K, B_{12}, potassium, sodium, calcium, nitrogen.
Salicylazosulfapyridine	Decreases absorption of folate.
Aminosalicylic acid	Decreases absorption of folate, vitamin B_{12}, iron, cholesterol, fat.
Chloramphenicol	Increases need for vitamins B_2, B_6, B_{12}.
Penicillin	Hypokalemia; renal potassium wasting.
Tetracycline	Decreases absorption of fat, amino acids, calcium, iron, magnesium, zinc.
Cycloserine	May decrease absorption of calcium, magnesium; may decrease serum folate, vitamins B_6, B_{12}; decreases protein synthesis.
Isoniazid	Vitamin B_6 deficiency.
Sulfonamides	Decrease absorption of folate; decrease serum folate, iron.
Nitrofurantoin	Decreases serum folate.
Antimitotics	
Methotrexate	Decreases absorption of folate, vitamin B_{12}.
Colchicine	Decreases absorption of vitamin B_{12}, carotene, fat, sodium, potassium, cholesterol, lactose, nitrogen.
Cathartics	
Phenolphthalein	Malabsorption, hypokalemia, deficiency of vitamin D, calcium.
Mineral oil	Malabsorption, decreased absorption of vitamins A, D, K.
Diuretics	Some cause hypokalemia, hypomagnesemia; may increase urinary excretion of vitamins B_1, B_6, calcium, magnesium, potassium.
Hypocholesterolemics	
Cholestyramine	Binds bile acids; decreases absorption of fat, carotene, vitamins A, D, K, B_{12}, folate, iron.
Clofibrate	Decreases absorption of carotene, vitamine B_{12}, iron, glucose.
Hypotensives	
Hydralazine	Vitamin B_6 deficiency.
Oral contraceptives	Vitamin B_6, folate deficiency; may increase the need for other nutrients.

*Reproduced, with permission, from Thiele VF: *Clinical Nutrition,* 2nd ed. Mosby, 1980.

(eg, anorexia, obstruction, malabsorption, hemorrhage, electrolyte losses) but also by the effects of treatment. Most cancer patients, therefore, need some dietary modifications depending upon the cancer site and the method of treatment. Enteral and parenteral nutritional preparations as well as oral feedings may be required to provide sufficient calories, protein, essential fatty acids, minerals, and vitamins to correct nutritional deficiencies. Periodic clinical and laboratory monitoring of the nutritional status of the cancer patient can help enhance the effects of treatment as well as maintain the patient's emotional well-being. Cancer patients in a good nutritional state are known to have fewer complications and can better tolerate treatment than those patients who are malnourished.

Diet & Carcinogenesis

Interest in the epidemiology of cancer has focused on the possible role of diet and nutrition in causing, altering susceptibility to, or preventing cancer. Dietary variables that have been considered include qualitative and quantitative characteristics of natural foodstuffs; influence of diet on gastrointestinal absorption, motility, and bacterial flora; preparation and serving of foodstuffs; chemical contamination of food; and food additives.

Chronic caloric restriction has been shown to inhibit carcinogenesis and tumor growth in experimental animals. Epidemiologic studies in humans have shown significant increase in the frequency of certain forms of cancer in obese individuals. Increased dietary fat consumption has also been correlated with a higher incidence of certain types of human cancer (eg, large bowel). Data regarding the alleged carcinogenicity of low-cholesterol (high–polyunsaturated fatty acid) diets are contradictory. Sources of nitrites may be of concern because of the potential conversion to carcinogenic nitrosamines. Diethylstilbestrol, red dye 2, artificial sweeteners, and certain other additives and contaminants are known to have carcinogenic properties in experimental animals, but there is little proof that they cause cancer in humans. Common sense, however, dictates avoiding the unnecessary alteration of foods with chemicals if safety factors are in question. It is apparent that further scientific studies are required to elucidate the possible role of the many dietary and nutritional factors in carcinogenesis.

Nutrition of the Older Patient

The rapidly growing population of individuals in the USA who are more than 65 years of age has led to increased interest in special problems pertaining to the nutritional status of older persons. Changes in dietary needs and habits occur for a wide variety of medical, social, and economic reasons. Although there is considerable individual variation, health factors that influence the nutrition of older persons may include the following alterations: poor appetite; defective oral health (eg, poor teeth, dry mouth); impairment of taste, smell, and vision; decreased gastrointestinal absorption and motility; decreased metabolism; impaired

mobility and decreased physical activity; pain and disease; use of multiple medications (including alcohol); psychologic problems; and intellectual deterioration. Social isolation, depression, and economic limitations frequently compound the problems of normal and abnormal changes associated with aging.

Nutrients most frequently deficient in diets of persons past 59 years of age are calcium, iron, and vitamin A. The most common nutritional problem is obesity, with a larger proportion of women than men in the overweight group. Low levels of hemoglobin and of serum albumin, vitamin D, ascorbic acid, and folate have been reported in many studies of elderly persons.

Identification and assessment of nutritional problems of the older patient must take into consideration the complex of medical and psychosocial problems and the functional status of each individual. Avoid rigid adherence to stereotyped concepts of geriatric nutrition that fail to take into account personal likes and dislikes.

Ames BN: Dietary carcinogens and anticarcinogens: Oxygen radicals and degenerative diseases. *Science* 1983;**221**:1256.

Boles JM et al: Nutritional status in intensive care patients: Evaluation in 84 unselected patients. *Crit Care Med* 1983; **11**:87.

Finch CA, Huchberg H: Perspectives in iron metabolism. *N Engl J Med* 1982;**306**:1520.

Goodwin JS, Goodwin JM, Garry PJ: Association between nutritional status and cognitive functioning in a healthy elderly population. *JAMA* 1983;**249**:2917.

Jackson AA: Aminoacids: Essential and non-essential? *Lancet* 1983;**1**:1034.

Manjarrez C, Bisser R: Nutrition and athletic performance. *Am Fam Physician* (Nov) 1983;**28**:105.

Meguid MM et al: Nutritional support in cancer. (Letter.) *Lancet* 1983;**2**:230.

Morgan MY: Alcohol and nutrition. *Br Med J* 1982;**38**:21.

Morrison SD: Nutrition and longevity. *Nutr Rev* 1983;**41**:133.

Munro HN: Nutritional requirements in the elderly. *Arch Intern Med* 1983;**143**:1200.

National Research Council: *Diet, Nutrition and Cancer*. National Academy Press, 1982.

Pariza MW: A perspective on diet, nutrition and cancer. *JAMA* 1984;**251**:1455.

Pollack ES et al: Prospective study of alcohol consumption and cancer. *N Engl J Med* 1984;**310**:617.

Prasad AS, Cossack ZT: Zinc supplementation and growth in sickle cell disease. *Ann Intern Med* 1984;**100**:367.

Rivlin RS, Shils ME, Sherlock P: Nutrition and cancer. *Am J Med* 1983;**75**:843.

Roe DA: Nutrient and drug interactions. *Nutr Rev* 1984;**42**:141.

Rosenberg IH, Solomons N (editors): Symposium: The biological availability of minerals and trace elements (2 parts). *Am J Clin Nutr* 1982;**35**:781, 1048.

Russell RM: Evaluating the nutritional status of the elderly. *Clin Nutr* 1983;**2**:4.

Russell RM, Cox ME, Solomons N: Zinc and the special senses. *Ann Intern Med* 1983;**99**:227.

Sidney S, Farquhar JW: Cholesterol, cancer and public health policy. *Am J Med* 1983;**75**:494.

Stein TP, Schluter MD, Diamond CE: Nutrition, protein turnover, and physical activity in young women. *Am J Clin Nutr* 1983;**38**:223.

Trace elements in human nutrition. *Dairy Council Dig* 1982;**53**:1.

Visocan BJ: Nutritional management of alcoholism. *J Am Diet Assoc* 1983;**83**:693.

Willet WC, MacMahon B: Diet and cancer. (2 parts.) *N Engl J Med* 1984;**310**:633, 697.

Winn DM et al: Diet and cancer. *Cancer Res* 1984;**44**:1216.

THERAPEUTIC DIETS*

Special diet therapy should be based upon sound scientific evidence rather than upon myth or tradition. In no aspect of medical therapeutics are there more bias, emotionalism, and inconclusive evidence than in the use of many of the so-called special diets.

There is little evidence to support the value of many classic or traditional diets (eg, Sippy diet for peptic ulcer, low-purine diet for gout, low-residue diet for ulcerative colitis). There is nothing to substantiate the extravagant claims made for most of the innumerable special diets proposed for the treatment of obesity, and in many instances these diets are nutritionally inadequate. It is not possible to comment individually on the numerous dietary fads that periodically sweep the USA except to say that they are regrettable.

There is good clinical and scientific evidence, however, to support the use of specific therapeutic diets in many gastrointestinal, cardiovascular, metabolic, and other disorders mentioned in this book. Allergy to certain foods may be very marked in some individuals, and in such instances, special nonallergenic diets may be of value. In many instances, however, such "allergies" may be more readily related to psychosocial factors.

Many special diets are nutritionally unbalanced, monotonous, expensive, difficult to procure, and difficult to adhere to. Consultation and cooperation with a professional dietitian will facilitate optimal use of special diets. The dietitian should be provided with certain information such as the nature of the illness; the type of diet desired by the physician; the total daily amount (in grams) of protein, carbohydrate, and fat; the size and frequency of feedings; the fluid intake desired; the patient's environmental and socioeconomic status; and the expected duration of therapy.

Clear Liquid Diet

This diet relieves thirst and supplies a few calories. It contains only water, sugar, nonresidue protein, and salts. Foods are limited to tea, coffee, broth, strained fruit juices, and carbonated beverages. This diet should be used—for short periods only—for patients with the following conditions: (1) immediate postoperative status, (2) acute semidebilitation, (3) constricting upper gastrointestinal lesions, and (4)

*Diabetic diets and hyperlipidemia diets are discussed in Chapter 20. The low-calorie obesity diet is discussed later in this chapter.

acute gastroenteritis. The diet is administered in 6 small feedings daily.

Full Liquid Diet

This diet does not require chewing and is nutritionally more adequate than the clear liquid diet, but it is still rather deficient in protein, B vitamins, and minerals. In addition to the clear liquid foods, other foods such as milk, eggnog, plain ice cream, gelatin, soft cereals, puddings, custards, proprietary liquid protein preparations, strained cream soups, and vitamin and mineral supplements are given. The diet is administered in 6 feedings daily as tolerated.

Soft Low-Residue Diet

This diet, which is nutritionally adequate, consists of low residue and easily assimilable proteins and carbohydrates. Permitted foods, in addition to those permitted in the liquid diets, include eggs; cottage cheese; ground or tender meat, fish, or chicken; white bread; soda crackers; refined cereals; boiled polished rice; potatoes (without skin); cooked and puréed vegetables; cooked fruits; ripe bananas; applesauce; gelatin desserts; plain puddings; plain cakes and cookies; marshmallows; and hard candies (melted in mouth).

Avoid corn, potato skins, fibrous vegetables, whole grain or bran cereals, raw fruit, and fried or highly seasoned foods.

Minimum Residue Diet

This diet contains foods from which most indigestible fiber has been removed. It is useful preoperatively to clear the operative site of the gastrointestinal tract of fecal residue.

A. Protein: Ground or tender beef, chicken, fish, lamb, liver, veal, crisp bacon, eggs. Avoid milk, milk products, cheeses of all kinds.

B. Carbohydrate: Soda crackers, French bread, melba toast, refined cereals, rice, strained oatmeal, cornflakes, puffed rice, plain cakes and cookies, macaroni, noodles, spaghetti, gelatin desserts, water ices, strained fruit juices, hard candies, marshmallows, sugar, syrup, honey, carbonated beverages, tomato juice.

C. Fat: Butter, margarine, mayonnaise.

D. Other Foods: Beverages such as coffee, tea, Sanka, Postum; salt, vinegar, gravies, spices, and herbs in moderation.

Soft ("Bland") Diet

This diet contains food soft in texture and mild in flavor, requiring minimal chewing. It may be useful for postsurgical patients and others recovering from gastrointestinal disturbances. Meals should be small and frequent and should be eaten slowly.

A. Protein: Adequate amounts of lean meats, broth, fish, eggs, cottage cheese, and milk.

B. Fats: Moderate amounts of butter, margarine, cream, and cream cheese. Polyunsaturated fats (soft margarines) are recommended in place of saturated types.

C. Carbohydrates: Only potatoes (white or sweet) and applesauce allowed during acute phase.

Restrict gastric secretagogues and irritants such as alcohol and caffeine (coffee, tea, cocoa, and cola beverages). *Avoid* chili powder, nutmeg, mustard seeds, cloves, and black pepper.

Low-Fat Diet (50–60 g daily)

Reduction of fat (10–25% less than usual intake) may be useful in controlling fatty acid diarrhea and other problems arising from abnormalities in the hydrolysis, absorption, or transport of fat (eg, chronic pancreatitis, intestinal bypass surgery, gastrectomy, short-gut syndrome). Small, frequent feedings are recommended.

A. Protein: Normal amounts of lean meats, fish, and poultry (with all visible fat removed); eggs as tolerated; low-fat or nonfat milk; yogurt; buttermilk; cottage cheese and mild cheddar cheeses; fat-free meat stock, bouillon, or broth.

B. Fats: One to 2 tbsp of butter, margarine, mayonnaise, and oils. Avoid cooking any food in fat.

C. Carbohydrates: Enriched or whole-grain breads and cereals; fresh, cooked, canned, or juices of all fruits and most vegetables; soft desserts or those made without added fat.

D. Beverages: Coffee, tea, fruit juices, carbonated beverages, and decaffeinated beverages may be given.

Low-Protein Diet (40–50 g daily)

A. Protein: Two oz meat, fish, or poultry; 1 cup milk; 1 egg or 1 oz cheese.

B. Carbohydrates: Fruits and juices as desired; cooked and raw vegetables as desired. Three servings of breads and cereals. One serving of potatoes, corn, etc. One serving of dessert. Sugar, hard candies, syrup, or honey as desired.

C. Fats: Butter, margarine, oils, and salad dressings as desired.

D. Salt: Restrict as indicated.

Note: Small, frequent feedings are recommended, with juices and fruits for between-meal snacks.

Low-Carbohydrate, High-Protein, High-Fat Diet

In this diet, simple sugars (sugars, syrups, honey, and fructose) are restricted and complex carbohydrates are limited to less than 140 g/d. The diet may be useful for the treatment of the hypoglycemic syndromes (see p 786). Small, frequent feedings are recommended.

A. Protein: Meat, fish, poultry, cheese, or nuts as desired.

B. Carbohydrates: Breads and cereals, not over 3 servings daily. Unsugared fruits and juices, not over 3 servings a day. Vegetables (raw or cooked), 3–6 servings a day. Starches such as potatoes, rice, or corn, 1 serving daily. No desserts containing sugar; artificially sweetened desserts or beverages in moderation.

C. Fats: Butter, margarine, oils, and salad dressings as desired.

Note: It is recommended that a higher protein intake be taken earlier in the day, with small, frequent feedings of cheese, nuts, etc, throughout the day.

High-Calorie, High-Protein, High-Vitamin Diet

This diet is useful in the treatment of pronounced weight loss due to chronic illness, prolonged inadequate food intake, and hypermetabolic states (eg, fever, body burns, hyperthyroidism).

Increase caloric value to 25–50% above normal. Increase protein to 90–100 g/d for adults. Select foods high in vitamin content, especially vitamin B complex. Provide foods in small, frequent feedings (6–8 a day).

A. Protein:

1. Milk–Up to 1 quart per day, as beverage or in or on foods.

2. Eggs–One or more, prepared in any way or added to other foods.

3. Cheeses–All kinds, as meat substitutes, added to sauces or dishes, or as between-meal snacks.

4. Meats, fish, poultry–Two to 3 portions daily (2–3 oz per serving), simply prepared by broiling, roasting, or stewing, or with cream or cheese sauces.

B. Fats: Two to 3 tbsp daily of butter, cream, margarine, mayonnaise, or oils.

C. Carbohydrates:

1. Bread and cereals–Four to 8 servings of any kind, but preferably whole grain or enriched white.

2. Fruits and fruit juices–Four to 6 servings (with added sugar) of any kind, fresh, cooked, or canned.

3. Vegetables–

a. Fresh or raw–Small portions 1–2 times daily with mayonnaise or dressings.

b. Cooked–One or 2 portions daily of green, white, red, or yellow vegetables.

4. Starches–One to 2 servings as potatoes, rice, etc, with added sauces, butter, gravies, or cream or cheese sauces.

5. Soups–Cream style or thick soups as desired.

6. Ice cream, sherbet, custard, pudding, plain cake, fruit dessert, gelatin, or cookies–One to 2 (or more) servings. Brown, white, or maple sugars; jellies, honey, syrups, 2–4 tbsp (or more).

7. Beverages–Coffee and tea in moderation; decaffeinated beverages, Postum, cocoa, eggnog, milk shakes, sweetened carbonated beverages, and fruit juices as desired. Wines and alcohol with discretion. Other milk-containing supplementary foods such as Metrecal, Meritene, Nutrament, or Sustagen can be used for meals or between-meal snacks.

Disaccharide Intolerance Diet
(Low in Lactose, Sucrose, Maltose, Galactose)

Indication: Those conditions that have been determined to be due to deficiencies of one or more enzymes such as lactase, invertase or sucrase, maltase and isomaltase, and galactase.

Omit all forms of milk, cheese, ice cream, frozen desserts containing milk, milk drinks, white breads and crackers, biscuits, muffins, cream soups, creamed dishes, and prepared foods containing milk. Also, omit some salad dressings, cold or luncheon meat products, cream substitutes, candies, health and geriatric products, and medications that may use lactose as a bulking agent, filler, or excipient.

Sucrase or invertase deficiency requires the omission of granulated sugar (cane or beet), syrups, jellies, molasses, cakes, cookies, puddings and candies, sorghum, pineapple, carrots, apricots, bananas, dates, melons, oranges, and peas. Some medications such as antibiotic syrups may also contain sucrose.

Isomaltase deficiency may occur in conjunction with invertase deficiency. Germinating cereals, malt, and probably wheat and potatoes should be restricted. Sucrose should also be avoided.

A rare disorder, glucose-galactose malabsorption, requires omission of all sources of sucrose, starch, and lactose. Special formulas and diets need to be devised.

Low-Gluten Diet

This diet eliminates gluten-containing foods such as wheat, oats, rye, barley, and buckwheat.

A. Protein: Meats, fish, poultry, eggs, cheese, and milk as desired. Substitutes such as beans, peas, or nuts may be taken as tolerated.

B. Fat: Butter, margarine, oils, salad dressings, and cream as desired or tolerated.

C. Carbohydrate: Fruits, vegetables, and sugars as desired; desserts such as gelatins, iced milk, and sherbet; cakes, cookies, puddings, or pastries made with corn, rice, potato, or soya starches or flours. (Most commercial or prepared mixes contain flours that should be omitted from this diet.) Breads made from gluten-free wheat starch or special baking mixes such as Paygel, Resource, or those made with corn, rice, potato, soya, or lima bean starches or flours. Cereals: rice, corn, cornflakes, Rice Krispies, corn meal.

D. Other Foods: Condiments, salt, vinegar, spices, and herbs as desired or tolerated.

Avoid beer and ale.

Sodium-Regulated Diets

When prescribing modification of dietary sodium, it is important to take into consideration not only the natural sodium content of foods but also the sodium content of prepared foods, local water supplies, and many types of medication. Drastic limitations on dietary sodium are not often necessary now that effective oral diuretic drugs are available. Correction of significant sodium depletion is best accomplished by oral or parenteral sodium chloride preparations.

A. High Content: ($\geq$ 125–1000 mg or 5.4–43.5 meq per average serving.) Cheese of all kinds, soda and graham crackers, condiments, relishes and sauces (soy, Worcestershire, ketchup, chili, barbecue), pick-

les, olives, cured and canned meats, fish, poultry, commercially prepared desserts, foods made with baking powder or baking soda, buttermilk, sauerkraut, tomato juice, vegetable juice cocktail, celery, potato chips, snack foods, pretzels, frozen meals or dinners, canned vegetables, canned soups, prepared cereals, frozen peas and lima beans and *any food that tastes salty*.

B. Medium High Content: (50–125 mg or 2.2–5.4 meq per average serving.) Commercial breads, butter, margarine, fresh fish and shellfish, milk, fresh meats, poultry, eggs, chocolate candies, ice cream, iced milk, sherbet, angel food cake, sponge cake, artichokes, beet greens, turnips, spinach, celery, carrots, beets, chard, kale, and cantaloupes.

C. Low Content: (< 50 mg or 2.2 meq per average serving.) All fruits (fresh, frozen, canned, dried), fruit juices, jellies, jams, syrups, honey, sugar (both white and brown), soybean curd, unsalted nuts, hard sugar candies, coffee, oil, tea, sweet or salt-free butter or margarine, herbs, plain gelatin, most fresh fruits and vegetables, puffed rice, puffed wheat, shredded wheat, Sugar Pops, nonenriched or quick-cooking cereals such as oatmeal, rolled wheat, cracked wheat, farina, corn meal, grits, rice, Ralston, Wheatena, or Wheathearts.

Potassium-Regulated Diets

When it is necessary to modify the potassium in the diet, one must consider not only the natural potassium content of foods but also the potassium content of special food preparations (eg, salt substitutes, low-salt milk) and certain medications (eg, penicillin G). A high intake is recommended when corticosteroids and certain diuretic drugs are being administered to the patient concurrently.

A. High Content: (300–500 mg or 7.7–12.8 meq per average serving.) All-Bran, milk of all kinds, yogurt, apricots (fresh and dried), avocados, bananas, dates, melons (casaba and honeydew), oranges (medium to large), peaches (dried), persimmons, raisins, prune juice, cooked chicken, beef, lamb, liver, ham, pork, veal, fish of all kinds, peanuts, pecan halves, artichokes (globe type), cooked dried white or red beans or black-eyed peas, lima beans, beet greens, raw carrots, celery, mushrooms, cooked chard, parsnips, white potatoes, radishes, cooked spinach, sweet potatoes, and raw tomatoes.

B. Medium High Content: (150–300 mg or 3.8–7.7 meq per average serving.) Fresh and canned peaches, orange juice, cantaloupe, nectarines, plums, watermelon, fresh and cooked asparagus, cabbage, cauliflower, greens, corn, rutabagas, squash of all kinds, tomato juice, turnips, shellfish, cured meats such as corned and dried beef, sausage and luncheon meats, and desserts containing dried raisins and nuts.

C. Low Content: (50–150 mg or 1.28–3.8 meq per average serving.) Cooked green and wax beans, beets, peas, broccoli, brussels sprouts, carrots, eggplant, mixed vegetables, onions, green peppers, raw lettuce and salad greens, berries of all kinds, bread of all kinds, rolls, buns, hot breads, cheeses of all kinds, cereals (cooked or dry prepared), eggs, canned soups, candies, desserts, and wines.

D. Little or No Content: (< 50 mg or 1.28 meq per average serving.) Beverages such as coffee, beer, gin, rum, vodka, whiskey, tea; hard sugar candies, butter, margarine, oils, and shortenings.

Low-Calcium Diet
(500–700 mg calcium, 1000–1200 mg phosphorus)
  A. Protein: (See Avoid list, below.)
  1. Meat, fish, or poultry–Only 4 oz cooked per day.
  2. Eggs–One per day; egg whites as desired.
  3. Milk–One cup (1/2 pint) daily; may use diluted whipping cream as milk substitute.
  4. Cheese–Cottage cheese, only 2 oz daily.
  B. Fat: Whipping cream, butter, margarine, salad dressings, and oils as desired.
  C. Carbohydrate: (See Avoid list, below.)
  1. Fruits–Three to 5 servings daily, including citrus.
  2. Vegetables, raw–Salads as desired.
  3. Vegetables, cooked–Two or 3 servings.
  4. Starches–Potatoes and corn, one or more servings.
  5. Breads, cereals, and pastas–Enriched white breads, rolls, crackers, nonenriched farina, cornflakes, corn meal, hominy grits, rice, Rice Krispies, puffed rice, macaroni, spaghetti, noodles.
  6. Desserts–Fruit pies, fruit ices, fruit gelatin, puddings made with allowed milk and egg, angel food cake, meringues, shortbreads, sugar, jellies, honey, sweetened beverages.

  Avoid organ meats such as brains, heart, liver, kidney, sweetbreads; sardines, fish roe; game such as pheasant, rabbit, deer; cheddar or other cheeses; rhubarb, beet greens, chard, collards, mustard greens, spinach, turnip greens, dried beans, peas, lentils, soybeans; whole-grain breads, cereals, and crackers; rye bread and all breads made with self-rising flour; oatmeal, brown and wild rice, bran, bran flakes, wheat germ, and any dry cereal not listed above; any milk-containing foods except as allowed; nuts, peanut butter, chocolate, and cocoa; condiments having a calcium or phosphate base.

High-Calcium Diet
  Indication: For conditions requiring the intake of over 1 g calcium per day.
  The normal well-balanced diet furnishes 800–1000 mg calcium per day, mostly from milk and cheese. Milk consumption of over 1 quart per day will provide 1150 mg calcium or more. Other foods that add to calcium intake are cheeses, particularly cheddar or American; leafy green vegetables such as "greens" (dandelion, beet, mustard, and turnip; kale), cabbage, broccoli, and brussels sprouts; dried beans and peas; nuts; and milk-containing desserts.
  If milk is not well tolerated, yogurt may some-

times be acceptable. Calcium gluconate or carbonate, 1–2 g daily, may be used as a supplement.

Antiflatulence Diet
  Because of the diverse physiologic and pathologic causes of flatulence, there is no single diet that is applicable to all or even any great number of patients with this common complaint (see p 355). A clear-cut rationale for dietary restrictions cannot always be identified, and individual tolerance of specific foods may vary considerably. Dietary origins of flatulence that deserve consideration include the following:
  (1) Foods containing excess air: Carbonated beverages, meringues, milk shakes, soufflés.
  (2) Lactose-containing foods: For lactose intolerance. (See low-lactose diet, p 801.)
  (3) Certain vegetables and fruits: Broccoli, brussels sprouts, cabbage, cauliflower, dried beans, cucumbers, green peppers, kohlrabi, lettuce, lima beans, nuts, onions, peas, radishes, raw apples, melons, prunes.
  (4) Diets high in fat: Fatty acids react with duodenal bicarbonate to produce carbon dioxide. (See Low-Fat Diet, p 801.)

Vegetarian Diets
  Foodstuffs of vegetable origin constitute most, if not all, of the diet of millions of people throughout the world. For people of the poorer nations, this is a matter of necessity; for a few, the vegetarian diet is one of choice. Strict vegetarians—those living entirely on fruits, vegetables, whole-grain cereals, legumes, and nuts—are less numerous than those who also eat dairy products (lactovegetarians) and those who in addition eat eggs (ovolactovegetarians). Diets devoid of all animal products—for economic, religious, cultist, or personal reasons—are nutritionally inadequate unless they are varied and provide all of the essential amino acids of proteins, vitamins, and minerals. Groups who are at particular risk on vegetarian diets are pregnant and lactating women, infants and children, and patients with diet-related diseases (eg, lactose intolerance). Clinicians should be aware of the nutritional characteristics of vegetable foodstuffs as it becomes apparent that human beings must rely increasingly on cereal grains, legumes, roots, tubers, and other vegetable sources of food in the not too distant future.
  The quantity and quality of protein are of major concern in all diets. Judicious combination of plant protein foods can provide the equivalent nutritional value of high-quality animal protein foods. Mixing of dietary cereal grains and legumes has maintained excellent health status for peoples throughout the world, and the supplementary effect of one plant food on another is well established.
  Two daily servings of high-protein meat substitutes such as legumes (eg, soybeans, beans, peas, lentils), high-protein nuts (eg, peanuts, almonds, cashews, walnuts), peanut butter, meat analogs (textured vegetable or soy protein products), or dairy products or eggs are recommended. The preschool

child in particular needs to be assured of an adequate intake of high-quality protein.

Although protein is of first importance in considering the adequacy of vegetarian diets, other nutrients that may be only marginally present in all-plant diets are calcium, iron, riboflavin, vitamin B_{12}, and, for children not exposed to sunlight, vitamin D.

The greatest risk of inadequacy in an all-plant diet comes from reliance on a single plant food source, eg, from a cereal grain or starchy root crop. Legumes, particularly soybeans, are rich in protein, B vitamins, and iron. Grains are good sources of carbohydrates, proteins, thiamine, iron, and trace minerals. Nuts and other seeds contribute fat, protein, B vitamins, and iron. Dark green, leafy vegetables are sources of calcium, riboflavin, and carotene (vitamin A precursors) and are good supplements to the grains and legumes in the total vegetarian diet.

Since plant foods do not contain vitamin B_{12}, some source needs to be supplied. Milk and eggs are satisfactory sources, but the total vegetarian diet can be supplemented with fortified soybean milk or vitamin B_{12} preparations. Infants and children may need supplementary vitamin D, particularly in winter months when exposure to sunlight is limited. Calcium and riboflavin can be obtained from a liberal intake of dark green, leafy vegetables or from fortified soy milk.

Dietary Fiber

Epidemiologic, clinical, and experimental evidence suggests that removal of fiber (a diverse group of plant constituents that are resistant to digestion by the human gastrointestinal tract) from the diet is directly or indirectly associated with certain diseases that are disproportionately common in industrialized countries of the world. The average diet in the USA provides 2–5 g of fiber per day. Disorders of the gastrointestinal tract that may be linked to decreased dietary fiber include functional constipation, gallbladder disease, appendicitis, diverticulitis, tumors of the colon and rectum, and hemorrhoids; cardiovascular disorders include coronary atherosclerosis, varicose veins, and deep vein thrombosis. These relationships, although conjectural, warrant serious consideration. Therapeutic implications, at least in the case of the mentioned gastrointestinal disorders, seem obvious and have already led to significant modification of older dietary concepts in the treatment of constipation, irritable bowel, ulcerative colitis, and colonic diverticulosis. (See Chapter 11.) Preventive aspects of diets high in fiber content with regard to the gastrointestinal and cardiovascular disorders are uncertain at present.

The following diet would provide the recommended 10 g of fiber daily:

One raw fresh fruit or one-half cup of dried fruit (cooked or uncooked).

One cup of raw fresh (especially carrots and turnips) or lightly cooked fresh vegetables. It is probably more convenient and desirable to eat some combination of several vegetables in smaller amounts each to add up to a cup total. The skins of fruits and vegetables should be eaten if they are edible.

Four to 6 slices of whole wheat berry bread, cracked-wheat bread, or rye bread.

Two to 4 tbsp of natural bran or ½ cup of All-Bran cereal, or a somewhat larger serving of less fibrous cereal (eg, 40% bran or raisin bran).

Snack foods that are good sources of fiber include peanuts, popcorn, graham crackers, raisins, almonds, walnuts, pecans, pumpkin seeds, and sunflower seeds.

Burton BT, Hirschman GH: Current concepts of nutritional therapy in chronic renal failure: An update. *J Am Diet Assoc* 1983;**82**:359.

Kolars JC et al: Yogurt: An autodigesting source of lactose. *N Engl J Med* 1984;**310**:1.

Truesdell DD, Whitney EN, Acosta PB: Nutrients in vegetarian foods. *J Am Diet Assoc* 1984;**84**:28.

Vahouny GV: Conclusions and recommendations of the symposium on "Dietary Fibers in Health and Disease," Washington DC, 1981. *Am J Clin Nutr* 1982;**35**:152.

Williams CA, Dickerson JWT: Vegetarianism. *The Physician* 1984;**2**:568.

Yaffe BH: Nutritional therapy of liver dysfunction. *Environ Nutr* 1983;**6**:1.

ENTERAL NUTRITION
(Tube Feeding, or Enteral Alimentation)

There are 3 general types of tube feedings: (1) blended, strained preparations made from common foods; (2) those with a milk base to which other foods may be added; and (3) commercial preparations, which may be preferred because of convenience and safety.

Tube feedings are employed when the patient is unable or unwilling to take food by mouth. Patients should be fed in the sitting position whenever possible. Feedings may be administered through a pliable polyethylene tube that may be passed intranasally and kept in place for prolonged periods. In some circumstances, a gastrostomy is necessary.

The tube feeding should supply the patient's requirements for carbohydrate, protein, fat, electrolytes, and water. It must pass through the tube without clogging. The feeding should be as close to the osmolality of blood plasma as possible.

A person of normal weight needs 30 kcal/kg. However, metabolic demands may necessitate an increase in caloric intake. Protein should make up about 20% of the calories. Carbohydrates (along with electrolytes) give the tube feeding its osmolality and should be limited to 35–40% of the calories. Fat will provide 30–45% of calories. A suitable concentration is 1 kcal/mL. An average normal adult requires about 2–2.5 L of water in 24 hours.

Feeding formulas may serve as excellent media for the growth of bacteria and must be refrigerated and not held for over 24 hours. To prevent the tube from clogging, each feeding should be followed with a small quantity of water. Measured volumes (150–200 mL) can be given every 2–4 hours.

Caution: (1) Begin with more dilute material and administer slowly. (2) The best rate is usually 3 L per 24 hours. (3) Most patients tolerate feedings best when not over 200 mL are given at a time. (4) If foods must be given rapidly, warm to body temperature. (5) If gastric distention is suspected, aspirate with a gastric tube and before each subsequent tube feeding if necessary. (6) Use with care in comatose patients to prevent aspiration. (7) If diarrhea occurs, add 15 mL of fluid pectin (Certo) to 1 quart of feeding, or liquid antidiarrheal drug in proper dose. (8) Prevent dehydration, hyperosmolality, and azotemia by providing adequate water to allow for the solute load and to permit normal excretion.

Blenderized (Blended) Tube Feeding Formula

The following formula supplies 1 kcal/mL in a volume of 2500 mL. The nutrient contents are as follows: protein, 20% or 125 g; fat, 45% or 125 g; carbohydrate, 35% or 220 g; calcium, 1312 mg; phosphorus, 1518 mg; iron, 24 mg; vitamin A, 7582 IU; thiamine, 2.675 mg; riboflavin, 3.746 mg; niacin, 27.91 mg; ascorbic acid, 163 mg; sodium, 2557 mg; potassium, 4159 mg.

Strained oatmeal	10 g
Dextri-Maltose	50 g
Instant nonfat dry milk	50 g
Strained liver	20 g
Strained beef	568 g
Strained applesauce	402 g
Strained green beans	484 g
Vegetable oil	85 mL
Orange juice	200 mL
Milk, homogenized	300 mL
Water	500 mL

Milk Base Tube Feeding Formula

The following formula supplies 1.4 kcal/mL in a volume of 1500 mL. The nutrient contents are as follows: protein, 100 g; fat, 110 g; carbohydrate, 190 g; sodium, 3565 mg; potassium, 3900 mg. *Note:* This formula is inadequate in iron.

Homogenized milk	800 mL
Half and half	600 mL
Eggnog powder	100 g
Instant nonfat dry milk	90 g
Salt	5.5 g
Vitamin preparation*	5 mL
Water to 1500 mL	

It has been recommended that pasteurized powdered egg or eggnog powder be substituted for raw egg because of the possibility of *Salmonella* infection. One tablespoon (15 g) of powdered egg is equivalent to one egg. Milk substitutes may be used for patients with lactose intolerance.

It is important to become familiar with some of the commercial enteral products for oral use and tube feeding. Many convenient commercial preparations

*Vitamin supplement contains 2 mg thiamine, 3 mg riboflavin, 30 mg niacin, and 100 mg ascorbic acid.

(eg, Ensure, Portagen, Sustacal, Vivonex) are available to meet general or specific nutritional needs. Factors to be considered in the selection of a product include palatability, composition (nitrogen, total carbohydrate, and lactose content), homogenization, viscosity, safety, and relative cost.

Gordon AM Jr: Enteral nutrition support. Guidelines for feeding product selection. *Postgrad Med* (July) 1982;**72**:72.

Heymsfield SB et al: Nutrient bioavailability from nasojejunally administered enteral formulas: Comparison to solid food. *Am J Clin Nutr* 1984;**38**:243.

TOTAL PARENTERAL NUTRITION (TPN)
(Intravenous Hyperalimentation)

When it is not possible to provide adequate nourishment by the normal alimentary route, all required nutrient substrates may be administered totally by parenteral means. Total parenteral nutrition may be used to meet usual and special metabolic needs for extended periods when adequate enteral intake is *impossible, improbable, inadvisable,* or *hazardous.* This has proved to be effective, even lifesaving, in severe alimentary disturbances and a wide variety of conditions such as multiple organ failure (renal, hepatic, and respiratory failure), extensive trauma, burns, overwhelming infection, and delayed postoperative function. The essential nutritional support provided by total parenteral nutrition may help to improve patient tolerance and increase therapeutic efficiency during cancer chemotherapy.

The total parenteral nutrition solution must provide sufficient calories, protein nitrogen, vitamins, and minerals to maintain basal metabolism, meet activity requirements, and promote growth and tissue healing. The basic nutrient solution for the average adult consists of 25–30% dextrose, 4–5% synthetic amino acid solution (FreAmine II, Aminosyn), and electrolytes to meet individual needs. Multivitamins and trace elements (zinc, copper, manganese, and chromium) are added to the basic solution as needed. Iron and iodine are also required for long-term treatment. Anabolic requirements per 1000 kcal include approximately 50–60 meq sodium, 40 meq potassium, 15–30 meq phosphate, 4–10 meq calcium, and 12–24 meq magnesium. Intralipid, a lipid soybean emulsion (10% solution) containing essential fatty acids and 1.1 kcal/mL, is given twice weekly to prevent fatty acid deficiency. The basic solution must be modified to meet specific individual requirements, especially for patients with diabetes, hepatic failure, renal failure, and electrolyte disorders.

Total parenteral nutrition should be administered under the close supervision of persons with expertise in the method; this often requires a team approach of several medical disciplines. Strict adherence to sterile technique and catheter protocol are required. The route of parenteral administration is dependent upon the patient's energy needs and the expected duration of treatment. Nutrition provided by peripheral veins causes fewer complications for those patients with lower caloric needs, but problems arise when relatively large volumes of fluid are required to deliver adequate calories. When caloric needs are great, central venous alimentation can provide the higher caloric density. Patients can be maintained in good nitrogen balance with weight gain and clinical improvement for months or years. This form of nutrition may satisfactorily support the patient before, during, and after definitive treatment of the primary medical or surgical problem. In selected patients who might otherwise have required repeated or prolonged hospital care for malnutrition, total parenteral nutrition can be employed successfully in the home.

Potential complications of intravenous hyperalimentation include physical injury to structures impinged upon by the catheter (eg, pleura, lungs, brachial plexus, heart), local and systemic infection, hypophosphatemia, metabolic acidosis, hypokalemia, anemia, hyperammonemia, essential fatty acid deficiency, hypoglycemia (following sudden withdrawal of the solution), and hyperosmolar hyperglycemic dehydration. The possibility of such complications can be reduced by proper antiseptic, aseptic, and catheterization technique, proper selection and modification of nutrient solutions, careful rate of infusion, use of insulin when needed, and careful clinical and biochemical monitoring.

AMA Department of Foods and Nutrition: Guidelines for essential trace element preparation for parenteral use. *JAMA* 1979; **241**:2051.

Copeland EM III: Intravenous alimentation: An update. *JPEN* 1982;**6**:236.

Darbinian JA, Coulston AM: Parenteral nutrition in cancer therapy: A useful adjunct? *J Am Diet Assoc* 1983;**82**:493.

Phillips GD, Odgers CL: *Parenteral and Enteral Nutrition: A Practical Guide,* 2nd ed. Flinders Univ Press (Australia), 1982.

Silberman H, Eisenberg D: *Parenteral and Enteral Nutrition for the Hospital.* Appleton-Century-Crofts, 1982.

Weinsier RL, Bacon J, Butterworth CE Jr: Central venous alimentation: A prospective study of the frequency of metabolic abnormalities among medical and surgical patients. *JPEN* 1982;**6**:421.

VITAMINS & VITAMIN DISORDERS

The body's requirement for vitamins may vary considerably, depending upon age, sex, physical activity, diet, metabolic rate, state of health, drug therapy, individual habits such as smoking, use of alcohol, use of contraceptives, and other factors affecting vitamin absorption, utilization, and excretion. Vitamin deficiencies are almost always multiple, although a particular symptom complex may predominate.

Early signs of vitamin deficiency are usually nonspecific, vague, and mild and are easily misinterpreted or missed entirely.

The treatment of multiple vitamin deficiencies consists of giving an adequate, balanced, high-protein, high-vitamin diet with vitamin supplementation as indicated. Vitamins used therapeutically for specific deficiencies are usually given in 5–10 times the amounts required for daily maintenance.

Vitamin dependencies, which are of hereditary origin, should be distinguished from the acquired vitamin deficiencies. Almost a dozen vitamin-dependent genetic diseases, involving 5 different vitamins (thiamine, nicotinamide, pyridoxine, vitamin B_{12}, and vitamin D), have been described. The vitamin dependencies do not respond to physiologic replacement therapy but only to large (pharmacologic) doses of the needed vitamin. At the other extreme, in the case of at least one vitamin (vitamin D), predisposed patients may react adversely to doses below the recommended prophylactic requirement.

Large doses of some vitamins (eg, vitamins A, D, K, niacin, pyridoxine) are toxic and may cause illness, particularly when continued for long periods. For this reason alone, the current popularity of so-called megavitamin therapy for a variety of imperfectly understood disorders (eg, schizophrenia) is not rational and is potentially hazardous.

Alhadeff L, Gualtieri CT, Lipton M: Toxic effects of water-soluble vitamins. *Nutr Rev* 1984;**42**:33.

Dubick MA, Rucker RB: Dietary supplements and health aids: A critical evaluation. 1. Vitamins and minerals. *J Nutr Educ* 1983;**15**:47.

Rivlin RS, Young EA (editors): Symposium on evidence relating selected vitamins and minerals to health and disease in the elderly population in the United States. *Am J Clin Nutr* 1982; **36(Suppl)**:986.

Rudman D, Williams PJ: Megadose vitamins: Use and misuse. *N Engl J Med* 1983;**309**:488.

FAT-SOLUBLE VITAMINS

1. VITAMIN A

Vitamin A is an alcohol of high molecular weight that is stored in the liver. Most of it is derived from conversion of beta-carotene in foods to vitamin A, mainly by the mucosa of the small intestine but also by the liver. It is necessary for normal function and structure of all epithelial cells and for the synthesis of visual purple in the retinal rods (hence for vision in dim light). The recent epidemiologic observation that dietary carotene intake is inversely related to the incidence of lung cancer—perhaps owing to the vitamin's role in maintaining epithelial integrity—is of great potential significance and requires further evaluation. Carotene only is present in leafy green and yellow fruits and vegetables; vitamin A and, at times, carotene are present in whole milk, butter, eggs, fish, and liver oil. Actually, vitamin A itself is quite rare in foods;

therefore, most is derived from carotene-bearing plant sources. The recommended daily allowances for adults are 5000 IU (or USP units) for men and 4000 IU for women; during pregnancy and lactation, 5000–6000 IU.

Hypovitaminosis A

A. Clinical Findings: Mild or early manifestations consist of dryness of the skin, tunnel vision, night blindness, and follicular hyperkeratosis. Severe or late manifestations are xerophthalmia, atrophy and keratinization of the skin, and keratomalacia.

B. Tests for Deficiency: Dark adaptation is impaired. A low serum value ($< 20 \mu g/dL$) of vitamin A may be found but is not diagnostic. A therapeutic test with 25,000–75,000 IU daily for 4 weeks may be helpful.

C. Treatment: Give oleovitamin A, 15–25 thousand units once or twice daily. If an absorption defect is present, it may be necessary to administer bile salts with the vitamin A or to give the same dosage in oil intramuscularly (50,000 units/mL in sesame oil). Skin lesions or profound malnutrition (eg, kwashiorkor) may require more treatment.

Hypervitaminosis A

This disorder is rare in adults, but it may occur as a result of chronic excessive ingestion of vitamin A. Current enthusiasm for large doses of vitamins is expected to increase the incidence of vitamin A toxicity. The minimal toxic adult dose is about 75–100 thousand units daily for 6 months; when ingested over a period of 8 years, a daily dose of 40,000 units may cause toxicity in adults.

A. Clinical Findings: Anorexia, loss of weight, dry and fissured skin, brittle nails, hair loss, gingivitis, cheilosis, hypercalcemia, hyperostosis and periosteal elevation of bone, bony resorption, hepatomegaly, cirrhosis, splenomegaly, anemia, and central nervous system manifestations.

B. Tests of Excess: Serum levels of vitamin A over $400 \mu g/dL$ are found (normal, $20–80 \mu g/dL$).

C. Treatment: Withdraw the medicinal source.

Goodman DS: Vitamin A and retinoids in health and disease. *N Engl J Med* 1984;**310**:1023.
Herbert V: Toxicity of 25,000 IU vitamin A supplements in "health" food users. *Am J Clin Nutr* 1982;**36**:185.
Willett WC et al: Relation of serum vitamins A and E and carotenoids to the risk of cancer. *N Engl J Med* 1984; **310**:436.

2. VITAMIN D

Vitamin D is the generic name for a family of about 10 sterols that have varying degrees of antirachitic potency. The 2 most important of these sterols are ergocalciferol (vitamin D_2) and cholecalciferol (vitamin D_3). The human body can synthesize provitamin D_3 (7-dehydrocholesterol), which can be converted photochemically to vitamin D_3 by ultraviolet irradiation of the skin. Natural sources of vitamin D include liver and viscera of fish, livers of fish-eating animals, egg yolks, and butter.

The daily allowances for adults are not known. For infants and children and for women during pregnancy and lactation—as well as for other individuals of both sexes to age 22—the recommended daily allowance is 400 units.

It is the current belief that vitamin D_3 must be transformed in the body to biologically much more active metabolites, 25-hydroxyvitamin D_3 and 1,25-dihydroxyvitamin D_3. These compounds, formed by the sequential hydroxylation of cholecalciferol by the liver and kidneys, are considerably more potent than the parent vitamin.

Vitamin D or its metabolites, together with parathyroid hormone and calcitonin, play an essential hormonal role in calcium homeostasis. The D vitamins maintain normal blood calcium and phosphorus levels by stimulating normal calcium transport in the intestine, mobilizing calcium from and to the bones, and controlling urinary phosphorus excretion.

Impaired metabolism of vitamin D or altered sensitivity of target tissues (intestine and bone) to the vitamin has been described in a wide variety of bone diseases and other disorders associated with abnormal calcium metabolism, eg, malabsorption, liver disease, renal failure, rickets, parathyroid disorders, and sarcoidosis.

There is, therefore, a wide spectrum of responsiveness to vitamin D. Some patients may require more than 50 times the therapeutic dose to correct manifestations of vitamin D deficiency (eg, vitamin D–resistant rickets), whereas others (eg, those with hyperparathyroidism) are hypersensitive even to doses below the recommended requirement.

Hypovitaminosis D

Hypovitaminosis D is usually due to inadequate dietary intake, lack of sunlight, or an intestinal absorption defect (eg, pancreatitis, sprue), hepatic disease, or renal disease.

A. Clinical Findings: Deficiency of vitamin D leads to osteomalacia in children (rickets) or infantile tetany. Some cases of adult osteomalacia appear to be associated with gastrointestinal disorders and with increased requirements of vitamin D.

B. Tests for Deficiency: Serum calcium and phosphorus may be normal or decreased, and serum alkaline phosphatase is generally increased. The urinary calcium is usually low.

C. Treatment: See Osteomalacia (p 720). Simple dietary increase of vitamin D is relatively ineffective in treating the deficiencies encountered in the malabsorption syndromes and in biliary cirrhosis.

Hypervitaminosis D

This disorder is usually caused by prolonged ingestion of 5–150 thousand units of the drug form daily.

A. Clinical Findings: The manifestations of

hypercalcemia are present and may progress to renal damage and metastatic calcification.

B. Tests of Excess: Serum calcium elevation (> 11.5 mg/dL) occurs if large doses of vitamin D are taken. (Always consider other causes of hypercalcemia.)

C. Treatment: Withdraw the medicinal source. Complete recovery, although it may be slow, will occur if overtreatment is discontinued in time. Prednisone will dramatically reduce hypercalcemia that is due to vitamin D intoxication. Treatment of hypercalcemia may be required (see p 1057).

Bikle DD: The vitamin D endocrine system. *Adv Intern Med* 1982;**27**:45.

Fraser DR: The physiological economy of vitamin D. *Lancet* 1983;**1**:969.

Manolagas SC, Deftos LJ: The vitamin D endocrine system and the hematolymphopoietic tissue. *Ann Intern Med* 1984;**100**:144.

Marel GM, Frame B, Norman AW: Symposium: Vitamin D in health and disease. *Ann Intern Med* 1982;**96**:674.

Parfitt AM et al: Vitamin D and bone health in the elderly. *Am J Clin Nutr* 1982;**36**:1225.

3. VITAMIN K

The K vitamins are fat-soluble chemical compounds necessary for the synthesis by the liver of blood coagulation factors II (prothrombin), VII, IX, and X. The similarity of the chemical structure of vitamin K to that of coenzyme Q suggests that the K vitamins may also be involved in the oxidative phosphorylation process in cellular mitochondria.

Vitamin K is widely distributed in foods. The naturally occurring form is called vitamin K_1. Vitamin K is also synthesized by microorganisms in the intestines and, since it differs from K_1 somewhat in chemical structure, is referred to as vitamin K_2. A third form of the vitamin, prepared synthetically, is known as vitamin K_3 (menadione).

The daily requirement of vitamin K is not known, but it is felt that it must be quite small. Vitamin K depletion due to dietary deficiency alone is extremely rare.

Hypovitaminosis K

Hypovitaminosis K may result from biliary obstruction or medical or surgical disorders of the small bowel that interfere with the absorption of fat. Long-term therapy with antibiotics or nonabsorbable sulfonamides that interfere with microorganism synthesis of vitamin K may also cause vitamin K deficiency.

A bleeding tendency or uncontrollable hemorrhage may occur. The coagulation defect may be aggravated by ingestion of drugs that depress prothrombin synthesis (eg, coumarins, salicylates). Prolongation of the prothrombin time as well as abnormal tests for coagulation factors VII, IX, and X may be demonstrated.

Successful treatment of the defective coagulation is dependent upon a functioning hepatic parenchyma, and vitamin K therapy is of no avail if liver disease is severe.

Hypervitaminosis K

Large doses of water-soluble vitamin K (derivative of K_3; menadione) to infants—particularly premature infants—may cause hemolytic anemia, hyperbilirubinemia, hepatomegaly, and even death. In adults with G6PD deficiency, ordinary doses of menadione or derivatives may cause hemolytic reactions.

Olson KE: The function and metabolism of vitamin K. *Ann Rev Nutr* 1984;**4**:281.

4. VITAMIN E
(Tocopherol)

Vitamin E is a natural antioxidant that plays a role in the normal physiology of animals and probably also of humans, although its exact role in humans is unclear. It is nontoxic. Hemolytic anemia due to vitamin E deficiency occurs in small premature infants who are given artificial formulas containing iron and high concentrations of unsaturated fatty acids. Vitamin E deficiency has been reported in malabsorption and maldigestion disorders of different types including chronic exocrine pancreatic insufficiency, advanced hepatobiliary disease, and intestinal resection. Deficiency may also occur in retinitis pigmentosa, myopathies, neuropathies, cystic fibrosis, and hereditary abetalipoproteinemia. The antitoxidant property of vitamin E has been utilized to counteract the harmful effects of excess of free radicals or pro-oxidants that occur in certain hereditary metabolic disorders or as a result of body stresses such as hyperoxia, ionizing radiation, and exposure to various drugs and toxins. The vitamin is widely held to be a panacea for a great variety of disorders; these claims cannot be scientifically substantiated. Recommended daily allowances for adults (based upon the usual range of intake of vitamin E) are 10 mg of α-tocopherol for men and 8 mg of α-tocopherol for women, with 10 mg of α-tocopherol during pregnancy and lactation. The requirement of the vitamin may be related to the polyunsaturated fatty acid content in body tissue.

Bieri JG, Corash L, Hubbard VS: Medical uses of vitamin E. *N Engl J Med* 1983;**308**:1063.

Muller DPR, Lloyd J, Wolff OH: Vitamin E and neurological function. *Lancet* 1983;**1**:398.

WATER-SOLUBLE VITAMINS: VITAMIN B COMPLEX

The members of the vitamin B complex are intimately associated in occurrence in food as well as in function (eg, as coenzymes). As a result of this close interrelationship, it is doubtful that a deficiency of a single B vitamin ever exists except under experimental conditions. Deficiency of a single member of the B complex would probably lead to impaired metabolism of the others. Hence, although certain clinical features may predominate in the absence of a single member of the complex, this does not mean that the deficiency can be entirely corrected by replacing that factor alone. Therefore, "specific therapy" always consists of providing adequate dietary or parenteral sources of all members of the B complex.

1. VITAMIN B₁
(Thiamine Hydrochloride)

Vitamin B_1 is a constituent of the enzyme that decarboxylates the alpha-keto acids (pyruvic acid and alpha-ketoglutaric acid). It is important, therefore, for normal carbohydrate oxidation. Dietary sources are liver, lean pork, kidney, and whole grain cereals. Steaming or exposure to moist heat reduces the thiamine content of foods. The daily dietary allowances are about 1.2–1.4 mg/d.

Hypovitaminosis B₁ (Beriberi)

Hypovitaminosis B_1 results from an inadequate intake due usually to idiosyncrasies of diet or excessive cooking or processing of foods. The increased need for vitamin B_1 during fever, high carbohydrate intake, alcoholism, or thyrotoxicosis may lead to deficiency.

A. Clinical Findings: Mild or early manifestations consist of vague multiple complaints suggestive of neurasthenia and include anorexia, formication, muscle cramps, calf tenderness, paresthesias, and hyperactivity followed later by hypoactivity of knee and ankle jerks.

Severe or late manifestations (beriberi) are anorexia, polyneuritis, serous effusions, subcutaneous edema, paralyses (particularly in the extremities), and cardiac insufficiency manifested by tachycardia, dyspnea, edema, and normal or decreased circulation time, elevated venous pressure, and nonspecific electrocardiographic changes.

A particularly virulent form of beriberi heart disease, probably associated with metabolic acidosis, is referred to as Shoshin beriberi in the Orient.

B. Treatment: Give thiamine hydrochloride, 20–50 mg orally, intravenously, or intramuscularly daily in divided doses for 2 weeks and then 10 mg daily orally. The clinical response to thiamine injection within 24–48 hours is one of the best criteria for a diagnosis of thiamine deficiency. An alternative is to give dried yeast tablets (brewer's yeast), 30 g 3 times daily. Give a well-balanced diet of 2500–4500 kcal/d when tolerated.

Goldfrank LR: A vitamin for an emergency [thiamine]. *Emerg Med* (Sept 30) 1982;**14**:113.

Iber FL et al: Thiamin in the elderly: Relation to alcoholism and to neurological degenerative disease. *Am J Clin Nutr* 1983; **36**:1067.

2. RIBOFLAVIN (VITAMIN B₂)

Riboflavin serves principally as a coenzyme for hydrogen transfer in the electron transport system of the respiratory chain. It is abundant in milk and milk products, leafy green vegetables, liver, kidneys, and heart. The daily dietary allowances for adults are 1.5–1.8 mg; in pregnancy and lactation, 1.5–2 mg.

Hypovitaminosis B₂ (Ariboflavinosis)

The etiologic factors in ariboflavinosis are similar to those in thiamine deficiency, but inadequate intake of milk is an important contributing factor. Riboflavin deficiency has been reported in women taking oral contraceptives. The manifestations of deficiency are highly variable and usually occur along with those of thiamine and niacin deficiency but may occur earlier.

A. Clinical Findings: Mild or early manifestations are oral pallor, superficial fissuring at the angles of the mouth, conjunctivitis and photophobia, lack of vigor, malaise, weakness, and weight loss. Severe or late manifestations consist of cheilosis (fissuring at the angles of the mouth), fissuring of the nares, magenta tongue, moderate edema, anemia, dysphagia, corneal vascularization and circumcorneal injection, and seborrheic dermatitis.

B. Treatment: Give riboflavin, 40–50 mg intravenously, intramuscularly, or orally daily until all symptoms have cleared. An alternative is to give dried yeast tablets (brewer's yeast), 30 g 3 times daily. A well-balanced diet consisting of 2500–4500 kcal daily should be given when tolerated.

Belke AZ et al: Effects of exercise on riboflavin requirements of young women. *Am J Clin Nutr* 1983;**37**:509.

Garry PJ et al: Nutritional status in a healthy elderly population: Riboflavin. *Am J Clin Nutr* 1982;**36**:902.

3. NICOTINIC ACID (Niacin)
& NICOTINAMIDE (Niacinamide)

Niacin and niacinamide function in important enzyme systems concerned with reversible oxidation and reduction by hydrogen transfer. They are present in liver, yeast, meat, whole-grain cereals, and peanuts. Nicotinic acid may be synthesized in the body from tryptophan. Therefore, a high-protein diet virtually assures adequate nicotinic acid. Sixty milligrams of tryptophan produce 1 mg of nicotinic acid.

The daily allowances for adults are 13–20 mg. Niacin may be used therapeutically as a vasodilating agent for headaches, myalgias, neurologic disorders, and edema of the labyrinth (100 mg or more daily in divided doses). Because niacin decreases the synthesis of low-density lipoprotein and lowers serum cholesterol, it has been recommended for the drug treatment of types II, III, IV, and V hyperlipoproteinemia. There is no good evidence that niacin or niacinamide in so-called megavitamin dosage is of value in the treatment of schizophrenia. Niacinamide does not possess the vasodilating effect of niacin.

Pellagra

The etiologic factors in deficiency of these components of the B complex are similar to those of thiamine deficiency. Niacin deficiency is the principal but not the only dietary defect in pellagra; low tryptophan content of some foods also plays a role.

A. Clinical Findings: Mild or early manifestations consist of multiple vague complaints; a reddened, roughened skin, and redness and hypertrophy of the papillae of the tongue. Severe or late manifestations are marked roughening of the skin when exposed to light and friction, diarrhea, abdominal distention, scarlet red tongue with atrophy of papillae, stomatitis, depression, mental dullness, rigidity, and peculiar sucking reactions.

B. Treatment: Give nicotinamide (niacinamide), 50–500 mg intravenously, intramuscularly, or orally daily until symptoms subside. Nicotinic acid (niacin) is less often used because of its vasodilating effect; the dosage is similar. Give therapeutic doses of thiamine, riboflavin, and pyridoxine also. An alternative is to give dried yeast tablets (brewer's yeast), 30 g 3 times daily.

A well-balanced diet consisting of 2500–4500 kcal/d and ample proteins should be given when tolerated. Dementia may require constant supervision.

Nicotinic Acid Poisoning

Large oral doses of nicotinic acid may cause flushing and burning of the skin and dizziness but are usually not harmful. After intravenous administration, hypotension may be severe. Anaphylaxis occurs rarely.

Kane JP et al: Normalization of low-density lipoprotein levels in heterozygous familial hypercholesterolemia with a combined drug regimen [colestipol and niacin]. *N Engl J Med* 1981; **304:**251.

WATER-SOLUBLE VITAMINS: VITAMIN C
(Ascorbic Acid)

Vitamin C is concerned with the formation and maintenance of intercellular supporting structures (dentine, cartilage, collagen, bone matrix). Its biochemical action is not clear. It may play a specific role in hydroxylation of proline in collagen, which may be related to connective tissue functioning and wound healing. Vitamin C may also play a role in the body's response to severe stress. Dietary sources include citrus fruits, tomatoes, paprika, bell peppers, and all leafy green vegetables. The ascorbic acid con-

tent of foods is markedly decreased by cooking, mincing, air contact, alkalies, and contact with copper utensils. The recommended allowance for adults in the USA is 45 mg daily; for pregnant or lactating women, 60 mg daily.

Ascorbic acid in doses of 0.5 g or more has been used in the prevention of neoplastic disease and in the treatment of certain poisonings, but proof of its value is lacking. It is used in dosages up to 200 mg daily orally to promote healing of wounds or ulcers or during recovery from protracted disease (eg, tuberculosis). Pharmacologic megadosages have been recommended for the prevention or palliation of the common cold, but recent studies suggest that massive vitamin C prophylaxis does not result in significantly fewer colds. Recent studies also suggest that large doses of vitamin C are not entirely free of undesirable side effects.

Hypovitaminosis C (Scurvy)

Scurvy is usually due to inadequate intake of vitamin C but may occur with increased metabolic needs. The disease is seen frequently in formula-fed infants, elderly bachelors and widowers, and food faddists. Vitamin C concentration in tissues has been reported to be decreased in healthy women taking oral contraceptives.

A. Clinical Findings: Mild or early manifestations are edema and hemorrhage of the gingivae, porosity of dentine, and hyperkeratotic hair follicles. Severe or late manifestations consist of severe muscle changes, swelling of the joints, rarefaction of bone, a marked bleeding tendency, extravasation of blood into fascial layers, anemia, loosening or loss of the teeth, and poor wound healing.

B. Tests for Deficiency: Capillary resistance is reduced, and x-rays of the long bones may show typical changes. Epiphyseal changes in children are pathognomonic. There is also a lowering of serum or white cell ascorbic acid levels.

C. Treatment: Give sodium ascorbate injection, 100–500 mg intramuscularly daily, or ascorbic acid, 100–500 mg orally daily, as long as deficiency persists.

Hodges RE: Vitamin C and cancer. *Nutr Rev* (Oct) 1982;**40:**289.
Vilter RW: Nutritional aspects of ascorbic acid: Uses and abuses. *West J Med* 1980;**133:**485.

OTHER VITAMINS

Many other vitamins have been described. Some are important in human nutrition and disease; others play an unknown role.

Pyridoxine Hydrochloride (Vitamin B_6)

Pyridoxine is important in transamination and decarboxylation of amino acids. Deficiency of the vitamin may result in an anemia with intramedullary hemolysis (see p 315). The recommended daily allowance for adults is about 2 mg. It may relieve nervous symptoms and weakness in pellagrins when niacin fails and may relieve glossitis and cheilosis when riboflavin fails. Its role (if any) in human atherosclerosis is uncertain. The therapeutic dosage is 10–50 mg intravenously or intramuscularly daily with other factors of the B complex. Severe sensory neuropathy has been described in association with pyridoxine megavitaminosis.

Schaumburg H et al: Sensory neuropathy from pyridoxine abuse: A new megavitamin syndrome. N Engl J Med 1983;**309**:445.

Folic Acid

Folic acid seems to be essential for the metabolism of cell nuclear materials. It is effective in the treatment of certain macrocytic anemias and in tropical sprue. The hematologic changes occur early in folic acid deficiency, because folate storage in the body lasts only 1–2 months. The recommended daily allowance for adults is 400 μg. This is increased to 800 μg in pregnancy and to 600 μg in lactation.

Body reserves of folate may be rapidly depleted in chronic alcoholism. Folate deficiency has been described in chronic alcoholism and in patients taking oral contraceptives and anticonvulsant drugs.

Rosenberg IH et al: Folate nutrition in the elderly. Am J Clin Nutr 1983;**36**:1060.

Cyanocobalamin (Vitamin B₁₂)

Vitamin B_{12} is an essential phosphorus- and cobalt-containing material isolated from purified liver extract; it is the effective principle (extrinsic factor), found only in animal food sources, that is lacking in pernicious anemia and certain other disorders of gastrointestinal absorption. (See Chapter 10.) Qualitative platelet abnormalities have been reported in cases of severe vitamin B_{12} deficiency. Hyperresponse with thrombosis in such cases may follow vitamin B_{12} therapy. Vitamin B_{12} deficiency of the body is rarely due to inadequate dietary intake, and often there is no primary intestinal disease. (See Pernicious Anemia.) The recommended daily allowance for adults is 3 μg.

Baker SJ, Mathan VI: Evidence regarding the minimum daily requirement of dietary vitamin B_{12}. Am J Clin Nutr 1981; **34**:2423.

PSEUDOVITAMINS

Laetrile, a substance derived from pulverized apricot pits, has been widely promoted for the prevention and treatment of cancer, but carefully controlled clinical trials have demonstrated that Laetrile is ineffective as an antineoplastic agent. The claim that the drug is a vitamin ("B₁₇") is also not borne out by any scientific investigation. The major component of Laetrile is amygdalin, a cyanide-containing glycoside capable of causing severe and even fatal poisoning.

Pangamic acid ("vitamin B-15"), a water-soluble compound sharing many of the biologic properties of diisopropylamine, is currently a popular item in health food stores. The FDA indicates that the drug has questionable vitamin properties, and no data are available on its effectiveness or safety.

Herbert V, Barrett S: Vitamins and Health Foods: The Great American Hustle. Stickley, 1981.
Moertel CG et al: A clinical trial of amygdalin (Laetrile) in the treatment of human cancer. N Engl J Med 1982;**306**:201.

• • •

OBESITY

Obesity is a complex disorder that may be defined as an increase in weight of over 10% above "normal," due to generalized deposition of fat in the body. "Normal" or "desirable" weight, however, is difficult to determine; the standard age, height, and weight tables ordinarily used for practical clinical purposes are not always acceptable to everyone (Callaway, 1984). Body build, musculature, familial tendencies, and socioeconomic factors must be taken into consideration. Social factors have a marked influence on the prevalence of obesity, and situational determinants have a great effect on the eating habits of obese persons. It is important to differentiate weight increase due to depot fat from the increase due to body water or lean body mass. Weight gain due to obesity should be distinguished from that due strictly to fluid retention in edematous states (eg, ascites, heart failure). Research techniques for evaluating total body fat are available but are not practical for clinical purposes. Since about 50% of adipose tissue is located subcutaneously, the measurement of skinfold thickness (triceps fat fold) has been reported to be a simple and fairly reliable method of identifying obesity among individuals in the medium range of body size. About 40–50% of the adult population of the USA are considered to be overweight.

From a metabolic point of view, all obesity has a common cause: intake of more calories than are required for energy metabolism. The reason for differences in the food intake energy utilizations of various individuals, which make it possible for one person to utilize calories more "efficiently" than another, are not always known. It has been suggested that there is a more effective absorption of foodstuffs from the gut in obese individuals than in lean ones. Many clinicians feel that the metabolic changes in obesity are a result of obesity rather than a cause of it.

Some studies suggest that there are 2 major types of obesity based upon the number as well as the size of the fat cells. Patients with so-called **hypertrophic** or adult-onset obesity usually have a normal fixed number of fat cells and gain weight by fatty deposition or hypertrophy of the normal number of cells. The patient with hypertrophic obesity is reasonably amenable to weight reduction. In the **hyperplastic-**

hypertrophic type of obesity, where both number and size of fat cells increase during childhood, weight reduction is difficult to achieve and to maintain. A high rate of weight reduction failure must be accepted, and particular effort must be made to minimize the metabolic consequences (eg, hyperglycemia) without inducing secondary physical disability and psychologic depression.

Although most cases of obesity are due to simple overeating resulting from emotional, familial, metabolic, and genetic factors, a few endocrine and metabolic disorders lead to specific types of obesity (eg, Cushing's syndrome and hypothalamic lesions). It is particularly difficult to explain the phenomena of fluid retention and fat mobilization and storage in obesity. Hypothyroidism is rarely a cause of obesity.

The association of obesity with increased morbidity and mortality rates is well known. Hypertension, diabetes mellitus, gallbladder disease, gout, and possibly coronary atherosclerosis are frequently associated with obesity. There is an unexplained increase in the incidence of certain types of cancer (breast, endometrium, gallbladder, colon) in obese individuals. Obesity presents special hazards in pregnancy and in surgical patients. The psychologic and cosmetic implications of obesity are also significant factors.

An obesity-hypoventilation syndrome has been described in extremely obese individuals who show little or no evidence of primary disease of the heart or lungs (see p 168).

Treatment

"Specific" weight-reducing chemical agents and hormones (eg, thyroid, chorionic gonadotropin), singly or in combination, are either ineffective or hazardous and have no place in the treatment of obesity. Juvenile-onset obesity is often very difficult to treat, possibly because of some ill-defined metabolic disorder, and it is important to institute a therapeutic program as early as possible.

A. Diet: Diet is the most important factor in the management of obesity. Preventive education about diet should be started during the formative years, at the time when eating habits are being established. The motivation to reduce caloric intake to normal levels is difficult to achieve in patients with long-standing overeating patterns. Diets that claim to offer easy weight reduction by reliance on certain "special" foods or unusual combinations of foods not only are invalid but may actually be harmful. There are a number of basic points to be considered in planning a diet for an obese patient.

1. Calories–In order to lose weight, it is necessary to decrease the intake to below the caloric requirements. An intake of 500 kcal per day less than the required calories should lead to an average weight loss of approximately 0.5 kg a week.

The number of calories per day to prescribe for a patient varies with age, occupation, temperament, and the urgency of the need for weight reduction. A daily caloric intake of 800–1200 kcal is satisfactory for a modest reducing diet. (Vitamin supplementation is advisable for patients with a daily intake of less than 1200 kcal.) An attempt should be made to maintain nitrogen balance, although this is not always possible. In these markedly restricted diets, ketonuria may appear; it is usually very slight after the first few days, however, and acidosis has never been observed. In addition, since the patients realize they are on a "diet," they often will adhere more willingly when they show rapid weight loss than when the results appear slowly. Patients should be informed that the "empty" calories in alcohol contribute to body weight but have no nutritive value.

Complications of rapid weight reduction are largely associated with severe or prolonged caloric restriction and occur most commonly in patients who were obese as children. Weakness, postural hypotension, ketosis, metabolic acidosis, hyperuricemia, urolithiasis, ulcerative colitis, and many other physical complications have been reported. Mental depression and even suicidal thoughts are not uncommon. The importance of careful medical and psychologic evaluation prior to weight reduction and periodic follow-up should be apparent.

2. Proteins–A protein intake of about 1 g/kg

Table 21–7. Low-calorie diets: Foods to be distributed into regular meals during the day.*

	800 kcal	1000 kcal	1200 kcal	1500 kcal
Breads, enriched white or whole-grain†	1/2 slice	1 slice	2 slices	3 slices
Fruit, unsugared (1/2 cup)	3 servings	3 servings	3 servings	3 servings
Eggs, any way but fried	One	One	One	One
Fats and oils, butter, margarine, mayonnaise, or oil	None	3 tsp	5 tsp	6 tsp
Milk (nonfat, skimmed, or buttermilk)	2 cups	2 cups	2 cups	2 cups
Meat, fish, or poultry, any way but fried‡	4 oz	5 oz	6 oz	6 oz
Vegetables, raw (salads) (1 serving = 1/2 cup)	2 servings	2 servings	2 servings	2 servings
Vegetables, cooked, green, yellow, or soup (1 serving = 1/2 cup)	2 servings	2 servings	3 servings	3 servings
Starch, potato, etc	None	None	None	1 serving
Artificial sweeteners	As desired	As desired	As desired	As desired

*See also Table 21–2.

†May substitute 1/2 cup cooked cereal or 1 cup dry prepared cereal for 1 slice bread.

‡May substitute 1/2 cup cottage cheese or 3 slices (3 oz) cheddar cheese for 3 oz meat.

Table 21—8. Caloric values of common "snack" foods.*

	Amount or Average Serving	Calorie Count		Amount or Average Serving	Calorie Count
Sandwiches			**Candies**		
Hamburger on bun	3-inch patty	500	Chocolate bars		
Peanut butter sandwich	2 tsp filling	200	Plain	1 bar (1¼ oz)	190
Cheese sandwich	1½ oz cheese	400	With nuts	1 bar	275
Ham sandwich	1½ oz ham	350	Chocolate covered bar	1 bar	250
Bread	1 slice	60	Chocolate cream, bonbon, fudge	1 piece 1-inch square	90
Beverages			Caramels, plain	1 piece ¾-inch cube	35
Carbonated drinks, soda, root beer, etc	6-oz glass	80	Chocolate nut caramels	1 piece	60
Cola beverages	12-oz glass (Pepsi)	150	**Desserts**		
Chocolate malted milk	10-oz glass (1¼ cups)	450	Pie		
Ginger ale	6-oz glass	60	Fruit (apple, etc)	⅙ pie	400
Tea or coffee, no cream or sugar	1 cup	0	Custard	⅙ pie	250
			Lemon meringue	⅙ pie	350
Tea or coffee, with 2 tbsp cream and 2 tsp sugar	1 cup	90	Pumpkin pie	⅙ pie	325
Hot chocolate	1 cup	200	Cookies, chocolate chip	1 (2-inch diameter)	50
Alcoholic Drinks			Cake		
Ale	8-oz glass	130	2 layers, iced white	1 serving	345
Beer	8-oz glass	110	Fruit, ¼-inch slice	1 serving	125
Highball (with ginger ale)	8-oz glass	140	Ice cream		
Manhattan	Average	175	Chocolate	½ cup	150
Martini	Average	160	Vanilla and other flavors	½ cup	130
Old-fashioned	Average	150	Milk sherbet	½ cup	120
Sherry	2-oz glass	80	Ice milk	½ cup	95
Scotch, bourbon, rye	1-oz jigger	80	Sundaes, small chocolate nut with whipped cream	Average	400
Fruits			Ice cream sodas, chocolate	10-oz glass	270
Apple	One 3-inch	90	**Late Snacks**		
Banana	One 6-inch	100	Cold potato	½ medium	65
Grapes	30 medium	75	Chicken leg	1 average	88
Orange	One 2¾-inch	80	Milk	7-oz glass	140
Pear	One	100	Mouthful of roast	½ × 2 × 3 inches	130
Salted Nuts			Piece of cheese	¼ × 2 × 3 inches	120
Almonds	10	130	Brownie	¾ × 1¾ × 2¼ inches	300
Cashews	10	60	Cream puff	4-inch diameter	450
Peanuts	10	60	Cheese cake	⅙ of 8-inch cake	480
Pecans	10 halves	150			

*Modified and reprinted by permission of Smith Kline & French Laboratories.

should be maintained. If it is necessary to add protein to the low-calorie diet, protein hydrolysate or casein (free of carbohydrate and fat) can be used.

3. Carbohydrate and fat–To reduce the intake of calories and the risk of ketosis, fats must be decreased. After the protein requirements have been met, the remaining calories may be supplied as half carbohydrate and half fat.

4. Vitamins and minerals–Most reducing diets are likely to be deficient in vitamins but adequate in minerals. Therefore, vitamins should be used to supply the average daily maintenance requirements during the time of weight reduction.

5. Sodium restriction–It has been shown that a normal person on a salt-free diet will lose up to 2–3 kg in a matter of days; this reduction is temporary, and the weight will return when salt is added to the diet. The same is true of the obese patient, and, although an apparently dramatic effect can be obtained with salt-free diets, it is of no permanent value.

6. Starvation regimens–Semistarvation and total starvation have been advocated for weight reduction. Although rapid loss of weight can be achieved by these methods, they are unphysiologic and can be quite hazardous. Several deaths have occurred. Total starvation results largely in breakdown of fat, but it may also lead to excessive protein breakdown, with fainting due to decrease in extracellular fluid volume because of sodium loss. Massive weight reduction can result in severe medical complications. Several deaths have been reported during and after total fasting due to intractable ventricular arrhythmias, lactic acidosis, hepatic failure, renal failure, and small bowel obstruction with complications. Periodic total fasting to the point of ketonemia has seemed to cause accelerated weight loss in patients who fail to lose significantly on 1000-kcal diets. This accelerated weight loss may be spurious, however, and often represents fluid loss due to ketonuria.

Some bizarre semistarvation and liquid protein

diets are hazardous because of inadequate intake of essential foodstuffs and may cause acute life-threatening hypokalemia and dysrhythmias in susceptible individuals.

B. Obesity Surgery: Jejunoileal shunt is being performed on selected patients whose massive or morbid obesity (ie, more than 2 times ideal weight) has *failed to respond to all conservative measures and is considered to be an imminent health hazard.* The procedure provides permanent weight reduction and alleviates many of the physiologic abnormalities associated with obesity but produces considerable chronic morbidity that seriously compromises its benefits. Complications are numerous, including intestinal malabsorption, fluid and electrolyte disturbances, hypocalcemia, osteopenia, renal calculi, renal failure, severe arthropathy, psychiatric disorders, cholelithiasis, hepatic dysfunction, and, more importantly, hepatic cirrhosis. *Many of the long-term effects are not known.*

Gastric bypass (gastric partition, gastroplasty) surgery that limits the amount of food that can be ingested is being employed as an alternative to jejunoileal bypass in many centers. Although this type of surgery would appear to be more physiologic and has fewer complications, results have been variable, *and long-term results and sequelae are not known.*

Patients who are being considered for surgery for morbid obesity should be given a thorough explanation of the risks and uncertainties as well as the possible benefits.

C. Medication:

1. Appetite suppressants–Amphetamines and other anorexigenic drugs may be of temporary value in aiding selected patients on reducing regimens by decreasing the appetite and giving a sense of well-being. However, their use is controversial because of their long-term inefficiency and the hazard of drug abuse (in the case of amphetamines), and the trend is definitely away from the use of these drugs.

2. Drugs to speed up metabolism–*Note:* There is no satisfactory drug to speed up metabolism. Thyroid has little or no place in the management of obesity. The low basal metabolic rate associated with obesity is merely due to the fact that the rate is a measurement of oxygen consumption in terms of body surface area. Tests that actually measure thyroid function (eg, T_3, T_4) are usually normal in obese patients. It has been shown that obese people with low basal metabolic rates can tolerate 0.2 g or more of thyroid per day without change in basal metabolic rate. Prolonged administration of thyroid may suppress normal thyroid secretion.

There is no scientific evidence to support the hypothesis that human chorionic gonadotropin exerts a physiologic antiobesity effect.

D. Exercise: Increase in physical activity is an important factor in long-range weight reduction and maintenance as well as for general psychologic and physical well-being. Although exercise increases the energy output, extreme exercise is necessary to alter body weight significantly. Caloric limitation must be

observed simultaneously with a planned exercise program.

E. Psychologic Factors: Overeating is largely a matter of habit and may be associated with varying degrees of emotional problems. Once significant obesity has been established, many secondary psychologic reactions occur relating to altered body image and changes in interpersonal relationships. Weight reduction is therefore essential for general psychologic as well as physical well-being. Mildly or moderately obese patients often respond to simple psychologic support, encouragement, dietary management, and situational adjustments. Relapses occur frequently and should be dealt with in an understanding manner. Conventional psychotherapy is seldom of lasting value in weight reduction in markedly obese patients. The patient must simply be convinced that lifelong eating habits must be modified permanently if desirable weight reduction is to be permanently maintained. Compulsive overeating is similar in some respects to addiction to tobacco or alcohol. Behavior modification therapy and self-help groups of obese patients are effective for some patients.

Note: Sudden weight reduction in emotionally unstable persons may have severe psychic consequences, eg, anorexia nervosa, psychotic reactions.

Alpers DH: Surgical therapy for obesity. (Editorial.) *N Engl J Med* 1983;**308**:1026.

Andersen T et al: Randomized trial of diet and gastroplasty compared with diet alone in morbid obesity. *N Engl J Med* 1984;**310**:352.

Boisaubin EV: Approach to obese patients. *West J Med* 1984;**140**:794.

Brownell KD: The psychology and physiology of obesity. *J Am Diet Assoc* 1984;**84**:406.

Callaway CW: Weight standards: Their clinical significance. (Editorial.) *Ann Intern Med* 1984;**100**:206.

Conn HL, de Felice EA, Kuo PT: *Health and Obesity.* Raven Press, 1983.

Felig P: Very-low-calorie protein diets. (Editorial.) *N Engl J Med* 1984;**310**:589.

Hocking MP et al: Jejunoileal bypass for morbid obesity: Late follow-up in 100 cases. *N Engl J Med* 1983;**308**:995.

Horton ES et al: Symposium on the regulation of energy balance in humans. *Am J Clin Nutr* 1983;**38**:972.

Hudiburgh NK: A multidisciplinary approach to weight control. *J Am Diet Assoc* 1984;**84**:447.

Newmark SR, Williamson B: Survey of very-low-calorie weight reducing diets. (2 parts.) *Arch Intern Med* 1983;**143**:1195, 1423.

Phinney SD et al: Normal cardiac rhythms during hypocaloric diets of varying carbohydrate content. *Arch Intern Med* 1983;**143**:2259.

Simopoulos AP, Van Itallie TB: Body weight, health and longevity. *Ann Intern Med* 1984;**100**:285.

Stewart AL, Brook RH: Effects of being overweight. *Am J Public Health* 1983;**73**:171.

Vaselli JR, Cleary MP, Van Itallie TB: Modern concepts of obesity. *Nutr Rev* 1983;**41**:361.

Wadden TA: The Cambridge diet. *JAMA* 1983;**250**:2833.

Wadden TA, Stunkard AJ, Brownell KD: Very low caloric diets: Their efficacy, safety and future. *Ann Intern Med* 1983;**99**:675.

ANOREXIA NERVOSA

Anorexia nervosa is a serious eating disorder that occurs principally in white females in the second and third decades of life and is manifested by extreme aversion to food, intense fear of gaining weight, and disturbance of body image. Amenorrhea and other metabolic changes are associated with the profound emaciation that occurs. The incidence in white adolescent females in Western countries is estimated to be 1:200–250.

The exact cause of anorexia nervosa is unknown. The illness appears to have its origin in complex psychologic problems including depression, obsessiveness, ineffectiveness, and unresolved conflict. It is not uncommon for the patient to have parents who are overly concerned with weight reduction, dietary matters, and exercise. The patient's anorexic behavior may follow a period of being overly sensitive about adolescent plumpness.

The relationship between the extreme malnutrition that occurs in anorexia nervosa and the neuroendocrine abnormalities that have been observed in the illness has not been clearly established. Involvement of the hypothalamic–anterior pituitary–gonadal axis is evident from defects of cyclic gonadotropin release, decreased estrogen production, amenorrhea, impaired thermoregulation, and alteration of appetite and satiety. Most evidence supports the theory that these endocrine abnormalities of anorexia nervosa are secondary to malnutrition, although it is possible that intrinsic hypothalamic malfunction may play a role.

The patient's persistent and morbid refusal to eat adequately, even in the face of real hunger, leads to profound weight loss and emaciation. Deceit will be practiced in order to lose weight, including misrepresentation of food intake, concealment of uneaten food, self-induced vomiting, and surreptitious purgation. Amenorrhea is a constant manifestation in women of childbearing age; it may rarely precede weight loss and may persist at times after weight loss has been corrected. Patients complain of intolerance to cold.

Physical findings include the appearance of cachexia (due to loss of at least 25% of ideal body weight), dry skin, increased body hair (lanugo), decreased body temperature, and acrocyanosis. The skin may have a yellowish tint due to hypercarotenemia. The pulse is slow, and the blood pressure is often low normal. Arrhythmias may be noted. There may be clinical and laboratory evidence of nutritional anemia, vitamin and mineral deficiencies, impaired renal function, electrolyte imbalance (particularly hypokalemia), hypothyroidism, and decreased gonadal function. Anorexia nervosa must be differentiated from panhypopituitarism (see p 691).

In the rare instances when anorexia nervosa occurs in males, the clinical picture is similar to that in females, with comparable psychologic problems and deficiency of male gonadal function.

Treatment of anorexia nervosa is difficult and is best carried out by individuals trained and experienced in the care of patients with the illness. The patient should be admitted to the hospital if weight loss is marked and unremitting, or if there is evidence of fluid and electrolyte abnormalities, intercurrent infection, or severe personal and family problems. Careful supervision and skilled nursing care are required during the weight gain process. The patient should not be left alone during meals and should be encouraged to eat by friendly persuasion and insistence. Punitive attitudes and forced feedings must be avoided, since they further aggravate the patient's lack of self-confidence and self-identity. When malnutrition is severe and life-threatening (eg, >40% weight loss), enteral and parenteral nutrition is essential. Adequate rest in the hospital must be ensured. Judicious use of tricyclic antidepressants for deeply depressed patients might be considered, although benefits are equivocal. Return of normal body weight is usually accompanied by an improvement of the patient's emotional status and sense of physical well-being.

Relapses and remissions are common. Long-term psychotherapy for the patient and the family (if necessary) and dietary management are usually required. Unless proper treatment is given, patients with anorexia nervosa may succumb from inanition, complicating infection, or suicide. The mortality rate may be as high as 30%.

Dempsey DT et al: Weight gain and nutritional efficacy in anorexia nervosa. *Am J Clin Nutr* 1984;**39:**236.

Herzog DB: Anorexia nervosa: A treatment challenge. *Drug Ther* 1982;**12:**103.

Humphries LL, Wrobel S, Weigert HT: Anorexia nervosa. *Am Fam Physician* (Nov) 1982;**26:**199.

Huse DM, Lucas AR: Dietary treatment of anorexia nervosa. *J Am Diet Assoc* 1983;**83:**687.

McSherry JA: The diagnostic challenge of anorexia nervosa. *Am Fam Physician* (Feb) 1984;**29:**141.

Provenzale JM: Anorexia nervosa: Thinness as illness. *Postgrad Med* (Oct) 1983;**74:**83.

BULIMIA
(Bulimarexia; Binge-Purge Syndrome)

Bulimia is a compulsive eating disorder in which the patient experiences recurrent uncontrollable urges to eat large quantities of high-calorie food in a short period of time. These gorging episodes (binges) are regularly followed by attempts to lose weight by self-induced vomiting or use of cathartics or diuretics. The disease occurs most frequently in young women from the middle and upper socioeconomic classes. High school and college students, models, and actresses seem to be particularly vulnerable.

Bulimia shares many features with anorexia nervosa, and the 2 disorders may overlap. The bulimic has an exaggerated fear of becoming fat and of the changing body shape, whereas the patient with anorexia is obsessed with becoming thin. The psychodynamics are unclear, but bulimic patients tend to be anxious, perfectionistic, and achievement-oriented.

Recognition of the disorder may be difficult because of the secretive nature of the binge eating. Patients must be questioned directly about preoccupation with food, eating habits, and purging activities that follow. Many bulimics are able to maintain a near-normal weight despite frequent weight fluctuations. A history of menstrual irregularities or amenorrhea is common. Clinical signs are those associated with the complications of vomiting or of laxative and diuretic abuse. These include chronic sore throat, painless parotid swelling, erosion of dental enamel, bowel irregularities, dehydration, and electrolytic disturbances.

Treatment consists of emotional support with individual, group, or family psychotherapy. The patient should be provided with adequate nutritional information and followed periodically to maintain health and prevent complications.

Bo-Linn GW et al: Purging and caloric absorption in bulimia patients and normal women. *Ann Intern Med* 1983;**99**:14.

Harris RT: Bulimarexia and related serious eating disorders with medical complications. *Ann Intern Med* 1983;**99**:800.

PROTEIN & CALORIE MALNUTRITION

Protein and calorie malnutrition occurs in a clinical continuum ranging from inadequate proteins with adequate calories (kwashiorkor) to inadequate proteins and calories (marasmus). These conditions constitute the most important problems in nutrition throughout the world.

Kwashiorkor

Kwashiorkor is a nutritional deficiency syndrome that usually occurs in weanling infants (usually age 2 years or older) at the birth of a sibling but may occur in children of any age and even in adults. It is attributed primarily to inadequate intake of proteins or perhaps of specific essential amino acids with adequate calories, but mineral and vitamin deficiencies may also play a role. It is prevalent in underprivileged sections of Africa, Asia, southern Europe, and Central and South America, in areas where the protein content of the diet is deficient in amount or of poor quality (vegetable protein). The condition may be precipitated by tropical infections, diarrhea, and extreme heat, which aggravate the nutritional deficiency by curtailing the intake, decreasing the absorption, and increasing the demand. The liver shows the most marked pathologic changes: hepatic enlargement and fatty infiltration that may progress to a condition resembling portal cirrhosis. There is also atrophy of the pancreatic acini, with loss of granules followed by fibrosis.

Kwashiorkor is characterized clinically by growth failure, irritability and apathy, skin changes (rash, desquamation, hyperpigmentation or depigmentation, ulceration), cheilosis, stomatitis, conjunctivitis, sparse or depigmented hair, anorexia, vomiting, diarrhea, hepatomegaly, muscular wasting, and edema. Blood changes include anemia, hypoalbuminemia, hyperglobulinemia, and low levels of urea, potassium, cholesterol, alkaline phosphatase, amylase, and lipase.

Prevention of the disease is a combined public health and socioeconomic problem and, in cases where personal or cultural food preferences prejudice the protein intake, an educational problem.

Treatment consists of supplying an adequate intake of protein (3–4 g/kg) of high biologic value (eg, milk, eggs, meat, soybeans). Patient and regular administration of skimmed or whole milk will often result in rather prompt recovery if the condition is not too far advanced. If oral feeding is a problem, tube feeding or intravenous hyperalimentation may be necessary. Vitamin supplements may be indicated. Intramuscular injection of the water-soluble palmitate has been recommended in severe vitamin A deficiency. Patients who are dehydrated as a result of vomiting or diarrhea, especially when critically ill, require appropriate oral or parenteral fluid and electrolyte replacement. Concomitant infections require simultaneous treatment. Whole blood or plasma transfusions may be necessary. During the recovery phase, attention should be paid to total calories as well as high protein intake.

Kwashiorkor syndromes occur in all degrees of severity, and the rate of recovery with proper treatment varies accordingly. Without treatment, the mortality rate in severe cases of this disorder is high.

Protein-Calorie Malnutrition

Marasmus, a condition caused by severe protein-calorie malnutrition in early life, is characterized by retarded growth and atrophy of muscles and viscera. There is no edema, nor are there skin changes as in kwashiorkor. Subcutaneous fat, however, is minimal or absent. The condition may be caused not only by unavailability of food but also by such factors as prematurity, diarrhea, cystic fibrosis, and mental retardation.

Protein-calorie malnutrition also occurs in older individuals, especially those who are poor, elderly, isolated, and chronically ill. Moderate or even severe degrees of protein-calorie malnutrition have surprisingly been observed in private patients in community hospitals. This may be due to inadequate food intake because of anorexia, prolonged nausea and vomiting, esophagitis, and malabsorption or to abnormal protein losses (eg, with burns or trauma). Awareness of some of the manifestations of semi-starvation—lethargy, anorexia, weight loss, decreased muscle mass, decreased strength, edema, hypoproteinemia, decreased iron-binding capacity, lymphopenia, and increased susceptibility to infection—can lead to timely corrective nutritional measures.

Treatment is similar to that for kwashiorkor. Failure to identify and treat protein-calorie malnutrition with oral, enteral, or total parenteral nutrition can contribute to the morbidity and mortality of many hospital patients.

Blackburn GL, Harvey KB: Nutritional assessment as a routine in clinical medicine. *Postgrad Med* (May) 1982;**71**:46.

Detsky AS et al: Evaluating the accuracy of nutritional assessment techniques applied to hospitalized patients: Methodology and comparison. *JPEN* 1984;**8**:153.

Gray DS, Kaminski MV Jr: Nutritional support of the hospitalized patient. *Am Fam Physician* (Sept) 1983;**28**:143.

Herbert VD, Hubbard VS (editors): Assessment of nutritional status. Selected papers: Conference on the assessment of nutritional status. *Am J Clin Nutr* 1982;**35(Suppl)**:1089.

Klidjian AM et al: Detection of dangerous malnutrition. *JPEN* 1982;**6**:119.

McIntosh EN, Laurent LL: Nutritional assessment of the hospitalized patient. *Am Fam Physician* (Jan) 1983;**27**:169.

Mendenhall CL et al: Protein-caloric malnutrition associated with alcoholic hepatitis. *Am J Med* 1984;**76**:211.

●　　●　　●

References

American Dietetic Association: *Handbook of Clinical Dietetics.* Yale Univ Press, 1981.

Anderson L et al: *Nutrition in Health and Disease,* 17th ed. Lippincott, 1982.

Blackburn GL, Grant IP, Young VR (editors): *Amino Acids: Metabolism and Medical Applications.* Wright, 1983.

Composition of Foods. Agriculture Handbook, 8–1 through 9, Agricultural Research Service, US Dept of Agriculture, Washington DC. Revised 1976 through 1982.

Davidson LSP, Passmore R: *Human Nutrition and Dietetics,* 7th ed. Churchill Livingstone, 1979.

Eisenstein AB: Nutritional and metabolic effects of alcohol. *J Am Diet Assoc* 1982;**81**:247.

Food and Nutrition Board, National Academy of Sciences–National Research Council: *Recommended Dietary Allowances,* 9th ed. Publication 1694, Washington DC, 1980.

Goodhart RS, Shils ME: *Modern Nutrition in Health and Disease: Dietotherapy,* 6th ed. Lea & Febiger, 1980.

Hertzler AA, Wenkam N, Standl B: Classifying cultural food habits and meanings. *J Am Diet Assoc* 1982;**80**:421.

Hodges RE: *Nutrition in Medical Practice.* Saunders, 1980.

Kart CS, Metress SP: *Nutrition, the Aged and Society.* Prentice-Hall, 1983.

Kohrs MB et al: Symposium on nutrition and aging. *Am J Clin Nutr* 1982;**36**:735.

Martin DW Jr, Mayes PA, Rodwell VW: *Harper's Review of Biochemistry,* 19th ed. Lange, 1983.

Neuberger A, Jukes TH (editors): *Human Nutrition: Current Issues and Controversies.* Burgess, 1982.

Nutrition Reviews: Present Knowledge in Nutrition, 5th ed. The Nutrition Foundation, 1984.

Pennington JAT, Church HN: *Bowes and Church's Food Values of Portions Commonly Used,* 13th ed. Lippincott, 1980.

Robinson CH, Weigley ES: *Basic Nutrition and Diet Therapy,* 5th ed. Macmillan, 1984.

Roe DA: *Handbook: Interaction of Selected Drugs and Nutrients in Patients,* 3rd ed. American Dietetic Association, 1982.

Taylor KB, Anthony LE: *Clinical Nutrition.* McGraw-Hill, 1983.

Thiele VF: *Clinical Nutrition,* 2nd ed. Mosby, 1980.

22 | Introduction to Infectious Diseases

Ernest Jawetz, MD, PhD, & Moses Grossman, MD

Infections can and do involve all human organ systems. In a book organized, as this one is, principally by organ system, many important infectious disease entities are discussed in the chapters devoted to specific anatomic areas. Thus, pneumonias are discussed in Chapter 7, infective endocarditis in Chapter 8, and urinary tract infections in Chapter 16. Other important infections are described under the headings of their etiologic agents in Chapters 23–28.

In this introductory chapter, we wish to focus on a few broad problems of infectious disease that touch upon many facets of diagnosis and treatment. To minimize duplication, we will refer to other areas of this book for more detailed or supplementary information.

FEVER OF UNDETERMINED ORIGIN (FUO)*

Fever of undetermined origin is defined as an illness of at least 3 weeks' duration with fever over 38 °C (100.4 °F) as the principal symptom. This "diagnosis" should not be entertained until diagnostic procedures, including repeated cultures of blood, tissues, and urine, skin and serologic tests, search for neoplasm or evidence of collagen vascular disease, etc, have failed to establish a specific etiologic diagnosis. Most cases of FUO are eventually found to represent atypical manifestations of common diseases rather than exotic illnesses.

Etiologic Considerations

It is important to proceed systematically in approaching this difficult diagnostic problem. Every effort should be made to identify infectious processes, obscure cancer, and autoimmune or collagen vascular diseases. Miscellaneous causes constitute a fourth major etiologic category.

A. Infectious Processes: It is well to consider systemic infections and localized infections separately. The former include tuberculosis, disseminated mycoses, infective endocarditis, infectious mononucleosis, cytomegalovirus infection, toxoplasmosis, brucellosis, salmonellosis, and many other less common diseases.

The most common form of localized infection is an obscure abscess. Liver, spleen, kidney, brain, and bone are organs where an abscess may be difficult to find. Likewise, a collection of pus may form in the peritoneal cavity or in the subdiaphragmatic, subhepatic, paracolonic, or other areas. Cholangitis, urinary tract infection, dental abscess, or a collection of pus in a paranasal sinus may cause prolonged fever before it is identified.

B. Neoplasms: Many cancers may present with obscure fever as a major symptom. The most common of these are lymphoma and leukemia.

C. Collagen Diseases: Juvenile rheumatoid arthritis is an excellent example of a disease in which fever continues for a long time as almost the only symptom. This may occur also in other collagen vascular disorders.

D. Miscellaneous Causes: Many other diseases can cause prolonged fever. Examples are sarcoidosis, other noncaseating granulomas, pulmonary embolization, chronic liver disease, and familial Mediterranean fever. At times the fever may be factitious or self-induced.

Approach to Diagnosis

The key to diagnosis often lies in careful daily physical examination of the patient, repeated review of the medical history, and dogged pursuit of any abnormal finding (eg, an enlarged lymph node, a questionable chest x-ray). Systematic scanning and x-ray surveys may yield a clue. Systematic examination by ultrasound, computed tomography (CT scan) and radionuclide scan may reveal abdominal or retroperitoneal lymphadenopathy or tumor or abscess in pelvis or abdomen. If these and other studies remain noncontributory, biopsy of a lymph node or of the liver may reveal abnormalities. Ultimately, exploratory laparotomy may be considered, although it rarely provides a diagnosis if the other mentioned studies were noncontributory.

If any tissue is obtained, optimal use of it must be made for touch preparations, microbiologic cultures, and histologic examinations.

It is most important to diagnose those diseases for which effective treatment is available and early institution of therapy may be curative.

With the passage of time, the true cause of fever

---

*This entity is discussed also in Chapter 1.

often becomes apparent; thus, it may be helpful to repeat tests that previously were noncontributory. About 10% of cases of FUO remain undiagnosed. Therapeutic trials without diagnosis are seldom indicated. There is little benefit (or harm) in suppressing the fever as such, but doing so may make the patient more comfortable.

Dinarello CA, Wolff SM: Molecular basis of fever in humans. *Am J Med* 1982;**72**:799.

Larson EB et al: Fever of undetermined origin: Diagnosis and follow-up of 105 cases, 1970–1980. *Medicine* 1982;**61**:269.

Pizzo PA et al: Prolonged fever in children: Review of 100 cases. *Pediatrics* 1975;**55**:468.

Quinn MJ et al: Computed tomography of the abdomen in evaluation of patients with fever of unknown origin. *Radiology* 1980; **136**:407.

INFECTIONS IN THE IMMUNODEFICIENT PATIENT

A description of the cellular basis of immune responses, the role of various host responses in maintaining health, and the methods used for detection of deficiencies in the immune system can be found in Chapter 34. Immunodeficiency may be congenital but more often is due to suppression of the immune system by diseases or drugs. Deficiencies of polymorphonuclear cells, T lymphocytes, or B lymphoctes tend to predispose the host to infection with different agents. Thus, polymorphonuclear cell deficiency predisposes particularly to infection with gram-negative enteric bacteria and staphylococci; B lymphocyte deficiency and hypogammaglobulinemia to infection with extracellular encapsulated organisms, eg, pneumococci or *Haemophilus* sp; and T lymphocyte deficiency to infection with intracellular bacteria (eg, mycobacteria, *Listeria*, *Legionella*), fungi (*Candida*, *Cryptococcus*, *Aspergillus*, etc), protozoa (*Pneumocystis carinii*, etc), and viruses (cytomegalovirus, herpes simplex, etc).

Many opportunistic organisms (ie, organisms that rarely produce invasive infections in an uncompromised host) do not produce disease except in the immunodeficient host. Such hosts are often infected with several opportunists simultaneously.

Infections caused by common organisms may present uncommon clinical manifestations. Determination of the specific infecting agents is essential for effective treatment.

Immunodeficient Hosts

Patients deficient in normal immune defenses fall into several groups:

(1) Congenital defects of cellular or humoral immunity or a combination of both, eg, Wiskott-Aldrich syndrome. These are usually children.

(2) Patients with cancer, particularly lymphoreticular cancer.

(3) Patients receiving immunosuppressive therapy. These include patients with neoplastic disease and transplant recipients who are receiving corticosteroids, other immunosuppressive drugs, or irradiation treatment.

(4) Patients who have very few polymorphonuclear cells ($< 500/\mu L$) or those whose polymorphonuclear cells do not function normally with respect to phagocytosis or the intracellular killing of phagocytosed microorganisms (eg, chronic granulomatous disease).

(5) A larger group of patients who are not classically immunodeficient but whose host defenses are seriously compromised by prior splenectomy, debilitating illness, diabetes mellitus, surgical or other invasive procedures (eg, intravenous drug abuse or intravenous hyperalimentation), burns, or massive antimicrobial therapy.

(6) Patients with variants of the acquired immunodeficiency syndrome (AIDS) (see p 824). This profound disturbance in T lymphocyte subpopulations is of unknown etiology and was recognized recently, particularly in male homosexuals, intravenous drug abusers, Haitian immigrants, some hemophiliacs receiving factor VIII concentrate, and some patients who received transfusion with blood from donors who have acquired immunodeficiency syndrome. It produces extreme susceptibility to opportunistic infections and to rapidly disseminating Kaposi's sarcoma and other neoplasms, with an exceedingly high death rate.

Infectious Agents

A. Bacteria: Any bacterium pathogenic for humans can infect the immunosuppressed host. Furthermore, noninvasive and nonpathogenic organisms (opportunists) may also cause disease in such cases. Examples include gram-negative bacteria—particularly *Pseudomonas*, *Serratia*, *Proteus*, *Providencia*, and *Nocardia*. Many come from the hospital environment and are resistant to antimicrobial drugs.

B. Fungi: *Candida*, *Aspergillus*, *Cryptococcus*, *Mucor*, and others can all cause disease in the immunosuppressed host. Candidiasis is the most common and is often found in patients receiving intensive antimicrobial therapy.

C. Viruses: Cytomegalovirus is the most common, but varicella-zoster and herpes simplex viruses are also important. Vaccinia virus may cause serious problems, and its use is contraindicated.

D. Protozoa: *Pneumocystis carinii* is an important cause of pneumonia in many immunodeficient patients. This diagnosis must be made early because reasonably effective therapy is available. *Toxoplasma gondii* is also important and is susceptible to therapy.

Cryptosporidium may cause chronic, severe diarrhea.

Approach to Diagnosis

A systematic approach is necessary, including the following steps:

(1) Review carefully the patient's current immune status, previous antimicrobial therapy, and *all* previous culture reports.

(2) Obtain pertinent cultures for bacteria, fungi, yeasts, and viruses.

(3) Consider which of the serologic tests for fungal, viral, and protozoal diseases are pertinent.

(4) Consider special diagnostic procedures, eg, lung biopsy or lung puncture or transbronchial biopsy to demonstrate *Pneumocystis*. Quantitation of T lymphocyte subpopulations by immunologic means (monoclonal antibodies in immunofluorescence tests) may be valuable.

(5) Consider whether the infection (eg, candidiasis) is superficial or systemic. Therapeutic considerations are quite different in each case.

Approach to Treatment

Caution: It is essential to avoid aggravating the patient's other problems and to avoid gross alterations of the host's normal microbial flora.

Provide general therapeutic measures to improve host defenses, correct electrolyte imbalance, offer adequate caloric intake, etc. Improve the patient's immune status whenever possible. This includes temporary decrease in immunosuppressive drug dosage in transplant patients and modification of chemotherapy in cancer patients.

Injection of immune globulin USP (human gamma globulin) at regular intervals can compensate for certain B cell deficiencies. Granulocyte transfusions are only rarely able to tide the patient over a prolonged period of neutropenia.

Antimicrobial drug therapy should be specific and lethal for the infecting agent. Combinations of chemotherapeutic agents may be necessary, since multiple infectious agents may be involved in some cases.

Thus, empiric combined therapy may have to be started promptly in the immunosuppressed patient with a pulmonary infiltrate. This often includes a cephalosporin (eg, cefoperazone or cefotaxime, 2 g every 4 hours in intravenous infusion) plus an aminoglycoside (eg, amikacin, 15 mg/kg/d) and even trimethoprim with sulfamethoxazole (16 tablets daily orally or appropriate doses intravenously) for possible *Pneumocystis* organisms. Amphotericin B may at times be started empirically on suspicion rather than on definitive proof of systemic candidiasis.

Love JL et al: Improved prognosis for granulocytopenic patients with gram negative bacteremia. *Am J Med* 1980;**68**:643.

Peterson PK et al: Infectious diseases in hospitalized renal transplant recipients. *Medicine* 1982;**61**:360.

Pizzo PA: Infectious complications in the child with cancer. 1. Pathophysiology of the compromised host and the initial evaluation and management of the febrile cancer patient. *J Pediatr* 1981;**98**:341.

Prober CG et al: Open lung biopsy in immunocompromised children with pulmonary infiltrates. *Am J Dis Child* 1984;**138**:60.

van der Meer JWM, van den Broek JP: Present status of the management of patients with defective phagocyte function. *Rev Infect Dis* 1984;**6**:107.

Young LS: Nosocomial infections in the immunocompromised adult. *Am J Med* 1981;**70**:398.

NOSOCOMIAL INFECTIONS

Nosocomial infections are by definition those acquired in the course of hospitalization. Classic examples of the distant past are "childbed fever" after delivery and wound gangrene after surgical operations. These were largely controlled by the development of aseptic techniques, the introduction of sterile materials and sterile surgical methods, and the rise of bacteriologic diagnosis.

At present in the USA, 3–7% of patients who enter the hospital free from infection acquire a nosocomial infection. Very rarely, a virulent, invasive, highly communicable organism such as Lassa fever virus is transmitted from an undiagnosed patient to others in the hospital. Much more commonly, patients acquire hospital infections with common organisms because of their own great susceptibility to infection or because of procedures carried out in the hospital.

Nosocomial infections can be attributed principally to one or more of the following features of contemporary medical care:

(1) Many hospitalized patients (especially in tertiary care hospitals, which have the highest nosocomial infection rate) are compromised because of deficiencies in their immunologic responses. These may be congenital but most commonly are acquired as a result of the administration of drugs for the treatment of cancer, for maintenance of transplants, or for suppression of autoimmune processes. The very young and the elderly are also particularly susceptible to infection.

(2) Many aspects of medical care now require the use of invasive techniques for diagnosis, monitoring, and therapy. Examples are the indwelling urinary catheter; intravascular lines used for measurements, infusions of fluids or drugs, or parenteral alimentation; drainage tubes; and shunts.

(3) Materials administered in intensive care may themselves be vectors of infection: Intravenous solutions or their containers may be contaminated; respirators and humidifiers may introduce microorganisms into particularly susceptible lungs; plastic tubing may carry infectious agents into the body, etc.

(4) The massive use of antimicrobial drugs contributes to the selection of drug-resistant microorganisms both in the individual patient and in the hospital environment. Thus, nosocomial infections are often attributable to members of the endogenous human microflora or free-living microorganisms that happen to be particularly resistant to antimicrobial drugs, presenting difficult management problems. Such organisms often are not established human "pathogens" but can be classed as "opportunists."

The principal anatomic sites of hospital-acquired infection are the urinary tract, surgical wounds, the respiratory tract, or skin sites where indwelling needles or tubes penetrate. Most notorious among nosocomial infections are those due to gram-negative bacteria, staphylococci, or mycotic organisms that develop in patients with granulocyte counts below 500–1000/μL as a result of cancer chemotherapy. In such patients, bloodstream invasion often occurs without a well-defined portal of entry. Patients with markedly depressed cell-mediated immunity may also develop viral infections in the hospital, eg, varicella-zoster, cytomegalovirus, hepatitis, and others. They are likewise open to opportunists like *Legionella, Nocardia* sp, and other bacteria and protozoa, eg, *Pneumocystis carinii.*

The management of the immunodeficient patient is outlined on p 819). In nosocomial infections, it is particularly important to be alert to the possibility of infection, maintain continuous surveillance of patients at high risk (eg, by use of nurse epidemiologists), and have a well-defined, regularly updated program for diagnosis and treatment (through the hospital infection control committee). Continuing education of all hospital personnel and information about possible sources of infection among personnel are essential to maintain awareness of the many problems. The high-risk areas of hospitals include the nursery (especially the intensive care nursery), operating and recovery rooms, intensive care and coronary care units, cancer chemotherapy areas, hemodialysis and transplantation units, and all areas where postoperative patients are cared for.

Dixon RE: Second International Conference on Nosocomial Infections. *Am J Med* 1981;**70**:379.

Garibaldi RA et al: Infections among patients in nursing homes. *N Engl J Med* 1981;**305**:731.

Maki DG: Nosocomial bacteremia: An epidemiologic overview. *Am J Med* 1981;**70**:719.

McGowan JE Jr: Antimicrobial resistance in hospital organisms and its relation to antibiotic use. *Rev Infect Dis* 1983;**5**:1033.

INFECTIONS OF THE CENTRAL NERVOUS SYSTEM

Infections of the central nervous system can be caused by almost any infectious agent but most commonly are due to pyogenic bacteria, mycobacteria, fungi, spirochetes, and viruses. Certain symptoms and signs are more or less common to all types of central nervous system infection: headache, fever, sensorial disturbances, neck and back stiffness, positive Kernig and Brudzinski signs, and cerebrospinal fluid abnormalities. In patients presenting with these manifestations, the possibility of central nervous system infection must be considered.

Such an infection constitutes a *medical emergency.* Immediate diagnostic steps must be instituted to establish the specific cause. Normally, these include the history, physical examination, blood count, blood culture, lumbar puncture with careful study and culture of the cerebrospinal fluid, and a chest film when the patient's condition permits. A nasopharyngeal culture is also helpful. The cerebrospinal fluid must be examined for cell count, glucose, and protein, and a smear must be stained for bacteria (and acid-fast smear when appropriate) and cultured for pyogenic organisms and for acid-fast organisms and fungi when indicated. Counterimmunoelectrophoresis and latex agglutination can detect antigens of encapsulated etiologic organisms. In bacterial meningitis, prompt therapy is essential to prevent death and minimize serious sequelae.

If a space-occupying lesion (brain abscess, subdural empyema) is suspected, its presence may be confirmed by CT scan, which ideally should precede lumbar puncture.

Etiologic Classification

Central nervous system infections can be divided into several categories that usually can be readily distinguished from each other by cerebrospinal fluid examination as the first step toward etiologic diagnosis (Table 22–1).

A. Purulent Meningitis: Due to infection with meningococci (40% of cases), pneumococci, streptococci, *Haemophilus influenzae,* staphylococci, and other pyogenic organisms. Postoperative meningitis is

Table 22–1. Typical cerebrospinal fluid findings in various central nervous system diseases.

Diagnosis	Cells/μL	Glucose (mg/dL)	Protein (mg/dL)	Opening Pressure
Normal[1]	0–5 lymphocytes	45–85	15–45	70–180 mm H_2O
Purulent meningitis (bacterial)[2]	200–20,000 polymorphonuclear neutrophils	Low (< 45)	High (> 50)	++++
Granulomatous meningitis (mycobacterial, fungal)[2,3]	100–1000, mostly lymphocytes	Low (< 45)	High (> 50)	+++
Aseptic meningitis, viral or meningoencephalitis[3,4]	100–1000, mostly lymphocytes	Normal	Moderately high (> 50)	Normal to +
Spirochetal meningitis[3]	25–2000, mostly lymphocytes	Normal or low	High (> 50)	+
"Neighborhood" reaction[5]	Variably increased	Normal	Normal or high	Variable

[1] Cerebrospinal fluid glucose must be considered in relation to blood glucose level. Normally, cerebrospinal fluid glucose is 20–30 mg/dL lower than blood glucose, or 50–70% the normal value of blood glucose.

[2] Organisms in smear or culture of cerebrospinal fluid; counterimmunoelectrophoresis or latex agglutination may be diagnostic.

[3] Polymorphonuclear neutrophils may predominate early.

[4] Viral isolation from cerebrospinal fluid early; antibody titer rise in paired specimens of serum.

[5] May occur in mastoiditis, brain abscess, epidural abscess, sinusitis, septic thrombus, brain tumor. Cerebrospinal fluid culture results usually negative.

often caused by staphylococci, gram-negative enteric bacteria, or fungi.

B. Granulomatous Meningitis: Due to *Mycobacterium tuberculosis; Coccidioides, Cryptococcus, Histoplasma,* and other fungi; or *Treponema pallidum* (meningovascular syphilis).

C. Aseptic Meningitis: Aseptic meningitis is a much more benign form of meningitis caused principally by viruses—epecially mumps virus, the enterovirus group (including coxsackieviruses and echoviruses), and herpesviruses. Poliomyelitis virus was a common cause of aseptic meningitis before the introduction of vaccination. Infectious mononucleosis may be accompanied by aseptic meningitis. Leptospiral infection is usually placed in the aseptic group because of the lymphocytic cellular response and its relatively benign course. This type of meningitis also occurs during secondary syphilis.

D. Encephalitis: Due to herpesviruses, arboviruses, and many other viruses. Produces disturbances of the sensorium, seizures, and many other manifestations. Cerebrospinal fluid may be entirely normal or may show some lymphocytes.

E. Partially Treated Bacterial Meningitis: Bacterial meningitis may present with the same course and some of the same cerebrospinal fluid findings as aseptic meningitis following partly effective antimicrobial therapy.

F. "Neighborhood" Reaction: As noted in Table 22–1, this term denotes a purulent infectious process in close proximity to the central nervous system that spills some of the products of the inflammatory process—pus or protein—into the cerebrospinal fluid. Such an infection might be a brain abscess, osteomyelitis of the vertebrae, epidural abscess, subdural empyema, etc.

G. Meningitis in the Neonate: In newborn infants, meningitis often accompanies sepsis and is most often caused by group B beta-hemolytic streptococci, gram-negative rods (most commonly *Escherichia coli*), Listeria monocytogenes, and *Haemophilus influenzae;* it fails to show the typical signs of meningitis present in children or adults. Fever and neck signs are often absent. Instead, the infant is irritable, lethargic, and anorexic. Antimicrobial therapy is directed to the enteric group of bacteria and the streptococci.

H. Noninfectious Meningeal Irritation: Meningismus, presenting with the classic signs of meningeal irritation with totally normal cerebrospinal fluid findings, may occur in the presence of other infections such as pneumonia, shigellosis, etc. Meningeal invasion by neoplastic cells may present not only with physical findings of meningeal irritation but also with increased cells and lowered cerebrospinal fluid glucose.

Treatment

Treatment consists of supporting circulation, ventilation, the airway, and other life-support functions that may be compromised by infection and resulting disturbance of the central nervous system. Increased

Table 22–2. Initial antimicrobial therapy for purulent meningitis of unknown cause.

Age Group	Optimal Therapy (Intravenous Dose/24 Hours)	
Adult*	Penicillin	24 million units
Child older than 7 years	Penicillin or ampicillin	360,000 units/kg 300 mg/kg
Infant and child up to 7 years	Ampicillin† *and* chloramphenicol	300 mg/kg 100 mg/kg
Neonate (up to 3 months)‡	Ampicillin *and* gentamicin	200 mg/kg 5–6 mg/kg

*In penicillin allergy, chloramphenicol is the best alternative therapy.
†Combination designed to include coverage of ampicillin-resistant *Haemophilus influenzae* meningitis. See p 864.
‡Moxalactam, cefoperazone, or cefotaxime may become drugs of choice for meningitis caused by gram-negative enteric bacteria.

intracranial pressure due to brain edema often requires therapeutic attention. In the case of purulent meningitis proper, antimicrobial treatment is imperative. Since the identity of the causative microorganism may remain unknown or doubtful for a few days, initial antibiotic treatment as listed in Table 22–2 should be directed against the microorganisms most common for each age group.

Landesman SH et al: Gram-negative bacillary meningitis: New therapy and changing concepts. *Arch Intern Med* 1982; **142**:939.
Peltola H: Meningococcal disease: Still with us. *Rev Infect Dis* 1983;**5**:71.
Schaad VB et al: Recrudescence and relapse in bacterial meningitis. *Pediatrics* 1981;**67**:183.

GRAM-NEGATIVE BACTEREMIA & SEPSIS

Overwhelming gram-negative bacteremia with high mortality was typical of the great pestilences of the past such as plague and typhoid. Although environmental control has greatly reduced this threat, the rare case of plague today (originating from infected rodents and their fleas) can be as devastating as in the past. More commonly, sporadic meningococcemia (originating in the respiratory tract of asymptomatic persons) requires emergency diagnosis and treatment and may nevertheless end in death within a few hours.

Recently, bacteremia and sepsis caused by gram-negative bacteria and fungi—especially in hospitals—have increased greatly in incidence and severity. Factors responsible for this shift are larger numbers of debilitated or immunodeficient patients; more extensive surgical procedures; greater use of invasive diagnostic and therapeutic procedures; and the relentless selection pressure of antimicrobial drugs within individual patients and within hospital populations, which favors the survival and proliferation of drug-resistant gram-negative bacteria, yeasts, and fungi in a hospital setting.

The following are among the most frequent events leading up to gram-negative bacteremia and sepsis:

(1) Urinary tract infection, cystoscopy, catheterization (especially with an indwelling catheter), and urologic surgery.

(2) Tracheostomy, use of respirators with aerosol, use of endotracheal tubes.

(3) Intravenous infusion (plastic catheter needle) without changing site frequently; thrombophlebitis; contaminated solutions; intravenous drug abuse by addicts.

(4) Postsurgical infection, especially during antimicrobial therapy.

(5) Infected burns, wounds; delivery or abortion; perforation of an abdominal viscus.

(6) Severe neutropenia, eg, due to cancer with or without chemotherapy.

Clinical Findings

A. Symptoms and Signs: The onset might be with a shaking chill followed by an abrupt rise of fever. Alternatively, the patient may only appear flushed and anxious, with moderate temperature elevation. Soon there may be a fall in blood pressure or even frank shock with greatly impaired organ perfusion (kidney, brain, heart), anuria, nitrogen retention, acidosis, circulatory collapse, and death.

Unless the sequence of clinical signs can be reversed early, the mortality rate may be 50% or higher.

B. Laboratory Findings: Initial leukopenia may be present and is often followed by moderate leukocytosis. Proteinuria may precede a drastic reduction in urine volume. There may be evidence of metabolic acidosis or respiratory alkalosis and of disseminated intravascular coagulation (see p 345).

Treatment

The consequences of irreversible gram-negative shock are so grave that the clinician must constantly be on guard (see list of predisposing factors, above). Whenever a suspicion of gram-negative bacteremia arises, immediate blood cultures must be taken and a survey of potential sources of infection (catheters, infusions, thrombophlebitis, abscesses) must be carried out. Prompt elimination of these sources is often the most important step in the management of bacteremic shock. Gram-positive bacteremia may occasionally also precipitate shock.

A. Antibiotic Drugs: Suspected or proved gram-negative bacteremia must be promptly and intensively treated with antimicrobial drugs. Selection of the best initial drug depends on the most likely source and type of organism and on the pattern of drug susceptibility that prevails in a given locality in a given year. In 1984, drugs used initially often include a new cephalosporin (eg, cefotaxime, cefoperazone, or moxalactam, 12 g/d) and an aminoglycoside (eg, tobramycin, 7 mg/kg/d). If *Bacteroides fragilis* or another anaerobe

is suspected of originating from bowel or the female genital tract, metronidazole, 500 mg 4 times daily, or cefoxitin, 12 g/d, might be a drug of choice.

B. Management of Shock: (See also discussion in Chapter 1.) Management of bacteremic shock is directed at maintenance of organ perfusion, ventilation, correction of acidosis, and improvement of cardiac function. Central venous pressure or pulmonary artery wedge pressure is monitored to prevent fluid overload (see p 10). Plasma volume expanders (blood plasma, dextran, electrolyte solutions) are given to maintain organ perfusion and correct the prominent lactic acidosis but avoid pulmonary edema. Cardiac output may be increased by drugs such as isoproterenol ($1-2$ μg/min by intravenous drip) and especially by dopamine. This sympathomimetic amine dilates mesenteric and renal vessels (and thus increases renal blood flow and urine output) in addition to increasing cardiac output if infused in doses of $2-10$ μg/kg/min. Vasoconstrictors such as norepinephrine may further restrict organ perfusion and are therefore used sparingly in the early treatment of bacteremic shock. Very large doses of corticosteroids (eg, $2-5$ g hydrocortisone intravenously) have been administered with claimed benefit. In one controlled human study (Schumer, 1976), methylprednisolone, 30 mg/kg injected in 20 minutes intravenously and repeated only once 4 hours later, markedly reduced the death rate from septic shock. Thus, a dose-related effect is possible. Heparinization may be considered in disseminated intravascular coagulation.

The opiate antagonist naloxone has been given experimentally to counteract the observed rise in endorphin blood levels during shock. There is evidence that antibody to the core glycolipid of gram-negative enteric bacteria can protect against shock and death in gram-negative sepsis. Antibody to *Pseudomonas aeruginosa* types may be beneficial in burn patients.

Prognosis

Persistent gram-negative bacteremia has a high mortality rate—often over 50%. Bad prognostic signs include hypothermia during bacteremia, severe underlying disease, azotemia, and shock. Failure to drain collections of pus adequately usually interferes with the response to antimicrobial therapy.

Guerrant RL et al: Campylobacteriosis in man: Pathogenic mechanisms and review of 91 blood stream infections. *Am J Med* 1978;**65**:584.

Kreger BE: Gram negative bacteremia. 4. Reevaluation of clinical features and treatment of 612 patients. *Am J Med* 1980;**68**:344.

Sheagren JN: Septic shock and corticosteroids. *N Engl J Med* 1981;**305**:456.

Yu VL: *Serratia marcescens:* Historical perspective and clinical review. *N Engl J Med* 1979;**300**:887.

Ziegler EJ et al: Treatment of gram-negative bacteremia and shock with human antiserum to a mutant *E coli*. *N Engl J Med* 1982;**307**:1225.

SYNDROMES OF PROBABLY INFECTIOUS ETIOLOGY

1. TOXIC SHOCK SYNDROME

Toxic shock syndrome is characterized by abrupt onset of high fever, vomiting, and watery diarrhea. Sore throat, myalgias, and headache are often complaints. Hypotensive shock with renal and cardiac failure are ominous manifestations in severe cases. A diffuse macular erythematous rash and nonpurulent conjunctivitis are common, and desquamation, especially of palms and soles, is typical as the victim recovers. Reported fatality rates range from 3.2 to 15%.

Although toxic shock syndrome has occurred in children 8–17 years old and in males, the great majority of cases (90% or more) have been reported in women of child-bearing age. Of these, 95% or more have begun within 5 days of the onset of a menstrual period in women who have used tampons. If a woman recovers from the syndrome, she should forgo use of tampons. Outbreaks have also developed in surgical patients.

Staphylococcus aureus has been isolated from various sites including the nasopharynx, vagina, or rectum or from wounds, but blood cultures are negative. It is probable that the cause is a toxin produced by some strains of staphylococci. Neither toxin C nor enterotoxin F has been definitely indicted.

Important aspects of treatment include rapid rehydration, antistaphylococcal drugs, and management of renal or cardiac insufficiency.

Bartlett P et al: Toxic shock syndrome associated with surgical wound infections. *JAMA* 1982;**247**:1448.

Bennett JV: Toxins and toxic shock syndrome. *J Infect Dis* 1981;**143**:631.

Schlech WF et al: Risk factors for development of toxic shock syndrome. *JAMA* 1982;**248**:835.

The toxic shock syndrome: Reports from a conference held by the Institute of Medicine, National Academy of Sciences. *Ann Intern Med* 1982;**96**:835.

2. KAWASAKI SYNDROME

Kawasaki syndrome, also called mucocutaneous lymph node syndrome, is a febrile illness of unknown cause. It occurs mainly in children under 5 years of age. Prominent features are prolonged fever, cracked lips, conjunctivitis, pharyngitis, strawberry tongue, a maculopapular red rash and edema of extremities with desquamation on hands and feet, lymphadenopathy, and angiitis of coronary arteries in up to 30% of cases. There may be thrombocytosis or electrocardiographic changes preceding a coronary occlusion or aneurysm formation.

First reported in Japan, outbreaks have also occurred in Hawaii, Massachusetts, and elsewhere. In these outbreaks, the majority of patients experienced antecedent respiratory illness.

Treatment is symptomatic and includes high doses of aspirin. One to 3% of patients have died.

Bell DM et al: Kawasaki syndrome: Description of two outbreaks in the United States. *N Engl J Med* 1981;**304**:1568.

Melish ME: Kawasaki syndrome. *Annu Rev Med* 1982;**33**:569.

3. ACQUIRED IMMUNODEFICIENCY SYNDROME (AIDS)

This entity has been recognized and defined only since 1979–1980. It has afflicted mainly young homosexual males with multiple sexual partners, abusers of intravenous drugs, Haitian immigrants, Central African natives and their close contacts, hemophiliacs receiving factor VIII concentrate, and a few recipients of blood by transfusion from persons afflicted with AIDS. Some children have been afflicted whose mothers were intravenous drug abusers or developed AIDS.

The onset may be insidious, with fatigue, weight loss, fever, diarrhea, and generalized lymphadenopathy; or acute, with an overwhelming opportunistic infection. Among the latter have been particularly *Pneumocystis carinii* pneumonia, *Mycobacterium avium-intracellulare*, herpesviruses, especially cytomegalovirus, several opportunistic fungi, *Toxoplasma gondii*, and *Cryptosporidium* diarrhea. Strikingly, Kaposi's sarcoma has a high incidence and disseminates rapidly, and other metastasizing neoplasms have occurred. The mortality rate of afflicted patients has been near 40% in 1–2 years of follow-up.

The etiology is not known, but an infectious agent transmitted by intimate (especially sexual) contact or by blood or blood products is suspected. Among the "candidate" agents is a human T cell leukemia-lymphoma virus (HTLV) to which many AIDS patients (but few others) have antibodies. Its etiologic role, if any, remains to be proved. The distribution of AIDS cases parallels that of hepatitis B infection. For that reason, precautions applicable to hepatitis B should be used in managing these patients and their blood specimens.

The immunologic disturbance is characterized by an abnormal ratio in T lymphocyte subpopulations and a low count of helper T lymphocytes. Such measurements employ monoclonal antibodies directed at T cell surface receptors. In normal persons, the ratio of OKT 4-reactive (inducer/helper) T cells to OKT 8-reactive (suppressor/killer) T cells is 1.5 or greater. In AIDS patients, that ratio has been 1 or less. The deficiency in cell-mediated immunity caused by a relative lack of helper T lymphocytes results in extreme susceptibility to opportunistic microorganisms or neoplastic cells. It also greatly hampers response to chemotherapeutic drugs. Until a way can be found to correct the immune deficiency, the prognosis for such patients—even if patients appear temporarily healthy—must be guarded.

Clumeck N et al: AIDS in African patients. *N Engl J Med* 1984;**310**:492.

Conte JE et al: Infection control guidelines for patients with AIDS. *N Engl J Med* 1983;**309**:740.

Curran JW et al: AIDS associated with transfusions. *N Engl J Med* 1984;**310**:69.

Davis KC et al: Acquired immunodeficiency syndrome in a patient with hemophilia. *Ann Intern Med* 1983;**98**:284.

Gallo RC et al: Frequent detection and isolation of cytopathic retroviruses (HTLV-III) from patients with AIDS and at risk for AIDS. *Science* 1984;**224**:500.

Harris C et al: Immunodeficiency in female sexual partners of men with AIDS. *N Engl J Med* 1983;**308**:1181.

Piot P et al: Acquired immunodeficiency syndrome in a heterosexual population in Zaire. *Lancet* 1984;**2**:65.

Pulmonary complications of the acquired immunodeficiency syndrome: Report of a National Heart, Lung, and Blood Institute Workshop. *N Engl J Med* 1984;**310**:1682.

Van de Perre P et al: Acquired immunodeficiency syndrome in Rwanda. *Lancet* 1984;**2**:62.

Viera J et al: Acquired immune deficiency in Haitians. *N Engl J Med* 1983;**308**:125.

NONTUBERCULOUS ATYPICAL MYCOBACTERIAL DISEASES

About 10% of mycobacterial infections seen in clinical practice are not caused by *Mycobacterium tuberculosis* but by "atypical" mycobacteria. These organisms have distinctive laboratory characteristics, occur in the environment, are not communicable from person to person, and are often strikingly resistant to antituberculosis drugs. Some representative species and clinical presentations are listed here. (See also p 150.)

Mycobacterium kansasii can produce pulmonary disease resembling tuberculosis, but the illness is less severe. Treatment is with ethambutol plus rifampin plus isoniazid, at least initially. *Mycobacterium marinum* produces skin granulomas but rarely systemic dissemination; initial treatment is with a tetracycline. *Mycobacterium scrofulaceum* and, less commonly, *Mycobacterium intracellulare* are prominent causes of cervical adenitis in children; excision is the management of choice. The *Mycobacterium avium-intracellulare* complex produces widespread asymptomatic infection and occasional pulmonary disease in the United States, Australia, and elsewhere. Most infected persons are well, but those who do become ill (especially immunodeficient persons) present a formidable treatment problem. Multiple drugs (rifampin, cycloserine, streptomycin, ethambutol) may be effective, and other drugs can be selected by sensitivity tests. Excisional surgery is sometimes successful. *Mycobacterium fortuitum* and similar organisms may produce skin ulcers after accidental inoculation and, rarely, lung disease. They are usually resistant to antimycobacterial drugs.

Diagnosis

Nontuberculous atypical mycobacterial disease is suspected when acid-fast bacilli are found on smear; however, the patient is not as ill as one might expect with tuberculosis, has no history of contact with tuberculosis, and nobody else in the family has the disease. Chest films may be negative, and the PPD-S is often less than 10 mm of induration. Specific diagnosis depends on cultural identification of the organism. This may take 1–4 weeks.

Treatment

The management of pulmonary disease is described on p 150. Cervical adenitis presumptively due to atypical mycobacteria is best managed by surgical excision, thus facilitating culture and histologic examination. The effective use of antimicrobial agents requires specific bacteriologic diagnosis and tests for drug sensitivity.

Schaad VB et al: Management of atypical mycobacterial lymphadenitis in childhood. *J Pediatr* 1979;**95**:384.

Wolinsky E: Nontuberculous mycobacteria and associated diseases. *Am Rev Respir Dis* 1979;**119**:107.

Zakowski P et al: Disseminated *Mycobacterium avium-intracellulare* infections in homosexual men dying of acquired immunodeficiency. *JAMA* 1982;**248**:2980.

ANAEROBIC INFECTIONS*

A large majority of the bacteria that make up the normal human flora are anaerobes. Prominent members of the normal microbial flora of the mouth (anaerobic spirochetes, *Bacteroides*, fusobacteria), the skin (anaerobic diphtheroids), the large bowel (*Bacteroides*, anaerobic streptococci, clostridia), and the female tract (*Bacteroides*, anaerobic streptococci, fusobacteria) may produce disease when displaced from their normal sites into tissues or closed body spaces.

Certain characteristics are suggestive of anaerobic infections: (1) They tend to involve mixtures of organisms, frequently several anaerobes. (2) They tend to form closed-space infections, either in discrete abscesses (lung, brain, pleura, peritoneum) or by burrowing through tissue layers. (3) Pus from anaerobic infections often has a foul odor. (4) Septic thrombophlebitis and metastatic suppurative lesions are frequent and often require surgical drainage in addition to antimicrobial therapy. (Most of the important anaerobes except *Bacteroides fragilis* are highly sensitive to penicillin G, but the diminished blood supply that favors proliferation of anaerobes because of reduced tissue oxygenation also interferes with the delivery of antimicrobials to the site of anaerobic infection.) (5) Bacteriologic examination may be negative or may yield only inconsequential aerobes unless rigorous anaerobic culture conditions are used, employing col-

*For clostridial infections, see Chapter 24. For pseudomembranous colitis, see p 392.

lection methods and media suitable for fastidious organisms.

The following is a brief listing of important types of infections that are most commonly caused by anaerobic organisms. Treatment of all of these infections consists of surgical exploration and judicious excision in conjunction with administration of antimicrobial drugs.

Upper Respiratory Tract

Bacteroides melaninogenicus together with anaerobic spirochetes is commonly involved in periodontal infections. These organisms, fusobacteria, and peptostreptococci are responsible for a substantial percentage of cases of chronic sinusitis and probably of peritonsillar abscess, chronic otitis media, and mastoiditis. Hygiene and drainage are usually more important in treatment than antimicrobials, but penicillin G is the drug of choice.

Chest Infections

Aspiration of saliva (which contains 10^8 anaerobic organisms per milliliter in addition to aerobes) may lead to pneumonitis, necrotizing pneumonia, lung abscess, and empyema. While polymicrobial infection is the rule, anaerobes—particularly *B melaninogenicus,* fusobacteria, and peptostreptococci—are common etiologic agents. All of these organisms are susceptible to penicillin G and tend to respond to drug treatment combined with surgical drainage when indicated.

While the relatively penicillin-resistant *Bacteroides fragilis* is found in about 20% of anaerobic chest infections, these still usually respond to penicillin G, 10 million units daily intravenously. Occasionally, clindamycin or chloramphenicol is required.

Central Nervous System

While anaerobes only rarely produce meningitis, they are a common cause of brain abscess, subdural empyema, or septic central nervous system thrombophlebitis. The organisms reach the central nervous system by direct extension from sinusitis, otitis, or mastoiditis or by hematogenous spread from chronic lung infections. Antimicrobial therapy (eg, penicillin, 20 million units intravenously, and chloramphenicol, 0.5 g orally every 6 hours) is an important adjunct to surgical drainage. Recent evidence suggests that some brain abscesses can be treated with metronidazole alone and may heal without surgical drainage.

Intra-abdominal Infections

In the colon there are up to 10^{11} anaerobes per gram of content—predominantly *B fragilis,* clostridia, and peptostreptococci. These organisms play a central etiologic role in most intra-abdominal abscesses following trauma to the colon, diverticulitis, appendicitis, or perirectal abscess and may also participate in hepatic abscess and cholecystitis, often in association with aerobic coliform bacteria. The gallbladder wall may be infected with clostridia as well. In infections associated with perforation of the lower bowel, penicillin G may be ineffective because of the resistance of *B fragilis;* chloramphenicol, clindamycin, or metronidazole may be the drugs of choice to aid in localization and supplement drainage.

Whereas the normal flora of the upper intestinal tract is more sparse than that of the colon, anaerobes comprise a large portion of it.

Female Genital Tract & Pelvic Infections

The normal flora of the vagina and cervix includes several species of *Bacteroides,* peptostreptococci, group B streptococci, lactobacilli, coliform bacteria, and, occasionally, spirochetes and clostridia. These organisms commonly cause genital tract infections and may disseminate from there.

While salpingitis is commonly caused by gonococci and chlamydiae, tubo-ovarian and pelvic abscesses are associated with anaerobes in a majority of cases. Postpartum infections may be caused by aerobic streptococci or staphylococci, but in most instances anaerobes are found, and the most severe cases of postpartum or postabortion sepsis are associated with clostridia and *Bacteroides.* These have a high mortality rate, and treatment requires both antimicrobials (penicillin, metronidazole, clindamycin) and abscess drainage or early hysterectomy.

Bacteremia & Endocarditis*

Anaerobes are probably responsible for 5–10% of cases of bacteremia seen in general hospitals. Most of these originate in the gastrointestinal tract and the female genital tract and—until now—have been associated with a high mortality rate. Endocarditis due to anaerobic and microaerophilic streptococci and *Bacteroides* originates in the same sites. Rigorous anaerobic cultures are essential in patients whose "routine" blood cultures in clinical endocarditis have remained negative in order to identify the causative organism and institute specific and adequate treatment. Most cases of streptococcal endocarditis can be effectively treated with 20–60 million units of penicillin G daily, but optimal therapy of other types of anaerobic bacterial endocarditis must rely on laboratory guidance. Anaerobic corynebacteria *(Propionibacterium),* clostridia, and *Bacteroides* occasionally cause endocarditis. *Bacteroides* bacteremia may cause disseminated intravascular coagulation.

Skin & Soft Tissue Infections

Anaerobic infections in the skin and soft tissue usually follow trauma, inadequate blood supply, or surgery and are commonest in areas that are contaminated by oral or fecal flora. There is often rapidly progressive tissue necrosis and a putrid odor.

Bacterial synergistic gangrene is a painful ulcerating lesion that commonly follows laparotomy performed as part of the management of intra-abdominal infections but produces little fever or systemic tox-

---

*See also fuller discussion in Chapter 8.

icity. It is usually caused by a mixture of anaerobic streptococci and *Staphylococcus aureus*. It requires wide excision of the discolored skin and (later) skin grafts, but recovery is the rule.

Synergistic necrotizing cellulitis progresses more rapidly, with high fever and often positive blood cultures for peptostreptococci, *Bacteroides*, and aerobic gram-negative bacteria. It occurs with greatest frequency on the perineum and the lower extremities and has a high mortality rate. Excision of necrotic tissue must be combined with antimicrobial drugs (eg, gentamicin plus clindamycin) in an effort at early control.

Necrotizing fasciitis is a mixed anaerobic or aerobic infection that rapidly dissects deep fascial planes and produces severe toxicity with a mortality rate up to 30%. Anaerobic streptococci and *S aureus* are the commonest etiologic organisms. Treatment requires extensive surgical incisions through fascial planes.

Nonclostridial crepitant cellulitis is an infection of subcutaneous or deeper tissues with peptostreptococci and coliform bacteria that leads to gas formation in tissue with minimal toxicity, lack of muscle involvement, and a good prognosis. Improved perfusion, incision and drainage, and antimicrobial drugs (eg, ampicillin) are often successful.

ANIMAL & HUMAN BITE WOUNDS

About 1% of emergency room visits in urban areas are for animal and human bites. Cats produce the highest percentage of bacterial infections (30–50%), many of which are caused by *Pasteurella multocida*. This organism is common to the oral microflora of animals and is susceptible to penicillin. Human bites are associated with bacterial infection in 15–20% of cases and dog bites in about 5% of cases. Tetanus prophylaxis must be considered in all bite wounds (see p 873) and rabies prophylaxis in animal bites (see p 847).

All bites, especially human bites, introduce a mixed complex anaerobic and aerobic flora into the wound. These wounds must be irrigated intensively and debrided. There is little evidence that "prophylactic" antimicrobial drugs are valuable. When bacterial infection is already evident, administration of penicillin G, warm soaks, and elevation and immobilization of the wounded area are advisable. Initial Gram stains and cultures from the wound may direct the choice of antibiotic. Clindamycin or cefoxitin may be desirable when lack of response suggests anaerobes, and nafcillin is indicated if lactamase-producing staphylococci are present. Hospitalization must be considered for major human bites to permit close observation, surgical intervention, or parenteral therapy.

Aghabanian RV, Conte JE: Mammalian bite wounds. *Ann Emerg Med* 1980;**9**:79.

Bartlett JG: Recent developments in the management of anaerobic infections. *Rev Infect Dis* 1983;**5**:235.

Dunn DL, Simmons RL: The role of anaerobic bacteria in intraabdominal infections. *Rev Infect Dis* 1984;**6**:5139.

Giuliano A et al: Bacteriology of necrotizing fasciitis. *Am J Surg* 1977;**134**:52.

Mathisen GE et al: Brain abscess and cerebritis. *Rev Infect Dis* 1984;**6**:5101.

Zaleznik DF, Kasper DL: The role of anaerobic bacteria in abscess formation. *Annu Rev Med* 1982;**33**:217.

SEXUALLY TRANSMITTED DISEASES

Some infectious diseases are transmitted most commonly—or most efficiently—by sexual contact. The frequency of some of these infections (eg, gonorrhea) has increased markedly in recent years as a result of changing patterns of sexual behavior. Others (eg, herpetic and chlamydial genital infections) are only now beginning to be appreciated as important systemic infections with a primarily sexual mode of transmission. Rectal and pharyngeal infections caused by these microorganisms are common as a result of varied sexual practices.

Most of the infectious agents that cause sexually transmitted diseases are fairly easily inactivated when exposed to a harsh environment. They are thus particularly suited to transmission by contact with mucous membranes. They may be bacteria (eg, gonococci), spirochetes (syphilis), chlamydiae (nongonococcal urethritis, cervicitis), viruses (eg, herpes simplex, hepatitis B virus, cytomegalovirus), or protozoa (eg, *Trichomonas*). In most infections caused by these agents, early lesions occur on genitalia or other sexually exposed mucous membranes; however, wide dissemination may occur, and involvement of nongenital tissues and organs may mimic many noninfectious disorders. All venereal diseases have subclinical or latent phases that may play an important role in long-term persistence of the infection or in its transmission from infected (but largely asymptomatic) persons to other contacts. Laboratory examinations are of particular importance in the diagnosis of such asymptomatic patients. Simultaneous infection by several different agents is common.

For each patient, there are one or more sexual contacts who require diagnosis and treatment. Finding a sexually transmitted disease in a child strongly suggests sexual abuse, and the case should be reported to the authorities. Several sexually transmitted diseases are reportable to public health authorities. The commonest sexually transmitted diseases are gonorrhea, syphilis, condyloma acuminatum, chlamydial genital infections, cytomegalovirus and herpesvirus genital infections, trichomoniasis, chancroid, granuloma inguinale, scabies, and lice. However, shigellosis, hepatitis, amebiasis, giardiasis, cryptosporidiasis, salmonellosis, and campylobacteriosis may also be transmitted by sexual (oral-anal) contact, especially in homosexual males (see p 828). In the same population, as in some other individuals, a dramatic acquired immunodeficiency syndrome (AIDS; see p 824) has been observed with increasing frequency and with a high mortality rate due to opportunistic infections or disseminating Kaposi's sarcoma. At present, the cause and the precise mode of transmission of AIDS are uncertain, but intimate sexual contact is one of the modes under consideration.

Clinical and epidemiologic details and methods of diagnosis and treatment are discussed for each infection separately elsewhere in this book (see Index).

Owen RL: Sexually transmitted diseases and traumatic problems in homosexual men. *Ann Intern Med* 1980;**92**:805.

Quinn TC et al: The etiology of anorectal infections in homosexual men. *Am J Med* 1981;**71**:395.

Sexually transmitted diseases: Treatment guidelines 1982. *Rev Infect Dis* 1982;**4**:S730.

INFECTIONS IN DRUG ADDICTS

The abuse of parenterally administered narcotic drugs has increased enormously. There are an estimated 250 thousand or more narcotic addicts in the USA, mostly in or near large urban centers. Consequently, many physicians and hospitals serving such urban and suburban populations are faced with the diagnosis and treatment of problems that are closely related to drug abuse. Infections are a large part of these problems.

Common Infections That Occur
With Greater Frequency in Drug Users

(1) Skin infections are associated with poor hygiene and multiple needle punctures, commonly due to *S aureus*.

(2) Hepatitis (see p 402) is nearly universal among habitual drug users and is transmissible both by the parenteral and by the fecal-oral route. Many addicts experience hepatitis twice.

(3) Aspiration pneumonia and its complications (lung abscess, empyema, brain abscess) are due to anaerobes, *Nocardia*, and other organisms.

(4) Pulmonary septic emboli may originate in venous thrombi or right-sided endocarditis.

(5) Sexually transmitted diseases are not directly related to drug abuse but, for social reasons, occur with greater frequency in population groups that are also involved in drug abuse.

(6) Acquired immunodeficiency syndrome has a high incidence among intravenous drug abusers (see p 824).

Infections Rare in USA Except in Drug Users

(1) Tetanus: Drug users now form a majority of cases of tetanus in the USA. Tetanus develops most commonly in the unimmunized female addict who injects drugs subcutaneously ("skin-popping").

(2) Malaria: Needle transmission occurs from addicts who acquired the infection in malaria-endemic areas outside of the USA.

(3) Melioidosis: This chronic pulmonary infection caused by *Pseudomonas pseudomallei* is occasionally seen in debilitated drug users.

Infective Endocarditis*

The organisms that cause infective endocarditis in those who use drugs intravenously are most commonly *S aureus*, *Candida* (especially *Candida parapsilosis*), *Streptococcus faecalis*, and gram-negative bacteria (especially *Pseudomonas* and *Serratia marcescens*).

Involvement of the left side of the heart is somewhat more frequent than involvement of the right side, and infection of more than one valve is not infrequent. Right-sided involvement, especially in the absence of murmurs, is often suggested by manifest pulmonary emboli. The diagnosis must be established by blood culture. Until the etiologic organism is known, treatment must be directed against the most probable organism—especially *S aureus* if the patient suffers from toxic delirium and petechial rashes in the presence of evidence of drug abuse.

Osteomyelitis†

Osteomyelitis involving vertebral bodies, sternoclavicular joints, and other sites usually results from hematogenous distribution of injected organisms or septic venous thrombi. Pain and fever precede roentgenologic changes by several weeks. *Serratia*, *Pseudomonas*, and other organisms rarely encountered in "spontaneous" bone or joint disease are found in addicts who use drugs intravenously.

Sapico FL, Montgomerie JZ: Vertebral osteomyelitis in intravenous drug abusers: Report of three cases and review of the literature. *Rev Infect Dis* 1980;**2**:196.

Scalcini MC, Sanders CV: Endocarditis from human to human transmission of *Staphylococcus aureus*. *Arch Intern Med* 1980;**140**:111.

DIAGNOSIS OF VIRAL INFECTIONS

In the diagnosis of viral infections, the current state of clinical knowledge and laboratory technology allows specific identification in the vast majority of cases. Diagnoses such as "viral syndrome," "viral diarrhea," or "flu syndrome" are not helpful.

Some viral illnesses present a clear-cut clinical syndrome (chickenpox, measles, mumps) that identifies the virus involved. Laboratory assistance is required only for confirmation in atypical cases or for the differential diagnosis of 2 syndromes that resemble each other.

In some instances, the clinical picture has a number of features that are suggestive of viral infection

*See also fuller discussion in Chapter 8.
†See fuller discussion in Chapter 15.

in general but could be caused by any one of a number of viruses. Such a "viral" picture is seen in aseptic meningitis, where the characteristic features are an initial polymorphonuclear pleocytosis in the cerebrospinal fluid which then shifts to a preponderance of mononuclear cells, normal cerebrospinal fluid glucose, and slight elevation of cerebrospinal fluid protein occurring a short time after the period of pleocytosis. It is the nature of the meningeal tissue response to viral invasion that differentiates this syndrome from the very different response to pyogenic bacteria. The viruses involved in aseptic meningitis include mumps and several enteroviruses; the specific viral diagnosis can only be made with laboratory assistance. In the case of the respiratory tract, viral infections also have certain features in common—widespread involvement of the respiratory epithelium with redness and clear nasal secretion, absence of a purulent response—and, if pneumonia is present, it is more apt to be interstitial pneumonia.

Sometimes the statistical predilection of one of the respiratory viruses for an anatomic site allows one to make an "educated guess." For example, respiratory syncytial virus is the most common cause of bronchiolitis, and parainfluenza virus is the most common cause of croup. However, specific identification of the virus involved can only be made in the laboratory.

At times, accurate diagnosis is of such import to the patient (rubella during pregnancy) or the community (hepatitis) that rapid laboratory confirmation of the suspected diagnosis is essential.

Diagnosis of viral illnesses requires the close collaboration of the clinician and the laboratory virologist. Knowing which specimens are most likely to be productive, when they should be obtained, and what to do with them in the laboratory depends on the virologist's understanding of the suspected diagnosis, the timetable of the illness, and the clinician's awareness of laboratory capabilities and limitations.

Laboratory Considerations

There are 3 basic laboratory techniques for making a viral diagnosis:

A. Isolation and Identification of the Virus: This requires prompt transport (best on wet ice) to the laboratory and inoculation of the appropriate specimen into a suitable tissue culture or into a live animal. A variety of techniques are then utilized to determine the presence and nature of the particular virus. At times this can be done very simply (eg, in the case of herpes simplex); at times it may be laborious, time-consuming, and expensive (eg, in the case of coxsackievirus). The isolation of virus from a specimen that is normally free of virus (eg, cerebrospinal fluid, lung biopsy) or from a pathologic lesion (herpes or varicella vesicle) has great diagnostic significance. However, finding a virus in the nasopharynx or in the stool may denote carriage rather than disease; in this case, additional evidence of a rise in antibody titer will be necessary before a specific diagnosis can be made.

B. Microscopic Methods: This entails the microscopic examination of cells, body fluids, or aspirates to demonstrate either the presence of the virus or specific cytologic changes peculiar to one virus or a group of viruses (eg, multinucleate giant cells at base of herpesvirus lesions; rotavirus structures seen in electron micrographs of diarrheal stools). Immunofluorescence methods are particularly useful in many viral illnesses (rabies, varicella, herpes simplex, etc) to identify antigen in cells from the patient. Viruses lead an obligately intracellular existence; therefore, it is important to examine scraped cells rather than exudates or transudates.

C. Serologic Methods: During viral illnesses, specific antibodies develop. The timing of rise in titer and persistence of antibodies varies. A 4-fold rise in antibody titer during the course of the illness is usually considered significant evidence of disease. Since a single serum titer is not particularly helpful, many laboratories will not do the test until paired sera (taken 2–3 weeks apart) are available. It is not practical to do serologic tests for a large number of viruses in any patient. Thus, the use of this method requires a specific suspicion of which virus might be involved.

Jawetz E, Melnick JL, Adelberg EA: *Review of Medical Microbiology,* 16th ed. Lange, 1984.
McIntosh K et al: Summary of a workshop on new and useful methods in viral diagnosis. *J Infect Dis* 1980;**142:**793.

HERPESVIRUSES OF HUMANS

This large group of DNA viruses shares common features that are important in the general clinical patterns manifested in humans. The better defined clinical pictures are described under the specific disease entities. The most important herpesviruses in human disease states are herpes simplex type 1, herpes simplex type 2, varicella-zoster, cytomegalovirus, and EB–infectious mononucleosis virus.

Each virus tends to produce subclinical primary infection more often than clinically manifest illness. Each tends to persist in a latent state (evidenced only by persistent immunologic reactivity) for the rest of the person's life. Reactivation producing a clinical recurrence of disease may follow a known or unrecognized triggering mechanism. In herpes simplex and varicella-zoster, the virus is latent in sensory ganglia, and reactivation is followed by the appearance of lesions in the distal sensory nerve distribution. As a result of the suppression of cell-mediated immunity by disease, drugs, or radiation, reactivation of virus may lead to widespread disseminated lesions on and within affected organs and the central nervous system. Severe or even fatal illness may also occur in the newborn or the immunodeficient child.

Herpesviruses can infect the fetus and induce serious congenital malformations. They have also been linked to neoplasia, but the relationship has not been definitely established. Primary or recurrent herpesvirus infections that involve surfaces of organs may lead to prolonged shedding of virus and its spread to contacts of the infected person.

Several drugs can inhibit replication of herpesviruses in laboratory models. Of these, idoxuridine and trifluorothymidine are effective in humans when applied topically to herpetic keratitis. However, they are too toxic for systemic use. Vidarabine (adenine arabinoside) and acyclovir (acycloguanosine) can be administered systemically. Vidarabine, 15 mg/kg/d intravenously, has been used in disseminated herpes simplex or herpetic encephalitis. If the diagnosis was made early, before onset of coma, the mortality rate from this otherwise very severe illness was significantly reduced. However, only 40% of survivors were sufficiently normal neurologically to resume normal activity. Vidarabine has also been employed in neonatal disseminated herpes and early in disseminating herpes zoster. Acyclovir (15 mg/kg/d) given intravenously is as effective as vidarabine and has very low toxicity. It is clearly beneficial in symptomatic primary genital herpes infections in females and in disseminating herpetic mucocutaneous lesions in immunosuppressed patients. Oral acyclovir has systemic antiherpes activity.

Topical acyclovir (5%) applied to primary genital herpetic lesions can reduce viral shedding and local pain and shorten healing time. It has no significant effect on recurrent lesions or on the recurrence rate. It is of benefit in treating mucocutaneous lesions in immunocompromised patients (see Chapter 29).

Photodynamic inactivation applied to mucocutaneous herpetic lesions has been discredited. (See also pp 69, 94, and 493 and Chapter 29.)

Balfour HH: Acyclovir and other chemotherapy for herpes group viral infections. *Annu Rev Med* 1984;**35**:279.
Corey L et al: A trial of topical acyclovir in genital herpes simplex virus infections. *N Engl J Med* 1982;**306**:1313.
Whitley RJ et al: Herpes simplex encephalitis: Clinical assessment. *JAMA* 1982;**247**:317.

SLOW VIRUSES

Several animal diseases (scrapie, visna) are caused by viruses that are definitely communicable but replicate in the host very slowly—for months without producing symptoms. Eventually, they produce progressive disease and death. At least 4 human degenerative diseases are believed to be caused by similar "slow" viruses.

Kuru and **Creutzfeldt-Jakob disease** are spongiform encephalopathies. The virus can be transmitted by brain or eye tissue, and perhaps by other forms of contact, to humans, chimpanzees, and monkeys. After many weeks or months, the diseases pursue an inexorable downhill course and end in death. Kuru is characterized by cerebellar ataxia, tremors, dysarthria, and emotional lability; Creutzfeldt-Jakob disease by progressive dementia, myoclonic fasciculations, ataxia,

and somnolence. Little is known about the characteristics of the causative viruses. There is no specific treatment, and prevention is limited to avoidance of specific risks (contamination by affected brain tissue, transplant of cornea from patient).

Subacute sclerosing encephalopathy (SSPE) is a slowly progressive demyelinating disorder of the central nervous system, ending in death. Viruses that are or resemble measles viruses have been grown from brain tissue, and the cerebrospinal fluid antibody to measles is high.

Progressive multifocal leukoencephalopathy (PML) is an extremely rare progressive demyelinating neurologic disease that occurs particularly in persons immunosuppressed by drugs or disease. From brain tissue of PML, certain papovaviruses (eg, JC virus) have been grown. However, a large percentage (60%) of a normal population has serum antibodies to the same virus, suggesting that disease production must have another determinant.

It is possible that other degenerative central nervous system diseases in humans (eg, multiple sclerosis) may be caused by "slow" viruses.

Johnson RT, ter Meulen V: Slow infections of the nervous system. *Adv Intern Med* 1978;**23**:353.

MISCELLANEOUS RESPIRATORY INFECTIONS

Infections of the respiratory tract are perhaps the most common human ailments. While they are a source of discomfort, disability, and loss of time for most average adults, they are a substantial cause of morbidity and serious illness in young children and in the elderly. As a result of advances in virologic techniques, specific associations of certain groups of viruses with certain disease syndromes have been established. Many of these viral infections run their natural course in older children and in adults, without specific treatment and without great risk of bacterial complications. In young infants and in the elderly, or in persons with impaired respiratory tract reserves, bacterial superinfection increases morbidity and mortality rates.

Several generalizations apply particularly to respiratory viral infections in children. Epithelium of different sites is often involved simultaneously with inflammatory reactions. Thus, there may be coexistent conjunctivitis, otitis, pharyngitis, tracheitis, or bronchitis. Symptoms often point mainly to an anatomic site of principal involvement rather than to a particular etiologic virus. Exceptions, however, exist: rhinoviruses are prominent in the common cold; respiratory syncytial virus is most likely to produce bronchiolitis; and parainfluenza virus tends to produce laryngotracheitis (croup). The incidence of both a specific virus infection and a particular symptom complex is sometimes age-related. Bronchiolitis occurs principally in children under age 2. The small diameter of the airway in the very young child predisposes to obstruction, necessitating frequent evaluation of symptoms, signs, and possible therapy. In the elderly individual, emphysema or bronchiectasis similarly contributes to poor ventilation and oxygenation, posing special problems in management.

In the following paragraphs, special entities, their recognition, and therapy are summarized briefly.

Croup (Laryngotracheobronchitis)

This is most commonly a parainfluenza virus infection of small children, with anatomic localization in the subglottal area. It produces hoarseness, a "seal bark" cough, and signs of upper airway obstruction with inspiratory stridor, xiphoid and suprasternal retraction, but no pain on swallowing. Treatment includes hydration, steam inhalation (hot or cold), and alertness to the possibility of complete airway obstruction. Should that emergency occur, intubation or tracheostomy is lifesaving.

Epiglottitis

This is a bacterial infection, usually due to *Haemophilus influenzae*. The epiglottis is markedly swollen and "cherry-red," producing an airway obstruction resembling viral croup but usually in an older child. The patient is often 1–6 years old (and occasionally is adult), febrile, appears toxic, and has pain on swallowing in addition to the "croupy cough." A lateral x-ray of the neck can help to establish swelling of the epiglottis. Direct laryngoscopy may result in complete obstruction and must therefore be performed only in a setting where intubation or tracheostomy can be performed immediately and expertly. Such airway maintenance is required in most patients in addition to antimicrobial therapy (currently ampicillin or chloramphenicol—or both—until laboratory results from culture are available).

Bronchiolitis

This viral infection is caused most often by respiratory syncytial virus in children under 2 years of age. It results in a "ball valve" obstruction to expiration at the level of the bronchiole, resembling bronchial asthma in pathophysiology. Clinical signs include low-grade fever, severe tachypnea (up to 100 respirations per minute), an expiratory wheeze, overinflation of lungs, depressed diaphragm, decreased air exchange, and greatly increased work of breathing. Foreign body aspiration and bronchial asthma may have to be considered in differential diagnosis.

Treatment consists of hydration, humidification of inspired air, and—with rising blood P_{CO_2}—the possible need for ventilatory support. In infants, the clinical course of respiratory syncytial viral infections can be favorably modified by use of aerosolized ribavirin.

Common Cold
(See also Chapter 6.)

This familiar syndrome is characterized mainly by nasal obstruction and discharge, sore throat, sneezing, hoarseness, and varying degrees of malaise, cough, sinusitis, and otitis. Fever is usually absent in adults but may be present in small children. Rhinoviruses, coronaviruses, parainfluenza viruses, and others may be the etiologic agents. All of these exist in multiple antigenic types, and recurrence of infection is common. Secondary bacterial infection is more common in children (15%) than in adults and may produce purulent sinusitis, otitis media, or tracheobronchitis.

Treatment is largely palliative, and its true merits are poorly established. Aspirin (0.6 g every 4–8 hours in adults) tends to act as an analgesic. Phenylephrine, 0.25% solution as nose drops 4 times daily, or methylhexamine or propylhexedrine inhalers may temporarily relieve nasal congestion. Sedative cough mixtures may suppress the annoying and incapacitating cough at some stages. There is no solid support for the claim that ascorbic acid (1–4 g daily) can prevent the common cold or markedly alter its severity. Antimicrobial drugs have no place in the management of the common cold unless secondary bacterial infection is unequivocally present. Antihistamines are of value only in allergic or vasomotor rhinitis.

Pneumonia

Upon first contact with a patient suspected of having acute pneumonitis, the physician must promptly undertake steps toward a specific etiologic diagnosis and arrive at a decision whether to administer antimicrobial drugs. Specific types of pneumonia are described elsewhere (pp 136–143); the general approach to the patient with pneumonitis of unknown cause acquired in the community is outlined here.

The principal initial differentiation must be between bacterial and nonbacterial pneumonias. Characteristically, bacterial pneumonia is associated with sudden onset, chills, high fever, pleuritic chest pain, tachypnea, blood-tinged or purulent sputum, and polymorphonuclear leukocytosis. None of these symptoms are common in viral or mycoplasmal pneumonia.

Diagnosis rests on history (aspiration or prior upper respiratory infection, rate of progression, pain); physical and x-ray findings of consolidation or pleural effusion; white blood cell count and differential; blood culture; and examination of sputum. The latter must include an immediate Gram stain (the possibility of many polymorphonuclear cells, many squamous epithelial cells [suggesting salivary admixture], prevalent microorganisms) and culture (normal flora versus one predominant type of pathogen). Unless a likely pathogen is found promptly in seriously ill pneumonia patients, transtracheal aspiration, fiberoptic bronchoscopy, or even lung biopsy must be considered to obtain an optimal specimen. This is especially important in immunocompromised hosts whose pneumonia is likely to be due to multiple, often opportunistic organisms.

Initial therapy is directed at the most probable pathogen. Since pneumococci account for 60–80% of typical bacterial pneumonia acquired outside the hospital, procaine penicillin G, 600,000 units intramuscularly twice daily, is often appropriate. Other prevailing causes of bacterial pneumonia are staphylococci in 5–15% and gram-negative bacteria in 15–20%. Therapeutic choices are given on pp 138–141. If the evidence favors nonbacterial etiology, antimicrobial drug treatment is generally not advisable.

For high-risk individuals, pneumococcal polysaccharide vaccines should be considered as prophylaxis.

Denny FW et al: Croup: An 11 year study in a pediatric practice. *Pediatrics* 1983;**71**:871.

Hall CB et al: Aerosolized ribavirin treatment of infants with respiratory syncytial viral infections. *N Engl J Med* 1983;**308**:1443.

Macfarlane JT et al: Hospital study of adult community-acquired pneumonia. *Lancet* 1982;**2**:255.

Murphy TF et al: Pneumonia: An 11 year study in pediatric practice. *Am J Epidemiol* 1981;**113**:12.

ACUTE GASTROINTESTINAL SYNDROMES: NAUSEA, VOMITING, & DIARRHEA

Acute disturbances of gastrointestinal function have a wide variety of causes. Often, however, they are associated with the acquisition of infectious agents or toxins produced by them. Many common causes of acute bacterial gastroenteritis, "food poisoning," and "traveler's diarrhea" are described—together with their etiologic agents—on pp 865–870 and listed in Table 24–1, and the epidemiologic setting and management of these disorders are briefly outlined.

Three categories of "infectious diarrheas" deserve mention, although there is much overlap between them.

(1) The first is induced by enterotoxins produced by microorganisms (*Staphylococcus aureus, Clostridium perfringens, Vibrio cholerae, Bacillus cereus, Escherichia coli,* etc). There is an absence of inflammation, and no leukocytes are found in feces. The principal site of involvement is the proximal small bowel; the incubation period between exposure and symptoms is brief; and there is generally no fever. Rotavirus diarrheas of small children and parvovirus (Norwalk viruses) or *Giardia lamblia* diarrheas of adults probably belong in the same category.

(2) A second category is caused by infectious agents that invade superficial tissues, penetrate epithelium of lower small bowel and colon, and induce an inflammatory response. Leukocytes and red blood cells are found in the feces. Fever is commonly present, but blood cultures tend to be negative. Etiologic agents include some *Shigella* spp and invasive *E coli* associated with dysentery, *Salmonella* spp and *Vibrio parahaemolyticus* associated with gastroenteritis, and *Campylobacter jejuni* and *Entamoeba histolytica* producing colitis.

(3) In a third category are invasive enteric fevers involving the distal small bowel, such as those caused

by *Salmonella typhi* or *Yersinia enterocolitica*. Frequently, there is a long incubation period, prolonged systemic illness, and positive blood cultures. Invasive *Entamoeba histolytica* with spread to visceral organs may fit here at times.

Other disorders, eg, antibiotic-associated colitis caused by a necrotizing toxin of *Clostridium difficile,* are distinct entities (see p 973). Enterovirus infections (eg, with poliovirus, coxsackieviruses, and echoviruses) often have diarrhea as a presenting symptom, and virus circulates in the blood, but the gastrointestinal localization is only part of a systemic viral dissemination. These are discussed on pp 836–852.

A broad ("gay bowel") syndrome of enterocolitis encountered especially in homosexual males has received much attention. It is transmitted as a result of oral-anal-genital sexual practices and includes a wide variety of infectious agents ranging from viruses (hepatitis, herpes simplex), chlamydiae (*Chlamydia trachomatis*), and bacteria (*Shigella, Salmonella, Campylobacter, Neisseria gonorrhoeae*) to protozoa (*G lamblia, E histolytica*), among others. Thus, it is necessary to consider the sexual practices of an individual who presents with an acute gastrointestinal tract syndrome to undertake proper diagnostic steps.

In all forms of acute gastrointestinal syndromes, restoration of fluid and electrolyte balance is an essential early therapeutic goal. When an etiologic diagnosis can be formulated, the decision to use antimicrobial or antiparasitic drugs depends on the clinical status of the patient and on the epidemiologic setting. In some disorders in categories (1) and (2), avoidance of antiinfective drugs is desirable (as discussed under individual headings in subsequent chapters).

ACTIVE IMMUNIZATION AGAINST INFECTIOUS DISEASES

Every individual—child or adult—should be adequately immunized against infectious diseases. The schedule of administration, dose, and recommended method of choice vary with each product and change often. Always consult the manufacturer's package insert and follow its recommendations.

The schedule for active immunizations in childhood (Table 22–3) is adapted from *Report,* 19th ed, by the Committee on Control of Infectious Diseases, American Academy of Pediatrics, 1982.

Recommended Immunization of Adults for Travel

Every adult, whether traveling or not, must be immunized with tetanus toxoid. Purified toxoid "for adult use" must be used to avoid reactions. Every adult should also receive primary or booster vaccination for poliomyelitis (oral live trivalent vaccine). Every traveler must fulfill the immunization requirements of the health authorities of different countries. These are

Table 22–3. Recommended schedule for active immunization of children.*

Normal Infants and Children[1]		Those Not Immunized in Infancy (7–18 Years)	
Age	Product Administered or Test Recommended	Schedule	Product Administered
2 months	DTP,[2] TOPV[3]	Initial	Td,[7] TOPV
4 months	DTP, TOPV	1 month later	Measles vaccine, mumps vaccine, rubella vaccine
6 months	DTP, TOPV[4]	2 months later	Td, TOPV
15–19 months	DTP, TOPV Measles vaccine, mumps vaccine, rubella vaccine;[5] tuberculin test[6]	6–12 months later	Td, TOPV
4–6 years (School entry)	DTP, TOPV; tuberculin test	14–16 years of age	Td
Every 10 years thereafter	Td[7]	Every 10 years thereafter	Td

*Follow manufacturer's directions for dose and precautions. A physician may choose to obtain informed consent for immunizations.

[1] A child who experiences any type of seizure after immunization should receive only diphtheria-tetanus (DT) vaccine subsequently.

[2] DTP. Toxoids of diphtheria and tetanus, aluminum-precipitated or aluminum hydroxide–adsorbed, combined with pertussis bacterial antigen. Three doses intramuscularly at 4- to 8-week intervals. Fourth dose intramuscularly about 1 year later. Not suitable for children over 7 years old.

[3] TOPV: Trivalent (types I, II, and III) oral live poliomyelitis virus vaccine. Inactivated trivalent vaccine (Salk type) preferred for immunodeficient children, children with immunodeficient members of the household, and for those initially immunized after age 18, but not recommended for others.

[4] Optional dose, if exposure to wild poliomyelitis virus is anticipated.

[5] These are live vaccines of attenuated viruses grown in cell culture. They may be administered as a mixture or singly at 1-month intervals. Persons who received measles vaccine (inactivated) before 1968 or before age 15 months should be reimmunized with measles vaccine. Some physicians prefer to give rubella vaccine to prepubertal females (age 10–14 years). These live vaccines are not recommended for severely immunodeficient children.

[6] It is desirable to give a tuberculin test prior to measles vaccination and at intervals thereafter, depending on probable risk of exposure.

[7] Td: Tetanus toxoid and diphtheria toxoid, purified, suitable for adults. It should be given every 7–10 years.

References:

Cody CL et al: Nature and rates of adverse reactions associated with DTP and DT immunization in infants and children.

Committee on Control of Infectious Diseases: *Report,* 19th ed. American Academy of Pediatrics, 1982.

General recommendations on immunization. *MMWR* (Jan 14) 1983;32:1.

listed in CDC Quarantine Division: *Health Information for International Travel.* Centers for Disease Control publication 81–8280, (Aug) 1981.

The following are suggestions for travel in different parts of the world.

Tetanus

Booster injection of 0.5 mL tetanus toxoid, for adult use, every 7–10 years, assuming completion of primary immunization. (All countries.)

Diphtheria

Because diphtheria is still prevalent in many parts of the world, a booster injection of diphtheria toxoid for adult use is indicated. This is usually given in combination with tetanus toxoid (Td) purified, for adults.

Smallpox

As of 1980, smallpox has been eradicated from the world. In 1982, a valid vaccination certificate was not required of travelers. Military personnel, however, continue to be vaccinated in the USA.

Traveler's Diarrhea

See p 870.

Typhoid

Suspension of killed *Salmonella typhi* can provide effective immunity. Two doses are given 4 weeks or more apart. A single booster dose is given every 3 years for probable exposure. (Many countries.)

Paratyphoid vaccines are probably ineffective and are not recommended at present.

Yellow Fever

Live attenuated yellow fever virus, 0.5 mL subcutaneously. WHO certificate requires registration of manufacturer and batch number of vaccine. Vaccination available in USA only at approved centers. Vaccination must be repeated at intervals of 10 years or less. (Africa, South America.)

Cholera

Suspension of killed vibrios, including prevalent antigenic types. Two injections are given intramuscularly 2–6 weeks apart. This must be followed by booster injections every 6 months during periods of possible exposure. Protection depends largely on booster doses. WHO certificate is valid for 6 months only. (Middle Eastern countries, Asia, occasionally others.) Benefit doubtful.

Plague

Suspension of killed plague bacilli given intramuscularly, 3 injections 4 or more weeks apart. A single booster injection 6 months later is desirable. (Some areas in South America, Southeast Asia, occasionally others.)

Typhus

Suspension of inactivated typhus rickettsiae can give some protection. However, no approved vaccine was available in the USA or Canada in 1984.

Measles

Persons born since 1957 who have not had live measles vaccine (after age 15 months) and who do not have a convincing history of clinical measles should receive measles vaccine (see above).

Hepatitis A

No active immunization available. Temporary passive immunity may be induced by the intramuscular injection of human gamma globulin, 0.02 mL/kg every 2–3 months, or 0.1 mL/kg every 6 months. Recommended for all parts of the world where environmental sanitation is poor and the risk of exposure to hepatitis A is high through contaminated food and water and contact with infected persons.

Hepatitis B

While not directly travel-related, postexposure prophylaxis against hepatitis is mentioned here. In 1982, an inactivated hepatitis B vaccine was licensed for use in persons at high risk who have no anti-HBs antibody. It might be considered for travelers to hyperendemic areas. (China, Southeast Asia.)

Pneumococcal Pneumonia

Elderly travelers, especially those with chronic obstructive respiratory disease or other chronic illnesses, may be given the 23-type pneumococcal vaccine, 0.5 mL intramuscularly once, several weeks before departure.

Meningococcal Meningitis

If travel is contemplated to an area where meningococcal meningitis is highly endemic or epidemic, polysaccharide vaccines from types A and C may be indicated. Follow manufacturer's dosage recommendations (Africa, South America).

Malaria

Take chloroquine phosphate, 500 mg once weekly, beginning 1 week prior to arrival in malaria-endemic area and continuing for 6 weeks after leaving it. Immunization not available. (In Southeast Asia, Africa, and South America, chloroquine-resistant *Plasmodium falciparum* may be present; pyrimethamine-sulfadoxine mixture may be required.)

Rabies

For travelers to areas where rabies is common in domestic animals (eg, India, parts of South America), preexposure prophylaxis with human diploid cell vaccine should be considered. It usually consists of 3 injections given 1 week apart, with a booster 3 weeks later. Such primary immunization can, very rarely, sensitize recipients to the vaccine.

Centers for Disease Control Quarantine Division: *Health Information for International Travel.* US Department of Health, Education, & Welfare Publication No. (CDC) 81-8280, (Aug) 1981.

1982. *MMWR* 1982;**31(Suppl).** [Entire issue.]

DuPont HL et al: Treatment of travelers' diarrhea with trimethoprim/sulfamethoxazole and with trimethoprim alone. *N Engl J Med* 1982;**307:**841.

Fulginiti VA (editor): *Immunization in Clinical Practice.* Lippincott, 1982.

Goodman RA, Orenstein WA, Hinman AR: Vaccination and disease prevention for adults. *JAMA* 1982;**248:**1607.

Immunization for travelers. *Med Lett Drugs Ther* 1979;**21:**57.

Rubella prevention. *MMWR* 1981;**30:**34.

Schiff GM: Active immunizations for adults. *Annu Rev Med* 1980;**31:**441.

HYPERSENSITIVITY TESTS & DESENSITIZATION

Tests for Hypersensitivity

Before injecting antitoxin, materials derived from animal sources, or drugs (eg, penicillin) to which a patient has reacted in the past, test for hypersensitivity. If both tests described below are negative, desensitization is not necessary, and a full dose of the material may be given. If any test is positive, desensitization is necessary or alternative drugs should be used.

A. Intradermal Test: Inject 0.1 mL of a 1:10 dilution of the antitoxin (or other material) intradermally on the flexor surface of the forearm. A large wheal and surrounding areola appearing within 5–20 minutes constitute a positive test.

B. Conjunctival Test: Instill 1 drop of a 1:10 dilution of the antitoxin into the conjunctival sac of one eye as a test dose and 1 drop of physiologic saline into the other eye as a control. Conjunctival redness, itching, and lacrimation appearing within 5–20 minutes in the test eye constitute a positive test if the control is negative.

Desensitization

A. Precautionary Measures:

1. If extreme hypersensitivity is suspected, it is advisable to perform desensitization or use an alternative drug.

2. An antihistaminic drug should be administered before beginning desensitization in order to lessen any reaction that might occur. An airway device must be available.

3. Epinephrine, 1 mL of 1:1000 solution, must be ready for immediate administration.

B. Desensitization Method: The following plan may be used in desensitization. Give doses of antitoxin intramuscularly at 30-minute intervals and observe closely for reactions.

First dose: 0.1 mL (1:10 dilution)
Second dose: 0.2 mL (1:10 dilution)
Third dose: 0.5 mL (1:10 dilution)
Fourth dose: 0.1 mL (undiluted)
Fifth dose: 0.2 mL (undiluted)
Sixth dose: 0.5 mL (undiluted)
Seventh dose: 1 mL (undiluted)
Eighth and subsequent doses: 1 mL (undiluted) every 30 minutes until the total amount of antitoxin is given.

Treatment of Reactions

A. Mild: If a mild reaction occurs, drop back to the next lower dose and continue with desensitization. If a severe reaction occurs, administer epinephrine (see below) and discontinue the antitoxin unless treatment is urgently needed. If desensitization is imperative, continue slowly, increasing the dosage of the antitoxin more gradually.

B. Severe: If manifestations of a severe reaction appear, give 0.5–1 mL of 1:1000 epinephrine into an intravenous drip of 5% dextrose in water at once. The symptoms include urticaria, angioneurotic edema, dyspnea, coughing, choking, and shock. Observe the patient closely and repeat epinephrine as necessary (see p 15).

Corticosteroids may be used (eg, hydrocortisone, 100 mg intravenously), but their effect begins only after 18 hours.

Norman PS: Specific therapy in allergy. *Med Clin North Am* 1974;**58**:111.

Sherman WB: *Hypersensitivity: Mechanism and Management.* Saunders, 1968.

●   ●   ●

References

Centers for Disease Control: Sexually transmitted diseases: Treatment guidelines 1982. *MMWR* (Aug 20) 1982;**31**:35S.

Dupont ML, Pickering LK: *Infections of the Gastrointestinal Tract.* Plenum Medical Book Co, 1980.

Feigin RD, Cherry JD: *Textbook of Pediatric Infectious Diseases.* Saunders, 1981.

Jawetz E, Melnick JL, Adelberg EA: *Review of Medical Microbiology,* 16th ed. Lange, 1984.

Mandell GL, Douglas RG Jr, Bennett JE: *Principles and Practice of Infectious Disease.* Wiley, 1979.

23 | Infectious Diseases: Viral & Rickettsial

Moses Grossman, MD, & Ernest Jawetz, MD, PhD

VIRAL DISEASES*

MEASLES
(Rubeola)

Essentials of Diagnosis

- Prodrome of fever, coryza, cough, conjunctivitis, photophobia, Koplik's spots.
- Rash: brick-red, irregular, maculopapular; onset 3 days after onset of prodrome; face to trunk to extremities.
- Leukopenia.
- Exposure 10–14 days previously.

General Considerations

Measles is an acute systemic viral (paramyxovirus) infection transmitted by inhalation of infective droplets. Its highest incidence is in young children. One attack confers permanent immunity. Communicability is greatest during the preeruptive stage but continues as long as the rash remains.

Clinical Findings

A. Symptoms and Signs: Fever is often as high as 40–40.6 °C (104–105 °F). It persists through the prodrome and rash (about 7 days), but may remit briefly at the onset of rash. Malaise may be marked. Coryza resembles that seen with upper respiratory infections (nasal obstruction, sneezing, and sore throat). Cough is persistent and nonproductive. There is conjunctivitis, with redness, swelling, photophobia, and discharge.

Koplik's spots are pathognomonic of measles. They appear about 2 days before the rash and last 1–4 days as tiny "table salt crystals" on the dull red mucous membranes of the cheeks and often on inner conjunctival folds and vaginal mucous membranes. The pharynx is red, and a yellowish exudate may appear on the tonsils. The tongue is coated in the center; the tip and margins are red. Moderate generalized lymphadenopathy is common. Splenomegaly occurs occasionally.

The rash usually appears first on the face and behind the ears 4 days after the onset of symptoms. The

*For herpesviruses, see p 829.

initial lesions are pinhead-sized papules which coalesce to form the brick-red, irregular, blotchy maculopapular rash and which may further coalesce in severe cases to form an almost uniform erythema on some areas of the body. By the second day, the rash begins to coalesce on the face as it appears on the trunk. On the third day, the rash is confluent on the trunk, begins to appear on the extremities, and begins to fade on the face. Thereafter, it fades in the order of its appearance. Hyperpigmentation remains in fair-skinned individuals and severe cases. Slight desquamation may follow.

Atypical measles is a syndrome occurring in children, adolescents, or adults who have received inactivated measles vaccine or who received live measles vaccine before age 12 months and as a result have developed hypersensitivity rather than protective immunity. When they are infected with wild measles virus, such individuals develop high fever, unusual rashes (papular, hemorrhagic), headache, arthralgias and pneumonitis, often with severe illness and a substantial mortality rate.

B. Laboratory Findings: Leukopenia is usually present unless secondary bacterial complications exist. Febrile proteinuria is present. Virus can be recovered from nasopharyngeal washings and from blood. A 4-fold rise in serum antibody supports the diagnosis.

Complications

A. Central Nervous System Complications: Encephalitis occurs in approximately 1:1000 to 1:2000 cases. Its onset is usually 3–7 days after the rash. Vomiting, convulsions, coma, and a variety of severe neurologic signs and symptoms develop. Treatment is symptomatic and supportive. There is an appreciable mortality rate, and many patients are left with permanent sequelae. Subacute sclerosing panencephalitis is a very late form of central nervous system complication, the measles virus acting as a "slow virus" to produce this degenerative central nervous system disease years after the initial infection.

B. Respiratory Tract Disease: Early in the course of the disease, bronchopneumonia or bronchiolitis due to the measles virus may occur and result in serious difficulties with ventilation.

C. Secondary Bacterial Infections: Immediately following measles, secondary bacterial infection—particularly cervical adenitis, otitis media, and pneumonia—occurs in about 15% of patients.

D. Tuberculosis: Measles produces temporary anergy to the tuberculin skin test; there may be exacerbations in patients with tuberculosis.

Prevention

Attenuated live virus vaccine can greatly reduce the incidence of measles. Its use has virtually eliminated endemic measles in the USA. It is important to immunize all children, including children in those areas of the world where the incidence and mortality rate of measles remain high. Combined virus vaccines (measles-mumps-rubella) are available and effective. Measles immunity is lasting if the vaccine is given at age 15 months or older. Complications of vaccination are negligible (see Table 22–3).

When susceptible individuals are exposed to measles, the live virus vaccine can prevent disease if given within 24 hours of exposure. This is rarely feasible in a household. Later, gamma globulin (0.25 mL/kg [0.1 mL/lb] body weight) can be injected for prevention of clinical illness. This must be followed by active immunization 3 months later.

Treatment

A. General Measures: Isolate the patient for the week following onset of rash and keep at bed rest until afebrile. Give aspirin, saline eye sponges, vasoconstrictor nose drops, and a sedative cough mixture as necessary.

B. Treatment of Complications: Secondary bacterial infections are treated with appropriate antimicrobial drugs. Postmeasles encephalitis can only be treated symptomatically.

Prognosis

The mortality rate of measles in the USA is 0.2%, but it may be as high as 10% in underdeveloped areas. Deaths are due principally to encephalitis (15% mortality rate) and bacterial pneumonia.

Amler RW et al: Imported measles in the United States. *JAMA* 1982;**248**:2129.
International Symposium on Measles Immunization. *Rev Infect Dis* 1983;**5**:389.
Martin DB et al: Atypical measles in adolescents and young adults. *Ann Intern Med* 1979;**90**:877.

EXANTHEM SUBITUM
(Roseola Infantum)

Although this illness is commonly diagnosed in clinical practice, laboratory confirmation is not available. Rotaviruses have been implicated as etiologic agents. The disease has been transmitted by blood filtrates.

The typical clinical picture is sudden development of very high fever (up to 41 °C [106 °F]) and irritability in a young child (age 6 months to 3 years).

Febrile convulsions occur commonly. The physical findings are limited to postoccipital and postauricular lymphadenopathy. It is essential to rule out other causes of high fever. The febrile state continues for 3 days. As the temperature drops, an evanescent, very transient maculopapular rash appears. The white blood count may be slightly elevated initially, but as the disease progresses, leukopenia is invariably present.

Treatment is purely symptomatic. Aspirin and tepid sponges will serve to keep the temperature down. Convulsions are usually very brief but may require anticonvulsant medication.

The prognosis is excellent. There are no reported deaths, and no sequelae occur.

RUBELLA
(German Measles)

Essentials of Diagnosis

- No prodrome; mild symptoms (fever, malaise, coryza) coinciding with eruption.
- Posterior cervical and postauricular lymphadenopathy.
- Fine maculopapular rash of 3 days' duration; face to trunk to extremities.
- Leukopenia.
- Exposure 14–21 days previously.
- Arthralgia, particularly in young women.

General Considerations

Rubella is a systemic viral disease transmitted by inhalation of infective droplets. It is only moderately communicable. One attack usually confers permanent immunity. The incubation period is 14–21 days (average, 16 days). The disease is transmissible for 1 week before the rash appears.

The clinical picture of rubella is difficult to distinguish from other viral illnesses such as infectious mononucleosis, echovirus infections, and coxsackievirus infections. Definitive diagnosis can only be made by isolating the virus or by serologic means.

The principal importance of rubella lies in the devastating effect this virus has on the fetus in utero, producing teratogenic effects and a continuing congenital infection.

Clinical Findings

A. Symptoms and Signs: Fever and malaise, usually mild, accompanied by tender suboccipital adenitis, may precede the eruption by 1 week. Mild coryza may be present. Joint pain (polyarthritis) occurs in about 25% of adult cases. These symptoms usually subside in less than 7 days.

Posterior cervical and postauricular lymphadenopathy is very common. Erythema of the palate and throat, sometimes blotchy, may be noted. A fine, pink maculopapular rash appears on the face, trunk, and extremities in rapid progression (2–3 days) and fades quickly, usually lasting 1 day in each area. Rubella without rash may be at least as common as the exan-

Table 23–1. Diagnostic features of some acute exanthems.

Disease	Prodromal Signs and Symptoms	Nature of Eruption	Other Diagnostic Features	Laboratory Tests
Measles (rubeola)	3–4 days of fever, coryza, conjunctivitis, and cough.	Maculopapular, brick-red; begins on head and neck; spreads downward. In 5–6 days rash brownish, desquamating. See atypical measles.	Koplik's spots on buccal mucosa.	White blood count low. Virus isolation in cell culture. Antibody tests by hemagglutination inhibition or neutralization.
Atypical measles	Same as measles.	Maculopapular centripetal rash, becoming confluent.	History of measles vaccination.	Measles antibody present in past, with titer rise during illness.
Rubella (German measles)	Little or no prodrome.	Maculopapular, pink; begins on head and neck, spreads downward, fades in 3 days. No desquamation.	Lymphadenopathy, postauricular or occipital.	White blood count normal or low. Serologic tests for immunity and definitive diagnosis (hemagglutination inhibition).
Chickenpox (varicella)	0–1 day of fever, anorexia, headache.	Rapid evolution of macules to papules, vesicles, crusts; all stages simultaneously present; lesions superficial, distribution centripetal.	Lesions on scalp and mucous membranes.	Specialized complement fixation and virus neutralization in cell culture. Fluorescent antibody test of smear of lesions.
Scarlet fever	½–2 days of malaise, sore throat, fever, vomiting.	Generalized, punctate, red; prominent on neck, in axilla, groin, skinfolds; circumoral pallor; fine desquamation involves hands and feet.	Strawberry tongue, exudative tonsillitis.	Group A hemolytic streptococci cultures from throat; antistreptolysin O titer rise.
Exanthem subitum	3–4 days of high fever.	As fever falls by crisis, pink maculopapules appear on chest and trunk; fade in 1–3 days.		White blood count low.
Erythema infectiosum	None. Usually in epidemics.	Red, flushed cheeks; circumoral pallor; maculopapules on extremities.	"Slapped face" appearance.	White blood count normal.
Meningococcemia	Hours of fever, vomiting.	Maculopapules, petechiae, purpura.	Meningeal signs, toxicity, shock.	Cultures of blood. Cerebrospinal fluid. High white blood count.
Rocky Mt. spotted fever	3–4 days of fever, chills, severe headaches.	Maculopapules, petechiae, initial distribution centripetal (extremities to trunk).	History of tick bite.	Agglutination (OX19, OX2), complement fixation.
Typhus fevers	3–4 days of fever, chills, severe headaches.	Maculopapules, petechiae, initial distribution centrifugal (trunk to extremities).	Endemic area, lice.	Agglutination (OX19), complement fixation.
Infectious mononucleosis	Fever, adenopathy, sore throat.	Maculopapular rash resembling rubella, rarely papulovesicular.	Splenomegaly, tonsillar exudate.	Atypical lymphocytes in blood smears; heterophil agglutination. Monospot test.
Enterovirus infections	1–2 days of fever, malaise.	Maculopapular rash resembling rubella, rarely papulovesicular or petechial.	Aseptic meningitis.	Virus isolation from stool or cerebrospinal fluid; complement fixation titer rise.
Drug eruptions	Occasionally fever.	Maculopapular rash resembling rubella, rarely papulovesicular.		Eosinophilia.
Eczema herpeticum	None.	Vesiculopustular lesions in area of eczema.		Herpes simplex virus isolated in cell culture. Multinucleate giant cells in smear of lesion.
Kawasaki disease	Fever, adenopathy, conjunctivitis.	Cracked lips, strawberry tongue, maculopapular polymorphous rash, peeling skin on fingers and toes.	Edema of extremities. Angiitis of coronary arteries.	Thrombocytosis, electrocardiographic changes.

thematous disease. Diagnosis can be suspected when there is epidemiologic evidence of the disease in the community but requires laboratory confirmation.

B. Laboratory Findings: Leukopenia may be present early and may be followed by an increase in plasma cells. Virus isolation and serologic tests of immunity (rubella virus hemagglutination inhibition and fluorescent antibody tests) are available. Defini-

tive diagnosis is based on a 4-fold rise in the antibody titer.

Complications

A. Complications in Pregnancy: It is important to know whether rubella antibodies are present at the beginning of pregnancy.

If a pregnant woman is exposed to a possible case

of rubella, an immediate hemagglutination-inhibiting rubella antibody level should be obtained. If antibodies are found, there is no reason for concern. If no antibodies are found, careful clinical and serologic follow-up is essential. If the occurrence of rubella in the expectant mother can be confirmed, therapeutic abortion may be considered. Judgment in this regard is tempered by personal, religious, legal, and other considerations. The risk to the fetus is highest in the first trimester but continues into the second as well.

B. Congenital Rubella: An infant acquiring the infection in utero may be normal at birth but more likely will have a wide variety of manifestations, including growth retardation, maculopapular rash, thrombocytopenia, cataracts, deafness, congenital heart defects, organomegaly, and many other manifestations. Viral excretion in the throat and urine persists for many months despite high antibody levels. The diagnosis is confirmed by isolation of the virus. A specific test for IgM rubella antibody is very useful for making this diagnosis in the neonate. Treatment is directed to the many anomalies.

Prevention

Live attenuated rubella virus vaccine (eg, RA 27/3) should be given to all girls before the menarche. When adult women are immunized, they must not be pregnant, and the absence of antibodies should be established. (In the USA, about 80% of 20-year-old women are immune to rubella.) Birth control must be practiced for at least 3 months after the use of the vaccine. Arthritis may follow administration of rubella vaccine.

Treatment

Give aspirin as required for symptomatic relief. Encephalitis and thrombocytopenic purpura can only be treated symptomatically.

Prognosis

Rubella (other than the congenital form) is a mild illness and rarely lasts more than 3–4 days. Congenital rubella, on the other hand, has a high mortality rate, and the congenital defects associated with it require many years of medical and surgical management.

Chantler JK, Ford DK, Tingle AJ: Persistent rubella infection and rubella associated arthritis. *Lancet* 1982;**1**:1323.

Hinman AR et al: Rational strategy for rubella vaccination. *Lancet* 1983;**1**:39.

Mann JM et al: Assessing risks of rubella vaccine during pregnancy: A standardized approach. *JAMA* 1981;**245**:1647.

Polk BF et al: An outbreak of rubella among hospital personnel. *N Engl J Med* 1980;**303**:541.

CYTOMEGALOVIRUS DISEASE

The vast majority of cytomegalovirus infections are clinically inapparent. The virus (human herpesvirus 5) can be cultured from the salivary glands of 10–25% of healthy individuals, from the cervix of 10% of healthy women, and from the urine of 1% of all newborns. Cytomegalovirus infection occurs in 85–95% of homosexual men and is sexually transmitted. In such individuals, cytomegalovirus infection may result in immunosuppression. In immunocompetent individuals, cytomegalovirus infection results in clinical disease in only a minority of cases.

Clinical Findings

A. Classification: Three important clinical entities are recognized.

1. Perinatal disease–Intrauterine infection results in serious disease characterized by jaundice, hepatosplenomegaly, purpura, thrombocytopenia, and many other findings. Sequelae include microcephaly, mental retardation (up to 30%), and hearing loss (around 15%). Infection acquired soon after birth is asymptomatic but may induce neurologic deficits later.

2. Acute acquired cytomegalovirus disease–The clinical picture is that of infectious mononucleosis with fever, malaise, muscle and joint pains, generalized lymphadenopathy, and an enlarged liver. Pharyngitis and respiratory symptoms are not pronounced. Laboratory findings include atypical lymphocytes and abnormal liver function tests. In contrast to Epstein-Barr herpesvirus infection, the heterophil antibody test is negative. This disease is common after massive blood transfusions, including those given to infants. In intensive care nurseries, up to 30% of infants acquire cytomegalovirus infection.

3. Disease in the immunosuppressed host–In immunocompromised persons, cytomegalovirus can cause an opportunistic severe pneumonia. Cytomegalovirus infection itself can result in immunosuppression and may provide a favorable environment for spread of other opportunistic pathogens (eg, *Pneumocystis carinii* pneumonia, disseminated herpes simplex lesions). Most male homosexuals with multiple sexual contacts have cytomegalovirus infection, including those who develop AIDS (see p 824). Some such persons have repeated infections with different strains.

B. Laboratory Findings: (In addition to those listed above.) In neonatal infections, urine often shows typical "owl eye" cells, which are renal epithelial cells with intranuclear inclusions. From urine, cervical secretions, semen, saliva, blood, and various tissues, cytomegalovirus can be grown in cell culture. Serologic tests are used to determine the incidence of infection in various groups. A significant titer rise is the only indication of recent infection.

Treatment

There is no specific treatment. Control fever, pain, and convulsions with appropriate drugs. The value of specific antiviral chemotherapy has not been established.

Medical Perspective: Cytomegalovirus pathogenicity, immunology, and vaccine initiatives. *J Infec Dis* 1981;**143**:618.

Panjrani ZFK, Hanshaw JB: Cytomegalovirus in the perinatal period. *Am J Dis Child* 1981;**135**:56.

Stagno S et al: Congenital cytomegalovirus infection: The relative importance of primary and recurrent maternal infection. *N Engl J Med* 1982;**306**:945.

Urmacher C et al: Outbreak of Kaposi's sarcoma and cytomegalovirus infection in young homosexual men. *Am J Med* 1982;**72**:569.

VARICELLA (Chickenpox) & HERPES ZOSTER (Shingles)*

Essentials of Diagnosis

- Fever and malaise just before or with eruption.
- Rash: pruritic, centripetal, papular, changing to vesicular, pustular, and finally crusting.
- Leukopenia.
- Exposure 14–20 days previously.

General Considerations

Varicella is a viral (human herpesvirus 3) disease spread by inhalations of infective droplets or contact with lesions. Most cases occur in children. One attack confers permanent immunity. The incubation period of varicella is 10–20 days (average, 14 days).

Herpes zoster is caused by the same virus and occurs in individuals who were infected with chickenpox earlier.

Clinical Findings

A. Varicella:

1. Symptoms and signs–Fever and malaise are usually mild in children and more severe in adults. Itching is characteristic of the eruption. Vesicular lesions, quickly rupturing to form small ulcers, may appear first in the oropharynx. The rash is most prominent on the face, scalp, and trunk but to a lesser extent commonly involves the extremities (centripetal). Maculopapules change in a few hours to vesicles that quickly become pustular and eventually form crusts. New lesions may erupt for 1–5 days, so that all stages of the eruption are generally present simultaneously. The crusts usually slough in 7–14 days. The vesicles and pustules are superficial, elliptic, and have slightly serrated borders.

The distribution and evolution of varicella distinguish it from herpes zoster.

2. Laboratory findings–Leukopenia is common. Multinucleated giant cells may be found in scrapings of the base of the vesicles. Virus isolation is possible.

B. Herpes Zoster:

This syndrome is caused by the same virus as varicella. Usually a single, unilateral dermatome is involved. Pain, sometimes very severe, may precede the appearance of the skin lesions. The lesions follow the distribution of a nerve root. Thoracic and lumbar roots are most common, but cervical roots and the trigeminal nerve may be involved. The skin lesions are similar to those of chickenpox and develop in the same way from maculopapules to vesicles to pustules. Antibody levels are higher and more persistent in zoster than they are in varicella.

Complications

Secondary bacterial infection of the lesions is common and may produce a pitted scar. Cellulitis, erysipelas, and surgical scarlet fever may occur.

Pneumonia of the interstitial type occurs more often in adults and may lead to alveolar capillary block, hypoxia, and sometimes death.

Encephalitis occurs infrequently. It tends to exhibit cerebellar signs—ataxia and nystagmus. Most patients recover without sequelae.

Varicella in immunosuppressed patients (eg, children with leukemia receiving antileukemic drugs or children with kidney transplants) is often very severe and may be fatal. Chickenpox contracted during the first or second trimester of pregnancy carries a small risk of a distinctive pattern of congenital malformations in the fetus.

In immunosuppressed patients, herpes zoster may disseminate, producing skin lesions beyond the dermatome, visceral lesions, and encephalitis. This is a serious, sometimes fatal complication.

Prevention

Varicella-zoster immune globulin (VZIG)* is effective in preventing chickenpox in exposed susceptible immunosuppressed children. Plasma from zoster patients can also be used but carries a risk of hepatitis. A live attenuated vaccine for immunocompromised susceptible children is under investigation.

Treatment

A. General Measures: Isolate the patient until primary crusts have disappeared, and keep at bed rest until afebrile. Hospital patients with varicella-zoster should be placed in isolation rooms, and personnel entering the room should wear gowns, gloves, and masks. Keep the skin clean by means of frequent tub baths or showers when afebrile. Calamine lotion locally and antihistaminics may relieve pruritus.

B. Treatment of Complications: Secondary bacterial infection of local lesions may be treated with bacitracin-neomycin ointment; if lesions are extensive, penicillin may be given intramuscularly. Varicella encephalitis and varicella pneumonia are treated symptomatically. Corticosteroids may have a beneficial effect in the latter. Bacterial pneumonia is treated with appropriate antibiotics.

In the management of varicella and zoster in the immunosuppressed host, vidarabine (adenine arabinoside) or acyclovir can be beneficial (see Chapter 29) when administered during the first 5 days of disease.

---

*See also p 69.

*VZIG may be obtained by calling the nearest regional Red Cross Blood Center or the Centers for Disease Control, Atlanta; central number: (404) 329–3311.

Zoster immune globulin is not helpful for clinical therapy but only for prevention.

Prognosis

The total duration from onset of symptoms to the disappearance of crusts rarely exceeds 2 weeks. Fatalities are rare except in immunosuppressed patients.

Grose C: Variation on a theme by Fenner: The pathogenesis of chickenpox. *Pediatrics* 1981;**68**:735.

Orenstein WO et al: Prophylaxis of varicella in high risk children: Dose response of zoster immune globulin. *J Pediatr* 1981; **98**:368.

Weller T: Varicella and herpes zoster. (2 parts.) *N Engl J Med* 1983;**309**:1362, 1434.

Whitley R et al: Vidarabine therapy of varicella in immunosuppressed patients. *J Pediatr* 1982;**101**:125.

VARIOLA
(Smallpox, Variola Major)

Smallpox was a highly contagious viral (poxvirus) disease characterized by severe headache, fever, and prostration and accompanied by a centrifugal rash developing from macules to papules to vesicles to pustules.

Immunization with vaccinia virus culminating in a worldwide effort by WHO has apparently succeeded in eradicating smallpox from the world as of 1979. While no more cases are expected, an isolated case may occur as a result of infection from laboratory-stored variola virus. If a case is suspected, the nearest public health facility must be contacted as an emergency measure, so that the diagnosis can be promptly established and the necessary methods of containment initiated.

VACCINIA

The efficacy of vaccination was the essential factor in the eradication of smallpox. Since the world has been declared free of smallpox, civilian vaccination is now indicated only for laboratory workers working with smallpox virus or closely related viruses. Vaccination is still practiced among military forces. Smallpox vaccination is no longer required for international travel.

Types of Reaction

Vaccinia is the cutaneous and sometimes generalized reaction that occurs following the deliberate introduction of vaccinia virus as an immunizing agent.

A **major reaction** involves the appearance of a papule followed by an umbilicated vesicle and subsequently by a pustule and crusting. Duration of this process depends on whether it is a primary vaccination (12 days) or a revaccination (6 days). Any reaction that does not produce a vesicle and ulcer is considered to be **equivocal** and does not indicate immunity.

Contraindications to Vaccination

Any form of immunosuppression, whether congenital or due to the presence of disease or the use of drugs, is an absolute contraindication to smallpox vaccination. Eczema in the patient or family member (including a past history of eczema), other forms of dermatitis, and burns also contraindicate vaccination. Smallpox vaccine should *never* be used "therapeutically."

Complications of Vaccination

Complications range from minor rashes to life-threatening complications such as postvaccinal encephalitis, vaccinia necrosum, and eczema vaccinatum. Vaccinia can be transmitted from military personnel and their families to contacts. Assistance with the management of such complications may be obtained through the Centers for Disease Control.*

US Public Health Service Advisory Committee on Immunization Practices: Smallpox vaccine. *MMWR* (Sept 5) 1980;**29**:417.

MUMPS
(Epidemic Parotitis)

Essentials of Diagnosis

- Painful, swollen salivary glands, usually parotid.
- Orchitis, meningoencephalitis, pancreatitis.
- Cerebrospinal fluid lymphocytic pleocytosis in meningoencephalitis.
- Exposure 14–21 days previously.

General Considerations

Mumps is a viral (paramyxovirus) disease spread by respiratory droplets that usually produces inflammation of the salivary glands and, less commonly, orchitis, meningoencephalitis, pancreatitis, and oophoritis. Most patients are children. The incubation period is 14–21 days (average, 18 days). Infectivity precedes the symptoms by about 1 day, is maximal for 3 days, and then declines until the swelling is gone.

Clinical Findings

A. Symptoms and Signs: Fever and malaise are variable but are often minimal in young children. High fever usually accompanies orchitis or meningoencephalitis. Pain and swelling of one or both (75%) of the parotid or other salivary glands occurs, usually in succession 1–3 days apart. Occasionally, one gland subsides completely (usually in 7 days or less) before others become involved. Orchitis occurs in 25% of men. Headache and lethargy suggest meningoencephalitis. Upper abdominal pain and nausea and vomiting suggest pancreatitis. Lower abdominal pain in females suggests oophoritis.

Tender parotid swelling is the commonest physical finding. Edema is occasionally marked. Swelling

*Centers for Disease Control (Atlanta); central number: (404) 329–3311.

and tenderness of the submaxillary and sublingual glands are variable. The orifice of Stensen's duct may be reddened and swollen. Neck stiffness and other signs of meningeal irritation suggest meningoencephalitis. Testicular swelling and tenderness (unilateral in 75%) denote orchitis. Epigastric tenderness suggests pancreatitis. Lower abdominal tenderness and ovarian enlargement may be noted in mumps oophoritis, but the diagnosis is often difficult. Salivary gland involvement must be differentiated from lymph node involvement in the anterior cervical space.

B. Laboratory Findings: Relative lymphocytosis may be present, but the blood picture is not typical. Serum amylase is commonly elevated with or without pancreatitis. Lymphocytic pleocytosis of the cerebrospinal fluid is present in meningoencephalitis, which may be asymptomatic. The diagnosis is confirmed by isolating mumps virus from saliva or demonstrating a 4-fold rise in complement-fixing antibodies in paired sera.

Differential Diagnosis

Swelling of the parotid gland may be due to causes other than mumps; calculi in the parotid ducts and a reaction to iodides may produce such swelling. Parotitis may also be produced by pyogenic organisms, particularly in debilitated individuals. Swelling of the parotid gland has to be differentiated from inflammation of the lymph nodes that are located more posteriorly and inferiorly than the parotid gland.

Complications

The "complications" of mumps are simply other manifestations of the disease less common than inflammation of the salivary glands. These usually follow the parotitis but may precede it or occur without salivary gland involvement: meningoencephalitis (30%), orchitis (25% of adult males), pancreatitis, oophoritis, thyroiditis, neuritis, myocarditis, and nephritis.

Aseptic meningitis is common during the course of mumps, often occurs without salivary gland involvement, and is the most common viral meningitis. This is a very benign self-limited illness. Occasionally, however, encephalitis develops. This is associated with cerebral edema, serious neurologic manifestations, and sometimes death. Deafness may develop (rarely) as a result of eighth nerve neuritis.

Prevention

Mumps live virus vaccine is safe and highly effective. It is recommended for routine immunization for children over age 1 year, either alone or in combination with other virus vaccines. Its use has markedly decreased the incidence of mumps in the USA. The mumps skin test is less reliable in determining immunity than are serum neutralization titers. Mumps hyperimmune globulin may be considered for passive protection of certain exposed susceptibles. However, its effectiveness is uncertain.

Treatment

A. General Measures: Isolate the patient until swelling subsides and keep at bed rest during the febrile period. Give aspirin or codeine for analgesia as required and alkaline aromatic mouthwashes.

B. Treatment of Complications:

1. Meningoencephalitis–The treatment of aseptic meningitis is purely symptomatic. The management of encephalitis requires attention to cerebral edema, the airway, and maintenance of vital functions.

2. Orchitis–Suspend the scrotum in a suspensory or toweling "bridge" and apply ice bags. Incision of the tunica may be necessary in severe cases. Give codeine or morphine as necessary for pain. Pain can also be relieved by injection of the spermatic cord at the external inguinal ring with 10–20 mL of 1% procaine solution. Reduce inflammatory reaction with hydrocortisone sodium succinate, 100 mg intravenously, followed by 20 mg orally every 6 hours for 2–3 days.

3. Pancreatitis–Symptomatic relief only and parenteral fluids if necessary.

4. Oophoritis–Symptomatic treatment only.

Prognosis

The entire course of the infection rarely exceeds 2 weeks. Fatalities (due to encephalitis) are very rare.

Orchitis often makes the patient very uncomfortable but very rarely results in sterility.

Koplan JP, Preblud SR: A benefit-cost analysis of mumps vaccine. *Am J Dis Child* 1982;136:362.
Mumps vaccine: Recommendations of Immunization Practices Advisory Committee. *Ann Intern Med* 1980;92:803.

POLIOMYELITIS

Essentials of Diagnosis

- Muscle weakness, headache, stiff neck, fever, nausea and vomiting, sore throat.
- Lower motor neuron lesion (flaccid paralysis) with decreased deep tendon reflexes and muscle wasting.
- Cerebrospinal fluid shows excess cells. Lymphocytes predominate; rarely more than $500/\mu L$.

General Considerations

Poliomyelitis virus (enterovirus) is present in throat washings and stools, and infection probably can be acquired by the respiratory droplet route or by ingestion. Since the introduction of effective vaccine, poliomyelitis has become a rare disease in developed areas of the world.

Three antigenically distinct types of poliomyelitis virus (I, II, and III) are recognized, with no cross-immunity between them.

The incubation period is 5–35 days (usually 7–14 days). Infectivity is maximal during the first week, but virus is excreted in stools for several weeks.

Clinical Findings

A. Symptoms and Signs:

1. Abortive poliomyelitis–The symptoms are fever, headache, vomiting, diarrhea, constipation, and sore throat.

2. Nonparalytic poliomyelitis–Headache, neck, back, and extremity pain; fever, vomiting, abdominal pain, lethargy, and irritability are present. Muscle spasm is always present in the extensors of the neck and back and often in hamstring and other muscles. The muscles may be tender to palpation.

3. Paralytic poliomyelitis–Paralysis may occur at any time during the febrile period. Tremors, muscle weakness, constipation, and ileus may appear. Paralytic poliomyelitis may be divided into 2 forms, which may coexist: (1) spinal poliomyelitis, with weakness of the muscles supplied by the spinal nerves; and (2) bulbar poliomyelitis, with weakness of the muscles supplied by the cranial nerves and variable "encephalitis" symptoms. Bulbar symptoms include diplopia (uncommon), facial weakness, dysphagia, dysphonia, nasal voice, weakness of the sternocleidomastoid and trapezius muscles, difficulty in chewing, inability to swallow or expel saliva, and regurgitation of fluids through the nose. The most life-threatening aspect of bulbar poliomyelitis is respiratory paralysis.

Paralysis of the neck flexors is manifested by "neck drop" on lifting the shoulders from the bed. Paralysis of the shoulder girdle often precedes intercostal and diaphragmatic paralysis, which leads to diminished chest expansion and decreased vital capacity. Cyanosis and stridor may appear later as a result of hypoxia. Paralysis may quickly become maximal or may progress over a period of several days until the temperature becomes normal.

Deep tendon reflexes are diminished or lost, often asymmetrically, in areas of involvement.

In bulbar poliomyelitis there may be loss of gag reflex, loss of movement of palate and pharyngeal muscles, pooling of secretions in the oropharynx, deviation of tongue, and loss of movement of the vocal cords. However, the patient can usually take deep breaths on command.

Lethargy or coma may be due to encephalitis or hypoxia, most often caused by hypoventilation.

Hypertension, hypotension, and tachycardia may occur. Convulsions are rare.

B. Laboratory Findings: The white blood cell count may be normal or mildly elevated. Cerebrospinal fluid pressure and protein are normal or slightly increased; glucose not decreased; cells are usually less than $500/\mu L$ (predominantly lymphocytes; polymorphonuclear cells may be elevated at first). Cerebrospinal fluid is normal in 5% of patients. The virus may be recovered from throat washings (early) and stools (early and late). Neutralizing and complement-fixing antibodies appear during the first or second week of illness.

Differential Diagnosis

Nonparalytic poliomyelitis is very difficult to distinguish from other forms of aseptic meningitis due to other enteroviruses. Muscle tenderness and spasm point to poliomyelitis. Otherwise, the distinction is made by laboratory means. Acute infectious polyneuritis (Guillain-Barré) and paralysis from a tick bite may initially resemble poliomyelitis but are easily distinguishable on the basis of clinical and laboratory findings.

Complications

Urinary tract infection, atelectasis, pneumonia, myocarditis, and pulmonary edema may occur.

Prevention

Oral live trivalent virus vaccine (Sabin) is easily administered, safe, and very effective in providing local gastrointestinal immunity as well as a good level of circulating antibody. It is essential for primary immunization of all infants. Routine immunization of adults in the USA is not recommended because of the low incidence of the disease. However, adults who are exposed to poliomyelitis or plan to travel to endemic areas should receive oral poliovaccine. Inactivated ("killed") poliomyelitis virus vaccine (Salk) should be given to immunodeficient or immunosuppressed individuals and members of their households.

Treatment

Cranial nerve involvement must be detected promptly. Maintain comfortable but changing positions in a "polio bed": firm mattress, foot board, sponge rubber pads or rolls, sandbags, and light splints. Change of position, hot packs for the extremities, and analgesic drugs usually control muscle spasm and pain. Fecal impaction and urinary retention (especially with paraplegia) must be managed. In cases of respiratory paralysis or weakness, intensive care is needed. Maintain a clear airway, remove secretions, and maintain ventilation—if necessary by intubation and mechanical assistance.

To prevent future deformity, active exercise is avoided during fever but passive range-of-motion exercises are carried out, as well as frequent changes in position. As soon as the fever has subsided, early mobilization and active exercise under skilled direction is begun. Early bracing and splinting may be helpful.

Prognosis

During the febrile period, paralysis may develop or progress. Mild weakness of small muscles is more likely to regress than severe weakness of large muscles. Bulbar poliomyelitis may occur in 5–30% of paralytic cases and carries the highest mortality rate (up to 50%).

Fox JP: Eradication of poliomyelitis in the United States: A commentary on the Salk reviews. *Rev Infect Dis* 1980;**2**:277.

Nightingale EO: Recommendations for a national policy on poliomyelitis vaccination. *N Engl J Med* 1977;**297**:249.

ENCEPHALITIS

Essentials of Diagnosis

- Fever, malaise, stiff neck, sore throat, and nausea and vomiting, progressing to stupor, coma, and convulsions.
- Signs of an upper motor neuron lesion (exaggerated deep tendon reflexes, absent superficial reflexes, pathologic reflexes, spastic paralysis).
- Cerebrospinal fluid protein and pressure often increased, with lymphocytic pleocytosis.

General Considerations

A. Viral Encephalitis: While arboviruses (Table 23–2) are the principal causes, many other viruses may produce encephalitis. Herpes simplex produces "masslike" lesions in the temporal lobes. Rabies virus invariably produces encephalitis; mumps virus, poliovirus, and other enteroviruses can cause aseptic meningitis or meningoencephalitis.

B. Encephalitis Accompanying Exanthematous Diseases of Childhood: This may occur in the course of measles, varicella, infectious mononucleosis, and rubella.

C. Encephalitis Following Vaccination: Encephalitis may follow use of certain immunizing agents. These include vaccines against smallpox, rabies, and pertussis.

D. Toxic Encephalitis: Toxic encephalitis due to drugs, poisons, or bacterial toxins (*Shigella dysenteriae* type 1) may be clinically indistinguishable from infectious encephalitis.

E. Reye's Syndrome: See p 849.

Clinical Findings

A. Symptoms and Signs: The symptoms are fever, malaise, sore throat, nausea and vomiting, lethargy, stupor, coma, and convulsions. Signs include stiff neck, signs of meningeal irritation, tremors, convulsions, cranial nerve palsies, paralysis of extremities, exaggerated deep reflexes, absent superficial reflexes, and pathologic reflexes.

B. Laboratory Findings: The white blood cell count is variable. Cerebrospinal fluid pressure and protein content are often increased; glucose is normal; lymphocytic pleocytosis may be present (polymorphonuclears may predominate early in some forms). The virus may sometimes be isolated from blood or, rarely, from cerebrospinal fluid. Serologic tests of blood may be diagnostic in a few specific types of encephalitis. A CT scan of the brain may reveal the temporal lobe lesions indicative of herpesvirus.

Differential Diagnosis

Mild forms of encephalitis must be differentiated from aseptic meningitis, lymphocytic choriomeningitis, and nonparalytic poliomyelitis; severe forms from cerebrovascular accidents, brain tumors, brain abscess, and poisoning.

Complications

Bronchial pneumonia, urinary retention and infection, and decubitus ulcers may occur. Late sequelae are mental deterioration, parkinsonism, and epilepsy.

Prevention

Effective measures include vigorous mosquito control and active immunization against childhood infectious diseases. Special inactivated virus vaccines have been prepared for high-risk persons.

Treatment

Although specific therapy for the majority of causative entities is not available, a variety of treatment measures and procedures may contribute significantly to a more successful outcome. Such measures include reduction of intracranial pressure (by the use of mannitol or a urea–invert sugar preparation and glucocorticoids), the control of convulsions, maintenance of the airway, administration of oxygen, and attention to adequate nutrition during periods of prolonged coma. After 72 hours of conventional intravenous nutrition, a nasogastric tube must be inserted and intestinal feedings begun.

Prevention or early treatment of decubiti, pneumonia, and urinary tract infections is important. Give anticonvulsants as needed.

Vidarabine (adenine arabinoside) or acyclovir may be effective antiviral drugs for biopsy-proved herpes simplex encephalitis if administered early in the disease before onset of coma, but they have no effect on other viral encephalitides (see Chapter 29).

Prognosis

The prognosis should always be guarded, especially in younger children. Sequelae may become ap-

---

Table 23–2. Arbovirus (arthropod-borne) encephalitis.

Disease	Geographic Distribution	Vector; Reservoir	Comment
California encephalitis	Throughout USA	Mosquitoes; small mammals	Mainly in children
Eastern (equine) encephalitis	Eastern part of North, Central, and South America	Mosquitoes; birds, small rodents	Often occurs in horses in the area
St. Louis encephalitis	Western and central USA, Florida	Mosquitoes; birds (including domestic fowl)	
Venezuelan encephalitis	South America	Mosquitoes	Rare in USA
Western (equine) encephalitis	Throughout western hemisphere	Mosquitoes; birds	Often occurs in horses in the area; particularly affects young children

parent late in the course of what appears to be a successful recovery.

Kennard C, Swash M: Acute viral encephalitis: Its diagnosis and outcome. *Brain* 1981;**104**:129.

Whitley RJ et al: Herpes simplex encephalitis: Vidarabine therapy and diagnostic problems. *N Engl J Med* 1981;**304**:313.

LYMPHOCYTIC CHORIOMENINGITIS

Essentials of Diagnosis

- "Influenzalike" prodrome of fever, chills, malaise, and cough, followed by meningitis with associated stiff neck.
- Kernig's sign, headache, nausea, vomiting, and lethargy.
- Cerebrospinal fluid: slight increase of protein, lymphocytic pleocytosis (500–1000/μL).
- Complement-fixing antibodies within 2 weeks.

General Considerations

Lymphocytic choriomeningitis is a viral (arenavirus) infection of the central nervous system. The reservoir of infection is the infected house mouse, although naturally infected guinea pigs, monkeys, dogs, and swine have been observed. Pet hamsters may be a source of infection. The virus is shed by the infected animal via oronasal secretions, urine, and feces, with transmission to humans probably through contaminated food and dust. The incubation period is probably 8–13 days to the appearance of systemic manifestations and 15–21 days to the appearance of meningeal symptoms. The disease is not communicable from person to person. Complications are rare.

This disease is principally confined to the eastern seaboard and northeastern states of the USA.

Clinical Findings

A. Symptoms and Signs: The prodromal illness is characterized by fever, chills, headache, myalgia, cough, and vomiting; the meningeal phase by headache, nausea and vomiting, and lethargy. Signs of pneumonia are occasionally present during the prodromal phase. During the meningeal phase there may be neck and back stiffness and a positive Kernig sign (meningeal irritation). Severe meningoencephalitis may disturb deep tendon reflexes and may cause paralysis and anesthesia of the skin.

The prodrome may terminate in complete recovery, or meningeal symptoms may appear after a few days of remission.

B. Laboratory Findings: Leukocytosis may be present. Cerebrospinal fluid lymphocytic pleocytosis (total count is often 500–3000/μL) may occur, with slight increase in protein and normal glucose. Complement-fixing antibodies appear during or after the second week. The virus may be recovered from the blood and cerebrospinal fluid by mouse inoculation.

Differential Diagnosis

The influenzalike prodrome and latent period help distinguish this from other aseptic meningitides, meningismus, and bacterial and granulomatous meningitis. A history of exposure to mice is an important diagnostic clue.

Treatment

Treat as for encephalitis.

Prognosis

Fatality is rare. The illness usually lasts 1–2 weeks, although convalescence may be prolonged.

Biggar RJ et al: Lymphocytic choriomeningitis outbreak associated with pet hamsters. *JAMA* 1975;**232**:494.

DENGUE
(Breakbone Fever, Dandy Fever)

Essentials of Diagnosis

- Sudden onset of high fever, chills, severe aching, headache, sore throat, prostration, and depression.
- Biphasic fever curve: initial phase, 3–4 days; remission, few hours to 2 days; second phase, 1–2 days.
- Rash: maculopapular, scarlatiniform, morbilliform, or petechial; on extremities to torso, occurring during remission or second phase.
- Leukopenia.

General Considerations

Dengue is a viral (group B arbovirus, togavirus) disease transmitted by the bite of the *Aedes* mosquito. It may be caused by one of several serotypes widely distributed between latitudes 25° north and 25° south. It occurs only in the active mosquito season (warm weather). The incubation period is 3–15 days (usually 5–8 days).

Clinical Findings

A. Symptoms and Signs: Dengue begins with a sudden onset of high fever (often of the saddleback type), chilliness, and severe aching ("breakbone") of the head, back, and extremities, accompanied by sore throat, prostration, and depression. There may be conjunctival redness and flushing or blotching of the skin. The initial febrile phase lasts 3–4 days, typically but not inevitably followed by a remission of a few hours to 2 days. The skin eruption appears in 80% of cases during the remission or during the second febrile phase, which lasts 1–2 days and is accompanied by similar but usually milder symptoms than in the first phase. The rash may be scarlatiniform, morbilliform, maculopapular, or petechial. It appears first on the dorsum of the hands and feet and spreads to the arms, legs, trunk, and neck but rarely to the face. The rash lasts 2 hours to several days and may be followed by desquamation. Petechial rashes and gastrointestinal hemorrhages occur in a high proportion of cases (mosquito-borne hemorrhagic fever) in Southeast Asia. These probably involve an immunologic reaction (immune complex disease).

Before the rash appears, it is difficult to distinguish dengue from malaria, yellow fever, or influenza. With the appearance of the eruption, which resembles rubella, the diagnosis is usually clear.

B. Laboratory Findings: Leukopenia is characteristic. Thrombocytopenia occurs in the hemorrhagic form of the disease. Virus may be recovered from the blood during the acute phase. Serologic diagnosis must consider the several viruses that can produce this clinical syndrome.

Complications

Depression, pneumonia, iritis, orchitis, and oophoritis are rare complications. Shock occurs in hemorrhagic dengue.

Prevention

Available prophylactic measures include control of mosquitoes by screening and insect repellents. An effective vaccine has been developed but has not been produced commercially.

Treatment

Treat shock by expanding circulating blood volume. Give salicylates as required for discomfort. Permit gradual restoration of activity during prolonged convalescence.

Prognosis

Fatalities are rare. Convalescence is slow.

Halstead SB: The pathogenesis of dengue: Molecular epidemiology in infectious disease. *Am J Epidemiol* 1981;**114**:632.

Morens DM: Dengue fever and dengue shock syndrome. *Hosp Pract* (July) 1982;**17**:103.

RIFT VALLEY FEVER

Rift Valley fever is a viral disease of sheep and cattle, chiefly in Africa, transmitted to humans probably by mosquito bites. It is not contagious. The clinical manifestations are closely similar to those of dengue: acute prostration, fever (often saddleback in type), myalgia and arthralgia, gastrointestinal distress, and sometimes hepatitis. The course is usually brief and self-limited.

There is no effective treatment. Complete recovery is the rule.

Meegan JM, Shope RE: Emerging concepts in Rift Valley fever. *Perspect Virol* 1981;**11**:267.

COLORADO TICK FEVER

Essentials of Diagnosis

- Fever, chills, myalgia, headache, prostration.

- Leukopenia.
- Second attack of fever after remission lasting 2–3 days.
- Onset 3–6 days following tick bite.

General Considerations

Colorado tick fever is an acute viral (orbivirus) infection transmitted by *Dermacentor andersoni* bites. The disease is limited to the western USA and is most prevalent during the tick season (March to August). The incubation period is 3–6 days.

Clinical Findings

A. Symptoms and Signs: The onset of fever (to 38.9–40.6 °C [102–105 °F]) is abrupt, sometimes with chills. Severe myalgia, headache, photophobia, anorexia, nausea and vomiting, and generalized weakness are prominent symptoms. Abnormal physical findings are limited to an occasional faint rash. Fever continues for 3 days, followed by a remission of 2–3 days and then by a full recrudescence lasting 3–4 days. In an occasional case there may be 2 or 3 bouts of fever.

Influenza, Rocky Mountain spotted fever, and other acute leukopenic fevers must be differentiated.

B. Laboratory Findings: Leukopenia (2000–3000/μL) with a shift to the left occurs. Viremia may be demonstrated by inoculation of blood into mice or by fluorescent antibody staining of the patient's red cells (with adsorbed virus). Complement-fixing antibodies appear during the third week after onset of the disease.

Complications

Aseptic meningitis or encephalitis occurs rarely. Asthenia may follow, but fatalities are very rare.

Treatment

No specific treatment is available. Aspirin or codeine may be given for pain.

Prognosis

The disease is self-limited and benign.

Goodpasture HC et al: Colorado tick fever: Clinical, epidemiologic and laboratory aspects of 228 cases in Colorado in 1973–74. *Ann Intern Med* 1978;**88**:303.

HEMORRHAGIC FEVERS

This is a diverse group of illnesses resulting from virus infections and perhaps immunologic responses to them. The common clinical features include high fever; hemorrhagic diathesis with petechiae or purpura; and bleeding from the nose, gastrointestinal tract, and genitourinary tract, with thrombocytopenia, leukopenia, and marked toxicity, often leading to shock and death. The viruses may be tick-borne (eg, Omsk hemorrhagic fever, Russia; Kyasanur Forest hemorrhagic fever, India), mosquito-borne (eg,

Chikungunya hemorrhagic fever, yellow fever, dengue), or zoonotic (often derived from rodents, eg, Junin hemorrhagic fever, Argentina; Machupo hemorrhagic fever, Bolivia; Lassa hemorrhagic fever, Nigeria). Into the last (zoonotic) group fall Marburg hemorrhagic fever (in persons who come into contact with vervet monkeys from Africa) and Ebola hemorrhagic fever occurring in Zaire and Sudan from an uncertain source.

Persons who present with symptoms compatible with those of hemorrhagic fever and who have traveled from a possible endemic area should be strictly isolated for diagnosis and symptomatic treatment. Conclusive diagnosis may be made by growing the virus from blood obtained early in the disease or by showing a significant specific antibody titer rise. Isolation is particularly important, because some of these infections are highly transmissible to close contacts, including medical personnel, and carry a mortality rate of 50–70%.

Although there is no specific treatment at present, it is all the more important to differentiate hemorrhagic fever from such easily treated entities as meningococcemia and Rocky Mountain spotted fever.

Gear JHS: Hemorrhagic fevers with special reference to recent outbreaks in Southern Africa. *Rev Infect Dis* 1979;**1**:571.

Simpson DIH: Viral haemorrhagic fevers of man. *Bull WHO* 1978;**56**:819.

Viral hemorrhagic fever: Initial management of suspected and confirmed cases. *MMWR* 1983;**32**:275.

Zweighaft RM et al: Lassa fever: Response to an imported case. *N Engl J Med* 1977;**297**:803.

RABIES

Essentials of Diagnosis

- Paresthesia, hydrophobia, rage alternating with calm.
- Convulsions, paralysis, thick tenacious saliva.
- History of animal bite.

General Considerations

Rabies is a viral (rhabdovirus) encephalitis transmitted by infected saliva that gains entry into the body by a bite or an open wound. Bats, skunks, and foxes are extensively infected. Dogs and cats may be infected. Rodents are unlikely to have rabies. The virus gains entry into the salivary glands of dogs 5–7 days before their death from rabies, thus limiting their period of infectivity. The incubation period may range from 10 days to 2 years but is usually 3–7 weeks. The virus travels in the nerves to the brain, multiplies there, and then migrates along the efferent nerves to the salivary glands.

Rabies is almost uniformly fatal. The most common clinical problem confronting the physician is the management of a patient bitten by an animal. (See Prevention.)

Clinical Findings

A. Symptoms and Signs: There is usually a history of animal bite. Pain appears at the site of the bite, followed by tingling. The skin is quite sensitive to changes of temperature, especially air currents. Attempts at drinking cause extremely painful laryngeal spasm, so that the patient refuses to drink (hydrophobia). The patient is restless and behaves in a peculiar manner. Muscle spasm, laryngospasm, and extreme excitability are present. Convulsions occur, and blowing on the back of the patient's neck will often precipitate a convulsion. Large amounts of thick tenacious saliva are present.

B. Laboratory Findings: Biting animals who are apparently well should be kept under observation. Sick or dead animals should be examined for rabies. The diagnosis of rabies in the brain of a rabid animal may be made rapidly by the fluorescent antibody technique.

Prevention

Since the disease is almost always fatal, prevention is the only available approach. Immunization of household dogs and cats and active immunization of persons with an unusual degree of exposure (eg, veterinarians) are important. However, the most important common decisions concern handling animal bites.

A. Local Treatment of Animal Bites and Scratches: Thorough and repeated flushing and cleansing of wounds with soap and water are important. If rabies immune globulin or antiserum is to be used, a portion should be infiltrated locally around the wound (see below). Wounds caused by animal bites should not be sutured.

B. The Biting Animal: A dog or cat should be captured, confined, and observed by a veterinarian for 7–10 days. A wild animal, if captured, should be sacrificed and the head shipped on ice to the nearest laboratory qualified to examine the brain for rabies. When the animal cannot be examined, skunks, bats, coyotes, foxes, and raccoons should be presumed to be rabid. The rabies potential of bites by other animals must be evaluated individually.

C. Postexposure Immunization: The physician must reach a decision based on the recommendations of the USPHS Advisory Committee but should also be influenced by the circumstances of the bite, the extent and location of the wound, the presence of rabies in the region, the type of animal responsible for the bite, etc.* Treatment includes both passive antibody and vaccine. The optimal form of passive immunization is human rabies immune globulin (20 IU/kg). Up to 50% of the globulin should be used to infiltrate the wound; the rest is administered intramuscularly. If the human gamma globulin is not available, equine rabies antiserum (40 IU/kg) can be used after appropriate tests

*Consultation is provided by the Rabies Investigation Unit, Centers for Disease Control, Atlanta; central number: (404) 329-3311.

for horse serum sensitivity. Two inactivated preparations of rabies vaccine are currently licensed. The human diploid cell rabies vaccine is preferred. It is given as 5 injections intramuscularly on days 0, 3, 7, 14, and 28 after exposure. The vaccine effectively produces a regular antibody response. Few side effects have occurred. The vaccine can be obtained through state health departments.

Only if diploid cell vaccine is not available should duck embryo vaccine be used. It must be given as a series of 23 injections during the 2 weeks after exposure, as indicated in the package insert. Its efficacy is probably low. When duck embryo vaccine is used, rabies immune globulin must be given concurrently.

Preexposure prophylaxis with 3 injections of diploid cell vaccine is recommended for persons at high risk of exposure (veterinarians, animal handlers, etc).

Treatment

This very severe illness with an almost universally fatal outcome requires skillful intensive care with attention to the airway, maintenance of oxygenation, and control of seizures.

Prognosis

Once the symptoms have appeared, death almost inevitably occurs after 2–3 days as a result of cardiac or respiratory failure or generalized paralysis.

Bahnmanyar M et al: Successful protection of humans exposed to rabies infection. *JAMA* 1976;**236**:2751.

Compendium of animal rabies vaccines, 1984: Recommendations for immunization procedures. *MMWR* 1983;**32**:665.

Houff SA et al: Human-to-human transmission of rabies virus by corneal transplant. *N Engl J Med* 1979;**300**:603.

Plotkin SA, Wiktor T: Vaccination of children with human cell culture rabies vaccine. *Pediatrics* 1979;**63**:219.

Recommendation of the Immunization Practices Advisory Committee: Rabies prevention—United States, 1984. *MMWR* 1984;**33**:393.

Warrell DA et al: Pathophysiologic studies in human rabies. *Am J Med* 1976;**60**:180.

YELLOW FEVER

Essentials of Diagnosis

- Sudden onset of severe headache, aching in legs, and tachycardia. Later, bradycardia, hypotension, jaundice, hemorrhagic tendency (''coffee-ground'' vomitus).
- Proteinuria, leukopenia, bilirubinemia, bilirubinuria.
- Endemic area.

General Considerations

Yellow fever is a viral (group B arbovirus, togavirus) infection transmitted by the *Aedes* and jungle mosquitoes. It is endemic to Africa and South America (tropical or subtropical), but epidemics have extended far into the temperate zone during warm seasons. The mosquito transmits the infection by first biting an individual having the disease and then biting a susceptible individual after the virus has multiplied within the mosquito's body. The incubation period in humans is 3–6 days.

Clinical Findings

A. Symptoms and Signs:

1. Mild form—Symptoms are malaise, headache, fever, retro-orbital pain, nausea, vomiting, and photophobia. Bradycardia may be present.

2. Severe form—Symptoms are the same as in the mild form, with sudden onset and then severe pains throughout the body, extreme prostration, bleeding into the skin and from the mucous membranes (''coffee-ground'' vomitus), oliguria, and jaundice. Signs include tachycardia, erythematous face, and conjunctival redness during the congestive phase, followed by a period of calm (on about the third day) with a normal temperature and then a return of fever, bradycardia, hypotension, jaundice, hemorrhages (gastrointestinal tract, bladder, nose, mouth, subcutaneous), and later delirium. The short course and mildness of the icterus distinguish yellow fever from leptospirosis. The mild form is difficult to distinguish from infectious hepatitis.

B. Laboratory Findings: Leukopenia occurs, although it may not be present at the onset. Proteinuria is present, sometimes as high as 5–6 g/L, and disappears completely with recovery. With jaundice there are bilirubinuria and bilirubinemia. The virus may be isolated from the blood by intracerebral mouse inoculation (first 3 days). Antibodies appear during and after the second week.

Differential Diagnosis

It may be difficult to distinguish yellow fever from leptospirosis and other forms of jaundice on clinical evidence alone.

Prevention

Transmission is prevented through mosquito control. Live virus vaccine is highly effective and should be provided for persons living in or traveling to endemic areas. (See Immunization, p 832.)

Treatment

Treatment consists of giving a liquid diet, limiting food to high-carbohydrate, high-protein liquids as tolerated; intravenous glucose and saline as required; analgesics and sedatives as required; and saline enemas for obstipation.

Prognosis

The mortality rate is high in the severe form, with death occurring most commonly between the sixth and the ninth days. In survivors, the temperature returns to normal by the seventh or eighth day. The prognosis in any individual case should be guarded at the onset, since sudden changes for the worse are common. Hiccup, copious black vomitus, melena, and anuria are unfavorable signs.

INFLUENZA

Essentials of Diagnosis

- Abrupt onset with fever, chills, malaise, cough, coryza, and muscle aches.
- Aching, fever, and prostration out of proportion to catarrhal symptoms.
- Leukopenia.

General Considerations

Influenza (orthomyxovirus) is transmitted by the respiratory route. Although sporadic cases occur, epidemics and pandemics appear at varying intervals, usually in the fall or winter. Antigenic types A and B produce clinically indistinguishable infections, whereas type C is usually a minor illness. The incubation period is 1–4 days.

It is difficult to diagnose influenza in the absence of a classic epidemic. The disease resembles many other mild febrile illnesses but is always accompanied by a cough.

Clinical Findings

A. Symptoms and Signs: The onset is usually abrupt, with fever, chills, malaise, muscular aching, substernal soreness, headache, nasal stuffiness, and occasionally nausea. Fever lasts 1–7 days (usually 3–5). Coryza, nonproductive cough, and sore throat are present. Signs include mild pharyngeal injection, flushed face, and conjunctival redness.

B. Laboratory Findings: Leukopenia is common. Proteinuria may be present. The virus may be isolated from the throat washings by inoculation of embryonated eggs or cell cultures. Complement-fixing and hemagglutination-inhibiting antibodies appear during the second week.

Complications

Influenza causes necrosis of the respiratory epithelium, which predisposes to secondary bacterial infections. Frequent complications are acute sinusitis, otitis media, purulent bronchitis, and pneumonia.

Pneumonia is commonly due to bacterial infection with pneumococci or staphylococci and rarely to the influenza virus itself. The circulatory system is not usually involved, but pericarditis, myocarditis, and thrombophlebitis sometimes occur.

Reye's syndrome is a rare and severe complication of influenza and other viral diseases (eg, parainfluenza virus, coxsackievirus, echovirus), particularly in young children. It consists of rapid development of hepatic failure and encephalopathy, and there is a 30% fatality rate. The pathogenesis is unknown; aspirin may be a risk factor. Hypoglycemia, elevation of serum transaminases and blood ammonia, prolonged prothrombin time, and change in mental status all occur within 2–3 weeks after onset of the virus infection. Histologically, the periphery of liver lobules shows striking fatty infiltration and glycogen depletion. Treatment is supportive and directed to the management of cerebral edema.

Prevention

Polyvalent influenza virus vaccine given twice (1–2 weeks apart) exerts moderate temporary protection. Partial immunity lasts a few months to 1 year. The vaccine for 1984–1985 is composed of type A/Philippines 82 (H3N2), type A/Chile 83 (H1N1), and type B/USSR 83 strains that are expected to prevail in the next season. Vaccination is recommended every year for persons with chronic respiratory insufficiency, cardiac disease, or other debilitating illness. Effective chemoprophylaxis for epidemiologically or virologically confirmed influenza A consists of amantadine hydrochloride, 200 mg orally daily. This markedly reduces the incidence of infection in individuals exposed to influenza A if begun immediately and continued for 10 days. The drug does not prevent other types of influenza or other viral diseases.

Treatment

Bed rest to reduce complications is important. Analgesics and a sedative cough mixture may be used. Antibiotics should be reserved for treatment of bacterial complications.

Prognosis

The duration of the uncomplicated illness is 1–7 days, and the prognosis is excellent. Purulent bronchitis and bronchiectasis may result in chronic pulmonary disease and fibrosis that persist throughout life. Most fatalities are due to bacterial pneumonia. Pneumococcal pneumonia is most common, but staphylococcal pneumonia is most serious. In recent epidemics, the mortality rate has been low except in debilitated persons—especially those with severe heart disease.

If the fever persists more than 4 days, if the cough becomes productive, or if the white blood cell count rises to about 12,000/μL, secondary bacterial infection should be ruled out or verified and treated.

Baine WB et al: Severe illness with influenza B. *Am J Med* 1980; **68**:181.

Gregg MB et al: Influenza-related mortality. *JAMA* 1978; **239**:115.

Hirsch MS, Swartz MN: Drug therapy: Antiviral agents. *N Engl J Med* 1980;**302**:903.

CAT-SCRATCH DISEASE

Essentials of Diagnosis

- A primary infected ulcer or papule-pustule at site of inoculation (30% of cases).
- Regional lymphadenopathy that often suppurates.
- History of scratch by cat at involved area.
- Positive intradermal test.

General Considerations

This is an acute infection that occurs worldwide and is more common in children and young adults in contact with cats or dogs. It may be transmitted by a scratch or other injury, but some proved cases lack such a history. The cause (on the basis of morphologic and immunologic evidence presented in 1983) appears to be a small gram-negative bacterium seen in lesions, especially on the walls of capillaries and inside macrophages.

Clinical Findings

A. Symptoms and Signs: A few days after the scratch, about one-third of patients develop a primary lesion at the site of inoculation. This primary lesion appears as an infected, scabbed ulcer or a papule with a central vesicle or pustule. One to 3 weeks later, symptoms of generalized infection appear (fever, malaise, headache), and the regional lymph nodes become enlarged without evidence of lymphangitis. The nodes may be tender and fixed, with overlying inflammation; or nontender, discrete, and without evidence of surrounding inflammation. Suppuration may occur, with the discharge of sterile pus.

Lymph node enlargement must be differentiated from that of lymphoma, tuberculosis, lymphogranuloma venereum, and acute bacterial infection.

B. Laboratory Findings: The sedimentation rate is elevated, the white blood cell count is usually normal, and the pus from the nodes is sterile. Intradermal skin testing with antigen prepared from the pus is positive (tuberculinlike reaction) in most cases. Lymph node morphology is fairly characteristic; excisional biopsy confirms the diagnosis.

Complications

Encephalitis occurs rarely. Macular or papular rashes and erythema nodosum are occasionally seen.

Treatment

There is no specific treatment. Available antimicrobial drugs are ineffective. Surgical removal of a large node or aspiration of liquid contents usually produces an amelioration of symptoms and fever.

Prognosis

The disease is benign and self-limiting. Symptoms may continue for 5 days to 2 weeks.

Torres JR et al: Cat-scratch disease causing reversible lymphadenopathy. *JAMA* 1978;**240:**1628.

INFECTIOUS MONONUCLEOSIS

Essentials of Diagnosis

- Fever, sore throat, malaise, lymphadenopathy.
- Frequently splenomegaly, occasionally maculopapular rash.
- Positive heterophil agglutination test (Monospot).
- "Atypical" large lymphocytes in blood smear; lymphocytosis.
- Hepatitis frequent, and occasionally myocarditis, neuritis, encephalitis.

General Considerations

Infectious mononucleosis is an acute infectious disease due to the Epstein-Barr (EB) herpesvirus (human herpesvirus 4). It is universal in distribution and may occur at any age but usually occurs between the ages of 10 and 35, either in an epidemic form or as sporadic cases. Its mode of transmission is probably by saliva. The incubation period is probably 5–15 days.

Clinical Findings

A. Symptoms and Signs: Symptoms are varied but typically include fever; discrete, nonsuppurative, slightly painful, enlarged lymph nodes, especially those of the posterior cervical chain; and, in approximately half of cases, splenomegaly. Sore throat is often present, and toxic symptoms (malaise, anorexia, and myalgia) occur frequently in the early phase of the illness. A maculopapular or occasionally petechial rash occurs in less than 50% of cases. Exudative pharyngitis, tonsillitis, or gingivitis may occur.

Common manifestations of infectious mononucleosis are hepatitis with hepatomegaly, nausea, anorexia, and jaundice; central nervous system involvement with headache, neck stiffness, photophobia, pains of neuritis, and occasionally even Guillain-Barré syndrome; pulmonary involvement with chest pain, dyspnea, and cough; and myocardial involvement with tachycardia and arrhythmias.

The varying symptoms of infectious mononucleosis—especially sore throat, hepatitis, rash, and lymphadenopathy—raise difficult problems in differential diagnosis.

B. Laboratory Findings: Initially, there is a granulocytopenia followed within 1 week by a lymphocytic leukocytosis. Many lymphocytes are atypical, ie, are larger than normal adult lymphocytes, stain more darkly, and frequently show vacuolated, foamy cytoplasm and dark chromatin in the nucleus.

The mononucleosis spot test and the heterophil (sheep cell agglutination) test usually become positive in infectious mononucleosis before the fourth week after onset of the illness. Titer rises in antibodies directed at several EB virus antigens can be detected by immunofluorescence. During acute illness, there is always a rise in antibody to EB virus capsid antigen (VCA). A false-positive VDRL or RPR test (see p 885) occurs in 10% of cases.

In central nervous system involvement, the cerebrospinal fluid may show increase of pressure, abnormal lymphocytes, and protein.

With myocardial involvement, electrocardiographic studies may show abnormal T waves and prolonged PR intervals.

Liver function tests are commonly abnormal.

Differential Diagnosis

Causes of pharyngitis with exudate include diphtheria and adenovirus, herpes simplex, gonococcal, and streptococcal infections. Cytomegalovirus infection may be indistinguishable from infectious mononucleosis due to EB virus, but the heterophil antibody and Monospot tests are negative. The same applies to toxoplasmosis and rubella.

Complications

These usually consist of secondary throat infections, often streptococcal, and (rarely) rupture of the spleen or hypersplenism. Very rarely, there may be a variety of neurologic involvements, eg, myelitis.

Treatment

A. General Measures: No specific treatment is available. The patient requires support and reassurance because of the frequent feeling of lassitude and duration of symptoms. Symptomatic relief can be afforded by the administration of aspirin, and hot saline or 30% glucose throat irrigations or gargles 3 or 4 times daily. In severely ill patients, symptomatic relief can be obtained through a short course of corticosteroids. Diagnosis must be well established.

B. Treatment of Complications: Hepatitis, myocarditis, and encephalitis are treated symptomatically. Rupture of the spleen requires emergency splenectomy. Frequent vigorous palpation of the spleen is unwise.

Prognosis

In uncomplicated cases, fever disappears in 10 days and lymphadenopathy and splenomegaly in 4 weeks. The illness sometimes lingers for 2–3 months.

Death is uncommon; when it does occur it is usually due to splenic rupture or hypersplenic phenomena (severe hemolytic anemia, thrombocytopenic purpura) or to encephalitis.

There are usually no sequelae.

Bird AG, Britton S: The relationship between Epstein-Barr virus and lymphoma. *Semin Hematol* 1982;**19**:285.

Fleisher GR et al: Intrafamilial transmission of EB virus infections. *J Pediatr* 1981;**98**:16.

Grose C et al: Primary EBV infection in acute neurologic diseases. *N Engl J Med* 1975;**292**:392.

Lymphoma in organ transplant recipients. (Editorial.) *Lancet* 1984;**1**:601.

Rapp CE, Hewetson JF: Infectious mononucleosis and the Epstein-Barr virus. *Am J Dis Child* 1978;**132**:78.

Sugden B: Epstein-Barr virus: A human pathogen inducing lymphoproliferation in vivo and in vitro. *Rev Infect Dis* 1982;**4**:1048.

COXSACKIEVIRUS INFECTIONS

Coxsackievirus infections cause several clinical syndromes. As with other enteroviruses, infections are most common during the summer. Two groups, A and B, are defined by their differing behavior after injection into suckling mice. There are more than 50 serotypes.

Clinical Findings

A. Symptoms and Signs: The clinical syndromes associated with coxsackievirus infection may be described briefly as follows:

1. Summer grippe (Coxsackie A and B) – A febrile illness, principally of children, which lasts 1–4 days; minor symptoms and respiratory tract infection are often present.

2. Herpangina (Coxsackie A2, 4, 5, 6, 7, 10) – Sudden onset of fever, which may be as high as 40.6 °C (105 °F), sometimes with febrile convulsions; headache, myalgia, vomiting; and sore throat, characterized early by petechiae or papules on the soft palate that become shallow ulcers in about 3 days and then heal.

3. Epidemic pleurodynia (Coxsackie B1, 2, 3, 4, 5) – Sudden onset of recurrent pain in the area of diaphragmatic attachment (lower chest or upper abdomen); fever is often present during attacks of pain; headache, sore throat, malaise, nausea; tenderness, hyperesthesia, and muscle swelling of the involved area; orchitis, pleurisy, and aseptic meningitis may occur. Relapse may occur after recovery.

4. Aseptic meningitis (Coxsackie A2, 4, 7, 9, 10, 16; B viruses) – Fever, headache, nausea, vomiting, stiff neck, drowsiness, cerebrospinal fluid lymphocytosis without chemical abnormalities; rarely, muscle paralysis. See also Viral Meningitis.

5. Acute nonspecific pericarditis (Coxsackie B types) – Sudden onset of anterior chest pain, often worse with inspiration and in the supine position; fever, myalgia, headache; pericardial friction rub appears early; pericardial effusion with paradoxic pulse, increased venous pressure, and increase in heart size may appear; electrocardiographic and x-ray evidence of pericarditis is often present. One or more relapses may occur.

6. Myocarditis (Coxsackie B3, 4, and others) – Heart failure in the neonatal period may be the result of myocarditis associated with infection acquired in utero. Adult heart disease may be caused by coxsackievirus group B.

7. Hand, foot, and mouth disease – Coxsackievirus type A16 and several other types produce an illness characterized by stomatitis and a vesicular rash on the hands and feet. This may take an epidemic form.

B. Laboratory Findings: Routine laboratory studies show no characteristic abnormalities. Neutralizing antibodies appear during convalescence. The virus may be isolated from throat washings or stools inoculated into suckling mice.

Treatment & Prognosis

Treatment is symptomatic. With the exception of myocarditis, all of the syndromes caused by coxsackieviruses are benign and self-limited.

Centers for Disease Control: Enteroviral disease in the United States, 1970–79. *J Infect Dis* 1982;**146**:103.

Schiff GM: Coxsackievirus B epidemic at a boys' camp. *Am J Dis Child* 1979;**133**:782.

ECHOVIRUS INFECTIONS

Echoviruses are enteroviruses that produce several clinical syndromes, particularly in children. Infection is most common during the summer.

Over 20 serotypes have been demonstrated. Types 4, 6, and 9 cause aseptic meningitis, which may be associated with rubelliform rash. Types 9 and 16 cause an exanthematous illness (Boston exanthem) characterized by a sudden onset of fever, nausea, and sore throat, and a rubelliform rash over the face and trunk that persists 1–10 days. Orchitis may occur. Type 18 causes epidemic diarrhea, characterized by a sudden onset of fever and diarrhea in infants. Types 18 and 20 cause common respiratory disease (see Chapter 6). Myocarditis has also been reported.

As is true of the other enterovirus infections also, the diagnosis is best established by correlation of the clinical, epidemiologic, and laboratory evidence. The virus produces cytopathic effects in tissue culture and can be recovered from the feces, throat washings, blood, and cerebrospinal fluid. A 4-fold rise in antibody titer signifies systemic infection.

Treatment is purely symptomatic. The prognosis is excellent, although occasional mild paralysis has been reported following central nervous system infection.

Jarvis WR et al: Echovirus type 7 meningitis in young children. *Am J Dis Child* 1981;**135**:1009.

ADENOVIRUS INFECTIONS

Adenoviruses (there are more than 30 antigenic types) produce a variety of clinical syndromes. These infections are self-limited and most common among military recruits, although sporadic cases occur in civilian populations. The incubation period is 4–9 days.

There are 5 clinical types of adenovirus infection:

(1) The common cold: Many infections produce rhinitis, pharyngitis, and mild malaise without fever and are indistinguishable from other infections that produce the common cold syndrome.

(2) Acute undifferentiated respiratory disease, nonstreptococcal exudative pharyngitis: Fever lasts 2–12 days and is accompanied by malaise and myalgia. Sore throat is often manifested by diffuse injection, a patchy exudate, and cervical lymphadenopathy. Cough is sometimes accompanied by rales and x-ray evidence of pneumonitis (primary atypical pneumonia) (especially with types 4 and 7 in military recruits). Conjunctivitis is often present.

(3) Pharyngoconjunctival fever: Fever and malaise, conjunctivitis (often unilateral), and mild pharyngitis.

(4) Epidemic keratoconjunctivitis (shipyard eye): Unilateral conjunctival redness, mild pain, and tearing, with a large preauricular lymph node. Keratitis leads to subepithelial opacities (especially with types 8, 19, or 37).

(5) Acute hemorrhagic cystitis in children: (Often associated with type 11.)

Vaccines are not available for general use. Live oral vaccines containing attenuated type 4 and type 7 have been used in military personnel.

Treatment is symptomatic.

Fox JP et al: Observations of adenovirus infections. *Am J Epidemiol* 1977;**105**:362.

INFECTIOUS HEPATITIS
(See p 402.)

RICKETTSIAL DISEASES (RICKETTSIOSES)

The rickettsioses are a group of febrile diseases caused by infection with rickettsiae. Rickettsiae, once thought to be viruses, are small obligate intracellular bacteria that are parasites of arthropods. In arthropods, rickettsiae grow in the cells lining the gut, often without harming the host. Human infection results either from the bite of the specific arthropod or from contamination with its feces. In humans, rickettsiae grow principally in endothelial cells of small blood vessels, producing vasculitis, necrosis of cells, thrombosis of vessels, skin rashes, and organ dysfunctions.

Different rickettsiae and their vectors are endemic in different parts of the world, but 2 or more types may coexist in the same geographic area. A summary of epidemiologic features is given in Table 23–3. The clinical picture is variable but usually includes a prodromal stage followed by fever, rash, and prostration. Isolation of rickettsiae from the patient is cumbersome and difficult and can be undertaken only by specialized laboratories. Laboratory diagnosis relies on the development of nonspecific antibodies to certain *Proteus* strains (Weil-Felix reaction) and of specific antibodies detected by complement fixation or immunofluorescence tests.

Prevention & Treatment

Preventive measures are directed at control of the vector, specific immunization when available, and (occasionally) drug chemoprophylaxis. All rickettsiae can be inhibited by tetracyclines or chloramphenicol. All early clinical infections respond in some degree to treatment with these drugs. Treatment usually consists of giving either tetracycline hydrochloride or chloramphenicol, 0.5 g orally every 4–6 hours for 4–10 days (50 mg/kg daily). In seriously ill patients, initial treatment may consist of 1 g of tetracycline or chloramphenicol intravenously. Supportive measures may include parenteral fluids, sedation, oxygen, and skin care. The vector (louse, tick, mite) must be removed from patients by appropriate measures.

Table 23–3. Rickettsial diseases.*

Disease	Rickettsia	Geographic Area of Prevalence	Insect Vector	Mammalian Reservoir	Weil-Felix Agglutination		
					OX19	OX2	OXK
Typhus group							
Epidemic typhus	Rickettsia prowazekii	South America, Africa, Asia	Louse	Humans	++	±	–
Murine typhus	Rickettsia typhi	Worldwide; small foci	Flea	Rodents	++	–	–
Scrub typhus	Rickettsia tsutsugamushi	Southeast Asia, Japan	Mite†	Rodents	–	–	++
Spotted fever group							
Rocky Mountain spotted fever (RMSF)	Rickettsia rickettsii	Western hemisphere	Tick†	Rodents, dogs	+	+	–
Fièvre boutonneuse Kenya tick typhus South African tick fever Indian tick typhus	Rickettsia conorii	Africa, India, Mediter- ranean countries	Tick†	Rodents, dogs	+	+	–
Queensland tick typhus	Rickettsia australis	Australia	Tick†	Rodents, marsupials	+	+	–
North Asian tick typhus	Rickettsia sibirica	Siberia, Mongolia	Tick†	Rodents	+	+	–
Rickettsialpox	Rickettsia akari	USA, Korea, USSR	Mite†	Mice	–	–	–
RMSF-like	Rickettsia canada	North America	Tick†	Rodents	?	?	–
Other							
Q fever	Coxiella burnetii	Worldwide	None‡	Cattle, sheep, goats	–	–	–
Trench fever	Rochalimaea quintana	Rare	Louse	Humans	?	?	?

*Reproduced, with permission, from Jawetz E, Melnick JL, Adelberg EA: *Review of Medical Microbiology,* 16th ed. Lange, 1984.
†Also serve as arthropod reservoir by maintaining rickettsiae through transovarian transmission.
‡Human infection results from inhalation of dust.

EPIDEMIC LOUSE-BORNE TYPHUS

Essentials of Diagnosis

- Prodrome of malaise and headache followed by abrupt chills and fever.
- Severe, intractable headaches, prostration, persisting high fever.
- Maculopapular rash appears on the fourth to seventh days on the trunk and in the axillas, spreading to the rest of the body but sparing the face, palms, and soles.
- Laboratory confirmation by *Proteus* OX19 agglutination and specific serologic tests.

General Considerations

Epidemic louse-borne typhus is due to infection with *Rickettsia prowazekii,* a parasite of the body louse that ultimately kills the louse. Transmission is greatly favored by crowded living conditions, famine, war, or any circumstances that predispose to heavy infestation with lice. When the louse sucks the blood of a person infected with *R prowazekii,* the organism becomes established in the gut of the louse and grows there. When the louse is transmitted to another person (through contact or clothing) and has a blood meal, it defecates simultaneously, and the infected feces are rubbed into the itching bite wound. Dry, infectious louse feces may also enter the respiratory tract and result in human infection. A deloused and bathed typhus patient is no longer infectious for other humans.

In a person who recovers from clinical or subclin-

ical typhus infection, *R prowazekii* may survive in lymphoid tissues for many years. Years later, such a person may have recrudescence of disease without exogenous exposure to lice or to the infectious agent. Such a recrudescence (Brill's disease) can serve as a source of infection for lice. Recently, cases of *R prowazekii* infection have occurred in the USA after contact with flying squirrels or their ectoparasites.

Clinical Findings

A. Symptoms and Signs: Prodromal malaise, cough, headache, and chest pain begin after an incubation period of 10–14 days. There is then an abrupt onset of chills, high fever, and prostration, with "influenzal symptoms" progressing to delirium and stupor. The headache is intractably severe, and the fever is unremitting for many days.

Other findings consist of conjunctivitis, flushed face, rales at the lung bases, and often splenomegaly. A macular rash (that soon becomes papular) appears first in the axillas and then over the trunk, spreading to the extremities but rarely involving the face, palms, or soles. In severely ill patients, the rash becomes hemorrhagic, and hypotension becomes marked. There may be renal insufficiency, stupor, and delirium. In spontaneous recovery, improvement begins 13–16 days after onset with rapid drop of fever.

B. Laboratory Findings: The white blood cell count is variable. Proteinuria and hematuria commonly occur. Serum obtained 5–12 days after onset of symptoms usually shows agglutinating antibodies for *Proteus* OX19 (rarely also OX2)—*R prowazekii* shares antigens with these *Proteus* strains—and specific antibodies for *R prowazekii* antigens demonstrated by complement fixation, microagglutination, or immunofluorescence. A titer rise is most significant. In primary rickettsial infection, early antibodies are IgM; in recrudescence (Brill's disease), early antibodies are predominantly IgG, and the Weil-Felix test is negative.

C. X-Ray Findings: X-rays of the chest may show patchy consolidation.

Differential Diagnosis

The prodromal symptoms and the early febrile stage are not specific enough to permit diagnosis in nonepidemic situations. The rash is usually sufficiently distinctive for diagnosis, but it may be missing in 5–10% of cases and may be difficult to observe in dark-skinned persons. A variety of other acute febrile diseases may have to be considered.

Brill's disease (recrudescent epidemic typhus) has a more gradual onset than primary *R prowazekii* infection, fever and rash are of shorter duration, and the disease is milder and rarely fatal.

Complications

Pneumonia, vasculitis with major vessel obstruction and gangrene, circulatory collapse, myocarditis, and uremia may occur.

Prevention

Prevention consists of louse control with insecticides, particularly by applying chemicals to clothing or treating it with heat, and frequent bathing. Immunization with vaccines consisting of inactivated egg-grown *R prowazekii* gives some protection against severe disease although the efficacy is limited. This vaccine is not available in the USA or Canada in 1984. An improved cell culture vaccine is being developed. Live attenuated (strain E) vaccine is under investigation.

Treatment

See p 852.

Prognosis

The prognosis depends greatly upon age and immunization status. In children under age 10, the disease is usually mild. The mortality rate is 10% in the second and third decades but may reach 60% in the sixth decade. Effective vaccination can convert a potentially serious disease into a relatively mild one.

Duma RJ et al: Epidemic typhus in the United States associated with flying squirrels. *JAMA* 1981;**245**:2318.

Ormsbee R et al: Serologic diagnosis of epidemic typhus fever. *Am J Epidemiol* 1977;**105**:261.

Philip RN et al: Immunofluorescence test for the serologic study of Rocky Mountain spotted fever and typhus. *J Clin Microbiol* 1976;**3**:51.

ENDEMIC FLEA-BORNE TYPHUS
(Murine Typhus)

Rickettsia typhi (R mooseri) is transmitted from rat to rat through the rat flea (rarely, the rat louse). Humans acquire the infection when bitten by an infected flea, which releases infected feces while sucking blood.

Flea typhus resembles Brill's disease (recrudescent epidemic typhus) in that it has a gradual onset and the fever and rash are of shorter duration (6–13 days) and the symptoms less severe than in louse-borne typhus. The rash is maculopapular, concentrated on the trunk, and fades fairly rapidly. Even without antibiotic treatment, flea typhus is a mild disease. Pneumonia or gangrene is rare. Fatalities are rare and limited to the elderly.

Complement-fixing or immunofluorescent antibodies can be detected in the patient's serum with specific *R typhi* antigens. There is a rising titer of agglutinating antibodies to *Proteus* OX19.

Preventive measures are directed at control of rats and their ectoparasites. Insecticides are first applied to rat runs, nests, and colonies, and the rats are then poisoned or trapped. Finally, buildings must be made ratproof. Antibiotic treatment need not be intensive because of the mildness of the natural disease. An experimental vaccine was fairly effective, but it is not commercially available now.

SPOTTED FEVERS
(Tick Typhus)

Tick-borne rickettsial infections occur in many different regions of the world and have been given regional or local names, eg, Rocky Mountain spotted fever in North America, Queensland tick typhus in Australia, boutonneuse fever in North Africa, Kenya tick typhus, etc. The causative agents are all antigenically related to *Rickettsia rickettsii*, and all are transmitted by hard (ixodid) ticks and have cycles in nature that involve dogs, rodents, or other animals. Rickettsiae are often transmitted from one generation of ticks to the next (transovarian transmission) without passage through a vertebrate host. Patients infected with spotted fevers usually develop antibodies to *Proteus* OX19 and OX2 in low titer, in addition to specific rickettsial antibodies, detected best by immunofluorescence, microagglutination, or complement fixation.

Control of spotted fevers involves prevention of tick bites, specific immunization when available, and antibiotic treatment of patients.

1. ROCKY MOUNTAIN SPOTTED FEVER

Essentials of Diagnosis

- Exposure to tick bite in endemic area.
- "Influenzal" prodrome followed by chills, fever,

severe headache, widespread aches and pains, restlessness, and prostration; occasionally, delirium and coma.

- Red macular rash appears between the second and sixth days of fever, first on the wrists and ankles and then spreading centrally; it may become petechial.
- Laboratory confirmation by agglutination of *Proteus* OX19 and OX2 and by specific antibodies with complement fixation and immunofluorescence.

General Considerations

The causative agent, *Rickettsia rickettsii,* is transmitted to humans by the bite of the wood tick, *Dermacentor andersoni,* in the western USA and by the bite of the dog tick, *Dermacentor variabilis,* in the eastern USA. Other hard ticks transmit the rickettsia in the southern USA and in Central and South America and are responsible for transmitting it among rodents, dogs, porcupines, and other animals. Most human cases occur in late spring and summer. In the USA, most cases occur in the eastern third of the country.

Clinical Findings

A. Symptoms and Signs: Three to 10 days after the bite of an infectious tick, anorexia, malaise, nausea, headache, and sore throat occur. These progress, with chills; fever; aches in bones, joints, and muscles; abdominal pain; nausea and vomiting; restlessness; insomnia; and irritability. Delirium, lethargy, stupor, and coma may appear. The face is flushed and the conjunctivas infected. Between days 2 and 6 of fever, a rash appears first on the wrists and ankles, spreading centrally to the arms, legs, and trunk. The rash is initially small, red, and macular but becomes larger and petechial. It spreads for 2–3 days. In some cases there is splenomegaly, hepatomegaly, jaundice, gangrene, myocarditis, or uremia.

B. Laboratory Findings: Leukocytosis, proteinuria, and hematuria are common. Rickettsiae can sometimes be isolated in special laboratories from blood obtained in the first few days of illness. A rise in antibody titer during the second week of illness can be detected by specific complement fixation, immunofluorescence, and microagglutination tests or by the Weil-Felix reaction with *Proteus* OX19 and OX2. Antibody response may be suppressed if antimicrobial drugs are given very early.

Differential Diagnosis

The early signs and symptoms of Rocky Mountain spotted fever are shared with many other infections. The rash may be confused with that of measles, typhoid, or meningococcemia. The suspicion of the latter requires blood cultures and cerebrospinal fluid examination.

Prevention

Protective clothing, tick-repellent chemicals, and the removal of ticks at frequent intervals are helpful.

Vaccines of inactivated *R rickettsii* grown in eggs or in cell culture have given moderate protection but are not commercially available in the USA or Canada in 1983.

Treatment & Prognosis

In mild, untreated cases, fever subsides at the end of the second week. The response to chloramphenicol or tetracycline (see Chapter 29) is prompt if the drugs are started early.

The mortality rate for Rocky Mountain spotted fever varies strikingly with age. In untreated elderly persons it may be 70%; in children, less than 20%.

D'Angelo LJ et al: Rocky Mountain spotted fever in the United States, 1975–77. *J Infect Dis* 1978;**138**:273.

Donohue JF: Lower respiratory involvement in Rocky Mountain spotted fever. *Arch Intern Med* 1980;**140**:223.

Hattwick MAW: Rocky Mountain spotted fever: Epidemiology of an increasing problem. *Ann Intern Med* 1976;**84**:732.

Hechemy KE: Laboratory diagnosis of Rocky Mountain spotted fever. *N Engl J Med* 1979;**300**:859.

Philip RN et al: A comparison of serologic methods for diagnosis of Rocky Mountain spotted fever. *Am J Epidemiol* 1977;**105**:56.

2. OTHER SPOTTED FEVERS

Tick-borne rickettsial infections in Africa, Asia, and Australia may resemble Rocky Mountain spotted fever but cover a wide spectrum from very mild to very severe. In many cases, a local lesion develops at the site of the tick bite (eschar), often with painful enlargement of the regional lymph nodes.

RICKETTSIALPOX

Rickettsia akari is a parasite of mice, transmitted by mites *(Allodermanyssus sanguineus)*. Upon close contact of mice with humans, infected mites may transmit the disease to humans. Rickettsialpox has an incubation period of 7–12 days. The onset is sudden, with chills, fever, headache, photophobia, and disseminated aches and pains. The primary lesion is a red papule that vesicates and forms a black eschar. Two to 4 days after onset of symptoms, a widespread papular eruption appears that becomes vesicular and forms crusts that are shed in about 10 days. Early lesions may resemble those of chickenpox.

Leukopenia and a rise in antibody titer with rickettsial antigen in complement fixation tests are often present. However, the Weil-Felix test is negative.

Treatment with tetracycline produces rapid improvement, but even without treatment the disease is fairly mild and self-limited. Control requires the elimination of mice from human habitations after insecticide has been applied to suppress the mite vectors.

Brettman LR et al: Rickettsialpox: Report of an outbreak and contemporary review. *South Afr Med J* 1981;**60**:363.

Wong B et al: Rickettsialpox: Case report and epidemiologic review. *JAMA* 1979;**242**:1998.

SCRUB TYPHUS
(Tsutsugamushi Disease)

Essentials of Diagnosis

- Exposure to mites in endemic area of Southeast Asia, the western Pacific, and Australia.
- Black eschar at site of bite, with regional and generalized lymphadenopathy.
- Conjunctivitis and a short-lived macular rash.
- Frequent pneumonitis, encephalitis, and cardiac failure.
- Laboratory confirmation with agglutinins to *Proteus* OXK and specific antibodies by immunofluorescence.

General Considerations

Scrub typhus is caused by *Rickettsia tsutsugamushi (R orientalis)*, which is principally a parasite of rodents transmitted by mites. The infectious agent can be transmitted from one generation of mites to the next (transovarian transmission) without a vertebrate host. The mites may spend much of their life cycle on vegetation but require a blood meal to complete maturation. At that point, humans coming in contact with infested vegetation are bitten by mite larvae and are infected.

Clinical Findings

A. Symptoms and Signs: After an incubation period of 1–3 weeks, there is a nonspecific prodrome, with malaise, chills, severe headache, and backache. At the site of the mite bite a papule develops that vesicates and forms a flat black eschar. The regional lymph nodes are enlarged and tender, and there may be generalized adenopathy. Fever rises gradually, and a generalized macular rash appears at the end of the first week of fever. The rash is most marked on the trunk and may be fleeting or may last for a week. The patient appears obtunded, confused, and out of contact with the environment. During the second or third week pneumonitis, myocarditis, and cardiac failure may develop.

B. Laboratory Findings: Blood obtained during the first few days of illness may permit isolation of the rickettsia by mouse inoculation in specialized laboratories. The Weil-Felix test usually shows a rising titer to *Proteus* OXK during the second week of illness. The complement fixation test is often unsatisfactory, but immunofluorescence with specific antigens is diagnostic.

Differential Diagnosis

Leptospirosis, typhoid, dengue, malaria, and other rickettsial infections may have to be considered. When the rash is fleeting and the eschar not evident, laboratory results are the best guide to diagnosis.

Prevention

Efforts must be made in endemic areas to minimize contact between humans and infected mites. Repeated application of long-acting miticides can make endemic areas safe. When this is not possible, insect repellents on clothing and skin provide some protection. For short exposure, chemoprophylaxis with chloramphenicol can prevent the disease but permits infection. No effective vaccines are available at present.

Treatment & Prognosis

Without treatment, fever may subside spontaneously after 2 weeks, but the mortality rate may be 10–30%. Early treatment with chloramphenicol or tetracyclines can virtually eliminate deaths.

TRENCH FEVER

Trench fever is a self-limited, louse-borne relapsing febrile disease caused by *Rochalimaea (Rickettsia) quintana*. This organism grows extracellularly in the louse intestine and is excreted in feces. Humans are infected when infected louse feces enter defects in skin. No animal reservoir except humans has been demonstrated.

This disease has occurred in epidemic forms in louse-infested troops and civilians during wars, and in endemic form in Central America. Onset is abrupt, with fever lasting 3–5 days, often followed by relapses. The patient becomes weak and complains of severe pain behind the eyes and in the back and legs. Lymphadenopathy and splenomegaly may appear, as well as a transient maculopapular rash. Subclinical infection is frequent, and a carrier state may occur. The differential diagnosis includes dengue, leptospirosis, malaria, relapsing fever, and typhus fever.

R quintana is the only rickettsia that has been grown on artificial media without living cells. The organism can be cultivated on agar containing 10% fresh blood and has been recovered from blood cultures of patients. In volunteers, such agar-grown rickettsiae caused typical disease. The Weil-Felix test is negative, but a specific complement fixation test and a specific enzyme immunoassay are available.

The illness is self-limited, and recovery regularly occurs without treatment.

Hollingdale MR et al: Enzyme immunoassay of antibody to *Rochalimaea quintana*. J Infect Dis 1978;**137:**578.

Q FEVER

Essentials of Diagnosis

- An acute or chronic febrile illness with severe headache, cough, prostration, and abdominal pain.
- Extensive pneumonitis, hepatitis, or encephalopathy; rarely endocarditis.

General Considerations

Coxiella burnetii is unique among rickettsiae in that it is usually transmitted to humans not by arthropods but by inhalation of infectious aerosols or ingestion of infected milk. It is a parasite of cattle, sheep, and goats, in which it produces mild or subclinical infection. It is excreted by cows and goats principally through the milk and placenta and by sheep through feces, placenta, and milk. Dry feces and milk, dust contaminated with them, and the tissues of these animals contain large numbers of infectious organisms that are spread by the airborne route. Inhalation of contaminated dust and of droplets from infected animal tissues is the main source of human infection. *Coxiella* is resistant to heat and drying, perhaps because the organism forms endosporelike structures. Thus, it survives in dust, on the fleece of infected animals, or in inadequately pasteurized milk. Spread from one human to another does not seem to occur even in the presence of florid pneumonitis, but fetal infection can occur.

Clinical Findings

A. Symptoms and Signs: After an incubation period of 1–3 weeks, a febrile illness develops with headache, prostration, and muscle pains, occasionally with a nonproductive cough, abdominal pains, or jaundice. Physical signs of pneumonitis are slight. Hepatitis may be severe. Endocarditis occurs rarely. At times, signs of encephalopathy are present. The clinical course may be acute or chronic and relapsing.

B. Laboratory Findings: Laboratory examination often shows leukopenia and a diagnostic rise in specific complement-fixing antibodies to *Coxiella* phase 2. The Weil-Felix test is negative. Liver function tests are often abnormal. Special laboratories may attempt isolation of the organism from blood, but it is rarely present in sputum.

C. X-Ray Examination: Chest x-ray shows marked pulmonary infiltration.

Differential Diagnosis

Viral, mycoplasmal, and bacterial pneumonias; viral hepatitis; brucellosis; tuberculosis; psittacosis; and other animal-borne diseases must be considered. The history of exposure to animals or animal dusts or animal tissues (eg, in slaughterhouses) should lead to appropriate specific serologic tests.

Prevention

Prevention must be based on detection of the infection in livestock, reduction of contact with infected animals or dusts contaminated by them, special care during contact with animal tissues, and effective pasteurization of milk. A vaccine of inactivated *Coxiella* is being developed for persons at high risk of infection.

Treatment & Prognosis

Treatment with tetracyclines can suppress symptoms and shorten the clinical course but does not always eradicate the infection. Even in untreated patients, the mortality rate is usually low, except with endocarditis.

Haldane EV et al: Endocarditis due to Q fever in Nova Scotia. *J Infect Dis* 1983;**148**:978.

Janigan DT et al: An inflammatory pseudotumor of the lung in Q fever pneumonia. *N Engl J Med* 1983;**308**:86.

Kimbrough RC et al: Q fever endocarditis in the United States. *Ann Intern Med* 1979;**91**:400.

Meiklejohn G et al: Cryptic epidemic of Q fever in a medical school. *J Infect Dis* 1981;**144**:107.

Tobin MJ et al: Q fever endocarditis. *Am J Med* 1982;**72**:396.

24 | Infectious Diseases: Bacterial

Moses Grossman, MD, & Ernest Jawetz, MD, PhD

SEREPTOCOCCAL SORE THROAT; STREPTOCOCCAL SKIN INFECTIONS

Essentials of Diagnosis

- Abrupt onset of sore throat, fever, malaise, nausea, and headache.
- Throat red and edematous, with or without exudate; cervical nodes tender.
- Scarlatiniform rash or pyoderma or erysipelas.
- Diagnosis confirmed by leukocytosis, throat or skin culture, and rise in antibody titer.

General Considerations

Beta-hemolytic group A streptococci are the most common bacterial cause of exudative pharyngitis, and they also cause skin infections. Respiratory infections are transmitted by droplets; skin infections are transmitted by contact. Either may be followed by suppurative and nonsuppurative (rheumatic fever, glomerulonephritis) complications. If group A streptococci produce erythrogenic toxin, they may cause scarlet fever rashes in susceptible persons.

Beta-hemolytic group B streptococci are often carried in the female genital tract and thus may infect the newborn. Group B streptococci are a common cause of neonatal sepsis, meningitis, and pneumonia.

Clinical Findings

A. Symptoms and Signs:

1. Streptococcal sore throat–"Strep throat" is characterized by a sudden onset of fever, sore throat, severe pain on swallowing, enlarged and tender cervical lymph nodes, malaise, and nausea. Children may vomit or convulse. The pharynx, soft palate, and tonsils are red and edematous, and there may be a purulent exudate. If scarlet fever rash occurs, the skin is diffusely erythematous, with superimposed fine red papules. The rash is most intense in the groin and axillas, blanches on pressure, and may become petechial. It fades in 2–5 days, leaving a fine desquamation. In scarlet fever, the face is flushed, with circumoral pallor; and the tongue is coated, with protrusion of enlarged red papillae (strawberry tongue).

2. Streptococcal skin lesions–Impetigo begins as a papule that rapidly becomes a vesicle and a pustule

with a thick, amber-colored crust. There is little redness, and the crusts appear "stuck on" the skin. Pyoderma is often chronic but produces little discomfort. It may become progressive in hot, humid climates.

Streptococci may enter the skin and subcutaneous tissues through abrasions or wounds and may produce progressive erysipelas (fever, chills, rapidly progressive edema and erythema, with a sharp advancing margin) or "surgical scarlet fever"—ie, wound infection with streptococci that produce erythrogenic toxin in a patient without antitoxin, who then develops signs of scarlet fever.

3. Neonatal group B streptococcal infectons–Group B streptococci are often part of the normal vaginal flora and thus may infect the newborn, particularly if the mother lacks specific antibody. Group B streptococcal infection during the first month of life may present as fulminant sepsis, meningitis, or respiratory distress syndrome. Group B streptococci may be inhibited but not killed by penicillin, and such "tolerance" may prevent their eradication from the mother or infant.

B. Laboratory Findings: Leukocytosis with an increase in polymorphonuclear neutrophils is a regular early finding, and the sedimentation rate may be elevated. The urine often contains protein and a few red cells. Cultures from the throat or from the material under impetigo crusts or wounds yield large numbers of hemolytic group A streptococci (95% inhibited by a bacitracin disk). In 1–3 weeks after onset of infection, there is a rise in antibodies, particularly to streptolysin O, hyaluronidase, streptokinase, deoxyribonuclease, and other streptococcal antigenic products. Elevated antibody levels may continue for months after the infection. In pyoderma, antihyaluronidase is the most commonly elevated antibody; in streptococcal pharyngitis, it is antistreptolysin O (ASO). Group B streptococcal infections in neonates are identified by culture of blood, cerebrospinal fluid, or respiratory tract specimens; latex agglutination can identify the antigen.

Complications

The suppurative complications of streptococcal sore throat include sinusitis, otitis media, mastoiditis, peritonsillar abscess, and suppuration of cervical lymph nodes, among others. Streptococcal skin infections (erysipelas; see Chapter 4) may lead to bacteremia and sepsis.

The outstanding nonsuppurative complications are rheumatic fever (0.05–3%) and glomerulonephritis (0.2–20%). Rheumatic fever may follow recurrent infections with any type of group A streptococci and begins 1–4 weeks after the onset of streptococcal sore throat. Glomerulonephritis follows a single infection with a nephritogenic strain of *Streptococcus* group A (eg, types 4, 12, 2, 49, and 60), more commonly on the skin than in the throat, and begins 1–3 weeks after the onset of the infection.

Differential Diagnosis

Streptococcal sore throat resembles (and cannot be reliably distinguished clinically from) the pharyngitis caused by adenoviruses; herpesviruses; and other agents, including gonococci. It may be confused with infectious mononucleosis, characterized by generalized and prominent adenopathy, splenomegaly, abnormal lymphocytes, and a positive serologic (heterophil) test; diphtheria, characterized by a more confluent pseudomembrane; candidiasis, which shows white patches of exudate and less erythema; and necrotizing ulcerative gingivostomatitis (Vincent's fusospirochetal disease), characterized by shallow ulcers in the mouth. The petechial rash of scarlet fever must be distinguished from that of meningococcemia; the typical scarlet fever rash resembles the rash of sunburn, drug reactions, rubella, echovirus infections, and toxic shock syndrome.

Prevention

Benzathine penicillin G, 1.2 million units as a single intramuscular injection every 4 weeks, is the method of choice to prevent reinfection with group A streptococci in persons who have suffered an initial attack of rheumatic fever. Prophylaxis with sulfadiazine, 1 g orally daily, or penicillin G, 200,000–400,000 units orally daily, is also acceptable but offers less reliable prophylaxis against rheumatic fever recurrences than benzathine penicillin G given intramuscularly. These regimens are administered continuously for 5 or more years.

There is no definite prophylaxis against glomerulonephritis except the very early eradication of nephritogenic streptococci, especially in contacts.

Treatment

A. Specific Measures: Antimicrobial treatment is often given without proof of streptococcal origin if fever and leukocytosis accompany a sore throat with tender cervical adenopathy.

1. Benzathine penicillin G, 1.2 million units intramuscularly as a single dose, is optimal therapy and usually eradicates the streptococci.

2. Penicillin V, 400,000 units orally 3 times daily, must be taken for 10 days, and this regimen is not easily enforced, since the patient becomes asymptomatic in 2–4 days. Penicillin lozenges are worthless. Topical treatment of skin infections is undesirable.

3. Patients hypersensitive to penicillin may be treated with erythromycin, 0.5 g 4 times daily (40 mg/kg/d) for 10 days.

B. General Measures: Aspirin and gargling with warm saline solution relieves sore throat. Bed rest is desirable until the patient is afebrile. Diet may be modified to reduce discomfort, and fluids may be forced during fever.

C. Treatment of Complications: The suppurative complications usually respond promptly to antistreptococcal treatment, and incision and drainage of abscesses is rarely needed. Rheumatic fever is best prevented by prompt treatment of severe streptococcal infections. Its treatment is discussed in Chapter 8.

The treatment of glomerulonephritis is discussed in Chapter 16.

Prognosis

Most streptococcal infections are self-limited. Severe illness or death is rare today except in untreated streptococcal pneumonia or sepsis. Treatment with antimicrobials shortens the course of sore throat, fever, and systemic symptoms to some extent. If adequate penicillin or erythromycin levels are maintained for 10 days, group A streptococci will be eliminated. This can prevent rheumatic fever if treatment is started during the first week after infection. In the USA, rheumatic fever now follows only 0.05% of group A streptococcal infections even without antistreptococcal treatment. Glomerulonephritis can sometimes be prevented if antistreptococcal drugs are given on epidemiologic grounds, ie, before onset of renal signs or symptoms in contacts of patients infected with nephritogenic strains. The mortality rate is high in neonates with group B streptococcal infection, and relapses occur after penicillin treatment.

Kaplan EL: The group A streptococcus upper respiratory tract carrier state: An enigma. *J Pediatr* 1980;**97**:337.

Nelson JD: The effect of penicillin therapy on the symptoms and signs of streptococcal pharyngitis. *Pediatr Infect Dis* 1984;**3**:10.

Pass MA, Gray BM, Dillon HC: Puerperal and perinatal infections with group B streptococci. *Am J Obstet Gynecol* 1982;**143**:147.

Wannamaker LW: Changes and changing concepts in the biology of group A streptococci and in the epidemiology of streptococcal infections. *Rev Infect Dis* 1979;**1**:967.

DIPHTHERIA

Essentials of Diagnosis

- Tenacious gray membrane at portal of entry.
- Sore throat, nasal discharge, hoarseness, malaise, fever.
- Myocarditis, neuritis.
- Smear and culture confirm the diagnosis.

General Considerations

Diphtheria is an acute infection, caused by *Corynebacterium diphtheriae,* that usually attacks the respiratory tract but may involve any mucous membrane or skin wound. The organism usually gains entry through the respiratory tract and is spread chiefly by respiratory secretions from patients with active disease or healthy carriers. The incubation period is 2–7 days. Myocarditis and late neuritis caused by an exotoxin are also characteristic.

Clinical Findings
A. Symptoms and Signs:
1. Pharyngeal diphtheria–Characteristically, a tenacious gray membrane forms from the tonsil onto the pillars and pharyngeal walls, surrounded by a narrow zone of erythema and a wider zone of edema. Early manifestations are mild sore throat, fever, and malaise, followed rapidly by severe signs of toxemia and prostration. Associated edema of the pharynx may add to the difficulty of breathing and swallowing.

If myocarditis develops, there is a rapid thready pulse along with indistinct heart sounds, cardiac arrhythmia, and, finally, cardiac decompensation with falling blood pressure, hepatic congestion, and associated nausea and vomiting.

In toxic neuritis the cranial nerves are involved first, causing nasal speech, regurgitation of food through the nose, diplopia, strabismus, and inability to swallow, resulting in pooling of saliva and respiratory secretions. The neuritis may progress to involve the intercostal muscles and those of the extremities. Sensory manifestations are much less prominent than motor weakness.

2. Nasal diphtheria–An occasional case will be limited to nasal infection only, producing a serosanguineous discharge but few constitutional symptoms.

3. Laryngeal diphtheria–This may occur as an extension of pharyngeal disease or separately. The signs and symptoms are those of upper airway obstruction in a progressively more toxic patient.

4. Cutaneous diphtheria–This occurs more commonly in tropical countries; lesions resemble impetigo.

B. Laboratory Findings:
Polymorphonuclear leukocytosis may be present. Bacterial culture will confirm the diagnosis. Throat smears are often unreliable. Albuminocytologic dissociation of the cerebrospinal fluid is noted in postdiphtheritic neuritis. Proteinuria as a result of toxic nephritis is not uncommon.

C. Electrocardiographic Findings:
In myocarditis, the ECG may show an arrhythmia, PR prolongation, heart block, and inversion of T waves.

Differential Diagnosis
Diphtheria must be differentiated from streptococcal pharyngitis, infectious mononucleosis, adenovirus infection, Vincent's infection, and candidiasis. A presumptive diagnosis of diphtheria must be made on clinical grounds without waiting for laboratory verification, since emergency treatment is needed.

Complications
The most common and most serious complications are myocarditis and toxic neuritis, the latter often producing paralysis of the soft palate and external muscles of the eyes as well as limb muscles.

Prevention
Active immunization with diphtheria toxoid is part of routine childhood immunization (usually as DTP) with appropriate booster injections.

Adults tend to have severe reactions to the usual childhood toxoid. Therefore, only "adult type" toxoid (Td) is used, which contains a smaller amount of diphtheria toxoid.

Susceptibility to diphtheria can be determined by intradermal injection of 0.1 mL of a solution containing a standard amount of diphtheria toxin (Schick test).

Exposed susceptibles should receive a booster dose of toxoid (start active immunization if not previously immune), full doses of erythromycin or penicillin, and daily throat inspections.

Treatment
A. Specific Measures:
1. Diphtheria antitoxin–Antitoxin must be given in all cases when diphtheria cannot be ruled out. The intravenous route is preferable in all but patients who are sensitive to horse serum. Conjunctival and skin tests for serum sensitivity should be done in all cases and desensitization carried out if necessary.

The exact dose of antitoxin is purely empiric: for mild early pharyngeal or laryngeal disease, 20–40 thousand units; for moderate nasopharyngeal disease, 40–60 thousand units; for severe, extensive, or late (3 days or more) disease, 80–100 thousand units.*

2. Antimicrobial therapy–Antibiotics are a useful adjunct to antitoxin, suppressing *C diphtheriae* and eliminating hemolytic streptococci, which are frequent secondary invaders. Penicillin and erythromycin are equally effective if given for 7–10 days.

3. Corticosteroids–Corticosteroids may be appropriate in 2 situations: (a) to diminish edema or obstruction in acute laryngeal diphtheria; and (b) to reduce the severity or incidence of acute myocarditis.

B. General Measures:
The patient should remain at absolute bed rest for at least 3 weeks until the danger of developing myocarditis has passed.

Give a liquid to soft diet as tolerated, hot saline or 30% glucose throat irrigations 3–4 times daily, and aspirin or codeine as required for relief of pain.

C. Treatment of Complications:
1. Myocarditis–No definitive treatment is known. Oxygen by tent or mask may be needed. Hypertonic glucose solution, 100 mL of 20% solution daily, may be of value. Digitalis and quinidine should be reserved for arrhythmias with rapid ventricular rate. It may be necessary to treat for shock as outlined in Chapter 1.

2. Neuritis–Nasal feeding should be attempted

*Diphtheria equine antitoxin can be obtained from the Centers for Disease Control (central number: [404] 329-3311).

if paralysis of deglutition is present. Tracheostomy and the use of a mechanical respirator may be necessary. Corrective splinting and physical therapy may be of value.

3. Respiratory tract obstruction–Croupy cough, stridor, and dyspnea suggest laryngeal obstruction. Suction of membrane and secretions under direct laryngoscopy may help. Intubation or tracheostomy should be performed before the appearance of cyanosis.

4. A chronic skin ulceration due to *C diphtheriae* is particularly apt to occur in warm, humid climates and can be followed by myocarditis and neuritis. Treatment is as for pharyngeal disease.

D. Treatment of Carriers: Eradication of organisms from a carrier is difficult. Erythromycin followed by a course of penicillin may be successful. Tonsillectomy is a last resort.

Prognosis

The mortality rate varies between 10 and 30%; it is higher in older people and when treatment has been delayed. Myocarditis that appears early is often fatal. A conduction disturbance or the appearance of an arrhythmia implies a poor prognosis. Neuritis is rarely fatal unless respiratory muscle paralysis occurs. Myocarditis and neuritis will subside slowly but completely if the patient survives.

Dobie RA, Tobey DN: Clinical features of diphtheria in the respiratory tract. *JAMA* 1979;**242**:2197.

Hodes HL: Diphtheria. *Pediatr Clin North Am* 1979;**26**:445.

PERTUSSIS
(Whooping Cough)

Essentials of Diagnosis

- Paroxysmal cough ending in a high-pitched inspiratory "whoop."
- Two-week prodromal catarrhal stage of malaise, cough, coryza, and anorexia.
- Predominantly in infants under age 2 years.
- Absolute lymphocytosis.
- Culture confirms diagnosis.

General Considerations

Pertussis is an acute infection of the respiratory tract caused by *Bordetella (Haemophilus) pertussis*. It is transmitted by respiratory droplets from infected individuals, now often adults with mild illness. The incubation period is 7–17 days. Infectivity is greatest early in the disease and decreases until the organisms disappear from the nasopharynx (after about 1 month). Infants are most commonly infected; half of all cases occur before age 2 years.

Clinical Findings

A. Symptoms and Signs: Physical findings are minimal or absent. Fever, if present, is low-grade. The symptoms of classic pertussis last about 6 weeks and are divided into 3 consecutive stages.

1. Catarrhal stage–The onset is insidious, with lacrimation, sneezing, and coryza, anorexia and malaise, and a hacking night cough that tends to become diurnal.

2. Paroxysmal stage–This follows the beginning of the catarrhal stage by 10–14 days and is characterized by rapid consecutive coughs usually followed by a deep, hurried, high-pitched inspiration (whoop). Paroxysms may involve 5–15 coughs before a breath is taken and may occur up to 50 times in 24 hours. Stimuli such as fright or anger, crying, sneezing, inhalation of irritants, and overdistension of the stomach may produce the paroxysms. The cough is productive of copious amounts of thick mucus. Vomiting is common during the paroxysms.

3. Convalescent stage–This stage usually begins 4 weeks after the onset of the illness with a decrease in the frequency and severity of paroxysms of cough.

B. Laboratory Findings: The white count is usually 15–20 thousand/μL (rarely, to 50,000), 60–80% lymphocytes. The clinical diagnosis can be confirmed by taking the culture with a nasopharyngeal wire swab and planting it on fresh special media. A specific immunofluorescent stain of the nasopharyngeal swab dried onto a slide may aid in the diagnosis. The organism is recovered in only about half of clinically diagnosed patients.

Differential Diagnosis

Pertussis must be differentiated from aspiration of a foreign body in children and from viral pneumonia, influenza, and acute bronchitis in older individuals. The lymphocytosis may suggest acute leukemia.

Several types of adenovirus and *Haemophilus* can produce a clinical picture essentially indistinguishable from that caused by *B pertussis*. Respiratory chlamydial infections may produce a syndrome resembling pertussis in infants under age 4 months (see p 881).

Complications

Asphyxia, the most common complication, occurs most frequently in infants and may lead to convulsions and brain damage. The increased intracranial pressure during a paroxysm may also lead to brain damage by causing cerebral hemorrhage. Pneumonia, atelectasis, interstitial and subcutaneous emphysema, and pneumothorax may occur as a result of damaged respiratory mucosa, inspissated mucus, or increased intrathoracic pressure.

Prevention

Active immunization with pertussis vaccine is recommended for all infants, usually combined with diphtheria and tetanus toxoids (DTP). The newborn derives little or no immunity from the mother. Because of the mildness of the disease in older individuals, neither primary nor booster immunization is recommended after age 6 years. Occasionally, neurologic disturbances may occur after DTP injection. Such rare individuals should subsequently receive DT immunization without the pertussis component (see Chapter 22).

Infants and young children or susceptible adults with significant exposure to pertussis should receive antimicrobial prophylaxis with erythromycin (40 mg/kg/d). Those previously immunized should receive a booster dose of vaccine. For persons not previously immunized, pertussis hyperimmune globulin (human) may be considered (see below).

Treatment
A. Specific Measures:
1. Antibiotics–Give erythromycin, 50 mg/kg daily orally for 10 days. Erythromycin may shorten the course of carriage. Antibiotics are of doubtful value at the paroxysmal coughing stage.

2. Hyperimmune gamma globulin (human), 2.5 mL intramuscularly, has been used in the treatment of small infants for 20 years, but proof of its efficacy is lacking.

3. Corticosteroids–In severe pertussis, corticosteroids given for 4–6 days may diminish the intensity of paroxysms.

B. General Measures:
1. Nutrition–Frequent small feedings may be necessary. Feeding can be repeated if vomiting occurs shortly after a meal. Parenteral fluids may be used to ensure adequate fluid intake in severe cases.

2. Cough–Sedative and expectorant cough mixtures are of only slight benefit.

3. Nursing care–In very young infants, a paroxysm will often terminate with an apneic spell instead of a whoop. Careful observation, skilled nursing care, and avoidance of stimuli that trigger paroxysms are most important in the young infant.

C. Treatment of Complications:
Pneumonia, usually due to secondary invaders, should be treated with erythromycin, ampicillin, or other appropriate antibiotic, depending upon specific bacteriologic diagnosis. Oxygen is often required.

Convulsions may require sedation, 100% oxygen inhalation, lumbar puncture, and anticonvulsive medication.

Prognosis
In children under age 1 year, the mortality rate until recently was over 20%; this rate has been reduced to 1–2% with antibacterial therapy. Bronchiectasis is a fairly common sequela, and brain damage may result.

Broome CV et al: Epidemiology of pertussis, Atlanta, 1977. *J Pediatr* 1981;**98**:362.

Cherry JD: The epidemiology of pertussis and pertussis immunization in the United Kingdom and the United States: A comparative study. *Curr Probl Pediatr* 1984;**16**(No. 2). [Entire issue.]

Cody CL et al: Nature and rates of adverse reactions associated with DTP and DT immunizations in infants and children. *Pediatrics* 1981;**68**:650.

MENINGITIS*

1. MENINGOCOCCAL MENINGITIS

Essentials of Diagnosis
- Fever, headache, vomiting, confusion, delirium, convulsions.
- Petechial rash of skin and mucous membranes.
- Neck and back stiffness with positive Kernig and Brudzinski signs.
- Purulent spinal fluid with gram-negative intracellular and extracellular organisms.
- Culture of cerebrospinal fluid, blood, or petechial aspiration confirms the diagnosis.
- Shock and disseminated intravascular clotting may occur.

General Considerations
Meningococcal meningitis is caused by *Neisseria meningitidis* of groups A, B, C, Y, and sometimes others. A varying (15–40%) segment of the population are nasopharyngeal carriers of meningococci, but relatively few develop disease. Infection is transmitted by droplets, and many factors probably play a role in determining clinical illness—including prior immunity, physical stress, and immediately antecedent viral infections. The clinical illness may take the form of meningococcemia (a fulminant form of septicemia without meningitis), both meningococcemia and meningitis, or predominantly meningitis. The development of meningococcal disease is favored by complement deficiencies (especially C7–C9).

Clinical Findings
A. Symptoms and Signs: High fever, chills, and headache; back, abdominal, and extremity pains; and nausea and vomiting are present. In severe cases, rapidly developing confusion, delirium, and coma occur. Twitchings or frank convulsions may also be present.

Nuchal and back rigidity are present, with positive Kernig and Brudzinski signs. A petechial rash is found in most cases. Petechiae may vary from pinhead-sized to large ecchymoses or even areas of skin gangrene that may later slough if the patient survives. These petechiae are found in any part of the skin, mucous membranes, or the conjunctiva but never in the nail beds, and they usually fade in 3–4 days. The increased intracranial pressure will cause the anterior fontanelle to bulge (if not closed) and may produce Cheyne-Stokes or Biot's respiration.

Shock due to the effects of endotoxin may be present and is a bad prognostic sign.

B. Laboratory Findings: Leukocytosis is usually marked and occurs very early in the course of the disease. The urine may contain protein, casts, and red cells. Lumbar puncture reveals a cloudy to frankly purulent cerebrospinal fluid, with elevated pressure, increased protein, and decreased glucose content. The fluid usually contains more than 100 cells/μL, with

*For approach to central nervous system infections, see p 821.

polymorphonuclear cells predominating and containing gram-negative intracellular diplococci. The absence of organisms in a gram-stained smear of the cerebrospinal fluid sediment does not rule out the diagnosis. The capsular polysaccharide can often be demonstrated in cerebrospinal fluid or urine by counterimmunoelectrophoresis or latex agglutination. The organism is usually demonstrated by smear or culture of the cerebrospinal fluid, oropharynx, blood, or aspirated petechiae.

Disseminated intravascular clotting is an important complication of meningococcal infection. Measurement of factor V and factor VIII activity (low), of fibrin split products (elevated), and of platelet count (low) help in establishing this diagnosis.

Differential Diagnosis

Meningococcal meningitis must be differentiated from other meningitides. In small infants, the clinical manifestations of meningeal infection may be erroneously diagnosed as upper respiratory infection or other acute infections.

Other bacterial infections (*Haemophilus*, pneumococcal, staphylococcal) or rickettsial or echovirus infection may also produce a petechial rash.

Complications

Arthritis, cranial nerve damage (especially the eighth nerve, with resulting deafness), and hydrocephalus may occur as complications. Myocarditis, nephritis, and intravascular coagulation may occur in severe cases.

Prevention

An effective polysaccharide vaccine for groups A and C meningococci is available. It has reduced the incidence of meningococcus groups A and C infection among military recruits. This vaccine is effective for control of epidemics in civilian populations.

Outbreaks in closed populations are best controlled by administering antimicrobials that reduce meningococcal carriage. Sulfonamides are not useful because many strains of meningococci are sulfonamide-resistant. Penicillin and ampicillin do not eliminate carriage. Rifampin (600 mg twice a day for 2 days for adults; 10 mg/kg twice a day for 2 days for children 1 month to 12 years; 5 mg/kg twice a day for 2 days for infants) is the drug of first choice, but it permits emergence of resistant strains. Minocycline (200 mg immediately for adults, then 100 mg every 12 hours for 5 days) is equally effective in eliminating the organisms, but it has a high incidence of vestibular side effects.

Exposed contacts. There is an increased risk to household members, who may be given rifampin for 2 days. Day-care center contacts are treated in the same manner. School and work contacts should not be treated. Hospital contacts should be treated only if intensive and intimate exposure has occurred, eg, giving mouth-to-mouth resuscitation.

Accidentally discovered carriers, without known close contact with a case of meningococcal disease, are generally not given prophylactic antimicrobials.

Treatment

A. Specific Measures: Antimicrobial therapy by the intravenous route must be started immediately. If meningococcus is established or strongly suspected as the infectious agent, aqueous penicillin G is the agent of choice (24 million units/24 h for adults; 400,000 units/kg/24 h for children). One-fourth of the dose is given rapidly intravenously and the rest by continuous drip or in divided doses every 4 hours. If the possibility of *Haemophilus influenzae* meningitis has not been ruled out, treat as discussed on p 864. If the patient is allergic to penicillin, chloramphenicol, 100 mg/kg daily, is the preferred alternative drug. The older cephalosporins are unsuitable in meningitis, but newer ones (eg, moxalactam, cefoperazone, cefotaxime) are effective. Treatment should be continued for 7–10 days by the intravenous route or until the patient is afebrile for 5 days and has normal cerebrospinal fluid glucose and no more than 30–50 cells/μL (mostly lymphocytes) in the cerebrospinal fluid.

B. General Measures: Hypovolemic shock is the most serious complication of meningococcal infections. Volume expansion with isotonic electrolyte solution is the initial approach while monitoring central venous pressure. Isoproterenol or dopamine is added to the infusion if the patient fails to respond.

Vital signs must be monitored. Ventilatory assistance may be required. If cerebral edema is present — and particularly if herniation of the brain through the foramen magnum is imminent — intravenous mannitol (2 g/kg) or urea (0.5 g/kg) may temporarily decrease the intracranial pressure.

Corticosteroids have no established role in the management of meningitis. In the presence of shock, high-dose (30 mg/kg) prednisone may be beneficial.

Heparinization should be considered if there is evidence of intravascular clotting. An initial dose of 50 units/kg intravenously is given; thereafter, an attempt is made to keep the clotting time at 20–30 minutes.

Prognosis

If the patient survives the first day, the prognosis is excellent. Sequelae are less common than in other forms of purulent meningitis.

Edwards MS, Baker CJ: Complications and sequelae of meningococcal infections in children. *J Pediatr* 1981;**99:**540.

Ellison RT et al: Prevalence of congenital or acquired complement deficiency in patients with sporadic meningococcal disease. *N Engl J Med* 1983;**308:**913.

Lepow ML, Gold R: Meningococcal A and other polysaccharide vaccines: A five-year progress report. *N Engl J Med* 1983;**308:**1158.

Mohammed I, Zaruba K: Control of epidemic meningococcal meningitis by mass vaccination. *Lancet* 1981;**2:**80.

2. PNEUMOCOCCAL, STREPTOCOCCAL, & STAPHYLOCOCCAL MENINGITIS

The symptoms are similar to those of meningococcal meningitis, but a preceding infection is usually present, and a focus is often demonstrable in the lungs (pneumococcal), the middle ear, or sinuses. The cerebrospinal fluid must be cultured and examined to determine the causative agent.

Specific treatment of pneumococcal and streptococcal meningitis consists of aqueous penicillin, 1 million units added every 2 hours to a continuous intravenous infusion.

Staphylococcal meningitis is treated with intravenous nafcillin (12 g/24 h or 300 mg/kg/24 h) in divided doses. When the organism is definitely penicillin-sensitive, penicillin G is preferred. The duration of therapy must be between 2 and 4 weeks. Complications, including ventriculitis, arachnoiditis, cerebrospinal fluid block, and hydrocephalus, are more common in these forms of meningitis than in meningococcal meningitis.

Tugwell P et al: Pneumococcal meningitis: A clinical and laboratory study. Q J Med 1976;**45:**583.

3. *HAEMOPHILUS INFLUENZAE* MENINGITIS

Haemophilus influenzae meningitis occurs most frequently in children under age 6 years. It may present for several days as an apparent respiratory infection; however, headache, irritability, fever, malaise, vomiting, unexplained leukocytosis, and nuchal and back rigidity should suggest meningitis. Lumbar puncture may reveal gram-negative pleomorphic rods in the purulent spinal fluid smear or culture. Counterimmunoelectrophoresis of cerebrospinal fluid or the latex agglutination test may confirm the presence of specific *Haemophilus influenzae* type b capsular polysaccharide. If culture is positive, assay for beta-lactamase production is necessary. It is not possible to distinguish *Haemophilus influenzae* meningitis from other purulent meningitides on the basis of the symptoms and signs. Identification of the organism is necessary for optimal treatment.

Prevention

No vaccine effective for children under age 2 years is available. An experimental *H influenzae* type b capsular polysaccharide vaccine protected children 3–5 years old in Finland.

Close contacts in the household or day-care center under 4 years of age should receive antimicrobial prophylaxis with rifampin (20 mg/kg/d for 4 days).

Treatment

A. Specific Measures: The rising prevalence of ampicillin-resistant strains (5 to >20%) requires that 2 antimicrobial drugs be used initially—sodium ampicillin, 300 mg/kg/d intravenously (one-fourth of the dose given immediately and the remainder in divided doses every 4 hours), and chloramphenicol, 100 mg/kg/d intravenously. The antibiotics should be given separately and not in a mixed injection. As soon as the antibiotic susceptibility of the *H influenzae* isolate has been established (the test for β-lactamase production is best and fastest), one of the 2 antibiotics should be stopped and the remaining agent continued for 10–14 days until the patient is clinically well, cerebrospinal fluid glucose is normal, and the cerebrospinal fluid cell count drops below 50/μL. Moxalactam, 150–200 mg/kg/d and other newer cephalosporins are equally effective and are drugs of choice when the *H influenzae* is resistant to both ampicillin and chloramphenicol.

B. General Measures: Management is similar to that described above for meningococcal meningitis. Shock is less likely to occur, but subdural effusion and other complications are more common.

Prognosis

The case fatality rate is about 5%. One must aim not only at survival but at prevention of sequelae, including the more subtle forms of central nervous system damage.

Dajani AS et al: Systemic *Haemophilus influenzae* disease: An overview. J Pediatr 1979;**94:**355.

Daum RS: Rifampin chemoprophylaxis of household contacts of patients with invasive infections due to *Haemophilus influenzae.* J Pediatr 1981;**98:**485.

Feldman WE et al: Relation of concentrations of *Haemophilus* type b in spinal fluid to late sequelae of patients with meningitis. J Pediatr 1982;**100:**209.

Kaplan SL et al: Moxalactam treatment of serious infections due to *Haemophilus influenzae* type b in children. Pediatrics 1983;**71:**187.

4. TUBERCULOUS MENINGITIS

Essentials of Diagnosis

- Gradual onset of listlessness, irritability, and anorexia.
- Headache, vomiting, coma, convulsions; neck and back rigidity.
- Tuberculous focus may be evident elsewhere.
- Cerebrospinal fluid shows several hundred lymphocytes, low glucose, and high protein.

General Considerations

Tuberculous meningitis is caused by hematogenous spread of tubercle bacilli from a focus usually in the lungs or the peritracheal, peribronchial, or mesenteric lymph nodes, or it may be a consequence of miliary spread. Its greatest incidence is in children age 1–5 years.

Clinical Findings

A. Symptoms and Signs: The onset is usually gradual, with listlessness, irritability, anorexia, and fever, followed by headache, vomiting, convulsions, and coma. In older patients, headache and behavioral changes are prominent early symptoms.

Nuchal rigidity, opisthotonos, and paralysis occur as the meningitis progresses. Paralysis of the extraocular muscles is common. Ophthalmoscopic examination may show choroid tubercles. General physical examination may reveal evidence of tuberculosis elsewhere. The tuberculin skin test may be negative in miliary tuberculosis.

B. Laboratory Findings: The spinal fluid is frequently yellowish, with increased pressure; 100–500 cells/μL (early, polymorphonuclear neutrophils; later, lymphocytes); increased protein; and decreased glucose. On standing, the cerebrospinal fluid may form a web and pellicle from which organisms may be demonstrated by smear and culture. Moderate leukocytosis is common. Chest x-ray often reveals a tuberculous focus.

Differential Diagnosis

Tuberculous meningitis may be confused with any other type of meningitis, but the gradual onset and evidence of tuberculosis elsewhere often point to the diagnosis.

Fungal and other granulomatous meningitides or rare neoplasms must be considered also.

Complications

Residual brain damage may result in motor paralysis, convulsive states, mental impairment, and abnormal behavior. The incidence of these complications increases the later therapy is started.

Prevention

Early identification of tuberculin converters and children with primary tuberculosis, and treatment with isoniazid at that stage, is the key to preventing tuberculous meningitis.

Treatment

A. Specific Measures: Give isoniazid, 10 mg/kg/d (up to a total of 300 mg/d); rifampin, 600 mg/d; and ethambutol, 15 mg/kg/d. All are given orally, and each can be given as a single daily dose. Treatment should be continued for 18–24 months. In addition, give streptomycin, 1 g intramuscularly daily for 2 weeks, and then continue twice weekly for 60–90 days. Corticosteroid treatment (60 mg of prednisone or equivalent daily) is used initially until improvement is established and then gradually discontinued.

Caution: Ethambutol rarely causes retinal neuropathy. Visual acuity should be tested monthly with a Snellen chart. Peripheral neuropathy due to isoniazid can be prevented by giving pyridoxine, 50 mg orally daily. The incidence of isoniazid hepatitis increases with age.

B. General Measures: Treat symptoms as they arise and maintain good nutrition and adequate fluid intake. Treat hyponatremia due to inappropriate antidiuretic hormone secretion that may be present.

Prognosis

The natural course of the untreated disease is death within 6–8 weeks. With early diagnosis and treatment, the recovery rate may reach 90%; if treatment is not instituted until the disease has reached the late stage, the survival rate is 25–30%. Serious neurologic sequelae are frequent.

Kennedy DH et al: Tuberculous meningitis. *JAMA* 1979; **241**:264.

McKenzie MS et al: Drug treatment of tuberculous meningitis in childhood. *Clin Pediatr* 1979;**18**:75.

SALMONELLOSIS

Salmonellosis includes infection by any of approximately 1600 serotypes of salmonellae. Three general clinical patterns are recognized: (1) enteric fever, the best example of which is typhoid fever, due to *Salmonella typhi;* (2) acute enterocolitis, caused by *Salmonella typhimurium* and many other types; and (3) the "septicemic" type, characterized by bacteremia and focal lesions, exemplified by infection with *Salmonella choleraesuis.* Any serotype may cause any of these clinical patterns. All are transmitted by ingestion of the organism in contaminated food or drink.

1. TYPHOID FEVER

Essentials of Diagnosis

- Gradual onset of malaise, headache, sore throat, cough, and finally "pea soup" diarrhea or constipation.
- Slow (stepladder) rise of fever to maximum and then slow return to normal.
- Rose spots, relative bradycardia, splenomegaly, and abdominal distension and tenderness.
- Leukopenia; blood, stool, and urine culture positive for *Salmonella typhi* (group D).
- Elevated or rising specific agglutination titers.

General Considerations

Typhoid fever is caused by the gram-negative rod *Salmonella typhi,* which enters the patient via the gastrointestinal tract, where it penetrates the intestinal wall and produces inflammation of the mesenteric lymph nodes and the spleen. Bacteremia occurs, and the infection then localizes principally in the lymphoid tissue of the small intestine (particularly within 60 cm of the ileocecal valve). Peyer's patches become inflamed and may ulcerate, with involvement greatest during the third week of disease. The organism may become localized in the lungs, gallbladder, kidneys, or central nervous system, with resulting inflammation. Infection is transmitted by consumption of contaminated food or drink. The sources of most infections are chronic carriers with persistent gallbladder or urinary tract infections. The incubation period is 5–14 days.

Clinical Findings

A. Symptoms and Signs: The onset is usually insidious but may be abrupt, especially in children, with chills and a sharp rise in temperature. The course of classic untreated typhoid fever can be divided into 3 stages.

1. Prodromal stage–During the period of invasion, the patient develops increasing malaise, headache, cough, general body aching, sore throat, and epistaxis. Frequently there is abdominal pain, constipation or diarrhea, and vomiting. During this period, the fever ascends in a stepladder fashion, the maximum temperature on each day being slightly higher than on the preceding day. The temperature is generally higher in the evening than in the morning.

2. Fastigium–After about 7–10 days, the fever stabilizes, varying less than 1.1 °C (2 °F) during the day, and the patient becomes quite sick. "Pea soup" diarrhea or severe constipation or marked abdominal distension is common. In severe cases the patient lies motionless and unresponsive, with eyes half-shut, appearing wasted and exhausted (the "typhoid state"), but can usually be aroused to carry out simple commands.

3. Stage of defervescence–If the patient survives the severe toxemia of the second stage of the disease and develops no complications, improvement occurs gradually. Fever declines in a stepladder fashion to normal in 7–10 days. The patient becomes more alert, and abdominal symptoms disappear. However, relapse may occur as late as 1–2 weeks after the temperature has returned to normal. This relapse is usually milder than the original infection.

During the early prodrome, physical findings are slight. Later, splenomegaly, abdominal distension and tenderness, relative bradycardia, dicrotic pulse, and occasionally meningismus, systolic murmur, and gallop rhythm appear. The rash (rose spots) commonly appears during the second week of disease. The individual spot, found principally on the trunk, is a pink papule 2–3 mm in diameter that fades on pressure. It disappears over a period of 3–4 days.

B. Laboratory Findings: Blood cultures may be positive in the first week and remain positive for a variable period thereafter. Stools are positive for the organism after the first week; the urine may be positive at any time.

During the second week, antibodies appear in the blood and continue to rise in titer until the end of the third week. If an anamnestic response to other infectious diseases or recent vaccination is ruled out, an O (somatic) antibody titer of 1:160 is presumptively diagnostic; a rising titer (as demonstrated by 2 specimens taken approximately a week apart) is diagnostic.

Moderate anemia and leukopenia are the rule.

Differential Diagnosis

This enteric form of infection can be produced by other *Salmonella* species (eg, *Salmonella paratyphi*).

Typhoid fever must be distinguished from other prolonged fevers associated with normal or depressed white count. Examples include tuberculosis, viral pneumonia, psittacosis, infective endocarditis, brucellosis, Q fever, and campylobacteriosis. *Yersinia enterocolitica* infection can produce enteritis with fever, diarrhea, vomiting, abdominal pain, and mesenteric adenitis. *Yersinia* infection may mimic appendicitis.

Complications

Complications occur in about 30% of untreated cases and account for 75% of all deaths. Intestinal hemorrhage is most likely to occur during the third week and is manifested by a sudden drop in temperature, rise in pulse, and signs of shock followed by dark or fresh blood in the stool. Intestinal perforation is most likely to occur during the third week. Sudden rigor, drop in temperature, and increase in pulse rate, accompanied by abdominal pain and tenderness, may be noted. Less frequent complications are urinary retention, pneumonia, thrombophlebitis, myocarditis, psychosis, cholecystitis, nephritis, spondylitis (typhoid spine), and meningitis.

Prevention

Active immunization should be provided for household contacts of a typhoid carrier, for travelers to endemic areas, and during epidemic outbreaks.

Typhoid vaccine is administered in 2 injections subcutaneously, not less than 4 weeks apart. The usual procedure is to revaccinate twice only at 4-year intervals. (See Chapter 22.) An experimental live attenuated vaccine has given very promising results.

Environmental hygiene control requires protection of food and water and adequate waste disposal.

Carriers must not be permitted to work as food handlers.

Treatment

A. Specific Measures: Give ampicillin, 100 mg/kg daily intravenously or 6 g daily in divided doses every 4 hours by mouth; or chloramphenicol, 1 g every 6 hours orally or intravenously until fever disappears and then 0.5 g every 6 hours for 2 weeks (children, 50 mg/kg daily). Some strains of *S typhi* from Central and South America are resistant to ampicillin or chloramphenicol or both. Sensitivity studies must guide the choice of antibiotic. Infections caused by drug-resistant salmonellae often respond to trimethoprim-sulfamethoxazole given orally or intravenously.

B. General Measures: Give a high-calorie, low-residue diet. Hydrocortisone, 100 mg intravenously every 8 hours, may tide over severely toxic patients. Maintain skin care.

Parenteral fluids may be necessary to supplement oral intake and maintain urine output. Abdominal distention may be relieved by abdominal stupes. Vasopressin and neostigmine must be used with great caution because of the danger of perforation. Strict linen, stool, and urine isolation must be observed.

C. Treatment of Complications: Secondary pneumonia may be treated with antibiotics, depending on the etiologic agent.

Transfusions should be given as required for hemorrhage. If perforation occurs, immediate surgery is required; anticipate and treat shock (see Chapter 1) before it becomes manifest.

D. Treatment of Carriers: Chemotherapy is usually ineffective in abolishing the carrier state. However, a trial of ampicillin first and then chloramphenicol is worthwhile. Cholecystectomy may be effective.

Prognosis

The mortality rate of typhoid fever is about 2% in treated cases. Elderly or debilitated persons are likely to do poorly. The course is milder in children.

With complications, the prognosis is poor. Relapses occur in up to 15% of cases. A residual carrier state frequently persists in spite of chemotherapy.

2. SALMONELLA ENTEROCOLITIS

By far the most common form of salmonellosis is acute enterocolitis. The commonest causative serotypes are *Salmonella typhimurium, Salmonella derby, Salmonella heidelberg, Salmonella infantis, Salmonella newport, Salmonella agona,* and *Salmonella enteritidis.* The incubation period is 8–48 hours after ingestion of contaminated food or liquid.

Symptoms and signs consist of fever (often with chills), nausea and vomiting, cramping abdominal pain, and diarrhea, which may be bloody. The disease persists over a course of 3–5 days. Differentiation must be made from viral gastroenteritis, food poisoning, shigellosis, amebic dysentery, acute ulcerative colitis, and acute surgical abdominal conditions. Leukocytosis is usually not present. The organisms can be cultured from the stools, but not from blood.

The disease is usually self-limited, but bacteremia with localization in joints or bones may occur, especially in young infants and in patients with sickle cell disease.

Treatment in the uncomplicated case of enterocolitis is symptomatic only. Antimicrobial therapy may prolong the carriage of salmonellae in the gastrointestinal tract. Young or malnourished infants, severely ill patients, those with sickle cell disease, and those in whom bacteremia is suspected should be treated with ampicillin (100 mg/kg intravenously or orally) or chloramphenicol (50–100 mg/kg orally).

Nelson JD et al: Treatment of salmonella gastroenteritis with ampicillin, amoxicillin or placebo. *Pediatrics* 1980;**65:**1125.

3. SEPTICEMIC SALMONELLOSIS

Rarely, *Salmonella* infection may be manifested by prolonged or recurrent fever accompanied by bacteremia and by localization and abscess formation in one or more sites—such as the bones, joints, pleura,

pericardium, endocardium, meninges, and lungs. Treatment is as for typhoid fever and should include drainage of accessible lesions.

Davis RC: *Salmonella* sepsis in infancy. *Am J Dis Child* 1981;**135:**1096.

Hoffman SL et al: Reduction of mortality in chloramphenicol-treated severe typhoid fever by high-dose dexamethasone. *N Engl J Med* 1984;**310:**82.

Hornick RB, Greisman S: Pathogenesis of typhoid fever. *Arch Intern Med* 1978;**138:**357.

Meals RA: Paratyphoid fever. *Arch Intern Med* 1976;**136:**1422.

Ryder RW, Blake PA: Typhoid fever in the United States, 1975–1976. *J Infect Dis* 1979;**139:**124.

"FOOD POISONING" & ACUTE ENTEROCOLITIS
(For full discussion, see p 832.)

Food poisoning is a nonspecific term often applied to the syndrome of acute anorexia, nausea, vomiting, or diarrhea that is attributed to food intake, particularly if it afflicts groups of people and is not accompanied by fever. The actual cause of such acute gastrointestinal upsets might be emotional stress, viral or bacterial infections, food intolerance, inorganic (eg, sodium nitrite) or organic (eg, mushroom, shellfish) poisons, or drugs (eg, antimicrobials). More specifically, food poisoning may refer to toxins produced by bacteria growing in food (staphylococci, clostridia, *Bacillus cereus*) or to acute food infections with short incubation periods and a mild course (*Salmonella* enterocolitis [see above]; infection with enterotoxigenic *Escherichia coli*, shigellae, or vibrios *(Vibrio cholerae,* El Tor vibrios, marine vibrios including *Vibrio parahaemolyticus, Vibrio vulnificus). Campylobacter jejuni* and *Yersinia enterocolitica* may produce similar clinical enterocolitis and can be identified only by special stool culture methods. *E coli* O157:H7 is an infrequent cause of hemorrhagic colitis. Some prominent features of some of these "food poisonings" are listed in Table 24–1. In general, the diagnosis must be suspected when groups of people who have shared a meal develop acute vomiting or diarrhea. Food and stools must be secured for bacteriologic and toxicologic examination. In febrile patients blood cultures are indicated.

Treatment usually consists of replacement of fluids and electrolytes and, very rarely, management of hypovolemic shock and respiratory embarrassment. If botulism is suspected (see p 874), polyvalent antitoxin must be administered.

Antimicrobial drugs are not indicated unless a specific microbial agent producing progressive systemic involvement can be identified. Antimicrobial drugs may in fact aggravate anorexia and diarrhea and may prolong microbial carriage and excretion.

Note: Iodochlorhydroxyquin (Entero-Vioform, Vioform) is not useful for prophylaxis or treatment of any of these disorders and may be harmful.

Blacklow NR, Cukor G: Viral gastroenteritis. *N Engl J Med* 1981;**304**:397.

Blaser MJ, Reller LB: *Campylobacter* enteritis. *N Engl J Med* 1981;**305**:1444.

Fekety R: Recent advances in management of bacterial diarrheas. *Rev Infect Dis* 1983;**5**:246.

Marks MI et al: *Yersinia enterocolitica* gastroenteritis: A prospective study of clinical, bacteriologic and epidemiologic features. *J Pediatr* 1980;**96**:26.

Terranova W, Blake PA: *Bacillus cereus* food poisoning. *N Engl J Med* 1978;**298**:143.

Thomas M et al: Hospital outbreak of *Clostridium perfringens* food poisoning. *Lancet* 1977;**1**:1046.

CHOLERA

Essentials of Diagnosis

- Sudden onset of severe, frequent diarrhea, up to 1 L per hour.
- The liquid stool (and occasionally vomitus) is gray, turbid, and without fecal odor, blood, or pus ("rice water stool").
- Rapid development of marked dehydration, acidosis, hypokalemia, and hypotension.
- History of sojourn in endemic area or contact with infected person.
- Positive stool cultures and agglutination of vibrios with specific sera.

General Considerations

Cholera is an acute diarrheal disease caused by *Vibrio cholerae* or related vibrios. A pandemic of cholera is in progress. The infection is acquired by the ingestion of food or drink contaminated by feces from cases or carriers containing large numbers of vibrios. The infective dose is near 10^7-10^9 vibrios. The vibrios grow in the small intestine (particularly the ileum) and produce a powerful exotoxin. The toxin activates adenylate cyclase, resulting in increased concentration of cyclic adenosine monophosphate in the gut wall. This produces massive hypersecretion of water and chloride into the gut lumen and reduces reabsorption of sodium. This results in massive diarrhea of up to 15 L/24 h, which is fatal in 50% of patients if untreated. The incubation period is 1–5 days. Only a small minority of exposed persons become ill.

Clinical Findings

A. Symptoms and Signs: The spectrum of severity of illness is wide. Typical cases have an explosive onset of frequent, watery stools that soon lose all fecal appearance and odor. They are grayish, turbid, and liquid, containing degenerated epithelium and mucus but few leukocytes or red blood cells. A typical stool may be 7 L/24 h containing Na+, 125 meq/L; K+, 20 meq/L; and HCO3−, 45 meq/L. Vomiting may also occur early. As a result, the patient rapidly becomes dehydrated and acidotic, with sunken eyes, hypotension, subnormal temperature, rapid and shallow breathing, muscle cramps, oliguria, shock, and coma.

B. Laboratory Findings: Blood studies reveal marked hemoconcentration, with rising specific gravity of plasma, metabolic acidosis, and often elevation of nonprotein nitrogen. The serum potassium may be normal in spite of severe potassium loss.

The vibrios can be easily grown from the stool—never from blood—and can be identified by agglutination with known specific serum.

Differential Diagnosis

Cholera must be distinguished from other causes of severe diarrhea and dehydration, particularly diarrheas due to shigellae, enterotoxigenic *E coli*, viruses, and protozoa in endemic areas.

Prevention

Cholera vaccine gives only limited protection and is of no value in controlling outbreaks. The vaccine is given in 2 injections 1–4 weeks apart (see package insert). A booster dose is given every 6 months when cholera is a hazard. Better vaccines, including toxoids, are being investigated. At present, cholera vaccination is not required of travelers entering the USA.

In endemic areas, all water, other drinks, food, and utensils must be boiled or avoided. Effective decontamination of excreta is essential, but strict isolation of patients is unnecessary and quarantine is undesirable. In countries with high standards of sanitation and public health, the importation of cholera rarely leads to outbreaks of significant size.

Treatment

Water and electrolyte losses must be restored promptly and continuously, and acidosis must be corrected. Diarrheal loss and hemoconcentration must be measured continuously. In moderately ill patients, it may be possible to provide replacement by oral fluids given in the same volume as that lost. A suitable oral solution contains NaCl, 4 g/L; NaHCO3, 4 g/L; KCl, 1–2 g/L; and glucose, 21 g/L. In more severely ill patients or those unable to take fluids by mouth, replacement must be by intravenous fluids. A suitable intravenous solution contains Na+, 133 meq/L; Cl−, 98 meq/L; K+, 13 meq/L; and HCO3−, 48 meq/L. Initially, this solution is infused at a rate of 50–100 mL/min until circulating blood volume and blood pressure are restored. It may then be given more slowly to replace lost stool volume. In children, more potassium and less sodium is lost, and potassium must be replaced. An older method relied on the degree of hemoconcentration to direct fluid replacement: For every 0.001 increase in plasma specific gravity above 1.025, 4 mL/kg of mixed isotonic sodium lactate and saline (1:2 ratio) were infused.

Tetracycline, 0.5 g orally every 6 hours for 3–5 days, and perhaps doxycycline, 200 mg orally as a single dose, suppresses vibrio growth in the gut and shortens the time of vibrio excretion.

Whenever cholera is suspected, the Health Department must be notified by telephone.

Table 24–1. Acute bacterial diarrheas and "food poisoning."

Organism	Incubation Period (Hours)	Vomiting	Diarrhea	Fever	Epidemiology	Pathogenesis	Clinical Features
Staphylococcus	1–8, rarely up to 18	+++	+	−	Staphylococci grow in meats, dairy, bakery products and produce enterotoxin.	Enterotoxin acts on receptors in gut that transmit impulse to medullary centers.	Abrupt onset, intense vomiting for up to 24 hours, regular recovery in 24–48 hours. Occurs in persons eating the same food. No treatment usually necessary except to restore fluids and electrolytes.
Bacillus cereus	1–8, rarely up to 18	+++	++	−	Reheated fried rice causes vomiting or diarrhea.	Enterotoxins formed in food or in gut from growth of B cereus.	After 1–6 hours, mainly vomiting. After 8–16 hours, mainly diarrhea. Both self-limited to less than 1 day.
Clostridium perfringens	8–16	±	+++	−	Clostridia grow in rewarmed meat dishes and produce enterotoxin.	Enterotoxin produced in food and in gut causes hypersecretion in small intestine.	Abrupt onset of profuse diarrhea; vomiting occasionally. Recovery usual without treatment in 1–4 days. Many clostridia in cultures of food and feces of patients.
Clostridium botulinum	24–96	±	Rare	−	Clostridia grow in anaerobic foods and produce toxin.	Toxin absorbed from gut blocks acetylcholine at neuromuscular junction.	Diplopia, dysphagia, dysphonia, respiratory embarrassment. Treatment requires clear airway, ventilation, and intravenous polyvalent antitoxin (see p 874). Toxin present in food and serum. Mortality rate high.
Escherichia coli (some strains)	24–72	±	++	−	Organisms grow in gut and produce toxin. May also invade superficial epithelium.	Toxin* causes hypersecretion in small intestine ("traveler's diarrhea").†	Usually abrupt onset of diarrhea; vomiting rare. A serious infection in neonates. In adults, "traveler's diarrhea" is usually self-limited in 1–3 days. Use diphenoxylate (Lomotil) but no antimicrobials.
Vibrio parahaemolyticus	6–96	+	++	±	Organisms grow in seafood and in gut and produce toxin, or invade.	Hypersecretion in small intestine; stools may be bloody.	Abrupt onset of diarrhea in groups consuming the same food, especially crabs and other seafood. Recovery is usually complete in 1–3 days. Food and stool cultures are positive.
Vibrio cholerae (mild cases)	24–72	+	+++	−	Organisms grow in gut and produce toxin.	Toxin* causes hypersecretion in small intestine. Infective dose: $10^7–10^9$ organisms.	Abrupt onset of liquid diarrhea in endemic area. Needs prompt replacement of fluids and electrolytes (see p 868) IV or orally. Tetracyclines shorten excretion of vibrios. Stool cultures positive.
Shigella spp (mild cases)	24–72	±	++	+	Organisms grow in superficial gut epithelium and gut lumen and produce toxin.	Organisms invade epithelial cells, blood, mucus, and PMNs in stools. Infective dose: $10^2–10^3$ organisms.	Abrupt onset of diarrhea, often with blood and pus in stools, cramps, tenesmus, and lethargy. Stool cultures are positive. In severe cases, give trimethoprim-sulfamethoxazole, ampicillin, or chloramphenicol. Do not give opiates. Restore fluids. Often mild and self-limited.
Salmonella spp	8–48	±	++	+	Organisms grow in gut. Do not produce toxin.	Superficial infection of gut, little invasion. Infective dose: 10^5 organisms.	Gradual or abrupt onset of diarrhea and low-grade fever. No antimicrobials unless systemic dissemination is suspected. Stool cultures are positive. Prolonged carriage is frequent.
Clostridium difficile	?	−	+++	+	Associated with antimicrobial drugs, eg, clindamycin.	Toxin causes epithelial necrosis in colon; pseudomembranous colitis (see p 392).	Especially after abdominal surgery; abrupt bloody diarrhea, and fever. Toxin in stool. Oral vancomycin useful in therapy.
Campylobacter jejuni	2–10 days	−	+++	+	Organism grows in jejunum and ileum.	Invasion and toxin production uncertain.	Fever, diarrhea; PMNs and fresh blood in stool, especially in children. Usually self-limited. Special media needed for culture at 43 °C. Erythromycin in severe cases with invasion. Usual recovery in 5–8 days.
Yersinia enterocolitica	?	±	++	+	Fecal-oral transmission (occasionally). Food-borne. ?In pets.	Gastroenteritis or mesenteric adenitis. Occasional bacteremia. Toxin† produced.	Severe abdominal pain, diarrhea, fever; PMNs and blood in stool; polyarthritis, erythema nodosum in children. If severe, give tetracycline or gentamicin. Keep stool at 4 °C before culture.

*Toxin stimulates adenylate cyclase activity and increases cAMP concentration in gut; this increases secretion of chloride and water and reduces reabsorption of sodium.

†Heat-stable toxin activates guanylate cyclase and results in hypersecretion.

Prognosis

The untreated disease lasts 3–5 days, with a mortality rate ranging from 20% to 80%. With prompt and competent treatment, the mortality rate is 1%.

Kelly MT et al: Cholera on the Texas Gulf coast. *JAMA* 1982; **247**:1598.

BACILLARY DYSENTERY
(Shigellosis)

Essentials of Diagnosis

- Diarrhea, often with blood and mucus.
- Cramps.
- Fever, malaise, prostration, clouded sensorium.
- Pus in stools; organism isolated on stool culture.

General Considerations

Shigella dysentery is a common disease, often self-limited and mild but occasionally serious, particularly in the first 3 years of life. Poor sanitary conditions promote the spread of *Shigella*. *Shigella sonnei* is the leading cause of this illness in the USA, followed by *Shigella flexneri*. *Shigella dysenteriae* causes the most serious form of the illness. Shigellae are invasive organisms: The infective dose is 10^2–10^3 organisms. Recently, there has been a rise in strains resistant to multiple antibiotics.

Clinical Findings

A. Symptoms and Signs: The illness usually starts abruptly, with diarrhea, lower abdominal cramps, and tenesmus. The diarrheal stool often is mixed with blood and mucus. Systemic symptoms are fever (in young children, up to 40 °C [104 °F]), chills, anorexia and malaise, headache, lethargy, and, in the most severe cases, meningismus, coma, and convulsions. As the illness progresses, the patient becomes progressively weaker and more dehydrated. The abdomen is tender. Sigmoidoscopic examination reveals an inflamed, engorged mucosa with punctate, sometimes large areas of ulceration.

B. Laboratory Findings: The white blood count shows an increase in polymorphonuclear cells with a pronounced shift to the left. The stool shows many leukocytes (even gross pus and mucus) and many red blood cells (or gross blood). Stool culture is positive for shigellae in most cases.

Differential Diagnosis

Bacillary dysentery must be distinguished from *Salmonella* enterocolitis (see p 867), enterotoxigenic *E coli*, *Campylobacter* enteritis, *Y enterocolitica* and vibrio infections, and viral diarrhea (caused by rotaviruses in young children and Norwalk viruses in adults). Amebic dysentery may be similar clinically and is diagnosed by finding amebas in the fresh stool specimen. Ulcerative colitis in the adolescent and adult is an important cause of bloody diarrhea.

Complications

Dehydration, acidosis, and electrolyte imbalance occur in infancy. Temporary disaccharidase deficiency may follow the diarrhea. Arthritis is an uncommon complication.

Treatment

A. Specific Measures: Treatment of shock, restoration of circulating blood volume, and renal perfusion are lifesaving in severe cases. The current antimicrobial agent of choice is trimethoprim-sulfamethoxazole, ampicillin (100 mg/kg/d), or chloramphenicol. Shigellae resistant to ampicillin and chloramphenicol are increasing in frequency. Drugs should not be continued beyond the beginning of marked improvement even if stool cultures remain positive. At times, single doses of tetracycline (2 g orally) or ampicillin (100 mg/kg) have given satisfactory results. Since the majority of cases are mild and self-limited, the use of even mildly toxic antibiotics cannot be justified.

B. General Measures: Parenteral hydration and correction of acidosis and electrolyte disturbances are essential in all moderately or severely ill patients. After the bowel has been at rest for a short time, clear fluids are given for 2–3 days. The diet should then be soft, easily digestible, and given in small frequent feedings, avoiding whole milk and high-residue and fatty foods.

Antispasmodics (eg, tincture of belladonna) are helpful when cramps are severe. Drugs that inhibit intestinal peristalsis (paregoric, diphenoxylate with atropine [Lomotil]) may ameliorate symptoms but prolong fever, diarrhea, and excretion of *Shigella* in feces. The patient should be placed on effective stool isolation precautions both in the hospital and in the home to limit spread of infection.

Prognosis

The prognosis is excellent in all but very young or debilitated patients if intravenous rehydration is available. The recent importation of the more virulent *S dysenteriae* from Central America—which may be ampicillin- and chloramphenicol-resistant—may make this illness a greater threat.

Butler T et al: Algorithms in the diagnosis and management of exotic diseases. 27. Shigellosis. *J Infect Dis* 1977;**136**:465.

Gilman RH et al: Single-dose ampicillin therapy for severe shigellosis in Bangladesh. *J Infect Dis* 1981;**143**:164.

TRAVELER'S DIARRHEA

Whenever a person travels from one country to another, particularly if the change involves a marked difference in climate, social conditions, or sanitation standards and facilities, diarrhea is likely to develop within 2–10 days. There may be up to 10 or even more loose stools per day, often accompanied by abdominal cramps, nausea, occasionally vomiting, and, rarely, fever. The stools do not usually contain mucus or blood, and, aside from weakness, dehydration, and occasionally acidosis, there are no systemic manifestations of infection. The illness usually subsides spontaneously within 1–5 days; rarely, it lasts 2–3 weeks.

Bacteriologic cultures of stools rarely reveal salmonellae or shigellae. Contributory causes may at times include unusual food and drink, change in living habits, occasional viral infections (enteroviruses or rotaviruses), and change in bowel flora. A significant number of cases of traveler's diarrhea are caused by acquisition of strains of *Escherichia coli* that produce a potent enterotoxin. This enterotoxin is released by the organisms growing in the small intestine, attaches to ganglioside receptors on intestinal villi, stimulates adenylate cyclase, and increases cyclic adenosine monophosphate concentration in the gut wall. As a result, there is hypersecretion of water and electrolytes into the gut, distension, and massive diarrhea. Strains of *E coli* that elaborate a heat-labile enterotoxin and are prevalent in a given environment appear to be particularly responsible, but heat-stable toxins (which activate guanylate cyclase) can also be involved. Some individuals do not permit unrestricted multiplication of these organisms; others are perhaps resistant to the enterotoxin because of prior exposure.

For most individuals the affliction is short-lived, and its effects may be further reduced by opiates or diphenoxylate with atropine (Lomotil). Antimicrobial drugs generally are not indicated and, indeed, may aggravate the diarrhea. For prophylaxis, bismuth subsalicylate suspension (Pepto-Bismol), 60 mL 4 times daily, has been suggested; or doxycycline, 200 mg on the first day of travel followed by 100 mg daily for 5–10 days. However, the risk of favoring colonization by drug-resistant *Shigella* or *Salmonella* is recognized. Many travelers might prefer to use caution in food and drink and take 160 mg trimethoprim plus 800 mg sulfamethoxazole daily for 3–5 days if traveler's diarrhea should develop. In all cases, water and electrolyte balance must be restored.

Carpenter C: Mechanisms of bacterial diarrheas. *Am J Med* 1980;**68**:313.

DuPont HL, Ericsson CD, Murray BE: Traveler's diarrhea: Can it be eluded? (Editorial.) *JAMA* 1983;**249**:1193.

DuPont HL et al: Treatment of travelers' diarrhea with trimethoprim/sulfamethoxazole and with trimethoprim alone. *N Engl J Med* 1982;**307**:841.

Ryder RW et al: Traveler's diarrhea in Panamanian tourists in Mexico. *J Infect Dis* 1981;**144**:442.

Sack DA et al: Prophylactic doxycycline for traveler's diarrhea. *N Engl J Med* 1978;**298**:758.

The traveler's diarrhea. *Med Lett Drugs Ther* (Dec 11) 1981; **23**:105.

BRUCELLOSIS

Essentials of Diagnosis

- Insidious onset: easy fatigability, headache, arthralgia, anorexia, sweating, irritability.
- Intermittent fever, especially at night, which may become chronic and undulant.
- Cervical and axillary lymphadenopathy; hepatosplenomegaly.
- Lymphocytosis, positive blood culture, elevated agglutination titer.

General Considerations

The infection is transmitted from animals to humans. *Brucella abortus* (cattle), *Brucella suis* (hogs), and *Brucella melitensis* (goats) are the main agents. Transmission to humans occurs by contact with infected meat (slaughterhouse workers), placentae of infected animals (farmers, veterinarians), or ingestion of infected unpasteurized milk or cheese. Organisms may enter through abraded skin or mucous membranes or via the respiratory tract. The incubation period varies from a few days to several weeks. The disorder may become chronic and persist for years. In the USA, brucellosis is very rare except in the midwestern states (from *B suis*) and in occasional outbreaks associated with consumption of goat cheese from Mexico.

Clinical Findings

A. Symptoms and Signs: The onset may be acute, with fever, chills, and sweats, but often the disease begins so insidiously that it may be weeks before the patient seeks medical care for weakness and exhaustion upon minimal activity. Symptoms also include headache, abdominal pains with anorexia and constipation, and arthralgia, sometimes associated with periarticular swelling but not local heat. The fever may be septic, sustained, low-grade, or even absent but is more often of the intermittent type preceded by chilliness, rising during the evening hours and falling with a sweat (night sweat) in the early morning hours. The chronic form may assume an undulant nature, with periods of normal temperature between acute attacks, and the above symptoms plus emotional instability and weight loss may persist for years, either continuously or intermittently.

Physical findings are minimal. Half of cases have peripheral lymph node enlargement and splenomegaly; hepatomegaly is less common.

B. Laboratory Findings: The white count is usually normal to low, with a relative or absolute lymphocytosis. Early in the course of infection, the organism can be recovered from the blood, cerebrospinal fluid, urine, and bone marrow; later, this may be difficult. An agglutination titer greater than 1:100 (and especially a rising titer) supports the diagnosis. A prozone phenomenon (serum agglutinates in high but not in low dilution) is common. IgG antibody indicates active disease, whereas IgM antibody may persist after recovery. The intradermal skin test is of no value. Liver enzyme levels are often elevated.

Differential Diagnosis

Brucellosis must be differentiated from any other acute febrile disease, especially influenza, tularemia, Q fever, and enteric fever. In its chronic form it resembles Hodgkin's disease, tuberculosis, and malaria. The chronic form may also simulate psychoneurosis, so that the latter is sometimes incorrectly given a diagnosis of chronic brucellosis.

Complications

The most frequent complications are bone and joint lesions such as spondylitis and suppurative arthritis (usually of a single joint), subacute infective endocarditis, encephalitis, and meningitis. Less common complications are pneumonitis with pleural effusion, hepatitis, and cholecystitis. Abortion in humans is no more common with this disease than with any other acute bacterial disease during pregnancy. Pancytopenia is rare.

Prevention

Prevention is by destruction of infected dairy animals, immunization of susceptible animals, and pasteurization of milk and milk products.

Treatment

A. Specific Measures: Tetracycline, 2 g orally daily for 21 days, is the treatment of choice. Streptomycin, 0.5 g intramuscularly every 12 hours, is occasionally given at the same time as tetracycline. Relapse may require re-treatment. Ampicillin may be effective. Trimethoprim-sulfamethoxazole has been used effectively in early cases.

B. General Measures: Place patient at bed rest during the acute febrile stage; maintain adequate nutrition.

Prognosis

In a few cases, brucellosis may remain active for many years as an intermittent illness, but about 75% of patients recover completely within 3–6 months, and fewer than 20% have residual disease after 1 year. Treatment has considerably shortened the natural course of the disease. Brucellosis is rarely fatal in either the acute or the chronic form.

Wise RI: Brucellosis in the United States: Past, present and future. *JAMA* 1980;**244**:2318.

GAS GANGRENE
(See also p 826.)

Essentials of Diagnosis

- Sudden onset of pain and edema in an area of wound contamination.
- Brown to blood-tinged watery exudate, with skin discoloration of surrounding area.
- Gas in the tissue by palpation or x-ray.
- Organisms in culture or smear of exudate.
- Prostration and systemic toxicity.

General Considerations

Gas gangrene or clostridial myositis is produced by entry of one of several clostridia (*Clostridium per-*

fringens, Clostridium ramosum, Clostridium bifermentans, Clostridium histolyticum, Clostridium novyi, etc) into devitalized tissues. It grows and produces toxins under anaerobic conditions, resulting in shock, hemolysis, and myonecrosis. Alpha toxin (lecithinase) of *C perfringens* is the most potent. *Clostridium difficile*, an infrequent member of the normal gut flora, produces a toxin that can lead to pseudomembranous colitis, especially after antibiotic administration (see Chapter 22).

Clinical Findings

A. Symptoms and Signs: The onset of gas gangrene is usually sudden, with rapidly increasing pain in the affected area accompanied by a fall in blood pressure, and tachycardia. The temperature may be elevated, but not proportionate to the severity of the inflammation. In the last stages of the disease, severe prostration, stupor, delirium, and coma occur.

The wound becomes swollen, and the surrounding skin is pale as a result of fluid accumulation beneath it. This is followed by a discharge of a brown to blood-tinged, serous, foul-smelling fluid from the wound. As the disease advances, the surrounding tissue changes from pale to dusky and finally becomes deeply discolored, with coalescent, red, fluid-filled vesicles. Gas may be palpable in the tissues. In clostridial sepsis, hemolysis and jaundice are common, often complicated by acute renal failure.

B. Laboratory Findings: Gas gangrene is a clinical rather than a bacteriologic diagnosis. Culture of the exudate confirms the diagnosis, and stained smears of the exudate showing the typical gram-positive rods (usually as part of a mixed flora) are valuable. Neither demonstration of clostridia in the smear from the wound nor the presence of gas is sufficient to make this diagnosis. The clinical picture must be present.

C. X-Ray Findings: X-ray may show gas in the soft tissues spreading along fascial planes.

Differential Diagnosis

Other types of infection can cause gas formation in the tissue, eg, *Enterobacter, Escherichia,* and mixed anaerobic infections including *Bacteroides* and peptostreptococci. Clostridia may produce serious puerperal infection with hemolysis.

Treatment

A. Specific Measures: Give penicillin, 2 million units every 3 hours as a bolus into an intravenous infusion. Polyvalent gas gangrene antitoxin is available but of dubious benefit.

B. Surgical Measures: Adequate surgical debridement and exposure of infected areas is essential. Radical surgical excision may be necessary. Hyperbaric oxygen therapy, if available, may be beneficial when used in conjunction with other measures. A tetanus toxoid booster injection should be given.

Prognosis

Without treatment, the mortality rate is very high.

Darke SG et al: Gas gangrene and related infection: Classification, clinical features and aetiology, management and mortality: A report of 88 cases. *Br J Surg* 1977;**64**:104.

TETANUS
(See also p 825.)

Essentials of Diagnosis

- Jaw stiffness followed by spasms of jaw muscles (trismus).
- Stiffness of the neck and other muscles, dysphagia, irritability, hyperreflexia.
- Finally, painful convulsions precipitated by minimal stimuli.
- History of wound and possible contamination.

General Considerations

Tetanus is an acute intoxication by the neurotoxin elaborated by *Clostridium tetani*. Spores of this organism are ubiquitous in soil. When introduced into a wound in the presence of necrotic tissue and impaired circulation, the spores germinate. Spores may enter clean wounds. In the newborn, infection enters through the umbilical stump. The vegetative bacteria elaborate a toxin, tetanospasmin, that blocks the action of inhibitory mediators at spinal synapses and also interferes with neuromuscular transmission. As a result, minor stimuli result in uncontrolled spasms, and reflexes are enormously exaggerated. The incubation period is 5 days to 15 weeks, with the average being 8–12 days.

In the USA today, female heroin users are particularly at risk.

Clinical Findings

A. Symptoms and Signs: Occasionally, the first symptom is pain and tingling at the site of inoculation, followed by spasticity of the group of muscles nearby, and this may be all that happens. More frequently, however, the presenting symptoms are stiffness of the jaw, neck stiffness, dysphagia, and irritability. Hyperreflexia develops later, with spasms of the jaw muscles (trismus) or facial muscles and rigidity and spasm of the muscles of the abdomen, neck, and back. Painful tonic convulsions precipitated by minor stimuli are common. The patient is awake and alert during the entire course of the illness. During convulsions the glottis and respiratory muscles go into spasm, so that the patient is unable to breathe and cyanosis and asphyxia may ensue. The temperature is only slightly elevated.

B. Laboratory Findings: The diagnosis of tetanus is made clinically. There is usually a polymorphonuclear leukocytosis.

Differential Diagnosis

Tetanus must be differentiated from various acute central nervous system infections. Trismus may occasionally develop with the use of phenothiazines. Strychnine poisoning should also be considered.

Complications

Airway obstruction and anoxia are common. Urinary retention and constipation may result from spasm of the sphincters. Respiratory arrest and cardiac failure are late, life-threatening events.

Prevention

Active immunization with tetanus toxoid should be universal. It is an essential part of childhood immunization, usually given as DTP (see p 833). For adults, give Td toxoid as recommended by manufacturers. Booster doses of toxoid should be given about every 10 years or at the time of a major injury.

Passive immunization should be used in nonimmunized individuals and those whose immunization status is uncertain whenever the wound is contaminated, major, or likely to have devitalized tissue. Tetanus immune globulin, 250 units intramuscularly, is the preferred agent. Tetanus antitoxin (equine or bovine) in a dose of 3000–5000 units should be used (after testing for serum hypersensitivity) only if tetanus immune globulin is not available. Active immunization with tetanus toxoid should be started concurrently. Table 24–2 provides a guide to prophylactic management.

Adequate debridement of wounds is an essential preventive measure. In suspect cases, benzathine penicillin G, 1.2 million units intramuscularly, may be a reasonable adjunctive measure.

Treatment

A. Specific Measures: Give tetanus immune globulin, 5000 units intramuscularly; this antitoxin does not cause sensitivity reactions. If tetanus immune globulin is not available, give tetanus antitoxin, 100,000 units intravenously, after testing for horse serum sensitivity. The value of antitoxin treatment has been questioned.

B. General Measures: Place the patient at bed rest and minimize stimulation. Sedation and anticonvulsant therapy are essential. Experience from areas of high incidence suggests that most convulsions can be eliminated by treatment with chlorpromazine (50–100

Table 24–2. Guide to tetanus prophylaxis in wound management.*

History of Tetanus Immunization	Clean, Minor Wounds		All Other Wounds	
	Td†	TIG‡	Td†	TIG‡
Uncertain, or less than 2 doses	Yes	No	Yes	Yes
Three or more doses; last dose within 10 years	No	No	Yes§	No

*Reproduced and modified, with permission, from *Ann Intern Med* 1981;**95**:726.

†Td = tetanus toxoid and diphtheria toxoid, adult form. Use only this preparation (Td-adult) in children older than 6 years.

‡TIG = tetanus immune globulin.

§Unless last Td dose was within the past year.

mg 4 times daily) or diazepam combined with a sedative (amobarbital, phenobarbital, or meprobamate). Mild cases of tetanus can be controlled with one or the other rather than both. Only rarely is general curarization required. Other recommended anticonvulsant regimens are tribromoethanol, 15–25 mg/kg rectally every 1–4 hours as needed; and amobarbital sodium, 5 mg/kg intramuscularly as needed. Paraldehyde, 4–8 mL intravenously (2–5% solution), may be combined with barbiturates. Penicillin is of value but should not be substituted for antitoxin.

Give intravenous fluids as necessary. Tracheostomy may be required for laryngeal spasm. Assisted respiration is required in conjunction with curarization. Hyperbaric oxygen therapy is of no established value.

Prognosis

The mortality rate is higher in very small children and very old people; with shorter incubation periods; with shorter intervals between onset of symptoms and the first convulsion; and with delay in treatment. If trismus develops early, the prognosis is grave. The overall mortality rate is about 40%. Contaminated lesions about the head and face are more dangerous than wounds on other parts of the body.

If the patient survives, recovery is complete.

Edmondson RS, Flowers MW: Intensive care in tetanus: Management, complications and mortality in 100 cases. *Br Med J* 1979;**1**:1401.

Immunization Practices Advisory Committee, Centers for Disease Control: Diphtheria, tetanus, and pertussis: Guidelines for vaccine prophylaxis and other preventive measures. *Ann Intern Med* 1981;**95**:723.

BOTULISM

Essentials of Diagnosis

- Sudden onset of cranial nerve paralysis, diplopia, dry mouth, dysphagia, dysphonia, and muscle weakness progressing to respiratory paralysis.
- History of recent ingestion of home-canned, smoked, or unusual foods.
- Demonstration of toxin in serum or food.

General Considerations

Botulism is food poisoning caused by ingestion of the toxin (usually type A, B, or E) of *Clostridium botulinum,* a strict anaerobic spore-forming bacillus found widespread in soil. Canned, smoked, or vacuum-packed anaerobic foods are involved—particularly home-canned vegetables, smoked meats, and vacuum-packed fish. The toxins block the release of acetylcholine from nerve endings. Clinically, there is early nervous system involvement leading to respiratory paralysis. The mortality rate in untreated cases is high. Botulism may follow wound infection.

Clinical Findings

A. Symptoms and Signs: Twelve to 36 hours after ingestion of the toxin, visual disturbances appear, particularly diplopia and loss of power of accommodation. Other symptoms are dry throat and mouth, dysphagia, and dysphonia. There may be nausea and vomiting, particularly with type E. Muscle weakness is prominent. The edrophonium (Tensilon) test gives typical results, and respiration is impaired, but the sensorium remains clear and the temperature normal. Progressive respiratory paralysis may lead to death unless mechanical assistance is provided.

Infant botulism. Infants in the first few months of life may present with weakness, generalized hypotonicity, and electromyographic findings compatible with botulism. Both botulinus organisms and toxin are found in the stool but not in serum. The cause of this syndrome is not known, but honey fed to infants has been incriminated.

B. Laboratory Findings: Most routine determinations are within normal limits. Toxin in the patient's serum and in suspected foods may be shown by mouse inoculation and identified with specific antiserum.

Differential Diagnosis

Cranial nerve involvement suggests bulbar poliomyelitis, myasthenia gravis, stroke, infectious neuronitis, or tick paralysis. Nausea and vomiting may suggest intestinal obstruction or other types of food poisoning.

Complications

The dysphagia may cause aspiration pneumonia; such infection and respiratory paralysis are the usual causes of death.

Prevention

Home-canned vegetables must be sterilized to destroy spores. Sterilization standards for commercial canned or vacuum-packed foods must be strictly enforced. Boiling food for 20 minutes can inactivate the toxin, but punctured or swollen cans or jars with defective seals should be discarded. Early and adequate treatment of wounds prevents wound botulism.

Treatment

As soon as the clinical diagnosis of botulism is suspected, the Centers for Disease Control should be consulted (central number: [404] 329–3311). That agency can ship pentavalent (A, B, C, D, E) botulinus antitoxin by air or can request release of trivalent (A, B, E) antitoxin from one of several regional quarantine centers in the USA. The Centers for Disease Control can also assay for toxin in the patient's serum or stool, as well as the suspect food item. Two vials of antitoxin are administered to the patient if tests for hypersensitivity are negative.

Adequate ventilation and oxygenation must be maintained by good respiratory drainage (elevate foot of bed), removal of respiratory obstruction by aspiration or tracheostomy, and mechanical respirator if necessary.

Parenteral fluids or alimentation are given as

necessary. Give nothing by mouth while swallowing difficulty persists. If pneumonitis develops, appropriate antimicrobials are used.

Guanidine hydrochloride, 15–35 mg/kg/d orally, has been used experimentally with occasional benefit.

The removal of unabsorbed toxin from the gut may be attempted if it can be done very soon after ingestion of the suspected toxin. Any remnants of suspected foods must be saved for analysis. Persons who might have eaten the suspected food must be located and observed.

Prognosis

If good ventilation can be maintained and the toxin promptly neutralized, the mortality rate may be substantially lower than the 30–70% that is to be expected in untreated patients. If the patient survives the attack of botulism, there are no neurologic residua.

Dowell VR: Botulism and tetanus: Selected epidemiologic and microbiologic aspects. *Rev Infect Dis* 1984;**6**:5202.

Simpson LL: The action of botulinal toxin. *Rev Infect Dis* 1979; **1**:656.

Thompson JA et al: Infant botulism: Clinical spectrum and epidemiology. *Pediatrics* 1980;**66**:936.

ANTHRAX

Anthrax is a disease of sheep, cattle, horses, goats, and swine caused by *Bacillus anthracis,* a gram-positive spore-forming aerobe transmitted to humans by entry through broken skin or mucous membranes or, less commonly, by inhalation. Human infection is rare. It is most apt to occur in farmers, veterinarians, and tannery and wool workers. Several clinical forms have been observed. Rarely, other gram-positive spore-forming bacilli (eg, *Bacillus cereus*) are found in sepsis, meningitis, or endocarditis. *B cereus* produces an enterotoxin (see p 867).

Clinical Findings

A. Symptoms and Signs:

1. Cutaneous anthrax ("malignant pustule")–An erythematous papule appears on an exposed area of skin and becomes vesicular, with a purple to black center. The area around the lesion is swollen or edematous and surrounded by vesicles. The center of the lesion finally forms a necrotic eschar and sloughs. Regional adenopathy, variable fever, malaise, headache, and nausea and vomiting may be present. After the eschar sloughs, hematogenous spread and sepsis may occur, at times manifested by shock, cyanosis, sweating, and collapse. Hemorrhagic meningitis may also occur.

Anthrax sepsis sometimes develops without a skin lesion.

2. Pulmonary anthrax ("woolsorter's disease")–This follows the inhalation of spores from hides, bristles, or wool. It is characterized by fever, malaise, headache, dyspnea, and cough; congestion of the nose, throat, and larynx; and evidence of pneumonia or mediastinitis. Very rarely, gram-positive spore-forming aerobic bacilli other than *B anthracis* (eg, *B cereus*) can produce a similar disease.

B. Laboratory Findings: The white count may be elevated or low. Sputum or blood culture may be positive for *B anthracis*. Smears of skin lesions show gram-positive encapsulated rods, and cultures should be attempted. Antibodies may be detected by an indirect hemagglutination test.

Treatment

Give penicillin G, 10 million units intravenously daily; or, in mild, localized cases, tetracycline, 0.5 g orally every 6 hours.

Prognosis

The prognosis is excellent in the cutaneous form of the disease if treatment is given early. Sepsis and pulmonary anthrax have a grave prognosis. Bacteremia is a very unfavorable sign.

LaForce FM: Woolsorters' disease in England. *Bull NY Acad Med* 1978;**54**:956.

TULAREMIA

Essentials of Diagnosis

- Fever, headache, nausea, and prostration.
- Papule progressing to ulcer at site of inoculation.
- Enlarged regional lymph nodes.
- History of contact with rabbits, other rodents, and biting arthropods (eg, ticks in summer) in endemic area.
- Confirmed by culture of ulcer, lymph node aspirate, or blood.

General Considerations

Tularemia is an infection of wild rodents— particularly rabbits and muskrats—with *Francisella (Pasteurella) tularensis*. It is transmitted from animals to humans by contact with animal tissues (eg, trapping muskrats, skinning rabbits); by the bite of certain ticks and biting flies; by consumption of infected, undercooked meat; or by drinking contaminated water. Infection in humans often produces a local lesion and widespread organ involvement but may be entirely asymptomatic. The incubation period is 2–10 days.

Clinical Findings

A. Symptoms and Signs: Fever, headache, and nausea begin suddenly, and a local lesion—a papule at the site of inoculation—develops and soon ulcerates. Regional lymph nodes become enlarged and tender and may suppurate. The local lesion may be on the skin of an extremity (ulceroglandular) or in the eye. Pneumonia may develop from hematogenous spread of the organism or may be primary after inhalation of infected aerosols. Following ingestion of infected meat or water, an enteric form (typhoidal) may be manifested by enteritis, stupor, and delirium. In any type of involvement, the spleen may be enlarged and tender and there may be rashes, generalized aches, and prostration. Asymptomatic infection is not rare.

B. Laboratory Findings: The white blood count is slightly elevated or normal. Culture of blood, an ulcerated lesion, or lymph node aspirate yields the organisms in special culture media early in the illness. A positive agglutination test (more than 1:80) develops in the second week after infection and may persist for several years. A delayed type skin test (read in 48 hours) becomes positive within a few days after infection; about 50% of patients have a positive skin test when first seen. The skin test (positive is more than 5 mm induration) is highly specific; it remains positive longer after infection than does the agglutination test, but skin test material is rarely available.

Differential Diagnosis

Tularemia must be differentiated from rickettsial and meningococcal infections, cat-scratch disease, infectious mononucleosis, and various pneumonias and fungal diseases. Epidemiologic considerations, positive skin tests, and rising agglutination titers are the chief differential points.

Complications

Hematogenous spread to any organ may produce severe problems, particularly meningitis, perisplenitis, pericarditis, and pneumonia.

Treatment

Streptomycin, 0.5 g intramuscularly every 6–8 hours, together with tetracycline, 0.5 g orally every 6 hours, is administered until 4–5 days after the patient becomes afebrile. Chloramphenicol may be substituted for tetracycline in the same dosage. Adequate fluid intake is essential, and oxygen may be required. Suppurating lymph nodes may be aspirated but should not be incised during the first week if the process is still localized. Later in the disease, drainage of fluctuant nodes may be needed and is safe after proper chemotherapy for several days.

Prognosis

The mortality rate of untreated ulceroglandular tularemia is 5%; that of tularemic pneumonia, 30%. Early chemotherapy is promptly effective and prevents fatalities. Skin tests and agglutination tests suggest that subclinical infection is common in outbreaks of tularemia.

Prevention

Awareness of the risk of infection through contact with potentially infected rodents, biting insects, or water supply is helpful.

Mason WL et al: Treatment of tularemia, including pulmonary tularemia, with gentamicin. *Am Rev Respir Dis* 1980;**121**:39.

Teutsch SM et al: Pneumonic tularemia on Martha's Vineyard. *N Engl J Med* 1979;**301**:826.

PLAGUE

Essentials of Diagnosis

- Sudden onset of high fever, malaise, muscular pains, and prostration.
- Axillary or inguinal lymphadenitis (bubo).
- Bacteremia, sepsis, and pneumonitis may occur.
- History of exposure to rodents in endemic area.
- Positive smear and culture from bubo and positive blood culture.

General Considerations

Plague is an infection of wild rodents with *Yersinia (Pasteurella) pestis,* a small gram-negative rod. It is transmitted from one rodent to another and from rodents to humans by the bites of fleas. Plague bacilli grow in the gut of the flea and obstruct it. When the hungry flea sucks blood, it regurgitates organisms into the bite wound. Feces of fleas may also transmit the infection. If a plague victim develops pneumonia, the infection can be transmitted by droplets to other persons and an epidemic may be started in this way. The incubation period is 2–10 days.

Following the flea bite, the organisms spread through the lymphatics to the lymph nodes, which become greatly enlarged (bubo). They may then reach the bloodstream to involve all organs. When pneumonia or meningitis develops, the outcome is often fatal.

Clinical Findings

A. Symptoms and Signs: The onset is usually sudden, with high fever, malaise, tachycardia, intense headache, and generalized muscular aches. The patient appears profoundly ill and very anxious. Delirium may ensue. If pneumonia develops, tachypnea, productive cough, blood-tinged sputum, and cyanosis also occur. Meningeal signs may develop. A pustule or ulcer at the site of inoculation and signs of lymphangitis may occur. Axillary, inguinal, or cervical lymph nodes become enlarged and tender and may eventually suppurate and drain. With hematogenous spread, the patient may rapidly become toxic and comatose, with purpuric spots (black plague) appearing on the skin.

Primary plague pneumonia results from the inhalation of bacilli in droplets coughed up by another patient with plague pneumonia. This is a fulminant pneumonitis with bloody, frothy sputum and sepsis and is usually fatal in unimmunized persons unless treatment is started within a few hours of onset.

B. Laboratory Findings: Peripheral white counts range from 12 to 20 thousand/μL. The plague bacillus may be found in smears from aspirates of buboes examined with Gram's or immunofluorescent stain. Cultures from bubo aspirate or pus and blood are positive but may grow slowly. In convalescing patients, an antibody titer rise may be demonstrated by agglutination tests.

C. X-Ray Findings: Pulmonary infiltration in a person suspected of having plague implies a grave prognosis and should lead to strict isolation.

Differential Diagnosis

The lymphadenitis of plague is most commonly mistaken for the lymphadenitis accompanying staphylococcal or streptococcal infections of an extremity, venereal diseases such as lymphogranuloma venereum or syphilis, and tularemia. The systemic manifestations resemble those of enteric or rickettsial fevers, malaria, or influenza. The pneumonia resembles other severe gram-negative or staphylococcal pneumonias.

Prevention

Periodic surveys of rodents and their ectoparasites in endemic areas provide guidelines for the need for extensive rodent and flea control measures. Total eradication of plague from wild rodents in an endemic area ("sylvatic plague") is rarely possible.

Drug prophylaxis may provide temporary protection for persons exposed to the risk of plague infection, particularly by the respiratory route. Tetracycline hydrochloride, 500 mg orally 1–2 times daily for 5 days, can accomplish this.

Plague vaccines—both live and killed—have been used for many years, but their efficacy is not clearly established. The USP formol-killed suspension gives some protection. It is given as directed by the manufacturer, usually in 2 doses 4 weeks apart, followed by a booster dose. For continued exposure, subsequent boosters are given every 6–12 months.

Treatment

Therapy must be started promptly when plague is suspected. Give streptomycin, 1 g intramuscularly, immediately, and then 0.5 g intramuscularly every 6–8 hours. Tetracycline, 2 g daily orally (parenterally if necessary), is given at the same time. Intravenous fluids, pressor drugs, oxygen, and tracheostomy are used as required.

Prognosis

If the diagnosis can be made and treatment started relatively early, most patients with bubonic plague will recover. In untreated cases, the mortality rate may range from 20 to 60%. When gross sepsis, pneumonia, and shock supervene, the outlook is poor. Primary pneumonic plague is almost invariably fatal unless treated intensively within hours of onset.

Mann JM et al: Peripatetic plague. *JAMA* 1982;**247**:47.

Washington RL et al: Septicemic plague that mimics Reye's syndrome. *Am J Dis Child* 1979;**133**:434.

LEPROSY

Essentials of Diagnosis

- Pale, anesthetic macular—or nodular and erythematous—skin lesions.
- Superficial nerve thickening with associated sensory changes.
- History of residence in endemic area in childhood.
- Acid-fast bacilli in skin lesions or nasal scrapings, or characteristic histologic nerve changes.

General Considerations

Leprosy is a chronic infectious disease caused by the acid-fast rod *Mycobacterium leprae*. The mode of transmission is unknown but probably involves prolonged exposure in childhood. Only rarely have adults become infected (eg, by tattooing). The disease is endemic in tropical and subtropical Asia, Africa, Central and South America and the Pacific regions, and the southern USA.

Clinical Findings

A. Symptoms and Signs: The onset is insidious. The lesions involve the cooler body tissues: skin, superficial nerves, nose, pharynx, larynx, eyes, and testicles. Skin lesions may occur as pale, anesthetic macular lesions 1–10 cm in diameter; discrete erythematous, infiltrated nodules 1–5 cm in diameter; or a diffuse skin infiltration. Neurologic disturbances are manifested by nerve infiltration and thickening, with resultant anesthesia, neuritis, paresthesia, trophic ulcers, and bone resorption and shortening of digits. In untreated cases, disfigurement due to the skin infiltration and nerve involvement may be extreme.

The disease is divided clinically and by laboratory tests into 2 distinct types: lepromatous and tuberculoid. In the lepromatous type, the course is progressive and malignant, with nodular skin lesions; slow, symmetric nerve involvement; abundant acid-fast bacilli in the skin lesions; and a negative lepromin skin test. The patient has impaired cellular immunity. In the tuberculoid type, the course is benign and nonprogressive, with macular skin lesions, severe asymmetric nerve involvement of sudden onset with few bacilli present in the lesions, and a positive lepromin skin test. Intermediate ("borderline") cases are frequent. Eye involvement (keratitis and iridocyclitis), nasal ulcers, epistaxis, anemia, and lymphadenopathy may occur.

B. Laboratory Findings: Laboratory confirmation of leprosy requires the demonstration of acid-fast bacilli in scrapings from slit skin smears or the nasal septum. Biopsy of skin or of a thickened involved nerve also gives a typical histologic picture.

M leprae has not been grown in culture media, but it multiplies in experimentally injected mouse foot pads and in armadillos.

Differential Diagnosis

The skin lesions of leprosy often resemble those of lupus erythematosus, sarcoidosis, syphilis, erythema nodosum, erythema multiforme, and vitiligo. Nerve involvement, sensory dissociation, and resulting deformity may require differentiation from syringomyelia and scleroderma.

Complications

Intercurrent pulmonary tuberculosis is common in the lepromatous type, probably because of deficient cellular immunity. Amyloidosis may occur with long-standing disease.

Prevention

Experimental vaccines made from animal-grown *M leprae* are promising for the immunization of children. Drugs and vaccines are being tested for prophylaxis in family contacts of patients with lepromatous leprosy.

Treatment

Drugs should be given cautiously, with slowly increasing doses, and must be withheld when they induce an exacerbation called "lepra reaction": fever, progressive anemia with or without leukopenia; severe gastrointestinal symptoms, allergic dermatitis, hepatitis, or mental disturbances; or erythema nodosum. It is important, therefore, to observe temperature, blood counts, and biopsy changes in lesions at regular intervals. Corticosteroids are valuable in lepra reactions. The duration of treatment must be guided by progress, preferably as judged by biopsy. Treatment must be continued for several years or indefinitely, because recrudescence may occur after cessation of therapy. No isolation procedures are warranted for patients under treatment.

Dapsone (DDS) is given orally, 50–100 mg/d. It is widely used because of efficacy, low cost, and low toxicity. DDS-resistant *M leprae* is found in 10–30% of patients on long-term treatment and occasionally in untreated persons. The likelihood of DDS resistance is reduced if rifampin is given simultaneously. If fever, granulocytopenia, or jaundice develops, DDS is discontinued and clofazimine is given. Rifampin, 10 mg/kg/d up to 600 mg/d orally, is given together with a second drug (eg, DDS). Rifampin is effective but costly. Clofazimine, 1–4 mg/kg/d orally, is given mainly in DDS-resistant lepromatous leprosy. Thalidomide, 100–400 mg/d orally, is valuable for management of erythema nodosum of leprosy (ENL) in nonpregnant patients. Corticosteroids are also useful. Surgical care of extremities can prevent deformity.

Prognosis

Untreated lepromatous leprosy is progressive and fatal in 10–20 years. In the tuberculoid type, spontaneous arrest usually occurs in 1–3 years; it may, however, produce crippling deformities.

With treatment, the lepromatous type regresses slowly (over a period of 3–8 years). Recovery from the tuberculoid type is more rapid. Recrudescences are always possible, and it may be safe to assume that the bacilli are never eradicated. Deformities persist after complete recovery and may markedly interfere with function and appearance.

Grove DI et al: Algorithms in the diagnosis and management of exotic diseases: Leprosy. *J Infect Dis* 1976;**134:**205.

Levy L, Noordene SK, Sansarri CQ: Increase in prevalence of leprosy caused by dapsone-resistant *Mycobacterium leprae*. *MMWR* (Jan 8) 1982;**30:**637.

CHANCROID

Chancroid is an acute localized venereal disease caused by the short gram-negative bacillus *Haemophilus ducreyi*. Infection occurs by sexual contact, although nonvenereal inoculation has occurred in medical personnel through contact with chancroid patients. The incubation period is 3–5 days.

The initial lesion at the site of inoculation is a vesicopustule that breaks down to form a painful, soft ulcer with a necrotic base, surrounding erythema, and undermined edges. Multiple lesions—started by auto-inoculation—and inguinal adenitis often develop. The adenitis is usually unilateral and consists of tender, matted nodes of moderate size with overlying erythema. The nodal mass softens, becomes fluctuant, and may rupture spontaneously. With lymph node involvement, fever, chills, and malaise may develop. These signs occur more commonly in men, whereas no external signs may be evident in women, although they can serve as sources of infection for contacts.

Swabs from lesions are best cultured on chocolate agar with 1% Isovitalex and vancomycin, 3 μg/mL, to yield *Haemophilus ducreyi*. The chancroid skin test may become positive and remain positive for life. Mixed venereal infection is very common (including syphilis and herpes), as is infection of the ulcer with fusiforms, spirochetes, and other organisms.

Balanitis and phimosis are frequent complications.

Chancroid must be differentiated from other genital ulcers. The chancre of syphilis is clean and painless, with a hard base.

Treat with erythromycin or tetracycline, 0.5 g orally 4 times daily for 10 days, or with trimethoprim-sulfamethoxazole for the same period. Cleaning the ulcers with soap and water promotes healing. Fluctuant buboes may be aspirated by needle. Chancroid usually responds to treatment and tends to be self-limited.

Hafiz S et al: Chancroid in Sheffield: A report of 22 cases diagnosed by isolating *Haemophilus ducreyi* in a modified medium. *Br J Vener Dis* 1981;**57:**382.

GONORRHEA

Essentials of Diagnosis

- Purulent urethral discharge, especially in men, with dysuria, yielding positive smear.
- Cervicitis with purulent discharge, or asymptomatic, yielding positive culture.
- Epididymitis, prostatitis, periurethral inflammation, proctitis in men.
- Vaginitis, salpingitis, proctitis in women.
- Fever, arthritis, skin lesions, conjunctivitis, pharyngitis.
- Gram-negative intracellular diplococci seen in a smear from the male urethra or cultured from any site, particularly the urethra, cervix, and rectum.

General Considerations

Gonorrhea is the most prevalent reportable communicable disease in the USA, with an estimated 2.5 million or more infectious cases annually. It is caused by *Neisseria gonorrhoeae,* a gram-negative diplococcus typically found inside polymorphonuclear cells. It is most commonly transmitted during sexual activity and has its greatest incidence in the 15- to 29-year-old age group. The incubation period is usually 2–8 days.

Clinical Findings

A. Symptoms and Signs:

1. Men–Initially, there is burning on urination and a serous or milky discharge. One to 3 days later, the urethral pain is more pronounced and the discharge becomes yellow, creamy, and profuse, sometimes blood-tinged. Without treatment, the disorder may regress and become chronic or progress to involve the prostate, epididymis, and periurethral glands with acute, painful inflammation. This in turn becomes chronic, with prostatitis and urethral strictures. Rectal infection is common in homosexual men. Unusual sites of primary infection (eg, the pharynx) must always be considered. Systemic involvement is listed below. Asymptomatic infection is common.

2. Women–Dysuria, frequency, and urgency may occur, with a purulent urethral discharge. Vaginitis and cervicitis with inflammation of Bartholin's glands are common. Most often, however, the infection is asymptomatic, with only slightly increased vaginal discharge and moderate cervicitis on examination. Infection may remain as a chronic cervicitis—a main reservoir of gonococci in any community. It may progress to involve the uterus and tubes with acute and chronic salpingitis and with ultimate scarring of tubes and sterility. In pelvic inflammatory disease, anaerobes often accompany gonococci. Rectal infection is common both as spread of the organism from the genital tract and as a result of infection by anal coitus. Systemic involvement is listed below.

B. Laboratory Findings:
Smears of urethral discharge in men, especially during the first week after onset, usually show typical gram-negative diplococci in polymorphonuclear leukocytes. Smears are less often positive in women. Cultures are essential in all cases where gonorrhea should be suspected and gonococci cannot be shown in gram-stained smears. This applies particularly to cervical, rectal, pharyngeal, and joint specimens. Specimens of pus or secretions are streaked on a selective medium such as Thayer-Martin or Transgrow. The latter is suitable for transport if a laboratory is not immediately available. The medium must be 20 °C when inoculated and must be incubated at 37 °C in a 10% CO_2 atmosphere (closed Transgrow bottle; Thayer-Martin in candle jar). Colonies are identified by oxidase test, Gram's stain, or immunofluorescence. No good serologic test is available.

Differential Diagnosis

The chief alternatives to acute gonococcal urethritis or cervicitis are nongonococcal urethritis; cervicitis or vaginitis due to *Chlamydia trachomatis, Gardnerella (Haemophilus) vaginalis, Trichomonas, Candida,* and many other agents associated with sexually transmitted diseases; pelvic inflammatory disease, arthritis, proctitis, and skin lesions. Often, several such agents coexist in a patient. Reiter's disease (urethritis, conjunctivitis, arthritis) may mimic gonorrhea or coexist with it.

Complications

The forms of local extension of the initial infection have been described. Systemic complications follow the dissemination of gonococci from the primary site (eg, genital tract) via the bloodstream. Gonococci that produce bacteremia and dissemination are resistant to serum but usually very sensitive to penicillin. They belong to certain nutritionally deficient auxotypes. In contrast, strains producing local gonorrhea are susceptible to the bactericidal action of serum but often drug-resistant. Gonococcal bacteremia is associated with intermittent fever, arthralgia, and skin lesions ranging from maculopapular to pustular or hemorrhagic. Rarely, gonococcal endocarditis or meningitis develops. Arthritis and tenosynovitis are common complications, particularly involving the knees, ankles, and wrists. Several joints are commonly involved. Gonococci can be isolated from less than half of patients with gonococcal arthritis. In the others, some immunologic reaction may be responsible. Gonococcal arthritis may be accompanied by iritis or conjunctivitis, with negative cultures. The most common form of eye involvement is direct inoculation of gonococci into the conjunctival sac. This may occur during passage through an infected birth canal, leading to ophthalmia neonatorum, or by autoinoculation of a person with genital infection. The purulent conjunctivitis may rapidly progress to panophthalmitis and loss of the eye unless treated promptly.

Prevention

Prevention is based on education, mechanical or chemical prophylaxis, and early diagnosis and treatment. The condom, if properly used, can reduce the risk of infection. Effective drugs taken in therapeutic doses within 24 hours of exposure can abort an infection, but prophylaxis with penicillin is no longer effective; in fact, penicillin prophylaxis contributes to the selection of penicillinase-producing gonococci. Intensive search for sex contacts by public health agencies must rely on physician reporting. Contacts are sometimes given full treatment for gonorrhea on epidemiologic grounds, without individual diagnosis, to reduce the reservoir of infection.

Ophthalmic infection of the newborn is prevented by the instillation of an adequate prophylactic agent (1% silver nitrate solution or 1% tetracycline ointment or erythromycin ointment) into each conjunctival sac immediately after birth.

Treatment

A. Uncomplicated Gonorrhea (Urethral, Cer-

vical, Pharyngeal, Rectal): (For both men and women.) Aqueous procaine penicillin G, 4.8 million units injected intramuscularly into 2 or more sites at one visit, together with 1 g probenecid orally given prior to injections. This treatment can also be effective in aborting syphilis within 2 weeks after infection.

An alternative treatment—particularly if coexistent chlamydial infection is suspected—consists of tetracycline hydrochloride, 500 mg orally 4 times daily for 7 days. Another alternative is amoxicillin, 3 g orally, together with 1 g of probenecid orally, just once, followed by tetracycline as above.

B. Penicillin-Resistant Gonorrhea: β-Lactamase-producing gonococci now exist in many countries. Their incidence is particularly high in West Africa and Southeast Asia but still relatively low in the USA. For such infections, the drug of choice is either spectinomycin, 2 g intramuscularly, or cefoxitin, 2 g intramuscularly, with probenecid, 1 g orally, or cefotaxime, 1 g intramuscularly, just once. Pharyngeal infections with β-lactamase-producing gonococci should be treated with a single daily dose of 9 tablets of trimethoprim-sulfamethoxazole for 5 days.

C. Follow-up Treatment: It is probable that multiple-dose oral treatment has much lower patient compliance than single-dose parenteral treatment. Urethral, rectal, or pharyngeal specimens should be obtained from men 7 days after completion of treatment. Cervical, rectal, or pharyngeal specimens should be obtained from women 7–14 days after the end of treatment. Serologic tests for syphilis are desirable 1 and 3 months later.

D. Treatment of Complications: In general, salpingitis, prostatitis, epididymitis, bacteremia, arthritis, eye infections, and other complications are treated with penicillin G, 10 million units daily for 3–4 days or until improved, and then amoxicillin, 0.5 g orally 4 times daily to complete 10 days of treatment. Postgonococcal urethritis and chlamydial urethritis exhibit persisting signs and symptoms after adequate therapy for gonorrhea and no further evidence of gonococci. Treatment should be with tetracycline, 0.5 g orally, or erythromycin, 0.5 g orally, 4 times daily for 10 days. Gonococcal ophthalmia requires topical in addition to systemic penicillin. For pelvic inflammatory disease occurring during infection with penicillinase-producing gonococci, cefoxitin, 2 g intravenously every 6 hours for 5–10 days, has been recommended.

Additional supportive treatment is needed for most complications. Prostatitis may be relieved by hot sitz baths or diathermy; acute epididymitis requires bed rest, cold and support to the scrotum, and analgesics. Acute salpingitis requires bed rest during the acute stage, and surgical evaluation if chronic pain and signs of inflammation continue. Aspiration of joints may be necessary to relieve high pressure; physical therapy should be instituted when inflammation subsides.

Prognosis

The regimens given above cure 95% of acute gonococcal infections, although the steady rise in resistance to drugs is responsible for an increasing number of relapses that require re-treatment. The complications of gonorrhea may cause irreversible damage (urethral stricture, persistent tubo-ovarian abscess, valve destruction in endocarditis, peritoneal adhesions with intestinal obstruction, sterility, etc) requiring surgical treatment.

Follow-up examinations cannot distinguish failures of chemotherapy from reinfection. Futhermore, the patient with acute gonorrhea may have undetected syphilis, genital herpes, or chlamydial infection from the same exposure or from more than one infected source. All of these must be detected by laboratory procedures in repeated follow-up. The recommended parenteral penicillin schedule is probably curative for most cases of coexisting syphilis. Patients treated with other antimicrobials will require additional penicillin treatment if serologic tests for syphilis become positive during 4 months following treatment for gonorrhea.

Brooks GF et al: Repeated gonorrhea: An analysis of importance and risk factors. *J Infect Dis* 1978;**137**:161.

Centers for Disease Control: *Sexually Transmitted Diseases Treatment Guidelines, 1982. MMWR* (Aug 20) 1982;**31**:35S.

Jaffe HW et al: Infections due to penicillinase-producing *Neisseria gonorrheae* in the United States. *J Infect Dis* 1981; **144**:191.

Tice AW, Rodriguez MVL: Pharyngeal gonorrhea. *JAMA* 1981; **246**:2717.

Treatment of sexually transmitted diseases. *Med Lett Drugs Ther* 1984;**26**:5.

GRANULOMA INGUINALE

Granuloma inguinale is a chronic, relapsing granulomatous anogenital infection due to *Calymmatobacterium (Donovania) granulomatis,* which is related to *Klebsiella* and occurs intracellularly. The pathognomonic cell, found in tissue scrapings or secretions, is large (25–90 μm) and contains intracytoplasmic cysts filled with bodies (Donovan bodies) that stain deeply with Wright's stain.

The incubation period is 8 days to 12 weeks.

The onset is insidious. The lesions occur on the skin or mucous membranes of the genitalia or perineal area. They are relatively painless infiltrated nodules that soon slough. A shallow, sharply demarcated ulcer forms, with beefy-red friable base of granulation tissue. The lesion spreads by contiguity. The advancing border has a characteristic rolled edge of granulation tissue. Large ulcerations may advance onto the lower abdomen and thighs. Scar formation and healing may occur along one border while the opposite border advances. The process may become indolent and stationary.

The characteristic Donovan bodies are found in scrapings from the ulcer base or on histologic sections. The microorganism may also be cultured on special media. A specific complement fixation test is not widely available.

Superinfection with spirochete-fusiform organisms is common. The ulcer then becomes purulent, painful, foul-smelling, and extremely difficult to treat. Other venereal diseases may coexist. Rare complications include superimposed malignancy and secondary elephantoid swelling of the genitalia.

Initial treatment consists of tetracycline or ampicillin, 2 g orally daily for 2 weeks.

With antimicrobial therapy, most cases can be cured. In resistant or untreated cases, massive extension of the lesion may occur, with resulting anemia, cachexia, and death.

Washing the genitalia with soap and water immediately after intercourse may reduce the likelihood of infection. A serologic test for syphilis must be performed to rule out the existence of this disease.

Kuberski T: Granuloma inguinale. *Sex Transm Dis* 1980;7:29.

BARTONELLOSIS
(Oroya Fever, Carrión's Disease)

Bartonellosis, an acute or chronic infection that occurs in the high Andean valleys of Colombia, Ecuador, and Peru, is caused by a gram-negative, very pleomorphic bacterium (*Bartonella bacilliformis*), which is transmitted to humans by the bite of *Phlebotomus*. The organism is parasitic in humans in red cells and cells of the reticuloendothelial system. The initial stage (Oroya fever) exhibits intermittent or remittent fever, malaise, headache, and bone and joint pains. The disease becomes more apparent with the rapid progression of severe macrocytic anemia, hemorrhagic lymph nodes, and hepatosplenomegaly. Masses of organisms fill the cytoplasm of vascular endothelial cells, resulting in occlusion and thrombosis. In favorable cases, Oroya fever lasts 2–6 weeks and subsides. In those who survive, the eruptive stage of the disease (verruga peruana) commonly begins 2–8 weeks later. Verruga may also appear in the absence of Oroya fever, possibly because of a mild, subclinical first stage. Multiple miliary and nodular hemangiomas appear in crops, particularly on the face and limbs. The lesions bleed easily, sometimes ulcerate, usually persist for 1–12 months, finally heal without scar formation, and produce little systemic reaction. In early Oroya fever, the organisms are best demonstrated by blood culture. Later, *Bartonella* organisms appear in red cells in large numbers. The severe macrocytic, hypochromic anemia (hemoglobin as low as 3–5 g) of Oroya fever is accompanied by jaundice, marked reticulocytosis, and numerous megaloblasts and normoblasts. In verrugous lesions, the organisms may be demonstrated in endothelial cells.

Chloramphenicol or a tetracycline, 2 g daily orally, has been effective and has reduced the mortality rate in these patients. Transfusion may be necessary if the anemia is severe. The *Phlebotomus* vector should be controlled.

Dooley JR: Haemotropic bacteria in man. *Lancet* 1980;2:1237.

Schultz MG: A history of bartonellosis (Carrión's disease). *Am J Trop Med Hyg* 1968;17:503.

CHLAMYDIAL INFECTIONS

Chlamydiae are a large group of obligate intracellular parasites closely related to gram-negative bacteria. They are assigned to 2 species—*Chlamydia psittaci* and *Chlamydia trachomatis*—on the basis of intracellular inclusions, sulfonamide susceptibility, antigenic composition, and disease production. *C psittaci* causes psittacosis in humans and many animal diseases. *C trachomatis* causes many different human infections involving the eye (trachoma, inclusion conjunctivitis), the genital tract (lymphogranuloma venereum, nongonococcal urethritis, cervicitis, salpingitis), or the respiratory tract (pneumonitis). A few specific diseases are described.

LYMPHOGRANULOMA VENEREUM

Essentials of Diagnosis

- Evanescent primary genital lesion.
- Lymph node enlargement, softening, and suppuration, with draining sinuses.
- Proctitis and rectal stricture in women or homosexual men.
- Systemic, joint, eye, and central nervous system involvement may occur.
- Positive complement fixation test and sometimes positive skin test.
- Elevated serum globulin.

General Considerations

Lymphogranuloma venereum is an acute and chronic sexually transmitted disease caused by *Chlamydia trachomatis* types L_1–L_3. After the genital lesion disappears, the infection spreads to lymph channels and lymph nodes of the genital and rectal areas. The disease is acquired during intercourse or through contact with contaminated exudate from active lesions. The incubation period is 5–21 days. Inapparent infections and latent disease are not uncommon in promiscuous individuals.

Clinical Findings

A. Symptoms and Signs: In men, the initial vesicular or ulcerative lesion (on the external genitalia) is evanescent and often goes unnoticed. Inguinal buboes appear 1–4 weeks after exposure, are often bilateral, and have a tendency to fuse, soften, and break down to form multiple draining sinuses, with extensive scarring. Proctoscopic examination is important for diagnosis and in evaluating therapy. In women, the genital lymph drainage is to the perirectal glands. Early anorectal manifestations are proctitis with tenesmus and bloody purulent discharge; late manifestations are chronic cicatrizing inflammation of the rectal and perirectal tissue. These changes lead to obstipation and rectal stricture and, occasionally, rectovaginal and perianal fistulas. They are also seen in homosexual men.

Systemic invasion may occur, causing fever, arthralgia, arthritis, skin rashes, conjunctivitis, and iritis. Nervous system invasion causes headache and meningeal irritation.

B. Laboratory Findings: The intradermal skin test (Frei test) and the complement fixation test may be positive, but cross-reaction with other chlamydiae occurs. A positive reaction may reflect an old (healed) infection; however, high complement fixation titers usually imply active infection. Specific immunofluorescence tests for antibody can be performed. Skin tests with commercial antigens are unreliable. The serum globulin levels are greatly elevated in chronic lymphogranuloma venereum. A false-positive nontreponemal test for syphilis (VDRL) may be present.

Differential Diagnosis

The early lesion of lymphogranuloma venereum must be differentiated from the lesions of syphilis, genital herpes, and chancroid; lymph node involvement must be distinguished from that due to tularemia, tuberculosis, plague, neoplasm, or pyogenic infection; rectal stricture must be differentiated from that due to neoplasm and ulcerative colitis.

Complications

Lymphatic involvement and blocking may cause marked disfiguration of the external genitalia (elephantiasis) as well as extensive scarring. Rectal stricture resists treatment and may require colostomy.

Treatment

A. Specific Measures: The antibiotics of choice are the tetracyclines, 0.25–0.5 g orally 4 times daily, or minocycline, 0.1 g twice daily for 10–20 days. Sulfadiazine, 1 g 3 times daily for 2–3 weeks or longer, has little effect on the chlamydial infection but reduces bacterial complications.

B. Local and General Measures: Place the patient at bed rest, apply warm compresses to buboes, and give analgesics. Aspirate fluctuant nodes with aseptic care. Plastic operations may be necessary in the chronic anorectal form of the disease. Rectal strictures should be treated by prolonged gentle dilatation, although in some cases this may be impossible, and colon shunting procedures may be necessary.

Prognosis

Prompt early treatment will cure the disorder and prevent late complications; the longer treatment is delayed, the more difficult it is to eradicate the infection and to reverse the pathologic changes. There may be a higher incidence of rectal carcinoma in persons with anorectal lymphogranuloma venereum.

Quinn TC et al: *Chlamydia trachomatis* proctitis. *N Engl J Med* 1981;**305**:195.
Sowmini CN et al: Minocycline in the treatment of lymphogranuloma venereum. *J Am Vener Dis Assoc* 1976;**2**:19.
Walzer PD, Armstrong D: Lymphogranuloma venereum presenting as supraclavicular and inguinal lymphadenopathy. *Sex Transm Dis* 1977;**4**:12.

CHLAMYDIAL GENITAL & NEONATAL INFECTIONS

Some males develop symptomatic or asymptomatic anterior urethritis from which gonococci cannot be isolated by available laboratory tests. This is referred to as nongonococcal urethritis. *Chlamydia trachomatis* immunotypes D–K can be isolated in about 50% of such cases by appropriate techniques. In other cases, a mycoplasma, *Ureaplasma urealyticum,* can be grown as a possible etiologic agent. In still others, gonococcal urethritis is diagnosed and treated; afterwards, gonococci can no longer be found, but postgonococcal urethritis persists. Some of the latter cases can be attributed to chlamydiae or mycoplasmas that were present originally in a mixed infection. Occasionally, epididymitis, prostatitis, or proctitis is caused by chlamydial infection.

The female sexual partners of men with chlamydial nongonococcal urethritis often are infected with the same organisms symptomatically or asymptomatically. Chlamydiae are often recovered from the cervix, and there may be overt cervicitis, salpingitis, or pelvic inflammatory disease. Males or females with genital chlamydial infection may infect the eye through finger contact and develop a follicular conjunctivitis ("inclusion conjunctivitis") that may become chronic and lead to pannus formation.

If a pregnant woman has chlamydial genital tract infection, the baby often acquires chlamydiae during passage through the birth canal. This may remain asymptomatic or may lead to the appearance of neonatal inclusion conjunctivitis (see p 96) during the first 2 weeks after birth. This conjunctivitis in the newborn may regress spontaneously, after topical treatment of the eye, or may remain chronic and lead to permanent changes in the conjunctiva or cornea.

The newborn infected with chlamydiae may also develop involvement of the respiratory tract with chlamydial pneumonitis appearing during the first 2–6 months of life. This chlamydial pneumonitis (see p 143) is often afebrile and associated with eosinophilia, hyperinflation of the lungs, and marked hypoxia. Chlamydial pneumonitis has also been seen in immunosuppressed adults.

The diagnosis of chlamydial infection relies on the isolation of chlamydiae in specially treated cell cultures or on the demonstration of chlamydial particles by immunofluorescence (with monoclonal antibodies) in secretions or surface scrapings. Occasionally, there is a significant rise in specific antibodies in serum or secretions. Neonatal pneumonitis produces high titers of antichlamydial IgM antibody.

Proof or strong suspicion of chlamydial genital infection should lead to antimicrobial treatment of both sex partners. Drugs of choice are tetracycline HCl, 0.5 g 2–4 times daily for 2 weeks, or erythromycin, 0.5 g 2–3 times daily for 2 weeks. The latter is employed in pregnant females. Neonatal inclusion conjunctivitis can be managed by topical tetracycline into the conjunctival sac, but systemic erythromycin, 40 mg/kg/d, may be preferred if there is suspicion of active chlamydial pneumonitis.

Nongonococcal urethritis not caused by chlamydiae but associated with *Ureaplasma* has been linked to infertility. It may be treated with trimethoprim-sulfamethoxazole, 2 tablets twice daily, or doxycycline, 0.1 g twice daily, for 2 weeks.

Alexander ER, Harrison MR: Role of *Chlamydia trachomatis* in perinatal infection. *Rev Infect Dis* 1983;**5**:713.

Bowie WR et al: Etiology of nongonococcal urethritis. *J Clin Invest* 1977;**59**:735.

Jones RB et al: Subacute chlamydial endocarditis. *JAMA* 1982;**247**:655.

Mardh PA et al: *Chlamydia trachomatis* in patients with salpingitis. *N Engl J Med* 1977;**296**:1377.

Mordhorst CH et al: Childhood trachoma in a nonendemic area. *JAMA* 1978;**239**:1765.

Oriel JD et al: Chlamydial infections of the uterine cervix with *Chlamydia trachomatis*. *J Infect Dis* 1978;**137**:443.

Schachter J: Chlamydial infections. (3 parts.) *N Engl J Med* 1978; **298**:428, 490, 540.

Taylor-Robinson D, McCormack WM: The genital mycoplasmas. (2 parts.) *N Engl J Med* 1980;**302**:1003, 1063.

Tipple MA et al: Clinical characteristics of the afebrile pneumonia associated with *C trachomatis* infection in infants less than 6 months of age. *Pediatrics* 1979;**63**:192.

PSITTACOSIS
(Ornithosis)

Essentials of Diagnosis

- Fever, chills, malaise, prostration; cough, epistaxis; occasionally, rose spots and splenomegaly.
- Slightly delayed appearance of signs of pneumonitis.
- Isolation of chlamydiae or rising titer of complement-fixing antibodies.
- Contact with infected bird (psittacine, pigeons, many others) 7–15 days previously.

General Considerations

Psittacosis is acquired from contact with birds (parrots, parakeets, pigeons, chickens, ducks, and many others). Human-to-human spread is rare.

Clinical Findings

A. Symptoms and Signs: The onset is usually rapid, with fever, chills, headache, backache, malaise, myalgia, epistaxis, dry cough, and prostration. Signs include those of pneumonitis, alteration of percussion note and breath sounds, and rales. Pulmonary findings may be absent early. Rose spots, splenomegaly, and meningismus are occasionally seen. Delirium, constipation or diarrhea, and abdominal distress may occur. Dyspnea and cyanosis may occur later.

B. Laboratory Findings: The white count is normal or decreased, often with a shift to the left. Proteinuria is frequently present. The organism may be isolated from the blood and sputum by inoculation of mice or cell cultures. Antibodies appear during the second week and can be demonstrated by complement fixation or immunofluorescence. Antibody response may be suppressed by early chemotherapy.

C. X-Ray Findings: The x-ray findings in psittacosis are those of central pneumonia that later becomes widespread or migratory. Psittacosis is indistinguishable from viral pneumonias by x-ray.

Differential Diagnosis

This disease can be differentiated from acute viral, mycoplasmal, or rickettsial pneumonias only by the history of contact with potentially infected birds and by laboratory tests. Rose spots and leukopenia suggest typhoid fever.

Complications

Myocarditis, secondary bacterial pneumonia.

Treatment

Treatment consists of giving tetracycline, 0.5 g orally every 6 hours or 0.5 g intravenously every 12 hours for 14–21 days. Give oxygen and sedation as required.

Prognosis

Psittacosis may vary from a mild respiratory infection (especially in children) to a severe, protracted illness. The mortality rate with early treatment is very low.

Byrum NP et al: Fulminant psittacosais. *Lancet* 1979;**1**:353.

Schachter J et al: Psittacosis: The reservoir persists. *J Infect Dis* 1978;**137**:44.

● ● ●

25 | Infectious Diseases: Spirochetal

Moses Grossman, MD, & Ernest Jawetz, MD, PhD

SYPHILIS

NATURAL HISTORY & PRINCIPLES OF DIAGNOSIS & TREATMENT

Syphilis is a complex infectious disease caused by *Treponema pallidum,* a spirochete capable of infecting any organ or tissue in the body and causing protean clinical manifestations. Transmission occurs most frequently during sexual contact, through minor skin or mucosal lesions; sites of inoculation are usually genital but may be extragenital. The organism is extremely sensitive to heat and drying but can survive for days in fluids; therefore, it can be transmitted in blood from infected persons. Syphilis can be transferred via the placenta from mother to fetus after the tenth week of pregnancy (congenital syphilis).

The immunologic response to infection is complex, but it provides the basis for most clinical diagnoses. The infection induces the synthesis of a number of antibodies, some of which react specifically with pathogenic treponemes and some with components of normal tissues (see below). If the disease is untreated, sufficient defenses develop to produce a relative resistance to reinfection; however, in most cases these immune reactions fail to eradicate existing infection and may contribute to tissue destruction in the late stages. Patients treated early in the disease are fully susceptible to reinfection.

The natural history of acquired syphilis is generally divided into 2 major clinical stages: (1) early, or infectious, syphilis and (2) late syphilis. The 2 stages are separated by a symptom-free latent phase during the first part of which (early latency) the infectious stage is liable to recur. Infectious syphilis includes the primary lesions (chancre and regional lymphadenopathy); the secondary lesions (commonly involving skin and mucous membranes, occasionally bone, central nervous system, or liver); relapsing lesions during early latency; and congenital lesions. The hallmark of these lesions is an abundance of spirochetes; tissue reaction is usually minimal. Late syphilis consists of so-called benign (gummatous) lesions involving skin, bones, and viscera; cardiovascular disease (principally aortitis); and a variety of central nervous system and ocular syndromes. These forms of syphilis are not contagious. The lesions contain few demonstrable spirochetes, but tissue reactivity (vasculitis, necrosis) is severe and suggestive of hypersensitivity phenomena.

Intensive public health efforts during and after World War II resulted in a marked reduction in infectious syphilis. Subsequently, however, this emphasis on sexually transmitted diseases declined, and funds for their control were markedly reduced. As a consequence, in the late 1950s, there again developed a rising incidence of early syphilis and other sexually transmitted diseases. In the 1960s, the incidence of early infectious syphilis declined, perhaps as a result of extensive use of penicillin during the ongoing gonorrhea epidemic. In the late 1970s, the frequency of reported early infectious syphilis increased again, perhaps as a result of more responsible reporting by physicians and more vigorous case-finding by public health agencies attempting to bring untreated patients to therapy. In the 1980s, the incidence of infectious syphilis is particularly high among homosexual males. Reinfection in treated persons is common. No appreciable rise in the incidence of congenital syphilis has been reported yet.

No vaccine against syphilis exists now or is likely to become available soon.

Laboratory Diagnosis

Since the infectious agent of syphilis cannot be cultured in vitro, diagnostic measures are confined principally to serologic testing, microscopic detection of *T pallidum* in lesions, and other examinations (biopsies, lumbar puncture, x-rays) for evidence of tissue damage.

A. Serologic Tests for Syphilis: There are 2 general categories of serologic tests for syphilis: (1) nontreponemal tests, which use a component of normal tissue (eg, beef heart cardiolipin) as an antigen to measure nonspecific antibodies (reagin) formed in the blood of patients with syphilis; and (2) treponemal tests, which employ live or killed *T pallidum* as antigen to detect antibodies specific for pathogenic treponemes.

1. Nontreponemal antigen tests–Commonly employed nontreponemal antigen tests are of 2 types:

(1) flocculation (VDRL, RPR) and (2) complement fixation (Kolmer, Wassermann). The flocculation tests are easy, rapid, and inexpensive to perform and are therefore used primarily for routine (often automated) screening for syphilis. Quantitative expression of the reactivity of the serum, based upon titration of dilutions of serum, may be valuable in establishing the diagnosis and in evaluating the efficacy of treatment.

The VDRL test (the nontreponemal test in widest use) generally becomes positive 4–6 weeks after infection, or 1–3 weeks after the appearance of a primary lesion; it is almost invariably positive in the secondary stage. The VDRL titer is usually high (> 1:32) in secondary syphilis and tends to be lower (< 1:4) or even negative in late forms of syphilis. A falling titer in treated early or latent syphilis suggests satisfactory response to treatment. These serologic tests are not highly specific and must be closely correlated with other clinical and laboratory findings. The tests are positive in patients with nonvenereal treponematoses (see below). More importantly, "false-positive" serologic reactions are frequently encountered in a wide variety of nontreponemal states including collagen diseases, infectious mononucleosis, malaria, many febrile diseases, leprosy, vaccination, drug addiction, old age, and possibly pregnancy. False-positive reactions are usually of low titer and transient and may be distinguished from true positives by specific treponemal antibody tests. The rapid plasma reagin (RPR) test is a simple, rapid, and reliable substitute for the traditional VDRL test and gives comparable results. It is suitable for automated screening tests.

2. Treponemal antibody tests–The fluorescent treponemal antibody absorption (FTA-ABS) test is the most widely employed treponemal test. It measures antibodies capable of reacting with killed *T pallidum* after absorption of the patient's serum with extracts of nonpathogenic treponemes. The FTA-ABS test is of value principally in determining whether a positive nontreponemal antigen test is "false-positive" or is indicative of syphilis. Because of its great sensitivity, particularly in the late stages of the disease, the FTA-ABS test is also of value when there is clinical evidence of syphilis but the routine serologic test for syphilis is negative. The test is positive in most patients with primary and in virtually all with secondary syphilis, and it usually remains positive permanently in spite of successful treatment. False-positive FTA-ABS tests occur rarely in systemic lupus erythematosus and in other disorders associated with abnormal globulins. A treponemal passive hemagglutination (TPHA) test is comparable in specificity and sensitivity to the FTA-ABS test but may become positive somewhat later in infection.

Final decision about the significance of the results of serologic tests for syphilis must be based upon a total clinical appraisal.

B. Microscopic Examination: In infectious syphilis, *T pallidum* may be shown by darkfield microscopic examination of fresh exudate from lesions or material aspirated from regional lymph nodes. The darkfield examination requires considerable experience and care in the proper collection of specimens and in the identification of pathogenic spirochetes by characteristic morphology and motility. Repeated examinations may be necessary. Spirochetes usually are not found in late syphilitic lesions by this technique.

An immunofluorescent staining technique for demonstrating *T pallidum* in dried smears of fluid taken from early syphilitic lesions is available. Slides are fixed and treated with fluorescein-labeled antitreponemal antibody that has been preabsorbed with nonpathogenic treponemes. The slides are then examined for fluorescing spirochetes in an ultraviolet microscope. Because of its simplicity and convenience to physicians (slides can be mailed), this technique has replaced darkfield microscopy in most health departments and medical center laboratories.

C. Spinal Fluid Examination: The cerebrospinal fluid findings in neurosyphilis usually consist of elevation of total protein and gamma globulins, increase in the cell count, and a positive reagin test (VDRL). False-positive reagin tests rarely occur in the cerebrospinal fluid. Improvement of the cerebrospinal fluid findings is of great prognostic value.

Cerebrospinal fluid examination is mandatory in all cases of secondary syphilis or latent syphilis not previously adequately treated. Asymptomatic neurosyphilis (ie, positive cerebrospinal fluid findings without symptoms) requires prolonged penicillin treatment as given for symptomatic neurosyphilis. Adequate treatment is indicated by gradual decrease in cerebrospinal fluid cell count, protein concentration, and VDRL titer. Rarely, serologic tests of cerebrospinal fluid may remain positive for years after adequate treatment of neurosyphilis even though all other parameters have returned to normal. In the presence of high-titer serum FTA-ABS, there may be a positive FTA test on cerebrospinal fluid without evidence of neurosyphilis.

Treatment
A. Specific Measures:
1. Penicillin, as benzathine penicillin G or aqueous procaine penicillin G, is the drug of choice for all forms of syphilis and other spirochetal infections. Effective tissue levels must be maintained for several days or weeks because of the spirochete's long generation time. Penicillin is highly effective in early infections and variably effective in the late stages. The principal contraindication is hypersensitivity to the penicillins. The recommended treatment schedules are included below in the discussion of the various forms of syphilis.

2. Other antibiotic therapy–Oral tetracyclines and erythromycins are effective in the treatment of syphilis for patients who are sensitive to penicillin. Tetracycline, 30–40 g, or erythromycin, 30–40 g, is given over a period of 10–15 days in early syphilis; twice as much is recommended for syphilis of more than 1 year's duration. Since experience with these antibiotics in the treatment of syphilis is limited, careful follow-up is necessary.

B. Local Measures (Mucocutaneous Lesions): Local treatment is usually not necessary. No local antiseptics or other chemicals should be applied to a suspected syphilitic lesion until specimens for microscopy have been obtained.

C. Public Health Measures: Patients with infectious syphilis must abstain from sexual activity until rendered noninfectious by antibiotic therapy. All cases of syphilis must be reported to the appropriate public health agency for assistance in identifying, investigating, and treating all contacts.

D. Epidemiologic Treatment: Patients who have been exposed to infectious syphilis within the preceding 3 months, as well as others who on epidemiologic grounds present a high risk for syphilis, should be treated as for early syphilis. Every effort should be made to establish a diagnosis in these persons.

Complications of Specific Therapy

The Jarisch-Herxheimer reaction is ascribed to the sudden massive destruction of spirochetes by drugs and release of toxic products and is manifested by fever and aggravation of the existing clinical picture. It is most likely to occur in early syphilis. Treatment should not be discontinued unless the symptoms become severe or threaten to be fatal or unless syphilitic laryngitis, auditory neuritis, or labyrinthitis is present, since the reaction may cause irreversible damage in these circumstances.

The reaction may be prevented or modified by simultaneous administration of corticosteroids. It usually begins within the first 24 hours and subsides spontaneously within the next 24 hours of penicillin treatment.

Follow-Up

Patients who receive treatment for early syphilis should be followed clinically and with periodic quantitative VDRL tests for at least 1 year. Patients with all other types of syphilis should be under similar observation for 2 or more years.

Prevention

Avoidance of sexual contact is the only reliable method of prophylaxis but is an impractical public health measure for obvious reasons.

A. Mechanical: The standard rubber condom is effective but protects covered parts only. The exposed parts should be washed with soap and water as soon after contact as possible. This applies to both sexes.

B. Antibiotic: If there is known exposure to infectious syphilis, abortive penicillin therapy may be used. Give 2.4 million units of procaine penicillin G intramuscularly in each buttock once. Treatment of gonococcal infection with penicillins is probably effective against incubating syphilis in most cases. However, other antimicrobial agents (eg, spectinomycin) may be ineffective in aborting preclinical syphilis. In view of the increasing use of antibiotics other than

penicillin for gonococcal disease, patients treated for gonorrhea should have a serologic test for syphilis 3–6 months after treatment.

C. Vaccine: An effective vaccine against syphilis is not yet available.

Course & Prognosis

The lesions associated with primary and secondary syphilis are self-limiting and resolve with few or no residua. Late syphilis may be highly destructive and permanently disabling and may lead to death. With treatment, the nontreponemal serologic tests usually return to negative in early syphilis. In late latent and late syphilis, serofastness is not uncommon even after adequate treatment. In broad terms, if no treatment is given, about one-third of people infected with syphilis will undergo spontaneous cure, about one-third will remain in the latent phase throughout life, and about one-third will develop serious late lesions.

Centers for Disease Control: Sexually transmitted diseases: Treatment guidelines 1982. *MMWR* (Aug 20) 1982;**31**:35S.

Fiumara NJ: Treatment of primary and secondary syphilis: Serological response. *JAMA* 1980;**243**:2500.

Jaffe HW et al: Tests for treponemal antibody in CSF. *Arch Intern Med* 1978;**138**:252.

Johnson RC: The spirochetes. *Annu Rev Microbiol* 1977;**31**:89.

Lee TJ, Sparling PF: Syphilis: An algorithm. *JAMA* 1979;**242**:1187.

CLINICAL STAGES OF SYPHILIS

1. PRIMARY SYPHILIS

Essentials of Diagnosis

- History of sexual contact (often unreliable).
- Painless ulcer on genitalia, perianal area, rectum, pharynx, tongue, lip, or elsewhere 2–6 weeks after exposure.
- Nontender enlargement of regional lymph nodes.
- Fluid expressed from lesion contains *T pallidum* by immunofluorescence or darkfield microscopy.
- Serologic test for syphilis often positive.

General Considerations

This is the stage of invasion and may pass unrecognized. The typical lesion is the chancre at the site or sites of inoculation, most frequently located on the penis, labia, cervix, or anorectal region. Anorectal lesions are especially common among male homosexuals. The primary lesion occurs occasionally in the oropharynx (lip, tongue, or tonsil) and rarely on the breast or finger. The chancre starts as a small erosion 10–90 days (average, 3–4 weeks) after inoculation that rapidly develops into a painless superficial ulcer with a clean base and firm, indurated margins, associated with enlargement of regional lymph nodes, which are rubbery, discrete, and nontender. Bacterial infection of the chancre may occur and may lead to pain. Healing occurs without treatment, but a scar may form, especially with secondary infection.

Laboratory Findings

The serologic test for syphilis is usually positive 1–2 weeks after the primary lesion is noted; rising titers are especially significant when there is a history of previous infection. Immunofluorescence or dark-field microscopy shows treponemes in at least 95% of chancres. The spinal fluid is normal at this stage.

The syphilitic chancre may be confused with chancroid, lymphogranuloma venereum, genital herpes, or neoplasm. Any lesion on the genitalia should be considered a possible primary syphilitic lesion.

Treatment

Give benzathine penicillin G, 1.2 million units in each buttock for a total dose of 2.4 million units once. Sometimes a dose of the same size is given twice more at weekly intervals, especially when a typical lesion was not observed by the physician. Other regimens of penicillin, or other drugs, are less desirable.

Fiumara NJ: Treatment of seropositive primary syphilis: An evaluation of 196 patients. *Sex Transm Dis* 1977;**4**:92.

2. SECONDARY SYPHILIS

Essentials of Diagnosis

- Generalized maculopapular skin rash.
- Mucous membrane lesions, including patches and ulcers.
- Weeping papules (condylomas) in moist skin areas.
- Generalized nontender lymphadenopathy.
- Fever.
- Meningitis, hepatitis, osteitis, arthritis, iritis.
- Many treponemes in scrapings of mucous membrane or skin lesions by immunofluorescence or darkfield microscopy.
- Serologic tests for syphilis always positive.

General Considerations & Treatment

The secondary stage of syphilis usually appears a few weeks (or up to 6 months) after development of the chancre, when sufficient dissemination of *T pallidum* has occurred to produce systemic signs (fever, lymphadenopathy) or infectious lesions at sites distant from the site of inoculation. The most common manifestations are skin and mucosal lesions. The skin lesions are nonpruritic, macular, papular, pustular, or follicular (or combinations of any of these types), although the maculopapular rash is the most common. The skin lesions usually are generalized; involvement of the palms and soles is especially suspicious. Annular lesions simulating ringworm are observed in blacks. Mucous membrane lesions range from ulcers and papules of the lips, mouth, throat, genitalia, and anus ("mucous patches") to a diffuse redness of the pharynx. Both skin and mucous membrane lesions are highly infectious at this stage. Specific lesions — **condylomata lata**—are fused, weeping papules on the moist areas of the skin and mucous membranes.

Meningeal, hepatic, renal, bone, and joint invasion with resulting cranial nerve palsies, jaundice, nephrotic syndrome, and periostitis may occur. Alopecia (moth-eaten appearance), iritis, and iridocyclitis may also occur. A transient myocarditis may be manifested by temporary electrocardiographic changes.

All serologic tests for syphilis are positive in almost all cases. The cutaneous and mucous membrane lesions often show *T pallidum* on microscopic examination. There is usually a transient cerebrospinal fluid involvement, with pleocytosis and elevated protein, although only 5% of cases have positive serologic cerebrospinal fluid reactions. There may be evidence of hepatitis or nephritis (immune complex type).

Skin lesions may be confused with the infectious exanthems, pityriasis rosea, and drug eruptions. Visceral lesions may suggest nephritis or hepatitis due to other causes. The diffusely red throat may mimic other forms of pharyngitis.

Treatment is as for primary syphilis unless central nervous system disease is present, in which case treatment is as for neurosyphilis (see below). Isolation of the patient is important.

Fiumara NJ: Treatment of secondary syphilis: An evaluation of 204 patients. *Sex Transm Dis* 1977;**4**:96.

Gamble CN, Readan JB: Immunopathology of syphilitic glomerulonephritis. *N Engl J Med* 1975;**292**:449.

3. RELAPSING SYPHILIS

The essentials of diagnosis are the same as in secondary syphilis.

The lesions of secondary syphilis heal spontaneously, but secondary syphilis may relapse if undiagnosed or inadequately treated. These relapses may include any of the findings noted under secondary syphilis: skin and mucous membrane, neurologic, ocular, bone, or visceral. Unlike the usual asymptomatic neurologic involvement of secondary syphilis, neurologic relapses may be fulminating, leading to death. Relapse is almost always accompanied by a rising titer in quantitative serologic tests; indeed, a rising titer may be the first or only evidence of relapse. About 70% of relapses occur during the first year after infection.

Treatment is as for primary syphilis unless central nervous system disease is present.

4. LATENT ("HIDDEN") SYPHILIS

Essentials of Diagnosis

- No physical signs.
- History of syphilis with inadequate treatment.
- Positive treponemal serologic tests for syphilis.

General Considerations & Treatment

Latent syphilis is the clinically quiescent phase during the interval after disappearance of secondary lesions and before the appearance of tertiary symptoms. Early latency is defined as the first 4 years after infection, during which time infectious lesions may recur ("relapsing syphilis"); after 4 years, the patient is said to be in the late latent phase. Transmission to the fetus, however, can probably occur in any phase. There are (by definition) no clinical manifestations during the latent phase, and the only significant laboratory findings are positive serologic tests. A diagnosis of latent syphilis is justified only when the cerebrospinal fluid is entirely negative, x-ray and physical examination shows no evidence of cardiovascular involvement, and false-positive tests for syphilis have been ruled out. The latent phase may last from months to a lifetime.

It is important to differentiate latent syphilis from a false-positive serologic test for syphilis, which can be due to the many causes listed above.

Treatment is with benzathine penicillin G, 2.4 million units 3 times at 7-day intervals. If there is evidence of cerebrospinal fluid involvement, treat as for neurosyphilis. Only a small percentage of serologic tests will be appreciably altered by treatment with penicillin. The treatment of this stage of the disease is intended to prevent the late sequelae.

Ducas J, Robson HG: Cerebrospinal fluid penicillin levels during therapy for latent syphilis. *JAMA* 1981;**246**:2583.

5. LATE (TERTIARY) SYPHILIS

Essentials of Diagnosis

- Infiltrative tumors of skin, bones, liver (gummas).
- Aortitis, aneurysms, aortic insufficiency.
- Central nervous system disorders, including meningovascular and degenerative changes, paresthesias, shooting pains, abnormal reflexes, dementia, or psychosis.

General Considerations

This stage may occur at any time after secondary syphilis, even after years of latency. Late lesions probably represent, at least in part, a delayed hypersensitivity reaction of the tissue to the organism and are usually divided into 2 types: (1) a localized gummatous reaction, with a relatively rapid onset and generally prompt response to therapy ("benign late syphilis"); and (2) diffuse inflammation of a more insidious onset that characteristically involves the central nervous system and large arteries, is often fatal if untreated, and is at best arrested by treatment. Gummas may involve any area or organ of the body but most often the skin or long bones. Cardiovascular disease is usually manifested by aortic aneurysm, aortic insufficiency, or aortitis. Various forms of diffuse or localized central nervous system involvement may occur.

Late syphilis must be differentiated from neoplasms of the skin, liver, lung, stomach, or brain; other forms of meningitis; and primary neurologic lesions.

Treatment is as for latent syphilis. Reversal of positive serologic tests does not usually occur. A second course of penicillin therapy may be given if necessary. There is no known method for reliable eradication of the treponeme from humans in the late stages of syphilis. Viable spirochetes are occasionally found in the eyes, in cerebrospinal fluid, and elsewhere in patients with "adequately" treated syphilis, but claims for their capacity to cause progressive disease are speculative.

Although almost any tissue and organ may be involved in late syphilis, the following are the most common types of involvement.

Skin

Cutaneous lesions of late syphilis are of 2 varieties: (1) multiple nodular lesions that eventually ulcerate or resolve by forming atrophic, pigmented scars; and (2) solitary gummas that start as painless subcutaneous nodules, then enlarge, attach to the overlying skin, and eventually ulcerate.

Mucous Membranes

Late lesions of the mucous membranes are nodular gummas or leukoplakia, highly destructive to the involved tissue.

Skeletal

Bone lesions are destructive, causing periostitis, osteitis, and arthritis with little or no associated redness or swelling but often marked myalgia and myositis of the neighboring muscles. The pain is especially severe at night.

Eyes

Late ocular lesions are gummatous iritis, chorioretinitis, optic atrophy, and cranial nerve palsies, in addition to the lesions of central nervous system syphilis.

Respiratory System

Respiratory involvement by late syphilis is caused by gummatous infiltrates into the larynx, trachea, and pulmonary parenchyma, producing discrete pulmonary densities. There may be hoarseness, respiratory distress, and wheezing secondary to the gummatous lesion itself or to subsequent stenosis occurring with healing.

Gastrointestinal System

Gummas involving the liver produce the usually benign, asymptomatic **hepar lobatum.** Infiltration into the stomach wall causes "leather bottle" stomach with epigastric distress, inability to eat large meals, regurgitation, belching, and weight loss. Occasionally a picture resembling Laennec's cirrhosis is produced by liver involvement.

Cardiovascular System
(See also p 261.)

Cardiovascular lesions (10–15% of late syphilitic lesions) are often progressive, disabling, and life-threatening. Central nervous system lesions are often present also. Involvement usually starts as an arteritis in the supracardiac portion of the aorta and progresses to cause one or more of the following: (1) Narrowing of the coronary ostia with resulting decreased coronary circulation, angina, cardiac insufficiency, and acute myocardial infarction. (2) Scarring of the aortic valves, producing aortic insufficiency with its water-hammer pulse, aortic diastolic murmur, frequently aortic systolic murmur, cardiac hypertrophy, and eventually congestive heart failure. (3) Weakness of the wall of the aorta, with saccular aneurysm formation and associated pressure symptoms of dysphagia, hoarseness, brassy cough, back pain (vertebral erosion), and occasionally rupture of the aneurysm. Recurrent respiratory infections are common as a result of pressure on the trachea and bronchi.

Treatment of cardiac problems requires first consideration, after which penicillin G is given as for latent syphilis.

Neurosyphilis

Neurosyphilis (15–20% of late syphilitic lesions; often present with cardiovascular syphilis) is, like cardiovascular syphilis, a progressive, disabling, and life-threatening complication. It develops more commonly in men than in women and in whites than in blacks. There are 4 clinical types.

(1) Asymptomatic neurosyphilis: This form is characterized by spinal fluid abnormalities (positive spinal fluid serology, increased cell count, occasionally increased protein) without symptoms or signs of neurologic involvement.

(2) Meningovascular syphilis: This form is characterized by meningeal involvement or changes in the vascular structures of the brain (or both), producing symptoms of low-grade meningitis (headache, irritability); cranial nerve palsies (basilar meningitis); unequal reflexes; irregular pupils with poor light and accommodation reflexes; and, when large vessels are involved, cerebrovascular accidents. The cerebrospinal fluid shows increased cells (100–1000/μL), elevated protein, and usually a positive serologic test for syphilis. The symptoms of acute meningitis are rare in late syphilis.

(3) Tabes dorsalis: This type of neurosyphilis is a chronic progressive degeneration of the parenchyma of the posterior columns of the spinal cord and of the posterior sensory ganglia and nerve roots. The symptoms and signs are impairment of proprioception and vibration sense, Argyll Robertson pupils (which react poorly to light but well to accommodation), and muscular hypotonia and hyporeflexia. Impairment of proprioception results in a wide-based gait and inability to walk in the dark. Paresthesias, analgesia, or sharp recurrent pains in the muscles of the leg ("shooting" or "lightning" pains) may occur. Crises are also common in tabes: gastric crises, consisting of sharp abdominal pains with nausea and vomiting (simulating an acute abdomen); laryngeal crises, with paroxysmal cough and dyspnea; urethral crises, with painful bladder spasms; and rectal and anal crises. Crises may begin suddenly, last for hours to days, and cease abruptly. Neurogenic bladder with overflow incontinence is also seen. Painless trophic ulcers may develop over pressure points on the feet. Joint damage may occur as a result of lack of sensory innervation (Charcot joint). The cerebrospinal fluid may have a normal or increased cell count (3–200/μL) and elevated protein, with variable results of serologic tests.

(4) General paresis: This is a generalized involvement of the cerebral cortex. The onset of clinical manifestations is insidious. There is usually a decrease in concentrating power, memory loss, dysarthria, tremor of the fingers and lips, irritability, and mild headaches. Most striking is the change of personality; the patient becomes slovenly, irresponsible, confused, and psychotic. Combinations of the various forms of neurosyphilis (especially tabes and paresis) are not uncommon. The cerebrospinal fluid findings resemble those of tabes dorsalis.

Special considerations in treatment of neurosyphilis. It is most important to prevent neurosyphilis by prompt diagnosis, adequate treatment, and followup of early syphilis. Involvement of the central nervous system must be considered in all cases except those that are treated early and effectively and followed. Lumbar puncture should be performed on all patients with syphilis in the secondary or later stages. In the presence of definite cerebrospinal fluid or neurologic abnormalities, treat for neurosyphilis. The pretreatment clinical and laboratory evaluation should include detailed neurologic, ocular, psychiatric, and cerebrospinal fluid examinations.

There is no simple established treatment schedule for neurosyphilis. The minimum acceptable therapy is as given for latent syphilis, but acute or treatment-resistant neurosyphilis is often treated with larger doses of short-acting penicillin (eg, aqueous penicillin G, 20 million units intravenously daily for 10–14 days).

All patients must have spinal fluid examinations at 3-month intervals for the first year and every 6 months for the second year following completion of antisyphilis therapy. The adequacy of response is at times difficult to evaluate (especially during a short period of observation), but it may be gauged by clinical improvement and effective and persistent reversal of cerebrospinal fluid changes. A second course of penicillin therapy may be given if necessary. Not infrequently, there is progression of neurologic symptoms and signs despite high and prolonged doses of penicillin. It has been postulated that these treatment failures are related to the unexplained persistence of viable *T pallidum* in central nervous system or ocular lesions in at least some cases.

Luxon L, Lees AJ, Greenwood RJ: Neurosyphilis today. *Lancet* 1979;**1**:90.

Tramont EC: Persistence of *T pallidum* following penicillin G therapy. *JAMA* 1976;**236**:2206.

6. SYPHILIS IN PREGNANCY

All pregnant women should have a nontreponemal serologic test for syphilis at the time of the first prenatal visit. Seroreactive patients should be evaluated promptly. Such evaluation includes the history (including prior therapy), a physical examination, a quantitative nontreponemal test, and a confirmatory treponemal test. If the FTA-ABS test is nonreactive and there is no clinical evidence of syphilis, treatment may be withheld. Both the quantitative nontreponemal test and the FTA-ABS test should be repeated in 4 weeks. If the diagnosis of syphilis cannot be excluded with reasonable certainty, the patient should be treated as outlined below.

Patients for whom there is documentation of adequate treatment for syphilis in the past need not be re-treated unless there is clinical or serologic evidence of reinfection (eg, 4-fold rise in titer of a quantitative nontreponemal test).

In women suspected of being at increased risk for syphilis, a second nontreponemal test should be performed during the third trimester.

The preferred treatment is with penicillin in dosage schedules appropriate for the stage of syphilis (see above). Penicillin prevents congenital syphilis in 90% of cases, even when treatment is given late in pregnancy.

For patients definitely known to be allergic to penicillin, the drug of second choice is erythromycin (base, stearate, or ethylsuccinate) in dosage schedules appropriate for the stage of syphilis. Such treatment is safe for the mother and the child, but the efficacy is not clearly established. Therefore, the documentation of penicillin allergy is particularly important before a decision is made not to use the first-choice drug. Erythromycin estolate and tetracycline are not recommended because of potential adverse effects on the mother and the fetus.

The infant should be evaluated immediately, as noted below, and at 6–8 weeks of age.

Centers for Disease Control: Sexually transmitted diseases: Treatment guidelines 1982. *MMWR* (Aug 20) 1982;**31**:35S.

Harter CA, Benirschke K: Fetal syphilis in the first trimester. *Am J Obstet Gynecol* 1976;**124**:705.

Jones JE Jr, Harris RE: Diagnostic evaluation of syphilis during pregnancy. *Obstet Gynecol* 1979;**124**:705.

7. CONGENITAL SYPHILIS

Congenital syphilis is a transplacentally transmitted infection that occurs in infants of untreated or inadequately treated mothers. The physical findings at birth are quite variable: The infant may have many or only minimal signs or even no signs until 6–8 weeks of life (delayed form). The most common findings are on the skin and mucous membranes—serous nasal discharge (snuffles), mucous membrane patches, maculopapular rash, condylomas. These lesions are infectious; *T pallidum* can easily be found microscopically, and the infant must be isolated. Other common findings are hepatosplenomegaly, anemia, or osteochondritis. These early active lesions subsequently heal, and if the disease is left untreated it produces the characteristic stigmas of syphilis—interstitial keratitis, Hutchinson's teeth, saddle nose, saber shins, deafness, and central nervous system involvement.

The serologic evaluation for syphilis in newborn infants is complicated by the transplacental acquisition of maternal antibody (IgG). Evaluation of a newborn suspected of having congenital syphilis includes the history of maternal therapy, a careful physical examination, hematocrit (for possible anemia), and x-rays of long bones. An FTA-ABS-IgM test detects the infant's own IgM antibody but is not invariably proof of treponemal activity in the infant. It is particularly important to follow the infant every 2–3 weeks over a period of 4 months to watch for developing physical signs; a sustained rise or fall in VDRL titer during this time will reveal the need for treatment.

Infants should be treated at birth if maternal treatment was inadequate, unknown, or done with drugs other than penicillin or if adequate follow-up of the infant cannot be assured.

Infants with congenital syphilis should always have a cerebrospinal fluid examination before therapy. If the diagnosis of congenital neurosyphilis cannot be excluded, the infant should be treated with aqueous penicillin G, 50,000 units/kg intramuscularly or intravenously daily in 2 divided doses for 10 days, or with aqueous procaine penicillin G, 50,000 units/kg intramuscularly daily for a minimum of 10 days. If the cerebrospinal fluid is perfectly normal, the infant may be treated with benzathine penicillin G, 50,000 units/kg intramuscularly in a single dose. Antibiotics other than penicillin are not recommended for congenital syphilis.

The quantitative nontreponemal test (VDRL) should be repeated 3, 6, and 12 months after therapy to establish falling titers.

Borobio MV, Nogales MC, Palomares JC: Value of serological diagnosis in congenital syphilis: Report of nine cases. *Br J Vener Dis* 1980;**56**:377.

Bryan EM, Nicholson E: Congenital syphilis. *Clin Pediatr* 1981; **20**:81.

NONVENEREAL TREPONEMATOSES

A variety of treponemal diseases other than syphilis occur endemically in many tropical areas of the world. They are distinguished from disease caused by *T pallidum* by their nonvenereal transmission, their relatively high incidence in certain geographic areas and among children, and their tendency to produce less severe visceral manifestations. As in syphilis, organisms can be demonstrated in infectious lesions with darkfield microscopy or immunofluorescence but cannot be cultured in artificial media; the serologic tests for syphilis are positive; the diseases have primary, secondary, and sometimes tertiary stages; and penicillin is the drug of choice. There is evidence that infection with these agents may provide partial resistance to syphilis and vice versa. Treatment with penicillin in doses appropriate to primary syphilis (eg, 2.4 million units of benzathine penicillin G intramuscularly) is generally curative in any stage of the nonvenereal treponematoses. In cases of penicillin hypersensitivity, tetracycline is usually the recommended alternative.

YAWS
(Frambesia)

Yaws is a contagious disease largely limited to tropical regions that is caused by *Treponema pertenue*. It is characterized by granulomatous lesions of the skin, mucous membranes, and bone. Yaws is rarely fatal, although if untreated it may lead to chronic disability and disfigurement. Yaws is acquired by direct nonvenereal contact, usually in childhood, although it may occur at any age. The "mother yaw," a painless papule that later ulcerates, appears 3–4 weeks after exposure. There is usually associated regional lymphadenopathy. Six to 12 weeks later, similar secondary lesions appear and last for several months or years. Painful ulcerated lesions on the soles are frequent and are called "crab yaws." Late gummatous lesions may occur, with associated tissue destruction involving large areas of skin and subcutaneous tissues. The late effects of yaws, with bone change, shortening of digits, and contractions, may be confused with similar changes occurring in leprosy. Central nervous system, cardiac, or other visceral involvement is rare.

Hopkins DR: Yaws in the Americas, 1950–1975. *J Infect Dis* 1977;**136**:548.

PINTA

Pinta is a nonvenereal spirochetal infection caused by *Treponema carateum*. It occurs endemically in rural areas of Latin America, especially in Mexico, Colombia, and Cuba, and in some areas of the Pacific. A nonulcerative, erythematous primary papule spreads slowly into a papulosquamous plaque showing a variety of color changes (slate, lilac, black). Secondary lesions resemble the primary one and appear within a year after it. These appear successively, new lesions together with older ones; are commonest

on the extremities; and later show atrophy and depigmentation. Some cases show pigment changes and atrophic patches on the soles and palms, with or without hyperkeratosis, that are indistinguishable from "crab yaws." Very rarely, central nervous system or cardiovascular disease is observed late in the course of infection.

ENDEMIC SYPHILIS
(Bejel, Skerljevo, Etc)

Endemic syphilis is an acute and chronic infection caused by an organism indistinguishable from *T pallidum*. It has been reported in a number of countries, particularly in the eastern Mediterranean area, often with local names: bejel in Syria and Iraq; skerljevo in Bosnia; and dichuchwa, njovera, and siti in Africa. It also occurs in Southeast Asia. The local forms have distinctive features. Moist ulcerated lesions of the skin or oral or nasopharyngeal mucosa are the most common manifestations. Generalized lymphadenopathy and secondary and tertiary bone and skin lesions are also common. Cardiovascular and central nervous system involvement is rare.

MISCELLANEOUS SPIROCHETAL DISEASES

RELAPSING FEVER

Relapsing fever is endemic in many parts of the world. The main reservoir is rodents, which serve as the source of infection for ticks (eg, *Ornithodoros*). The distribution and seasonal incidence of the disease are determined by the ecology of the ticks in different areas. In the USA, infected ticks are found throughout the West, especially in mountainous areas, but clinical cases are uncommon in humans.

The infectious organism is a spirochete, *Borrelia recurrentis*. It may be transmitted transovarially from one generation of ticks to the next. The spirochetes occur in all tissues of the tick, and humans can be infected by tick bites or by rubbing crushed tick tissues or feces into the bite wound. Tick-borne relapsing fever is endemic but is not transmitted from person to person. Different species (or strain) names have been given to *Borrelia* in different parts of the world where the organisms are transmitted by different ticks.

When an infected person harbors lice, the lice become infected with *Borrelia* by sucking blood. A few days later, the lice serve as a source of infection for other persons. Large epidemics may occur in louse-infested populations, and transmission is favored by crowding, malnutrition, and cold climate.

Clinical Findings
A. Symptoms and Signs: There is an abrupt

onset of fever, chills, tachycardia, nausea, vomiting, arthralgia, and severe headache. Hepatomegaly and splenomegaly may develop, as well as various types of rashes. Delirium occurs with high fever, and there may be various neurologic and psychic abnormalities. The attack terminates, usually abruptly, after 3–10 days. After an interval of 1–2 weeks, a relapse occurs, but often it is somewhat milder. Three to 10 relapses may occur before recovery.

B. Laboratory Findings: During episodes of fever, large spirochetes are seen in blood smears stained with Wright's or Giemsa's stain. The organisms can be cultured in special media but rapidly lose pathogenicity. The spirochetes can multiply in injected rats or mice and can be seen in their blood.

A variety of anti-*Borrelia* antibodies develop during the illness; sometimes the Weil-Felix test and nontreponemal serologic test for syphilis may also be positive. Cerebrospinal fluid abnormalities occur in patients with meningeal involvement. Mild anemia and thrombocytopenia are common, but the white blood cell count tends to be normal.

Differential Diagnosis

The manifestations of relapsing fever may be confused with malaria, leptospirosis, meningococcemia, yellow fever, typhus, or rat-bite fever.

Prevention

Prevention of tick bites (as described for rickettsial diseases, p 854) and delousing procedures applicable to large groups (see p 853) can prevent illness. Arthropod vectors should be controlled if possible.

An effective means of chemoprophylaxis has not been developed.

Treatment

A single dose of 0.5 g tetracycline or erythromycin orally or a single dose of 600,000 units of procaine penicillin G intramuscularly probably constitutes adequate treatment. Jarisch-Herxheimer reactions may occur and must be managed.

Prognosis

The overall mortality rate is usually about 5%. Fatalities are most common in old, debilitated, or very young patients. With treatment, the initial attack is shortened and relapses are largely prevented.

Butler T et al: *Borrelia recurrentis* infection. *J Infect Dis* 1978; **137:**573.

Edell TA et al: Tick-borne relapsing fever in Colorado. *JAMA* 1979;**241:**2279.

Malison MD: Relapsing fever. *JAMA* 1979;**241:**2819.

RAT-BITE FEVER
(Spirillary Rat-Bite Fever, Sodoku)

Rat-bite fever is an uncommon acute infectious disease caused by *Spirillum minor*. It is transmitted to

humans by the bite of a rat. Inhabitants of rat-infested slum dwellings and laboratory workers are at greatest risk.

Clinical Findings

A. Symptoms and Signs: The original rat bite, unless secondarily infected, heals promptly, but 1 or several weeks later the site becomes swollen, indurated, and painful; assumes a dusky purplish hue; and may ulcerate. Regional lymphangitis and lymphadenitis, fever, chills, malaise, myalgia, arthralgia, and headache are present. Splenomegaly may occur. A sparse, dusky-red maculopapular rash appears on the trunk and extremities in many cases, and there may be frank arthritis.

After a few days, both the local and systemic symptoms subside, only to reappear again in a few more days. This relapsing pattern of fever of 24–48 hours alternating with an equal afebrile period may persist for weeks. The other features, however, usually recur only during the first few relapses.

B. Laboratory Findings: Leukocytosis is often present, and the nontreponemal test for syphilis is often falsely positive. The organism may be identified in darkfield examination of the ulcer exudate or aspirated lymph node material; more commonly, it is observed after inoculation of a laboratory animal with the patient's exudate or blood. It has not been cultured in artificial media.

Differential Diagnosis

Rat-bite fever must be distinguished from the rat bite-induced lymphadenitis and rash of streptobacillary fever. Reliable differentiation requires an increasing titer of agglutinins against *Streptobacillus moniliformis* or identification of the causative organism. Rat-bite fever may also be distinguished from tularemia rickettsial disease, *Pasteurella multocida* infections, and relapsing fever by identification of the causative organism.

Treatment

Treat with procaine penicillin G, 300,000 units intramuscularly every 12 hours; or tetracycline hydrochloride, 0.5 g every 6 hours for 2–3 days. Give supportive and symptomatic measures as indicated.

Prognosis

The reported mortality rate is about 10%, but this should be markedly reduced by prompt diagnosis and antimicrobial treatment.

Cole JS et al: Rat-bite fever. *Ann Intern Med* 1969;**71:**979.

LEPTOSPIROSIS

Leptospirosis is an acute and often severe infection that frequently affects the liver or other organs and is caused by any of several *Leptospira* species (or of serogroups of *Leptospira interrogans*). The 3 most common serogroups and their reservoirs of infection are *Leptospira icterohaemorrhagiae* of rats, *Leptospira canicola* of dogs, and *Leptospira pomona* of cattle and swine. Several other varieties can also cause the disease, but *L icterohaemorrhagiae* causes the most severe illness. The disease is worldwide in distribution, and the incidence is higher than usually supposed. The Leptospirae are often transmitted to humans by the ingestion of food and drink contaminated by the urine of the reservoir animal. The organism may also enter through minor skin lesions and probably via the conjunctiva. Many infections have followed bathing in contaminated water. The disease is an occupational hazard among sewer workers, rice planters, and farmers. The incubation period is 2–20 days.

Clinical Findings

A. Symptoms and Signs: There is a sudden onset of fever to 39–40 °C (102.2–104 °F), chills, abdominal pains, vomiting, and myalgia especially of the calf muscles. Extremely severe headache is usually present. The conjunctiva is markedly reddened. The liver may be palpable, and in about 50% of cases (most commonly in *L icterohaemorrhagiae* infections ["Weil's disease"]) jaundice is present on about the fifth day and may be associated with nephritis. Capillary hemorrhages and purpuric skin lesions may also appear. The illness is often biphasic. After initial improvement, the second phase develops at the time that IgM antibodies appear. It manifests itself often as "aseptic meningitis" with intense headache, stiff neck, and pleocytosis. Nephritis and hepatitis may also recur until the illness resolves.

Pretibial fever occurred during World War II at Fort Bragg, USA. In pretibial fever, there is patchy erythema on the skin of the lower legs or generalized rash occurring with fever.

Leptospirosis with jaundice must be distinguished from hepatitis, yellow fever, and relapsing fever.

B. Laboratory Findings: The leukocyte count may be normal or as high as 50,000/μL, with neutrophils predominating. The urine may contain bile, protein, casts, and red cells. Oliguria is not uncommon, and in severe cases uremia may occur. In cases with meningeal involvement, organisms may be found in the cerebrospinal fluid. The organism may be identified by darkfield examination of the patient's blood (during the first 10 days) or by culture on a semisolid medium (eg, Fletcher's EMJH) for 1–6 weeks. The organism may also be grown from the urine from the tenth day to the sixth week. Specific agglutination titers develop after 7 days and may persist at high levels for many years; specific serologic tests are of particular value in diagnosis of the milder, anicteric forms and of aseptic meningitis. Serum CPK is usually elevated in leptospirosis patients and normal in hepatitis patients.

Complications

Myocarditis, aseptic meningitis, renal failure,

and massive hemorrhage are not common but are the usual causes of death. Iridocyclitis may occur.

Treatment

Various antimicrobial drugs, including penicillin and tetracyclines, show antileptospiral activity. Penicillin has been given, but its therapeutic effect is in doubt, despite observed Jarisch-Herxheimer reactions. Observe for evidence of renal failure, and treat as necessary. Effective prophylaxis consists of doxycycline, 200 mg orally, given once weekly during the risk of exposure.

Prognosis

Without jaundice, the disease is almost never fatal. With jaundice, the mortality rate is 5% for those under age 30 and 30% for those over age 60.

Martone WJ, Kaufmann AF: Leptospirosis in humans in the United States, 1974–1978. *J Infect Dis* 1979;**140:**1020.

Takafuji ET et al: An efficacy trial of doxycycline chemoprophylaxis against leptospirosis. *N Engl J Med* 1984;**310:** 497.

Wong ML et al: Leptospirosis: Childhood disease. *J Pediatr* 1977;**90:**532.

LYME DISEASE

This illness, named after the town of Lyme, Connecticut, occurs typically in summer. It presents with the unique skin lesion erythema chronicum migrans, often accompanied by headache, stiff neck, fever, myalgias, arthralgias, or lymphadenopathy. Weeks or months later, some patients have neurologic symptoms and frank arthritis, which may recur for several years. The disease occurs also in Europe and Australia.

The disease is transmitted by a small ixodid tick, often *Ixodes dammini,* that carries spirochetes (*Borrelia burgdorferi*). The same spirochetes have been recovered from the blood and cerebrospinal fluid of patients, who also develop specific IgM antibodies to the spirochetes 3–6 weeks after onset of illness. In patients with arthritis and other complications, high titers of IgG antibody are found, and it is probable that the late complications are a manifestation of antigen-antibody complex deposition.

Penicillin or tetracycline given early in the acute illness terminates it abruptly and prevents late arthritis and other complications.

Benach JL et al: Spirochetes isolated from the blood of two patients with Lyme disease. *N Engl J Med* 1983;**308:**740.

Campagna J et al: Lyme disease in northern California. *West J Med* 1983;**139:**319.

Hardin JA et al: Immune complexes and the evolution of Lyme arthritis. *N Engl J Med* 1979;**301:**1358.

Meyerhoff J: Lyme disease. *Am J Med* 1983;**75:**663.

Steere AC et al: Treatment of the early manifestations of Lyme disease. *Ann Intern Med* 1983;**99:**22.

26 | Infectious Diseases: Protozoal

Robert S. Goldsmith, MD, MPH, DTM&H

AMEBIASIS

Essentials of Diagnosis

- Mild to moderate amebic colitis: recurrent diarrhea and abdominal cramps, sometimes alternating with constipation. Mucus may be present but no blood.
- Severe amebic colitis: semiformed to liquid stools streaked with blood and mucus, fever, colic, prostration. In fulminant cases, ileus, perforation, peritonitis, hemorrhage.
- Hepatic amebiasis: hepatic enlargement, pain, and tenderness; fever.
- Laboratory findings: amebas in stools or in abscess aspirate. Serologic tests positive with severe colitis or hepatic abscess. Radiologic methods show size and location of abscess.

General Considerations

Amebiasis is caused by the protozoan parasite *Entamoeba histolytica*. The organisms either live as commensals in the lumen of the large intestine without causing disease (the asymptomatic chronic carrier) or invade the colon wall causing acute dysentery or chronic diarrhea of variable severity. The organisms may also be carried by the blood to the liver, where they produce hepatic abscesses. Rarely, they are carried to the lungs, brain, or other organs or invade the perianal skin.

E histolytica exists as 2 forms in feces: cysts (10–14 μm) and motile trophozoites (12–50 μm). In the absence of diarrhea, trophozoites encyst in the large bowel. Trophozoites passed into the environment die rapidly, but cysts remain viable in soil and water for several weeks to months at appropriate temperature and humidity.

The infection is present worldwide but is most prevalent and severe in tropical areas, where rates may exceed 40% under conditions of crowding, poor sanitation, and poor nutrition. In temperate areas, amebiasis tends to be a mild, chronic disease that often remains undiagnosed. In the USA, seropositive rates of 2–5% have been reported in various studies in normal populations.

Humans are the only known host and are universally susceptible. Only cysts are infectious, the source of infection being persons who eliminate cysts in their feces—asymptomatic carriers and those with chronic diarrhea. On ingestion, cysts survive gastric acidity, but trophozoites are destroyed.

Transmission generally occurs through ingestion of cysts from fecally contaminated food or water. Flies and other arthropods also serve as mechanical vectors; to an undetermined degree, transmission results from contamination of food by the hands of food handlers. Where human excrement is used as fertilizer, it is often a source of food contamination. Person-to-person contact is important in transmission; therefore, all household members as well as an infected person's sexual partner should have their stools examined. Amebiasis is rarely epidemic, but urban outbreaks have occurred because of common-source water contamination. Sexual transmission of *E histolytica* and other intestinal protozoa has reached epidemic proportions among male homosexuals in some urban areas. In closed institutions such as mental institutions, prevalence rates as high as 50% have been reported.

It is undetermined whether strains differ with regard to invasiveness, or whether all strains under the right conditions can become invasive. Present evidence favors the latter view, but the circumstances under which commensals become invasive is little understood. Malnutrition probably predisposes to enhanced virulence. Corticosteroids and other immunosuppressive drugs often convert a commensal infection to an invasive one. Women in late pregnancy and the puerperium are especially susceptible. Tissue invasion elicits both humoral (IgM and IgG) antibodies and a cellular immune response, but humoral antibody titers do not correlate with protective immunity.

The characteristic intestinal lesion is the amebic ulcer, which can occur anywhere in the large bowel (including the appendix) and sometimes in the terminal ileum but predominates in the cecum, descending colon, and the rectosigmoid colon—areas of greatest fecal stasis. Trophozoites invade the colonic mucosa by means of their ameboid movement and proteolytic secretions and induce necrosis to form the characteristic flask-shaped ulcers. Usually the ulcers are limited to the outer muscular layer, but when this has been penetrated to the serous layer, perforation may result and lead to local abscess or generalized peritonitis. In fulminating cases, the ulceration may be extensive, and the bowel becomes thin and friable. Hepatic abscesses range in size from a few millimeters to 15 cm or larger, usually are single but may be multiple, occur more often in the right lobe and in the upper portion of that lobe, and are more common in men.

Clinical Findings

A. Symptoms and Signs: Amebiasis has protean clinical manifestations that can be classified into intestinal and extraintestinal lesions and further subdivided into the clinical syndromes described below. Some patients have an acute onset of intense diarrhea as early as 8 days (commonly 2–4 weeks) after infection. Others may have an asymptomatic intestinal infection for months to several years before coming down with either intestinal symptoms or a liver abscess. Transition may occur from one type of intestinal infection to another, and each may give rise to hepatic abscess, or the intestinal infection may clear spontaneously.

1. Intestinal amebiasis–

a. Asymptomatic infection–In most infected persons, the organism lives as a commensal, and the patient is without symptoms.

b. Mild to moderate colitis (nondysenteric colitis)–This may follow acute disease or be the initial manifestation. The patient passes only a few stools a day, which are semiformed and have a strong fetid odor; mucus may be present, but the stools are free of blood. There may be abdominal cramps, flatulence, chronic fatigue, and weight loss. Characteristically, there are periods of remission and recurrence that may last days to weeks or longer, and during remission the patient may have constipation. Abdominal examination may show hyperperistalsis and tenderness and fullness due to gaseous distention of the colon. Occasionally in chronic infection, a palpable, thickened colon may be found, particularly over the cecum and descending colon.

c. Severe colitis (dysenteric colitis)–As the severity of intestinal infection increases, the number of stools increases, and they change from semiformed to liquid with an unpleasant odor, and streaks of blood and mucus begin to appear. With larger numbers of stools, 10–20 or more, little fecal material is present, but blood (fresh or dark), mucus, and bits of necrotic tissue become increasingly evident. With increasing severity, the patient may become prostrate and show signs of toxicity, with fever up to 40.5 °C (105 °F), and have colic, tenesmus, vomiting, generalized abdominal tenderness, and nonspecific hepatic enlargement and tenderness. Rare complications include appendicitis, bowel perforation (followed by peritonitis, pericolonic abscess, retroperitoneal fecal cellulitis, fistula to the abdominal surface), and fulminating colitis (with paralytic ileus, hypotension, dehydration with electrolyte changes, massive mucosal sloughing, and hemorrhage). Death may follow.

d. Localized ulcerative lesions of the colon– Sometimes the bowel ulcerations are limited to the rectal area, which may result in the passage of formed stools with bloody exudate. Bowel ulcerations limited to the cecum may cause pain with little diarrhea and simulate acute appendicitis. Amebic appendicitis itself, in which the appendix is extensively involved but not the remainder of the large bowel, is rare.

e. Localized granulomatous lesions of the colon (ameboma)–This occurs as a result of excessive production of granulation tissue in response to amebic infection, either in the course of dysentery or slowly in chronic intestinal infection. These masses may present as an irregular tumor (single or multiple) that projects into the bowel or as an annular constricting mass up to several inches in length. Clinical findings (pain, obstructive symptoms, and hemorrhage) and x-ray findings may simulate bowel carcinoma or lymphogranuloma venereum. At endoscopy, the mass is deep red and bleeds easily, and biopsy specimens show granulation tissue and *E histolytica.* Surgical removal of the lesion without anti-amebic treatment is likely to result in the death of the patient.

f. Postdysenteric colitis–This is an uncommon sequela of severe amebic colitis. Following adequate treatment, diarrhea continues and the mucosa may be reddened and edematous, but no ulcers or organisms are found. Most such cases are self-limited, with permanent remission in weeks to months. However, the diarrhea may be profound and unremitting and in some instances probably represents ulcerative colitis triggered by the amebic infection.

2. Extraintestinal amebiasis–

a. Hepatic amebiasis–Amebic liver abscess, although a relatively infrequent consequence of intestinal amebiasis, is not uncommon given the large number of intestinal infections. A large percentage of patients with liver abscess do not have concurrent intestinal symptoms nor can they recall having had chronic intestinal symptoms. The onset of symptoms can be sudden or gradual, ranging from a few days to many months. Cardinal manifestations are fever (often high), pain (continuous, stabbing, or pleuritic, and sometimes severe), and an enlarged and tender liver. Patients may also experience malaise or prostration, sweating, chills, anorexia, and weight loss. The liver enlargement may present subcostally, in the epigastrium, as a localized bulging of the rib cage, or, as a result of enlargement against the dome of the diaphragm, it may produce coughing and findings at the right lung base (dullness to percussion, rales, and diminished breath sounds). Intercostal tenderness is common. Localizing signs may be an area of edema or a point of maximum tenderness. Without prompt treatment, the hepatic abscess may rupture into the pleural, peritoneal, or pericardial space or other contiguous organs, and death may follow.

b. Nonspecific hepatic enlargement–A low-grade, nonspecific enlargement of the liver—in which amebic liver infection is not present—may accompany invasive amebic bowel disease. It disappears with eradication of the amebic bowel infection but without use of specific drugs required to eradicate an amebic liver infection.

3. Other extraintestinal infections–Metastatic

infections may rarely occur throughout the body, particularly in the lungs and brain. Other rare sites of infection are the perianal skin and genitals.

B. Laboratory Findings: *E histolytica* trophozoites and cysts in stool specimens are difficult to detect. Three specimens obtained under optimum conditions and tested by skilled personnel in appropriate laboratories will probably detect only 80% of amebic infections. Three additional tests will raise the diagnosis rate to about 90%. Trophozoites predominate in liquid stools, and cysts predominate in formed stools.

A standard procedure is to collect 3 specimens at 2-day intervals or longer, with one of the 3 obtained after a laxative. They should be collected in a clean container without having come in contact with urine or toilet water. Because trophozoites rapidly autolyze, specimens should be examined within about 30 minutes or should immediately be mixed with a preservative. Polyvinyl alcohol is commonly used but is a poison; therefore, a child-proof bottle should be provided and labeled as such.

If the patient has received specific therapy, antibiotics, antimalarials, antidiarrheal preparations containing bismuth or kaolin, magnesium hydroxide, barium, or mineral oil, specimen collection should be delayed 10–14 days.

In mild intestinal amebiasis, there are usually no findings by sigmoidoscopy. In severe disease, sigmoidoscopy commonly aids diagnosis by permitting detection of ulcerative lesions (from 1 mm to 2 cm) with intact intervening mucosa and collection of exudate for examination. Exudate should be collected with a glass pipette (not cotton) or obtained by scraping with a metal instrument. The colon should not be cleansed before sigmoidoscopy, since this washes exudate from ulcers and destroys trophozoites. In some centers, rectal biopsy has enhanced diagnosis; the specimens are best examined by immunofluorescent methods. Where possible, in vitro culture of amebas can be attempted.

Finding trophozoites that contain ingested red blood cells is diagnostic for invasive *E histolytica*, but they may be confused with the occasional macrophage also containing red blood cells. *E histolytica* cysts and trophozoites must be differentiated from the other pathogenic intestinal protozoa: *Giardia lamblia, Dientamoeba fragilis, Balantidium coli, Sarcocystis* sp, and *Isospora belli;* and from the nonpathogens: *Endolimax nana, Entamoeba coli, Entamoeba polecki, Entamoeba hartmanni, Iodamoeba bütschlii, Trichomonas hominis, Chilomastix mesnili,* and other flagellates. Leukocytes and macrophages are relatively scarce (in contrast to bacillary dysentery) unless there is concomitant bacillary infection. Charcot-Leyden crystals may be present.

In dysentery, the white blood cell count can reach 20,000 or higher, but it is not elevated in mild colitis. A low-grade eosinophilia is occasionally present. Serologic testing for amebiasis is specific and usually positive if there has been substantial tissue invasion (as occurs in liver amebic abscess or severe intestinal infection); with relatively little tissue invasion (as in mild or asymptomatic intestinal infection), only a few patients are positive. The indirect hemagglutination test is sensitive and apparently produces no false-positive reactions. Positive titers persist for several years after successful treatment. Test results from central laboratories may not be available for 1–3 weeks, but immunodiffusion tests can provide results in hours to 2 days. The antibody detected by immunodiffusion tests disappears within several months after successful treatment.

In amebic liver abscess, serologic tests will be positive, but the stools may or may not contain the parasite. The white count ranges from 15,000 to 25,000/μL (25% < 10,000; 10% > 25,000). Eosinophilia is not present. Liver function test abnormalities, when present, are usually low-grade. In many patients, aspiration is indicated for diagnosis and, if the abscess is large, for therapy as well as to prevent rupture. The risks are hemorrhage and bacterial infection; therefore, aspiration should be done under strict aseptic conditions. Divide the aspirate into serial 30- to 50-mL aliquots, but examine only the last sample. Add 10 units of streptodornase per milliliter, mix, incubate for 30 minutes at 37 °C, centrifuge for 5 minutes at 1000 rpm, and then examine for trophozoites.

Procedures used to locate and define liver lesions include chest x-ray and fluoroscopy, radioisotope scanning, ultrasound, CT scans, and sometimes arteriography.

Differential Diagnosis

Amebiasis should be considered in persons residing in or in travelers returning from endemic areas and in individuals intimately associated with known cases. Amebiasis should be included in the differential diagnosis of most cases of acute and chronic diarrhea (including persons with only mild changes in bowel habits who have an exposure history), liver abscess, annular lesions of the colon, and skin lesions in the perianal area. All patients with inflammatory bowel disease should be tested by stool examination and serology, because of the risk of overwhelming amebic disease if steroid therapy were given.

Treatment

Amebiasis may present in many different clinical forms (see above). The choice of drug depends on the clinical presentation and the site of drug action. Treatment may require the concurrent or sequential use of several drugs. Table 26–1 outlines a preferred and an alternative method of treatment for each clinical type of amebiasis. No drugs are recommended as safe or effective for chemoprophylaxis.

The **tissue amebicides** dehydroemetine and emetine act on organisms in the bowel wall and in other tissues but not on amebas in the bowel lumen. Chloroquine is active principally against amebas in the liver. The **luminal amebicides** diloxanide furoate, iodoquinol, and paromomycin act on organisms in the bowel lumen but are ineffective against amebas in the bowel wall or other tissues. Oral tetracycline inhibits

Table 26—1. Treatment of amebiasis.

	Drug(s) of Choice	Alternative Drug(s)
Asymptomatic intestinal infection	Diloxanide furoate[1,2]	Iodoquinol[3] or Paromomycin[7]
Mild to moderate intestinal infection (nondysenteric colitis)	(1) Metronidazole[4] plus (2) Diloxanide furoate[2] or iodoquinol[3]	(1) Diloxanide[2] or iodoquinol[3] plus (2) A tetracycline[5] followed by (3) Chloroquine[6] or (1) Paromomycin[7] followed by (2) Chloroquine[6]
Severe intestinal infection (dysenteric colitis)	(1) Metronidazole[8] plus (2) Diloxanide furoate[2] or iodoquinol[3] **If parenteral therapy is needed initially** (1) Intravenous metronidazole[9] until oral therapy can be started (2) Then give oral metronidazole[8] plus diloxanide furoate[2] or iodoquinol[3]	(1) A tetracycline[5] plus (2) Diloxanide furoate[2] or iodoquinol[3] followed by (3) Chloroquine[10] or (1) Dehydroemetine[1,11] or emetine followed by (2) A tetracycline[5] plus diloxanide furoate[2] or iodoquinol[3] followed by (3) Chloroquine[10]
Hepatic abscess	(1) Metronidazole[8,9] followed by (2) Diloxanide furoate[2] or iodoquinol[3] plus (3) Chloroquine[10]	(1) Dehydroemetine[1,12] or emetine plus (2) Chloroquine[13] plus (3) Diloxanide furoate[2] or iodoquinol[3]
Ameboma or extraintestinal infection	As for hepatic abscess, but not including chloroquine	As for hepatic abscess, but not including chloroquine

[1] Available in the USA only from the Parasitic Disease Drug Service, Centers for Disease Control, Atlanta 30333. Telephone requests may be made by calling (404) 329–3670 days; (404) 329–2888 nights, weekends, and holidays.

[2] Diloxanide furoate, 500 mg 3 times daily for 10 days.

[3] Iodoquinol, 650 mg 3 times daily for 21 days.

[4] Metronidazole, 750 mg 3 times daily for 10 days.

[5] A tetracycline, 250 mg 4 times daily for 10 days; in severe dysentery, give 500 mg 4 times daily for the first 5 days, then 250 mg 4 times daily for 5 days.

[6] Chloroquine, 500 mg (salt) daily for 7 days.

[7] Paromomycin, 25–30 mg/kg (maximum 3 g) daily in 3 divided doses for 5–10 days.

[8] Metronidazole, 750 mg 3 times daily for 5–10 days.

[9] An intravenous metronidazole is available; change to oral medication as soon as possible. See manufacturer's recommendation for dosage.

[10] Chloroquine, 500 mg (salt) daily for 14 days.

[11] Dehydroemetine, 1 mg/kg IM or subcut daily for the least number of days necessary to control severe symptoms (usually 3–5 days) (maximum daily dose 90 mg).

[12] Dehydroemetine, 1 mg/kg IM or subcut daily for 8–10 days (maximum daily dose 90 mg) or emetine.

[13] Chloroquine, 500 mg (salt) twice daily for 2 days and then 500 mg daily for 21 days.

the bacterial associates of *E histolytica* and thus has an indirect effect on amebas in the bowel lumen and bowel wall but not in other tissues. Given parenterally, antibiotics have little antiamebic activity at any site. Metronidazole is unique in that it is effective both in the bowel lumen and in the bowel wall and other tissues. However, metronidazole when used alone for bowel infections is not sufficient as a luminal amebicide, for it fails to cure up to 50% of infections.

A. Asymptomatic Intestinal Infection: Cure rates with a single course of diloxanide furoate or iodoquinol are 80–85%. Other alternatives for treatment or re-treatment are paromomycin plus iodoquinol or metronidazole plus iodoquinol or diloxanide furoate. Usually in asymptomatic infection, a tissue amebicidal drug is not given to prevent liver infection.

B. Mild to Moderate Intestinal Infection: When iodoquinol is used, concomitant use of a tetracycline probably increases intestinal cure rates. It is less well established that adding a tetracycline to diloxanide furoate therapy increases effectiveness. Chloroquine is used to destroy trophozoites carried to the liver or to eradicate an undetected early-stage amebic liver abscess; the minimum dose needed to accomplish this is not known. In endemic areas where intestinal infection and reinfection are common yet hepatic abscess is rare (eg, in urban communities where intestinal amebiasis is sexually transmitted among male homosexuals but hepatic amebiasis is uncommon), it is probably unnecessary to use chloroquine in the treatment of mild intestinal disease.

C. Severe Intestinal Infection: Fluid and electrolyte therapy and opiates to control bowel motility are necessary adjuncts in severe amebic dysentery.

D. Hepatic Abscess: When metronidazole is given for 10 days, early or late treatment failure occurs rarely. If a satisfactory clinical response has not occurred within 2–3 days, especially if the abscess has been adequately drained, therapy should be changed to the alternative mode of treatment: dehydroemetine (or emetine) plus chloroquine. When the clinical response to metronidazole is adequate, it is suggested that a 2-week course of chloroquine follow to prevent late failures. The need for adding this course of chloroquine remains to be evaluated.

Since a comparative trial of metronidazole with and without aspiration has not been reported, the indications for therapeutic aspiration are still controversial. Aspiration is clearly indicated, however, when the diagnosis is in doubt, if rupture of a large abscess is impending, or if there is a lack of response to therapy.

E. Adverse Drug Reactions: Dehydroemetine and emetine are general protoplasmic poisons having adverse effects on many tissues and a narrow range between therapeutic and toxic effects; dehydroemetine may be the safer of the 2 drugs. Metronidazole has been found to induce neoplasms in rodents and to be mutagenic in the *Salmonella* test system and thus may be carcinogenic. However, based on current evidence, some authorities consider the drug to be essentially free of cancer risk. The other nitroimidazoles have similar mutagenic action in the *Salmonella* test system. The halogenated hydroxyquinolines have been increasingly implicated in the production of neurotoxicity. The tetracyclines should not be used for children under age 8 years; use erythromycin stearate instead, even though it is somewhat less effective.

Follow-Up Care

Follow-up examination consists of study of at least 3 stools at 2- to 3-day intervals, starting 2–4 weeks after the end of treatment. For some patients, sigmoidoscopy and reexamination of stools within 3 months may be indicated.

Prevention & Control

Prevention is effected through education about personal hygiene, sanitary disposal of human feces, protection of rural and urban water supplies against fecal contamination, separation of fresh water lines and sewer lines, and by fly control and protection of foods against contamination by flies.

Prognosis

The mortality rate from untreated amebic dysentery or hepatic abscess may be high. With modern chemotherapy instituted early in the course of the disease, the prognosis is good.

Adams EB, MacLeod IN: Invasive amebiasis. 1. Amebic dysentery and its complications. 2. Amebic liver abscess and its complications. *Medicine* 1977;**56:**315, 325.

Harries J: Amoebiasis: A review. *J R Soc Med* 1982;**75:**190.

Idiosyncratic neurotoxicity: Clioquinol and bismuth. (Editorial.) *Lancet* 1980;**1:**857.

Knight R: The chemotherapy of amebiasis. *J Antimicrob Chemother* 1980;**6:**577.

Krogstad DJ, Spencer HC Jr, Healy GR: Current concepts in parasitology: Amebiasis. *N Engl J Med* 1978;**298:**262.

Ralls PW et al: Patterns of resolution in successfully treated hepatic amebic abscess: Sonographic evaluation. *Radiology* 1983;**149:**541.

Ravdin JI, Guerrant RL: A review of the parasite cellular mechanisms involved in the pathogenesis of amebiasis. *Rev Infect Dis* 1982;**4:**1185.

Roe FJC: Toxicologic evaluation of metronidazole with particular reference to carcinogenic, mutagenic, and teratogenic potential. *Surgery* 1983;**93:**158.

PRIMARY AMEBIC MENINGOENCEPHALITIS

Primary amebic meningoencephalitis is a fulminating, purulent meningoencephalitis that is rapidly fatal. The disease is rare but probably has worldwide distribution. More than 100 cases have been recognized in the past 15 years, mostly in children and young adults. The responsible organisms are free-living ameboflagellates of the genus *Naegleria;* most cases have been due to *Naegleria fowleri.*

N fowleri is a thermophilic organism found in fresh, warm lake water, domestic water supplies, swimming pools, thermal water, and sewers. Most patients give a history of exposure to fresh water, eg, swimming in surface water or in swimming pools. Dust is also a possible source of infection. Nasal and throat swabs have shown a human carrier state, and serologic surveys suggest that inapparent infections occur.

The organism apparently invades the central nervous system along the olfactory nerves and may then spread to other tissues. The incubation period is not established but appears to vary from 1 day to 2 weeks. Early symptoms include headache, fever, and lethargy, often associated with rhinitis and pharyngitis. Vomiting, disorientation, and other signs of meningoencephalitis develop within 1 or 2 days, followed by coma and then death on the fifth or sixth day. A few victims have been shown at autopsy to have a nonspecific myocarditis.

Specific diagnosis depends on finding amebas— sometimes hematophagous—in the cerebrospinal fluid. Amebas must be differentiated from mononuclear cells (1) by examination of a fresh, wet preparation and (2) by staining with Gram's stain and other stains such as trichrome and iron-hematoxylin. The wet mount is examined by standard microscopy with the aperture restricted or the condenser wound down to enhance refractility and contrast; a warm stage is not required. *Naegleria* are far more motile than mononuclear cells and demonstrate eruptive pseudopodal formation. The cerebrospinal fluid is purulent and contains hundreds to thousands of white blood cells—mostly neutrophils—per microliter, but examination for bacteria and fungi is negative. Spinal fluid pressure may be increased, protein is usually moderately elevated, glucose may be low, and red cells are usually present—up to several thousand per microliter. Culture and mouse inoculation should be performed for isolation and identification. Serologic testing for antibody and circulating antigen is experimental.

Only 2 well-documented survivors are reported in the literature. One patient was treated with intravenous and intrathecal amphotericin B in large doses and the other with a combination of amphotericin B, miconazole, and rifampin. Recent experimental studies have shown a marked synergistic effect in vitro and in vivo between amphotericin B and either tetracycline or rifampin.

Precise species identification of the free-living ameba is based on morphology, demonstration of flagellate transformation (*Naegleria* only), immunofluorescent antibody studies, immunoelectrophoretic antigen patterns, and isoenzyme studies. The presence of cysts or mitotic division in tissue section may be pathognomonic of *Acanthamoeba* infection.

Acanthamoeba Infections

Free-living amebas of the genus *Acanthamoeba* (*Hartmannella*) are found in soil and in fresh, brackish, and thermal water. They have been recognized only recently as human pathogens, causing a number of poorly defined syndromes: (1) a subacute and chronic focal granulomatous encephalitis that invariably has led to death, (2) skin lesions, (3) granulomatous dissemination to many tissues, and (4) uveitis and corneal ulceration leading to blindness. Portals of entry may include the skin, eyes, or respiratory tract. A commensal nasal carrier state is established, and immunocompromised patients may have increased susceptibility. In the encephalitis syndrome, cerebrospinal fluid lymphocytes have been described.

There is no effective treatment at present. In vitro studies show that some strains are sensitive to sulfonamides, clotrimazole, pentamidine, paromomycin, flucytosine, and other drugs but not to amphotericin B.

Dorsch MM, Cameron AS, Robinson BS: The epidemiology and control of primary amoebic meningoencephalitis with particular reference to South Australia. *Trans R Soc Trop Med Hyg* 1983;**77**:372.

John DT: Primary amebic meningoencephalitis and the biology of *Naegleria fowleri. Annu Rev Microbiol* 1982;**36**:101.

Key SN et al: Keratitis due to *Acanthamoeba castellani:* Clinico-

pathologic case report. *Arch Ophthalmol* 1980;**98**:475.

Martinez AJ: Is *Acanthamoeba* encephalitis an opportunistic infection? *Neurology* 1980;**30**:567.

Martinez AJ et al: Primary amebic meningoencephalitis. Pages 225–250 in: *Pathology Annual.* Vol 12, part 2. Sommers SC, Rosen PP (editors). Appleton-Century-Crofts, 1977.

Thong YH: Primary amoebic meningoencephalitis: Fifteen years later. *Aust Med J* 1980;**1**:352.

BABESIOSIS
(Piroplasmosis)

Babesia are tick-borne protozoal parasites that affect wild and domestic animals worldwide. Babesiosis in humans is a rare intraerythrocytic infection caused by 2 *Babesia* species and characterized by fever, chills, myalgia, and hemolytic anemia. The infection has been recognized only in Europe (*Babesia divergens*) and North America (*Babesia microti*), with most infections reported from the northeastern coastal region of the USA. Humans are infected as a result of *Ixodes* tick bites, but transmission from blood transfusion has also been reported. The parasite apparently enters the red blood cells without passing through an exoerythrocytic stage. Multiplication, cell rupture, and infection of other cells can result in hemolytic anemia, hemoglobinuria, and acute renal necrosis. Splenectomized persons are apparently more susceptible to infection and more severe illness.

The clinical spectrum of babesiosis ranges from asymptomatic to lethal infection. The incubation period is 1–4 weeks, but patients usually do not recall the tick bite. *B microti* infection lasts a few weeks to a month; the illness is characterized by irregular fever, chills, diaphoresis, myalgia, and fatigue but is without malarialike periodicity of symptoms. Most patients have a moderate hemolytic anemia and occasionally hepatosplenomegaly. Although parasitemia may continue for months, with or without malaise, the disease is self-limited and patients recover without sequelae.

The few reported infections with *B divergens* have been in patients who have undergone splenectomy. These infections progress rapidly with high fever, severe hemolytic anemia, jaundice, hemoglobinuria, and renal failure; death usually follows.

Diagnosis is by identification of the intraerythrocytic parasite on Giemsa-stained thick or thin blood smears; no gametocytes and no intracellular pigment are seen. The organism must be differentiated from malarial parasites, particularly *Plasmodium falciparum*. Isolation of the parasite can be attempted by inoculating patient blood into hamsters or gerbils. Serologic tests are available.

Exchange transfusion is effective in reversing the disease process. Drug treatment is unsatisfactory. Chloroquine is no longer thought to be effective. Pentamidine isethionate, 4 mg/kg daily intramuscularly for 10 days, can be tried. A recent report describes potential efficacy for clindamycin and quinine.

Clindamycin and quinine treatment for *Babesia microti* infections. *MMWR* 1983;**32**:65.

Gombert ME et al: Human babesiosis: Clinical and therapeutic considerations. *JAMA* 1982;**248**:3005.

Rosner F et al: Babesiosis in splenectomized adults: Review of 22 reported cases. *Am J Med* 1984;**76**:696.

Ruebush TK II: Human babesiosis in North America. *Trans R Soc Trop Med Hyg* 1980;**74**:149.

MALARIA

Essentials of Diagnosis

- Paroxysms (often periodic) of chills, fever, and sweating.
- Splenomegaly, anemia, leukopenia.
- Delirium, coma, convulsions, gastrointestinal disorders, jaundice.
- Characteristic parasites in erythrocytes, identified in thick or thin blood films.

General Considerations

Four species of the genus *Plasmodium* are responsible for human malaria. Although the infection is generally limited to the tropics and subtropics, many imported cases occur in the USA and other countries free of malaria transmission. Malaria is known to exist in parts of Mexico, Haiti, Central and South America, Africa, the Middle East, Turkey, the Indian subcontinent, Southeast Asia, China, the Malay archipelago, and Oceania. The most common parasites, *Plasmodium vivax* and *Plasmodium falciparum*, are found through the malaria belt. *Plasmodium malariae* is widely distributed but is less common. *Plasmodium ovale* is rare, but in West Africa it seems to replace *P vivax*.

Malaria is transmitted from human to human by the bite of infected female *Anopheles* mosquitoes. Congenital transmission and transmission by blood transfusion or the use of contaminated needles by drug abusers also occur.

The mosquito becomes infected by taking blood containing the sexual forms of the parasite (micro- and macrogametocytes). After a developmental phase in the mosquito, sporozoites develop that are inoculated into humans when the mosquito next feeds. The first stage of development in humans, the exoerythrocytic stage, takes place in the liver. Subsequently, parasites escape from the liver into the bloodstream, invade red blood cells, multiply, and 48 hours later (or 72 with *P malariae*) cause the red cells to rupture, releasing a new crop of parasites. This cycle of invasion, multiplication, and red cell rupture may be repeated many times. Symptoms do not appear until several of these erythrocytic cycles have been completed. The incubation period varies considerably, depending upon the species and strain of parasite, the intensity of the infection, and the immune status of the host. The usual incubation period is 8–20 days for *P falciparum*, and almost all cases will develop within 2 months of infection; 12–18 days for *P vivax* and *P ovale*, but initial attacks may occur up to 8 months after infection; and 24–30 days for *P malariae*. If untreated, *P falciparum* infections usually terminate spontaneously in 6–8 months but can persist for up to 3 years; *P vivax* and *P ovale* infections can persist without treatment for as long as 5 years; *P malariae* infections have lasted for as long as 40 years.

P falciparum and *P malariae* have only one cycle of liver cell invasion and multiplication. Liver infection ceases spontaneously in less than 4 weeks; thereafter, multiplication is confined to the red cells. Thus, treatment that eliminates these species from the red cells will cure the infection. *P vivax* (and presumably *P ovale*) have, however, a dormant hepatic stage (the hypnozoite) that is responsible for subsequent relapses. Cure of *P vivax* and *P ovale* infections, therefore, requires treatment to eradicate parasites both from the red cells and from the liver.

Clinical Findings

A. Symptoms and Signs: The paroxysms of malaria are closely related to events in the bloodstream. The chill, lasting from 15 minutes to an hour, begins as a generation of parasites rupture their host red cells and escape into the blood. Nausea, vomiting, and headache are common at this time. The succeeding hot stage, lasting several hours, is accompanied by a spiking fever, sometimes reaching 40 °C (104 °F) or higher. During this stage, the parasites presumably invade new red cells. The third, or sweating stage, concludes the episode. The fever subsides and the patient frequently falls asleep, to awake feeling relatively well. In *P vivax* (benign tertian malaria), *P ovale,* and *P falciparum* (malignant tertian malaria) infections, red cells are ruptured and paroxysms occur every 48 hours. In *P malariae* infections (quartan malaria), the cycle takes 72 hours. Early, the cycles are frequently asynchronous and the fever patterns irregular. As the disease progresses, splenomegaly and, to a lesser extent, hepatomegaly appear.

P falciparum infection is more serious than the others because of the high frequency of severe or fatal complications. *P falciparum* malaria may also be more difficult to recognize clinically. It often presents as a flulike illness with nonspecific symptoms of fever, headache, myalgia, nausea, diarrhea, and abdominal pain or discomfort. The fever may be low-grade, continuous, or with daily spikes and may occur without chills or rigors. Parasites are sometimes difficult to find on blood smears.

B. Laboratory Findings: The thick and thin blood film, stained with Giemsa's stain, is the mainstay of malaria diagnosis. The thin film is used primarily for species differentiation after the presence of an infection is detected on a thick film. Because the level of parasitemia varies from hour to hour, especially for *P falciparum* infections, blood should be examined several times a day for 2–3 days. In all but falciparum infections, the number of red cells infected seldom exceeds 2% of the total cells. Very high red cell infection rates may occur with falciparum infection

(20–30% or more). For this reason, anemia is frequently much more severe in falciparum malaria. The anemia is normocytic, with poikilocytosis and anisocytosis. During paroxysms, there may be transient leukocytosis; leukopenia develops subsequently, with a relative increase in large mononuclear cells. During attacks, hepatic function tests often become abnormal, but the tests revert to normal with treatment or spontaneous recovery. Hemolytic jaundice and thrombocytopenia may develop in severe infections.

There are no specific blood chemical findings. In *P malariae* infections, a form of nephrosis, with protein and casts in the urine, sometimes occurs in children. Severe falciparum infections may cause renal damage.

Serologic tests are not used in the diagnosis of acute malaria but may be of value occasionally in the diagnosis of low-level infections that are long-standing and relapsing. A titer of 1:64 in the indirect immunofluorescence test indicates that the patient has acquired malaria at some time in the past.

Differential Diagnosis

Uncomplicated malaria, particularly when modified by partial immunity, must be distinguished from a variety of other causes of fever, splenomegaly, anemia, or hepatomegaly. Some diseases often considered in the diagnosis of malaria in the tropics include urinary tract infections, typhoid fever, infectious hepatitis, dengue, kala-azar, influenza, amebic liver abscess, leptospirosis, and relapsing fever. Examination of multiple blood films is essential to differentiate atypical malaria from some of the above.

Complications

Serious complications of malaria occur primarily in falciparum infections, particularly in persons who have experienced repeated attacks with inadequate treatment. These complications include cerebral malaria with headache, convulsions, delirium, and coma; hyperpyrexia, closely resembling heat hyperpyrexia; gastrointestinal disorders resembling cholera or acute bacillary dysentery; and algid malaria, which resembles acute adrenal insufficiency. Blackwater fever must be considered apart from other falciparum complications. This acute intravascular hemolytic condition develops in patients with long-standing falciparum infections and a history of irregular quinine dosage. The principal findings are profound anemia, jaundice, fever, and hemoglobinuria. The mortality rate may be as high as 30%, primarily as a result of anuria and uremia.

Treatment & Prophylaxis

A. Drug Classification: The antimalarial drugs can be classified according to their selective action on different phases of the parasite's life cycle. Except for the action of pyrimethamine and proguanil (chlorguanide) to prevent maturation of the pre-erythrocytic schizonts of *P falciparum*, none of the drugs prevent infection (ie, are true causal prophylactic drugs), but they do prevent attacks or effect cure. The schizonticidal drugs, which destroy circulating plasmodia and thus prevent attacks, include quinine; the 4-aminoquinolines, chloroquine and amodiaquine; and the antifolate drugs, pyrimethamine and proguanil. Primaquine destroys the persisting liver stage (the hypnozoite) of *P vivax* and *P ovale,* preventing relapses from these parasites; primaquine is also used to destroy the gametocytes of *P falciparum.* Drug combinations that have come into use to treat falciparum malaria resistant to chloroquine include Fansidar (pyrimethamine plus sulfadoxine) and Maloprim* (pyrimethamine plus dapsone).

B. Prophylaxis: Adults and children at whatever age, including breast-fed infants, require prophylaxis, but no method is 100% effective. Travelers to malarious areas must be warned that if they develop fever, even when taking prophylactics regularly, malaria is a possible diagnosis. Travelers should also be reminded of the need to use other protective measures against mosquito bites, such as wearing long sleeves and trousers during hours when mosquitoes are biting and using space sprays, mosquito nets, and screens.

Questions about malaria prophylaxis can be directed to state health departments or to the Parasitic Diseases Division, Center for Infectious Diseases, Centers for Disease Control, Atlanta 30333; telephone (404) 329–3670 (for emergencies only; nights and weekends, call [404] 329–2888).

C. Parasite Resistance to Drugs: *P falciparum* resistance to pyrimethamine and proguanil is common in most endemic areas, but the degree and distribution of resistance are not accurately known.

Strains of *P falciparum* resistant to chloroquine have been reported in Central and South America from Panama, Brazil, Ecuador, Guyana, Surinam, French Guiana, Bolivia, Peru, Colombia, and Venezuela; in South and Southeast Asia from Laos, Vietnam, Thailand, Kampuchea, Timor, Borneo, the Philippines, Indonesia, Malaysia, Burma, Assam, Nepal, Sri Lanka, Bangladesh, and Hainan Island and the southern provinces of China; in Oceania from Papua New Guinea, Vanuatu, and the Solomon Islands; and in Africa from Kenya, Tanzania, Uganda, Mozambique, Madagascar, the Comoro Islands, Sudan (central), Zambia, Zaire (northeast), Burundi, and Rwanda.

Strains of *P falciparum* resistant to pyrimethamine-sulfadoxine (Fansidar) have been established or suspected in Thailand, Papua New Guinea, Irian Jaya, Indonesia, Kenya, Colombia, Kampuchea, Tanzania, and parts of Brazil.

Strains of *P falciparum* in Thailand have shown decreased sensitivity to quinine. In many areas of the world, particularly in Southeast Asia, *P vivax* is resistant to pyrimethamine, including the pyrimethamine-containing drugs Fansidar and Maloprim. Radical cure of *P vivax* with primaquine requires a larger dosage (22.5 mg [base] for 14 days) in areas of the southwest Pacific and for many strains in Thailand.

*Not available in the USA.

Table 26—2. Chemoprophylaxis and treatment of malaria in nonimmune populations.

CHEMOPROPHYLAXIS

Chemoprophylaxis of all species (except chloroquine-resistant P falciparum)

Prevention of attacks while in endemic area

Chloroquine phosphate, 500 mg (salt)[1,2] once weekly.

Prevention of attacks after leaving endemic area

Chloroquine phosphate, 500 mg (salt) once weekly for 6 weeks *plus* primaquine diphosphate, 26.3 mg (salt)[4,5] daily for 14 days,

or

Chloroquine phosphate, 500 mg (salt), *plus* primaquine diphosphate, 78.9 mg (salt)[4,5] once weekly for 8 weeks.

Chemoprophylaxis of chloroquine-resistant P falciparum

Prevention of attacks while in endemic area

Pyrimethamine, 25 mg, *plus* sulfadoxine, 500 mg (Fansidar)[2,3] weekly, *plus* chloroquine phosphate, 500 mg (salt)[1,2] weekly to prevent attacks due to *P vivax* and *P malariae.*

Prevention of attacks after leaving endemic area

Pyrimethamine, 25 mg, *plus* sulfadoxine, 500 mg (Fansidar),[3] once weekly for 6 weeks,

plus

Chloroquine and primaquine by one of the 2 methods in the left-hand column to eradicate *P vivax* and *P malariae* infection.

TREATMENT

Treatment of all species (except chloroquine-resistant P falciparum)

Oral treatment

Chloroquine phosphate, 1 g (600 mg base) as initial dose, then 0.5 g in 6 hours, then 0.5 g daily for the next 2 days,

followed by

Primaquine diphosphate, 26.3 mg (salt)[4] daily for 14 days if the infection is due to *P vivax* or *P ovale.*

Parenteral treatment of severe attacks

Quinine dihydrochloride.[6,7] Start oral chloroquine therapy as soon as possible; follow with primaquine if the infection is due to *P vivax* or *P ovale.*

or

Chloroquine hydrochloride,[6] 250 mg (salt) (200 mg base), intramuscularly; repeat every 6 hours, but start oral chloroquine therapy as soon as possible; follow with primaquine if the infection is due to *P vivax* or *P ovale.*

Treatment of chloroquine-resistant P falciparum

Oral treatment

Quinine sulfate, 650 mg 3 times daily for 3 days; on the fourth day, give pyrimethamine, 75 mg, and sulfadoxine, 1500 mg (Fansidar),[3]

or

Quinine sulfate, 650 mg 3 times daily for 3 days, *plus* pyrimethamine, 25 mg twice daily for 3 days, and sulfadiazine, 500 mg 4 times daily for 5 days,

or

Quinine sulfate, 650 mg 3 times daily for 3 days, *plus* either tetracycline, 250 mg 4 times daily for 7 days, or clindamycin, 900 mg 3 times daily for 3 days.

Parenteral treatment of severe attacks

Quinine dihydrochloride.[6,7] Start oral therapy with quinine plus a second drug (see above) as soon as possible.

---

[1] 500 mg chloroquine phosphate salt = 300 mg chloroquine base.

[2] Before leaving home, patients should take a test dose to detect possible idiosyncratic reactions. The first dose of the drug should be started 1 week before entering the endemic area. It is essential that the drug be continued weekly for 6 weeks after leaving the endemic area.

[3] Available in the USA and generally can be obtained in the endemic area.

[4] 26.3 mg primaquine diphosphate salt = 15 mg primaquine base.

[5] Chloroquine alone, when taken for 6 weeks after leaving the endemic area, is curative for *P falciparum* and *P malariae,* but primaquine is needed to eradicate the persistent exoerythrocytic (liver) stages of *P vivax* and *P ovale.* Start primaquine only after returning home, continue chloroquine weekly until that time and during primaquine therapy. Only travelers likely to be exposed to infection require primaquine (see text). Patients should be screened for G6PD deficiency before use of primaquine.

[6] Parenteral chloroquine and quinine are available in the USA from the Parasitic Disease Drug Service, Centers for Disease Control, Atlanta 30333, (404) 329—3670; after hours in emergencies, (404) 329—2888.

[7] Quinine dihydrochloride, 600 mg in 300 mL of normal saline intravenously slowly over 2 hours; repeat every 6—8 hours until oral therapy is possible, but not more often than 3 times in 24 hours. In an emergency, when parenteral quinine or chloroquine is unavailable, quinidine gluconate has been used; 800 mg is diluted in 250 mg of 5% dextrose and administered very slowly intravenously under electrocardiographic monitoring; widening of the QRS interval requires discontinuation of the drug.

D. Drugs of Choice (Except Where *P falciparum* Is Resistant to Chloroquine): (See Table 26–2.)

1. Chloroquine phosphate–Chloroquine (Aralen) is used in chemoprophylaxis to prevent attacks (to suppress symptoms) of all forms of malaria but does not prevent infection. *P falciparum* and *P malariae* infections are terminated (suppressive cure) if chloroquine is taken weekly for 6 weeks, because these infections have no persistent exoerythrocytic phase. However, in *P vivax* and *P ovale* infections, which have a persistent liver phase, delayed initial attacks or relapses may occur after stopping chloroquine; concurrent use of primaquine eradicates the liver phase.

Chloroquine is also the drug of choice for treating acute attacks of malaria, but cure occurs only with *P falciparum* and *P malariae*. Cure for *P vivax* and *P ovale* requires primaquine to eradicate the liver phase of the infections.

If symptoms caused by *P falciparum* do not begin to respond to chloroquine within about 48 hours, parasite resistance to this drug must be considered. Although capable of causing ocular damage when used in large doses for prolonged periods for collagen disease, chloroquine causes few toxic symptoms when used for malaria prophylaxis or treatment. Gastrointestinal symptoms, mild headache, pruritus, anorexia, malaise, and urticaria may occur; taking the drug after meals may reduce side effects. A total cumulative dosage of 60 g (base) theoretically may be critical in the development of ocular, ototoxic, and myopathic effects. A recent WHO paper, however, presented the view that weekly administration of 0.5 g (of salt) chloroquine could continue for up to 7 years. Pregnancy is not a contraindication to chloroquine.

Certain antacids and antidiarrheal agents (kaolin, calcium carbonate, and magnesium trisilicate) have been shown to interfere with absorption of chloroquine and should not be taken within about 4 hours of chloroquine.

If patients cannot absorb the drug rapidly because of vomiting or severe diarrhea, or if they are comatose or have a high parasite count (100,000/μL), give chloroquine hydrochloride intramuscularly. An effective blood level is usually rapidly attained after intramuscular injection. Start oral medication as soon as possible. Do not use chloroquine for severely ill patients whose infections originated in an endemic region where *P falciparum* is resistant to chloroquine.

2. Primaquine phosphate–This drug has been shown to be the most effective agent against the liver forms of *P vivax* and *P ovale*. It is employed to prevent relapse of disease by eliminating liver parasites (''radical cure'') in patients who have had an acute attack and for individuals returning from an endemic area who have probably been exposed to malaria. Although opinion differs, in persons with a low probability of exposure it is generally preferable to depend on extended follow-up for the detection of such malarial infections and to avoid the toxicity of primaquine. This drug is also used occasionally to eliminate gameto-

cytes of *P falciparum* from patients and thus prevent their transmission to mosquitoes; the dosage is either 45 mg (base) once or 15 mg/d for 5 days.

All patients should be tested for glucose-6-phosphate dehydrogenase (G6PD) deficiency before therapy is begun and should be followed carefully during treatment, because severe hemolytic reactions occur in some individuals whose red blood cells are deficient in G6PD. This deficiency is most common among blacks, persons from the Mediterranean littoral, and persons of Asian extraction. For individuals deficient in G6PD, give primaquine phosphate, 78.9 mg (45 mg base), and chloroquine phosphate, 0.5 g (0.3 g base) weekly, for 8 weeks. However, for persons suspected of having the Mediterranean or Canton forms of G6PD deficiency, it may be preferable not to give primaquine but to treat attacks of malaria with chloroquine as they occur. Other occasional side effects of the drug are gastrointestinal disturbances, neutropenia, and dizziness; methemoglobinemia can occur in G6PD-deficient persons. Primaquine should not be used in pregnancy.

3. Quinine–Parenteral quinine (quinine dihydrochloride) is used in the treatment of severe attacks of malaria due to *P falciparum* strains sensitive or resistant to chloroquine. It should be used with extreme caution and only for patients who cannot take the medication orally; appropriate oral therapy should be started as soon as possible. The intravenous infusions should be given slowly over 2 hours; blood pressure and ECG should be monitored frequently. Quinine toxicity (cinchonism) includes nausea and vomiting, diarrhea, tinnitus, blurred vision, and, less often, fever and hypotension. Severe toxicity, with coma, convulsions, and blindness, occurs only rarely.

Oral quinine (quinine sulfate) is used in prophylaxis where *P falciparum* has become resistant to both chloroquine and pyrimethamine-sulfadoxine (Fansidar). Oral quinine is also used to treat malaria due to chloroquine-resistant strains of *P falciparum*. Although quinine alone will control an acute attack, in many infections, particularly with strains from Southeast Asia, it fails to prevent recurrence. Addition of pyrimethamine-sulfadoxine or other drugs (see Table 26–2) lowers the rate of recurrence.

E. Alternative Drugs (Except Where *P falciparum* Is Resistant to Chloroquine):

1. Amodiaquine* (Basoquin,* Camoquin*) is a congener of chloroquine. Prophylactically, the dosage is 520 mg (400 mg base) once weekly while in the endemic area and then weekly for 6 weeks after leaving. Therapeutically, the initial dose in an acute attack is 780 mg (600 mg base), followed by 520 mg (400 mg base) daily for 2 days. In prophylaxis and treatment, primaquine is needed to eradicate *P vivax* and *P ovale* infections.

2. Pyrimethamine (Daraprim, Malocide*), an antifolic compound, is effective in prophylaxis where strains are sensitive but is not used in treatment be-

*Not available in the USA.

cause of its slow action. Give 25–50 mg weekly (according to local advice) and for 6 weeks after leaving the endemic area. Primaquine is needed to eradicate *P vivax* and *P ovale* infections. Pyrimethamine toxicity is very low; the drug has the advantage of being tasteless and is available in a syrup form. Its disadvantage is that wherever it has been extensively used by itself, drug-resistant strains of *P vivax* and *P falciparum* have usually appeared. Pyrimethamine is contraindicated in pregnancy, because teratogenic effects occurred when it was tested in rats; however, in humans no teratogenic effects have been attributed to the drug after 30 years of extensive usage.

3. Proguanil* (chlorguanide,* Paludrine*) is an antifolic compound similar to pyrimethamine and has very low toxicity. It is the drug of choice for malaria prophylaxis in many parts of the world. The prophylactic dose, 200 mg daily, should be continued for 6 weeks after leaving the endemic area. However, wherever proguanil is extensively used, drug-resistant strains of *P vivax* and *P falciparum* usually appear. To eradicate the relapsing malarias, primaquine is used. Proguanil is not advised in treatment of acute attacks of malaria.

F. Drugs of Choice Where *P falciparum* Is Resistant to Chloroquine: Chloroquine resistance is usually (not always) associated with cross-resistance to amodiaquine, quinacrine, and sometimes to quinine along with concomitant resistance to pyrimethamine and proguanil. In the past 3 years, there have been increasing reports of concomitant resistance to Fansidar and Maloprim.

1. Quinine–In the treatment of acute illness due to *P falciparum* strains resistant to chloroquine, both quinine (see above) and pyrimethamine-sulfadoxine (see below) are required, because pyrimethamine-sulfadoxine acts too slowly when used alone. In the presence of hepatic dysfunction, the daily dose of quinine should be reduced. For severe infections in Thailand and Kampuchea, a loading dose of quinine of 20 mg/kg during the first 4 hours has been suggested, followed by maintenance doses thereafter.

2. Pyrimethamine-sulfadoxine (Fansidar)–For both prophylaxis and treatment in most areas of the world where *P falciparum* is resistant to chloroquine, the drug of choice is a synergistic combination of a long-acting sulfonamide with a folic acid antagonist (eg, pyrimethamine or trimethoprim). Current experience has led to the combination of pyrimethamine, 25 mg, and sulfadoxine, 500 mg, as the drug of choice. This fixed-dose combination is available in the USA under the trade name Fansidar and in other countries as Fansidar and Falcidar.

Serious side effects to Fansidar are rare. Pyrimethamine in high doses for prolonged periods has caused megaloblastic anemia due to folate deficiency, but this has not happened when the drug has been used for weekly prophylaxis for malaria. The antifolate effect may be exacerbated by poor nutrition, concur-

rent use of antimicrobials (including sulfonamides), and pregnancy. Periodic hemograms are recommended to monitor patients using the drug longer than 6 months. Adverse effects of sulfonamides include hypersensitivity reactions, blood dyscrasias, hepatitis, toxic nephrosis, and central nervous system symptoms. Pyrimethamine-sulfadoxine is contraindicated in pregnancy.

For chemoprophylaxis of falciparum malaria resistant to chloroquine, pyrimethamine-sulfadoxine is given weekly while the patient is in the endemic area; it is essential that it be continued weekly for 6 weeks after leaving to provide suppressive cure. Since in many areas of the world *P vivax* and *P ovale* are resistant to the pyrimethamine, chloroquine is recommended for concurrent use with pyrimethamine-sulfadoxine to provide chemoprophylaxis for these parasites. After the patient has left the endemic area, primaquine can be given according to the guidelines presented above to provide radical cure of *P vivax* and *P ovale* infection.

G. Alternative Drugs Where *P falciparum* Is Resistant to Chloroquine: For treatment, quinine plus either tetracycline or clindamycin may be used in the dosages presented in Table 26–2. For prophylaxis (but not for treatment), Maloprim* may be given (each tablet contains pyrimethamine, 12.5 mg, plus dapsone, 100 mg). The dosage is 2 tablets per week before entering the endemic area, 1 tablet weekly while exposed, and 1 tablet weekly for 6 weeks after leaving. Hemolytic anemia, methemoglobinemia, agranulocytosis, and bone marrow red cell aplasia have rarely been associated with dapsone used as an antimalarial; periodic hemograms are recommended when Maloprim is used for longer than 6 months. Some persons sensitive to sulfonamides may also be sensitive to dapsone. *P falciparum* resistant to Maloprim has been reported from Kenya and Tanzania. Another combination available in some countries for prophylaxis is pyrimethamine-sulfalene (Matakelfin*).

Mefloquine* is a new quinoline methanol derivative. It has minimal side effects and is effective against all strains of plasmodia, including those resistant to chloroquine and quinine. Although resistance can also develop to mefloquine, no resistance has been reported to the combination of quinine and mefloquine. Mefloquine is not available commercially.

H. Drugs of Choice Where *P falciparum* Is Resistant to Both Chloroquine and Fansidar: Combined resistance has been reported from eastern Thailand and Papua New Guinea and in instances also from other areas of Thailand, Kampuchea, Indonesia, Brazil, Colombia, and East Africa. For selected areas and patients, quinine sulfate, 325 mg twice daily and for 6 weeks after leaving the endemic area, may be indicated for prophylaxis. Chloroquine is not taken concurrently. The guidelines for taking primaquine to eradicate *P vivax* are as described above. Tetracy-

---

clines have been recommended by some authorities for prophylaxis in eastern Thailand.

In treatment, quinine, 650 mg 3 times daily for 3 days, plus tetracycline, 250 mg 4 times daily for 7 days, has usually been effective.

I. General Measures: Corticosteroids were recently shown to be deleterious in cerebral malaria and should no longer be used. The WHO 1973 Expert Report suggests the following measures: ". . . some workers advocate the use of heparin as an antithrombotic agent, but this compound must be given with caution in the presence of deep jaundice. In some patients with severe falciparum malaria, anuria and consequent nitrogen retention may occur. Dialysis is indicated in these cases if the facilities are available; the same considerations apply to mannitol diuresis. Severe anemia is an indication for blood transfusion.''

Prognosis

The uncomplicated and untreated primary attack of *P vivax*, *P ovale*, or *P falciparum* malaria usually lasts 2–4 weeks; that of *P malariae* about twice as long. Each type of infection may subsequently relapse (once or many times) before the infection terminates spontaneously. With modern antimalarial drugs, the prognosis is good for most malaria infections, but in *P falciparum* infections, when complications such as cerebral malaria and blackwater fever develop, the prognosis is poor even with treatment.

Bruce-Chwatt LJ (editor): *Chemotherapy of Malaria,* 2nd ed. World Health Organization Monograph Series 27. World Health Organization, 1981.

Bygbjerg IC et al: Mefloquine resistance of falciparum malaria from Tanzania enhanced by treatment. *Lancet* 1983;**1:**774.

Centers for Disease Control: Prevention of malaria in travelers, 1982. *MMWR* 1982;**31(Suppl 1).** [Entire issue.]

Chongsuphajaisiddhi T: Pathophysiology of malaria. *Southeast Asian J Trop Med Public Health* 1981;**12:**298.

Chongsuphajaisiddhi T, Sabchareon A, Attanath P: Treatment of quinine resistant falciparum malaria in Thai children. *Southeast Asian J Trop Med Public Health* 1983;**14:**357.

Cohen S (editor): *Malaria.* British Medical Bulletin. Churchill Livingstone, 1982.

Hall AP: The treatment of severe falciparum malaria. *Trans R Soc Trop Med Hyg* 1977;**71:**367.

Hess U, Timmermans PM, Jones M: Combined chloroquine/Fansidar–resistant falciparum malaria appears in east Africa. *Am J Trop Med Hyg* 1983;**32:**217.

Kreier JP (editor): *Malaria.* Vol 1: *Epidemiology, Chemotherapy, Morphology, and Metabolism.* Vol 2: *Pathology, Vector Studies, and Culture.* Vol 3: *Immunology and Immunization.* Academic Press, 1980.

Peters W: Current trends in malaria chemoprophylaxis and treatment. *Bull Soc Path Ex* 1983;**76:**446.

Pinichpongse S et al: An evaluation of five regimens for the outpatient therapy of falciparum malaria in Thailand 1980–81. *Bull WHO* 1982;**60:**907.

Public Health Laboratory Service Malaria Reference Laboratory: Malaria prophylaxis. *Br Med J* 1983;**286:**787; 1983;**287:** 1454; 1984;**288:**1216.

Quinine in chloroquine-resistant falciparum malaria. (Editorial.) *Lancet* 1983;**1:**452.

Reacher M et al: Drug therapy for *Plasmodium falciparum* malaria resistant to pyrimethamine-sulfadoxine (Fansidar). A study of alternate regimens in Eastern Thailand. *Lancet* 1981;**2·**1066.

Sassani JW et al: Progressive chloroquine retinopathy. *Ann Ophthalmol* 1983;**15:**19.

Warrell DA et al: Dexamethasone proves deleterious in cerebral malaria: A double-blind trial in 100 comatose patients. *N Engl J Med* 1982;**306:**313.

Wyler DJ: Malaria: Resurgence, resistance, and research. (2 parts.) *N Engl J Med* 1983;**308:**875, 934.

AFRICAN TRYPANOSOMIASIS
(Sleeping Sickness)

Essentials of Diagnosis

- Minor inflammation at site of bite.
- Fever, tachycardia, splenomegaly, lymphadenopathy.
- Trypanosomes seen in thick blood films or lymph node aspirates in early stage, or in cerebrospinal fluid in late stage.

Gambian trypanosomiasis:
- Slow progression, with personality changes, headache, apathy, somnolence, tremors, speech and gait disturbances, anorexia, coma, death.

Rhodesian trypanosomiasis:
- Rapid progression of above events.

General Considerations

Rhodesian and Gambian trypanosomiasis are caused by *Trypanosoma brucei rhodesiense* and *Trypanosoma brucei gambiense,* respectively, both hemoflagellates morphologically indistinguishable from the third member of the group, *Trypanosoma brucei brucei,* a pathogen of animals but not of humans. All are transmitted by bites of tsetse flies (*Glossina* sp). Rhodesian sleeping sickness is primarily a zoonosis of game animals, transmitted by *Glossina* living in savannah. Cattle and sheep may also serve as incidental reservoirs. Within the sylvatic cycle, humans are only infected sporadically; but epidemics have occurred in which the transmission cycle is probably human to fly to human. Gambian sleeping sickness is a human disease with human-to-fly-to-human transmission paramount and humans serving as reservoir hosts. Pigs and dogs may serve as reservoirs, but *T brucei gambiense* has not been isolated from naturally infected animals. The *Glossina* vectors inhabit shaded areas along streams and rivers. Sleeping sickness in humans occurs focally throughout tropical Africa from south of the Sahara to about 20 degrees south latitude. *T brucei gambiense* infections are limited to west and central Africa up to the eastern Rift Valley and are particularly important in Zaire. *T brucei rhodesiense* occurs to the east of the Rift Valley and is most active in Tanzania and Zambia.

Clinical Findings

A. Symptoms and Signs: The first stage of infection, the trypanosomal chancre, is a local inflammatory reaction that appears about 48 hours after the tsetse fly bite. Many patients give no history of such a reaction; in others the lesions are painful or pruritic for up to 3 weeks. The second stage, invasion of the bloodstream and reticuloendothelial system, usually begins several weeks later. Symptoms may appear at once, particularly in rhodesiense infections, or after several years. An irregular fever pattern with persistent tachycardia is characteristic. Transient rashes, often circinate, and scattered areas of firm edema may appear. There may be myalgias and arthralgias and delayed sensation to pain, with deep hyperesthesia. The spleen is usually enlarged. Enlarged, rubbery, and painless lymph nodes, particularly those of the posterior cervical group (Winterbottom's sign) are commonly found in gambiense infection; lymph nodes are not often enlarged in rhodesiense infection. Signs of myocardial involvement appear early in Rhodesian trypanosomiasis. The patient may succumb to myocarditis before signs of central nervous system invasion appear. Central nervous system manifestations appear within a few weeks or months of onset in rhodesiense infection. Gambian sleeping sickness differs from the acute and virulent Rhodesian form in that it develops more insidiously, starting 6 months to several years from onset. Personality changes, apathy, and headaches are among the early findings. Tremors, disturbances of speech and gait, mania, somnolence, and anorexia appear late. The patient becomes severely emaciated, and finally comatose. Death often results from secondary infection.

B. Laboratory Findings: Definitive diagnosis is made by finding the organism in blood, lymph node and bone marrow aspirate, or cerebrospinal fluid. Although trypanosomes are often difficult to find in peripheral blood, multiple specimens should be examined (1) for motile organisms in wet films, (2) after staining thick and thin films, and (3) after concentration by centrifugation of heparinized blood (the buffy coat is examined). Aspirate lymph nodes that are still soft (not yet fibrosed) by the "massage" technique; organisms on wet films or stained smears are seen more often with infections due to *T brucei gambiense* than in those due to *T brucei rhodesiense*. Other diagnostic techniques with blood include Millipore filtration, DEAE cellulose separation of trypanosomes, and inoculation of mice or rats. The cerebrospinal fluid contains increased cells (lymphocytes) and an elevated protein. Examination of wet films and stained smears of centrifuged cerebrospinal fluid specimens may show trypanosomes in advanced cases of trypanosomiasis; inoculate spinal fluid into an experimental animal. The immunofluorescence and ELISA serologic tests may be useful, but false-negative results may occur. Blood for serologic testing can be collected and stored on filter paper.

Other laboratory findings include anemia, increased sedimentation rate, reduced total serum protein, increased serum globulin, and an elevated IgM level. The serum IgM level begins to rise shortly after infection and may reach 10–20 times normal. Normal or low levels of IgM in acute disease probably rule out the infection. An elevated IgM in the cerebrospinal fluid is nearly pathognomonic and differentiates trypanosomiasis from other diseases causing elevated serum IgM levels.

Differential Diagnosis

Trypanosomiasis may be mistaken for a variety of other diseases, including malaria, kala-azar, tuberculosis, cerebral tumors, encephalitis, and cerebral syphilis. Serologic tests for syphilis may be falsely positive in trypanosomiasis. Malaria, suggested by fever and splenomegaly, may be ruled out by blood examinations; kala-azar can usually be ruled out clinically without resorting to spleen or marrow puncture. Other central nervous system conditions are differentiated by neurologic examination and lumbar puncture findings.

Prevention

Pentamidine is the drug of choice for chemoprophylaxis of sleeping sickness, but it is effective with certainty only against the Gambian type. In Rhodesian infection, pentamidine may lead to suppression of early symptoms, resulting in recognition of the disease too late in its course for effective treatment. Excretion of pentamidine isethionate from the body is slow; one intramuscular injection (4 mg/kg, maximum 300 mg) will protect against gambiense infection for 6 months. The drug is potentially toxic and should only be used for persons at high risk.

Treatment

A. Specific Measures: Only patients positive for trypanosomes should receive treatment. Suramin and pentamidine do not cross the blood-brain barrier and therefore can only be used in the early stage of the disease. (In the USA, the following drugs are available only from the Parasitic Disease Drug Service, Centers for Disease Control, Atlanta 30333. Call [404] 329–3670.)

1. Early disease: hemolymphatic stage –

a. Suramin sodium is the drug of choice in the early stages of trypanosomiasis before the central nervous system is invaded. This organic urea compound is administered intravenously in freshly prepared 10% solution in distilled water. Start treatment with a test dose of 100 mg; then give 20 mg/kg body weight (maximum, 1 g) every 5–7 days. The usual course is 5 injections, and it should not exceed 7. Because of occasional renal toxicity, frequent urinalyses are essential during therapy. Discontinue if red blood cells, casts, or significant amounts of protein occur in the urine. Dermatitis, gastrointestinal disturbances, and many other side effects are also reported. The drug is contraindicated in renal disease.

b. Pentamidine isethionate, a diamidine, is a somewhat less effective alternative to suramin in treating early Gambian trypanosomiasis. It is administered as a 2% solution intramuscularly. The drug may induce a sudden fall in blood pressure or hypoglycemia if given intravenously. Use with caution in renal disease. Administer in doses of 3–4 mg (base)/kg; the powder must be freshly dissolved in 2–3 mL of water and given intramuscularly daily or every other day for 7–10 injections.

2. Late disease: central nervous system involvement –

a. Melarsoprol (Mel B) is the trivalent arsenical melarsen oxide coupled with dimercaprol (BAL) to reduce toxicity. It is the drug of choice in treating gambiense and rhodesiense infections of the central nervous system, but drug resistance does occur. The drug has only a narrow margin of safety; in approximately 10% of cases, reactive and hemorrhagic encephalopathy develops and may be fatal. The drug is prepared as a 3.6% solution in propylene glycol and must be given intravenously. A recommended schedule is 3 series of 3 daily injections, each series separated by an interval of at least 1 week. Each injection is 3.6 mg/kg (maximum 200 mg). If the patient is a poor risk, start with 1.8 mg/kg and increase over the first 3 days. For *T brucei rhodesiense* infections, a course of suramin is given concurrently with melarsoprol. For *T brucei gambiense* infections, it is preferable that 2–3 injections of suramin precede melarsoprol.

Melarsonyl potassium (Mel W) is a water-soluble alternative compound effective against *T brucei gambiense*, but the results against *T brucei rhodesiense* have been inconclusive.

b. Nitrofurazone may be tried when melarsoprol has not been successful. It is given in a dosage of 0.5 g 3–4 times daily for 5–7 days. Side effects include polyneuropathy.

B. General Measures: Good nursing care, treatment of anemia and concurrent infections, and correction of malnutrition are essential in the management of patients with advanced African trypanosomiasis. Following treatment, patients should be monitored for signs of central nervous system involvement at regular intervals for 1–2 years.

Prognosis

If untreated, most cases of African trypanosomiasis are fatal. With treatment the prognosis is excellent, even in Rhodesian infection, if therapy is started before onset of central nervous system symptoms; if started late, irreversible brain damage or death is common.

Apted FIC: Present status of chemotherapy and chemoprophylaxis of human trypanosomiasis in the eastern hemisphere. *Pharmacol Ther* 1980;**11**:391.

Foulkes JR: Human trypanosomiasis in Africa. *Br Med J* 1981;**283**:1172.

Symposium on Pathogenesis of Trypanosomiasis. Royal Society of Tropical Medicine and Hygiene. *Trans R Soc Trop Med Hyg* 1980;**74**:706.

WHO Expert Committee: *The African Trypanosomiases*. Technical Report Series No. 635. World Health Organization, 1979.

AMERICAN TRYPANOSOMIASIS
(Chagas' Disease)

Essentials of Diagnosis

- Unilateral palpebral and facial edema and conjunctivitis (Romaña's sign).
- Hard, edematous, red, and painful cutaneous nodule (chagoma).
- Intermittent fever, lymphadenitis, hepatomegaly, signs and symptoms of acute or chronic myocarditis or meningoencephalitis.
- Trypanosomes in blood, isolation by animal inoculation, or positive serologic tests.

General Considerations

Chagas' disease is caused by *Trypanosoma cruzi*. The organism is a protozoan parasite of humans and wild and domestic animals and is transmitted by many species of triatomine bugs. *T cruzi* occurs only in the Americas; it is found in wild animals from southern South America to northern Mexico, Texas, and the southwestern USA. Human infection is less widespread. The triatomine bugs become infected by ingesting blood with circulating trypanosomes from infected animals or humans. Multiplication occurs in the digestive tract of the bug; infective forms are eliminated in feces. Infection in humans is through "contamination" with bug feces; the parasite penetrates the skin (generally through the bite wound) or through the conjunctiva. Transmission can also occur by blood transfusion or in utero.

In the vertebrate host, the trypanosomes first multiply close to the point of entry, assuming a leishmanial form. They then enter the bloodstream as trypanosomes and later invade the heart and other tissues, where they assume a leishmanial form. Multiplication causes cellular destruction, inflammation, and fibrosis. Infection continues for many years, probably for life.

Clinical Findings

A. Symptoms and Signs: The earliest finding in the acute infection is either the chagoma or Romaña's sign. In heavily endemic areas, initial infection commonly occurs in childhood. The acute form of the disease may be fatal, particularly in infants and young children. In addition to intermittent fever, local lymphadenitis, and hepatomegaly, there may be splenomegaly, psychologic changes, focal neurologic symptoms, convulsions, tachycardia, cardiac enlargement, arrhythmias, and cardiac failure. Myocardial damage dominates the chronic form of the disease. Clinical findings range from arrhythmias and heart block to congestive heart failure (mainly right-sided) and thromboembolic phenomena. Sudden cardiac arrest in young persons may occur. Symptomatic chronic central nervous system infection is rare. Megacolon and megaesophagus, caused by damage to nerve plexuses in the bowel or esophageal wall, occur in some areas of Chile, Argentina, and Brazil.

B. Laboratory Findings: Appropriate selection

of tests allows a parasitologic diagnosis in most acute cases and in up to 40% of chronic ones. Trypanosomes should be looked for in the blood of all patients by the following methods but are usually found only in the acute stage of infections: examination of wet (fresh) blood films, stained thick and thin films, and stained films of buffy coat after centrifugation of 5–10 mL of heparinized blood. *Trypanosoma rangeli,* a non-pathogenic blood trypanosome also found in humans in Central America and northern South America, must not be mistaken for *T cruzi.* In the acute stage, trypanosomes may also be found in lymph node aspirates; on occasion, lymph node biopsy has been helpful. Blood should also be cultured in Nicolle-Novy-MacNeal medium or inoculated into laboratory mice or rats 3–10 days old. In chronic infections, xenodiagnosis, which consists of permitting uninfected reduviids to feed on the patient and then examining their intestinal contents for trypanosomal infection, may establish the diagnosis. Various serologic tests are of presumptive diagnostic value when positive; the complement fixation test is most commonly used. A specific immune globulin demonstrated for chagasic myocardiopathy is known as endothelial-vascular immunoglobulin (EVI). Antibodies of the IgM class are usually elevated in the acute stage but normal in the chronic stage. The most important electrocardiographic abnormalities are complete right bundle branch block, conduction defects, and arrhythmias.

Differential Diagnosis

The early acute infection, with Romaña's sign, might be confused with trichinosis, but palpebral and facial edema is unilateral, not bilateral, and there is no eosinophilia. The chagoma may be mistaken for any of a variety of tropical skin lesions. Kala-azar resembles Chagas' disease in some respects (intermittent fever, hepatomegaly, splenomegaly), but in the former the spleen is much larger, there are no central nervous system symptoms, and cardiac symptoms usually appear only after anemia becomes severe. Chronic infection in adults, usually myocardial, is not clinically characteristic.

Treatment

Treatment of Chagas' disease is unsatisfactory; no drug is established as both safe and effective. Nifurtimox (Bayer 2502, Lampit), a nitrofuran, has effected cures in 75–90% of patients treated during the acute phase of illness. The drug should be tried in the chronic stage, but it is doubtful if it can eradicate intracellular parasites in all cases at doses patients can tolerate. Although parasitemia disappears, serologic reactivity remains for years. Side effects include anorexia, weight loss, vomiting, headache, vertigo, insomnia, and convulsions, especially in adults. Children tolerate the drug well. Mutagenicity and carcinogenicity are properties of some nitro compounds and thus are possible risk factors in treatment with nifurtimox. The dosage is 8–10 mg/kg daily for 90 days in acute infections and for 120 days in chronic infections. It is

available in the USA only from the Parasitic Disease Drug Service, Centers for Disease Control, Atlanta 30333; call (404) 329–3670.

Primaquine phosphate may also be tried at a dosage of 26.3 mg (salt) for 7–10 days. Benznidazole, a nitroimidazole, continues to undergo clinical trials in acute and chronic infections; its adverse reactions include skin rashes, peripheral polyneuropathy, and blood dyscrasias.

Prognosis

Acute infections in infants and young children are often fatal, particularly when the central nervous system is involved. Adults with chronic cardiac infections also may ultimately succumb to the disease. Mortality rates are not known because infections are often unrecognized.

Brener Z: Present status of chemotherapy and chemoprophylaxis of human trypanosomiasis in the Western Hemisphere. *Pharmacol Ther* 1979;**7**:71.

Brener Z: Recent developments in the field of Chagas' disease. *Bull WHO* 1982;**60**:463.

McCabe RE et al: Ketoconazole protects against infection with *Trypanosoma cruzi* in a murine model. *Am J Trop Med Hyg* 1983;**32**:960.

Miles MA: The epidemiology of South American trypanosomiasis: Biochemical and immunological approaches and their relevance to control. *Trans R Soc Trop Med Hyg* 1983; **77**:5.

Peralta JM et al: Autoantibodies and chronic Chagas' heart disease. *Trans R Soc Trop Med Hyg* 1981;**75**:568.

LEISHMANIASIS

The leishmaniae are intracellular protozoal parasites. The leishmanial diseases are caused by different species of *Leishmania* in different parts of the world and often result in significant morbidity and mortality rates. The clinical manifestations of leishmaniasis may be classified as (1) visceral, (2) cutaneous, and (3) mucocutaneous. The disease is a zoonosis transmitted by bites of sandflies (*Phlebotomus* sp) from wild or domestic animal reservoirs to humans, except in the case of Indian kala-azar, which is transmitted directly from human to human. The leishmaniae have 2 distinct forms in their life cycle: (1) In infected mammalian hosts, the parasite is found in its amastigote form (2–3 μm in length) within mononuclear phagocytes; (2) in the sandfly vector, the parasite converts to and is then transmitted as a flagellated extracellular promastigote.

Belehu A et al: Immunopathological aspects of leishmaniasis. *Springer Semin Immunopathol* 1980;**2**:399.

Chance ML: Leishmaniasis. *Br Med J* 1981;**283**:1245.

Lainson R: Leishmaniasis. Pages 41–103 in: *Parasitic Zoonoses. CRC Handbook Series in Zoonoses.* Vol 11. CRC Press, 1982.

Marsden PD: Current concepts in parasitology: Leishmaniasis. *N Engl J Med* 1979;**300**:350.

Pearson RD et al: The immunobiology of leishmaniasis. *Rev Infect Dis* 1983;**5**:907.

1. VISCERAL LEISHMANIASIS
(Kala-Azar)

Essentials of Diagnosis

- Insidious or acute onset with fever.
- Marked splenomegaly, hepatomegaly.
- Anemia, leukopenia, and wasting.
- Pigmentation of skin on forehead and hands.
- Leishman-Donovan bodies in splenic or sternal puncture smears.
- Elevated serum globulins (IgG) and total proteins.

General Considerations

Visceral leishmaniasis is geographically widespread. It is caused mainly by 2 species: *Leishmania donovani* in the Indian region and *Leishmania infantum* in the USSR, China, Middle East, Mediterranean basin, and Africa. It also occurs in South America, where the agent has been tentatively designated *Leishmania chagasi*. In each locale, the disease has its own peculiar clinical and epidemiologic features, and in some places it may also occur in epidemics. Although humans are the major reservoir, animal reservoirs such as the dog are important. The incubation period varies from weeks to months.

Clinical Findings

A. Symptoms and Signs: A local lesion at the site of the bite may precede systemic manifestations but usually is inapparent. The onset may be acute or insidious. Fever often peaks twice daily with chills and sweats, weakness, weight loss, cough, or diarrhea. Usually there is marked enlargement of the spleen, with discomfort in the left hypochondrium, and the liver is somewhat enlarged.

Eventually the spleen becomes huge, hard, and nontender. Generalized lymphadenopathy is common. Hyperpigmentation of skin, especially on hands, feet, abdomen, and forehead is marked in light-skinned patients (Kala-azar = black sickness). In blacks, there may be warty eruptions or skin ulcers. There may be bleeding from nose and gums, jaundice, ascites, and wasting; death is often due to intercurrent infections.

Post-kala-azar dermal leishmaniasis may appear 1–2 years after apparent cure (up to 10 years in India and China). This may simulate leprosy as multiple hypopigmented macules or nodules develop on preexisting lesions. Erythematous patches may appear on the face. Leishmanias are present in the skin. The condition responds well to additional courses of antimony.

B. Laboratory Findings: There is usually progressive leukopenia (seldom over $3000/\mu L$ after the first 1–2 months), with lymphocytosis and monocytosis. Occasional leukocytosis, due to concurrent sepsis, may be confusing. Associated with the hypersplenism is a normochromic anemia and a low platelet count. Diagnosis must always be confirmed by demonstrating Leishman-Donovan bodies in blood or in aspirates of sternal marrow, liver, or spleen by

stained smears; by culture in Nicolle-Novy-MacNeal medium; or by inoculation into hamsters. Buffy coat preparations of centrifuged blood may also show the organism. Serologic tests are useful, for they seldom give false-negative results. Some cross-reactions do occur. Diagnosis is supported by an increase in total serum proteins up to and greater than 10 g/dL, mainly hypergammaglobulinemia due to increased IgG. The leishmania skin test is negative in active visceral leishmaniasis but becomes positive after recovery.

Differential Diagnosis

Acute or subacute kala-azar may resemble enteric fever (but there is no toxemia) or malaria (response to antimalarial therapy may aid the diagnosis, since concomitant malaria parasites may be present in the blood in kala-azar) and other causes of splenomegaly, eg, brucellosis and lymphoma.

Chronic cases may also be confused with infectious mononucleosis, leukemia, anemias due to other causes, and tuberculosis. Post-kala-azar dermatitis may resemble leprosy.

Treatment

Visceral leishmaniasis in India usually responds well to pentavalent antimonials or pentamidine, but the former is usually necessary in areas where *L infantum* or *L chagasi* is the causative agent. The Sudanese, East African, and South American forms are generally less susceptible to drug therapy, and childhood kala-azar is occasionally completely resistant to treatment. Amphotericin B may be used as the last resort for such patients.

When giving antimonials, fresh solutions only should be used, and the ampules must be stored away from heat. Intravenous injection must be given slowly over 5 minutes through a 22- to 23-gauge needle.

(1) Antimony sodium gluconate (sodium stibogluconate), 0.2-g test dose followed by 10 mg/kg/d (maximum 600 mg/d) as 5% solution intramuscularly or intravenously for 10 days. In China, India, and Sudan, one 6- to 10-day course is usually sufficient, but in other regions (such as Kenya) several courses may be needed. Formerly, rest intervals of 2–4 weeks were advocated between courses. Recent work suggests (1) that rest periods are not only unnecessary but may increase the likelihood of relapse and of induced drug resistance; and (2) that higher doses are well tolerated. Available in the USA only from the Parasitic Disease Drug Service, Centers for Disease Control, Atlanta 30333.

(2) Pentamidine isethionate, 2–4 mg/kg intravenously or (preferably) intramuscularly, daily or on alternate days, up to 15 injections. Pentamidine is not available in the USA for this indication.

(3) Stilbamidine isethionate is used only in antimony-resistant cases and must be given with great care because it is unstable and may produce immediate reactions or delayed trigeminal hyperesthesia. The initial adult dose is 25 mg intravenously daily, increasing by 10–20 mg daily to 2 mg/kg daily. The most that

should be given is about 10 injections or a total of about 15 mg/kg.

(4) Amphotericin B is dissolved in 500 mL of 5% dextrose and injected slowly intravenously over 6 hours on alternate days. The initial dose is 0.5 mg/kg/d, which is gradually increased to 1 mg/kg/d until a total of about 30 mg/kg is given. Patients must be closely monitored in hospital, because side effects may be severe.

(5) Allopurinol is undergoing clinical trials for the treatment of kala-azar resistant to antimony sodium gluconate.

Prognosis

Without treatment, kala-azar is usually fatal. Therapy is usually effective, but relapses may occur after 2 or more years and require additional courses of therapy. Keep the patient under observation for at least 12 months; the spleen, blood studies, and body weight should return to normal.

See also references above.

Chulay JD et al: A comparison of 3 dosage regimens of sodium stibogluconate in the treatment of visceral leishmaniasis in Kenya. *J Infect Dis* 1983;**148**:148.

Jha TK: Evaluation of diamidine compound (pentamidine isethionate) in the treatment of resistant cases of kala-azar occurring in North Bihar, India. *Trans R Soc Trop Med Hyg* 1983;**77**:167.

Rassam MB, Al-Mudhaffar SA: Comparative diagnostic study of kala azar. *Ann Trop Med Parasitol* 1980;**74**:283.

2. CUTANEOUS LEISHMANIASIS

Cutaneous leishmaniasis may present as self-healing ulcers (Oriental sore), chronic mutilating ulcers, or, rarely, as disseminated cutaneous leishmaniasis that is nonulcerating and resembles lepromatous leprosy.

Cutaneous leishmaniasis is caused by *Leishmania tropica* in the USSR, India, Middle East, Mediterranean basin, and Africa; by *Leishmania aethiopica* in Ethiopia and Kenya; by *Leishmania mexicana* subspecies in Mexico and Guatemala ("chiclero's ulcer") and in South America; by *Leishmania peruviana* (uta) in the Peruvian and Argentinian highlands; and by *Leishmania braziliensis* subspecies in South and Central America. *L tropica major* is a rural acute disease characterized by a wet, rapidly ulcerating sore; *L tropica minor* is a chronic urban disease that produces a dry sore which ulcerates only slowly or not at all.

Disseminated cutaneous leishmaniasis is a rare syndrome caused by *L mexicana* subspecies in the Amazon region of Brazil and in Venezuela. It appears to be incurable. Long-standing nodular, nonulcerative skin lesions are widely disseminated. As in the case of leprosy, there is a state of impaired cell-mediated immunity, and parasites are usually abundant in smears and sections. The Montenegro skin test is negative. A form of diffuse cutaneous leishmaniasis also occurs in Ethiopia and the Sudan.

In cutaneous leishmaniasis, cutaneous swellings appear about 2–8 weeks after bites of sandflies. The swellings may ulcerate and discharge pus, or they may remain dry. Dry and moist forms are caused by locally distinct leishmanias, with the dry forms having longer incubation periods.

Lesions tend to heal spontaneously over a period of months to 2 years, but secondary infection may lead to gross extension and disfigurement, especially if the lesion is on the face.

Leishmanias cannot be detected in purulent discharge but may be seen in stained scrapings from the cleaned edge of the ulcer or in material aspirated after the injection of saline under the margin of the ulcer. Under sterile conditions, aspirate may be inoculated into NNN medium or into hamsters. The skin test is positive early. Serologic tests may be helpful.

Single lesions of Old World leishmaniasis (Oriental sore) may be cleaned, covered, and left to heal spontaneously. Local heat often helps the healing process. Carbon dioxide snow, infrared therapy, the intralesional installation of a pentavalent antimony compound or quinicrine, or radiotherapy is often effective. Antibiotics may be required for secondary infections. Antimony sodium gluconate as for visceral leishmaniasis may be effective with indolent ulcers. Metronidazole and cycloguanil pamoate have given variable results. Rifampin and ketoconazole are being tested.

Lesions caused by *L aethiopica* have been treated only with pentamidine in the past, because of poor response to conventional doses of pentavalent antimonials; however, high-dose antimonial therapy has recently been reported as effective.

The milder forms of solitary nodules and ulcers due to *L mexicana* from Mexico and Central America seldom require treatment. Metronidazole at dosage levels used to treat amebiasis, or cycloguanil pamoate, 5 mg/kg as a single repository injection, may be tried to speed healing. If necessary, use antimony sodium gluconate, 10 mg/kg/d (maximum 600 mg/d) intramuscularly or intravenously for 6–10 days. If there is any suspicion that a lesion is caused by *L braziliensis*, it should be treated with antimony sodium gluconate.

See also references above.

Chulay JD et al: High-dose sodium stibogluconate treatment of cutaneous leishmaniasis in Kenya. *Trans R Soc Trop Med Hyg* 1983;**77**:717.

Currie M: Treatment of cutaneous leishmaniasis by curettage. *Br Med J* 1983;**287**:1099.

Evan-Paz Z et al: Rifampicin treatment of cutaneous leishmaniasis. *Int J Dermatol* 1982;**21**:110.

Hendricks L, Wright N: Diagnosis of cutaneous leishmaniasis by in vitro cultivation of saline aspirates in Schneider's Drosophila Medium. *Am J Trop Med Hyg* 1979;**28**:962.

Mayrink W et al: American cutaneous leishmaniasis: Disappearance of amastigotes from lesions during antimonial therapy. *Rev Inst Med Trop Sao Paulo* 1983;**25**:265.

Weinrauch L et al: Efficacy of ketoconazole in cutaneous leishmaniasis. *Arch Dermatol Res* 1983;**275**:353.

3. MUCOCUTANEOUS (NASO-ORAL) LEISHMANIASIS

Leishmania braziliensis causes severe naso-oral lesions (espundia) in many lowland forest areas of South America and Central America. The initial lesion, single or multiple, is on exposed skin; it is initially papular (can be pruriginous or painful), then nodular, and later may ulcerate. Nonulcerating tumors may become wartlike or papillomatous. Healing follows with scarring within several months to a year. Naso-oral involvement is either by direct extension or, more often, metastatically to the mucosa; it may appear concurrently with the initial lesion, shortly after healing, or after many years. The mucosa of the anterior part of the nasal septum is generally the first area to be involved. Extensive destruction of the soft tissues and cartilage of the nose, oral cavity, and lips may follow and may extend to the larynx and pharynx. Gross and hideous destruction and marked suffering can result. Severe bacterial infection is common. Regional lymphangitis, lymphadenitis, fever, weight loss, keratitis, and anemia may be present. In blacks, large polypoid masses may affect the lips and cheeks. Death may result from inanition or bacterial infection.

Diagnosis is by finding Leishman-Donovan bodies in scrapings, biopsy specimen, or aspirated tissue juice; the organism also grows with difficulty in Novy-MacNeal-Nicolle medium or after hamster inoculation. The Montenegro skin test is useful. If an injection of a suspension of killed leptomonads produces a fully developed papule in 2–3 days that disappears after a week, the diagnosis is fairly certain. Antibodies are detectable in most cases and disappear with radical cure.

Specific treatment should be combined, if necessary, with local or systemic antibiotics or sulfonamides. Give antimony sodium gluconate, 10 mg/kg/d (maximum 600 mg/d) intramuscularly or intravenously for 6–10 days. Established naso-oral lesions are often difficult to cure. Two additional courses can be given. If initial treatment fails, use amphotericin B, 0.25–1 mg/kg, by slow intravenous infusion daily or every 2 days for up to 8 weeks. In some areas, pyrimethamine, 50 mg/d for 15 days, plus folinic acid, 6 mg/d, has appeared promising; the course is repeated up to 4 times, with 15-day intervals between courses. Ethylstibamine can be tried as for visceral leishmaniasis. Nifurtimox (Lampit) is undergoing clinical trials.

See also references above.

Crofts MAJ: Use of amphotericin B in mucocutaneous leishmaniasis. *J Trop Med Hyg* 1976;**79**:111.

Marsden PD et al: Mucocutaneous leishmaniasis: An unsolved clinical problem. *Trop Doct* 1977;**7**:7.

GIARDIASIS

Essentials of Diagnosis

- Most infections are asymptomatic.
- In some cases, acute or chronic diarrhea, mild to severe, with bulky, greasy, frothy, malodorous stools, free of blood and pus. Lassitude.
- Upper abdominal discomfort, cramps, distension, and excessive flatus.
- Cysts and occasionally trophozoites in stools.
- Trophozoites in duodenal fluid.

General Considerations

Giardiasis is a protozoal infection of the upper small intestine caused by the flagellate *Giardia lamblia*. Often the infection is asymptomatic, but it may present as acute or chronic diarrhea or rarely as a malabsorption syndrome. The parasite occurs worldwide, and the infection is considered the most common intestinal protozoal pathogen in the USA and Europe. Persons of all ages are affected, but occurrence is particularly high among children. Prevalence rates of up to 20% have been reported in lower economic groups, and giardiasis is a well recognized problem in special groups including travelers, campers, male homosexuals, and persons with impaired immune states.

The organism occurs in feces as a symmetric, heart-shaped flagellated trophozoite measuring 10–25 μm × 6–12 μm and as a cyst measuring 8–13 μm × 6–11 μm. Only the cyst form is infectious by the oral route; trophozoites are destroyed by gastric acidity. Most infections are sporadic, resulting from cysts transmitted by person-to-person contact, by anal-oral sexual contact, or as a result of fecal contamination of water or food. Multiple infections are common in households, and outbreaks occur in nursery schools and mental institutions and as a result of contamination of water supplies. Humans are the reservoir for *Giardia*, but dogs and beavers have been implicated as a source of infection.

After the cysts are ingested, trophozoites emerge in the duodenum and jejunum. They can cause epithelial damage, atrophy of villi, hypertrophic crypts, and extensive cellular infiltration of the lamina propria by lymphocytes, plasma cells, and neutrophils. It is likely that hypogammaglobulinemia, low secretory IgA levels in the gut, achlorhydria, and malnutrition favor the development of illness. Serum antibodies have been demonstrated, usually in association with symptomatic disease.

Clinical Findings

A. Symptoms and Signs: The clinical forms of giardiasis are (1) asymptomatic infection, (2) acute diarrhea, (3) chronic diarrhea, and (4) malabsorption syndrome. A large proportion of patients remain asymptomatic cyst carriers, and their infection clears spontaneously. The incubation period is usually 1–3 weeks but may be longer. The illness may begin gradually or be sudden and severe. The acute phase may last days or weeks, but it is usually self-limited, although cyst excretion may continue. In a few patients, the disorder may become chronic and last for years, but it does not appear to last indefinitely.

In both the acute and chronic forms of the disease, diarrhea ranges from mild to severe; most often it is mild. There may be no complaints other than of one bulky, loose bowel movement a day, often after breakfast. With larger numbers of movements, the stools become increasingly watery and may contain mucus but are usually free of blood and pus; they are copious, frothy, malodorous, and greasy, tending to float in the toilet bowl. The diarrhea may be continuous or recurrent; if it is recurrent, stools may be normal to mushy during intervening days, or the patient may be constipated. Other less common gastrointestinal symptoms are anorexia, nausea and vomiting, midepigastric discomfort and cramps (often after meals), belching, flatulence, borborygmus, and abdominal distension. Weight loss and weakness are common, but low-grade fever is less common; headache, urticaria, and myalgia are rare.

A malabsorption syndrome develops in a few patients, either in the acute phase, when diarrhea persists for more than a few weeks, or in the chronic phase. There may be rapid and marked weight loss and debility, particularly in the acute stage. Malabsorption that is reversible with treatment has been confirmed for fat- and protein-losing enteropathy and vitamin B_{12}, D-xylose, and lactase deficiency. Other reversible disturbances occur less frequently.

With treatment and successful eradication of the infection, there are no sequelae. Without treatment, severe malabsorption may rarely contribute to death from other causes.

B. Laboratory Tests: Diagnosis is achieved through identifying cysts or trophozoites in feces or duodenal fluid. Detecting the organism can be difficult, because the number of cysts passed in the feces varies considerably from day to day, and at the onset of infection, patients may have symptoms for about a week before organisms can be detected.

If clinically warranted, diagnostic accuracy can be increased by proceeding as follows: (1) routine stool examinations → (2) examination of upper intestinal fluid by the duodenal string test (Entero-Test) or by duodenal aspiration → (3) duodenal biopsy. Three stool specimens should be examined at intervals of 2 days or longer. Unless they can be submitted within an hour, specimens should be preserved immediately in a fixative. Stool specimens obtained with a purge do not increase the sensitivity of parasite detection. Use of barium, antibiotics, antacids, kaolin products, or oily laxatives may temporarily reduce the number of parasites or interfere with detection, requiring a delay in further examination for about 10 days.

Negative stool examinations may necessitate sampling duodenal contents by the duodenal string test or by duodenal aspiration. Duodenal aspirate should be concentrated by centrifugation at 500 rpm for 5 min-utes. Mucus or aspirate should be examined by wet mount after permanent staining.

The final diagnostic procedure for occasional patients is biopsy at the duodenojejunal junction, combined with aspiration. The biopsy specimens should first be pressed onto a slide to obtain a mucosal imprint for staining and then be sectioned for histologic examination. Procedures are being developed to detect *Giardia* antigen in feces.

Serologic tests are not available for diagnosis. The hemogram is usually normal. Eosinophilia is rare. Radiologic examination of the small bowel is usually normal in asymptomatic and mildly ill persons but may show nonspecific findings of altered motility, thickened mucosal folds, and barium column segmentation in patients with marked symptoms.

Treatment

A. Specific Measures: Symptomatic patients should be treated; asymptomatic patients should usually be treated, since they can transmit the infection to others and may occasionally become symptomatic themselves. In selected instances of asymptomatic infection, it is often best to wait a few weeks before starting treatment to see if the infection will clear spontaneously.

Treatment can be carried out effectively using the nitroimidazole compounds tinidazole and metronidazole or with quinacrine or furazolidone. Occasional treatment failures require re-treatment with an alternative drug. Tinidazole, where available, is the drug of choice, based on recent reports that it is effective as a single dose. Furazolidone is the least effective but in the USA the most convenient pediatric preparation.

All of these drugs occasionally have unpleasant side effects. In addition, furazolidone induces mammary tumors in rats, metronidazole increases the rate of naturally occurring tumors in rodents, and both metronidazole and tinidazole are mutagens in the *Salmonella* test system. These findings suggest that these drugs may carry risk factors for carcinogenicity.

1. Tinidazole (Fasigyn) (not available in the USA), 2 g given once, has had reported cure rates of 90–100%. The drug was formerly given in a dosage of 150 mg twice daily for 7 days. Adverse reactions consist of mild gastrointestinal side effects in about 10% of patients; headache and vertigo are less common.

2. Metronidazole (Flagyl)–Adults receive 250 mg 3 times daily for 5–10 days; children receive 5 mg/kg 3 times daily for 5 days. Cure rates are generally between 85 and 95%. Metronidazole may cause gastrointestinal symptoms, headache, and a metallic taste. Patients must be warned that alcohol may cause a disulfiramlike reaction. Liquid suspensions for pediatric use are available only outside the USA.

3. Quinacrine (mepacrine, Atabrine)–For adults and children over 8 years of age, give 100 mg 3 times daily after meals for 5–7 days; for younger children, give 2 mg/kg 3 times daily (maximum 300 mg/d) for 5–7 days. (The drug has a bitter taste, and young children tend to tolerate it poorly.) Cure rates are 80–95%. Gastrointestinal symptoms, headache, and dizziness are common; harmless yellowing of the skin is infrequent. Toxic psychosis and exfoliative dermatitis are rare. Quinacrine is contraindicated in psoriasis or in persons with a history of psychosis.

4. Furazolidone (Furoxone) –Adults receive 100 mg 4 times daily for 10 days; children receive 1.25 mg/kg 4 times daily for 10 days. Cure rates range from 72 to 90%. The drug is prepared as a pediatric suspension. Gastrointestinal symptoms, fever, headache, rash, and a disulfiramlike reaction with alcohol occur. Furazolidone can cause mild hemolysis in glucose-6-phosphate dehydrogenase–deficient persons. Hypersensitivity reactions have occurred rarely, including hypotension, urticaria, and serum sickness.

In follow-up, it is best to wait about 2 weeks before rechecking 2 or more stools at weekly intervals.

B. Prevention and Control: There is no effective chemoprophylaxis for giardiasis. Individual treatment of small quantities of water with iodine tablets or drops probably makes drinking water safe, except in the case of very cold water.

Battles against giardia in gut mucosa. (Editorial.) *Lancet* 1982; **2**:527.

Davidson RA: Issues in clinical parasitology: The treatment of giardiasis. *Am J Gastroenterol* 1984;**79**:256.

Gillon J: Giardiasis: Review of epidemiology: Pathogenetic mechanisms and host responses. *Q J Med* 1984;**209**:29.

Jokipii L, Jokipii AMM: Single-dose metronidazole and tinidazole as therapy for giardiasis: Success rates, side effects, and drug absorption and elimination. *J Infect Dis* 1979;**140**:984.

Pickering LK et al: Occurrence of *Giardia lamblia* in children in day care centers. *J Pediatr* 1984;**104**:522.

Smith JW, Wolfe MS: Giardiasis. *Annu Rev Med* 1980;**31**:373.

Visvesvara GS: Giardiasis in children. *J Pediatr Gastroenterol Nutr* 1982;**1**:463.

BALANTIDIASIS

Balantidium coli is a large ciliated intestinal protozoon found throughout the world, particularly in the tropics. Infection results from ingestion of viable cysts passed in stools of humans or swine, the reservoir hosts. In the new host, the cyst wall dissolves, and the trophozoite may invade the mucosa and submucosa of the large bowel and terminal ileum, causing abscesses and irregularly rounded ulcerations. Many cases are asymptomatic and probably need not be treated. Chronic recurrent diarrhea, alternating with constipation, is the most common clinical manifestation, but attacks of severe dysentery with bloody mucoid stools, tenesmus, and colic may occur intermittently. Diagnosis is made by finding trophozoites in liquid stools and cysts in formed stools. The treatment of choice is tetracycline hydrochloride, 500 mg 4 times daily for 10 days. The alternative drug is iodoquinol (diiodohydroxyquin), 650 mg 3 times daily for 21 days. Occasional success has also been reported with met-

ronidazole, 750 mg 3 times daily for 10 days; paromomycin, ampicillin, and carbarsone.

In properly treated mild to moderate symptomatic cases, the prognosis is good, but in spite of treatment, fatalities have occurred in severe infections as a result of intestinal perforation or hemorrhage.

Knight R: Giardiasis, isosporiasis and balantidiasis. *Clin Gastroenterol* 1978;**7**:31.

TOXOPLASMOSIS

Toxoplasma gondii, an obligate intracellular parasite, is found worldwide in humans and in many species of animals and birds. The parasite is a coccidian of cats, the definitive host, and exists in 3 forms: The trophozoite (tachyzoite) is the rapidly proliferating form seen in the tissues and body fluids in the acute stage. The trophozoites can enter and multiply in most mammalian nucleated cells. The cyst (cystozoite), containing viable trophozoites, is the latent form that can persist indefinitely in the host in the chronic stage and is found particularly in muscle and nerve tissue. The oocyst is the form passed only in the feces of the cat family. In the intestinal epithelium of cats, a sexual cycle occurs, with subsequent release of oocysts. Human infection occurs by ingestion of oocysts, by ingestion of cysts in raw or undercooked meat, by transplacental transmission, or, rarely, by direct inoculation of trophozoites, as in blood transfusion.

The clinical manifestations of toxoplasmosis may be grouped into 4 syndromes: acquired toxoplasmosis in the normal host, congenital infection, retinochoroiditis, and acquired or reactivated disease in the immunologically compromised host. (1) In the latter, toxoplasmosis may present as a disseminated disease, particularly in patients given immunosuppressive drugs or patients with lymphoreticular, hematologic, or other cancers or with the acquired immunodeficiency syndrome. Encephalitis is the most common manifestation; pneumonitis and myocarditis may also occur. (2) Most patients with acquired toxoplasmosis are probably asymptomatic. In the adult age group in most populations, a large proportion have been infected and are seropositive. Mild infections present commonly with a syndrome resembling infectious mononucleosis. It includes fever, malaise, myalgia, headache, sore throat, generalized lymphadenopathy, and maculopapular rashes. Hepatosplenomegaly may occur. Rarely, severe cases include pneumonitis, meningoencephalitis, hepatitis, myocarditis, and retinochoroiditis. Atypical lymphocytes may be present, but there is no heterophil antibody. Symptoms may fluctuate over months, but most patients recover spontaneously. (3) Congenital transmission occurs only as a result of acute infection during pregnancy and may occur in any trimester. Infection has been detected in up to 1% of women during pregnancy; approximately 20–40% of such infections are transmitted to the fetus, but only a small percentage result in abortions or stillbirths or in active disease in live-born infants. Signs of congenital toxoplasmosis may be present at birth or progress during the first months of life: microcephaly, internal hydrocephalus, seizures, mental retardation, hepatosplenomegaly, pneumonitis, rash, fever, retinochoroiditis, and cerebral calcification. (4) The retinochoroiditis form of toxoplasmosis is usually a late sequela of congenital infection, with symptoms being first noted in the second or third decade of life.

Diagnosis depends principally on serologic test results. However, toxoplasmosis can be diagnosed occasionally by histologic examination of tissue or isolation of the parasite in mice or tissue culture. The organism may be directly identified by staining bone marrow aspirates; cerebrospinal fluid sediment; sputum, blood, and other tissue or body fluids; or placental tissue. However, the demonstration of cysts does not establish a causal relationship to clinical illness, since cysts may be found in both acute and chronic illness. Only isolation from blood or body fluids confirms acute infection; isolation from tissues could represent chronic infection.

Serologic tests—the Feldman-Sabin dye test, the complement fixation test, ELISA, and indirect immunofluorescence and other tests—can be conducted on blood, cerebrospinal fluid, and other body fluids. In acute acquired toxoplasmosis, the diagnosis is established serologically by a 4-fold rise in serologic titers by any test or by a single high titer (1:160) of IgM antibodies. A presumptive diagnosis is supported by a single very high titer ($\geq$ 1:1000) of IgG antibodies; however, these antibodies may persist for years. In immunocompetent persons, a negative Feldman-Sabin dye test virtually excludes the diagnosis of acute toxoplasmosis, but high titers can persist for years after recovery. For the IgM indirect fluorescent antibody test, however, negative results can occur in up to 25% of acute cases. In the acquired immunodeficiency syndrome and in patients with cancer, serologic methods for diagnosis of reactivated toxoplasmosis may give false-negative results. The diagnosis of congenital infection is supported by a high titer of IgM antibodies in cord blood; the presence of specific IgM antibody is diagnostic. The presence of IgG antibodies may indicate only transplacental passage from the mother.

Where available, the following new methods may be useful in diagnosis: Testing for antigenemia has been used to demonstrate acute infection, and lymphocyte transformation to *Toxoplasma* antigens has provided a specific and sensitive indicator of prior infection.

Acute toxoplasmosis in immunologically normal persons, whether asymptomatic or mildly symptomatic, usually does not require treatment. Treatment is indicated, however, in persistent (over 1–2 weeks) or severe infection, active retinochoroiditis, congenitally infected infants with or without symptoms, infection in the immunologically compromised patient, and in pregnancy. Treatment of toxoplasmosis acquired at any time during pregnancy decreases but does not eliminate the chance of a congenitally infected infant.

Opinions vary on appropriate treatment of maternal toxoplasmosis.

The treatment of choice is pyrimethamine (25 mg/d in divided doses for 1 month) plus either trisulfapyrimidine (2–6 g/d in 4 divided doses) or sulfadiazine (100 mg/kg/d [maximum 6 g/d] in 2 divided doses). In the treatment of severe disease in immunodeficient patients, the dose of pyrimethamine may be increased to 50 mg/d. Other sulfonamides are not used. The usual sulfonamide precautions must be observed, and folinic acid, 10 mg/d in divided doses, is given to avoid the hematologic effects of folate deficiency. Pyrimethamine in the first trimester of pregnancy may be inadvisable, because it has been shown to be teratogenic in animals. Corticosteroids may be required in the management of ocular disease. Spiramycin is in use in Europe at a dosage of 100 mg/kg/d in 4 divided doses for 10–14 days and is safe during pregnancy. Trimethoprim-sulfamethoxazole is being used but with unreliable results. Clindamycin is also being tested; because it is concentrated in the ocular choroid, it has been used in the treatment of ocular disease.

Pregnant women should have their serum examined for toxoplasma antibody. If the IgM test is negative and the conventional tests less than 1:1000, no further evaluation is necessary. Those with negative titers by conventional tests should take measures to prevent infection—preferably by having no further contact with cats and not eating raw meats. Vegetables and fruits should be thoroughly washed or cooked and the hands washed after handling raw meat.

Freezing of meat to −20 °C for 2 days kills cysts in tissues. Under appropriate environmental conditions, oocysts passed in cat feces can remain infective for a year or more.

Henderson JB et al: The evaluation of new services: Possibilities for preventing congenital toxoplasmosis. *Int J Epidemiol* 1984;**13**:65.

Lakhanpal V et al: Clindamycin in the treatment of toxoplasmic retinochoroiditis. *Am J Ophthalmol* 1983;**95**:605.

McCabe RE, Remington JS: The diagnosis and treatment of toxoplasmosis. *Eur J Clin Microbiol* 1983;**2**:95.

McCarthy M: Of cats and women. (Letter.) *Br Med J* 1983;**287**:445.

Ryning FW, Mills J: *Pneumocystis carinii, Toxoplasma gondii,* cytomegalovirus and the compromised host. *West J Med* 1979;**130**:18.

COCCIDIOSIS: ISOSPORIASIS, CRYPTOSPORIDIASIS, SARCOCYSTIASIS

Coccidiosis is an intestinal infection usually accompanied by diarrhea and abdominal discomfort and caused by coccidia of 3 genera: *Isospora, Cryptosporidium,* and *Sarcocystis.* Rarely, sarcocystiasis also presents as transient painful muscular and subcutaneous swellings. Although these infections occur worldwide, they are recognized only sporadically.

Clinical Findings

A. Isosporiasis: Isosporiasis, caused by *Isospora belli*, is considered host-specific for humans, with transmission directly from person to person. Infection is by the fecal-oral route following ingestion of oocysts. Sporozoites excyst and invade jejunal and duodenal epithelial cells, in which they undergo both a sexual and an asexual cycle, resulting in the liberation of unsporulated oocysts, $23-33 \times 12-14$ μm, into the feces.

The incubation period is 7–11 days. Some patients remain asymptomatic. Most symptomatic infections follow a benign, self-limited course lasting a few weeks or months. The principal findings are diarrhea, abdominal pain, flatulence, low-grade fever, malaise, and anorexia. Infrequently, the disease is protracted or recurrent; when severe, there may be intense diarrhea, steatorrhea, malabsorption, and weight loss. Several deaths have been reported.

The diagnosis is made by finding the parasite in feces or duodenal aspirates or by duodenal biopsy. Diagnosis by stool examination is often difficult, for the organisms may be scanty even in the presence of significant symptoms. The laboratory should be notified of the need to search for the organisms, so that special concentration techniques will be used. Because of their buoyancy, oocysts must be looked for just beneath the coverslip of the preparation. Although the peroral duodenal string test or duodenal aspiration may also assist in diagnosis, frequently diagnosis can be made only after duodenal biopsy and search of multiple serial sections. Some patients have marked steatorrhea, and up to 50% of patients with isosporiasis have eosinophilia.

B. Cryptosporidiasis: Fewer than 100 cases of cryptosporidiasis have been reported in humans since its recognition as a human pathogen in 1976, about half in immunologically competent persons and half in immunosuppressed persons. However, information is accumulating to show that the infection may be an unrecognized cause of mild gastroenteritis worldwide, and this is of possible special importance for young children in developing countries. The organism has been described in many animal species, and fecal-oral transmission from animals to humans may be an important mode of infection. Human-to-human transmission is presumed to occur. Infective oocysts (4 μm in diameter) shed in feces by a host proliferate sexually and asexually in the new host. The organisms attach to the microvillous borders of enterocytes of the small and large bowel and are also found free within mucosal crypts. Other epithelial surfaces are sometimes infected, including the gallbladder and respiratory tract, but the parasite is not invasive. Clinically, in immunocompetent persons, a diarrheal disease occurs, with low-grade fever and abdominal cramps, that is self-limited within a few days to about 2 weeks. In immunologically deficient patients, however, especially those with acquired immunodeficiency syndrome (AIDS), an illness characterized by chronic profuse, watery diarrhea, fever, marked weight loss, and lymphadenopathy can occur that may lead to death. Diagnosis is by detection of oocysts in stool by a variety of flotation, concentration, and staining methods or by mucosal biopsy. An immunofluorescent serologic test is being developed. No therapeutic agent is available, but spiramycin shows promise.

C. Sarcocystiasis: *Sarcocystis* is a 2-host coccidian. Human disease occurs as 2 syndromes, both rare: an enteric infection in which humans are the definitive host, and a muscle infection in which humans are an intermediate host. In the enteric form of the disease, sporocysts passed in human feces are not infective for humans but must be ingested by cattle or pigs. Humans become infected by eating poorly cooked beef or pork containing oocysts of *Sarcocystis bovihominis* or *Sarcocystis suihominis*, respectively. (Formerly, the causative agent was known as *Isospora hominis*.) Organisms enter intestinal epithelial cells and are transformed into oocysts that release sporocysts into the feces. The fecal stage of the parasite is more mature than that of *I belli*—the oocyst has lost its wall and appears as single or paired sporocysts. Clinically, the intestinal infection is often asymptomatic or causes mild, protracted diarrhea.

The muscle form of sarcocystiasis results when humans ingest sporocysts in feces from an infected carnivore that has eaten prey which harbored sarcocysts. The sporocysts liberate sporozoites that invade the intestinal wall and are disseminated to skeletal muscle. This results in subcutaneous and muscular inflammation lasting several days to 2 weeks and the finding of swellings at these sites, sometimes associated with eosinophilia. Sarcocysts are often asymptomatic, however, such as those found incidentally at autopsy in cardiac muscle.

Treatment

There is no satisfactory drug for coccidiosis. Instances of effective treatment for isosporiasis have been described using (1) sulfadiazine, 4 g, and pyrimethamine, 35–75 mg, in 4 divided doses daily for 3 weeks; or (2) trimethoprim-sulfamethoxazole, 2–8 tablets daily for 3 weeks (tablets contain trimethoprim, 80 mg, and sulfamethoxazole, 400 mg). No treatment has been effective in cryptosporidiasis.

Beaver PC, Gadgil K, Morera P: *Sarcocystis* in man: A review and report of five cases. *Am J Trop Med Hyg* 1979;**28**:819.

Cryptosporidiosis. (Editorial.) *Lancet* 1984;**1**:492.

Pitlik SD et al: Human cryptosporidiosis: Spectrum of disease: Report of six cases and review of the literature. *Arch Intern Med* 1983;**143**:2269.

Update: Treatment of cryptosporidiosis in patients with acquired immunodeficiency syndrome (AIDS). *MMWR* 1984;**33**:117.

Westerman EL, Christensen RP: Chronic *Isospora belli* infection treated with co-trimoxazole. *Ann Intern Med* 1979;**91**:413.

PNEUMOCYSTOSIS
(*Pneumocystis carinii* Pneumonia)

Pneumocystosis is an acute interstitial plasma cell pneumonia caused by *Pneumocystis carinii*. The disease occurs worldwide; although rare in the general population, it occurs in larger numbers among 2 groups: (1) as epidemics among 2- to 6-month-old infants, and (2) as sporadic cases among older children and adults who have an abnormal or altered immune status. In infants, outbreaks of primary infection occur among undernourished marasmic children living in nursing homes. Most childhood-adult cases are assumed to be due to reactivation of latent infection in the presence of immunosuppression; they occur generally in debilitated adults, patients treated with immunosuppressive drugs or irradiation for the management of organ transplants and cancer, patients receiving adrenocorticosteroid therapy, and patients with acquired immunodeficiency syndrome (AIDS) (see Chapter 22). In the USA, *Pneumocystis* pneumonia occurs in about 60% of AIDS patients and is a major cause of death in patients with the syndrome.

The organism appears to be a protozoan with intra- and extracellular stages. One- to 2-μm sporozoites are found in cysts that rupture to release 2- to 5-μm trophozoites. Antibodies to *P carinii* are found in a large proportion of normal children, which suggests that many asymptomatic and latent infections occur early in life. Although the mode of transmission in primary infection is unknown, some evidence suggests airborne transmission. The organism has been found in lung tissue of many wild and domestic animals.

In the sporadic form of the disease associated with deficient cell-mediated immunity, the onset is abrupt, with high fever, tachypnea, mild cough, intercostal retractions, and cyanosis. Without treatment, the course usually is one of rapid deterioration and death. In the infantile form of the disease, the patient is generally free of fever and may show eosinophilia.

With rare exceptions, pathologic findings are limited to the pulmonary parenchyma. Pulmonary physical findings may be slight (including no rales) and disproportionate to the degree of illness and to the radiologic findings. X-ray findings include bilateral or asymmetric alveolar infiltrates, pulmonary consolidation, nodular infiltrates in the periphery, and other atypical findings. The blood gases usually show impaired diffusion and severe hypoxemia with minimal (or no) CO_2 retention, resulting in uncompensated respiratory alkalosis.

Specific diagnosis depends on morphologic demonstration of the organism in clinical specimens using specific stains. Sputum, transtracheal aspirates, bronchial washings, and bronchial brushing provide relatively low yields of the organisms, in contrast with the approximately 80% yields using procedures that sample the parenchymal compartments—bronchoalveolar lavage, transbronchial biopsy, transthoracic aspiration, and open lung biopsy. Gallium citrate Ga 67 localizes in the lungs with many pathologic conditions;

diffuse gallium accumulation on chest x-ray may provide early recognition of *P carinii* infection. Serologic tests are not helpful in diagnosis at present.

The treatment of choice for *Pneumocystis* pneumonia is trimethoprim-sulfamethoxazole. Trimethoprim, 20 mg/kg, plus sulfamethoxazole, 100 mg/kg, is given daily by mouth in 4 equal doses for at least 10–14 days or longer. When possible, blood levels should be monitored for adequacy of absorption. If necessary, corresponding intravenous dosage is available (follow the manufacturer's directions). Sulfonamide precautions must be observed. Patients with AIDS have a high frequency of hypersensitivity reactions to trimethoprim-sulfamethoxazole—fever, rashes (sometimes severe), malaise, and leukopenia. Because of the hypoxia usually associated with this disease, oxygen therapy may be indicated to maintain the P_{O_2} at 70 mm Hg or higher.

Pentamidine, which is more toxic than trimethoprim-sulfamethoxazole, is used to treat patients who have had adverse reactions or who fail to respond to the latter drug. Pentamidine causes side effects in nearly 50% of patients, including severe renal reactions, hypoglycemia, hypotension, liver function abnormalities, and reactions at the injection site. Pentamidine is administered intramuscularly as a single daily dose for 12–14 days. Two types of the salt are manufactured; although efficacy and toxicity are similar, dosages are calculated differently—the daily dose of pentamidine isethionate is 4 mg (of salt) per kilogram, while that of pentamidine methanesulfonate is 2.3 mg (of base) per kilogram. In the USA, pentamidine is available as the methanesulfonate salt and only from the Parasitic Disease Drug Service, Centers for Disease Control, Atlanta 30333.

Chemoprophylaxis for high-risk immunocompromised patients consists of oral trimethoprim-sulfamethoxazole in one-fourth of the therapeutic dose. Persons with G6PD deficiency should not receive such prophylaxis.

The fatality rate for the endemic infantile form of pneumocystosis is 20–50%. For the sporadic form in immunodeficient persons, the fatality rate may approach 100% in the absence of early and adequate treatment. Susceptibility to recurrence varies with the immunologic status of the individual. Resistance to trimethoprim occurs sometimes during recurrence.

Haverkos HW (coordinator): Assessment of therapy for *Pneumocystis carinii* pneumonia. *Am J Med* 1984;**76**:501.

Hughes WT: Trimethoprim-sulfamethoxazole therapy for *P carinii* pneumonitis in children. *Rev Infect Dis* 1982;**4**:602.

Jaffe HS et al: Complications of cotrimoxazole in treatment of AIDS-associated *Pneumocystis carinii* pneumonia in homosexual men. *Lancet* 1983;**2**:1109.

Kaye SB: *Pneumocystis* pneumonia. *Br Med J* 1983;**286**:479.

Levin M et al: *Pneumocystis* pneumonia: Importance of gallium scan for early diagnosis and description of a new immunoperoxidase technique to demonstrate *Pneumocystis carinii*. *Am Rev Respir Dis* 1983;**128**:182.

Smith JW, Bartlett MS: Laboratory diagnosis of *Pneumocystis carinii* infection. *Clin Lab Med* 1982;**2**:393.

• • •

References

Adams ARD, Maegraith BG: *Clinical Tropical Diseases,* 6th ed. Blackwell, 1976.

Barrett-Connor E: Drugs for the treatment of parasitic infection. *Med Clin North Am* 1982;**66:**245.

Beaver PC, Jug RC, Cupp EW: *Clinical Parasitology,* 9th ed. Lea & Febiger, 1984.

Brown HW, Neva FA: *Basic Clinical Parasitology,* 5th ed. Appleton-Century-Crofts, 1983.

Drugs for parasitic infections. *Med Lett Drugs Ther* 1982;**26:**27.

Ginger CD: Antiparasitic agents. *Annu Reports Medicinal Chem* 1982;**17:**129.

Hoskins DW: Drugs for intestinal parasitism. In: *Drugs of Choice.* Modell W (editor). Mosby, 1984.

Immunology of parasitic infections: Report of a workshop. *Am J Trop Med Hyg* 1977;**26(Suppl):**Part 2.

Janssen PA, van den Bossche H: Treatment of helminthiasis. *Scand J Infect Dis* [Suppl] 1982;**36:**52.

Jelliffe DB, Stanfield JP (editors): *Diseases of Children in the Subtropics and Tropics,* 3rd ed. Arnold, 1978.

Knight R et al: Progress report: Intestinal parasites. *Gut* 1973;**14:**145.

Manson-Bahr PEC, Apted FIC: *Manson's Tropical Diseases,* 18th ed. Baillière Tindall, 1982.

Marchalonis JJ (editor): Immunobiology of parasites and parasitic infections. *Contemp Top Immunobiol* 1984;**12.** [Entire issue.]

Marcial-Rojas RA (editor): *Pathology of Protozoal and Helminthic Diseases With Clinical Correlation.* Williams & Wilkins, 1971.

Marsden PD: The treatment and control of parasitic diseases. *Rev Infect Dis* 1982;**4:**885.

Most H: Treatment of parasitic infections of travelers and immigrants. *N Engl J Med* 1984;**310:**298.

Pearson RD, Hewlett EL, Guerrant RL: *Tropical Diseases in North America.* Year Book, 1984.

Schönfeld H (volume editor): *Antiparasitic Chemotherapy.* Karger, 1981.

Steck EA: The chemotherapy of protozoal infections in man. *J Protozool* 1981;**28:**10.

Steele JH (editor-in-chief): *CRC Handbook Series in Zoonoses. Section C: Parasitic Zoonoses.* Vol 3. Hillyer GV, Hopla CE (volume editors). CRC Press, 1982.

Strickland GT: *Hunter's Tropical Medicine,* 6th ed. Saunders, 1984.

Stürchler D: Chemotherapy of human intestinal helminthiases: A review, with particular reference to community treatment. *Adv Pharmacol Chemother* 1982;**19:**129.

Walls KW, Wilson M: Immunoserology in parasitic infections. *Lab Res Methods Biol Med* 1983;**8:**191.

Warren KS, Mahmoud AAF: *Tropical and Geographic Medicine.* McGraw-Hill, 1984.

WHO Scientific Group: Intestinal protozoan and helminthic infections. Technical Report Series 666. World Health Organization, 1981.

Wolfe JS: The treatment of intestinal protozoan infections. *Med Clin North Am* 1982;**66:**707.

27 | Infectious Diseases: Helminthic

Robert S. Goldsmith, MD, MPH, DTM&H

TREMATODE (FLUKE) INFECTIONS

SCHISTOSOMIASIS
(Bilharziasis)

Essentials of Diagnosis
- Transient erythematous, pruritic skin rash.
- Fever, malaise, urticaria, eosinophilia, and hepatosplenomegaly.
- Either (1) diarrhea, dysentery, abdominal pain, anorexia, weight loss, splenomegaly, and ascites; or (2) terminal hematuria, urinary frequency, urethral and bladder pain.

General Considerations

Three blood flukes, or trematodes, are responsible for this worldwide complex of diseases. *Schistosoma mansoni,* the cause of intestinal schistosomiasis, is widespread in Egypt and is common locally in tropical Africa, eastern South America, and the Caribbean (including Puerto Rico but not Cuba). Vesical or urinary schistosomiasis, caused by *Schistosoma haematobium,* is common in Egypt and other parts of Africa and in parts of the Middle East. Asiatic intestinal schistosomiasis, due to *Schistosoma japonicum* infection, is important in China, Japan, and the Philippines.

Various species of snails, the intermediate hosts, are infected by larvae hatched from eggs reaching fresh water in feces or urine. After development, infective larvae (cercariae) leave the snails and penetrate human skin or mucous membranes that come in contact with water. Immature *S mansoni* organisms migrate to branches of the inferior mesenteric veins in the large bowel wall. Here the adults mature, mate, and deposit eggs. Many eggs reach the bowel lumen and are passed in the feces; others lodge in the bowel wall and induce inflammation, fibrosis, ulceration, and granuloma or polyp formation. Eggs may be carried to the liver, where similar changes occur, provoking periportal cirrhosis. Portal hypertension results in splenomegaly and ascites. Eggs may lodge ectopically in the lungs, spinal cord, or other tissues.

S japonicum adults lie in branches of the superior and inferior mesenteric veins in the small and large bowel walls. Eggs are passed in the stool or lodge in the bowel wall, provoking changes similar to those noted above. Because greater numbers of eggs are produced by *S japonicum,* the resulting disease is more extensive and severe. Eggs are frequently carried to the liver (and occasionally to the central nervous system), and cirrhosis and portal hypertension are common.

The adult *S haematobium* matures in the venous plexuses of the bladder, prostate, and uterus. Eggs are passed in the urine or retained in the tissues, particularly the bladder wall and the female genital organs. In addition to fibrosis, ulceration, and granuloma and papilloma formation, bladder wall calcification, chronic cystitis, pyelitis, or pyelonephritis often occurs. Bladder cancer is common in advanced cases in Egypt.

A number of animal schistosomes sometimes infect humans. *Schistosoma intercalatum* causes human disease in central Africa, and *Schistosoma mekongi* has recently been recognized in humans in a limited area along the Mekong River in Thailand, Cambodia, and Laos.

Clinical Findings

A. Symptoms and Signs: The first sign of infection, an itchy erythematous or petechial rash at sites of penetration of cercariae, lasts about 2–5 days. A second clinical stage occurs 4–5 weeks later as the immature flukes migrate through the blood vessels of various organs. Symptoms at this time are primarily allergic and vary greatly in severity. In addition to fever, urticaria, malaise, and respiratory symptoms, the liver and spleen may be temporarily enlarged. The patient again becomes asymptomatic in 2–8 weeks. The final clinical stage begins 6 months to several years after infection as lesions develop around eggs embedded in the tissues. The course and severity of the disease depend upon the number of adult worms present, the number of eggs produced, and the sites of the lesions they provoke. Diarrhea, dysentery, and abdominal pain are common in the early stages of intestinal infections. Anorexia, weight loss, polypoid intestinal tumors, and signs of portal hypertension and hepatic insufficiency appear as the disease progresses. Death commonly results from intercurrent infection. The symptoms of urinary tract disease (particularly terminal hematuria, frequency, and pain) depend upon the extent of the pathologic changes described above. Ureteral and renal damage may result in fatal uremia, or the patient may die of bladder carcinoma many years after first being infected. Advanced schistosomiasis usually develops only after repeated reinfections.

B. Laboratory Findings: Definitive diagnosis is made by finding characteristic eggs in excreta or by mucosal or liver biopsy. In *S haematobium* infection, eggs may be found in the urine, in tissues obtained from the vesicle mucosa, or less frequently in stools. Eggs are sought in urine specimens collected between 9:00 AM and 2:00 PM or in 24-hour collections. They are processed by either examination of the sediment or preferably by membrane filtration. In *S mansoni* and *S japonicum* infections, eggs may be found in stool specimens by direct examination, but some form of concentration is usually necessary; repeated examinations are often needed to find eggs in light infections. If results are negative, proceed to rectal mucosal biopsy of suspicious lesions or take biopsy specimens at 2–3 sites of normal mucosa. Biopsy specimens should be examined as crush preparations between 2 glass slides. The Kato thick smear or membrane filtration method is useful to quantitate fecal egg output in order to estimate severity of infection and to follow response to therapy. When eggs are found, their viability should be determined, since dead eggs are retained in the tissues for months. For an occasional patient, a liver biopsy may be necessary to achieve diagnosis.

Screening for infection is possible by skin testing or serology. Serologic tests become positive a few weeks after infection, but both false-positive and false-negative reactions may occur. Microscopic hematuria may be present in *S haematobium* infection, and in advanced disease, lower abdominal x-rays may show calcification of the bladder wall or ureters. Eosinophilia is common during the migration of the immature flukes, but the count usually returns to normal later.

Differential Diagnosis

Schistosomiasis mansoni or japonicum should be considered in all unresponsive gastrointestinal disorders in persons who have been in endemic areas. Early intestinal schistosomiasis may be mistaken for amebiasis, bacillary dysentery, or other causes of diarrhea and dysentery. Later, the various causes of portal hypertension or of bowel papillomas and polyps must be considered. Vesical schistosomiasis must be differentiated from other causes of hematuria, prostatic disease, genitourinary tract cancer, and bacterial infections of the urinary tract.

Complications

Among the many complications of these diseases are transverse myelitis (*S mansoni* eggs in the spinal cord), seizures, optic neuritis, paralysis, mental disorders (*S japonicum* eggs in the brain), liver failure *(S mansoni, S japonicum)*, ruptured esophageal varices due to portal hypertension, uremia and bladder neoplasms *(S haematobium)*, and chronic pulmonary disease (periarteritis and endarteritis, primarily due to *S mansoni* eggs).

Treatment

A. General Considerations: The development of the new drugs metrifonate, oxamniquine, and praziquantel now makes it possible to treat infections caused by all schistosome species without the concern for serious side effects that was experienced with the older drugs.

In less advanced disease states, there is evidence of reversibility of some pathologic features—shrinkage or elimination of bladder and bowel ulcerations and granulomas—following drug therapy. In long-standing disease, the damage is not reversible. In selected instances, corrective surgery may be indicated for removal of papillomas, polyps, and early carcinoma; splenectomy, shunt procedures, craniotomy, and other neurosurgical procedures may also be needed.

After treatment, periodic laboratory follow-up is essential, starting at 3 months and continuing at intervals for 1 year. The decision to repeat treatment depends on the intensity of live ova output and on whether reinfection is likely. Some authorities believe that worm burdens in which fewer than 50 eggs per gram of stool are passed do not require treatment.

B. Specific Measures: Treatment should be given only if live ova are identified. The drugs of choice for the treatment of *S haematobium* are metrifonate or praziquantel; for *S mansoni*, oxamniquine or praziquantel; and for *S japonicum, S mekongi*, and *S intercalatum*, praziquantel. Alternative drugs for all 3 parasites, but less satisfactory because of their potential toxicity, are niridazole and stibocaptate. Tartar emetic, the most toxic, is a third alternative for the treatment of *S japonicum* infections.

1. Praziquantel, a pyrazino isoquinoline compound, is given orally and has the unique characteristic of being effective against all human schistosome species. The drug is effective in adults and children and is well tolerated by patients in the hepatosplenic stage of advanced schistosomiasis; its safety in children under 4 years of age, however, has not been established. More than 10,000 patients were treated in 31 study groups at various dosage schedules; cure rates at 6 months for *S haematobium, S mansoni*, and *S japonicum* infections were 87%, 80%, and 84%, respectively, with marked reduction in ovum counts in those not cured.

The manufacturer's recommended dosage to treat all forms of schistosomiasis is 20 mg/kg 3 times daily for 1 day. Lower dosages have been reported to be highly effective in some parts of the world and for some species. Tablets are taken after a meal with water and should not be chewed. The interval between doses should be no less than 4 and no more than 6 hours.

The drug is free of embryologic toxicity and mutagenic or carcinogenic potential. There are no laboratory test abnormalities. Mild and transient side effects persisting for hours to 1 day are common includ-

Table 27–1. Drugs for the treatment of helminthic infections.*

Infecting Organism	Drug of Choice	Alternative Drugs
Roundworms (nematodes)		
Ascaris lumbricoides (roundworm)	Pyrantel pamoate	Piperazine, mebendazole, levamisole,[1] or bephenium[1]
Trichuris trichiura (whipworm)	Mebendazole	Oxantel pamoate[1,2] or hexylresorcinol[1] by retention enema
Necator americanus (hookworm) *Ancylostoma duodenale* (hookworm)	Pyrantel pamoate[2] or mebendazole	Bephenium,[1] tetrachloroethylene, or thiabendazole
Strongyloides stercoralis (threadworm)	Thiabendazole	Mebendazole,[3,4] niridazole,[4] pyrvinium pamoate,[3,4] or levamisole[1,4]
Enterobius vermicularis (pinworm)	Mebendazole or pyrantel pamoate	Pyrvinium pamoate
Trichinella spiralis (trichinosis)	ACTH, corticosteroids, and thiabendazole[4] or mebendazole[3,4]	None
Trichostrongylus species	Pyrantel pamoate[3] or mebendazole[2]	Bephenium,[1] levamisole,[1] or thiabendazole[3]
Cutaneous larva migrans (creeping eruption)	Thiabendazole	Diethylcarbamazine[4,5]
Visceral larva migrans	Thiabendazole[4]	Diethylcarbamazine[4,5]
Angiostrongylus cantonensis	Levamisole[1,4]	None
Wuchereria bancrofti (filariasis) *Brugia malayi* (filariasis) Tropical eosinophilia *Loa loa* (loiasis)	Diethylcarbamazine[5]	None
Onchocerca volvulus (onchocerciasis)	Suramin[6] plus diethylcarbamazine[5]	None
Dracunculus medinensis (guinea worm)	Niridazole[6] or metronidazole[3]	Thiabendazole[3]
Intestinal capillariasis	Mebendazole	Thiabendazole
Flukes (trematodes)		
Schistosoma haematobium (bilharziasis)	Metrifonate[6] or praziquantel	Niridazole[6] or stibocaptate[6] (see antimony compounds)
Schistosoma mansoni	Oxamniquine or praziquantel	Niridazole[6] or stibocaptate[6] (see antimony compounds)
Schistosoma japonicum	Praziquantel	Niridazole,[6] tartar emetic, or stibocaptate[6] (see antimony compounds)
Clonorchis sinensis (liver fluke) *Opisthorchis* species	Praziquantel	None
Paragonimus westermani (lung fluke)	Bithionol[6] or praziquantel	
Fasciola hepatica (sheep liver fluke)	Bithionol[6]	Emetine, dehydroemetine,[6] or metronidazole[3,4]
Fasciolopsis buski (large intestinal fluke)	Praziquantel, tetrachloroethylene, or niclosamide	Hexylresorcinol,[1] dichlorophen,[1,4] or bephenium[1]
Heterophyes heterophyes, Metagonimus yokogawai and other small intestinal flukes	Tetrachloroethylene or niclosamide	Hexylresorcinol,[1] bephenium,[1] or praziquantel[2,4]
Tapeworm (cestodes)		
Taenia saginata (beef tapeworm)	Niclosamide	Praziquantel,[2] dichlorophen,[1] paromomycin,[3] or mebendazole[3,4]
Diphyllobothrium latum (fish tapeworm)	Niclosamide	Praziquantel[2] or dichlorophen[1]
Taenia solium (pork tapeworm)	Niclosamide	Praziquantel[2] or mebendazole[3,4]
Cysticercosis (pork tapeworm larval stage)	Praziquantel[2,3]	None
Hymenolepis nana (dwarf tapeworm)	Praziquantel	Niclosamide or paromomycin[3]
Hymenolepis diminuta (rat tapeworm) *Dipylidium caninum*	Niclosamide	Praziquantel
Echinococcus granulosus (hydatid disease) *Echinococcus multilocularis*	Mebendazole[2,3,4]	None

*Reproduced, with permission, from Katzung BG (editor): *Basic & Clinical Pharmacology,* 2nd ed. Lange, 1984.

[1] Not available in the USA.

[2] Undergoing clinical investigation.

[3] Available in the USA but not approved for this indication.

[4] Effectiveness not established.

[5] Available in the USA only from Lederle Laboratories. Telephone (914) 753–5000.

[6] Available in the USA only from the Parasitic Disease Drug Service, Centers for Disease Control, Atlanta 30333. Telephone (404) 329–3670 during the day, (404) 329–2888 nights, weekends, and holidays.

ing malaise, headache, dizziness, and anorexia. Less frequent are fatigue, drowsiness, nausea, vomiting, generalized abdominal pain, loose stools, pruritus, urticaria, arthralgia and myalgia, and low-grade fever. The drug should not be used in pregnancy, and because of drug-induced dizziness, patients should not drive and should be cautioned if their work requires physical coordination or alertness. In areas where cysticercosis may coexist with an infection being treated with praziquantel, treatment is best carried out in a hospital.

2. Metrifonate is a highly effective oral drug and a drug of choice for the treatment of *S haematobium* infections, but it is not effective against *S mansoni* or *S japonicum*. The drug is a cholinesterase inhibitor and at therapeutic dosages in humans produces prolonged depression of blood cholinesterase activity, which is not known to be associated with any significant disturbance of organ structure or function. In the treatment of *S haematobium* infections, the dosage is 7.5–10 mg/kg (maximum 600 mg) once and then repeated twice at 2-week intervals. Cure rates at this schedule in various clinical trials ranged from 44 to 93%. Those not cured showed marked reduction in ovum counts. Some studies reported no side effects; others noted mild and transient findings (up to 12 hours), including gastrointestinal symptoms, headache, bronchospasm, weakness, and vertigo. One case of organophosphate poisoning following a standard dose has been reported. In the USA, metrifonate is available only from the Parasitic Disease Drug Service, Centers for Disease Control, Atlanta 30333 ([404] 329–3670).

3. Oxamniquine is a highly effective oral drug and a drug of choice for the treatment of *S mansoni* infections and is both safe and effective in the advanced (hepatosplenic) form of the disease. The drug is not effective against *S haematobium* or *S japonicum*. It is a tetrahydroquinoline derivative. The dosage for strains of *S mansoni* in the western hemisphere is 12–15 mg/kg given once; for children under 30 kg, 20 mg/kg is given in 2 divided doses in 1 day, with an interval of 2–8 hours between doses. Cure rates are 70–95% with a marked reduction in egg excretion in those not cured. For most African strains, the total dosage for adults and children varies by region from 40 to 60 mg/kg in divided doses over 2–3 days. Dizziness persisting for about 6 hours is common. Less frequent side effects are drowsiness, nausea and vomiting, diarrhea, abdominal pain, and headache. An orange or red discoloration of the urine may occur. Rarely reported side effects are central nervous system stimulation with behavioral changes, hallucinations, or seizures; patients should be observed for 2 hours after ingestion of the drug for appearance of these findings. Since the drug makes some patients dizzy or drowsy, it should be used with caution in patients whose work or activity requires mental alertness. The drug has shown mutagenic and embryocidal effects and is contraindicated in pregnancy.

4. Niridazole, a nitrothiazole derivative, is an effective oral drug for treating *S mansoni* and *S haematobium* infections and may be tried against *S japonicum*. It should be administered only under close medical supervision. High cure rates have been achieved with oral doses of 25 mg/kg body weight (maximum, 1.5 g) daily in 2 divided doses for 7 days. (In the treatment of *S japonicum*, continue for 10 days if possible.) Phenobarbital, 100–150 mg daily, should be given because it reduces the incidence of central nervous system reactions. Drug side effects include occasional nausea, vomiting, anorexia, headache, T wave depression, and possible temporary suppression of spermatogenesis. Deep brown coloration of the urine disappears after treatment. Antihistamines may be useful in controlling infrequent allergic manifestations (skin rashes, pruritus) caused by the release of foreign proteins from disintegrating worms. The main toxic effects, which are neuropsychiatric, occur in 1–2% of all patients but in up to 21% of patients with advanced liver disease. If marked mood changes, slurred speech, confusional states, or epilepsy occurs, the drug should be discontinued. The drug should not be given to patients with advanced liver disease due to schistosomiasis or other causes, renal or cardiac disease, a history of epilepsy or psychiatric disorder, or hypertension and should not be given with isoniazid. Patients should be checked for G6PD deficiency. In animal experiments, niridazole has shown mutagenic and carcinogenic properties and has had deleterious effects on the hemopoietic system. Mutagenic activity has also been found in the urine of patients treated with niridazole. This drug is available in the USA only from the Parasitic Disease Drug Service, Centers for Disease Control, Atlanta 30333; the FDA requires that all patients receiving the drug be hospitalized for observation.

5. Sodium antimony dimercaptosuccinate (Astiban, stibocaptate) is an intramuscular preparation that can be administered on an outpatient basis and used as an alternative drug for the treatment of *S haematobium, S mansoni,* and *S japonicum* infections. The total dose is 40 mg/kg body weight (maximum, 2.5 g), to be divided into 5 equal intramuscular injections given once a week over a period of 5 weeks. After each injection, the patient should rest for 30 minutes. Stibocaptate is available in the USA only from the Parasitic Disease Drug Service, Centers for Disease Control, Atlanta 30333.

Mild side effects include gastrointestinal symptoms, headache, weakness, skin rashes, pain at the injection site, and arthralgia. More severe reactions are infrequent but are an indication for stopping treatment: progressive proteinuria, fever, precordial pain, hematuria, thrombocytopenia, or hemolytic anemia. Sudden deaths due to cardiac arrhythmias and shock occur very rarely. Renal, cardiac, and nonschistosomal hepatic disease contraindicate use.

6. Antimony potassium (or sodium) tartrate (tartar emetic) is effective but is the most toxic of the antimonial drugs. It is used mainly as a third alternative drug for treatment of *S japonicum* infections. The patient must be hospitalized and be at bed rest during treatment. The drug is administered intravenously very slowly through a fine needle over a 10-minute period, taking care to avoid leakage into the perivascular tissues. The initial dose is 8 mL of a freshly prepared 0.5% solution. Subsequent doses of 12, 16, 20, 24, and 28 mL are given on alternate days. Thereafter, continue 28 mL on alternate days until a total of 360 mL (1.8 g) has been given.

Common side effects include nausea, vomiting, diarrhea, abdominal pain, syncope, tachycardia, dyspnea, paroxysmal coughing, and erythematous rashes. More severe toxic effects include exfoliative dermatitis, toxic liver necrosis, and toxic myocarditis. Cardiac, pulmonary, renal, hepatic, central nervous system, and febrile diseases are contraindications to use of this drug.

7. Surgery—As a last resort in patients who have repeated episodes of variceal bleeding, splenorenal anastomosis is done rather than portacaval shunts, which are associated with a high level of chronic portal systemic encephalopathy. Filtering of *S mansoni* adults from the portal system should be considered whenever splenectomy is contemplated. A single dose of tartar emetic allows most worms to be washed back into the portal venous system, whence they are filtered by tapping the portal vein via the splenic and returning filtered blood to the saphenous vein. Thousands of worms have been removed in this way from a single patient.

Prognosis

With treatment, the prognosis is good in early and light infections if reinfection does not occur. In advanced disease with extensive involvement of the intestines, liver, bladder, or other organs, the outlook is poor even with treatment.

Classen HG, Schramm V (editors): Praziquantel (Embay 8440, Biltricide). (Given at the Biltricide Symposium on African Schistosomiasis, Nairobi, February 24–26, 1980.) *Drug Res* 1981;**31**:535.

Damian RT: Immunity in schistosomiasis: A holistic view. *Contemp Top Immunobiol* 1984;**12**:359.

Jewsbury JM: Metrifonate in schistosomiasis. *Acta Pharmacol Toxicol* 1981;**49(Suppl 5)**:123.

Jordan P, Rosenfield PL: Schistosomiasis control: Past, present, and future. *Annu Rev Public Health* 1983;**4**:311.

Katz N et al: Clinical trial with oxamniquine and praziquantel in the acute and chronic phases of *Schistosomiasis mansoni*. *Rev Inst Med Trop Sao Paulo* 1983;**5**:173.

Lambertucci JR et al: A double blind trial with oxamniquine in chronic schistosomiasis. *Trans R Soc Trop Med Hyg* 1982;**76**:751.

McMahon JE: A comparative trial of praziquantel, metrifonate and niridazole against *Schistosoma haematobium*. *Ann Trop Med Parasitol* 1983;**77**:139.

Minggang C et al: A retrospective survey on side effects of praziquantel among 25,693 cases of *Schistosomiasis japonica*. *Southeast Asian J Trop Med Public Health* 1983;**14**:495.

Nash TE et al: Schistosome infections in humans: Perspectives and recent findings. (NIH conference.) *Ann Intern Med* 1982;**97**:740.

Nash TE et al: Treatment of *Schistosoma mekongi* with

praziquantel: A double-blind study. *Am J Trop Med Hyg* 1982;**31**:977.

Obeid FN et al: Bilharzial portal hypertension. *Arch Surg* 1983;**118**:702.

Warren KS: Schistosomiasis: Host-pathogen biology. *Rev Infect Dis* 1982;**4**:771.

FASCIOLOPSIASIS

The large intestinal fluke, *Fasciolopsis buski*, is a common parasite of humans and pigs in central and south China, Taiwan, Southeast Asia, Indonesia, eastern India, and Bangladesh. When eggs shed in stools reach water, they hatch to produce free-swimming larvae that penetrate and develop in the flesh of snails. Cercariae escape from the snails and encyst on various water plants. Humans are infected by eating these plants uncooked, usually water chestnuts, bamboo shoots, or caltrops. Adult flukes live in the small intestine attached to the mucosa or buried in mucous secretions and mature in about 3 months.

After an incubation period of several months, manifestations of gastrointestinal irritation appear in all but light infections. Symptoms in severe infections include upper abdominal pain, diarrhea, intermittent constipation, anorexia, and nausea. Edema of the face and body and ascites may occur later. Intestinal stasis, ileus, and partial obstruction have been described. Death may result from cachexia or intercurrent infection.

Leukocytosis with moderate eosinophilia is common. The diagnosis depends on finding characteristic eggs or, occasionally, flukes in the stools. No serologic test is available. Absence from the endemic area for 6 months or longer makes the diagnosis unlikely.

The drug of first choice will probably become praziquantel, but sufficient data are not yet available. A recommended dosage is 20 mg/kg given once. Alternative drugs are tetrachloroethylene, administered as for hookworm disease, and niclosamide, administered as for taeniasis but given every other day for 3 doses. Where available, dichlorophen or bephenium can also serve as alternative drugs.

In rare cases—particularly in children—heavy infections with severe toxemia have resulted in death in spite of treatment to remove the flukes. With these rare exceptions, the prognosis is good with proper treatment.

Bunnag D, Radomoyos P, Harinasuta T: Field trial on the treatment of fasciolopsiasis with praziquantel. *Southeast Asian J Trop Med Public Health* 1983;**14**:216.

Idris M et al: The treatment of fasciolopsiasis with niclosamide and dichlorophen. *J Trop Med Hyg* 1980;**83**:71.

FASCIOLIASIS

Infection by *Fasciola hepatica*, the sheep liver fluke, results from ingestion of encysted metacercariae on watercress or other aquatic vegetables or ingesting the encysted metacercariae with water. A wide range of herbivorous mammals can become infected. The illness in humans is prevalent in sheep-raising countries, particularly where raw salads are eaten. Eggs of the worm, passed in host feces, release a miracidium that infects snails; the snails subsequently release cercariae that in turn encyst to complete the life cycle.

There are 3 clinical syndromes: acute, chronic latent, and chronic obstructive. The acute illness, lasting up to several months, may be associated with serious symptoms. During this period, the immature larvae migrate through the liver to mature in the bile ducts. Cardinal features of the acute phase are an enlarged and tender liver, high fever, leukocytosis, and high eosinophilia. Pain may be present in the epigastrium or right upper quadrant, and the patient may experience headache, anorexia, and vomiting. In severe illnesses, the patient may be prostrated, wasted, and jaundiced. A variety of allergic symptoms, including myalgia and urticaria, may be present. Anemia may occur, plus leukocytosis up to 35,000, with eosinophilia to 90%. Hypergammaglobulinemia is common; other liver function tests may be abnormal. Early diagnosis is difficult in the acute phase, because ova are not found in the feces for 3–4 months. In the chronic latent phase, many infected persons are relatively free of symptoms. Others have variable degrees of pain in the epigastrium or right upper quadrant, vomiting or diarrhea, and hepatomegaly. Leukocytosis, eosinophilia, and altered liver function are sometimes seen. The chronic obstructive phase takes place if the extrahepatic bile ducts are occluded, producing a clinical picture similar to that of choledocholithiasis.

Diagnosis is made by detecting characteristic eggs in the feces; repeated examinations may be necessary. Sometimes the diagnosis can only be made by finding eggs in biliary drainage and, in rare instances, only after liver biopsy or at surgical exploration. In some regions of the world, spurious infections are common (but transient) as a result of ingestion of egg-containing cow or sheep liver. Serologic tests are often useful in diagnosis.

Bithionol, given as for paragonimiasis, is the drug of choice. Side effects occur in up to 40% of patients but are generally mild and transient; gastrointestinal symptoms and headache are the most common symptoms. If bithionol is not available, use emetine hydrochloride, 1 mg/kg body weight intramuscularly up to a maximum of 65 mg daily for 10 days. Dehydroemetine may be less toxic than emetine; the dosage is 1 mg/kg intramuscularly or subcutaneously for 10 days (maximum daily dose, 90 mg). For any of the drugs, the destruction of parasites followed by release of antigen in sensitized patients may evoke clinical symptoms.

Reports on the effectiveness of praziquantel have been variable. Although ineffective when used for 1–2 days, it may be useful when continued for 3–5 days.

Bithionol and dehydroemetine are available in the USA only from the Parasitic Disease Drug Service, Centers for Disease Control, Atlanta 30333.

In endemic areas, aquatic plants should not be eaten raw; washing does not destroy the metacercariae, but cooking will. Drinking water must be boiled or purified.

Jones EA et al: Massive infection with *Fasciola hepatica* in man. *Am J Med* 1977;**63**:836.

CLONORCHIASIS & OPISTHORCHIASIS

Infection by *Clonorchis sinensis,* the liver fluke, is endemic in areas of Japan, Korea, China, Formosa, and Southeast Asia. Imported cases are seen in the USA. Certain snails are infected as they ingest eggs shed into water in human or animal feces. Larval forms escape from the snails, penetrate the flesh of various freshwater fish, and encyst. Fish-eating mammals, including dogs and cats, are of great importance in maintaining the natural cycle. Human infection results from eating such fish, either raw or undercooked. In humans the ingested parasites excyst in the duodenum and ascend the bile ducts into the bile capillaries, where they mature and remain throughout their lives, shedding eggs in the bile. In the chronic stage of infection, there is progressive bile duct thickening, periductal fibrosis, dilatation, biliary stasis, and secondary infection. Little fibrosis occurs in the portal tracts. Occasionally, adults inhabit the pancreatic duct.

Most patients harbor few parasites and are asymptomatic. Among symptomatic patients, both acute and chronic syndromes occur. Acute symptoms follow entry of immature worms into the biliary ducts and may persist for several months. Symptoms include malaise, low-grade fever, high leukocytosis and eosinophilia, an enlarged, tender liver, and pain in the hepatic area or epigastrium. The acute syndrome is difficult to diagnose, since ova may not appear in the feces until 3–4 weeks after onset of symptoms.

In chronic clonorchiasis, findings include weakness, anorexia, epigastric pain, diarrhea, prolonged low-grade fever, progressive hepatomegaly, and intermittent episodes of right upper quadrant pain and localized hepatic area tenderness. Cholangiocarcinoma has been linked with late *Clonorchis* infection.

Complications of clonorchiasis are usually localized. Intrahepatic bile duct calculi may develop, leading to recurrent pyogenic cholangitis, biliary abscess, or endophlebitis of the portal-venous branches. Although focal initially, recurrent pyogenic cholangitis gradually results in destruction of the liver parenchyma, fibrosis, and, in a few patients, cirrhosis with ascites, anasarca, and jaundice. Rarely, a severe form of pancholangitis has been described. Flukes may also enter the pancreatic duct, causing acute pancreatitis.

The diagnosis is established by finding characteristic eggs in stools or duodenal aspirate. During the chronic stage of infection, leukocytosis varies according to intensity of infection; eosinophilia may be present. In advanced disease, liver function tests will indicate parenchymal damage. Transhepatic cholangiograms may show alternating stricture and dilatation of the biliary tree. Serologic tests are sometimes available.

The drug of choice is praziquantel. At a dosage of 25 mg/kg 3 times daily after meals, cure rates for clonorchiasis and opisthorchiasis range from 88 to 100%, with marked reduction in ova counts in those not cured. (See under Schistosomiasis for side effects, p 919.) Chloroquine is no longer recommended because of its potential toxicity and lack of efficacy.

Clonorchiasis is rarely fatal, but patients with advanced infections and impaired liver function may succumb more readily to other diseases. The prognosis is good for light to moderate infections.

Pickling, smoking, or drying may not suffice to kill the metacercariae in fish.

Chen M-G et al: Praziquantel in 237 cases of clonorchiasis sinensis. *Chin Med J* 1983;**96:**935.

Löscher T et al: Praziquantel in clonorchiasis and opisthorchiasis. *Tropenmed Parasitol* 1981;**32:**234.

Koompirochana C et al: Opisthorchiasis: A clinicopathologic study of 154 autopsy cases. *Southeast Asian J Trop Med Public Health* 1978;**9:**60.

Rim H-J et al: Clinical evaluation of the therapeutic efficacy of praziquantel (Embay 8440) against *Clonorchis sinensis* infection in man. *Ann Trop Med Parasitol* 1981;**75:**27.

PARAGONIMIASIS

Paragonimus westermani, the lung fluke, commonly infects humans throughout the Far East, and foci are present in West Africa, South Asia, Indonesia and New Guinea, Central America, and northern South America. Many carnivores and omnivores in addition to humans serve as reservoir host for the adult fluke. A number of other *Paragonimus* species can also infect humans. Eggs reaching water, either in sputum or feces, hatch in 3–6 weeks. The miracidia penetrate snails and develop, and the emergent cercariae encyst in the tissues of crabs and crayfish. When these crustaceans are eaten raw or pickled—or when crabs are crushed and food vessels or fingers are contaminated by metacercariae that are later ingested— immature flukes excyst in the small intestine and penetrate the peritoneal cavity. Most migrate through the diaphragm and enter the peripheral lung parenchyma; some may lodge in the peritoneum, the intestinal wall, the liver, or other tissues but usually fail to mature. Rarely, they may migrate to the brain or spinal cord. A capsule of fibrous and inflammatory tissue forms around the parasite as it matures and later swells and ruptures into a bronchiole. Fluid containing eggs, blood, and inflammatory cells is released and expectorated in the sputum.

The infection is asymptomatic until the flukes mature and begin producing eggs. The insidious onset is marked by low-grade fever, cough, or hemoptysis. The cough is dry at first; later a rusty or blood-flecked viscous sputum is produced. Pleuritic chest pain is common. The condition is chronic and slowly progressive. Dyspnea, signs of bronchitis and bronchiectasis, weakness, malaise, and weight loss are apparent in heavy infections. Many patients with light infections do not appear seriously ill. Parasites in the peritoneal cavity or intestinal wall may cause abdominal pain, diarrhea, or dysentery. Those in the central nervous system, depending on their location, may provoke seizures, palsies, or meningoencephalitis.

Diagnosis is by finding characteristic eggs in sputum, feces, or pleural fluid. Various serologic tests are available. Eosinophilia and low-grade leukocytosis are common. Chest x-rays may show a patchy infiltrate, nodular shadows, calcified spots, or pleural thickening or effusion. Cerebral paragonimiasis can result in intracranial calcifications.

Praziquantel is a drug of choice for the treatment of pulmonary infections at a dosage of 25 mg/kg after meals 3 times daily for 2 days. Cure rates of about 90% can be anticipated. (See under Schistosomiasis for side effects, p 919.) Bithionol remains a second drug of choice; 30–50 mg/kg body weight should be given on alternate days for 10–15 doses (20–30 days). The daily dose should be divided into a morning and evening dose. Cure rates of over 95% have been reported. Side effects are frequent but generally mild and transient. Gastrointestinal symptoms, particularly diarrhea, occur in most patients. Liver function should be tested serially. Antibiotics may be necessary to control secondary pulmonary infection. Bithionol is available in the USA only from the Parasitic Disease Drug Service, Centers for Disease Control, Atlanta 30333.

In the acute stages of cerebral paragonimiasis, particularly meningitis, bithionol may be effective. In the chronic stage, when the drug by itself is unlikely to be effective, surgical removal is indicated when possible, as well as chemotherapy.

Some authorities believe that surgery should be attempted only in "active" cases simulating brain tumors and that a marked increase in gamma globulin may be useful in differentiating cerebral paragonimiasis from brain tumors.

Chung HL et al: Recent progress in studies of *Paragonimus* and paragonimiasis control in China. *Chin Med J* 1981;**94:**483.

Johnson RJ et al: Successful praziquantel treatment of paragonimiasis following bithionol failure. *Am J Trop Med Hyg* 1983;**32:**1309.

Rim H-J et al: Clinical evaluation of praziquantel (Embay 8440; Biltricide) in the treatment of *Paragonimus westermani*. *Korean J Parasitol* 1981;**19:**27.

CESTODE INFECTIONS

TAPEWORM INFECTIONS
(See also Echinococcosis)

Essentials of Diagnosis

- Finding segments in clothing or bedding.
- Most infections asymptomatic; occasionally diarrhea or vague abdominal pains.
- Characteristic eggs or segments in the stool.
- Rarely (in cysticercosis), seizures, mental deterioration, signs and symptoms of internal hydrocephalus.

General Considerations

A number of species of adult tapeworms have been recorded as human parasites, but only 6 infect humans frequently. *Taenia saginata,* the beef tapeworm, and *Taenia solium,* the pork tapeworm, are cosmopolitan and common. *T solium* is no longer transmitted in the USA. The fish tapeworm, *Diphyllobothrium latum,* is found in cold or temperate lake regions in many areas of the world, particularly in Europe, the USA, and Japan, but also in the Middle East, in central and southern Africa, and in Chile. The dwarf tapeworms, *Hymenolepis nana* and *Hymenolepis diminuta,* are cosmopolitan. The dog tapeworm, *Dipylidium caninum,* is occasionally reported in children in Europe and the Americas.

The adult tapeworm consists of a head (scolex), which is a simple attachment organ, a neck, and a chain of individual segments (proglottids). *H nana* adults are rarely more than 2.5–5 cm long. Beef, pork, and fish tapeworms often exceed 300 cm in length. Gravid segments of *T saginata* and *T solium* detach themselves from the chain and are passed in the feces. Gravid segments of *D latum* consistently release eggs in the feces and sometimes *T solium* and *T saginata* rupture and release eggs. In the case of *T saginata,* the most common tapeworm found in humans in the USA, eggs are expelled from the segments after they pass from the host. The eggs hatch when ingested by cattle, releasing embryos that encyst in muscles as cysticerci. Humans are infected by eating undercooked beef containing viable cysticerci. In the human intestine, the cysticercus develops into an adult worm.

The life cycle of *T solium* is similar except that the pig is the normal host of the larval stage, and humans are infected by eating undercooked pork. However, if a person accidentally ingests *T solium* eggs, the larvae find their way to many parts of the body and encyst as cysticerci. Transmission of ova may occur from person to person or by autoinfection.

The intermediate hosts of the fish tapeworm are various species of freshwater crustaceans and fish. Eggs passed in human feces are taken up by crustaceans that in turn are eaten by fish. Human infection results from eating raw or poorly cooked fish.

The *H nana* life cycle is unusual in that both larval and adult stages of the worms are found in the human intestine. Adult worms expel infective eggs in the intestinal lumen. Newly hatched larvae invade the mucosa, where they develop for a time before returning to the lumen to mature. *H nana,* requiring no intermediate host, can be transmitted directly from person to person. A similar dwarf tapeworm, *H diminuta,* is a common parasite of rodents. Many arthropods, such as rat fleas, beetles, and cockroaches, serve as intermediate hosts. Humans are infected by accidentally swallowing the infected arthropods, usually in cereals or stored products. Multiple dwarf tapeworm infections are the rule, whereas a person rarely harbors more than one or 2 of the larger adult tapeworms.

Dipylidium caninum infections generally occur in young children living in close association with infected dogs or cats. Transmission results from swallowing the infected intermediate hosts, fleas or lice.

Sparganosis is infection by larval stages of several species of diphyllobothriid tapeworms (not including *D latum*) that are widespread in frogs, reptiles, birds, and some mammals. Rarely they may cause in humans subcutaneous nodules 2 × 3 cm in size that often are tender, pruritic, and painful, or ocular sparganosis characterized by marked edema of the lids and intense pain, which may progress to corneal ulceration, infection, and unilateral blindness. One form proliferates, resulting in hundreds of larvae distributed throughout the body. Infections are acquired by using frog or other meat poultices, by eating the raw flesh of small animals, or by ingesting infected copepods in water. The diagnosis is usually made after surgical removal.

Clinical Findings

A. Symptoms and Signs: Adult taeniae in the human intestine ordinarily cause no symptoms. Heavy infections with *H nana* may, however, cause diarrhea, abdominal pain, anorexia, weight loss, and irritability, particularly in children. In 1–2% of those harboring the fish tapeworm, a macrocytic anemia of considerable severity may be found accompanied by glossitis, lethargy, and signs of nerve damage. In nonanemic carriers, common complaints are fatigue, dizziness, a sensation of hunger, diarrhea, and numbness of the extremities. For unknown reasons, the anemia occurs mostly in Finland. In cysticercosis, most larvae lodge in muscles or connective tissues, where they remain silent and eventually calcify. In the brain, however, they may cause a wide variety of manifestations: epileptic seizures, mental deterioration, personality disturbances, and internal hydrocephalus with headache, giddiness, papilledema, and nerve palsies.

B. Laboratory Findings: Infection by a beef or pork tapeworm is often discovered by the patient finding one or more segments in stool, clothing, or bedding. To determine the species of worm, segments must be flattened between glass slides and examined microscopically for anatomic detail. Enzyme electrophoresis of glucose phosphate isomerase is also able to distinguish between *T saginata* and *T solium*. The presence of eggs in the stools is infrequent, but the perianal swab test with cellophane tape, as used to diagnose pinworm, is sometimes useful in detecting the eggs of *T saginata*. The eggs look alike and do not differentiate between the species.

In cysticercosis, x-rays often reveal calcified cysticerci in muscles, but those in the central nervous system calcify less frequently. A search should be made for subcutaneous nodules. When cysticerci lodge in the fourth ventricle, the cerebrospinal fluid pressure may be abnormal and the fluid may show increased numbers of mononuclear cells. Skin and serologic tests are also available as aids in diagnosis of cysticercosis.

The diagnosis of fish tapeworm is by finding characteristic operculated eggs in stool; repeat examinations may be necessary. Proglottids are passed occasionally, and their internal morphology is also diagnostic. In fish tapeworm–induced macrocytic anemia, the marrow may be megaloblastic, and hydrochloric acid is usually present in the stomach. This anemia is attributed to the affinity of the worm for dietary vitamin B_{12}.

The diagnosis of *H nana* and *H diminuta* is by finding characteristic eggs in feces; proglottids are usually not seen, because they disintegrate in the bowel. *D caninum* is usually diagnosed following detection of proglottids in feces or after their active migration through the anus.

Serologic tests are not available for diagnosis of intestinal tapeworm infections.

Differential Diagnosis

Fish tapeworm anemia may mimic pernicious anemia, but the presence of gastric hydrochloric acid and positive stool examinations will establish the diagnosis. Cysticercosis should be considered in all cases of epilepsy in patients who have lived in an endemic area for the pork tapeworm.

Complications

Pork tapeworm infection may be complicated by cysticercosis if the patient's hands are contaminated and eggs are unknowingly transferred to the mouth. For such a patient, vomiting is also a hazard in that eggs may be propelled up the small intestine into the stomach, where they may hatch.

Treatment

Niclosamide is the drug of choice for the treatment of all of the adult tapeworm infections except *H nana* infection, for which it is an alternative drug. Other alternative drugs are praziquantel, paromomycin, dichlorophen, and mebendazole. Quinacrine and aspidium oleoresin are no longer recommended, because of their potential toxicity.

The drug of choice for the treatment of *H nana* infection and cysticercosis is praziquantel.

A. Specific Measures for the Treatment of Adult Tapeworm Infections: Pre- and posttreatment purges are no longer used for any of the following drugs, except for the treatment of *T solium*.

1. Niclosamide–For *T saginata, T solium,* and *D latum* infections, only a single treatment is required and results in over 95% cure rates. The drug should be administered in the morning before the patient has eaten. The adult dosage is 4 tablets (2 g). Children weighing more than 34 kg are given 3 tablets; children 11–34 kg, 2 tablets. The tablets *must be chewed thoroughly* and swallowed with water. Eating may be resumed in 2 hours. For *T solium* infection, an effective purge (such as magnesium or sodium sulfate, 15–30 g) should be given 1–2 hours after treatment to eliminate mature segments before they disintegrate and release eggs; the patient should be followed closely to ensure that prompt evacuation of the bowel occurs.

For *H nana* and *H diminuta* infections, one mode of therapy is to treat with niclosamide daily for 5–7 days; some workers repeat the course in 5 days. Cure rates are about 75%.

Niclosamide rarely causes side effects.

2. Praziquantel–*H nana* infections are treated only once with 15–25 mg/kg; 86% of 473 persons were cured when treated with 15 mg/kg; 94% of 521 persons were cured when treated with 25 mg/kg.

T saginata and *T solium* infections treated with a single 10 mg/kg dose of praziquantel resulted in cure rates over 97%. Although 10 mg/kg will probably be satisfactory in the treatment of *D latum* infection, in reports to date, a single dose of 25 mg/kg resulted in 95% cure rates.

3. Paromomycin, an antibiotic not appreciably absorbed from the gastrointestinal tract, is effective for the treatment of *T saginata* in an adult dosage of 1 g every 15 minutes for 4 doses. For children give 11 mg/kg every 15 minutes for 4 doses. In the USA, paromomycin is considered an investigational drug for the treatment of tapeworm infections. The treatment course for *H nana* is 45 mg/kg daily (to a maximum of 4 g) for 5–7 days. Gastrointestinal side effects are common but not severe. Because vomiting may occur, it is better not to use the drug to treat *T solium* infections.

4. Dichlorophen given for 2 days is also an effective drug for *T saginata, T solium,* and *D latum*. The dosage is 75 mg/kg (to a maximum of 6 g) taken on an empty stomach in the morning without prior dietary restrictions (except for avoiding alcohol) or purgatives. Breakfast may follow in 2 hours. Because of the risk of drug-induced vomiting, it is preferable to use an alternative drug in the treatment of *T solium* infection. Dichlorophen is not available in the USA.

5. Mebendazole, at a dosage of 300 mg twice daily for 3 days, appears to be effective therapy for *T solium;* the drug has a theoretic advantage over niclosamide in that proglottids are expelled intact after therapy. Reports have varied on the effectiveness of the drug for *T saginata*.

B. Follow-Up Care: Except following mebendazole administration, a disintegrating worm is usually passed within 24–48 hours of treatment. Since efforts are not generally made to recover and identify the scolex, cure can be presumed only if regenerated segments have not reappeared 3–5 months later. If it is preferred that parasitic cure be established immediately, the head (scolex) must be found in post-treatment stools. A laxative is given 2 hours after treatment, and stools are collected in a preservative for 24 hours. To facilitate examination, toilet paper must be disposed of separately.

C. Neurocysticercosis: Praziquantel is the first drug to be useful in the treatment of neurocysticercosis. In many (not all) cases, therapy has resulted in reduction in cerebral hypertension, amelioration of seizures, or disappearance of lesions on cerebral tomograms. The dosage of praziquantel is 50 mg/kg in 2–3 divided doses for 15 days. Corticosteroids (dexamethasone, 4–16 mg/kg, or equivalent) must be administered concurrently and for 3 days afterward to decrease or block cerebral and meningeal tissue inflammatory reactions and edema that result from dying parasites. The following clinical findings occur in many patients, are usually mild (rarely severe), and generally subside within 48–72 hours: increased intracranial pressure, headache, vomiting, mental changes, and convulsions. A few deaths from intracranial hypertension, meningitis, or complications due to ventricular blockage have occurred during or shortly after treatment.

Prognosis

Because the prognosis is often poor in cerebral cysticercosis, the eradication of a *T solium* infection is a matter of much greater urgency than that of the other tapeworm infections, which are usually benign.

Flisser A et al (editors): *Cysticercosis: Present State of Knowledge and Perspectives.* Academic Press, 1982.

Friedman J, Mates S: Praziquantel therapy for cysticercosis. *Arch Neurol* 1983;**40**:257.

Hamrick HJ et al: Two cases of dipylidiasis (dog tapeworm infection) in children: Update on an old problem. *Pediatrics* 1983;**72**:114.

Jones WE: Niclosamide as a treatment for *Hymenolepis diminuta* and *Dipylidium caninum* infection in man. *Am J Trop Med Hyg* 1979;**28**:300.

Loo L, Braude A: Cerebral cysticercosis in San Diego: A report of 23 cases and a review of the literature. *Medicine* 1982;**61**:341.

Ruttenber AJ et al: Diphyllobothriasis associated with salmon consumption in Pacific coast states. *Am J Trop Med Hyg* 1984;**33**:455.

Sotelo J et al: Therapy of parenchymal brain cysticercosis with praziquantel. *N Engl J Med* 1984;**310**:1001.

Von Bonsdorff B: *Diphyllobothriasis in Man.* Academic Press, 1977.

ECHINOCOCCOSIS/HYDATIDOSIS
(Hydatid Disease)

Human echinococcosis results from parasitism by the larval stage of 2 *Echinococcus* species: *Echinococcus granulosus* (cystic hydatid disease) and *Echinococcus multilocularis* (alveolar hydatid disease).

Very rarely, *Echinococcus oligarthrus* (polycystic hydatid disease) has been reported from northern South America and Panama. Echinococcosis is a zoonosis in which humans are an intermediate host of the larval stage of the parasite. The definitive host is a carnivore that harbors the adult tapeworm in the small intestine; the carnivore becomes infected by ingesting the larval form in tissue of the intermediate host. The intermediate hosts, including humans, become infected by ingesting tapeworm eggs passed in carnivore feces. The larval stages are referred to as hydatid cysts.

1. CYSTIC HYDATID DISEASE
(Unilocular Hydatid Disease)

Essentials of Diagnosis

- Cystic tumor of liver, lung, or, infrequently, bone, brain, or other organs as detected by radiologic and nuclear medicine procedures.
- Positive serologic tests.
- History of exposure to dogs associated with livestock in a hydatid-endemic region.

General Considerations

Human infection with *E granulosus* occurs principally where dogs are used to herd grazing animals, particularly sheep. The disease is common throughout southern South America, the Mediterranean littoral, the Middle East, central Asia, and East Africa. Foci of endemicity are in eastern Europe, Iceland, Russia, Australasia, India, and the United Kingdom. In North America, endemic foci have been reported from California, Utah, the lower Mississippi Valley, Alaska, and northwestern Canada and autochthonous cases have been reported from other states in the USA.

There are at least 2 geographic strains of the parasite. The pastoral strain—which is more pathogenic to humans—has a transmission cycle in which dogs are the definitive host and usually sheep, but also cattle, hogs, and other domestic livestock, are intermediate hosts. The sylvatic, or northern, strain is maintained in wolves and wild ungulates (moose and reindeer) in northern Alaska, Canada, Scandinavia, and Eurasia.

Human infection occurs when eggs passed in dog feces are accidentally swallowed. Embryos liberated from the eggs penetrate the intestinal mucosa, enter the portal bloodstream, and are carried to the liver where they are trapped and become hydatid cysts (65% of all cysts). Some larvae reach the lung (25%) and develop into pulmonary hydatids. Infrequently, cysts form in the brain, bones, skeletal muscles, kidneys, spleen, or other tissues. Cysts of the sylvatic strain tend to localize in the lungs.

The wall of the cyst has 3 layers. The inner germinal layer gives rise within the cyst to scoleces, brood capsules, and daughter cysts. The supporting intermediate layer is an acellular laminated membrane. These 2 layers are derived from the parasite. The outer, granulomatous adventitial layer is produced by the host. The disease becomes evident because of cyst pressure or release of cyst contents. In the liver, cysts may increase in size 1–5 cm in diameter per year and become enormous, but symptoms generally do not develop until they reach about 10 cm. Some cysts die spontaneously. Part or all of the adventitial layer may calcify, which does not necessarily mean cyst death. Calcification may also occur in some splenic cysts.

Clinical Findings

A. Symptoms and Signs: A liver cyst may remain silent for 10–20 or more years until it becomes large enough to be palpable, to be visible as an abdominal swelling, to produce pressure effects, or to produce symptoms due to leakage or rupture. There may be right upper quadrant pain, nausea, and vomiting. The effects of pressure may result in cholangitis, obstructive jaundice, cirrhosis, portal hypertension, and secondary infection; the latter can progress to hepatic abscess. If a cyst ruptures suddenly, anaphylaxis and death may occur. Fluid and hydatid particles may escape slowly, resulting in allergic manifestations, including a rise in the eosinophil count. Rupture can occur into the pleural or pericardial cavity, the duodendum, colon, renal pelvis, peritoneum, or pleural space, and dissemination of scoleces may be followed by the development of multiple secondary cysts. A characteristic clinical syndrome may follow intrabiliary extrusion of cyst contents—jaundice, biliary colic, and urticaria.

Pulmonary cysts cause no symptoms until they leak; become large enough to obstruct a bronchus, causing segmental collapse; or erode a bronchus and rupture. Brain cysts produce symptoms earlier and may cause seizures or symptoms of increased intracranial pressure. Cysts in the bone marrow or spongiosa do not have an adventitial layer, are irregular in shape, erode osseous tissue, and may present as pain or as spontaneous fracture. The bones most often affected are the vertebrae; many of these cases develop epidural extension with compression of the spinal cord and paraplegia. Because 20% of patients have multiple cysts, each patient should be screened for cysts in the liver, spleen, kidneys, lungs, brain, bones, skin, tongue, vitreous, and other tissues.

B. Laboratory and X-Ray Findings: Scintillation scan, CT scan, and ultrasound examination are used to detect a cystic mass in the liver. The mass can be further defined by angiography, which may show the "halo" sign. X-rays of the abdomen may show spotty calcified densities or a calcified cyst wall in the liver or spleen. Chest x-ray may show a pulmonary lesion (calcification of the cyst wall usually does not occur in the lungs). An intravenous urogram or full body or bone scan may detect other cysts at other sites.

Two or 3 serologic tests should be done. The finding of an arc-5 in the immunoelectrophoresis test and a high titer in the indirect hemagglutination test is particularly useful to confirm the diagnosis. But up to 50% of intact lung cysts may give a negative serologic result. The disappearance within about a year of arc-5

or seroconversion from positive to negative in the complement fixation or immunofluorescent tests is indicative of complete surgical removal of a cyst. Because of its poor specificity, the Casoni intracutaneous skin test should probably be abandoned.

Eosinophilia is uncommon except after cyst rupture. Liver function tests are usually normal. Diagnostic aspiration of suspected hydatid cysts should never be undertaken because of the danger of leakage or rupture. Confirmation of the diagnosis is possible only by examination of cyst contents after surgical removal.

Differential Diagnosis

Hydatid cysts of the liver need to be differentiated from bacterial and amebic abscesses. Hydatid cysts in any site may be mistaken for a variety of malignant and nonmalignant tumors. In the lung, a cyst may be confused with an advanced tubercular lesion. Allergic symptoms arising from cyst leakage may resemble those associated with many other diseases.

Treatment

A. Surgical Treatment: The current definitive treatment is surgical removal of cysts where their location permits it. All lung cysts should be removed but not all liver cysts. Operative treatment of liver cysts involves 2 major problems: (1) selection of a method to sterilize and remove cyst contents without spillage, and (2) management of the remaining cavity. Germicidal solutions include cetrimide, hypertonic saline, silver nitrate, and sodium hypochlorite. Curettage, lavage, and instillation of chemical sterilization substances are indicated treatment of bone cysts.

B. Drug Treatment: In some cases because of the extent or location of cysts or the patient's general condition, surgery may not be indicated. Under such conditions, mebendazole may be tried. When used at high doses for several months, marked regression and apparent death of cysts has occurred in some patients. In other patients, however, cysts were either stable or continued to grow and if removed were viable. A suggested dosage of mebendazole is 50 mg/kg/d in 3 divided doses for 3 months, with many patients requiring repeated courses. When possible, mebendazole levels should be monitored; serum levels in excess of 100 mg/kg 1–2 hours after an oral dose may be necessary for parasite killing. In unresponsive cases, it is possible that plasma levels of mebendazole are insufficient; some researchers, therefore, give up to 200 mg/kg/d. Occasional side effects with treatment include pruritus, rash, alopecia, reversible leukopenia, gastric irritation, musculoskeletal pain, fever, and acute pain in cyst area; 6 cases of glomerulonephritis and 3 of agranulocytosis (with one death) have been reported.

Prophylactic treatment of pet dogs is with 5 mg/kg of praziquantel at monthly intervals.

Prognosis

Patients may live for years with relatively large hydatid cysts before the condition is diagnosed. Liver and lung cysts often can be removed surgically without great difficulty, but in patients with cysts in less accessible sites the prognosis is less favorable. Surgical mortality varies from 2 to 10%, and postoperative recurrence of cysts may be seen in some patients. The prognosis is always grave in secondary echinococcosis. About 15% of patients eventually die because of the disease or its complications.

2. ALVEOLAR HYDATID DISEASE
(Multilocular Hydatid Disease)

Alveolar hydatid disease results from infection by the larval form of *Echinococcus multilocularis*. The life cycle involves foxes as definitive host and microtine rodents as intermediate host. Domestic dogs and cats can also become infected with the adult tapeworm when they eat infected wild rodents. Human infection is by accidental ingestion of tapeworm eggs passed in fox or dog feces. The disease in humans has been reported in parts of central Europe, much of the USSR, the northwestern part of Canada, and western Alaska. The primary localization of alveolar cysts is in the liver, where they may extend locally or metastasize to other tissues. The larval mass has poorly defined borders and behaves like a neoplasm; it infiltrates and proliferates indefinitely by exogenous budding of the germinative membrane, producing an alveoluslike pattern of microvesicles, ie, irregular, thin, peripheral layers of dense fibrous tissue, necrotic cavities containing an amorphous material, and focal calcification. X-ray shows hepatomegaly and characteristic scattered areas of radiolucency often outlined by 2- to 4-mm calcific rings. Serologic tests are the same as for cystic hydatid disease and cannot distinguish between the species. Treatment is by surgical removal of the entire larval mass, when possible. Long-term mebendazole therapy (40 mg/kg/d) inhibits growth of the parasite and has extended patient survival, but larval tissue is not completely destroyed.

Beggs I: The radiological appearances of hydatid disease of the liver. *Clin Radiol* 1983;**34**:555.

Kammerer WS, Schantz PM: Long-term follow-up of human hydatid disease *(Echinococcus granulosus)* treated with a high-dose mebendazole regimen. *Am J Trop Med Hyg* 1984;**33**:132.

Morris DL: Chemotherapy of hydatid disease. *J Antimicrob Chemother* 1983;**11**:494.

Rickard MD, Williams JF: Hydatidosis/cysticercosis: Immune mechanisms and immunization against infection. *Adv Parasitol* 1982;**21**:229.

Saidi F: *Surgery of Hydatid Disease.* Saunders, 1976.

Wilson JF, Rausch RL: Mebendazole and alveolar hydatid disease. *Ann Trop Med Parasitol* 1982;**76**:165.

NEMATODE (ROUNDWORM) INFECTIONS

ANGIOSTRONGYLIASIS

1. *ANGIOSTRONGYLUS CANTONENSIS* (Eosinophilic Meningoencephalitis)

A nematode of rats, *Angiostrongylus cantonensis*, is the causative agent of a form of eosinophilic meningoencephalitis reported from Hawaii and other Pacific islands, south and east Asia, Australia, and Madagascar. Human infection results from the ingestion of infected larvae contained in raw food—either infected mollusks, the intermediate host, or transport hosts (crabs, shrimp, fish) that have ingested mollusks. Drinking water can also become contaminated with infective larvae, as can fingers during the collection and preparation of snails for cooking.

The larvae usually invade the central nervous system, producing signs and symptoms of meningoencephalitis, including headache, fever, neck stiffness, nausea and vomiting, and multiple neurologic findings, particularly asymmetric transient paresthesias and cranial nerve palsies. A characteristic feature is spinal fluid pleocytosis, consisting largely of eosinophils. Occasionally, the parasite can be recovered from spinal fluid. Peripheral eosinophilia is common. Serologic and skin tests have been developed but are not specific. Ocular infection has been reported from Thailand.

No specific treatment is available. Corticosteroids have not influenced the course of the disease. The illness usually persists for weeks to months, the parasite dies, and the patient then recovers spontaneously without sequelae. However, fatalities have been recorded.

2. *ANGIOSTRONGYLUS COSTARICENSIS*

Angiostrongylus costaricensis has been identified in humans in Mexico, Central America, Venezuela, and Brazil, but the known geographic range of the parasite in rats extends from northern South America to Texas. The normal definitive hosts are rat species, and the intermediate host is a slug that contaminates the food of humans with the infective third-stage larvae. Adult worms mature in the mesenteric vessels, where they cause arteritis, thrombosis, and ischemic necrosis; their eggs give rise to eosinophilic granulomas. The granulomas are most commonly localized in the appendix but may also be found in the terminal ileum, the cecum, the first part of the ascending colon, and the regional lymph nodes. Patients have fever, right lower quadrant abdominal pain and a mass, leukocytosis, and eosinophilia. Incomplete or complete obstruction, infarction, and an inflammatory reaction are the most common complications. A serologic test has been described but is not very useful.

There is no specific treatment. Operative treatment is frequently necessary.

Ko RC et al: First report of human angiostrongyliasis in Hong Kong diagnosed by computerized axial topography (CAT) and enzyme-linked immunosorbent assay. *Trans R Soc Trop Med Hyg* 1984;**78**:354.

Kuberski T, Wallace GD: Clinical manifestations of eosinophilic meningitis due to *Angiostrongylus cantonensis*. *Neurology* 1979;**29**:1566.

Loria-Cortes R, Lobo-Sanahuja JF: Clinical abdominal angiostrongylosis: A study of 116 children with intestinal eosinophilic granuloma caused by *Angiostrongylus costaricensis*. *Am J Trop Med Hyg* 1980;**29**:538.

Morera P et al: Visceral larva migrans–like syndrome caused by *Angiostrongylus costaricensis*. *Am J Trop Med Hyg* 1982;**31**:67.

ASCARIASIS

Essentials of Diagnosis

- Pneumonitis with fever, cough, hemoptysis, urticaria, and accompanying eosinophilia.
- Vague abdominal discomfort and colic.
- Inflammatory reactions in organs and tissues invaded by wandering adult worms.
- Characteristic ova in the stool; larvae in the sputum.

General Considerations

Ascaris lumbricoides, a large intestinal roundworm, is the most common of the intestinal helminths of humans. It is cosmopolitan in distribution, although it flourishes best in warm, humid climates. In temperate regions it is generally associated with low standards of personal hygiene. The adult worms live in the small intestine. After fertilization, the female produces enormous numbers of characteristic eggs that are carried out to the soil in feces. Under suitable conditions the eggs become infective, containing an active larva, in 2–3 weeks. Humans are infected by ingestion of the mature eggs in fecally contaminated food and drink. The eggs hatch in the small intestine, releasing motile larvae that penetrate the wall of the small intestine and reach the right heart via the mesenteric venules and lymphatics. From the heart they move to the lung, burrow through the alveolar walls, and migrate up the bronchial tree into the pharynx, down the esophagus, and back to the small intestine. The larvae mature and female egg production begins about 60–75 days after ingestion of the infective eggs. The large adult worms, which are 20–40 cm long, may live for 1 year or more.

Clinical Findings

A. Symptoms and Signs: No symptoms arise from the early migration of the larvae after hatching. In the lung, however, they damage capillary and alveolar walls as they force their way through. Hemorrhage may result from this trauma, and accumulations of leukocytes and serous exudates in and around the air spaces may lead to consolidation. Pneumonitis occasionally develops with heavy infections. Symptoms and signs include fever, cough, hemoptysis, rales, and other evidences of lobular involvement. Eosinophilia is usual at this stage, and urticaria is not uncommon. After passage through the lungs, it is believed that (rarely) the larvae may go astray, lodging in the brain, kidney, eye, spinal cord, or skin. Many bizarre symptoms may result from such invasions.

Small numbers of adult worms in the intestine usually produce no symptoms. With heavy infection, vague abdominal discomfort and colic may occur, particularly in children. *Ascaris* infection in childhood may contribute to protein and other nutritional deficiencies when a high parasite load is associated with a low protein intake. When the infection is heavy, and particularly if the worms are stimulated by certain oral medications or anesthetics, wandering may occur. Adult worms may be coughed up, vomited, or passed out through the nose. They may also force themselves into the common bile duct, the pancreatic duct, the appendix, diverticula, and other sites. Mechanical blockage and inflammation usually result. With very heavy infestations, masses of worms may cause intestinal obstruction, volvulus, or intussusception; during typhoid fever, bowel perforation may occur. It is important that *Ascaris* infections be cured prior to bowel surgery because the worms have been known to break open suture lines postoperatively.

B. Laboratory Findings: The diagnosis usually depends upon finding the characteristic eggs in stool specimens. Occasionally a spontaneously passed adult worm reveals a previously unsuspected infection. There are no characteristic alterations of the blood picture during the intestinal phase. Skin tests are of no value in diagnosis. During the pulmonary phase there may be eosinophilia, and larvae may occasionally be found in the sputum. Occasionally, the diagnosis may be established by chance, when radiologic examination of the abdomen (with or without barium) shows characteristic findings.

Differential Diagnosis

Ascariasis must be differentiated from allergic disorders such as urticaria, Löffler's syndrome, and asthma. The pneumonitis associated with ascariasis is similar to other types of pneumonitis, especially that occurring with hookworm or *Strongyloides* infection. *Ascaris*-induced pancreatitis, appendicitis, diverticulitis, etc, must be differentiated from other causes of inflammation of these tissues.

Complications & Sequelae

Bacterial pneumonia may be superimposed upon pneumonitis resulting from larval migration. During the migratory stage, allergic manifestations may be severe. Because anesthesia stimulates the worms to become hypermotile, they should be removed in advance for patients undergoing elective surgery.

Treatment

Pyrantel pamoate is the drug of choice in treatment of ascariasis. Piperazine and mebendazole are effective alternative drugs available in the USA; levamisole and bephenium are also effective and available in other countries. None of the drugs require pre- or posttreatment purges. Stools should be rechecked at 2 weeks and patients re-treated until all ascarids are removed. Ascariasis, hookworm, and trichuriasis infections, which often occur together, may be treated simultaneously by mebendazole. Ascariasis and hookworm combined may be treated with pyrantel pamoate or bephenium.

A. Pyrantel pamoate is highly effective when administered as a single oral dose of 10 mg of base per kg body weight (maximum, 1 g). In various studies, cure rates of 85–100% have been reported. It may be given before or after meals. Infrequent side effects include vomiting, diarrhea, headache, dizziness, drowsiness, and rash. Experience with this drug is limited in children under age 2 years.

B. Piperazine: Many brands of syrups and tablets of piperazine salts are available; in solution, all form piperazine hexahydrate. Usually, each milliliter of syrup contains the equivalent of 100 mg of piperazine hexahydrate; tablets usually contain 250 or 500 mg. The dosage for piperazine (as the hexahydrate) is 75 mg/kg body weight (maximum, 3.5 g) for 2 days in succession, giving the drug orally before or after breakfast. For heavy infestations, treatment should be continued for 4 days in succession or the 2-day course should be repeated after 1 week.

Gastrointestinal symptoms and headache occur occasionally with piperazine; central nervous system symptoms, including temporary ataxia and exacerbation of seizures, are rarely reported. Allergic symptoms have been attributed to piperazine. The drug should not be used for patients with hepatic or renal insufficiency or with a history of seizures or chronic neurologic disease. Piperazine may be used in the last trimester of pregnancy.

C. Mebendazole is effective when given in a dosage of 100 mg twice daily before or after meals for 3 days. Gastrointestinal side effects are infrequent, but worms may appear occasionally at the nose or mouth of children under age 5. The drug is contraindicated in pregnancy, and experience is limited in children under age 2 years.

D. Levamisole: This drug is highly effective (with cure rates of 86–100%) as a single oral dose of 150 mg; children should receive a single dose of 3 mg/kg. Levamisole is the levorotatory isomer of tetramisole. Side effects from levamisole—nausea, vomiting, abdominal cramps, headache, and dizziness—are mild and transient and occur in some patients. The drug has immunomodulating and immunostimulating properties that are currently under investigation.

E. Bephenium Hydroxynaphthoate: Bephenium is less effective than the other drugs and has more side effects. Reported cure rates after one dose (5 g for older children and adults; 2.5 g for children under 22 kg) vary from 30 to 82%. However, a 3-day course, as

for hookworm infection, may be effective for mixed infections with both parasites. Bephenium is no longer marketed in the USA.

Prognosis

The complications caused by wandering adult worms, plus the possibility of intestinal obstruction, require that all *Ascaris* infections be treated and completely eradicated.

Carrera E, Nesheim MC, Crompton DWT: Lactose maldigestion in *Ascaris*-infected preschool children. *Am J Clin Nutr* 1984;**39**:255.

Moens J et al: Levamisole in ascariasis: A multicenter controlled evaluation. *Am J Trop Med Hyg* 1978;**27**:897.

Pawlowski ZS: Ascariasis. *Clin Gastroenterol* 1978;**7**:157.

Pawlowski ZS: Ascariasis: Host-pathogen biology. *Rev Infect Dis* 1982;**4**:806.

CUTANEOUS LARVA MIGRANS
(Creeping Eruption)

Creeping eruption, prevalent throughout the tropics and subtropics, is caused by the larvae of the dog and cat hookworms, *Ancylostoma braziliense* and *Ancylostoma caninum;* a number of other animal hookworms have rarely been implicated. It is a common infection of humans in the southeastern USA, particularly where people come in contact with moist sandy soil (beaches, children's sand piles) contaminated by dog or cat feces. The larvae may invade any skin surface, but the hands or feet are usually affected. The larvae may remain active in the skin for several weeks or months, slowly advancing but rarely moving more than 1 cm from the penetration site. Eventually, if not killed by treatment, the larvae die and are absorbed.

Soon after invasion of the skin, minute itchy erythematous papules appear at the sites of entry. Two or 3 days later, characteristic serpiginous eruptions begin to form as larval migration starts. Hundreds of lesions may occur on a single patient. These intensely pruritic lesions may persist for several months as migration continues. The parasite usually lies slightly ahead of the advancing border of the eruption. Vesiculation and crusting commonly occur in the later stages. Eosinophilia is common.

Simple transient cases may not require treatment. The larvae must be killed to provide relief in severe or persistent cases. Thiabendazole, given as for strongyloidiasis, is very effective and the drug of choice. Progression of the lesions and itching are usually stopped within 48 hours, but if active lesions are still present at that time, repeat treatment. Thiabendazole cream (15% in a hygroscopic base) applied topically daily for 5 days may also be effective. Antihistamines are helpful in controlling pruritus, and antibiotic ointments may be necessary to treat secondary infections.

Winter PAD, Fripp PJ: Treatment of cutaneous larva migrans (sandworm disease). (Correspondence.) *S Afr Med J* 1978; **54**:556.

DRACUNCULIASIS
(Guinea Worm Infection, Dracunculosis, Dracontiasis)

Dracunculus medinensis is a nematode parasite of humans found through northern and central Africa, southern Asia, and northeastern South America. It occurs in the Caribbean but is not seen in the USA except in imported cases. Humans are infected by swallowing water containing the infected intermediate host, the crustacean *Cyclops,* which is common in wells and ponds in the tropics. Larvae escape from the crustacean in the human host and mature in the connective tissues. After mating, the male worm dies and the gravid female, now 1 meter or more in length, moves to the surface of the body. The head of the worm reaches the skin surface, a blister develops and ruptures, and the uterus discharges great numbers of larvae whenever the ulcer comes in contact with water. Larval discharge continues intermittently, for as long as 3 weeks, until the uterus is empty. The female worm then dies and is either extruded or absorbed. In the absence of secondary infection, the ulcer heals in 4–6 weeks following onset.

Clinical Findings
A. Symptoms and Signs:
Clinical effects are produced only by the female worm. Multiple infections occur, but the uuual infection is with a single worm. Several hours before the head appears at the skin surface, local erythema and tenderness often develop in the area where emergence is to take place. In some patients there may be systemic symptoms at this time, including urticaria, generalized pruritus, nausea, vomiting, and dyspnea. As the blister forms and ruptures, these symptoms subside. The tissues surrounding the ulceration that remains after rupture of the blister frequently become indurated, reddened, and tender; and since 90% of the lesions appear on the leg or foot, the patient often must give up walking and work. Uninfected ulcers heal in 4–6 weeks, but secondary infection is common and prolongs the course.

Calcified guinea worms are occasionally revealed as chance findings during x-ray examination of persons in endemic areas.

B. Laboratory Findings:
When a worm is not visible in the ulcer, the diagosis may be made by detection of larvae in fluid expressed from the moistened ulcer. A skin test is available, but its value as a diagnostic aid is not established. Eosinophilia of about 10% often accompanies the symptoms before blister formation.

Complications
Secondary infection is the rule and may cause an abscess that eventually involves deep structures. Ankle and knee joint infection and deformity is a common complication in some areas. If the worm is broken during removal, sepsis almost always results, leading to cellulitis, abscess formation, or septicemia. The worm rarely reaches ectopic sites. Epidural localization has resulted in abscesses leading to paraplegia.

Treatment
A. General Measures:
The patient should be at bed rest with the affected part elevated. Cleanse the lesion and control secondary infection with antibiotics.

B. Specific Measures:
Three drugs are now used to facilitate rapid resolution of symptoms, expulsion or removal of worms, and healing of ulcers. The relative merits of the 3 drugs—metronidazole, niridazole, and thiabendazole—require further comparative, controlled clinical trials. The incidence of significant side effects is metronidazole < thiabendazole < niridazole. Give metronidazole, 750 mg 3 times daily for 10 days; or niridazole, 25 mg/kg in divided doses daily for 7 days; or thiabendazole, 25 mg/kg twice daily for 2 days. Mebendazole has also been tried, with conflicting results. The ulcers should be dressed daily and the emerging worms eased out by applying gentle traction to the stick around which they are wound. The extraction process may require several days. The procedure can be hazardous if part of the worm is in deep fascia or is wound around tendons.

C. Surgical Removal:
If necessary, following chemotherapy, make multiple incisions under local anesthesia along the worm tract and remove the entire worm carefully. Injection of a contrast medium in the tract, followed by x-ray, may facilitate locating the worm. Give antihistamines preoperatively to control allergic symptoms arising from manipulation or rupture of the worm.

Hopkins DR: Dracunculiasis: An eradicable scourge. *Epidemiol Rev* 1983;5:208.

Kale OO, Elemile T, Enahoro F: Controlled comparative trial of thiabendazole and metronidazole in the treatment of dracontiasis. *Ann Trop Med Parasitol* 1983;77:151.

Muller R: Guinea worm disease: Epidemiology, control, and treatment. *Bull WHO* 1979;57:683.

ENTEROBIASIS
(Pinworm Infection)

Essentials of Diagnosis
- Perianal pruritus, usually nocturnal, associated with insomnia and restlessness.
- Vague gastrointestinal symptoms.
- Eggs on skin of perianal area.

General Considerations
Enterobius vermicularis, a short spindle-shaped roundworm often called the pinworm, is worldwide in distribution and the most common cause of helminthic infection of humans in the USA. Humans are the only host for the parasite. Children are affected more often than adults. The adult worms inhabit the cecum and adjacent bowel areas, lying with their heads loosely attached to the mucosa. When the fertilized female worms become gravid they migrate down the colon

and out onto the skin, where eggs are deposited in large numbers. The females die after oviposition. The eggs become infective in a few hours and may then infect humans if transferred to the mouth by contaminated food, drink, or hands. Retroinfection occasionally occurs when the eggs hatch on the perianal skin and the larvae migrate through the anus into the large intestine. After being swallowed, the infective eggs hatch in the duodenum and the larvae migrate down to the cecum, molting twice en route. The development of a mature ovipositing female from an ingested egg requires about 2 months.

Clinical Findings

A. Symptoms and Signs: A large number of patients are asymptomatic. The most common and most important symptom is pruritus of the perianal area, particularly at night. This must be distinguished from similar pruritus due to mycotic infections, allergies, and psychologic disorders. Insomnia, restlessness, enuresis, and irritability are common symptoms, particularly in children. Many mild gastrointestinal symptoms—abdominal pain, nausea, vomiting, diarrhea, anorexia—have also been attributed to enterobiasis, although the association is difficult to prove. At night, worms may occasionally be seen near the anus. Rarely, ectopic disease (vulvovaginitis, urethritis, appendicitis, and other disorders) may occur.

B. Laboratory Findings: Except for a modest eosinophilia (4–12%), blood counts are usually normal. The diagnosis depends upon finding adult worms in the stool or eggs on the perianal skin; eggs are seldom found on stool examination. The most reliable diagnostic technique consists of applying a short strip of sealing cellulose pressure-sensitive tape (eg, Scotch Tape) to the perianal skin and spreading the tape on a slide for study. Three such preparations made on consecutive mornings before bathing or defecation will establish the diagnosis in about 90% of cases. Before the diagnosis can be ruled out, 5–7 such examinations are necessary.

Complications

It has been postulated that the presence of large numbers of worms in the cecum may predispose to appendicitis, but the evidence for this is inconclusive. Worms occasionally migrate into the vagina, uterus, and uterine tubes, where they may produce an intense vaginitis. Granulomas rarely occur when worms enter tissue.

Treatment

A. General Measures: Symptomatic patients should be treated, and in some situations all members of the patient's household should be treated concurrently, since for each overt case there are usually several inapparent cases. However, treatment of all nonsymptomatic cases is not necessary. Careful washing of hands with soap and water after defecation and again before meals is important. Fingernails should be kept trimmed close and clean, scratching of the peri-

anal area avoided, and the hands kept away from the mouth. Ordinary washing of bedding will usually kill pinworm eggs. Recurrence is frequent in children because of continued exposure outside the home.

B. Specific Measures:
Since eggs deposited in a moist environment remain infective for 2–3 weeks, the following drugs (except piperazine) are recommended every 2 weeks for 3 doses (only 2 doses has been the standard approach to therapy).

1. Pyrantel pamoate is a highly effective drug (with cure rates of over 95%) and a drug of choice. It is administered in a single oral dose of 10 mg of the base per kilogram body weight (maximum, 1 g); repeat after 2 and 4 weeks. It may be given before or after meals. Infrequent side effects include vomiting, diarrhea, headache, dizziness, drowsiness, and rash. Experience with this drug is still limited in children under age 2.

2. Mebendazole is highly effective and also a drug of choice. It is administered as a single 100-mg oral dose, irrespective of body weight. It may be given with or without food and should be chewed for best effect. Repeat treatment after 2 and 4 weeks. Gastrointestinal side effects are infrequent. The drug has not yet been adequately studied in children under age 2 and should not be used in pregnancy.

3. Pyrvinium pamoate in syrup is given as a single dose of 5 mg/kg body weight (maximum, 0.25 g) and is repeated after 2 and 4 weeks. Pyrvinium is well tolerated, but it may cause gastrointestinal symptoms and dizziness in some persons, particularly older children and adults. Posttreatment stools are often stained red for several days, and the tablets must be swallowed intact to avoid temporary staining of the teeth. For these reasons it is viewed as an alternate drug in enterobiasis treatment.

4. Other drugs–Piperazine citrate is no longer recommended in this text for the treatment of pinworms because the course of treatment requires 1 week. **Thiabendazole** is not recommended because of its frequent side effects, which in rare cases may be severe.

Prognosis

Although annoying, the infection is benign. Cure is readily attainable with one of several effective drugs, but reinfection is common.

Chandrasoma PT, Mendis KN: *Enterobius vermicularis* in ectopic sites. *Am J Trop Med Hyg* 1977;**26**:644.

Wagner ED, Eby WC: Pinworm prevalence in California elementary school children, and diagnostic methods. *Am J Trop Med Hyg* 1983;**32**:998.

FILARIASIS

Essentials of Diagnosis

- Recurrent attacks appearing at irregular intervals of lymphangitis, lymphadenitis, fever, orchitis.

- Hydrocele, chyluria, elephantiasis of legs, arms, genitalia, or breasts.
- Characteristic microfilariae in the blood.
- Eosinophilia; positive skin or complement fixation tests.

General Considerations

Filariasis is caused by infection with one of 2 filarial nematodes, *Wuchereria bancrofti* and *Brugia malayi*. Infective larvae of *B malayi* are transmitted to humans by the bite of certain *Mansonia* and *Anopheles* mosquitoes of south India, Ceylon, south China, and Southeast Asia. *W bancrofti,* widely distributed in the tropics and subtropics of both hemispheres and on Pacific islands, is transmitted by certain *Culex* and *Aedes* mosquitoes. Over months, adult worms mature in or near superficial and deep lymphatics and lymph nodes. For a period of about 1 year, females produce large numbers of motile larvae (microfilariae), which appear in the peripheral blood. Microfilariae of *W bancrofti* are found in the blood chiefly at night (nocturnal periodicity), except for a nonperiodic variety in the South Pacific. *B malayi* microfilariae are usually nocturnally periodic but may be semiperiodic (present at all times, with a slight nocturnal rise). While humans are the only vertebrate hosts for *W bancrofti,* cats, monkeys, and other animals may harbor *B malayi*. Several other species of filarial worms infect humans, usually without causing important signs or symptoms. The microfilariae of *Dipetalonema* species (African and South American Tropics) and *Mansonella ozzardi* (West Indies and South America) must be differentiated from those of the pathogenic species. Several *Dirofilaria* species have been reported to occasionally cause signs and symptoms in humans, including painful subcutaneous nodules and coin lesions in the lung.

Clinical Findings

A. Symptoms and Signs: The early clinical manifestations are inflammatory; those of the later stages are obstructive. Episodes of fever, with or without inflammation of lymphatics and nodes, occur at irregular intervals in typical early cases. Persistent lymph node enlargement is most common in *B malayi* but occurs in some *W bancrofti* infections. Funiculitis and orchitis are common, and abscesses may form at sites of lymphatic inflammation. Such episodes may occur intermittently for months or years before the first obstructive signs appear. The number and severity of these attacks, and the extent of the later changes, depend primarily upon the intensity of the infection, which in turn is related to the length of residence in an endemic area. Obstructive phenomena, arising from interference with normal lymphatic flow, include hydrocele, scrotal lymphedema, lymphatic varices, and elephantiasis. Chyluria may result from rupture of distended lymphatics into the urinary tract. In the early stages of elephantiasis, the tissues of the affected part are edematous and soft; later, with skin hypertrophy and subcutaneous connective tissue proliferation, the part becomes hard. As the swelling enlarges, sometimes to enormous size, the skin surface folds and fissures. Bancroftian elephantiasis frequently involves the legs and genitalia, less often the arms and breasts; in *B malayi* infections, elephantiasis of the legs below the knees is most common and the genitals are rarely affected.

Hydrocele and elephantoid tissue changes in persons residing in endemic areas are usually filarial in origin. Elephantiasis in those who have visited endemic areas only briefly is rarely due to filariasis. Many infections are asymptomatic and detected only by blood examination.

B. Laboratory Findings: Diagnosis is by finding microfilariae in the blood. They are rare in the first 2–3 years after infection, abundant as the disease progresses, and again rare in the advanced obstructive stage. Both day and night (9:00 PM) anticoagulated blood specimens should be examined initially by wet film for motile larvae and by Giemsa-stained thick smears for specific morphology; if these are negative, the blood specimens should be concentrated by the Knott concentration or membrane filtration technique. If all of these are negative, the oral administration of 100 mg of diethylcarbamazine often produces positive blood specimens when examined in 1 hour. Microfilariae may also be found in hydrocele, lymphatic, ascitic, and pleural fluids.

Skin testing (using an antigen prepared from *Dirofilaria immitis*) and serologic tests may be helpful in diagnostic screening, but false-positive and false-negative reactions occur. An indirect hemagglutination titer of 1:128 and a bentonite flocculation titer of 1:5 in combination are considered significant titers. Most active clinical cases have higher titers. Lymphangiography is helpful in differential diagnosis. Removal of nodes for diagnosis may further impair drainage from the affected area and is contraindicated.

Differential Diagnosis

Diagnosis of the early febrile and inflammatory episodes may be difficult, particularly when the patient has moved away from an endemic area, because attacks of lymphangitis, adenitis, and fever are transitory and microfilariae may be rare in the blood. Filarial funiculitis, orchitis, and epididymitis may suggest gonococcal infection, but there is no urethral discharge in the uncomplicated case. Among the late manifestations, elephantiasis may be confused with hernia, Milroy's disease, multiple lipomatosis, severe congestive heart failure, venous thrombosis, and obstructive lesions of the lymphatics, which may produce nonfilarial elephantiasis of the extremities. The last 3 named can be distinguished readily from filariasis. Multiple lipomas may produce a massive soft lumpy swelling of the proximal part of a limb. In contrast, the filarial lesion starts distally and becomes hard as it enlarges. Milroy's congenital elephantiasis usually involves both legs below the knees. The skin is smooth, there is no eosinophilia, and the patient often has never visited the tropics.

Treatment

A. General Measures: Patients with attacks of lymphangitis should be treated during a quiescent period between attacks; bed rest is indicated during the inflammatory episodes. Antibiotics should be given for secondary infections, particularly abscesses over inflamed nodes. Suspensory bandaging is a valuable palliative measure for orchitis, epididymitis, and scrotal lymphedema. Treat mild edema of a limb with rest, elevation, and use of an elastic stocking. Chyluria usually requires no treatment except rest.

B. Surgical Measures: Surgical removal of the elephantoid scrotum, vulva, or breast is relatively easy, and results are usually satisfactory. Surgery for limb elephantiasis is difficult; results are often disappointing.

C. Specific Measures: Diethylcarbamazine rapidly kills microfilariae in the blood but only slowly kills adult worms or injures them, reducing their ability to reproduce. *W bancrofti* infections are treated with diethylcarbamazine (salt), 2 mg/kg orally 3 times a day after meals for 2–4 weeks. To reduce the incidence of allergic reactions from dying microfilariae, a single dose (2 mg/kg) is administered on the first day, 2 doses on the second day, and 3 doses on the third day and thereafter. For *B malayi,* the same schedule should be used, but individual doses should start at 1 mg/kg once on the first day and gradually increase to 2 mg/kg 3 times daily by the fourth to fifth day.

Antihistamines may be given for the first 4–5 days of diethylcarbamazine therapy to reduce the incidence of "allergic" reactions. Start corticosteroids and temporarily lower or interrupt doses of diethylcarbamazine if severe reactions occur.

Blood should be checked for microfilariae several weeks after treatment is completed; if any are still present, a course may be repeated at intervals of 3–4 weeks. However, since the initial treatment does not kill all adult worms, microfilariae may reappear in 3–12 months. Cure may require subsequent courses of treatment over 1–2 years.

Only a few mild side effects can be attributed directly to the drug: headache, malaise, anorexia, and weakness are most frequent. Reactions to dying microfilariae are usually mild or absent for *W bancrofti* and more intense for *B malayi.* Nevertheless, even in *W bancrofti* infection, about 25% of patients experience generalized reactions including headache, gastrointestinal symptoms, cough, chest pains, muscle or joint pain, malaise, fever, and papular rash. Local reactions may occur around dying adult or immature worms, including lymphangitis, lymphadenitis, and lymph abscess. These reactions are most common from the third day of treatment onward and may last as long as 10 days.

In prophylaxis of filariasis caused by *W bancrofti* and *B malayi,* 50 mg of diethylcarbamazine monthly has been recommended.

Prognosis

In early and mild cases, the prognosis is good with treatment and if the patient avoids reinfection. Drug treatment will not significantly influence the course of advanced filariasis.

Awadzi K: Therapy of tropical diseases—filariasis. Page 449 in: *Clinical Pharmacology and Therapeutics.* Proceedings of the First World Conference, 1980.

Muylle L et al: Usefulness of apheresis to extract microfilarias in management of loiasis. *Br Med J* 1983;**287**:519.

Nelson GS: Current concepts in parasitology: Filariasis. *N Engl J Med* 1979;**300**:1136.

Paroxysmal inflammatory filariasis: Filarial fevers. (Editorial.) *Arch Intern Med* 1983;**143**:1523.

GNATHOSTOMIASIS

Gnathostomiasis is an infection due to the nematode parasite *Gnathostoma spinigerum,* which is found only in eastern and southern Asia. A single migratory subcutaneous swelling is the most common manifestation. The usually painless swelling caused by the migrating worm is firm, pruritic, and variable in size. It may appear anywhere on the body surface, remain in that area for days or weeks, or wander continually. Internal organs, the eye, and the cervix may also be invaded. Occasionally the worm becomes visible under the skin.

Spontaneous pneumothorax, leukorrhea, hematuria, hemoptysis, paroxysmal coughing, and edema of the pharynx with dyspnea have been reported as complications. A myeloencephalitis may occur.

A high eosinophilia accompanies the infection. Specific skin-testing antigens are available as a diagnostic aid, but final diagnosis usually rests upon identification of the worm.

Surgical removal of the worm when it appears close to the skin surface is the only effective treatment. Chemotherapy has not proved successful, although symptoms may be relieved by the use of diethylcarbamazine as for filariasis, and thiabendazole should be tried. Courses of quinine or prednisolone have provided temporary relief of symptoms.

Daengsvang S: Gnathostomiasis in Southeast Asia. *Southeast Asian J Trop Med Public Health* 1981;**12**:319.

HOOKWORM DISEASE

Essentials of Diagnosis

- Weakness, fatigue, pallor, palpitation, dyspnea associated with a hypochromic, microcytic anemia.
- Diarrhea, flatulence, abdominal discomfort, weight loss.
- Transient episodes of coughing, with sore throat and bloody sputum.
- Pruritic, erythematous, maculopapular or vesicular dermatitis.
- Characteristic eggs in the stool; guaiac-positive stool.

General Considerations

Hookworm disease, widespread in the tropics and subtropics, is caused by *Ancylostoma duodenale* and *Necator americanus*. In the western hemisphere and tropical Africa, *Necator* was the prevailing species, and in the Far East and the Mediterranean, *Ancylostoma* was prevalent. Both species have now become widely distributed throughout the tropics and subtropics. The adult worms, approximately 1 cm long, attach themselves to the mucosa of the small intestine, where they suck blood and mucosal substances. Symptomatology and pathology are proportionate to the number of worms infecting the patient. A burden of at least 100 worms is necessary to produce anemia and symptoms in an adult. Eggs produced by the female worms are passed in the stool, which must fall on warm, moist soil if larval development is to take place. Infective larvae remain in the soil until they come in contact with human skin. After penetrating the skin, the larvae migrate through the lungs and eventually reach the small intestine, where final development into adult worms takes place. Experimental evidence indicates that *Ancylostoma* infections can probably also be acquired by ingestion of the larvae.

Clinical Findings

A. Symptoms and Signs: Ground itch, the first manifestation of hookworm infection, is a pruritic erythematous dermatitis, either maculopapular or vesicular, associated with the invasion of infective larvae. *Strongyloides* infection and creeping eruption caused by nonhuman hookworm species must be considered in the differential diagnosis at this stage. The severity of the dermatitis is a function of the number of invading larvae and the sensitivity of the host. The pulmonary phase of the disease is a transient reaction to larval migration through the lungs. Bloody sputum and cough result from damage caused by larvae breaking into alveoli from small blood vessels. Two or more weeks after the skin invasion, and depending upon the number of worms present, abdominal discomfort, flatulence, diarrhea, and other symptoms of intestinal irritation may appear as worms begin to attach themselves to the mucosa. When dietary intake of iron is inadequate to meet the demands of the hookworm, patients become anemic. The severity of the anemia depends upon the worm burden. Protein loss may also be significant. In chronic infections, a host-parasite balance may occur that limits the level of infection.

B. Laboratory Findings: The diagnosis depends upon demonstration of characteristic eggs in the feces. The stool usually contains occult blood; the severity of the hypochromic microcytic anemia will depend upon the worm burden, which can be estimated by quantitative egg counts: light infections, up to 2000 ova per gram of feces; moderate, 2000–5000; heavy, over 5000. Eosinophilia is usually present in the early months of the infection but may not be marked in the chronic stages.

Complications

The skin lesions may become secondarily infected. In highly sensitive individuals the allergic reaction to the invading and migrating larvae may be severe. With profound anemia there may be cardiac decompensation with edema and ascites, mental retardation, stunting of growth, and impaired renal function. In heavy infections, hypoproteinemia may also be present. Malabsorption has been described in some cases.

Treatment

A. General Measures: Estimation of the need for treatment can be based on semiquantitative or quantitative counts of eggs in stools. Clinically significant infections requiring treatment have about 5000 ova per gram, which is about equivalent to 4–5 ova per low-power microscopic field of unconcentrated stool. Light infections in asymptomatic patients do not require treatment, since the worms do not multiply in the host, the presence of a few worms does not result in injury to the host, and iron loss is replaced by dietary intake. Remaining worms will be passed in a few years. Stools should be checked 2 weeks after treatment. If the ova count is still moderate to heavy, a course of the treatment should be repeated. (Some workers argue that all of the worms should be eradicated.) If anemia is present, provide iron medication and a high-protein diet. In severe anemia, blood transfusion with packed red cells may be necessary.

If ascariasis and hookworm infections are both present, either give mebendazole for the combined infection or piperazine first to eradicate *Ascaris,* followed by a drug to eradicate hookworms.

B. Specific Measures:

1. Pyrantel pamoate is one of the drugs of first choice. In *Ancylostoma duodenale* infections, pyrantel given as a single dose, 10 mg of the base per kilogram body weight (maximum 1 g), produces cures in 76–98% of cases and a marked reduction in the worm burden in the remainder. However, for *Necator americanus* infections a single dose may give a satisfactory cure rate in light infection, but for moderate or heavy infection a 3-day course is necessary. If the species is unknown, treat as for necatoriasis. Side effects are infrequent, mild, and transient, including gastrointestinal symptoms, drowsiness, and headache. The drug is given before or after meals, without purges.

2. Mebendazole is also a drug of choice for treatment of *Necator* and *Ancylostoma* infections. When it is given at a dosage of 100 mg twice daily for 3 days, reported cure rates for both species range from 35 to 95%. The drug is given before or after meals, without purges. Therapy is remarkably free of side effects; gastrointestinal symptoms occur infrequently. The drug should not be used in pregnancy, and experience with the drug in children under 2 years is limited.

3. Bephenium hydroxynaphthoate is used only as an alternative drug for hookworm infection because it may cause nausea and vomiting and has a bitter taste. The drug is given on an empty stomach, and food is then withheld for 2 hours. For young children, however, the taste may be disguised when mixed with a flavored vehicle such as chocolate milk or orange juice. For *Ancylostoma* infections, give 5 g of the granules (2.5 g base) twice daily for 1 day, repeating in 2 weeks if necessary. For children weighing less than 22 kg, give half this dose. Do not use in pregnancy. *Necator* is generally more resistant to bephenium, but the same dose for 3 days may reduce the worm load to acceptable levels. *Do not follow with a purge.* Bephenium is no longer marketed in the USA.

4. Tetrachloroethylene is an effective alternative drug for *Necator* and may be used for *Ancylostoma*. **Caution:** Be sure to correct severe anemia before giving this drug. Tetrachloroethylene is contraindicated in patients with alcoholism, chronic gastrointestinal disorders, severe constipation, or hepatic disease and in patients undergoing heavy metal therapy. It is generally recommended that ascarids be removed from the intestinal tract before tetrachloroethylene is used. Eliminate fatty food for 24 hours before and 3 days after medication. Give tetrachloroethylene, 0.12 mL/kg body weight (not more than 5 mL) in soluble gelatin capsules containing 1 mL, in the morning on an empty stomach. The patient should be kept at bed rest for 4 hours after treatment, and then may resume eating. Side effects may be reduced by giving the drug at bedtime, also on an empty stomach. Two or more treatments at 4-day intervals may be required. Saline purgation following treatment is no longer recommended. Note that the drug may deteriorate if not adequately refrigerated at ambient tropical temperatures.

Prognosis

If the disease is recognized before serious secondary complications appear, the prognosis is favorable. With iron therapy, improved nutrition, and administration of an anthelmintic, complete recovery is the rule. The persistence of a few eggs in the stool of an asymptomatic person who is not anemic is not an indication for repeated treatments.

Gilman RH: Hookworm disease: Host-pathogen biology. *Rev Infect Dis* 1982;**4**:824.

Miller TA: Hookworm infection in man. *Adv Parasitol* 1979; **17**:315.

Sharma S, Charles ES: Chemotherapy of hookworm infections. *Prog Drug Res* 1982;**26**:9.

INTESTINAL & HEPATIC CAPILLARIASIS

Fatal infections by the liver parasite *Capillaria hepatica* have been recorded, but the syndrome of intestinal capillariasis recently recognized in the northern Philippines is a new clinical entity. It has also been reported from Thailand. The parasite, *Capillaria philippinensis,* is found in the mucosa of the small intestine, especially the jejunum. Infection is charac-

terized by an intractable diarrhea associated with a severe protein-losing enteropathy and malabsorption; many deaths have occurred. Adult nematodes and eggs can be found in the stool. Mebendazole, which is free from side effects, has become the drug of first choice and is given at a dosage of 100 mg 4 times daily for 20 or more days. Treatment with thiabendazole in a dosage of 12 mg/kg orally twice daily for 30 days has been successful but causes marked side effects. In some cases, relapses have occurred when the drug was discontinued.

Pereira VG, Franca LCM: Successful treatment of *Capillaria hepatica* infection in an acutely ill adult. *Am J Trop Med Hyg* 1983;**32**:1272.

Singson CN et al: Mebendazole in the treatment of intestinal capillariasis. *Am J Trop Med Hyg* 1975;**24**:932.

LOIASIS

Loiasis is a common and distinctive disease of tropical Africa caused by the filarial nematode *Loa loa*. The intermediate host, *Chrysops,* a biting fly, carries the infection from human or monkey to human. Infective larvae, introduced by the biting fly, develop into adult worms in about 12 months. It is the adult worms migrating through subcutaneous tissues that cause the symptoms of loiasis, not the larval microfilariae in the bloodstream.

Many infected individuals remain symptom-free; others develop severe allergic reactions to the infection. The first definite signs of the disease are the appearance of Calabar swelling or the migration of a worm beneath the conjunctiva of the eye. The swelling, which may be painful, is a temporary subcutaneous edematous reaction, often several inches in diameter. The overlying and surrounding skin is often erythematous and pruritic. The swelling may migrate a few inches before disappearing; more often it remains in one place for several days and then subsides. The reaction occurs most frequently on the hands, forearms, and around the eyes, but it may appear anywhere. Some patients experience Calabar swellings at infrequent intervals, others as often as twice a week.

Migrating worms are sometimes visible in subcutaneous tissues, and migration across the eye produces a foreign body sensation, often with considerable irritation. The parasite has also been found in cerebrospinal fluid associated with a meningoencephalitis. Generalized urticaria, edema of a whole limb, extensive erythema, and generalized pruritus have been reported in some patients.

The adult worm may be recovered from the eye or skin (rarely), or microfilariae may be found in daytime blood films (20–30% of patients). Complement fixation and skin tests are often useful in diagnosis. The eosinophil count is elevated, varying between 10 and 40% or more.

Although surgical removal of adult worms is sometimes possible, it is not recommended. The most satisfactory treatment is with diethylcarbamazine, which kills both microfilariae and adults. Give 1 mg/kg once on the first day and gradually increase to 2 mg/kg 3 times daily by the fourth or fifth day; continue treatment up to a total of 72 mg/kg. The drug should be given after meals. The gradual increase will reduce the risk of allergic reactions (fever, urticaria, rashes, pruritis, encephalitis), which are common as a result of the rapid killing of microfilariae. Allergic reactions are more likely to be severe in patients with pretreatment microfilariae counts greater than 50 per microliter of blood. Antihistamines given for the first 4–5 days may reduce the incidence of such reactions, but corticosteroids should be started and the doses of diethylcarbamazine lowered temporarily if severe reactions occur. Adult worms tend to appear under the skin, where they die, form small nodules, and are gradually absorbed.

The prognosis is good with treatment. A second course may be required. Without treatment, loiasis is annoying and uncomfortable but rarely life-endangering. Fatal encephalitis rarely occurs.

Paleologo FP, Neafie RC, Connor DH: Lymphadenitis caused by *Loa loa. Am J Trop Med Hyg* 1984;**33**:395.

Stanley SL Jr, Kell O: Ascending paralysis associated with diethylcarbamazine treatment for *M loa loa* infection. *Trop Doct* 1982;**12**:16.

ONCHOCERCIASIS

Humans and *Simulium* black flies are the natural hosts of *Onchocerca volvulus,* a filarial nematode found in many parts of tropical Africa and in localized areas of Yemen, southern Mexico, Guatemala, Venezuela, Colombia, and northern Brazil. Nearly 40 million persons are afflicted, and an estimated half million are blind from the infection. The biting fly introduces infective larvae that develop slowly in the cutaneous and subcutaneous tissues of humans. Flies are infected in turn by picking up microfilariae while biting. Adult worms may live for years, frequently in fibrous nodules. Microfilariae, motile and migratory, may be found in the skin, subcutaneous tissues, and lymphatics, in the conjunctiva and other structures of the eye, and occasionally in the blood, urine, and cerebrospinal fluid. The life span of the female worms is up to 15 years and that of microfilariae as long as 30 months.

Clinical Findings

A. Symptoms and Signs: Intensity of infection determines the extent and severity of the clinical picture. After an incubation period of several months to 1 year, skin manifestations appear in up to 40% of patients. Localized or generalized pruritus is common and may be severe, causing scratching, skin excoriation, and lichenification. Depending on the part of the world where it occurs and on the stage of the disease, a variety of pigmentary changes, papules, focal edema, dryness with scaling, atrophy, and acute inflammation resembling erysipelas may appear. Subcutaneous nodules consisting of fibrous tissue surrounding one or more adult worms appear at a later stage of infection. Few patients have more than 3–6 palpable nodules. These are painless, freely movable, and between 0.5 and 1 cm in diameter. An unknown proportion are deeply situated and are not palpable. Common sites are over bony prominences on the trunk, thighs, shoulders, arms, and head. In Africa, nodules are commonly distributed around the pelvis, but in Central America about 50% are on the head. The severity of eye lesions and the development of blindness are related to the intensity of infection, especially the density of microfilariae found in the head region and near the eye. The types of eye lesions seen are "fluffy" corneal opacities, sclerosing keratitis, anterior uveitis (with the secondary glaucoma and secondary cataract that may result), chorioretinitis, optic neuritis, and postneuritic optic atrophy. The following factors indicate greater risk of blindness: (1) head nodules, (2) 10 (or possibly 5) microfilariae per milligram of skin snip taken from the outer canthus of the eye, (3) more than 50 microfilariae in the cornea or more than 20 in the anterior chamber, and (4) night blindness, contraction of visual fields, mild uveitis, and edema of the optic disk or retina. Lymphadenopathy, elephantiasis, hanging groin, weight loss, and hernia, which may develop as late sequelae of the infection, can be incapacitating.

B. Laboratory Findings: The diagnosis is made by demonstrating microfilariae in skin snips or shavings. The snips are performed by tenting the skin with a needle and cutting off a bit of skin above the needle tip with a razor. Blood-free shavings may be cut with a razor blade from the top of a ridge of skin firmly pressed between thumb and forefinger. The snip or shaving is examined in a drop of saline under a coverslip on a slide, for many microfilariae emerge from the snip within 30 minutes. Shavings or snips should be taken from several sites over bony prominences of the scapular region, hips, and thighs and should be of such thickness that the outer parts of the dermal papillae—the level where microfilariae are most likely to be found—are included. A variety of punches are available that facilitate the procedure. In west Africa, *Onchocerca* microfilariae must be distinguished from *Dipetalonema perstans* microfilariae that are also found in the skin. In removal of skin fragments, care must be taken to prevent bleeding, or the specimen may be contaminated by blood microfilariae. The 2 types of microfilariae can be distinguished by staining.

The Mazotti challenge test, using a small dose of diethylcarbamazine (12.5–25 mg), may be useful in diagnosis in patients in whom microfilariae are not found. A skin reaction begins in 15 minutes to 24 hours. In addition, in 2–4 hours microfilariae may appear and should be looked for in the blood and urine. The test should be used only in selected patients and with appropriate safeguards because severe reactions may occur.

Aspiration of nodules will often reveal microfilariae, and adult worms may be demonstrated in excised nodules. In patients with eye lesions, microfilariae can sometimes be seen in the anterior chamber by slit lamp examination. Eosinophilia of 15–50% is common. Serologic tests are usually positive, but cross-reactions occur with other forms of filariasis.

Treatment

The preferred treatment of onchocerciasis consists of surgical removal of accessible nodules (particularly those on the head), the use of suramin in selected patients to kill adult worms, and use of diethylcarbamazine before and after suramin to slowly destroy microfilariae.

A. Surgical Removal: As many nodules as possible should be excised surgically, particularly when nodules are located close to the eyes. Some are deep in the subcutaneous tissues and cannot be detected by palpation.

B. Diethylcarbamazine: This drug kills the microfilariae of onchocerciasis but not the adult worms. Only a few mild, occasional side effects can be attributed directly to the drug: headache, malaise, weakness; less often, vomiting. However, mild to severe allergic symptoms are frequent owing to release of foreign protein from dying microfilariae and may start within 30 minutes. Severe reactions are more likely if microfilariae are producing symptoms in the skin, if microfilariae or nodules are close to the eyes, and if skin concentrations of microfilariae are high (over 100/mg). Treatment should begin with low doses and increase progressively. The following is one type of dosage schedule for heavy infections, with the drug to be given after meals: Initially, give 25 mg once and wait several days for the reaction to subside; then give 25 mg daily for 2 days; then 50 mg twice daily for 2 days; then 100 mg twice daily for 2 days; then 200 mg twice daily for 7 days. When reactions to diethylcarbamazine have nearly ceased, suramin treatment is started and is continued weekly until completed.

About 3–4 weeks after completing the course of suramin, remaining microfilariae in the skin are killed by giving a course of diethylcarbamazine, 200 mg twice daily for 3–5 days, and repeating the course at 3- to 4-week intervals until pruritic skin reactions no longer occur.

In mild infections, symptomatic relief may be provided by antihistamines and analgesics. However, all patients with heavy infections, skin reactions, or ocular complications should receive corticosteroids starting 1 day before treatment and continuing for 3–7 days, at which time the dosage is to be reduced gradually.

Use of diethylcarbamazine in the form of ocular inserts and as 1% lotion applied locally to the skin is under clinical study.

C. Suramin sodium is effective in eradicating infection by killing the adult worms, but it has potential renal toxicity (proteinuria, casts, red cells) and can produce a variety of other serious side effects. Fatal reactions have occurred. Its usage requires hospitalization, expert consultation, and close attention to cautions and contraindications. Before starting suramin,

all patients should have a course of diethylcarbamazine to eliminate most microfilariae. Then an initial dose of 0.1 g of suramin is given intravenously slowly over 3 minutes. If tolerated, subsequent dosages are 1 g given intravenously weekly for 4–7 weeks depending upon the severity of the disease. Suramin is available in the USA only from the Parasitic Disease Drug Service, Centers for Disease Control, Atlanta 30333.

Prognosis

With chemotherapy, progression of the disease usually can be checked. The prognosis is unfavorable only for those patients who are seen for the first time with already far advanced ocular onchocerciasis.

Awadzi K et al: The chemotherapy of onchocerciasis. 7. The effect of prednisone on the Mazzotti reaction. *Ann Trop Med Parasitol* 1982;**76**:331.

Connor DH: Onchocerciasis. *N Engl J Med* 1978;**298**:379.

Greene BM et al: Ocular and systemic complications of diethylcarbamazine therapy for onchocerciasis: Association with circulating immune complexes. *J Infect Dis* 1983;**147**:890.

Scharlau G: Onchocerciasis-chemotherapy: A risk-approach. *Trop Doct* 1981;**11**:8.

STRONGYLOIDIASIS

Essentials of Diagnosis

- Pruritic dermatitis at sites of larval penetration.
- Diarrhea, epigastric pain, nausea, malaise, weight loss.
- Cough, rales, transient pulmonary infiltrates.
- Eosinophilia; characteristic larvae in stool specimens, duodenal aspirate, or sputum.

General Considerations

Strongyloidiasis is an infection caused by the small nematode *Strongyloides stercoralis*. The major symptoms result from adult parasitism, principally in the duodenum and jejunum, or from larval migration through the pulmonary and cutaneous tissues. *Strongyloides*, unlike other helminths infecting humans, multiplies within the host; this can result in persistence of infection at a low level as well as in overwhelming infection (hyperinfection syndrome) with severe intestinal ulceration, malabsorption, and other complications that can lead to death.

The parasite is an infection of humans, but dogs, cats, and primates have been found naturally infected with strains indistinguishable from those of humans. The disease is endemic in tropical and subtropical areas; although prevalence is generally low, in some areas rates exceed 25%. In temperate areas, including the USA, the disease occurs sporadically. Multiple infections in households are common, and prevalence in institutions, particularly mental institutions, may be high. Hospital staff should be protected from contact with feces and sputum from infected patients.

The parasite is uniquely capable of maintaining its life cycle both within the human host and in soil.

Infection occurs when filariform larvae penetrate the skin, enter the bloodstream, and are carried to the lungs, where they escape from capillaries into alveoli and ascend the bronchial tree to the glottis. The larvae are then swallowed and carried to the duodenum and upper jejunum, where maturation to the adult stage takes place. The parasitic female, generally held to be parthenogenetic, matures and lives embedded in the mucosa, where its eggs are laid and hatch. Rhabditiform larvae, which are noninfective, emerge, and most migrate into the intestinal lumen to leave the host via the feces. The time from skin penetration to egg-laying by the mature adult is about 4 weeks. The life span of the adult worm may be as long as 5 years.

In the soil, the rhabditiform larvae metamorphose into the infective (filariform) larvae. However, the parasite also has a free-living cycle in soil, in which some rhabditiform larvae develop into adults that produce eggs from which rhabditiform larvae emerge to continue the life cycle.

Autoinfection, which probably occurs at a low rate in most infections, is an important factor in determining worm burden and is responsible for persistence of asymptomatic or symptomatic strongyloidiasis in individuals for many years after they leave an endemic area. Internal autoinfection takes place in the lower bowel when some rhabditiform larvae, instead of passing with the feces, develop into filariform larvae that penetrate the intestinal mucosa, enter the intestinal lymphatic and portal circulation, are carried to the lungs, and return to the small bowel to complete the cycle. This process is accelerated by constipation and other conditions that reduce bowel motility. In addition, an external autoinfection cycle can occur as a result of fecal contamination of the perianal area.

In the hyperinfection syndrome, autoinfection is greatly increased, resulting in a marked increase in the intestinal worm burden and in massive dissemination of filariform larvae to the lungs and most other tissues. Occasionally, in the lungs and elsewhere, larvae metamorphose into adults. Hyperinfection is generally initiated under conditions of depressed host cellular immunity, especially in debilitated, malnourished persons and in patients receiving immunosuppressive therapy, particularly corticosteroids. However, the syndrome can occur in individuals who show no obvious predisposing cause.

Mucosal histologic changes include congestion, excessive mucus secretion, microulcerations, and edema. In heavy long-standing infection there may be spruelike mucosal atrophy, flattening of the villi, and inflammatory reactions with granuloma formation and fibrosis. In hyperinfection, larvae that gain access to the systemic circulation may be carried to any tissue where they can cause local inflammatory reactions and granuloma formation. Penetration of the bowel wall by filariform larvae can result in gram-negative septicemia.

Clinical Findings

A. Signs and Symptoms: The time from penetra-tion of the skin by filariform larvae until rhabditiform larvae appear in the feces is 3–4 weeks. The severity of disease ranges from asymptomatic to fatal. Although an acute syndrome can sometimes be recognized in which cutaneous symptoms are followed by pulmonary and then intestinal symptoms, most patients have chronic symptoms that continue for years or sometimes for life. Symptoms may be continuous, or exacerbations may recur at irregular intervals.

1. Cutaneous manifestations–In acute infection, filariform larvae usually invade the skin of the feet. The reaction in unsensitized patients may be minimal, with only a macule or papule, but in sensitized patients there may be focal edema, inflammation, petechiae, serpiginous or urticarial tracts, and intense itching. In chronic infections, stationary urticaria may be present, or larva currens, characterized by transient eruptions that migrate in serpiginous tracts, may occur; the latter are seen particularly in the perianal area of the buttocks.

2. Intestinal manifestations–Symptoms range from mild to severe, the most common being diarrhea, abdominal pain, and flatulence. Anorexia, nausea, vomiting, and epigastric tenderness may be present. The diarrhea may alternate with constipation, and in severe cases the feces contain mucus and blood. The pain is often epigastric in location and may mimic the burning, dull cramp, or ache of duodenal ulcer. Malabsorption or a protein-losing enteropathy can result from a large intestinal worm burden.

3. Pulmonary manifestations–With migration of larvae through the lungs, bronchi, and trachea there may be a dry cough and throat irritation without further difficulty, or a low-grade fever, bronchitis, dyspnea, wheezing, asthma, and hemoptysis. As the disease becomes more marked, bronchopneumonia and pleural effusion can occur, accompanied by progressive dyspnea; the cough may become productive of an odorless, mucopurulent sputum; miliary abscesses can develop.

4. Other findings–Severe infection may present with fever, malaise, and weakness leading to prostration and emaciation.

5. Hyperinfection syndrome–Massive increase in the intestinal worm burden with intense dissemination of larvae to the lungs and other tissues can result in the following complications: severe diarrhea with generalized abdominal pain and distention, bronchopneumonia, pleural effusion, pericarditis and myocarditis, hepatic granulomas, cholecystitis, ulcerating lesions at all levels of the gastrointestinal tract, paralytic ileus, perforation and peritonitis, gram-negative septicemia, meningitis, cachexia, shock, and death.

B. Laboratory Findings: Eggs are seldom found in feces. Diagnosis is by finding the larval stages in feces or duodenal fluid. Rhabditiform larvae may be found in recently passed stool specimens; filariform larvae will be present in specimens held in the laboratory for some hours or if the specimen is processed by stool culture. Three specimens, preserved or unpreserved, should be collected at 2-day intervals or longer, since the number of larvae in feces may vary considerably from day to day. Each specimen should be examined by direct microscopy, and in addition, to increase sensitivity of testing, one or more should be processed by culture, using the Baermann concentration method. Stool specimens used in the Baermann procedure must be unpreserved; they can be received in the laboratory up to 48 hours after passage if held at refrigerated but nonfreezing temperatures.

Although larvae cannot be found in the stools of 25% or more of infected patients, the diagnosis can often be made by examination of duodenal mucus for rhabditiform larvae or ova. Mucus is obtained by means of the duodenal string test or by duodenal intubation and aspiration. Duodenal biopsy is seldom indicated but will confirm the diagnosis in most patients. Occasionally, filariform larvae can be detected in sputum during the pulmonary phase of the disease.

In chronic low-grade intestinal strongyloidiasis, the white blood cell count is often normal, with a slightly elevated percentage of eosinophils. However, with increasing larval migration, eosinophilia may reach 50% and leukocytosis 20,000/μL. Mild anemia may be present. Serum IgE immunoglobulins may be elevated. The complement fixation test is not satisfactory because of cross-reactions with filariasis. In the hyperinfection syndrome, there may be findings of hypoproteinemia, malabsorption, and abnormal liver function. Ova and rhabditiform and filariform larvae may be present in sputum, and filariform larvae in the urine; eosinopenia, when present, is thought to be a poor prognostic sign.

Small bowel x-rays early in the disease may show inflammation and irritability, with prominent mucosal folds; there may be a dilatation, delay, and ulcerative duodenitis. Later in the disease, the findings can resemble those in nontropical and tropical sprue, or there may be narrowing, rigidity, and diminished peristalsis. During pulmonary migration of larvae, fine nodulation or irregular patches of pneumonitis may be seen.

Differential Diagnosis

Because of varied signs and symptoms, the diagnosis of strongyloidiasis is often difficult, especially in nonendemic areas. The disease should always be considered in patients with unexplained eosinophilia. Eosinophilia plus one or more of the following factors should further enhance consideration of the diagnosis: endemic area exposure, duodenal ulcer-like pain, persistent or recurrent diarrhea, recurrent coughing or wheezing, and transient pulmonary infiltrates. The duodenitis and jejunitis of strongyloidiasis can mimic giardiasis, cholecystitis, and pancreatitis. Transient pulmonary infiltrates must be differentiated from tropical pulmonary eosinophilia and Löffler's syndrome. The diagnosis should be considered among the many causes of malabsorption in the tropics.

Treatment

Since *Strongyloides* can multiply in humans, treatment should continue until the parasite is eradi-

cated. Patients receiving immunosuppressive therapy should be examined for the presence of the infection before and probably at intervals during treatment. In concurrent infection with *Strongyloides* and *Ascaris* or hookworm (which is common), eradicate *Ascaris* and hookworms first and *Strongyloides* subsequently.

A. Thiabendazole: Thiabendazole is the drug of choice. An oral dose of 25 mg/kg (maximum, 1.5 g) is given after meals twice daily for 2–3 days. A 5- to 7-day course of treatment is needed for disseminated infections. Tablet and liquid formulations are available; tablets should be chewed. Side effects, including headache, weakness, vomiting, vertigo, and decreased mental alertness, occur in as many as 30% of patients and may be severe. These symptoms are lessened if the drug is taken after meals. Other potentially serious side effects occur rarely. Erythema multiforme and the Stevens-Johnson syndrome have been associated with thiabendazole therapy; in severe cases, fatalities have occurred.

B. Alternative Drugs: If thiabendazole cannot be tolerated, mebendazole (500 mg 3 times daily for 14 days), cambendazole (5 mg/kg once), pyrvinium pamoate (2–6.4 mg/kg), or levamisole can be tried, but their efficacy is based on limited trials.

Prognosis

The prognosis is favorable except in the hyperinfection syndrome. Infections associated with emaciation, advanced liver disease, cancer, immunologic disorders, or the use of immunosuppressive drugs may be difficult to treat. In selected instances, a 2-day course of treatment with thiabendazole once monthly can be tried to control infections that cannot be eradicated.

Bicalho SA, Leao OJ, Pena Q Jr: Cambendazole in the treatment of human strongyloidiasis. *Am J Trop Med Hyg* 1983; **32:**1181.

Davidson RA, Fletcher RH, Chapman LE: Risk factors for strongyloidiasis: A case-control study. *Arch Intern Med* 1984; **144:**321.

Marcial-Rojas RA: Strongyloidiasis. Chapter 37 in: *Pathology of Protozoal and Helminthic Diseases With Clinical Correlation.* Marcial-Rojas RA (editor). Williams & Wilkins, 1971.

Scowden EB, Schaffner W, Stone WJ: Overwhelming strongyloidiasis: An unappreciated opportunistic infection. *Medicine* 1978;**57:**527.

Strongyloidiasis. Pages 451–473 in: *The Radiology of Tropical Disease with Epidemiological, Pathological, and Clinical Correlation.* Reeder MM, Palmer PES (editors). Williams & Wilkins, 1981.

Wilson KH, Kauffman CA: Persistent *Strongyloides stercoralis* in a blind loop of the bowel: Successful treatment with mebendazole. *Arch Intern Med* 1983;**143:**357.

TRICHINOSIS
(Trichiniasis, Trichinellosis)

Essentials of Diagnosis

- First week: diarrhea, cramps, malaise.
- Second week to 1–2 months: muscle pain and

tenderness, fever, periorbital and facial edema, conjunctivitis.

- Eosinophilia and elevated serum enzymes.
- Positive skin and serologic tests.
- History of ingestion of raw or inadequately cooked pork (including boar) or bear meat.

General Considerations

Trichinosis is caused by the nematode *Trichinella spiralis*. Adult worms live in the intestines of humans, pigs, bears, rats, and most carnivores, including marine animals; fowl are resistant to infection. Larvae liberated by the females enter striated muscle, are encysted, and live for years; in the natural life cycle, these larvae develop into a new generation of adults when parasitized muscle is ingested by a new host. Pigs generally become infected by feeding on uncooked food scraps or, less often, by eating infected rats.

Gastric juices liberate the encysted larvae, which rapidly mature and mate. The adult female burrows into the mucosa of the small intestine. Within 4–5 days, she begins to discharge larvae that are disseminated via the lymphatics and bloodstream to most body tissues. Although larvae that reach striated muscle encyst and remain viable for several years, those that reach other tissues are rapidly destroyed.

Humans usually acquire the infection by eating encysted larvae in raw or undercooked pork or pork products. Cases occur sporadically or in outbreaks. Sometimes the source of infection is the flesh of wild animals, particularly bear or walrus in far northern areas or bush pigs in Africa. Ground beef has also been contaminated by adulteration with pork or inadvertently in common meat grinders. Although the disease is present wherever pork is eaten, trichinosis is a greater problem in many temperate areas than in the tropics. In the USA, there has been a marked reduction in the prevalence of trichinosis both in humans and in pigs. Nevertheless, the annual incidence of infection is estimated to be over 150,000 cases, although most are asymptomatic or so mild as to elude diagnosis.

Clinical Findings

A. Symptoms and Signs: The clinical picture varies considerably in severity, depending upon the number of larvae disseminated, the tissues invaded, the immune status of the host, the age of the host (children have less severe infections), and, perhaps, the strain of the parasite. Infection ranges from (1) asymptomatic, in which eosinophilia may be recognized only by chance; to (2) a mild febrile illness in which there may be one or more mild, short-lasting symptoms; to (3) a severe disease with multiple system involvement that rarely progresses to a fulminating fatal illness. The intensity of infection at the level of 1–10 larvae per gram of muscle ordinarily does not produce symptoms; 50–100 larvae per gram may result in severe symptoms. The incubation period is generally from 2 to 12 days but can be as long as 28 days or begin within 12 hours if the infection is heavy.

In the pathogenesis of the disease, 3 clinical stages can be differentiated: the intestinal stage, the stage of muscle invasion, and the stage of convalescence. The intestinal stage can be asymptomatic or symptomatic and lasts from 1 to 7 days. Diarrhea, abdominal cramps, and malaise are the major findings; nausea and vomiting occur less frequently; and constipation is occasionally present. Fever and leukocytosis are rarely found during the first week.

The stage of muscular invasion, which is the result of larval migration and muscle penetration, begins at the end of the first week. It lasts about 6 weeks, corresponding with the death of the worms. Symptoms and findings include fever (low-grade to marked); muscle pain (especially upon movement) and muscle tenderness, edema, and spasm; periorbital and facial edema; sweating; photophobia and conjunctivitis; weakness or prostration; pain on swallowing; dyspnea, coughing, and hoarseness; subconjunctival, retinal, and nail splinter hemorrhages; and rashes and formication. The most frequently parasitized muscles and sites of findings are the masseters, the tongue, the diaphragm, the intercostal muscles, and the extraocular, laryngeal, paravertebral, nuchal, deltoid, pectoral, gluteus, biceps, and gastrocnemius muscles. Inflammatory reactions around larvae that reach tissues other than muscle may result in a broad range of symptoms and findings, including the development of meningitis, encephalitis, myocarditis, bronchopneumonia, nephritis, and peripheral and cranial nerve disorders. Death may occur between 4 and 8 weeks.

The stage of convalescence generally begins in the second month but in severe infections may not begin before 3 months or longer. Vague muscle pains and malaise may persist for several more months. Permanent muscular atrophy has been reported.

B. Laboratory Findings: The diagnosis is supported or confirmed by findings of eosinophilia, positive serologic tests, and detection of larvae in muscle biopsy specimens.

Leukocytosis and eosinophilia appear during the second week after ingestion of infected meat. The proportion of eosinophils rises to a maximum of 20–75% in the third or fourth week and then slowly declines to normal. In severe cases, the eosinophilia may disappear entirely.

Serologic tests can detect most clinically manifest cases but are not sufficiently sensitive to detect low-level infections involving only a few larvae per gram of muscle. More than one test should be used and then repeated, since it is important to observe seroconversion from a negative to a positive titer or to a rising titer. The bentonite flocculation test (positive titer, ≥ 1:5) is highly sensitive and is considered nearly 100% specific. It becomes positive in the third or fourth week and reaches a maximum titer at about 2 months. The immunofluorescence test (positive titer ≥ 16), which is also highly positive and specific, may become positive in the second week. A variety of other tests are available at some laboratories.

In most persons with moderate infections, the

bentonite flocculation test is negative within 2–3 years after infection; after 5 years, two-thirds of these persons may give negative responses to a variety of tests. The intradermal test, which becomes positive within 3 weeks, is no longer recommended. Since the test may remain positive for years, and since batches of antigen vary in potency, poor-to-good correlation of the skin and serologic tests in studies may result.

Adult worms may be looked for in feces, although they are seldom found. In the second week, there are occasional larvae in blood, duodenal washings, and, rarely, in spinal fluid. In the third to fourth weeks, definitive diagnosis becomes possible through biopsy of skeletal muscle (particularly gastrocnemius and pectoralis), preferably at a site of swelling or tenderness. Portions of the specimen should be examined microscopically by compression between glass slides, by digestion, and by preparation of many histologic sections. If biopsy is done too early, there are 2 possible risks: larvae may not be detectable because they have not yet coiled, and young larvae may be digested in the course of the digestion test. Myositis in the absence of larvae is a significant finding.

Nonspecific laboratory findings include elevation of serum enzymes (creatinine phosphokinase, lactate dehydrogenase, and serum transaminases). Serum aldolase may be very high. The sedimentation rate remains low, but there may be a marked hypergammaglobulinemia with reversal of the albumin/globulin ratio.

C. X-Ray Findings: Chest x-rays during the acute phase may show disseminated or localized infiltrates, although calcified cysts are not detectable radiologically.

D. Electrocardiographic Findings: ECGs should be done to look for signs of myocarditis.

Complications

The more important complications are allergic granulomatous reactions in the lungs, encephalitis, and cardiac failure.

Differential Diagnosis

Mild infections and those with atypical symptoms are often difficult to diagnose; because of its protean manifestations, trichinosis may resemble many other diseases. Eosinophilia, muscle pain and tenderness, and fever should lead the physician to consider dermatomyositis and polyarteritis nodosa.

Prevention

Public health measures to prevent feeding of uncooked garbage to hogs and animal inspection by various techniques have significantly reduced the frequency and intensity of infection in the USA and other countries. However, animal and human infections do continue to occur in the USA. The chief safeguard against trichinosis is adequate cooking of pork at the newly recommended temperature of 77 °C (170 °F). Alternatively, larvae can be made nonviable by freezing meat at −15 °C (5 °F) for 20 days. Recent reports

indicate that *T spiralis* in arctic sylvatic animals is resistant to that temperature.

Treatment

The treatment of trichinosis is principally supportive, since most cases recover spontaneously without sequelae. If the patient is still in the intestinal phase of the disease (the adults live up to 6 weeks), thiabendazole is indicated at an oral dosage of 25 mg/kg (maximum 1.5 g) twice daily after meals for 3–5 days. Side effects may occur (see under Strongyloidiasis, above). Corticosteroids are contraindicated in the intestinal phase.

In the stage of larval invasion of muscle, severe infections require hospitalization and high doses of corticosteroids for 24–48 hours, followed by lower doses for several days or weeks to control symptoms. Thiabendazole has been tried in the muscle stage with equivocal relief of muscle pain or tenderness or lysis of fever. However, further trials are recommended.

Initial reports suggest some success for mebendazole efficacy against adult worms in the intestinal tract, migrating larvae, and larvae in muscle using the following schedule: 200–400 mg 3 times daily for 3 days, followed by 400–500 mg 3 times daily for 10 days. Daily doses should be given in 3 divided portions.

Prognosis

Death may rarely occur in 2–3 weeks in overwhelming infections; more often, it occurs in 4–8 weeks from a major complication such as cardiac failure or pneumonia.

Campbell WC (editor): Trichinella *and Trichinosis.* Plenum Press, 1983.

Horstmann RD et al: Observations on mebendazole vs thiabendazole in the treatment of human trichinellosis. *Tropenmed Parasitol* 1982;**33**:191.

Levin ML: Treatment of trichinosis with mebendazole. *Am J Trop Med Hyg* 1983;**32**:980.

TRICHURIASIS
(Trichocephaliasis)

Essentials of Diagnosis

- Most infections are silent; heavy infections may cause abdominal pain, distention, flatulence, diarrhea, and rectal prolapse.
- Characteristic barrel-shaped eggs in stool.

General Considerations

Trichuris trichiura is a common intestinal parasite of humans throughout the world, particularly in the subtropics and tropics. The small slender worms, 30–50 mm in length and often called whipworms, attach themselves to the mucosa of the large intestine, particularly the cecum. The worms cause symptoms only when present in very large numbers. Eggs passed in the feces require 2–4 weeks for larval development after reaching the soil before becoming infective. New infections are acquired by direct ingestion of the infective eggs.

Clinical Findings

A. Symptoms and Signs: Light (fewer than 10,000 ova per gram of feces) to moderate infections rarely cause symptoms. Heavy infections (usually 50,000 or more ova per gram of feces) may be accompanied by a variety of symptoms arising from irritation of the mucosa. Among the most common of these are abdominal pain, tenesmus, diarrhea, distention, flatulence, nausea, vomiting, and weight loss. In heavy infections, most often found in malnourished young children, blood loss may be significant and rectal prolapse may occur.

B. Laboratory Findings: Detection of whipworm eggs in the stool is essential for diagnosis. Eosinophilia (5–20%) is common with all but light infections, and severe hypochromic anemia may be present with heavy infections.

Treatment

A. Mebendazole: Patients with asymptomatic light infections do not require treatment. For those with heavier or symptomatic infections, give mebendazole, 100 mg twice daily before or after meals for 3 days. It may be therapeutically advantageous for the tablets to be chewed before swallowing. Cure rates of 60–80% and higher are reported after one course of treatment, with marked reduction in ova counts in the remaining patients. For severe trichuriasis, a longer course of treatment (up to 6 days) or a repeat course will often be necessary. Gastrointestinal side effects from the drug are rare. The drug is contraindicated in pregnancy, and experience with it is limited in children under age 2.

B. Oxantel Pamoate: Oxantel pamoate is an analog of pyrantel pamoate and acts only on *T trichiura*. Cure rates of 57–100% have been reported in various trials. One treatment schedule is 15 mg/kg (base) daily for 2 days for patients with mild to moderate intensity of infection. For patients with severe infection, give 10 mg/kg (base) daily for 5 days. Oxantel pamoate (Telopar) is also marketed in combination with pyrantel pamoate (Combantrin) as oxantel-pyrantel (Quantrel), which combines the efficacy of both drugs to provide broad-spectrum anthelmintic action against trichuriasis, hookworm, ascariasis, pinworm, and trichostrongyliasis infections. Neither oxantel nor oxantel-pyrantel is available in the USA.

C. Hexylresorcinol: If mebendazole is not available, hexylresorcinol by enema may be used. A soapsuds cleansing enema is followed by a 0.2% hexylresorcinol enema (volume, 20–30 mL/kg up to 1200 mL). The enema should be retained for 30 minutes if possible; retention is facilitated by taping the buttocks together. If necessary, use a small saline enema to initiate expulsion. Perianal skin irritation is prevented by the application of a film of petrolatum. Hexylresorcinol is not available in the USA.

D. Thiabendazole should *not* be used, because it is not effective and is potentially toxic.

Blechman MG, Chavarria AP, Diermissen AG: A double-blind study of flubendazole in the treatment of *Trichuris trichiura* infections. *Clin Res Rev* 1982;**2**:115.
Cabrera BD, Cruz AC: Clinical trial of oxantel-pyrantel (Quantrel) against trichuriasis. *Acta Med Philippina* 1980;**16**:95.

VISCERAL LARVA MIGRANS
(Toxocariasis)

Visceral larva migrans is caused by the larval form of the dog and cat ascarids *Toxocara canis* and *Toxocara cati*. Infection usually occurs in young children as a result of eating soil contaminated by animal feces containing *Toxocara* ova. Puppies are a more important source of infection than cats, because prenatal infection occurs only in dogs. Direct contact with animals as a source of infection is uncommon, because the ova require a prolonged extrinsic incubation period before becoming infective. The larvae, unable to mature in an abnormal host, migrate through the body and lodge in various organs, particularly the lungs, liver, and brain, where they produce eosinophilic granulomas. Because the disease is difficult to diagnose, its distribution is not well known, but it is probably cosmopolitan.

Clinical Findings

A. Acute Infection: Fever, cough, hepatomegaly, and nervous symptoms are the commonest clinical findings. A variety of other symptoms may occur when such organs as the heart, eyes, and kidneys are invaded. Many infections are asymptomatic. Eosinophil counts of 30–80% and marked leukocytosis are common. The white count may exceed 100,000/μL. Hyperglobulinemia occurs when the liver is extensively invaded and is a useful clue in diagnosis.

Serologic tests were formerly lacking in sensitivity and specificity, but the new ELISA antibody technique is more effective in differentiating toxocariasis from ascariasis and filariasis. Additionally, the nonspecific isohemagglutinin titer is usually greater than 1:1024. No parasitic forms can be found by stool examination.

Specific diagnosis can only be made by liver biopsy to search for *Toxocara* larvae, but the procedure is seldom justified.

There is no specific treatment, but thiabendazole or levamisole should be tried. The cortisones, antibiotics, antihistamines, and analgesics may be needed to provide symptomatic relief. Symptoms may persist for months but generally clear within 1–2 years, and the ultimate prognosis is usually good.

B. Ocular Toxocariasis: The principal pathologic entity is eosinophilic granuloma of the retina that resembles retinoblastoma; until the recent development of the ELISA test, this resulted in the enucleation of many eyes. The most common findings are chronic endophthalmitis with retinal detachment, posterior pole granuloma, and peripheral granuloma. The majority of reported cases are in children who present with visual loss. If doubt exists whether a patient with a positive serum ELISA result has retinoblastoma along with a toxocaral reaction, the finding of a high vitreous ELISA favors toxocariasis. Treatment includes corticosteroids (subconjunctival applications may be preferable to oral usage), vitrectomy for vitreous traction, laser photocoagulation, and an anthelmintic drug.

Disease in humans is best prevented by periodic treatment of puppies and nursing bitches, starting at 2 weeks postpartum, repeating at weekly intervals for 3 weeks and then biannually. *Toxocara* ova in the soil may continue to be a source of infection for years.

Kielar RA: *Toxocara canis* endophthalmitis with low ELISA titer. *Ann Ophthalmol* 1983;**15:**447.

Molk R: Ocular toxocariasis: A review of the literature. *Ann Ophthalmol* 1983;**15:**216.

Schantz PM, Glickman LT: Toxocaral visceral larva migrans. *N Engl J Med* 1978;**298:**436.

●　　●　　●

References
(See also p 917.)

Kagan I: Serodiagnosis in parasitic diseases. Page 724 in: *Manual of Clinical Microbiology,* 3rd ed. Lennette EH (editor). American Society for Microbiology, 1980.

Reeder MM, Palmer PE (editors): *The Radiology of Tropical Disease With Epidemiological, Pathological, and Clinical Correlation.* Williams & Wilkins, 1980.

Schönfeld H (volume editor): *Antiparasitic Chemotherapy.* Karger, 1981.

WHO Expert Committee: *Parasitic Zoonoses.* Technical Report Series, No. 637. World Health Organization, 1979.

WHO Scientific Group: *Intestinal Protozoan and Helminthic Infections.* Technical Report Series, No. 666. World Health Organization, 1981.

Wilcocks C, Manson-Bahr PEC: *Manson's Tropical Diseases,* 18th ed. Williams & Wilkins, 1981.

Woodruff AW (editor): *Medicine in the Tropics.* Churchill Livingstone, 1974.

28 | Infectious Diseases: Mycotic*

Carlyn Halde, PhD

COCCIDIOIDOMYCOSIS

Essentials of Diagnosis

- Influenzalike illness with malaise, fever, backache, headache, and cough.
- Pleural pain.
- Arthralgia and periarticular swelling of knees and ankles.
- Erythema nodosum or erythema multiforme.
- Dissemination (rare) may result in meningitis or granulomatous lesions in any or all organs.
- X-ray findings vary widely from pneumonitis to cavitation.
- Positive skin test, serologic tests useful; sporangia containing endospores demonstrable in sputum or tissues.

General Considerations

Coccidioidomycosis should be considered in the diagnosis of any obscure illness in a patient who has lived in or visited an endemic area.

Infection results from the inhalation of arthroconidia of *Coccidioides immitis*, a mold that grows in soil in certain arid regions of the southwestern United States, Mexico, and in Central and South America.

About 60% of infections are subclinical and unrecognized other than by the subsequent development of a positive coccidioidin skin test. In the remaining cases, symptoms may be of severity warranting medical attention. Fewer than 1% show dissemination, but among these patients the mortality rate is high.

Clinical Findings

A. Symptoms and Signs: Symptoms of primary coccidioidomycosis occur in about 40% of infections. These vary from mild to severe and prostrating and resemble those due to viral, bacterial, or other mycotic infections. The onset (after an incubation period of 10–30 days) is usually that of a respiratory tract illness with fever and occasionally chills. Pleural pain is common and usually severe. Muscular ache, backache, and headache may be severe. Nasopharyngitis may be followed by bronchitis accompanied by a dry or slightly productive cough. Weakness and anorexia may become marked, leading to prostration. A morbilliform rash may appear 1–2 days after the onset of symptoms.

Arthralgia accompanied by periarticular swellings, often of the knees and ankles, is common. Erythema nodosum may appear 2–20 days after onset of symptoms. Erythema multiforme may appear on the upper extremities, head, or thorax. Breath sounds may become bronchial in nature, especially in the severely ill patient. Persistent pulmonary lesions, varying from cavities and abscesses to parenchymal nodular densities or bronchiectasis, occur in about 5% of diagnosed cases.

About 0.1% of white and 1% of nonwhite patients are unable to localize or control infection caused by *C immitis*. Symptoms in progressive coccidioidomycosis depend upon the site of dissemination. Any or all organs may be involved. Pulmonary findings usually become more pronounced, with mediastinal and hilar lymph node enlargement, cough, and increased sputum production. Pulmonary abscesses may rupture into the pleural space, producing an empyema. Extension to bones and skin may take place, and pericardial and myocardial extension is not unusual.

Lesions in the bones are often in the bony prominences and the ends of long bones. The ankle, wrist, and elbow joints are commonly involved. Meningitis occurs in 30–50% of disseminated cases. Subcutaneous abscesses and verrucous skin lesions are especially common in fulminating cases. Lymphadenitis may occur and may progress to suppuration. Mediastinal and retroperitoneal abscesses are not uncommon.

B. Laboratory Findings: In primary coccidioidomycosis, there may be a moderate leukocytosis and eosinophilia. The sedimentation rate is elevated, returning to normal as the infection subsides. If the sedimentation rate persists or increases, there is a danger of progressive disease. A coccidioidin skin test becomes positive within 1–3 weeks after onset of symptoms. Precipitin antibodies appear in most symptomatic infections but disappear after 1–6 months. Complement-fixing antibodies appear later but persist longer. An initial eosinophilia of 15% or higher together with a persistent rising complement fixation titer is a bad prognostic sign. A rising complement fixation titer may herald dissemination weeks before it is otherwise evident. Demonstrable antibodies in spinal fluid are pathognomonic for coccidioidal meningitis. Spinal fluid findings include increased cell count with lymphocytosis and reduced sugar. Sporangia filled with endospores may be found in clinical specimens. These should be cultured only by trained techni-

---

*Superficial mycoses are discussed in Chapter 4.

cians using safety precautions because of the danger of laboratory infection.

C. X-Ray Findings: X-ray findings vary, but patchy and nodular infiltrations are the most common. Hilar lymphadenopathy may be visible. There may be primary pleural effusion and thin-walled cavities.

Complications

Pulmonary infiltrations persisting for 6 or more weeks should be suspected of possible progression, especially with increase in area, enlargement of mediastinal and hilar nodes, cavity enlargement, and hemoptysis. Progressive disease is more likely to appear in blacks, Filipinos, and Mexicans. Immunodeficient patients or pregnant women of any race are also more vulnerable to dissemination.

Treatment

Bed rest is the most important therapeutic measure for the primary infection. This should be continued until there is a complete regression of fever, a normal sedimentation rate, clearing or stabilization of pulmonary radiologic findings, and a lowering of the complement fixation titer. These precautions are especially important for patients in whom the rate of dissemination is high. General symptomatic therapy is given as needed.

There is no specific therapy for patients with disseminated disease. Amphotericin B has proved effective in some patients and should be tried. The drug is suspended in 500 mL of 5% dextrose in distilled water (not saline) and administered intravenously over a 4-hour period. Toxic properties (including renal toxicity) suggest that the adult dose should not exceed 0.5–1 mg/kg. Therapy should begin with 1 mg/d, increasing by 5-mg increments to 25–35 mg/d or to 40–60 mg/d in the acutely ill. As the illness stabilizes, continue at 25–35 mg/d, decreasing with poor tolerance or increasing with poor clinical response. Therapy should continue to a total dose of 2.5–3 g. (See p 975 for precautions in the use of this drug.) Coccidioidal meningitis has been controlled with oral ketoconazole, 800–1200 mg/d, with or without intrathecal amphotericin B. Ketoconazole, at a lower dose, is continued indefinitely.

The best monitor of renal function is a creatinine clearance test done before treatment and once a week during treatment. Determine the blood urea nitrogen periodically.

Thoracic surgery is indicated for giant, infected, or ruptured cavities. Surgical drainage is also useful for subcutaneous abscesses. Excisional surgery may be used to remove any focus of proliferating sporangia. Amphotericin B is advisable following extensive surgical manipulation of infected tissue.

Prognosis

The prognosis is good, but persistent pulmonary cavities may present complications. Nodules, cavities, and fibrotic residuals may rarely progress after long periods of stability or regression. Oral ketoconazole,

200–800 mg daily 1–2 hours before breakfast, is used in amphotericin B failure; however, therapy must be continued for 6 months or longer after recovery in order to prevent relapse.

Bayer AS: Fungal pneumonias; pulmonary coccidioidal syndromes. 1. Primary and progressive primary coccidioidal pneumonias; diagnostic, therapeutic, and prognostic considerations. 2. Miliary, nodular, and cavitary pulmonary coccidioidomycosis; chemotherapeutic and surgical considerations. *Chest* 1981;**79**:575, 686.

Bouza E et al: Coccidioidal meningitis: An analysis of 31 cases and a review of the literature. *Medicine* 1981;**60**:139.

Catanzaro A et al: Treatment of coccidioidomycosis with ketoconazole: An evaluation utilizing a new scoring system. (In: Symposium on ketoconazole therapy.) *Am J Med* 1983;**74** (**Suppl 1B**):64.

Craven PC et al: High-dose ketoconazole for treatment of fungal infections of the central nervous system. *Ann Intern Med* 1983;**98**:160.

Hermans PE, Keys TF: Antifungal agents used for deep-seated mycotic infections. *Mayo Clin Proc* 1983;**58**:223.

HISTOPLASMOSIS

Essentials of Diagnosis

- Asymptomatic to severe respiratory symptoms with malaise, fever, cough, and chest pain.
- Ulceration of naso- and oropharynx.
- Hepatomegaly, splenomegaly, and lymphadenopathy.
- Anemia and leukopenia.
- Diarrhea in children.
- Positive skin test; positive serologic findings; small budding fungus cells found within reticuloendothelial cells; culture confirms diagnosis.

General Considerations

Histoplasmosis is caused by *Histoplasma capsulatum,* a mold that has been isolated from soil in endemic areas (central and eastern United States, eastern Canada, Mexico, Central America, South America, Africa, and Southeast Asia). Infection takes place presumably by inhalation of spores. These convert into small budding cells that are engulfed by phagocytic cells in the lungs. The organism proliferates and may be carried by the blood to other areas of the body.

Clinical Findings

A. Symptoms and Signs: Most cases of histoplasmosis are asymptomatic or mild and so are unrecognized. Past infection is recognized by the development of a positive histoplasmin skin test and occasionally by pulmonary and splenic calcification. Symptomatic infections may present mild influenzalike characteristics, often lasting 1–4 days. Signs and symptoms of pulmonary involvement are usually absent even in patients who subsequently show areas of calcification on chest x-ray. Moderately severe infections are frequently diagnosed as atypical pneumonia.

These patients have fever, cough, and mild chest pain lasting 5–15 days. Physical examination is usually negative. X-ray findings are variable and nonspecific.

Severe infections have been divided into 3 groups: (1) Acute histoplasmosis frequently occurs in epidemics. It is a severe disease with marked prostration, fever, and occasional chest pain but no particular symptoms relative to the lungs even when x-rays show severe disseminated pneumonitis. The illness may last from 1 week to 6 months but is almost never fatal. (2) Acute progressive histoplasmosis is usually fatal within 6 weeks or less. Symptoms usually consist of fever, dyspnea, cough, loss of weight, and prostration. Diarrhea is usually present in children. Ulcers of the mucous membranes of the oropharynx may be present. The liver and spleen are nearly always enlarged, and all the organs of the body are involved. (3) Chronic progressive histoplasmosis may continue for years. It is usually seen in older patients with chronic obstructive lung disease. The lungs show chronic progressive changes, often with cavities. The disease closely resembles chronic tuberculosis, and occasionally the patient has both diseases. Chronic histoplasmosis appears to be primarily confined to the lungs, but all organs of the body are involved in the terminal stage.

B. Laboratory Findings: In the moderately to severely ill patient, the sedimentation rate is elevated. Leukopenia is present, with a normal differential count or neutropenia. Most patients with progressive disease show a progressive hypochromic anemia. Immunodiffusion and complement-fixing antibodies can be demonstrated, and a change in titer is of use in prognosis.

Treatment

There is no specific therapy. Bed rest and supportive care are indicated for the primary form. Normal activities should not be resumed until fever has subsided. Resection of lung tissue containing cavities has been useful. Amphotericin B (as for coccidioidomycosis) in a low total dose (150–500 mg) has given excellent results in severe acute pulmonary disease. Chronic histoplasmosis rarely relapses after a total dose of 2500 mg. In clinical trials, oral ketoconazole, 200 mg 30 minutes before breakfast, appeared useful for treatment of disseminated or progressive cavitary histoplasmosis in the host that is not compromised but was not effective in the compromised host.

Prognosis

The prognosis is excellent for primary pulmonary histoplasmosis and poor in untreated generalized infection. Most cavities resolve with time and therapy.

Goodwin RA et al: Histoplasmosis in normal hosts. *Medicine* 1981;**60:**231.

Lowell JR, McLarty JW: Factors relating to recurrence of chronic pulmonary histoplasmosis following treatment with amphotericin B. *Am J Med Sci* 1983;**285:**13.

Slama TG: Treatment of disseminated and progressive cavitary histoplasmosis with ketoconazole. (In: Symposium on ketoconazole therapy.) *Am J Med* 1983;**74(Suppl 1B):**70.

BLASTOMYCOSIS

Blastomyces dermatitidis causes this chronic systemic fungus infection. The disease occurs more often in men and in a geographically delimited area of central and eastern United States and Canada. A few cases have been found in Mexico and Africa.

Mild or asymptomatic cases are rarely found. When dissemination takes place, lesions are most frequently seen on the skin, in bones, and in the urogenital system, although any or all organs or tissues of the body may be attacked.

Little is known concerning the mildest pulmonary phase of this disease. Cough, moderate fever, dyspnea, and chest pain are evident in symptomatic patients. These may disappear or may progress to a marked degree, with bloody and purulent sputum production, pleurisy, fever, chills, loss of weight, and prostration. Even serious pulmonary disease may be self-limiting. Radiologic studies usually reveal massive densities projecting irregularly from the mediastinal nodes, which are markedly enlarged. Raised, verrucous cutaneous lesions that have an abrupt downward sloping border are usually present in disseminated blastomycosis. The surface is covered with miliary pustules. The border extends slowly, leaving a central atrophic scar. In some patients, only cutaneous lesions are found. These may persist untreated for long periods, with a gradual decline in the patient's health. Bones—often the ribs and vertebrae—are frequently involved. These lesions appear both destructive and proliferative on x-ray. Epididymitis, prostatitis, and other involvement of the male urogenital system may occur. Central nervous system involvement is not a common complication. The viscera may be invaded, but rarely the gastrointestinal tract.

Laboratory findings usually include leukocytosis, hypochromic anemia, and elevated sedimentation rate. The organism is found in clinical specimens as a 5- to 20-μm, thick-walled cell that may have a single bud. It grows readily on culture. Complement-fixing antibody titer is variable but useful for prognosis.

There is no specific therapy for blastomycosis. Amphotericin B (as for coccidioidomycosis) in a total dose of 1.5–2 g appears to be the best drug available for treatment. Both ketoconazole and 2-hydroxystilbamidine have a greater relapse rate but are less toxic. Large abscesses or bronchopleural fistulas require drainage or correction, but resection of residual lung cavities is not indicated.

Careful follow-up for early evidence of relapse should be made for several years so that therapy may be resumed or another drug instituted. Patients whose disease is limited to localized cutaneous lesions have the best prognosis in that they show a better immunologic response to their infection.

Ismail MA, Lerner SA: Disseminated blastomycosis in a pregnant woman: Review of amphotericin B usage during pregnancy. *Am Rev Respir Dis* 1982;**126:**350.

Sarosi GA, Davies SF: State of the art: Blastomycosis. *Am Rev Respir Dis* 1979;**120**:911.

Short KL et al: The use of ketoconazole to treat systemic blastomycosis presenting as acute epididymitis. *J Urol* 1983; **129**:382.

PARACOCCIDIOIDOMYCOSIS
(South American Blastomycosis)

Paracoccidioides brasiliensis infections have been found only in patients who have resided in South or Central America or Mexico. Ulceration of the naso- and oropharynx is usually the first symptom. Papules ulcerate and enlarge both peripherally and deeper into the subcutaneous tissue. Extensive coalescent ulcerations may eventually result in destruction of the epiglottis, vocal cords, and uvula. Extension to the lips and face may occur. Eating and drinking are extremely painful. Skin lesions, usually on the face, may occur. Variable in appearance, they may have a necrotic central crater with a hard hyperkeratotic border. Lymph node enlargement may follow mucocutaneous lesions, eventually ulcerating and forming draining sinuses. Lymph node enlargement may be the presenting symptom, with subsequent suppuration and rupture through the skin. In some patients, gastrointestinal disturbances are first noted. Although the liver and spleen become enlarged, there is a lack of specific gastrointestinal symptoms. Cough, sometimes with sputum, indicates pulmonary involvement, but the signs and symptoms are often mild, even though x-ray findings indicate severe parenchymatous changes in the lungs.

The extensive ulceration of the upper gastrointestinal tract prevents sufficient intake and absorption of food. Most patients become cachectic early. Death may result from respiratory failure or malnutrition.

Laboratory findings include elevated sedimentation rate, leukocytosis with a neutrophilia showing a shift to the left, and sometimes eosinophilia and monocytosis. Serologic results are variable. A high titer usually indicates progressive disease; a descending titer is a favorable sign. The fungus is found in clinical specimens as a spherical cell that may have many buds arising from it. Colonial and cellular morphology are typical on culture.

The prognosis for paracoccidioidomycosis treated with amphotericin B and sulfonamides has been poor, with 32% mortality after 1–2 years. Trials with oral ketoconazole, 200–400 mg daily 1–2 hours before breakfast, show a clinical response within 1 month and effective control after 6 months. The rare relapse responded to resumed ketoconazole therapy. No deaths and 91.6% sustained remissions were observed in 24 patients in the following 1–2 years.

Restrepo A et al: Treatment of paracoccidioidomycosis with ketoconazole: A three-year experience. (In: Symposium on ketoconazole therapy.) *Am J Med* 1983;**74(Suppl 1B)**:48.

Sugar AM, Restrepo A, Stevens DA: Paracoccidioidomycosis in the immunosuppressed host: Report of a case and review of the literature. *Am Rev Respir Dis* 1984;**129**:340.

SPOROTRICHOSIS

Sporotrichosis is a chronic fungal infection caused by *Sporothrix schenckii*. It is worldwide in distribution; most patients are people whose occupation brings them in contact with soil, plants, or decaying wood. Infection takes place when the organism is introduced by trauma into the skin—usually on the hand, arm, or foot.

The most common form of sporotrichosis begins with a hard, nontender subcutaneous nodule. This later becomes adherent to the overlying skin, ulcerates (chancriform), and may persist for a long time. Within a few days to weeks, similar nodules usually develop along the lymphatics draining this area, and these may ulcerate. The lymphatic vessels become indurated and are easily palpable. The infection usually ceases to spread before the regional lymph nodes are invaded, and blood-borne dissemination is rare. The general health of the patient is not affected. Some patients complain of considerable pain. Skin infection may not spread through the lymphatics but may appear only as warty or papular, scaly lesions that may become pustular.

Pulmonary sporotrichosis presents no characteristic findings. Patients may be asymptomatic, although pleural effusion, hilar adenopathy, fibrosis, caseous nodularity, and cavitation have been reported.

Disseminated sporotrichosis presents a picture of multiple, hard subcutaneous nodules scattered over the body. These become soft but rarely rupture spontaneously. Lesions may also develop in the bones, joints, muscles, and viscera.

Cultures are needed to establish diagnosis. A skin test with heat-killed vaccine or sporotrichin is positive.

Potassium iodide taken orally in increasing dosage promotes rapid healing, although the drug is not fungicidal. Give as the saturated solution, 5 drops 3 times a day, after meals, increasing by 1 drop per dose until 40 drops 3 times a day are being given. Continue until signs of the active disease have disappeared. The dosage is then decreased by 1 drop per dose until 5 drops are being given, and then is discontinued. Care must be taken to reduce the dosage if signs of iodism appear. Oral ketoconazole has been effective in isolated cases of lymphocutaneous infection. Amphotericin B intravenously (as for coccidioidomycosis) and miconazole have been effective in systemic infection. Surgery is usually contraindicated except for simple aspiration of secondary nodules.

The prognosis is good for all forms of sporotrichosis except the disseminated type.

Smith PW et al: Disseminated cutaneous sporotrichosis: Three illustrative cases. *Arch Dermatol* 1981;**117**:143.

CHROMOBLASTOMYCOSIS

Chromoblastomycosis is a chronic, principally tropical cutaneous infection caused by several species of closely related black molds (*Fonsecaea* spp and *Phialophora* sp). In nature, these fungi grow as filamentous saprophytes in soil and on decaying vegetation.

The disease progresses slowly before the development of clinically characteristic lesions.

Lesions occur most frequently on a lower extremity but may occur on the hands, arms, and elsewhere. The lesion begins as a papule or ulcer. Over a period of months to years the lesions enlarge to become vegetating, papillomatous, verrucous, elevated nodules with a cauliflowerlike appearance or widespread dry verrucous plaques. The latter lesions spread peripherally with a raised, verrucous border, leaving central atrophic scarring. The surface of the active border contains minute abscesses. Satellite lesions may appear along the lymphatics. There may be extensive secondary bacterial infection, with a resulting foul odor. Some patients complain of itching. Elephantiasis may result if there are marked fibrosis and lymph stasis in the limb.

The fungus is seen as brown, thick-walled, spherical, sometimes septate cells in pus. The type of reproduction found in culture determines the species.

Oral flucytosine, 150 mg/kg/d, thiabendazole, 25 mg/kg/d, and ketoconazole have proved effective. Surgical excision and skin grafting may be useful.

Prolonged topical heat therapy or intralesional amphotericin B have been successful.

McGinnis MR: Chromoblastomycosis and phaeohyphomycosis: New concepts, diagnosis, and mycology. *J Am Acad Dermatol* 1983;**8**:1.

MYCETOMA
(Maduromycosis & Actinomycotic Mycetoma)

Maduromycosis is the term used to describe mycetoma caused by the true fungi. Actinomycotic mycetoma is caused by *Nocardia* and *Actinomadura* sp. The many species of causative agents are found in soil. Organisms are introduced by trauma in barefoot people. Mycetoma may occur on the hands and other parts of the body also. With time, the subcutaneous lesions develop sinuses that drain to the surface as well as deep into muscle and bone. Granules (dense colonies of the agent in tissue) drain out in the pus.

The disease begins as a papule, nodule, or abscess that over months to years progresses slowly to form multiple abscesses and sinus tracts ramifying deep into the tissue. The entire area becomes indurated, and the skin becomes discolored. Open sinuses or atrophic scars are scattered over its surface. Secondary bacterial infection may result in large open ulcers. X-rays show destructive changes in the underlying bone. Extensive fibrosis in the tissue causes elephantiasis. Pain is not a serious complaint until the disease is far advanced.

The agents occur as white, yellow, red, or black granules in the tissue or pus. Microscopic examination assists in the diagnosis. The granules of *Nocardia* and *Actinomadura* consist of delicate, gram-positive branching filaments 1 μm in diameter. Maduromycosis caused by the true fungi has granules consisting of filaments 5 μm in diameter sometimes cemented to large thick-walled cells.

The prognosis is good for patients with actinomycotic mycetoma, since they usually respond well to sulfonamides and sulfones, especially if treated early. Give trimethoprim-sulfamethoxazole, 2 tablets twice a day. Dapsone (Avlosulfon), 100 mg twice daily after meals, and other sulfones have been reported to be effective. All of these medications must be taken for long periods of time and continued for several months after clinical cure to prevent a relapse. Surgical procedures such as drainage assist greatly in healing.

There is no specific therapy for maduromycosis, and at present the prognosis is poor. Sulfones have been reported to be effective in isolated cases. Surgical excision of early lesions may prevent spread. Amputation is necessary in far-advanced cases.

Tight RR, Bartlett MS: Actinomycetoma in the United States. *Rev Infect Dis* 1981;**3**:1139.

ACTINOMYCOSIS*

Actinomyces israelii and other species of *Actinomyces* occur in the normal flora of the mouth and tonsillar crypts. *A israelii* and related species play a role in the production of normal dental plaque and also grow in tonsillar crypts. They are anaerobic, gram-positive, branching filamentous bacteria (1 μm in diameter) that may fragment into bacillary forms. In diseased tissue, these filaments are seen as a compact mass called a "sulfur granule." When introduced into traumatized tissue and associated with other anaerobic bacteria, these actinomycetes become pathogens. Hard, indurated, granulomatous suppurative lesions develop that give rise to sinus tracts.

The most common site of infection is the cervicofacial area (about 60% of cases), and infection typically follows extraction of a tooth or other trauma. Lesions may develop in the gastrointestinal tract or lungs following ingestion or aspiration of the fungus from its endogenous source in the mouth.

Cervicofacial actinomycosis develops slowly. The area becomes markedly indurated, and the overlying skin becomes reddish or cyanotic. The surface is irregular. Abscesses developing within and eventually draining to the surface persist for long periods. Sulfur granules may be found in the pus. There is usually little pain unless there is marked secondary infection. Trismus indicates that the muscles of mastication are involved. X-ray reveals eventual involvement of the bone, with rarefaction as well as some proliferation of the underlying bone.

---

*Included in this chapter by convention, since these organisms were thought for many years to be fungi.

Abdominal actinomycosis usually causes pain in the ileocecal region, spiking fever and chills, intestinal colic, vomiting, and weight loss. Irregular masses in the ileocecal area or elsewhere in the abdomen may be palpated. Pelvic inflammatory disease caused by actinomycetes is associated with prolonged use of an intrauterine contraceptive device. Sinuses draining to the exterior may develop. X-ray may reveal the mass or enlarged viscera. Vertebrae and pelvic bones may be invaded.

Thoracic actinomycosis begins with fever, cough, and sputum production. The patient becomes weak, loses weight, and may have night sweats and dyspnea. Pleural pain may be present. Multiple sinuses may extend through the chest wall, to the heart, or into the abdominal cavity. Ribs may be involved. X-ray shows massive areas of consolidation, frequently at the bases of the lungs.

The sedimentation rate may be elevated in patients with progressive disease. Anemia and leukocytosis are usually present. The anaerobic, gram-positive organism may be demonstrated as a granule or as scattered branching gram-positive filaments in the pus. Anaerobic culture is necessary to distinguish *Actinomyces* species from *Nocardia* species. Specific identification by culture is necessary to avoid confusion with nocardiosis, because specific therapy differs radically.

Penicillin G is the drug of choice. Ten to 20 million units are given via a parenteral route for 4–6 weeks. Continue treatment with penicillin V orally. Prolonged massive therapy is necessary in order to push effective levels of the drug into the abscesses where the organism is found. Sulfonamides may be added to the regimen, as well as streptomycin, which will control associated gram-negative organisms. Broad-spectrum antibiotics should be considered only if sensitivity tests show that the organism is resistant to penicillin. Immediate amelioration of symptoms or prompt improvement cannot be expected because of the chronic nature of this disease. Therapy should be continued for weeks to months after clinical manifestations have disappeared in order to ensure cure. Surgical procedures such as drainage and resection are of great benefit.

With penicillin and surgery, the prognosis is good. The difficulties of diagnosis, however, may permit extensive destruction of tissue before therapy is started.

Valicenti JF et al: Detection and prevalence of IUD-associated *Actinomyces* colonization and related morbidity: A prospective study of 69,925 cervical smears. *JAMA* 1982;**247**:1149.

OPPORTUNISTIC FUNGUS INFECTIONS

Debilitating diseases and often the drugs used in their treatment (corticosteroids, antibiotics, antimetabolites), as well as pregnancy and other altered physiologic states, may render a patient susceptible to invasion by many species of fungi that ordinarily are unable to cause disease. These factors may also cause infections due to the pathogenic fungi to be more serious.

1. CANDIDIASIS

Candida albicans may be cultured in small numbers from the mouth, vagina, and feces of most people. It is more frequent in debilitated individuals. Thrush, vaginitis, cutaneous lesions (frequently in intertriginous areas), onychia, and paronychia are common. These are discussed elsewhere in this book. Yeasts are frequent secondary invaders in other infections. Patients most susceptible to the development of systemic candidiasis are (1) those with hematologic cancer, (2) those immunosuppressed by disease or therapy, (3) postoperative patients, and (4) those who have undergone prolonged antibiotic therapy.

Systemic infection is of 2 types. Endocarditis, which almost always affects previously damaged heart valves, usually follows heart surgery or inoculation by contaminated needles or catheters. Splenomegaly and petechiae are usual, and emboli are common. In the other type of systemic infection, upper gastrointestinal tract candidiasis is usually the source. Dissemination follows antibiotic or cytotoxic chemotherapy for serious debilitating disease; the eyes, kidneys, spleen, lungs, liver, and heart are most commonly involved. Fungiuria is usual in renal disease; however, especially in older persons, *Candida* organisms can be found in the bladder or as a urethral saprophyte.

Bronchial or pulmonary infection is nearly always superimposed on other serious underlying disease.

Candida albicans is seen as gram-positive budding cells (2.5–6 μm) and as a pseudomycelium. It grows readily in culture. It is the most common cause of systemic disease, but *Candida tropicalis, Candida parapsilosis,* and *Torulopsis glabrata* are not uncommon. Many species may cause endocarditis. Serologic tests aid in diagnosis and prognosis.

Intravenous administration of amphotericin B (as for coccidioidomycosis) is necessary in serious systemic infections. When combined with flucytosine (Ancobon), 150 mg/kg/d orally, lower doses of this toxic drug may be used and still prevent emergence of resistant organisms. Associated oral, gastrointestinal, and cutaneous lesions should be treated with clotrimazole, nystatin, or miconazole mouthwash, tablets, and lotions. Gentian violet, 1%, in 10–20% alcohol, is also effective for oral, cutaneous, and vaginal lesions. Antibiotic therapy should be discontinued if possible. The correction of underlying factors may be sufficient to control candidiasis without specific therapy. Management of the severely immunocompromised patient includes prophylaxis with ketoconazole, clotrimazole, or nystatin.

Response to chemotherapy is poor in endocarditis. Valve replacement is usually necessary. In other systemic infections, the prognosis is good only if the underlying predisposing factors are corrected.

Henderson DK et al: Hematogenous *Candida* endophthalmitis in patients receiving parenteral hyperalimentation fluids. *J Infect Dis* 1981;**143**:655.

Meunier-Carpenter F et al: Fungemia in the immunocompromised host: Changing patterns, antigenemia, high mortality. *Am J Med* 1981;**71**:363.

2. CRYPTOCOCCOSIS

Cryptococcus neoformans, an encapsulated budding yeast that has been found worldwide in soil and on dried pigeon dung, causes cryptococcosis. Disseminated infection usually involves the central nervous system.

Infections are acquired by inhalation. In the lung the infection may remain localized, heal, or disseminate. Upon dissemination, lesions may form in any part of the body, but involvement of the central nervous system is most common and is the usual cause of death. Generalized meningoencephalitis occurs more frequently than localized granuloma in the brain or spinal cord. Solitary localized lesions may develop in the skin and, rarely, in the bones and other organs.

Spontaneous resolution of some pulmonary cases of cryptococcosis has been reported. The incidence of fatal cases, on the other hand, is increasing as a result of increased numbers of infections in susceptible debilitated individuals (especially in leukemia and lymphoma).

In pulmonary cryptococcosis there are no specific signs or symptoms, and many patients are nearly asymptomatic. The patient may present with a subacute respiratory infection with low-grade fever, pleural pain, and cough. There may be sputum production. Physical examination usually reveals signs of bronchitis or pulmonary consolidation. X-rays commonly show a solitary, moderately dense infiltration in the lower half of the lung field, with little or no hilar enlargement. More diffuse pneumonic infiltration, also in the lower lung fields, or extensive peribronchial infiltration or miliary lesions, may also occur.

Central nervous system involvement usually presents a history of recent upper respiratory or pulmonary infection. Increasingly painful headache is usually the first and most prominent symptom. Vertigo, nausea, anorexia, ocular disorders, and mental deterioration develop. Nuchal rigidity is present, and Kernig's and Brudzinski's signs are positive. Patellar and Achilles reflexes are often diminished or absent.

Acneiform lesions enlarge slowly and ulcerate, often coalescing with other lesions to cover a large area. Bone lesions are painful, and the area is often swollen. Eye involvement may result from direct extension along the subarachnoid space into the optic nerve.

A mild anemia, leukocytosis, and increased sedimentation rate are found. Spinal fluid findings include increased pressure, many white cells (usually lymphocytes), budding encapsulated fungus cells, increased protein and globulin, and decreased sugar and chlorides. Cryptococcal antigen in cerebrospinal fluid may be the only evidence for establishing a diagnosis in a living patient. Marked depletion of serum opsonins and complement occurs during fungemia.

A combination of amphotericin B (0.3 mg/kg/d administered as for coccidioidomycosis) and flucytosine (Ancobon), 150 mg/kg/d divided into 4 equal doses and given every 6 hours, may be curative in a 6-week regimen with a more rapid sterilization of cerebrospinal fluid. Experimental studies in mice show the combination of oral flucytosine and ketoconazole to be superior in cryptococcal meningitis. Oral ketoconazole is effective for nonmeningeal cryptococcosis. Surgical resection of pulmonary granulomas has been successful.

Craven PC, Graybill JR: Combination of oral flucytosine and ketoconazole as therapy for experimental cryptococcal meningitis. *J Infect Dis* 1984;**149**:584.

Kerkering TM, Duma RJ, Shadomy S: The evolution of pulmonary cryptococcosis. Clinical implications from a study of 41 patients with and without compromising host factors. *Ann Intern Med* 1981;**94**:611.

3. NOCARDIOSIS*

Nocardia asteroides and *Nocardia brasiliensis,* aerobic filamentous soil bacteria, cause pulmonary and systemic nocardiosis. Bronchopulmonary abnormalities predispose to colonization, but infection is unusual without underlying immunosuppressive disease.

Pulmonary involvement usually begins with malaise, loss of weight, fever, and night sweats. Cough and production of purulent sputum are the chief complaints. X-ray shows massive areas of consolidation, usually at the base of both lungs. Small areas of rarefaction caused by abscess formation within these consolidated masses may lead to multiple cavities. The lesions may penetrate to the exterior through the chest wall, invading the ribs. Pleural adhesions are common.

Dissemination may involve any organ. Lesions in the brain or meninges are most frequent, and such dissemination may occur following any minor pulmonary symptoms. Dissemination is common in immunocompromised patients.

An increased sedimentation rate and leukocytosis with increase in neutrophils are found in systemic nocardiosis. *N asteroides* is usually found as delicate, branching, gram-positive filaments that may be partially acid-fast. Identification is made by culture.

Give trimethoprim-sulfamethoxazole, 2–8 tablets twice a day orally, depending on the patient's weight and renal function and the severity of disease.

---

*Included in this chapter by convention, since these organisms were thought for many years to be fungi.

Sensitivity tests should be used to determine the appropriate antibiotic, which should be administered concurrently if needed. Response is slow, and therapy should be continued for months after all clinical manifestations have disappeared. Surgical procedures such as drainage and resection may be urgently required.

The prognosis in systemic nocardiosis is poor when diagnosis and therapy are delayed.

Smego RA et al: Trimethoprim-sulfamethoxazole therapy for *Nocardia* infections. *Arch Intern Med* 1983;**143**:711.

4. ASPERGILLOSIS

Aspergillus fumigatus is the usual cause of aspergillosis, although many species may cause a wide spectrum of disease. Burn eschar and detritus in the external ear canal are often colonized by these fungi. Mere colonization of an ectatic bronchus to form a compact mass of mycelium ("fungus ball") is usually associated with some immunity, and the fungus rarely adheres to or penetrates the wall of the bronchus. A pulmonary toilet regimen appears the most effective management for patients with *Aspergillus*-colonized cavities.

Allergic bronchopulmonary aspergillosis results from colonization but leads to bronchiectasis and pulmonary fibrosis. Early diagnosis and effective steroid therapy are extremely important. Steroids may work by inhibiting toxic antigen-antibody reactions, which reduces the volume of bronchial sputum, making a less suitable culture medium for the growth of the fungus in the bronchi.

Invasive aspergillosis is a serious form of the disease in patients with cancer and marked granulocytopenia. First growing in necrotic tissue or pulmonary cavities produced by other causes, the hyphae most commonly invade pulmonary parenchyma, with subsequent hematologic dissemination to kidney and other organs. Early diagnosis by biopsy or serologic study is crucial. Amphotericin B instituted within 96 hours of onset of clinical infection has achieved the most favorable outcome. Daily doses as high as 0.8–1 mg/kg for the first 2 weeks have been used for fulminant infections. Concurrent flucytosine therapy is sometimes helpful. Management requires reduction of corticosteroid and cytotoxic chemotherapy, if possible.

Thoracotomy with wedge resection is done for relapsing or medically recalcitrant lesions.

Aspergillus is recognized in tissue and sputum as dichotomously branched, septate hyphae. Serologic tests may be helpful in diagnosis.

Rinaldi MG: Invasive aspergillosis. *Rev Infect Dis* 1983;**5**:1061.
Weiland D et al: Aspergillosis in 25 renal transplant patients: Epidemiology, clinical presentation, diagnosis and management. *Ann Surg* 1983;**198**:622.

5. MUCORMYCOSIS

The term "mucormycosis" (zygomycosis, phycomycosis) is applied to opportunistic infections caused by members of the genera *Rhizopus, Mucor, Absidia,* and *Cunninghamella*. These appear in tissues as broad, branching nonseptate hyphae that may show a special affinity for blood vessels. Biopsy is almost always required for diagnosis. Sinus, orbit, and brain infections are most often associated with acidosis (usually diabetic). Pulmonary disease occurs in patients with leukemia or lymphoma or those who are seriously compromised in other ways (transplant patients). Cutaneous lesions occur as complications of burn wounds and as nosocomial infections from contaminated surgical tape. High-dosage amphotericin B therapy initiated early, control of diabetes or other underlying condition, and extensive surgical removal of necrotic, nonperfused tissue are essential features of good management. The prognosis is poor.

Lehrer RI et al: Mucormycosis. *Ann Intern Med* 1980;**93**:93.

6. MYCOTIC KERATITIS

Candida albicans, Fusarium, or *Aspergillus* is most often responsible for mycotic keratitis. Trauma to the cornea followed by corticosteroid and antibiotic therapy is often a predisposing factor. Prompt withdrawal of corticosteroids, removal of the infected necrotic tissue, and application of natamycin or ketoconazole are useful in management. Amphotericin B and flucytosine are used for fungal endophthalmitis. Natamycin does not penetrate corneal epithelium adequately for treatment of deep fungal keratitis or intraocular infections.

•   •   •

References

Dismukes WE et al: Treatment of systemic mycoses with ketoconazole: Emphasis on toxicity and clinical response in 52 patients. *Ann Intern Med* 1983;**98**:13.
Drugs for treatment of systemic fungal infections. *Med Lett Drugs Ther* 1984;**26**:36.
Hann IM et al: Ketoconazole versus nystatin plus amphotericin B for fungal prophylaxis in severely immunocompromised patients. *Lancet* 1982;**1**: 826.
Jones BR et al: Recognition and chemotherapy of oculomycosis.

In: Symposium on antifungal therapy. Cartwright RY (editor). *Postgrad Med J* 1979; **55**:625.
Laham MN, Carpenter JL: *Aspergillus terreus*, a pathogen capable of causing infective endocarditis, pulmonary mycetoma, and allergic bronchopulmonary aspergillosis. *Am Rev Respir Dis* 1982;**125**:769.
Rippon JW: *Medical Mycology*, 2nd ed. Saunders, 1982.
Salaki JS, Louria DB, Chmel H: Fungal and yeast infections of the central nervous system. *Medicine* 1984;**63**:108.

29 | Anti-infective Chemotherapeutic & Antibiotic Agents

Ernest Jawetz, MD, PhD

Some Rules for Antimicrobial Therapy

Antimicrobial drugs are used on a very large scale, and their proper use gives striking therapeutic results. On the other hand, they can create serious untoward reactions and should therefore be administered only upon proper indication.

Drugs of choice and second-line drugs are presented in Table 29–4.

The following steps merit consideration in each patient.

A. Etiologic Diagnosis: Formulate an etiologic diagnosis based on clinical observations. It is evident that microbial infections are best treated early. Therefore, the physician must attempt to decide on clinical grounds (1) whether the patient has a microbial infection that can probably be influenced by antimicrobial drugs and (2) the most probable kind of microorganisms causing such infection ("best guess").

B. "Best Guess": Select a specific antimicrobial drug on the basis of past experience for empiric therapy. Based on a "best guess," the physician should choose a drug that is likely to be effective against the suspected microorganism.

C. Laboratory Control: Before beginning antimicrobial drug treatment, obtain meaningful specimens for laboratory examination to determine the causative infectious organism and, if desirable, its susceptibility to antimicrobial drugs.

D. Clinical Response: Based on the clinical response of the patient, evaluate the laboratory reports and consider the desirability of changing the antimicrobial drug regimen. Laboratory results should not automatically overrule clinical judgment. The isolation of an organism that reinforces the initial clinical impression is a useful confirmation. Conversely, laboratory results may contradict the initial clinical impression and may force its reconsideration. If the specimen was obtained from a site that is normally devoid of bacterial flora and not exposed to the external environment (eg, blood, cerebrospinal fluid, pleural fluid, joint fluid), the recovery of a microorganism is a significant finding even if the organism recovered is different from the clinically suspected etiologic agent, and this may force a change in antimicrobial treatment. On the other hand, the isolation of unexpected microorganisms from the respiratory tract, gut, or surface lesions (sites that have a complex flora) must be criti-

cally evaluated before drugs are abandoned that were judiciously selected on the basis of an initial "best guess" for empiric treatment.

E. Drug Susceptibility Tests: Some microorganisms are fairly uniformly susceptible to certain drugs; if such organisms are isolated from the patient, they need not be tested for drug susceptibility. For example, group A hemolytic streptococci and most pneumococci and clostridia respond predictably to penicillin. On the other hand, some kinds of microorganisms (eg, enteric gram-negative rods) are sufficiently variable in their response to warrant drug susceptibility testing when they are isolated from a significant specimen.

Antimicrobial drug susceptibility tests may be done on solid media as "disk tests," in broth in tubes,

Table 29–1. Blood levels of some commonly used antibiotics at therapeutic dosages in adults.

	Route	Daily Dose	Expected Mean Concentration per mL Blood or per gram Tissue
Penicillin	IM	0.6–1 million units	1 unit
	Oral	0.6 million units	0.2 unit
Nafcillin	IV	6–12 g	5–30 μg
Dicloxacillin	Oral	2–4 g	3–12 μg
Ampicillin	Oral	2–3 g	3–4 μg
	IV	4–6 g	10–40 μg
Amoxicillin	Oral	2 g	8–10 μg
Carbenicillin	IV	30 g	100–200 μg
Ticarcillin	IV	18 g	100–200 μg
Cephalothin	IV	8–12 g	10–20 μg
Cefazolin	IV	4–6 g	20–60 μg
Cefoxitin, cefamandole	IV	8–12 g	50–80 μg
Cefotaxime, moxalactam	IV	8–12 g	40–80 μg
Tetracyclines	Oral	2 g	6–8 μg
Chloramphenicol	Oral	2 g	8–10 μg
Erythromycin	Oral	2 g	0.5–2 μg
Amikacin	IM	1 g	20–30 μg
Gentamicin, tobramycin	IM	0.3 g	3–6 μg
Vancomycin	IV	2 g	10–20 μg
Clindamycin	IV	2.4 g	3–6 μg

or in wells of microdilution plates. The latter method yields results expressed as MIC (minimal inhibitory concentration), and the technique can be modified to give MBC (minimal bactericidal concentration) results. In some infections, the MIC or MBC permits a better estimate of the amount of drug required for therapeutic effect in vivo.

Disk tests usually indicate whether an isolate is susceptible or resistant to drug concentrations achieved in vivo with conventional dosage regimens, thus providing valuable guidance in selecting therapy. When there appear to be marked discrepancies between test results and clinical response of the patient, the following possibilities must be considered:

1. Choice of inappropriate drug, dosage, or route of administration.

2. Failure to drain a collection of pus or to remove a foreign body.

3. Failure of a poorly diffusing drug to reach the site of infection (eg, central nervous system) or to reach intracellular phagocytosed bacteria.

4. Superinfection in the course of prolonged chemotherapy. After suppression of the original infection or of normal flora, a second type of microorganism may establish itself against which the originally selected drug is ineffective.

5. Emergence of drug-resistant or tolerant organisms.

6. Participation of 2 or more microorganisms in the infectious process, of which only one was originally detected and used for drug selection.

F. Adequate Dosage: To determine whether the proper drug is being used in adequate dosage, a serum assay can be performed. Two days after a drug regimen is established, serum is obtained from the patient 1–2 hours after a drug dose. Dilutions of this serum are set up against the microorganism originally isolated from the patient's infection and the antibacterial activity estimated. If an adequate dose of a proper drug is being employed, the serum should be markedly bactericidal ($> 1:5$) in vitro. In infections limited to the urinary tract, the antibacterial activity of urine can be estimated. In persons with renal insufficiency, the dose or frequency of administration must be adjusted. This can

Table 29–2. Examples of incompatibilities between antimicrobial drugs and other agents.

Antimicrobial Drug	Other Agent	Results
In vitro incompatibilities when mixed for intravenous administration*		
Amphotericin B	Benzylpenicillin, tetracyclines, aminoglycosides, 0.9% NaCl	Precipitate
Cephalosporins	Calcium gluconate or calcium chloride, polymyxin B, erythromycin, tetracyclines	Precipitate
Chloramphenicol	Polymyxin B, tetracyclines, vancomycin, hydrocortisone, B complex vitamins	Precipitate
Gentamicin, tobramycin	Carbenicillin, ticarcillin	Inactivation in vitro
Nafcillin	Any acidic solution, B complex vitamins	Inactivation in 12 hours
Novobiocin	Aminoglycosides, erythromycins	Insoluble precipitate
Oxacillin	Any acidic solution, B complex vitamins	Inactivation in 12 hours
Penicillin G	Any acidic solution, B complex vitamins, amphotericin B, chloramphenicol, tetracyclines, vancomycin, metaraminol, phenylephrine, carbohydrate at pH > 8.0	Inactivation in 12 hours, precipitate
Tetracyclines, lincomycin	Calcium-containing solutions, amphotericin B, cephalosporins, heparin, hydrocortisone, polymyxin B, chloramphenicol, any divalent cations, iron	Chelation, inactivation, precipitate
Vancomycin	Heparin, penicillins, hydrocortisone, chloramphenicol	Precipitate
Physiologic drug interactions*		
Aminoglycosides, polymyxins	Other aminoglycosides, vancomycin	Increased nephrotoxicity; ototoxicity, neurotoxicity
Amphotericin B	Digitalis, curare	Increased digitalis and curare effects
Chloramphenicol	Phenytoin, tolbutamide, dicumarol, ethanol	Increased blood concentration of these drugs
Rifampin	Quinidine, digoxin	Decreased quinidine and digoxin effect
Griseofulvin, rifampin	Anticoagulants	Decreased anticoagulant effect
Sulfonamides, chloramphenicol, tetracyclines, nalidixic acid	Anticoagulants	Increased anticoagulant effect (probably due to inhibition of intestinal flora)
Metronidazole	Phenobarbital	Reduced metronidazole levels
Miconazole	Coumarin drugs	Increased anticoagulant effect
Sulfonamides, chloramphenicol	Sulfonylurea	Hypoglycemia
Sulfonamides (oral)	Methenamine (oral)	Insoluble HCOH-sulfonamide compound in urine

*Many other incompatibilities may occur.

sometimes be done by reference to dosage nomograms or rules; however, it is best to directly measure the drug level (Table 29–1) in the patient's serum, particularly in the case of drugs that can be oto-, nephro-, or neurotoxic when given in excessive doses.

G. Duration of Antimicrobial Therapy: Generally speaking, effective antimicrobial treatment results in reversal of the clinical and laboratory parameters of active infection and marked clinical improvement within a very few days. However, treatment may have to be continued for varying periods to effect cure. A few examples of timing are illustrative:

Streptococcal pharyngitis requires 10 days of effective penicillin levels to eradicate the organism. Acute uncomplicated gonorrhea can be eradicated in males by 24 hours of effective drug levels. Endocarditis caused by viridans streptococci is curable in 3 weeks; that caused by staphylococci usually requires 5–6 weeks of treatment. Acute cystitis in women often responds in just 1–3 days of treatment. Pneumococcal pneumonia and meningococcal meningitis require penicillin for only 3 days after complete defervescence.

In bacterial meningitis due to *Haemophilus influenzae*, effective antimicrobial drugs should be continued until the cerebrospinal fluid glucose has returned to near normal. Many months of treatment are required in mycobacterial or fungal infections.

To minimize untoward reactions from drugs and the likelihood of superinfection, treatment should be continued only as long as necessary to eradicate the infectious agent.

H. Adverse Reactions: The administration of antimicrobial drugs is commonly associated with untoward reactions. (1) Hypersensitivity: The most common hypersensitivity reactions are fever and skin rashes. Hematologic or hepatic disorders and anaphylaxis are rare. (2) Direct toxicity: Most common are nausea, vomiting, and diarrhea. More serious toxic reactions are impairment of renal, hepatic, or hematopoietic functions or damage to the eighth nerve. (3) Suppression of normal microbial flora and "superinfection" by drug-resistant microorganisms, or continued infection with the initial pathogen through the emergence of drug-resistant variants.

In each case, the physician must evaluate the desirability of continuing a given drug regimen against the risk of discontinuing it. The severity and prognosis of each untoward reaction must be evaluated and a choice made between continuing a probably offending drug and discontinuing the drug but risking uncontrolled infection. An effective antimicrobial drug regimen that evokes hypersensitivity reactions can sometimes be continued with the simultaneous use of corticosteroids. In the presence of impaired renal function, reduction in dosage or frequency of medication is often necessary (Table 29–3).

I. Oral Antibiotics: The absorption of oral

Table 29–3. Use of antibiotics in patients with renal failure.

	Principal Mode of Excretion or Detoxification	Approximate Half-Life in Serum		Proposed Dosage Regimen in Renal Failure		Significant Removal of Drug by Dialysis (H = Hemodialysis; P = Peritoneal Dialysis)
		Normal	Renal Failure*	Initial Dose†	Give Half of Initial Dose at Interval of	
Penicillin G	Tubular secretion	0.5 h	6 h	4 g IV	8–12 h	H, P no
Ampicillin	Tubular secretion	1 h	8 h	6 g IV	8–12 h	H yes, P no
Carbenicillin, ticarcillin	Tubular secretion	1.5 h	16 h	3–4 g IV	12–18 h	H, P yes
Nafcillin	Liver 80%, kidney 20%	0.5 h	2 h	2 g IV	4–6 h	H, P no
Cephalothin	Tubular secretion	0.8 h	8 h	4 g IV	18 h	H, P yes
Cephalexin, cephradine	Tubular secretion and glomerular filtration	2 h	15 h	2 g orally	8–12 h	H, P yes
Cefazolin	Kidney	2 h	30 h	2 g IM, IV	24 h	H yes, P no
Cefoxitin, cefamandole	Tubular secretion and glomerular filtration	1–1.5 h	16–20 h	2 g IV	12–18 h	H, P yes
Cefotaxime, moxalactam	Tubular secretion and liver	1–2 h	20–30 h	2 g IV	24 h	H, P yes
Amikacin	Glomerular filtration	2.5 h	2–3 d	15 mg/kg IM	3 d	H, P yes
Tobramycin, gentamicin	Glomerular filtration	2.5 h	2–4 d	3 mg/kg IM	2–3 d	H, P yes‡
Vancomycin	Glomerular filtration	6 h	6–9 d	1 g IV	5–8 d	H, P no
Tetracycline	Glomerular filtration	8 h	3 d	1 g orally or 0.5 g IV	3 d	H, P no
Chloramphenicol	Mainly liver	3 h	4 h	1 g orally or IV	8 h	H, P no
Erythromycin	Mainly liver	1.5 h	5 h	1 g orally or IV	8 h	H, P no
Clindamycin	Glomerular filtration and liver	2.5 h	4 h	600 mg IV or IM	8 h	H, P no

*Considered here to be marked by creatinine clearance of 10 mL/min or less.

†For a 60-kg adult with a serious systemic infection. The "initial dose" listed is administered as an intravenous infusion over a period of 1–8 hours, or as 2 intramuscular injections during an 8-hour period, or as 2–3 oral doses during the same period.

‡Aminoglycosides are removed irregularly in peritoneal dialysis. Gentamicin is removed 60% in hemodialysis.

penicillins, cephalosporins, macrolides, tetracyclines, lincomycins, etc, is impaired by food. Therefore, these oral drugs must be given between meals.

J. Intravenous Antibiotics: When an antibiotic must be administered intravenously (eg, for life-threatening infection or for maintenance of very high blood levels), the following cautions should be observed:

(1) Give in neutral solution (pH 7.0–7.2) of sodium chloride (0.9%) or dextrose (5%) in water.

(2) Give alone without admixture of any other drug in order to avoid chemical and physical incompatibilities (which can occur frequently).

(3) Administer by intermittent (every 2–6 hours) addition to the intravenous infusion ("bolus injection") to avoid inactivation (by temperature, changing pH, etc) and prolonged vein irritation from high drug concentration, which favors thrombophlebitis.

(4) The infusion site must be changed every 48 hours to reduce the chance of superinfection.

Bennett WM et al: Drug therapy in renal failure. *Ann Intern Med* 1980;**93:**62.

Calderwood SB, Moellering RC: Common adverse effects of antibacterial agents on major organ systems. *Surg Clin North Am* 1980;**60:**65.

Mills J, Barriere SL, Jawetz E: Clinical use of antimicrobials. Chapter 52 in: *Basic & Clinical Pharmacology,* 2nd ed. Katzung BG (editor). Lange, 1984.

Neu HC (guest editor): Impact of the patient at risk on current and future antimicrobial therapy. *Am J Med* 1984;**76(No. 5A).** [Entire issue.]

PENICILLINS

The penicillins are a large group of antimicrobial substances, all of which share a common chemical nucleus (6-aminopenicillanic acid) which contains a β-lactam ring essential to their biologic activity. All β-lactam antibiotics inhibit formation of microbial cell walls. In particular, they block the final transpeptidation reaction in the synthesis of cell wall mucopeptide (peptidoglycan), and they activate autolytic enzymes in the cell wall. These reactions result in cell death.

Antimicrobial Activity

The initial step in penicillin action is the binding of the drug to receptors, penicillin-binding proteins, some of which are transpeptidation enzymes. The penicillin-binding proteins of different organisms differ in number and in affinity for a given drug. After penicillins have attached to receptors, peptidoglycan synthesis is inhibited, because the activity of transpeptidation enzymes is blocked. The final bactericidal action is the removal of an inhibitor of the autolytic enzymes in the cell wall, which activates the enzymes and results in cell lysis. Organisms that are defective in autolysin function are inhibited but not killed by β-lactam antibiotics ("tolerance"). Organisms that produce β-lactamases (penicillinases) are resistant to some penicillins because the β-lactam ring is broken

and the drug inactivated. Only organisms that are actively synthesizing peptidoglycan (in the process of multiplication) are susceptible to β-lactam antibiotics. Nonmultiplying organisms or those lacking cell walls (L forms) are not susceptible but may act as "persisters."

One million units of penicillin G equals 0.6 g. Other penicillins are prescribed in grams. A blood level of $0.01–1$ μg/mL of penicillin G or ampicillin is lethal for a majority of susceptible microorganisms. Most β-lactamase-resistant penicillins are 5–50 times less active.

Penicillins can be arranged into groups:

1. Highest activity against gram-positive organisms but susceptible to hydrolysis by β-lactamases, eg, penicillin G, benzathine penicillin.

2. Relatively resistant to β-lactamases but less active against gram-positive organisms and inactive against gram-negative ones, eg, nafcillin.

3. Relatively high activity against both gram-positive and gram-negative organisms but destroyed by β-lactamases (penicillinases), eg, ampicillin, amoxicillin, carbenicillin, ticarcillin, piperacillin.

4. Stable to gastric acid and suitable for oral administration, eg, penicillin V, cloxacillin, ampicillin.

Resistance

Resistance to penicillins falls into several categories:

1. Production of β-lactamases, eg, by staphylococci, gonococci, *Haemophilus,* coliform organisms.

2. Lack of penicillin receptors (eg, resistant pneumococci) or impermeability of cell envelope so that penicillins cannot reach receptors (eg, metabolically inactive bacteria).

3. Failure of activation of autolytic enzymes in the cell wall; "tolerance," eg, in staphylococci, group B streptococci.

4. Cell wall-deficient (L) forms or mycoplasmas, which do not synthesize peptidoglycans.

Absorption, Distribution, & Excretion

After parenteral administration, absorption of most penicillins is complete and rapid. Because of the irritation and consequent local pain produced by the intramuscular injection of large doses, administration by the intravenous route (intermittent bolus addition to a continuous infusion) is often preferred. After oral administration, only a portion of the dose is absorbed—from 5 to 35%, depending upon acid stability, binding to foods, and the presence of buffers. In order to minimize binding to foods, oral penicillins should not be preceded or followed by food for at least 1 hour.

After absorption, penicillins are widely distributed in body fluids and tissues. This varies to some extent with the degree of protein binding exhibited by different penicillins. Penicillin G and ampicillin are moderately protein-bound (40–60%), whereas cloxacillin and nafcillin are highly protein-bound (95–98%). With parenteral doses of 3–6 g (5–10 million units) of penicillin G per 24 hours, injected in divided doses intramuscularly or added to intravenous infusions, average serum levels of the drug reach 1–10 units (0.6–6 μg)/mL. A rough relationship of 6 g given parenterally per day yielding serum levels of 1–6 μg/mL also applies to other penicillins. The highly serum-bound penicillins yield, on the average, lower levels of free drug than less strongly bound penicillins.

Special dosage forms of penicillin have been designed for delayed absorption to yield low blood and tissue levels for long periods. The outstanding example is benzathine penicillin G. After a single intramuscular injection of 0.75 g (1.2 million units), serum levels in excess of 0.03 unit/mL are maintained for 10 days and levels in excess of 0.005 unit/mL for 3 weeks. The latter is sufficient to protect against beta-hemolytic streptococcal infection; the former, to treat an established infection with these organisms. Procaine penicillin also has delayed absorption, yielding levels for 24 hours.

In many tissues, penicillin concentrations are equal to those in serum. Lower levels are found in the eye, prostate, and central nervous system. However, with active inflammation of the meninges, as in bacterial meningitis, penicillin levels in the cerebrospinal fluid exceed 0.2 μg/mL with a daily parenteral dose of 12 g. Thus, pneumococcal and meningococcal meningitis may be treated with systemic penicillin, and intrathecal injection is contraindicated. Penetration into inflamed joints is likewise sufficient for treatment of infective arthritis caused by susceptible organisms.

Most of the absorbed penicillin is rapidly excreted by the kidneys into the urine; small amounts are excreted by other channels. About 10% of renal excretion is by glomerular filtration and 90% by tubular secretion, to a maximum of about 2 g/h in an adult. Tubular secretion can be partially blocked by probenecid (Benemid) to achieve higher systemic levels. Renal clearance is less efficient in the newborn, so that proportionately smaller doses result in higher systemic levels and are maintained longer than in the adult. Individuals with impaired renal function likewise tend to maintain higher penicillin levels longer.

Renal excretion of penicillin results in very high levels in the urine. Thus, systemic daily doses of 6 g of penicillin may yield urine levels of 500–3000 μg/mL—enough to suppress not only gram-positive but also many gram-negative bacteria in the urine (provided they produce little β-lactamase).

Penicillin is also excreted into sputum and milk to levels of 3–15% of those present in the serum. This is the case in both humans and cattle. The presence of penicillin in the milk of cows treated for mastitis presents a problem in allergy.

Indications, Dosages, & Routes of Administration

The penicillins are by far the most effective and the most widely used antimicrobial drugs. All oral penicillins must be given 1 hour away from meal times to reduce binding and acid inactivation. Blood levels of all penicillins can be raised by giving probenecid, 0.5 g (10 mg/kg) every 6 hours orally.

A. Penicillin G: This is the drug of choice for infections caused by pneumococci, streptococci, meningococci, non-β-lactamase-producing staphylococci and gonococci, *Treponema pallidum* and many other spirochetes, *Bacillus anthracis* and other gram-positive rods, clostridia, *Actinomyces, Listeria,* and *Bacteroides* (except *Bacteroides fragilis*).

1. Intramuscular or intravenous–Most of the above-mentioned infections respond to aqueous penicillin G in daily doses of 0.6–5 million units (0.36–3 g) administered by intermittent intramuscular injection every 4–6 hours. Much larger amounts (6–50 g daily) can be given by intermittent addition (every 2–6 hours) to an intravenous infusion in serious or complicated infections due to these organisms. Sites for such intravenous administration are subject to thrombophlebitis and superinfection and must be rotated every 2 days and kept scrupulously aseptic. In enterococcal endocarditis, an aminoglycoside is given simultaneously with large doses of a penicillin.

2. Oral–Penicillin V is indicated only in minor infections (eg, of the respiratory tract or its associated structures) in daily doses of 1–4 g (1.6–6.4 million units). About one-fifth of the oral dose is absorbed, but oral administration is subject to so many variables that it should not be relied upon in seriously ill patients.

3. Intrathecal–With high serum levels of penicillin, adequate concentrations reach the central nervous system and cerebrospinal fluid for the treatment of central nervous system infection. Therefore, and because injection of more than 10,000 units of penicillin G into the subdural space may cause convulsions, intrathecal injection has been virtually abandoned.

4. Topical–Penicillins have been applied to skin, wounds, and mucous membranes by compress, ointment, and aerosol. These applications are highly sensitizing and seldom warranted. Rarely, solutions of penicillin (eg, 100,000 units/mL) are instilled into joint or pleural space infected with susceptible organisms.

B. Benzathine Penicillin G: This penicillin is a salt of very low water solubility. It is injected intramuscularly to establish a depot that yields low but prolonged drug levels. A single injection of 1.2 million units intramuscularly is satisfactory for treatment of beta-hemolytic streptococcal pharyngitis. An injection of 1.2–2.4 million units every 3–4 weeks provides satisfactory prophylaxis for rheumatics against reinfection with group A streptococci. Early syphilis can be treated with benzathine penicillin, 2.4 million units intramuscularly 1–3 times at weekly intervals. There is no indication for using this drug by mouth. Procaine penicillin G is another repository form for maintaining drug levels for up to 24 hours. For highly susceptible infections, 600 thousand units intramuscularly are given once daily. For uncomplicated gonorrhea, 4.8 million units of procaine penicillin are given once intramuscularly with probenecid, 1 g orally.

C. Ampicillin, Amoxicillin, Carbenicillin,

Ticarcillin, Piperacillin, Mezlocillin, Azlocillin: These drugs have greater activity against gram-negative aerobes than penicillin G but are destroyed by penicillinases (β-lactamases).

Ampicillin, 500 mg orally every 6 hours, is used to treat common urinary tract infections with gram-negative coliform bacteria or mixed secondary bacterial infections of the respiratory tract (eg, sinusitis, bronchitis, otitis). Ampicillin, 300 mg/kg/d intravenously, is a current choice for bacterial meningitis in children, especially if the disease is caused by *H influenzae*. However, β-lactamase-producing *Haemophilus* organisms are appearing more frequently, and for that reason chloramphenicol remains essential.

Ampicillin is ineffective against *Enterobacter, Pseudomonas,* and indole-positive *Proteus* infections. In *Salmonella* infections, ampicillin, 6–12 g intravenously, can suppress signs and symptoms and may eliminate organisms from some carriers. In typhoid and paratyphoid infections, ampicillin is an alternative to chloramphenicol. However, it usually has no beneficial effect in simple *Salmonella* gastroenteritis. In severely malnourished children with salmonellosis, ampicillin, 100 mg/kg/d intramuscularly, was effective.

Amoxicillin (500 mg orally every 8 hours) is better absorbed than ampicillin. The spectrum, activity, and side effects are comparable. Bacampicillin and pivampicillin have therapeutic effects comparable to those of ampicillin but can be administered orally every 12 hours (400–800 mg) to achieve adequate tissue concentrations.

Carbenicillin resembles ampicillin but has more marked activity against *Pseudomonas* and *Proteus,* although *Klebsiella* organisms are usually resistant. Ticarcillin resembles carbenicillin but gives higher tissue levels. In susceptible populations of *Pseudomonas* organisms, resistance to these drugs may emerge rapidly. Therefore, in *Pseudomonas* sepsis (eg, burns, leukemia), carbenicillin, 30 g/d (300–500 mg/kg/d), or ticarcillin, 18 g/d (200–300 mg/kg/d), intravenously is usually combined with tobramycin, 5–7 mg/kg/d, to delay emergence of resistance and perhaps to obtain synergistic effects. Carbenicillin indanyl sodium is acid-stable and can be given orally in urinary tract infections.

Piperacillin, mezlocillin, and azlocillin all resemble ticarcillin but are somewhat more active against some gram-negative aerobes, especially *Pseudomonas*. Hetacillin is converted to ampicillin in vivo and has no advantage.

D. β-Lactamase-Resistant Penicillins: Methicillin, oxacillin, cloxacillin, dicloxacillin, nafcillin, and others are relatively resistant to destruction by β-lactamase. The only indication for the use of these drugs is infection by β-lactamase-producing staphylococci.

1. Oral–Oxacillin, cloxacillin, dicloxacillin, or nafcillin may be given in doses of 0.25–0.5 g every 4–6 hours in mild or localized staphylococcal infections (50–100 mg/kg/d for children). Food must not be given within an hour of these doses because it interferes with absorption.

2. Intravenous–For serious systemic staphylococcal infections, nafcillin, 6–12 g, is administered intravenously, usually by injecting 1–2 g during 20–30 minutes every 2–4 hours into a continuous infusion of 5% dextrose in water or physiologic saline solution. The dose for children is nafcillin, 50–100 mg/kg/d. Eighty percent of nafcillin is excreted into the biliary tract, and only 20% is cleared by tubular secretion. Thus, the action of nafcillin is little affected by renal failure.

Adverse Effects

The penicillins undoubtedly possess less direct toxicity than any other antibiotics. Most of the serious side effects are due to hypersensitivity.

A. Allergy: All penicillins are cross-sensitizing and cross-reacting. Any preparation containing penicillin may induce sensitization, including foods or cosmetics. In general, sensitization occurs in proportion to the duration and total dose of penicillin received in the past. The responsible antigenic determinants appear to be degradation products of penicillins, particularly penicilloic acid and products of alkaline hydrolysis (minor antigenic determinants) bound to host protein. Skin tests with penicilloyl-polylysine, with minor antigenic determinants, and with undegraded penicillin can identify many hypersensitive individuals. Among positive reactors to skin tests, the incidence of subsequent immediate severe penicillin reactions is high. Although many persons develop IgG antibodies to antigenic determinants of penicillin, the presence of such antibodies is not correlated with allergic reactivity (except rare hemolytic anemia), and serologic tests have little predictive value. A history of a penicillin reaction in the past is not reliable; however, in such cases the drug should be administered with caution (airway, 0.1% epinephrine in syringe, competent personnel available, intravenous fluids running), or a substitute drug should be given.

Allergic reactions may occur as typical anaphylactic shock, typical serum sickness type reactions (urticaria, fever, joint swelling, angioneurotic edema, intense pruritus, and respiratory embarrassment occurring 7–12 days after exposure), and a variety of skin rashes, oral lesions, fever, interstitial nephritis, eosinophilia, hemolytic anemia, other hematologic disturbances, and vasculitis. The incidence of hypersensitivity to penicillin is estimated to be 1–5% among adults in the USA but is negligible in small children. Acute anaphylactic life-threatening reactions are fortunately very rare (0.05%). Ampicillin produces maculopapular skin rashes more frequently than other penicillins, but some ampicillin rashes are not allergic in origin. Methicillin and other penicillins can induce nephritis with primary tubular lesions, associated with anti-basement membrane antibodies. Nafcillin is less nephrotoxic than methicillin.

Individuals known to be hypersensitive to penicillin can at times tolerate the drug during corticosteroid administration. "Desensitization" is only infrequently warranted.

B. Toxicity: Since the action of penicillin is directed against a unique bacterial structure, the cell wall, it is virtually without effect on animal cells. The toxic effects of penicillin G are due to the direct irritation caused by intramuscular or intravenous injection of exceedingly high concentrations (eg, 1 g/mL). Such concentrations may cause local pain, induration, thrombophlebitis, or degeneration of an accidentally injected nerve. All penicillins are irritating to the central nervous system. There is no indication for intrathecal administration at present. In rare cases, a patient receiving more than 50 g of penicillin G daily parenterally exhibits signs of cerebrocortical irritation as a result of the passage of unusually large amounts of penicillin into the central nervous system. With doses of this magnitude, direct cation toxicity (Na^+, K^+) can also occur. Potassium penicillin G contains 1.7 meq of K^+ per million units (2.8 meq/g), and potassium may accumulate in renal failure. Carbenicillin contains 4.7 meq of Na^+ per gram—a risk in heart failure.

Large doses of penicillins given orally may lead to gastrointestinal upset, particularly nausea and diarrhea. This is most pronounced with the broad-spectrum penicillins—ampicillin or amoxicillin—and may be accompanied by luxuriant overgrowth of staphylococci, *Pseudomonas,* clostridia, or yeasts, leading to enteritis. Superinfections in other organ systems may occur with penicillins as with any other antibiotic. Methicillin and carbenicillin can cause granulocytopenia. Carbenicillin and ticarcillin can produce hypokalemic alkalosis and elevation of serum transaminases and can damage platelets or induce hemostatic defects leading to bleeding tendency.

Barza M: Antimicrobial spectrum, pharmacology and therapeutic uses of penicillins. *Am J Hosp Pharm* 1977;**34:**57.

Brown CH et al: The hemostatic defect produced by carbenicillin. *N Engl J Med* 1974;**291:**265.

Erffmeyer JE: Adverse reactions to penicillin. *Ann Allergy* 1981; **47:**288.

Finegold SM et al: Comparative trial of bacampicillin and amoxicillin in bacterial infections of the lower respiratory tract. *Rev Infect Dis* 1981;**3:**150.

Nolan CM, Abernathy RS: Nephropathy associated with methicillin therapy. *Arch Intern Med* 1977;**137:**997.

Parker CS: Drug allergy. (3 parts.) *N Engl J Med* 1975;**292:**511, 732, 957.

CEPHALOSPORINS

Cephalosporins and cephamycins are β-lactam drugs related to penicillins. In place of 6-aminopenicillanic acid, they have a nucleus of 7-aminocephalosporanic acid. Their mode of action is similar to that of penicillins; there is limited cross allergenicity; and they are resistant to β-lactamases in varying degrees. New semisynthetic derivatives are appearing in profusion, with the cost of each successive "generation" higher than the last, but the claims for individual advantages are not always well established.

Antimicrobial Activity

The mechanism of action of cephalosporins is analogous to that described for penicillins. The bacterial receptors are similar or identical to penicillin-binding proteins, but different drugs may bind to different penicillin-binding proteins. Cephalosporins resist inactivation by β-lactamases in varying degrees. Resistance to cephalosporins may be a function of the absence of receptors, of permeability of bacteria, and of the type and amount of β-lactamases produced. Resistance can emerge during therapy and may not be easily detected in vitro. Enterococci and methicillin-resistant staphylococci are virtually always resistant to cephalosporins.

The earlier cephalosporins were active against gram-positive and some gram-negative bacteria, including *Escherichia coli, Klebsiella* sp, and *Proteus* sp, but not against more resistant bacteria. Subsequent cephalosporins had somewhat broader activity against gram-negative organisms (including *Haemophilus* sp and *Enterobacter*) and anaerobes (eg, *Bacteroides*). The latest cephalosporins are active against many enteric bacteria, including *Pseudomonas* sp, *Serratia* sp, and anaerobes, and they tend to reach the central nervous system, although their activity against gram-positive pathogens is greatly reduced. There are substantial differences between individual drugs, and testing for the susceptibility of individual isolates is particularly important, since resistance to drugs is emerging with excessive drug use.

Absorption, Distribution, & Excretion

Cephalexin, cephradine, cefadroxil, and cefaclor are absorbed from the gut to a limited extent, and therapeutic urine levels are reached after oral doses. Concentrations in other tissues are variable and usually low. Most other cephalosporins are not significantly absorbed from the gut. After parenteral (usually intravenous) injection, they are distributed widely in tissues, and 40–80% of drug in serum is protein-bound. The earlier cephalosporins do not reach the central nervous system and cerebrospinal fluid in significant concentration after intravenous dosage and are ineffective in meningitis. However, moxalactam, cefotaxime, cefuroxime, cefoperazone, and perhaps other newer cephalosporins do reach the central nervous system and can be effective in meningitis caused by gram-negative rods.

The serum half-life of cephalosporins ranges from 1 to 2.5 hours with normal renal function and from 16 to 30 hours in renal failure. Excretion is primarily by tubular excretion and to some extent by the liver. Cefoperazone is excreted largely into the bile.

**Indications, Dosages, & Routes
of Administration**

A. Oral: Cephalexin or cephradine, 0.5 g orally 4 times daily (30 mg/kg/d), can be used in urinary or respiratory tract infections and some soft tissue infections due to susceptible organisms. Urine levels reach

50–500 μg/mL. Cefadroxil (1 g every 12 hours) has similar indications. Cefaclor may be beneficial in otitis media because of its activity against *H influenzae*.

B. Intravenous: Typically, a portion of the daily dose is added as a bolus every 4–8 hours to an intravenous infusion. Cefazolin, 4 g/d (50–100 mg/kg/d) has been used for surgical prophylaxis because it gives high and prolonged serum levels. Cephalothin, 6–12 g/d (50–200 mg/kg/d) yields somewhat lower serum levels but is highly resistant to destruction by staphylococcal β-lactamases. Cephapirin (4–10 g/d) is similar. Cefamandole (6–12 g/d) and cefuroxime (5–9 g/d) are often active against *Klebsiella, Enterobacter,* and some anaerobes, with varying efficacy. They do not reach the central nervous system and are used for similar indications. Cefoxitin (3–12 g/d) is particularly effective against *Bacteroides fragilis* and in mixed anaerobic infections. It (as well as cefuroxime) is an effective alternative drug for β-lactamase-producing *Neisseria gonorrhoeae* infections.

Cefotaxime (4–12 g/d; 50–200 mg/kg/d), ceftizoxime (4–12 g/d), moxalactam (4–12 g/d), and cefoperazone (6–12 g/d) are newer cephalosporins that are reported to have broader spectrum and greater clinical efficacy. All of them can be effective against a variety of gram-negative enteric rods and against anaerobes to varying degrees. They should be considered mainly in hospital-acquired infections due to bacteria likely to be resistant to other less expensive drugs. *None* of them should be used in gram-positive coccal infections, and *none* are suitable for surgical prophylaxis. It is important to note, however, that these newer drugs are effective in the treatment of meningitis due to gram-negative enteric bacteria or to *H influenzae*, with or without sepsis. None of the earlier cephalosporins were appropriate for central nervous system infections.

C. Intramuscular: Cefazolin, 0.5–1 g every 4 hours, provides adequate levels for treating less ill patients for the same indications or for surgical (24-hour) prophylaxis. Cephapirin, 1 g every 4–6 hours, is equivalent, although it produces somewhat lower levels in serum.

Adverse Effects

A. Allergy: Cephalosporins are sensitizing, and a variety of hypersensitivity reactions occur, including anaphylaxis, fever, skin rashes, nephritis, granulocytopenia, and hemolytic anemia. The frequency of cross-allergy between cephalosporins and penicillins is unsettled (6–18%). Persons with documented penicillin hypersensitivity are 4 times more likely to react to a cephalosporin than persons without such a history; however, many tolerate a cephalosporin without reaction.

B. Toxicity: Local pain after intramuscular injection or thrombophlebitis after intravenous injection can occur. Several newer cephalosporins can cause hypoprothrombinemia requiring vitamin K administration, and disulfiramlike effects. Cephaloridine is nephrotoxic and is no longer used.

C. Superinfection: Several of the newer cephalosporins have diminished activity against gram-positive organisms, particularly·enterococci and staphylococci. Consequently, superinfection with such organisms may occur during treatment of gram-negative bacterial infections.

Landesman SH et al: Past and current roles for cephalosporin antibiotics in treatment of meningitis. *Am J Med* 1981;**71**: 693.

Neu HC: The new β-lactamase-stable cephalosporins. *Ann Intern Med* 1982;**97**:408.

Petz LD: Immunologic cross-reactivity between penicillins and cephalosporins: A review. *J Infect Dis* 1978;**137(Suppl)**:S74.

Rahal JJ: Moxalactam therapy for gram-negative bacillary meningitis. *Rev Infect Dis* 1982;**4**:606.

Swedish Study Group: Cefuroxime versus ampicillin and chloramphenicol in the treatment of bacterial meningitis. *Lancet* 1982;**1**:295.

Yu VL: Enterococcal superinfection after therapy with moxalactam. *Ann Intern Med* 1981;**94**:784.

ERYTHROMYCIN GROUP
(Macrolides)

The erythromycins are a group of closely related compounds characterized by a macrocyclic lactone ring to which sugars are attached. There are several different members of the group.

Erythromycins inhibit protein synthesis and are bacteriostatic or bactericidal for gram-positive organisms—especially pneumococci, streptococci, and corynebacteria—in concentrations of 0.02–2 μg/mL. Chlamydiae, mycoplasmas, *Legionella*, and *Campylobacter* are also susceptible. Activity is enhanced at alkaline pH. There is complete cross-resistance among all members of the erythromycin group. Absorption of these drugs varies greatly. Basic erythromycins are destroyed by stomach acids. Erythromycin stearate is acid-resistant. The propionyl ester of erythromycin (erythromycin estolate) is among the best-absorbed oral preparations. Oral doses of 2 g/d result in blood levels of up to 2 μg/mL, and there is wide distribution of the drug in all tissues except the central nervous system. Erythromycins are excreted largely in bile; only 5% of the dose is excreted into the urine.

Erythromycins are drugs of choice in corynebacterial infections (diphtheria, diphtheroid sepsis, erythrasma); in respiratory, genital, or ocular chlamydial infections; and in pneumonias caused by *Mycoplasma* and *Legionella* (see Chapter 7). The erythromycins are useful as substitutes for penicillin in persons with streptococcal and pneumococcal infections who are allergic to penicillin. In rheumatic persons taking penicillin, erythromycin can be given prior to dental procedures as prophylaxis.

Dosages

A. Oral: Erythromycin base, stearate, succinate, or estolate, 0.5 g every 6 hours (for children, 40 mg/kg/d). A combination of erythromycin and sulfisoxazole is available for acute otitis media in children. Sometimes erythromycin is given orally together with neomycin for preoperative preparation of the colon.

B. Intravenous: Erythromycin lactobionate or gluceptate, 0.5 g every 12 hours.

Adverse Effects

Nausea, vomiting, and diarrhea may occur after oral intake. Erythromycins, particularly the estolate, can produce acute cholestatic hepatitis (fever, jaundice, impaired liver function), probably as a hypersensitivity reaction. Most patients recover from this, but hepatitis recurs if the drug is re-administered.

Ginsburg CM, Eichenwald HF: Erythromycin: Review of its uses in pediatrics. *J Pediatr* 1976;**89**:872.

TETRACYCLINE GROUP

The tetracyclines are a large group of drugs with common basic chemical structures, antimicrobial activity, and pharmacologic properties. Microorganisms resistant to this group show extensive cross-resistance to all tetracyclines.

Antimicrobial Activity

Tetracyclines are inhibitors of protein synthesis and are bacteriostatic for many gram-positive and gram-negative bacteria. They are strongly inhibitory for the growth of mycoplasmas, rickettsiae, chlamydiae, and some protozoa (eg, amebas). Equal concentrations of all tetracyclines in blood or tissue have approximately equal antimicrobial activity. However, there are great differences in the susceptibility of different strains of a given species of microorganism, and laboratory tests are therefore important. Because of the emergence of resistant strains, tetracyclines have lost some of their former usefulness. *Proteus* and *Pseudomonas* are regularly resistant; among coliform bacteria, *Bacteroides,* pneumococci, staphylococci, streptococci, shigellae, and vibrios, strains resistant to tetracyclines are increasingly common.

Absorption, Distribution, & Excretion

Tetracyclines are absorbed somewhat irregularly from the gut. Absorption is limited by the low solubility of the drugs and by chelation with divalent cations, eg, Ca^{2+} or Fe^{2+}. A large proportion of orally administered tetracycline remains in the gut lumen, modifies intestinal flora, and is excreted in feces. With full systemic doses (2 g/d), levels of active drug in serum reach 5–8 μg/mL. The drugs are widely distributed in tissues and body fluids, but the levels in central nervous system, cerebrospinal fluid, and joint fluids are only 3–10% of serum levels. Tetracyclines are specifically deposited in growing bones and teeth, bound to calcium.

Absorbed tetracyclines are excreted mainly in bile and urine. Up to 20% of oral doses may appear in the urine after glomerular filtration. Urine levels may be 5–50 μg/mL or more. With renal failure, doses of tetracyclines must be reduced or intervals between doses increased. Up to 80% of an oral dose appears in the feces.

Demeclocycline, methacycline, minocycline, and doxycycline are well absorbed from the gut but are excreted more slowly than other drugs in the tetracycline group. This may lead to accumulation and prolonged blood levels. Renal clearance ranges from 9 mL/min for minocycline to 90 mL/min for oxytetracycline. Doxycycline does not accumulate greatly in renal failure and can be used in uremia. Minocycline appears in respiratory secretions.

Indications, Dosages, & Routes of Administration

At present, tetracyclines are drugs of choice in cholera, mycoplasmal pneumonia, and chlamydial and rickettsial infections. They may be used in various susceptible bacterial infections and in amebiasis. Minocycline is effective for chemoprophylaxis of meningococcal disease (200 mg daily for 5 days).

A. Oral: Tetracycline hydrochloride and oxytetracycline are dispensed in 250-mg capsules. Give 0.25–0.5 g orally every 6 hours (for children, 20–40 mg/kg/d). In acne vulgaris, 0.25 g once or twice daily for many months is prescribed by dermatologists. Tetracycline hydrochloride, 2 g/d orally for 7 days, can eradicate acute gonorrhea and also be effective against chlamydial infections. Doxycycline, 100 mg twice daily, can accomplish the same effect. Usually, however, chlamydial infections are treated for longer periods (eg, 14 days). A single 200-mg dose of doxycycline may stop the shedding of vibrios in cholera, and a single 2.5-g dose of tetracycline hydrochloride may control enteric infection due to *Shigella.* Doxycycline, 200 mg once weekly, is effective prophylaxis against leptospirosis.

Demeclocycline and methacycline are long-acting tetracyclines available in capsules containing 50 or 150 mg. Give 0.15–0.3 g orally every 6 hours (for children, 12–20 mg/kg/d). Doxycycline and minocycline are available in capsules containing 50 or 100 mg or as powder for oral suspension. Give doxycycline, 100 mg every 12 hours on the first day and 100 mg/d for maintenance. Give minocycline, 200 mg for the first dose and then 100 mg every 12 hours.

B. Intramuscular or Intravenous: Several tetracyclines (eg, rolitetracycline) are formulated for intramuscular or intravenous injection. Give 0.1–0.5 g every 6–12 hours in individuals unable to take oral medication (for children, 10–15 mg/kg/d).

C. Topical: Topical tetracycline, 1%, in ointment, can be applied to conjunctival infections.

Adverse Effects

A. Allergy: Hypersensitivity reactions with fever or skin rashes are uncommon.

B. Gastrointestinal Side Effects: Gastrointestinal side effects, especially diarrhea, nausea, and anorexia, are common. These can be diminished by reducing the dose or by administering tetracyclines with food or carboxymethylcellulose, but sometimes they force discontinuance of the drug. After a few days of oral use, the gut flora is modified so that drug-resistant bacteria and yeasts become prominent. This may cause functional gut disturbances, anal pruritus, and even enterocolitis with shock and death.

C. Bones and Teeth: Tetracyclines are bound to calcium deposited in growing bones and teeth, causing fluorescence, discoloration, enamel dysplasia, deformity, or growth inhibition. Therefore, tetracyclines should not be given to pregnant women or children under age 6 years.

D. Liver Damage: Tetracyclines can impair hepatic function or even cause liver necrosis, particularly during pregnancy, in the presence of preexisting liver damage, or with doses of more than 3 g intravenously.

E. Kidney Damage: Outdated tetracycline preparations have been implicated in renal tubular acidosis and other forms of renal damage. Tetracyclines may increase blood urea nitrogen when diuretics are administered.

F. Other: Tetracyclines, principally demeclocycline, may induce photosensitization, especially in blonds. Intravenous injection may cause thrombophlebitis, and intramuscular injection may induce local inflammation with pain. Minocycline induces vestibular reactions (dizziness, vertigo, nausea, vomiting), with a frequency of 35–70% after doses of 200 mg daily. Demeclocycline inhibits antidiuretic hormone.

Barza M, Schiefe RT: Antimicrobial spectrum, pharmacology and therapeutic use of antibiotics. 1. Tetracyclines. *Am J Hosp Pharm* 1977;**34**:49.

Pickering LK et al: Single-dose tetracycline therapy for shigellosis in adults. *JAMA* 1978;**239**:853.

CHLORAMPHENICOL

Chloramphenicol is a potent inhibitor of bacterial protein synthesis; in concentrations of 0.5–10 μg/mL, it inhibits the growth of many bacteria and rickettsiae. Resistant strains of organisms produce an enzyme that inactivates the drug. This enzyme is under control of a transmissible plasmid. There is no cross-resistance with other drugs.

After oral administration, chloramphenicol is rapidly and completely absorbed. Administration of 2 g/d orally to adults results in blood levels of 5–10 μg/mL. In children, chloramphenicol palmitate, 50 mg/kg/d orally, is hydrolyzed in the gut to yield free chloramphenicol and gives a blood level of 10 μg/mL. Chloramphenicol succinate, 25–50 mg/kg/d intramuscularly or intravenously, yields free chloramphenicol by hydrolysis and gives blood levels comparable to those achieved by oral administration. After absorption, chloramphenicol is widely distributed to all tissues, including the eye and the central nervous system, where drug levels are similar to serum levels. It penetrates cells readily. Chloramphenicol is metabolized either by conjugation with glucuronic acid in the liver or by reduction to inactive aryl amines. In hepatic insufficiency, the drug may accumulate to toxic levels. Only 10% of active drug is excreted into the urine.

Because of its potential toxicity, chloramphenicol is at present a possible drug of choice only in the following cases: (1) Symptomatic *Salmonella* infection, eg, typhoid fever (some strains in Central and South America are now resistant). (2) *H influenzae* meningitis, laryngotracheitis, or pneumonia that does not respond to ampicillin. Initial therapy of childhood bacterial meningitis consists of both ampicillin and chloramphenicol. The latter is discontinued if the causative *Haemophilus* organism fails to produce β-lactamase. (3) Meningococcal infection in patients hypersensitive to penicillin. (4) Anaerobic or mixed infections in the central nervous system, eg, brain abscess. (5) Severe rickettsial infections. (6) It is occasionally used topically in ophthalmology (0.5% solution) but is not effective in chlamydial infections.

In serious systemic infection, give 0.5 g orally every 4–6 hours (for children, 30–50 mg/kg/d) for 7–21 days. Similar amounts are given intravenously.

Adverse Effects

Nausea, vomiting, and diarrhea occur infrequently. The most serious adverse effects pertain to the hematopoietic system. Adults taking chloramphenicol in excess of 50 mg/kg/d regularly exhibit disturbances in red cell maturation after 1–2 weeks of blood levels above 25 μg/mL. There is anemia, rise in serum iron concentration, reticulocytopenia, and the appearance of vacuolated nucleated red cells in the bone marrow. These changes regress when the drug is stopped and are not related to the rare aplastic anemia.

Serious aplastic anemia is a rare consequence of chloramphenicol administration and represents a specific, probably genetically determined individual defect. It is seen more frequently with prolonged or repeated use. It tends to be irreversible. It has been estimated that fatal aplastic anemia occurs in one of 25–40 thousand courses of chloramphenicol treatment. Hypoplastic anemia may be followed by the development of leukemia.

Chloramphenicol inhibits the metabolism of certain drugs. Thus, it may prolong the action and raise blood concentration of tolbutamide, phenytoin, chlorpropamide, and warfarin sodium (Coumadin).

Chloramphenicol is specifically toxic for newborns, particularly premature infants. Because they lack the mechanism for detoxification of the drug in the liver, the drug may accumulate, producing the highly fatal "gray syndrome," with vomiting, flaccidity, hypothermia, and collapse. Chloramphenicol should rarely be used in infants, and the dose should be limited to less than 50 mg/kg/d in full-term infants and less than 30 mg/kg/d in prematures. Serum levels should be monitored if possible.

Gump DW: Chloramphenicol: A 1981 view. *Arch Intern Med* 1981; **141**:573.

AMINOGLYCOSIDES

Aminoglycosides are a group of bactericidal drugs sharing chemical, antimicrobial, pharmacologic, and toxic characteristics. At present, the group includes streptomycin, neomycin, kanamycin, amikacin, gentamicin, tobramycin, sisomicin, netilmicin, and others. All these agents inhibit protein synthesis in bacteria by attaching to and inhibiting the function of the 30S subunit of the bacterial ribosome. Resistance is based on (1) a deficiency of the ribosomal receptor (chromosomal mutant); (2) the enzymatic destruction of the drug (plasmid-mediated transmissible resistance of clinical importance) by acetylation, phosphorylation, or adenylylation; or (3) a lack of permeability to the drug molecule or failure of active transport across cell membranes. The last-named form of resistance can be chromosomal (eg, streptococci are relatively impermeable to aminoglycosides), or it may be plasmid-mediated (clinically significant resistance among gram-negative enteric bacteria). Anaerobic bacteria are often resistant to aminoglycosides because transport across the cell membrane is an oxygen-dependent energy-requiring process.

All aminoglycosides are more active at alkaline than at acid pH. All are potentially ototoxic and nephrotoxic, though to different degrees. All can accumulate in renal failure; therefore, dosage adjustments must be made in uremia.

Aminoglycosides are used most widely against gram-negative enteric bacteria or when there is a suspicion of sepsis. In the treatment of bacteremia or endocarditis caused by fecal streptococci or by some gram-negative bacteria, the aminoglycoside is given together with a β-lactam drug to enhance permeability and facilitate the entry of the aminoglycoside. Aminoglycosides are selected according to recent susceptibility patterns in a given area or hospital until susceptibility tests become available on a specific isolate. All (positively charged) aminoglycosides and polymyxins are inhibited in blood cultures by sodium polyanetholesulfonate and other polyanionic detergents. Some aminoglycosides (especially streptomycin) are useful as antimycobacterial drugs.

Streptomycin is the oldest of the aminoglycosides, and its pharmacologic properties are very well known. Neomycin is now limited to topical use, and kanamycin is used mainly in small children. Among the newer aminoglycosides, gentamicin, tobramycin, and amikacin are preferred, whereas sisomicin, netilmicin, and others are not as well established.

General Properties of Aminoglycosides

Because of the similarities of the aminoglycosides, a summary of properties is presented briefly before each drug is taken up individually for a discussion of its main clinical uses.

A. Physical Properties: Aminoglycosides are water-soluble and stable in solution. If they are mixed in solution with β-lactam antibiotics, they may form complexes and lose some activity.

B. Absorption, Distribution, Metabolism, and Excretion: Aminoglycosides are well absorbed after intramuscular or intravenous injection, but they are not absorbed from the gut. They are distributed widely in tissues and penetrate into pleural, peritoneal, or joint fluid in the presence of inflammation. Except in small infants, they diffuse poorly into the eye, prostate, bile, central nervous system, or spinal fluid after parenteral injection. For treatment of central nervous system infection of adults, they must be injected intrathecally or intraventricularly.

There is no significant metabolic breakdown of aminoglycosides. The serum half-life is 2–3 hours. Excretion is almost entirely by glomerular filtration. Some representative mean blood or tissue concentrations following commonly used doses are shown in Table 29–1. Urine levels usually are 10–50 times higher. The protein binding level is below 10% for all aminoglycosides except streptomycin (35%). Aminoglycosides are removed fairly effectively by hemodialysis but irregularly by peritoneal dialysis.

C. Dose and Effect of Impaired Renal Function: In persons with normal renal function, the dose of kanamycin or amikacin is 15 mg/kg/d; that for gentamicin or tobramycin is 3–7 mg/kg/d, usually injected in 3 equal amounts every 8 hours.

In persons with impaired renal function, excretion is diminished and there is the danger of drug accumulation with increased side effects. Therefore, if the interval is kept constant, the dose has to be reduced, or the interval must be increased if the dose is kept constant (see Table 29–3). Nomograms have been constructed relating serum creatinine levels to adjustments of treatment regimens. One widely used formula uses a multiplication factor (kanamycin or amikacin = 9, gentamicin = 8, tobramycin = 6) times the serum creatinine value (mg/dL) to give the interval between doses in hours. However, there is considerable variation in aminoglycoside levels in different patients with similar creatinine values. Therefore, it is highly desirable to monitor drug levels in blood whenever possible to avoid severe toxicity when renal functional capacity is rapidly changing.

D. Adverse Effects: All aminoglycosides can cause varying degrees of ototoxicity and nephrotoxicity. Ototoxicity can present either as hearing loss (cochlear damage) that is noted first with high-frequency tones, or as vestibular damage, evident by vertigo, ataxia, and loss of balance. Nephrotoxicity is evident with rising serum creatinine levels or reduced creatinine clearance.

In very high doses, aminoglycosides can be neurotoxic, producing a curarelike effect with neuromuscular blockade that results in respiratory paralysis. Neostigmine can be an antidote to this reaction. Rarely, aminoglycosides cause hypersensitivity and local reactions.

Table 29—4. Drug selection, 1984—1985.

Suspected or Proved Etiologic Agent	Drug(s) of First Choice	Alternative Drug(s)
Gram-negative cocci		
Gonococcus	Penicillin,[1] ampicillin, tetracycline[2]	Spectinomycin, cefoxitin
Meningococcus	Penicillin[1]	Chloramphenicol, sulfonamide
Gram-positive cocci		
Pneumococcus *(Streptococcus pneumoniae)*	Penicillin[1]	Erythromycin,[3] cephalosporin[4]
Streptococcus, hemolytic groups A, B, C, G	Penicillin[1]	Erythromycin,[3] cephalosporin[4]
Streptococcus viridans	Penicillin[1] + aminoglycoside(?)[5]	Cephalosporin,[4] vancomycin
Staphylococcus, nonpenicillinase-producing	Penicillin[1]	Cephalosporin,[4] vancomycin
Staphylococcus, penicillinase-producing	Penicillinase-resistant penicillin[6]	Vancomycin, cephalosporin[4]
Streptococcus faecalis (enterococcus)	Ampicillin + aminoglycoside[5]	Vancomycin
Gram-negative rods		
Acinetobacter (Mima-Herellea)	Aminoglycoside[5]	Minocycline
Bacteroides (except *B fragilis*)	Penicillin,[1] chloramphenicol	Clindamycin, cephalosporin[4]
Bacteroides fragilis	Metronidazole, clindamycin	Cefoxitin, chloramphenicol
Brucella	Tetracycline[2] + streptomycin	Streptomycin + sulfonamide[7]
Enterobacter	Aminoglycoside,[5] new cephalosporin[8]	Chloramphenicol
Escherichia		
Escherichia coli sepsis	Aminoglycoside[5]	New cephalosporin,[8] ampicillin
Escherichia coli urinary infection (first attack)	Sulfonamide,[9] TMP-SMX[10]	Ampicillin, cephalosporin[4]
Haemophilus (meningitis, respiratory infections)	Chloramphenicol + ampicillin	New cephalosporin[8]
Klebsiella	New cephalosporin,[8] aminoglycoside[5]	Chloramphenicol
Legionella pneumophila (pneumonia)	Erythromycin[3]	Tetracycline,[2] rifampin
Pasteurella (Yersinia) (plague, tularemia)	Streptomycin, tetracycline[2]	Sulfonamide,[7] chloramphenicol
Proteus		
Proteus mirabilis	Ampicillin	New cephalosporin,[8] aminoglycoside[5]
Proteus vulgaris and other species	Aminoglycoside[5]	Chloramphenicol
Pseudomonas		
Pseudomonas aeruginosa	Aminoglycoside[5] + ticarcillin	New cephalosporin,[8] polymyxin
Pseudomonas pseudomallei (melioidosis)	Tetracycline,[2] TMP-SMX[10]	Chloramphenicol
Pseudomonas mallei (glanders)	Streptomycin + tetracycline[2]	Chloramphenicol
Salmonella	Chloramphenicol, ampicillin	TMP-SMX[10]
Serratia, Providencia	Aminoglycoside[5]	TMP-SMX[10] + polymyxin
Shigella	TMP-SMX,[10] chloramphenicol	Ampicillin, tetracycline[2]
Vibrio (cholera)	Tetracycline[2]	TMP-SMX[10]
Gram-positive rods		
Actinomyces	Penicillin[1]	Tetracycline[2]
Bacillus (eg, anthrax)	Penicillin[1]	Erythromycin
Clostridium (eg, gas gangrene, tetanus)	Penicillin[1]	Tetracycline,[2] cephalosporin[4]
Corynebacterium	Erythromycin	Penicillin,[1] cephalosporin[4]
Listeria	Ampicillin + aminoglycoside[5]	Tetracycline[2]
Acid-fast rods		
Mycobacterium tuberculosis	INH + rifampin, INH + ethambutol[11]	Other antituberculosis drugs
Mycobacterium leprae	Dapsone + rifampin, clofazimine	Amithiozone
Mycobacteria, atypical	Rifampin + ethambutol + INH	Combinations
Nocardia	Sulfonamide[7]	Minocycline
Spirochetes		
Borrelia (relapsing fever)	Tetracycline[2]	Penicillin[1]
Leptospira	Penicillin[1]	Tetracycline[2]
Treponema (syphilis, yaws)	Penicillin[1]	Erythromycin, tetracycline[2]
Mycoplasma	Tetracycline[2]	Erythromycin
Chlamydia trachomatis, Chlamydia psittaci	Tetracycline[2]	Erythromycin
Rickettsiae	Tetracycline[2]	Chloramphenicol

[1] Penicillin G is preferred for parenteral injection; penicillin V for oral administration. Only highly sensitive microorganisms should be treated with oral penicillin.

[2] All tetracyclines have similar activity against microorganisms and comparable therapeutic activity and toxicity. Dosage is determined by the rates of absorption and excretion of different preparations.

[3] Erythromycin estolate is the best-absorbed oral form but carries greatest risk of hepatitis. Also erythromycin stearate, erythromycin ethylsuccinate.

[4] Cefazolin, cephapirin, cephalothin, cefamandole, and cefoxitin are older parenteral cephalosporins; cephalexin and cephradine the best oral forms.

[5] Aminoglycoside: Gentamicin, tobramycin, amikacin, netilmicin, selected by local pattern of susceptibility.

[6] Parenteral nafcillin or oxacillin. Oral dicloxacillin, cloxacillin, or oxacillin.

[7] Trisulfapyrimidines and sulfisoxazole have the advantage of greater solubility in urine over sulfadiazine for oral administration; sodium sulfadiazine is suitable for intravenous injection in severely ill persons.

[8] New cephalosporins (1984): Cefotaxime, moxalactam, cefoperazone, cefuroxime, etc.

[9] For previously untreated urinary tract infection, a highly soluble sulfonamide such as sulfisoxazole or trisulfapyrimidines is the first choice. TMP-SMX[10] is acceptable.

[10] TMP-SMX is a mixture of 1 part trimethoprim + 5 parts sulfamethoxazole.

[11] Either or both.

1. STREPTOMYCIN

Streptomycin is bactericidal for both gram-positive and gram-negative bacteria. However, resistance emerges so rapidly and has become so widespread that only a few specific indications for this drug remain. Serum levels reach 20 μg/mL when 0.5 g is injected intramuscularly every 6–8 hours (20–40 mg/kg/d).

Principal indications for streptomycin at present are (1) plague and tularemia; (2) endocarditis caused by *S faecalis* or *Streptococcus viridans,* used in conjunction with a penicillin; (3) serious active tuberculosis, used with other antituberculosis drugs; (4) acute brucellosis, used with tetracycline.

Streptomycin exhibits all the adverse effects typically associated with the aminoglycosides. It should not be given concurrently with other aminoglycosides, because excessive ototoxicity may occur. Dihydrostreptomycin is no longer used, because of severe ototoxicity.

2. NEOMYCIN & KANAMYCIN

These aminoglycosides are closely related, with similar activity and complete cross-resistance. The related paromomycin is used in amebiasis. These drugs are stable and are not absorbed from the gut. They are now severely limited in systemic use because of oto- and nephrotoxicity.

Neomycin is now limited to topical and oral use. Ointments containing 1–5 mg/g neomycin, often combined with bacitracin and polymyxin, can be applied to infected superficial skin lesions. The drug mixture covers most staphylococci and gram-negative bacteria likely to be present, but the efficacy of such topical treatment is in doubt. Solutions of neomycin, 1–5 mg/mL, have been used for irrigation of infected joints or wounds. The total amount of drug must be kept below 15 mg/kg/d, because absorption can lead to systemic toxicity.

In preparation for elective bowel surgery, 1 g of neomycin or kanamycin is given orally every 4–6 hours for 1–2 days (often combined with erythromycin) to reduce aerobic bowel flora. Action on gram-negative anaerobes is negligible. In hepatic coma, the coliform bacteria can be suppressed for prolonged periods by oral neomycin or kanamycin, 1 g every 6–8 hours, during reduced protein intake. This results in diminished ammonia production and intoxication. Similar doses of neomycin or kanamycin may suppress invasive enteropathogenic *Escherichia coli* but not other enteric pathogens.

Kanamycin is somewhat less toxic than neomycin. It is used for the same indications and in the same doses as neomycin for topical application and oral intake. In addition, kanamycin, 15–20 mg/kg/d, continues to be given intramuscularly or intravenously to newborns with suspected sepsis. Intrathecal or intraventricular doses of 10–20 mg/d have been used in gram-negative bacillary meningitis.

In addition to oto- and nephrotoxicity, which can result from systemic absorption of neomycin or kanamycin, these drugs can give rise to allergic reactions when applied topically to skin or eye. Respiratory arrest has followed the instillation of 3–5 g of neomycin or kanamycin into the peritoneal cavity after colonic surgery; this can be overcome by neostigmine.

3. AMIKACIN

Amikacin is a semisynthetic derivative of kanamycin. It is relatively resistant to several of the enzymes that inactivate gentamicin and tobramycin and therefore can be employed against some microorganisms resistant to these drugs. However, bacterial resistance due to impermeability to amikacin is increasing. Many gram-negative enteric bacteria—including many strains of *Proteus, Pseudomonas, Enterobacter,* and *Serratia*—are inhibited by 1–20 μg/mL of amikacin in vitro. After the injection of 500 mg amikacin intramuscularly every 12 hours (15 mg/kg/d), peak levels in serum are 10–30 μg/mL. Some infections caused by gram-negative bacteria resistant to gentamicin respond to amikacin. Central nervous system infections require intrathecal or intraventricular injection of 1–10 mg daily.

Like all aminoglycosides, amikacin is nephrotoxic and ototoxic (particularly for the auditory portion of the eighth nerve). Its levels should be monitored in patients with renal failure.

Meyer RD: Drugs five years later: Amikacin. *Ann Intern Med* 1981;**95**:328.

Sarubbi FA, Hull JH: Amikacin serum concentrations: Prediction of levels and dosage guidelines. *Ann Intern Med* 1978; **89**:612.

4. GENTAMICIN

Gentamicin is a widely used aminoglycoside antibiotic. In concentrations of 0.5–5 μg/mL, gentamicin is bactericidal not only for staphylococci and coliform organisms but also for many strains of *Pseudomonas, Proteus,* and *Serratia.* Enterococci are resistant. With doses of 3–7 mg/kg/d, serum levels reach 3–8 μg/mL. Gentamicin may be synergistic with carbenicillin or ticarcillin against *Pseudomonas.* However, the 2 drugs cannot be mixed in vitro because they inactivate each other. Sisomicin resembles the C1a component of gentamicin.

Indications, Dosages, & Routes of Administration

Gentamicin is used in severe infections caused by gram-negative bacteria. Included are sepsis, infected burns, pneumonia, and other serious infections due to coliform organisms, *Klebsiella-Enterobacter, Proteus, Pseudomonas,* and *Serratia.* The dosage is 3–7 mg/kg/d intramuscularly (or intravenously) in 3 equal doses for 7–10 days. In urinary tract infections caused by these organisms, 0.8–1.2 mg/kg/d is given intramuscularly for 10 days or longer. In renal failure, the suggested dose is 1 mg/kg intramuscularly every (8 × serum creatinine level in milligrams per deciliter) hours. However, serum levels should be monitored by laboratory assay. About 2–3% of patients develop vestibular dysfunction and loss of hearing when peak serum levels exceed 10 μg/mL. For infected burns or skin lesions, creams containing 0.1% gentamicin are used. Such topical use should be restricted to avoid favoring the development of resistant bacteria in hospitals. In meningitis due to gram-negative bacteria, 1–10 mg of gentamicin have been injected daily intrathecally or intraventricularly in adults. However, in neonatal gram-negative bacillary meningitis the benefit of either of these routes is in doubt, and intraventricular gentamicin is toxic.

McCracken GH et al: Intraventricular gentamicin therapy in gram-negative bacillary meningitis of infants. *Lancet* 1980; **1**:787.

5. TOBRAMYCIN

Tobramycin is an aminoglycoside that greatly resembles gentamicin in antibacterial activity and pharmacologic properties and exhibits partial cross-resistance. Tobramycin may be effective against some gentamicin-resistant gram-negative bacteria, especially *Pseudomonas*. A daily dose of 3–5 mg/kg is given in 3 equal amounts intramuscularly at intervals of 8 hours. In uremia, the suggested dose is 1 mg/kg intramuscularly every (6 × serum creatinine level [in mg/dL]) hours. However, blood levels should be monitored. Tobramycin is somewhat less nephrotoxic than gentamicin, but the ototoxicity of the 2 is similar.

Smith CR et al: Double blind comparison of the nephrotoxicity and auditory toxicity of gentamicin and tobramycin. *N Engl J Med* 1980; **302**:1106.

6. NETILMICIN

Netilmicin became available in the USA in 1983. It shares many characteristics with gentamicin and tobramycin. However, it is expected that netilmicin will not be inactivated by many gentamicin-resistant and tobramycin-resistant bacteria.

The dosage (5–7 mg/kg/d) and the routes of administration are the same as for gentamicin. The principal indication for netilmicin may be iatrogenic infections in immunocompromised and severely ill patients at very high risk for gram-negative bacterial sepsis in the hospital setting.

Netilmicin may prove to be less ototoxic and possibly less nephrotoxic than the other aminoglycosides.

7. SPECTINOMYCIN

Spectinomycin is an aminocyclitol antibiotic (related to aminoglycosides) for intramuscular administration. Its sole application is in the treatment of gonococci producing β-lactamase or of persons with gonorrhea who are hypersensitive to penicillin. One injection of 2 g (40 mg/kg) is given. About 5–10% of gonococci are probably resistant. There is usually pain at the injection site, and there may be nausea and fever.

Rettig PJ et al: Spectinomycin therapy for gonorrhea in prepubertal children. *Am J Dis Child* 1980; **134**:359.

POLYMYXINS

The polymyxins are a group of basic polypeptides bactericidal for most gram-negative bacteria except *Proteus* and especially useful against *Pseudomonas*. Only 2 drugs are used: polymyxin B sulfate and colistin (polymyxin E) methanesulfonate.

Polymyxins are not absorbed from the gut. They are distributed in some tissues after parenteral injection, but they do not reach the central nervous system, cerebrospinal fluid, joints, or ocular tissues unless injected locally. Blood levels usually do not exceed 1–4 μg/mL. Polymyxins are excreted into the urine, where concentrations of 25–300 μg/mL may be reached. Excretion is impaired in renal insufficiency.

Indications, Dosages, & Routes of Administration

With the availability of other drugs, polymyxins are now only rarely indicated in serious infections due to gram-negative bacteria resistant to aminoglycosides. Polymyxins may be synergistic with trimethoprim-sulfamethoxazole against *Serratia*.

A. Intramuscular: The injection of polymyxin B is painful. Therefore, colistimethate, which contains a local anesthetic and is more rapidly excreted in the urine, has been given intramuscularly, 2.5–5 mg/kg/d, for urinary tract infection.

B. Intravenous: Polymyxin B sulfate, 2.5 mg/kg/d, can be injected by continuous intravenous infusion in gram-negative bacterial sepsis.

C. Intrathecal: In cases of confirmed *Pseudomonas* meningitis, administer polymyxin B sulfate, 2–10 mg once daily for 2–3 days and then every other day for 2–3 weeks.

D. Topical: Solutions of polymyxin B sulfate, 1 mg/mL, can be applied to infected surfaces; injected into joint spaces, intrapleurally, or subconjunctivally; or inhaled as aerosols. Ointments containing 0.5 mg/g polymyxin B sulfate in a mixture with neomycin or bacitracin are often applied to infected skin lesions. Solutions containing polymyxin B, 20 mg/L, and neomycin, 40 mg/L, can be used for continuous irrigation of the bladder with an indwelling catheter and a closed drainage system. Purulent exudates inactivate polymyxins.

Table 29—5. Examples of empiric choice of antimicrobials in acutely ill adults pending identification of causative organism.

Suspected Clinical Diagnosis	Likely Etiologic Agents	Drugs of Choice	Alternative Drugs
(a) Meningitis, bacterial	Pneumococcus, meningococcus	Penicillin G, 2 million units IV every 2 hours	Chloramphenicol, 0.5 g IV every 6 hours
(b) Meningitis, postoperative or posttraumatic	*Staphylococcus aureus,* pneumococcus, gram-negative bacteria	Penicillin G as in (a) + nafcillin, 1.5 g IV every 4 hours, + gentamicin,* 1.7 mg/kg IV every 8 hours	Vancomycin, 0.5 g IV every 6 hours, + moxalactam, 2 g IV every 4 hours
(c) Brain abscess	Mixed anaerobes, pneumococci, streptococci	Penicillin G as in (a) + chloramphenicol as in (a)	Chloramphenicol as in (a), or 0.5 g orally every 4 hours
(d) Pneumonia, acute, acquired in community, severe	Pneumococcus	Penicillin G, 1 million units IV every 8 hours	Erythromycin, 0.5 g orally 4 times daily
(e) Pneumonia, postoperative, or in chronic lung disease	Pneumococcus, *S aureus, Klebsiella,* mixed anaerobes	Nafcillin as in (b) + gentamicin* as in (b) + clindamycin	Cefotaxime,† 2 g IV every 4 hours, + gentamicin as in (b)
(f) Endocarditis, acute (including prosthetic or intravenous drug user)	*S aureus, Streptococcus faecalis,* gram-negative aerobic bacteria	Penicillin G as in (a) + nafcillin as in (b) + cefotaxime† as in (e)	Gentamicin* as in (b) + vancomycin as in (b)
(g) Septic thrombophlebitis (eg, intravenous tubing, intravascular shunts)	Same as (f)	Same as (f)	Same as (f)
(h) Intra-abdominal sepsis (eg, abortion, surgery)	*Bacteroides,* gram-negative bacteria, streptococci, clostridia	Gentamicin* as in (b) + clindamycin, 7 mg/kg IV every 6 hours, + penicillin G as in (a)	Cefotaxime† as in (f) + clindamycin, 7 mg/kg every 6 hours
(i) Osteomyelitis	*S aureus*	Nafcillin as in (b)	Vancomycin as in (b)
(j) Septic arthritis	*S aureus, Neisseria gonorrhoeae,* gram-negative bacteria	Nafcillin as in (b) + gentamicin* as in (b)	Cefotaxime† as in (f) + vancomycin as in (b)
(k) Urinary tract infection, first episode with little fever, acquired in community	*Escherichia coli*	Sulfisoxazole, 1 g orally 4 times daily for 1—3 days	Ampicillin, 0.5 g orally 4 times daily for 1—3 days
(l) Urinary tract infection, pyelonephritis, with flank pain (recurrent) and fever	*E coli, Proteus, Klebsiella, Pseudomonas, Enterobacter*	Prevailing aminoglycosides, eg, gentamicin* as in (b)	Prevailing cephalosporin, eg, cefotaxime, 2 g IV every 6 hours
(m) Suspected sepsis in granulocytopenic patients receiving cancer chemotherapy	*S aureus, Pseudomonas, Klebsiella, E coli*	Ticarcillin, 12 g IV daily, + gentamicin* as in (b)	Nafcillin as in (b) + amikacin, 7.5 mg/kg IM every 12 hours
(n) Acute cholecystitis	Enteric gram-negative and gram-positive aerobes and anaerobes	Ampicillin + tobramycin	Cefoxitin + gentamicin*
(o) Peritonitis (eg, perforated viscus)	Gram-negative enteric anaerobes and aerobes, streptococci, clostridia	Cefoxitin + tobramycin	Ticarcillin, amikacin, clindamycin

*Depending on local drug susceptibility patterns, use tobramycin, 5—7 mg/kg/d, or amikacin, 15 mg/kg/d, in place of gentamicin.
†Cefotaxime or moxalactam or cefoperazone, depending on drug susceptibility patterns.

Adverse Effects

The toxicities of polymyxin B and colistimethate are similar. With the usual blood levels there are paresthesias, dizziness, flushing, and incoordination. These disappear when the drug has been excreted. With unusually high levels, respiratory arrest and paralysis can occur. This may be reversible by administration of calcium gluconate. Depending upon the dose, all polymyxins are nephrotoxic. Kidney function must be monitored and the regimen adjusted (Table 29–3).

Davis SD: Polymyxins, colistin, vancomycin and bacitracin. In: Kagan BM (editor): *Antimicrobial Therapy,* 3rd ed. Saunders, 1980.

ANTITUBERCULOSIS DRUGS

Singular problems exist in the treatment of tuberculosis and other mycobacterial infections. They tend to be exceedingly chronic but may give rise to hyperacute lethal complications. The organisms are frequently intracellular, have long periods of metabolic inactivity, and tend to develop resistance to any one drug. Combined drug therapy is usually employed to delay the emergence of this resistance. "First-line" drugs, often employed together in tuberculous meningitis, miliary dissemination, or severe pulmonary disease, are isoniazid, ethambutol, rifampin, and streptomycin. A series of "second-line" drugs will be mentioned only briefly. Most patients become noninfectious within 2–4 weeks after effective drug therapy is instituted. In active pulmonary tuberculosis without complications, treatment schedules including isonia-zid and rifampin for 6–9 months are satisfactory.

Addington WW: Treatment of pulmonary tuberculosis: Current options. *Arch Intern Med* 1979;**139**:1391.

Dutt AK, Stead WW: Present chemotherapy for tuberculosis. *J Infect Dis* 1982;**146**:698.

Guidelines for short-course tuberculosis chemotherapy. (2 parts.) *MMWR* 1980;**29**:97, 183.

Lester TW: Drug-resistant and atypical mycobacterial disease: Bacteriology and treatment. *Arch Intern Med* 1979;**139**:1399.

1. ISONIAZID (INH)

Isoniazid is the hydrazide of isonicotinic acid (INH), the most active antituberculosis drug. Isoniazid in a concentration of 0.2 μg/mL or less inhibits and kills most tubercle bacilli. However, some "atypical" mycobacteria are resistant. In susceptible large populations of *Mycobacterium tuberculosis*, isoniazid-resistant mutants occur. Their emergence is delayed in the presence of a second drug. There is no cross-resistance between isoniazid, streptomycin, etham-butol, and rifampin.

Isoniazid is well absorbed from the gut and dif-fuses readily into all tissues, including the central nervous system, and into living cells. The inactivation of isoniazid—particularly its acetylation—is under genetic control. However, the speed of isoniazid acety-lation has little influence over the selection of drug regimens. Isoniazid and its conjugates are excreted mainly in the urine.

Indications, Dosages, & Routes of Administration

(See also Table 7–3.)

Isoniazid is the most widely used drug in tuber-culosis. It should not be given as the sole drug in active tuberculosis. This favors emergence of resistance (up to 30% in some countries). In active, clinically man-ifest disease, it is given in conjunction with rifampin or ethambutol. The initial dose is 8–10 mg/kg/d orally (up to 20 mg/kg/d in smaller children); later, the dos-age is reduced to 5–7 mg/kg/d. Dosage needs to be reduced only for very severe renal failure.

Children (or young adults) who convert from a negative to a positive tuberculin test but who have no evidence of an active lesion may be given 10 mg/kg/d (maximum: 300 mg/d) for 1 year as prophylaxis against the 5–15% risk of meningitis or miliary dis-semination. For this "prophylaxis," isoniazid is given as the sole drug. Such isoniazid prophylaxis is also indicated in adults with positive tuberculin test results who must be immunosuppressed by cancer chemo-therapy or for organ transplant.

Toxic reactions to isoniazid include insomnia, restlessness, fever, myalgia, hyperreflexia, and even convulsions and psychotic episodes. Some of these are attributable to a relative pyridoxine deficiency and peripheral neuritis and can be prevented by the admin-istration of pyridoxine, 100 mg/d. Isoniazid can induce hepatitis. Progressive liver damage occurs rarely in patients under age 20; in 1.5% of persons between 30 and 50 years of age; and in 2.5% of older individuals. The risk of hepatitis is greater in alcoholics and in rapid rather than in slow acetylators of isoniazid and is an important determinant in the prophylactic use of isoniazid. Isoniazid can reduce the metabolism of phenytoin, increasing its blood level and toxicity.

Wolinsky E: Nontuberculous mycobacteria and associated dis-eases. *Am Rev Respir Dis* 1979;**119**:107.

2. ETHAMBUTOL

This is a synthetic, water-soluble, heat-stable compound, dispensed as the hydrochloride.

Many strains of *M tuberculosis* and of "atypical" mycobacteria are inhibited in vitro by ethambutol, 1–5 μg/mL. The mechanism of action is not known.

Ethambutol is well absorbed from the gut. About 20% of the drug is excreted in feces and 50% in the urine, in unchanged form. Excretion is delayed in renal failure. About 15% of absorbed drug is metabolized by oxidation and conversion to a dicarboxylic acid. In meningitis, ethambutol appears in the cerebrospinal fluid.

Resistance to ethambutol emerges fairly rapidly among mycobacteria when the drug is used alone. Therefore, ethambutol, 15 mg/kg, is usually given as a single daily dose in combination with isoniazid.

Hypersensitivity to ethambutol occurs infre-quently. It may cause a rise in the serum uric acid. The commonest side effects are visual disturbances: reduc-tion in visual acuity, optic neuritis, and perhaps retinal damage occur in some patients receiving ethambutol, 25 mg/kg/d for several months. Most changes are reversible, but periodid visual acuity testing is manda-tory. With doses of 15 mg/kg/d, side effects are rare.

Doster B et al: Ethambutol in the initial treatment of pulmonary tuberculosis. *Am Rev Respir Dis* 1973;**107**:177.

3. RIFAMPIN

Rifampin is a semisynthetic derivative of rifamy-cin. Rifampin, 1 μg/mL or less, inhibits many gram-positive cocci, meningococci, and mycobacteria in vitro. Gram-negative organisms are often more resis-tant. Highly resistant mutants occur frequently in sus-ceptible microbial populations.

Rifampin binds strongly to DNA-dependent bacterial RNA polymerase and thus inhibits RNA synthesis in bacteria. Rifampin penetrates well into phagocytic cells and can kill intracellular organisms. Rifampin sometimes enhances the activity of am-photericin B against various fungi.

Rifampin given orally is well absorbed and widely distributed in tissues. It is excreted mainly through the liver and to a lesser extent in the urine.

With oral doses of 600 mg, serum levels exceed 5 μg/mL for 4–6 hours, and urine levels may be 3–20 times higher.

In the treatment of tuberculosis, a single oral dose of 600 mg (10–20 mg/kg) is given daily. In order to delay the rapid emergence of resistant microorganisms, combined treatment with isoniazid or ethambutol is required. Rifampin is effective for treatment of leprosy (see below). Rifampin, 600 mg twice daily for 2 days, can terminate the meningococcal carrier state, but strains with up to 10% resistance emerge. Close contacts of children with manifest *H influenzae* infection (eg, in family or day-care center) can receive rifampin, 20 mg/kg/d for 4 days, as prophylaxis. Occasionally, rifampin combined with trimethoprim-sulfamethoxazole can eradicate staphylococcal infections of bone, heart, or carriage sites. Rifampin should never be given alone in bronchial or urinary tract infections.

Rifampin imparts an orange color to urine and sweat. Occasional adverse effects include rashes, thrombocytopenia, impaired liver function, light chain proteinuria, and some impairment of immune response. In intermittent administration, rifampin must be given at least twice weekly to avoid a "flu syndrome," anemia, and other adverse affects. Rifampin increases the dose requirement for warfarin in anticoagulation and increases urinary methadone excretion.

Cox F et al: Rifampin prophylaxis for contacts of *Haemophilus influenzae* type B disease. *JAMA* 1981;**245**:1043.
Farr B, Mandell GL: Rifampin. *Med Clin North Am* 1982; **66**:157.

4. STREPTOMYCIN

The general pharmacologic features and toxicity of streptomycin are described above. Streptomycin, 1–10 μg/mL, is inhibitory and bactericidal for most tubercle bacilli, whereas most "atypical" mycobacteria are resistant. All large populations of tubercle bacilli contain some streptomycin-resistant mutants, which tend to emerge during prolonged treatment with streptomycin alone and result in "treatment resistance" within 2–4 months. Therefore, streptomycin is employed only in combination with another antituberculosis drug.

Streptomycin penetrates poorly into cells and exerts its action mainly on extracellular tubercle bacilli. Since at any moment 90% of tubercle bacilli are intracellular and thus unaffected by streptomycin, treatment for many months is required.

For combination therapy in tuberculous meningitis, miliary dissemination, and severe organ tuberculosis, streptomycin is given intramuscularly, 1 g daily (30 mg/kg/d for children) for weeks or months. This is followed by streptomycin, 1 g intramuscularly 2–3 times a week for months. In tuberculous meningitis, intrathecal injections (1–2 mg/kg/d) are sometimes given in addition.

Prolonged streptomycin treatment may impair vestibular function and result in inability to maintain equilibrium. Later, some compensation usually occurs, so that patients can function fairly well.

5. SHORT-COURSE THERAPY

For uncomplicated pulmonary tuberculosis, treatment for only 6–9 months can be satisfactory *provided that* both isoniazid and rifampin are administered. In adults, isoniazid, 300 mg, and rifampin, 600 mg, are given daily for 2–8 weeks, depending on the speed of sputum conversion and on the clinical and x-ray evidence of response. Subsequently, isoniazid, 15 mg/kg, and rifampin, 600 mg, can be given twice weekly. Ethambutol, 15 mg/kg/d, is given in addition if the patient resides in or has come from an area with a high level of initial drug resistance. Other regimens have been proposed.

6. ALTERNATIVE DRUGS IN TUBERCULOSIS TREATMENT

The drugs listed alphabetically below are usually considered only in cases of drug resistance (clinical or laboratory) to "first line" drugs and when expert guidance is available to deal with toxic side effects.

Aminosalicylic acid (PAS), closely related to p-aminobenzoic acid, inhibits most tubercle bacilli in concentrations of 1–5 μg/mL but has no effect on other bacteria. Resistant *M tuberculosis* will emerge rapidly unless another antituberculosis drug is present.

Aminosalicylic acid is readily absorbed from the gut. Doses of 8–12 g/d orally give blood levels of 10 μg/mL. The drug is widely distributed in tissues (except the central nervous system) and rapidly excreted into the urine. To avoid crystalluria, the urine should be kept alkaline.

Common side effects include anorexia, nausea, diarrhea, and epigastric pain. These may be diminished by taking the drug with meals and with antacids, but peptic ulceration may occur. Sodium aminosalicylate may be given parenterally. Hypersensitivity reactions include fever, skin rashes, granulocytopenia, lymphadenopathy, and arthralgias.

Capreomycin, 0.5–1.5 g/d intramuscularly, can perhaps substitute for streptomycin in combined therapy. It is nephrotoxic and ototoxic.

Cycloserine, 0.5–1 g/d orally, has been used alone or with isoniazid. It can induce a variety of central nervous system dysfunctions and psychotic reactions. These may be controlled by phenytoin, 100 mg/d orally. In smaller doses (15–20 mg/kg/d) it has been used in urinary tract infections.

Ethionamide, 0.5–1 g/d orally, has been used in combination therapy but produces marked gastric irritation.

Pyrazinamide, 0.75 g twice daily orally, has been used in combination therapy but may produce serious liver damage.

Viomycin, 2 g intramuscularly every 3 days, can occasionally substitute for streptomycin in combination therapy. It is nephrotoxic and ototoxic.

SULFONAMIDES & ANTIFOLATE DRUGS

Since the demonstration, in 1935, of the striking antibacterial activity of sulfanilamide, the molecule has been drastically altered in many ways. More than 150 different sulfonamides have been marketed at one time or another, the modifications being designed principally to achieve greater antibacterial activity, a wider antibacterial spectrum, greater solubility, or more prolonged action. Because of their low cost and their relative efficacy in some common bacterial infections, sulfonamides are still used widely. However, the increasing emergence of sulfonamide resistance (eg, among streptococci, gonococci, meningococci, and shigellae) and the higher efficacy of other antimicrobial drugs have curtailed the number of specific indications for sulfonamides as drugs of choice. The present indications for the use of these drugs can be summarized as follows:

(1) First (previously untreated) infection of the urinary tract: Many coliform organisms, which are the most common causes of urinary infections, are still susceptible to sulfonamides or to trimethoprim-sulfamethoxazole.

(2) *Chlamydia trachomatis* infections of eye and genital tract: Sulfonamides may effectively suppress clinical activity, particularly in acute infections. They are ineffective in psittacosis.

(3) Parasitic diseases: The combination of a sulfonamide with trimethoprim is often effective for prophylaxis and treatment of *Pneumocystis carinii* pneumonia in immunodeficient individuals. The combination is also sometimes effective in falciparum malaria. The combination of a sulfonamide with pyrimethamine is employed in the treatment of toxoplasmosis.

(4) Bacterial infections: Sulfonamides are the drugs of choice in nocardiosis. In underdeveloped parts of the world, sulfonamides, because of their availability and low cost, may still be useful for the treatment of pneumococcal or staphylococcal infections; bacterial sinusitis, bronchitis, or otitis media; bacillary *(Shigella)* dysentery; and meningococcal infections. In many developed countries, however, sulfonamide resistance of the respective etiologic organisms is widespread.

Trimethoprim-sulfamethoxazole is a choice in *Pneumocystis* pneumonia, *Shigella* enteritis, systemic *Salmonella* infections, *Serratia* sepsis, recurrent urinary tract infections, and many other infections.

(5) Leprosy: Certain sulfones are the drugs of choice in leprosy.

Antimicrobial Activity

The action of sulfonamides is bacteriostatic and is reversible upon removal of the drug or in the presence of an excess of *p*-aminobenzoic acid (PABA). Susceptible microorganisms require extracellular PABA in order to synthesize folic acid, an essential step in the formation of purines. Sulfonamides are structural analogs of PABA and can enter into the reaction in place of PABA, competing for the enzyme involved, so that nonfunctional analogs of folic acid are formed. As a result, further growth of the microorganism is inhibited. Animal cells and some sulfonamide-resistant microorganisms are unable to synthesize folic acid from PABA but depend on exogenous sources of preformed folic acid.

Trimethoprim, a substituted pyrimidine, is a folate antagonist. It inhibits dihydrofolate reductase of bacteria 50,000 times more efficiently than it inhibits the same enzyme of mammalian cells. In concentrations of 0.1–5 μg/mL it inhibits many gram-negative enteric bacteria found in urinary tract infections. A mixture of one part trimethoprim plus 5 parts sulfamethoxazole can result in sequential blocking of steps in the synthesis of purines. Some organisms carry plasmids that make them resistant to trimethoprim.

Pharmacologic Properties

The soluble sulfonamides are readily absorbed from the gut, distributed widely in tissues and body fluids, and excreted primarily by glomerular filtration into the urine. Varying amounts of sulfonamides are acetylated by the liver or bound to plasma protein. A portion of the drug in the urine is acetylated, but enough active drug remains in the urine to permit effective treatment of urinary tract infections (usually 10–20 times the concentration present in the blood). In order to be therapeutically effective for systemic therapy, a sulfonamide must achieve a concentration of 8–12 mg/dL of blood. This is accomplished by full systemic doses listed below.

"Long-acting" sulfonamides (eg, sulfamethoxypyridazine) are readily absorbed after oral intake, but excretion is very slow, resulting in prolonged blood levels. These compounds are more convenient but cause more toxic reactions than short-acting sulfonamides.

"Insoluble" sulfonamides (eg, phthalylsulfathiazole) are absorbed to only a slight extent after oral administration and are largely excreted in the feces. Their action is limited to temporary suppression of intestinal flora.

For parenteral (usually intravenous) administration, sodium salts of several sulfonamides are used because of their greater solubility. Their distribution and excretion are similar to those of the orally administered, absorbed sulfonamides. Trimethoprim concentrates by nonionic diffusion in prostatic and vaginal fluids, which are more acidic than serum.

Dosages & Routes of Administration

A. Topical: The application of sulfonamides to skin, wounds, or mucous membranes is undesirable because of the high risk of allergic sensitization or reaction and the low antimicrobial activity. Exceptions are the application of sodium sulfacetamide solution (30%) or ointment (10%) to the conjunctiva, and mafenide acetate cream (Sulfamylon) or silver sulfadiazine to control the flora of the burn wound.

B. Oral: For systemic disease, the soluble, rapidly excreted sulfonamides (eg, sulfadiazine, sulfisoxazole) are given in an initial dose of 2–4 g (40 mg/kg) followed by a maintenance dose of 0.5–1 g (20 mg/kg) every 4–6 hours. Trisulfapyrimidines USP may be given in the same total doses. Urine must be kept alkaline.

For urinary tract infections (first attack, not previously treated), trisulfapyrimidines or sulfisoxazole, highly soluble in urine, is given in somewhat lower doses than shown above. Following one course of sulfonamides, resistant organisms usually prevail. Trimethoprim, 100 mg orally every 12 hours, gives sufficiently high urine levels to inhibit organisms causing urinary tract infections. Simultaneous administration of sulfamethoxazole, 1600 mg/d orally, and trimethoprim, 320 mg/d orally (4 tablets), may be more effective in urinary tract infections than sulfonamide alone. Half a tablet of the combination 3 times weekly serves as prophylaxis for recurrent urinary tract infections in some women.

For "intestinal surgery prophylaxis," insoluble sulfonamides (eg, phthalylsulfathiazole), 8–15 g/d, are given for 5–7 days before operations on the bowel. Salicylazosulfapyridine (sulfasalazine), 6 g/d, has been given in ulcerative colitis. The drug is split in the gut to yield sulfapyridine and salicylate. The latter may have anti-inflammatory action.

C. Intravenous: Sodium sulfadiazine can be injected intravenously in 0.5% concentration in 5% dextrose in water or physiologic saline solution in a total dose of 6-8 g/d (120 mg/kg/d). This is reserved for comatose individuals or those unable to take oral medication. The intravenous form of trimethoprim-sulfamethoxazole contains 80 mg of trimethoprim and 400 mg of sulfamethoxazole per 5-mL ampule in 40% propylene glycol, to be diluted with 125 mL of 5% dextrose in water. Up to 5 such ampules are given in *Pneumocystis carinii* pneumonia or gram-negative bacterial sepsis caused by susceptible organisms.

Adverse Effects

Sulfonamides produce a wide variety of side effects—due partly to hypersensitivity, partly to direct toxicity—that must be considered whenever unexplained symptoms or signs occur in a patient who may have received these drugs. Except in the mildest reactions, fluids should be forced, and—if symptoms and signs progressively increase—the drugs should be discontinued. Precautions to prevent complications (below) are important.

A. Systemic Side Effects: Fever, skin rashes, urticaria; nausea, vomiting, or diarrhea; stomatitis, conjunctivitis, arthritis, exfoliative dermatitis; bone marrow depression, thrombocytopenia, hemolytic (in G6PD deficiency) or aplastic anemia, granulocyto-

penia, leukemoid reactions; hepatitis, polyarteritis nodosa, vasculitis, Stevens-Johnson syndrome; psychosis; and many others.

Trimethoprim can evoke similar side effects. It may precipitate folate deficiency.

Application of mafenide to burns may cause severe pain.

B. Urinary Tract Disturbances: Sulfonamides may precipitate in urine, especially at neutral or acid pH, producing hematuria, crystalluria, or even obstruction. They have also been implicated in various types of nephritis and nephrosis. Sulfonamides and methenamine salts should not be given together.

Precautions in the Use of Sulfonamides

(1) There is cross-allergenicity among all sulfonamides. Obtain a history of past administration or reaction. Observe for possible allergic responses.

(2) Keep the urine volume above 1500 mL/d by forcing fluids. Check urine pH—it should be 7.5 or higher. Give alkali by mouth (sodium bicarbonate or equivalent, 5–15 g/d). Examine fresh urine for crystals and red cells every 2–4 days.

(3) Check hemoglobin, white blood cell count, and differential count once weekly to detect possible disturbances early in high-risk patients.

Lawson DH, Jick H: Adverse reactions to co-trimoxazole in hospitalized medical patients. *Am J Med Sci* 1978;**275**:53.

Rubin RH, Swartz MN: Trimethoprim-sulfamethoxazole. *N Engl J Med* 1980;**303**:426.

Towner KJ et al: Increasing importance of plasmid-mediated trimethoprim resistance in enterobacteria. *Br Med J* 1980; **280**:517.

SULFONES USED IN THE TREATMENT OF LEPROSY

A number of drugs closely related to the sulfonamides (eg, dapsone; diaminodiphenylsulfone, DDS) have been used effectively in the long-term treatment of leprosy. The clinical manifestations of both lepromatous and tuberculoid leprosy can often be suppressed by treatment extending over several years. It appears that 5–30% of *Mycobacterium leprae* organisms are resistant to dapsone in 1984. Consequently, initial combined treatment with rifampin is advocated (see p 969).

Absorption, Metabolism, & Excretion

All of the sulfones are well absorbed from the intestinal tract, are distributed widely in all tissues, and tend to be retained in skin, muscle, liver, and kidney. Skin involved by leprosy contains 10 times more drug than normal skin. Sulfones are excreted into the bile and reabsorbed by the intestine. Consequently, blood levels are prolonged. Excretion into the urine is variable, and the drug occurs in urine mostly as a glucuronic acid conjugate. Some persons acetylate sulfones slowly and others rapidly, and this requires dosage adjustment.

Adverse Effects

The sulfones may cause any of the side effects listed above for sulfonamides. Anorexia, nausea, and vomiting are common. Hemolysis, methemoglobinemia, or agranulocytosis may occur. If sulfones are not tolerated, clofazimine or amithiozone can be substituted.

SPECIALIZED DRUGS AGAINST BACTERIA

1. BACITRACIN

This polypeptide antibiotic is selectively active against gram-positive bacteria, including penicillinase-producing staphylococci, in concentrations of 0.1–20 units/mL. Bacitracin is absorbed to only a slight extent from gut, skin, wounds, or mucous membranes. Topical application results in local effects without significant toxicity. Bacitracin, 500 units/g in ointment base, is often combined with polymyxin or neomycin for the suppression of mixed bacterial flora in surface lesions. Systemic administration of bacitracin has been abandoned because of its severe nephrotoxicity.

2. LINCOMYCIN & CLINDAMYCIN

These drugs resemble erythromycin (although different in structure) and are active against gram-positive organisms (except enterococci). Lincomycin, 0.5 g orally every 6 hours (30–60 mg/kg/d for children), or clindamycin, 0.15–0.3 g orally every 6 hours (10–40 mg/kg/d for children) yields serum concentrations of 2–5 μg/mL. The drugs are widely distributed in tissues. Excretion is through the bile and urine. The drugs are alternatives to erythromycin as substitutes for penicillin. Clindamycin is effective against most strains of *Bacteroides* and is a drug of choice in anaerobic infections, sometimes in combination with an aminoglycoside. Seriously ill patients are given clindamycin, 600 mg (20–30 mg/kg/d) intravenously during a 1-hour period every 8 hours. Success has also been reported in staphylococcal osteomyelitis. These drugs are ineffective in meningitis.

Common side effects are diarrhea, nausea, and skin rashes. Impaired liver function and neutropenia have been noted. If 3–4 g are given rapidly intravenously, cardiorespiratory arrest may occur. Bloody diarrhea with pseudomembranous colitis has been associated with clindamycin administration and has caused some fatalities. This appears to be due to a necrotizing toxin produced by *Clostridium difficile*. This organism is clindamycin-resistant and increases in the gut with the selection pressure exerted by administration of this drug. The organism is sensitive to vancomycin, and the colitis rapidly regresses during oral treatment with vancomycin (see below).

Bartlett JG: Anti-anaerobic antibacterial agents. *Lancet* 1982; **2**:478.

Larson HE et al: *Clostridium difficile* and the etiology of pseudomembranous colitis. *Lancet* 1978;**1**:1063.

3. METRONIDAZOLE

This is an antiprotozoal drug (see p 897) used for trichomonal and amebic infections. It also has striking antibacterial effects in anaerobic infections, in which the dose is 500–750 mg orally 3 or 4 times daily. In trichomoniasis and in *Gardnerella (Haemophilus)* vaginitis, 250 mg orally 3 times daily for 10 days is used. Metronidazole may also be effective for preparation of the colon before bowel surgery, though it has not yet been approved for this purpose because of possible carcinogenic effects. Metronidazole can be given intravenously (7.5 mg/kg in 1 hour 4 times daily), but this route is seldom needed, since similar doses given by rectal suppository are well absorbed and give therapeutically active levels. Simultaneous administration of barbiturates reduces the half-life of metronidazole. Metronidazole reaches high levels in brain tissue. In encapsulated anaerobic brain abscess, metronidazole is sometimes curative without surgical drainage.

Adverse effects including stomatitis, nausea, diarrhea, and vestibular reactions may occur with prolonged use of higher dosages.

Goldman P: Metronidazole. *N Engl J Med* 1980;**303**:1212.

Warner JF et al: Metronidazole therapy of anaerobic bacteremia, meningitis, and brain abscess. *Arch Intern Med* 1979; **139**:167.

4. VANCOMYCIN

This drug is bactericidal for most gram-positive organisms, particularly staphylococci and enterococci, in concentrations of 0.5–10 μg/mL. Resistant mutants are very rare, and there is no cross-resistance with other antimicrobial drugs. Vancomycin is not absorbed from the gut. It is given orally (2 g/d) only for the treatment of antibiotic-associated enterocolitis. For systemic effect the drug must be administered intravenously, and for meningitis intrathecally. After intravenous injection of 0.5 g over a period of 20 minutes, blood levels of 10 μg/mL are maintained for 1–2 hours. Vancomycin is excreted mainly via the kidneys but may accumulate also in liver failure. In renal insufficiency, the half-life may be up to 8 days. Thus, only one dose of 0.5–1 g may be given every 4–8 days to a uremic individual undergoing hemodialysis.

The only indications for parenteral vancomycin are serious staphylococcal infection or enterococcal endocarditis untreatable with penicillins. Vancomycin, 0.5 g, is injected intravenously over a 20-minute period every 6–8 hours (for children, 20–40 mg/kg/d). Against streptococci, synergism with an aminoglycoside can occur. Vancomycin, 0.5 g 4 times daily orally, is very effective in enterocolitis.

Vancomycin is irritating to tissues; chills, fever, and thrombophlebitis sometimes follow intravenous injection. The drug is somewhat ototoxic and perhaps nephrotoxic.

Tedesco F et al: Oral vancomycin for antibiotic-associated pseudomembranous colitis. *Lancet* 1978;**2**:226.
Wise RI: The Vancomycin Symposium: Summary and comments. *Rev Infect Dis* 1981;**3(Suppl)**:S293.

URINARY ANTISEPTICS

These drugs exert antimicrobial activity in the urine but have little or no systemic antibacterial effect. Their usefulness is limited to urinary tract infections.

1. NITROFURANTOIN

Nitrofurantoin is bacteriostatic and bactericidal for both gram-positive and gram-negative bacteria in concentrations of 10–500 μg/mL. The activity of nitrofurantoin is greatly enhanced at pH 6.5 or less.

Nitrofurantoin is rapidly absorbed from the gut. The drug is bound so completely to serum protein that it has no systemic antibacterial activity. In kidney tubules, the drug is separated from carrier protein and excreted in urine, where concentrations may be 200–400 μg/mL. In renal failure, there is virtually no excretion into the urine and no therapeutic effect.

The average daily dose in urinary tract infections is 100 mg orally 4 times daily (for children, 5–10 mg/kg/d), taken with food. If oral medication is not feasible, nitrofurantoin can be given by continuous intravenous infusion, 180–360 mg/d.

Oral nitrofurantoin often causes nausea and vomiting. Hemolytic anemia occurs in G6PD deficiency. Hypersensitivity may produce skin rashes and pulmonary infiltration.

2. NALIDIXIC ACID & OXOLINIC ACID

Nalidixic acid is a synthetic urinary antiseptic that inhibits many gram-negative bacteria in concentrations of 1–50 μg/mL but has no effect on *Pseudomonas*. In susceptible bacterial populations, resistant mutants emerge fairly rapidly.

Nalidixic acid is readily absorbed from the gut. In the blood, virtually all drug is firmly bound to protein. Thus, there is no systemic antibacterial action. About 20% of the absorbed drug is excreted in the urine in active form to give urine levels of 10–150 μg/mL, which may produce false-positive tests for glucose.

The dose in urinary tract infections is 1 g orally 4 times daily (for children, 30–60 mg/kg/d). Adverse reactions include nausea, vomiting, rash, drowsiness, visual hallucinations, excitement, and, rarely, increased intracranial pressure with convulsions.

Oxolinic acid is similar to nalidixic acid.

Brumfitt W, Hamilton-Miller JMT: Sulfonamides, nalidixic acid, oxolinic acid, methenamine and nitrofurans. In: *Antimicrobial Therapy,* 3rd ed. Kagan BM (editor): Saunders, 1980.

3. METHENAMINE MANDELATE & METHENAMINE HIPPURATE

These are salts of methenamine and mandelic acid or hippuric acid. The action of the drug depends on the liberation of formaldehyde and of acid in the urine and is enhanced by acetohydroxamic acid. The urinary pH must be below 5.5, and sulfonamides must not be given at the same time. The drug inhibits a variety of different microorganisms except those (eg, *Proteus*) that liberate ammonia from urea and produce strongly alkaline urine. The dosage is 2–6 g orally daily.

4. ACIDIFYING AGENTS

Urine with a pH below 5.5 tends to be antibacterial. Many substances can acidify urine and thus produce antibacterial activity. Ammonium chloride, ascorbic acid, methionine, and mandelic acid are sometimes used. The dose must be established for each patient by testing the urine for acid pH with test paper at frequent intervals.

SYSTEMICALLY ACTIVE DRUGS IN URINARY TRACT INFECTIONS

Many antimicrobial drugs are excreted in the urine in very high concentration. For this reason, low and relatively nontoxic amounts of aminoglycosides, polymyxins, and cycloserine (see above) can produce effective urine levels. Many penicillins, cephalosporins, aminoglycosides, and trimethoprim-sulfamethoxazole can reach very high urine levels and can thus be effective in urinary tract infections.

Jawetz E: Urinary antiseptics. Chapter 51 in: *Basic & Clinical Pharmacology,* 2nd ed. Katzung BG (editor). Lange, 1984.
Lohr JA et al: Prevention of recurrent urinary tract infections in girls. *Pediatrics* 1977;**59**:562.
Souney P, Polk BF: Single-dose therapy for urinary tract infections in women. *Rev Infect Dis* 1982;**4**:29.

ANTIFUNGAL DRUGS

Most antibacterial substances have no effect on pathogenic fungi. Only a few drugs are known to be therapeutically useful in mycotic infections. Penicillins are used to treat actinomycosis; sulfonamides have been employed in nocardiosis.

1. AMPHOTERICIN B

Amphotericin B, 0.1–0.8 μg/mL, inhibits in vitro several organisms producing systemic mycotic disease in humans, including *Histoplasma, Cryptococcus, Coccidioides, Candida, Blastomyces, Sporothrix,* and others. This drug can be used for treatment of these systemic fungal infections. Intrathecal administration is necessary for the treatment of meningitis.

Amphotericin B solutions in 500 mL 5% dextrose in water are given intravenously over a 4- to 8-hour period. The initial dose is 1–5 mg/d, increasing daily by 5-mg increments until a final dosage of 0.4–0.8 mg/kg/d (25–60 mg/d) is reached. This is usually continued daily or on alternate days for many weeks. In fungal meningitis, amphotericin B, 0.5 mg, is injected intrathecally 3 times weekly; continuous treatment (many weeks) with an Ommaya reservoir is sometimes employed. Relapses of fungal meningitis occur commonly. Combined treatment with flucytosine may be beneficial. Amphotericin B can also be effective in *Naegleria* meningoencephalitis.

Amphotericin B is 85% protein-bound and is little removed by hemodialysis.

In impaired renal function, the amphotericin dose need not be reduced initially. However, if the drug further depresses renal function, the amphotericin dose is temporarily lowered (or even stopped for a few days) until renal function returns to its pretreatment level.

The intravenous administration of amphotericin B usually produces chills, fever, vomiting, and headache. Tolerance may be enhanced by temporary lowering of the dose or administration of aspirin, diphenhydramine, phenothiazines, and corticosteroids. Therapeutically active amounts of amphotericin B commonly impair kidney and liver function and produce anemia (impaired iron utilization by bone marrow). Electrolyte disturbances (hypokalemia, distal tubular acidosis), shock, and a variety of neurologic symptoms also occur.

Drutz DJ, Catanzaro A: Coccidioidomycosis. *Am Rev Respir Dis* 1978;**117**:727.

Medoff G, Kobayashi GS: Strategies in the treatment of systemic fungal infections. *N Engl J Med* 1980;**302**:145.

2. GRISEOFULVIN

Griseofulvin is an antibiotic that can inhibit the growth of some dermatophytes but has no effect on bacteria or on the fungi that cause deep mycoses. Absorption of griseofulvin microsize, 1 g/d, gives blood levels of 0.5–1.5 μg/mL. The absorbed drug has an affinity for skin and is deposited there, bound to keratin. Thus, it makes keratin resistant to fungal growth, and the new growth of hair or nails is first free of infection. As keratinized structures are shed, they are replaced by uninfected ones. The bulk of ingested griseofulvin is excreted in the feces. Topical application of griseofulvin has little effect.

Give oral doses of 0.5–1 g/d (for children, 15 mg/kg/d) for 3–5 weeks if only the skin is involved and for 3–6 months or longer if the hair and nails are involved. Griseofulvin is most successful in severe dermatophytosis, particularly if caused by *Trichophyton rubrum*. Some strains of fungi are resistant.

An ultramicrosize particle formulation is better absorbed (Gris-PEG). The adult dose is 0.25–0.5 g orally daily.

Side effects include headache, nausea, diarrhea, photosensitivity, fever, skin rashes, and disturbances of hepatic, nervous, and hematopoietic systems. Griseofulvin increases the metabolism of coumarin anticoagulants, so that higher doses are needed. It is teratogenic and carcinogenic in rodents.

3. NYSTATIN

Nystatin inhibits *Candida* species upon direct contact. The drug is not absorbed from mucous membranes or gut. Nystatin in ointments, suspensions, etc, can be applied to buccal or vaginal mucous membranes to suppress a local *Candida* infection. After oral intake of nystatin, *Candida* in the gut is suppressed and the drug is excreted in feces. The only indication for the use of nystatin orally is in leukemic immunosuppression.

4. FLUCYTOSINE

5-Flucytosine inhibits some strains of *Candida, Cryptococcus, Aspergillus, Torulopsis,* and other fungi. Flucytosine is effectively removed during hemodialysis. Dosages of 3–8 g daily (150 mg/kg/d) orally have produced good serum (50 μg/mL) and cerebrospinal fluid levels and clinical remissions in cases of meningitis or sepsis. Resistant organisms may appear, and toxic effects (bone marrow depression, abnormal liver function, loss of hair) occur. The side effects may be caused by conversion of flucytosine to 5-fluorouracil in the body. The value of combined use of flucytosine and amphotericin B in *Candida* sepsis and cryptococcosis has been suggested.

Bennett JE et al: A comparison of amphotericin alone and combined with flucytosine in the treatment of cryptococcal meningitis. *N Engl J Med* 1979;**301**:126.

5. NATAMYCIN

Natamycin is a polyene antifungal drug effective against many different fungi in vitro. When combined with appropriate surgical measures, topical application of 5% ophthalmic suspension may be beneficial in the treatment of keratitis caused by *Fusarium, Cephalosporium,* or other fungi. The drug may also be effective in the treatment of oral or vaginal candidiasis. The toxicity after topical application appears to be low.

6. ANTIFUNGAL IMIDAZOLES

These antifungal drugs increase membrane permeability and inhibit lipid and enzyme synthesis. **Clotrimazole,** taken orally in 10-mg troches 5 times daily, can suppress oral candidiasis. It is too toxic for systemic use. **Miconazole** is used as a 2% cream in dermatophytosis and vaginal candidiasis. When used intravenously (30 mg/kg/d) it produced many serious side effects and was only moderately effective in controlling systemic mycoses.

Ketoconazole inhibits synthesis of sterols in fungal cell membranes, among other effects. It can be given orally in a single dose, 200–400 mg daily, preferably with food. It is well absorbed and reaches serum levels of 2–4 μg/mL, and it is degraded in vivo, requiring no renal or biliary excretion. Thus, the dose is unchanged in renal failure.

Ketoconazole dramatically improves chronic mucocutaneous candidiasis, vaginal candidiasis, and paracoccidioidomycosis. It also has therapeutic benefits in noncavitary pulmonary coccidioidomycosis and histoplasmosis but not in meningitis due to these fungi. In disease of moderate severity, this oral antifungal drug has given encouraging results.

Adverse effects include nausea, vomiting, skin rashes, and occasional elevations in transaminase levels. Ketoconazole blocks the synthesis of adrenal steroids and can cause gynecomastia.

Pont A et al: Ketoconazole blocks adrenal steroid synthesis. *Ann Intern Med* 1982;**97:**370.

Restrepo A, Stevens DA, Utz JP (editors): Symposium on ketoconazole. *Rev Infect Dis* 1980;**2:**519.

Ross JB et al: Ketoconazole for treatment of chronic pulmonary coccidioidomycosis. *Ann Intern Med* 1982;**96:**440.

ANTIMICROBIAL DRUGS USED IN COMBINATION

Indications

Possible reasons for employing 2 or more antimicrobials simultaneously instead of a single drug are as follows:

(1) Prompt treatment in desperately ill patients suspected of having a serious microbial infection. A good guess about the most probable 2 or 3 pathogens is made, and drugs are aimed at those organisms. Before such treatment is started, adequate specimens must be obtained for identifying the etiologic agent in the laboratory. Suspected gram-negative or staphylococcal sepsis and bacterial meningitis in children are the foremost indications in this category at present.

(2) To delay the emergence of microbial mutants resistant to one drug in chronic infections by the use of a second or third non–cross-reacting drug. The most prominent examples are active tuberculosis of one or more organs, with large microbial populations.

(3) Mixed infections, particularly those following massive trauma or those involving vascular structures. Each drug is aimed at an important pathogenic microorganism.

(4) To achieve bactericidal synergism (see below). In a few infections, eg, enterococcal sepsis, a combination of drugs is more likely to eradicate the infection than either drug used alone. Unfortunately, such synergism is unpredictable, and a given drug pair may be synergistic for only a single microbial strain. Occasionally, simultaneous use of 2 drugs permits significant reduction in dose and thus avoids toxicity but still provides satisfactory antimicrobial action.

Disadvantages

The following disadvantages of using antimicrobial drugs in combinations must always be considered:

(1) The doctor may feel that since several drugs are already being given, everything possible has been done for the patient. This attitude leads to relaxation of the effort to establish a specific diagnosis. It may also give a false sense of security.

(2) The more drugs are administered, the greater the chance for drug reactions to occur or for the patient to become sensitized to drugs.

(3) The cost is unnecessarily high.

(4) Antimicrobial combinations usually accomplish no more than an effective single drug.

(5) On very rare occasions, one drug may antagonize a second drug given simultaneously. Antagonism resulting in higher morbidity and mortality rates has been observed mainly in bacterial meningitis when a bacteriostatic drug (eg, tetracycline or chloramphenicol) was given with a bactericidal drug (eg, a penicillin or aminoglycoside). However, antagonism is usually limited by time-dose relationships and is overcome by an excess dose of one of the drugs in the pair and is therefore a very infrequent problem in clinical therapy.

Synergism

Antimicrobial synergism can occur in several types of situations. Synergistic drug combinations must be selected by complex laboratory procedures.

(1) Sequential block of a microbial metabolic pathway by 2 drugs. Sulfonamides inhibit the use of extracellular *p*-aminobenzoic acid by some microbes for the synthesis of folic acid. Trimethoprim or pyrimethamine inhibits the next metabolic step, the reduction of dihydro- to tetrahydrofolic acid. The simultaneous use of a sulfonamide plus trimethoprim is effective in some bacterial infections (eg, urinary tract, enteric) and in some parasitic infections (*Pneumocystis* infection, malaria). Pyrimethamine plus a sulfonamide is used in toxoplasmosis.

(2) One drug may greatly enhance the uptake of a second drug and thereby greatly increase the overall bactericidal effect. Penicillins enhance the uptake of aminoglycosides by enterococci. Thus, a penicillin plus an aminoglycoside may be essential for the eradication of *S faecalis* or *Streptococcus* group B infec-

tions, particularly in sepsis or endocarditis. Similarly, ticarcillin plus gentamicin may be synergistic against some strains of *Pseudomonas.* Cell wall inhibitors (penicillins and cephalosporins) may also enhance the entry of aminoglycosides into other gram-negative bacteria and thus produce synergistic effects.

(3) One drug may affect the cell membrane and facilitate the entry of the second drug. The combined effect may then be greater than the sum of its parts. Polymyxins have been synergistic with trimethoprim-sulfamethoxazole or rifampin against *Serratia,* and amphotericin has been synergistic with flucytosine against certain fungi.

(4) One drug prevents the inactivation of a second drug by microbial enzymes. Thus, inhibitors of β-lactamase (eg, clavulanic acid) can protect amoxicillin from inactivation by β-lactamase–producing *H influenzae* and other organisms.

Jawetz E: The doctor's dilemma. In: *Current Clinical Topics in Infectious Diseases.* Remington JS, Swartz MN (editors). McGraw-Hill, 1981.

Rahal JJ: Antibiotic combinations: The clinical relevance of synergy and antagonism. *Medicine* 1978;**57:**179.

ANTIMICROBIAL CHEMOPROPHYLAXIS

Anti-infective chemoprophylaxis implies the administration of antimicrobial drugs to prevent infection. In a broader sense, it also includes the use of antimicrobial drugs soon after the acquisition of pathogenic microorganisms (eg, after compound fracture) but before the development of signs of infection.

Useful chemoprophylaxis is limited to the action of a specific drug on a specific organism. An effort to prevent all types of microorganisms in the environment from establishing themselves as the cause of a resulting infection only selects the most drug-resistant organisms as the cause of a resulting infection. In all proposed uses of prophylactic antimicrobials, the risk of the patient's acquiring an infection must be weighed against the toxicity, cost, inconvenience, and enhanced risk of superinfection resulting from the "prophylactic" drug.

Prophylaxis in Persons of Normal Susceptibility Exposed to a Specific Pathogen

In this category, a specific drug is administered to prevent one specific infection. Outstanding examples are the prevention of reinfection with group A hemolytic streptococci in rheumatic patients; the injection of benzathine penicillin G, 1.2 million units intramuscularly once every 3–4 weeks; prevention of meningitis by eradicating the meningococcal carrier state with rifampin, 600 mg orally twice daily for 2 days, or minocycline, 100 mg every 12 hours for 5 days; prevention of *H influenzae* disease in contacts of patients with rifampin, 20 mg/kg/d for 4 days; prevention of syphilis by the injection of benzathine penicillin G, 2.4 million units intramuscularly, within 24 hours of expo-

sure; prevention of plague pneumonia with tetracycline, 0.5 g twice daily for 5 days, when exposed to infectious droplets; and prevention of clinical rickettsial disease (but not of infection) by the daily ingestion of 1 g of tetracycline during exposure.

Early treatment of an asymptomatic infection is sometimes called "prophylaxis." Thus, administration of isoniazid, 6–10 mg/kg/d (maximum, 300 mg daily) orally for 6–12 months, to an asymptomatic person who converts from a negative to a positive tuberculin skin test may prevent later clinical active tuberculosis.

Prophylaxis in Persons of Increased Susceptibility

Certain anatomic or functional abnormalities predispose to serious infections. It may be feasible to prevent or abort such infections by giving a specific drug for short periods. Some important examples are listed below:

A. Heart Disease: Persons with congenital or acquired abnormalities of the heart valves are unusually susceptible to implantation of microorganisms circulating in the bloodstream. This bacterial endocarditis can sometimes be prevented if the proper drug can be used during periods of bacteremia. Viridans streptococci enter the bloodstream from the upper respiratory tract. Large numbers of these organisms are pushed into the circulation during dental procedures and operations on the mouth or throat. At such times, the increased risk warrants the use of a prophylactic antimicrobial drug aimed at viridans streptococci, eg, an oral penicillin given one hour before and for one day after the procedure (see American Heart Association recommendations in Kaplan et al reference, 1977a, below). It may be that an aminoglycoside should be given together with penicillin for optimal bactericidal effect. In persons hypersensitive to penicillin or those receiving daily doses of penicillin for prolonged periods (for rheumatic fever prophylaxis), erythromycin, 2 g daily orally, can be substituted to cover penicillin-resistant viridans streptococci in the throat.

Enterococci cause 5–15% of cases of bacterial endocarditis. They reach the bloodstream from the urinary or gastrointestinal tract or from the female genital tract. During surgical procedures in these areas, persons with heart valve abnormalities can be given prophylaxis directed against enterococci, eg, penicillin G, 5 million units, plus gentamicin, 3 mg/kg intramuscularly daily, beginning on the day of surgery and continuing for 2 days.

During and after cardiac catheterization, blood cultures may be positive in 10–20% of patients. Many of these persons also have fever, but very few acquire endocarditis. Prophylactic antimicrobials do not appear to influence these events.

B. Respiratory Tract Disease: Persons with functional and anatomic abnormalities of the respiratory tract—eg, emphysema or bronchiectasis—are subject to attacks of "recurrent chronic bronchitis." This is a recurrent bacterial infection, often precipitated by acute viral infections and resulting in respiratory decompensation. The most common organisms are pneumococci and *H influenzae*. Chemoprophylaxis consists of giving tetracycline or ampicillin, 1 g daily orally, during the "respiratory disease season." This is successful only in patients who are not hospitalized; otherwise, superinfection with *Pseudomonas, Proteus,* or yeasts is common. Similar prophylaxis of bacterial infection has been applied to children with mucoviscidosis who are not hospitalized. In spite of this, such children contract complicating infections caused by *Pseudomonas* and staphylococci. Trimethoprim-sulfamethoxazole is effective as a prophylactic against *Pneumocystis* pneumonia in immunocompromised persons.

C. Recurrent Urinary Tract Infection: In certain women who are subject to frequently recurring urinary tract infections, the oral intake of nitrofurantoin, 200 mg, or trimethoprim (40 mg)–sulfamethoxazole (200 mg), daily or 3 times weekly, can markedly reduce the frequency of symptomatic recurrences over periods of many months—perhaps years—until resistant microorganisms appear.

Certain women frequently develop symptoms of cystitis after sexual intercourse. The ingestion of a single dose of antimicrobial drug (200 mg nitrofurantoin, 250 mg cephalexin, etc) can prevent this postcoital cystitis by early inhibition of growth of bacteria moved into the proximal urethra or bladder from the introitus during intercourse.

D. Opportunistic Infections in Severe Granulocytopenia: Patients with leukemia or neoplasm develop profound leukopenia while being given antineoplastic chemotherapy. When the neutrophil count falls below $500/\mu L$, they become unusually susceptible to opportunistic infections, most often gram-negative sepsis. In some cancer centers, such individuals are given a drug combination (eg, vancomycin, gentamicin, cephalosporin) directed at the most prevalent opportunists at the earliest sign—or even without clinical evidence—of infection. This is continued for several days until the granulocyte count rises again. Retrospective studies suggest that there is some benefit to this procedure.

In other centers, such patients are given oral insoluble antimicrobials (neomycin + polymyxin + nystatin) during the period of granulopenia to reduce the incidence of gram-negative sepsis. Some benefit has been reported from this approach.

Prophylaxis in Surgery

A major portion of all antimicrobial drugs used in hospitals is employed on surgical services with the stated intent of "prophylaxis." The administration of antimicrobials before and after surgical procedures is sometimes viewed as "banning the microbial world" both from the site of the operation and from other organ systems that suffer postoperative complications. Regrettably, the provable benefit of antimicrobial prophylaxis in surgery is much more limited.

Several general features of "surgical prophylaxis" merit consideration.

(1) In clean elective surgical procedures (ie, procedures during which no tissue bearing normal flora is traversed, other than the prepared skin), the disadvantages of "routine" antibiotic prophylaxis (allergy, toxicity, superinfection) generally outweigh the possible benefits.

(2) Prophylactic administration of antibiotics should generally be considered only if the expected rate of infectious complications approaches or exceeds 5%. An exception to this rule is the elective insertion of prostheses (cardiovascular, orthopedic), where a possible infection would have a catastrophic effect.

(3) If prophylactic antimicrobials are to be effective, a sufficient concentration of drug must be present at the operative site to inhibit or kill bacteria that might settle there. Thus, it is essential that drug administration begin 1–3 hours before operation.

(4) Prolonged administration of antimicrobial drugs tends to alter the normal flora of organ systems, suppressing the susceptible microorganisms and favoring the implantation of drug-resistant ones. Thus, antimicrobial prophylaxis should last only 1–3 days after the procedure to prevent superinfection.

(5) Systemic antimicrobial levels usually do not prevent wound infection, pneumonia, or urinary tract infection if physiologic abnormalities or foreign bodies are present.

In major surgical procedures, the administration of a "broad-spectrum" bactericidal drug from just before until 1 day after the procedure has been found effective. Thus, cefazolin, 1 g intramuscularly or intravenously given 2 hours before gastrointestinal, gallbladder, or orthopedic operations and again at 2, 10, and 18 hours after the end of the operation, results in a lowering of the risk of deep infections at the operative site. Similarly, in cardiovascular surgery, antimicrobials directed at the commonest organisms producing infection are begun just prior to the procedure and continued for 2 or 3 days thereafter. While this prevents drug-susceptible organisms from producing endocarditis, pericarditis, or similar complications, it may favor the implantation of drug-resistant bacteria or fungi.

Other forms of surgical prophylaxis attempt to reduce normal flora or existing bacterial contamination at the site. Thus, the colon is routinely prepared not only by mechanical cleansing through cathartics and enemas but also by the oral administration of insoluble drugs (eg, neomycin, 1 g, plus erythromycin base, 0.5 g, every 6 hours) for 1–2 days before operation. In the case of a perforated viscus resulting in peritoneal contamination, there is little doubt that immediate treatment with an aminoglycoside, a penicillin, or clindamycin reduces the impact of seeded infection. Similarly, grossly infected compound fractures or war wounds benefit from a penicillin or cephalosporin plus an aminoglycoside. In all these instances, the antimicrobials tend to reduce the likelihood of rapid and early invasion of the bloodstream and tend to help localize the infectious process—although they generally are incapable of preventing it altogether. The surgeon must be watchful for the selection of the most resistant members of the flora, which tend to manifest themselves 2 or 3 days after the beginning of such "prophylaxis"—which is really an attempt at very early treatment.

In all situations where antimicrobials are administered with the hope that they may have a "prophylactic" effect, the risk from these same drugs (allergy, toxicity, selection of superinfecting microorganisms) must be evaluated daily, and the course of prophylaxis must be kept as brief as possible.

Topical antimicrobials (intravenous tube site catheter, closed urinary drainage, within a surgical wound, acrylic bone cement, etc) may have limited usefulness but must always be viewed with suspicion.

Baum ML et al: A survey of clinical trials of antibiotic prophylaxis in colon surgery. *N Engl J Med* 1981;**305**:795.

Hughes WT et al: Successful chemoprophylaxis for *Pneumocystis carinii* pneumonitis. *N Engl J Med* 1977;**297**:1419.

Jackson GG: Considerations of antibiotic prophylaxis in nonsurgical high risk patients. *Am J Med* 1981;**70**:467.

Kaplan EL et al: AHA Committee Report: Prevention of bacterial endocarditis. *Circulation* 1977a;**56**:A139.

Kaplan EL et al: AHA Committee Report: Prevention of rheumatic fever. *Circulation* 1977b;**55**:S1.

Sandusky WR: Use of prophylactic antibiotics in surgical patients. *Surg Clin North Am* 1980;**60**:83.

Storring RA et al: Oral non-absorbed antibiotics prevent infection in acute non-lymphoblastic leukemia. *Lancet* 1977;**2**:837.

ANTIVIRAL CHEMOTHERAPY

Several compounds can influence viral replication and the development of viral disease.

Amantadine hydrochloride, 200 mg orally daily for 2–3 days before and 6–7 days after influenza A infection, reduces the incidence and severity of symptoms. It deserves wider use as a prophylactic in persons at high risk. The most marked untoward effects are insomnia, nightmares, and ataxia, especially in the elderly. Amantadine may accumulate and be more toxic in renal insufficiency. Rimantadine is equally effective and perhaps less toxic.

Idoxuridine, 0.1% solution or 0.5% ointment, can be applied topically every 2 hours to acute dendritic herpetic keratitis to enhance healing. It is also used, with corticosteroids, for stromal disciform lesions of the cornea to reduce the chance of acute epithelial herpes. Because of its toxicity for the cornea, it must not be used for more than 2–3 weeks. **Trifluridine** ointment (1%) is more effective than idoxuridine in herpetic keratitis but also more expensive.

Vidarabine (adenine arabinoside), 3% administered topically, is very effective in herpetic keratitis. Vidarabine, 15 mg/kg/d intravenously, provides systemic treatment for some herpesvirus infections. In immunocompromised patients it can reduce the dissemination of herpes zoster if begun before the

fifth day of the skin eruption. In herpes simplex encephalitis it can reduce the mortality rate significantly if begun before the patient becomes comatose and continued for 10 days. About 40% of the survivors of herpes simplex encephalitis may resume a normal life, while the remainder suffer major neurologic sequelae. In neonatal herpes it can limit the spread of lesions. However, the incidence of cytomegalovirus pneumonia in recipients of bone marrow transplants or kidney transplants has not been reduced by prophylactic vidarabine. Topical vidarabine likewise has no effect on local herpetic lesions of skin or mucous membranes.

The untoward effects of vidarabine include rashes, gastrointestinal disturbances, and neurologic abnormalities including tremors, ataxia, abnormal electroencephalogram, paresthesias, and encephalopathy. All these appear to be enhanced in the presence of renal failure.

Methisazone, 2–4 g orally given within 2 days after exposure to smallpox, protects against clinical disease. The drug is also effective against complications of vaccinia. The most serious toxic effect is profuse vomiting.

Photodynamic inactivation has been widely used as topical therapy for skin and mucous membrane lesions caused by herpes simplex in recent years. Controlled clinical studies have failed to show a significant benefit from this treatment. There is no justification for its use.

Acyclovir (acycloguanosine) has been effective against several herpesvirus infections in humans and is the least toxic antiviral drug. In herpes-infected cells, it is selectively active against viral DNA polymerase and thus inhibits virus proliferation. Given intravenously (15 mg/kg/d or 250 mg/m^2 every 8 hours), it can prevent or limit mucocutaneous herpes simplex in immunocompromised patients and can reduce pain and accelerate healing of herpes zoster and primary genital herpes simplex (in females), but it affects neither the establishment of latent infection nor the frequency of recurrence. Trials in herpetic encephalitis and in neonatal herpetic dissemination promise efficacy at least equal to that of vidarabine. There is no significant effect on cytomegalovirus or EB virus infections, but acyclovir can arrest the progression of varicella and herpes zoster in immunocompromised patients.

Oral acyclovir, 200 mg 5 times daily, has therapeutic effects similar to intravenous administration, particularly in primary genital herpes simplex infections.

Topical 5% acyclovir ointment can be applied to mucocutaneous lesions caused by herpes simplex virus. It can shorten the period of pain and viral shedding in mucocutaneous oral lesions in immunosuppressed persons but not in patients with normal immunity. It can also be of benefit in primary but not recurrent genital herpetic lesions by decreasing healing time of lesions and reducing pain.

Ribavirin aerosols sprayed into the respiratory tract early in influenza B infection of young adults or respiratory syncytial virus infections of small children resulted in a reduction of symptoms and more rapid recovery.

Human interferons have been prepared from stimulated lymphocytes or other cells and, more recently, by recombinant DNA technology. If given intravenously, 10^6–10^9 units daily prevented dissemination of early herpes zoster in immunocompromised patients, prevented or delayed reaction of herpes simplex after trigeminal root section, and suppressed viremia with hepatitis B virus. Interferons may have an adjunctive role in managing certain neoplasms or virus infections. Such preparations exhibit moderate antineoplastic and antiviral effects and, in high doses, significant toxicity. Possible practical use of this material is not yet evident.

Balfour HH et al: Acyclovir halts progression of herpes zoster in immunocompromised patients. *N Engl J Med* 1983;**308**:1448.

Bryson YB et al: Treatment of first episodes of genital herpes simplex virus infection with oral acyclovir. *N Engl J Med* 1983;**308**:916.

Corey L et al: A trial of topical acyclovir in genital herpes simplex virus infections. *N Engl J Med* 1982;**306**:1313.

Dolin R et al: A controlled trial of amantadine and rimantadine in the prophylaxis of influenza A infection. *N Engl J Med* 1982; **307**:580.

Hirsch MS, Schooley RT: Treatment of herpesvirus infections. (2 parts.) *N Engl J Med* 1983;**309**:963, 1034.

Kaufman RH et al: Treatment of genital herpes simplex infection with photodynamic inactivation. *Am J Obstet Gynecol* 1979; **132**:861.

McClung HW et al: Ribavirin aerosol treatment of influenza B infection. *JAMA* 1983;**249**:2671.

Reichman RC et al: Topically administered acyclovir in the treatment of recurrent herpes simplex genitalis. *J Infect Dis* 1983;**147**:336.

Reichman RC et al: Treatment of recurrent genital herpes simplex infections with oral acyclovir. *JAMA* 1984;**251**:2103.

Saral R et al: Acyclovir prophylaxis against herpes simplex infection in patients with leukemia. *Ann Intern Med* 1983;**99**:773.

Wade JC et al: Intravenous acyclovir to treat mucocutaneous herpes simplex virus infections after marrow transplantation. *Ann Intern Med* 1982;**96**:265.

Whitley RJ et al: Neonatal herpes simplex virus infection: Follow-up evaluation of vidarabine therapy. *Pediatrics* 1983;**72**:778.

●   ●   ●

References

Barrett SP, Watt PJ: Antibiotics and the liver. *J Antimicrob Chemother* 1979;**5**:337.

Blair JE, Lennette EH, Truant JP: *Manual of Clinical Microbiology*, 3rd ed. American Society of Microbiology, 1980.

Committee on Infectious Diseases: *Report*, 19th ed. American Academy of Pediatrics, 1982.

Grieco MH: Use of antibiotics in the elderly. *Bull NY Acad Med* 1980;**56**:197.

Handbook of Antimicrobial Therapy. Med Lett Drugs Ther, 1982.

Jawetz E, Melnick JL, Adelberg EA: *Review of Medical Microbiology*, 16th ed. Lange, 1984.

Kagan BM: *Antimicrobial Therapy*, 3rd ed. Saunders, 1980.

Katzung BG (editor): *Basic & Clinical Pharmacology*, 2nd ed. Lange, 1984.

Disorders Due to Physical Agents | 30

Milton J. Chatton, MD

DISORDERS DUE TO COLD

There is considerable individual variation in cold tolerance. Factors that increase the possibility of injury by exposure to cold include poor general physical condition, nonacclimatization, advanced age, systemic illness, anoxia, and use of alcohol and other sedative drugs. High wind velocity (the windchill factor) may markedly increase the severity of cold injury at low temperatures.

Cold Urticaria

Some persons have a familial or acquired hypersensitivity to cold and may develop urticaria upon even limited exposure to a cold wind. The urticaria usually occurs only on exposed areas, but in markedly sensitive individuals the response can be generalized. Immersion in cold water may result in severe systemic symptoms, including shock. Familial cold urticaria, manifested as a burning sensation of the skin occurring about 30 minutes after exposure to cold, does not seem to be a true urticarial disorder. In some patients with acquired cold urticaria, the disorder may be due to an underlying disease (eg, collagen disease, lymphoma, multiple myeloma) associated with cryoglobulinemia, which may result in purpura, Raynaud's phenomenon, and leg ulceration. Cold urticaria may also be associated with cold hemoglobinuria as a complication of syphilis. In the majority of cases of acquired cold urticaria, the cause cannot be determined. The diagnosis of cold urticaria can usually be confirmed by application of an ice cube to the skin. Histamine and other mediators released in the cold urticaria response are similar to those found in allergic reactions. Antihistamines, however, are of limited value in preventing or treating attacks of cold urticaria.

Raynaud's Phenomenon (See p 287.)

ACCIDENTAL SYSTEMIC HYPOTHERMIA

Accidental systemic hypothermia may result from exposure (atmospheric or immersion) to prolonged or extreme cold. The condition may arise in otherwise healthy individuals in the course of occupational or recreational exposure or in victims of accidents and other misfortunes. Acute alcoholism is commonly a predisposing cause.

Systemic hypothermia may follow exposure even to comparatively ordinary temperatures when there is altered homeostasis due to debility or disease. In colder climates, elderly and inactive individuals living in inadequately heated housing are particularly susceptible. Patients with cardiovascular or cerebrovascular disease, mental retardation, myxedema, and hypopituitarism are more vulnerable to accidental hypothermia. Sedative and tranquilizing drugs may be contributing factors. Administration of large amounts of refrigerated stored blood (without rewarming) can cause systemic hypothermia.

Clinical Findings

Early manifestations of hypothermia are not characteristic. There may be weakness, drowsiness, irritability, confusion, and impaired coordination. A lowered body temperature may be the sole finding.

The internal (core) body temperature in accidental hypothermia may range from 25 to 35 °C (77–95 °F). Oral temperatures are useless, so a special rectal thermometer that reads as low as 25 °C is required. At rectal temperatures below 35 °C, the patient may become delirious, may be drowsy or comatose, and may stop breathing. Metabolic acidosis, pneumonia, ventricular fibrillation, hypoglycemia or hyperglycemia, and renal failure may occur. Myocardial irritability and conduction defects are important hemodynamic effects of cold. A progression of electrocardiographic abnormalities includes the pathognomonic "J" waves of Osborn. Death in systemic hypothermia usually results from cardiac arrest or ventricular fibrillation.

Treatment

Patients with mild hypothermia (rectal temperature greater than 33 °C) who have been otherwise physically healthy usually respond well to a warm bed or to rapid rewarming with a warm bath or warm packs and blankets. A conservative approach is also usually employed in treating elderly or debilitated patients, using an electric blanket kept at 37 °C (98.6 °F).

Patients with moderate or severe hypothermia (core temperatures of less than 32 °C [89.6 °F]) do not have the thermoregulatory shivering mechanism and so require active rewarming with individualized supportive care. The methods and rate of active rewarming are controversial. Aggressive rewarming should be attempted only by those experienced in the methods. Cardiopulmonary resuscitation may be necessary. The need for oxygen therapy, endotracheal intubation, controlled ventilation, warmed intravenous fluids, and treatment of metabolic acidosis should be dictated by careful clinical, physiologic, and laboratory monitoring during the rapid rewarming process. It should be kept in mind that active rewarming is hazardous.

Active external rewarming methods. These are sometimes preferred when the hypothermia is of an acute nature (eg, sudden, brief immersion in cold water). Although relatively simple and generally available, active external warming methods may cause marked peripheral dilatation that predisposes to ventricular fibrillation and hypovolemic shock. Either heated blankets or warm baths may be used for active external rewarming. Rewarming by a warm bath is best carried out in a tub of stirred water at 40–42 °C (104–107.6 °F) with a rate of rewarming of about 1–2 °C/h. It is easier to monitor the patient and to carry out diagnostic and therapeutic procedures when heated blankets are used for active rewarming.

Active internal (core) rewarming methods. Internal rewarming is suggested for patients with profound hypothermia of long duration, but the indications or preferred methods are not clearly established. Repeated peritoneal dialysis may be employed with 2 L of warm (43 °C) potassium-free dialysate solution exchanged at intervals of 10–12 minutes until the rectal temperature is raised to about 35 °C. The administration of heated, humidified air through a face mask or endotracheal tube may be useful, either alone or as an adjunct to other rewarming techniques. Warm gastrointestinal irrigations and warm intravenous fluids are of some, but limited, value. Extracorporeal blood rewarming methods (eg, with femoral arteriovenous shunts) are effective but necessarily limited to medical centers.

Prognosis

With proper early care, more than 75% of otherwise healthy patients may survive moderate or severe systemic hypothermia. The risk of aspiration pneumonia is great in comatose patients. After obtaining at least one blood culture, consider use of antimicrobial drugs (see p 142). The prognosis is grave if there are underlying predisposing causes or treatment is delayed.

COLD INJURY OF THE EXTREMITIES

In the normal individual, exposure of the extremities to cold produces immediate localized vasoconstriction followed by generalized vasoconstriction. When the skin temperature falls to 25 °C (77

°F), tissue metabolism is slowed, but the demand for oxygen is greater than the slowed circulation can supply, and the area becomes cyanotic. At 15 °C (59 °F), tissue metabolism is markedly decreased and the dissociation of oxyhemoglobin is reduced; this gives a deceptive pink, well-oxygenated appearance to the skin. Tissue damage occurs at this temperature. Tissue death may be caused by ischemia and thromboses in the smaller vessels or by actual freezing. Freezing (frostbite) does not occur until the skin temperature drops to −10 to −4 °C (14–24.8 °F) or even lower, depending on such factors as wind, mobility, venous stasis, malnutrition, and occlusive arterial disease.

Prevention

"Keep warm, keep moving, and keep dry." Individuals should wear warm, dry clothing, preferably several layers, with a windproof outer garment. Wet clothing, socks, and shoes should be removed as soon as possible and replaced with dry ones. Extra socks, mittens, and insoles should always be carried in a pack when a person is in cold or icy areas. Cramped positions, constricting clothing, and prolonged dependency of the feet are to be avoided. Arms, legs, fingers, and toes should be exercised to maintain circulation. Wet and muddy ground and exposure to wind should be avoided. Good nutrition and skin cleanliness are necessary. Tobacco and alcohol should be avoided when the danger of frostbite is present.

CHILBLAIN
(Pernio)

Chilblains are red, itching skin lesions, usually on the extremities, caused by exposure to cold without actual freezing of the tissues. They may be associated with edema or blistering and are aggravated by warmth. With continued exposure, ulcerative or hemorrhagic lesions may appear and progress to scarring, fibrosis, and atrophy.

Treatment consists of elevating the affected part slightly and allowing it to warm gradually at room temperature. Do not rub or massage injured tissues or apply ice or heat. Protect the area from trauma and secondary infection.

FROSTBITE

Frostbite is injury of the superficial tissues due to freezing. In mild cases, the symptoms are numbness, prickling, and itching. With increasing severity, there may be paresthesia and stiffness. Thawing causes tenderness and burning pain. The skin is white or yellow, loses its elasticity, and becomes immobile. Edema, blisters, necrosis, and gangrene may appear.

Treatment

A. Immediate Treatment: Treat the patient for associated systemic hypothermia.

1. Rewarming—Superficial frostbite (frostnip) of extremities in the field can be treated by firm steady pressure with the warm hand (without rubbing), by placing fingers in the armpits, and, in the case of the toes or heels, by removing footwear, drying feet, rewarming, and covering with adequate dry socks or other protective footwear.

Rapid thawing at temperatures slightly above body heat may significantly decrease tissue necrosis. If there is any possibility of refreezing, the frostbitten part should not be thawed, even if this might mean prolonged walking on frozen feet. Refreezing results in increased tissue necrosis. It has been suggested that rewarming is best accomplished by immersing the frozen portion of the body for several minutes in water heated to 40–42 °C (104–107.6 °F) *(not warmer)*. This temperature range of the water feels warm but not hot to the normal hand. Dry heat (eg, stove or open fire) is more difficult to regulate and is not recommended. After thawing has occurred and the part has returned to normal temperature (usually in about 30 minutes), discontinue external heat. Never permit rewarming by exercise or thawing by rubbing with snow or ice water.

2. Protection of the part—Avoid trauma, eg, pressure or friction. Physical therapy is contraindicated in the early stage. Keep the patient at bed rest with the affected parts elevated and uncovered at room temperature. Do not apply casts, dressings, or bandages.

3. Anti-infective measures—Prevention of infection after the rewarming process is of great importance. Protect skin blebs from physical contact. Local infections may be treated with mild soaks of soapy water or povidone-iodine (Betadine). Whirlpool therapy at temperatures slightly below body temperature twice daily for 15–20 minutes for a period of 3 or more weeks helps cleanse the skin and debrides superficial sloughing tissue. Antibiotics may be required for deep infections.

4. Anticoagulants—Early administration of heparin for prevention of secondary thromboses is of questionable value.

B. Follow-Up Care: Gentle, progressive physical therapy to promote circulation is important as healing progresses. Buerger's exercises should be instituted as soon as tolerated. Vasodilating agents are of questionable value.

C. Surgery: Early regional sympathectomy (within 36–72 hours) has been reported to protect against the sequelae of frostbite, but the value of this measure is controversial. In general, other surgical intervention is to be avoided. *Amputation should not be considered until it is definitely established that the tissues are dead.* Tissue necrosis (even with black eschar formation) may be quite superficial, and *the underlying skin may sometimes heal spontaneously even after a period of months.*

Prognosis

Recovery from the frostbite injury is most often complete, but there may be increased susceptibility to discomfort in the involved extremity upon reexposure to cold.

IMMERSION SYNDROME
(Immersion Foot or Trench Foot)

Immersion foot (or hand) is caused by prolonged immersion in cool or cold water or mud. The affected parts are first cold and anesthetic. They become hot with intense burning and shooting pains during the hyperemic period and pale or cyanotic with diminished pulsations during the vasospastic period; blistering, swelling, redness, heat, ecchymoses, hemorrhage, or gangrene and secondary complications such as lymphangitis, cellulitis, and thrombophlebitis follow later.

Treatment is best instituted during the stage of reactive hyperemia. Immediate treatment consists of protecting the extremities from trauma and secondary infection and gradual rewarming by exposure to cool air (not ice or heat). Do not massage or moisten the skin or immerse the part in water. Bed rest is required until all ulcers have healed. Keep the affected parts elevated to aid in removal of edema fluid, and protect pressure sites (eg, heels) with pillows. Antibiotics should be used if infection develops. Later treatment is as for Buerger's disease (see p 285).

Bangs CC: Caught in the cold. *Emerg Med* (Dec 15) 1982;**14**:29.

Collins KJ, Exton-Smith AN, Doré C: Urban hypothermia: Preferred temperature and thermal perception in old age. *Br Med J* 1981;**282**:175.

Dembert ML: Medical problems from cold exposure. *Am Fam Physician* (Jan) 1982;**25**:99.

McCauley RL et al: Frostbite injuries: A rational approach based on the pathophysiology. *J Trauma* 1983;**23**:143.

Reed G: Emergency: Accidental hypothermia. *Hosp Med* (Feb) 1984;**20**:13.

Reuler JB: Hypothermia: Pathophysiology, clinical settings and management. *Ann Intern Med* 1978;**89**:519.

White JD: Hypothermia: The Bellevue experience. *Ann Emerg Med* 1982;**11**:417.

Wong KC: Physiology and pharmacology of hypothermia. *West J Med* 1983;**138**:227.

DISORDERS DUE TO HEAT

Exposure to excessive heat results in prompt peripheral vasodilatation, increased cardiac output, and sweating.

Fluid loss through sweating may amount to 3–4 L/h with heavy work at high temperatures. The salt content of sweat increases to 0.2–0.5% with rising temperatures.

Acclimatization usually results after 8–10 days of exposure to high temperatures, but even a fully acclimatized person may suffer a disorder in the event of excessive fatigue; severe infection; alcohol intoxication; use of belladonnalike drugs; or failure to maintain hydration, salt intake, or caloric intake. Elderly or obese persons and those with chronic debilitating diseases are most susceptible to disorders due to sustained climatic heat. Breakdown may be due to circulatory failure or failure of the sweating mechanism. Cessation of sweating may indicate stroke or collapse.

The 4 main physical disorders due to environmental heat stress are (in the order of increasing severity): heat syncope, heat cramps, heat exhaustion, and heat stroke.

Prevention

Avoid unnecessary exposure to heat and maintain adequate fluid and salt intake, using 0.1% saline as drinking water or salt tablets and water. Activity should be increased slowly until one is acclimatized. Clothing should be loose-fitting (preferably white) and permeable to moisture. Avoid alcoholic indulgence, excessive fatigue, and infections. Maintain good nutrition.

HEAT SYNCOPE

Simple fainting may occur suddenly after exertion in the heat. The patient's skin is cool and moist, the pulse is weak, and there is transient hypotension. The patient usually responds promptly to rest in a recumbent position, cooling, and liquids by mouth.

HEAT CRAMPS

Heat cramps are due primarily to salt depletion and are painful spasms of the voluntary (skeletal) muscles of the abdomen and extremities. The skin is moist and cool, and muscle twitchings may be present. The temperature is normal or only slightly increased. Laboratory studies reveal hemoconcentration and low serum sodium.

Sodium chloride, 1 g every 30–60 minutes with large amounts of water, or physiologic saline solution given by mouth or intravenously usually relieves the attack promptly. Place the patient in a cool place and massage sore muscles gently. Rest should be continued for 1–3 days depending upon the severity of the attack.

HEAT EXHAUSTION

Heat exhaustion is a systemic reaction to prolonged heat exposure (hours to days) and is due to sodium depletion, dehydration, or a combination of both of these factors.

When heat exhaustion is due predominantly to water depletion (usually when the water supply is inadequate), the patient complains of intense thirst and weakness and has marked central nervous system symptoms, including muscular incoordination, psy-

chosis, hyperthermia, delirium, and coma. If circulatory failure or major seizures occur, the condition may rapidly progress to heat stroke.

Individuals not acclimatized to heat may develop systemic symptoms of heat exhaustion predominantly as a result of salt depletion. This condition will occur when thermal sweating is replaced by an adequate intake of water but no salt. The patient complains of muscular cramps, as in the case of heat cramps, but there is also associated weakness, nausea, vomiting, and diarrhea. The patient is not thirsty, so administration of water without salt serves only to aggravate the symptoms. Pale skin, tachycardia, and hypotension are evident. The body temperature is usually not elevated. Serum sodium levels are low.

Initial treatment measures include placing the patient in a cool place and providing adequate cool water and salted fruit drinks or salt tablets according to the estimated relative water and salt depletion. If the patient is unable to take oral fluids or salt, administer either physiologic saline or isotonic glucose intravenously based upon clinical and laboratory findings. If there is marked hyponatremia with water intoxication, intravenous hypertonic saline may be required.

HEAT STROKE

Heat stroke is a *medical emergency* characterized by sudden loss of consciousness and by failure of the heat-regulating mechanism, as manifested by high fever and cessation of sweating. Heat stroke usually follows excessive exposure to heat or strenuous physical activity under hot atmospheric conditions, although the condition may develop in elderly, infirm, or otherwise susceptible individuals in the absence of unusual exposure to heat. In exertion-induced heat stroke, increased cardiac output and decreased systemic vascular resistance are normal circulatory adjustments to dissipate the heat load. In elderly patients, this fails to occur, and there is an unexplained decreased cardiac output and increased peripheral resistance. Cardiovascular disease, alcoholism, obesity, prior febrile illness, and debility are predisposing factors. Diuretics, sedatives, and antipsychotic and anticholinergic drugs may also be contributing factors. The extreme heat that develops in the disorder may cause widespread direct damage to body tissues, with rhabdomyolysis. Morbidity and death result from cerebral, cardiovascular, hepatic, and renal destruction.

There may be premonitory headache, dizziness, nausea, confusion, convulsions, and visual disturbances, which then progress to coma. The skin is hot, flushed, and usually dry; the pulse is strong and very rapid; the blood pressure is at first mildly elevated but later falls below normal. The rectal temperature may be as high as 43 °C (109.4 °F). Hyperventilation may cause an initial respiratory alkalosis, but this is often followed by metabolic acidosis. Laboratory findings may include hemoconcentration, decreased blood coagulation, and evidence of disseminated intravascular coagulation; a scanty concentrated urine containing protein, tubular casts, and myoglobin; decreased serum potassium, calcium, and phosphorus; and increased serum transaminase.

Treatment is aimed first at prompt reduction of temperature. As a first aid measure, place the patient in a shady, cool place and remove all clothing. Sprinkle the patient's entire body with cold water or daub the skin generously with rubbing alcohol and cool by fanning. Give chlorpromazine, 25–50 mg intramuscularly, to control shivering and delirium and to make cooling treatment more tolerable for the conscious patient. As soon as possible, immerse the patient in a tub of cold water or use cold wet sheets or ice packs. Once the rectal temperature drops to 39 °C (102.2 °F), do not lower temperature too rapidly. Continued temperature monitoring is required. If the temperature starts to rise again, resume the cooling process.

Maintain an adequate airway and administer oxygen in high concentration to combat hypoxia. Monitor arterial blood gases and pH and central venous pressure or pulmonary artery wedge pressure. Maintain blood pressure and urine output with intravenous crystalloids and inotropic agents as needed. (See Chapter 1.) Observe carefully for evidence of complications (eg, renal failure, rhabdomyolysis, cardiac arrhythmias, disseminated intravascular coagulation, and hepatic failure). If Pa_{O_2} falls below 65 mm Hg, endotracheal intubation is usually required. Administer 1–2 L of cold physiologic saline or lactated Ringer's injection in accordance with clinical, hemodynamic, and laboratory findings. Inotropic agents (eg, dopamine) may be indicated for shock (see p 12). For treatment of acute renal failure, see p 560.

With early diagnosis and proper care, 80–90% of otherwise healthy patients may survive heat stroke. Extreme hyperpyrexia (over 41 °C [105.8 °F] rectally), coma of more than 2 hours' duration, and marked hypertransaminasemia and hyperkalemia are unfavorable prognostic signs.

Patients with heat stroke should avoid immediate reexposure to heat. Hypersensitivity to high temperatures may remain for a considerable time.

American College of Sports Medicine: Position Statement: Prevention of thermal injuries during distance running. *Physician Sportsmed* (July) 1984;**12:**49.

Beyer CB: Heat stress and the young athlete: Recognizing and reducing the risks. *Postgrad Med* (July) 1984;**76:**109.

Costrini AM et al: Cardiovascular and metabolic manifestations of heat stroke and severe heat exhaustion. *Am J Med* 1979; **66:**296.

England AC et al: Preventing severe heat injury in runners: Suggestions from the 1979 Peachtree Road Race experience. *Ann Intern Med* 1982;**97:**196.

Johnson LW: Preventing heat stroke. *Am Fam Physician* (July) 1982;**26:**137.

Jones TS et al: Morbidity and mortality associated with the July 1980 heat wave in St. Louis and Kansas City, Mo. *JAMA* 1982;**247:**3327.

Kilbourne EM et al: Risk factors for heatstroke: A case control study. *JAMA* 1982;**247:**3332.

Sprung CL et al: The metabolic and respiratory alterations of heat stroke. *Arch Intern Med* 1980;**140:**665.

BURNS*

It is estimated that there are 2,000,000 injuries, 60,000 hospitalizations, and 8000 deaths due to burns each year in the USA. The tragedy is that burns are largely preventable. The National Center for Health Statistics (1979) indicates that burns are the second leading cause of death in children.

Scalds are a common form of thermal injury to children and the elderly. They can be partially prevented by regulating water heater temperature (Table 30–1). Enforcement of the Flammable Fabric Act in the USA has reduced flame injury to children. However, loose-fitting clothing of the elderly is a hazard near an open flame. Carelessness with burning cigarettes is a common cause of dwelling fires. Smoke alarms and other fire safety measures have helped to save lives and prevent injury, but further safety legislation and public education are needed.

Table 30–1. Temperatures at which tap water scalds may occur at various exposure times.

Skin Temperature (°C)	(°F)	Time For Second-Degree Scald (seconds)
65.6	150	Any
60.0	140*	1.5*
54.4	130	12
51.7	125	42
48.9	120	300

*Note the risk at this common household temperature.

CLASSIFICATION

Burns are classified by extent, depth, patient age, and associated illness or injury.

Extent

The "rule of nines" (Fig 30–1) is useful for rapid assessment of extent of burn by the physician. More detailed charts based on age are available when the patient reaches the burn unit. Errors in determining the extent of burns are common. It is important to view the entire patient after cleaning soot to make an accurate assessment.

Depth

Judgment of depth of injury is difficult. The **first-degree burn** is red or gray but will demonstrate excellent capillary refill. The first-degree burn is not

*By R. Laurence Berkowitz, MD.

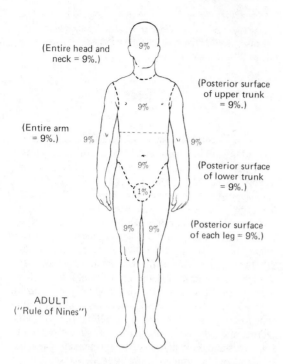

(Entire head and neck = 9%.)

9%

(Posterior surface of upper trunk = 9%.)

(Entire arm = 9%.)

9%

9%

9%

9%

(Posterior surface of lower trunk = 9%.)

1%

9%   9%

(Posterior surface of each leg = 9%.)

ADULT
("Rule of Nines")

Figure 30–1. Estimation of body surface area in burns.

calculated into the estimate of total burn surface area (TBSA), as it does not represent a significant injury in terms of fluid resuscitation. First-degree burns are not blistered initially. If the wound is blistered, this represents a partial-thickness injury to the dermis, or a **second-degree burn.** However, a deep second-degree burn may have lost its blister and may actually appear hyperemic from fixed hemoglobin in the tissue. This

redness will not have good refill and will not be as exquisitely sensitive as the hyperemia of the first-degree burn. The line between the partial- and full-thickness injury, or **third-degree burn,** may be rather indefinite. The initial vasoconstriction of a second-degree burn may make it appear more severe at first. Concerning healing properties of any second- or third-degree burn, the critical factors are blood supply and appendage population. In areas rich in vascularity, hair follicles, and sweat glands, the prospects for reepithelialization are good. Otherwise, even when the dermis is healthy, epithelialization may be slow and more scarring will result.

Age of the Patient

As much as extent and depth of the burn, age of the victim plays a critical part. Even a relatively small burn in an elderly patient or infant may be fatal, as demonstrated in Fig 30–2.

Associated Injuries & Illnesses

An injury commonly associated with burns is smoke inhalation. The products of combustion, not heat, are responsible for lower airway injury. Certain toxic substances from plastic products produce hydrochloric acid and hydrocyanic acid. Electrical injury as a cause of burn may also produce cardiac arrhythmias that require immediate attention. Premorbid physical and psychosocial disorders that complicate recovery from burn injury include cardiac or pulmonary disease, diabetes, alcoholism, drug abuse, and psychiatric illness.

Special Burn Care Units & Facilities

The American Burn Association has recommended that major burns be treated in specialized burn care facilities. It also advocates that moderate burns be

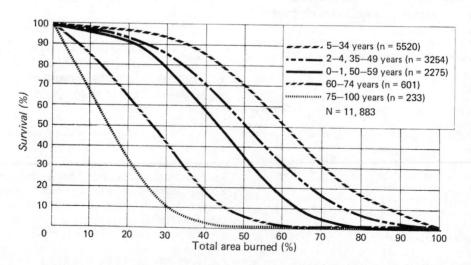

Legend:
- - - - - 5–34 years (n = 5520)
- · - · - 2–4, 35–49 years (n = 3254)
——— 0–1, 50–59 years (n = 2275)
- - - - 60–74 years (n = 601)
·········· 75–100 years (n = 233)
N = 11, 883

Survival (%) axis: 0, 10, 20, 30, 40, 50, 60, 70, 80, 90, 100
Total area burned (%) axis: 0, 10, 20, 30, 40, 50, 60, 70, 80, 90, 100

Figure 30–2. Sigmoid curves showing survival of humans as a function of total percentage of body surface burned and age. Survival curves estimated by probit analysis for 5 different age categories. (Reproduced, with permission, from Feller I, Flora JD Jr, Bawol R: Baseline results of therapy for burned patients. *JAMA* 1976;**236**:1943. Copyright 1976, American Medical Association.)

treated in a specialized facility or hospital where personnel with expertise in burn care are available. The American Burn Association has classified burn injuries as follows:

A. Major Burn Injuries:

1. Partial-thickness burns over more than 25% of body surface area in adults or 20% in children.

2. Full-thickness burns over more than 10% of surface area in any age group.

3. Burns involving the hands, face, eyes, ears, feet, or perineum.

4. Burns complicated by inhalation injury.

5. Electrical and chemical burns.

6. Burns complicated by fractures and other major trauma.

7. Burns in poor-risk patients (extremes of age or intercurrent disease).

B. Moderate Uncomplicated Burn Injuries:

1. Partial-thickness burns over 15–25% of body surface area in adults or 10–20% of body surface area in children.

2. Full-thickness burns over 2–10% of body surface area.

3. Burns not involving the specific conditions listed above.

C. Minor Burn Injuries:

1. Partial-thickness burns over less than 15% of body surface area in adults or 10% in children.

2. Full-thickness burns over less than 2% of body surface area.

INITIAL MANAGEMENT

Airway

The physician or emergency medical technician should proceed as with any other trauma. The first priority is establishment of an airway, then evaluation of the cervical spine and head injuries, and then stabilization of fractures. *The burn wound itself is a lower priority.* At some point during the initial management, intubation should be considered for most major burn cases, regardless of the area of the body involved, for as fluid resuscitation proceeds, generalized edema develops, including the soft tissues of the upper airway and perhaps the lungs as well. *Tracheostomy is rarely indicated for the burn victim,* unless dictated by other circumstances. Inhalation injuries should be followed by serial arterial blood gases, spirometry, and xenon clearance studies. The use of corticosteroids is controversial but generally not recommended because of potential immunosuppression.

Cooling the Wound

Cooling the victim for up to 20 minutes following the burn has been shown to reduce the depth of injury. Saline soaks at room temperature or cooler should be used. At the scene of an injury, a hose can be used for this purpose. Fire extinguishers and ice are not recommended, as crystallizing of tissues may occur.

History

As soon as possible, obtain a detailed history of the circumstances of the injury including locale, substances involved, and length of burning. The initial history may be extremely valuable. Medications, mental disturbances, confusion resulting from the injury, or the presence of an endotracheal tube may later prevent the recording of an accurate history. A rapid assessment of the extent of injury is more important than the depth, as fluid calculation is based on the collective area of second- and third-degree burns.

Vascular Access

Simultaneously with the above procedures, venous access must be sought. The victim of a major burn is in hypovolemic shock. The great veins are frequently depleted, and *large-bore cannulas in the region of the neck and thorax are hazardous and ill-advised* in the initial phase of management. These sites, in fact, should be spared, as they will be critical in later periods. *A well-secured peripheral cutdown or femoral vein puncture is the preferred route of fluid administration.* A burn eschar, since it has been flame-sterilized, is an acceptable location for the initial cutdown; it is best to save unburned regions for later use. Femoral lines also provide rapid, safe access. They can be replaced as soon as the patient is stable. An arterial line may also be useful for monitoring mean arterial pressure. The line may be placed initially in the femoral artery and later changed (as peripheral resistance decreases) to a safer site such as the dorsalis pedis, temporal, or radial arteries. Swan-Ganz catheter placement is indicated in patients with preexisting cardiopulmonary disease or in the management of severe burn cases to determine cardiac output and peripheral resistance. Once these parameters have been established, this catheter is usually removed.

FLUID RESUSCITATION

Crystalloids

Generalized capillary leak results from burn injury over more than 25% of the total body surface area. This often necessitates replacement of a large volume of fluid. An intravenous line is recommended in the management of burns that cover more than 20% of total body surface area in the adult and 10% in the child.

There are many formulas for fluid resuscitation, eg, Evans, Brooke, hypertonic saline (Monafo), and Parkland (Baxter). All of these fluids deliver approximately 0.5–0.6 meq of sodium per kilogram of body weight per percent of body surface area burned. The total amount of fluid in all but the hypertonic saline formula is roughly the same but differs in distribution. The Parkland formula is currently the most widely used in the USA. It relies upon the use of lactated Ringer's injection, which is available in every emergency room. For adults and children, the fluid requirement is estimated as 3–5 mL/kg body weight

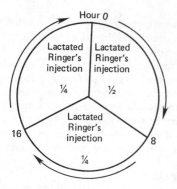

Figure 30–3. Half of the calculated crystalloid formula (lactated Ringer's injection [4 mL/kg wt/% TBSA]) is given in the first 8 hours, beginning at the time of the injury. The remainder is given evenly over the ensuing 16 hours.

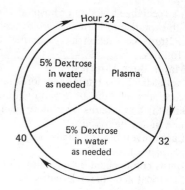

Figure 30–4. The colloid formula (aged plasma or 5% normal serum albumin [0.3–0.5 mL/kg wt/% TBSA]) is given as calculated between hours 24 and 32. In the remaining 16-hour period, 5% dextrose in water is given as needed to maintain a urine output of no less than 30 mL/h.

per percent of body surface area burned (Fig 30–3). In the elderly or those with lesser burns, the smaller amount would be used. In children (who have a larger relative surface-to-volume ratio) and for treatment of deep electrical burns, the larger amount would be used. Begin with 4 mL/kg body weight per percent of body surface area burned, and vary this amount according to the patient's response. *Remember that a formula is only a guideline and that blind adherence to any set of numbers can result in disaster.*

Half of the calculated fluid is given in the first 8-hour period. The remaining fluid, divided into 2 equal parts, is delivered over the next 16 hours. An extremely large volume of fluid may be required. For example, an injury over 40% of the total body surface area in a 70-kg victim may require 13 L *in the first 24 hours.* Calculate the first 8-hour period from the hour of injury, and catch up to that point if necessary.

Colloids

After 24 hours, capillary leaks have sealed in the majority of cases, and plasma volume may be restored with colloids (plasma or albumin). The Parkland formula calls for 0.3–0.5 mL/kg body weight per percent of body surface area burned to be given over the first 8-hour period of the second 24 hours. Fluids given in the following 16 hours consist of dextrose in water in quantities sufficient to maintain adequate urine output (Fig 30–4). It is hoped that during the second 24-hour period the vascular system will hold colloids and draw off edema fluid, resulting in diuresis.

Adequacy of Resuscitation

Guidelines for adequacy of fluid resuscitation are mental alertness, urinary output, and the vital signs. Mental alertness is the most important because it is the best indicator of adequate cerebral perfusion. Overmedication may cloud the sensorium during the resuscitation phase. Analgesics in the form of small doses of intravenous morphine should be used judiciously so as

not to interfere with diagnosis. Renal perfusion is judged by urinary output. Adequate urinary output is 30–50 mL/h in adults and 1 mL/kg body weight/h in children. A smaller output represents inadequate renal perfusion. However, a larger output is unnecessary, and overloading results in edema in every organ. Keep edema at a minimum by maintaining a careful balance between input and output.

Monitoring Fluid Resuscitation

A Foley catheter is essential for monitoring urinary output. *Diuretics have no part in this phase of patient management.* The use of mannitol may be indicated in the resuscitation of an electrical burn victim in whom myoglobin in the urine may precipitate in the kidneys. It should be used only until the urine is clear, and then discontinued.

Escharotomy

As edema fluid accumulates, ischemia may develop under any constricting eschar of an extremity. Similarly, an eschar of the thorax or abdomen may limit respiratory excursion. Escharotomy incisions (Fig 30–5) through the anesthetic eschar can save life and limb. *The penalty for failing to perform escharotomy can be great.*

THE BURN WOUND

Treatment of the burn wound is based on several basic principles: (1) Prevent or delay infection. (2) Protect from desiccation and further injury those burned areas that will spontaneously reepithelialize in 7–10 days. (3) Excise and graft those burned areas that cannot spontaneously reepithelialize during this period.

Prophylactic Antibiotics

Regardless of the severity of the burn, prophylac-

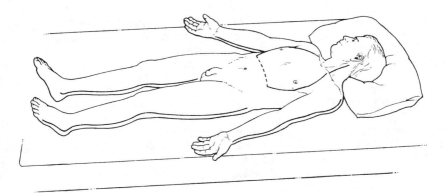

Figure 30–5. Proper placement of escharotomy incisions. Notice that the incisions must cross affected joints. (Reproduced, with permission, from McDougal WS, Slade CL, Pruitt BA Jr: *Manual of Burns.* Springer-Verlag, 1978.)

tic systemic antibiotics are usually not recommended. Their effectiveness is unproved, and they have the disadvantage of favoring the growth of resistant organisms.

Topical Antibiotics

Topical antibiotics delay or prevent infection. The ideal agent is one that would readily penetrate the burn wound eschar, be effective against both gram-negative and gram-positive microorganisms as well as *Candida,* be painless and inexpensive, and have no deleterious side effects. Such an ideal agent does not currently exist. Silver sulfadiazine (Silvadene) is currently the recommended topical agent. It is painless, easy to apply, effective against most *Pseudomonas,* and a good penetrator of eschar, but some microorganisms are resistant to it, and it may cause leukopenia or fever and delay epithelialization.

Mafenide (Sulfamylon), which penetrates eschars better than silver sulfadiazine and is more effective against *Pseudomonas,* inhibits carbonic anhydrase when used as a 10% solution, which may be painful to the patient and result in metabolic acidosis; it also delays epithelialization. When diluted to a 5% solution, pain and metabolic side effects are lessened. It is useful primarily for deep burns, eg, electrical burns and burns of the ear or nose where cartilage is close to the surface, and when silver sulfadiazine is ineffective. It is best to limit the use of mafenide to no more than 10% of the total body surface area at any given time.

Povidone-iodine is especially useful against *Candida* and both gram-positive and gram-negative microorganisms. However, it penetrates eschar poorly, is very desiccating to the wound surface, and is painful. Also, significantly high blood iodine levels have been demonstrated in patients receiving this agent.

Gentamicin and silver nitrate are no longer recommended as topical agents.

Wound Closure

The goal of therapy after fluid resuscitation is closure of the wound. Nature's own blister is the best cover to protect wounds that spontaneously epithelialize in 7–10 days (ie, superficial second-degree burns). The serum in the blister nurses the surface of the **zone of stasis** until epithelialization takes place (Fig 30–6). Where the blister has been disrupted, human amnion, porcine heterografts (preferably fresh, or frozen and meshed), or collagen composite dressings (Biobrane) can substitute. Cadaver homograft can also serve this purpose if available.

Wounds that will not heal spontaneously in 7–10 days (ie, deep second-degree or third-degree burns) are best treated by excision and autograft; otherwise, granulation and infection may develop. Granulation is nature's signal that attempts to close the wound have

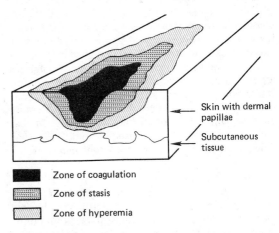

Skin with dermal papillae

Subcutaneous tissue

■ Zone of coagulation
▨ Zone of stasis
▧ Zone of hyperemia

Figure 30–6. The burn wound has 3 general zones of tissue death. The zone of necrosis or coagulation involves irreversible skin death. The intermediate zone of capillary stasis is vulnerable to desiccation and infection that can convert potentially salvageable tissue to full-thickness destruction and irreversible skin death. There is minimal cell involvement in the outermost hyperemic zone. (Modified from Zawacki BE: Reversal of capillary stasis and prevention of necrosis in burns. *Ann Surg* 1974;**180**:98. Redrawn, with permission, from Artz CP, Moncrief JA, Pruitt BA: *Burns: A Team Approach.* Saunders, 1979.)

failed. A "skin equivalent"—a patient's own skin cells grown in culture into multilayered sheets of epithelium—may provide an adjunct or alternative to traditional skin graft methods in the near future.

PATIENT SUPPORT

During the wound closure phase, the patient must be supported in many ways. Most important is adequate nutrition. Enteral feedings may begin once the ileus of the resuscitation period is relieved, which usually coincides with the subsidence of edema. The large nasogastric sump tube used to decompress stomach contents during resuscitation may now be replaced with a smaller, preferably soft Silastic tube. This will aid in delivering the 4000–6000 kcal/d that may be required during the wound closure period. The metabolic demands are immense. A useful guide is to provide 25 kcal/kg body weight plus 40 kcal per percent of burn surface area. Fat emulsions (Intralipid) given intravenously are useful during the resuscitation period to span the period of ileus.

Many enteral formulas are available. Eggs are a readily available source of protein and calories that are well tolerated by the patient. More than 30 eggs per day are desirable in many cases. Early enteral feedings reduce the need for antacids and lessen the likelihood of Curling's ulcer, a life-threatening complication of burn injury. Careful monitoring of pH and hourly antacid delivery during the resuscitation phase are necessary. Cimetidine is also used to reduce acid production; however, undesirable side effects such as leukopenia and confusion in the elderly may result.

Pain plays a major role during the wound closure phase. The patient is more aware of pain during dressing changes and postsurgical periods. Hydrotherapy aids in dressing removal and joint range of motion, but it can be a source of wound contamination. Analgesics are essential, but overuse or underuse may be harmful. Intravenous morphine, meperidine, fentanyl, nitrous oxide, and ketamine all may play a role during dressing changes but require close patient monitoring. Methadone given on a regular basis in some cases has reduced the need for other intravenous narcotics.

The Burn Team

The burn team consists of a group of highly skilled professionals—nurses, dietitians, physical therapists, occupational therapists, and counselors—who work closely with the physician in providing comprehensive services for the victim from the period of intensive care through recovery and rehabilitation. During the intensive care period, the burn nurse plays a pivotal role, working closely with the dietitian and other members of the team. As the burn victim emerges from the overwhelming physical insult, the burn nurse must attend to the patient's rehabilitative needs. The occupational therapist splints the extremities to minimize deformity and especially looks after the burned hand, which alternately requires splinting and joint range of motion. Later, the occupational therapist assists the patient in returning to the activities of daily living. The physical therapist assists the patient in regaining range of motion in the larger joints and in beginning to walk. The therapists, under the guidance of a physiatrist, are the key to patient management after leaving the hospital as well. They are responsible for proper measurement and fitting of splints and elastic garments, which attempt to break the will of scar tissue by means of pressure.

The psychosocial and vocational needs of the patient are often as overwhelming as the physical insult, and it is often necessary to have the social worker and psychologist work closely with the patient, the patient's family, and the hospital staff. The psychiatrist is useful in management of psychosis, pain control, and psychotropic medications when indicated. A clergyman may be called upon for spiritual support and guidance.

Many of the residual physical and emotional problems in burn patients, eg, body disfigurement, impaired mobility, persistent itching, decreased ability to perspire, and decreased skin sensitivity with impairment of sexual enjoyment, may require special individualized attention.

Group therapy—sessions with other burn patients—may be invaluable in helping a victim with a devastating injury readjust to society.

Demling RH: Fluid resuscitation after major burns. *JAMA* 1983;**250**:1438.

Demling RH: Improved survival after massive burns. *J Trauma* 1983;**23**:179.

Fein A, Leff A, Hopewell PC: Pathophysiology and management of the complications resulting from fire and the inhaled products of combustion. *Crit Care Med* 1980;**8**:2.

Fisher SV, Helm PA: *Rehabilitation of the Burn Patient.* Williams & Wilkins, 1984.

Gallico GG III et al: Permanent coverage of large burn wounds with autologous cultured human epithelium. *N Engl J Med* 1984;**311**:448.

Gillespie RW: The burn at first sight. *Emerg Med* (Feb 29) 1984;**16**:141.

Lockhart SP et al: Topical silver sulphadiazine: Side effects and urinary excretion. *Burns* 1984;**10**:1.

Monafo WW, Crabtree JH, Galster AD: Hemodynamics and metabolic support of the severely burned patient. In: Shoemaker WC, Thompson WL, Holbrook PR (editors): *The Society of Critical Care Medicine: Textbook of Critical Care.* Saunders, 1984.

Munster AM: The early management of thermal burns. *Surgery* 1980;**87**:29.

Supportive therapy in burn care. *J Trauma* 1981;**21**(Suppl 8):665. [Entire issue.]

Wachtel TL, Kahn V, Frank HA (editors): *Current Topics in Burn Care.* Aspen, 1983.

ELECTRIC SHOCK

The possibility of life-threatening electrical injury exists in all electrified areas—home, school, industry, agriculture, recreation, and even in hospitals. Electric shock may result from carelessness, ignorance, faulty appliances and equipment, or from an act of nature—lightning. Dry skin provides a high-resistance barrier to ordinary levels of external electric current. Skin moistened with water, sweat, saline solution, or urine, however, has greatly reduced resistance to electric current. The effect of electric current may be a local unpleasant tingling or a painful sensation. The amount and type of current, the duration and area of exposure, and the pathway of the current through the body determine the degree of damage. If the current passes through the heart or brain stem, death may occur immediately owing to ventricular fibrillation or apnea. Current passing through skeletal muscle can cause contractions severe enough to result in bone fracture.

Direct current is much less dangerous than alternating current. Alternating current of high voltage with a very high number of cycles per second (hertz, Hz) may be less dangerous than a low voltage with fewer cycles per second. With alternating currents of 25–300 Hz, low voltages (below 220) tend to produce ventricular fibrillation; high voltages (over 1000), respiratory failure; intermediate voltages (220–1000), both. Domestic house current (AC) of 100 volts with low cycles (about 60 Hz) is, accordingly, dangerous to the heart, since it may cause ventricular fibrillation.

Electrical burns are of 3 distinct types: flash (arcing) burns, flame (clothing) burns, and the direct heating effect of tissues by the electric current. The latter lesions are usually sharply demarcated, round or oval, painless gray areas with inflammatory reaction. The superficial appearance of many burns is deceptive when they are discrete, and operation frequently discloses more extensive destruction than anticipated. Little happens to them for several weeks; sloughing then occurs slowly over a fairly wide area.

Electric shock may produce momentary or prolonged loss of consciousness. With recovery there may be muscular pain, fatigue, headache, and nervous irritability. The physical signs vary according to the action of the current. With ventricular fibrillation, no heart sounds or pulse can be found and the patient is unconscious. The respirations continue for a few minutes, becoming exaggerated as asphyxia occurs and then ceasing as death intervenes. With respiratory failure, respirations are absent and the patient is unconscious; the pulse can be felt, but there is a marked fall in blood pressure and the skin is cold and cyanotic.

Electric shock may be a hazard in routine hospital equipment that is usually considered to be harmless (eg, electrocardiographs, suction machines, electrically operated beds, x-ray units). Proper installation, utilization, and maintenance of equipment by qualified personnel should minimize this hazard. Battery-operated devices provide the maximum protection from accidental electric shock. Electrochemical cutaneous burns have been reported with direct current voltages as low as 3 volts.

Treatment

A. Emergency Measures: Free the victim from the current at once. This may be done in many ways, but the rescuer must be protected. Turn off the power, sever the wire with a dry wooden-handled axe, make a proper ground to divert the current, or drag the victim carefully away by means of dry clothing or a leather belt.

If breathing and pulses are absent, institute cardiopulmonary resuscitation immediately (see p 1109) and continue until spontaneous breathing and cardiac function return or rigor mortis is noted.

B. Hospital Measures: Hospitalize the patient when revived and observe for shock, sudden cardiac dilatation, secondary hemorrhage, acidosis, or myoglobinuria.

Treat tissue burns conservatively. The direction and extent of tissue injury may not be apparent for weeks. Infection is usually not a problem early. Patience and delay are important in treatment; allow granulation tissue to be well established before attempting surgery. Hemorrhage may occur late and may be severe.

The unpredictable damage to deep tissues in electrical burns makes it difficult to assess the fluid requirements for patients who are in shock.

Prognosis

Complications may occur in almost every part of the body. The most common cause of death in those who survive the original electric shock is systemic infection.

Christensen JA et al: Delayed neurologic injury secondary to high-voltage current with recovery. *J Trauma* 1980;**20:**166.

Dixon GF: The evaluation and management of electrical injuries. *Crit Care Med* 1983;**11:**384.

Electrocution of a truck driver—West Virginia. *MMWR* (Jan) 1984;**33:**14.

Fraser-Darling A: Electrocution, drowning, and burns. *Br Med J* 1981;**282:**530.

Hunt JL et al: Acute electric burns: Current diagnostic and therapeutic approaches to management. *Arch Surg* 1980;**115:**434.

Lazarus HM, Hutto W: Electric burns and frostbite: Patterns of vascular injury. *J Trauma* 1982;**22:**581.

Monies-Chass I et al: How can electrical accidents in the operating room be prevented? *Ann Plast Surg* 1982;**8:**264.

Sances A Jr et al: Electrical injuries. *Surg Gynecol Obstet* 1979;**149:**97.

IRRADIATION REACTIONS

The effects of radiation on the body have been observed in clinical use of x-rays and radioactive agents, after occupational or accidental exposure, and following the use of atomic weaponry. The harmful effects of radiation are determined by the extent of exposure, which in turn depends not only on the quantity of radiation delivered to the body but also the type of radiation (x-rays, neutrons, gamma rays, alpha or beta particles) to which tissues are exposed, and the duration of exposure.

Tolerance to radiation is difficult to define, and there is no firm basis for evaluating radiation effects for all types and levels of radiation. The National Committee on Radiation Protection has set the maximum permissible radiation exposure for occupationally exposed workers over age 18 at 0.1 rem* per week for the whole body (but not to exceed 5 rem per year) and 1.5 rem per week for the hands. (For purposes of comparison, routine chest x-rays deliver from 0.1–0.2 rem.) If recommended limits for radiation safety in occupational workers or in clinical practice are exceeded, serious radiation injury may occur (see below).

Death after acute lethal radiation exposure is usually due to hematopoietic failure, gastrointestinal mucosal damage, central nervous system damage, or widespread vascular injury. Four hundred to 600 rads of x-ray or gamma radiation applied to the entire body at one time may be fatal within 60 days; death is usually due to hemorrhage, anemia, and infection secondary to hematopoietic injury. Levels of 1000–3000 rads to the entire body destroy gastrointestinal mucosa; this leads to toxemia and death within 2 weeks. Total body doses above 3000 rads cause widespread vascular damage, cerebral anoxia, hypotensive shock, and death within 48 hours.

ACUTE (IMMEDIATE) RADIATION EFFECTS ON NORMAL TISSUES

Clinical Findings

A. Injury to Skin and Mucous Membranes: Irradiation may cause erythema, epilation, destruction of fingernails, or epidermolysis.

B. Injury to Deep Structures:

1. Hematopoietic tissues–Injury to the bone marrow may cause diminished production of blood elements. Lymphocytes are most sensitive, polymorphonuclear leukocytes next most sensitive, and erythrocytes least sensitive. Damage to the blood-forming organs may vary from transient depression of one or more blood elements to complete destruction.

2. Cardiovascular–Pericarditis with effusion or constrictive carditis may occur after a period of months or even years. Myocarditis is less common. Smaller vessels (the capillaries and arterioles) are more readily damaged than larger blood vessels.

*In radiation terminology, a rad is the unit of absorbed dose and a rem is the unit of any radiation dose to body tissue in terms of its estimated biologic effect. Roentgen (R) refers to the amount of radiation dose delivered to the body. For x-ray or gamma ray radiation, rems, rads, and roentgens are virtually the same. For particulate radiation from radioactive materials, these terms may differ greatly (eg, for neutrons, 1 rad = 10 rems). In the Système Internationale (SI) nomenclature, the rad has been replaced by the gray (Gy), and 1 rad = 0.01 Gy. The SI replacement for the rem is the Sievert (Sv), and 1 rem = 0.01 Sv.

3. Gonads–In males, small single doses of radiation (200–300 R) cause aspermatogenesis, and larger doses (600–800 R) may cause sterility. In females, single doses of 200 R may cause temporary cessation of menses, and 500–800 R may cause permanent castration. Moderate to heavy radiation of the embryo in utero results in injury to the fetus or in embryonic death and abortion.

4. Respiratory tract–High or repeated moderate doses of radiation may cause pneumonitis, often delayed for weeks or months.

5. The salivary glands may be depressed by radiation, but relatively large doses may be required.

6. Mouth, pharynx, esophagus, and stomach–Mucositis with edema and painful swallowing of food may occur within hours or days after onset of radiation. Gastric secretion may be temporarily (occasionally permanently) inhibited by moderately high doses of radiation.

7. Intestines–Inflammation and ulceration may follow moderately large doses of radiation.

8. Endocrine glands and viscera–Hepatitis and nephritis may be delayed effects of therapeutic radiation. The normal thyroid, pituitary, pancreas, adrenals, and bladder are relatively resistant to low or moderate doses of radiation.

9. The brain and spinal cord may be damaged by high doses of radiation because of impaired blood supply.

10. Peripheral and autonomic nerves are highly resistant to radiation.

C. Systemic Reaction (Radiation Sickness): The basic mechanisms of radiation sickness are not known. Anorexia, nausea, vomiting, weakness, exhaustion, lassitude, and in some cases prostration may occur, singly or in combination. Radiation sickness associated with x-ray therapy is most likely to occur when the therapy is given in large dosage to large areas over the abdomen, less often when given over the thorax, and rarely when therapy is given over the extremities. With protracted therapy, this complication is rarely significant. The patient's psychologic reaction to the illness or its treatment plays an important role in aggravating or minimizing such effect.

Prevention

Persons handling radiation sources can minimize exposure to radiation by recognizing the importance of time, distance, and shielding. Areas housing x-ray and nuclear materials must be properly shielded. Inadequately trained personnel should not be permitted to work with x-ray and nuclear radiation. Any unnecessary exposures, diagnostic or therapeutic, should be avoided. X-ray equipment should be periodically checked for reliability of output, and proper filters should be employed. When feasible, it is advisable to shield the gonads, especially of young persons. Fluoroscopic examination should be performed as rapidly as possible, using an optimal combination of beam characteristics and filtration; the tube-to-table distance should be at least 45 cm, and the beam size should be kept to a minimum required by the examination. Special protective clothing may be necessary to protect against contamination with radioisotopes. In the event of accidental contamination, removal of all clothing and vigorous bathing with soap and water should be followed by careful instrument (Geiger counter) check for localization of ionizing radiation.

No safe and effective radioprotectant drugs are as yet available.

Emergency Treatment for Radiation Accident Victims

The need for emergency radiation accident care has grown because of the proliferation of radiation equipment and nuclear reactor plants and the increased transportation of radioactive materials. Hospitals have been asked to develop plans for management of patients accidentally exposed to ionizing radiation or to spillage or contamination with radioactive materials. The plans should provide for effective emergency care and disposition of victims and materials with the least possible risk of spreading radioactive contamination to personnel and facilities. Clinicians should be at least aware of the complexity of the problems involved. (See Leonard and USERDA references, below.)

Treatment

The success of treatment of local radiation effects depends upon the extent, degree, and location of tissue injury. Treatment of systemic reactions is symptomatic and supportive. No truly effective antinauseant drug is available for the distressing nausea that frequently occurs. Chlorpromazine, 25–50 mg given deeply intramuscularly every 4–6 hours as necessary or 10–50 mg orally every 4–6 hours as necessary, may be of value. Dimenhydrinate, 100 mg, or perphenazine, 4–8 mg, 1 hour before and 1 and 4 hours after radiation therapy has been recommended. Simple, palatable foods and emotional support may help.

When radiation dosage levels are sufficient to cause damage to gastrointestinal mucosa, bone marrow, and other important tissues, good medical and nursing care may be lifesaving. Blood transfusions, bone marrow transplants, antibiotics, fluid and electrolyte maintenance, and other medical measures may support patients not too severely injured by radiation. Recovery obviously depends upon the severity of the injury. Patients with fulminant high-dose radiation syndrome—with cerebral anoxia and shock—fail to respond to treatment, and death occurs in 1–2 days.

CHRONIC (DELAYED) EFFECTS OF EXCESSIVE DOSES OF IONIZING RADIATION

The risk of radiation exposure is a subject of much interest and controversy. There are concerns about possible delayed effects of exposure to medical radiation as well as those due to accidental environmental contamination. The chronic effects of radiation may be difficult to evaluate, because they take many years to become apparent. Furthermore, it is difficult to differentiate effects presumed to be due to radiation from abnormal conditions known to occur spontaneously in the population at large.

Skin scarring, atrophy and telangiectasis, obliterative endarteritis, pericarditis, pulmonary fibrosis, hepatitis, intestinal stenosis, nephritis, and other late effects of radiation are known to occur.

The incidence of neoplastic disease, including leukemia, is increased in persons exposed to excessive radiation. The latency period between radiation therapy and the development of cancer may be 30 years or longer. Much of our knowledge of radiation-induced cancer in humans has been derived from follow-up studies of the survivors of the bombings in Japan during World War II. There is an increased incidence of thyroid cancer in patients who have received radiation therapy to the thymus.

Microcephaly and other congenital abnormalities may occur in children exposed in utero, especially if the fetus was exposed during early pregnancy.

Note: See also references below dealing with medical implications of low-level radiation and nuclear war.

Abrams HL, Von Kaenel WE: Medical problems of survivors of nuclear war: Infection and the spread of communicable disease. *N Engl J Med* 1981;**305:**1226.

Cassel C, Jameton A: Medical responsibility and the thermonuclear war. *Ann Intern Med* 1982;**97:**426.

Chacko DC: Considerations in the diagnosis of radiation injury. *JAMA* 1981;**245:**1256.

Finnerty NA, Buzdar AU, Blumenschein GR: Radiation-induced breast cancer. *Arch Intern Med* 1984;**144:**1217.

Fleming MF, Archer VE: Ionizing radiation: Health hazards of medical uses. *Consultant* (Jan) 1984;**28:**167.

Goldman M: Ionizing radiation and its risks. *West J Med* 1982;**137:**540.

Health Policy Committee, American College of Physicians: The medical consequences of radiation accidents and nuclear war. *Ann Intern Med* 1982;**97:**447.

Health and Public Policy Committee, American College of Physicians: Low-level radioactive waste management. *Ann Intern Med* 1984;**100:**912.

Hendee WR: Real and perceived risks of medical radiation exposure. *West J Med* 1983;**138:**380.

Hiatt HH: The final epidemic: Prescriptions for prevention. *JAMA* 1984;**252:**635.

Johnson CT: Cancer incidence in an area of radioactive fallout downwind from the Nevada test site. *JAMA* 1984;**251:**230.

Larsen PR et al: Thyroid hypofunction after exposure to fallout from a hydrogen bomb explosion. *JAMA* 1982;**247:**1571.

Leonard RB: Emergency department radiation accident protocol. *Ann Emerg Med* 1980;**9:**462.

McKenna G, Glatstein E: When radiation therapy causes heart disease. *J Resp Dis* (June) 1984;**100:**912.

Smith JS, Fisher JH: Three Mile Island: The silent disaster. *JAMA* 1981;**245:**1656.

United States Energy Research and Development Administration: Emergency handling of radiation accident cases. Publication No. ERDA-17, 1975.

Watson GM: The nature of radiation injury. *Pathology* 1980; **12:**155.

DROWNING

Drowning is the fourth leading cause of accidental death in the USA. The number of deaths due to drowning could undoubtedly be significantly reduced if adequate preventive and first aid instruction programs were instituted.

The asphyxia of drowning is usually due to aspiration of fluid, but it may result from airway obstruction caused by laryngeal spasm while the victim is gasping under water. About 10% of victims develop laryngospasms after the first gulp and never aspirate water ("dry drowning"). The rapid sequence of events after submersion—hypoxemia, laryngospasm, fluid aspiration, ineffective circulation, brain injury, and brain death—may take place within 5–10 minutes. This sequence may be delayed for longer periods if the victim, especially a child, has been submerged in very cold water or if the victim has ingested significant amounts of barbiturates. Immersion in cold water can also cause a rapid fall in the victim's core temperature, so that systemic hypothermia and death may occur before actual drowning.

Past emphasis on differences in the pathophysiology of drowning in fresh water (hypotonic) and sea water (hypertonic), based upon observations in animal models, is of limited clinical significance in humans, since the amount of fluid aspirated is usually small. The primary effect in both cases is perfusion of poorly ventilated alveoli. The clinical presentation in both types of drowning is similar, and *cardiopulmonary resuscitation is the immediate requirement of rescue*.

A number of circumstances or primary events may precede near drowning and must be taken into consideration in management: (1) use of alcohol or other drugs (a contributing factor in an estimated 25% of adult drownings), (2) extreme fatigue, (3) intentional hyperventilation, (4) sudden acute illness (eg, epilepsy, myocardial infarction), (5) head or spinal cord injury sustained in diving, (6) venomous stings by aquatic animals, and (7) decompression sickness in deep water diving.

When first seen, the near-drowning victim may present with a wide range of clinical manifestations. Spontaneous return of consciousness often occurs in otherwise healthy individuals when submersion is very brief. Many other patients respond promptly to immediate ventilation. Other patients, with more severe degrees of near drowning, may have frank pulmonary failure, pulmonary edema, shock, anoxic encephalopathy, cerebral edema, and cardiac arrest. A few patients may be deceptively asymptomatic during the recovery period, only to deteriorate or die as a result of acute respiratory failure within the following 12–24 hours.

Clinical Findings

A. Symptoms and Signs: The patient may be unconscious, semiconscious, or awake but apprehensive, restless, and complaining of headaches or chest pain. Vomiting is common. Examination may reveal cyanosis, trismus, apnea, tachypnea, and wheezing. A pink froth from the mouth and nose indicates pulmonary edema. Cardiovascular manifestations may include tachycardia, arrhythmias, hypotension, cardiac arrest, and circulatory shock.

B. Laboratory Findings: Urinalysis shows proteinuria, hemoglobinuria, and acetonuria. There is usually a leukocytosis. The P_{aO_2} is usually decreased and the P_{aCO_2} increased or decreased. The blood pH is decreased as a result of metabolic acidosis. Chest x-rays may show pneumonitis or pulmonary edema.

Treatment

A. First Aid: Immediate measures to combat hypoxemia at the scene of the incident—with sustained effective ventilation, oxygenation, and circulatory support—are critical to survival with complete recovery.

1. If the victim is not breathing, clear the mouth and pharynx with the fingers, extend the victim's head, and institute immediate mouth-to-mouth or mouth-to-nose breathing.

2. Check carotid and femoral pulses. If pulses cannot be detected, institute cardiopulmonary resuscitation without delay (see p 1109).

3. Do not waste time attempting to drain water from the victim's lungs, since this measure is most often of no value. The Heimlich maneuver of subdiaphragmatic pressure may clear the airway in a few persons, especially those who have gagged or vomited while aspirating water.

4. All near-drowning patients, with or without aspiration, should be hospitalized at least overnight for observation, chest x-rays, and serial arterial blood gas determinations. It may take 24 hours for pneumonitis or pulmonary edema to become evident. Call for assistance in moving the victim to the nearest hospital.

5. Do not discontinue basic life support for seemingly "hopeless" patients. Complete recovery has been reported after prolonged resuscitation efforts even when victims have had wide, fixed pupils.

B. Hospital Care: Careful observation of the patient; continuous monitoring of cardiorespiratory function; serial determination of arterial blood gases, pH, and electrolytes; and measurement of urinary output are required.

1. Ensure optimal ventilation and oxygenation—The danger of hypoxemia exists even in the alert, conscious patient who appears to be breathing normally. The proper assessment of oxygen requirements must be based upon initial and serial determination of arterial blood gases and pH. If the initial arterial blood gases and pH are within normal limits, there has probably been little or no alveolar damage due to aspiration, and full recovery usually occurs promptly. Chest x-ray is normal.

Endotracheal intubation is necessary for patients unable to maintain an open airway or normal blood gases and pH. If the victim does not have spontaneous respirations, intubation is required.

Initiate intermittent mandatory oxygen therapy with a volume ventilator. Positive end-expiratory pressure (PEEP) should be considered when the patient is unable to achieve a P_{aO_2} greater than 55 mm Hg when receiving less than 50% oxygen. Ventilatory support should be continued until normal arterial blood gases and pH have been established and can be maintained while the patient is breathing room air. Serial physical examinations and chest x-rays should be carried out to detect possible pneumonitis, atelectasis, and pulmonary edema. Bronchospasm due to aspirated material may require use of bronchodilators. Antibiotics should be given when there is x-ray or laboratory evidence of pneumonitis and other infections.

2. Cardiovascular support–Hypoxemia, acidosis, and hypothermia may cause myocardial depression, ventricular fibrillation, and cardiac arrest. Central venous pressure (or, preferably, pulmonary artery wedge pressure) monitoring may be used as a guide for determining needs of vascular fluid replacement and cardiac drug therapy. If low cardiac output persists after adequate intravascular volume replacement, inotropic substances (eg, dopamine) should be considered. An increasing left ventricular pressure may indicate pulmonary edema and the need for fluid restriction, ventilatory modification, diuretics, and vasodilator drugs.

3. Correction of blood pH and electrolyte abnormalities–Metabolic acidosis is almost invariably present in near-drowning victims. Many authorities feel that patients who have been pulseless should routinely be given intravenous sodium bicarbonate, 1 meq/kg, upon admission. This is advisable, but all subsequent bicarbonate administration should be based upon arterial blood gas and pH findings. Alkalosis is dangerous and should be avoided.

4. Cerebral injury–Some near-drowning patients may progress to irreversible central nervous system damage despite apparently adequate treatment of hypoxia and shock. Several types of measures to prevent cerebral injury have been employed with varying degrees of success—hypothermia, barbiturates, corticosteroids, osmolar agents (eg, mannitol), and readjustment of ventilatory assistance.

Course & Prognosis

Victims of near drowning who have had prolonged hypoxemia should remain under close hospital observation for 2–3 days after all supportive measures have been withdrawn and clinical and laboratory findings have been stable. Residual complications of near drowning may include intellectual impairment, convulsive disorders, and pulmonary or cardiac disease.

Chipman C, Adelman R, Sexton G: Criteria for cessation of CPR in the emergency department. *Ann Emerg Med* 1981;**10**:11.
Martin TG: Neardrowning and cold water immersion. *Ann Emerg Med* 1984;**13**:263.
Oakes DD et al: Prognosis and management of victims of near-drowning. *J Trauma* 1982;**22**:544.
Redding JS: Drowning and near drowning: Can the victim be saved? *Postgrad Med* (July) 1983;**74**:85.
Smith DS: Notes on drowning: The misunderstood, preventable tragedy. *Physicians Sportsmed* (July) 1984;**12**:66.

OTHER DISORDERS DUE TO PHYSICAL AGENTS

DECOMPRESSION SICKNESS
(Caisson Disease, Bends)

Decompression sickness has long been known as an occupational hazard for professional divers who are involved in deep-water exploration, rescue, salvage, or construction, and professional divers and their surface supporting teams are familiar with the prevention, recognition, and treatment of this disease. In recent years, the sport of scuba diving has become very popular, and a large number of untrained individuals are exposed to the hazards of decompression sickness.

At low depths the greatly increased pressure (eg, at 30 meters [100 ft] the pressure is 4 times greater than at the surface) compresses the respiratory gases into the blood and other tissues. During ascent from depths greater than 9 meters, gases dissolved in the blood and other tissues escape as the external pressure decreases. The appearance of symptoms is dependent upon the depth and duration of submersion, the degree of physical exertion, the age, weight, and physical condition of the diver, and the rate of ascent. The size and number of gas bubbles (notably nitrogen) escaping from the tissues are dependent upon the difference between the atmospheric pressure and the partial pressure of the gas dissolved in the tissues. It is the release of gas bubbles, and particularly the location of their release, that determines the symptoms.

Decompression sickness may also occur in rapid ascents from sea level to high altitudes when there is no adequate pressurizing protection. Deep-sea and scuba divers may be vulnerable to air embolism if airplane travel is attempted too soon (within a few hours) after diving.

The onset of symptoms occurs within 30 minutes in half of cases and almost invariably within 6 hours. Symptoms, which are highly variable, include pain (largely in the joints), pruritic rash, visual disturbances, weakness or paralysis, dizziness or vertigo, headache, dyspnea, paresthesias, aphasia, and coma.

Early recognition and prompt treatment are extremely important. Continuous administration of oxygen is indicated as a first aid measure, whether or not cyanosis is present. Aspirin may be given for pain, but narcotics should be used very cautiously, since they may obscure the patient's response to recompression. Rapid transportation to a treatment facility for recompression, hyperbaric oxygen, hydration treatment of plasma deficits, and supportive measures is necessary not only to relieve symptoms but also to prevent permanent impairment. The physician should be familiar with the nearest compression center. The local public health department or nearest naval facility should be able to provide such information. Hypothermia may also be indicated.

Davis JC et al: Altitude decompression sickness: Hyperbaric therapy results in 145 cases. *Aviat Space Environ Med* 1977; **48**:722.
Kizer KW: Delayed treatment of dysbarism: A retrospective review of 50 cases. *JAMA* 1982;**247**:2555.
Kizer KW: Disorders of the deep. *Emerg Med* (June 30) 1984;**16**:18.

MOUNTAIN SICKNESS

Modern, rapid means of transportation have increased the number of unacclimatized individuals who are exposed to the effects of high altitude. Lack of sufficient time for acclimatization, increased physical activity, and varying degrees of health may be responsible for the acute and chronic disturbances that result from hypoxia at altitudes greater than 2000 meters. Marked individual differences in tolerance to hypoxia exist. Patients with sickle cell disease are at high risk of painful crises from altitude-induced hypoxemia; if they have had no previous mountain exposure, they should be advised to avoid mountains.

Acute Mountain Sickness

Initial manifestations include dizziness, headache, lassitude, drowsiness, chilliness, nausea and vomiting, facial pallor, dyspnea, and cyanosis. Later, there is facial flushing, irritability, difficulty in concentrating, vertigo, tinnitus, visual (retinal hemorrhages may occur) and auditory disturbances, anorexia, insomnia, increased dyspnea and weakness on exertion, increased headaches (due to cerebral edema), palpitations, tachycardia, Cheyne-Stokes breathing, and weight loss. Voluntary, periodic hyperventilation may relieve symptoms. In most individuals, symptoms clear within 24–48 hours, but in some instances, if the symptoms are sufficiently persistent or severe, return to lower altitudes is required. Administration of oxygen will often relieve acute symptoms. Judicious use of sedatives may be of value for some adults with irritability and insomnia. Preventive measures include adequate rest and sleep the day before travel, reduced food intake, and avoidance of alcohol, tobacco, and unnecessary physical activity during travel. Acetazolamide (Diamox), 250 mg every 8 hours one day before, during, and several days after ascent, may prevent symptoms of acute mountain sickness or alleviate its severity.

Acute High-Altitude Pulmonary Edema

This serious complication usually occurs at levels above 3000 meters. Early symptoms of pulmonary edema may appear within 6–36 hours after arrival at a high-altitude area—dry, incessant cough, dyspnea at rest, and substernal oppression. Later, wheezing, orthopnea, and hemoptysis may occur. Recognition of the early symptoms may enable the patient to climb down (or be assisted) to lower altitudes before incapacitating pulmonary edema develops. An early descent of even 500 or 1000 meters may result in improvement of symptoms. Physical findings include tachycardia, mild fever, tachypnea, cyanosis, and rales and rhonchi. The patient may become confused or even comatose, and the entire clinical picture may resemble severe pneumonia. Microthrombi are often found in the pulmonary capillaries. The white count is often slightly elevated, but the blood sedimentation rate is usually normal. Chest x-ray findings vary from irregular patchy exudate in one lung to nodular densities bilaterally or with transient prominence of the central pulmonary arteries. Transient, nonspecific electrocardiographic changes, occasionally showing right ventricular strain, may occur. Pulmonary arterial blood pressure is elevated, whereas pulmonary wedge pressure is normal. Treatment, which must often be given under field conditions, consists of rest in the semi-Fowler position and administration of 100% oxygen by mask at a rate of 6–8 L/min for 15–20 min. To conserve oxygen, lower flow rates may be used for the next 24–48 h until the victim recovers or can be evacuated to a lower altitude. Assistance for prompt descent (eg, by helicopter) may be lifesaving. Treatment for acute respiratory distress syndrome (see p 167) may be required for some patients who have a prolonged course of pulmonary edema. Rapid digitalization and use of diuretics, corticosteroids, and other drugs have been recommended but are of no proved value. If bacterial pneumonia exists, appropriate antibiotic therapy should be given.

Preventive measures include education of prospective mountaineers regarding the possibility of serious pulmonary edema, optimal physical conditioning before travel, gradual ascent to permit acclimatization, and a period of rest and inactivity for 1–2 days after arrival at high altitudes. Acetazolamide (Diamox), 250 mg orally every 8 hours beginning the day before ascent and continuing for 3–4 days after arrival at high altitudes, may reduce the incidence and severity of pulmonary edema. Prompt medical attention with rest and high-flow oxygen if respiratory symptoms develop may prevent progression to frank pulmonary edema. Persons with a history of high-altitude pulmonary edema should be hospitalized for further observation if possible. Mountaineering parties at levels of 3000 meters or higher, if hospital facilities are not available, should carry a supply of oxygen and equipment sufficient for several days. Persons with symptomatic cardiac or pulmonary disease should avoid high altitudes.

Subacute Mountain Sickness

This occurs most frequently in unacclimatized individuals and at altitudes above 4500 meters. Symptoms, which are probably due to central nervous system anoxia without associated alveolar hyperventilation, are similar to but more persistent and severe than those of acute mountain sickness. There are additional problems of dehydration, skin dryness, and pruritus.

The hematocrit may be elevated, and there may be electrocardiographic and chest x-ray evidence of right ventricular hypertrophy. Treatment consists of rest, oxygen administration, and return to lower altitudes.

Chronic Mountain Sickness (Monge's Disease)

This uncommon condition of chronic alveolar hypoventilation, which is encountered in residents of high-altitude communities who have lost their acclimatization to such an environment, is difficult to differentiate clinically from chronic pulmonary disease. The disorder is characterized by somnolence, mental depression, hypoxemia, cyanosis, clubbing of fingers, polycythemia (hematocrit often $> 75\%$), signs of right ventricular failure, electrocardiographic evidence of right axis deviation and right atrial and ventricular hypertrophy, and x-ray evidence of right heart enlargement and central pulmonary vessel prominence. There is no x-ray evidence of structural pulmonary disease. Pulmonary function tests usually disclose alveolar hypoventilation and elevated CO_2 tension but fail to reveal defective oxygen transport. There is a diminished respiratory response to CO_2. Almost complete disappearance of all abnormalities eventually occurs when the patient returns to sea level.

Blume FD et al: Impaired osmoregulation at high altitude: Studies on Mt. Everest. *JAMA* 1984;**252**:524.

Claster S, Godwin MJ, Embury SH: Risk of altitude exposure in sickle cell disease. *West J Med* 1981;**135**:364.

Hackett PH: Acute mountain sickness: The clinical approach. *Adv Cardiol* 1980;**27**:6.

Houston CS: Altitude illness: The dangers of heights and how to avoid them. *Postgrad Med* (July) 1983;**74**:231.

Larson EB et al: Acute mountain sickness and acetazolamide: Clinical efficacy and effect on ventilation. *JAMA* 1982;**248**:328.

Meehan RT, Zavala DC: The pathophysiology of acute high-altitude illness. *Am J Med* 1982;**73**:395.

MEDICAL EFFECTS OF AIR TRAVEL & SELECTION OF PATIENTS FOR AIR TRAVEL

The decision about whether or not it is advisable for a patient to travel by air depends not only upon the nature and severity of the illness but also upon such factors as the duration of flight, the altitude to be flown, pressurization, the availability of supplementary oxygen and other medical supplies, the presence of attending physicians and trained nursing attendants, and other special considerations. Air carriers in the USA cannot legally allow the use of personal (passenger-supplied) oxygen containers, but most major airlines will supply oxygen upon advance written request from the passenger's physician. Airline policies, charges, and other details must be checked with each carrier. Medical hazards or complications of modern air travel are remarkably uncommon; unless there is some specific contraindication (Table 30–2),

Table 30–2. Contraindications to commercial air travel.*

Cardiovascular
 Within 4 weeks after myocardial infarction†
 Within 2 weeks after cerebrovascular accident
 Severe hypertension
 Decompensated cardiovascular disease or restricted cardiac reserve‡

Bronchopulmonary
 Pneumothorax
 Congenital pulmonary cysts
 Vital capacity less than 50%

Eye, ear, nose, and throat
 Recent eye surgery
 Acute sinusitis or otitis media
 Surgical mandibular fixation (permanent wiring of jaw)

Gastrointestinal tract
 Less than 10–14 days after abdominal surgery
 Acute diverticulitis or ulcerative colitis
 Acute esophageal varices
 Acute gastroenteritis

Neuropsychiatric
 Epilepsy (unless well controlled medically and cabin altitude does not exceed 8000 ft)
 Previous violent or unpredictable behavior
 Recent skull fracture
 Brain tumor

Hematologic
 Anemia (hemoglobin < 8.5 g/dL or red blood cell count of 3 million/μL in an adult)
 Sickle cell disease (except below 68-m [22,500-foot] altitude)
 Blood dyscrasias with active bleeding (hemophilia, leukemia)

Pregnancy
 Beyond 240 days or with threatened miscarriage

Miscellaneous
 Need for intravenous fluids or special medical apparatus†

*Slightly modified and reproduced, with permission, from *Mod Med* (June) 1982;**50**:196. Based on recommendations of the American Medical Association in *JAMA* 1982;**247**:1009.
†Consultation with an airline flight surgeon is suggested.
‡In some cases, low-altitude flights can be made without supplemental oxygen in accordance with recommendations of the American College of Chest Physicians.

air transportation may actually be the best means of moving patients. The Air Transport Association of America defines an incapacitated passenger as "one who is suffering from a physical or mental disability and who, because of such disability or the effect of the flight on the disability, is incapable of self-care; would endanger the health or safety of such person or other passengers or airline employees; or would cause discomfort or annoyance of other passengers."

Cardiovascular Disease

A. Cardiac Decompensation: Patients in congestive failure should not fly until they are compensated by appropriate treatment, or unless they are in a pressurized plane with 100% oxygen therapy available during the entire flight.

B. Compensated Valvular or Other Heart Disease: Patients should not fly over 2400–2800 meters unless the aircraft is pressurized and oxygen is administered at altitudes of 2400 meters or higher.

C. Acute Myocardial Infarction, Convalescent and Asymptomatic: At least 4 weeks of convalescence are recommended even for asymptomatic patients if flying is contemplated. Ambulatory, stabilized, and compensated patients tolerate air travel well. Oxygen should be available.

D. Angina Pectoris: Air travel is inadvisable for patients with severe angina. In mild to moderate cases of angina, air travel may be permitted, especially in pressurized planes. Oxygen should be available.

Respiratory Disease

A. Nasopharyngeal Disorders: Nasal allergies and infections predispose to development of aerotitis. Chewing gum, nasal decongestants, and appropriate anti-infective treatment may prevent barotitis.

B. Asthma: Patients with mild asthma can travel without difficulty. Patients with status asthmaticus should not be permitted to fly.

C. Congenital Pulmonary Cysts: Patients should not travel unless cleared by physician.

D. Tuberculosis: Patients with active, communicable tuberculosis or pneumothorax should not be permitted to travel by air.

E. Other Pulmonary Disorders: Patients may be flown safely unless there is marked impairment of pulmonary function (vital capacity < 50%).

Anemia

If hemoglobin is less than 8–9 g/dL, oxygen should be available. Patients with severe anemia should not travel until hemoglobin has been raised to a reasonable level. Patients with sickle cell anemia appear to be particularly vulnerable.

Diabetes Mellitus

Diabetics who do not need insulin or who can administer their own insulin during flight may fly safely. "Brittle" diabetics who are subject to frequent episodes of hypoglycemia should be in optimal control before flying and should carry sugar or candy in case hypoglycemic reactions occur.

Contagious Diseases

Patients with contagious diseases are not permitted to travel by scheduled passenger airlines at any time.

Patients With Surgical Problems

Patients convalescing from thoracic or abdominal surgery should not fly until 10 days after surgery, and then only if their wound is healed and there is no drainage.

Colostomy patients may be permitted to travel by air providing they are nonodorous and colostomy bags are emptied before flight.

Patients with large hernias unsupported by a truss or binder should not be permitted to fly in nonpressurized aircraft because of an increased danger of strangulation.

Postsurgical or posttraumatic eye cases require pressurized cabins and oxygen therapy to avoid retinal damage due to hypoxia.

Psychiatric Disorders

Severely psychotic, agitated, or disturbed patients should not be permitted to fly on scheduled airlines even when accompanied by a medical attendant.

Extremely nervous or apprehensive patients may travel by air if they receive adequate sedatives or tranquilizers before and during flight.

Motion Sickness

Patients subject to motion sickness should receive sedatives or antihistamines (eg, dimenhydrinate or meclizine), 50 mg 4 times daily, before and during the flight. Small meals of easily digested food before and during flight may reduce the tendency to nausea and vomiting.

Pregnancy

Pregnant women may be permitted to fly during the first 8 months of pregnancy unless there is a history of habitual abortion or premature birth. During the ninth month of pregnancy, a statement must be furnished that delivery is not due within 72 hours of destination time. Infants less than 1 week old should not be flown at high altitudes or for long distances.

AMA Commission on Emergency Medical Services: Medical aspects of transportation aboard commercial aircraft. *JAMA* 1982;**247:**1007.

Kusumi RK: Medical aspects of air travel. *Am Fam Physician* (June) 1981;**23:**125.

Mills FJ, Harding RM: Fitness to travel by air. 2. Specific medical considerations. *Br Med J* 1983;**286:**1340.

Schley WS: Barotrauma during air travel. *Hosp Med* (July) 1983;**19:**119.

Schwartz JS, Bencowitz HZ, Moser KM: Air travel hypoxemia with chronic obstructive pulmonary disease. *Ann Intern Med* 1984;**100:**473.

Voss MW: Air travel for the chronically ill and the elderly. *Am Fam Physician* (March) 1983;**27:**235.

Poisoning | 31

*Robert H. Dreisbach, MD, PhD**

DIAGNOSIS OF POISONING

The diagnosis of poisoning, when not obvious, depends in great measure upon considering the possibility that poisoning has occurred. Once poisoning is included in the differential diagnosis, the physician will be more likely to take the necessary steps to confirm or reject this possibility.

In general, the steps leading to a diagnosis of poisoning are as follows:

(1) Question the patient, relatives and roommates, coworkers, etc, carefully concerning the presence of poisons in the environment or possible bites by venomous animals or insects.

(2) Take a careful history and perform a complete physical examination. Be aware that the history is likely to be unreliable, especially in attempted suicide.

(3) Take samples for laboratory evaluation of damage to specific organs and to confirm or rule out exposure to specific poisons. Gastric contents usually have the highest concentration of poison and can be used to indicate the possibility but not the seriousness of poisoning.

Cases of poisoning generally fall into 3 specific categories: (1) exposure to a known poison, (2) exposure to an unknown substance that may be a poison, and (3) disease of undetermined cause in which poisoning must be considered as part of the differential diagnosis. For further information on the diagnosis and treatment of poisoning, consult the books listed on this page and in the bibliography at the end of the chapter.

Call Poison Information Center

Obtain the telephone number of the nearest poison information center, and record it for ready reference. Poison information centers are in most cases able to identify the ingredients of trade-named mixtures, give some estimate of their toxicity, suggest the necessary treatment, and make referrals to experienced toxicologists.

*Prepared with the help of Kent R. Olson, MD, Program Director, San Francisco Bay Area Regional Poison Control Center, and Assistant Clinical Professor of Medicine, University of California School of Medicine (San Francisco).

EXPOSURE TO KNOWN POISONS

In many cases of poisoning, the agent responsible is known and the physician's only problem is to determine whether the degree of exposure is sufficient to require more than emergency or first aid treatment. The exact quantity of poison absorbed by the patient will probably not be known, but the physician may be able to estimate the greatest amount the patient could have absorbed by examining the container from which the poison was obtained and comparing the missing quantity with the known fatal dose. Reported minimum lethal doses (MLD) are useful indications of the relative hazards of poisonous substances, but the fatal dose may vary greatly. If the poison is known to cause serious or fatal poisoning, treatment for exposure to any quantity must be vigorous.

EXPOSURE TO SUBSTANCES THAT MAY BE POISONOUS

If a patient has been exposed to a substance whose ingredients are not known, the physician must identify the contents without delay. In addition to the regional poison information center, the following sources are suggested for identifying the contents of trade-named mixtures.

Books

Since available proprietary mixtures number in the hundreds of thousands, it is impractical to include all of these names in a single reference work. However, a number of books are useful in determining the contents of mixtures and should be available to every physician:

(1) Gosselin RE et al: *Clinical Toxicology of Commercial Products,* 5th ed. Williams & Wilkins, 1984. (Lists ingredients of 17,500 products.)

(2) *The Merck Index,* 9th ed. Merck, 1976.

(3) *American Drug Index* (annual publication). Lippincott.

(4) *Physicians' Desk Reference* (annual publication). Medical Economics, Inc. (Tablet and capsule identification guide.)

(5) Dreisbach RH: *Handbook of Poisoning: Prevention, Diagnosis, & Treatment,* 11th ed. Lange,

1983. (Lists 6000 poisons and trade-named mixtures.)

(6) Griffenhagen GB (editor): *Handbook of Non-Prescription Drugs* (annual publication). American Pharmaceutical Association.

(7) Berg GL (editor): *Farm Chemical Handbook* (annual publication). Meister.

Other Sources of Information

(1) Rumack BH (editor): Poisindex. National Center for Poison Information, Denver, CO 80204. A microfiche information system. Revised quarterly.

(2) Likes KE (editor): Toxifile. Chicago Micro Corporation, Chicago, IL 60625. A microfiche information system.

(3) The manufacturer or the local representative. Another way to identify the contents of a substance is to telephone the manufacturer or the local distributor, who will be able to provide information concerning the type of toxic hazard to be expected from the material in question and what treatment should be given.

(4) Poisoning hotlines to manufacturers. Call the poison control center for the telephone number.

DIFFERENTIAL DIAGNOSIS OF DISEASES THAT MAY BE THE RESULT OF POISONING

In any disease state of questionable origin, poisoning by one or more substances must be considered as part of the differential diagnosis. For example, the high incidence of cases of lead poisoning discovered in a few medical centers in recent years indicates that many cases must go unrecognized. Some patients had symptoms for more than a year and had been seen by several physicians before the diagnosis was made. Admittedly, the diagnosis of lead poisoning is difficult, but the possibility of this disorder must be considered before steps can be taken to confirm the diagnosis. The most important confirmatory steps in any case of poisoning are the discovery of a source of the poison and a history of exposure to it.

Intentional self-administration of drugs or chemicals for suicidal, "mind-altering," or therapeutic purposes should be included as possible sources of poisoning. The patient may not admit such use until the physician can find suggestive evidence, either by laboratory examination of blood, urine, or gastric contents or by other means. The willingness of some individuals to ingest or inject substances without knowing what they are causes frequent bizarre episodes. Street drugs are sometimes adulterated with potent agents, including strychnine, with fatal results.

In making the differential diagnosis of a disease that may be the result of poisoning, the number of poisons that must be considered in any particular case can be reduced by classifying exposure possibilities. A convenient classification based on exposure consists of the following groups: (1) household, (2) medicinal, (3) industrial, (4) agricultural, and (5) natural.

SYSTEM EXAMINATION

A carefully taken history and physical examination are essential for therapeutic purposes and may also provide valuable information for determining the cause and extent of a poisoning. Below are commonly seen symptoms and signs and poisons that may be causative.

Vital Signs

Tachycardia: Amphetamines, cocaine, atropine, iron, theophylline, antidepressants.

Bradycardia: Digitalis, oleander, organophosphates, clonidine, beta blockers.

Hyperthermia: Amphetamines, cocaine, phencyclidine (PCP), atropine, salicylates, pentachlorophenol.

Hypothermia: Barbiturates, ethanol, narcotics, sedatives, insulin-induced hypoglycemia.

Hyperventilation: Salicylates, methanol, ethylene glycol, caffeine, theophylline.

Respiratory depression: Barbiturates, narcotics, sedatives, ethanol, antidepressants, organophosphates.

Hypertension: Amphetamines, cocaine, phenylpropanolamine, nicotine, phencyclidine (PCP).

Hypotension: Iron, nitrites, narcotics, antihypertensives, antidepressants, barbiturates, theophylline.

Skin

Cyanosis: Methemoglobinemia (nitrites, chlorates, aniline), cyanide, carbon monoxide (more common than flushing), apnea.

Flushing or redness: Ethanol, cyanide, atropine.

Jaundice: *Amanita phalloides* mushrooms, acetaminophen, carbon tetrachloride and other halogenated hydrocarbons.

Dry skin and mucous membranes: Atropine, antihistamines, antidepressants.

Sweaty skin: Organophosphates, nicotine, amphetamines, cocaine, phencyclidine (PCP).

Mouth

Dry mouth: Atropine, antihistamines, antidepressants.

Salivation: Organophosphates, mercury, lead.

Characteristic breath odors: Ethanol, ammonia, camphor, paraldehyde, garlic (arsenic, organophosphates, arsine), bitter almond (cyanide), rotten eggs (hydrogen sulfide), peanuts (rat poisons).

Eyes

Ptosis: Botulism, thallium, cholinergic excess, elapid type snakebite.

Dilated pupils: Atropine, amphetamines, cocaine, LSD.

Constricted pupils: Narcotics, clonidine, phenothiazines, organophosphates, pilocarpine.
Oculogyric crises: Antipsychotics.

Ears

Tinnitus, deafness, vestibular disturbances (see p 106).

Abdomen

Abdominal pain: Black widow spider bite, lead, arsenic, organophosphates, *Amanita phalloides* mushrooms.
Hematemesis: Corrosives, anticoagulants, iron, fluoride.

Neuromuscular System

Headache: Nitrites, carbon monoxide, lead, solvent inhalation.
Delirium, hallucinations: Ethanol (including withdrawal), cocaine, amphetamines, phencyclidine (PCP), atropine, LSD, salicylates.
Convulsions: Antidepressants, theophylline, isoniazid, phenothiazines, antihistamines, camphor, amphetamines, cocaine, lindane, organophosphates, ethanol and sedative withdrawal.
Rigidity and cramps: Strychnine, heatstroke, tetanus, black widow spider bite, phencyclidine (PCP).

Laboratory, ECG, & X-Ray Studies

Urine occult blood (eg, Hematest) positive: Hemoglobinuria (naphthalene, arsine, chlorates, favism); myoglobinuria (phencyclidine [PCP], amphetamines, convulsants, heatstroke); hematuria (anticoagulants).
Urine Phenistix positive: Salicylates, phenothiazines.
Urine oxalate crystals: Ethylene glycol, soluble oxalates.
Proteinuria: Arsenic, mercury, phosphorus.
Hypoglycemia: Salicylates, ethanol.
ECG: (1) Ventricular arrhythmias—amphetamines, cocaine, antidepressants, theophylline, digitalis preparations, quinidine; (2) AV block—antidepressants, digitalis, beta blockers, calcium channel blockers, quinidine.
X-rays of abdomen (radiopaque pills or toxins): Disk batteries, chloral hydrate, heavy metals, iodide, phenothiazines, antidepressants, sodium chloride, enteric coated tablets.

SPECIAL LABORATORY TESTS

Special chemical examinations for lead or other heavy metals, pesticides, cholinesterase, depressants, tranquilizers, alkaloids, etc, may be necessary in the differential diagnosis of poisoning. The following laboratories are suggested. It is wise to make prior arrangements with laboratory personnel to make certain they will accept samples for analyses.

(1) Private toxicology laboratories: Most will do comprehensive screening of blood, urine, and gastric samples.
(2) County coroner's laboratory: Metals, blood alcohol, barbiturates, alkaloids.
(3) City, county, or state police laboratory: Blood alcohol, barbiturates, other poisons.
(4) State toxicologist's office: As under (1). Analyses in connection with criminal poisonings.
(5) Federal Bureau of Investigation Laboratory, Washington DC (only through local police).
(6) State departments of public health will usually perform analyses relating only to cases of occupational poisoning: insecticides, metals.
(7) County hospital laboratory: Lead, barbiturates, alkaloids, blood alcohol.
(8) Technical Development Laboratory, United States Public Health Service, PO Box 769, Savannah, GA 31402: Insecticides in blood, body fat, blood cholinesterase. (Send weighed, frozen sample, with patient identification and history. Specify pesticide.)

PRINCIPLES OF TREATMENT OF POISONING

(See also First Aid Measures, below.)

In emergency treatment of any suspected poisoning, the following general procedures should be carried out: (1) Support vital functions. Maintain airway and respiration. Combat shock, convulsions, and other specific manifestations as they arise. (2) Place large-bore intravenous catheter, and draw blood for complete blood count; glucose, electrolyte, and renal function tests; liver function tests; and tests for specific suspected toxins or toxicologic screening. (3) Give specific antidote if one exists. (4) Remove poison by emesis or lavage, catharsis, and administration of activated charcoal as soon as possible.

Supportive & Symptomatic Measures

The victim of acute poisoning must be kept under close observation in order to anticipate the immediate and delayed complications of the poisoning. Suicidal patients need special surveillance and should be seen by a psychiatrist.

A. Respiratory Abnormalities: Obtain arterial blood gases to measure adequacy of ventilation and oxygenation as soon as is feasible.

1. Respiratory obstruction—Correct by positioning, oropharyngeal airway, or endotracheal intubation.

2. Respiratory depression—Remove from toxic atmosphere. Administer artificial respiration as

---

First Aid Measures in Poisoning

The following summary is provided for the physician's use in giving instructions for first aid treatment in response to an emergency inquiry. With the exceptions noted under Ingested Poison, anyone can carry out these procedures. The rescuer should avoid self-contamination.

If respirations are depressed, give artificial respiration by direct mouth-to-mouth resuscitation or bag-valve-mask inflation. Remove any objects or vomitus from the victim's mouth, hold the jaw forward and tip the head backward, and blow into the mouth until the chest rises. Repeat 10–15 times per minute. Obtain help immediately.

Ingested Poison
Lay persons should *not* attempt treatment (other than maintaining respirations) if the patient is convulsing or unconscious. If the patient has ingested petroleum products (eg, kerosene, gasoline, paint thinner) or corrosives (acid or alkali), do *not* induce emesis. Water or milk may be given to patients who have ingested a corrosive substance.
1. Induce emesis: Give 30 mL (½ oz) syrup of ipecac. Follow with ½ glass of water. *(Not effective after charcoal.)*
2. Give activated charcoal after emesis.
3. Conserve body warmth by applying blankets. Avoid external heat.

Inhaled Poisons
1. Carry the victim to fresh air immediately; loosen tight clothing.
2. Administer oxygen as soon as possible. Assist respiration if needed.

Skin Contamination
1. Drench skin with water in tub or shower.
2. Direct a stream of water onto the skin while removing the patient's clothing.
3. Do *not* use chemical antidotes.

Eye Contamination
1. Holding the lids apart, wash the eye for 5 minutes or longer with running water at eye fountain or with a gentle stream of water from a hose or tap (see p 94).
2. Do *not* use chemical antidotes.

Snake, Insect, or Arachnid Bite
1. Immobilize the patient immediately.
2. Do *not* apply a tourniquet.
3. If the patient must be moved, carry on a stretcher as gently as possible.
4. Seek medical attention as soon as possible. Specific antivenin may be indicated (see text).

Identification of Unknown Toxic Agent
The following information is useful in attempting to identify a toxic agent. It should be available when calling the Poison Information Center.
1. Physical state (solid, liquid, gas).
2. Odor.
3. Trade name.
4. Use.
5. Presence of poison label.
6. Inflammability warning.

---

needed. Stimulants (analeptic drugs) are of no value in poisoning.

3. Methemoglobinemia: Give 100% oxygen by mask, and methylene blue, 0.1 mL/kg of 1% solution slowly intravenously, in the presence of symptoms or if methemoglobin level is over 30%.

B. Circulatory Failure:

1. Shock–(See p 8.) The principal measures include recumbent position, warmth, and parenteral fluids. Give saline in 200-mL boluses up to 1–2 L.

2. Cardiac failure–(See p 244.) When hypotension does not respond to 1–2 L of saline and is due to the cardiac depressant effects of toxins, administration of dopamine or dobutamine is recommended. A pulmonary artery catheter is useful in guiding the use of fluids and pressors in critically ill patients.

3. Pulmonary edema–Give oxygen by mask. The oxygen concentration should not exceed 50% to avoid lung injury. Ventilatory assistance, including positive end expiratory pressure (PEEP), may be needed to maintain adequate arterial oxygen saturation. Furosemide and mannitol diuresis may be helpful.

C. Coma:

1. Give 50% glucose, 1 mL/kg intravenously after blood sample for serum glucose has been drawn. In alcoholic or malnourished patients, also give 100 mg of thiamine intramuscularly to prevent Wernicke's syndrome.

2. Give naloxone (Narcan), 0.01–0.05 mg/kg intravenously. Up to 0.2 mg/kg is occasionally required for massive narcotic overdose.

D. Convulsions:

1. Give diazepam, 0.1-0.2 mg/kg intravenously over 1–2 minutes.

2. Give phenytoin, 15–20 mg/kg intravenously at a rate no faster than 0.5 mg/kg/min.

3. If these are unsuccessful, phenobarbital, pentobarbital, or other anticonvulsants may be useful (obtain neurologic consultation).

E. Start Electrocardiographic Monitoring: Obtain 12-lead ECG, noting rate, rhythm, presence of arrhythmias, and PR, QRS, and QT intervals. Attach continuous monitor for at least 6 hours if irregularities are present or overdose of tricyclic antidepressants is suspected.

Removal of Poison
Caution: Do not use stomach tubes or emetics in poisonings due to corrosive agents; further injury may result. Some tablets and capsules may form masses of drug in the stomach, requiring gastrotomy for removal.

A. Emesis: This is the quickest and most effective way to evacuate gastric contents.

1. Indications–For removal of poison in conscious, cooperative patients and for promptness, since ipecac can be given in the home in the first few minutes after poisoning.

2. Contraindications–(1) Drowsy, unconscious, or convulsing patients. (2) Ingestion of kerosene or other hydrocarbons (danger of aspiration of stomach contents). (3) Ingestion of corrosive poisons. (4) Ingestion of rapidly acting convulsants.

3. Technique–Give syrup of ipecac, 30 mL (15 mL in children), followed by ½ glass of water (120 mL). Repeat in 20 minutes if necessary. Dose should be 10 mL of syrup of ipecac in patients under 1 year of age. *Ipecac is not effective after charcoal has been given.*

B. Adsorption: Activated charcoal is effective for adsorbing almost all poisons. One satisfactory preparation is Charcoaid, available from the Requa Manufacturing Company, 1 Seneca Place, Greenwich, CT 06830. Each Charcoaid container contains activated charcoal, 30 g, in 150 mL of sorbitol solution. This preparation keeps well, it resuspends easily, the sorbitol does not interfere with adsorption, and the sorbitol counteracts the constipating effect of the charcoal. Give 60–90 g orally after emesis, or use as lavage fluid.

C. Gastric Aspiration and Lavage:

1. Indications–(1) For removal of ingested poisons when emesis is refused, contraindicated, or unsuccessful. (2) For collection and examination of gastric contents for identification of poison. (3) For convenient administration of antidotes. Danger of aspiration pneumonia is reduced by tracheal intubation.

2. Contraindications–(1) Corrosion of tissues by poison. (2) Stuporous or comatose patients with absent gag reflex, unless endotracheally intubated prior to lavage. (3) Kerosene or other hydrocarbons.

3. Technique–Gently insert a lubricated, soft but noncollapsible stomach tube (at least 37–40F) through the mouth or nose into the stomach. Aspirate and save contents; then lavage repeatedly with 50–100 mL of fluid until return is clear. Always remove excess lavage fluid.

Collect and save washings in clean containers for toxicologic examination when indicated. In forensic cases, seal with sealing wax and place in a locked refrigerator; deliver to toxicologist personally and get a signed receipt.

4. Gastric lavage fluids–(1) Warm tap water or saline. (2) Activated charcoal: Use 50 g in 400 mL water and stir or shake until completely wet. The suspension should have a slightly thickened consistency.

D. Catharsis:

1. Indications–For removal of unabsorbed poisons, especially those that have passed into the intestine.

2. Contraindications–Do not use mineral oil or other oil-based cathartics. Avoid sodium-based cathartics in hypertension, renal failure, and conges-

tive heart failure. Avoid magnesium-based cathartics in renal failure.

3. Materials–Sodium sulfate 10%, 1–2 mL/kg; magnesium sulfate 10%, 2–3 mL/kg; or sorbitol 70%, 1–2 mL/kg. Combine with activated charcoal, 60–90 g.

4. Technique–A single dose is usually given. Repeated doses of activated charcoal, 20–30 g in water, or 15–20 mL of sorbitol may hasten elimination of some drugs (eg, digitoxin, theophylline, phenobarbital).

Inactivation by Demulcents

Demulcents precipitate metals and also help to limit the absorption of many poisons. These bland agents are also soothing to inflamed mucous membranes. Use whites of 3 or 4 eggs beaten in 500 mL of milk or water, evaporated milk, or thin flour or starch solution (boiled, if possible). Follow with lavage.

Antidotes

Give "specific" antidotes when there is reasonable certainty of a specific diagnosis (Table 31–1). To effectively negate the physiologic effects of the toxic agent, the antidote must be given promptly. Keep in mind, however, that antidotes frequently have serious side effects of their own. The indications and dosages for specific antidotes are discussed in the respective sections for specific toxins.

Increased Drug Removal

A. Diuretics: Osmotic diuretics (eg, mannitol, urea, hypertonic glucose) or saluretic agents (eg, ethacrynic acid, furosemide) may increase drug excretion in cases of serious poisoning with drugs primarily excreted by the kidney (eg, salicylates and phenobarbital). Osmotic diuretics may also relieve cerebral edema (eg, in lead poisoning). Forced diuresis requires an adequate osmotic load and appropriate parenteral fluids and is hazardous. Basic drugs (eg, amphetamines, strychnine) are best excreted by maintaining an acid urine. Acidic drugs (eg, salicylates, phenobarbi-

Table 31–1. Some toxic agents for which there are "specific" antidotes.

Toxic Agent	Specific Antidote
Acetaminophen	Acetylcysteine
Anticholinergics (eg, atropine)	Physostimine
Anticholinesterases (eg, organophosphate pesticides, physostigmine)	Atropine
Carbon monoxide	Oxygen
Cyanide	Sodium nitrite, sodium thiosulfate
Heavy metals (eg, lead, arsenic, mercury, iron)	Specific chelating agents
Hydrogen sulfide	Sodium nitrite
Isoniazid	Pyridoxine
Methanol (methyl alcohol)	Ethanol (ethyl alcohol)
Narcotics	Naloxone (Narcan)
Snake venom	Specific venom antisera

Table 31–2. Toxic agents for which hemoperfusion or hemodialysis may be indicated.

Sedative-hypnotics: Barbiturates (long-acting), ethchlorvynol.
Alcohols: Methanol, ethylene glycol.
Analgesics: Acetaminophen, salicylates, phenacetin.
Cardioactive agents: Digitoxin, disopyramide.
Metals: Arsenic and mercury after dimercaprol, lead after edetate, iron after deferoxamine, lithium, potassium.
Halides: Bromide, fluoride, iodide.
Miscellaneous: Anilines, nitrobenzenes, borates, boric acid, nitrofurantoin, theophylline, thiocyanates.

tal) are best excreted with an alkaline urine. Contraindications to osmotic diuresis include renal insufficiency, pulmonary edema, cardiac insufficiency, and persistent severe hypotension despite adequate fluid replacement. Acidification is contraindicated in the presence of rhabdomyolysis or myoglobinuria.

B. Dialysis: The indications for dialysis are as follows: (1) Known or suspected potentially lethal amounts of a dialyzable drug (Table 31–2). (2) Poisoning with deep coma, apnea, severe hypotension, fluid and electrolyte or acid-base disturbance, or extreme body temperature changes which cannot be corrected by conventional measures. (3) Poisoning in patients with severe renal, cardiac, pulmonary, or hepatic disease who will not be able to eliminate the toxin by usual mechanisms.

Constant monitoring of vital signs, central venous pressure, and frequent laboratory determinations of fluids, electrolytes, and blood gases are required.

Peritoneal dialysis may be employed for acute poisonings when hemodialysis is not available, but it is very inefficient.

Dialysis should usually augment rather than replace well-established emergency and supportive measures.

C. Hemoperfusion: Many of the substances that cannot be removed effectively by aqueous dialysis (Table 31–2) can be removed by hemoperfusion through resin or coated charcoal columns. Indications are the same as for dialysis.

Bayer NJ, Rumack B, Wanke L: *Toxicologic Emergencies.* Brady, 1984.
Driggers DA: Pediatric poisoning: The first thirty minutes. *Postgrad Med* (Aug) 1982;**72**:52.
Goldfrank LR: *Toxicologic Emergencies.* Appleton-Century-Crofts, 1982.
Haddad LM, Winchester JF (editors): *Clinical Management of Poisoning and Drug Overdosage.* Saunders, 1983.
Marcum LN, Berve MO: Prehospital management of the poisoned patient. *Crit Care Q* 1982;**4**:25.
Saxena K, Kingston R: Acute poisoning: Management protocol. *Postgrad Med* (May) 1982;**71**:67.

TREATMENT OF COMMON SPECIFIC POISONINGS
(Alphabetical Order)

ACETAMINOPHEN

Acetaminophen is available in many over-the-counter and prescription items. Ingestion of 150 mg/kg or more in a single dose by an adult may cause liver damage within the first 12 hours, but symptoms and signs of liver damage may not appear for 24–48 hours. Peak plasma levels do not occur until 4 or more hours after ingestion. Patients with 4-hour plasma acetaminophen levels above 150 μg/mL are at risk of developing severe hepatic necrosis.

Treatment

Treatment should be started immediately in any patient with a 4-hour level > 150 μg/mL and is probably useless after 12 hours. Removal of the drug is by emesis or gastric lavage. *Do not use activated charcoal, since it may hinder antidotal treatment!*

Give the specific antidote acetylcysteine (Mucomyst), 140 mg/kg orally of a 20% solution diluted to 5% in fruit juice or soda as a loading dose. Follow with 70 mg/kg orally every 4 hours for 3 days or until the plasma acetaminophen level is zero. If a dose is vomited within 1 hour, it should be repeated. It may be necessary to give the drug by duodenal tube. Discontinue acetylcysteine if hepatic encephalopathy occurs.

Davis AM et al: Severe hepatic damage after acetaminophen use in psittacosis. *Am J Med* 1983;**74**:349.
Rumack BH et al: Acetaminophen overdose: 662 cases with evaluation of acetylcysteine treatment. *Arch Intern Med* 1981; **141**:380.

ACIDS, CORROSIVE

The strong mineral acids exert primarily a local corrosive effect on the skin and mucous membranes. In severe burns, circulatory collapse may result. Symptoms include severe pain in the throat and upper gastrointestinal tract, marked thirst, bloody vomitus; difficulty in swallowing, breathing, and speaking; discoloration and destruction of skin and mucous membranes in and around the mouth; and shock.

The MLD is 1 mL of concentrated acid.

Inhalation of volatile acids, fumes, or gases such as chlorine, fluorine, bromine, or iodine causes severe irritation of the throat and chest with paroxysmal coughing and inhibition of respiration and may be followed by pulmonary edema.

Treatment

A. Ingested: Dilute immediately by giving 200

Table 31—3. Chronic toxicity of ethyl alcohol.

Psychoneurologic effects
  Acute alcoholism
    Intoxication, excitement, coma
  Withdrawal effects
    Hallucinosis, convulsions, delirium tremens
  Nutritional disorders
    Wernicke-Korsakoff syndrome, pellagra

Gastrointestinal effects
  Acute and chronic gastritis, malabsorption syndrome,
    fatty liver, cirrhosis, acute and chronic pancreatitis

Hematologic effects
  Anemia due to acute or chronic blood loss
  Cytoplasmic vacuolization of erythroid precursors
  Megaloblastic marrow alterations (inhibition of folate
    metabolism) with anemia
  Sideroblastic marrow abnormalities
  Stomatocytic erythrocyte changes
  Hemolytic anemia, thrombocytopenia
  Defective granulocyte mobilization
  Pancytopenia with hypocellular bone marrow

Neuromuscular effects
  Peripheral polyneuropathy
  Acute and chronic alcoholic myopathy

Cardiovascular effects
  Cardiomyopathy, elevated blood pressure

Metabolic effects
  Lactic acidosis, hypoglycemia, hypomagnesemia, hypo-
    uricemia, hyperlipidemia

Pulmonary effects
  Pulmonary aspiration, respiratory infections.
    Lung volumes, airway resistance, diffusion, gas ex-
    change all adversely affected.

Conditions aggravated by alcohol
  Traumatic encephalopathy, epilepsy, Hodgkin's disease,
    porphyria, peptic ulcer, pancreatitis

Drugs that contraindicate concomitant use of alcohol
  Disulfiram, sedatives, hypnotics, tranquilizers, phenformin

mL of milk or water to drink. Do not give bicarbonate or carbonates.

Relieve pain and treat shock (see p 9). Perform esophagoscopy promptly to determine the presence of injury but do not attempt to pass beyond the injury. Perforation, peritonitis, and major bleeding are indications for surgery.

B. Skin Contact: Flood with water for 15 minutes. Use no chemical antidotes; the heat of the reaction may cause additional injury. Relieve pain and treat shock. For hydrofluoric acid burns, inject 0.5 mL of 10% calcium gluconate with local anesthetic per square centimeter under the burned area.

C. Eye Contact: Flood with water for 15 minutes, holding the eyelids open. Check pH with pH 6–8 test paper, and repeat irrigation, using normal saline, until pH is 7. Arrange for slit lamp examination.

D. Inhalation: Remove from further exposure to fumes or gas. Check skin and clothing. Treat pulmonary edema.

Penner GE: Acid ingestion: Toxicology and treatment. *Ann Emerg Med* 1980;**9**:374.
Trevino MA et al: Treatment of severe hydrofluoric acid exposures. *J Oral Med* 1983;**25**:861.

ALCOHOL, ETHYL
(See also p 670.)

The principal manifestations of ethyl alcohol poisoning are central nervous system depression and gastric irritation, with nausea and vomiting. Hypoglycemia is indicated by seizures, hypothermia, conjugate deviation of the eyes, extensor rigidity, positive Babinski reflexes, and trismus. Use by pregnant women causes irreversible fetal brain injury.

Differentiate alcohol poisoning from depressant poisoning, head injury, mental disorders, and insulin hypoglycemia.

The MLD is 300 mL or 1 mL/kg in small children. The potentially lethal blood level is 3 mg/mL.

Treatment of Severe Alcoholic Intoxication

A. Emergency Measures: Remove unabsorbed alcohol by gastric lavage with tap water. Ipecac-induced emesis is useful in patients who are awake. Naloxone, 0.01 mg/kg intravenously, has been reported to have an arousal effect in acute alcohol coma.

B. General Measures: (Similar to those for barbiturate poisoning.)

1. Maintain the airway and adequate oxygenation and ventilation (determine arterial P_{O_2} and P_{CO_2}). Keep the patient warm.

2. If the patient is comatose and areflexic, treat as for barbiturate poisoning.

3. Determine blood alcohol and glucose levels.

4. Give glucose orally or intravenously for hypoglycemia or ketoacidosis.

5. Give thiamine, 100 mg intramuscularly, concurrently with glucose administration.

6. Dialysis is rarely necessary.

Eckardt MJ et al: Health hazards associated with alcoholism. *JAMA* 1981;**246**:648.
Smile DH: Acute alcohol withdrawal complicated by supraventricular tachycardia: Treatment with intravenous propranolol. *Ann Emerg Med* 1984;**13**:53.
West LJ et al: Alcoholism. *Ann Intern Med* 1984;**100**:405.

ALCOHOL, METHYL

Methyl alcohol is a central nervous system depressant that is metabolized to formic acid, which produces specific damage to the retinal cells and metabolic acidosis. The MLD is 30–60 mL. Symptoms include headache, abdominal pain, dyspnea, nausea, vomiting, and blindness. Examination reveals flush or cyanosis, excitement or depression, delirium, coma, and convulsions. The serum osmolality is often elevated. Methanol can be detected in the serum and urine.

Treatment

Determine blood P_{O_2}, P_{CO_2}, and pH. Give intravenous fluids and sodium bicarbonate to combat metabolic acidosis. Give ethyl alcohol, orally or intravenously, 7.5 mL/kg of a 10% solution as a loading dose, followed by 2.5 mL/kg of the 10% solution every hour for 3–4 days, to block the metabolism of methyl alcohol until it is excreted. Maintain blood ethanol level at 1 mg/mL. Dialysis is useful and is recommended when the serum methanol level exceeds 40 mg/dL (0.4 mg/mL).

Martens J et al: Recovery without sequelae from severe methanol intoxication. *Postgrad Med J* 1982;**58**:454.
Sejersted OM et al: Formate concentrations in plasma in patients poisoned with methanol. *Acta Med Scand* 1983;**213**:105.

ALKALIES

The strong alkalies are common ingredients of household cleaning compounds and may be detected by their "soapy" texture. Those with solutions above pH 12 are corrosive. Clinitest tablets and disk batteries are also a source. Alkalies exert a local corrosive effect on mucous membranes and may produce circulatory failure. Symptoms include burning pain in the upper gastrointestinal tract, nausea, vomiting, and difficulty in swallowing and breathing. Examination reveals destruction and edema of the affected skin and mucous membranes and bloody vomitus and stools. X-ray will reveal the presence of disk batteries in the gastrointestinal tract.

The MLD is 1 g.

Treatment

A. Ingested: Dilute immediately with 200 mL of water or milk.

Immediate endoscopy is recommended to evaluate the extent of damage.

The use of corticosteroids to prevent stricture formation is controversial and is definitely contraindicated if there is evidence of esophageal perforation.

If x-ray reveals the location of ingested disk batteries in the esophagus, immediate endoscopic removal is mandatory.

B. Skin Contact: Wash with running water until the skin no longer feels soapy. Relieve pain and treat shock.

C. Eye Contact: Wash with water continuously for 30 minutes, holding the lids open. Check pH with pH 6–8 test paper, and repeat irrigation, using normal saline, for additional 30-minute periods until pH is 7. Have the eye examined by an ophthalmologist to determine the extent of damage.

Mofenson HC et al: Ingestion of small flat disc batteries. *Ann Emerg Med* 1983;**12**:88.

ANTICOAGULANTS

Dicumarol, ethyl biscoumacetate, phenindione, and warfarin are used medically to inhibit the clotting mechanism by inhibiting prothrombin formation in the liver. Abnormal bleeding occurs only after prolonged administration. The MLD of dicumarol and warfarin is 0.1 g; of phenindione, 0.2 g; of ethyl biscoumacetate, 0.6 g. The pathologic findings consist of numerous gross and microscopic hemorrhages.

Clinical Findings

Anticoagulants cause bleeding: hemoptysis, hematuria, bloody stools, hemorrhages into organs, widespread bruising, and bleeding into joint spaces. Phenindione may also cause jaundice, hepatomegaly, skin rash, and agranulocytosis. The prothrombin concentration is lowered after administration of anticoagulants. Gross or microscopic hematuria may be present. The red cell count may also be reduced. The white count may be decreased after phenindione administration.

Treatment

Discontinue the drug at the first sign of bleeding. If ingestion of more than 10 times a daily therapeutic dose is discovered within 2 hours, remove by gastric lavage and catharsis. Obtain blood prothrombin time (PT). Give phytonadione, 5–10 mg orally. For more rapid effect, give 0.1 mg/kg intramuscularly as the diluted emulsion. Give transfusions of fresh blood, fresh plasma, or fresh frozen plasma if hemorrhage is severe. Absolute bed rest must be maintained to prevent further hemorrhages.

O'Reilly RA: Drugs used in disorders of coagulation. Chapter 32 in: *Basic & Clinical Pharmacology,* 2nd ed. Katzung BG (editor). Lange, 1984.

ARSENIC

Arsenic is found in pesticides and industrial chemicals. Symptoms of poisoning usually appear within 1 hour after ingestion but may be delayed as long as 12 hours. They include abdominal pain, difficulty in swallowing, persistent vomiting, diarrhea, urinary suppression, and skeletal muscle cramps. Later findings are severe thirst and shock. In chronic poisoning, symptoms can be vague.

The MLD of inorganic arsenic is 1 mg/kg. The MLD of alkyl methanearsonates is 0.1–0.5 g/kg.

Treatment

A. Emergency Measures: Induce vomiting. Follow with 50 mL of milk. Lavage with 2–4 L of warm tap water.

B. Antidote: For symptomatic patients or those with massive overdose, give dimercaprol injection (BAL), 10% solution in oil. Give immediately 2.5 mg/kg dimercaprol intramuscularly, then 2 mg/kg intramuscularly every 4 hours for 2 days. The side effects include nausea, vomiting, headache, generalized aches, and burning sensations around the head and face. These usually subside in 30 minutes. An antihistamine such as diphenhydramine, 25–50 mg orally, will reduce the side effects if given 30 minutes before dimercaprol.

Follow BAL with oral penicillamine, 100 mg/kg/d in 4 divided doses (maximum 1 g/d) for 1 week. If urinary arsenic excretion is above 50 μg in 24 hours, give penicillamine for an additional week.

C. General Measures: Relieve pain and treat diarrhea. Hemodialysis will speed the removal of arsenic combined with dimercaprol if renal failure is present.

Hutton JT: Source, symptoms and signs of arsenic poisoning. *J Fam Pract* 1983;**17**:423.

ATROPINE & ANTICHOLINERGICS

Atropine, scopolamine, belladonna, Lomotil, *Datura stramonium, Hyoscyamus niger,* some mushrooms, tricyclic antidepressants, and antihistamines are parasympathetic depressants with variable central nervous system effects. The patient complains of dryness of the mouth, thirst, difficulty in swallowing, and blurring of vision. The physical signs include dilated pupils, flushed skin, tachycardia, fever (although hypothermia has been reported), delirium, delusions, ileus, and flushed appearance of the face, neck, and upper trunk. Antidepressants and antihistamines may induce convulsions.

The MLD of atropine is 2–10 mg.

Treatment

Remove the poison by lavage and catharsis, and attempt to calm the patient.

A. Emergency Measures: Induce vomiting or lavage with 2–4 L of water, preferably containing activated charcoal. Follow lavage with sodium sulfate, 30 g in 200 mL of water.

B. General Measures: Treat respiratory difficulty as for barbiturate poisoning. Cold-water sponge baths are indicated to control high temperatures. Maintain blood pressure. If symptoms are severe (eg, hyperthermia or excessively rapid tachycardia), give physostigmine salicylate, 1 mg slowly intravenously over 5 minutes, with electrocardiographic monitoring, until symptoms are controlled. Arrhythmias and convulsions are a hazard with physostigmine administration, and it should not be used with antidepressant overdose.

LaCouture PG, Lovejoy FH Jr, Mitchell AA: Acute hypothermia associated with atropine. *Am J Dis Child* 1983;**137**:291.

BARBITURATES & OTHER DEPRESSANTS
(Sedative-Hypnotics & Tranquilizers)

The barbiturates are among the most common offenders in accidental as well as suicidal poisoning. Other (or multiple) sedative-hypnotic drugs—particularly alcohol—may be involved (see p 675). Obtain data on the drug and its dosage and time of ingestion from the patient, relatives, friends, or attending physician when possible.

Features of mild poisoning include drowsiness, mental confusion, and nystagmus. There may be euphoria or irritability. Moderate or severe poisoning causes stupor, shallow and slow respirations, circulatory collapse, cold clammy skin, cyanosis, pulmonary edema, dilated and nonreacting pupils, hyporeflexia, coma, and death.

The MLD is 0.5–2 g. The lethal serum level in unsupported patients who have taken short-acting barbiturates is about 3.5 mg/dL; and with long-acting barbiturates, the lethal level is about 8 mg/dL. The analytical method used must be specific for the unmetabolized drug.

Treatment

Note: The critical factor in the management of barbiturate poisoning is constant medical and nursing attendance to maintain physiologic responses until the danger of respiratory failure and circulatory depression has passed.

A. Mild Poisoning: Empty the stomach with vomiting or lavage and give symptomatic and supportive nursing care. Give activated charcoal. Keep the patient under observation until the danger is past. Place suicidal patients under psychiatric care.

B. Moderate or Serious Poisoning: Most patients will survive even days of unconsciousness if the airway is protected (usually with cuffed endotracheal tube) and if artificial respiration is maintained with intermittent positive pressure breathing or other mechanical ventilating apparatus. Oxygen concentration should not exceed 50% unless arterial oxygen saturation is inadequate with ventilatory assistance. The patient should be hospitalized and antishock measures instituted. Examine the patient and record the following at intervals of 1–4 hours (or oftener if the patient's condition is very poor): temperature, pulse, respiration, and blood pressure; mental status or state of consciousness, skin color (cyanosis or pallor), lung bases (pulmonary edema), reflexes (corneal, pupillary, gag, patellar), and sensation (response to pain).

1. Airway–Aspirate mucus, pull tongue forward, and insert oropharyngeal airway. Intratracheal intubation and mechanical assistance to respiration with constant supervision may be required. Serial determination of blood gases is essential.

2. Lavage with 2–4 L of warm tap water, preferably containing activated charcoal. Repeated administration of activated charcoal, 30–50 g, can increase the elimination of barbiturates. Give a saline cathartic to speed the elimination of the charcoal. In drowsy or comatose patients, liquids should be given only by stomach tube with the airway protected. *Caution:* The danger of aspiration pneumonia is great in stuporous or comatose patients.

3. Insert an indwelling catheter, and save urine for toxicologic quantitation.

4. Parenteral fluids–Monitor central venous pressure. Serum sodium should also be monitored in order to control the sodium content of parenteral fluids. If cardiac failure is absent and renal function is adequate, give 1 L of 0.45% sodium chloride solution and 1–2 L of 5% dextrose solution intravenously daily to maintain a daily urine output of 1–1.5 L. Unless fluid loss has been excessive, restrict fluids to 2–3 L during the first 24 hours to reduce the danger of pulmonary edema. In the event of shock, give plasma or other fluids intravenously in order to maintain a satisfactory blood pressure. (See treatment of shock, p 9.) Vasopressors may be useful if fluid replacement is ineffective in maintaining blood pressure. Hypothermia commonly occurs and may cause intractable hypotension until the temperature is restored to normal.

5. Central nervous system stimulants (analeptics or convulsant drugs) are contraindicated. They cause hyperthermia, cardiac arrhythmias, and convulsions.

6. Hemodialysis or hemoperfusion is usually reserved for patients with severe intoxication and unstable vital signs who cannot be stabilized with supportive measures. Dialysis or hemoperfusion is of no value for poisoning with drugs with very large volumes of distribution (eg, glutethimide).

Goldberg MJ, Berlinger WG: Treatment of phenobarbital overdose with activated charcoal. *JAMA* 1982;**247**:2400.

McCarron MM et al: Short-acting barbiturate overdosage: Correlation of intoxication score with serum barbiturate concentration. *JAMA* 1982;**248**:55.

BEE, YELLOW JACKET, WASP, & HORNET STINGS

Stings of these common insects, although locally painful, usually cause only mild symptoms of brief duration. Local cold compresses, application of baking soda solution, and oral salicylates or antihistamines are sufficient treatment. Multiple stings may cause a shocklike reaction with hemoglobinuria. Sensitive individuals may develop an acute allergic or even fatal anaphylactic response after a single sting. Prior venom desensitization is possible.

Treatment

See p 15. Acute allergic or anaphylactic reactions should be treated with epinephrine, 0.005 mg/kg subcutaneously, intravenous fluids, and close observation.

BROMIDES

Bromides are central nervous system depressants still found in some over-the-counter preparations. Acute poisoning is rare. The symptoms include anorexia, constipation, drowsiness, apathy, and hallucinations. The physical examination reveals dermatitis, conjunctivitis, foul breath, furred tongue, sordes, unequal pupils, ataxia, abnormal reflexes (often bizarre), toxic psychosis, delirium, and coma. The serum chloride level may be falsely elevated.

The MLD is 10 g or more.

Treatment

A. Emergency Measures: Lavage copiously with saline to remove unabsorbed bromides and later to remove those excreted into the stomach. Follow with sodium sulfate, 30 g in 200 mL of water for catharsis.

B. General Measures: Give sodium chloride in addition to the regular dietary salt intake: (1) 1000 mL of physiologic saline intravenously once or twice daily; or (2) 1–2 g as salt tablets every 4 hours orally. Continue until the blood bromide level is below 50 mg/dL. With chloride loading, diuretics will aid excretion of bromide.

Force fluids to 4 L daily.

CARBON MONOXIDE

Carbon monoxide poisoning results from unvented or inadequately vented combustion devices. Voluntary inhalation of carbon monoxide in exhaust fumes is often used for suicidal purposes. The gas exerts its toxic effect by combining with hemoglobin to form a relatively stable compound (carboxyhemoglobin) which secondarily causes tissue anoxia. Manifestations are headache, faintness, giddiness, tinnitus, vomiting, vertigo, loss of memory, fainting, collapse, paralysis, unconsciousness, and electrocardiographic changes. Skin color varies from normal (more than half) to flushed, cyanotic, or, uncommonly, cherry-pink. Blisters and bullous lesions may also occur. Subclinical toxicity has been reported in dense traffic situations. Hyperexcitability and convulsions can occur during the recovery period after severe poisoning. After apparent recovery, persistent neurologic complications are common.

Treatment

Remove the patient from the toxic atmosphere. Clothing must be loosened and the patient kept warm and at rest. Give artificial respiration with 100% oxygen by tight-fitting mask or endotracheal tube for at least 1 hour. Maintain body warmth and blood pressure. Reduce hyperthermia by cooling applications. Diazepam, 5–10 mg orally, may be necessary for excitability during the recovery period.

Burney RE, Wu SC, Nemiroff MJ: Mass carbon monoxide poisoning: Clinical effects and results of treatment in 184 victims. *Ann Emerg Med* 1982;**11**:394.
Jones CTA, MacKay HAF: Carbon monoxide poisoning in a former mining community. *Br Med J* 1983;**286**:603.
O'Sullivan BP: Carbon monoxide poisoning in an infant exposed to a kerosene heater. *J Pediatr* 1983;**103**:249.

CARBON TETRACHLORIDE

Carbon tetrachloride is a local irritant and cellular poison which when ingested, inhaled, or absorbed through the skin may severely damage the heart, liver, and kidneys. The effects are increased by ingestion of alcohol. Manifestations include headache, hiccup, nausea, vomiting, diarrhea, abdominal pain, drowsiness, visual disturbances, neuritis, and intoxication. Early signs are jaundice, liver tenderness, oliguria, and uremia. Nephrosis and cirrhosis may occur later. Ingested carbon tetrachloride may be visible on x-ray. The MLD is 3 mL.

Treatment

A. Emergency Measures: The patient should be removed from exposure and kept recumbent and warm. For poisoning due to ingestion, lavage copiously with tap water and give activated charcoal and a cathartic. Do not give alcoholic beverages or stimulants.

B. General Measures: Give inhalations of 100% oxygen by mask and artificial ventilation if respirations are depressed. Treat cardiac, hepatic, and renal complications symptomatically. Maintain urine output at 4 L daily by osmotic diuresis if renal function is normal. Hemodialysis and total parenteral nutrition may be of value.

Fogel RP et al: Carbon tetrachloride poisoning treated with hemodialysis and total parenteral nutrition. *Can Med Assoc J* 1983;**128**:560.

CHLORINATED INSECTICIDES
(Chlorophenothane [DDT], Lindane, Toxaphene, Chlordane, Aldrin, Endrin)

DDT and other chlorinated insecticides are central nervous system stimulants that can cause poisoning by ingestion, inhalation, or direct contact. The MLD is about 20 g for DDT, 3 g for lindane, 2 g for toxaphene, 1 g for chlordane, and less than 1 g for endrin and aldrin. Poisoning following ingestion of DDT solution usually results from the organic solvent, whereas fatalities from the other chlorinated insecticides have resulted from the insecticide alone. The manifestations of poisoning are tired and aching limbs, nervous irritability, mental sluggishness, muscle twitchings, convulsions, and coma.

Treatment
A. Emergency Measures: (Avoid epinephrine, which may cause ventricular fibrillation.) Give activated charcoal at once if available, lavage with large quantities of warm tap water, and give a cathartic.

B. General Measures: For convulsions give diazepam, 0.1 mg/kg slowly intravenously. Maintain the airway and give oxygen. Do not give stimulants.

Telch J, Jarvis DA: Acute intoxication with lindane (gamma benzene hexachloride). *Can Med Assoc J* 1982;**126**:662.

CYANIDES: HYDROCYANIC ACID
(Prussic Acid, Rat Poison, Cyanogas, Cyanogen, Laetrile)

Hydrocyanic acid and the cyanides cause death by inactivation of the respiratory enzyme, preventing utilization of oxygen by the tissues. The clinical combination of cyanosis, asphyxia, and the odor of bitter almonds on the breath is diagnostic. Respiration is first stimulated and later depressed. A marked drop in blood pressure may occur.
The MLD is 0.05 g.

Treatment
A. Emergency Measures: *Act quickly.* Use nitrites to form methemoglobin, which combines with cyanide to form nontoxic cyanmethemoglobin. Then give thiosulfates to convert the cyanide released by dissociation of cyanmethemoglobin to thiocyanate.

1. Poisoning by inhalation–Place patient in open air in recumbent position. Remove contaminated clothing. Give artificial respiration.

2. Poisoning by ingestion–Induce vomiting immediately with a finger down the patient's throat. Do not wait until lavage tube has arrived; death may occur within a few minutes.

3. Give amyl nitrite inhalations for 15–30 seconds every 2 minutes until intravenous antidotes are given.

B. Antidote: Administration of antidotes must be based on hemoglobin level. At 14 g/dL hemoglobin, give 0.4 mL/kg of 3% sodium nitrite intravenously and 1–2 mL/kg of 25% sodium thiosulfate intravenously. At lower hemoglobin levels, reduce dosage in exact proportion. Further administration of nitrite should not exceed 40% methemoglobinemia. Inject sodium nitrite over 10–15 minutes, monitoring blood pressure during administration.

C. General Measures: Combat shock, and give 100% oxygen by forced ventilation.

Litovitz PL et al: Cyanide poisoning treated with hyperbaric oxygen. *Am J Emerg Med* 1983;**1**:94.

CYCLIC ANTIDEPRESSANTS*
(Amitriptyline, Amoxapine, Doxepin, Desipramine, Imipramine, Nortriptyline, Protriptyline)

These prescription drugs are not only widely available for accidental or suicidal ingestion but are also being used as drugs of abuse. Overdoses cause anxiety, agitation, delirium, tachycardia, convulsions, hypotension, pyrexia, dilated pupils, and coma. Death occurs most often from cardiac rhythm disturbances, including extrasystole, wandering pacemaker, atrioventricular or intraventricular block, and ventricular fibrillation. The toxic dose is approximately 15–20 mg/kg. Significant toxicity is usually accompanied by widening of the QRS interval on the ECG (> 100 ms), but this may be absent with newer drugs such as amoxapine.

Treatment

Remove ingested drug by emesis, gastric lavage with activated charcoal, and catharsis. Continue gastric charcoal administration to interrupt enterohepatic reabsorption of drug. Monitor ECG for 24 hours after all signs disappear. Control convulsions with diazepam, 0.1 mg/kg slowly intravenously, and phenytoin, 0.5 mg/kg/min intravenously to a loading dose of 15 mg/kg. Arrhythmias may respond to sodium bicarbonate, 0.5 meq/kg slowly intravenously, repeated as needed to maintain the serum pH at 7.4–7.5. Any of the following may initiate or exacerbate the cardiac rhythm disturbances: physostigmine, quinidine, propranolol, procainamide, disopyramide, corticosteroids, or atropine. Some exacerbate hypotension. Ventricular pacing may be necessary.

Knudsen K, Heath A: Effects of self poisoning with maprotiline. *Br Med J* 1984;**288**:601.

Rogol AB et al: Generalized convulsions as the presenting sign of amoxapine intoxication. *Clin Pediatr* 1984;**23**:235.

Sawyer WT et al: A case of severe acute desipramine overdose. *Am J Psychiatry* 1984;**141**:122.

DIGITALIS

Because digitalis, digitoxin, and related drugs have a prolonged action, poisoning is most likely to occur when large doses are given to patients who have previously received digitalis drugs. Digitalizing doses should therefore be given only to patients who have not received digitalis for at least 1 week.

Clinical Findings

The principal manifestations of digitalis poisoning are vomiting and irregular pulse. Other signs include anorexia, nausea, diarrhea, yellow vision, delirium, slow pulse, fall of blood pressure, and ventricular fibrillation. The ECG may show lengthened PR

*See p 640.

interval, heart block, ventricular extrasystoles, ventricular tachycardia, and a depressed ST segment. With acute ingestion of an overdose, toxicity is accompanied by hyperkalemia. With chronic intoxication, in contrast, the potassium level is usually depressed.

The toxic serum level of digoxin is 1.7 ng/mL; for digitalis, 25 ng/mL.

Treatment

A. Emergency Measures: Discontinue digitalis and diuretics. Remove ingested digitalis by emesis or lavage. Repeated administration of activated charcoal or cholestyramine resin can be used as an intestinal binding agent for digitoxin. Do not give epinephrine or other stimulants. These may induce ventricular fibrillation.

B. General Measures: In the presence of hypokalemia, give potassium chloride slowly intravenously during electrocardiographic monitoring until the ECG shows improvement or evidence of potassium intoxication. Serum potassium must be determined before and during potassium administration. Hyperkalemia can be corrected by intravenous sodium bicarbonate, glucose with insulin, oral Kayexalate, or hemodialysis. Hyperkalemia (> 5 meq/L) is usually an indication for digitalis-specific antibodies (see below). Phenytoin, propranolol, or procainamide can be used to control arrhythmias. Ventricular defibrillation and ventricular pacing may be required. The use of digoxin-specific Fab antibody fragments is now possible. Call the nearest regional poison control center for information on availability.

Bowman K: Digitalis intoxication in geriatric in-patients. *Acta Med Scand* 1983;**214**:345.

Smith TW et al: Treatment of life-threatening digitalis intoxication with digoxin-specific Fab antibody fragments: Experience in 26 cases. *N Engl J Med* 1982;**307**:1357.

FLUORIDES SOLUBLE IN WATER
(Insect Powders)

Acute symptoms include vomiting, diarrhea, salivation; shallow, rapid, and difficult respirations; convulsive seizures, rapid pulse, coma, and cyanosis. Fluoride is corrosive, lowers the serum calcium level, and has direct toxicity to cellular processes. Overdose may result in death due to respiratory failure.

The MLD of fluoride is 6 mg/kg. Fluoride toothpaste contains 0.1% fluoride.

Chronic fluoride poisoning is manifested by weakness, weight loss, general ill health, joint stiffness, brittle bones, discoloration of teeth (during tooth formation), and anemia.

Treatment

A. Emergency Measures: Lavage with 1% calcium chloride, calcium lactate, or calcium gluconate;

or large quantities of milk to form insoluble calcium fluoride. Give calcium gluconate, 10%, 10–20 mL intravenously; or calcium chloride, 5%, 10–20 mL intravenously for convulsions. Give magnesium sulfate, 30 g, in 200 mL of water as cathartic, and egg whites in milk as demulcent.

B. General Measures: Treat shock and give supportive measures. Diuresis and dialysis are useful.

Zogt RL et al: Acute fluoride poisoning associated with an on-site fluoridator in a Vermont elementary school. *Am J Public Health* 1982;**72:**1168.

IRON

Iron salts are used extensively as antianemic agents in a large number of prescription and over-the-counter "blood tonic" drugs. They are responsible for many instances of mild to severe acute poisoning as well as chronic poisoning.

Acute poisoning is manifested by lethargy, nausea, vomiting, tarry stools, diarrhea, fast and weak pulse, hypotension, dehydration, acidosis, hyperglycemia, and coma within ½–1 hour following ingestion of iron salts. If this is not fatal, the symptoms may clear in a few hours and the patient may be asymptomatic for 6–12 hours. Symptoms then return, with cyanosis, pulmonary edema, shock, convulsions, anuria, hypoglycemia, and death in coma within 24–48 hours. Late sequelae include hepatic failure and pyloric stenosis. Doses exceeding 60 mg/kg of elemental iron are associated with fatalities in young children, and serious toxicity can occur at doses of 30 mg/kg or serum levels above 350 μg/dL.

Chronic poisoning may occur after prolonged excess dosage of parenteral iron, causing exogenous hemosiderosis with damage to the liver and pancreas.

Treatment

When a large amount of iron has been ingested (> 60 mg/kg, or > 30 mg/kg with evidence of toxicity), give deferoxamine mesylate (Desferal), 80 mg/kg (maximum 2 g) intramuscularly, unless the patient is in shock. If the patient is in shock, give deferoxamine, 15 mg/kg/h intravenously (maximum 80 mg/kg per 12 hours); maintain adequate blood volume; and utilize other therapy (see p 10). In patients not in shock or coma, induce emesis with syrup of ipecac if the patient has not vomited. Follow with gastric lavage using sodium bicarbonate, 1–5%. If an x-ray film of the abdomen reveals a significant number of iron pills not removed by repeated emesis or lavage, consider gastrotomy. Draw blood for hemoglobin, white count, serum iron, total iron-binding capacity, electrolyte concentrations, blood typing, glucose, and serum iron test. Start an infusion of isotonic saline or dextrose solution to correct electrolyte disturbance and dehydration and maintain urinary output.

Repeat deferoxamine after 12 hours if symptoms and iron determination warrant. Monitor blood pressure during administration of deferoxamine and reduce the rate of administration if blood pressure falls. In the presence of renal failure, dialysis must accompany deferoxamine use.

Lacouture PG et al: Emergency assessment of severity in iron overdose by clinical and laboratory methods. *J Pediatr* 1981;**99:**89.

Robotham JL, Lietman PS: Acute iron poisoning. *Am J Dis Child* 1980;**134:**875.

LEAD

Lead poisoning may occur by ingestion (eg, bone meal) or by inhalation of lead dust or fumes. Poisoning is manifested by a metallic taste, anorexia, irritability, apathy, abdominal colic, vomiting, diarrhea, constipation, headache, leg cramps, black stools (lead sulfide), oliguria, stupor, convulsions, palsies, and coma. Chronic lead poisoning causes variable involvement of the central nervous system, the blood-forming organs, and the gastrointestinal tract.

Diagnostic laboratory tests include blood lead (> 50 μg/dL), blood erythrocyte protoporphyrin (EPP) > 100 μg/dL, urine coproporphyrin (> 500 μg/L), urine δ-aminolevulinic acid (> 13 mg/L), x-ray of abdomen (radiopaque paint), and x-ray of long bones (lead line). Blood lead level over 10 μg/dL indicates excessive exposure to lead. Levels above 50 μg/dL are consistent with serious intoxication.

The MLD is 0.5 g of absorbed lead.

Treatment

A. Acute Poisoning:

1. Establish adequate urine flow (0.5–1 mL/min). Give dextrose in water (10%, 10–20 mL/kg body weight) over 1–2 hours, or mannitol solution (20%) at a rate of 1 mL/min until 10 mL/kg have been given. Daily urine output should be 350–500 mL/m². If adequate urine flow is not obtained, hemodialysis should accompany the use of antidotes.

2. Control convulsions with diazepam, 0.1 mg/kg intravenously. Barbiturates are best for long-term control of convulsions after the acute phase is under control.

3. For symptomatic children with blood lead levels above 70 μg/dL, including those with lead encephalopathy, give dimercaprol (BAL) and calcium disodium edetate (EDTA) as follows: Begin first with dimercaprol, 4 mg/kg intramuscularly, and repeat every 4 hours for 5 days (30 doses). Four hours after the first dimercaprol injection, give EDTA, 12.5 mg/kg (20% solution, with 0.5% procaine added) intramuscularly, in a different site from dimercaprol. Repeat every 4 hours for 5 days (30 doses). If symptoms have not improved by the fourth day, extend treatment to 7 days (42 doses each of both dimercaprol and EDTA). If blood lead is still above 70 μg/dL 14 days later, repeat the 5-day course of both drugs. If blood lead level is 50–70 μg/dL, give EDTA alone.

4. For asymptomatic children, if blood lead is

above 70 μg/dL, give a 5-day course of dimercaprol-EDTA as above. If blood lead is below this level, give EDTA intramuscularly alone every 6 hours for a 5-day course (20 injections) if EDTA lead mobilization test is positive (24-hour urinary excretion exceeds 1 μg of lead per milligram of EDTA after giving EDTA, 25 mg/kg intramuscularly [maximum 1 g]).

5. For adults with encephalopathy, painful neuropathy, or abdominal symptoms, give dimercaprol-EDTA intramuscularly as above, or, if the patient is dimercaprol-intolerant, give 50 mg/kg EDTA intravenously as 0.5% solution over not less than 8 hours.

6. Follow-up therapy (all cases)–Give penicillamine (Cuprimine) orally daily in 3 doses one-half hour before meals. The daily dosage is 100 mg/kg up to a maximum total of 1 g. Therapy should be continued for 1–2 months for adults and for 3–6 months for children. Blood lead should be below 50 μg/dL at the end of treatment.

B. Chronic Poisoning: Remove permanently from exposure and give an adequate diet with vitamin supplements. Courses of oral penicillamine as for acute poisoning may be employed, especially when hematologic complications have occurred.

Mielke HW et al: Lead concentrations in inner-city soils as a factor in the child lead problem. *Am J Public Health* 1983; **73**:1366.

MERCURY

Acute poisoning (by ingestion or inhalation) is manifested by a metallic taste, salivation, thirst, a burning sensation in the throat, discoloration and edema of oral mucous membranes, abdominal pain, vomiting, bloody diarrhea, anuria, and shock. Chronic poisoning causes weakness, ataxia, intention tremors, irritability, depression, and muscle cramps. Chronic intoxication in children may be a cause of acrodynia. Exposure to high concentrations of mercury vapor causes bronchitis and pneumonitis. Exposure to alkyl (organic) mercury derivatives from contaminated fish or fungicides used on seeds causes ataxia, tremors, and convulsions.

The MLD is about 70 mg of mercury bichloride.

Treatment

A. Acute Poisoning: Give dimercaprol (BAL) at once, as for arsenic poisoning. Ingested inorganic salts may be precipitated with egg whites or milk. Remove by emesis, lavage, and cathartic. Penicillamine, 100 mg/kg orally in divided doses (maximum 1 g/d), is also effective. Maintain urine output. Treat oliguria and anuria if they occur. Hemodialysis can be used to speed the removal of mercury combined with dimercaprol.

B. Chronic Poisoning: Remove from exposure.

Jaffe KM et al: Survival after acute mercury vapor poisoning. *Am J Dis Child* 1983;**137**:749.

MUSHROOMS

The most dangerous species of mushrooms are *Amanita phalloides, Amanita verna, Amanita virosa, Gyromitra esculenta,* and the *Galerina* species, all of which contain amanitin, a potent cytotoxin. Ingestion of part of one mushroom of a dangerous species may be sufficient to cause death. The true incidence of morbidity and mortality from mushroom poisoning is unknown.

The pathologic finding in fatalities from amanitin-containing mushroom poisoning is acute necrosis of the liver, kidneys, heart, and skeletal muscles.

Clinical Findings

The principal manifestations of acute mushroom poisoning are vomiting, diarrhea, and jaundice.

A. Symptoms and Signs:

1. Amanitin type cyclopeptides (*Amanita phalloides, Amanita verna, Amanita virosa,* and *Galerina* species)–After a latent interval of 12–24 hours, severe abdominal cramps and vomiting begin and progress to profuse diarrhea, bloody vomitus and stools, painful tenderness and enlargement of the liver, oliguria or anuria, jaundice, pulmonary edema, mental confusion and depression, hypoglycemia, and signs of cerebral injury with coma or convulsions. The fatality rate is about 20%.

2. Gyromitrin type (*Gyromitra* and *Helvella* species)–Vomiting, diarrhea, hepatic necrosis, convulsions, coma, hemolysis. The fatality rate is 15–20%.

3. Muscarine type (*Inocybe* and *Clitocybe* species)–Vomiting, diarrhea, bradycardia, hypotension, salivation, miosis, bronchospasm, lacrimation. Cardiac arrhythmias may occur. The fatality rate is less than 5%.

4. Anticholinergic type (eg, *Amanita muscaria, Amanita pantherina*)–This type causes a variety of symptoms that may be atropinelike, including excitement, delirium, flushed skin, dilated pupils, and muscular tremors, beginning 1–2 hours after ingestion. Fatalities are rare.

5. Gastrointestinal irritant type (eg, *Boletus, Cantharellus*)–Nausea, vomiting, diarrhea, and malaise may last up to 1 week. Fatalities are rare.

6. Disulfiram type (*Coprinus* species)–Vomiting, diarrhea, cardiac arrhythmias, and disulfiramlike sensitivity to alcohol that may persist for several days. Fatalities are rare.

7. Hallucinogenic type (*Psilocybe* and *Panaeolus* species)–Mydriasis, ataxia, weakness, disorientation, abdominal pain, and nausea and vomiting. Fatalities are rare.

B. Laboratory Findings: Increase in creatinine and blood urea. Effects on the liver are revealed by increased transaminase and bilirubin levels. The blood glucose should be monitored daily or as required.

Treatment

A. Emergency Measures: After the onset of

symptoms, efforts to remove the toxic agent are probably useless. However, induction of emesis is recommended for any ingestion of an unidentified or potentially toxic mushroom. Activated charcoal and a cathartic should be given.

B. Antidote:

1. A variety of unproved antidotes have been suggested for amanitin type mushroom poisoning. The administration of thioctic acid has been recommended, but the drug is not readily available and results are equivocal. Administration of penicillin G and dexamethasone are also of unproved value. Aggressive fluid replacement for diarrhea and intensive supportive care for hepatic failure are the mainstay of treatment.

2. For mushrooms producing predominantly muscarinic-cholinergic symptoms, give atropine, 0.01 mg/kg orally or subcutaneously; repeat as needed.

3. For gyromitrin poisoning, give pyridoxine, 25 mg/kg intravenously.

4. For *Coprinus* ingestion, avoid alcohol. Treat alcohol reaction with fluids and supine position.

C. General Measures:

1. Careful control of fluid and electrolyte balance, with avoidance of hypoglycemia, must be continued for 5–10 days. In severely poisoned patients, liver function has been known to begin to return 6–8 days after exposure, followed by eventual complete recovery.

2. Repeated hemodialysis or charcoal hemoperfusion has been reported to be successful in bringing about recovery in cases of *A phalloides* poisoning. If renal function is normal, forced diuresis (eg, with furosemide) for 24–36 hours has been suggested. Interruption of the enterohepatic circulation of the amanitin toxin by the administration of oral charcoal and laxatives may be of value. However, by the time these methods are employed most of the amanitin has already caused cellular damage and has already been excreted. Their use remains questionable.

3. Give 5–10% dextrose, 4–5 L intravenously every 24 hours, if the urine output is adequate. Give vitamin K and fresh-frozen plasma for bleeding.

4. As soon as fluids can be given by mouth, give fruit juices fortified by glucose, 120 g/L, up to 4–5 L orally daily.

5. Control convulsions with diazepam.

DiPalma JR: Mushroom poisoning. *Am Fam Physician* (May) 1981;**23:**169.

Hanrahan JP, Gordon MA: Mushroom poisoning. *JAMA* 1984;**251:**1057.

Olson KR et al: *Amanita phalloides*–type mushroom poisoning. *West J Med* 1982;**137:**282.

Schumacher T, Høiland K: Mushroom poisoning caused by species of the genus *Cortinarius Fries. Arch Toxicol* 1983; **53:**87.

OPIOID NARCOTICS
(Morphine, Heroin, Etc)
(See p 673.)

PARAQUAT

Paraquat is used as a herbicide. Concentrated solutions of paraquat are corrosive to the esophagus. The fatal dose after absorption may be as small as 4 mg/kg. Paraquat causes pulmonary edema and fibrosis with respiratory insufficiency, and renal damage with anuria. A urinary excretion rate over 1 mg/h indicates severe poisoning. Patients with plasma paraquat levels above 0.2 mg/L at 24 hours are likely to die.

Treatment

Remove by emesis, gastric lavage, and catharsis. Clay (bentonite or fuller's earth) and activated charcoal are effective adsorbents. Gut perfusion with a solution containing 6 g sodium chloride, 0.75 g potassium chloride, and 3 g sodium bicarbonate per liter at a rate of 1 mL/kg/min by gastric tube has been suggested. Administer 200 mL of 20% mannitol into the gastric tube each hour and 60 g of fuller's earth by gastric tube every 2 hours. Forced diuresis may also be helpful. Hemoperfusion over activated charcoal, 8 hours per day for 2–3 weeks, has been reported to be lifesaving. For further information and for rapid determination of paraquat levels, call the Chevron Poison Information Service, (415) 233-3737.

Landrigan PJ et al: Paraquat and marihuana: Epidemiologic risk assessment. *Am J Public Health* 1983;**73:**784.

Tungsanga K et al: Paraquat poisoning: Evidence of systemic toxicity after dermal exposure. *Postgrad Med J* 1983;**59:** 338.

CHOLINESTERASE INHIBITOR PESTICIDES
(Organophosphates: Parathion, TEPP, Malathion, Thimet, Phosdrin, Systox, HETP, EPN, OMPA, Etc; Carbamates: Carbaryl, Aldicarb, Benomyl)

Inhalation, skin absorption, or ingestion of organophosphorus or carbamate pesticides causes marked depression of cholinesterase, resulting in continuous and excessive stimulation of the parasympathetic nervous system. Manifestations of acute poisoning appear within hours after exposure and include headache, sweating, salivation, lacrimation, vomiting, diarrhea, muscular twitchings, convulsions, dyspnea, and blurred vision. Pulse and blood pressure can be extremely variable. Constricted pupils with the above symptoms and signs and a history of exposure during the past 24 hours warrant therapy.

The MLD is 0.02–1 g.

Treatment

A. Emergency Measures: Maintain airway and give artificial respiration. If the material has been ingested, remove poison by induced vomiting or gastric lavage with tap water. Remove from the skin (especially the hair and under the fingernails) by copious washing. Remove and isolate contaminated clothing. Emergency personnel must avoid contamination. Counteract parasympathetic stimulation by giving atropine sulfate, 0.05 mg/kg intramuscularly or intravenously every 3–8 minutes until symptoms are relieved or signs of atropinization (dilated pupils, dry mouth) appear. Repeat as necessary to maintain complete atropinization. As much as 12 mg of atropine has been given safely in the first 2 hours. Give pralidoxime (Protopam), 25 mg/kg (maximum dose 1 g) slowly intravenously in aqueous solution. Repeat after 30 minutes if respiration does not improve.

B. General Measures: Give 40% oxygen under positive pressure if pulmonary edema or respiratory difficulty appears. Prolonged artificial respiration may be necessary. Take a blood sample for determination of red cell cholinesterase levels. (This is of no practical value in immediate diagnosis or treatment of the acute episode but aids in confirmation of the diagnosis.)

Lotti M et al: Occupational exposure to the cotton defoliants DEF and merphos. *J Occup Med* 1983;**25**:517.

Stuart LD, Oehme FW: Organophosphorus delayed neurotoxicity: A neuromyelopathy of animals and man. *Vet Hum Toxicol* 1982;**24**:107.

PETROLEUM DISTILLATES
(Petroleum Ether, Charcoal Lighter Fluid, Kerosene, Paint Thinner, Benzine, Gasoline, Etc)

Petroleum distillate toxicity occurs almost entirely as a result of pulmonary aspiration during or after ingestion. The intratracheal toxicity is 100 times the gastric toxicity. Gasoline or other volatile hydrocarbons can also cause poisoning by inhalation. Acute manifestations are vomiting, coughing, and bronchial pneumonia. Vertigo, muscular incoordination, weak and irregular pulse, neuropathy, twitchings, and convulsions occur with serious poisoning and may be due to hypoxemia or the systemic effects of some agents (eg, camphor). Chronic poisoning also causes headache, drowsiness, dim vision, cold and numb hands, weakness, loss of memory, loss of weight, tachycardia, mental dullness or confusion, sores in the mouth, dermatoses, and anemia.

Treatment

Remove the patient to fresh air. Since aspiration is the primary danger, use of lavage or emesis induced by syrup of ipecac is controversial. Removal of ingested hydrocarbon is only suggested if the amount exceeds 50 mL or if the preparation contains toxic solutes. If lavage is done, use a cuffed endotracheal tube to prevent aspiration. Use warm saline for lavage and follow with sodium sulfate, 30 g in 200 mL of water. Watch the victim closely for 3–4 days for symptoms of respiratory involvement. Treat pulmonary edema by positive pressure oxygen administration. Oxygen concentration should not exceed 40%. If fever occurs, give specific antibiotic. Ventilatory assistance may be necessary.

Banner W Jr, Walson PD: Systemic toxicity following gasoline aspiration. *Am J Emerg Med* 1983;**1**:292.

Wasserman GS: Hydrocarbon poisoning. *Crit Care Q* 1982;**4**:33.

PHENCYCLIDINE

Phencyclidine (PCP) was until recently one of the most commonly abused street drugs—second only to alcohol as a cause of emergency room visits for drug intoxication in many cities. It occurs under a variety of names or is misrepresented as other psychotomimetic agents. The drug has a wide range of toxic manifestations. Doses under 5 mg (adults) cause hyperactivity, horizontal and vertical nystagmus, inability to speak, incoordination, diaphoresis, flushing, rigidity, peripheral anesthesia, rhabdomyolysis with myoglobinuria, and wild movements. Doses over 10 mg cause, in addition, seizures, coma, hypertension, fever, and decreased or absent reflexes. Children are more susceptible. Convulsions and respiratory arrest occur at 1 mg/kg. Apnea occurs at serum levels of 0.3 μg/mL. Symptoms may persist for several days, with a cyclic course resulting from excretion of the drug into the stomach and reabsorption from the intestinal tract. The EEG reveals slowed delta rhythm and rhythmic to dysrhythmic theta activity.

Treatment

Maintain a quiet, calm atmosphere. Sedate the agitated patient with diazepam, 0.1 mg/kg intravenously, or haloperidol, 0.05–0.1 mg/kg intramuscularly. Intubate if necessary and maintain respiration. After gastric lavage and administration of a cathartic, restrict sensory input, prevent injuries, monitor vital signs, and maintain gastric suction. Repeated administration of activated charcoal, 30 g in sorbitol, may prevent reabsorption of PCP. In patients with coma, convulsions, or respiratory depression, maintain respiration and control convulsions by giving diazepam, 10 mg slowly intravenously. Control hypertension by giving nitroprusside, 0.5–5 μg/kg/min intravenously. Alkalinization of the urine aids in preventing renal deposition of myoglobin, but in renal failure, hemodialysis is necessary in patients whose serum creatinine levels are high and rising.

Lowering blood pH removes PCP from the central nervous system by ion trapping but is hazardous and may promote myoglobinuric renal failure.

Kaufman KR et al: Phencyclidine in umbilical cord blood: Preliminary data. *Am J Psychiatry* 1983;**140**:450.

Krenzelok EP: Phencyclidine: A contemporary drug of abuse. *Crit Care Q* 1982;**4**:55.

Martin BR et al: Pharmocokinetics and mechanism of action of phencyclidine. *Fed Proc* 1983;**42**:2559.

PHENOLS & DERIVATIVES

The phenols are present in carbolic acid, Lysol, cresol, and creosote. Hexachlorophene—2,2'-methylenebis(3,4,6-trichlorophenol)—is a widely used antiseptic (pHisoHex, etc). Pentachlorophenol is used as a wood preservative, and dinitrophenols are used as pesticides. They are local corrosives and also have marked systemic effects (after oral or dermal absorption) on the nervous and circulatory systems. Manifestations include burning in the upper gastrointestinal tract, thirst, nausea and vomiting, erosion of mucous membranes, dark vomitus, oliguria, muscle spasms, circulatory collapse, and respiratory failure. Pentachlorophenol and dinitrophenols, in addition, cause hyperthermia by interfering with oxidative phosphorylation.

The MLD is 2 g. Hexachlorophene orally (250 mg/kg) was fatal to a child.

Treatment

A. Ingestion: Delay absorption by giving tap water, milk, or activated charcoal and then remove by repeated gastric lavage with tap water or by inducing vomiting. Then give activated charcoal and cathartic. Some authorities recommend castor oil or olive oil to retard absorption of phenol. Do not give mineral oil, and do not use alcohol for lavage. Give supportive measures as outlined on pp 1001–1004.

B. External Burns: Wash with olive oil or soap and water (or both). Remove contaminated clothing.

Brancato DJ: Recognizing potential toxicity of phenol. *Vet Hum Toxicol* 1982;**24**:29.

Wood S et al: Pentachlorophenol poisoning. *J Oral Med* 1983;**25**:527.

PHENOTHIAZINE TRANQUILIZERS
(Chlorpromazine, Promazine, Prochlorperazine, Etc)

Chlorpromazine and related drugs are synthetic chemicals derived in most instances from phenothiazine. They are used as antiemetics and psychic inhibitors and as potentiators of analgesic and hypnotic drugs.

The acute fatal dose for these compounds appears to be above 50 mg/kg.

Clinical Findings

A. Symptoms and Signs: Minimum doses induce drowsiness and mild hypotension in as many as 50% of patients. Larger doses cause drowsiness, severe postural hypotension, tachycardia, dryness of the mouth, nausea, ataxia, anorexia, nasal congestion, fever, constipation, tremor, blurring of vision, stiffness of muscles, seizures, and coma. Intravenous injection of solutions containing more than 25 mg/mL of these drugs causes thrombophlebitis and cellulitis in a small number of patients.

Prolonged administration may cause pigment deposition in the eye, toxic amblyopia, jaundice, and generalized maculopapular eruptions. Some patients develop an acute extrapyramidal reaction similar to paralysis agitans, with spasmodic contractions of the face and neck muscles, extensor rigidity of the back muscles, carpopedal spasm, and motor restlessness.

B. Laboratory Findings: Leukopenia and agranulocytosis can occur. Liver function tests occasionally indicate an obstructive type of jaundice.

Treatment

Remove overdoses by emesis or gastric lavage. Follow with activated charcoal and cathartic. For severe hypotension, treatment with fluids and pressor agents may be necessary. Control convulsions cautiously with diazepam, 0.1 mg/kg intravenously. Avoid other depressant drugs.

For intolerable extrapyramidal signs, give diphenhydramine, 0.5–1 mg/kg intravenously. When agranulocytosis is complicated by infection, give antibiotic therapy. No measures have been helpful for jaundice other than discontinuing the drug.

May DC et al: Neuroleptic malignant syndrome: Response to dantrolene sodium. *Ann Intern Med* 1983;**98**:183.

PHOSPHORUS, INORGANIC
(Rat Paste, Fireworks, Matches)

Phosphorus poisoning may result from contact, ingestion, or inhalation. Phosphorus is a local irritant and systemic toxin that acts on the liver, kidneys, muscles, bones, and cardiovascular system. Toxicity is manifested early by a garlic taste and breath odor, pain in the upper gastrointestinal tract, vomiting, and diarrhea. Other symptoms and signs are headache, pleuritis, extreme weakness, jaundice, oliguria, petechiae, prostration, and cardiovascular collapse.

The MLD is 50 mg.

Treatment

A. Emergency Measures: Lavage with 5–10 L of tap water or induce emesis. Give sodium sulfate, 30 g in 200 mL of water, and activated charcoal, 50–100 g. Give whites of eggs beaten in milk as demulcent.

B. General Measures: Observe carefully for several days, and treat as for acute hepatitis if signs of jaundice or liver involvement appear.

McCarron MM, Gaddis GP, Trotter AT: Acute yellow phosphorus poisoning from pesticide pastes. *Clin Toxicol* 1981;**18**:693.

SALICYLATE POISONING

Salicylate poisoning is most commonly caused by aspirin ingestion. Effects include acid-base disturbances, hypoprothrombinemia, hyperthermia, pulmonary and cerebral edema, and gastroenteritis. The acid-base disturbances are the most dangerous. Respiratory alkalosis appears first, followed by metabolic acidosis. Severe poisoning after acute overdose is associated with initial serum salicylate levels above 100 mg/dL. To determine initial level, the disappearance half-time must be calculated from serial serum salicylate determinations.

Salicylates stimulate the respiratory center, producing hyperpnea, CO_2 loss, a falling serum CO_2 content, and a normal or high arterial blood pH; this combination represents respiratory alkalosis. In an effort to compensate, the kidneys excrete increased amounts of bicarbonate, potassium, and sodium but retain chloride. The chief dangers to the patient during this stage are hypokalemia and dehydration. Salicylates also interfere with carbohydrate metabolism, which results in the formation of fixed acids and ketones. Aspirin administration during certain viral infections (eg, varicella, influenza) is suspected of being a risk factor in the occurrence of Reye's syndrome (see p 849).

When first seen, the patient may be in alkalosis or acidosis. Diagnosis and treatment depend upon determination of serum CO_2 content, potassium, sodium, and chloride and arterial pH. Testing urine pH is an unreliable indication of acidosis or alkalosis.

The clinical picture includes a history of salicylate ingestion, hyperpnea, flushed face, hyperthermia, tinnitus, abdominal pain, vomiting, dehydration, spontaneous bleeding, twitchings, convulsions, pulmonary edema, uremia, and coma. Salicylates may give a false-positive ketonuria and glycosuria, or true ketonuria and glycosuria may be present. The Phenistix or ferric chloride test aids in diagnosis of salicylate ingestion.

The MLD for acute overdose is 150 mg/kg. However, repeated overmedication with only slightly supratherapeutic doses of salicylate may lead to severe intoxication. This so-called chronic or therapeutic intoxication often goes unrecognized initially and carries high morbidity and mortality rates.

Treatment

A. Emergency Measures: At any time, empty the stomach by giving ipecac or other emetic. If emesis is not thorough, aspirate the gastric contents without using additional fluids, and then lavage with 2–4 L of warm tap water containing activated charcoal. Follow with activated charcoal and cathartic. Treat shock (see p 9).

B. General Measures: Salicylate poisoning can only be treated adequately with knowledge of the blood or serum pH and the serum salicylate, sodium, potassium, and chloride. Hydration in the first hour should begin with 400 mL/m² of intravenous fluid

prepared as follows: To each liter of 5% dextrose, add 50 meq of sodium chloride (17 mL of 3 meq/mL) and 25 meq of sodium bicarbonate (28 mL of 7.5%). After the first hour, modify this solution according to indicated electrolyte needs, and continue at one-third the initial rate until urine flow begins, dehydration is corrected, or evidence of renal insufficiency appears (rising blood urea nitrogen). The goal of rehydration is to establish a normal urine output; forced diuresis is not necessary, and overhydration may contribute to cerebral or pulmonary edema. After urine flow is established, up to 50% of the sodium in the above solution can be replaced by potassium citrate (use 3 meq/mL), depending on the measured potassium deficit. Treat acidosis and alkalinize the urine with sodium bicarbonate, 7.5% solution (44.6 meq/50 mL), 3 meq/kg (3.3 mL) orally, diluted in 5% dextrose. Repeat every 30 minutes until the urine is alkaline or acidosis is corrected. Maintenance of alkaline urine greatly speeds the excretion of salicylates but is difficult and dangerous to perform in seriously ill patients, especially those with chronic intoxication. Serious potassium deficit can be corrected by giving potassium orally or intravenously.

Phytonadione, 0.1 mg/kg intramuscularly, should be given once for hypoprothrombinemia. Hemodialysis may be lifesaving for critically ill patients with high serum salicylate concentrations, intractable acidosis or electrolyte abnormalities, persistent convulsions, or renal insufficiency.

Reduce fever with cold water (10 °C [50 °F]) sponge baths.

Prescott LF et al: Diuresis or urinary alkalinisation for salicylate poisoning? *Br Med J* 1982;**285**:1383.

Proudfoot AT: Toxicity of salicylates. *Am J Med* (Nov 14) 1983 (Suppl):99.

Young RSK et al: Reye's syndrome associated with long-term aspirin therapy. *JAMA* 1984;**251**:754.

SNAKE BITES

The venom of poisonous snakes and lizards may be predominantly neurotoxic (coral snake) or predominantly cytolytic (pit viper). Neurotoxins cause respiratory paralysis; cytolytic venoms cause tissue destruction by digestion and hemorrhage due to hemolysis and destruction of the endothelial lining of the blood vessels. The manifestations of cytolytic envenomation (eg, rattlesnake venom) are local pain, thirst, perspiration, nausea, vomiting, local redness, swelling, extravasation of blood, and collapse. In about half of bites by venomous snakes, no envenomation occurs.

Treatment

A. Emergency Measures: Immobilize the patient and the bitten part in a horizontal position immediately. Avoid manipulation of the bitten area. Transport the patient to a medical facility for definitive treatment. Do not give alcoholic beverages or stimulants; do not apply ice; do not use incision or suction. The trauma to underlying structures resulting from incision and suction performed by unskilled people is probably not justified in view of the small amount of venom that can be recovered in this way (10% at most). Cryotherapy increases tissue loss.

B. Specific Antidote and General Measures:

1. Pit viper (eg, rattlesnake) envenomation–With local signs such as swelling, pain, and ecchymosis but no systemic symptoms, give 4–5 vials of polyvalent crotalid antivenin by intravenous drip. (This should be preceded by skin testing for horse serum sensitivity with the kit supplied.) For more serious envenomation with marked local effects and systemic toxicity (eg, hypotension, coagulopathy), 10–20 vials may be required. Epinephrine should be available for immediate use in the event of an allergic reaction. Specific antiserum therapy is less effective after 4–6 hours and probably useless more than 24 hours after the bite. Monitor vital signs and the blood coagulation profile. Type and cross-match blood. Adequacy of venom neutralization is indicated by improvement in signs and symptoms, and the rate of swelling slows. In delayed serum sickness reactions, give prednisone, 45–60 mg daily in divided doses.

2. Coral snake envenomation–Give 1–2 vials of specific coral snake antivenom as soon as possible, since venom is fixed to neural tissues before symptoms occur.

To locate antisera for exotic snakes, call Poison Information Center, Oklahoma City, OK; (405) 271–5454.

Otten EJ, McKimm D: Venomous snakebite in a patient allergic to horse serum. *Ann Emerg Med* 1983;**12**:624.

Sivaprasad R, Cantini EM: Western diamondback rattlesnake (*Crotalus atrox*) poisoning. *Postgrad Med* (June) 1982; **71**:223.

SPIDER BITES & SCORPION STINGS

The toxin of the less venomous species of spiders and scorpions causes only local pain, redness, and swelling. That of the more venomous species, including black widow spiders (*Latrodectus mactans*), causes generalized muscular pains, muscle spasms and rigidity, and nausea and vomiting. The brown recluse spider (*Loxosceles reclusa*) causes progressive local necrosis as well as hemolytic reactions (rare). Stings by most scorpions cause only local pain. Stings by the more toxic *Centruroides* species (found in the Southwestern USA) may cause muscle cramps, throat tightness, twitching and jerking, respiratory difficulty, and occasionally convulsions.

Treatment

A. Black Widow Spider Bites: Pain may be relieved with parenteral narcotics or muscle relaxants (eg, methocarbamol, 15 mg/kg). Calcium gluconate 10%, 0.1–0.2 mL/kg intravenously, may relieve mus-

cle rigidity. Antivenin is rarely indicated, usually only for very young or elderly patients who do not respond to the above measures. Horse serum sensitivity testing is required.

B. Brown Recluse Spider Bites: Because bites occasionally progress to extensive local necrosis, some authorities recommend early excision of the bite site, whereas others use oral corticosteroids. Recently, interest has focused on the use of dapsone and colchicine. All of these treatments remain of unproved value.

C. Scorpion Stings: No specific treatment is available. For *Centruroides* stings, some toxicologists use a specific antivenom, but this is neither approved nor widely available.

Anderson PC: Necrotizing spider bites. *Am Fam Physician* (Sept) 1982;**26**:198.

King LE Jr, Rees RS: Dapsone treatment of a brown recluse bite. *JAMA* 1983;**250**:648.

STRYCHNINE

Strychnine poisoning may result from ingestion or injection. The manifestations are tetanic muscle rigidity, convulsions, opisthotonos, dyspnea, foaming at the mouth, and asphyxia. Although victims appear to be convulsing, they are usually awake.

Treatment

A. Emergency Measures: Control tetanic rigidity or convulsions with succinylcholine or pancuronium (the patient must be endotracheally intubated and will require mechanical ventilation). In less severe cases, give diazepam, 0.05–0.2 mg/kg (maximum 10 mg) slowly intravenously, and repeat at 30-minute to 4-hour intervals. If possible, lavage gently with activated charcoal before symptoms appear. Activated charcoal given orally in 70% sorbitol or another cathartic may also prevent or delay absorption. Do not induce emesis, and do not lavage after twitching or convulsions have appeared unless succinylcholine or another neuromuscular blocker is being given. Severe metabolic acidosis, rhabdomyolysis, and myoglobinuria may occur. The urine should be alkalinized to prevent renal myoglobin deposition.

B. General Measures: Keep the patient quiet in a darkened room; avoid sudden stimuli.

Boyd RE et al: Strychnine poisoning: Recovery from profound lactic acidosis, hyperthermia, and rhabdomyolysis. *Am J Med* 1983;**74**:507.

THEOPHYLLINE, CAFFEINE

Overdoses occur most commonly from the therapeutic use of caffeine as a stimulant in newborns or theophylline (aminophylline, oxytriphylline) to improve respiration or circulation in older patients. Massive overdose may occur in cases of suicide. Manifestations of overdose are tachypnea, tremor, hypotension, arrhythmias, hypokalemia, cardiac arrest, or convulsions. Serious symptoms can occur at 25 mg/kg and fatalities at 50–100 mg/kg. Fatalities occur at plasma theophylline levels over 60 μg/mL. Convulsions are often difficult to control with diazepam and phenytoin, and their persistence is an indication for hemoperfusion.

Treatment

Remove ingested drug by emesis, lavage with activated charcoal, and catharsis. Remove rectally administered theophylline by enema. Control convulsions with diazepam, 0.1–0.2 mg/kg slowly intravenously, phenytoin, 0.5 mg/kg/min intravenously to a total of 15 mg/kg, or both. Treat hypotension with intravenous fluids. Tachycardia and hypotension may respond to propranolol, 0.03–0.06 mg/kg intravenously. Hemoperfusion is extremely effective and should be used if severe toxicity is present.

Mountain RD, Neff TA: Oral theophylline intoxication. *Arch Intern Med* 1984;**144**:724.

Stewart MF et al: Risk of giving intravenous aminophylline to acutely ill patients receiving maintenance treatment with theophylline. *Br Med J* 1984;**288**:450.

TREATMENT OF LESS COMMON SPECIFIC POISONINGS

(Alphabetical Order)

Acetaldehyde (Industrial)

Inhalation of vapors causes severe irritation of mucous membranes with coughing and then pulmonary edema, followed by narcosis. Ingestion causes narcosis and respiratory failure. The MLD in adults is about 5 g.

Remove from exposure or remove ingested poison by gastric lavage or emesis followed by catharsis. Give oxygen for respiratory difficulty. Treat pulmonary edema.

Akee (Tree)

Manifestations are abdominal discomfort, vomiting, convulsions, coma, hypothermia, hypoglycemia, and fall of blood pressure. Jaundice may appear during the recovery phase.

Remove ingested akee by gastric lavage or emesis followed by catharsis. Control convulsions. Give carbohydrates as 5% glucose intravenously or as sugar dissolved in fruit juice orally to protect from liver damage.

Aminopyrine, Antipyrine, Phenylbutazone (Analgesics)

Manifestations are dizziness, cyanosis, coma, and convulsions. Prolonged administration causes epigastric pain, urticaria, leukopenia, liver damage, exfoliative dermatitis, gastric or duodenal erosion, and adrenal necrosis. The MLD is 5–30 g.

Treat acute poisoning as for salicylates. Treat chronic poisoning by discontinuing the drug.

Bury RW et al: Acute phenylbutazone poisoning in a child. *Med J Austral* 1983;**1**:478.

Amphetamine, Methamphetamine, Dextroamphetamine, and Ephedrine (Sympathomimetics)

Manifestations are tachycardia, dilated pupils, blurred vision, spasms, convulsions, gasping respirations, cardiac arrhythmias, psychosis, hyperthermia, and respiratory failure. The blood pressure is elevated initially but below normal later. The MLD is 120 mg.

Remove ingested drug by emesis or gastric lavage followed by catharsis. Give artificial respiration if cyanosis is present. Maintain blood pressure in cardiovascular collapse by the administration of fluids. Give diazepam, 0.1–0.2 mg/kg intravenously over 2 minutes, and repeat as needed. Nitroprusside (see p 209), or phentolamine (see p 757) may be useful to control severe hypertension.

Aniline (Industrial or cloth-marking ink)

Manifestations are cyanosis, shallow respirations, fall of blood pressure, convulsions, and coma. Blood methemoglobin, as determined photometrically, may reach 60% or more of total hemoglobin. The MLD is 1 g.

Remove aniline from skin by washing thoroughly with soap and water or, if ingested, remove by emesis, gastric lavage, and catharsis. Give fluids and oxygen if respiration is shallow or if there is evidence of air hunger. For methemoglobinemia, give methylene blue, 0.1 mL/kg of 1% solution intravenously over a 10-minute period.

Antimony (Paint)

Manifestations are severe diarrhea with mucus followed by blood, hemorrhagic nephritis, and hepatitis. The MLD is 100 mg.

Remove ingested poison by gastric lavage, emesis, and catharsis. Treat as for arsenic poisoning.

Arsine Industrial)

(See also Arsenic, p 1006.)

Manifestations are pyrexia, cough, abdominal pain, hemolytic anemia, hemoglobinuria, anuria, methemoglobinemia, and diarrhea.

Alkalinize urine as for fava bean poisoning. Give blood transfusions if anemia is severe. Treat anuria.

Barium (Rodenticide)

Manifestations are tightness of the muscles of the face and neck, fibrillary muscular tremors, weakness, profound hypokalemia, difficulty in breathing, irregularity of the heart, convulsions, and cardiac and respiratory failure. The MLD is 1 g.

Give 30 g sodium sulfate in 200 mL of water orally or by gastric tube, and repeat in 1 hour, to form insoluble barium sulfate.

Benzene (Solvent)

Manifestations are visual blurring, tremors, shallow and rapid respirations, ventricular irregularities, unconsciousness, and convulsions. Repeated exposure results in aplastic anemia and abnormal bleeding. The TLV is 1 ppm.

Remove patient from contaminated air and give artificial respiration with oxygen. Induce emesis or perform gastric lavage if more than 1 mL/kg was ingested. Aspiration pneumonitis is a potential complication.

Arp EW Jr et al: Lymphocytic leukemia and exposures to benzene and other solvents in the rubber industry. *J Oral Med* 1983;25:598.

Beryllium (Industrial)

Manifestations include acute pneumonitis, chest pain, bronchial spasm, fever, dyspnea, cough, and cyanosis. Right heart failure may occur. Pulmonary granulomatosis with weight loss and marked dyspnea may occur years after initial exposure. X-ray examination reveals diffuse increase in density of the lung fields or snowstorm appearance. No degree of exposure is safe.

Place the patient at complete bed rest and administer 60% oxygen by mask for cyanosis. Calcium disodium edetate has been suggested. The administration of corticosteroid or related drugs gives symptomatic relief but is not curative.

Beta-Adrenergic Blocking Agents

Overdose with β-adrenergic blocking agents such as propranolol results in hypotension, bradycardia, and variable heart block. Central nervous system toxicity includes coma, convulsions, and respiratory depression. Hypoglycemia and hyperkalemia may occur.

Treatment includes gastric emptying and administration of activated charcoal. Symptomatic bradycardia or heart block may respond to atropine, isoproterenol, or intracardiac pacing. Hypotension may respond to intravenous fluids, dopamine, or norepinephrine. However, because of intense β-adrenergic receptor blockade, catecholamines may be ineffective. Glucagon activates adenylate cyclase and increases heart rate and myocardial contractility independently of β-adrenergic receptors. It has successfully reversed beta-blocker overdose in doses of 50–70 μg/kg intravenously.

Salzberg MR, Gallagher EJ: Propranolol overdose. *Ann Emerg Med* 1980;9:26.

Bleaching Solutions (Household)

Clorox, Purex, Sani-Clor, etc, cause irritation and corrosion of mucous membranes with edema of the pharynx and larynx. Severe burns or perforation of the esophagus or stomach is rare. The MLD is 15 mL.

Because most ingestions involve small quantities of dilute products, injury is rare and no treatment is needed. For massive ingestion, gastric lavage with tap water is recommended. *Caution:* Do not use acid antidotes.

Boric Acid (Antiseptic)

Manifestations from ingestion or skin application are fever, anuria, and flushing followed by desquamation, lethargy, and convulsions. The MLD is 5–15 g.

Remove ingested boric acid by emesis or gastric lavage followed by catharsis. Maintain urine output by giving liquids orally or, in the presence of vomiting, by giving 5% dextrose intravenously. Control convulsions. Remove circulating boric acid by dialysis.

O'Sullivan K, Taylor M: Chronic boric acid poisoning in infants. *Arch Dis Child* 1983;58:737.

Bromates (Cold wave neutralizer)

Manifestations are vomiting, abdominal pains, oliguria, coma, convulsions, fall of blood pressure, hematuria, proteinuria, and renal failure. The MLD is 4 g.

Remove poison by gastric lavage with 1–2% bicarbonate solution, emesis, and catharsis. Give sodium thiosulfate, 1–5 g intravenously as a 10% solution. Treat shock by administration of fluids.

Cadmium (Metal plating)

Ingestion causes diarrhea, vomiting, muscular aches, salivation, and abdominal pain. Inhalation causes shortness of breath, pain in the chest, foamy or bloody sputum, muscular aches. Chronic exposure produces anemia, and x-ray indicates lung consolidation. A sulfosalicylic acid–precipitable protein is present in the urine. The MLD is about 10 mg.

Treat pulmonary edema and give calcium disodium edetate. Remove ingested poison by emesis or gastric lavage followed by catharsis.

Calcium Entry-Blocking Agents

Overdose with calcium channel-blocking agents may result in hypotension, bradycardia, and atrioventricular heart block. The various agents (verapamil, diltiazem, nifedipine) have differing effects on cardiac conduction and peripheral vascular resistance that may account for variable clinical manifestations of overdose.

Treatment includes gastric emptying followed by administration of activated charcoal. Atrioventricular block and bradycardia may be managed with atropine, isoproterenol, or intracardiac pacing. Hypotension may respond to supine positioning, intravenous fluids, and pressor agents. Intravenous calcium has been used successfully to reverse the effects of verapamil toxicity and may be given in doses of 10–20 mg/kg of calcium chloride.

Morris DL, Goldschlager N: Calcium infusion for reversal of adverse effects of intravenous verapamil. *JAMA* 1983;**249:** 3212.

Camphor (Stimulant)

Manifestations are a feeling of tension, dizziness, irrational behavior, rigidity, tachycardia, twitching of the facial muscles, and generalized convulsions. The MLD is 1 g.

Remove ingested poison by gastric lavage or emesis followed by catharsis. Control convulsions with diazepam.

Cantharidin (Irritant)

Manifestations are severe vomiting, diarrhea, fall of blood pressure, hematuria, and death in respiratory failure or uremia. The MLD is 10 mg.

Remove ingested poison by gastric lavage or emesis followed by catharsis. Treat cardiovascular collapse by blood transfusions and intravenous saline. Treat anuria.

Castor Beans (Plant)

Manifestations are vomiting, diarrhea, severe abdominal pain, cyanosis, circulatory collapse, and oliguria. Urine may show protein, casts, red blood cells, and hemoglobin. The MLD is 1 bean.

Remove ingested beans by gastric lavage or emesis followed by catharsis. Maintain blood pressure by blood transfusions. Alkalinize urine by giving 5–15 g of sodium bicarbonate daily to prevent precipitation of hemoglobin or hemoglobin products in the kidneys. Treat anuria.

Chloramine-T (Disinfectant)

Manifestations are cyanosis, frothing at the mouth, and respiratory failure within a few minutes to 1 hour after ingestion. The MLD is 0.5 g.

Remove ingested chloramine-T by gastric lavage or emesis followed by catharsis.

Chlorates (Disinfectant)

Manifestations are cyanosis, hemolysis, anuria, and convulsions. The MLD is 15 g. Laboratory findings include methemoglobinemia, hemolytic type anemia, and elevation of serum potassium level.

Remove ingested chlorate by gastric lavage or emesis followed by catharsis. Treat methemoglobinemia. Force fluids to 2–4 L daily to remove chlorate if urine output is adequate.

Steffen C, Seitz R: Severe chlorate poisoning: Report of a case. *Arch Toxicol* 1981;**48:**281.

Chlorinated Hydrocarbons

For volatile chlorinated hydrocarbons, see Carbon Tetrachloride; for nonvolatile chlorinated hydrocarbons, see Chlorophenothane (DDT).

Chlorinated Naphthalene (Insulator)

The principal manifestation is a papular acneiform eruption that progresses to pustule formation. Jaundice, enlargement of the liver, and weakness also occur. Impairment of hepatic cell function is revealed by appropriate tests.

Treat liver damage as outlined under carbon tetrachloride poisoning.

Chromium & Chromate (Rustproofing)

Ingestion causes abdominal pain, vomiting, shock, and oliguria or anuria. Skin contact leads to incapacitating eczematous dermatitis and ulceration. Ulceration and perforation of the nasal septum also occur. Acute hepatitis has been observed. Examination of the urine reveals proteinuria and hematuria. The MLD of soluble chromate is 5 g.

Remove ingested chromate by gastric lavage, emesis, and catharsis. Treat oliguria and liver damage.

Clonidine (Hypotensive)

Overdose of clonidine causes bradycardia, hypotension, respiratory depression, and coma. Hypertension occasionally occurs.

Maintain airway and respiration. Symptomatic treatment is usually sufficient even in massive overdose. Maintain blood pressure with intravenous fluids. Dopamine can also be used.

Yagupoky P, Gorodischer R: Massive clonidine ingestion with hypertension in a 9-month-old infant. *Pediatrics* 1983;**72:** 500.

Cocaine (Local anesthetic)

Manifestations are restlessness, excitability, hallucinations, irregular respirations, convulsions, and circulatory failure. The MLD is sometimes said to be 1.2 g, but death has resulted from intravenous injection of as little as 20 mg.

Maintain airway and oxygenation. Control convulsions with diazepam and phenytoin. Propranolol, 0.02–0.06 mg/kg slowly intravenously, may be useful for tachyarrhythmias.

Caruana BS et al: Cocaine-packet ingestion: Diagnosis, management and natural history. *Ann Intern Med* 1984;**100:**73.

Jonsson S et al: Acute cocaine poisoning: Importance of treating seizures and acidosis. *Am J Med* 1983;**75:**1061.

Colchicine (Gout remedy)

Manifestations are burning in the throat, watery to bloody diarrhea, cardiovascular collapse, and oliguria. The MLD is 6 mg.

Remove ingested poison by emesis or gastric lavage followed by catharsis. Give oxygen for respiratory difficulty. Treat oliguria.

Detergents (Soaps, detergents, antiseptics)

A. Cationic Detergents: These include the antiseptics of the quaternary ammonium type (Diaparene, Zephiran, benzalkonium chloride). Manifestations are severe vomiting, shock, convulsions, and death within 1–4 hours. The MLD is 1–3 g.

Remove unabsorbed detergent by emesis or gastric lavage. Ordinary face soap is an effective antidote for unabsorbed cationic detergent but is not effective against the systemic effects. Treat respiratory embarrassment or shock with appropriate measures. Control convulsions with short-acting barbiturates.

B. Anionic or Nonionic Detergents: These compounds, which are present in general laundry detergents and dishwashing liquids, cause only nausea, vomiting, and diarrhea. Certain laundry compounds and electric dishwasher detergents may contain alkalies, however, and their ingestion requires immediate treatment for caustic poisoning (see p 1006). Poisoning with certain phosphate additives to some detergents requires treatment with parenteral calcium.

Dioxane (Solvent)

Prolonged exposure may lead to kidney and liver damage and pulmonary edema.

Remove from further exposure and treat symptomatically.

Disulfiram (Antabuse) Plus Alcohol
(Alcohol sensitizer)

Manifestations are flushing, sweating, tachycardia, postural hypotension, cardiac arrhythmias, air hunger, and cardiac pain.

Maintain airway and respiration. Place the patient in the supine or Trendelenburg position, and give intravenous fluids to reverse hypotension.

Ergotamine (Migraine remedy)

Manifestations are rise or fall of blood pressure, weak pulse, convulsions, and loss of consciousness. Prolonged administration causes numbness and coldness of the extremities, tingling, pain in the chest, contractions of the facial muscles, and convulsions. Impending gangrene has resulted from 40 mg given over 5 days. The maximum safe dose is 6 mg/d.

Remove ingested drug by emesis or gastric lavage followed by catharsis. Treat convulsions. Severe arterial vasoconstriction should be treated with intra-arterial vasodilators and heparin.

Ethylene Chlorohydrin (Fumigant)

Manifestations are abdominal pain, excitability, delirium, respiratory slowing, fall of blood pressure, twitching of muscles, cyanosis, and coma with respiratory and circulatory failure. The MLD is 5 mL.

Remove from further exposure and remove ingested poison by emesis, gastric lavage, and catharsis. Treat as for methyl bromide poisoning.

Ethylene Glycol (Antifreeze)

The initial symptoms in massive dosage (over 100 mL in a single dose) are those of alcoholic intoxication. These symptoms then progress to stupor, anuria, and unconsciousness with convulsions. Smaller amounts (10–30 mL) result in anuria beginning 24–72 hours after ingestion. There is anion-gap metabolic acidosis and an elevation of the measured serum osmo-

lality. The urine may show calcium oxalate crystals, protein, red cells, and casts.

Remove ingested glycol by gastric lavage or emesis and catharsis. Give calcium gluconate, 10 mL of 10% solution intravenously, for symptomatic hypocalcemia. Give artificial respiration, using oxygen for depressed respiration. In the absence of renal impairment, force fluids to 4 L or more daily to increase excretion of glycol. Correct acidosis with sodium bicarbonate intravenously. Give ethyl alcohol as in methyl alcohol poisoning. Dialysis is mandatory for significant intoxication.

Brown CG et al: Ethylene glycol poisoning. *Ann Emerg Med* 1983;**12**:501.

Fava Beans (Plant)

Manifestations are hemolysis, fever, jaundice, dark urine, oliguria, and pallor. The urine may show the presence of hemoglobin.

Give blood transfusions until anemia is corrected. Alkalinize urine with 5–15 g of sodium bicarbonate every 4 hours to prevent the precipitation of hemoglobin in the kidneys. In the presence of normal kidney function, maintain urine output by giving 2–4 L of fluid daily orally or intravenously. Give cortisone, 25–100 mg daily. Treat anuria.

Fluoroacetate (Rodenticide)

Symptoms begin within minutes to hours with vomiting, excitability, convulsions, irregularity of the heartbeat, and depression of respiration. The fatal dose is estimated to be 5 mg/kg.

Remove ingested poison by emesis, gastric lavage, and catharsis. Control convulsions.

Formaldehyde (Disinfectant)

Ingestion causes corrosive damage resulting in severe abdominal pain followed by cardiovascular collapse, loss of consciousness, anuria, and circulatory failure. Metabolic acidosis is not uncommon. The MLD is 60 mL.

Remove ingested poison by gastric lavage or emesis followed by catharsis, preferably with 1% ammonium carbonate solution. Treat shock by administration of fluids; treat acidosis with bicarbonate; and consider hemodialysis to remove formaldehyde and its metabolite, formate.

Main DM, Hogan TJ: Health effects of low-level exposure to formaldehyde. *J Oral Med* 1983;**25**:896.

Gold Salts (Antirheumatic)

Manifestations are skin rash, itching, eruptions, metallic taste, hepatitis, granulocytopenia, and aplastic anemia. Give dimercaprol (BAL).

Hydralazine (Hypotensive)

Chronic use may cause fever, diffuse erythematous facial dermatitis, lymph gland enlargement, splenomegaly, arthralgia, and simulated disseminated lupus erythematosus. Acute overdose causes hypotension and tachycardia.

Discontinue further use at the first indication of joint involvement or rash. Give aspirin, 1–3 g daily, or cortisone, 50–150 mg daily, until symptoms regress. For acute overdose, treat with the supine position and intravenous fluids. Monitor the ECG.

Hydrogen Sulfide & Carbon Disulfide (Fumigants)

Manifestations are painful conjunctivitis, appearance of a halo around lights, anosmia, pulmonary edema, restlessness, blurred vision, unconsciousness, and paralysis of respiration. Prolonged exposure causes persistent low blood pressure, impaired gait and balance, memory loss, mental depression, and parkinsonian tremor. The TLV is 10 ppm. Rapid olfactory fatigue occurs with higher levels of hydrogen sulfide.

Remove from exposure. Treat acute hydrogen sulfide poisoning with nitrites, as described for cyanide. However, do not use sodium thiosulfate. Treat pulmonary edema.

Iodine (Disinfectant)

Manifestations include a characteristic stain of the mouth and odor of the breath, yellow or bluish vomitus, pain and burning in the pharynx and esophagus, marked thirst, diarrhea (stools may be bloody), weakness, dizziness, syncope, and convulsions. The MLD is 2 g.

Give 15 g cornstarch or flour in 500 mL of water or, if available, 250 mL of 1% sodium thiosulfate in water. Follow with an emetic or remove by lavage with sodium thiosulfate solution, 1%, and repeat until evidence of iodine has disappeared from the gastric contents. Then give milk or beaten eggs. Maintain blood pressure and respiration.

Ipecac, Emetine (Emetics)

Ipecac syrup contains only small quantities of emetine and is not toxic in usual doses. However, poisoning may occur after massive overdose or after chronic daily use (eg, bulimic patients who induce emesis after each meal). Manifestations are fatigue, dyspnea, tachycardia, low blood pressure, unconsciousness, and death from heart failure. The ECG reveals depressed T waves and arrhythmias. The MLD of emetine is 1 g.

Management of poisoning with these agents consists of removing ingested poison by gastric lavage or emesis followed by catharsis. Cautious digitalization may be helpful for myocardial weakness.

Iproniazid, Isocarboxazid, Pheniprazine, Nialamide, Phenelzine (Stimulants)

Overdoses cause ataxia, stupor, excitement, fall of blood pressure, tachycardia, and convulsions. Repeated administration may cause weakness, hallucinations, mania, urine retention, liver injury with nausea, and vomiting. The MLD is 5 g.

Remove ingested drug by gastric lavage, emesis,

and catharsis. Give artificial respiration if respiration is depressed. Maintain blood pressure. Do not give stimulants. Pyridoxine, 5 g intravenously, may be effective in controlling convulsions. Discontinue administration at the first appearance of jaundice. Treat liver impairment as for carbon tetrachloride poisoning.

Isoniazid (Tuberculosis remedy)

Overdose causes convulsions, acidosis, coma, and cardiorespiratory depression.

Remove ingested drug with emesis, gastric lavage, activated charcoal, and catharsis. Treat convulsions with diazepam or phenytoin. Pyridoxine, 5 g intravenously, may control convulsions and has been suggested as a specific antidote.

Magnesium Salts (Cathartic)

Manifestations of toxicity include watery diarrhea, gastrointestinal irritation, vomiting, tenesmus, flaccid paralysis, and, in the presence of impaired renal function, severe fall of blood pressure. The MLD is 30–60 g.

Dilute orally or rectally administered magnesium sulfate by giving tap water. Give artificial respiration if necessary. Give calcium gluconate, 10 mL of 10% solution intravenously slowly, as a specific antidote.

Manganese (Industrial)

Ingestion causes lethargy, edema, and symptoms of extrapyramidal tract lesions. Inhalation causes bronchitis, pneumonia, and liver enlargement. Signs of parkinsonism also occur. Hepatic cell function tests may be impaired. The MAC is 6 mg/m^3.

Remove from further exposure. Give calcium disodium edetate.

Meprobamate (Sedative)

Manifestations are drowsiness and incoordination progressing to coma with cyanosis and respiratory depression. The MLD is 12 g.

Remove ingested drug by gastric lavage or emesis followed by catharsis. Use resuscitative measures as for barbiturates if respiratory depression is present.

Metaldehyde (Snail bait)

Manifestations are severe vomiting, abdominal pains, temperature elevation, muscular rigidity, convulsions, coma, and death from respiratory failure up to 48 hours after ingestion. The MLD for adults is about 5 g.

Treat as for acetaldehyde poisoning, but note that snail bait sometimes contains arsenic. Gastric lavage with 5% sodium bicarbonate will slow the rate of conversion of metaldehyde to acetaldehyde. Activated charcoal is effective.

Longstreth WT Jr, Pierson DJ: Metaldehyde poisoning from slug bait ingestion. *West J Med* 1982;**137**:134.

Metal Fumes (Industrial)

Inhalation of zinc oxide or other metal fumes

causes fever, cough, chills, muscular aches, and weakness. Pulmonary edema may follow (rare).

Treat pulmonary edema. Bed rest and administration of analgesics will ordinarily relieve generalized symptoms within 12 hours.

Methyl Bromide & Methyl Chloride
(Fumigants)

Manifestations are dizziness, drowsiness, fall of blood pressure, coma, convulsions, and pulmonary edema after a latent period of 1–4 hours.

Treat convulsions. Treat pulmonary edema.

Methyl Sulfate (Industrial)

Ingestion or contact causes corrosion equivalent to that from sulfuric acid. Vapor exposure causes irritation and erythema of the eyes, pulmonary edema, proteinuria, and hematuria. The MLD for adults is about 1 g.

Treat as for corrosive acid poisoning.

Methysergide Maleate (Sansert)
(Migraine remedy)

Methysergide may cause fibrotic disorders involving primarily the retroperitoneal areas (retroperitoneal fibrosis) but also suggestive fibrotic changes affecting the aorta, heart valves, and lungs. Manifestations include chest pain, dyspnea, fever, pleural effusion; pain in the back, abdomen, and pelvis; hydronephrosis, renal insufficiency, intermittent claudication, and edema of the lower extremities.

Cessation of methysergide therapy results in partial or complete remission of the disorder. Surgical removal of adhesions may be necessary.

Naphthalene (Mothballs)

Manifestations are vomiting and diarrhea. Hemolysis may result in jaundice, pain on urination, and anuria. The MLD for adults is about 2 g. (*Note:* The usual moth repellent is paradichlorobenzene, which may cause seizures but does not cause hemolysis.)

Remove ingested naphthalene by gastric lavage or emesis followed by catharsis. Alkalinize urine by giving sodium bicarbonate, 5 g orally every 4 hours or as necessary to maintain alkaline urine. Give repeated small blood transfusions until hemoglobin is 60–80% of normal.

Naphthol (Industrial)

Acute poisoning is the same as that which occurs with phenol. Prolonged contact may cause bladder tumors, hemolytic anemia, and cataracts. Addition of ferric chloride to acidified urine gives a violet or blue color indicating the presence of a phenolic compound. The MLD for naphthol is 2 g.

Treat as for phenol poisoning.

Naphthylamine (Industrial)

Repeated exposure may cause skin sensitivity reactions with weeping and crusting. Exposure to large amounts may cause methemoglobinemia with cyanosis.

Remove from further exposure. Treat cyanosis as for aniline poisoning.

Nickel Carbonyl (Industrial)

Immediate symptoms are cough, dizziness, and weakness. Delayed reactions are characterized by dyspnea, cyanosis, rapid pulse, and respiratory embarrassment. The TLV is 0.05 ppm.

Treat cyanosis and dyspnea by giving 100% oxygen by mask. Treat pulmonary edema. Give sodium diethyldithiocarbamate, 50–100 mg/kg orally or intramuscularly.

Nicotine (Tobacco)

Manifestations are respiratory stimulation, nausea, diarrhea, tachycardia, elevation of blood pressure, salivation, and, with large doses, rapid progression to prostration, convulsions, respiratory slowing, cardiac irregularity, and coma. The fatal dose of pure nicotine is approximately 1 mg/kg. The MLD of tobacco is 5 g.

Remove nicotine from skin by scrubbing or, if ingested, remove by thorough gastric lavage after activated charcoal administration.

Nitrites (Food preservatives,
recreational inhalants)

Manifestations are flushing of the skin, vomiting, dizziness, marked fall of blood pressure, cyanosis, and respiratory paralysis. The MLD is 2 g.

Remove ingested poison by gastric lavage or emesis followed by catharsis. Treat shock (see p 9). Treat methemoglobinemia by the administration of methylene blue, 0.1 mL/kg of 1% solution intravenously over 10 minutes.

Nitrophenols (Herbicide)

Manifestations are fever, prostration, thirst, excessive perspiration, difficulty in breathing, muscular tremors, and coma. Cataracts occur after repeated exposure. The MLD is 100 mg.

Remove ingested poison by emesis, gastric lavage, and catharsis. If the body temperature is elevated, reduce to normal by immersion in cold water or by applying cold packs.

Oxalic Acid (Component of some bleaches)

Oxalic acid is a corrosive that also precipitates ionized calcium. Manifestations are burning in the mouth and throat, violent abdominal pains, bloody vomitus, dyspnea, tremors, oliguria, and circulatory collapse. The MLD is 4 g.

Give one of the following to precipitate as insoluble calcium oxalate: calcium lactate or other calcium salt, 30 g in 200 mL of water or large amounts of milk. Give whites of eggs beaten in milk as demulcent. Give calcium gluconate or calcium lactate, 10 mL of 10% solution intravenously, and calcium orally, 1–2 g 4 times daily. Institute supportive measures as required.

Paraldehyde (Hypnotic)

Manifestations are deep sleep with ordinary doses and respiratory or cardiac depression occasionally with doses over 10 mL. There is a characteristic pungent odor.

Treat as for acetaldehyde or barbiturate poisoning.

Permanganate (Antiseptic)

Ingestion of solid or concentrated permanganate causes laryngeal edema, necrosis of oral mucosa, slow pulse, and cardiovascular collapse. Anuria may occur. The MLD is 10 g.

Protect and maintain a patent airway. Remove ingested poison by gastric lavage or emesis followed by catharsis. Treat shock (see p 9) and anuria.

Phenacetin & Acetanilid (Analgesics)

Acute poisoning may cause hemolysis and methemoglobinemia. Prolonged administration leads to renal impairment, cyanosis, hemolytic anemia, and skin eruptions. The MLD is 5–20 g.

Treat phenacetin as for acetaminophen poisoning. Treat methemoglobinemia by giving methylene blue, 0.1 mL/kg of 1% solution slowly intravenously.

Dubach UC, Rosner B, Pfister E: Epidemiologic study of abuse of analgesics containing phenacetin: Renal morbidity and mortality (1968–1979). *N Engl J Med* 1983;**308**:357.

Phenolphthalein (Laxative)

Manifestations are erythematous, itching skin rash, purging, collapse, and fall of blood pressure.

Prevent further use. Treat blood pressure fall by administration of fluids.

Physostigmine, Neostigmine, & Related Drugs (Parasympathomimetics)

Manifestations are tremors, marked peristalsis, involuntary defecation and urination, pinpoint pupils, difficult breathing, arrhythmias, convulsions, and severe respiratory difficulty. The MLD is 6 mg.

Give atropine sulfate, 2 mg intravenously or intramuscularly every 2–4 hours as necessary to relieve respiratory difficulty and other symptoms.

Poison Hemlock (Plant)

Manifestations are gradually increasing muscular weakness followed by paralysis with respiratory failure. Proteinuria also occurs.

Treat respiratory failure by artificial respiration with oxygen. Remove ingested poison by gastric lavage or emesis followed by catharsis.

Poison Ivy, Poison Oak (Plants)

Local effects begin after a delay of hours to days and include itching, swelling, vesiculation, generalized edema, proteinuria, and microscopic hematuria.

Minimize skin contamination by washing with strong soap and water. Remove ingested plant material by gastric lavage or emesis followed by saline catharsis. Treat exudative stage by exposure to air or with wet dressings of 1% aluminum acetate. Generalized reactions may be treated with corticosteroids to relieve symptoms.

Procaine, Lidocaine (Local anesthetics)

Manifestations are dizziness, weakness, fall of blood pressure, muscular tremors, convulsions, and cardiovascular collapse. The injected MLD is 1 g.

Treat as for cocaine poisoning.

Propylthiouracil (Antithyroid)

Manifestations are skin rash, urticaria, joint pains, fever, and leukopenia.

Treat agranulocytosis (see p 337).

Quinidine (Antifibrillatory)

Manifestations of toxicity are tinnitus, diarrhea, dizziness, severe fall of blood pressure, arrhythmias, syncope, respiratory failure, thrombocytopenic purpura after prolonged use, urticaria, and anaphylactoid reactions. The ECG may show widening of QRS complex, lengthened QT interval, premature ventricular beats, and lengthened PR interval. The MLD is 1 g.

Remove ingested drug by gastric lavage or emesis followed by catharsis. Raise blood pressure by intravenous saline or blood transfusions or with levarterenol. The administration of sixth-molar sodium lactate solution intravenously is said to reduce the cardiotoxic effects of quinidine.

Swiryn S, Kim SS: Quinidine-induced syncope. *Arch Intern Med* 1983;**143**:314.

Quinine, Quinacrine, Chloroquine (Antimalarials)

Manifestations are progressive tinnitus, blurring of vision, weakness, fall of blood pressure, anuria, and cardiac irregularities. Repeated ingestion of quinine causes visual loss associated with pallor of optic disks, narrowing of retinal vessels, and papilledema. Quinacrine causes hepatitis, aplastic anemia, psychosis, and jaundice. Chloroquine causes dizziness and blurred vision. The urine may show red cells, protein, and casts. The MLD is 1 g.

Remove ingested drug by lavage or emesis followed by catharsis. Treat shock (see p 9). Give 2–4 L of fluids daily to promote renal excretion. Treat anuria.

Shellfish ("Red tide")

Manifestations are numbness and tingling of lips, tongue, face, and extremities, respiratory weakness or paralysis, and convulsions.

Remove ingested shellfish by gastric lavage or emesis followed by catharsis. Give artificial respiration with oxygen, and maintain blood pressure.

Silver Nitrate (Antiseptic)

Silver nitrate is a protein precipitant. Poisoning is manifested by nausea, vomiting, diarrhea, bloody stools, blue discoloration about the mouth, and shock.

Lavage with saline solution to precipitate silver chloride. Give whites of eggs beaten in milk as demulcent, and sodium sulfate, 30 g in 200 mL of water, as cathartic. Institute supportive measures.

Dimercaprol has not proved effective.

Stibine (Industrial)

Manifestations are weakness, jaundice, anemia, and weak pulse. The TLV is 0.1 ppm.

Treat by blood transfusion and alkalinization of the urine.

Sulfonamides (Antibacterial)

Manifestations are skin eruptions, fever, hematuria, and oliguria or anuria with azotemia. The urine shows crystals, red cells, and protein.

If kidney function is normal, force fluids to 4 L daily to speed excretion of sulfonamides. Treat anuria.

Talc (Dusting powder)

Prolonged inhalation causes fine fibrosis of the lungs and calcification of the pericardium.

Remove from further exposure. Treat as for silicosis.

Tetrachloroethane (Solvent)

Manifestations are irritation of the eyes and nose, headache, nausea, abdominal pain, jaundice, and anuria. Hepatic cell impairment may be revealed by appropriate tests. The urine may show proteins, red cells, or casts. The MLD is 1 g.

Treat as for carbon tetrachloride poisoning.

Thallium (Rodenticide)

Thallium poisoning is characterized by slow onset of ataxia, pains and paresthesias of the extremities, bilateral ptosis, loss of hair, fever, and abdominal pains. More severe poisoning is indicated by lethargy, jumbled speech, tremors, convulsions and cyanosis, pulmonary edema, and respiratory difficulty. The MLD is 1 g.

Remove ingested poison by emesis; perform gastric lavage with Prussian blue (ferric ferrocyanide), 125 mg, and cathartic. Give Berlin blue (Antidotum Thallii Heyl), 1 g orally 3 times daily for 2–3 weeks, as a thallium-trapping agent. Furosemide and mannitol forced diuresis, hemoperfusion, or hemodialysis can remove up to 40% of absorbed thallium. Maintain blood pressure.

McCormack J, McKinney W: Thallium poisoning in a group assassination attempt. *Postgrad Med* (Dec) 1983;**74**:239.

Thanite (Insecticide)

Respiratory difficulty and convulsions occur.

Remove ingested poison by emesis or gastric lavage. Treat convulsions as for strychnine poisoning.

Thiocyanates (Insecticides)

Manifestations are disorientation, weakness, low blood pressure, psychotic behavior, and convulsions.

Remove ingested thiocyanate by gastric lavage or emesis followed by catharsis. Give 2–4 L of fluid orally or intravenously daily to maintain adequate urine output. Remove thiocyanate by peritoneal dialysis or by hemodialysis if necessary.

Thyroid (Medicinal)

Manifestations are fever, tachycardia, hypertension, and cardiovascular collapse at doses of 0.3 g/kg. Symptoms may be delayed for 2–5 days after ingestion of thyroid preparations.

Empty the stomach with emesis or lavage and follow with activated charcoal.

Trichloroethylene (Solvent)

Manifestations are dizziness, headache, excitement, and loss of consciousness. Irregular pulse may occur. The MLD is 5 mL.

Remove patient to fresh air, and give artificial respiration. Avoid epinephrine or other stimulants.

Trinitrotoluene (Explosive)

Manifestations include jaundice, dermatitis, cyanosis, pallor, loss of appetite, and oliguria or anuria. The liver may be enlarged or atrophic. Hepatic cell injury may be revealed by appropriate tests. The MLD is 1 g.

Remove from skin by thorough washing with soap and water. Remove swallowed trinitrotoluene by gastric lavage or emesis and catharsis. Protect the liver by giving 10 mL of 10% calcium gluconate intravenously 3 times daily and a high-carbohydrate, high-calcium diet, including at least 1 quart of skimmed milk daily. Give vitamin D in high doses daily.

Tri-orthocresyl Phosphate (Plasticizer)

After 1–30 days' delay, weakness of the distal muscles develops, with footdrop, wristdrop, and loss of plantar reflex. Death may occur from respiratory muscle paralysis. The MLD for adults is about 5 g.

Remove by gastric lavage or emesis followed by catharsis. Maintain respiration.

Veratrum, Zygadenus (Plants)

Manifestations are nausea, severe vomiting, muscular weakness, slow pulse, and low blood pressure. Excessive amounts may cause marked rise in blood pressure initially.

Remove ingested poison by gastric lavage or emesis followed by catharsis. Atropine, 2 mg subcutaneously, will block the reflex fall of blood pressure and the bradycardia. Elevation of blood pressure is treated with phentolamine hydrochloride, 25 mg subcutaneously repeated every 4 hours.

Volatile Anesthetics: Ether, Chloroform, Halothane, Divinyl Ether, Cyclopropane, Ethyl Chloride, Ethylene, Nitrous Oxide

Manifestations are excitement, unconsciousness, depression, and paralysis of respiration. Cardiac irregularities occur with cyclopropane, chloroform, and halothane. Severe fall of blood pressure or cardiac arrest may also occur. The MLD is 1–30 mL.

Remove volatile anesthetic by artificial respiration. Maintain blood pressure (see p 10). Prevent hypoxia by administering oxygen.

Volatile Oils: Turpentine, Pine Oil, Menthol, Absinthe, Savin, Pennyroyal, Eucalyptus

Manifestations are vomiting, diarrhea, unconsciousness, shallow respiration, hematuria, and convulsions. The MLD is 15 g.

Give 60–120 mL of liquid petrolatum or castor oil and then remove oils by gastric lavage, taking care to prevent aspiration. Follow with a saline cathartic. Give artificial respiration if necessary. If kidney function is normal, give fluids, 2–4 L daily, after the danger of pulmonary edema has passed.

Zinc Sulfate (Astringent)

Manifestations are burning pain in the mouth and throat, vomiting, diarrhea, anuria, and cardiovascular collapse. The MLD is 30 g.

Give milk or starch drinks to dilute the poison and remove by gastric lavage. Replace fluid loss with 5% dextrose in saline. Relieve pain by giving morphine sulfate, 10 mg.

· · ·

AIR POLLUTION & SMOKING

There is considerable evidence that the present levels of atmospheric contaminants that exist in many larger urban areas are sufficient to cause discomfort or significantly impair health. Toxicologic and epidemiologic studies suggest that the noxious nature of the atmosphere is usually due to a complex mixture of pollutants and to meteorologic factors.

Air pollutants are usually divided into 2 broad classes: (1) particulates (smoke, dust, ash, mists, and fumes that exist in the atmosphere in either a solid or liquid state) and (2) gases (eg, carbon monoxide, sulfur oxides, hydrogen sulfide, nitrogen oxides, and carbon compounds—particularly those reacting in the atmosphere to form photochemical smog).

The irritating effects of air pollution on the eye and upper respiratory tract are well known. Inhalation of irritant materials may interfere with lung function, aggravating chronic bronchitis, chronic constrictive ventilatory disease, pulmonary emphysema, and bronchial asthma. The particulate fraction contains a number of carcinogenic substances, and these could play a part in the rapidly changing incidence of different cancers.

The ill effects of atmospheric pollution are most obvious during acute episodes of unusually high pollution. Marked increases in the incidence of illnesses and deaths due to cardiorespiratory damage were reported in the Meuse Valley in Belgium in 1930; in Donora,

Pennsylvania, in 1948; and in London in 1952 and 1962.

Evidence of the adverse effect on human health of self-administered air pollution by tobacco smoking is overwhelming. Seventy-five thousand people die of lung cancer in the USA annually, and almost all of these deaths are due to smoking or exposure to secondary tobacco smoke. Pneumoconioses such as asbestosis are almost entirely limited to those people who smoke during exposure to the dust. Smoking plays a role in cardiovascular disease deaths and other cancer deaths, but the role cannot be so clearly stated as in lung cancer. Several hazardous contaminants are present in tobacco smoke at concentrations far beyond those allowed in industrial or community air. Cigarette smoke contains 200–650 ppm of nitrogen oxides and 40,000 ppm of carbon monoxide. Carcinogenic polynuclear aromatic hydrocarbons are also present in excessive concentration.

ENVIRONMENTAL HAZARDS

A number of substances used in industry or as pesticides are under investigation for long-term low-concentration toxicity or carcinogenicity. Some of these agents are stable and persist as contaminants for months to years after use. A list of some of these substances and their suspected effects follows.

Asbestos—Pulmonary effects and mesotheliomas.

Chloroform—Liver cancer.

Chloromethyl methyl ether—Lung cancer.

4,4'-Diaminodiphenyl methane—Toxic hepatitis.

Formaldehyde—Respiratory damage, cancer.

n-Hexane—Neuropathy.

Kepone—Neurologic effects.

Methyl butyl ketone (MBK)—Neuropathy.

Mirex—Liver cancer.

α-Naphthylthiourea—Bladder tumors.

Polybrominated biphenyl (PBB)—Birth defects, liver cancer.

Polychlorinated biphenyl (PCB)—Birth defects, liver cancer, melanoma.

Tetrachlorodibenzodioxin (TCDD, dioxin)— Birth defects, chloracne.

Vinyl chloride—Angiosarcoma of the liver.

Adams L et al: Respiratory impairment induced by smoking in children in secondary schools. Br Med J 1984;**288**:891.

Calesnick B: Dioxin and agent orange. Am Fam Physician (Feb) 1984;**29**:303.

Casey PH, Collie WR: Severe mental retardation and multiple congenital anomalies of uncertain cause after extreme parental exposure to 2,4-D. J Pediatrics 1984;**104**:313.

Couri D, Milk M: Toxicity and metabolism of the neurotoxic hexacarbons, n-hexane 2-hexanone, 2,5-hexane dione. Annu Rev Pharmacol Toxicol 1982;**22**:145.

Friedman GD: Prevalence and correlates of passive smoking. Am J Public Health 1983;**73**:401.

Halperin WE et al: Nasal cancer in a worker exposed to formaldehyde. JAMA 1983;**249**:510.

Hunninghake GW, Crystal RG: Cigarette smoking and lung destruction. *Am Rev Respir Dis* 1983;**128**:833.

Jacobson JL et al: The transfer of polychlorinated biphenyls (PCBs) and polybrominated biphenyls (PBBs) across the human placenta and into maternal milk. *Am J Public Health* 1984;**74**:378.

Keogh AM et al: Exacerbation of Goodpasture's syndrome after inadvertent exposure to hydrocarbon fumes. *Br Med J* 1984;**288**:188.

Kotin P: Carcinogenesis: Problems and paradoxes. *J Occup Med* 1982;**24**:290.

Kuratsune M et al: PCB poisoning in Japan and Taiwan. *Am J Industr Med* 1984;**5**:1.

Langauer-Lewowicka H et al: Vinyl chloride disease: Neurological disturbances. *Int Arch Occup Environ Health* 1983;**52**:151.

Levine RJ et al: Superiority of reproductive histories to sperm counts in detecting infertility at a dibromochloropropane manufacturing plant. *J Oral Med* 1983;**25**:591.

McCallum RI et al: Lung cancer associated with chloromethyl methyl ether manufacture: An investigation at two factories in the United Kingdom. *Br J Ind Med* 1983;**40**:384.

Moses M et al: Health status of workers with past exposure to 2,3,7,8-tetrachlorodibenzo-p-dioxin in the manufacture of 2,4,5-trichlorophenoxy acidic acid. *Am J Industr Med* 1984;**5**:161.

Schwartz EM, Rae WA: Effect of polybrominated biphenyls (PBB) on developmental abilities in young children. *Am J Public Health* 1983;**73**:277.

Sexton M, Hebel JR: Clinical trial of change in maternal smoking and its effect on birth weight. *JAMA* 1984;**251**:911.

Smith AB et al: Metabolic and health consequences of occupational exposure to polychlorinated biphenyls. *Br J Ind Med* 1982;**39**:361.

Stevens RD, Moolgavkar SH: A cohort analysis of lung cancer and smoking in British males. *Am J Epidemiol* 1984;**119**:624.

Tager IB et al: Longitudinal study of the effects of maternal smoking on pulmonary function in children. *N Engl J Med* 1983;**309**:699.

Ware JH et al: Passive smoking, gas cooking, and respiratory health of children living in six cities. *Am Rev Respir Dis* 1984; **129**:366.

•   •   •

References

Adverse Reactions. A monthly report of adverse reactions to drugs and therapeutic devices by the Adverse Reactions Branch, Food and Drug Administration, US Department of Health and Human Services, Washington DC.

Adverse Reactions Titles. Excerpta Medica (monthly bibliography).

Baselt RC: *Disposition of Toxic Drugs and Chemicals in Man.* Biomedical Publications, 1982.

Clayton GD, Clayton FE (editors): *Patty's Industrial Hygiene and Toxicology,* 3rd ed. 4 vols. Wiley, 1981, 1982.

Clin-Alert. A weekly to fortnightly serial publication of all adverse drug reactions reported in the international medical literature. Science Editors, Inc., Louisville, Kentucky.

Dangerous Properties of Industrial Materials Report. Van Nostrand Reinhold. Bimonthly serial.

Doull J, Klaassen C, Amdur M (editors): *Casarett and Doull's Toxicology: The Basic Science of Poisons,* 2nd ed. Macmillan, 1980.

Dreisbach RH: *Handbook of Poisoning: Prevention, Diagnosis, & Treatment,* 11th ed. Lange, 1983.

Dukes MNG (editor): *Meyler's Side Effects of Drugs,* 9th ed. Excerpta Medica, 1980.

FDA Clinical Experience Abstracts. Food and Drug Administration (monthly). US Department of Health and Human Services, Washington DC.

FDA Drug Bulletin. Food and Drug Administration (monthly). US Department of Health and Human Services, Washington DC.

Gee JBL, Morgan WKC, Brooks SM: *Occupational Lung Disease.* Raven Press, 1984.

Gilman AG, Goodman LS, Gilman A (editors): *Goodman and Gilman's The Pharmacological Basis of Therapeutics,* 6th ed. Macmillan, 1980.

Haddad LM, Winchester JF (editors): *Clinical Management of Poisoning and Drug Overdose.* Saunders, 1983.

Hayes AW: *Principles and Methods of Toxicology.* Raven Press, 1984.

Katzung BG (editor): *Basic & Clinical Pharmacology,* 2nd ed. Lange, 1984.

Key MM et al (editors): *Occupational Diseases: A Guide to Their Recognition.* NIOSH Publication No. 77–181. US Department of Health, Education, and Welfare, 1977.

Mills J, Ho MT, Trunkey DD (editors): *Current Emergency Diagnosis & Treatment.* Lange, 1983.

National Institute of Occupational Safety and Health: *Registry of Toxic Effects of Chemical Substances.* US Government Printing Office. (Annual publication.)

Polson CJ, Green MA, Lee MR: *Clinical Toxicology.* Lippincott, 1983.

Rom WN: *Environmental and Occupational Medicine.* Little, Brown, 1983.

Sax NI: *Dangerous Properties of Industrial Materials,* 5th ed. Van Nostrand Reinhold, 1979.

Sittig M: *Handbook of Toxic and Hazardous Chemicals.* Noyes, 1981.

Skoutakis VA: *Clinical Toxicology of Drugs.* Lea & Febiger, 1982.

32 | Medical Genetics

Margaret S. Kosek, MD

The rapid advance of the science of genetics in recent years has so many applications to clinical medicine that a knowledge of basic genetic principles is now a necessity for diagnostic purposes. Many cases of mental retardation, infertility, dwarfism, habitual abortion, and multiple congenital anomalies are associated with specific chromosomal defects. Cells of certain tumors have an abnormal chromosomal composition, in some instances a specific one. Many of the metabolic disorders are hereditary, and even in the case of some drug reactions the problem lies not only with the drug but also with the patient who has inherited an enzymatic defect that prevents normal detoxification. Future genetic investigation promises to increase our understanding of the causes and the mechanisms of individual responses to disease.

GENERAL CONSIDERATIONS

Inherited characteristics are carried from generation to generation by the **chromosome**, a complex nucleic acid structure in the nucleus of the cell. Humans normally have 46 chromosomes, which are arranged in 23 pairs. One of these pairs determines the sex of the individual; these are the **sex chromosomes,** which are designated as XX (female) and XY (male). The remaining 22 pairs are called **autosomes** (not sex determiners). Pairs of autosomes are **homologous,** ie, each member of a pair has the same configuration and genetic material as the other member of the pair. The sex chromosomes, on the other hand, are **heterologous,** ie, the X chromosome differs in both size and total function from the Y chromosome.

The X chromosome is roughly 5 times the size of the Y chromosome. Both the X and Y chromosomes have a genetic as well as sex-determining aspect, but the genetic information is more extensive on the X chromosome. The very small amount of genetic information on the Y chromosome has only recently been discovered.

GENES

Chromosomes are composed of thousands of **genes,** which are the basic units of heredity. The gene is the information area for the transmission of an inherited trait. The genes are arranged in a linear fashion on the chromosomes. The exact location of a gene on a chromosome is its **locus.** Each chromosome has thousands of loci arranged in a definite manner, and the number and arrangement of genes on homologous chromosomes are identical. Genes that occupy homologous loci are **alleles,** or partner genes. Each individual, therefore, has 2 of each kind of gene, one on each chromosome of a pair of chromosomes.

Although genes usually remain stable from generation to generation, it is possible for them to undergo a change, or **mutation,** and thereby to transmit a new or altered trait. This change will then be transmitted to future generations. Mutation may occur spontaneously or may be induced by such environmental factors as radiation, medication, or viral infections. Both advanced maternal and paternal age favor mutation. In women, trisomy 21 is the classic example. In men over 30, fresh gene mutation accounts for sporadic cases of achondroplasia, hemophilia A, and Marfan's syndrome.

The human genome is estimated to contain 50–100 thousand genes. Approximately 3400 genes are known. Combined information from family linkage studies, somatic cell hybridization, and gene dosage studies now permits human gene mapping, with 400 genes assigned to specific parts of specific chromosomes. Mapping has been of use in disease diagnosis, identification of heterozygotes, and prenatal diagnosis. Linkage studies can already reveal in utero mendelian disorders that are not biochemically identifiable. Another application is understanding gene interaction and regulation within the cell, for in human development it is important to understand the control mechanism that turns genes on and off.

Comings DE (editor): Human gene map. *Am J Hum Genet* 1983;**35**:134.

THE CHEMICAL BASIS OF HEREDITY (THE GENETIC CODE)

Chromosomes are composed of many deoxyribonucleic acid (DNA) molecules, each of which is a gene. DNA has 2 functions. First, it is able to synthesize, or **replicate,** itself, thereby assuring the integrity of hereditary transmission to future generations. Second, the sequential order of the bases (cytosine, guanine, adenine, thymine) of DNA acts as the **genetic code** that determines the development and metabolism of cells. DNA accomplishes this by directing the synthesis of its alter ego, messenger RNA (mRNA), which carries the genetic message out of the nucleus to the cytoplasm where it becomes associated with the ribosomes that are the site of protein synthesis. Here the messenger RNA forms the template for sequencing particular amino acids. With the help of another RNA, transfer RNA (tRNA), the amino acids are incorporated into a polypeptide chain and then synthesized into specific proteins and enzymes. (See Fig 32–1.)

MODES OF INHERITANCE

1. MENDELIAN INHERITANCE

The essential definitions of modes of inheritance can be illustrated by studying the inheritance of a **single** characteristic carried by only **one** gene and not influenced by environmental factors.

Syndactyly (webbed fingers or toes) is a clinical example of this. Fig 32–2 illustrates a family tree with the abnormality. The gene for syndactyly is represented as **D** and the gene for normal interdigital spaces as **d.**

Each parent is represented by 2 genes, each of

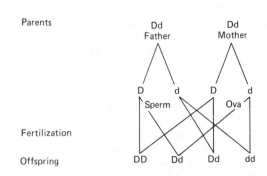

Figure 32–2. Mode of inheritance of syndactyly.

which they received from their mother and father, respectively. Their genetic constitution has arbitrarily been designated Dd. The male parent (Dd) will be able to produce sperms that are either D or d. The female parent will be able to produce ova that are either D or d. The possible offspring are DD, Dd, or dd.

If we examine the parents and offspring for the presence of syndactyly, we find it in both parents (Dd and Dd) and 3 (DD, Dd, Dd) of the 4 offspring. Since these people have the same physical characteristic, ie, syndactyly, they are said to have the same **phenotype.** Their genetic composition, or **genotype,** is different, for it may be either Dd or DD. The genotype, therefore, may be the same as the phenotype, but it does not have to be. Since syndactyly is present if D is one gene of a pair of genes (Dd) as well as both genes (DD), it is a **dominant** trait. Normal digital spaces (d) are present only if d is on both genes (dd) and is a **recessive** trait. If an individual's genetic constitution for syndactyly contains similar genes (DD, dd), the person is a **homozygote;** if it contains dissimilar genes (Dd), the person is a **heterozygote.**

Besides dominant and recessive inheritance, an intermediate, or **codominant, inheritance** may also occur. With codominance, the 2 characteristics are expressed in the heterozygote. Hemoglobin S disease is an example of this. The S homozygote (SS) has sickle cell anemia; the S heterozygote (AS) has sickle cell trait, with characteristics of hemoglobin A and hemoglobin S, and the person without S is normal.

Inheritance is either **autosomal** or **X-linked (sex-linked)** depending on the chromosomal location of the gene. In investigating family trees for genetic disease, certain inheritance patterns with distinct features become evident. **Autosomal dominant inheritance** (Fig 32–2) has 3 criteria: (1) every affected person has an affected parent; (2) every affected person who marries a normal person has a 1:2 chance of having each offspring affected; and (3) every normal child of an affected person will have normal offspring. With **autosomal recessive inheritance,** the following characteristics are present: The vast majority of affected persons have parents who are normal in all outward appearances. In affected families, each child has a 1:4 chance of having a genetic defect. When an affected person and a normal person marry, their off-

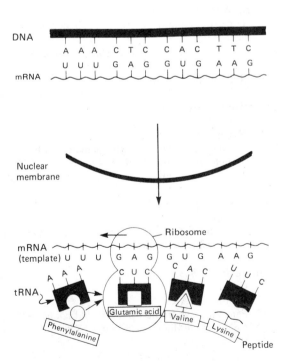

Figure 32–1. Diagrammatic representation of the way in which genetic information is translated into protein synthesis. (Reproduced, with permission, from Emery AEH: *Elements of Medical Genetics,* 6th ed. Churchill Livingstone, 1983.)

spring will be normal in most cases. If their offspring is affected, the "normal" parent is a heterozygote. When 2 affected persons marry, all their children will be affected. Lastly, the rarer the defect, the more likely it is that there is consanguinity in the family tree.

With **X-linked recessive inheritance,** there are 2 main characteristics: the defect is carried by women and exhibited by men, and affected men can pass the disease only through their daughters. Hemophilia A is an important clinical example of this (Fig 32–3). The female with her two X chromosomes must have the gene for hemophilia present in each X chromosome to have this recessive disease. Since the frequency of this gene in the population is low, the chances of 2 affected X chromosomes occurring together, although possible, is highly unlikely. Therefore, hemophilia is very rare in females. Males, with their XY chromosome composition, need the hemophilia gene present only on one chromosome (the X) to have it expressed clinically, for there is no homologous locus on the Y chromosome to neutralize the effect of the hemophiliac gene. Since the Y chromosome has to come from the father, the affected X chromosome is from the mother, thereby giving the "mother-to-son" inheritance pattern. In the case of **X-linked dominant inheritance,** no fully dominant X-linked gene has been discovered in humans.

Genes do not always have an "all or none" action. A certain number of offspring may fail to show expression of a gene even though the gene may be a dominant or homozygous recessive. **Penetrance** is the statistical concept that refers to the frequency with which a gene or genotype is morphologically manifest in the offspring. A comparable term, **expressivity,** refers to the degree of phenotypic expression of a trait (ie, forme fruste versus full expression). These variables make genetic analysis far more difficult.

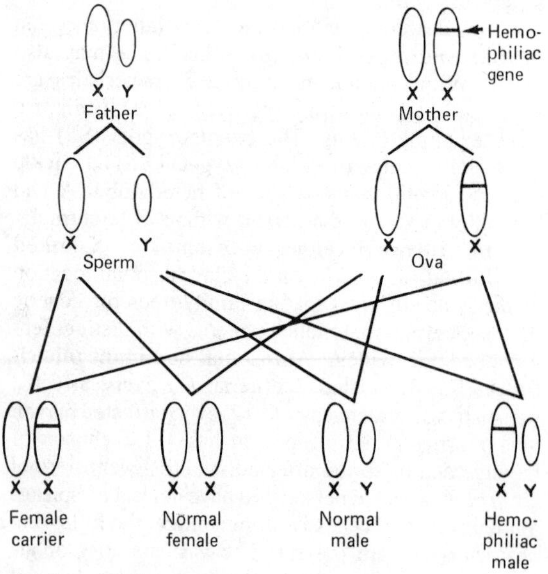

The genetic disorders carried by a single gene have been most completely studied. They frequently have a characteristic somatic or biochemical defect that can be readily traced in many generations. Of the 3 distinct patterns of inheritance, there are 800 known dominant conditions, 550 known recessive conditions, and 100 known sex-linked conditions. On the whole, these genetic disorders are rare. Perhaps 1% of all liveborn children will be affected with an autosomal disorder at some time in their life. It is much more difficult to determine the mode of inheritance of the common diseases of possible genetic background (eg, arteriosclerosis), because the disease may be the result not only of genetic constitution but also of environmental factors (eg, diet).

Some Diseases With Known Modes of Inheritance

AD = Autosomal dominant
AR = Autosomal recessive
XD = X-linked (sex-linked) dominant
XR = X-linked (sex-linked) recessive

Central Nervous System
A. Diffuse cerebral sclerosis (Pelizaeus-Merzbacher type): XD?, XR?
B. Diffuse cerebral sclerosis (Sholz type): XD?, XR?
C. Retinoblastoma: AD

Digestive System
A. Cystic fibrosis of the pancreas: AR
B. Hyperbilirubinemia:
1. Congenital nonhemolytic jaundice with kernicterus (Crigler-Najjar): AR
2. Familial nonhemolytic jaundice (Gilbert's disease): AD
3. Chronic idiopathic jaundice (Dubin-Johnson): Probably AD
4. Chronic familial nonhemolytic jaundice (Rotor's syndrome): AD

Genitourinary System
A. Cystinosis: AR
B. Cystinuria: AR
C. Fanconi's syndrome (infantile and adult): AR
D. Nephrogenic diabetes insipidus: XR
E. Renal glycosuria: AD
F. Vitamin D-resistant rickets: XD

Skin
A. Albinism: AR
B. Anhidrotic ectodermal dysplasia: AR?
C. Xeroderma pigmentosum: AR

Figure 32–3. The inheritance of hemophilia from a female carrier, illustrating "mother-to-son" inheritance of X-linked recessive disease.

Hematologic System

A. Cell Disorders:
  1. Congenital nonspherocytic hemolytic anemia (pyruvate kinase deficiency): AR
  2. Sickle cell disease (homozygous hemoglobin S): AD
  3. Sickle cell trait (heterozygous hemoglobin S): AD
  4. Spherocytosis: AD
  5. Thalassemia major (homozygous): AD
  6. Thalassemia minor (heterozygous): AD

B. Plasma Disorders:
  1. Congenital agammaglobulinemia: XR
  2. Congenital afibrinogenemia: AR
  3. Hemophilia A (factor VIII deficiency): XR
  4. Hemophilia B (factor IX deficiency): XR
  5. Hemophilia C (factor XI deficiency): AD
  6. Deficiency of factor XII: AR
  7. Deficiency of factor V: AR
  8. Deficiency of factor VII: AR
  9. Deficiency of factor X: AR
  10. Von Willebrand's disease (deficiencies of factor VIII procoagulant [VIII:C], factor VIII-related antigen [VIIIR:Ag], and factor VIII-related ristocetin cofactor [VIIIR:WF or VIIIR:Rcf]): AD

Musculoskeletal System

A. Severe generalized familial muscular dystrophy (Duchenne's pseudohypertrophic muscular dystrophy): XR
B. Muscular dystrophy (facioscapulohumeral syndrome of Landouzy-Déjérine): AD
C. Progressive dystrophia ophthalmoplegica: AD
D. Myotonia atrophica: AD
E. Progressive muscular dystrophy (tardive type of Becker): XR
F. Charcot-Marie-Tooth peroneal muscular atrophy: AD, AR
G. Pseudohypoparathyroidism: XR
H. Periodic paralysis:
  1. Hyperkalemic: AD
  2. Hypokalemic: AD
  3. Normokalemic: AD

Endocrine System

A. Pituitary:
  1. Pituitary diabetes insipidus: AD
B. Thyroid:
  1. Familial cretinism with goiter–
    a. Iodide trapping defect: AR
    b. Iodide organification defect: AR?, AD?
    c. Iodotyrosyl coupling defect: AR?
    d. Deiodinase defect: AR
    e. Abnormal serum iodoprotein: AR
C. Adrenal:
  1. Congenital virilizing adrenal hyperplasia: AR

Metabolic Disorders

A. Carbohydrate:
  1. Diabetes mellitus: AR
  2. Galactosemia: AR
  3. Glycogen storage disease (types I, II, III, IV, V, VI) (Von Gierke's disease): AR
  4. Gargoylism (lipochondrodystrophy) (Hurler's disease): AR, XR
  5. Hyperoxaluria: AR
  6. Hereditary lactose intolerance: AR
  7. Mucopolysaccharidoses–
    a. Type I–Hurler's disease: AR
    b. Type II–Hunter's disease: XR
    c. Type III–Sanfilippo syndrome (heparitinuria): AR
    d. Type IV–Morquio's disease: AR
    e. Type V–Scheie's syndrome: AR
    f. Type VI–Maroteaux-Lamy syndrome: AR

B. Fat:
  1. The primary hyperlipidemias–
    a. Type I–Familial hyperchylomicronemia (lipoprotein lipase deficiency): AR
    b. Type II–Familial hyperbetalipoproteinemia (essential familial hypercholesterolemia): AD
    c. Type III–Hyperlipidemia (broad beta disease): AD
    d. Familial combined hyperlipidemia (multiple lipoprotein type): AD
    e. Familial hypertriglyceridemia: AD
  2. Familial high-density lipoprotein disease (Tangier disease): AR
  3. Gaucher's disease (cerebroside lipidosis): AR
  4. Niemann-Pick disease (sphingomyelin lipidosis): AR
  5. Tay-Sachs disease (infantile amaurotic idiocy): AR

C. Protein:
  1. Amino acids–
    a. Homocystinuria: AR
    b. Phenylketonuria: AR
  2. Porphyrias–
    a. Congenital erythropoietic porphyria: AR
    b. Erythropoietic porphyria: AR
    c. Acute intermittent porphyria: AD
    d. Porphyria cutanea tarda hereditaria: AD
  3. Other–
    a. Deficiency of pseudocholinesterase: AR
    b. Deficiency of glucose-6-phosphate dehydrogenase: XD
    c. Alkaptonuria: AR
    d. Hyperuricemia: AD
    e. Hereditary orotic aciduria: AR

D. Minerals:
  1. Hepatolenticular degeneration (Wilson's disease): AR
  2. Hemochromatosis: AD, AR

McKusick VA: *Mendelian Inheritance in Man: Catalogs of Autosomal Dominant, Autosomal Recessive, and X-linked Phenotypes*, 6th ed. Johns Hopkins Univ Press, 1983.

2. POLYGENIC OR MULTIFACTORIAL INHERITANCE

A study of *single* common malformations reveals familial clustering, varying frequencies in different racial or ethnic groups, and a higher frequency in monozygotic than in dizygotic twins. The inheritance pattern does not follow simple mendelian laws, and risks are calculated on an empirical basis from family studies carried out in particular populations. Studies suggest a significant genetic component in addition to unspecified environmental conditions.

Some examples are gout, atherosclerosis, and congenital dislocation of the hip.

CYTOGENETICS

Cytogenetics is the study of the chromosomal structure of cells. Because of the constancy of chromosomal number and morphology, classification of chromosomes is possible. The basic characteristics of chromosomes are (1) total length, (2) position of the centromere, (3) the length of the arms, (4) the presence or absence of satellites, and (5) the banding pattern (Fig 32–14).

The 2 halves of the chromosome are called **chromatids.** A palely staining cross-over point or primary constriction called the **centromere** (centrosome) divides the chromosome into 2 arm lengths. Chromosomes are described according to the position of the centromere. If the centromere is at the middle of the chromosome, it is a **metacentric** chromosome; if near the middle of the chromosome, it is **submetacentric;** and if near the end of the chromosome, it is **acrocentric.** On some chromosomes there is a secondary constriction. The chromosomal material distal to this constriction is called a **satellite.**

In the Denver classification, chromosomes are arranged in 7 groups according to descending total length: group A (chromosomes 1–3); group B (chromosomes 4, 5); group C (chromosomes 6–12); group D (chromosomes 13–15); group E (chromosomes 16–18); group F (chromosomes 19, 20); and group G (chromosomes 21, 22). The X chromosome is in group C and the Y chromosome is in group G. Staining techniques—quinacrine (Q), Giemsa (G), terminal (T), constitutive heterochromatin (C), and reverse (R)—disclose banded regions on each chromosome (Fig 32–14) that are unique and allow absolute identification of the chromosome. These banded patterns vary with the stain and produce complementary rather than redundant information.

The chromosomal analysis is recorded by a uniform system of notation. First, there is the total chromosome count, followed by the sex chromosomes, and then any abnormalities thereafter. The autosomes are all designated by their numbers (1–22), and if the autosomes cannot be identified, the involved chromosome group is identified by its letter (A–G). A plus (+) or minus (−) sign indicates, respectively, a gain or loss of chromosomal material. The letter p represents the short arm of the chromosome, and the letter q represents the long arm. Other common symbols are i for isochromosome; r for ring chromosome; s for satellite; ins for insertion; inv for inversion; mar for marker; del for deletion; [:] for chromosomal break; [::] for chromosomal break and join; and end for endoreduplication. Translocations of material from one chromosome to another are identified by t followed by the numbers of the involved chromosomes in parentheses; the chromosome bands in which the breaks occur are identified in a second set of parentheses. *Examples:* The normal male is 46,XY; a girl with Down's syndrome is 47,XX,21$^+$; a boy with cri du chat syndrome is 46,XY,5p$^-$. A patient with chronic myelogenous leukemia is t(9;22)(q34;q11).

A modification of the Paris Conference nomenclature allows classification of the 900–1000 bands now identified by prometaphase studies. The short arm (p) and the long arm (q) of each chromosome is divided into regions, bands, and subbands each of which is numbered from the centromere outward. A decimal point is placed between the band and subband designations. For example, 5p31.2 is chromosome 5, short arm, region 3, band 1, subband 2.

An international system for human cytogenetic nomenclature: High-resolution banding (1981) ISCN (1981). *Cytogenet Cell Genet* 1981;**31:**1. [Entire issue.]

Methods of Cellular Division

Cells divide in one of 2 ways: by **mitosis** (Fig 32–4) or by **meiosis** (Fig 32–7). In mitosis, a mother cell divides longitudinally to produce 2 daughter cells of exactly the same chromosomal number and composition as the mother cell. This type of cellular division is purely multiplicative (1 cell → 2 cells → 4 cells → 8 cells, etc). Meiosis occurs in the ovary or testis and involves 2 separate steps. The first step is **reduction-division,** in which the germ cell with a **diploid (2n)** number of chromosomes (46) produces 2 cells with a **haploid (n)** number of chromosomes (23). During this step, chromosomal material is exchanged between like chromosomes, thereby accounting for the random distribution of maternal and paternal genes. Crossovers do not normally occur between the X and Y chromosome or between the Y chromosome and the autosomes. The second step is **equational division,** in which 4 daughter cells with a haploid number of chromosomes are formed by longitudinal division of the chromosomes produced in the first step of meiotic division. In the male, the 4 haploid cells are sperms. In the female, one of the 4 haploid cells is large and matures to eventually form an ovum. The other 3 haploid cells are small cells called **polar bodies,** and they undergo spontaneous degeneration.

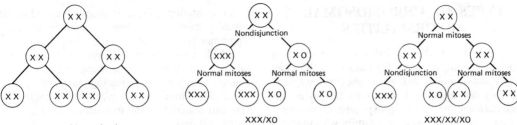

Figure 32–4. Normal mitoses (female).

Figure 32–5. Formation of mosaic with 2 stem cells.

Figure 32–6. Formation of mosaic with 3 stem cells.

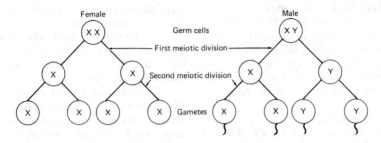

Figure 32–7. Normal meiosis.

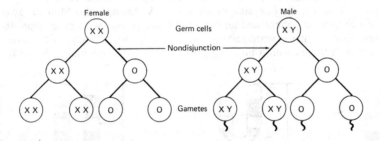

Figure 32–8. Formation of abnormal gametes by nondisjunction in first meiotic division.

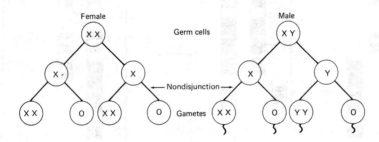

Figure 32–9. Formation of abnormal gametes by nondisjunction in second meiotic division.

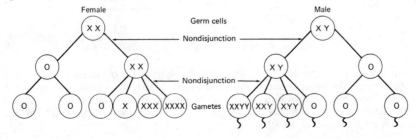

Figure 32–10. Formation of abnormal gametes by nondisjunction in first and second meiotic division.

TYPES OF CHROMOSOMAL ABNORMALITIES

Chromosomal abnormalities can be those of number, structure, or a combination of both. They affect the autosomes as well as the sex chromosomes. Often they are associated with such factors as advanced parental age, radiation exposure, certain viral infections, and membership in a family with multiple cytogenetic defects. Once produced, these abnormalities are capable of perpetuating themselves.

These major structural changes may occur in a **balanced** or an **unbalanced** form. In the latter, there is a gain or loss of genetic material. In the former, there is no change in the amount of genetic material but only a rearrangement of it. It is possible, though not proved, that at the sites of breaks and new attachments of chromosome fragments there has been permanent structural or functional damage to a single gene.

Abnormalities of Morphology

A. Nondisjunction: (See Figs 32–4 to 32–10.) Nondisjunction is failure of a chromatid pair to separate in a dividing cell. If it occurs in either the first or second divisions of meiosis, this results in gametes with abnormal chromosomal patterns. If it occurs in mitosis, **mosaic** patterns occur, ie, one area of an organism will have one genetic pattern and another area of the same organism another genetic pattern.

In medical practice, patients with a mosaic ge-netic constitution present an incomplete and variable clinical picture with features of each of the genetic syndromes represented in the mosaic.

B. Translocation: (See Fig 32–11.) In simple translocation, there is an exchange of chromosomal material between 2 nonhomologous chromosomes.

C. Deletion: In deletion, there is a loss of chromosomal material owing to breakage of a chromatid during cell division.

D. Duplication: If breakage occurs in a chromatid during cell division, the broken portion may realign itself so that many loci are duplicated on one chromosome and are entirely absent from the other member of the pair of chromosomes.

E. Occurrence of Isochromosomes: An isochromosome is a chromosome in which the arms on either side of the centromere have the same genetic material in the same order.

F. Inversion: Inversion occurs if, after fracture of a chromatid, the fragment reattaches itself to the same chromosome in an upside down manner. The same genetic material is present but is distributed in a different order.

Abnormalities of Chromosomal Number (Aneuploidy) (See Table 32–1.)

A. Aneuploidy: More or fewer than 46 chromosomes. A cell with more than 46 chromosomes is hyperdiploid, and one with fewer than 46 chromosomes is hypodiploid. If there is a balanced gain or loss

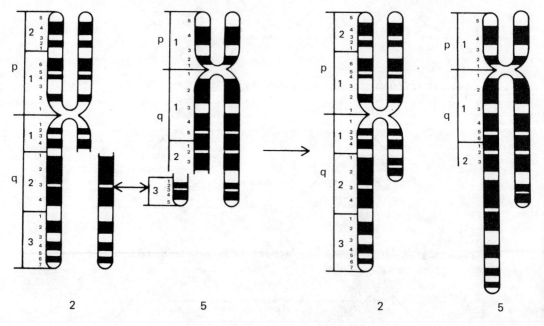

Figure 32–11. Reciprocal translocations. 46,XY,t(2;5)(q21;q31). Breakage and union have occurred at bands 2q21 and 5q31 in the long arms of chromosomes 2 and 5, respectively. The segments distal to these bands have been exchanged between the 3 chromosomes. Note that the derivative chromosome with the lowest number (ie, No. 2) is designated first. (Reproduced, with permission, from Stanbury JE, Wyngaarden JB, Fredrickson DS [editors]: *The Metabolic Basis of Inherited Disease,* 4th ed. McGraw-Hill, 1978.)

Table 32–1. Numerical abnormalities of sex chromosomes.*†

Pheno-type	Sex Chromatin	Sex Chromosome	Chromosome Number	Incidence In Newborn	Clinical Picture
Female	Positive	XX	46		Normal female.
Female	Few smaller than normal Barr bodies (7%)	Xx (partial deletion)	46	0.05–0.15/1000	Streak gonads. No secondary sex charac-teristics. Amenorrheic.
Female	Negative	XO	45	0.1–0.3/1000	Turner's syndrome.
Female	Positive for 2 Barr bodies	XXX	47	0.7/1000	Usually normal appearing female with mental retardation. Occasional menstrual disturbances and absence of secondary sex characteristics.
Female	Positive for 3 Barr bodies	XXXX	48	Rare	Normal female with mental retardation.
Female	Positive for 4 Barr bodies	XXXXX	49	Rare	Mental retardation with mongoloid fa-cies and simian palmar crease. Skeletal defects similar to those of 49,XXXXY.
Hermaph-rodite	Positive	XX	46	Rare	Variable phenotype. Both testicular and ovarian tissue in gonads.
Male	Negative	XY	46		Normal male.
Male	Positive for 1 Barr body	XXY	47	1/1000	Klinefelter's syndrome.
Male	Negative	XYY	47	1/1000	Undescended testes, ± mental retarda-tion, irregularity of teeth. Tall (>6 feet). Radioulnar synostosis.
Male	Negative	XYYY	48	Rare	Mild psychomotor retardation, inguinal hernia, undescended testes, pulmonary stenosis, simian lines, dental dysplasia.
Male	Positive for 1 Barr body	XXYY	48	1/25,000	Klinefelter's syndrome.
Male	Positive for 2 Barr bodies	XXXY	48	Rare	Klinefelter's syndrome with more men-tal retardation and testicular atrophy.
Male	Positive for 3 Barr bodies	XXXXY	49	Rare	Mental retardation, hypoplastic external genitals, and skeletal defects. Facies sug-gestive of Down's syndrome.

*Normal male and normal female included for comparison.

†Reference: Pitcher DC: Sex chromosome disorders. *CRC Crit Rev Clin Lab Sci* 1981;13:241.

of chromosomes or structural rearrangements, the cell is pseudodiploid.

B. Monosomy: (Chromosomal number is 45.) In monosomy, only one member of a pair of chromosomes is present. *Example:* Stillborns, monosomy 21–22.

C. Trisomy: (Chromosomal number is 47.) Trisomy is caused by nondisjunction of a chromosome pair during the first meiotic division, with the result that 3 chromosomes are present instead of the usual 2. *Example:* Trisomy 13; 18; 21.

D. Polysomy: (Chromosomal number is 48 or more.) Polysomy occurs when one chromosome is represented 4 or more times. *Example:* XXXXY.

E. Complex Aneuploidy: In complex aneu-ploidy, 2 or more chromosomes have an abnormal variation in number; the structure of these chromo-somes is normal. *Example:* Trisomy 21 and XXX in the same patient.

METHODS OF STUDY OF CHROMOSOMAL ABNORMALITIES

Several laboratory tests are available for the study of patients with known or suspected chromosomal aberrations: (1) the study of cells for the presence of

sex chromatin bodies in their nuclei; (2) chromosomal analysis; and (3) DNA analysis for gene-specific probes or linkage mapping. The first test is easily obtainable and relatively inexpensive and is used for screening. The chromosomal and DNA analyses are reliable but expensive tests performed by highly trained personnel, usually at medical centers.

Sex Chromatin Analysis (See Fig 32–12.)

A. The X Chromosome: The sex chromatin

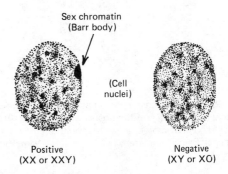

Figure 32–12. Normal chromatin pattern. (Redrawn and re-produced, with permission, from Eggen RR: Cytogenetics: Review of newest advances in a new field of clinical pathol-ogy. *Am J Clin Pathol* 1963;39:3.)

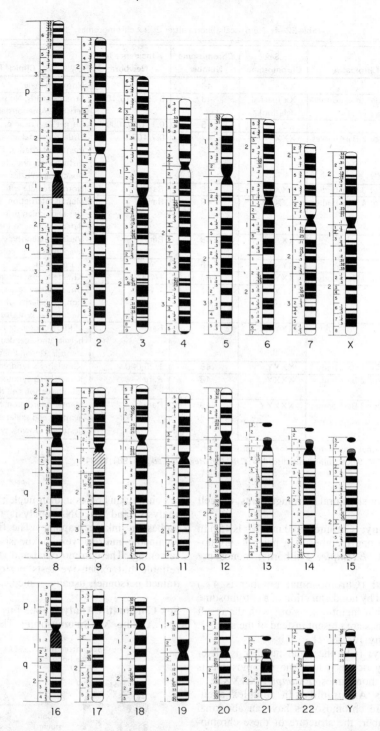

Figure 32–13. Schematic representation and nomenclature of chromosomes at 850-band stage. (Reproduced, with permission, from Yunis JJ: Chromosomes and cancer: New nomenclature and future directions. *Hum Pathol* 1981;**12**:494. Slightly modified, in order to conform with the new International System of Chromosome Nomenclature, from Yunis JJ, Ramsey N: Familial occurrence of the aniridia–Wilms' tumor syndrome with deletion 11p13 –14.1. *J Pediatr* 1980;**96**:1027.)

(Barr) body is a solid, well-defined planoconvex mass, approximately 1 μm in diameter, which is near or at the inner surface of the nuclear membrane. It is visible by light microscopy and, with proper staining, can be identified in all tissues of the body. The most frequent source of specimens for study is in the desquamated cells—buccal, vaginal, and amniotic. The sex chromatin body represents the heterochromatic X chromosome. The number of these chromatin bodies in a cell is one less than the number of X chromosomes in that cell. Females have an incidence of 40–60% and are "chromatin positive." Males do not possess the sex chromatin bodies and are therefore "chromatin negative." For an unknown reason, sex chromatin bodies are diminished in the first few days of life and during treatment with corticotropin, corticosteroids, testosterone, and progesterone. Diethylstilbestrol, on the other hand, causes a significant increase in sex chromatin bodies. The sex chromatin can be seen in the trophoblast at the 12th day, and in the embryo itself at the 16th day. Analysis of amniotic cells for sex chromatin can predict the sex of the unborn child.

B. The Y Chromosome: Quinacrine mustard (QM), a fluorescent material, binds itself to chromosomal DNA and gives each chromosome a characteristic pattern. Since the fluorescence of the distal portion of the Y chromosome is characteristically the brightest, it can be reliably and easily identified. In XYY individuals, 2 of these fluorescent bodies are seen. This technique is applicable to all cells of the body. Those cells most frequently used are peripheral leukocytes, sperm, and buccal mucosa.

Chromosomal Analysis

Chromosome analyses are done by growing cells from biopsy in tissue culture; chemically inhibiting their mitoses; and then sorting, counting, and staining the chromosomes. Specimens are most often taken from the peripheral blood, bone marrow, skin, and testes. A statistically significant number of cells must be counted. Stains that reveal the banding patterns of chromosomes provide so much more useful information than other stains that they should be used if available. The results of these analyses appear in the literature as the **karyotype,** which is a drawing or photograph of a systematized array of chromosomes of a single cell (Fig 32–13).

The present indications for these highly technical procedures are as follows: (1) Patients with malformations consistent with autosomal trisomy or deletion syndromes. (2) Parents of patients with a trisomy syndrome if the mother is younger than 30 years of age or if there are other similarly affected siblings. (3) Parents of all children with Down's syndrome who are found to be of the translocation or mosaic type. (4) Patients with an abnormality on sex chromatin analysis. (5) Children who are grossly retarded physically or mentally, especially if there are associated anomalies. (6) All cases of intersex. (7) All females with evidence of Turner's syndrome, whether they are chromatin positive or chromatin negative. (8) All males with Klinefelter's

syndrome, whether they are chromatin positive or chromatin negative. (9) Tall males (over 6 feet) with behavioral disorders. (10) Couples with multiple spontaneous abortions of unknown cause (see below). (11) Girls with primary amenorrhea and boys with delayed pubertal development. Up to 25% of patients with primary amenorrhea have a chromosomal abnormality. (12) Certain malignant and premalignant diseases (see pp 1040–1044). (13) Certain families and populations who have chromosomal variants (polymorphism) that are valuable for linkage and genealogic studies. (14) Persons exposed to large amounts of radiation or those whose parents may have been exposed to chemical mutagens. The number, type, and duration of chromosomal abnormalities correlate well with the amount of radiation. (15) Infertile couples.

DNA Analysis

The DNA of every somatic cell in the body is identical. The DNA can be extracted and chemically denatured, so that a single DNA strand can be obtained. Bacterial enzymes called **restriction endonucleases** have the ability to cleave the DNA strand. A few of the cleaved fragments have been identified, and some are known to be associated with disease.

A. Gene-Specific Probes: In a few diseases (eg, sickle cell disease), the primary genetic defect has been identified at the nucleotide level. Because it is known that cytosine pairs with guanine and thymine with adenine, a complementary sequence of the primary genetic defect can be made, labeled with a radioactive isotope, and used as a probe to investigate a patient's DNA for the primary genetic defect.

A Y-specific DNA probe is available for fetal sex determination.

B. DNA Linkage Analysis: In many genetic diseases, the molecular basis of the defect has not been identified. In some of these diseases, linkage mapping is possible (ie, DNA sequences are examined to detect possible links between a polymorphic genetic marker and a locus known to cause disease). Every individual has DNA polymorphism, ie, a condition in which one or 2 normal but different nucleotide sequences can exist at a specific site. These inherited variations act as markers. If these markers are detected near a locus known to cause a certain disease, then the potential for that disease is assumed to be present. The closer the marker to the locus known to cause disease, the more accurate the diagnosis (eg, Duchenne's muscular dystrophy is loosely linked to one marker; classic PKU is closely linked to another one).

PRENATAL DIAGNOSIS

Each year, great strides are made in prenatal diagnosis of genetic diseases. It is now possible to diagnose approximately 100 inborn errors of metabolism, more than 30 monogenic disorders, and an increasing number of structural defects.

Amniocentesis is by far the most frequently used procedure for prenatal diagnosis. During this procedure, which is performed during the 12th–16th weeks of pregnancy, 10–30 mL of amniotic fluid is withdrawn via the transabdominal approach. Sonography is done prior to amniocentesis to determine (1) if there is a missed abortion and therefore no need for the procedure or (2) if there is a multiple pregnancy, so that each amniotic sac can be sampled. Both cells and fluid are analyzed; in most diagnosable inherited metabolic disorders, specific enzyme defects are detected in the cultured cells. Autosomal and sex chromosomal disorders are diagnosed by cytogenetic analysis, either by direct analysis or by cell culture. High-resolution techniques for analysis of amniotic cell chromosomes are now available. Abnormal elevation of chemicals in amniotic fluid is sometimes a nonspecific indicator of an inherited disorder (eg, alpha-fetoprotein in open neural tube defects).

Recently, recombinant DNA technology has been used in analysis of amniotic cells. Gene-specific probes and DNA-linkage analysis now make it possible to diagnose several genetic diseases prenatally (see above). The current indications for amniocentesis are as follows:

(1) Advanced maternal age. *Example:* Down's syndrome. The risk of Down's syndrome increases from 1:2000 live births at maternal age 20, to 1:300 at age 35, to 1:100 at age 40, and to 1:40 at age 45.

(2) Carrier of X-linked disease. *Example:* Hemophilia A, Duchenne's muscular dystrophy. Male fetuses have a 50% chance of being affected and could be aborted if that is the parents' wish.

(3) Known or possible carrier of a biochemical disease. *Example:* Tay-Sachs disease. Enzymatic studies on cultured amniotic fluid cells identify over 80 inborn errors of metabolism. Before these complicated studies are undertaken, it should be established that both parents are heterozygotes.

(4) Positive family history of a chromosomal defect. This includes a documented chromosomal defect in a parent, a family history of a chromosomal defect, or a previous child or conceptus with a defined or undefined chromosomal defect. *Example:* a parent who is a translocation carrier of Down's syndrome, an abortus with a proved trisomy.

(5) Open neural tube defects. *Examples:* Anencephaly, meningomyelocele. Maternal serum alpha-fetoprotein levels and sonography can be used to diagnose most open neural tube defects. If these tests are not definitive, alpha-fetoprotein levels in amniotic fluid can be measured as a nonspecific predictor.

In several thousand reported cases, the morbidity rate associated with amniocentesis is approximately 1%. For the mother, the problem is infection and bleeding. Maternal blood group sensitization is avoided by giving RhoGAM to an Rh-negative mother whose mate is Rh-positive. For the fetus, the risk is abortion, puncture, and possibly induced malformation. Abortion is less likely as the physician becomes more experienced with the puncture technique.

Amniocentesis cannot be performed until the second trimester, and this means prolonged uncertainty and, in positive diagnoses, the physical and emotional trauma of a second-trimester abortion. Recently, **chorion biopsy** has been attempted during the 8th–12th weeks. A sample of chorionic villi is obtained by endoscopic needle aspiration under ultrasound guidance. These trophoblastic cells have the same genetic makeup as the fetus and can be analyzed in the same way as amniotic cells. In 85 pregnancies in which chorion biopsy was performed, there was a 6% fetal loss; however, the spontaneous abortion rate is 5% of all pregnancies, so some fetal deaths would have occurred anyway and were not due to the procedure.

Many mendelian disorders and most multifactorially inherited congenital disorders occur without demonstrated cytogenetic or biochemical abnormalities. **Ultrasonic scanning,** a safe procedure, can diagnose gross skeletal malformations as well as bony malformations known to be associated with specific diseases (*example:* Ellis-van Creveld syndrome). It can detect certain fluid-containing abnormalities such as polycystic kidneys and gastrointestinal obstruction, for there is a large contrast difference between the fluid and surrounding tissues. It is the solid mass lesions of the fetus that are clearly more difficult to diagnose. In **fetography** and **amniography,** contrast medium placed in the amniotic fluid permits diagnosis of soft tissue malformations as well as some gastrointestinal tract abnormalities. **Fetoscopy,** in which an endoscope is introduced into the uterus, can diagnose gross anomalies, sample fetal blood, and permit skin biopsies. Antenatal diagnosis is possible for hemophilia, hemoglobinopathies, hemolytic anemias, chronic granulomatous disease, the homozygous state of α_1-antitrypsin deficiency, epidermolysis bullosa, and ichthyosiform erythroderma. Since the procedure entails a 5% risk of inducing abortion, it is recommended only for entities of significant severity and risk.

Of parents with indications for antenatal genetic diagnosis, 95% will be reassured that their baby does not have a genetic problem. Few of the conditions diagnosed are treatable; with many, however, appropriate management can be started on the first day of life.

Epstein CJ et al: Recent developments in prenatal diagnosis of genetic diseases and birth defects. *Annu Rev Genet* 1983;**17**:49.

Ferguson-Smith MA (editor): Early prenatal diagnosis. *Br Med Bull* 1983;**39**:301. [Entire issue.]

Finley SC, Finley WH, Flowers CE Jr (editors): Birth defects: Clinical and ethical considerations. *Birth Defects: Original Article Series* 1983;**19**. [Entire issue.]

CHROMOSOMAL DISORDERS

Frequency

Chromosomal anomalies occur surprisingly often. In live newborns, the incidence of gross chromosomal defects is 0.5%; in live prematures, 2.5%; in stillbirths, 6.9%; and in spontaneous abortions, about 30%. The most frequent chromosomal defects are trisomy 18, triploidy, and 45,XO. With live births, trisomy of the sex chromosomes is most frequent. The XXX genotype is 1:1000 female births and the XXY is 2:1000 male births. Down's syndrome (trisomy 21) is the most frequent autosomal anomaly. Its incidence is 1:2000 if the mother is age 25 and 1:100 if the mother is age 40 or over. Advanced paternal age accounts for one-fourth of cases. Trisomy 13 and 18 rates are 0.3:1000 and 0.2:1000 live births, respectively.

Chromosomal studies done on abortuses, stillbirths, and tissues of infants who die in the neonatal period can provide valuable information for explaining habitual abortions, monitoring a subsequent pregnancy, and furnishing genetic counseling.

DISORDERS DUE TO ABNORMALITIES OF THE X & Y CHROMOSOMES

Most disorders of the sex chromosomes (Table 32–1) are compatible with life and do not display marked phenotypic abnormalities. They are primarily due to an excess number of sex chromosomes, but there are 2 important exceptions: Turner's syndrome (XO) and fragile X syndrome, a form of X-linked mental retardation. The latter was discovered in 1980 and, next to Down's syndrome, is the most common cause of mental retardation that can be specifically diagnosed. Its frequency is approximately one half that of Down's syndrome. Before adolescence, the patient has nonspecific mental retardation, but after puberty, a significant portion of affected males have macroorchidism, with testicular volumes 3–4 times normal size. A prominent jaw, large ears, and normal to enlarged head circumference may also be present. Female carriers for fragile X syndrome may be normal, but a significant proportion have mental retardation of a less severe nature. Cytogenetically, the fragile site is at Xq27. Prenatal diagnosis is possible by chromosomal analysis of amniotic fluid cells.

Patients with sex chromosome abnormalities have diverse clinical features (see p 1035). The more frequent syndromes—XXY (Klinefelter's), XYY, and XO (Turner's)—do not have serious malformations associated with them. Longitudinal studies of patients with Klinefelter's syndrome reveal minor skeletal differences, a reduction in testicular volume, and, in one-third of cases, gynecomastia. Otherwise, there is a definite but small lowering of IQ (from the mean of 104 to 96), a slight but definite increase in abnormalities measured by behavioral and personality tests, and a definite increase in reading and more general learning disabilities. Unselected data on XYY males and XO females reveal a similar picture. In sex chromosomal syndromes prior to birth, additional or deficient genetic material is associated with growth retardation except where an extra Y chromosome is present. After birth, sex chromosomes behave differently. When there is additional X or (especially) Y material, individuals tend to be tall. In patients with only one X chromosome (Turner's syndrome), the average height is less than 1.5 m (5 ft); patients with multiple Y syndromes have an average height of over 1.8 m (6 ft). As the number of X and Y chromosomes increases, the disability increases. These include (singly or in combination) such problems as mental retardation, sterility, abnormal sex characteristics, and skeletal abnormalities.

At present, there are far more patients with multiple X syndromes than with multiple Y syndromes. This may only reflect the fact that screening procedures for the X chromosomes have been available for over 20 years, whereas methods of screening for the Y chromosome have been available for only a few years.

The **Lyon hypothesis** states that for patients with multiple X chromosome constitutions (including the normal female), only one X chromosome is genetically active and capable of transmitting its information; the others became genetically inactive early in embryonic formation by an unknown mechanism. The same is suspected to be true for the multiple Y chromosome states, but there is no evidence to support this as yet.

Hogge WA et al: Prenatal diagnosis of the fragile (X) syndrome. *Obst Gynecol* 1984;**63**:195.

Long-term outlook for children with sex chromosome abnormalities. (Editorial.) *Lancet* 1982;**2**:27.

AUTOSOMAL DISORDERS

Although autosomes far outnumber sex chromosomes, very few disorders were attributed to autosomal aberrations until staining techniques revealed a characteristic pattern for each autosome. Initially, patients with clinically identifiable syndromes—trisomy 13, 18, and 21—demonstrated severe growth defects and mental retardation in addition to multiple congenital defects and died early. The mean survival time for trisomy 13 is 130 days and for trisomy 21, 30 years. As more cases were found, it was apparent that the physical appearance became less characteristic with survival beyond the first few months. Now, with the use of banding techniques, hundreds of case reports are available describing partial deletions and partial trisomies for almost every chromosome. Identifiable cases include those with mental retardation and minor congenital anomalies as well as those with normal intelligence and minor defects, previously described as variations of normal. Patients now range in age from newborns to 50 years.

Correlation of autosomal defects and clinical findings is now possible and is facilitated by several International Registries of Chromosomal Variations in Man.

In addition, identification of carriers of balanced translocations allows genetic counseling and prenatal diagnosis to prevent recurrences.

The most prevalent autosomal disorder is Down's syndrome, or mongolism. Ninety-five percent of cases are due to trisomy 21, and the remaining 5% are due to translocations of D/21, 21/21, and 22/21 types. The trisomy 21 cases have an increasing frequency with advancing parental ages. Advanced maternal age accounts for 75% of cases and advanced paternal age for the remainder. The translocation cases account for the carrier state of Down's syndrome, for familial Down's syndrome, and for the occurrence of Down's syndrome in younger mothers. Physical examination cannot distinguish between trisomy and translocation Down's syndrome.

Recently, family studies showed that depressive disorders segregate with HLA, suggesting that the HLA locus is on the long arm of chromosome 6. This is one of the few identified relationships between chromosomal defects and psychiatric disorders.

Borgaonkar DS: *Chromosomal Variation in Man: A Catalogue of Chromosomal Variants and Anomalies,* 3rd ed. Liss, 1981.
Weitkamp LR et al: Depressive disorders and HLA: A gene on chromosome 6 that can affect behavior. *N Engl J Med* 1981; **305**:301.

CANCER

Studies of cancer patients indicate that genetic factors play a role in only a small percentage of cases. With carcinoma of the stomach, breast, colon, prostate, and endometrium, a hereditary factor with a site-specific basis is operating, for relatives of patients with these types of cancer have a 3-fold higher risk of having the same type of cancer. Only rarely do the mendelian laws of inheritance appear. The classic examples are polyposis of the colon, Recklinghausen's neurofibromatosis, hereditary adenomatosis, basal cell nevus syndrome, and some cases of retinoblastoma. In general, the majority of cases of cancer are of unknown cause.

Chromosomes & Cancer

In the past 2 decades, there has been a search for the relationships between chromosomal abnormalities and cancer. The chromosomal abnormalities of cancer are nonrandom. In hematologic malignant disease, over 90% of all types of acute leukemia exhibit some form of chromosomal defect. The chromosomal abnormalities involve specific segments of only a limited number of chromosomes, with preferential involvement of 5, 7, 8, 15, 17, and 21. Deletions are prevalent in chromosomes 5 and 7 following exposure to either industrial or cytotoxic chemicals and are suggestive of an epidemiologic role in leukemias associated with such exposures. In solid tumors, the chromosomal studies are not so complete, primarily for technical reasons. Tissue culture is often not successful or may not yield metaphases suitable for reliable analysis.

In 1982, **oncogenes,** genes with tumorigenic activity, were discovered in the Rous sarcoma virus and soon in many other cancer-causing viruses. These same oncogenes are present in the cells of humans and all animal species. Because oncogenes have been preserved throughout evolution, it is felt they play an essential role in an important process such as normal cell division or differentiation. When these genes fulfill their normal function, they are called **proto-oncogenes.** It is postulated that proto-oncogenes are transformed into oncogenes by viral action, aging, mutation due to a chemical agent or ionizing radiation, or chromosomal rearrangement. Neoplasia could then result from several mechanisms: (1) when suppression of a given gene by a contiguous gene is removed; (2) when a translocation could place the oncogene next to a DNA-activating sequence; and (3) when there is gene amplification (ie, many extra copies of a gene are present in a given chromosome). Under these circumstances, the gene products could be expressed in altered form, in abnormal amounts, or at abnormal times.

A few oncogene products have been isolated. Rous sarcoma virus oncogenes produce protein kinase, an enzyme that plays an important role in cell growth and proliferation, and simian virus oncogenes produce a platelet-derived growth factor. These discoveries suggest that rational mechanisms exist by which genes produce cancer. Whatever the mechanism, the process is complex, involving the interaction of many genes.

Fragile sites may also be important in the development of cancer. Fragile sites are chromosome gaps or breaks that occur when cultured cells are grown in a media deficient in thymidine or folic acid. It appears that the fragile site has a unique DNA structure, and when its precursor substances are missing, the cell is prone to rearrangement. So far, 15 heritable fragile sites have been identified, 8 of which are located near chromosomal rearrangements known to be associated with leukemia and lymphoma. These fragile sites occur at a frequency of 0.2% and are inherited as simple mendelian codominant traits.

A. Solid Tumors: Cytogenetic information in solid tumors is limited because of technical difficulties. Only 10–15% of human solid tumors have suitable chromosomal preparations with direct technique or short-term culture. From these studies, certain generalities emerge.

1. Abnormalities in chromosomal number and structure–Banding techniques reveal that most primary tumors have numerical rather than structural abnormalities. Their modal number is pseudodiploid or hyperdiploid (fewer than 60 chromosomes). Only a few marker chromosomes are present. Metastatic cells, on the other hand, have near triploid or near tetraploid modes. So many marker chromosomes are present in such a large number of chromosomes that it is impossible to determine the origin of the markers.

Interestingly, tumors originating in the same organ and with the same pathologic diagnosis may have remarkably different karyotypes.

2. Nonrandom chromosome involvement – In solid tumors, aberrations of chromosomes 1, 3, 6, 8, and 14 are common, and involvement of chromosomes 5, 7, 13, 17, and 22 is less common. Later in tumor development, trisomy 1q and other chromosomal aberrations often occur. These probably indicate the locations of genes causing uncontrolled growth.

3. Rare and unusual chromosomal findings – Human and experimentally produced tumors may have chromosomes with 2 unusual morphologic characteristics: homogeneously staining regions (HSR) and double minutes (DM). HSR are long unbanded regions that may occur on many chromosomes; DM are small paired chromosome structures that are reiterations of identical sequences of dark-light bands. Recently, both HSR and DM have been shown to be sites of gene amplification. HSR regions are present in human neuroblastomas, with amplification of the c-myc oncogene. The degree of malignancy of these tumors is directly related to the amount of gene amplification.

Solid tumors may develop as early as the stage of embryogenesis. Two such tumors, retinoblastomas and Wilms' tumor with associated aniridia, may provide insight into the importance of chromosomal changes in tumors. There are 3 types of retinoblastomas; unilateral, bilateral, and those associated with mental retardation or congenital defects (1%). In unilateral and bilateral tumors, which are autosomal dominant, partial deletion of the long arm of one chromosome of the chromosome 13 pair (del 13q14) occurs in tumor cells. In the third type, this deletion occurs in tumor cells and all cells of the body. This suggests that alterations at gene site 13q14 are important for the development of retinoblastoma. About 2% of Wilms' tumors have associated bilateral aniridia. These patients have a characteristic deletion of the short arm of chromosome 11 (del 11p13); this probably indicates that genes associated with the development of aniridia and Wilms' tumor are located near each other and that a chromosomal deletion is the cause of both conditions.

Genetic instability appears to contribute to the development of solid tumors. Phenotypic females with an XY complement have a 25% greater risk of developing ovarian carcinoma. This is true whether or not mosaicism is present or the Y chromosome is intact or partially deleted. Tumors that develop in these patients are of different types, with gonadoblastoma occurring most frequently, sometimes as early as age 3. XXY males (Klinefelter's syndrome) have a 30-fold increase in the incidence of breast cancer as well as predisposition to acute nonlymphocytic leukemia. Patients with trisomy 21 or sex chromosome aneuploidy (XXX or XXY) have an increased incidence of retinoblastoma. Chromosomal translocations have been found in several solid tumors, eg, Ewing's sarcoma, mixed tumor

Table 32–2. Nonrandom translocations characterizing human leukemias and cancers.*†

Translocation	Condition
t(9;22)(q34;q11)	CML, acute leukemias (AML, ALL)
t(8;21)(q22;q22)	AML (M2 with Auer bodies)
t(4;11)(q21;q23)	ALL
t(8;14)(q23;q32)	ALL (L3), Burkitt's lymphoma, other lymphomas
t(15;17)(q24;q21)	APL(M3)
t(11;C)(q21–23;C)‡	ANLL
t(3;8)(p25;q21)	Mixed tumor of parotid
t(6;14)(q21;q24)	Serous cystadenocarcinoma of ovary
t(9;11)(p21;q23)	Acute monoblastic leukemia (M5)
t(11;21)(q22;q21)	Myeloproliferative disorders, ANLL
t(6;12)(q15;p13)	Prolymphocytic leukemia
t(6;9)(p23;q24)	ANLL (M2 without Auer bodies)
t(15;18)?	Bladder cancer

*Reproduced, with permission, from Sandberg AA: Chromosomes in human neoplasia. *Curr Probl Cancer* 1983;**8**:11.

†ALL, acute lymphoblastic leukemia; AML, acute myeloblastic leukemia; ANLL, acute nonlymphocytic leukemia; APL, acute promyelocytic leukemia; CML, chronic myelocytic leukemia.

‡C = Chromosomes 6, 9, 10, 17, 19.

of the parotid, serous cystadenoma of the ovary, and familial renal cell carcinoma.

Of the remaining types of solid tumors, meningiomas have undergone the most study. Over 95% of the 267 reported cases are associated with monosomy 22. Other tumors associated with nonmorphologic chromosome changes are cancer of the bladder, endometrium, breast, and cervix; seminoma; malignant melanoma; neuroblastoma; and small cell cancer of the lung.

B. Leukemia and Lymphoma: Trisomy 21 is the only chromosomal syndrome in which a clear relationship to leukemia has been established. Children with trisomy 21 have a 20-fold increased risk of developing acute leukemia.

1. Chronic myelogenous leukemia (CML) – In chronic myelogenous leukemia, 95% of patients show an abnormal chromosome (Ph[1] or Philadelphia) in their leukemic cells in the peripheral blood and bone marrow during the preleukemic stage as well as before and after treatment. This change may be present in a small percentage or in 100% of the leukemic cells. It also occurs in red cell precursors, megakaryocytes, and macrophages, but not in the lymphocyte series or skin fibroblasts. In 95% of cases, the Ph[1] chromosome (22q⁻) is due to a balanced reciprocal translocation [(9;22) (q34;q11)] between the long arm of chromosome 22 and the long arm of chromosome 9. In the remaining cases, and without apparent difference in the clinical and hematologic pattern, the translocation is from chromosome 22 to chromosomes 2, 6, 11, 12, 13, 14, 16, 17, 19, 21, or 22. At present, CML patients can be divided into 2 groups on the basis of the Philadelphia chromosome. Those with the chromosomal defect (Ph[1+]) show the clinical and hematologic features of typical chronic myelogenous leukemia:

Table 32–3. Nonrandom morphologic chromosome changes in human cancer and leukemia.*†

Chromosome	Condition
1p−	Malignant melanoma
1p−(p32→pter)	Neuroblastoma
1p−,i(1q)	Endometrial cancer
1q+	Breast cancer
3p−(p14→p23)	Small cell cancer of lung
3p−,3q−,5q−,7q−	Complicating leukemia
5q−	Refractory anemia; ANLL (EL and AML), cervical cancer
6q−	Lymphoma, ALL, malignant melanoma
i(6p)	Malignant melanoma
7q−	ANLL (EL and AML)
9p−	T-cell ALL
11q	ANLL (AMoL and AMMoL), cervical cancer
i(12p)	Seminoma
12q−	Complicating acute leukemia, adenocàrcinoma of large bowel
14q+	Lymphoma, ALL, CLL
14q+(q32)	Adult T-cell leukemia
i(16q)	Bladder cancer
i(17q)	CML (BP)
20q−	PV
21q−	Preleukemia, ANLL, thrombocythemia?
22q−	CML, meningioma

*Reproduced, with permission, from Sandberg AA: A chromosomal hypothesis of oncogenesis. *Cancer Genet Cytogenet* 1983; 8:278.

†ALL, acute lymphoblastic leukemia; AML, acute myeloblastic leukemia; AMMoL, acute myelomonocytic leukemia; AMoL, acute monocytic leukemia; ANLL, acute nonlymphocytic leukemia; BP, blastic phase; CLL, chronic lymphocytic leukemia; CML, chronic myelocytic leukemia; EL, erythroleukemia; PV, polycythemia vera.

they respond rapidly to chemotherapy and are easily controlled therapeutically. They have an equal sex distribution, a median age of 48, and a median survival of 42 months. The Ph¹-negative (Ph¹⁻) patients, who constitute 15% of all patients, have normal karyotypes. Clinically and hematologically, they represent a heterogeneous group. They are predominantly males with a median age of 66 who respond poorly to treatment and die in the first year of their disease.

In the chronic phase of Ph¹⁺ CML, 10% of the patients have additional chromosomal abnormalities, such as an extra 8, second Ph¹, and, in 1% of cases, loss of the Y chromosome. These patients do not have a poorer prognosis than patients who have the 46 Ph¹⁺ pattern. When patients with CML enter their terminal blast phase, 80–90% have other chromosomal abnormalities superimposed on the Ph¹⁺ cell line. Since virtually all of these patients have been treated, it is difficult to say whether or not therapy affects the pattern of chromosomal abnormalities. Their modal chromosomal numbers range from 47 to 52. There is a distinct nonrandom involvement of chromosomes 8, 17, 19, and 22. The isochromosome for the long arm of chromosome 17 [i(17q)] appears to be a reliable

marker for the impending blast phase. The blast cells may have either lymphoid or myeloid characteristics. Patients with blasts of lymphoid morphology may respond to vincristine and prednisone therapy and have a median survival rate of 5 months, whereas those with myeloid morphology do not respond to this therapy and have a median survival rate of 3 months. The change in karyotype may precede the blast phase by 2–4 months. Some patients in the blast phase have received autologous bone marrow transplantation after total body irradiation and high-dose cyclophosphamide therapy. Since they receive their own circulating stem cells that were harvested and stored during the chronic phase of disease, they again had Ph¹⁺ abnormality. Patients who received allogeneic bone marrow transplantation from healthy histocompatible donors have remained hematologically and cytogenetically normal over follow-up periods of more than 4 years.

2. Other leukemias–Acute leukemias are classified on the basis of morphologic and cytochemical methods by the 1980 modification of the French-American-British (FAB) Study Group. The acute nonlymphocytic leukemias (ANLL) include the acute myeloblastic leukemias (AML, FAB M1 and M2), acute promyelocytic leukemia (APL, FAB M3 and M3 variant), acute myelomonocytic leukemia (AMML, FAB M4), acute monocytic leukemia (AMoL, FAB M5), and acute erythroleukemia (AEL, FAB M6). With high-resolution banding techniques, 96% of ANLL patients demonstrate a chromosomal abnormality; this indicates that the FAB subgroups are heterogeneous. Prognosis is aided by use of chromosomal analysis in addition to the FAB classification.

Certain trends are apparent in the ANLL studies. Most patients have a recurrent defect. These changes are present before treatment and disappear during remission, and the same karyotype recurs during relapse.

Table 32–4. Nonrandomness of missing or extra chromosomes in human cancer and leukemia.*†

Chromosome	Condition
−5	ANLL (EL and AML), complicating acute leukemia
−7	ANLL (EL and AML), complicating acute leukemia
+7	Adenocarcinoma of large bowel
+8	ANLL, CML (BP), polyps of colon, bladder cancer
+12	Hematologic conditions, especially CLL, seminoma
+21	ALL
−22	Meningioma
±3, −5, 7, ±12, ±17	Complicating leukemia

*Reproduced, with permission, from Sandberg AA: A chromosomal hypothesis of oncogenesis. *Cancer Genet Cytogenet* 1983; 8:278.

†ALL, acute lymphoblastic leukemia; AML, acute myeloblastic leukemia; ANLL, acute nonlymphocytic leukemia; BP, blastic phase; CLL, chronic lymphocytic leukemia; CML, chronic myelocytic leukemia; EL, erythroleukemia.

Occasionally, in relapse, additional chromosomal changes are superimposed on the original aberration. The modal number is in the diploid range (45–47) in 85% of patients. Survival studies of ANLL patients indicate that the prognosis is better in those with some normal karyotypes in bone marrow cells at the time of diagnosis. Patients with all normal metaphases at the time of diagnosis had a 13-month median survival rate, while those with all abnormal metaphases had an 8-month median survival rate. Patients with both normal and abnormal metaphases had an intermediate survival time. Certain karyotypes were valuable in prognosis. The highest rate of complete remission occurred in patients with 4 chromosomal abnormalities: t(8;21), +21, t(15;17), and hypoploidy. The median survival rate was longest in patients with 3 chromosomal abnormalities: $^{-}7$ or $7q^{-}$, t(15;17), and hypoploidy. Patients with abnormalities of chromosome 5 generally did poorly. It is interesting to note that patients with no chromosomal abnormalities did not respond better or live longer.

Certain structural rearrangements seem to be related to specific types of leukemia. Leukemias with an abnormal clone are associated with a poor prognosis, except for the 8:21 translocation of AML. In **acute myeloblastic leukemia** (AML), 5–30% of aneuploid patients have translocation of the long arms of 8 and 21. These patients have the same survival rate as those with normal karyotypes, unless there is an associated loss of either sex chromosome. Then the survival time shortens from 15 months to 5 months. The frequency of the t(8;21) type varies geographically, with a 30% incidence in Japan, a 24% incidence in Chicago, and a 3% incidence in Europe. About 40% of patients with **acute promyelocytic leukemia** have a 15 and 17 translocation that is specific for this disease. It is a poor prognostic factor. If APL patients have no chromosomal abnormality, they have a 45% complete remission rate and a 4-month median survival rate, while if the t(15;17) abnormality is present, there is only a 26% complete remission rate and a 1-month median survival rate. Clinically, patients with the t(15;17) defect have a high incidence of disseminated intravascular coagulation (DIC) due to massive cell lysis during induction therapy. Again, there is a remarkable geographic variation in the frequency of this finding. In **acute monocytic** (AMoL) and **acute myelomonocytic leukemia** (AMMoL), high-resolution chromosomal studies identify a specific chromosomal abnormality with reciprocal translocations involving 11q23. An additional chromosomal defect in AMMoL was discovered in 1983 (see 1983 LeBeau reference at end of chapter). In 18 of 308 newly diagnosed patients, there was inversion of chromosome 16 [inv(16)(p13q22)]. These patients also had abnormal eosinophils in marrow. This group responded well to intensive therapy, with complete remission occurring in 13 of the 17 treated patients; 10 of the 13 have continued to remain in complete remission. Sandberg has identified another subgroup in AML, a translocation occurring between chromosomes 6 and 9 [t(6;9)(p23;q34)]. Its relationship to clinical course, response to therapy, and survival rates has not yet been determined. In **acute erythroleukemia** (AEL), the frequent chromosomal abnormalities are bizarre, random, and of poor prognosis. **ANLL as a second cancer** has been observed in patients treated for Hodgkin's disease, non-Hodgkin's lymphoma, and other solid tumors as well as after renal transplant (one case). The median time of onset of leukemia is 4–5 years after the time of diagnosis of the original disease. These patients have had exposure to environmental mutagens and either radiotherapy or chemotherapy or both. Their bone marrows contain an abnormal clone of cells, usually with a hypodiploid modal number and a nonrandom loss of chromosomes 3, 5, 7, and 17. These same findings are present in patients with ANLL de novo who have had exposure to chemical solvents, pesticides, and petroleum products, but they are not present in childhood ANLL. Rowley proposes that these particular chromosomal changes may identify acute leukemia associated with exposure to mutagens. These patients go rapidly downhill and are unresponsive to therapy.

In **acute lymphoblastic leukemia** (ALL), the chromosomes have poorly defined morphologic features and indistinct bands, making accurate karyotypic analysis difficult. In a recent review of 330 children and adults with untreated ALL, 66% had clonal abnormalities. Pseudodiploidy was the most common. In 53%, the modal chromosome number was 46. Translocations were present in one-third, with t(9;22), the Ph[1] chromosome; t(4;11); and t(8;14) being the most common. The incidence of clonal abnormalities varied with cell type: 100% for B cell ALL, 70% with non–B cell, non–T cell ALL, and 39% with T cell ALL. Karyotype correlated with the achievement of remission, duration of remission, and survival. Patients without chromosomal abnormalities or with only a $6q^{-}$ did well. Those with a modal number over 50 responded best to chemotherapy and, if children, often had long-term survival or cures. Patients with translocations responded poorly to therapy and had the shortest survival time. Karyotypic abnormalities had a different prognosis in children than in adults, but when a specific subset of ALL was compared, such as t(8;14), the prognosis was the same. Sandberg recently reported a characteristic abnormality in **prolymphocytic leukemia** (PML), [t(6;12)(q15;p13)]. In **chronic lymphocytic leukemia** (CLL), there is such a low mitotic index that no conclusive studies have been done. Surface marker studies indicate that 90% of CLL cells are of B cell origin. Recent studies reveal trisomy 12 to be the most frequent abnormal karyotype. The presence of any abnormal karyotype was associated with advanced clinical stage and shortened survival time.

3. Lymphomas and related diseases–Far less cytogenetic information is available about lymphomas than about leukemia. In Hodgkin's disease, studies have been limited by the low yield of dividing cells and low number of clear-cut aneuploid clones, so that complete chromosomal analyses with banding are available for far fewer patients with Hodgkin's disease than for any other lymphoma. In Hodgkin's disease, the modal chromosomal number tends to be triploid or tetraploid. About one-third of the samples have a 14q+ chromosome. In non-Hodgkin's lymphomas, a new high-resolution technique of chromosome analysis has a 95% success rate. The modal number tends to be diploid. In 3 situations, the chromosomal aberration correlates with the histologic type: In follicular lymphomas of small cleaved cell, mixed cell, and large cell types there is a translocation between chromosomes 18 and 14; in lymphomas of the small noncleaved cell or large cell immunoblastic types, there is a translocation between chromosomes 8 and 14; and in small cell lymphocytic leukemia, there is a trisomy 12. The few patients with near tetraploidy had the highest median survival rate (69 months), while patients with t(14;18) had the lowest survival rate (12 months). In Burkitt's lymphoma, a solid tumor of B cell origin, 90% of patients have a translocation between the long arm of chromosome 8 (8q⁻) and the long arm of chromosome 14 (14q⁻). The remaining 10% have a t(8;2) or t(8;22). The translocated gene segment of chromosome 8, which contains the oncogene c-myc, is transposed directly into immunoglobulin loci on chromosome 2, 14, and 22. These translocations occur in every Burkitt's lymphoma, whether it is of the African or non-African type, and whether it is Epstein-Barr virus (EBV)-positive or -negative. In multiple myeloma, a 14q+ anomaly is present but does not appear to involve 8.

The constancy of the break point of chromosome 14q32 in both Burkitt's and non-Burkitt's lymphoma suggests that an abnormality at this site confers proliferative advantage to the malignant cell.

4. Other related hematologic disorders–There are limited cytogenetic studies of other hematologic disorders that have a recognized propensity for neoplastic transformation. In **preleukemia**, patients with any abnormal karyotype have a poor prognosis, since 60% have a fatal outcome compared with 30% of patients with a normal karyotype. These patients usually progress to overt ANLL. Their chromosomal changes are nonspecific. The most consistent specific chromosomal abnormality in **refractory anemia with excess blasts** (RAEB) is a deletion of the long arm of chromosome 5 (5q⁻). The presence of this chromosomal anomaly corresponds to slower development of the illness and rare transformation into acute leukemia. In **polycythemia vera,** 26% of untreated patients have both numerical and structural abnormalities in their bone marrow. Aneuploidy is the most common, with hyperdiploid states more common than hypodiploid. The chromosomes most commonly affected are 1, 8, 9, and 20. It is the partial deletion of the long arm of chromosome 20 (20q⁻) that is the most consistent specific finding. It has no prognostic value, but its presence can distinguish between primary and secondary polycythemia. The chromosomal changes, however, do not indicate which patients progress to leukemia. The information in **acute and chronic myelofib-**

rosis is limited because of technical difficulties in obtaining adequate preparations. About 40% of these patients have nonspecific chromosomal abnormalities. If patients have normal chromosomes at the time of diagnosis, 92% respond to androgen therapy, while only 22% of patients with chromosomal abnormalities respond to this therapy. In a study of 27 patients with **acquired idiopathic sideroblastic anemia (AISA),** 40% of cases had a variety of chromosomal disturbances, primarily heteroploidy and disturbances in the F chromosomes. The results of the chromosomal banding studies were strikingly similar to those in polycythemia vera, a fact of great interest, since both diseases may transform to leukemia. In **chronic myelomonocytic leukemia,** no specific chromosomal abnormalities have been noted.

5. Chromosomal breakage diseases–Six autosomal recessive diseases—Bloom's syndrome, Fanconi's anemia, ataxia-telangiectasia, glutathione reductase deficiency, Kostmann's agranulocytosis, and pernicious anemia—tend toward chromosomal breakage and rearrangement in vitro. In addition, each of these diseases has a relatively high incidence of neoplasia, primarily leukemia and lymphoma. In studies of patients with ataxia-telangiectasia, the anomalous clone in most cases is a structural rearrangement in 14. Most often it is a translocation involving 14, 7, 6, and X.

Kaneko Y: Prognostic implications of karyotype and morphology in patients with non-Hodgkin's lymphoma. *Int J Cancer* 1983;**32:**683.

Marx JL: What do oncogenes do? *Science* 1984;**223:**673.

Molecular biology and lymphoma. (Editorial.) *Lancet* 1984; **1:**26.

Sandberg AA: Chromosomes in human neoplasia. *Curr Probl Cancer* 1983;**8:**3.

Sandberg AA: Fourth International Workshop on Chromosomes in Leukemia: A prospective study of acute nonlymphocytic leukemia (1982). *Cancer Genet Cytogenet* 1984;**11:**249.

Sandberg AA et al: Chromosome analysis in hematologic disorders: The leukemias. *Am J Med* 1984;**76:**971.

Wolman SR: Cytogenetics and cancer. *Arch Pathol Lab Med* 1984;**108:**15.

Yunis JJ: The chromosomal basis of human neoplasia. *Science* 1983;**221:**227.

Yunis JJ: Fragile sites and a predisposition to leukemia and lymphoma. *Cancer Genet Cytogenet* 1984;**12:**85.

Yunis JJ: Recurrent chromosomal defects are found in most patients with acute nonlymphocytic leukemia. *Cancer Genet Cytogenet* 1984;**11:**125.

Yunis JJ et al: Distinctive chromosomal abnormalities in histologic subtypes of non-Hodgkin's lymphoma. *N Engl J Med* 1982;**307:**1231.

CHROMOSOMES & IONIZING RADIATION

The major problem of ionizing radiation is not the danger of lethal doses but of small doses that allow the cells to multiply after permanent alteration of their genetic material.

Detectable chromosomal changes occur after diagnostic and therapeutic x-ray as well as with beta and gamma radiation (^{131}I, ^{32}P). These usually persist for a few hours to several weeks. In vitro studies reveal a direct relationship between the dose of ionizing radiation and the number of chromosomal abnormalities.

VIRUSES, CHEMICALS, & CHROMOSOMES

For more than half a century, viruses and chemicals have been known to induce chromosomal aberrations in plants and animals. Only in the past decade have human chromosomal defects been proved to be caused by these agents. The measles, chickenpox, hepatitis, and rubella viruses may cause chromosomal aberrations in the leukocytes that may persist for several months after the clinical illness. Drugs such as ozone, analogous and intermediary metabolites of nucleic acids, and alkylating agents have deleterious effects on chromosomes. Studies of workers exposed to chemical solvents, insecticides, petroleum products, and anesthetic gases reveal an increased number of structural chromosomal abnormalities in their peripheral blood cells. Their nonrandom chromosomal abnormalities were primarily one of 4 changes: 5^-, 7^-, 8^+, and 21^+. Different carcinogens have different clonal abnormalities. Follow-up is being done to determine the incidence of fetal malformation and wastage as well as leukemia in these groups.

It is hoped that these new findings will add to our understanding of "spontaneous" chromosomal changes as well as chemical carcinogenesis.

Sandberg AA (editor): Correlation of karyotype and occupational exposure to potential mutagenic/carcinogenic agents in acute nonlymphocytic leukemia. *Cancer Genet Cytogenet* 1984;**11**:326.

GENETIC COUNSELING

With our new scientific tools for the detection of genetic disease by amniocentesis and biochemical identification of heterozygotes, the clinician will face the problem of transmitting this information to the patient in a meaningful manner. The National Foundation has a list of genetic counseling centers where adequately trained personnel can assist with or perform this function.

In undertaking genetic counseling, the physician needs the following specific information: (1) An accurate diagnosis, since closely related disorders — especially biochemical defects — may have a markedly different prognosis and mode of inheritance. (2) A detailed family history with an accurate pedigree showing the affected and nonaffected members. (3) A knowledge of the behavior of the disorder from the literature. With this information at hand, the risk of recurrence can be estimated.

In informing the family of the chances of recurrence, the counselor must use terms and analogies the parents can understand. The parents must be aware of the range of possible defects involved; only then can they decide whether or not to have more children.

An aspect of counseling that is frequently neglected is the extension of counseling to other members of the family. This involves not only informing and instructing high-risk relatives but also reassuring low-risk relatives.

Lynch HT et al (editors): *International Directory of Genetic Services*, 7th ed. Birth Defects Series. The National Foundation, New York, 1983.

SELECTED HEREDITARY METABOLIC DISEASES

Garrod's original description in 1908 of 4 inborn errors of metabolism was regarded with interest, but these disorders were largely considered to be rare medical curiosities of little clinical importance. The several hundred hereditary metabolic disorders about which we now have at least some knowledge include common and uncommon, benign and serious diseases, metabolic disturbances involving almost every class of biochemical substance, and diseases of all organs and tissues of the body. Newly recognized metabolic disorders are being reported at a rapid rate, and this information has contributed greatly to the study of the molecular biology of humans and animals.

Information about metabolic abnormalities is not only important in furthering our understanding of hitherto obscure disease processes but also fundamental to a proper therapeutic approach to them. Old concepts of hereditary transmission of physical traits simply as dominant or recessive have had to be modified to explain the "asymptomatic carriers" of hereditary traits. Biochemical studies on relatives of patients with hereditary metabolic disorders may reveal deficiencies not clinically manifest. Recognition of the heterozygote carrier may be of extreme value from a eugenic point of view (in preventing potentially incompatible matings) and from the standpoint of the health of the individual (eg, in suggesting special dietary control, appropriate medication, and avoidance of drug idiosyncrasies).

Determination of the genetic basis of metabolic disorders is based on the family history and appropriate biochemical studies of the patient and available relatives. Biochemical studies may include the determination of essential blood constituents, abnormal protein molecules, specific enzymes, abnormal metabolites, electrolytes, renal transport mechanisms, and tolerance or restriction tests with food or chemicals.

Several of the hereditary metabolic disorders (eg, diabetes mellitus, hyperlipidemia, gout) as they relate to specific organ systems are discussed in other sections of this book.

ABNORMALITY OF MOLECULAR STRUCTURE OF PROTEIN: METHEMOGLOBINEMIA

Congenital methemoglobinemia is a disease caused either by a deficiency of erythrocyte NADH dehydrogenase required in converting methemoglobin to hemoglobin or by the presence of one of 5 different abnormal hemoglobins, each designated as an M hemoglobin. The former is the more frequent form and is inherited as an autosomal recessive trait; the latter is autosomal dominant. Clinically, the disease is manifested by a persistent gray cyanosis not associated with cardiac or respiratory abnormality, and by easy fatigability, dyspnea, tachycardia, and dizziness with exertion. The venous blood is brown; the oxygen capacity of arterial blood is reduced, and excessive amounts of methemoglobin are present in the blood.

Oral administration of riboflavin, 120 mg/d, significantly decreases methemoglobin in the disease caused by enzyme deficiency. In addition, in some cases, continuous administration of methylene blue, 240 mg/d orally, will relieve the symptoms and cyanosis.

The prognosis for life is good. Pregnancies are not compromised. Heterozygotes can be identified by assays of enzyme activity. Toxic agents such as nitrites and aniline derivatives create a special hazard for NADH dehydrogenase-deficient patients. They cause a sudden increase in methemoglobin, which is tolerated poorly and may be fatal.

Hirano M et al: Congenital methaemoglobinaemia due to NADH methaemoglobin reductase deficiency: Successful treatment with oral riboflavin. *Br J Haematol* 1981;**47**:353.

DISORDERS OF AMINO ACIDS

Albinism

Albinism is a term that covers many clinical syndromes exhibiting hypomelanosis of the skin and eye due to inherited metabolic defects. Their incidence is 1:20,000. There are 3 forms of albinism: **ocular,** which is a sex-linked recessive trait as well as an autosomal recessive trait; **oculocutaneous,** which is autosomal dominant; and **cutaneous,** which is autosomal dominant. In the ocular form, the eye defect occurs alone. Clinical manifestations are photophobia, nystagmus, defective vision, and absence of binocular vision. The metabolic defect of ocular albinism is unknown. In the oculocutaneous form, defects in hair and skin pigmentation occur in addition to the ocular defects. The hypopigmented skin acquires folds and wrinkles easily when exposed to solar radiation. There is a high frequency of solar keratosis, basal cell carcinoma, and squamous cell carcinoma. Biochemically, patients with oculocutaneous albinism are divided into tyrosinase-positive and tyrosinase-negative, but the biochemical distinction does not separate the

patients clinically. In both the ocular and oculocutaneous forms, there are abnormal optic pathways as well as rearrangements in the geniculocortical projections that account for the absence of binocular vision. The cutaneous form is a partial albinism or piebaldism that affects only the skin and hair. There is localized loss of melanocytes. Some patients have associated deafness.

There is no specific treatment. Sunlight should be avoided. Sunscreen preparations are useful. Dark glasses will help patients with photophobia.

Alkaptonuria

Alkaptonuria is a rare autosomal recessive disease caused by a deficiency of the enzyme homogentisic oxidase. Since this enzyme is necessary in the intermediate metabolism of phenylalanine and tyrosine, its precursor, homogentisic acid, increases and is deposited in the connective tissues of the body to give them, grossly, a blue-black color and, microscopically, an ochre color (hence, ochronosis).

The cardinal features of alkaptonuria are pigmentation of the cartilage and other connective tissues, arthritis in later life, and signs of homogentisic acid in the urine. The blue-black pigmentation, not usually noticeable until age 20–30 years, is most apparent in the scleras of the eyes and pinnas of the ears. The arthritis may resemble rheumatoid arthritis clinically. The large joints of the body—mainly hips, knees, lumbosacral spine, and shoulders—may undergo acute inflammation followed by limitation of motion and ankylosis. In the urine, the homogentisic acid causes a dark color (particularly when the urine is alkaline), and since it has reducing properties, it may give a false-positive result in Benedict's test for sugar.

Diagnosis rests on the identification of homogentisic acid in the urine by means of paper chromatography.

Since the disease has a prolonged, benign course, no attempts have been made to control phenylalanine and tyrosine in the diet. Degenerative arthritis is treated symptomatically. Vitamin C, a reducing agent, has been suggested as a means of decreasing pigment formation and deposition. There is no method for detection of the heterozygote.

Phenylketonuria

Phenylketonuria (PKU) is one of the milestone diseases of medicine, for it was this disease in which the first biochemical cause of mental retardation was discovered and in which dietary treatment proved to be effective; prevention was thus made possible through early identification and treatment. It is an autosomal recessive disease whose incidence varies from 1:5000 in Irish persons and Scots to 1:300,000 in blacks, Ashkenazic Jews, and Finns. Clinically, the classic picture is represented by a blond, blue-eyed child with fair skin, eczema, and mental retardation. Seizures and behavioral problems are often present.

Since screening of newborns is widespread, the presenting problem is hyperphenylalaninemia in a healthy newborn infant. But hyperphenylalaninemia is no longer synonymous with phenylketonuria, for mass screening has revealed multiple causes of hyperphenylalaninemia. Thus far, 3 causes of hyperphenylalaninemia severe enough to require treatment have been defined. First, there is classic phenylketonuria due to phenylalanine hydroxylase deficiency. This form, accounting for 97% of cases, requires and responds to dietary treatment (to prevent mental retardation). The remaining 3% of cases are due to defects in 2 other enzymes that are involved not only in phenylalanine metabolism but also in biosynthesis of neurotransmitters such as dopamine, norepinephrine, and serotonin. Adequate therapy for this group requires BH_4, sepiapterin, levodopa, carbidopa, and 5-hydroxytryptophan in addition to the dietary regimen in order to prevent progressive neurologic degeneration.

Therapy consists of a restricted phenylalanine diet, with enough phenylalanine present to support adequate growth without causing mental impairment. Weekly blood levels are checked to keep the blood levels between 3 and 10 mg/dL. All agree that the diet should be maintained for 3–6 years, and some investigators feel it should be maintained for life. After age 6, it can be used to modify such symptoms as hyperkinesis, seizures, learning disorders, and eczema. The diet will not reverse or improve existing mental retardation, but if it is instituted before age 2 months, the child has a statistically significant chance of attaining normal intelligence.

Genetics plays an important role in prevention. Once a patient is identified, the entire family and any subsequent offspring should be checked for phenylketonuria. If the mother has classic phenylketonuria, she can bear a normal infant, but there is an increase both in the rate of abortion and in the risk of bearing offspring with nonphenylketonuric mental retardation, microcephaly, and congenital heart disease. In 34 cases in which phenylalanine-restricted diets were used in pregnancy, the outcomes varied from mental normality with no associated fetal defects to neonatal deaths due to congenital heart disease. The current recommendation is to initiate therapy prior to conception.

The heterozygote can be identified and is free of any signs or symptoms of phenylketonuria. In 1984, prenatal diagnosis of phenylketonuria by DNA linkage studies was successfully done. With the marker chromosome used, probably 75% of the PKU families can be identified.

Lenke RR, Levy HL: Maternal phenylketonuria and hyperphenylalaninemia: An international survey of the outcome of untreated and treated pregnancies. N Engl J Med 1980;303: 1202.

Homocystinuria

Homocystinuria, an autosomal disease with considerable genetic heterogeneity, is the second most common inborn error of amino acid metabolism. Its incidence is 1:200,000 live births. The vast majority of cases are due to a deficiency in the liver enzyme cystathionine synthase, thereby causing an increased amount of methionine and other metabolites in blood and other body tissues. The cardinal signs and symptoms are due to defective collagen formation and occur in the eye, skeletal system, central nervous system, and cardiovascular system. Lens ectopia is typically present and may cause secondary glaucoma, myopia, retinal detachment, and cataract. The skeletal system consistently shows osteoporosis and genu valgum, and frequently there are chest, vertebral, and foot deformities. Mental retardation is present in half of cases. Major motor seizures are frequently present. The lethal complication is in the cardiovascular system, where multiple arterial and venous thromboses occur as a result of enhanced platelet stickiness. Occasionally, an abdominal aortic aneurysm may be present.

If ectopic lens is present, patients with homocystinuria may be wrongly diagnosed as having Marfan's syndrome. Diagnosis is suspected by a combination of clinical findings and excessive urinary homocysteine excretion, but definitive diagnosis requires the demonstration of reduced cystathionine synthase activity.

Treatment to achieve biochemical control should start as soon as the disease is diagnosed, for most clinical complications are irreversible. About half of patients repond to massive doses of pyridoxine. A daily dose of 500–1000 mg of pyridoxine, when effective, will cause a biochemical response in a few days; it should then be lowered until a minimum effective dose is found. A recent study of pyridoxine-resistant patients treated with betaine, 6 g/d, in addition to folate and pyridoxine showed biochemical improvement in all 10 patients and clinical improvement in 6. Studies in animals have shown that the vascular injury is induced by homocystine. A single dose of dipyridamole, 100 mg, combined with aspirin, 1 g, has also been reported to be effective in decreasing the incidence of thrombotic episodes.

Identification of heterozygotes is possible. Prenatal diagnosis is feasible but has not been reported.

Weilcken DE et al: Homocystinuria: The effects of betaine in the treatment of patients not responsive to pyridoxine. N Engl J Med 1983;309:448.

DISORDERS OF CARBOHYDRATE METABOLISM

Essential Fructosuria

Essential fructosuria is a rare metabolic disease (1:130,000) that is inherited as an autosomal recessive trait. It is an asymptomatic, harmless condition that is usually suspected by the finding of nonglucose-reducing sugar on routine urinalysis. Definitive diagnosis is made by means of paper chromatography of the urine.

Hereditary Fructose Intolerance

Hereditary fructose intolerance is an autosomal recessive disease caused by the absence of the enzyme fructose-1-phosphate aldolase in the jejunum. As a result, fructose 1-phosphate accumulates in the liver and in the proximal tubules of the kidney. Hypoglycemia results not from hyperinsulinism but rather from failure of glucose release from the liver cells. Renal damage causes failure of acidification of the urine, as well as albuminuria and aminoaciduria. These derangements of liver and kidney function are reversible.

Clinically, the presenting symptoms are those of hypoglycemia and vomiting after the ingestion of fructose. In infants, the disease may progress to hepatosplenomegaly, failure to thrive, cachexia, and death. If the chronic state occurs, children and adults characteristically avoid sweets and fruits, and their teeth are in excellent condition. Studies reveal normal intelligence in spite of frequent hypoglycemic attacks.

Diagnosis is made by demonstrating a marked and prolonged fall of glucose and serum inorganic phosphorus during an intravenous fructose tolerance test.

Therapy consists entirely of avoiding fructose in fruits, vegetables, and sucrose-containing foods. Lack of recognition of the large amounts of fructose present in potatoes has resulted in some common failures in treatment. In hospitalized patients, intravenous fluids containing fructose must be avoided.

Disorders of Galactose Metabolism

Galactosemia is a disturbance of galactose metabolism caused by an enzyme deficiency. The 3 enzymes involved are transferase, which accounts for 90% of cases; galactokinase, which accounts for 10% of cases; and a newly described variant, epimerase.

In transferase deficiency, the toxicity syndrome is characterized by failure to thrive, vomiting, liver disease, cataracts, and mental retardation. Galactokinase deficiency, which is rarer, is mild and is mainly evidenced by cataracts. Epimerase deficiency involves only red cells, has no associated galactosemia, and is a benign disorder that is detected by screening procedures. The diagnosis is suggested by the detection of galactose in blood and urine and is confirmed by demonstration of enzyme deficiency in the peripheral red cells.

The disorder is treated by avoidance of galactose in foods. Nutramigen and soybean milks are effective substitutes for cow's milk. This diet is not harmful to the body, and it results in a striking regression of signs and symptoms: the cataracts get smaller, liver and renal abnormalities disappear, and growth returns. Mental retardation, which is usually mild to moderate, is probably not altered.

Genetic studies play a highly significant role in these disorders. Since the heterozygotes can be identified by blood studies and the affected fetus identified by amniotic fluid or fetal blood analysis, a maternal diet free of galactose can be maintained during the pregnancy. In transferase deficiency, Donnell and others have reported 10 normal children and one with cataracts when this diet was used by mothers.

Idiopathic Lactase Deficiency

Human infants have a high concentration of lactase at birth. This concentration falls rapidly in the first 4–5 years, and in many populations it reaches very low levels in adolescent and adult life. It is deficient in 3–19% of the adult white population, 70% of American blacks, 90% of American Indians, and in virtually all Orientals.

Clinically, the characteristic history is that of a patient with a normal diet in infancy and childhood who begins to dislike or avoid milk in adolescence or adulthood. The symptoms range from bloating and flatulence to crampy abdominal pain and diarrhea. Repeated oral sugar tolerance tests are useful, but confirmation of the diagnosis requires demonstration of the enzyme deficiency by means of intestinal biopsy. Withdrawal of dietary lactose causes prompt disappearance of symptoms.

It is important to rule out secondary lactase deficiencies caused by intestinal disorders (eg, irritable colon, sprue, nonspecific intestinal injury, kwashiorkor), since these diseases are treatable.

Glycogen Storage Diseases (GSD)

Glycogen storage diseases now constitute 12 separate entities, all of which are clinically and biochemically identifiable. Each has deficient activity of specific enzymes involved in the synthesis and degradation of glycogen, causing an accumulation of abnormal glycogen in any or all of the tissues of the liver, heart, skeletal muscle, kidney, and brain. The inheritance pattern is probably autosomal recessive (with the exception of type IXB, which is X-linked recessive).

Clinically, there is a wide range of symptoms and findings, varying from type IIA—which causes death in infancy—to type X—which, without therapy, is found in patients with hepatomegaly. In liver findings, the cardinal feature is hepatomegaly, which can be asymptomatic or associated with hypoglycemia and hyperlipidemia. Cardiac findings are those of a large, failing heart. If muscle involvement is present, there can be marked hypotonia or complaints of muscle pain and cramps on exercise. Kidney changes include bilateral enlargement, renal stones, and symptoms of hyperuricemia, as well as excess excretion of amino acids, phosphate, glucose, and galactose. Central nervous system involvement may include delayed motor and mental development, ataxia, hypotonia, spasticity, rigidity, and death.

Diagnosis, treatment, and prognosis depend on the exact definition of the biochemical defect by tissue evaluation. Many new (and as yet unproved) therapy procedures require precise diagnosis.

Prenatal diagnosis is indicated in types II and IVA, but in types I, II, VI, IX, and X, prenatal diagnosis is probably not indicated, because the conditions are compatible with normal life.

DISORDERS OF LIPID METABOLISM

Gaucher's Disease

Gaucher's disease is a lysosomal storage disease caused by a deficiency of the enzyme glucosylceramide β-glucosidase. Its substrate, glycocerebroside, accumulates in phagocytic cells throughout the body, primarily those of the liver, spleen, and bone marrow. Its incidence ranges from 1 per 5000 to 1 per 10,000 among Jews of Eastern European origin.

Clinically, it presents in 3 forms. The adult form, or type I, is characterized by splenomegaly, hepatomegaly, anemia, thrombocytopenia, and erosion of the cortices of long bones. Some adults may succumb as early as the third decade, but many are symptom-free until the seventh or eighth decade. Neurologic symptoms are rare. In type II, the infantile form, there is pronounced neurologic and little visceral involvement. Symptoms may occur by age 3 months, and death usually occurs by age 2. The third form, type III, or juvenile, has a wide variety of clinical signs and symptoms, including both neurologic and visceral involvement. These patients survive longer than do those with type II. Each clinical type is inherited as an autosomal recessive trait and "breeds true" (ie, is passed to the next generation without alteration).

Laboratory studies reveal an elevated serum acid phosphatase, but definitive diagnosis of this disorder requires the demonstration of a diminished leukocyte β-glucosidase level (7–15% of normal) or demonstration of Gaucher cells in the bone marrow by electron microscopy.

Treatment is supportive. Splenectomy is indicated only when hypersplenism occurs. Attempts at enzyme replacement by transplantation of a kidney and a spleen seemed encouraging initially, but both patients died within a year of transplantation. Infusion enzyme replacement therapy shows some success but has not been tried on a long-term basis.

Desnick RJ, Gatt S, Grabowski GA: Gaucher's disease: A century of delineation and research. *Prog Clin Biol Res* 1982; **95**:309.

Niemann-Pick Disease (Sphingomyelin Lipidosis)

Niemann-Pick disease is a rare autosomal recessive disorder characterized by the excessive storage of phospholipids, especially sphingomyelin, in the reticuloendothelial system. Manifestations occur early in infancy and consist primarily of hepatosplenomegaly and central nervous system involvement, with mental retardation and convulsions. Other symptoms and signs include diffuse pulmonary infiltration, cutaneous lesions, a cherry-red macular spot, gastrointestinal bleeding, lymph node enlargement, thrombocytopenia, anemia, and foam cells in hepatic or marrow biopsies. Definitive diagnosis is established by demonstrating sphingomyelinase deficiency in white blood cells and cultured skin fibroblasts.

Treatment is supportive. Death usually occurs during childhood.

G$_{M2}$ Gangliosidoses (Tay-Sachs Disease)

Tay-Sachs disease is an autosomal recessive disease that is clinically apparent by age 5–6 months and invariably leads to death by age 3–4 years. The enzyme hexosaminidase A is absent, resulting in an accumulation of G_{M2} ganglioside in the ganglion cells. The destruction of the ganglion cells is accompanied by glial proliferation and myelin degeneration. Clinically, psychomotor retardation, hypotonia, dementia, and blindness (associated with the cherry-red spot on the retina) occur. There are 2 rare variants, each with the same clinical and pathologic course but with different hexosaminidase defects.

The current application of genetic principles to this disease may well make it a model for genetic counseling for inborn errors of metabolism: the disease occurs primarily in Jews who have emigrated from northeastern Europe. With the advent of blood tests for hexosaminidase activity, discernment of the magnitude of the disease and identification of heterozygotes and affected fetuses are possible. In New York City, the Jewish population has a carrier rate of 1:30 and the non-Jewish population 1:300. With the help of synagogues, education and mass screening of this at-risk Jewish population have been undertaken, and genetic counseling has been given to the carriers. No specific therapy is available. Enzyme replacement is not available.

DISORDERS OF PORPHYRIN METABOLISM

The porphyrins are cyclic compounds that are the precursors of heme and other important enzymes and pigments. Enzymatic defects in the heme synthetic pathways cause a group of disorders, the porphyrias, which may be either hereditary or acquired. These diseases have long been of interest because of their unusual range of clinical symptoms as well as the relative ease of identifying small amounts of porphyrin in the urine.

The porphyrias are classified into 2 main categories, depending on whether the excessive porphyrin production takes place in the liver or in bone marrow. The classification is as follows:

Hepatic porphyrias
Acute intermittent porphyria
Variegate porphyria
Hereditary coproporphyria
Porphyria cutanea tarda

Erythropoietic porphyrias
Congenital porphyria
Erythropoietic protoporphyria

Hepatic Porphyria

The hepatic porphyrias are a group of chemically and biochemically distinct diseases whose site of abnormal porphyrin metabolism is the liver.

A. Acute Intermittent Porphyria: This is an autosomal dominant disease with worldwide distribution. Its biochemical defect, a decrease in uroporphyrinogen-1-synthase, seems to be generalized, for it has been reported in liver cells, erythrocytes, fibroblasts, and lymphocytes. The disease is clinically latent throughout adult life in about 90% of the people who inherit the gene defect. For the remaining 10%, it is at puberty or shortly thereafter that the first symptoms occur. Characteristically, intermittent abdominal and neurologic manifestations occur with variable severity. The abdominal symptoms are often the presenting complaint. They may be mild, such as nausea, vomiting, and colicky pain, but often they are severe enough to present as an acute abdomen without fever or leukocytosis. There may be multiple surgical scars on the abdomen. Neurologic findings are just as variable, including paresthesia, hypesthesia, neuritic pain, wristdrop and footdrop, psychoses, convulsions, and quadriplegia. Significantly, there is no associated cutaneous sensitivity. Four exogenous factors may convert the latent disease to a manifest disease: drugs, steroids, starvation, and infection. The drugs include barbiturates, sulfonamides, and griseofulvin, and the steroids include estrogens. No doubt endogenous factors also play a role in precipitating an attack. Death due to respiratory paralysis may occur in 25% of patients with acute attacks.

Diagnosis is suspected by noting that freshly voided urine left standing in light and air turns dark. Definitive diagnosis is made by demonstrating increased porphobilinogens (PBG) and aminolevulinic acid (ALA) in the urine. A limited number of laboratories are able to demonstrate the enzymatic defect in erythrocytes.

B. Variegate Porphyria: This is an autosomal dominant disease first recognized in the Afrikaners of South Africa but now known in people in Sweden, Holland, England, and the USA. Its biochemical defect is a deficiency of protoporphyrinogen oxidase. Clinical symptoms do not appear until the third decade. In addition to acute abdominal and neurologic manifestations such as those that occur in acute intermittent porphyria, cutaneous manifestations also appear, characterized by increased sensitivity of exposed skin to minor mechanical trauma and to light. Barbiturates and sulfonamides can induce the condition. Diagnosis rests on demonstration of continuous excretion of protoporphyrins and coproporphyrins in the feces.

C. Hereditary Coproporphyria: This autosomal dominant disease resembles variegate porphyria in its photosensitivity, abdominal and neurologic manifestations, and exacerbations. However, it is a much milder disease, and latent cases are frequent. The distinction is a biochemical one: in hereditary coproporphyria, there is a steady excretion of large amounts of coproporphyrin in the feces and, to a lesser extent, the urine. The enzymatic defect, a decrease in coproporphyrinogen oxidase, can be demonstrated in erythrocytes.

D. Porphyria Cutanea Tarda: Porphyria cutanea tarda, the most common form of porphyria, is an autosomal dominant disease caused by partial deficiency of the enzyme uroporphyrinogen decarboxylase. Family studies indicate it can present as an overt, subclinical, or latent disorder. Although its distribution is worldwide, it is most common among the Bantu of Africa. It occurs more often in males, at middle age, with symptoms limited to the skin. Abdominal and neurologic manifestations do not occur. Photosensitivity is the major clinical finding, but hypertrichosis of the forehead and hyperpigmentation of the exposed skin are also prevalent. Estrogens, busulfan, barbiturates, phenytoin, and tolbutamide can induce the condition. For unknown reasons, all patients have evidence of liver dysfunction. This may be due to concomitant diseases (eg, alcoholic cirrhosis, tuberculosis, intestinal disease) as well as to overproduction of uroporphyrin, which in itself may be toxic to the liver. When the disease is of long duration, there is increased risk of hepatocellular carcinoma. Pathologically, there is hepatic parenchymal iron overload caused by increased saturation of iron-binding protein with iron. Biochemical evaluation indicates increased excretion of uroporphyrins with a variable amount of fecal porphyrins. A new method of measuring plasma porphyrins appears useful in diagnosis as well as in following the effectiveness of therapy.

A toxic form of this disease became apparent in 1956 when there was an explosive outbreak of porphyria in eastern Turkey. The chronic ingestion of hexachlorobenzene, a fungicidal agent used in wheat, inhibited hepatic uroporphyrinogen decarboxylase, thus causing the disease. No genetic factors were involved.

Erythropoietic Porphyrias

A. Congenital Porphyria: Congenital erythropoietic porphyria is a very rare autosomal recessive disease with worldwide distribution. It is caused by an enzyme defect in the erythroid series of the bone marrow that results in an excess deposition of porphyrins in the tissues. Clinically, it presents as a well-defined syndrome in the newborn period or shortly thereafter. There is photosensitivity, erythrodontia (seen most readily with a Wood lamp), and fluctuating red urine that is usually associated with hemolytic anemia. The skin changes, occurring primarily on the hands and face, present as vesicles and bullae and progress to scarring and mutilation. The disease is slowly progressive, and death results from the hemolytic anemia or intercurrent infection. Splenectomy may be effective in decreasing hemolysis. Few patients survive beyond age 40. The clinical diagnosis is confirmed biochemically by demonstrating the porphyrinuria, especially of uroporphyrin I.

B. Erythropoietic Protoporphyria: Erythropoietic protoporphyria is an autosomal dominant disease with partial penetrance. Many latent forms exist, and these may be more common. The disease is mild, with clinical manifestations limited to the skin. It appears in childhood or early adolescence as a fluctuating solar urticaria or solar eczema. Intense painful itching, erythema, and edema occur and progress to chronic skin changes, particularly on the hands. Occasionally, there is mild hemolytic anemia. Liver disease due to porphyrin deposition occasionally occurs and may progress to cirrhosis. Cholelithiasis due to precipitated protoporphyrins may be present. Fluorescence microscopy confirms the diagnosis by demonstrating the excess protoporphyrin in the red cells.

Treatment of Porphyrias

Preventive medicine is the most important feature in the long-term management of patients with porphyria. This includes a careful discussion of precipitating factors as well as information about prenatal diagnosis. Precipitating factors include infection, emotional stress, "crash" diets, and the use of drugs such as alcohol, estrogens, and barbiturates. Women who have acute attacks at the time of menstruation will be helped by contraceptives that prevent ovulation. Patients with photosensitivity should avoid direct sunlight or should use dermatologic sunscreen preparations. The oral sun protective agent β-carotene (Solatene) in doses of 15–180 mg/d is effective.

Symptomatic treatment is important in the management of abdominal and neurologic manifestations. Mild abdominal symptoms can be controlled with the use of chlorpromazine or other phenothiazines; propoxyphene can be used in pain in the extremities; meperidine is effective in severe pain. Propranolol can stop persistent sinus tachycardia. Observation must be continuous, since progressive paralysis can cause respiratory failure, which in turn requires respiratory assistance. Physical therapy should be used to prevent secondary complications of neuropathy.

The acute attack of porphyria should be terminated as quickly as possible to prevent lasting neuronal damage. Hematin is the drug of first choice. At the dosage level of 3–4 mg/kg intravenously, there is a report of a dramatic recovery in 25 of 31 attacks in 20 patients, without any side effects. In 1978, there was a case report of the successful use of hematin prophylactically. Another method—high carbohydrate intake achieved with levulose, 400–500 mg/d intravenously—is also successful in treating acute attacks of porphyria. The clinical response is variable, and a rebound phenomenon with symptoms of a mild acute attack may occur 24–48 hours after infusion. Both hematin and high-carbohydrate intake act by suppressing hepatic aminolevulinic synthase, thus reducing the overproduction of α-aminolevulinic acid and porphobilinogen.

Recent isolated case reports indicate that large doses of propranolol also can be effective therapy for acute porphyria.

In cutaneous erythropoietic porphyria, hematin therapy, with its marked repressive effect on porphyrin synthesis, has produced remissions lasting several years. Splenectomy, which is helpful in the management of hemolytic anemia, may also reduce photosensitivity and porphyrin excretion.

In porphyria cutanea tarda, phlebotomy lowers urinary uroporphyrin excretion and induces the remission of skin lesions. This is probably related to the depletion of hepatic iron stores. In a series of 15 patients, chloroquine therapy, 250 mg daily for 5 days, produced clinical improvement in 10 patients and full remission in 7 others. Clinical response did not correlate with uroporphyrin levels, but in 6 patients it did correlate positively with immunofluorescence tests on skin biopsy. In some cases, plasmapheresis was effective.

In protoporphyria, a case report reveals a 15-month remission of photosensitivity symptoms after several transfusions with washed, packed red blood cells. The early recognition of liver disease in protoporphyria is important, for it may prove fatal. Cholestyramine, 4 g 3 times daily before meals, may reverse hepatic disease by binding protoporphyrin in the intestines and interrupting its enterohepatic circulation.

Abramowicz M (editor): Hemin infusions in acute intermittent porphyria. *Med Lett Drugs Ther* 1984;**26**:42.

Del Batlle AM (editor): Porphyrins and porphyria: Etiopathogenesis, clinics and treatment. *Int J Biochem* 1980;**12**:1.

Schmid R: The hepatic porphyrias. *Semin Liver Dis* 1982;**2**:1.

Spiva D: Erythrocytapheresis and plasma exchange in the management of the porphyrias. *Prog Clin Biol Res* 1982;**106**:331.

Tsega E et al: Chloroquine in the treatment of porphyria cutanea tarda. *Trans R Soc Trop Med Hyg* 1981;**75**:401.

OTHER METABOLIC DISORDERS

Cystic Fibrosis

Cystic fibrosis of the pancreas is one of the common inherited diseases among whites of European ancestry. This autosomal recessive disease has an incidence of 1:1500 white births and 1:17,000 black births in the USA. Its unknown defect involves all exocrine glands, causing high-protein, highly viscous secretions that readily obstruct the ducts of the body. These obstructions cause the major clinical manifestations of the disease.

Initially, cystic fibrosis was recognized only in infants and children, in whom it presented as meconium ileus in the newborn period or as chronic pulmonary and gastrointestinal disease in growth-retarded children. With the improvement of diagnostic tests, as well as with vigorous treatment, patients are now alive and functioning well in their mid 40s.

The major clinical signs and symptoms involve the gastrointestinal and pulmonary tracts. Pancreatic insufficiency with steatorrhea and azotorrhea is present in 95% of patients, but in adults, in contrast to children, it is rarely symptomatic. Twenty-five percent of adults have a meconium ileus equivalent (abnormal fecal accumulation) causing partial intestinal obstruction and intussusception. Generalized biliary cirrhosis, cholelithiasis (12%), and rectal prolapse may occur. These gastrointestinal complications contribute to the malnutrition and growth retardation in pediatric patients.

It is the disease in the pulmonary tract, however, that determines the life of the patient. It occurs in 97% of patients and is the major cause of morbidity and mortality. The tenacious secretions and their secondary infections cause sinusitis, chronic bronchitis, recurrent pneumonias, bronchiectasis, hyperaeration, and cor pulmonale. Elsewhere, the sweat glands—with increased sodium and chloride secretion—can cause a depletion syndrome, especially in hot weather. The salt in the sweat may have a corrosive effect on metal and leather ornaments and clothing in direct contact with the skin. With respect to the reproductive tract, women can be fertile, whereas all affected men are sterile; atresia of the vas deferens and an abnormality in the exocrine glands cause sterility in the presence of spermatogenesis. Women who do not have pancreatic insufficiency tolerate pregnancy without undue hazard. Those with pancreatic insufficiency may have permanent deterioration of pulmonary function.

Diagnosis is readily and easily made in the presence of clinical symptoms by a demonstration of a sodium and chloride concentration greater than 60 meq/L in sweat induced by pilocarpine iontophoresis. The specimen should be 125–375 mg (average, 250 mg); a sweat sample of less than 40 mg is inadequate for accurate assay.

Therapy should be vigorous and continuous, for recent studies have shown that adequately treated adult patients can have a successful intellectual, socioeconomic, and marital life. A high-calorie, low-fat diet with multivitamin supplementation is necessary, since absorption is incomplete. The adequate dose of pancreatic enzyme replacement (Cotazyme, Viokase) is determined by the clinical response of a good growth pattern, an improvement in stool consistency, and a decrease in the number of bowel movements. If the enzyme replacements are given with cimetidine, 20 mg/kg body weight/24 h, or sodium bicarbonate, 15 g/m²/24 h, there is a significant decrease in fat and nitrogen excretion, presumably due to the prevention of acid-peptide destruction of the pancreatic enzymes in the stomach. A new form of pancrelipase supplement, enteric-coated microspheres in a gelatin capsule (Pancrease), passes intact through the stomach to the intestines, where it enhances fat absorption and allows a more normal diet. The daily average dose is about 5 tablets. The treatment of meconium ileus is, of course, surgical. The intussusception and fecal accumulation in adults require enemas of diatrizoate sodium (Gastrografin or Hypaque). Supplementary salt is needed, especially during hot weather, febrile episodes, and physical exertion; adults require over 4 g/d. For the respiratory tract, attention is directed to adequate drainage and prevention of infection. Adequate hydration, daily pulmonary percussion and drainage, bronchodilators, expectorants, and daily antibiotics are used in management. Patients with thick, tenacious sputum can use acetylcysteine (Mucomyst) for treatment, but this agent should not be used for prophylaxis. Many medical centers prescribe mist tents, but the efficacy of this method has not yet been proved. In managing the many complications of cystic fibrosis, a positive therapeutic environment should be provided in order to minimize the patient's anxiety and depression.

Genetic counselors are able to respond only with statistical answers to questions about risks to patients and their parents, for there is no reproducible biochemical marker of the mutant gene.

Matson JA, Capen CV: Pregnancy in the cystic fibrosis patient: An update. *J Reprod Med* 1982;**27**:373.

Park RW Grand RJ: Gastrointestinal manifestations of cystic fibrosis: A review. *Gastroenterology* 1981;**81**:1143.

Primary Hyperoxaluria

Primary hyperoxaluria is an autosomal recessive disease characterized by continuous excessive synthesis of oxalic acid, leading to increased excretion of oxalates in the urine as well as to deposition of calcium oxalate in the tissues, especially the kidneys, synoviums, and myocardium. Biochemically, there are 2 types, each with its own enzyme defect; clinically, they are indistinguishable.

The disease presents in childhood, usually before age 5 years. There is either asymptomatic gross hematuria or typical renal colic due to calcium oxalate stones. Rarely, there are symptoms of renal tubular acidosis. The clinical course is one of progressive renal insufficiency, leading to death by age 20 years. Extrarenal manifestations are arthritis and cardiac disease. The disease can be simulated in animals and humans by pyridoxine deficiency.

Diagnosis depends on demonstration of excess renal oxalic acid excretion (normal, 60 mg of oxalic acid/1.73 m²) in the absence of pyridoxine deficiency and ileal disease. The 2 types of the disease can be distinguished by measuring the amounts of glyoxylic, glycolic, and L-glyceric acid in the urine.

There is no specific treatment for primary hyperoxaluria at present. Pyridoxine, 100 mg 4 times daily, can reduce oxalate excretion, but the effect is not striking. In some cases, pyridoxine in high doses (1 g/24 h) decreased oxalate excretion by 60–70%, with corresponding clinical benefit. Thiazide diuretics, such as bendroflumethiazide, 2.5–5 mg daily, are helpful in stone prophylaxis, because they decrease the Ca:Mg ratio. All measures that reduce the risk of renal stones should be used, including forced fluids, a high-phosphate regimen, oral magnesium oxide, and allopurinol. Terminal renal failure is managed by chronic hemodialysis. In most cases, renal transplantation has not been successful, because oxalate crystals quickly accumulate in the transplanted kidney. There are rare cases of 3-year survivals. All siblings should be screened for hyperoxaluria, because early treatment of the asymptomatic patient decreases the morbidity of the disease.

Hallson PC, Rose GA, Sulaiman S: Magnesium reduces calcium oxalate crystal formation in human whole urine. *Clin Sci* 1982;**62:**17.

Marfan's Syndrome

Marfan's syndrome is a generalized disorder of the connective tissue, inherited as an autosomal dominant trait. In its classic form, it has a prevalence of 4–6 cases per 100,000 population, with no racial or ethnic predeliction. Its biochemical basis remains unknown. Clinically, it is manifested in the skeletal system, the eye, and the cardiovascular system, but in a given case there is such great variability in clinical expression that manifestations may not be present in all 3 systems.

The skeletal system characteristically shows extraordinarily long tubular bones, causing arachnodactyly and anomalous skeletal proportions. The patient is usually taller than might be expected on the basis of age and family background, but the excessive length of the arms and legs in relation to the trunk is even more indicative. Other skeletal anomalies include "tower skull," kyphoscoliosis, hyperextensibility of the joints, and genu recurvatum.

In the eye, 50–80% of the patients have lens dislocation that is bilateral, probably occurs in utero, and rarely progresses. Myopia and detached retinas are also described.

An elastin abnormality accounts for the weakness of the aortic media, leading to aortic regurgitation or aortic dilatation or dissection. Prolapse of the posterior mitral valve leaflet is present in 80% of cases. All patients are at risk for endocarditis.

Treatment is directed at the cardiovascular system, for it accounts for 95% of the deaths. Echocardiography is the most sensitive means of detecting early aortic changes. Patients are examined yearly to follow the course of the slow but progressive aortic dilatation. In adults, when the aortic diameter reaches 5.5 cm, the life-threatening complications of aortic rupture—dissection or aortic regurgitation—may occur. Prophylactic repair of the ascending aorta is now performed with a mortality rate of less than 10%. In addition, aortic valves have been successfully replaced. Medical management involves treatment with propranolol or reserpine to reduce the abruptness of ventricular ejections in the hope of protecting the aorta. With skeletal defects, treatment is primarily for scoliosis, which is the most deforming and disabling complication. Eyes are examined annually to diagnose refractive errors, prevent amblyopia, and detect early retinal detachment. The lens rarely requires removal.

Women with Marfan's syndrome have an increased rate of early spontaneous abortions. If patients have minimal cardiovascular disease, the risk of maternal death is low, but patients with preexisting aortic regurgitation, aortic root dilatation, or other severe cardiovascular disease have significant risk of death from aortic dissection. Counseling regarding pregnancy risk requires evaluation of cardiovascular status, including echocardiographic determination of aortic root diameter.

In 1979, before cardiovascular surgery was available, the average survival age was 32 years. Survivors aged 82 years have also been reported.

Abraham PA et al: Marfan syndrome: Demonstration of abnormal elastin in aorta. *J Clin Invest* 1982;**70:**1245.

Pyeritz RE: Maternal and fetal complications of pregnancy in the Marfan's disease. *Am J Med* 1981;**71:**784.

● ● ●

References

(For additional references, see Chapter 21.)

Baraitser M: *Oxford Monographs of Medical Genetics: The Genetics of Neurologic Disorders.* Oxford Univ Press, 1982.

Emery AEH: *Elements of Medical Genetics,* 6th ed. Churchill Livingstone, 1983.

Emery AEH, Rimoin DL: *The Principles and Practice of Medical Genetics.* 2 vols. Churchill Livingstone, 1983.

Feingold M, Pashayan HM: *Genetics and Birth Defects in Clinical Practice.* Little Brown, 1983.

Garrod AE: *Inborn Errors in Metabolism.* Oxford Univ Press, 1963.

Goodman RM, Gorlin RJ: *Atlas of the Face in Genetic Disorders,* 2nd ed. Mosby, 1977.

Harper PS: *Practical Genetic Counselling.* Univ Park Press, 1981.

Harris H, Hirschhorn K (editors): *Advances in Human Genetics.* Plenum Press. [Annual.]

LeBeau MM et al: Association of an inversion of chromosome 16 with abnormal marrow eosinophils in acute myelomonocytic leukemia: A unique cytogenetic-clinicopathological association. *N Engl J Med* 1983;**309:**630.

Prenatal Diagnosis. [All issues; publication began in Jan 1981.]

Roman HL et al (editors): *Annual Review of Genetics.* Annual Reviews, Inc. [Annual.]

Simpson JL et al: *Genetics in Obstetrics and Gynecology.* Grune & Stratton, 1982.

Smith DW: *Recognizable Patterns of Human Malformation,* 3rd ed. Saunders, 1982.

Stanbury JB et al (editors): *The Metabolic Basis of Inherited Disease,* 5th ed. McGraw-Hill, 1983.

Steinberg AG, Bearn AG: *Progress in Medical Genetics.* Grune & Stratton. [Annual.]

Winick M: *Nutritional Management of Genetic Disorders.* Wiley Interscience, 1980.

33 | Malignant Disorders

Sydney E. Salmon, MD

Neoplastic disorders of specific organ systems are discussed elsewhere in this book. It is nonetheless worth emphasizing here that early diagnosis through screening is important for several specific neoplasms: cervical Papanicolaou smears should be obtained at least every 2 years in women, and breast self-examination should be carried out monthly. Mammograms should be obtained starting at age 45–50 and repeated regularly in women who have had prior breast cancer or have a strong family history of breast cancer. Rectal examination and tests for occult blood in feces should be done annually after age 40. The major features of this chapter are medical aspects of cancer, including (1) unusual symptoms and syndromes that may be important in the diagnosis and management of cancer, (2) the diagnosis and treatment of emergency problems and complications of cancer, (3) cancer chemotherapy for advanced disease, and (4) adjuvant chemotherapy for micrometastases of primary cancers.

THE PARANEOPLASTIC SYNDROMES

The clinical manifestations of cancer are usually due to pressure effects of local tumor growth; to infiltration or metastatic deposition of tumor cells in a variety of organs in the body; or to certain systemic symptoms. Except in the case of functioning tumors such as those of the endocrine glands, systemic symptoms of cancer usually are not specific, often consisting of weakness, anorexia, and weight loss. In the paraneoplastic syndromes ("beyond tumor growth"), clinical findings may resemble those of primary endocrine, metabolic, hematologic, or neuromuscular disorders. At present, the mechanisms for such remote effects can be classed in 3 groups: (1) effects initiated by a tumor product (eg, carcinoid syndrome), (2) effects of destruction of normal tissues by tumor (eg, hypercalcemia with osteolytic skeletal metastases), and (3) effects due to unknown mechanisms (eg, osteoarthropathy with bronchogenic carcinoma). In paraneoplastic syndromes associated with ectopic hormone production, tumor tissue itself secretes the hormone that produces the syndrome. Ectopic hormones secreted by neoplasms are often "prohormones" of higher molecular weight than those secreted by the more differentiated normal endocrine cell.

The paraneoplastic syndromes are of considerable clinical importance for the following reasons:

(1) They sometimes accompany relatively limited neoplastic growth and may provide the clinician with an early clue to the presence of certain types of cancer. In some cases, early diagnosis may favorably affect the prognosis.

(2) The pathologic (metabolic or toxic) effects of the syndrome may constitute a more urgent hazard to the patient's life than the underlying cancer (eg, hypercalcemia, hyponatremia).

(3) Effective treatment of the tumor should be accompanied by resolution of the paraneoplastic syndrome, and, conversely, recurrence of the cancer may be heralded by return of the systemic symptoms.

Not all endocrine or metabolic syndromes associated with cancer are necessarily "paraneoplastic." In some instances, the secretory product or syndrome results from continuation of function of the normal precursor cell type that became malignant. The function of the cell may be a normal one greatly exaggerated (eg, adrenal carcinoma, insulinoma, carcinoid syndrome) by the greater number of functioning cells. Although the details of the mechanisms of some metabolic effects are not known, in some instances the identical symptom complex (eg, hypercalcemia) may be induced by entirely different mechanisms. Hypercalcemia may be due to secretions of parathyroid hormone, an osteoclast-activating factor, prostaglandins, or other hormone secretion by the tumor or to direct invasion of the skeleton by metastases. In each situation, effective antitumor treatment usually results in return of serum calcium to normal, although supportive measures may also be of benefit.

Common paraneoplastic syndromes and endocrine secretions associated with functional cancers are summarized in Table 33–1.

Mundy GR et al: The hypercalcemia of cancer: Clinical implications and pathogenic mechanisms. *N Engl J Med* 1984;**310:** 1718.

Table 33—1. Paraneoplastic syndromes and certain endocrine secretions associated with cancer.

Hormone Excess or Syndrome	Broncho-genic Carcinoma	Breast Carcinoma	Renal Carcinoma	Adrenal Carcinoma	Hepa-toma	Multiple Myeloma	Lym-phoma	Thy-moma	Prostatic Carcinoma	Pancreatic Carcinoma	Chorio-carcinoma
Hypercalcemia	++	++++	++	++	+	++++	+	+	++	+	+
Cushing's syndrome	+++		+	+++				++	+	++	
Inappropriate ADH secretion	+++						+			+	
Hypoglycemia				+	++		+				
Gonadotropins	+					+					++++
Thyrotropin											+++
Polycythemia			+++	+	++						
Erythroid aplasia								++			
Fever			+++		++		+++	++		+	
Neuromyopathy	++	+						++	+	+	
Dermatomyositis	++	+								+	
Coagulopathy	+	++			+	+			+++	+++	
Thrombophlebitis			+						+	+++	
Immunologic deficiency						+++	+++	+++			

Slungaard A et al: Pulmonary carcinoma with eosinophilia: Demonstration of a tumor-derived eosinophilopoietic factor. *N Engl J Med* 1983;**309**:778.

Stolinsky DC: Paraneoplastic syndromes. *West J Med* 1980; **132**:189.

DIAGNOSIS & TREATMENT OF EMERGENCIES & COMPLICATIONS OF MALIGNANT DISEASE

Cancer is a chronic disease, but acute emergency complications may occur as a consequence of local accumulations of tumor (spinal cord compression, superior vena cava syndrome, malignant effusions, etc) or of more generalized systemic effects of cancer (hypercalcemia, septicemia and opportunistic infections, disseminated intravascular coagulation, hyperuricemia, carcinoid syndrome, etc). Prompt and effective treatment of such complications is one of the most important aspects of management of the patient with advanced cancer.

Yarboro JW (editor): Oncologic emergencies. *Semin Oncol* 1978;**5**:123. [Entire issue.]

SPINAL CORD COMPRESSION

Spinal cord compression by tumor mass is manifested by progressive weakness and sensory changes in the lower extremities, back pain, and blockage of contrast material as shown by myelography. It occurs as a complication of lymphoma or multiple myeloma, carcinomas of the lung, prostate, breast, and colon, and certain other neoplasms. Back pain at the level of the lesion occurs in over 80% of cases and may be aggravated by lying down, weight bearing, sneezing, or coughing. Since involvement is usually extradural, a mixture of nerve root and spinal cord symptoms often develops.

The initial findings of impending cord compression may be quite subtle, and there should be a high index of suspicion when cancer patients develop weakness of the lower extremities or back pain. Prompt diagnosis and therapy are essential to prevent permanent residual or spinal cord damage. Once paralysis develops, it is usually irreversible, whereas patients who are treated promptly may have complete return of function and may respond favorably to subsequent anticancer therapy.

Spinal cord compression may require a team approach to management: The medical oncologist usually coordinates the diagnostic and therapeutic program with the help of the radiologist, radiotherapist, and neurosurgeon. While bone films usually show evidence of vertebral metastases, they are not a substitute for myelography. When the symptoms and neurologic examination are at all suggestive of a diagnosis of cord compression, an emergency myelogram should be performed, usually by a neurosurgeon, who then follows the patient in case decompression laminectomy becomes necessary. If a block is demonstrated on myelography, the contrast medium is often left in the spinal canal so that alleviation of the block can subsequently be demonstrated on follow-up x-rays after treatment. Contrast-enhanced CT scans can also be useful in diagnosing spinal cord compression. CT scans are particularly useful in patients with paravertebral soft tissue masses, and they can also demonstrate the exact route of tumor extension through the vertebral bone.

Emergency treatment: Radiation therapy to the involved area of the block and 2 adjacent vertebrae above and below represents the treatment of choice. The addition of chemotherapy is occasionally of use in treating lymphomas.

Emergency surgery is indicated as the primary treatment if the patient is not known to have cancer. Aside from this, decompression laminectomy is indicated only in patients with extremely rapid progression of signs and symptoms. Patients must be followed closely, as occasional patients may require operation if disease continues to progress despite treatment or if spinal instability is a problem.

When the block is relieved, the flow of contrast in the rest of the canal should be assessed, as blocks due to tumor (especially lymphoma) often are multiple. Surgery for spinal cord compression may also be useful with recurrent symptoms of cord compression at the same site after a long, symptom-free interval.

Rodicho LD et al: Early diagnosis of spinal epidural metastases. *Am J Med* 1981;**70**:1181.

SUPERIOR VENA CAVA SYNDROME

Superior vena cava syndrome is a potentially fatal complication of bronchogenic carcinoma, lymphomas, and certain other neoplasms that metastasize to the mediastinum. It is characterized by brawny edema and flushing of the head and neck and dilated neck and arm veins, and it often develops gradually over 2–3 weeks. Partial syndromes may result from subclavian vein obstruction. The onset of symptoms is acute or subacute. Venous pressure in the upper extremities is increased, and bilateral brachial venography or sodium pertechnetate Tc 99m scanning demonstrates a block to the flow of contrast material into the right heart as well as large collateral veins. The patient is often in a state of low cardiac output and is at risk of sudden death from cardiovascular collapse. Although the underlying carcinoma is usually incurable when the condition develops, emergency therapy for this syndrome, which is not necessarily a terminal event, can provide effective palliation for prolonged periods of time (particularly in small cell carcinoma,

for which continued chemotherapy can be quite effective). Therapy should be initiated within hours of recognition. Treatment is sometimes indicated even when the diagnosis of cancer has not been confirmed histologically, since the syndrome is almost always due to cancer, and thoracotomy or mediastinoscopy may lead to death. In such unproved cases of cancer, the block should be unequivocally demonstrated angiographically, and other signs of tumor should be present on chest x-ray as well.

Emergency treatment consists of (1) administration of intravenous cyclophosphamide (1 g/m²) or freshly mixed mechlorethamine (0.4 mg/kg) through a lower extremity vein (to initiate tumor shrinkage); (2) intravenous injection of a potent parenteral diuretic (eg, ethacrynic acid) to relieve the edematous component of vena caval compression; and (3) mediastinal irradiation, starting within 24 hours, with a treatment plan designed to give a high daily dose but a short total course of therapy to rapidly shrink the local tumor even further. Intensive combined therapy will reverse the process in up to 90% of patients. In patients with a subacute presentation, radiation therapy alone usually suffices.

The ultimate prognosis depends on the nature of the primary neoplasm. Even in non-small cell bronchogenic carcinoma, occasional patients have slowly growing tumors that may not cause further symptoms for considerable periods of time.

Perez CA, Presant CA, Van Amburg AL III: Management of superior vena cava syndrome. *Semin Oncol* 1978;**5**:123.

MALIGNANT EFFUSIONS

The development of effusions in closed compartments such as the pleural, pericardial, and peritoneal spaces presents significant diagnostic and therapeutic problems in patients with advanced neoplasms. Most malignant effusions are not acute emergencies, but they can be if they accumulate rapidly or occur in the pericardial space. Although direct involvement (thickening) of the serous surface with tumor appears to be the most frequent initiating factor in such cases, not all effusions in cancer patients are malignant. Benign processes such as congestive heart failure, pulmonary embolus, trauma, and infection (eg, tuberculosis) may be responsible, mimicking the effects of a neoplasm. Bloody effusions are usually malignant but occasionally are due to embolus with infarction or trauma. Chylous effusions may be associated with thoracic duct obstruction or may result from mediastinal lymph node enlargement in lymphoma. Cytologic or cell block examination of the fluid—or hook needle biopsy (eg, with the Cope pleural biopsy needle)—should be used to prove that the effusion is truly neoplastic before local therapy is used to prevent recurrence. Pericardial effusions should be tapped with continuous electrocardiographic monitoring with a V lead attached to the pericardiocentesis needle so that the epicardium will be detected should it be contacted, or alternatively with the aid of ultrasonic localization. Pericardiocentesis is ideally carried out in a cardiac catheterization laboratory.

The management of malignant effusions should be appropriate to the severity of involvement. Effusions due to lung, ovarian, and breast carcinoma often require more than simple drainage. In other neoplasms, simple drainage is sometimes sufficient, especially if it coincides with the initiation of effective systemic chemotherapy. Drainage of a large pleural effusion can be accomplished rapidly and with relative safety with a closed system using a disposable phlebotomy set connected to a vacuum phlebotomy bottle after the needle has been passed through the skin of the thorax. Thoracentesis performed in this fashion requires very little manipulation of the patient and prevents inadvertent pneumothorax associated with multiple changes of a stopcock connected to a syringe. Ultrasonography may facilitate removal of localized or loculated effusions. For recurrent effusions, closed water-seal drainage with a chest tube for 3–4 days is an effective way to seal off the pleural space. Post-tap films are always indicated after thoracentesis to assess the results and rule out pneumothorax.

Recurrent effusions that do not respond to repeated taps or a chest tube may often be controlled by instillation of tetracycline, bleomycin, quinacrine, or mechlorethamine. These agents will eliminate or suppress effusion due to carcinoma in two-thirds of patients. The alkylating agent thiotepa and the antibiotic bleomycin appear to be preferable for suppression of ascites, since they produce less local pain and discomfort in the peritoneum than do other agents.

The procedure is as follows: Most of the pleural, ascitic, or pericardial fluid is withdrawn. While a free flow of fluid is still present, tetracycline (200 mg), mechlorethamine (20–30 mg), thiotepa (30 mg), or bleomycin (60 mg) is instilled into the cavity. The solution should be freshly mixed at the time of injection. After the drug is injected and the needle withdrawn, the patient is placed in a variety of positions in order to distribute the drug throughout the cavity. On the following day, the remaining fluid is withdrawn from the body cavity. Inasmuch as at least half of the instilled drug is absorbed systemically from the cavity, use of alkylating agents is not advised for patients who already have significant pancytopenia or bone marrow depression due to chemotherapy. In such cases, bleomycin, quinacrine, or tetracycline is indicated, as these agents do not depress the bone marrow. Quinacrine is usually administered in a dose of 200 mg/d for 5 days, with daily drainage of residual fluid. Two or more daily doses of tetracycline are also frequently required.

Nausea and vomiting commonly follow the instillation of mechlorethamine but can often be controlled with prophylactic administration of an antiemetic agent prior to the procedure and at intervals afterward. Pleural pain and fever may occur after intracavitary administration of alkylating agents, tetracycline, or

quinacrine but are more common with the latter compounds. Narcotic analgesics are indicated for pain during the acute period; however, the need for these usually abates within several days. Bleomycin instillation may cause fever but generally is unassociated with significant toxicity. Recent tumor cloning studies have shown that when cytotoxic anticancer drugs are instilled locally and lead to resolution of malignant effusions, they are generally exerting a specific cytotoxic effect. Far higher local concentrations of these drugs are attained than when they are administered systemically. Such effusions can also act as "sanctuaries" in which viable tumor stem cells are protected from systemic chemotherapy. Once a pleural space or other potential space has been effectively sealed with such drug treatments, recurrent effusion is usually not a problem.

Theologides A: Neoplastic cardiac tamponade. *Semin Oncol* 1978;5:181.

HYPERCALCEMIA

Hypercalcemia secondary to cancer is a fairly common medical emergency, particularly in breast carcinoma and multiple myeloma but also with a variety of other cancers. Bone metastasis is not an essential feature of the syndrome. Typical findings in addition to elevated serum calcium are anorexia, nausea and vomiting, constipation, muscular weakness and hyporeflexia, confusion, psychosis, tremor, and lethargy. However, a wide range of symptom complexes may be observed, and in some cases elevated serum calcium is the only abnormal finding. Electrocardiography often shows a shortening of the QT interval. When the serum calcium rises above 12 mg/dL, sudden death due to cardiac arrhythmia or asystole may occur. The tragic consequences of untreated hypercalcemia are best illustrated in the instance of the young mother with breast cancer who dies of unrecognized hypercalcemia. Inasmuch as the underlying cancer can often be palliated for many years after an episode of hypercalcemia, this complication of cancer need not indicate a poor prognosis and should be treated as a medical emergency.

In the absence of signs or symptoms of hypercalcemia, a laboratory report of elevated serum calcium should be repeated immediately to exclude the possibility of error.

Emergency treatment consists of (1) intravenous fluids, 3–4 L daily (including saline infusions); (2) low-calcium diet; (3) prednisone, 60–80 mg/d orally for 4–5 days, followed by tapering; (4) intravenous administration of a potent diuretic (such as furosemide) once saline infusion has been initiated; (5) calcitonin intramuscularly or intravenously; and (6) for severe hypercalcemia (greater than 15 mg/dL) or refractory cases, mithramycin (Mithracin), 25 μg/kg intravenously every other day for 2–4 doses. Although mithramycin therapy is often effective in relieving hypercalcemia and can be used less frequently for chronic management, the drug has significant toxicities, including potential hemorrhagic syndrome. In most instances, however, only a limited number of doses are required, and these complications are unlikely to occur. Mithramycin therapy should therefore be considered as part of the initial management of severe hypercalcemia and as an adjunctive agent in milder cases.

Once the acute hypercalcemic episode has been treated, it is usually appropriate to begin systemic chemotherapy. In the case of breast cancer, hypercalcemia may appear as a "flare" after initiation of estrogen or antiestrogen therapy. Recent evidence suggests that when flares occurring after antiestrogen therapy are suppressed with analgesics and hypocalcemic agents, the patient will often achieve excellent remission with continued therapy. If chronic hypercalcemia persists—even if only to a moderate degree—the patient should be treated with small doses of prednisone alone or with calcitonin or oral sodium phosphate supplements (1–2 g/d) and encouraged to maintain a high fluid intake in the hope of preventing renal damage. When phosphate is used, if no alternative source of phosphate is available, disposable Fleet's Phospho-Soda enemas can be given orally. (*Caution:* Excessive dosage will lead to diarrhea.) Intravenous sodium phosphate infusions are not advisable, since they are associated with extreme danger of metastatic calcification in addition to the hypernatremic effects. Chronic hypercalcemia that is refractory to the above measures can sometimes be managed with once-weekly mithramycin injection, 25 μg/kg intravenously. In most instances, when the cancer responds to chemotherapy, hypercalcemia subsides.

Mundy GR et al: The hypercalcemia of cancer: Clinical implications and pathogenic mechanisms. *N Engl J Med* 1984; **310:**1718.

HYPERURICEMIA & ACUTE URATE NEPHROPATHY

Increased blood levels of uric acid are often observed in patients with neoplasms who are receiving cancer chemotherapy. In this circumstance, hyperuricemia should be viewed as a preventable complication rather than as an acute emergency, inasmuch as uric acid formation can be inhibited with allopurinol. At present, hyperuricemia is most often a complication of treatment for hematologic neoplasms such as leukemia, lymphoma, and myeloma, but it may occur with any form of cancer that undergoes rapid destruction and release of nucleic acid constituents, and in some instances allopurinol will not have been given. Less commonly, certain rapidly proliferating neoplasms with a high nucleic acid turnover (eg, acute leukemia) may be present with hyperuricemia even in the absence of prior chemotherapy. If the patient is also receiving a thiazide diuretic, the

problem may be compounded by decreased urate excretion. Initial follow-up of patients receiving cancer chemotherapy should include measurements of serum uric acid and creatinine as well as complete blood counts. Rapid elevation of the serum uric acid concentration usually does not produce gouty arthritis in these patients but does present the danger of acute urate nephropathy. In this form of acute renal failure, uric acid crystallizes in the distal tubules, the collecting ducts, and the renal parenchyma. The danger of uric acid nephropathy is present when the serum urate concentration is above 15 mg/dL, and in some instances it may rise to as high as 80 mg/dL.

Prophylactic therapy consists of giving allopurinol, 100 mg orally 3 times daily, starting 1 day before initiation of chemotherapy. Allopurinol inhibits xanthine oxidase and prevents conversion of the highly soluble hypoxanthine and xanthine to the relatively insoluble uric acid. Patients who are to receive the purine antagonists mercaptopurine or azathioprine for cancer chemotherapy should be given only 25–35% of the calculated dose if they are also receiving allopurinol, inasmuch as the latter drug potentiates both the effects and toxicity of these drugs.

Emergency therapy for established severe hyperuricemia consists of (1) hydration with 2–4 L of fluid per day; (2) alkalinization of the urine with 6–8 g of sodium bicarbonate per day (to enhance urate solubility); (3) allopurinol, 200 mg 4 times daily orally; and (4) in severe cases, with serum urate levels above 25–30 mg/dL, emergency hemodialysis or peritoneal dialysis. *Caution:* Once the uropathy is established, items 1–3 are in fact dangerous until some means of getting rid of excess fluid is assured.

Since patients who suffer from this complication are often entering a stage of complete remission of the neoplasm, the prognosis is good if renal damage can be prevented.

BACTERIAL SEPSIS IN CANCER PATIENTS

Many patients with disseminated neoplasms have increased susceptibility to infection. In some instances, this results from impaired host defense mechanisms (eg, acute leukemia, Hodgkin's disease, multiple myeloma, chronic lymphocytic leukemia); in others, it results from the myelosuppressive and immunosuppressive effects of cancer chemotherapy or a combination of these factors. In patients with acute leukemia and in those with granulocytopenia (less than 600 granulocytes per microliter), infection is a medical emergency. Although fever alone does not prove the presence of infection, in these patients as well as in patients with multiple myeloma or chronic lymphocytic leukemia, fever is virtually pathognomonic of infection. While infections in patients with myeloma or chronic leukemia are often due to sensitive organisms, patients with leukemia or pancytopenia are less fortunate, as resistant gram-negative organisms are more often responsible. Appropriate cultures (eg, blood, sputum, urine, cerebrospinal fluid) should always be obtained before starting therapy; however, one usually cannot wait for results of these studies before initiating bactericidal antibiotic therapy. Gram-stained smears may show a predominant organism in sputum, urine, or cerebrospinal fluid.

Emergency Treatment

In the absence of granulocytopenia and in nonleukemic patients, the combination of a cephalosporin antibiotic with an aminoglycoside (tobramycin or gentamicin) has proved useful for patients with acute bacteremia. Combinations of this nature must be given judiciously, as they are of very broad spectrum; they should always be replaced by the most appropriate antibiotics as soon as culture data become available. In the current era of intensive chemotherapy of acute leukemia, *Pseudomonas* bacteremia is the most frequent infection in granulocytopenic patients and may be fulminant and fatal within 72 hours. Prompt institution of combination therapy with gentamicin and carbenicillin or ticarcillin may offer the best chance of curing *Pseudomonas* bacteremia in cancer patients. This combination is less effective against *Escherichia coli* sepsis and should not be used for that purpose. Initial treatment of febrile patients with acute leukemia and granulocytopenia should consist of 3 drugs: a cephalosporin, an aminoglycoside such as tobramycin, and carbenicillin. Amphotericin B should be added if the patient does not respond. If a causative organism is isolated, the combination is replaced with the best agent or agents; otherwise, the combination is continued until the infection has resolved.

Granulocyte transfusions are useful in the treatment of granulocytopenic cancer patients with sepsis, though the complexity of procurement methods has largely limited their availability to leukemia treatment centers. Normal ABO-compatible donors or patients with chronic myelogenous leukemia can serve as granulocyte donors for cancer patients with granulocytopenia. White cell collection is ideally carried out with a continuous or intermittent flow blood cell separator. White cells may also be collected by filtration leukapheresis; however, side reactions due to leukocyte damage in recipients are more frequent. Optimal use of normal granulocyte transfusion appears to require at least 4 daily transfusions (in addition to antibiotics) to localize infection.

Beutler SM et al: Preventing infection in neutropenic cancer patients. (Specialty conference.) *West J Med* 1983;**138**:690.
Higby DJ, Burnett D: Granulocyte transfusions: Current status. *Blood* 1980;**55**:2.

CARCINOID SYNDROME

Although tumors of argentaffin cells are rare and usually slow-growing, they synthesize and secrete a variety of vasoactive materials including serotonin, histamine, catecholamines, prostaglandins, and vasoactive peptides. These substances are capable of initiating acute severe vascular changes that may be fatal.

Carcinoid tumors usually arise from the ileum, stomach, or bronchi and tend to metastasize early.

The manifestations of carcinoid syndrome include facial flushing, edema of the head and neck (especially severe with bronchial carcinoid), abdominal cramps and diarrhea, asthmatic symptoms, cardiac lesions (pulmonary or tricuspid stenosis or insufficiency), telangiectases, and increased urinary 5-hydroxyindoleacetic acid (5-HIAA). Very severe acute symptoms occur in patients with bronchial carcinoids, beginning with disorientation and tremulousness followed by fever and flushing episodes that may last 3 or 4 days. Hypotension and pulmonary edema have also been observed. Even a small coin lesion in the lung may produce the entire syndrome, so that the lung tumor may not be identified until after the diagnosis of carcinoid has been established biochemically. Qualitative test for urinary 5-HIAA is positive in most instances and indicates that the patient is probably secreting 25–30 mg of 5-HIAA per day. False negatives may occur in patients receiving phenothiazines, and false positives have been observed after ingestion of serotonin-rich foods such as bananas or walnuts or in patients taking cough syrups containing glycerol guaiacolate. Ideally, all drugs should be withheld for several days prior to the urine collection.

A provocative test for induction of the flush can be performed by injecting 5 μg of epinephrine (0.5 mL of 1:1000 solution diluted 100 times) intravenously. If the test is positive, the facial flush and some dyspnea usually appear within several minutes.

Emergency therapy for patients with bronchial carcinoids and prolonged flushing episodes consists of giving prednisone, 15–30 mg orally daily. The effect is dramatic, and treatment is usually continued for prolonged periods. However, the flushing itself may be due to kinins rather than serotonin, and corticosteroids may have no effect on kinin-mediated features of the syndrome. Abdominal cramps and diarrhea can usually be managed with diphenoxylate with atropine (Lomotil), alone or in combination with an antiserotonin agent such as methysergide maleate.

The H_1 histamine receptor antagonist cyproheptadine, the H_2 receptor blocker cimetidine, and phenothiazines may prove useful in prevention of flushing. Cyproheptadine is particularly useful because it is also a serotonin antagonist.

Patients with intestinal carcinoids may do well for 10–15 years with supportive therapy, and cancer chemotherapy may not be indicated. Because bronchial lesions cause more severe symptoms, chemotherapy with doxorubicin plus cyclophosphamide or streptozocin should be considered if resection is not feasible or if metastases have occurred.

Moertel CG: Treatment of the carcinoid tumor and the malignant carcinoid syndrome. *J Clin Oncol* 1983;**1**:727.

CANCER CHEMOTHERAPY

Use of cytotoxic drugs and hormones has become a highly specialized and increasingly effective means of treating cancer.Treatment is optimally directed by a medical oncologist who either provides primary care for such patients or serves as consultant to the patient's personal physician. Selection of specific drugs or protocols for various types of cancer has traditionally been based on results of prior clinical trials; however, many patients have drug-resistant tumors. A new approach that is being applied in ovarian cancer and a variety of other neoplasms is the use of in vitro chemosensitivity testing with the clonogenic or "tumor stem cell assay." When done properly, this test is about 70% accurate at selecting effective drugs and over 95% accurate at identifying which agent will be ineffective in a given patient's cancer. It is likely that such chemosensitivity testing will gain wide use in the 1980s, both for tailoring treatment for specific patients and for aiding in the discovery of new anticancer drugs.

Cancer chemotherapy is usually curative in advanced stages of choriocarcinoma in women; in Burkitt's lymphoma and testicular tumors; and in some cases of acute leukemia, embryonal rhabdomyosarcoma, Hodgkin's disease, and diffuse histiocytic lymphoma. When combined with initial surgery and irradiation, chemotherapy also increases the cure rate in Wilms' tumor, and early data suggest that a similar approach may provide long-term control of breast cancer and osteogenic sarcoma. Combination chemotherapy provides significant palliation of symptoms along with prolongation of survival in many children with acute leukemia, Ewing's sarcoma, and retinoblastoma, and in adults with Hodgkin's disease, non-Hodgkin's lymphomas, mycosis fungoides, multiple myeloma, macroglobulinemia, carcinomas of the head and neck, thyroid, breast, stomach, ovary, endometrium, and prostate, small cell carcinoma of the lung, and various soft tissue sarcomas. Patients with carcinoma of the bladder or pancreas or chronic leukemia also achieve some relief of symptoms, although survival rates have not yet increased significantly. The results of currently available treatments are largely unsuccessful in squamous cancer of the lung as well as in metastatic melanoma and in adenocarcinomas of the colon or gallbladder.

A summary of the types of cancer responsive to chemotherapy and the current treatment of choice is offered in Table 33–2. In some instances (eg, Hodgkin's disease), optimal therapy may require a combination of therapeutic modalities, eg, radiation therapy plus chemotherapy rather than chemotherapy alone. All patients with stage I or II Hodgkin's disease should receive radiation therapy. Table 33–3 outlines the currently used dosage schedules and the toxicities of the cancer chemotherapeutic agents. The dosage schedules given are for single-agent therapy. Combination therapy, as now used in advanced Hodgkin's disease, testicular tumors, and certain other neoplasms, requires reductions of the dosages shown— otherwise, the combined toxicity would be prohibitive. Such combination therapy should be attempted only by specialists in centers where adequate supportive services are available.

Hormonal therapy also plays an important role in cancer management. Hormonal therapy or ablation is important in palliation of breast and prostatic carcinoma, while added progestins are useful in suppression of endometrial carcinoma. Studies have shown that the 30% of women with metastatic breast cancer who show objective improvement with hormonal therapy have tumors that contain cytoplasmic estrogen receptors (and probably progesterone receptors as well). Patients whose tumors lack these receptor proteins are unresponsive to hormonal management but frequently respond to cytotoxic chemotherapy. New antiestrogens (eg, tamoxifen) have substantial additive cytotoxic effects to oophorectomy (and sometimes adrenalectomy) in women whose tumors are estrogen or progesterone receptor–positive. Thus, estrogen and progesterone receptor status should be assessed on all breast cancers at the time of mastectomy and on biopsy material (if available) from patients who manifest metastatic breast cancer. Antiestrogens such as tamoxifen have far lower affinity for the estrogen receptor protein than do endogenous estrogens. Therefore, the drug is of lesser value in the presence of functional ovaries. Although chemotherapy with drugs such as cyclophosphamide may depress ovarian function, oophorectomy is far more definitive and should be considered for premenopausal women to be treated with tamoxifen alone or in combination with cytotoxic agents.

Nonspecific immunotherapy with BCG appears to have some limited value in ovarian carcinoma and nodular lymphomas. Interferon appears to have some antitumor activity in non-Hodgkin's lymphomas, multiple myeloma, and several other neoplasms.

MECHANISMS OF ACTION OF CANCER CHEMOTHERAPEUTIC AGENTS

Although the emphasis of this chapter is on the empirical applications of cancer chemotherapy, the cytokinetics and mechanisms of drug action should be discussed briefly. At the clinical level of detectability of tumors, growth characteristics vary considerably between tumors of different histologies or tissue of origin. The key cells in a cancer are the clonogenic **tumor stem cells,** which comprise less than 1% of cancer cells but provide for population renewal and serve as the seeds of metastasis. Soft agar culture to detect these cells and measure their drug sensitivity has recently been developed. Another useful concept is that of the "growth fraction"—the percentage of tumor cells that are proliferating at any given time. The

Table 33–2. Cancers responsive to chemotherapy.

Diagnosis	Current Treatment of Choice	Other Valuable Agents
Acute lymphocytic leukemia	Induction: vincristine plus prednisone. Remission maintenance: mercaptopurine, methotrexate, and cyclophosphamide in various combinations.	Asparaginase, daunorubicin, VM-26,* carmustine, doxorubicin, cytarabine, allopurinol,† craniospinal radiotherapy.
Acute myelocytic and myelo-monocytic leukemia	Combination chemotherapy: thioguanine, cytarabine, and daunorubicin; or doxorubicin, vincristine, cytarabine, prednisone.	Methotrexate, mercaptopurine, allopurinol,† azacytidine,* AMSA, mitoxantrone.*
Chronic myelocytic leukemia	Busulfan.	Vincristine, mercaptopurine, hydroxyurea, melphalan, cytarabine, allopurinol.†
Chronic lymphocytic leukemia	Chlorambucil and prednisone (if indicated).	Vincristine, androgens,† allopurinol,† doxorubicin.
Hodgkin's disease (stages III and IV)	Combination chemotherapy: mechlorethamine, vincristine, procarbazine, prednisone ("MOPP").	Doxorubicin, bleomycin, vinblastine, dacarbazine ("ABVD"); lomustine, VM-26*
Non-Hodgkin's lymphomas	Combination chemotherapy: cyclophosphamide, doxorubicin, vincristine, prednisone.	Bleomycin, lomustine, carmustine, VM-26,* BCG,* AMSA, mitoxantrone,* interferon.*
Multiple myeloma	Combination chemotherapy: melphalan, cyclophosphamide, doxorubicin, vincristine, carmustine.	Vincristine, vindesine,* interferon,* androgens.†
Macroglobulinemia	Chlorambucil.	Melphalan.
Polycythemia vera	Busulfan, chlorambucil, or cyclophosphamide.	
Carcinoma of lung	Cyclophosphamide, doxorubicin, methotrexate, and lomustine (depends on cell type).	Cisplatin, quinacrine,† mitomycin, vincristine, VP-16,* fluorouracil, vindesine*
"Head and neck" carcinomas	Cisplatin and fluorouracil.	Hydroxyurea, doxorubicin, vinblastine, methotrexate, bleomycin.
Carcinoma of endometrium	Doxorubicin plus cyclophosphamide.	Progestins, fluorouracil, vinblastine, cisplatin.
Carcinoma of ovary	Doxorubicin, cyclophosphamide, and cisplatin.	Melphalan, fluorouracil, vincristine, hexamethylmelamine,* bleomycin, BCG.*
Carcinoma of cervix	Mitomycin, bleomycin, vincristine, and cisplatin.	Lomustine, cyclophosphamide, doxorubicin, methotrexate.
Breast carcinoma	(1) Combination chemotherapy (see text) if lymph nodes are positive at mastectomy. (2) Combination chemotherapy; hormonal manipulation for late recurrence. (See text.)	Cyclophosphamide, doxorubicin, vincristine, methotrexate, fluorouracil, mitomycin, vinblastine, mitoxantrone,* quinacrine,† prednisone,† megestrol, androgens.
Choriocarcinoma (trophoblastic neoplasms)	Methotrexate, alone or in combination with vincristine, dactinomycin, and cyclophosphamide.	Vinblastine, mercaptopurine, chlorambucil, doxorubicin.
Carcinoma of testis	Combination therapy: cisplatin, vinblastine, bleomycin.	Methotrexate, dactinomycin, mithramycin, doxorubicin, cyclophsophamide, etoposide.
Carcinoma of prostate	Estrogens.	Doxorubicin plus cyclophosphamide, and cisplatin, estramustine, fluorouracil, progestins.
Wilms' tumor (children)	Vincristine plus dactinomycin after surgery and radiotherapy.	Methotrexate, cyclophosphamide, doxorubicin.
Neuroblastoma	Cyclophosphamide plus doxorubicin and vincristine.	Dactinomycin, daunorubicin, cisplatin.
Carcinoma of thyroid	Radioiodine (^{131}I), doxorubicin.	Bleomycin, fluorouracil, melphalan.
Carcinoma of adrenal	Mitotane.	Doxorubicin.
Carcinoma of stomach or pancreas	Fluorouracil plus doxorubicin and mitomycin.	Hydroxyurea, lomustine.
Carcinoma of colon	Fluorouracil.	Cyclophosphamide, mitomycin, carmustine.
Carcinoid	Doxorubicin plus cyclophosphamide.	Dactinomycin, methysergide,† streptozocin.
Insulinoma	Streptozocin.	Doxorubicin, fluorouracil, mitomycin.
Osteogenic sarcoma	Doxorubicin, or methotrexate with citrovorum rescue initiated after surgery.	Cyclophosphamide, dacarbazine.
Miscellaneous sarcomas	Doxorubicin plus dacarbazine.	Methotrexate, dactinomycin, cyclophosphamide, vincristine, vinblastine.
Melanoma	Dacarbazine and dactinomycin.	Lomustine, cisplatin, mitomycin, vinblastine.

*Investigational agent. Treatment available through qualified investigators and centers authorized by National Cancer Institute and Cooperative Oncology Groups.

†Supportive agent, not oncolytic.

Table 33–3. Dosage and toxicity of cancer chemotherapeutic drugs when used as single agents.

Chemotherapeutic Agent	Usual Adult Dosage	Acute Toxicity	Delayed Toxicity
Alkylating agents			
Mechlorethamine (nitrogen mustard, HN2, Mustargen)	0.4 mg/kg IV in single or divided doses.	Nausea and vomiting	Moderate depression of blood count. Excessive doses produce severe bone marrow depression with leukopenia, thrombocytopenia, and bleeding. Alopecia and hemorrhagic cystitis occur with cyclophosphamide (see p 1062), while busulfan occasionally causes pigmentation and other unusual toxicities (see p 1063). Acute leukemia may develop in 5–10% of patients receiving prolonged therapy with melphalan or chlorambucil.
Chlorambucil (Leukeran)	0.1–0.2 mg/kg/d orally; 6–12 mg/d.	None	
Cyclophosphamide	3.5–5 mg/kg/d orally for 10 days; 1 g/m² IV as single dose every 3–4 weeks.	Nausea and vomiting	
Melphalan (Alkeran)	0.25 mg/kg/d orally for 4 days every 6 weeks.	None	
Thiotepa	0.2 mg/kg IV for 5 days.	None	
Busulfan (Myleran)	2–8 mg/d orally; 150–250 mg/course.	None	
Carmustine (BCNU, bischloro-ethylnitrosourea)	200 mg/m² IV every 6 weeks.	Nausea and vomiting	Leukopenia and thrombocytopenia. Rarely hepatitis. Acute leukemia has been observed to occur in some patients receiving semustine.
Lomustine (CCNU) or semustine (methyl-CCNU)	130 mg/m² orally every 6 weeks.	Nausea and vomiting	
Procarbazine (N-methyl-hydrazine, Matulane)	50–300 mg/d orally.	Nausea and vomiting	Bone marrow depression, mental depression, monoamine oxidase inhibition.
Dacarbazine (dimethyl triazeno imidazole carboxamide, DTIC)	250 mg/m²/d for 5 days every 3 weeks.	Anorexia, nausea, vomiting	Bone marrow depression.
Cisplatin (Platinol)	50–100 mg/m² IV every 3 weeks.	Nausea and vomiting	Nephrotoxicity, mild otic and bone marrow toxicity, neurotoxicity.
Structural analogs or antimetabolites			
Methotrexate (amethopterin, MTX)	2.5–5 mg/d orally; 15 mg intrathecally weekly or every other week for 4 doses. 20–25 mg IM twice weekly is well tolerated and may be preferable.	None	Oral and gastrointestinal tract ulceration, bone and marrow depression, leukopenia, thrombocytopenia.
Mercaptopurine (Purinethol, 6-MP)	2.5 mg/kg/d orally.	None	Usually well tolerated. Larger dosages may cause bone marrow depression.
Thioguanine (6-TG)	2 mg/kg/d orally.	None	Usually well tolerated. Larger dosages may cause bone marrow depression.
Fluorouracil (5-FU)	15 mg/kg IV for 3–5 days, or 15 mg/kg weekly for at least 6 weeks.	None	Nausea, oral and gastrointestinal ulceration, bone marrow depression.
Cytarabine (Ara-C, Cytosar)	100 mg/m²/d for 5–10 days given by continuous IV infusion, or in divided doses subcut or IV every 8 hours.	None	Nausea and vomiting, bone marrow depression, megaloblastosis, leukopenia, thrombocytopenia.
Hormonal agents			
Androgens			
Testosterone propionate	100 mg IM 3 times weekly.	None	Fluid retention, masculinization. There is a 10% incidence of cholestatic jaundice with fluoxymesterone.
Fluoxymesterone (Halotestin)	20–40 mg/d orally.	None	
Estrogens			
Diethylstilbestrol	1–5 mg 3 times a day orally.	Occasional nausea and vomiting	Fluid retention, feminization, uterine bleeding.
Ethinyl estradiol (Estinyl)	3 mg/d orally.	None	
Antiestrogen			
Tamoxifen (Nolvadex)	20 mg/d orally.	None	None
Progestins			
Hydroxyprogesterone caproate (Delalutin)	1 g IM twice weekly.	None	Occasional fluid retention.
Medroxyprogesterone (Provera)	100–200 mg/d orally; 200–600 mg orally twice weekly.	None	
Megestrol acetate (Megace)	40 mg 4 times a day orally.	None	
Adrenocorticosteroids			
Prednisone	20–100 mg/d orally or, when effective, 50–100 mg every other day orally as single dose.	None	Fluid retention, hypertension, diabetes, increased susceptibility to infection, "moon facies," osteoporosis.

Table 33–3 (cont'd). Dosage and toxicity of cancer chemotherapeutic drugs when used as single agents.

Chemotherapeutic Agent	Usual Adult Dosage	Acute Toxicity	Delayed Toxicity
Natural products and miscellaneous agents			
Vinblastine (Velban)	0.1–0.2 mg/kg IV weekly.	Nausea and vomiting	Alopecia, loss of reflexes, bone marrow depression.
Vincristine (Oncovin)	1.5 mg/m^2 IV (maximum: 2 mg weekly).	None	Areflexia, muscle weakness, peripheral neuritis, paralytic ileus, alopecia (below).
Dactinomycin (actinomycin D, Cosmegen)	0.04 mg/kg IV weekly.	Nausea and vomiting	Stomatitis, gastrointestinal tract upset, alopecia, bone marrow depression.
Daunorubicin (daunomycin, rubidomycin)	30–60 mg/m^2 daily IV for 3 days, or 30–60 mg/m^2 IV weekly.	Nausea, fever, red urine (not hematuria)	Cardiotoxicity, bone marrow depression, alopecia.
Doxorubicin (Adriamycin)	60 mg/m^2 IV every 3 weeks to a maximum total dose of 550 mg/m^2.	Nausea, red urine (not hematuria)	Cardiotoxicity, alopecia, bone marrow depression, stomatitis.
Mithramycin (Mithracin)	25–50 μg/kg IV every other day for up to 8 doses.	Nausea and vomiting	Thrombocytopenia, hepatotoxicity.
Mitomycin (Mutamycin)	20 mg/m^2 every 6 weeks.	Nausea	Thrombocytopenia, leukopenia.
Bleomycin (Blenoxane)	Up to 15 mg/m^2 twice weekly to a total dose of 200 mg/m^2.	Allergic reactions, fever, hypotension	Fever, dermatitis, pulmonary fibrosis (see p 1063).
Hydroxyurea (Hydrea)	300 mg/m^2 orally for 5 days.	Nausea and vomiting	Bone marrow depression.
Mitotane (*o,p'*-DDD, Lysodren)	6–12 g/d orally.	Nausea and vomiting	Dermatitis, diarrhea, mental depression, muscle tremors.
Supportive agents			
Allopurinol (Zyloprim)	300–800 mg/d orally for prevention or relief of hyperuricemia.	None	Usually none. Enhances effects and toxicity of mercaptopurine when used in combination.
Quinacrine (Atabrine)	100–200 mg/d by intracavitary injection for 6 days.	Local pain and fever	None.

leukemias, certain lymphomas, and genital tract tumors have relatively high growth fractions and are quite susceptible to treatment with drugs that have specific toxicity for proliferating cells. These drugs include cytarabine, mercaptopurine, thioguanine, methotrexate, fluorouracil, azacytidine, vincristine, vinblastine, bleomycin, and certain steroid hormones. These drugs are therefore classed as **cell cycle specific (CCS)** agents, and their utility has proved to be greatest in tumors with high growth fractions such as those mentioned above. The sequential 4 phases of the cell cycle are G_1 (period of RNA and protein synthesis), S phase (period of DNA synthesis), G_2 (period of assembly of the mitotic spindle apparatus), and M (mitosis). Cytarabine is an excellent example of a drug with selective toxicity during just the S phase of the cell cycle, and its current use is virtually limited to the management of acute leukemia, in which it has had a major beneficial effect.

A second major group of drugs are classed as **cell cycle nonspecific (CCNS)** agents. Most of these drugs act by complexing with cellular DNA and are capable of doing this whether cells are proliferating or not. Examples are the alkylating agents (eg, mechlorethamine, cyclophosphamide, melphalan, carmustine),

other chemical agents (cisplatin), and antibiotics such as dactinomycin, doxorubicin, and mitomycin. Such drugs are useful in the treatment of a variety of so-called "solid tumors," which generally have low growth fractions at the clinical phase of disease; but they are also quite useful in high growth fraction tumors. Tumor kinetics are far from static, however, and our strategy in cancer chemotherapy is now undergoing radical revision to exploit our expanding knowledge of cytokinetics, pharmacokinetics, selective cell line sensitivity, etc.

For example, drugs that have had the greatest value in humans are those that produce a fractional kill of at least 5–6 logs (100,000-fold to 1 million-fold reduction in tumor cell number) in animal tumor systems. Because patients with human tumors present with 10^{10}–10^{12} tumor cells, use of effective combination chemotherapy should be given serious consideration after a major reduction in the body burden of tumor is first accomplished with surgery or irradiation. A new strategy that has already been proved effective in Hodgkin's disease is the use of alternating non-cross-resistant combinations of drugs (eg, "MOPP-ABVD") for induction of remission. This approach has yet to be tested in other types of cancer. A theoretic scheme of strategies in cancer chemotherapy is shown in Fig 33–1.

ADJUVANT CHEMOTHERAPY FOR MICROMETASTASES

One of the most important roles of cancer chemotherapy is undoubtedly as an "adjuvant" (to eradicate minimal residual disease) after "primary field" treat-

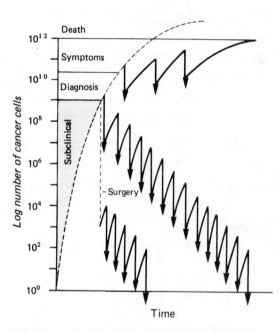

Figure 33–1. Relationship of tumor cell number to time of diagnosis, symptoms, treatment, and survival. Three alternative approaches to drug treatment are shown for comparison with the course of tumor growth when no treatment is given (dotted line). In the protocol diagrammed at top, treatment (indicated by the arrows) is given infrequently, and the result is manifested as prolongation of survival but with recurrence of symptoms between courses of treatment and eventual death of the patient. The combination chemotherapy treatment diagrammed in the middle section is begun earlier and is more intensive. Tumor cell kill exceeds regrowth, drug resistance does not develop, and "cure" results. In this example, treatment has been continued long after all clinical evidence of cancer has disappeared (1–3 years). This approach has been established as effective in the treatment of childhood acute leukemia, testicular cancers, and Hodgkin's disease. The recent introduction of the concept of "alternating non–cross-resistant" combination chemotherapy may further enhance this approach. In the treatment diagrammed near the bottom of the graph, early surgery has been employed to remove the primary tumor, and intensive adjuvant chemotherapy has been administered long enough (up to 1 year) to eradicate the remaining 10^3 tumor stem cells that comprise the remaining occult micrometastases. This approach is now widely applied and appears effective in the treatment of breast cancer, osteosarcoma, and Wilms' tumor.

ment with surgery or irradiation. Failures with primary field therapy are due principally to occult micrometastases of tumor stem cells outside the primary field. These distant micrometastases are usually present in patients with one or more positive lymph nodes at the time of surgery (eg, in breast cancer) and in patients with tumors having a known propensity for early hematogenous spread (eg, osteogenic sarcoma, Wilms' tumor). The risk of recurrent or metastatic disease in such patients can be extremely high (over 80%). Only systemic therapy can adequately attack micrometastases. Chemotherapeutic regimens that induce regression of advanced cancer may have curative potential (at the right dosage and schedule) when combined with surgery for high-risk "early" cancer. Studies in experimental animals have shown that chemotherapy can eradicate small numbers of residual cancer cells after surgery.

The efficacy of adjuvant chemotherapy is also well established in pediatric neoplasms, eg, Wilms' tumor and rhabdomyosarcoma, where substantial improvement in survival has been obtained with adjuvant therapy. Recent studies have shown significant prolongation of survival in both pre- and postmenopausal women with stage II breast cancer who received adjuvant chemotherapy. In breast cancer, women with positive lymph nodes at breast cancer surgery have had prolonged disease-free survival from combination chemotherapy. Several useful combination chemotherapy regimens for adjuvant therapy for breast cancer are "CMF" (cyclophosphamide-methotrexate-fluorouracil), alone or with the addition of vincristine and prednisone (CVFVP), and "D/C" (doxorubicin-cyclophosphamide). There is clear evidence of a dose-response effect of adjuvant cytotoxic chemotherapy, and low-dose protocols are generally ineffective. The antiestrogen tamoxifen has recently been shown to be a useful adjuvant in postmenopausal women with estrogen receptor–positive primaries. In osteogenic sarcoma and soft-tissue sarcomas of the extremities, doxorubicin alone and doxorubicin in combination with other drugs have proved useful as adjuvants. A recent report from the Gastrointestinal Tumor Study Group indicates that relapse-free survival is improved in patients with rectal cancer when they receive postoperative radiotherapy and the combination of fluorouracil plus semustine.

Although it is still early to assess the overall results of these regimens, adjuvant chemotherapy should be considered as part of standard and indicated therapy in the patient groups discussed above. Thus, adjuvant chemotherapy (with curative intent) should now be given serious consideration for patients who undergo primary surgical staging and therapy and are found to have a stage and histologic type of cancer known to be associated with a high risk of micrometastasis and for which effective chemotherapy is available. However, at present adjuvant therapy remains investigational and unproved for a number of common tumors, including non-small cell lung cancer, pancreatic cancer, and colon cancer. Adjuvant herapy is probably not indicated in early Hodgkin's disease or testicular carcinoma, since the cure rates with chemotherapy for these diseases when advanced and recurrent are high.

ones SE, Salmon SE (editors): *Adjuvant Therapy of Cancer IV.* Grune & Stratton, 1984. [Summarizes adjuvant therapy in major disease categories.]

TOXICITY & DOSE MODIFICATION OF CHEMOTHERAPEUTIC AGENTS

A number of cancer chemotherapeutic agents have cytotoxic effects on rapidly proliferating normal cells in bone marrow, mucosa, and skin. Still other drugs such as the *Vinca* alkaloids produce neuropathy, and the hormones often have psychic effects. Acute and chronic toxicities of the various drugs are summarized in Table 33–3. Early recognition of significant toxicity is important to make certain that the ratio of benefit to toxic effects of treatment remains favorable. Appropriate dose modification usually minimizes these side effects, so that therapy can be continued with relative safety.

Bone Marrow Toxicity

Depression of bone marrow is usually the most significant limiting toxicity in cancer chemotherapy.

Commonly used short-acting drugs that affect bone marrow are the oral alkylating agents (eg, cyclophosphamide, melphalan, chlorambucil), procarbazine, mercaptopurine, methotrexate, vinblastine, fluorouracil, dactinomycin, and doxorubicin. In general, it is preferable to use alkylating agents in intensive "pulse" courses every 3–4 weeks rather than to administer in continuous daily schedules. This allows for complete hematologic (and immunologic) recovery between courses rather than leaving the patient continuously suppressed with a cytotoxic agent. This approach reduces side effects but does not reduce therapeutic efficacy. The standard dosage schedules that produce tumor responses with these agents often do induce some bone marrow depression. In such instances, if the drug is not discontinued or its dosage reduced, severe bone marrow aplasia may result in pancytopenia, bleeding, or infection. Simple guidelines to therapy can usually prevent severe marrow depression.

White blood counts (and differential counts), hematocrit or hemoglobin, and platelet counts should be obtained frequently. With long-term chemotherapy, counts should be obtained initially at weekly intervals; the frequency of counts may be reduced only after the patient's sensitivity to the drug can be well predicted (eg, 3–4 months) and cumulative toxicity excluded.

In patients with normal blood counts as well as normal liver and kidney function, drugs should usually

be started at their full dosage and tapered if need be, rather than starting at a lower dose and escalating the dose to hematologic tolerance. When the dose is escalated, toxicity often cannot be adequately anticipated, especially if it is cumulative, and marrow depression is often more severe.

Drug dosage can usually be tapered on a fixed schedule as a function of the peripheral white blood count or platelet count (or both). In this fashion, smooth titration control of drug administration can usually be attained for oral alkylating agents or antimetabolites. A scheme for dose modifications is shown in Table 33–4. Alternatively, the interval between drug courses can be lengthened, thereby permitting more complete hematologic recovery.

Drugs with delayed hematologic toxicities do not always fit into such a simple scheme, and in general they should be administered by specialists familiar with the specific toxicities. Drugs requiring special precautions with respect to toxicity include doxorubicin, mitomycin, busulfan, cytarabine, bleomycin, mithramycin, carmustine, lomustine, semustine, and daunorubicin.

Chemotherapy-Induced Nausea & Vomiting

A number of cytotoxic anticancer drugs induce nausea and vomiting as side effects. In general, these symptoms are thought to originate in the central nervous system rather than peripherally. Parenteral administration of single agents such as doxorubicin and cyclophosphamide frequently is associated with mild to moderate nausea and vomiting, whereas parenteral administration of nitrosoureas and particularly cisplatin usually causes severe symptoms, which can limit patient acceptance of chemotherapy. Combination chemotherapy with agents including those listed above can also cause severe symptomatology. Recent advances in the study of antiemetics clearly reduce and often eliminate nausea and vomiting associated with drugs such as cisplatin. Cannabinoids (eg, tetrahydrocannabinol) were in vogue several years ago (supplied by the National Cancer Institute), but other agents now appear preferable and cause fewer side effects. Metoclopramide (Reglan) is a particularly useful agent, especially when administered parenterally at a dosage of 1 mg/kg, both 30 minutes before and again 30 minutes after the administration of chemotherapy. Dexamethasone has potent antiemetic effects when administered at a dosage of 10 mg at similar intervals. Both of these agents are significantly more potent than conventional agents such as pro-

Table 33–4. Scheme for dose modification of cancer chemotherapeutic agents.

Granulocyte Count (/µL)	Platelet Count (/µL)	Suggested Drug Dosage (% of full dose)
> 3000	> 100,000	100%
2000–3000	75,000–100,000	50%
< 2000	< 50,000	0%

chlorperazine (Compazine), diphenhydramine (Bena-dryl), and thiethylperazine (Torecan). Combinations of antiemetics (eg, metoclopramide along with dexa-methasone and other agents) is often more effective than maximal doses of any one agent for blocking cisplatin-induced vomiting. Inclusion of diazepam in such combinations is often useful for its sedating ef-fect. A patient receiving potent antiemetics along with chemotherapy on an outpatient basis must be escorted to and from the clinic, since the antiemetics often induce marked sedation and transient impairment of balance and reflexes.

Plezia PM et al: Immediate termination of intractable vomiting induced by cisplatin combination chemotherapy using an in-tensive five-drug antiemetic regimen. *Cancer Treat Rep* 1984;**68**. [In press.]

Gastrointestinal & Skin Toxicity

Since antimetabolites such as methotrexate and fluorouracil act only on rapidly proliferating cells, they damage the cells of mucosal surfaces such as the gas-trointestinal tract. Methotrexate has similar effects on the skin. These toxicities are at times more significant than those that have occurred in the bone marrow, and they should be looked for routinely when these agents are used.

Erythema of the buccal mucosa is an early sign of mucosal toxicity. If therapy is continued beyond this point, oral ulceration will develop. In general, it is wise to discontinue therapy at the time of appearance of early oral ulceration. This finding usually heralds the appearance of similar but potentially more serious ulceration at other sites lower in the gastrointestinal tract. Therapy can usually be reinstituted when the oral ulcer heals (1 week to 10 days). The dose of drug used may need to be modified downward at this point, with titration to an acceptable level of effect on the mucosa.

Miscellaneous Drug-Specific Toxicities

The toxicities of individual drugs have been summarized in Table 33–3; however, several of these warrant additional mention, since they occur with fre-quently administered agents, and special measures are often indicated.

A. Cyclophosphamide-Induced Hemorrhagic Cystitis: Metabolic products of cyclophosphamide that retain cytotoxic activity are excreted into the urine. Some patients appear to metabolize more of the drug to these active excretory products; if their urine is concentrated, severe bladder damage may result. In general, it is wise to advise patients receiving cy-clophosphamide to maintain a large fluid intake. Early symptoms include dysuria and frequency despite the absence of bacteriuria. Such symptoms develop in about 20% of patients who receive the drug. Should microscopic hematuria develop, it is advisable to stop the drug temporarily or switch to a different alkylating agent, to increase fluid intake, and to administer a urinary analgesic such as phenazopyridine. With se-vere cystitis, large segments of bladder mucosa may be

shed and the patient may have prolonged gross hematuria. Such patients should be observed for signs of urinary obstruction and may require cystoscopy for removal of obstructing blood clots. Patients with tumors responsive to cyclophosphamide who develop severe cystitis should stop taking all drugs until the syndrome clears and should then be given different alkylating agents (eg, chlorambucil, melphalan, mechlorethamine) that lack this toxicity, as they are likely to be equally effective against the tumor.

B. Vincristine Neuropathy: Neuropathy is a toxic side effect that is peculiar to the *Vinca* alkaloid drugs, especially vincristine. The peripheral neuropa-thy can be sensory, motor, autonomic, or a combina-tion of these effects. In its mildest form, it consists of paresthesias ("pins and needles") of the fingers and toes. Occasional patients develop acute jaw or throat pain after vincristine therapy. This may be a form of trigeminal neuralgia. With continued vincristine therapy, the paresthesias extend to the proximal inter-phalangeal joints, hyporeflexia appears in the lower extremities, and significant weakness develops in the quadriceps muscle group. At this point, it is wise to discontinue vincristine therapy until the neuropathy has subsided. A useful means of judging whether pe-ripheral motor neuropathy is significant enough to warrant stopping treatment is to have the patient at-tempt to do deep knee bends or get up out of a chair without using the arm muscles.

Constipation is the most common symptom of autonomic neuropathy associated with vincristine therapy. Patients receiving vincristine should be started on stool softeners and mild cathartics when therapy is begun; otherwise, severe impaction may result in association with an atonic bowel.

More serious autonomic involvement can lead to acute intestinal obstruction with signs indistinguish-able from those of an acute abdomen. Bladder neurop-athies are uncommon but may be severe.

These 2 complications are absolute contraindica-tions to continued vincristine therapy.

C. Methotrexate Toxicity and "Citrovorum Rescue": In addition to standard uses of methotrexate for chemotherapy, this drug has some use in a very high dosage that would lead to fatal bone marrow toxicity if it were given without an antidote. The bone marrow toxicity of methotrexate can be prevented by early administration of citrovorum factor (folinic acid, leucovorin). If an overdose of methotrexate is adminis-tered accidentally, folinic acid therapy should be initi-ated as soon as possible, preferably within 1 hour. Intravenous infusion should be employed for large overdosages, inasmuch as it is generally advisable to give citrovorum factor repeatedly. Up to 75 mg should be given in the first 12 hours, followed by 12 mg intramuscularly every 4 hours for at least 6 doses.

Intentional high-dosage methotrexate therapy with citrovorum rescue should only be considered for osteosarcoma patients with good renal function.

Vigorous hydration and bicarbonate loading also appear to be important in preventing crystallization of high-dose methotrexate in the renal tubular epithelium. Daily monitoring of the serum creatinine is mandatory because methotrexate metabolism is slowed by renal insufficiency and high-dosage methotrexate can itself cause renal injury. When high-dose methotrexate is used, folinic acid therapy should probably be started within 4 hours of the methotrexate dose and continued for 3 days (or longer if the creatinine level rises).

D. Busulfan Toxicity: The alkylating agent busulfan, frequently used for treatment of chronic myelogenous leukemia, has curious delayed toxicities including (1) increased skin pigmentation, (2) a wasting syndrome similar to that seen in adrenal insufficiency, and (3) progressive pulmonary fibrosis. Patients who develop either of the latter 2 problems should be switched to a different drug (eg, melphalan) when further therapy is needed. The pigmentary changes are innocuous and will usually regress slowly after treatment is discontinued; in this instance, change to a different compound is optional.

E. Bleomycin Toxicity: This antibiotic has found increasing application in cancer chemotherapy in view of activity in squamous cell carcinomas, Hodgkin's disease, non-Hodgkin's lymphomas, and testicular tumors. Bleomycin produces edema of the interphalangeal joints and hardening of the palmar and plantar skin as well as sometimes also inducing an anaphylactic or serum sickness–like reaction or a serious or fatal pulmonary fibrotic reaction (seen especially in elderly patients receiving a total dose of over 300 units). If nonproductive cough, dyspnea, and pulmonary infiltrates develop, discontinue the drug and institute antibiotic and high-dose corticosteroid therapy. Fever alone or with chills is an occasional complication of bleomycin treatment and is not an absolute contraindication to continued treatment. The fever may be avoided by prednisone administration at the time of injection. Moreover, fever alone is not predictive of pulmonary toxicity. About 1% of patients (especially those with lymphoma) may have a severe or even fatal hypotensive reaction after the initial dose of bleomycin. In order to identify such patients, it is wise to administer a test dose of 5 units of bleomycin first with adequate monitoring and emergency facilities available should they be needed. Patients exhibiting a hypotensive reaction should not receive further bleomycin therapy.

F. Doxorubicin-Induced Myocarditis: The anthracycline antibiotics doxorubicin and daunomycin both have delayed cardiac toxicity. The problem is greater with doxorubicin because it has a major role in the treatment of acute leukemia, sarcomas, breast cancer, lymphomas, and certain other solid tumors. Studies of left ventricular function and endomyocardial biopsies indicate that some changes in cardiac dynamics occur in most patients by the time they have received 300 mg/m^2. The *mu*ltiple-*ga*ted ("MUGA") radionuclide cardiac scan appears to be the most useful noninvasive test for assessing toxicity. Doxorubicin should not be used in elderly patients with significant intrinsic cardiac disease, and in general, patients should not receive a total dose in excess of 550 mg/m^2. Patients who have had prior chest or mediastinal radiotherapy may develop doxorubicin heart disease at lower total doses. The appearance of a high resting pulse may herald the appearance of overt cardiac toxicity. Unfortunately, toxicity may be irreversible and frequently fatal at dosage levels above 550 mg/m^2. At lower doses (eg, 350 mg/m^2), the symptoms and signs of cardiac failure generally respond well to digitalis, diuretics, and cessation of doxorubicin therapy. Recent evidence suggests that cardiac toxicity can be correlated with high peak plasma levels obtained with intermittent high-dose bolus therapy (eg, every 3–4 weeks). Use of weekly injections or low-dose continuous infusion schedules appears to delay the occurrence of cardiac toxicity. Current laboratory studies suggest that cardiac toxicity may be due to a mechanism involving the formation of intracellular free radicals in cardiac muscle.

G. Cisplatin Nephrotoxicity and Neurotoxicity: Cisplatin is effective in testicular, bladder, and ovarian cancer as well as in several other types of tumor. Nausea and vomiting are common, but nephrotoxicity and neurotoxicity are more serious. Vigorous hydration plus mannitol diuresis may substantially reduce nephrotoxicity. The neurotoxicity of this drug is delayed and manifested as a peripheral neuropathy of mixed sensorimotor type and may be associated with painful paresthesias. The neuropathy may be secondary to hypomagnesemia, which can be induced by cisplatin. Therefore, the serum magnesium should be measured if neuropathy develops, and treatment with parenteral magnesium sulfate should be tried. These supportive measures do not appear to reduce the therapeutic effectiveness of cisplatin.

EVALUATION OF TUMOR RESPONSE

Inasmuch as cancer chemotherapy can induce clinical improvement, significant toxicity, or both, it is extremely important to critically assess the beneficial effects of treatment to determine that the net effect is favorable. The most valuable signs to follow during therapy include the following:

A. Tumor Size: Significant shrinkage in tumor size can be demonstrated on physical examination, chest film or other x-ray, sonography, or radionuclide scanning procedure such as bone scanning (breast, lung, prostate cancer). CT scanning has assumed a significant role in evaluating tumor size and location for a wide variety of tumors and sites. Nuclear magnetic resonance (NMR) scanning appears to be the best noninvasive means of evaluating brain tumors, but CT scanning is also useful. Sonography has special utility in pelvic neoplasms.

B. Marker Substances: Significant decrease in the quantity of a tumor product or marker substance reflects a reduced amount of tumor in the body. Examples of such markers include paraproteins in the serum or urine in multiple myeloma and macroglobulinemia, chorionic gonadotropin in choriocarcinoma and testicular tumors, prostatic acid phosphatase in prostatic cancer, urinary steroids in adrenal carcinoma and paraneoplastic Cushing's syndrome, and 5-hydroxyindoleacetic acid in carcinoid syndrome. Tumor-secreted fetal antigens are becoming of increasing importance. These include alpha$_1$-fetoprotein in hepatoma, in teratoembryonal carcinoma, and in occasional cases of gastric carcinoma; ovarian tumor antigen (OC 125) in ovarian cancer; and carcinoembryonic antigen in carcinomas of the colon, lungs, and breast. Monoclonal antibodies are now used for measurement of a number of the tumor markers and offer the potential of delineating a number of additional markers for diagnostic purposes.

C. Organ Function: Return to normal function of organs that were previously impaired by tumor is a useful indicator of drug effectiveness. Examples of such improvement include the return to normal liver function (eg, increased serum albumin) in patients known to have liver metastases and improvement in neurologic findings in patients with cerebral metastases. Disappearance of the signs and symptoms of the paraneoplastic syndromes often falls in this general category and can be taken as an indication of tumor response.

D. General Well-Being and Performance Status: A valuable sign of clinical improvement is the general well-being of the patient. Although this finding is a combination of subjective and objective factors and may be partly a placebo effect, it nonetheless serves as a sign of clinical improvement in assessing some of the objective observations listed above. Factors included in the assessment of general well-being are improved appetite and weight gain and increased "performance status" (eg, ambulatory versus bedridden). Evaluation of factors such as activity status enables the physician to judge whether the net effect of chemotherapy is worthwhile palliation.

• • •

References

Alberts DS et al: In vitro clonogenic assay for predicting responses of ovarian cancer to chemotherapy. *Lancet* 1980;**2:**340.

Baum M et al: Controlled trial of tamoxifen as adjuvant agent in management of early breast cancer. *Lancet* 1983;**1:**257.

Bonadonna G, Valagussa P: Dose-response effect of adjuvant chemotherapy in breast cancer. *N Engl J Med* 1981;**304:**10.

Clark GM et al: Progesterone as a prognostic factor in stage II breast cancer. *N Engl J Med* 1983;**309:**1343.

Dean JC, Salmon SE, Griffith KS: Prevention of alopecia with scalp hypothermia. *N Engl J Med* 1979;**301:**1427.

DeVita VT Jr: Progress in cancer management. *Cancer* 1983;**51:**2401.

DeVita VT Jr, Hellman S, Rosenberg SA (editors): *Principles and Practice of Oncology.* Lippincott, 1982.

Dorr RT, Fritz WL: *Cancer Chemotherapy Handbook.* Elsevier, 1980.

Einhorn LH, Williams SD: Current concepts in cancer: The role of cis-platinum in solid-tumor therapy. *N Engl J Med* 1979;**300:**289.

Einhorn LH et al: The role of maintenance therapy in disseminated testicular cancer. *N Engl J Med* 1981;**305:**727.

Fisher B et al: Influence of tumor estrogen and progesterone receptor levels on the response to tamoxifen and chemotherapy in primary breast cancer. *J Clin Oncol* 1983;**1:**227.

Fisher B et al: Treatment of primary breast cancer with chemotherapy and tamoxifen. *N Engl J Med* 1981;**305:**1.

Frei E III: The National Cancer Chemotherapy Program. *Science* 1982;**217:**600.

Gale RP: Advances in the treatment of acute myelogenous leukemia. *N Engl J Med* 1979;**300:**1189.

Glucksberg H et al: Combination chemotherapy (CMFVP) versus L-phenylalanine mustard (L-PAM) for operable breast cancer with positive axillary nodes. *Cancer* 1982;**50:**423.

Goldie JH, Coldman AJ, Gudauskas GA: Rationale for the use of alternating non–cross-resistant chemotherapy. *Cancer Treat Rep* 1982;**66:**439.

Holland JF, Frei E III (editors): *Cancer Medicine,* 2nd ed. Lea & Febiger, 1982.

Ingle J et al: Randomized trial of diethylstilbestrol vs. tamoxifen in postmenopasual women with advanced cancer. *N Engl J Med* 1981;**304:**16.

Kaplan HS: *Hodgkin's Disease,* 2nd ed. Harvard Univ Press, 1980.

Lederman GS et al: Chemotherapy of refractory germ cell cancer with etoposide. *J Clin Oncol* 1983;**1:**706.

Leichman L et al: Preoperative chemotherapy for carcinoma of the esophagus: A potentially curative approach. *J Clin Oncol* 1984;**2:**75.

Miller TP, Jones SE: Chemotherapy of localized histiocytic lymphoma. *Lancet* 1979;**1:**358.

Moertel CG, Hanley JA, Johnson LA: Streptozotocin alone compared with streptozotocin plus fluorouracil in the treatment of advanced islet-cell carcinoma. *N Engl J Med* 1980;**303:**1189.

Oldham RK: Monoclonal antibodies in cancer therapy. *J Clin Oncol* 1983;**1:**582.

Oncology Committee, American College of Physicians: Oncology: An annotated bibliography of recent literature. *Ann Intern Med* 1982;**97:**630.

Perry MC: Toxicity of chemotherapy. *Semin Oncol* 1982;**9:**1. [Entire issue.]

Portlock CS, Goffinet DR: *Manual of Clinical Problems in Oncology.* Little Brown, 1980.

Posner JB: Neurological complications of cancer. *Disease-A-Month* (Feb) 1978;**25.**

Prosnitz LR, Kapp DS, Weissberg JB: Radiotherapy. *N Engl J Med* 1983;**309:**771.

Quesada JR et al: Alpha interferon for induction of remission in hairy cell leukemia. *N Engl J Med* 1984;**301:**15.

Rainey JM, Jones SE, Salmon SE: Combination chemotherapy for advanced breast cancer utilizing vincristine, Adriamycin and cyclophosphamide (VAC). *Cancer* 1979;**43:**66.

Rosenberg SA et al: The treatment of soft tissue sarcomas of the extremities: Prospective randomized evaluations of (1) limb-sparing surgery plus radiation therapy compared with amputation and (2) the role of adjuvant chemotherapy. *Ann Surg* 1982;**196**:305.

Salmon SE, Sartorelli AC: Cancer chemotherapy. Chap 58, pp 676–711, in: *Basic & Clinical Pharmacology,* 2nd ed. Katzung BG (editor). Lange, 1984.

Salmon SE, Trent JM: *Human Tumor Cloning.* Grune & Stratton, 1984.

Salmon SE et al: Alternating combination chemotherapy improves survival in multiple myeloma. *J Clin Oncol* 1983; **1**:453.

Salmon SE et al: Quantitation of differential sensitivity of human tumor stem cells to anticancer drugs. *N Engl J Med* 1978; **298**:1321.

Santoro A et al: Alternating drug combinations in the treatment of advanced Hodgkin's disease. *N Engl J Med* 1982;**306**:770.

Schimke RT: Gene amplification, drug resistance and cancer. *Cancer Res* 1984;**44**:1735.

Veronesi U et al: Comparing radical mastectomy with quadrantectomy, axillary dissection, and radiotherapy in patients with small cancers of the breast. *N Engl J Med* 1981;**305**:6.

Von Hoff DD et al: Prospective clinical trial of a human tumor cloning system. *Cancer Res* 1983;**43**:1926.

Weiss GR et al: Long-term hepatic arterial infusion of 5-fluoro-deoxyuridine for liver metastases using an implantable infusion pump. *J Clin Oncol* 1983;**1**:337.

Wilson CB: Current concepts in cancer: Brain tumors. *N Engl J Med* 1979;**300**:1469.

34 | Immunologic Disorders

Samuel Strober, MD, & F. Carl Grumet, MD

A wide variety of diseases in humans are now known to be associated with disorders of the immune response. Recent studies of immunoglobulin structure and function and of the cellular basis of immunity have resulted in a better understanding of these disorders. This chapter is designed to provide an approach to the patient with immunologic disease by outlining some of the advances that have significant clinical application. A discussion of immunologic deficiency disorders, HLA-linked diseases, autoimmunity, and the gammopathies will illustrate the practical uses of current concepts and techniques in clinical immunology.

IMMUNOGLOBULIN STRUCTURE & FUNCTION

The basic unit of all immunoglobulin molecules consists of 4 polypeptide chains linked by disulfide bonds. There are 2 identical heavy chains (molecular weight 53–75 thousand) and 2 identical light chains (molecular weight about 23,000). Both heavy and light chains have a C-terminal constant (C) region (constant amino acid sequence within a class or type) and an N-terminal variable (V) region, with considerable variation in amino acid sequence from molecule to molecule. The V regions of heavy and light chains together form the antibody combining site, which is responsible for the specific interaction with antigen. A schematic diagram of the basic immunoglobulin molecule is shown in Fig 34–1.

The class of heavy chain and the type of light chain are determined by the amino acid sequence in the constant region in the case of heavy chains and in both the constant and variable regions in the case of light chains. Researchers have identified 5 classes of heavy chains (γ, α, μ, δ, and ϵ) and 2 types of light chains (κ and λ). Either type of light chain can be associated with each of the heavy chain classes. Approximately 70% of human immunoglobulin molecules carry κ light chains and 30% carry λ light chains.

Immunoglobulin Classes

A. Immunoglobulin M (IgM): IgM is made up of 5 identical basic immunoglobulin units. Each unit has a μ heavy chain and a κ or λ light chain. These units are connected to each other by disulfide bond bridges and a small polypeptide known as J chain. The molecular weight of IgM is about 900,000, and the sedimentation coefficient is 19S. The IgM molecule is found predominantly in the intravascular compartment and does not cross the placenta.

B. Immunoglobulin A (IgA): IgA is present in high concentrations in the blood and in seromucous secretions such as saliva, colostrum, tears, and secretions of the bronchi and the gastrointestinal tract. IgA found in the serum is a single basic immunoglobulin unit with α heavy chains. Exocrine or secretory IgA is made up of 2 basic units connected to each other by J chain. A 60,000 molecular weight molecule called transport piece or T piece is attached to the Fc portion. The latter molecule is necessary for the transportation of IgA molecules into the lumens of exocrine glands. Secretory IgA appears to play an important role in host defense mechanisms against viral and bacterial infections. IgA does not cross the placenta.

C. Immunoglobulin G (IgG): IgG is a single basic immunoglobulin unit with γ heavy chains and comprises about 85% of total serum immunoglobulins. Its molecular weight is approximately 150,000, and its sedimentation coefficient is 7S. IgG is distributed in the extracellular fluid and crosses the placenta. Both IgG and IgM molecules bind complement via a receptor present in the constant region of the γ and μ heavy chains.

D. Immunoglobulin E (IgE): IgE is present in the serum in very low concentrations as a single basic immunoglobulin unit with ϵ heavy chains. Approximately 50% of patients with allergic diseases have increased serum IgE levels. IgE is a skin-sensitizing or reaginic antibody by virtue of a mast cell attachment site present on the constant region of the ϵ heavy chain. The specific interaction between antigen and IgE bound to the surface of mast cells results in the release of inflammatory mast cell products such as histamine and serotonin. A wheal and flare reaction or severe bronchospasm may be precipitated by such interactions in the tissues of the skin or lungs, respectively.

E. Immunoglobulin D (IgD): IgD is present in the serum in very low concentrations as a single basic immunoglobulin unit with δ heavy chains. IgD is found on the surface of the majority of immunoglobulin-bearing lymphocytes in association with IgM. The role of IgD is not yet known.

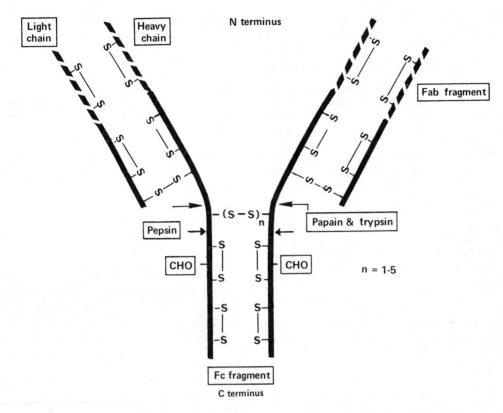

Figure 34–1. Structure of immunoglobulins. Electron microscopic studies have demonstrated that immunoglobulin molecules are Y-shaped. Solid lines indicate regions of constant amino acid sequences; broken lines indicate variable regions. Note symmetry in structure of molecule. One intrachain disulfide loop recurs for every 110–120 amino acid residues along heavy and light chains; about 60 residues are contained within each loop. From 1 to 5 inter–heavy chain disulfide bonds are present in each molecule depending on subclass of heavy chain. Points of cleavage of heavy chains by the proteolytic enzymes papain, trypsin, and pepsin, in relation to the inter–heavy chain disulfide bonds, are indicated. (Reproduced, with permission, from Freedman SO [editor]: *Clinical Immunology.* Harper, 1971.)

Dorrington KJ, Painter RH: Biological activity of the constant region of immunoglobulin G. *Prog Immunol* 1977;**3**:298.

Hood L, Weissman IL, Wood R: *Immunology.* Benjamin, 1978.

Immunoglobulin Genes

Recent investigations of genes that code for immunoglobulin light and heavy chain molecules have elucidated the mechanism by which rearrangements in the DNA of B cells result in the synthesis and expression of immunoglobulin molecules. Genes that code for all of the heavy chains, genes for the κ light chains, and genes for the λ light chains are on 3 different chromosomes. It is now clear that the single polypeptide heavy chains are coded for by as many as 4 different genetic regions on the same chromosome (V, D, J, C_H) that, in the germ line DNA, are quite distant from one another. During B cell development, one of a tandem series of a few hundred V genes is translocated along with the D and J genes close to a C_H gene. This DNA rearrangement produces a functional immunoglobulin heavy chain gene. The V, D, and J genes selected for translocation determine the amino acid sequence of the heavy chain variable region. The C_H gene selected determines the amino acid sequence of the heavy chain constant region. Eight C_H genes (C_μ, C_δ, $C_{\gamma 3}$, $C_{\gamma 1}$, $C_{\gamma 2a}$, $C_{\gamma 2b}$, C_ϵ, and C_α) coding for the 8 immunoglobulin classes, 6 J genes, and a few D genes have been identified in mouse germ line DNA. Functional κ and λ light chain genes are also formed by DNA rearrangements involving one of a series of V genes (different from heavy chain V genes), a J gene, and a C_λ or C_κ constant region gene.

Korsmeyer SJ, Waldmann TA: Immunoglobulins II: Gene organization and assembly. Chap 5, pp 43–54, in: *Basic & Clinical Immunology,* 5th ed. Stites DP et al (editors). Lange, 1984.

Sakano H et al: Two types of somatic recombination are necessary for the generation of complete immunoglobulin heavy-chain genes. *Nature* 1980;**286**:676.

CELLULAR BASIS OF IMMUNE RESPONSES

Development of T & B Lymphocytes

Lymphocytes are able to interact with antigens and initiate the immune responses of vertebrates. In avian species, 2 lines of lymphocytes have been identified: one derived from the thymus and the other from the bursa of Fabricius. The thymus-derived cells are involved in cellular immune responses; the bursa-derived cells are involved in humoral antibody responses. The lymphocytes of mammalian species can also be divided into 2 cell lines: T lymphocytes, which are analogous to the thymus-derived cells in birds; and B lymphocytes, which are analogous to the bursa-derived cells.

Both T and B lymphocytes are derived from precursor cells in the marrow. In the case of T lymphocytes, the precursor cells migrate to the thymus, where they develop some of the functional and cell surface characteristics of mature T cells. Thereafter, the cells migrate to the T-dependent areas of the peripheral lymphoid tissues (paracortical areas of lymph nodes and periarteriolar sheath of the spleen) and enter the pool of long-lived lymphocytes that recirculate from the blood to the lymph. Some maturation of T cells may occur in the peripheral tissues under the influence of a thymic humoral hormone (thymosin).

Two sequences of B cell maturation are now recognized: antigen-independent and antigen-dependent maturation. Antigen-independent maturation includes those stages of B cell development from precursor cells in the marrow through the virgin B cell (a cell which has not been exposed to antigen previously) found in the peripheral lymphoid tissues. Several developmental stages occur in the marrow, and others occur following migration to the solid lymphoid tissues in the periphery. The production and maturation of virgin B cells is an ongoing process even in adult animals. Antigen-dependent maturation occurs following the interaction of antigen with virgin B cells. Memory B cells and antibody-forming cells (plasma cells) are the final products of this developmental sequence. Many of the memory B cells are long-lived and recirculate from the blood to the lymph. Mature B cells in the periphery are found predominantly in the thymus-independent areas (primary follicles and germinal centers) of the lymph nodes and spleen.

Subpopulations of T Cells

T lymphocytes are heterogeneous with respect to their cell surface features (Table 34–1) and functional characteristics. At least 3 subpopulations of T cells are now recognized.

A. Helper or Cooperator Cells: These cells help to amplify the production of antibody-forming cells from B lymphocytes after interaction with antigen. The precise mechanism by which T cells cooperate with B cells has not been elucidated. Helper T cells also amplify the production of effector T cells for cell-mediated cytotoxicity.

B. Cytotoxic or Killer T Cells: These cells are generated after mature T cells interact with certain antigens such as those present on the surface of foreign cells. These cells are responsible for organ graft rejection and for cell-mediated killing of foreign cells in vitro.

Table 34–1. Surface markers commonly used in humans to identify T and B cells.

T Cells	B Cells
*Leu-4, OKT 3 antigen (all T cells)	Immunoglobulins
*Leu-3, OKT 4 antigen (helper subset)	C3 receptor (binds third component of complement)
*Leu-2, OKT 5/8 antigen (suppressor/cytotoxic subset)	Fc receptor (binds Fc portion of immunoglobulins)
Receptor for sheep red blood cells (all T cells)	HLA-D region antigen

*Antigens detected by monoclonal antibodies.

C. Suppressor T Cells: These cells suppress rather than amplify the formation of antibody-forming cells from B lymphocytes. Suppressor T cells are regarded as regulatory cells that modulate humoral antibody formation. Alterations in these cells may play an important role in those disease entities in which there is an overproduction (systemic lupus erythematosus or autoimmune thyroiditis) or an underproduction (common variable agammaglobulinemia) of immunoglobulin. Cell-mediated immunity (ie, organ graft rejection) is also regulated by suppressor cells. The mechanism of action of suppressor cells has not yet been elucidated.

Identification of T Cell Subpopulations With Monoclonal Antibodies

Monoclonal antibodies to T cell subpopulations have been produced by immunizing mice with human T cells and subsequently fusing the spleen cells of the mice with mouse myeloma cells to develop hybridoma cell lines. Several hybridoma lines have been found that secrete monoclonal antibodies which identify cell surface antigens common to all human T cells (Leu-4 antigen [same as OKT 3 antigen]) or surface antigens which identify subsets. The Leu-3 (same as OKT 4) antigen is present on the surface of helper T cells but not on suppressor or cytotoxic T cells. On the other hand, the Leu-2 (same as OKT 5/8) antigen is present on the surface of suppressor and cytotoxic T cells but not on helper T cells. Approximately 75% of the peripheral blood lymphocytes of normal individuals carry the Leu-4 antigen (all T cells), 50% carry the Leu-3 antigen (helper cells), and 25% carry the Leu-2 antigen (suppressor/cytotoxic cells).

Much literature has accumulated concerning changes in the helper and suppressor/cytotoxic T cell subsets identified by monoclonal antibodies (Table 34–1) in various autoimmune and immunodeficient disease states. Patterns of change reported in autoimmune diseases such as lupus erythematosus have been quite variable within a given disease entity. Thus, a specific pattern has not yet been shown to be diagnostic for a given autoimmune disease. In addition, efforts in understanding disease-related changes in T cell subsets have been hampered by the lack of a monoclonal antibody that clearly distinguishes cytotoxic and suppressor T cells. This has also limited the usefulness of subset monitoring in kidney transplant recipients, in whom changes in subsets may be critical in predicting rejection episodes. On the other hand, certain immunodeficiency diseases such as acquired immunodeficiency syndrome (AIDS) are characterized by a specific pattern of T cell subset changes that are helpful in diagnostic evaluation (see p 1084).

T Cell Lymphokines

Many T cell functions can be mediated by humoral factors (glycoproteins) secreted by T cells. These factors are called lymphokines, and they are usually secreted when T cells are activated by antigens or mitogens. Some of these factors are antigen-specific; others are non-antigen-specific and are regulatory molecules that control polyclonal T and B cell proliferation and differentiation. Antigen-specific helper and suppressor factors appear to mediate the function of antigen-specific T helper and suppressor cells that regulate the immune response to a given antigen. Table 34–2 lists examples of non-antigen-specific lymphokines and their function.

Lymphokines are currently being used in both diagnosis and treatment of disease. The secretion of macrophage inhibitory factor (MIF) by peripheral blood lymphocytes in vitro has been used as a test of T lymphocyte function in the workup of immunodeficiency diseases. Experimental trials of the administration of IL-2 or interferon to patients with acquired immunodeficiency syndrome are in progress.

T Cell Recognition of Antigen & the Major Histocompatibility Complex (MHC)

T cells interact with several different types of cells during the regulation and mediation of immune responses. Examples of T cell interactions with other cells include presentation of antigens to T cells by macrophages, T cell-induced differentiation of B cells into antibody-secreting cells, and T cell killing of a variety of virus-infected cells. In all of these cell-cell

Table 34–2. Non-antigen-specific T cell lymphokines.

Lymphokine	Function
T cell growth factor (TCGF, IL-2)	Promotes proliferation of T cells activated by antigens or mitogens
B cell growth factor (BCGF)	Promotes proliferation of B cells activated by antigens or mitogens
T cell replacing factor (TRF)	Induces activated B cells to differentiate into immunoglobulin secreting cells
Macrophage inhibitory factor (MIF)	Inhibits motility of macrophages
Macrophage activating factor (MAF)	Promotes killing of bacteria and tumor cells by macrophages
Gamma interferon	Inhibits viral replication

interactions, T cells recognize foreign antigens on the surface of the non-T cell in association with other cell surface antigens that are coded for by the major histocompatibility gene complex of the non-T cell. Therefore, the T cells must have cell surface receptors that can recognize at least 2 different molecules; one recognition site binds to any single foreign antigen (viral, bacterial, etc) and the other binds to major histocompatibility antigens. An example of this "dual recognition" is observed in the killing of virus-infected target cells by cytolytic T cells. Cytolytic T cells taken from animals immunized to a given virus will kill virus-infected target cells if the target cells carry the same histocompatibility antigens as the immunized animal. Virus-infected target cells carrying different histocompatibility antigens will not be killed.

A critical question raised by the above studies concerns host defense against viral infection in bone marrow transplant recipients who do not share the MHC (HLA) antigens of the marrow donors. After marrow transplantation, the donor T cells maturing in the host thymus are presumed to recognize foreign antigen in association with host-type histocompatibility antigens. However, most antigen-presenting cells will bear donor-type histocompatibility antigens; this may lead to a severe immunodeficiency state, with a completely mismatched marrow transplant. However, at the present time, almost all transplant recipients share at least one HLA haplotype with the donor.

T Cell Cloning

T cells that are activated by antigens in vivo or in vitro can be subsequently cultured in vitro for months to years. A critical requirement for the continued in vitro proliferation of T cells is the presence of T cell growth factor (IL-2) in the tissue culture medium. Proliferation is also dependent upon the presence of specific antigen in the tissue culture medium. Initially, the antigen-activated T cells cultured in vitro are polyclonal. However, single cells can be selected from these primary cultures and placed in secondary cultures in which all the cells are derived from a single cell. T cell cultures derived from single T cells are called T cell clones. The clones require antigenic stimulation or IL-2 (or both) for continued growth and viability. Each clone recognizes a specific antigenic determinant and will proliferate only when that determinant is present in the culture. The antigen must be presented to the T cell clone by macrophages or B lymphocytes added to the culture. In the absence of the latter cells, antigen added to the culture will not induce T cell proliferation or differentiation. In addition, the macrophage or B lymphocytes must carry the appropriate major histocompatibility complex antigen specifically recognized by the T cell clone. Antigen presented by macrophages or B lymphocytes carrying the inappropriate histocompatibility antigens will not induce cell proliferation. The advent of T cell cloning has provided important insights into the fine specificity of T cell recognition of antigen.

Fathman CG, Fitch FW (editors): *Isolation, Utilization, and Characterization of T Cell Clones.* Academic Press, 1982.

Ledbetter JA et al: Evolutionary conservation of surface molecules that distinguish T lymphocyte helper/inducer and T cytotoxic/suppressor subpopulations in mouse and man. *J Exp Med* 1981;**153**:310.

Rocklin RE: Mediators of cellular immunity. Chap 9, pp 97–108, in: *Basic & Clinical Immunology,* 4th ed. Stites DP et al (editors). Lange, 1982.

Subpopulations & Surface Markers of B Lymphocytes

Subpopulations of B cells that express different classes of surface markers are shown in Table 34–1. The majority of B cells in mice and humans express both IgM and IgD on the cell surface. The minority of cells express surface IgG. Most of the IgG-bearing cells in the mouse spleen express an additional class of surface immunoglobulin (either IgM or IgD). The mature IgM- and IgD-bearing B cells are derived from pre-B cells found mainly in the bone marrow. The latter have been shown to contain intracytoplasmic IgM but do not express surface immunoglobulin. The pre-B cells first synthesize μ heavy chains but no light chains. The subsequent synthesis of light chains is followed shortly by the appearance of surface IgM. Patients with congenital hypogammaglobulinemia frequently show a developmental arrest at the stage of the pre-B cell. The majority of patients with acquired hypogammaglobulinemia have a block of transition from the mature B cell to the plasma cell. Thus, most patients with acquired disease have normal numbers of circulating mature B cells.

Studies of the relationship between the immune function of B cell subpopulations and the expression of different classes of surface immunoglobulin have made use of a new technologic advance, the fluorescence-activated cell sorter (FACS). B cells are stained for the different surface immunoglobulins using standard immunofluorescent techniques and then separated into purified populations of positively or negatively stained cells on the FACS. Single cells contained in microdroplets pass in front of a laser beam, and those cells that fluoresce intensely are recognized by photoelectric receivers. The path of the positively stained cells is electronically deflected from that of the negatively stained cells, and the 2 populations are collected in different receptacles.

There is general agreement that the subpopulations of the IgG-bearing cells contain memory cells that give rise to a rapid secondary IgG antibody response after rechallenge with antigen. Virgin B cells bearing surface IgM have been shown to give rise to the primary IgM antibody response. However, there is ample evidence that there is no simple correlation between memory cells and surface IgG or between virgin cells and surface IgM. In addition, there is no clear correlation between the expression of a given class of immunoglobulin on the surface of a B cell and the class of antibody secreted by its progeny. For example, virgin and memory B cells bearing surface IgM but little or no IgG give rise to an early IgM antibody response followed by an IgG response. This "switching" of immunoglobulin classes by B cell clones has been shown to take place during the secretory phase of immunoglobulin synthesis. Thus, IgG-bearing cells rapidly give rise to IgG-secreting progeny, but IgM-bearing cells (IgG) give rise to a wave of IgM-secreting cells followed by a wave of IgG-secreting cells.

B cells have been commonly identified by other surface markers in addition to immunoglobulins. These include the receptor for the Fc piece of immunoglobulins, the receptor for the C3 component of complement, and surface antigens coded for by the HLA-D genetic region in humans (Table 34–1). All mature B cells bear surface immunoglobulin that is thought to be the antigen-specific receptor. Therefore, surface immunoglobulin does not mark a subpopulation of B cells. On the other hand, the other B cell markers (Ia antigen, Fc receptor, C3 receptor) are present on most but not all mature B cells. The subpopulations of B cells carrying these markers may differ in their function from those that do not. However, the role of these markers or receptors in the function of B cells in the immune response is unclear.

Other subpopulations of B lymphocytes have been defined by physical characteristics (electrical charge, cell density, cell size), by surface antigens at several non-MHC genetic loci, and by their ability to respond to thymus-dependent and thymus-independent antigens.

Other Cells Involved in Immune Responses

A. Macrophages: Macrophages are involved in the initial ingestion and processing of some antigens (especially particulate substances) before interaction with lymphocytes. They are thought to play an important role in allowing T and B lymphocytes to cooperate in the induction of humoral antibody responses. In addition, they appear to be effector cells for certain types of tumor immunity in that they can kill tumor cells in vitro.

B. NK (Natural Killer) Cells: These cells are thought to be lymphocytic (nonphagocytic) in origin but are not directly linked to the T or B cell lineage. They are capable of killing a foreign cell in vitro after they have been incubated with antibodies specifically directed against the foreign cells (antibody-dependent cell-mediated immunity). NK cells may play an important role in effector mechanisms in tumor immunity.

Role of T & B Lymphocytes, Macrophages, & Complement in Host Defense

Fig 34–2 shows some of the mechanisms by which humoral immunity provides a defense against bacterial infection. The neutralization of bacterial toxins by antibodies is an important feature of this defense, since the lethal effects of certain bacteria such as tetanus and diphtheria are dependent upon the function of these toxins. Antibodies that bind to the toxins

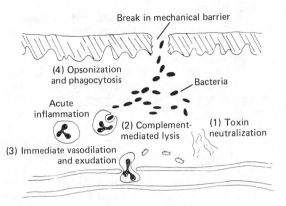

Figure 34–2. Antibody-mediated mechanisms of protection against bacterial infections. Bacterial infections may be resisted by each of the antibody-mediated immune mechanisms including (1) neutralization of bacterial toxins, (2) cytotoxic lysis by antibody and complement, (3) acute anaphylactic vascular events leading to immediate exudate of inflammatory cells and fluids, and (4) acute polymorphonuclear infiltration (Arthus reaction) and opsonization of bacteria leading to increased phagocytosis. (Reproduced, with permission, from Sell S: *Immunology, Immunopathology and Immunity,* 2nd ed. Harper & Row, 1975.)

neutralize their activity by blocking the ability of the toxin to bind to host cell receptors. Direct lysis of bacteria is also mediated by antibody usually of the IgM class. The latter antibodies bind to the polysaccharides of the bacterial cell wall and subsequently bind complement by virtue of the Fc portion of the immunoglobulin molecule. Activation of complement components on the bacterial cell wall results in interaction of the last complement components with the bacterial cell surface membrane, so that the membrane is disrupted and large holes are formed. These holes result in the rapid lysis of the bacteria.

Activation of complement on the bacterial cell wall also results in the local generation of mediators of inflammation, since many of the activated complement components are chemotactic factors that attract neutrophils and macrophages. In addition, activation of complement results in the local release of other mediators of inflammation such as histamine, which increase the permeability of capillaries to the traffic of neutrophils and macrophages. Certain classes of antibodies that bind to the bacterial cell wall do not activate complement but enhance the capacity of macrophages to phagocytize the bacteria. These antibodies are called opsonins, or opsonic antibodies, and they allow for more rapid removal of bacteria by the reticuloendothelial system of cells.

The role of T cells in host defense is not as well elucidated as that of antibodies. It is clear that T cells limit the extent of viral infections by virtue of direct cytolysis of the infected cells by killer T cells. However, the wide variety of lymphokines secreted by T cells appear to play important roles in limiting fungal, viral, bacterial, parasitic, and worm-caused infec-

tions. For example, the secretion of gamma interferon limits viral replication; macrophage inhibition factor allows for the accumulation of macrophages in the area of local microbial growth and invasion; and macrophage activation factor promotes the phagocytosis and intracellular killing of bacteria such as *Toxoplasma* and *Listeria*.

Hayward AR et al: *Developmental Immunobiology*. Elsevier-North Holland, 1977.
Hood LE, Weissman IL, Wood WB: *Immunology*. Benjamin/Cummings, 1978.

MECHANISMS OF AUTOIMMUNE DISEASE

Cell-Mediated Autoimmunity

Certain autoimmune diseases are mediated by T cells that have become specifically immunized to autologous tissues. Cytotoxic or killer T cells generated by this aberrant immune response attack and injure specific organs in the absence of serum autoantibodies. Autoimmune allergic encephalomyelitis and lymphocytic choriomeningitis are 2 examples of T cell–mediated autoimmune disease in animals.

Humoral Antibody–Mediated Autoimmunity

Several autoimmune diseases have been shown to be caused by humoral autoantibody in the absence of cell-mediated autoimmunity. The autoimmune hemolytic anemias, idiopathic thrombocytopenia, and Goodpasture's syndrome appear to be mediated solely by autoantibodies directed against autologous cell membrane constituents. In these diseases, antibody attaches to cell membranes, fixes complement, and thereby causes severe injury to the cell.

Immune Complex Disease

In this group of diseases (systemic lupus erythematosus, rheumatoid arthritis, some drug-induced hemolytic anemias and thrombocytopenias), autologous tissues are injured as "innocent bystanders." Autoantibodies are not directed against cellular components of the target organ but rather against autologous or heterologous antigens in the serum. The resultant antigen-antibody complexes bind nonspecifically to autologous membranes (eg, glomerular basement membrane) and fix complement. Fixation and subsequent activation of complement components produce a local inflammatory response that results in tissue injury.

Stites DP et al (editors): *Basic & Clinical Immunology*, 5th ed. Lange, 1984.

MECHANISM OF ACTION OF IMMUNOSUPPRESSIVE DRUGS

Therapies that suppress immune responses are used commonly to treat recipients of organ transplants and patients with autoimmune diseases. The most frequently used drugs and their modes of action are briefly summarized below.

(1) Corticosteroids. This group of drugs has potent anti-inflammatory effects and direct effects on immunocompetent cells. Suppression of immune responses is the result of both effects. Corticosteroids inhibit cell-mediated immune responses more severely than humoral responses, and little change is observed in the levels of serum immunoglobulins in short-term (several days) studies. The mechanisms by which corticosteroids inhibit T lymphocyte immune responsiveness in humans are not clear. Disruption of the interaction between T cells and macrophages appears to be an important mechanism, and corticosteroids have been shown to block the activation of T cells by interleukin-1 (IL-1) derived from macrophages. In addition, corticosteroids inhibit the expression of class II histocompatibility antigens on the macrophage surface, thereby interfering with presentation of antigen to T cells.

(2) Cytotoxic drugs. The most frequently used cytotoxic drugs are azathioprine and cyclophosphamide. Azathioprine is a nitroimidazole derivative of mercaptopurine, an antagonist of purine synthesis. Azathioprine is a phase-specific drug that kills rapidly replicating cells going through the S phase of the mitotic cycle. It inhibits proliferation of both T and B cells as well as cells mediating inflammation (ie, macrophages). Cyclophosphamide is an alkylating agent that damages cells by cross-linking DNA. Although this cycle-specific drug is most effective in killing cells going through the mitotic cycle, it can also cause intermitotic cell injury and death. Cyclophosphamide can inhibit both cell-mediated and humoral immunity as well as inflammation. Azathioprine and cyclophosphamide are effective inhibitors of the production of serum antibodies.

(3) Antimetabolites. The most commonly used antimetabolite is methotrexate, an inhibitor of folic acid synthesis. Methotrexate inhibits rapidly proliferating cells in S phase and suppresses both cell-mediated and humoral immunity as well as inflammation.

(4) Cyclosporine. This cyclic polypeptide derived from a fungus has been used recently as an immunosuppressive drug in organ transplant recipients. Cyclosporine interferes with the secretion of interleukin-2 (IL-2) by T lymphocytes. Since IL-2 is necessary for T cell replication, this drug is a potent inhibitor of T cell proliferation and thereby inhibits T cell-mediated immune responses. Little effect has been shown on direct B cell immune responses or on inflammation.

Salaman JR (editor): *Immunosuppressive Therapy.* MTP Press, 1981.

GENETIC CONTROL OF THE IMMUNE RESPONSE

In recent years it has become apparent that the ability to mount a specific immune response is under direct control by genes other than those which are the structural genes for the immunoglobulin light and heavy chains. The former genes are closely associated on the same chromosome with the structural genes for the major transplantation antigens. The major transplantation antigens are the cell surface glycoproteins (found on all tissues of the body), which elicit the strongest transplantation rejection reaction when tissues are exchanged between 2 members of a particular species. In humans, this genetic region has been designated the **human leukocyte antigen (HLA)** complex because these antigens were first detected on peripheral blood lymphocytes.

The classic transplantation antigens in humans are called class I HLA molecules and consist of a 44,000-MW membrane-bound glycoprotein heavy chain complexed to a 12,000-MW light chain (β_2-microglobulin). The 3 allelic series of class I antigens are highly polymorphic and are designated HLA-A (23 alleles), HLA-B (47 alleles), and HLA-C (8 alleles). In addition, B locus molecules each possess one of 2 possible public antigenic determinants, Bw4 or Bw6. Class I antigens are detected by serologic methods and are present on all nucleated cells and on platelets but are only weakly expressed on erythrocytes. Another series of transplantation antigens has also been identified, designated class II HLA molecules, which consists of membrane-bound glycoproteins with a 34,000-MW heavy chain and a 28,000-MW light chain. Class II antigen distribution is restricted primarily to B lymphocytes, monocytes, and activated (but not resting) T lymphocytes. Four class II antigen series are recognized: HLA-DR with 14 alleles, HLA-DP (formerly SB) with 6 alleles, HLA-DQ (formerly DC, MB, or MT) with 3 alleles, and HLA-D with 19 alleles.

Through study of families with intra-HLA recombinations and by use of somatic cell hybrids, the HLA region has been localized to chromosome 6, and the order of the different HLA loci is shown in Fig 34–3. Most (98%) of the time, the HLA complex is inherited intact as a haplotype, and, therefore, within any particular family, the number of different combinations found will be fairly small; eg, siblings have a 1:4 chance of being HLA-identical. In contrast, because of the great polymorphism of the HLA system, the number of antigen combinations among unrelated

```
      DQ   Bf
 —DP—DR—C2—B—C——A—
      D    C4
```

Figure 34–3. Genetic map of the HLA region. The centromere is to the left. Bf, C2, and C4 are genes for components of the complement system.

individuals is large, resulting in very low probabilities (less than one in several thousand, depending upon the phenotype involved) of finding HLA-compatible individuals in a random donor pool. This is particularly important when compatible donors are needed for allosensitized patients requiring platelet transfusions or organ transplantation; family members have the highest likelihood of being compatible donors, whereas unrelated individuals have only very low probabilities of being compatible with the patient. HLA-A, -B, and -C typing is utilized for selection of compatible donors for platelet transfusions to allosensitized, thrombocytopenic recipients. Typing for the class I antigens as well as for D, DQ, and DR antigens is important in determining compatibility for organ transplantation. Typing for all of the known HLA markers is of value in studying associations between the HLA system and genetic control of disease susceptibility.

A genetic region determining the structure of the mixed lymphocyte culture antigens and mapping within the major transplantation antigen complex of the mouse was identified several years ago. At the same time, it became apparent that a series of genes determining the ability to mount a specific immune response to a given antigen or antigenic determinant also mapped in the same region. The latter genes determining the ability to respond well or poorly to a particular antigen have been given the designation of immune response, or **Ir**, genes. Specific Ir genes identified in the mouse and rat control the ability to mount a strong or weak immune response to a wide variety of synthetic polypeptides, native proteins, viruses, thyroglobulin, and basic encephalitogenic proteins. In both humans and monkeys, the evidence indicates that Ir genes controlling immune responses to antigens such as ragweed allergen are closely linked to the major transplantation antigen gene complex. Presumably, in humans these Ir genes will map in the same region as the genes determining the class II antigens (Fig 34–3).

Although the exact mechanism of action of Ir genes is not yet known, it is clear that they affect the ability to recognize foreign antigens and to initiate the development of cellular and humoral immunity to these antigens. Genes with such a strong effect on specific immune responsiveness might be expected to have major effects on resistance or susceptibility to a wide variety of infectious, neoplastic, and autoimmune diseases.

This appears to be the case. Although methods are not yet available for Ir genotyping in humans, methods are available for HLA typing and for typing for particular HLA-D antigens in humans, and such typing procedures have revealed extraordinarily strong associations between these genes and particular human diseases.

Benacerraf B, McDevitt HO: Histocompatibility linked immune response genes. *Science* 1972;**175:**273.

Grumet FC: Relationship between diseases and the HLA system. Page 125 in: *Blood Group Antigens and Disease.* Garratty G (editor). AABB Publication, Arlington, VA, 1983.

CLINICAL IMMUNOLOGY LABORATORY TESTS

Procedures for Testing Cell-Mediated Immunity, or T Cell Function

A. Skin Testing: Cell-mediated immunity can be assessed qualitatively by evaluating skin reactivity following intradermal injection of a battery of antigens to which humans are frequently sensitized (ie, streptokinase, streptodornase, purified protein derivative, *Trichophyton, Dermatophyton,* or *Candida*). Skin painting with dinitrochlorobenzene is helpful if there is doubt about prior exposure to any of the above antigens, since dinitrochlorobenzene functions as both the sensitizing and the "test" antigen. Anergy or lack of skin reactivity to all of these substances indicates a marked depression of cell-mediated immunity.

B. In Vitro Stimulation of Peripheral Blood Lymphocytes With Phytohemagglutinin or Allogeneic Lymphocytes (Mixed Lymphocyte Culture, MLC): T but not B lymphocytes are transformed to blast cells upon short-term incubation with phytohemagglutinin or allogeneic lymphocytes in vitro. Quantitative determinations of blast transformation can be made by following the cellular uptake of ^{3}H-thymidine introduced into the culture medium. The in vitro uptake of ^{3}H-thymidine by human peripheral blood lymphocytes serves as an indicator of T cell function and correlates well with the manifestations of cell-mediated immunity as measured by skin reactivity.

Procedures for Measuring Humoral Immunity, or B Cell Function

There are 4 methods of assessing humoral immunity: (1) quantitative and qualitative determinations of serum immunoglobulins; (2) determination of isohemagglutinin and febrile agglutinin titers; (3) determination of antibody titers following primary or booster immunization with tetanus toxoid, diphtheria toxoid, and pertussis vaccines; and (4) determination of the percentage of peripheral blood lymphocytes bearing surface immunoglobulins by immunofluorescent staining techniques. The first method tests for the presence of serum immunoglobulins but not for the functional adequacy of the immunoglobulins. The second method tests for functional antibodies that are present in the serum of almost all individuals as a consequence of exposure to ubiquitous environmental antigens. The third method examines functional antibody activity in the serum after intentional immunization and is a more definitive test of specific humoral antibody formation. The fourth method tests for the presence of the precursors of cells that give rise to serum antibodies and is helpful in determining whether there has been a maturational arrest.

The 2 most commonly used tests of humoral immunity, which provide the first screening procedure for many immunodeficiency states, are immunoelectrophoresis and quantitative immunoglobulin determinations.

A. Immunoelectrophoresis: Immunoelectrophoresis is most useful as a screening device for semiquantitative estimates of the amounts of IgG, IgA, or IgM in the serum or urine and for identifying abnormal immunoglobulin molecules such as myeloma (M) proteins. The absence of certain immunoglobulin classes or the presence of abnormal immunoglobulin molecules in concentrations too low to be detected by serum electrophoresis will be readily apparent on immunoelectrophoresis.

Serum proteins are separated by their electrical charge and identified with appropriate antisera. The interaction between the class-specific antisera and the major serum immunoglobulin classes produces characteristic arcs on the plate. The density of each arc is a measure of the amount of immunoglobulin present. Abnormal immunoglobulins such as myeloma (M) proteins form a sharp arc that merges with the normal immunoglobulin arc of the same class. Once an abnormal immunoglobulin or immunoglobulin fragment (ie, light chain) is found in the serum or urine, further characterization with respect to the heavy chain class and light chain type should be performed using class- or type-specific antisera.

B. Quantitative Immunoglobulin Determinations; Radial Diffusion and Nephelometry Techniques: Quantitative determinations of the serum IgG, IgA, and IgM levels can be carried out quickly in the clinical laboratory using the radial diffusion technique. Circular wells are cut in a gel plate impregnated with a specific goat or horse antiserum directed against a single human immunoglobulin class. A circular precipitin ring will form after the human serum proteins placed in the well diffuse through the gel. The radius or diameter of the precipitin ring is proportionate to the concentration of serum immunoglobulin. The precise immunoglobulin level is determined by comparing the diameter of the unknown serum to that of a standard containing known levels of immunoglobulins.

Determinations of the serum concentrations of IgM, IgG, and IgA can also be made accurately and rapidly using the technique of nephelometry. Highly purified, optically clear, heterologous antibodies to each human immunoglobulin class are added to a sample of serum. A precipitate (heterologous antibody–human immunoglobulin complex) is formed in the fluid phase. The turbidity produced by the precipitate is related to the concentration of each class of human immunoglobulin. Accurate measurements of turbidity can be made with a nephelometer in which a sharply focused light source (frequently a laser beam) is passed through the solution. The precipitate scatters the light, and the extent of scatter is measured by a photoelectric detector. With appropriate standards, the light scatter measurements are accurately related to the concentration of each serum immunoglobulin.

Quantitative immunoglobulin measurements do not differentiate between normal and abnormal immunoglobulin molecules, as does the immunoelectrophoresis procedure. The normal serum concentrations of the 3 major immunoglobulin classes are as follows:

IgG 711–1536 mg/dL (92–207 IU/mL)
IgA 54–489 mg/dL (54–268 IU/mL)
IgM 37–212 mg/dL (69–287 IU/mL)

TECHNIQUES FOR IDENTIFICATION OF HUMAN T & B CELLS

B Cells

Cell surface characteristics found on B but not T cells include the following: (1) easily detectable surface immunoglobulin, (2) a receptor for complement (C3), and (3) a receptor for the Fc portion of immunoglobulins that have been aggregated or complexed with antigen (Table 34–1).

Surface immunoglobulin is commonly detected by direct fluorescence staining of live cell suspensions with fluorescein-conjugated heterologous antisera directed against human immunoglobulin. The receptor for complement is identified by incubating suspensions of live lymphocytes in vitro with sheep red blood cells coated with antibody and complement. The sensitized red cells adhere to the surface of the lymphocytes via the complement receptor and form rosettes that are identified under the light microscope. The receptor for aggregated immunoglobulin is identified by incubating lymphocytes in vitro with fluorescein-labeled IgG aggregates.

T Cells

Methods currently used to identify peripheral T lymphocytes in humans depend upon the presence of surface markers that are shared by human thymocytes and the absence of surface markers associated with B cells. T cell markers include T cell–specific surface antigens identified by heterologous antisera and a surface receptor that binds sheep red blood cells. Recently, monoclonal antisera have been used in both immunofluorescence staining and in vitro cytotoxicity assays to identify T cell subsets (Table 34–1). The receptor for sheep red blood cells is detected by incubating live suspensions of human lymphocytes in vitro with sheep red blood cells and monitoring the formation of spontaneous rosettes under the light microscope. Approximately 75% of human peripheral blood lymphocytes are T cells and up to 25% are B cells.

Hoffman RA et al: Simple and rapid measurement of human T lymphocytes and their subclasses in peripheral blood. *Proc Natl Acad Sci* 1980;**77**:4914.

Ledbetter JA et al: Evolutionary conservation of surface molecules that distinguish T lymphocyte help/inducer and T cytotoxic/suppressor subpopulations in mouse and man. *J Exp Med* 1981;**153**:310.

Null Cells

Approximately 5–10% of human peripheral blood lymphocytes are called ''null'' cells, since they do not carry many of the surface markers associated with T or B cells. Some of the null cells function as natural killer (NK) cells in antibody-dependent cell-mediated cytotoxicity; others may be immature T or B cells that have not yet acquired the full complement of developmental surface markers.

INTERPRETATION OF RESULTS OF T & B CELL TYPING

Immunodeficiency Diseases

Thymic hypoplasia is associated with a marked decrease in the percentage and absolute number of T cells in the peripheral blood. On the other hand, the absence of B cells in the blood is frequently found in X-linked agammaglobulinemia. Typing of peripheral blood T and B cells can help to establish the diagnosis of the above diseases in early childhood.

Lymphoproliferative Diseases

The presence of a marked increase in the percentage and absolute count of peripheral blood lymphocytes that bear immunoglobulin of a single heavy chain class and light chain type represents a monoclonal proliferation of cells. Almost all patients with chronic lymphocytic leukemia and non-Hodgkin's lymphoma with blood involvement show this picture. On the other hand, lymphocytosis secondary to viral or bacterial infection is associated with a normal percentage of B cells and the usual distribution of immunoglobulin classes on the cell surface.

A marked decrease in the percentage of B cells in the peripheral blood (> 5%) is seen in some cases of multiple myeloma but not in benign monoclonal gammopathy. This may provide a diagnostic tool for differentiating these disease states in the future.

TESTS FOR AUTOANTIBODIES ASSOCIATED WITH AUTOIMMUNE DISEASES

Assays for autoantibodies are similar to those used for detection of antibodies to heterologous antigens. Four of the more commonly used methods are discussed below:

Tanned Red Blood Cell Hemagglutination

Red cells (human, sheep, etc) are incubated with tannic acid, so that the cell surface becomes "sticky." The tanned cells are subsequently incubated with the specific antigen (eg, thyroglobulin), which is adsorbed to the cell surface. The antigen-coated cells are suspended in the unknown serum, and antibody is detected by red cell agglutination. Antigen-coated latex particles are substituted for red cells in the latex fixation test.

Radioimmune Precipitation

Specific antigen (eg, DNA) is radiolabeled, usually by iodination (^{125}I) or tritiation (^{3}H). Labeled antigen is incubated with the unknown serum to allow antigen-antibody complexes to form. Complexes are then precipitated by the addition of ammonium sulfate or anti-immunoglobulin. The amount of radioactivity in the supernatant or precipitate is related to the amount of antigen bound by specific antibody in the unknown serum.

Immunofluorescence Microscopy

This technique is most frequently used for detection of antinuclear antibody. Frozen sections of mouse liver are cut and placed on glass slides. Unknown serum is placed over the sections and washed away. A fluorescein-conjugated rabbit anti-human immunoglobulin is applied thereafter and washed. Antinuclear antibody specifically binds to the mouse cell nucleus, and the fluorescein conjugate binds to the human antibody. Fluorescence of the cell nucleus observed by fluorescence microscopy indicates a positive test.

Complement Fixation

Specific antigen, unknown serum, and complement are incubated together. Sheep red blood cells coated with anti-sheep cell antibody are subsequently added to the reaction mixture for 30 minutes at 37 °C. Lysis of sheep cells indicates that complement is present (attaches to sheep cell surface). Lack of lysis indicates that complement has been consumed by the in-

Table 34–3. Some autoimmune diseases and their associated antibodies.

Autoimmune Disease	Associated Autoantibodies
Autoimmune hemolytic anemia	Anti-blood group substance antibody
Autoimmune thyroiditis	Antithyroglobulin antibody
Chronic active hepatitis	Anti-smooth muscle, anticytoplasmic, antinuclear, anti-immunoglobulin (rheumatoid factor) antibody
Goodpasture's syndrome	Anti-basement membrane antibody
Idiopathic thrombocytopenic purpura	Antiplatelet antibody
Pemphigoid	Anti-basement membrane antibody
Pemphigus vulgaris	Anti-intercellular antibody
Pernicious anemia	Anti-parietal cell, anti-intrinsic factor antibody
Polymyositis	Antinuclear antibody
Primary biliary cirrhosis	Antimitochondrial antibody, antinuclear antibody
Rheumatoid arthritis	Anti-immunoglobulin (rheumatoid factor), antinuclear antibody
Scleroderma	Antinuclear antibody
Sjögren's syndrome	Anti-immunoglobulin, anti-salivary gland, antinuclear antibody
Systemic lupus erythematosus	Antinuclear, anti-DNA, anti-ENA (extractable nuclear antigen), anti-immunoglobulin, antilymphocyte, anti-red blood cell antibody

teraction of antibody in the unknown serum with the specific antigen. Lack of lysis is therefore interpreted as a positive test for the presence of specific antibody.

A list of autoimmune diseases and frequently associated autoantibodies is shown in Table 34–3. Many of the autoantibodies are not specific for a single disease entity (eg, antinuclear antibody, rheumatoid factor). Tests for the latter autoantibodies are best used as screening procedures in that a negative result makes the diagnosis of certain autoimmune diseases unlikely. For example, a negative antinuclear antibody test makes the diagnosis of systemic lupus erythematosus unlikely, since this antibody is detected in the serum of more than 95% of lupus patients.

MEASUREMENT OF SERUM COMPLEMENT LEVELS

Determination of the concentration of serum complement components is useful in the diagnosis and management of some diseases. In systemic lupus erythematosus, levels of C3, the third component of complement, have been correlated with the activity of glomerulonephritis. Decreased levels of C3 are thought to be a result of complement activation by immune complexes that circulate in the blood. During periods of active nephritis, the complement levels are frequently low, but during remissions, these levels return to normal. The immune complexes bind to and activate the first component of complement. The activated C1 begins a cascade in which C4, C2, and C3 are sequentially activated. The cleavage of C3 results in decreased C3 levels, which are commonly measured using anti-C3 antibodies in the radial diffusion assay. Reduction of C3 levels is also observed in certain forms of idiopathic glomerulonephritis (hypocomplementemic glomerulonephritis). The mechanism of complement consumption in this disease is unclear but may be related to circulating immune complexes. The level of C3 in joint fluid may be of value in distinguishing joint effusions caused by rheumatoid arthritis from other arthritides. In rheumatoid arthritis, the complement level is reduced presumably owing to activation by immune complexes in joint fluid (rheumatoid factor and IgG). In most other arthritides, the complement level is normal.

Measurement of the serum level of C4 is of value in the diagnosis of hereditary angioneurotic edema. In this disease, there is a genetic deficiency in the enzyme that inhibits C1 esterase activity. Increased esterase activity leads to excessive cleavage of C4 and a marked reduction in the C4 serum level. Thus, a decreased C4 level is suggestive of the disease, but a definitive diagnosis is based upon the absence or reduction of the C1 esterase inhibitor level in serum. The latter measurement is commonly performed by radioimmunoassay.

HLA TYPING

The standard method for detecting HLA-A, -B, and -C antigens is that of lymphocyte microcytotoxicity. Utilizing microliter quantities of reagents, 2000 lymphocytes isolated from peripheral blood or lymph nodes are added to each well of a typing tray that has been preloaded with sera containing the appropriate cytotoxic alloantibody. After allowing one-half hour for the alloantibodies to bind to target lymphocytes, a source of complement, generally fresh-frozen rabbit serum, is added. During the next hour, those cells to which antibody has been specifically bound will have complement activated at the cell surface, resulting in focal cell membrane damage and cell death or lysis. By addition of a suitable vital dye (eg, eosin, fluorescein diacetate, or trypan blue), viable and nonviable cells can readily be distinguished under the proper microscopic conditions. Thus, wells with little or no cell death lack antibodies recognizing antigens of the particular target cell and are negative tests, while wells with all or most cells killed are positive and indicate that the target cells possess specific antigen recognized by the reagent alloantibody in that particular well. Putting together the proper panel of test antisera, it is thus possible to type for all of the known HLA-A, -B, and -C specificities, while international exchanges of reagents regularly assure antigen standardization and uniform assignment among laboratories. At the present time, the best sources of alloantisera are parous women, 10–30% of whom routinely become sensitized during pregnancy to paternal antigens carried by the fetus. A small number of antibodies are also provided by individuals allosensitized by other causes, eg, transfusion or transplantation, and a few xenogeneic monoclonal antibodies have also begun to be used.

Typing for the class II antigens HLA-DR and -DQ is performed as described above, except that isolated or otherwise marked (eg, by fluoresceinated antibodies) B lymphocytes are used as targets rather than unseparated peripheral blood lymphocytes. Antigens of the HLA-D and -DP series, rather than being detected by serologic techniques, utilize in vitro cellular reactivity based upon the principle that lymphocytes of one individual will undergo DNA synthesis and proliferation upon encountering lymphocytes from another individual possessing foreign HLA-D or -DP antigens. To detect HLA-D antigens, cells of an individual selected for D homozygosity are irradiated or treated with mitomycin C to ablate their immune responsiveness. These "stimulator" cells are then mixed with peripheral blood lymphocytes of the test subject ("responder") in this mixed leukocyte culture (MLR). A responder lacking the stimulator's D antigen will respond by brisk DNA synthesis and proliferation that can readily be measured by methods such as DNA incorporation of tritiated thymidine. Responders possessing the D antigen of the stimulator will remain quiescent, thus permitting identification of particular D specificities.

HLA-DP antigens are identified by an extension of the MLR called primed lymphocyte typing. Following stimulation in a first MLR, the responder cells are restimulated in a secondary MLR by a different stimulator cell. If the 2 stimulator cells share a DP (or a D) antigen not possessed by the responder, the responder cells will demonstrate a brisk proliferative response.

Although technically demanding and requiring viable lymphoid cells and experienced laboratories, particularly for typing of class II antigens, HLA typing is available at most large medical centers or blood banks.

Grumet FC: HLA serology—1983. Pages 207–220 in: *Advances in Immunobiology: Blood Cell Antigens and Bone Marrow Transplantation.* McCullough J, Sandler SG (editors). Liss, 1984.

Jorgensen F: HLA-D typing by MLC with homozygous typing cells. Pages 57–70 in: *HLA Typing: Methodology and Clinical Aspects.* Vol 1. Ferrone S, Solheim BG (editors). CRC Press, 1982.

Moen T: Primed lymphocyte typing (PLT): Application in typing for HLA-D locus determinants. Pages 71–82 in: *HLA Typing: Methodology and Clinical Aspects.* Vol 1. Ferrone S, Solheim BG (editors). CRC Press, 1982.

Vellios F (editor): Laboratory diagnosis of immune and autoimmune reactions. *Am J Clin Pathol* 1977;**68(Suppl)**:633. [Entire issue.]

GAMMOPATHIES

The gammopathies include those disease entities in which there is a disproportionate proliferation of a single clone of antibody-forming cells that produce a homogeneous heavy chain, light chain, or complete immunoglobulin molecule. The amino acid sequence of the variable (V) regions is fixed, and only one type (κ or λ) of light chain is produced.

Benign Monoclonal Gammopathy

The diagnosis is made upon finding a homogeneous (monoclonal) immunoglobulin (with either κ or λ chains but not both) in immunoelectrophoresis of the serum of an otherwise normal individual. Screening of large populations in Sweden shows that the incidence of homogeneous immunoglobulins in the serum increases with age and may approach 3% in persons 70 years of age or older. Follow-up studies show that a small percentage of apparently normal persons with a homogeneous serum immunoglobulin will go on to develop multiple myeloma. Parameters that suggest a favorable prognosis in "benign" monoclonal gammopathy include the following: (1) concentration of homogeneous immunoglobulin < 1 g/dL, (2) no significant increase in the concentration of the homogeneous immunoglobulin from the time of diagnosis, (3) no decrease in the concentration of normal immunoglobulins, (4) absence of a homogeneous light chain in the urine (Bence Jones proteinuria), (5) normal hematocrit and serum albumin concentration.

Multiple Myeloma

This disease is characterized by the spread of neoplastic plasma cells throughout the bone marrow. Rarely, a single extraosseous plasmacytoma may be found. Anemia, hypercalcemia, increased susceptibility to infection, and bone pain are frequent findings. Certain diagnosis depends upon the presence of the following: (1) x-ray findings of osteolytic lesions or diffuse osteoporosis, (2) presence of a homogeneous serum immunoglobulin (myeloma protein) or a single type of light chain in the urine (Bence Jones proteinuria), (3) finding of an abnormal plasma cell infiltrate in the bone marrow biopsy.

Waldenström's Macroglobulinemia

Waldenström's macroglobulinemia is characterized by a proliferation of abnormal lymphoid cells that have the features of both lymphocytic and plasmacytic lines. These cells secrete a homogeneous macroglobulin (IgM) that is easily detected and characterized by immunoelectrophoresis. Bence Jones proteinuria is present in 10% of cases. Clinical manifestations frequently depend upon the physicochemical characteristics of the macroglobulin. Raynaud's phenomenon and peripheral vascular occlusions are associated with cold-insoluble proteins (cryoglobulins). Retinal hemorrhages, visual impairment, and transient neurologic deficits are not uncommon with high-viscosity serum. Bleeding diatheses and hemolytic anemia can occur when the macroglobulin complexes with coagulation factors or binds to the surface of red blood cells.

Amyloidosis

Amyloidosis is manifested by impaired organ function from extracellular infiltration of the tissue with insoluble protein fibrils. Variations in composition of the fibrils for the most part can be correlated with the clinical syndromes (Table 34–4).

One chemical type of amyloid occurs (1) in a primary form, or (2) in company with plasmacytosis in bone marrow or lymphoid tissues. The protein fibrils in these entities are composed of immunoglobulin light chains or fragments of light chains, particularly the V region. This form of amyloid has been designated AL.

A nonimmunoglobulin protein (AA) is the major component of amyloid fibrils that form secondary to infection (osteomyelitis, tuberculosis), inflammation, rheumatoid arthritis, Hodgkin's disease, regional enteritis, renal cell carcinoma, leprosy, and intravenous drug abuse. The hereditary systemic amyloidosis associated with familial Mediterranean fever is composed of AA protein. The source of the protein is obscure, but it may be derived from the acute-phase reactant SAA.

All varieties of amyloid fibrils contain about a 10% concentration of an α_1-glycoprotein known as "P" or plasma component.

Symptoms and signs of amyloid infiltration are related to malfunction of the organ involved, eg, nephrotic syndrome, chronic renal failure, car-

Table 34—4. Classification of amyloidosis.*

	Clinical Type	Common Sites of Deposition	Chemical Type of Fibril†
Familial	Amyloid polyneuropathy (Portuguese, dominant inheritance)	Peripheral nerves	AF$_p$ (prealbumin)
		Viscera	
	Familial Mediterranean fever (recessive)	Liver, spleen, kidneys, adrenals	AA
Generalized	Primary	Tongue, heart, gut, skeletal and smooth muscles, nerves, skin, ligaments	AL
	Associated with plasma cell dyscrasia	Liver, spleen, kidneys, heart, adrenals	AL
	Secondary (infection, inflammation, etc)	Any site	AA
Localized	Lichen amyloidosis	Skin	AD
	Endocrine-related (eg, thyroid medullary carcinoma, diabetes mellitus, Addison's disease)	Endocrine organ (thyroid)	AE (AE$_t$)
Senile		Heart	AS$_c$
		Brain	AS$_b$

*Modified and reproduced, with permission, from Stites DP et al (editors): *Basic & Clinical Immunology,* 5th ed. Lange, 1984.
†AA = amyloid A; AD = amyloid dermatologic; AE = amyloid endocrine; AF = amyloid familial; AL = amyloid light chain; AS = amyloid senile.

diomyopathy, cardiac conduction defects, intestinal malabsorption, intestinal obstruction, carpal tunnel syndrome, macroglossia, peripheral neuropathy, end-organ insufficiency of endocrine glands, respiratory failure, obstruction to ventilation, and capillary damage with ecchymosis. See Table 34–4 for a list of organs characteristically involved with each type of amyloid.

The diagnosis of amyloidosis is based first on a suspicion that it may be present, since clinical manifestations may be varied and atypical. The family history may reveal a hereditary origin. Preexisting long-standing infection or debilitating illness should suggest the possibility of its existence. Microscopic examination of biopsy (eg, gingival, renal, rectal) or surgical specimens after suitable staining procedures is diagnostic. It has been reported that fine-needle biopsy of subcutaneous abdominal fat is a simple and reliable method for diagnosing secondary systemic amyloidosis.

Treatment of localized amyloid "tumors" is by surgical excision. There is no effective treatment of systemic amyloidosis, and death usually occurs within 1–3 years. Treatment of the predisposing disease may cause a temporary remission or slow the progress of the disease, but it is unlikely that the established metabolic process is altered. Patients with plasma cell dyscrasia may occasionally respond to treatment with melphalan and prednisone. Colchicine may be of use in familial Mediterranean fever. Early and adequate treatment of pyogenic infections will probably prevent much secondary amyloidosis.

Heavy Chain Disease (α, γ, μ)

These are rare disorders in which the abnormal serum and urine protein is a part of a homogeneous α, γ, or μ heavy chain. The clinical presentation is more typical of lymphoma than multiple myeloma, and there are no destructive bone lesions. Alpha chain disease is frequently associated with severe diarrhea and infiltration of the lamina propria of the small intestine with abnormal plasma cells.

Block KJ et al: Gamma heavy chain disease. *Am J Med* 1973; **55**:61.

Franklin EC: Immunopathology of the amyloid diseases. *Hosp Pract* (Sept) 1980;**15**:70.

Glenner GG: Amyloid deposits and amyloidosis: The fibrilloses. (2 parts.) *N Engl J Med* 1980;**302**:1283, 1333.

Glenner GG, Page DL: Amyloid, amyloidosis, and amyloidogenesis. *Int Rev Exp Pathol* 1976;**15**:1.

Kyle RA: Monoclonal gammopathy of undetermined significance. *Am J Med* 1978;**64**:814.

Kyle RA: Multiple myeloma: Review of 869 cases. *Mayo Clin Proc* 1975;**50**:29.

Stites DP et al: *Basic & Clinical Immunology,* 5th ed. Lange, 1984.

Wright JR, Calkins E: Clinico-pathological differentiation of common amyloid syndromes. *Medicine* 1981;**60**:429.

IMMUNOLOGIC DEFICIENCY DISEASES

The primary immunologic deficiency diseases include congenital and acquired disorders of humoral immunity (B cell function) or cell-mediated immunity (T cell function). The most recent classification of immunodeficiency disorders recommended by WHO is shown below:

Infantile X-linked agammaglobulinemia (see below)

Selective immunoglobulin deficiency (see below)

Transient hypogammaglobulinemia of infancy

X-linked immunodeficiency with hyper-IgM

Thymic hypoplasia (pharyngeal pouch syndrome, DiGeorge's syndrome) (see below)

Immunodeficiency with normal serum globulins or hyperimmunoglobulinemia

Immunodeficiency with ataxia-telangiectasia (see below)

Immunodeficiency with thrombocytopenia and eczema (Wiskott-Aldrich syndrome) (see below)

Immunodeficiency with thymoma
Immunodeficiency with generalized hematopoietic hypoplasia
Severe combined immunodeficiency (see below):
(1) With dysostosis
(2) With adenosine deaminase deficiency
Variable immunodeficiency (common, largely unclassified) (see below)
Acquired immunodeficiency syndrome (AIDS) (see below)

Bergsma D et al (editors): *Immunodeficiency in Man and Animals.* (National Foundation–March of Dimes Original Article Series.) Sinauer Associates, 1975.
Cooper MD et al: Meeting report of the Second International Workshop on Primary Immunodeficiency Disease in Man. *Clin Immunol Immunopathol* 1974;**2**:416.
Stites DP et al (editors): *Basic & Clinical Immunology,* 5th ed. Lange, 1984.
Waldmann TA et al: Disorders of suppressor immunoregulatory cells in the pathogenesis of immunodeficiency and autoimmunity. *Ann Intern Med* 1978;**88**:226.

INFANTILE X-LINKED AGAMMAGLOBULINEMIA

This hereditary disorder results in a deficit in B cell function with essentially intact T cell function.

Clinical Findings

The diagnosis is based on the low IgG levels in serum, an X-linked pattern of heredity, intact cell-mediated immunity, and the absence of plasma cells in biopsy specimens of regional lymph nodes draining the site of recent antigenic stimulation such as DTP vaccine.

A. Symptoms and Signs: There are no symptoms during the first 9 months of life (probably due to presence of maternal antibody). During the second year, the infant shows increased susceptibility to pyogenic infections (gram-positive organisms) and *Haemophilus influenzae*, resulting in recurrent furunculosis, pneumonia, and meningitis. There is normal susceptibility to viral exanthematous infections such as rubella, measles, chickenpox, and varicella. Other characteristic findings are chronic sinusitis, bronchiectasis, and arthritis of the large joints, which has the appearance of rheumatoid arthritis.

B. Laboratory Findings: IgG levels in the serum are less than 100 mg/dL, serum IgA and IgM levels are less than 1% of normal, and isohemagglutinins are low or absent. The Schick test is positive, and antitoxin titers do not rise after vaccination with DTP vaccine. The peripheral lymphocyte count and skin reactivity to *Candida* antigen, purified protein derivative, and dinitrochlorobenzene are normal. There are no immunoglobulin-staining lymphocytes in the peripheral blood in most cases.

Treatment

Recurrent bacterial infections can be prevented by the administration of gamma globulin for an indefinite period of time. The gamma globulin is usually administered intramuscularly. The usual loading dose is 300 mg gamma globulin ($\sim$ 1.8 mL) per kg body weight in 3 equally divided injections. Thereafter, monthly injections of 0.6 mL/kg body weight are given to maintain an IgG level of at least 200 mg/dL.

THYMIC HYPOPLASIA
(DiGeorge's Syndrome)

DiGeorge's syndrome is due to failure of embryogenesis of the third and fourth pharyngeal pouches. This results in aplasia of the parathyroid and thymus glands. The syndrome presents as a pure T cell functional deficiency with intact B cell function.

Clinical Findings

A. Symptoms and Signs: The major manifestations are neonatal tetany, hypertelorism, and increased susceptibility to viral, fungal, and bacterial infections. Infections are frequently lethal.

B. Laboratory Findings: Serum immunoglobulin levels are normal. The humoral antibody response may be low or normal, depending on the antigen used for immunization. (A low response is thought to be due to lack of helper T cells.) Skin reactivity to intradermal injections of *Candida* antigen or skin painting with dinitrochlorobenzene is markedly depressed, as is blastogenesis of peripheral blood lymphocytes upon incubation with phytohemagglutinin or with allogeneic lymphocytes. Serum calcium and the peripheral lymphocyte count are low. Biopsy of lymph nodes shows normal germinal center formation but marked deficits in the thymus-dependent or paracortical areas. There are no T cells in peripheral blood.

Treatment

Transplantation of fetal thymic tissue has been successful in reversing the deficits in cell-mediated immunity and raising the peripheral lymphocyte count to normal. The thymus-dependent areas of the lymph nodes of transplant recipients are also repopulated.

SEVERE COMBINED IMMUNODEFICIENCY

Both T and B cell function are markedly decreased in this entity, which is inherited in an autosomal recessive or X-linked pattern. A sporadic appearance in families also occurs. Dysostosis and adenosine deaminase deficiency are associated with severe combined immunodeficiency in some cases.

Clinical Findings

A. Symptoms and Signs: Increased susceptibility to infection is noted at 3–6 months of age. Death usually occurs within 2 years. The period of infancy is marked by watery diarrhea, usually associated with

Salmonella or enteropathic *Escherichia coli* infections. Pulmonary infections, usually with *Pseudomonas* and *Pneumocystis carinii,* are common, as is candidiasis in the mouth and diaper areas. Common viral exanthems such as chickenpox and measles are often lethal.

B. Laboratory Findings: Serum immunoglobulin levels are usually less than 1% of normal, and antibodies do not form in response to vaccinations such as DTP. The peripheral lymphocyte count is less than 2000/μL. Decreased delayed hypersensitivity is manifested by lack of skin reactivity to painting with dinitrochlorobenzene or intradermal injection with *Candida* antigen. Lymph node biopsy shows no lymphocytes, plasma cells, or lymphoid follicles.

Treatment

Passive administration of gamma globulin is ineffective. Bone marrow transplantation has been successful, but the complications of graft-versus-host remains a serious problem.

IMMUNODEFICIENCY WITH THROMBOCYTOPENIA & ECZEMA
(Wiskott-Aldrich Syndrome)

This disorder is characterized by eczema, thrombocytopenia, and recurrent bacterial and viral infections. Inheritance is X-linked, and affected individuals rarely survive more than 10 years. There appears to be a combined T and B cell functional deficit. IgM levels are low and isohemagglutinins absent, but IgG and IgA levels are normal. Cell-mediated immunity is impaired as measured by decreased skin reactivity to common fungal antigens and decreased response to phytohemagglutinin stimulation in vitro.

IMMUNODEFICIENCY WITH ATAXIA-TELANGIECTASIA

The clinical presentation of ataxia-telangiectasia begins in infancy with ataxia and choreoathetoid movements. Telangiectasia of the conjunctiva, face, arms, and eyelids is first noted 5–10 years later. Chronic sinusitis and respiratory infections follow, and death due to intercurrent pulmonary infection or lymphoreticular neoplasm occurs in the second or third decade. Approximately 80% of affected individuals lack serum and secretory IgA. In addition, there is a marked deficit in T cell function associated with a hypoplastic or dysplastic thymus gland. The disease is inherited in an autosomal recessive pattern.

VARIABLE IMMUNODEFICIENCY

Primary Acquired Agammaglobulinemia

Onset is in adulthood, with increased susceptibility to pyogenic infections; recurrent sinusitis and

pneumonia progressing to bronchiectasis; spruelike syndrome with diarrhea, steatorrhea, malabsorption, and protein-losing enteropathy; and hepatosplenomegaly.

There is no arthritis of the type associated with congenital agammaglobulinemia. Autoimmune diseases are common. Laboratory study discloses serum IgG levels usually less than 500 mg/dL; serum IgA and IgM levels are subnormal (variable). Lymph node biopsy shows marked reduction in plasma cells. Noncaseating granulomas are frequently found in the spleen, liver, lungs, or skin.

Recent evidence suggests that suppressor T cells inhibit B cells from producing antibody-forming cells in certain cases of adult-onset agammaglobulinemia. The absolute B cell count in the peripheral blood in these cases is normal. Although therapy at present is similar to that of congenital agammaglobulinemia, newer therapeutic goals may include elimination of suppressor T cells.

SELECTIVE IMMUNOGLOBULIN DEFICIENCY

Absence of serum IgA with normal levels of IgG and IgM is found in a small percentage of normal individuals. Occasionally, a spruelike syndrome with steatorrhea has been associated with an isolated IgA deficit. Treatment with commercial gamma globulin (Cohn fraction II) is ineffective, since IgA and IgM are not present in this preparation. Frequent infusions of plasma (containing IgA) are hazardous, since anti-IgA antibodies may develop, resulting in systemic anaphylaxis or serum sickness.

ACQUIRED IMMUNODEFICIENCY SYNDROME (AIDS)

This recently described disorder is characterized clinically by pneumonia, fever, malaise, anorexia, weight loss, and lymphadenopathy associated with a variety of opportunistic infectious agents including cytomegalovirus, herpesvirus, *Pneumocystis,* and fungi. A concomitant of the disease is a markedly increased incidence of Kaposi's sarcoma. Populations at increased risk of the disease are homosexuals, intravenous drug abusers, hemophiliacs who frequently receive blood products, and Haitians. Immunologic tests reveal a severe deficiency of T lymphocyte function and number, with little alteration in B lymphocyte function and number. Patients are frequently anergic, as judged by skin test reactivity to a battery of antigens injected intradermally. In addition, in vitro tests of peripheral blood T cell function such as proliferative responses to antigens and mitogens are markedly reduced or absent. The absolute lymphocyte count is severely decreased (frequently < 500 cells/μL), and the ratio of helper to suppressor/cytotoxic T cells is considerably lower than normal (normal ratio is approximately 2). The change in the latter ratio is due to a greater reduction in the absolute number of helper T cells in the peripheral blood as compared to suppressor/cytotoxic cells. These changes in T cell number and function appear to be characteristic of the disease entity.

Although the pathogenesis of the disease is unknown, epidemiologic data suggest that a communicable agent plays an important role. Sexual and intravenous transmission, including transfusion with blood products, is suspected. The disease has been reported to be lethal in a high proportion of victims, especially those with Kaposi's sarcoma.

Gallo RC et al: Frequent detection and isolation of cytopathic retroviruses (HTLV-III) from patients with AIDS and at risk for AIDS. *Science* 1984;**224**:500.

Gottlieb MS et al: *Pneumocystis carinii* pneumonia and mucosal candidiasis in previously healthy homosexual men: Evidence of a new acquired immunodeficiency. *N Engl J Med* 1981;**305**:1425.

Masur H et al: An outbreak of community-acquired *Pneumocystis carinii* pneumonia: Initial manifestation of cellular immune dysfunction. *N Engl J Med* 1981;**305**:1431.

SECONDARY IMMUNODEFICIENCY

Deficiencies in cell-mediated immunity, humoral immunity, or both have been associated with many diseases. Two examples of altered immunity secondary to well-characterized underlying disease are discussed below.

Immunodeficiency Associated With Sarcoidosis

The immunodeficiency associated with sarcoidosis is characterized by a partial deficit in T cell function with intact B cell function. Patients with sarcoidosis show a greater incidence (50%) of nonreactivity to intradermal injections of common antigens (*Candida*, mumps, purified protein derivative) as compared to controls. However, complete lack of skin reactivity to a battery of skin tests is infrequent. In addition, reactivity is dependent upon the immunogenicity (potency) of the antigenic stimulus. For example, negative reactions may occur after skin painting with dinitrochlorobenzene, but skin painting with poison ivy extract regularly elicits a positive reaction. A similarly positive reaction to purified protein derivative is usually noted during active infection with *Mycobacterium tuberculosis* but is frequently absent after vaccination with BCG. Serum immunoglobulin levels are normal or high, and specific antibody formation is generally intact.

Immunodeficiency Associated With Hodgkin's Disease

A moderate to severe deficit in T cell function with intact B cell function is frequently found in Hodgkin's disease. Only 10–20% of patients with Hodgkin's disease show skin reactivity to mumps, *Candida*, or *Trichophyton* antigen, as compared to 70–90% of controls. Lack of reactivity to dinitrochlorobenzene is also common. Many patients show depressed responses to in vitro stimulation of peripheral blood lymphocytes with phytohemagglutinin. Serum immunoglobulins are normal, and specific antibody formation is intact except in agonal cases.

The clinical significance of depressed cell-mediated immunity in Hodgkin's disease is difficult to evaluate, since most patients are treated with potent immunosuppressive agents. Nevertheless, frequent infections with herpes zoster and *Cryptococcus* are probably related to immunodeficiency associated with the underlying disease.

AUTOIMMUNE DISEASES

The diagnosis and treatment of specific autoimmune diseases are described elsewhere in this book. Autoantibodies associated with certain autoimmune diseases do not appear to be implicated in the pathogenesis of tissue injury but are thought instead to be by-products of the injury (eg, autoimmune thyroiditis and antithyroglobulin antibody).

ASSOCIATIONS BETWEEN HLA ANTIGENS & SPECIFIC DISEASES

Analogous to animal models in which specific disease susceptibility genes are known to reside in the species MHC, in humans very striking associations are observed between particular HLA antigens and specific diseases. Proper evaluation of an HLA-disease relationship must take into account the following factors: (1) HLA antigen frequencies vary substantially among different ethnic groups, and therefore control populations must be carefully selected. (2) Appropriate statistical corrections must be made to compensate for the large number of variables (antigens) tested. (3) Accurate clinical definition of disease is necessary to avoid diluting an HLA-disease association by mixing together diseases that are pathogenetically different but clinically similar. (4) If the disease studied has a fatal outcome, then the proper disease phase must be selected to demonstrate associations. (5) Some quantitative measure of strength of association is necessary to compare different HLA-disease relationships. One such simple measure is that of relative risk (RR) = [(No. of patients antigen-positive) × (No. of controls antigen-negative)] ÷ [(No. of patients antigen-negative) × (No. of controls antigen-positive)].

Table 34–5 is a partial list of HLA-disease associations. The strongest is that between HLA-B27 and ankylosing spondylitis, which holds in all ethnic groups and is even more striking in Japanese people than in Caucasians. Other spondyloarthropathies (eg, Reiter's syndrome, arthritis following *Salmonella* or

Table 34—5. HLA and disease associations.

Disease	Antigen	Frequency Patients (%)	Controls (%)	Relative Risk
Ankylosing spondylitis				
Caucasians	B27	79–100	4–13	87
Japanese	B27	67–92	0–2	324
Reiter's disease	B27	65–100	4–14	37
Salmonella arthritis	B27	60–92	8–14	30
Rheumatoid arthritis	DR4	70	28	6
Psoriasis vulgaris	Cw6	87	33	13
Graves' disease				
Caucasians	Dw3	50–54	4–26	4
Japanese	Dw12	48	16	5
Diabetes mellitus	DR3 heterozygotes			3
Diabetes mellitus	DR4 heterozygotes			6
Diabetes mellitus	DR3/DR4 heterozygotes			33
Acute lymphocytic leukemia	A2	83	44	6
Systemic lupus erythematosus	DR4	73	33	5

Yersinia infection) are also strongly associated with B27, suggesting that despite apparently different causes the pathogeneses of these diseases share some common factor related to the B27 marker. B27 is not specific for all arthritis; eg, rheumatoid arthritis associates not with that antigen but with DR4. These data thus support the concept that ankylosing spondylitis and rheumatoid arthritis are distinct entities rather than variants of a single disease. Furthermore, disease associations are not restricted to just B and DR; eg, psoriasis vulgaris is associated with a C locus antigen and acute lymphocytic leukemia with an A locus antigen. Since both class I and class II antigens show disease associations, it is not unreasonable to assume that several different mechanisms may be required to explain the associations. Consistent with this suggestion is the phenomenon observed with diabetes mellitus in which heterozygote individuals possessing both the DR3 and the DR4 antigens have a relative risk of 33, far greater than expected by simple addition of risks for DR3 plus DR4. In addition to different mechanisms associating with different antigens, it appears that a single mechanism may associate with different antigens in different ethnic groups. Thus, among Caucasians in whom the Dw12 antigen is almost absent, Dw3 is associated with Graves' disease. Reciprocally, among Japanese people where Dw3 is almost completely lacking, Dw12 is associated with Graves' disease.

Whenever diseases of fatal outcome are studied, suitable steps must be taken to assure that patients have been tested at the proper phase of disease. Thus, among long-term survivors with acute lymphocytic leukemia, HLA-A2 stands out with a relative risk of 6. When typing is performed on all patients at the time of diagnosis, however, there is no significant difference of A2 frequency between patients and controls, implying that the A2 antigen is not associated with disease susceptibility but rather with greater survival, consistent with the previous suggestion that no single mecha-

nism can be invoked to explain all of the observed HLA-disease associations.

Another interesting phenomenon can be demonstrated by considering combinations of different antigens (ie, haplotypes) with regard to disease associations. For rheumatoid arthritis, individuals with DR4 have a relative risk of 5, individuals with Bw62 have a relative risk of 2.5, but individuals who have the extended haplotype (or "supratype") HLA-Bw62, -Cw3, -BfS, -C4A3, -C4B2.9, -DR4 have a relative risk of 16. These observations imply either interaction among different genes affecting susceptibility, or unusual linkage (ie, linkage disequilibrium) between the known HLA genes and some nearby gene actually responsible for the disease susceptibility.

Several mechanisms have been postulated to explain these associations: specific immune response genes linked to the HLA region, pathogens mimicking HLA antigens, and HLA antigens serving as pathogen receptors. Experimental data do not yet permit any of these hypotheses to be proved; however, steady improvement of HLA-typing capabilities along with better understanding of normal immune function and characterization of the actual HLA genes themselves hold promise of understanding of HLA-disease relationships in the near future. At present, in addition to their value as investigative tools, HLA and disease associations have clinical usefulness as a diagnostic aid (eg, B27 typing and ankylosing spondylitis) or in identifying individuals likely to have particularly good or bad (eg, hydralazine-induced lupus) responses to therapeutic regimens.

Bergsma D et al (editors): *Immunodeficiency in Man and Animals.* (National Foundation–March of Dimes Original Article Series.) Sinauer Associates, 1975.

Bobrove AM et al: Quantitation of T and B lymphocytes and cellular immune function in Hodgkin's disease. *Cancer* 1975; **36:**169.

Grumet FC: HLA and disease. *Clin Immunol Rev* 1983;**2:**123.

Herman PE et al: Idiopathic late-onset immunoglobulin deficiency: Clinical observations in fifty patients. *Am J Med* 1976; **61**:221.

Möller G (editor): HLA and disease susceptibility. *Immunol Rev* 1983;**70**:5. [Entire issue.]

Peterson RDA, Cooper MD, Good RA: Lymphoid tissue abnormalities associated with ataxia-telangiectasia. *Am J Med* 1966;**41**:342.

Rosen FS, Cooper MD, Wedgwood RJP: The primary immunodeficiencies. (2 parts.) *N Engl J Med* 1984;**311**:235, 300.

Samter M (editor): *Immunologic Diseases,* 3rd ed. Vol 2. Little, Brown, 1978.

Waldmann TA et al: The role of suppressor cells in the pathogenesis of common variable hypogammaglobulinemia and the immunodeficiency associated with myeloma. *Fed Proc* 1976;**35**:2067.

• • •

References

Bellanti JA: *Immunology.* Saunders, 1979.

Bodmer W: HLA structure and function: A contemporary view. *Tissue Antigens* 1981;**17**:9.

Freedman SO, Gold P (editors): *Clinical Immunology,* 2nd ed. Harper & Row, 1976.

Fudenberg HH et al: *Basic Immunogenetics,* 2nd ed. Oxford, 1978.

Gell PGH, Coombs RRA, Lachmann PJ (editors): *Clinical Aspects of Immunology,* 3rd ed. Blackwell, 1975.

Hood L, Weissman IL, Wood R: *Immunology.* Benjamin, 1978.

Martin DW Jr: Blood plasma and clotting. Pages 559–572 in: *Harper's Review of Biochemistry,* 19th ed. Martin DW Jr, Mayes PA, Rodwell VW. Lange, 1983.

Samter M (editor): *Immunological Diseases,* 3rd ed. 2 vols. Little, Brown, 1978.

Schwartz RS (editor): *Progress in Clinical Immunology.* 4 vols. Grune & Stratton, 1980.

Solomon A, McLaughlin CL: Immunoglobulin disturbances and their clinical significance. *Med Clin North Am* 1973;**57**:499.

Stites DP et al (editors): *Basic & Clinical Immunology,* 5th ed. Lange, 1984.

Appendix

TABLE OF CONTENTS

CHEMICAL CONSTITUENTS OF BLOOD & BODY FLUIDS

Validity of Numerical Values in Reporting Laboratory Results

The value reported from a clinical laboratory after determination of the concentration or amount of a substance in a specimen is not precisely accurate. It represents the best value obtainable with the method, reagents, instruments, and technical personnel involved in obtaining and processing the material.

Accuracy is the degree of agreement of the determination with the "true" value (eg, the known concentration in a control sample). **Precision** denotes the reproducibility of the analysis and is expressed in terms of variation among several determinations on the same sample. **Reliability** is a measure of the congruence of accuracy and precision.

Precision is not absolute but is subject to variation inherent in the complexity of the method, the stability of reagents, the accuracy of the primary standard, the sophistication of the equipment, and the skill of the technical personnel. Each laboratory should maintain data on precision (reproducibility) that can be expressed statistically in terms of the standard deviation from the mean value obtained by repeated analyses of the same sample. For example, the precision in determination of cholesterol in serum in a good laboratory may be the mean value ± 5 mg/dL. The 95% confidence limits are ± 2 SD, or ± 10 mg/dL. Thus, any value reported is "accurate" within a range of 20 mg/dL. Thus, the reported value 200 mg/dL means that the true value lies between 190 and 210 mg/dL. For the determination of serum potassium with a variance of 1 SD of ± 0.1 mmol/L, values ± 0.2 mmol could be obtained on the same specimen. A report of 5.5 could represent at best the range 5.3–5.7 mmol/L. That is, the 2 results—5.3 and 5.7 mmol/L—might be obtained on analysis of the same sample and still be within the limits of precision of the test.

Physicians should obtain from the laboratory the values for the variation of a given determination as a basis for deciding whether one reported value represents a change from another on the same patient.

Interpretation of Laboratory Tests

Normal values are those that fall within 2 standard deviations from the mean value for the normal population. This normal range encompasses 95% of the population. Many factors may affect values and influence the normal range; by the same token, various factors may produce values that are normal under the prevailing conditions but outside the 95% limits determined under other circumstances. These factors include **age; race; sex; environment; posture; diurnal** and **other cyclic variations; fasting** or **postprandial state, foods eaten; drugs;** and **level of exercise.**

Normal or reference values vary with the method employed, the laboratory, and conditions of collection and preservation of specimens. The normal values established by individual laboratories should be clearly expressed to ensure proper interpretation.

Interpretation of laboratory results must always be related to the condition of the patient. A low value may be the result of deficit or of dilution of the substance measured, eg, low serum sodium. Deviation from normal may be associated with a specific disease or with some drug consumed by the subject—eg, elevated serum uric acid levels may occur in patients with gout or may be due to treatment with chlorothiazides or with antineoplastic agents. (See Tables 2 and 3.)

Values may be influenced by the method of collection of the specimen. Inaccurate collection of a 24-hour urine specimen, variations in concentration of the randomly collected urine specimen, hemolysis in a blood sample, addition of an inappropriate anticoagulant, and contaminated glassware or other apparatus are examples of causes of erroneous results.

Table 1. Drugs interfering directly with chemical tests.*

Many drugs and metabolites react with ferric chloride and affect tests for ketone bodies, phenylpyruvic acid, homogentisic acid, and melanogen. Dyes (eg, methylene blue, phenazopyridine, BSP, phenolsulfonphthalein, indigo-carmine, indocyanine green, azure A) color plasma and urine; they affect most colorimetric procedures. Some drugs act as indicators (eg, phenolphthalein, vegetable laxatives) and affect tests carried out at a particular pH.

Test	Drug	Effect†	Cause
Bilirubin	Caffeine, theophylline.	−	Color reaction depressed.
Calcium	Edathamil (EDTA).	−	Interferes with dye-binding methods; no effect on flame methods.
Chloride	Bromide.	+	Reacts like chloride.
Cholesterol	Bromide.	+	Enhances color when iron reagent used.
	Metandienone.	+	Interferes with Zimmerman reaction.
Creatinine	Ascorbic acid, salicylates, barbiturates, methyldopa.	+	Interfere with alkaline picrate method.
Glucose	Dextran.	+	Copper complex in copper reduction methods.
Iron	Intravenous iron-dextran.	+	Total iron increased.
Iron-binding capacity (unsaturated)	Intravenous iron-dextran.	−	Available transferrin saturated.
Protein	Dextran.	−	Hemodilution.
Quinidine	Triamterene.	+	Interfering fluorescence.
Uric acid	Ascorbic acid, theophylline.	+	Phosphotungstic acid reduced.
Urine			
Catecholamines	Erythromycin, methyldopa, tetracyclines, quinine, quinidine, salicylates, hydralazine, B vitamins (high doses).	+	Interfering fluorescence.
Chloride	Bromide.	+	Reacts like chloride.
Creatinine	Nitrofuran derivatives.	+	React with color reagent.
Glucose	Some vaginal powders.	+	Contain glucose: urine contaminated.
(Benedict's test)	Drugs excreted as glucuronates.	+	Reduce Benedict's reagent.
	Salicylates.	+	Excreted as salicyluric acid.
	Ascorbic acid (high doses).	+	Reduces Benedict's reagent.
	Chloral hydrate.	+	Metabolites reduce.
	Nitrofuran derivatives.	+	Metabolites reduce.
	Cephalothin.	+	Black-brown color.
5-HIAA	Phenothiazines	−	Inhibit color reaction.
	Mephenesin, methocarbamol.	+	Similar color reaction.
17-Hydroxysteroids, 17-ketogenic steroids, 17-ketosteroids	Meprobamate, phenothiazines, spironolactone, penicillin G	+	Similar color reactions.
	Cortisone.	+	Mainly 17-hydroxy- and 17-ketogenic steroids.
Pregnanediol	Mandelamine.	+	Unknown.
Protein	Tolbutamide.	+	Metabolite precipitated by salicylsulfonic acid; by heat and acetic acid.
Phenolsulfonphthalein	Dyes and BSP.	+	Interfering colors.
Uric acid	Theophylline, ascorbic acid.	+	Phosphotungstic acid reduced.
Vanillylmandelic acid	Mandelamine.	+	Similar color.

*Slightly modified and reproduced, with permission, from Lubran M: The effects of drugs on laboratory values. *Med Clin North Am* 1969;**53**:211.

†Plus (+) indicates a false-positive or enhanced effect; minus (−), a false-negative or diminished effect.

Table 2. Drugs affecting prothrombin time (Quick one-stage test) of patients on anticoagulant therapy with coumarin or phenindione derivatives.*

Prothrombin Time Increased By	Prothrombin Time Decreased By
Acetaminophen	Antihistamines
Alcohol (in large amounts)	Barbiturates
Allopurinol	Carbamazepine
Amidopyrine	Digitalis (in cardiac failure)
Amiodarone	Diuretics
p-Aminosalicylic acid	Ethchlorvynol
Anabolic steroids	Glutethimide
Antibiotics (tetracyclines, some	Griseofulvin
cephalosporins, chloramphenicol, metronidazole, sulfonamides)	Mineral oil
	Oral contraceptives
Chloral hydrate	Phenytoin
Cholestyramine	Rifampin
Cimetidine	Thiopurines (azathioprine,
Clofibrate	mercaptopurine)
Glucagon	Vitamin K (in polyvitamin
Heparin	preparations and some
Hydroxyzine	diets)
Indomethacin	Xanthines (eg, caffeine)
Mefenamic acid	
Metandienone	
Methylthiouracil, propylthiouracil	
Phenylbutazone, oxyphenbutazone	
Phenyramidol	
Phenytoin	
Quinine, quinidine	
Salicylates (in excess of 1 g/d)	
Sulfinpyrazone	
Thyroid hormones	
D-Thyroxine	
Tricyclic antidepressants	

*Modified and reproduced, with permission, from Lubran M: The effects of drugs on laboratory values. *Med Clin North Am* 1969;**53**:211.

Note: Whenever an unusual or abnormal result is obtained, all possible sources of error must be considered before responding with therapy based on the laboratory report. Laboratory medicine is a specialty, and experts in the field should be consulted whenever results are unusual or in doubt.

Effect of Meals & Posture on Concentration of Substances in Blood

A. Meals: The usual normal values for blood tests have been determined by assay of "fasting" specimens collected after 8–12 hours of abstinence from food. With few exceptions, water is usually permitted as desired.

Few routine tests are altered from usual fasting values if blood is drawn 3–4 hours after breakfast. When blood is drawn 3–4 hours after lunch, values are more likely to vary from those of the true fasting state (ie, as much as +31% for glutamic-oxaloacetic transaminase [GOT], −5% for lactate dehydrogenase, and lesser variations for other substances). Valid mea-

surement of triglyceride in serum or plasma requires abstinence from food for 10–14 hours.

B. Posture: Plasma volume measured in a person who has been supine for several hours is 12–15% greater than in a person who has been up and about or standing for an hour or so. It follows that measurements performed on blood obtained after the subject has been lying down for an hour or more will yield lower values than when blood has been obtained after the same subject has been upright. An intermediate change apparently occurs with sitting.

Values in the same subject change when position changes from supine to standing as follows: increase in total protein, albumin, calcium, potassium, phosphate, cholesterol, triglyceride, glutamic-oxaloacetic transaminase (GOT), the phosphatases, total thyroxine, and hematocrit, erythrocyte count, and hemoglobin. The greatest change occurs in concentration of total protein and enzymes (+11%) and calcium (+3 to +4%). In a series of studies, change from the upright to the supine position resulted in the following decreases: total protein, −0.5 g; albumin, −0.4 to −0.6 g; calcium, −0.4 mg; cholesterol, −10 to −25 mg; total thyroxine −0.8 to −1.8 μg; hematocrit, −4 to −9%, reflecting hemodilution as interstitial fluid reenters the circulation.

A tourniquet applied for 1 minute instead of 3 minutes produced the following changes in reported values: total protein, +5%; iron, +6.7%; cholesterol, +5%; glutamic-oxaloacetic transaminase, +9.3%; and bilirubin, +8.4%. Decreases were observed for potassium, −6%; and creatinine, −2.3%.

Validity of Laboratory Tests*

The clinical value of a test is related to its specificity and sensitivity and the incidence of the disease in the population tested.

Specificity means percentage of negative results among people who do not have the disease. The test for phenylketonuria is highly specific: 99.9% of normal individuals give a negative result. In contrast, the carcinoembryonic antigen (CEA) test for carcinoma of the colon has a variable specificity: about 3% of nonsmoking individuals give a false-positive result (97% specificity), whereas in smokers 20% give positive results (80% specificity). The overlap of serum thyroxine levels between hyperthyroid patients and those taking oral contraceptives or those who are pregnant is an example of a change in specificity from that prevailing in a different set of individuals.

Sensitivity means percentage of positive results in patients with the disease. The test for phenylketonuria is highly sensitive: A positive result is ob-

*This section is an abridged version of an article by Krieg AF, Gambino R, Galen RS: Why are clinical laboratory tests performed? When are they valid? *JAMA* 1975;**233**:76. Reprinted from the Journal of the American Medical Association. Copyright 1975. American Medical Association. See also Galen RS, Gambino SR: *Beyond Normality: The Predictive Value and Efficiency of Medical Diagnosis.* Wiley, 1975.

tained in all who have the disease (100% sensitivity). The CEA test has low specificity: Only 72% of those with carcinoma of the colon provide a positive result when the disease is extensive, and only 20% are positive with early disease. Lower sensitivity occurs in the early stages of many diseases—in contrast to the higher sensitivity in well-established disease.

The **predictive value** of a positive test defines the percentage of positive results that are true positives. This is related fundamentally to the incidence of the disease. In a group of patients on a urology service, the incidence of renal disease is higher than in the general population, and the serum creatinine level will have a higher predictive value in that group than for the general population.

Formulas for definitions:

$$\text{Sensitivity} = \frac{\text{True positive}}{\text{True positive + false negative}} \times 100$$

$$\text{Specificity} = \frac{\text{True negative}}{\text{True negative + false positive}} \times 100$$

$$\text{Predictive value} = \frac{\text{True positive}}{\text{True positive + false positive}} \times 100$$

Before ordering a test, attempt to determine whether test sensitivity, specificity, and predictive value are adequate to provide useful information. To be useful, the result should influence diagnosis, prognosis, or therapy; lead to a better understanding of the disease process; and benefit the patient.

SI Units (Système International d'Unités)

A "coherent" system of measurement has been under development by an international organization designated the General Conference of Weights and Measures. An adaptation has been tentatively recommended by the Commission on Quantities and Units of the Section on Clinical Chemistry, International Union of Pure and Applied Chemistry. SI units are in use in some European countries, and the conversion to SI will continue if the system proves to be helpful in understanding physiologic mechanisms.

Eight fundamental measurable properties of matter (with authorized abbreviations shown in parentheses) were selected for clinical use.

length: metre (m)
mass: kilogram (kg)
amount of substance: mole (mol)
time: second (s)
thermodynamic temperature: kelvin (K)
electric current: ampere (A)
luminous intensity: candela (cd)
catalytic activity: katal (kat)

Derived from these are the following measurable properties:

mass concentration: kilogram/litre (kg/L)
mass fraction: kilogram/kilogram (kg/kg)
volume fraction: litre/litre (L/L)
volume: cubic metre (m^3); for clinical use, the unit will be the litre (L)
substance concentration: mole/litre (mol/L)
molality: mole/kilogram (mol/kg)
mole fraction: mole/mole (mol/mol)
pressure: pascal (Pa) = newton/m^2

Decimal factors are as follows:

Number	Name	Symbol
10^{12}	tera	T
10^9	giga	G
10^6	mega	M
10^3	kilo	k
10^2	hecto	h
10^1	deca	da
10^{-1}	deci	d
10^{-2}	centi	c
10^{-3}	milli	m
10^{-6}	micro	μ
10^{-9}	nano	n
10^{-12}	pico	p
10^{-15}	femto	f
10^{-18}	atto	a

"Per"—eg, "per second"—is often written as the negative exponent. Per second thus becomes $\cdot s^{-1}$; per meter squared, $\cdot m^{-2}$; per kilogram, $\cdot kg^{-1}$. *Example:* $cm/s = cm \cdot s^{-1}$; $g/m^2 = g \cdot m^{-2}$; etc.

In anticipation that the SI system may be adopted in the next several years, values are reported here in the traditional units with equivalent SI units following in parentheses.

COMMON CLINICAL VALUES IN TRADITIONAL & SI MEASUREMENTS*

Albumin, Serum: See Protein, serum.

Aldolase, Serum: Normal (varies with method): 3–8 units/mL (Sibley-Lehninger). Males, < 33 units; females, < 19 units (Warburg and Christian).

A. Precautions: Serum should be separated promptly. Avoid hemolysis. If there is to be any delay in the determination, the serum should be frozen.

B. Physiologic Basis: Aldolase, also known as zymohexase, splits fructose-1,6-diphosphate to yield dihydroxyacetone phosphate and glyceraldehyde-3-phosphate. Because it is present in higher concentra-

*The values listed below and in the following section have been gleaned from many sources. Values will vary with method and individual laboratory.

:ion in tissue cells than in serum, destruction of tissue results in elevation of serum concentration.

C. Interpretation: High levels in serum occur in myocardial infarction, muscular dystrophies, hemolytic anemia, metastatic prostatic carcinoma, leukemia, acute pancreatitis, and acute hepatitis. In obstructive jaundice or cirrhosis of the liver, serum aldolase is normal or only slightly elevated.

Aminotransferases, Serum: Normal AST (SGOT), 6–25 IU/L at 30 °C; SMA, 10–40 IU/L at 37 °C; SMAC, 0–41 IU/L at 37 °C. ALT (SGPT), 3–26 IU/L at 30 °C; SMAC, 0–45 IU/L at 37 °C.

A. Precautions: Avoid hemolysis. Remove serum from clot promptly.

B. Physiologic Basis: Aspartate aminotransferase (AST; SGOT), alanine aminotransferase (ALT; SGPT), and lactic dehydrogenase are intracellular enzymes involved in amino acid or carbohydrate metabolism. These enzymes are present in high concentrations in muscle, liver, and brain. Elevations of concentrations of these enzymes in the blood indicate necrosis or disease, especially of these tissues.

C. Interpretation:

1. Elevated after myocardial infarction (especially AST); acute infectious hepatitis (ALT usually elevated more than AST); cirrhosis of the liver; liver neoplasm, metastatic or primary; and in transudates associated with neoplastic involvement of serous cavities. SGOT is elevated in muscular dystrophy, dermatomyositis, and paroxysmal myoglobinuria.

2. Decreased with pyridoxine (vitamin B_6) deficiency (often as a result of repeated hemodialysis), renal insufficiency, and pregnancy.

D. Drug Effects on Laboratory Results: Elevated by a host of drugs, including anabolic steroids, androgens, clofibrate, erythromycin (especially estolate) and other antibiotics, isoniazid, methotrexate, methyldopa, phenothiazines, oral contraceptives, salicylates, acetaminophen, phenacetin, indomethacin, acetohexamide, allopurinol, dicumarol, carbamazepine, chlordiazepoxide, desipramine, imipramine, codeine, morphine, meperidine, tolazamide, propranolol, guanethidine, pyridoxine, and drugs that produce spasm of the sphincter of Oddi.

Ammonia, Blood: Normal (Conway): 80–110 μg/dL whole blood. (SI: 47–65 μmol/L.)

A. Precautions: Do not use anticoagulants containing ammonia. Suitable anticoagulants include potassium oxalate, calcium disodium edetate, and heparin that is ammonia-free. The determination should be done immediately after drawing blood. If the blood is kept in an ice-water bath it may be held for up to 1 hour.

B. Physiologic Basis: Ammonia present in the blood is derived from 2 principal sources: (1) In the large intestine, putrefactive action of bacteria on nitrogenous materials releases significant quantities of ammonia. (2) In the process of protein metabolism,

ammonia is liberated. Ammonia entering the portal vein or the systemic circulation is rapidly converted to urea in the liver. Liver insufficiency may result in an increase in blood ammonia concentration, especially if protein consumption is high or if there is bleeding into the bowel.

C. Interpretation: Blood ammonia is elevated in hepatic insufficiency or with liver bypass in the form of a portacaval shunt, particularly if protein intake is high or if there is bleeding into the bowel.

D. Drug Effects on Laboratory Results: Elevated by methicillin, ammonia cycle resins, chlorthalidone, spironolactone. Decreased by monoamine oxidase inhibitors, oral antimicrobial agents.

Amylase, Serum: Normal (varies with method): 80–180 Somogyi units/dL serum. (One Somogyi unit equals amount of enzyme that will produce 1 mg of reducing sugar from starch at pH 7.2.) 0.8–3.2 IU/L.

A. Precautions: If storage for more than 1 hour is necessary, blood or serum must be refrigerated.

B. Physiologic Basis: Normally, small amounts of amylase (diastase), molecular weight about 50,000, originating in the pancreas and salivary glands, are present in the blood. Inflammatory disease of these glands or obstruction of their ducts results in regurgitation of large amounts of enzyme into the blood and increased excretion via the kidney.

C. Interpretation:

1. Elevated in acute pancreatitis, pseudocyst of the pancreas, obstruction of pancreatic ducts (carcinoma, stone, stricture, duct sphincter spasm after morphine), mumps, occasionally in the presence of renal insufficiency, occasionally in diabetic acidosis, and occasionally with inflammation of the pancreas from a perforating peptic ulcer. Rarely, combination of amylase with an immunoglobulin produces elevated serum amylase activity (macroamylasemia) because the large molecular complex (molecular weight at least 160,000) is not filtered by the glomerulus.

2. Decreased in acute and chronic hepatitis, pancreatic insufficiency, and occasionally in toxemia of pregnancy.

D. Drug Effects on Laboratory Results: Elevated by morphine, codeine, meperidine, methacholine, pancreozymin, sodium diatrizoate, cyproheptadine, and perhaps by pentazocine and thiazide diuretics. Pancreatitis may be induced by indomethacin, furosemide, chlorthalidone, ethacrynic acid, corticosteroids, histamine, salicylates, and tetracyclines. Decreased by barbiturate poisoning.

Amylase, Urine: Normal: Varies with method. 40–250 Somogyi units/h.

A. Precautions: If the determination is delayed more than 1 hour after collecting the specimen, urine must be refrigerated.

B. Physiologic Basis: See Amylase, Serum. If renal function is adequate, amylase is rapidly excreted in the urine. A timed urine specimen (ie, 2, 6, or 24 hours) should be collected and the rate of excretion determined.

C. Interpretation: Elevation of the concentration of amylase in the urine occurs in the same situations in which serum amylase concentration is elevated. Urinary amylase concentration remains elevated for up to 7 days after serum amylase levels have returned to normal following an attack of pancreatitis. Thus, the determination of urinary amylase may be useful if the patient is seen late in the course of an attack of pancreatitis. An elevated serum amylase with normal or low urine amylase excretory rate may be seen in the presence of renal insufficiency or with macroamylasemia.

Bicarbonate, Serum or Plasma: Normal: 24–28 meq/L. (SI: 24–28 mmol/L.)

A. Precautions: Plasma or serum should be separated from blood cells and kept refrigerated in stoppered tubes.

B. Physiologic Basis: Bicarbonate–carbonic acid buffer is one of the most important buffer systems in maintaining normal pH of body fluids. Bicarbonate and pH determinations on arterial whole blood serve as a basis for assessing "acid-base balance."

C. Interpretation:

1. Elevated in–

(a) Metabolic alkalosis (arterial blood pH increased) due to ingestion of large quantities of sodium bicarbonate, protracted vomiting of acid gastric juice, accompanying potassium deficit.

(b) Respiratory acidosis (arterial blood pH decreased) due to inadequate elimination of CO_2 (leading to elevated P_{CO_2}) because of pulmonary emphysema, poor diffusion in alveolar membrane disease, heart failure with pulmonary congestion or edema, ventilatory failure due to any cause, including oversedation, narcotics, or inadequate artificial respiration.

2. Decreased in–

(a) Metabolic acidosis (arterial blood pH decreased) due to diabetic ketoacidosis, lactic acidosis, starvation, persistent diarrhea, renal insufficiency, ingestion of excess acidifying salts, methanol, or salicylate intoxication.

(b) Respiratory alkalosis (arterial blood pH increased) due to hyperventilation (decreased P_{CO_2}).

Bilirubin, Serum: Normal: Total 0.2–1.2 mg/dL (SI: 3.5–20.5 μmol/L). Direct (glucuronide), 0.1–0.4 mg/dL. Indirect (unconjugated), 0.2–0.7 mg/dL. (SI: direct, up to 7 μmol/L; indirect, up to 12 μmol/L.)

A. Precautions: The fasting state is preferred to avoid turbidity of serum. For optimal stability of stored serum, samples should be frozen and stored in the dark.

B. Physiologic Basis: Destruction of hemoglobin yields bilirubin, which is conjugated in the liver to the diglucuronide and excreted in the bile. Bilirubin accumulates in the plasma when liver insufficiency exists, biliary obstruction is present, or the rate of hemolysis increases. Rarely, abnormalities of enzyme systems involved in bilirubin metabolism in the liver (eg, absence of glucuronyl transferase) result in abnormal bilirubin concentrations.

C. Interpretation:

1. Direct and indirect forms of serum bilirubin are elevated in acute or chronic hepatitis; biliary tract obstruction (cholangiolar, hepatic, or common ducts); toxic reactions to many drugs, chemicals, and toxins; and Dubin-Johnson and Rotor's syndromes.

2. Indirect serum bilirubin is elevated in hemolytic diseases or reactions and absence or deficiency of glucuronyl transferase, as in Gilbert's disease and Crigler-Najjar syndrome.

3. Direct and total bilirubin can be significantly elevated in normal and jaundiced subjects by fasting 24–48 hours (in some instances even 12 hours) or by prolonged caloric restriction.

D. Drug Effects on Laboratory Results: Elevated by acetaminophen, chlordiazepoxide, novobiocin, acetohexamide. Many drugs produce either hepatocellular damage or cholestasis.

Calcium, Serum: Normal: 8.5–10.5 mg/dL or 4.2–5.2 meq/L. (Ionized, 4.2–5.2 mg/dL or 2.1–2.6 meq/L.) (SI: total, 2.1–2.6 mmol/L; ionized, 1.05–1.3 mmol/L.)

A. Precautions: Glassware must be free of calcium. The patient should be fasting. Serum should be promptly separated from the clot.

B. Physiologic Basis: Endocrine, renal, gastrointestinal, and nutritional factors normally provide for precise regulation of calcium concentration in plasma and other body fluids. Since some calcium is bound to plasma protein, especially albumin, determination of the plasma albumin concentration is necessary before the clinical significance of abnormal serum calcium levels can be interpreted accurately.

C. Interpretation:

1. Elevated in hyperparathyroidism, secretion of parathyroidlike hormone by malignant tumors, vitamin D excess, milk-alkali syndrome, osteolytic disease such as multiple myeloma, invasion of bone by metastatic cancer, Paget's disease of bone, Boeck's sarcoid, immobilization, and familial hypocalciuria. Occasionally elevated with hyperthyroidism and with ingestion of thiazide drugs.

2. Decreased in hypoparathyroidism, vitamin D deficiency (rickets, osteomalacia), renal insufficiency, hypoproteinemia, malabsorption syndrome (sprue, ileitis, celiac disease, pancreatic insufficiency), severe pancreatitis with pancreatic necrosis, and pseudohypoparathyroidism.

Calcium, Urine, Daily Excretion: Ordinarily there is a moderate continuous urinary calcium excretion of 50–150 mg/24 h, depending upon the intake. (SI: 1.2–3.7 mmol/24 h.)

A. Procedure: The patient should remain on a diet free of milk or cheese for 3 days prior to testing; for quantitative testing, a neutral ash diet containing about

150 mg calcium per day is given for 3 days. Quantitative calcium excretion studies may be made on a carefully timed 24-hour urine specimen.

B. Interpretation: On the quantitative diet a normal person excretes 125± 50 mg (1.8–4.4 mmol) of calcium per 24 hours. In hyperparathyroidism, the urinary calcium excretion usually exceeds 200 mg/24 h (5 mmol/d). Urinary calcium excretion is almost always elevated when serum calcium is high.

Ceruloplasmin and Copper, Serum: Normal: Ceruloplasmin, 25–43 mg/dL (SI: 1.7–2.9 μmol/L); copper, 100–200 μg/dL (SI: 16–31 μmol/L).

A. Precautions: None.

B. Physiologic Basis: About 5% of serum copper is loosely bound to albumin and 95% to ceruloplasmin, an oxidase enzyme that is an alpha$_2$ globulin with a blue color. In Wilson's disease, serum copper and ceruloplasmin are low and urinary copper is high.

C. Interpretation:

1. Elevated in pregnancy, hyperthyroidism, infection, aplastic anemia, acute leukemia, Hodgkin's disease, cirrhosis of the liver, and with use of oral contraceptives.

2. Decreased in Wilson's disease and accompanied by increased urinary excretion of copper, malabsorption, nephrosis, and copper deficiency that may accompany total parenteral nutrition.

Chloride, Serum or Plasma: Normal: 96–106 meq/L. (SI: 96–106 mmol/L.)

A. Precautions: Determination with whole blood yields lower results than those obtained using serum or plasma as the specimen. Always use serum or plasma.

B. Physiologic Basis: Chloride is the principal inorganic anion of the extracellular fluid. It is important in maintenance of acid-base balance even though it exerts no buffer action. When chloride as HCl or NH_4Cl is lost, alkalosis follows; when chloride is retained or ingested, acidosis follows. Chloride (with sodium) plays an important role in control of osmolarity of body fluids.

C. Interpretation:

1. Elevated in renal insufficiency (when Cl intake exceeds excretion), nephrosis (occasionally), renal tubular acidosis, hyperparathyroidism (occasionally), ureterosigmoid anastomosis (reabsorption from urine in gut), dehydration (water deficit), and overtreatment with saline solution.

2. Decreased in gastrointestinal disease with loss of gastric and intestinal fluids (vomiting, diarrhea, gastrointestinal suction), renal insufficiency (with salt deprivation), overtreatment with diuretics, chronic respiratory acidosis (emphysema), diabetic acidosis, excessive sweating, adrenal insufficiency (NaCl loss), hyperadrenocorticism (chronic K$^+$ loss), and metabolic alkalosis (NaHCO$_3$ ingestion; K$^+$ deficit).

Chloride, Urine:

Urine chloride content varies with dietary intake, acid-base balance, endocrine "balance," body stores of other electrolytes, and water balance. Relationships and responses are so variable and complex that there is little clinical value in urine chloride determinations other than in balance studies.

Cholesterol, Plasma or Serum: Normal: 150–280 mg/dL. (SI: 3.9–7.2 mmol/L.) See Table 3.

A. Precautions: The fasting state is preferred.

B. Physiologic Basis: Cholesterol concentrations are determined by metabolic functions, which are influenced by heredity, nutrition, endocrine function, and integrity of vital organs such as the liver and kidney. Cholesterol metabolism is intimately associated with lipid metabolism.

C. Interpretation:

1. Elevated in familial hypercholesterolemia (xanthomatosis), hypothyroidism, poorly controlled diabetes mellitus, nephrotic syndrome, chronic hepatitis, biliary cirrhosis, obstructive jaundice, hypoproteinemia (idiopathic, with nephrosis or chronic hepatitis), and lipidemia (idiopathic, familial).

2. Decreased in acute hepatitis and Gaucher's disease, occasionally in hyperthyroidism, acute infections, anemia, malnutrition, apolipoprotein deficiency.

D. Drug Effects on Laboratory Results: Elevated by bromides, anabolic agents, trimethadione, oral contraceptives. Decreased by cholestyramine resin, haloperidol, nicotinic acid, salicylates, thyroid hormone, estrogens, clofibrate, chlorpropamide, phenformin, kanamycin, neomycin, phenyramidol.

Table 3. Lipidemia: Ranges of USA population for serum concentrations of cholesterol (C), triglyceride (TG), low-density lipoprotein cholesterol (LDL-C) and high-density lipoprotein cholesterol (HDL-C).*

Age	C (mg/dL)	TG (mg/dL)	LDL-C (mg/dL) Upper Limit	HDL-C (mg/dL)	
				Male	Female
< 29	120–240	10–140	170		
30–39	140–270	10–150	190	45 ± 12	55 ± 12
40–49	150–310	10–160	190		
> 49	160–330	10–190	210		

*Reproduced, with permission, from Krupp MA et al: *Physician's Handbook*, 20th ed. Lange, 1982.

Creatine Kinase (CK) or Creatine Phosphokinase (CPK), Serum: Normal: Varies with method. 10–50 IU/L at 30 °C.

A. Precautions: The enzyme is unstable, and the red cell content inhibits enzyme activity. Serum must be removed from the clot promptly. If assay cannot be done soon after drawing blood, serum must be frozen.

B. Physiologic Basis: CPK splits creatine phosphate in the presence of ADP to yield creatine and

ATP. Skeletal and heart muscle and brain are rich in the enzyme.

C. Interpretation:

1. Elevated in the presence of muscle damage such as with myocardial infarction, trauma to muscle, muscular dystrophies, polymyositis, severe muscular exertion (jogging), hypothyroidism, and cerebral infarction (necrosis). Following myocardial infarction, serum CK concentration increases rapidly (within 3–5 hours), and remains elevated for a shorter time after the episode (2 or 3 days) than does AST or LDH.

2. Not elevated in pulmonary infarction or parenchymal liver disease.

Creatine Kinase Isoenzymes, Serum: See Table 4.

A. Precautions: As for CK, above.

B. Physiologic Basis: CK consists of 3 proteins separable by electrophoresis. Skeletal muscle is characterized by isoenzyme MM, myocardium by isoenzyme MB, and brain by isoenzyme BB.

C. Interpretation: CK isoenzymes are increased in serum. CK-MM is elevated in injury to skeletal muscle, myocardial muscle, and brain; in muscle disease (eg, dystrophies, hypothyroidism, dermatomyositis, polymyositis); in rhabdomyolysis; and after severe exercise. CK-MB is elevated soon (within 2–4 hours) after myocardial infarction and for up to 72 hours afterward (high levels are prolonged with extension of infarct or new infarction); also elevated in extensive rhabdomyolysis or muscle injury, severe muscle disease, Reye's syndrome, or Rocky Mountain spotted fever. CK-BB is occasionally elevated in severe shock, in some carcinomas (especially oat cell carcinoma or carcinoma of the ovary, breast, or prostate), or in biliary atresia.

Table 4. Creatine kinase isoenzymes.

Isoenzyme	Normal Levels % of Total
(Fastest) Fraction 1, BB	0
Fraction 2, MB	0–3
(Slowest) Fraction 3, MM	97–100

Creatine, Urine (24 Hours): Normal: See Table 5.

A. Precautions: Collection of the 24-hour specimen must be accurate. The specimen may be refrigerated or preserved with 10 mL of toluene or 10 mL of 5% thymol in chloroform.

B. Physiologic Basis: Creatine is an important constituent of muscle, brain, and blood; in the form of creatine phosphate, it serves as a source of high-energy phosphate. Normally, small amounts of creatine are excreted in the urine, but in states of elevated catabolism and in the presence of muscular dystrophies, the rate of excretion is increased.

C. Interpretation:

1. Elevated in muscular dystrophies such as progressive muscular dystrophy, myotonia atrophica, and

Table 5. Urine creatine and creatinine, normal values (24 hours).*

	Creatine	Creatinine
Newborn	4.5 mg/kg	10 mg/kg
1–7 months	8.1 mg/kg	12.8 mg/kg
2–3 years	7.9 mg/kg	12.1 mg/kg
4–4½ years	4.5 mg/kg	14.6 mg/kg
9–9½ years	2.5 mg/kg	18.1 mg/kg
11–14 years	2.7 mg/kg	20.1 mg/kg
Adult male	0–50 mg	25 mg/kg
Adult female	0–100 mg	21 mg/kg

*SI factors: creatine, mg/24 h × 7.63 = μmol/24 h; creatinine, mg/24 h × 8.84 = μmol/24 h.

myasthenia gravis; muscle wasting, as in acute poliomyelitis, amyotrophic lateral sclerosis, and myositis manifested by muscle wasting; starvation and cachectic states, hyperthyroidism, and febrile diseases.

2. Decreased in hypothyroidism, amyotonia congenita, and renal insufficiency.

Creatinine, Plasma or Serum: Normal: 0.7–1.5 mg/dL. (SI: 60–132 μmol/L.)

A. Precautions: None.

B. Physiologic Basis: Endogenous creatinine is excreted by filtration through the glomerulus and by tubular secretion at a rate about 20% greater than clearance of inulin. The Jaffe reaction measures chromogens other than creatinine in the plasma. Because the chromogens are not passed into the urine, the measurement of creatinine in the urine is about 20% less than chromogen plus creatinine in plasma, providing, fortuitously, a compensation for the amount secreted. Thus, inulin and creatinine clearances for clinical purposes are comparable and creatinine clearance is an acceptable measure of glomerular filtration rate except that with advancing renal failure, creatinine clearance exceeds inulin clearance owing to the secretion of creatinine by remaining renal tubules.

C. Interpretation: Creatinine is elevated in acute or chronic renal insufficiency, urinary tract obstruction, and impairment of renal function induced by some drugs. Materials other than creatinine may react to give falsely high results with the alkaline picrate method (Jaffe reaction): acetoacetate, acetone, β-hydroxybutyrate, α-ketoglutarate, pyruvate, glucose, bilirubin, hemoglobin, urea, and uric acid. Values below 0.7 mg/dL are of no known significance.

D. Drug Effects on Laboratory Results: Elevated by ascorbic acid, salicylates, barbiturates, sulfobromophthalein, methyldopa, and phenolsulfonphthalein, all of which interfere with the determination by the alkaline picrate method.

Creatinine, Urine: See Table 5 for normal values.

Glucose, Plasma, Serum: Normal: Fasting "true" glucose, 65–110 mg/dL. (SI: 3.6–6.1 mmol/L.)

A. Precautions: If determination is delayed beyond 1 hour, sodium fluoride, about 3 mg/mL blood, should be added to the specimen. The filtrates may be refrigerated for up to 24 hours. Errors in interpretation may occur if the patient has eaten sugar or received glucose solution parenterally just prior to the collection of what is thought to be a "fasting" specimen.

B. Physiologic Basis: The glucose concentration in extracellular fluid is normally closely regulated, with the result that a source of energy is available to tissues, and no glucose is excreted in the urine. Hyperglycemia and hypoglycemia are nonspecific signs of abnormal glucose metabolism.

C. Interpretation:

1. Elevated in diabetes, hyperthyroidism, adrenocortical hyperactivity (cortical excess), hyperpituitarism, and hepatic disease (occasionally).

2. Decreased in hyperinsulinism, adrenal insufficiency, hypopituitarism, hepatic insufficiency (occasionally), functional hypoglycemia, and by hypoglycemic agents.

D. Drug Effects on Laboratory Results: Elevated by corticosteroids, chlorthalidone, thiazide diuretics, furosemide, ethacrynic acid, triamterene, indomethacin, oral contraceptives (estrogen-progestin combinations), isoniazid, nicotinic acid (large doses), phenothiazines, and paraldehyde. Decreased by acetaminophen, phenacetin, cyproheptadine, pargyline, and propranolol.

γ-Glutamyl Transpeptidase or Transferase, Serum: Normal: Males, < 30 mU/mL at 30 °C. Females, < 25 mU/mL at 30 °C. Adolescents, < 50 mU/mL at 30 °C. ·

A. Precautions: Avoid hemolysis.

B. Physiologic Basis: γ-Glutamyl transferase (GGT) is an extremely sensitive indicator of liver disease. Levels are often elevated when transaminases and alkaline phosphatase are normal, and it is considered more specific than both for identifying liver impairment due to alcoholism.

The enzyme is present in liver, kidney, and pancreas and transfers C-terminal glutamic acid from a peptide to other peptides or L-amino acids. It is induced by alcohol.

C. Interpretation: Elevated in acute infectious or toxic hepatitis, chronic and subacute hepatitis, cirrhosis of the liver, intrahepatic or extrahepatic obstruction, primary or metastatic liver neoplasms, and liver damage due to alcoholism. It is elevated occasionally in congestive heart failure and rarely in postmyocardial infarction, pancreatitis, and pancreatic carcinoma.

Iron, Serum: Normal: 50–175 μg/dL. (SI: 9–31.3 μmol/L.)

A. Precautions: Syringes and needles must be iron-free. Hemolysis of blood must be avoided. The serum must be free of hemoglobin.

B. Physiologic Basis: Because of diurnal variation with highest values in the morning, fasting morning blood specimens are desirable. Iron concentration in the plasma is determined by several factors, including absorption from the intestine; storage in intestine, liver, spleen, and marrow; breakdown or loss of hemoglobin; and synthesis of new hemoglobin.

C. Interpretation:

1. Elevated in hemochromatosis, hemosiderosis (multiple transfusions, excess iron administration), hemolytic disease, pernicious anemia, hypoplastic anemias, often in viral hepatitis. Spuriously elevated if patient has received parenteral iron during the 2–3 months prior to determination.

2. Decreased in iron deficiency, with infections, nephrosis, and chronic renal insufficiency, and during periods of active hematopoiesis.

Iron-Binding Capacity, Serum: Normal: Total 250–410 μg/dL. (SI: 45–73 μmol/L.) Percent saturation, 20–55%.

A. Precautions: None.

B. Physiologic Basis: Iron is transported as a complex of the metal-binding globulin transferrin or siderophilin. Normally, this transport protein carries an amount of iron that represents about 30–40% of its capacity to combine with iron.

C. Interpretation of Total Iron-Binding Capacity:

1. Elevated in iron deficiency anemia, with use of oral contraceptives, in late pregnancy, occasionally with hepatitis, and in infants.

2. Decreased in association with decreased plasma proteins (nephrosis, starvation, cancer), chronic inflammation, hemosiderosis (transfusions, thalassemia).

D. Interpretation of Saturation of Transferrin:

1. Elevated in iron excess (iron poisoning, hemolytic disease, thalassemia, hemochromatosis, pyridoxine deficiency, nephrosis, and occasionally with hepatitis).

2. Decreased in iron deficiency, chronic infection, cancer, late pregnancy.

Lactate Dehydrogenase, Serum, Serous Fluids, Spinal Fluid, Urine: Normal: Serum, 55–140 IU/L at 30 °C; SMA, 100–225 IU/L at 37 °C; SMAC, 60–200 IU/L at 37 °C. Serous fluids, lower than serum. Spinal fluid, 15–75 units (Wroblewski); 6.3–30 IU/L. Urine, less than 8300 units/8 h (Wroblewski).

A. Precautions: Any degree of hemolysis must be avoided because the concentration of LDH within red blood cells is 100 times that in normal serum. Heparin and oxalate may inhibit enzyme activity. Remove serum from clot promptly.

B. Physiologic Basis: LDH catalyzes the interconversion of lactate and pyruvate in the presence of NADH or NADH$_2$. It is distributed generally in body cells and fluids.

C. Interpretation: Elevated in all conditions accompanied by tissue necrosis, particularly those involving acute injury of the heart, red cells, kidney, skeletal muscle, liver, lung, and skin. Marked elevations accompany hemolytic anemias, the anemias of vitamin B_{12} and folate deficiency, and polycythemia rubra vera. The course of rise in concentration over 3–4 days followed by a slow decline during the following 5–7 days may be helpful in confirming the presence of a myocardial infarction; however, pulmonary infarction, neoplastic disease, and megaloblastic anemia must be excluded. Although elevated during the acute phase of infectious hepatitis, enzyme activity is seldom increased in chronic liver disease.

D. Drug Effects on Laboratory Results: Decreased by clofibrate.

Lactate Dehydrogenase Isoenzymes, Serum: Normal serum levels are as shown in Table 6.

A. Precautions: As for LDH (see above).

B. Physiologic Basis: LDH consists of 5 separable proteins, each made of tetramers of 2 types, or subunits, H and M. The 5 isoenzymes can be distinguished by kinetics, electrophoresis, chromatography, and immunologic characteristics. By electrophoretic separation, the mobility of the isoenzymes corresponds to serum proteins α_1, α_2, β, γ_1, and γ_2. These are usually numbered 1 (fastest moving), 2, 3, 4, and 5 (slowest moving). Isoenzyme 1 is present in high concentrations in heart muscle (tetramer H H H H) and in erythrocytes and kidney cortex; isoenzyme 5, in skeletal muscle (tetramer M M M M) and liver.

C. Interpretation: In myocardial infarction, the α isoenzymes are elevated—particularly LDH 1—to yield a ratio of LDH 1:LDH 2 of > 1. Similar α isoenzyme elevations occur in renal cortex infarction and with hemolytic anemias.

LDH 5 and 4 are relatively increased in the presence of acute hepatitis, acute muscle injury, dermatomyositis, and muscular dystrophies.

D. Drug Effects on Laboratory Results: Decreased by clofibrate.

Table 6. Lactate dehydrogenase isoenzymes.

	Isoenzyme	Percentage of Total (and Range)
(Fastest)	1 (a_1)	28 (15–30)
	2 (a_2)	36 (22–50)
	3 (β)	23 (15–30)
	4 (γ_1)	6 (0–15)
(Slowest)	5 (γ_2)	6 (0–15)

Lipase, Serum: Normal: 0.2–1.5 units.

A. Precautions: None. The specimen may be stored under refrigeration up to 24 hours prior to the determination.

B. Physiologic Basis: A low concentration of fat-splitting enzyme is present in circulating blood. In the presence of pancreatitis, pancreatic lipase is released into the circulation in higher concentrations,

which persist, as a rule, for a longer period than does the elevated concentration of amylase.

C. Interpretation: Serum lipase is elevated in acute or exacerbated pancreatitis and in obstruction of pancreatic ducts by stone or neoplasm.

Magnesium, Serum: Normal: 1.8–3 mg/dL or 1.5–2.5 meq/L. (SI: 0.75–1.25 mmol/L.)

A. Precautions: None.

B. Physiologic Basis: Magnesium is primarily an intracellular electrolyte. In extracellular fluid it affects neuromuscular irritability and response. Magnesium deficit may exist with little or no change in extracellular fluid concentrations. Low magnesium levels in plasma have been associated with tetany, weakness, disorientation, and somnolence.

C. Interpretation:

1. Elevated in renal insufficiency and in overtreatment with magnesium salts.

2. Decreased in chronic diarrhea, acute loss of enteric fluids, starvation, chronic alcoholism, chronic hepatitis, hepatic insufficiency, excessive renal loss, and inadequate replacement with parenteral nutrition. May be decreased in and contribute to persistent hypocalcemia in patients with hypoparathyroidism (especially after surgery for hyperparathyroidism) and when large doses of vitamin D and calcium are being administered.

Phosphatase, Acid, Serum: Normal: 0.1–0.63 Sigma units. Values vary with method.

A. Precautions: Do not draw blood for assay for 24 hours after prostatic massage or instrumentation. For methods that measure enzyme activity, complete the determination promptly, since activity declines quickly; avoid hemolysis. For immunoassay methods, the enzyme is stable for 3–4 days when the serum is refrigerated or frozen.

B. Physiologic Basis: Phosphatases active at pH 4.9 are present in high concentration in the prostate gland, erythrocytes, platelets, reticuloendothelial cells, liver, spleen, and kidney. A variety of isoenzymes have been found in these tissues and serum and account for different activities operating against different substrates.

C. Interpretation: In the presence of carcinoma of the prostate, the prostatic fraction of acid phosphatase may be increased in the serum, particularly if the cancer has spread beyond the capsule of the gland or has metastasized. Palpation of the prostate will produce a transient increase. Total acid phosphatase may be increased in Gaucher's disease, malignant tumors involving bone, renal disease, hepatobiliary disease, and diseases of the reticuloendothelial system. Fever may cause spurious elevations.

Phosphatase, Alkaline, Serum: Normal: King-Armstrong, 5–13 units; Bessey-Lowry, children, 2.8–6.7 units; Bessey-Lowry, adults, 0.8–2.3 units. Adults, 24–71 IU/L at

30 °C; SMA, 30–85 IU/L at 37 °C; SMAC, 30–115 IU/L at 37 °C.

A. Precautions: Serum may be kept in the refrigerator for 24–48 hours, but values may increase slightly (10%). The specimen will deteriorate if it is not refrigerated. Do not use fluoride or oxalate.

B. Physiologic Basis: Alkaline phosphatase is present in high concentration in growing bone, in bile, and in the placenta. In serum it consists of a mixture of isoenzymes not yet clearly defined. The isoenzymes may be separated by electrophoresis; liver alkaline phosphatase migrates faster than bone and placental alkaline phosphatase, which migrate together.

C. Interpretation:

1. Elevated in–

a. Children (normal growth of bone).

b. Osteoblastic bone disease–Hyperparathyroidism, rickets and osteomalacia, neoplastic bone disease (osteosarcoma, metastatic neoplasms), ossification as in myositis ossificans, Paget's disease (osteitis deformans), and Boeck's sarcoid.

c. Hepatic duct or cholangiolar obstruction due to stone, stricture, or neoplasm.

d. Hepatic disease resulting from drugs such as chlorpromazine, methyltestosterone.

e. Pregnancy.

2. Decreased in hypothyroidism and in growth retardation in children.

D. Drug Effects on Laboratory Results: Elevated by acetohexamide, tolazamide, tolbutamide, chlorpropamide, allopurinol, sulfobromophthalein, carbamazepine, cephaloridine, furosemide, methyldopa, phenothiazine, and oral contraceptives (estrogen-progestin combinations).

Phosphorus, Inorganic, Serum: Normal: Children, 4–7 mg/dL. (SI: 1.3–2.3 mmol/L.) Adults, 3–4.5 mg/dL. (SI: 1–1.5 mmol/L.)

A. Precautions: Glassware cleaned with phosphate cleansers must be thoroughly rinsed. The fasting state is necessary to avoid postprandial depression of phosphate associated with glucose transport and metabolism.

B. Physiologic Basis: The concentration of inorganic phosphate in circulating plasma is influenced by parathyroid gland function, action of vitamin D, intestinal absorption, renal function, bone metabolism, and nutrition.

C. Interpretation:

1. Increased in renal insufficiency, hypoparathyroidism, and hypervitaminosis D.

2. Decreased in hyperparathyroidism, hypovitaminosis D (rickets, osteomalacia), malabsorption syndrome (steatorrhea), ingestion of antacids that bind phosphate in the gut, starvation or cachexia, chronic alcoholism (especially with liver disease), hyperalimentation with phosphate-poor solutions, carbohydrate administration (especially intravenously), renal tubular defects, use of thiazide diuretics, acid-base disturbances, diabetic ketoacidosis (especially during

recovery), genetic hypophosphatemia, and occasionally during pregnancy and with hypothyroidism.

Potassium, Serum or Plasma: Normal: 3.5–5 meq/L. (SI: 3.5–5 mmol/L.)

A. Precautions: Avoid hemolysis, which releases erythrocyte potassium. Serum must be separated promptly from the clot, or plasma from the red cell mass, to prevent diffusion of potassium from erythrocytes. Platelets and leukocytes are rich in potassium; if these elements are present in large numbers (eg, in thrombocytosis or leukemia), the potassium released during coagulation will increase potassium concentration in serum. If these are sources of artifact, plasma from heparinized blood should be employed.

B. Physiologic Basis: Potassium concentration in plasma determines neuromuscular and muscular irritability. Elevated or decreased concentrations impair the capability of muscle tissue to contract.

C. Interpretation: (See Precautions, above.)

1. Increased in renal insufficiency (especially in the presence of increased rate of protein or tissue breakdown); adrenal insufficiency (especially hypoaldosteronism); use of spironolactone; too rapid administration of potassium salts, especially intravenously; and use of triamterene or phenformin.

2. Decreased in–

a. Inadequate intake (starvation).

b. Inadequate absorption or unusual enteric losses–Vomiting, diarrhea, or malabsorption syndrome; use of sodium polystyrene-sulfonate resin.

c. Unusual renal loss–Secondary to hyperadrenocorticism (especially hyperaldosteronism) and to adrenocorticosteroid therapy, metabolic alkalosis, use of diuretics such as chlorothiazide and its derivatives and the mercurials; renal tubular defects such as the de Toni-Fanconi syndrome and renal tubular acidosis; treatment with antibiotics that are excreted as anions (carbenicillin, ticarcillin); use of degraded tetracycline, phenothiazines, amphotericin B, and drugs with high sodium content (eg, carbenicillin).

d. Abnormal redistribution between extracellular and intracellular fluids–Familial periodic paralysis, testosterone administration.

Proteins, Serum or Plasma (Includes Fibrinogen): Normal: See Interpretation, below.

A. Precautions: Serum or plasma must be free of hemolysis. Since fibrinogen is removed in the process of coagulation of the blood, fibrinogen determinations cannot be done on serum.

B. Physiologic Basis: Concentration of protein determines colloidal osmotic pressure of plasma. The concentration of protein in plasma is influenced by the nutritional state, hepatic function, renal function, occurrence of disease such as multiple myeloma, and metabolic errors. Variations in the fractions of plasma proteins may signify specific disease.

C. Interpretation:

1. Total protein, serum–Normal: 6–8 g/dL.

Table 7. Protein fractions as determined by electrophoresis.

	Percentage of Total Protein
Albumin	52–68
a_1 globulin	2.4–4.4
a_2 globulin	6.1–10.1
β globulin	8.5–14.5
γ globulin	10–21

Table 8. Gamma globulins by immunoelectrophoresis.

IgA	90–450 mg/dL
IgG	700–1500 mg/dL
IgM	40–250 mg/dL
IgD	0.3–40 mg/dL
IgE	0.006–0.16 mg/dL

Table 9. Some constituents of globulins.

Globulin	Representative Constituents
a_1	Thyroxine-binding globulin
	Transcortin
	Glycoprotein
	Lipoprotein
	Antitrypsin
a_2	Haptoglobin
	Glycoprotein
	Macroglobulin
	Ceruloplasmin
β	Transferrin
	Lipoprotein
	Glycoprotein
γ	γG γD
	γM γE
	γA

(SI: 60–80 g/L.) See albumin and globulin fractions, below.

2. Albumin, serum or plasma–Normal: 3.5–5.5 g/dL. (SI: 35–55 g/L.)

a. Elevated in dehydration, shock, hemoconcentration, administration of large quantities of concentrated albumin "solution" intravenously.

b. Decreased in malnutrition, malabsorption syndrome, acute or chronic glomerulonephritis, nephrosis, acute or chronic hepatic insufficiency, neoplastic diseases, and leukemia.

3. Globulin, serum or plasma–Normal: 2–3.6 g/dL. (SI: 20–36 g/L.)

a. Elevated in hepatic disease, infectious hepatitis, cirrhosis of the liver, biliary cirrhosis, and hemochromatosis; disseminated lupus erythematosus; plasma cell myeloma; lymphoproliferative disease; sarcoidosis; and acute or chronic infectious diseases, particularly lymphogranuloma venereum, typhus, leishmaniasis, schistosomiasis, and malaria.

b. Decreased in malnutrition, congenital agammaglobulinemia, acquired hypogammaglobulinemia, and lymphatic leukemia.

4. Fibrinogen, plasma–Normal: 0.2–0.6 g/dL. (SI: 2–6 g/L.)

a. Elevated in glomerulonephritis, nephrosis (occasionally), and infectious diseases.

b. Decreased in disseminated intravascular coagulation (accidents of pregnancy including placental ablation, amniotic fluid embolism, and violent labor; meningococcal meningitis; metastatic carcinoma of the prostate and occasionally of other organs; and leukemia), acute and chronic hepatic insufficiency, and congenital fibrinogenopenia.

Sodium, Serum or Plasma: Normal: 136–145 meq/L. (SI: 136–145 mmol/L.)

A. Precautions: Clean glassware completely.

B. Physiologic Basis: Sodium constitutes 140 of the 155 meq of cation in plasma. With its associated anions it provides the bulk of osmotically active solute in the plasma, thus affecting the distribution of body water significantly. A shift of sodium into cells or a loss of sodium from the body results in a decrease of extracellular fluid volume, affecting circulation, renal function, and nervous system function.

C. Interpretation:

1. Increased in dehydration (water deficit), central nervous system trauma or disease, and as a result of hyperaldosteronism or to corticosterone or corticosteroid excess.

2. Decreased in adrenal insufficiency; renal insufficiency, especially with inadequate sodium intake; renal tubular acidosis; as a physiologic response to trauma or burns (sodium shift into cells); unusual losses via the gastrointestinal tract, as in acute or chronic diarrhea, intestinal obstruction or fistula; and in unusual sweating with inadequate sodium replacement. In some patients with edema associated with cardiac or renal disease, serum sodium concentration is low even though total body sodium content is greater than normal; water retention (excess ADH) and abnormal distribution of sodium between intracellular and extracellular fluid contribute to this paradoxic situation. Hyperglycemia occasionally results in shift of intracellular water to the extracellular space, producing a dilutional hyponatremia. (Artifact: When measured by the flame photometer, serum or plasma sodium will be decreased in the presence of hyperlipidemia or hyperglobulinemia; in these disorders, the volume ordinarily occupied by water is taken up by other substances, and the serum or plasma will thus be "deficient" in water and electrolyte. In the presence of hyperglycemia, serum sodium concentration will be reduced by 1.6 meq/L per 100 mg/dL glucose above 200 mg/dL because of shifts of water into extracellular fluid.)

Thyroxine (T_4), Total, Serum: Normal: Radioimmunoassay (RIA), 5–14 μg/dL (SI: 64–180 nmol/L); competitive binding protein (CPB)

(Murphy-Pattee), 4–11 μg/dL (SI: 51–142 nmol/L).

A. Precautions: None.

B. Physiologic Basis: The total thyroxine level does not necessarily reflect the physiologic hormonal effect of thyroxine. Levels of thyroxine vary with the concentration of the carrier proteins (thyroxine-binding globulin and prealbumin), which are readily altered by physiologic conditions such as pregnancy and by a variety of diseases and drugs. Any interpretation of the significance of total T_4 depends upon knowing the concentration of carrier protein either from direct measurement or from the result of the erythrocyte or resin uptake of triiodothyronine (T_3) (see below). It is the concentration of free T_4 and of T_3 that determines hormonal activity.

C. Interpretation:

1. Elevated in hyperthyroidism, at times with active thyroiditis, acromegaly, and with elevation of thyroxine-binding proteins.

2. Decreased in hypothyroidism (primary or secondary) and with decreased concentrations of thyroxine-binding proteins.

D. Drug Effects on Laboratory Results: Increased by ingestion of excess thyroid hormone T_4. A variety of drugs alter concentration of thyroxine-binding proteins (see below), with parallel changes in total T_4 concentration. Decreased by ingestion of T_3, which inhibits thyrotropin secretion, with resultant decrease in T_4 secretion and concentration. T_4 synthesis may be decreased by aminosalicylic acid, corticosteroids, lithium, the thiouracils, methimazole, and sulfonamides. Total T_4 concentration may be reduced because of displacement from carrier protein-binding sites by aspirin, chlorpropamide, phenytoin, halofenate, and tolbutamide. Cholestyramine may reduce T_4 concentration by interfering with its enterohepatic circulation.

Thyroxine, Free, Serum (FT$_4$): Normal (equilibrium dialysis): 0.8–2.4 ng/dL. (SI: 0.01–0.03 nmol/L.) May be estimated from measurement of total thyroxine and resin T_3 uptake.

A. Precautions: None.

B. Physiologic Basis: The metabolic activity of T_4 is related to the concentration of free T_4. T_4 is apparently largely converted to T_3 in peripheral tissue. (T_3 is also secreted by the thyroid gland.) Both T_4 and T_3 seem to be active hormones.

C. Interpretation:

1. Elevated in hyperthyroidism and at times with active thyroiditis.

2. Decreased in hypothyroidism.

D. Drug Effects on Laboratory Results: Elevated by ingestion of excess thyroid hormone T_4. Decreased by T_3, thiouracils, and methimazole.

Thyroxine-Binding Globulin (TBG), Serum: Normal (radioimmunoassay): 2–4.8 mg/dL.

A. Precautions: None.

B. Physiologic Basis: TBG is the principal carrier protein for T_4 and T_3 in the plasma. Variations in concentration of TBG are accompanied by corresponding variations in concentration of T_4 with intrinsic adjustments that maintain the physiologically active free hormones at proper concentration for euthyroid function. The inherited abnormalities of TBG concentration appear to be X-linked.

C. Interpretation:

1. Elevated in pregnancy, in infectious hepatitis, and in hereditary increase in TBG concentration.

2. Decreased in major depleting illness with hypoproteinemia (globulin), nephrotic syndrome, cirrhosis of the liver, active acromegaly, estrogen deficiency, and hereditary TBG deficiency.

D. Drug Effects on Laboratory Results: TBG or binding capacity increased by pregnancy, estrogens and progestins (including oral contraceptives), chlormadinone, perphenazine, and clofibrate. Decreased by androgen, anabolic steroids, cortisol, prednisone, corticotropin, and oxymetholone.

Triiodothyronine Uptake: Resin (RT$_3$U) or Thyroxine-Binding Globulin Assessment (TBG Assessment): Normal: RT$_3$U, as percentage of uptake of ^{125}I-T_3 by resin, 25–36%; RT$_3$U ratio (TBG assessment) expressed as ratio of binding of ^{125}I-T_3 by resin in test serum/pooled normal serum, 0.85–1.15.

A. Precautions: None.

B. Physiologic Basis: When serum thyroxine-binding proteins are normal, more TBG binding sites will be occupied by T_4 in T_4 hyperthyroidism, and fewer binding sites will be occupied in hypothyroidism. ^{125}I-labeled T_3 added to serum along with a secondary binder (resin, charcoal, talc, etc) is partitioned between TBG and the binder. The binder is separated from the serum, and the radioactivity of the binder is measured for the RT$_3$U test. Since the resin takes up the non–TBG-bound radioactive T_3, its activity varies inversely with the numbers of available TBG sites, ie, RT$_3$U is increased if TBG is more nearly saturated by T_4 and decreased if TBG is less well saturated by T_4.

C. Interpretation:

1. RT$_3$U and RT$_3$U ratio are increased when available sites are decreased, as in hyperthyroidism, acromegaly, nephrotic syndrome, severe hepatic cirrhosis, and hereditary TBG deficiency.

2. RT$_3$U and RT$_3$U ratio are decreased when available TBG sites are increased, as in hypothyroidism, pregnancy, the newborn, infectious hepatitis, and hereditary increase in TBG.

D. Drug Effects on Laboratory Results: RT$_3$U and RT$_3$U ratio are elevated by excess T_4, androgens, anabolic steroids, corticosteroids, corticotropin, anticoagulant therapy (heparin and warfarin), oxymetholone, phenytoin, phenylbutazone, and large doses of salicylate. RT$_3$U and RT$_3$U ratio are decreased by T_3 therapy; by estrogens and progestins, including oral contraceptives; and by thiouracils, chlormadinone, perphenazine, and clofibrate.

Thyroxine Index: Calculation of "Corrected" T_4 From Values for Total T_4 (TT_4) and RT_3U or RT_3U Ratio: Normal (varies with method):

$$\text{Free thyroxine index} = RT_3U \text{ (in \%)} \times TT_4 \text{ in } \mu g/dL$$

or

$$\text{Corrected } T_4 = RT_3U \text{ ratio} \times TT_4 \text{ in } \mu g/dL$$

A. Precautions: None.

B. Physiologic Basis: This calculation yields a value for TT_4 corrected for altered TBG concentration. The concentration of free thyroxine (FT_4) per se depends on the equilibrium among FT_4, T_4 bound to TBG (T_4TBG), and unoccupied sites on TBG.

$$FT_4 + TBG \rightleftharpoons T_4TBG$$

The index FT_4I is more properly a value for T_4 "corrected" for variations in TBG.

C. Interpretation: FT_4I is increased over T_4 in conditions in which RT_3U ratio is increased (see Triiodothyronine Uptake).

FT_4I is decreased below T_4 in conditions in which RT_3U ratio is decreased.

D. Drug Effects on Laboratory Results: As for RT_3U and RT_3U ratio.

Triglycerides, Serum: Normal: < 165 mg/dL. (SI: < 1.65 g/L.) See also Table 3, p 1095.

A. Precautions: Subject must be in a fasting state (preferably for at least 16 hours). The determination may be delayed if the serum is promptly separated from the clot and refrigerated.

B. Physiologic Basis: Dietary fat is hydrolyzed in the small intestine, absorbed and resynthesized by the mucosal cells, and secreted into lacteals in the form of chylomicrons. Triglycerides in the chylomicrons are cleared from the blood by tissue lipoprotein lipase (mainly adipose tissue), and the split products absorbed and stored. Free fatty acids derived mainly from adipose tissue are precursors of the endogenous triglycerides produced by the liver. Transport of endogenous triglycerides is in association with β-lipoproteins, the very low density lipoproteins. (For further details, see Chapter 20.) In order to assure measurement of endogenous triglycerides, blood must be drawn in the postabsorptive state.

C. Interpretation: Concentration of triglycerides, cholesterol, and lipoprotein fractions (very low density, low-density, and high-density) is interpreted collectively. Disturbances in normal relationships of these lipid moieties may be primary or secondary in origin.

1. Elevated (hyperlipoproteinemia) –

a. Primary – Type I hyperlipoproteinemia (exogenous hyperlipidemia), type II hyperbetalipoproteinemia, type III broad beta hyperlipoproteinemia, type IV hyperlipoproteinemia (endogenous hyperlipidemia), and type V hyperlipoproteinemia (mixed hyperlipidemia).

b. Secondary – Hypothyroidism, diabetes mellitus, nephrotic syndrome, chronic alcoholism with fatty liver, ingestion of contraceptive steroids, biliary obstruction, stress.

2. Decreased (hypolipoproteinemia) –

a. Primary – Tangier disease (α-lipoprotein deficiency), abetalipoproteinemia, and a few rare, poorly defined syndromes.

b. Secondary – Malnutrition, malabsorption, and occasionally with parenchymal liver disease.

Urea Nitrogen & Urea, Blood, Plasma, or Serum: Normal: Blood urea nitrogen, 8–25 mg/dL (SI: 2.9–8.9 mmol/L). Urea, 21–53 mg/dL (SI: 3.5–9 mmol/L).

A. Precautions: *Do not use* ammonium oxalate or "double oxalate" as anticoagulant, for the ammonia will be measured as urea.

B. Physiologic Basis: Urea, an end product of protein metabolism, is excreted by the kidney. In the glomerular filtrate the urea concentration is the same as in the plasma. Tubular reabsorption of urea varies inversely with rate of urine flow. Thus, urea is a less useful measure of glomerular filtration than is creatinine, which is not reabsorbed. Blood urea nitrogen varies directly with protein intake and inversely with the rate of excretion of urea.

C. Interpretation:

1. Elevated in –

a. Renal insufficiency – Nephritis, acute and chronic; acute renal failure (tubular necrosis), urinary tract obstruction.

b. Increased nitrogen metabolism associated with diminished renal blood flow or impaired renal function – Dehydration from any cause, gastrointestinal bleeding (combination of increased protein absorption from digestion of blood plus decreased renal blood flow).

c. Decreased renal blood flow – Shock, adrenal insufficiency, occasionally congestive heart failure.

2. Decreased in hepatic failure, nephrosis not complicated by renal insufficiency, and cachexia.

D. Drug Effects on Laboratory Results: Elevated by many antibiotics that impair renal function, guanethidine, methyldopa, indomethacin, isoniazid, propranolol, and potent diuretics (decreased blood volume and renal blood flow).

Uric Acid, Serum or Plasma: Normal: Males, 3–9 mg/dL (SI: 0.18–0.53 mmol/L); females, 2.5–7.5 mg/dL (SI: 0.15–0.45 mmol/L).

A. Precautions: If plasma is used, lithium oxalate should be used as the anticoagulant; potassium oxalate may interfere with the determination.

B. Physiologic Basis: Uric acid, an end product of nucleoprotein metabolism, is excreted by the kidney. Gout, a genetically transmitted metabolic error, is characterized by an increased plasma or serum uric acid concentration, an increase in total body uric acid, and deposition of uric acid in tissues. An increase in uric acid concentration in plasma and serum may accompany increased nucleoprotein catabolism (blood dyscrasias, therapy with antileukemic drugs), use of thiazide diuretics, or decreased renal excretion.

C. Interpretation:

1. Elevated in gout, toxemia of pregnancy (eclampsia), leukemia, polycythemia, therapy with antileukemic drugs and a variety of other agents, renal insufficiency, glycogen storage disease (type I), Lesch-Nyhan syndrome (X-linked hypoxanthine-guanine phosphoribosyltransferase deficit), and Down's syndrome. The incidence of hyperuricemia is greater in Filipinos than in whites.

2. Decreased in acute hepatitis (occasionally), treatment with allopurinol, probenecid.

D. Drug Effects on Laboratory Results: Elevated by salicylates (low doses), thiazide diuretics, ethacrynic acid, spironolactone, furosemide, triamterene, and ascorbic acid. Decreased by salicylates (large doses), methyldopa, clofibrate, phenylbutazone, cinchophen, sulfinpyrazone, and phenothiazines.

Uric Acid, Urine: Normal: 350–600 mg/24 h on a standard purine-free diet. (SI: 2.1–3.6 mmol/24 h.) Normal urinary uric acid/creatinine ratio for adults is 0.21–0.59; maximum of 0.75 for 24-hour urine while on purine-free diet.

A. Precautions: Diet should be free of high-purine foods prior to and during 24-hour urine collection. Strenuous activity may be associated with elevated purine excretion.

B. Physiologic Basis: Elevated serum uric acid may result from overproduction or diminished excretion.

C. Interpretation:

1. Elevated renal excretion occurs in about 25–30% of cases of gout due to increased purine synthesis. Excess uric acid synthesis and excretion are associated with myeloproliferative disorders. Lesch-Nyhan syndrome (hypoxanthine-guanine phosphoribosyltransferase deficit) and some cases of glycogen storage disease are associated with uricosuria.

2. Decreased in renal insufficiency, in some cases of glycogen storage disease (type I), and in any metabolic defect producing either lacticacidemia or β-hydroxybutyricacidemia. Salicylates in doses of less than 2–3 g/d may produce renal retention of uric acid.

● ● ●

References

Friedman RB et al: Effects of diseases on clinical laboratory tests. *Clin Chem* 1980;**26(Suppl 4)**:1D.

Hansten PD: *Drug Interactions: Clinical Significance of Drug Interactions,* 4th ed. Lea & Febiger, 1979.

Hansten PD, Lybecker LA: Drug effects on laboratory tests. In: Katzung BG (editor): *Basic & Clinical Pharmacology,* 2nd ed. Lange, 1984.

Henry JB (editor): *Clinical Diagnosis and Management by Laboratory Methods,* 16th ed. Vols 1 and 2. Saunders, 1979.

Lippert H, Lehmann HP: *SI Units in Medicine: An Introduction to the International System of Units With Conversion Tables and Normal Ranges.* Urban & Schwarzenberg, 1978.

Powsner EK: SI quantities and units for American medicine. *JAMA* 1984;**252**:1737.

Scully RE et al: Normal reference laboratory values: Case records of the Massachusetts General Hospital. *N Engl J Med* 1980; **302**:37.

Sonnenwirth AC, Jarett L: *Gradwohl's Laboratory Methods and Diagnosis,* 8th ed. Vols 1 and 2. Mosby, 1980.

Young DS: "Normal laboratory values" (case records of the Massachusetts General Hospital) in SI units. *N Engl J Med* 1975;**292**:795.

NORMAL LABORATORY VALUES

(SI Values in Parentheses)

HEMATOLOGY

Bleeding time: Ivy method: 1–7 minutes (60–420 seconds). Template method: 3–9 minutes (180–540 seconds).

Cellular measurements of red cells: Average diameter = 7.3 μm (5.5–8.8 μm).
Mean corpuscular volume (MCV): Men, 80–94 fL; women, 81–99 fL (by Coulter counter).
Mean corpuscular hemoglobin (MCH): 27–32 pg.
Mean corpuscular hemoglobin concentration (MCHC): 32–36 g/dL red blood cells (32–36%).
Color, saturation, and volume indices: 1 (0.9–1.1).

Clot retraction: Begins in 1–3 hours; complete in 6–24 hours. No clot lysis in 24 hours.

Coagulation time (Lee-White): At 37 °C, 6–12 minutes; at room temperature, 10–18 minutes.

Fibrinogen split products: Negative > 1:4 dilution.

Fragility of red cells: Begins at 0.45–0.38% NaCl; complete at 0.36–0.3% NaCl.

Hematocrit (PCV): Men, 40–52%; women, 37–47%.

Hemoglobin: [B] Men, 14–18 g/dL (2.09–2.79 mmol/L as Hb tetramer); women, 12–16 g/dL (1.86–2.48 mmol/L). (Serum hemoglobin: 2–3 mg/dL.)

Partial thromboplastin time: Activated, 25–37 seconds.

Platelets: 150–400 thousand/μL (0.15–0.4 × 10^{12}/L).

Prothrombin: [P] 75–125%. Less than 2 seconds deviation from control.

Red blood count (RBC): Men, 4.5–6.2 million/μL (4.5–6.2 × 10^{12}/L); women, 4–5.5 million/μL (4–5.5 × 10^{12}/L).

Reticulocytes: 0.2–2% of red cells.

Sedimentation rate: Less than 20 mm/h (Westergren); 0–10 mm/h (Wintrobe).

White blood count (WBC) and differential: 5–10 thousand/μL (5–10 × 10^9/L).

Myelocytes	0 %
Juvenile neutrophils	0 %
Band neutrophils	0–5 %
Segmented neutrophils	40–60%
Lymphocytes	20–40%
Eosinophils	1–3 %
Basophils	0–1 %
Monocytes	4–8 %

Lymphocytes: Total, 1500–4000/μL.	
B cells	5–25%
T cells	60–88%
Suppressor	10–43%
Helper	32–66%
H:S	> 1

BLOOD (B), PLASMA (P), OR SERUM (S) CHEMICAL CONSTITUENTS

Below are listed the specimen used, the source—blood [B], plasma [P], or serum [S]—the fasting state, and the normal values. Values vary with the procedure employed.

Acetone and acetoacetate: [S] 0.3–2 mg/dL (3–20 mg/L).

Aldolase: [S] Values vary with method used.

α-Amino acid nitrogen: [S, fasting] 3–5.5 mg/dL (2.2–3.9 mmol/L).

Aminotransferases [S]:
Aspartate aminotransferase (AST; SGOT), 6–25 IU/L at 30 °C; SMA, 10–40 IU/L at 37 °C; SMAC, 0–41 IU/L at 37 °C.
Alanine aminotransferase (ALT; SGPT), 3–26 IU/L at 30 °C; SMAC 0–45 IU/L at 37 °C.

Ammonia: [B] 80–110 μg/dL (47–65 μmol/L) (diffusion method). Do not use anticoagulant containing ammonium oxalate.

Amylase: [S] 80–180 units/dL (Somogyi). Values vary with method used.

α_1-Antitrypsin: [S] > 180 mg/dL.

Ascorbic acid: [P] 0.4–1.5 mg/dL (23–85 μmol/L).

Base, total serum: [S] 145–160 meq/L (145–160 mmol/L).

Bicarbonate: [S] 24–28 meq/L (24–28 mmol/L).

Bilirubin: [S] Total, 0.2–1.2 mg/dL (3.4–20.4 μmol/L). Direct, 0.1–0.4 mg/dL (1.7–6.8 μmol/L).

Calcium: [S] 8.5–10.3 mg/dL; 4.2–5.1 meq/L (2.1–2.6 mmol/L). Values vary with protein concentration.

Calcium, ionized: [S] 4.25–5.25 mg/dL; 2.1–2.6 meq/L (1.05–1.3 mmol/L).

β-Carotene: [S, fasting] 50–300 μg/dL (0.9–5.58 μmol/L).

Ceruloplasmin: [S] 25–43 mg/dL (1.7–2.9 μmol/L).

Chloride: [S] 96–106 meq/L (96–106 mmol/L).

Cholesterol: [S] 150–280 mg/dL (3.9–7.28 mmol/L). (See Lipid Fractions.) Values vary with age.

Cholesteryl esters: [S] 65–75% of total cholesterol.

CO_2 content: [S or P] 24–29 meq/L (24–29 mmol/L).

Complement: [S] C3 ($β_{1C}$), 90–250 mg/dL; C4 ($β_{1E}$), 10–60 mg/dL. Total (CH_{50}), 75–160 mg/dL.

Copper: [S or P] 100–200 μg/dL (16–31 μmol/L).

Cortisol: [P] 8:00 AM: 5–25 μg/dL (138–590 nmol/L); 8:00 PM: < 10 μg/dL (275 nmol/L).

Creatine kinase: [S] 10–50 IU/L at 30 °C. Values vary with method used.

Creatine kinase isoenzymes: See p 1096.

Creatinine: [S] 0.7–1.5 mg/dL (62–132 μmol/L).

Epinephrine: [P,] Supine < 0.1 μg/L (< 0.55 nmol/L).

Ferritin: [S] Adult women, 20–120 ng/mL; men, 30–300 ng/mL. Child to 15 years, 7–140 ng/mL.

Folic acid: [S] 2–20 ng/mL (4.5–45 nmol/L); [RBC]> 140 ng/mL (>318 nmol/L).

Glucose: [S, fasting] 65–110 mg/dL (3.6–6.1 mmol/L).

Glucose tolerance: See p 765.

Haptoglobin: [S] 40–170 mg of hemoglobin-binding capacity.

Hemoglobin A_{1C} [B]: See p 765.

Iron: [S] 50–175 μg/dL (9–31.3 μmol/L).

Iron-binding capacity, total: [S] 250–410 μg/dL (44.7–73.4 μmol/L). Percent saturation: 20–55%.

Lactate: [B, special handling] Venous: 4–16 mg/dL (0.44–1.8 mmol/L).

Lactate dehydrogenase (SLDH): [S] 55–140 IU/L at 30 °C; SMA, 100–225 IU/L at 37 °C; SMAC, 60–200 IU/L at 37 °C.

Lipase: [S] 0.2–1.5 units (mL of 0.1 N NaOH).

Lipid fractions: [P, S] Desirable levels: HDL cholesterol, > 40 mg/dL; LDL cholesterol, < 180 mg/dL; VLDL cholesterol, < 40 mg/dL. (To convert to mmol/L, multiply by 0.026.)

Lipids, total: [S] 450–1000 mg/dL (4.5–10 g/L).

Magnesium: [P] 1.8–3 mg/dL (0.75–1.25 mmol/L).

Nonprotein nitrogen (NPN): [S] 15–35 mg/dL (14–21 mmol/L). Do not use anticoagulant containing ammonium oxalate.

Norepinephrine: [P] Supine, < 0.5 μg/L (< 3 nmol/L).

Osmolality: [S] 275–295 mosm/kg water.

Oxygen:
  Capacity: [B] 16–24 vol% (varies with hemoglobin concentration).
  Arterial content: [B] 15–23 vol% (varies with hemoglobin concentration).
  Arterial % saturation: 94–100% of capacity.
  Arterial P_{O_2} (Pa_{O_2}): 80–100 mm Hg (10.67–13.33 kPa) (sea level). (Values vary with age.)

Pa_{CO_2}: [B, arterial] 35–45 mm Hg (4.7–6 kPa).

pH (reaction): [B, arterial] 7.35–7.45 (H^+ 44.7–45.5 nmol/L).

Phosphatase, acid: [S] 1–5 units (King-Armstrong), 0.1–0.63 units (Bessey-Lowry). (See also p 1098.)

Phosphatase, alkaline: [S] 5–13 units (King-Armstrong); Adults, 0.8–2.3 (Bessey-Lowry); SMA, 30–85 IU/L at 37 °C; SMAC, 30–115 IU/L at 37 °C.

Phospholipid: [S] 145–200 mg/dL (1.45–2 g/L).

Phosphorus, inorganic: [S, fasting] 3–4.5 mg/dL (1–1.5 mmol/L).

Potassium: [S or P] 3.5–5 meq/L (3.5–5 mmol/L).

Protein:
  Total: [S] 6–8 g/dL (60–80 g/L).
  Albumin: [S] 3.5–5.5 g/dL (35–55 g/L).
  Globulin: [S] 2–3.6 g/dL (20–36 g/L).
  Fibrinogen: [P] 0.2–0.6 g/dL (2–6 g/L).
  Separation by electrophoresis: See Table 7.

Prothrombin clotting time: [P] By control.

Pyruvate: [B] 0.6–1 mg/dL (70–114 μmol/L).

Serotonin: [B] 0.05–0.2 μg/mL.

Sodium: [S] 135–145 meq/L (135–145 mmol/L).

Specific gravity:
  [B] 1.056 (varies with hemoglobin and protein concentration).
  [S] 1.0254–1.0288 (varies with protein concentration).

Sulfate: [P or S] as sulfur. 0.5–1.5 mg/dL (156–468 μmol/L).

Transferrin: [S] 200–400 mg/dL (23–45 μmol/L).

Triglycerides: [S] < 165 mg/dL (5.4 meq/L or 1.9 mmol/L). (See Lipid Fractions.)

Urea nitrogen: [S] 8–25 mg/dL (2.9–8.9 mmol/L). Do not use anticoagulant containing ammonium oxalate.

Uric Acid: [S] Men, 3–9 mg/dL (0.18–0.53 mmol/L); women, 2.5–7.5 mg/dL (0.15–0.45 mmol/L).

Vitamin A: [S] 15–60 μg/dL (0.53–2.1 μmol/L).

Vitamin B$_{12}$: [S] > 200 pg/mL (> 148 pmol/L).

Vitamin D: [S]. Cholecalciferol (D$_3$): 25-Hydroxycholecalciferol, 10–80 ng/mL (26–208 nmol/L); 1,25-dihydroxycholecalciferol, 21–45 pg/mL (50–108 pmol/L); 24,25-dihydroxycholecalciferol, 1–5 ng/mL (2.4–12 nmol/L).

Volume, blood (Evans blue dye method): Adults, 2990–6980 mL. Women, 46.3–85.5 mL/kg; men, 66.2–97.7 mL/kg.

Zinc: [S] 50–150 μg/dL (7.65–22.95 μmol/L).

HORMONES, SERUM OR PLASMA

Pituitary:
  Growth (hGH): [S] Adults, 1–10 ng/mL (by RIA) (46–465 pmol/L).
  Thyroid-stimulating (TSH): [S] < 10 μU/mL.
  Follicle-stimulating hormone (FSH): [S] Prepubertal, 2–12 mIU/mL; adult men, 1–15 mIU/mL; adult women, 1–30 mIU/mL; castrate or postmenopausal, 30–200 mIU/mL (by RIA).
  Luteinizing hormone (LH): [S] Prepubertal, 2–12 mIU/mL; adult men, 1–15 mIU/mL; adult women, < 30 mIU/mL; castrate or postmenopausal, > 30 mIU/mL.
  Corticotropin (ACTH): [P] 8:00–10:00 AM: up to 100 pg/mL (22 pmol/L).

Prolactin: [S] 0–20 ng/mL (0–8 nmol/L).
Somatomedin C: [P] 0.4–2 U/mL.
Antidiuretic hormone: [P] Serum osmolality 285 mosm/kg, 0–2 pg/mL; > 290 mosm/kg, 2–12 + pg/mL.

Adrenal:
  Aldosterone: [P] Supine, normal salt intake, 2–9 ng/dL (56–250 pmol/L); increased when upright.
  Cortisol: [S] 8:00 AM, 5–20 μg/dL (0.14–0.55 μmol/L); 8:00 PM, < 10 μg/dL.
  Deoxycortisol: [S] Baseline, 50–250 ng/dL (1.44–7.2 nmol/L); after metyrapone, > 7 μg/dL (> 0.2 μmol/L).
  Dopamine: [P] < 135 pg/mL.
  Epinephrine: [P] < 80 pg/mL.
  Norepinephrine: [P] < 400 pg/mL.
  Also see Miscellaneous Normal Values.

Thyroid:
  Thyroxine, free (FT$_4$): [S] 0.8–2.4 ng/dL (0.01–0.03 nmol/L).
  Thyroxine, total (TT$_4$): [S] 4–11 μg/dL (52–143 nmol/L) T$_4$ (by CPB); 5–12 μg/dL (65–154 nmol/L) (by RIA).
  Thyroxine-binding globulin: [S] 2–4.8 mg/dL (20–48 mg/L).
  Triiodothyronine: [S] 80–220 ng/dL (1.2–3.3 nmol/L).
  Reverse triiodothyronine: [S] Adult 30–80 ng/dL (0.45–1.2 nmol/L).
  Triiodothyronine uptake (RT$_3$U): [S] 25–36%; as TBG assessment (RT$_3$U ratio), 0.85–1.15.
  Calcitonin: [S] < 400 pg/mL (< 117 pmol/L).

Parathyroid: Parathyroid hormone levels vary with method and antibody. Correlate with serum calcium.

Islets:
  Insulin: [S] 4–25 μU/mL (29–181 pmol/L).
  C-peptide: [S] 0.9–4.2 ng/mL.
  Glucagon: [S] Fasting, 20–100 pg/mL.

Stomach:
  Gastrin: [S, special handling] Up to 100 pg/mL (47 pmol/L). Elevated, > 200 pg/mL.
  Pepsinogen I: [S] 25–100 ng/mL.

Kidney:
  Renin activity: [P, special handling] Normal sodium intake: Supine, 1–3 ng/mL/h; standing, 3–6 ng/mL/h. Sodium depleted: Supine, 2–6 ng/mL/h; standing, 3–20 ng/mL/h.

Gonad:
  Testosterone: [S] Prepubertal, < 100 ng/dL; adult men, 300–1000 ng/dL; adult women, 20–80 ng/dL; luteal phase, up to 120 ng/dL. Free testosterone: Men, 10–30 ng/dL; women, 0.3–2 ng/dL. (1 ng/dL = 0.035 nmol/L.)

Estradiol (E$_2$), RIA: [S, special handling] Men, 12–34 pg/mL; women, menstrual cycle 1–10 days, 24–68 pg/mL; 11–20 days, 50–186 pg/mL; 21–30 days, 73–149 pg/mL. (1 pg/mL = 3.6 pmol/L.)

Progesterone, RIA: [S] Follicular phase, 20–150 ng/dL; luteal phase, 300–2400 ng/dL; pregnancy, > 2400 ng/dL; men, < 100 ng/dL. (1 ng/dL = 30 pmol/L.)

Placenta:

Estriol (E$_3$), RIA: [S] Men and nonpregnant women, < 0.2 μg/dL (> 7 nmol/L).

Chorionic gonadotropin: Men, beta subunit: [S] < 9 mIU/mL; pregnancy after implantation, > 10 mIU/mL.

NORMAL CEREBROSPINAL FLUID VALUES

Appearance: Clear and colorless.

Cells: Adults, 0–5 mononuclears/μL. Infants, 0–20 mononuclears/μL.

Glucose: 50–85 mg/dL (2.8–4.7 mmol/L). (Draw serum glucose at same time.)

Pressure (reclining): Newborn, 30–80 mm water. Children, 50–100 mm water. Adults, 70–200 mm water (avg = 125).

Proteins, total: 20–45 mg/dL (200–450 mg/L) in lumbar cerebrospinal fluid. IgG: 2–6 mg/dL (0.02–0.06 g/L).

Specific gravity: 1.003–1.008.

RENAL FUNCTION TESTS

p-Aminohippurate (PAH) clearance (RPF): Men, 560–830 mL/min; women, 490–700 mL/min.

Creatinine clearance, endogenous (GFR): Approximates inulin clearance (see below).

Filtration fraction (FF): Men, 17–21%; women, 17–23%. (FF = GFR/RPF.)

Inulin clearance (GFR): Men, 110–150 mL/min; women, 105–132 mL/min (corrected to 1.73 m^2 surface area).

Maximal glucose reabsorptive capacity (Tm$_G$): Men, 300–450 mg/min; women, 250–350 mg/min.

Maximal PAH excretory capacity (Tmp$_{AH}$): 80–90 mg/min.

Osmolality: On normal diet and fluid intake: Range 500–850 mosm/kg water. Achievable range, normal kidney: Dilution 40–80 mosm; concentration (dehydration) up to 1400 mosm/kg water (at least 3–4 times plasma osmolality).

Specific gravity of urine: 1.003–1.030.

MISCELLANEOUS NORMAL VALUES
(Urine [U], Serum [S])

Addis urine sediment count: Maximum values per 24 hours are as follows:

Red cells, 1 million
White and epithelial cells, 2 million
Casts, 100 thousand
Protein, 30 mg

Adrenal hormones and metabolites:

Aldosterone: [U] 2–26 μg/24 h (5.5–72 nmol). Values vary with sodium and potassium intake.

Catecholamines: [U] Total < 100 μg/24 h. < 10 μg epinephrine (< 55 nmol); < 100 μg norepinephrine/ 24 h (< 591 nmol). Values vary with method used.

Cortisol, free: [U] 20–100 μg/24 h (0.55–2.76 μmol).

11,17-Hydroxycorticoids: [U] Men, 4–12 mg/24 h; women, 4–8 mg/24 h. Values vary with method used.

17-Ketosteroids: [U] Under 8 years, 0–2 mg/24 h; adolescents, 2–20 mg/24 h. Men, 10–20 mg/24 h; women, 5–15 mg/24 h. Values vary with method used.

Metanephrine: [U]< 1.3 mg/24 h (< 6.6 μmol) or < 2.2 μg/mg creatinine. Values vary with method used.

Vanillylmandelic acid (VMA): [U] Up to 7 mg/24 h (< 35 μmol).

Fecal fat: Less than 30% dry weight.

Lead: [U] < 0.12 mg/24 h (< 0.57 μmol).

Porphyrins: [U]
Delta-aminolevulinic acid: Adult, 1.5–7.5 mg/24 h (11.4–57.2 μmol).
Coproporphyrin: < 230 μg/24 h (< 345 nmol).
Uroporphyrin: < 50 μg/24 h (< 60 nmol).
Porphobilinogen: < 2 mg/24 h (< 8.8 μmol).

Urobilinogen: [U] 0–2.5 mg/24 h (< 4.23 μmol).

Urobilinogen, fecal: 40–280 mg/24 h (68–474 μmol).

Table 10. Therapeutic serum levels of some commonly used drugs.*

Drug	Therapeutic Range		Toxic Level
	Peak	Trough	
Antibiotics			
Amikacin	20–30 μg/mL	1–8 μg/mL	> 30 μg/mL
Kanamycin	20–30 μg/mL	1–8 μg/mL	> 30 μg/mL
Gentamicin	5–10 μg/mL	< 2 μg/mL	> 12 μg/mL
Tobramycin	5–10 μg/mL	< 2 μg/mL	> 12 μg/mL
Netilmicin	6–10 μg/mL	< 2 μg/mL	> 12 μg/mL
Chloramphenicol	15–20 μg/mL	. . .	> 25 μg/mL

Drug	Therapeutic Range	Toxic Level
Antiarrhythmics		
Digoxin	0.8–2 ng/mL	2.5 ng/mL
Digitoxin	10–22 ng/mL	35 ng/mL
Lidocaine	1.5–5 μg/mL	> 7 μg/mL
Procainamide	4–10 μg/mL	> 16 μg/mL
Procainamide + n-acetylprocainamide	10–30 μg/mL	> 30 μg/mL
Quinidine	2–5 μg/mL	> 10 μg/mL
Disopyramide	3–5 μg/mL	> 7 μg/mL
Antiepileptics		
Phenytoin	10–20 μg/mL	> 20 μg/mL
Phenobarbital	15–40 μg/mL	> 40 μg/mL
Primidone	5–12 μg/mL	> 15 μg/mL
Ethosuximide	40–100 μg/mL	> 150 μg/mL
Valproic acid	50–100 μg/mL	> 100 μg/mL
Carbamazepine	8–12 μg/mL	> 15 μg/mL
Antidepressants		
Amitriptyline	120–250 ng/mL	> 500 ng/mL
Desipramine	150–250 ng/mL	> 500 ng/mL
Imipramine	150–250 ng/mL	> 500 ng/mL
Nortriptyline	50–150 ng/mL	> 500 ng/mL
Lithium	0.6–1.4 meq/L	> 2 meq/L
Others		
Theophylline	10–20 μg/mL	> 20 μg/mL
Aspirin	100–250 μg/mL	> 300 μg/mL
Acetaminophen	. . .	> 250 μg/mL

*See also Holford NHG: Clinical interpretation of drug concentrations. Chapter 65 in: *Basic & Clinical Pharmacology*, 2nd ed. Katzung BG (editor). Lange, 1984.

CARDIOPULMONARY RESUSCITATION (CPR)

Basic Life Support

Time is a crucial factor in providing (1) emergency oxygenation and (2) circulation support. Prompt recognition of cardiac or respiratory arrest and rapid intervention are required. External support of respiration and circulation must be instituted just as soon as it can be established that the patient's unresponsiveness is due to apnea or apparent cardiac arrest. This necessitates rapid differentiation from other causes of sudden unconsciousness such as syncope, epilepsy, or choking on food. Delays of more than 3–4 minutes after the onset of respiratory or circulatory arrest decrease the chance of effective resuscitation and increase the possibility of permanent brain damage. Call for help but do not stop preparations for immediate resuscitation.

Step 1: Place patient supine on a firm surface (not a bed). A 1.2-× 1.8-m (4 × 6′) plywood sheet to be placed under the bed patient should be available in emergency care centers.

Step 2: Look and listen to determine if the patient is breathing. If the patient is not breathing, take immediate steps to open the airway. In unconscious patients, the tongue becomes lax and may fall backward, blocking the victim's airway. Gently tip the victim's head backward as far as possible by lifting up the neck, near the base of the skull, with one hand and pressing down on the forehead with the other hand. (See Fig 1.) Avoid hyperextending the victim's neck in accident cases when there is a possibility of neck fracture. In such an instance, keep mandible displaced forward by pulling strongly at the angle of the jaw ("chin-lift").

If Victim Is Not Breathing:

Step 3: Clear the mouth and pharynx of foreign material (eg, blood, vomitus) with the hooked index finger ("finger-sweep") but avoid undue probing. Do not remove dentures but leave them in the mouth to obtain a better seal around the lips.

Step 4: If steps 2–3 fail to open airway, forcibly blow air through mouth (keeping nose closed) or nose (keeping mouth closed) and quickly and fully inflate the lungs 4 times. Exhaled air contains 16–18% oxygen. Watch for chest movement. If this fails to clear the airway immediately, foreign body airway obstruction is possible; roll the patient onto one side and deliver a sharp blow between the shoulder blades. If this measure also fails, use the Heimlich maneuver (see p 1113) and if required use an endotracheal (preferably orotracheal) tube. Perform a cricothyrotomy or tracheostomy if other measures fail.

Step 5: Feel the carotid or femoral artery for pulsations.

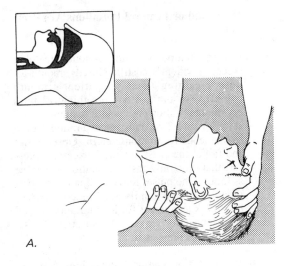

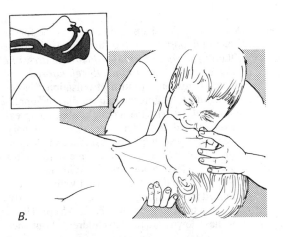

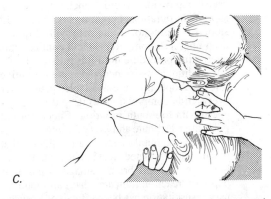

Figure 1. Proper performance of mouth-to-mouth resuscitation. *A:* Open airway by positioning neck anteriorly in extension. Inserts show airway obstructed when the neck is in resting flexed position and opening when neck is extended. *B:* Rescuer should close victim's nose with fingers, seal mouth around victim's mouth, and deliver breath by vigorous expiration. *C:* Victim is allowed to exhale passively by unsealing mouth and nose. Rescuer should listen and feel for expiratory air flow.

a. If Carotid or Femoral Pulsations Are Present:

Give lung inflation by mouth-to-mouth breathing (keeping patient's nostrils closed), mouth-to-nose breathing (keeping patient's mouth closed), or mouth-to-stoma breathing, 12 times per minute—allowing about 2 seconds for inspiration and 3 seconds for expiration—until spontaneous respirations return. Observe rise and fall of the chest, avoiding excessive pressure that may cause gastric dilatation. Continue as long as the pulses remain palpable and previously dilated pupils remain constricted. Bag-mask techniques for lung inflation should be reserved for experts. If pulsations cease, follow directions as in 5b, below.

b. If Carotid or Femoral Pulsations Are Absent:

Deliver a single, sharp, quick blow of the fist to the mid portion of the sternum (precordial thump) *in case of witnessed cardiac arrest in the electrocardiographically monitored patient.* If response (return of pulsations) is not immediate, begin external cardiac compression *without delay.* Alternate cardiac compression (closed heart massage) and pulmonary ventilation (as in 5a, above). Place the heel of one hand on the lower third of the sternum just above the level of the xiphoid. With the heel of the other hand on top of it and with fully extended arms, apply firm vertical pressure sufficient to force the sternum about 4–5 cm (1½–2 inches) downward (less in children) about once every second (60–80 per minute). There should be a slight pause at the maximal point of each compression. Avoid "quick jabs," which shorten the duration of compression.* After 15 sternal compressions, alternate with 2 quick, deep lung inflations. Repeat and continue this alternating procedure until it is possible to obtain additional assistance and more definitive care. If 2 operators are available, pause after every fifth compression while partner gives one mouth-to-mouth inflation. Check carotid pulse after 1 minute and every 5 minutes thereafter. Check pupils periodically. Pupils that remain widely dilated are an indication of cerebral hypoxia and brain damage. Return of pupillary reaction indicates that cardiopulmonary resuscitation has been effective. Resuscitation must be continuous during transportation to the hospital.

Advanced Life Support
Until spontaneous respiration and circulation are

*For children, use only one hand; for babies, use only 2 fingers of one hand, compressing 80–100 times per minute.

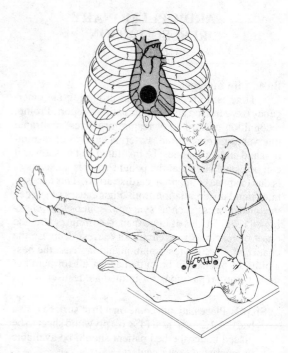

Figure 2. Technique of closed chest cardiac massage. Heavy circle in heart drawing shows area of application of force. Circles on supine figure show points of application of electrodes for defibrillation.

restored, there must be no interruption of artificial ventilation and cardiac massage while the attempt to (1) restart spontaneous circulation and (2) stabilize the cardiopulmonary circulation (steps 6–12 below) are being carried out. Three basic questions must be considered at this point: (1) What is the underlying cause, and is it correctable? (2) What is the nature of the cardiac arrest? If possible, determine the type of cardiac arrest by means of electrocardiography: (a) asystole, (b) shock or electromechanical dissociation (electrical activity without effective mechanical contraction), or (c) ventricular fibrillation. (3) What further measures will be necessary? Plan upon the assistance of a trained emergency resuscitation team with a cardiologist, anesthesiologist, and surgeon. Cardiac monitoring and assisted ventilation equipment, a DC defibrillator, emergency drugs, and adequate laboratory facilities are required.

Step 6: Provide for adequate prolonged oxygenation *as soon as possible* by intubation, administration of 100% oxygen, and mechanically assisted ventilation. Promptly establish a cutdown for long-term intravenous therapy and monitoring. Attach electrocardiographic leads and take the first of serial specimens for arterial blood gases and pH. Combat shock with intravenous fluids and vasoactive drugs (see pp 11 and 12).

Step 7: If a spontaneous effective heartbeat is not restored after 1–2 minutes of cardiac compression, have an assistant give epinephrine (adrenaline), 0.5–1 mg (adult dose) (0.5–1 mL of 1:1000 aqueous solution) diluted to 10 mL, intravenously every 5 minutes as indicated. Epinephrine may stimulate cardiac contractions and induce ventricular fibrillation that can then be treated by DC countershock (see below).

Step 8: If the victim is pulseless, immediately give 1 meq/kg sodium bicarbonate solution intravenously to combat metabolic acidosis. Do not interrupt cardiopulmonary resuscitation. Repeat no more than one-half the initial dose of bicarbonate every 10 minutes during cardiopulmonary resuscitation until spontaneous circulation is restored. Monitoring of arterial blood gas and pH is required throughout bicarbonate treatment to prevent hazardous alkalosis and severe hyperosmolar states.

Step 9: In case asystole and electromechanical dissociation persist, continue artificial respiration and external cardiac compression, epinephrine, and sodium bicarbonate as above. Rarely, a temporary pacemaker may restore an effective paced ventricular rhythm. Give also calcium chloride, 5 mL (0.5 g) of 10% solution intravenously every 10 minutes as indicated. (*Caution:* Do not give *with* bicarbonate.) Monitor blood pH, gases, and electrolytes.

Step 10: If electrocardiography demonstrates ventricular fibrillation, maintain respiration and external cardiac massage until just before giving an external defibrillating shock. Become familiar with the manufacturer's recommendations for each type of defibrillator. A DC countershock of 200–300 joules (watt-second) is given across the heart, ie, with one paddle electrode firmly applied to the skin over the apex of the heart and the other paddle applied just to the right of the upper sternum. If this fails, repeat the defibrillation attempt with a 200- to 300-joule shock. Monitor with electrocardiography. If cardiac function is still not restored, continue external support of respiration and circulation and give bicarbonate and epinephrine as above. Then make a third defibrillation attempt with no greater than a 360-joule countershock. If cardiac action is reestablished but remains weak, give calcium chloride as above. If fibrillation persists or recurs, give lidocaine, 75 mg bolus injection, and an additional 50 mg every 5 minutes, to a total of 225 mg if necessary. Procainamide, 100 mg intravenously every 5 minutes at a rate of 20 mg/min (to a total of 1 g if necessary), may be used if lidocaine fails to suppress the fibrillation. If lidocaine and procainamide fail to control the dysrhythmia, give bretylium, 5 mg/kg, as a bolus intravenously followed by electrical defibrillation. For refractory or recurrent ventricular tachycardia, give a loading dose of bretylium, 5–10 mg/kg intravenously, over 10 minutes; the maintenance dose can also be followed by a continuous infusion at a rate of 1–2 mg/min. It may be necessary to use a pacemaker to override the abnormal rhythm.

Step 11: In some instances of cardiac arrest with electrical sinus bradycardia (with a heart rate of < 60/min when associated with premature ventricular contractions or systolic blood pressure < 90 mm Hg) or cardiac arrest with sinus bradycardia associated with a high degree of atrioventricular block, atropine sulfate, 0.4–0.6 mg intravenously, may be of value. Isoproterenol may be the treatment of choice for patients with profound bradycardia with complete heart block, and it may also be useful for treatment of profound bradycardia refractory to atropine. Give isoproterenol, 1 mg in 500 mL of 5% dextrose in water by intravenous infusion at a rate of 0.03 mg/5 min, and adjust the dose to increase the heart rate to approximately 60 beats/min.

Step 12: Consider the use of assisted circulation in selected cases. A few patients who cannot be salvaged by conventional cardiopulmonary resuscitation may be saved by the addition of partial cardiopulmonary bypass measures.

Follow-Up Measures

When cardiac and pulmonary function have been reestablished and satisfactorily maintained, evaluation of central nervous system function deserves careful consideration. Decisions about the nature and duration of subsequent treatment must be individualized. Physicians must decide if they are "prolonging life" or simply "prolonging dying." Complete recovery, however, has been reported in a few patients unconscious up to a week after appropriate treatment.

Step 13: Support ventilation and circulation. Treat complications that might arise. Do not overlook the possibility of complications of external cardiac massage (eg, broken ribs, ruptured viscera).

Step 14: Meticulous postresuscitation care is required, particularly for the first 48 hours after recovery. Observe carefully for possible multiple cardiac arrhythmias, especially recurrent fibrillation or cardiac standstill.

Eisenberg MS, Hallstrom A, Bergner L: Long-term survival after out-of-hospital cardiac arrest. *N Engl J Med* 1982;**306:**1340.

Ewy GA: Current status of cardiopulmonary resuscitation. *Mod Concepts Cardiovasc Dis* 1984;**53:**43.

Graver K: New trends in the management of cardiac arrest. *Am Fam Physician* (Feb) 1984;**29:**223.

Longstreth WT et al: Neurologic recovery after cardiac arrest. *Ann Intern Med* 1983;**98(Part 1):**588.

Roth R et al: Out-of-hospital cardiac arrest: Factors associated with survival. *Ann Emerg Med* 1984;**13:**237.

Safar P: Cardiopulmonary-cerebral resuscitation. In: *Textbook of Critical Care.* Shoemaker WC et al (editors). Saunders, 1984.

Standards and guidelines for cardiopulmonary resuscitation (CPR) and emergency cardiac care (ECC). *JAMA* 1980;**244:**453.

Stueven H et al: Use of calcium in prehospital cardiac arrest. *Ann Emerg Med* 1983;**12:**136.

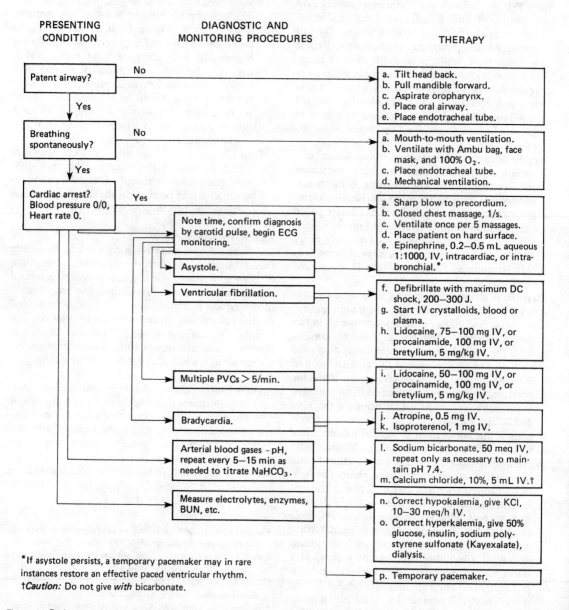

CARDIORESPIRATORY ARREST

| PRESENTING CONDITION | DIAGNOSTIC AND MONITORING PROCEDURES | THERAPY |

Patent airway? — No →
a. Tilt head back.
b. Pull mandible forward.
c. Aspirate oropharynx.
d. Place oral airway.
e. Place endotracheal tube.

Yes ↓

Breathing spontaneously? — No →
a. Mouth-to-mouth ventilation.
b. Ventilate with Ambu bag, face mask, and 100% O_2.
c. Place endotracheal tube.
d. Mechanical ventilation.

Yes ↓

Cardiac arrest? Blood pressure 0/0, Heart rate 0. — Yes →
a. Sharp blow to precordium.
b. Closed chest massage, 1/s.
c. Ventilate once per 5 massages.
d. Place patient on hard surface.
e. Epinephrine, 0.2–0.5 mL aqueous 1:1000, IV, intracardiac, or intra-bronchial.*

Note time, confirm diagnosis by carotid pulse, begin ECG monitoring.

Asystole.

Ventricular fibrillation. →
f. Defibrillate with maximum DC shock, 200–300 J.
g. Start IV crystalloids, blood or plasma.
h. Lidocaine, 75–100 mg IV, or procainamide, 100 mg IV, or bretylium, 5 mg/kg IV.

Multiple PVCs > 5/min. →
i. Lidocaine, 50–100 mg IV, or procainamide, 100 mg IV, or bretylium, 5 mg/kg IV.

Bradycardia. →
j. Atropine, 0.5 mg IV.
k. Isoproterenol, 1 mg IV.

Arterial blood gases – pH, repeat every 5–15 min as needed to titrate $NaHCO_3$. →
l. Sodium bicarbonate, 50 meq IV, repeat only as necessary to maintain pH 7.4.
m. Calcium chloride, 10%, 5 mL IV.†

Measure electrolytes, enzymes, BUN, etc. →
n. Correct hypokalemia, give KCl, 10–30 meq/h IV.
o. Correct hyperkalemia, give 50% glucose, insulin, sodium polystyrene sulfonate (Kayexalate), dialysis.

p. Temporary pacemaker.

*If asystole persists, a temporary pacemaker may in rare instances restore an effective paced ventricular rhythm.
†*Caution:* Do not give *with* bicarbonate.

Figure 3. Patient care algorithm for cardiopulmonary resuscitation. (Modified and reproduced, with permission, from Shoemaker WC: A patient care algorithm for cardiac arrest. *Crit Care Med* [May-June] 1976;4:157.)

EMERGENCY TREATMENT OF FOOD CHOKING & OTHER CAUSES OF ACUTE AIRWAY OBSTRUCTION

The diagnosis of life-threatening food choking should be suspected in every case of respiratory distress or loss of consciousness that occurs while the patient is eating. A bolus of food or other foreign object is usually lodged fairly high in the pharynx. Predisposing factors to acute airway obstruction include acute alcoholism, dentures, swallowing disorders due to any cause, and chronic obstructive pulmonary disease.

In a hospital setting, elderly or debilitated patients who are sedated and have poor dentition are particularly prone to asphyxiation from large chunks of food. The clinical picture of the choking patient is easily mistaken for that of acute myocardial infarction.

If the unconscious patient is not breathing but can be ventilated, proceed with mouth-to-mouth or mouth-to-nose ventilation. If there is no pulse, institute cardiopulmonary resuscitation (see p 1109).

Treatment (Act quickly!)

If airway obstruction is only partial, as evidenced by wheezing, forceful coughing, and adequate airway exchange, do *not* interfere with the patient's attempt to expel the foreign body. *If the patient is able to speak, even in a whisper, do not use the Heimlich procedure.*

If there is progressive or complete airway obstruction (ie, the *conscious patient is unable to speak, cough, or breathe* and often clutches the neck as a sign of choking distress) and it is not possible to ventilate the patient, the following should be performed in quick succession:

A. If Patient Is Sitting or Standing:

1. Deliver a rapid series of 4 hard, sharp blows with the heel of the hand to the interscapular portion of the patient's spine. If the back blows are ineffective, then

2. Wrap arms around patient's waist. Make a fist with one hand and grasp the fist with the other. Place thumb side of fist against patient's abdomen just above the navel and below the rib cage (see Fig 4). Then press fist into the abdomen with a firm, quick upward thrust (not simply a squeeze or bear hug). Repeat 8 times if necessary.*

3. If the above procedure is unsuccessful and the patient can open his or her mouth, try removing food or other object with fingers.

4. If obstruction still persists, repeat the 4 blows to the upper back.

5. Those properly trained may use direct visualization with tongue blade and flashlight or laryngoscope for direct forceps extraction.

*When it is difficult to encircle the abdomen (eg, marked obesity, pregnancy), it may be necessary to utilize an alternative technique of forceful chest thrusts.

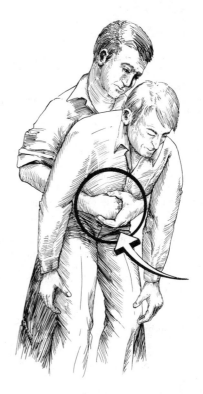

Figure 4. Heimlich procedure.

B. With Patient Lying Down: (When unconscious or when extremely tall or heavy.)

1. Roll the patient onto one side and deliver a rapid series of 4 hard, sharp blows with the heel of the hand to the interscapular portion of the spine. If the back blows are ineffective, then

2. Quickly turn the patient to supine position (on back) and straddle his or her body. With one hand atop the other on the abdomen slightly above the navel, press the heel of the bottom hand into the abdomen with quick upward thrusts, as above.

3. If patient vomits, turn quickly on side and clear mouth to prevent aspiration.

4. Attempt direct visualization and forceps extraction if necessary.

5. If the above measures fail, it is necessary for trained operators to perform emergency cricothyrotomy or tracheostomy. Fractured ribs have been reported in a few recipients of the Heimlich procedure.

Gann DS: Emergency management of the obstructed airway. (Commentary.) *JAMA* 1980;**243**:1141.

Hoffman JR: Treatment of foreign body obstruction of the upper airway. *West J Med* 1982;**136**:11.

Redding JS: The choking controversy: Critique of evidence on the Heimlich maneuver. *Crit Care Med* 1979;**7**:475.

Standards and guidelines for cardiopulmonary resuscitation (CPR) and emergency cardiac care (ECC). *JAMA* 1980;**244**:453.

Table 11. Schedules of controlled drugs.*

Schedule I: (All nonresearch use forbidden.)
  Narcotics: Heroin and many nonmarketed synthetic narcotics
  Hallucinogens:
    LSD
    MDA, STP, DMT, DET, mescaline, peyote, bufotenine, ibogaine, psilocybin
  Marihuana, tetrahydrocannabinols

Schedule II: (No telephone prescriptions, no refills.)
  Narcotics:
    Opium
    Opium alkaloids and derived phenanthrene alkaloids: Morphine, codeine, hydromorphone (Dilaudid), oxymorphone (Numorphan), oxycodone (dihydrohydroxycodeinone, a component of Percobarb, Percodan, Percocet, Tylox)
    Designated synthetic drugs: Meperidine (Demerol), methadone, levorphanol (Levo-Dromoran), fentanyl (ingredient in Innovar)
  Stimulants:
    Coca leaves and cocaine
    Amphetamine (Benzedrine)
    Biphetamine
    Dextroamphetamine (Dexedrine)
    Methamphetamine (Desoxyn)
    Phenmetrazine (Preludin)
    Methylphenidate (Ritalin)
    Above in mixtures with other controlled or uncontrolled drugs
  Depressants:
    Amobarbital (Amytal)
    Pentobarbital (Nembutal)
    Secobarbital (Seconal)
    Mixtures of above (eg, Tuinal)
    Phencyclidine (PCP) (veterinary drug only)

Schedule III: (Prescription must be rewritten after 6 months or 5 refills.)
  Narcotics: The following opiates in combination with one or more active nonnarcotic ingredients, provided the amount does not exceed that shown:
    Codeine and dihydrocodeine: Not to exceed 1800 mg/dL or 90 mg/tablet or other dose unit
    Dihydrocodeinone (hydrocodone and in Hycodan): Not to exceed 300 mg/dL or 15 mg/tablet
    Opium: 500 mg/dL or 25 mg/5 mL, or other dosage unit (paregoric)
  Narcotic antagonist: Nalorphine (Nalline)
  Stimulants:
    Benzphetamine (Didrex)
    Chlorphentermine (Pre-Sate)
    Phendimetrazine (eg, Dietabs, Plegine)
  Depressants:
    Schedule II barbiturates in mixtures with noncontrolled drugs or in suppository dose form

Depressants (cont'd):
    Aprobarbital (Alurate)
    Butabarbital (Butisol)
    Glutethimide (Doriden)
    Hexobarbital (Sombulex)
    Methyprylon (Noludar)
    Talbutal (Lotusate)
    Thiamylal (Surital)
    Thiopental (Pentothal)

Schedule IV: (Prescription must be rewritten after 6 months or 5 refills. Differs from Schedule III in penalties for illegal possession.)
  Narcotics:
    Pentazocine (Talwin)
    Propoxyphene (Darvon)
  Stimulants:
    Diethylpropion (Tenuate)
    Mazindol (Sanorex)
    Phentermine (Adipex)
    Fenfluramine (Pondimin)
  Depressants:
    Benzodiazepines:
      Alprazolam (Xanax)
      Chlordiazepoxide (Librium)
      Clonazepam (Clonopin)
      Clorazepate (Tranxene)
      Diazepam (Valium)
      Flurazepam (Dalmane)
      Halazepam (Paxipam)
      Lorazepam (Ativan)
      Oxazepam (Serax)
      Prazepam (Centrax)
      Temazepam (Restoril)
    Chloral hydrate
    Ethchlorvynol (Placidyl)
    Ethinamate (Valmid)
    Meprobamate (Equanil, Miltown, etc)
    Mephobarbital (Mebaral)
    Methohexital (Brevital)
    Paraldehyde
    Phenobarbital

Schedule V: (As any other [nonnarcotic] prescription drug; may also be dispensed without prescription unless additional state regulations apply.)
  Narcotics:
    Diphenoxylate (not more than 2.5 mg and not less than 0.025 mg of atropine per dosage unit, as in Lomotil)
    Loperamide (Imodium)
  The following drugs in combination with other active, nonnarcotic ingredients and provided the amount per 100 mL or 100 g does not exceed that shown:
    Codeine: 200 mg
    Dihydrocodeine: 100 mg
    Ethylmorphine: 100 mg

*Modified and reproduced, with permission, from Katzung BG (editor): *Basic & Clinical Pharmacology*, 2nd ed. Lange, 1984. Local or state laws may be at variance with federal schedules of controlled drugs.

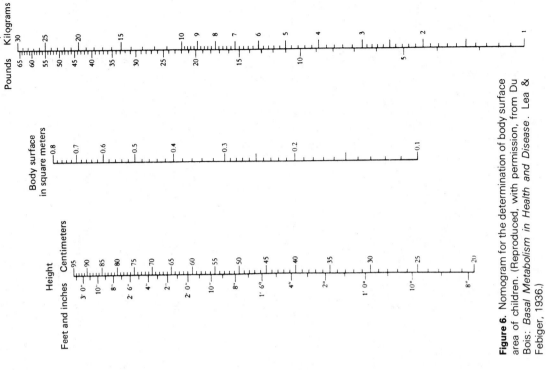

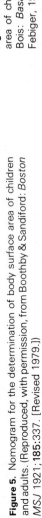

Figure 6. Nomogram for the determination of body surface area of children. (Reproduced, with permission, from Du Bois: *Basal Metabolism in Health and Disease*. Lea & Febiger, 1936.)

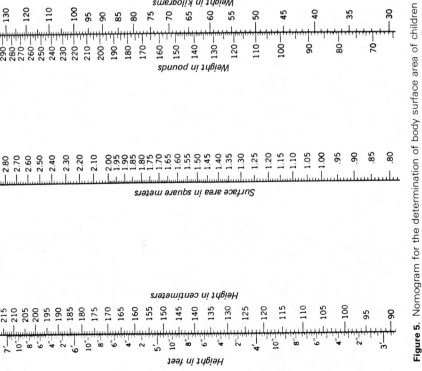

Figure 5. Nomogram for the determination of body surface area of children and adults. (Reproduced, with permission, from Boothby & Sandiford: *Boston MSJ* 1921;**185**:337. [Revised 1979.])

Table 12. The 10 leading causes of death according to age group and sex, 1979.*

	All Ages		Ages 1–14		Ages 15–34		Ages 35–54		Ages 55–74		Ages 75+	
	Male	Female	Male	Female	Male	Female	Male	Female	Male	Female	Male	Female
1.	Heart diseases 396,315	Heart diseases 336,806	Accidents 5933	Accidents 3106	Accidents 34,309	Accidents 8717	Heart diseases 40,848	Cancer 27,258	Heart diseases 190,298	Heart diseases 100,700	Heart diseases 161,718	Heart diseases 221,309
2.	Cancer 220,015	Cancer 183,380	Cancer 1226	Cancer 904	Homicide 10,195	Cancer 3434	Cancer 26,475	Heart diseases 12,853	Cancer 123,443	Cancer 91,347	Cancer 64,871	Cerebrovascular diseases 70,601
3.	Accidents 74,403	Cerebrovascular diseases 99,049	Congenital anomalies 858	Congenital anomalies 741	Suicide 8750	Homicide 2506	Accidents 14,150	Accidents 4521	Cerebrovascular diseases 25,767	Cerebrovascular diseases 23,650	Cerebrovascular diseases 39,506	Cancer 60,388
4.	Cerebrovascular diseases 70,439	Accidents 30,909	Homicide 390	Homicide 318	Cancer 3933	Suicide 2353	Cirrhosis of liver 7088	Cerebrovascular diseases 4026	Accidents 12,281	Diabetes 8103	Pneumonia, influenza 13,719	Pneumonia, influenza 15,552
5.	Pneumonia, influenza 23,725	Pneumonia, influenza 21,305	Heart diseases 287	Heart diseases 266	Heart diseases 2758	Heart diseases 1392	Suicide 5207	Cirrhosis of liver 3518	Chronic obstructive lung diseases 11,452	Accidents 6052	Chronic obstructive lung diseases 9335	Arteriosclerosis 15,262
6.	Chronic obstructive lung diseases 21,586	Diabetes 19,397	Pneumonia, influenza 248	Pneumonia, influenza 222	Cirrhosis of liver 903	Cerebrovascular diseases 639	Homicide 4905	Suicide 2458	Cirrhosis of liver 9949	Cirrhosis of liver 5232	Arteriosclerosis 8526	Diabetes 9568
7.	Suicide 20,256	Arteriosclerosis 17,375	Meningitis 133	Meningitis 106	Cerebrovascular diseases 687	Cirrhosis of liver 415	Cerebrovascular diseases 4312	Diabetes 1372	Pneumonia, influenza 7020	Chronic obstructive lung diseases 4555	Accidents 7117	Accidents 8047
8.	Cirrhosis of liver 19,369	Cirrhosis of liver 10,351	Cerebral palsy 130	Cerebral palsy 101	Congenital anomalies 613	Congenital anomalies 378	Pneumonia, influenza 1599	Homicide 1168	Diabetes 6832	Pneumonia, influenza 3828	Diabetes 4988	Nephritis 4174
9.	Homicide 17,628	Diseases of infancy 10,098	Suicide 104	Benign neoplasm 70	Pneumonia, influenza 511	Pneumonia, influenza 354	Diabetes 1589	Pneumonia, influenza 848	Aortic aneurysm 5175	Nephritis 2455	Nephritis 4155	Chronic obstructive lung diseases 3475
10.	Diabetes 13,795	Chronic obstructive lung diseases 8530	Anemias 87	Anemias 69	Diabetes 368	Diabetes 315	Chronic obstructive lung diseases 773	Nephritis 542	Suicide 4593	Arteriosclerosis 2042	Aortic aneurysm 4067	Aortic aneurysm 2591

*Taken from: Vital Statistics of the United States, 1979.

CONVERSION TABLES

Fahrenheit/Celsius Temperature Conversion
($^\circ F = 9/5\,^\circ C + 32;\ ^\circ C = 5/9\,[^\circ F - 32]$)

$^\circ F$		$^\circ C$	$^\circ F$		$^\circ C$	$^\circ F$		$^\circ C$
90	=	32.2	97	=	36.1	104	=	40.0
91	=	32.8	98	=	36.7	105	=	40.6
92	=	33.3	99	=	37.2	106	=	41.1
93	=	33.9	100	=	37.8	107	=	41.7
94	=	34.4	101	=	38.3	108	=	42.2
95	=	35.0	102	=	38.9	109	=	42.8
96	=	35.6	103	=	39.4			

Milliequivalent Conversion Factors

meq/L of:	Divide mg/dL or vol% by:
Calcium	2.0
Chloride (from Cl)	3.5
(from NaCl)	5.85
CO_2 combining power	2.222
Magnesium	1.2
Phosphorus	3.1 (mmol)
Potassium	3.9
Sodium	2.3

Approximate Length Equivalents

Metric System	US System
1 cm	0.4 in
1 m	39.4 in
1 km	3281 ft (0.6 mi)

Metric System Prefixes (Small Measurement)

In accordance with the decision of several scientific societies to employ a universal system of metric nomenclature, the following prefixes have become standard in many medical texts and journals.

k	kilo-	10^3
c	centi-	10^{-2}
m	milli-	10^{-3}
μ	micro-	10^{-6}
n	nano- (formerly millimicro, mμ)	10^{-9}
p	pico- (formerly micromicro, $\mu\mu$)	10^{-12}
f	femto-	10^{-15}
a	atto-	10^{-18}

Household Equivalents (Approximate)

1 tsp = 6 mL
1 tbsp = 15 mL
1 oz (eg, medicine glass) = 30 mL
1 cup = 8 fluid oz = 240 mL
1 quart = 946 mL

Apothecary Equivalents

Metric	Approximate Apothecary Equivalents	Metric	Approximate Apothecary Equivalents	Metric	Approximate Apothecary Equivalents
30 g	1 oz	0.12 g	2 gr	3 mg	1/20 gr
6 g	90 gr	0.1 g	1½ gr	2 mg	1/30 gr
5 g	75 gr	75 mg	1¼ gr	1.5 mg	1/40 gr
4 g	60 gr	60 mg	1 gr	1.2 mg	1/50 gr
3 g	45 gr	50 mg	3/4 gr	1 mg	1/60 gr
2 g	30 gr	40 mg	2/3 gr	0.8 mg	1/80 gr
1.5 g	22 gr	30 mg	1/2 gr	0.6 mg	1/100 gr
1 g	15 gr	25 mg	3/8 gr	0.5 mg	1/120 gr
0.75 g	12 gr	20 mg	1/3 gr	0.4 mg	1/150 gr
0.6 g	10 gr	15 mg	1/4 gr	0.3 mg	1/200 gr
0.5 g	7½ gr	12 mg	1/5 gr	0.25 mg	1/250 gr
0.4 g	6 gr	10 mg	1/6 gr	0.2 mg	1/300 gr
0.3 g	5 gr	8 mg	1/8 gr	0.15 mg	1/400 gr
0.25 g	4 gr	6 mg	1/10 gr	0.12 mg	1/500 gr
0.2 g	3 gr	5 mg	1/12 gr	0.1 mg	1/600 gr
0.15 g	2½ gr	4 mg	1/15 gr		

Pounds to Kilograms
(1 kg = 2.2 lb; 1 lb = 0.45 kg)

lb	kg	lb	kg	lb	kg	lb	kg	lb	kg
5	2.3	50	22.7	95	43.1	140	63.5	185	83.9
10	4.5	55	25.0	100	45.4	145	65.8	190	86.2
15	6.8	60	27.2	105	47.6	150	68.0	195	88.5
20	9.1	65	29.5	110	49.9	155	70.3	200	90.7
25	11.3	70	31.7	115	52.2	160	72.6	205	93.0
30	13.6	75	34.0	120	54.4	165	74.8	210	95.3
35	15.9	80	36.3	125	56.7	170	77.1	215	97.5
40	18.1	85	38.6	130	58.9	175	79.4	220	99.8
45	20.4	90	40.8	135	61.2	180	81.6		

Feet and Inches to Centimeters
(1 cm = 0.39 in; 1 in = 2.54 cm)

ft	in	cm	ft	in	cm	ft	in	cm	ft	in	cm	ft	in	cm
0	6	15.2	2	4	71.1	3	4	101.6	4	4	132.0	5	4	162.6
1	0	30.5	2	5	73.6	3	5	104.1	4	5	134.6	5	5	165.1
1	6	45.7	2	6	76.1	3	6	106.6	4	6	137.1	5	6	167.6
1	7	48.3	2	7	78.7	3	7	109.2	4	7	139.6	5	7	170.2
1	8	50.8	2	8	81.2	3	8	111.7	4	8	142.2	5	8	172.7
1	9	53.3	2	9	83.8	3	9	114.2	4	9	144.7	5	9	175.3
1	10	55.9	2	10	86.3	3	10	116.8	4	10	147.3	5	10	177.8
1	11	58.4	2	11	88.8	3	11	119.3	4	11	149.8	5	11	180.3
2	0	61.0	3	0	91.4	4	0	121.9	5	0	152.4	6	0	182.9
2	1	63.5	3	1	93.9	4	1	124.4	5	1	154.9	6	1	185.4
2	2	66.0	3	2	96.4	4	2	127.0	5	2	157.5	6	2	188.0
2	3	68.6	3	3	99.0	4	3	129.5	5	3	160.0	6	3	190.5

Desirable Weights (Pounds)*
(See p 811.)

Men (Ages 25–59)					Women (Ages 25–59)				
Height† Feet Inches		Small Frame	Medium Frame	Large Frame	Height† Feet Inches		Small Frame	Medium Frame	Large Frame
5	2	128–134	131–141	138–150	4	10	102–111	109–121	118–131
5	3	130–136	133–143	140–153	4	11	103–113	111–123	120–134
5	4	132–138	135–145	142–156	5	0	104–115	113–126	122–137
5	5	134–140	137–148	144–160	5	1	106–118	115–129	125–140
5	6	136–142	139–151	146–164	5	2	108–121	118–132	128–143
5	7	138–145	142–154	149–168	5	3	111–124	121–135	131–147
5	8	140–148	145–157	152–172	5	4	114–127	124–138	134–151
5	9	142–151	148–160	155–176	5	5	117–130	127–141	137–155
5	10	144–154	151–163	158–180	5	6	120–133	130–144	140–159
5	11	146–157	154–166	161–184	5	7	123–136	133–147	143–163
6	0	149–160	157–170	164–188	5	8	126–139	136–150	146–167
6	1	152–164	160–174	168–192	5	9	129–142	139–153	149–170
6	2	155–168	164–178	172–197	5	10	132–145	142–156	152–173
6	3	158–172	167–182	176–202	5	11	135–148	145–159	155–176
6	4	162–176	171–187	181–207	6	0	138–151	148–162	158–179

*With indoor clothing weighing 5 pounds for men and 3 pounds for women.
†With shoes with 1-inch heels.
Source of basic data: *Build Study, 1979.* Society of Actuaries and Association of Life Insurance Medical Directors of America, 1980.
Copyright © 1983 by the Metropolitan Life Insurance Company.

Index